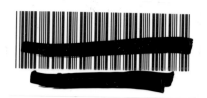

Neurodegenerative Diseases
Neurobiology, Pathogenesis and Therapeutics

Neurodegenerative diseases are among the major contributors to disability and disease, with Alzheimer's and Parkinson's diseases the most prevalent among many in this category. This major reference reviews the rapidly advancing knowledge of pathogenesis and treatment of neurodegenerative diseases in the context of a comprehensive survey of each disease and its clinical features. The editors and contributors are among the leading experts in the field internationally.

Covering basic science, diagnostic tools and therapeutic approaches, the book focuses on all aspects of neurodegenerative disease, including the normal aging process. The dementias, prion diseases, Parkinson's disease and atypical parkinsonisms, neurodegenerative ataxias, motor neuron diseases, degenerative diseases with chorea, iron and copper disorders, and mitochondrial diseases, are all methodically presented and discussed, with extensive illustrations. In each case the underlying genetics, neuropathological and clinical issues are fully reviewed, making this the most complete as well as the most authoritative reference available to clinicians and neuroscientists.

M. Flint Beal is Anne Parrish Titzell Professor and Chairman of the Department of Neurology and Neuroscience at the Weill Medical College of Cornell University, and Director of Neurology at the New York Presbyterian Cornell Campus. An internationally recognized authority on neurodegenerative disorders, his research has focused on the mechanism of neuronal degeneration in Alzheimer's disease, Huntington's disease, Parkinson's disease and amyotrophic lateral sclerosis.

Anthony E. Lang is Professor in the Department of Medicine, Division of Neurology, University of Toronto. A founding member of the Parkinson Study Group and the Movement Disorders Society, his research has included clinical trials of poorly recognized neurological disorders, clinical trials of new therapeutic modalities, and studies in molecular biology, neurophysiology, neuropsychology and imaging.

Albert C. Ludolph is Professor of Neurology, Chair of Neurology, and Chairman of the Neuroscience Center of the University of Ulm, Germany. A neurologist and psychiatrist, his major interest is in toxicological models of vulnerability and genetic models for the pathogenesis of neurodegenerative diseases.

Neurodegenerative Diseases

Neurobiology, Pathogenesis and Therapeutics

M. Flint Beal
Weill Medical College of Cornell University

Anthony E. Lang
University of Toronto

Albert C. Ludolph
University of Ulm

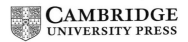

CAMBRIDGE UNIVERSITY PRESS
Cambridge, New York, Melbourne, Madrid, Cape Town, Singapore, São Paulo

Cambridge University Press
The Edinburgh Building, Cambridge CB2 2RU, UK

www.cambridge.org
Information on this title: www.cambridge.org/9780521811668

First published 2005

Printed in Thailand by Imago

A catalog record for this book is available from the British Library

Library of Congress Cataloging in Publication data

ISBN-13 978-0-521-81166-8 hardback
ISBN-10 0-521-81166-X hardback

Contents

Contributors

Editors

M. Flint Beal
The New York Hospital
525 E. 68th Street
New York
NY 10021
USA

Anthony E. Lang
Toronto Western Hospital
7 McLaughlin
Room 304, 11th floor
399 Bathhurst Street
Toronto
ON M5T 2S8
Canada

Albert C. Ludolph
Neurologische
Universitatsklinik Ulm
Steinhovelstrasse 9
89075 Ulm
Germany

List of contributors

Rocco Agostino
Department of Neurological Sciences and INM Neuromed
IRCCS
University of Rome "La Sapienza"
Viale de'll Universita 30
00185 Rome
Italy

Adriano Aguzzi
Institute of Neuropathology
Universitatsspital Zurich
Schmelzbergstrasse 12
Zurich CH-8091
Switzerland

Marilyn S. Albert
Department of Neurology (Meyer 6-113)
Johns Hopkins University School of
Medicine
600 N Wolfe Street
Baltimore
MD 21287
USA

Ammar Al-Chalabi
Department of Neurology
Institute of Psychiatry
London SE5 8AF
UK

Stanley H. Appel
Department of Neurology
Baylor College of Medicine
6501 Fannin, Suite NB302
Houston
TX

M. Flint Beal
Department of Neurology
Weill Medical College
Cornell University
New York
NY
USA

Alfredo Berardelli
Department of Neurological Sciences
University of Rome "La Sapienza"
Viale de'll Università 30
00185 Rome
Italy

Daniela Berg
Hertie Institute for Clinical Brain Research,
Hoppe–Seyler Strasse 3
D-72076 Tübingen,
Germany

Lars Bertram
Genetics and Aging Research Unit
Department of Neurology
Massachusetts General Hospital
114 16th Street
Charlestown
MA 02129
USA

Konrad Beyreuther
Centre for Molecular Biology
The University of Heidelberg
Heidelberg
Germany

Kailish P. Bhatia
Sobell Department of Movement
Neuroscience
Institute of Neurology
Queen Square
London WC1N 3BG
UK

Lars M. Bjorklund
Udall Parkinson's Disease Research
Center of Excellence
Neuroregeneration Laboratories
McLean Hospital/Harvard Medical
School
115 Mill Street
Belmont
MA 02478
USA

David R. Borchelt
Department of Pathology and Division
of Neuropathology
The Johns Hopkins University School
of Medicine
558 Ross Research Building
72 Rutland Avenue
Baltimore
MD 21205-2196
USA

Adam L. Boxer
Memory and Aging Center
Department of Neurology
University of California
350 Parnassus Ave
Suite 800, Box 1207
San Francisco
CA 94143-1207
USA

George J. Brewer
Department of Human Genetics and
Department of Internal Medicine
University of Michigan School of
Medicine
Ann Arbor
MI
USA

Robert H. Brown
Cecil B Day Neuromuscular Laboratory
Massachusetts General Hospital East
Bldg 114 The Navy Yard, 16th St, Rm
2125
Charlestown
MA 02129
USA

Ashley I. Bush
Laboratory for Oxidation Biology
Genetics and Aging Research Unit
Building 114, 16th Street
Charlestown
MA 02129-4404
USA
and
Mental Health Research Institute of
Victoria, and
Department of Pathology
University of Melbourne
Parkville
Victoria
Australia

Eva Chmielnicki
Department of Neurology and
Neuroscience
Cornell University Medical Center
1300 York Avenue, Room E607
New York
NY 10021
USA

Ji-Kyung Choi
Department of Radiology
Athinoula A Martinos Center for
Biomedical Imaging
Massachusetts General Hospital and
Harvard Medical School
Building 149, 13th Street Charlestown
MA 02129
USA

Alan Colchester
Kent Institute of Medicine and Health Sciences
University of Kent
Canterbury CT2 7PD
UK

Carlo Colosimo
Department of Neurology
University "La Sapienza"
I-00185 Rome
Italy

Marcus S. Cooke
Genome Instability Group
Departments of Cancer Studies and Genetics
University of Leicester
Leicester Royal Infirmary
University Hospitals of Leicester
NHS Trust
Leicester LE2 7LX
UK

Tom O. Crawford
Department of Neurology
Johns Hopkins University School of Medicine
600 N Wolfe Street
Baltimore
MD 21287-3923
USA

John P. Crow
Department of Pharmacology and Toxicology
University of Arkansas College of Medicine
Little Rock, AR
USA

Antonio Currà
Department of Neurological
Sciences and INM Neuromed
IRCCS
University of Rome "La Sapienza"
00185 Rome
Italy

Ted M. Dawson
Department of Neurology
Johns Hopkins University School of Medicine
600 N Wolfe Street, Pathol 2-210
Baltimore
MD 21205
USA

Valina L. Dawson
Department of Neurology
Johns Hopkins University School of
Medicine
600 N Wolfe Street, Pathol 2-210
Baltimore
MD 21205
USA

Vijay Dhawan
Institute for Medical Research
Long Shore – Long Island
Jewish Health System
350 Community Drive
Manhasset
NY 11030
USA

Dennis W. Dickson
Department of Pathology
Mayo Clinic Jacksonville
4500 San Pablo Road
Jacksonville
FL 32224
USA

David Eidelberg
Institute for Medical Research
North Shore – Long Island
Jewish Health System
350 Community Drive
Manhasset
NY 11030
USA

Lisa M. Ellerby
Buck Institute for Research
in Aging
8001 Redwood Blvd
Novato
CA 94945
USA

Andrew Feigin
Institute for Medical Research
Long Shore – Long Island
Jewish Health System
350 Community Drive
Manhasset
NY 11030
USA

John K. Fink
5214 CCGCB Box 0940
1500 E Medical Center Drive
Ann Arbor
MI 481099-0940
USA

Mark S. Forman
Center for Neurodegenerative Disease Research
Department of Pathology and Laboratory Medicine
University of Pennsylvania School of Medicine
HUP, Maloney Bldg, Room A009
Philadelphia
PA 19104-4283
USA

Avi L. Friedlich
Laboratory for Oxidation Biology
Genetics and Aging Research Unit
Building 114, 16th Street
Charlestown
MA 02190-4404
USA

Thomas Gasser
Department of Neurodegenerative Disorders
Hertie-Institute for Clinical Brain Research
Center of Neurology
University of Tübingen
Germany

Richard A. Gatti
Department of Pathology and Laboratory Medicine
David Geffen School of Medicine at
UCLA
Los Angeles
CA 90095-1732
USA

Felix Geser
Department of Neurology
University Hospital
A-6020 Innsbruck
Austria

Stuart L. Gibb
Department of Neurology
Massachusetts General Hospital
Harvard Medical School
16th Street, Bldg 114
Charlestown
MA 02129
USA

Jonathan D. Gitlin
Washington University School of Medicine
McDonnell Pediatric Research
Building
660 South Euclid Avenue
St Louis
MO 63110
USA

Christopher G. Goetz
Section of Movement Disorders
Department of Neurological Sciences
Rush University Medical Center
1725 W Harrison Street, Suite 755
Chicago
IL 60612
USA

Lawrence I. Golbe
Department of Neurology
97 Paterson Street
New Brunswick
NJ 08901
USA

Alfred L. Goldberg
Department of Cell Biology
Harvard Medical School
240 Longwood Ave
Boston
MA 02115
USA

Steven A. Goldman
Division of Cell and Gene Therapy
University of Rochester Medical
Center
601 Elmwood Avenue
MRBX, Box 645
Rochester
NY 14642
USA

J. Timothy Greenamyre
Pittsburgh Institute for Neurodegenerative Diseases
University of Pittsburgh
S-506 Biomedical Science Tower
203 Lothrop Street
Pittsburgh
PA 15213
USA

James G. Greene
Center for Neurodegenerative
Disease and Department of Neurology
Emory University
Whitehead Building
Room 505M
615 Michael Street
Atlanta
GA 30322
USA

John Hardy
Laboratory of Neurogenetics
National Institute on Aging
National Institutes of Health
Building 10, Room 6C103,
MSC1589
Bethesda
MD 20892
USA

Patrick Hof
Department of Neuroscience
Mount Sinai School of Medicine
One Gustave Levy Place
New York
NY 10029
USA

Hrissanthi Ikonomidou
Department of Pediatric Neurology
Carl Gustav Carus University
Fetscherstrasse 74
Dresden D-01307
Germany

Ole Isacson
Neuroregeneration Laboratories
McLean Hospital/Harvard Medical School
114 Mill Street
Belmont
MA 02478
USA

Bruce G. Jenkins
Department of Radiology
Athinoula A Martinos Center for Biomedical Imaging
Massachusetts General Hospital and
Harvard Medical School
Building 149, 13th Street Charlestown
MA 02129
USA

Julene Johnson

Keith A. Josephs
Mayo Alzheimer's Disease Research
Center
Department of Neurology
Mayo Clinic
200 First Street
SW Rochester
MN 55905-0001
USA

Kwang-Soo Kim
Udall Parkinson's Disease Research
Center of Excellence
Molecular Neurobiology Laboratory
McLean Hospital/Harvard Medical
School
115 Mill Street
Belmont
MA 02478
USA

Thomas Klockgether
Department of Neurology
University of Bonn
Sigmund-Freud-Str. 25
D-53105 Bonn
Germany

Michel Koenig
Institut de Génétique et de Biologie
Moléculaire et Cellulaire
1 rue Laurent Fries
BP 10142
674 Illkirch Cedex
France

Katie Kompoliti
Section of Movement Disorders
Department of Neurological
Sciences
Rush University Medical Center
1725 W Harrison Street, Suite 755
Chicago
IL 60612
USA

Satoshi Kono
Edward Mallinckrodt Department of
Pediatrics
Washington University School of
Medicine
St Louis
MO
USA and
First Department of Medicine
Hamamatsu University School of
Medicine
Hamamatsu
Japan

Christoph M. Kosinski
Department of Neurology
University Hospital Aachen
Pauwelsstrasse 30
Aachen 52074
Germany

Bernhard Landwehrmeyer
Department of Neurology
University of Ulm
Steinhoevelstrasse 9
Ulm 89079
Germany

Albert R. La Spada
Department of Laboratory Medicine
Medicine and Neurology
Centre for Neurogenetics and Neurotherapeutics
University of Washington Medical
Center
Box 357 110, Room NW120
Seattle
WA 98195-7110
USA

Michael K. Lee
Department of Pathology and Division of
Neuropathology
The Johns Hopkins University School of
Medicine
558 Ross Research Building
72 Rutland Avenue
Baltimore
MD 21205-2196
USA

Virginia M.-Y. Lee
Center for Neurodegenerative Disease
Research
Department of Pathology and
Laboratory Medicine
University of Pennsylvania School of
Medicine
HUP, Maloney Bldg, Room A009
Philadelphia
PA 19104-4283
USA

Frank Lehmann-Horn
Abteilung für Angewandte Physiologie
Albert-Einstein-Allee 11
Universität Ulm
D-89069
Germany

Nigel Leigh
Department of Clinical Neurology
Guy's, King's and St Thomas'
School of Medicine and Institute of
Psychiatry
DeCrespigny Park
London SE5 8AF
UK

Holger Lerche
Neurologischen Klinik und
Abteilung für
Angewandte Physiologie
Universität Ulm
Helmholtzstrasse 8/1
Ulm
D-89081
Germany

Peter A. LeWitt
Clinical Neuroscience Center
26400 West Twelve Mile Road
Suite 110
Southfield
MI 48034
USA

Albert C. Ludolph
Department of Neurology
University of Ulm
Germany

Jacques Mallet
Hôpital Pitié-Salpétrière (Batiment
CERVI)
83 Boulevard de l'Hôpital
75013 Paris
France

Alan S. Mandir
Department of Neurology
Johns Hopkins University School of
Medicine
600 N Wolfe Street, Path 219
Baltimore
MD 21287
USA

Stefan L. Marklund
Department of Medical Biosciences
Clinical Chemistry
Umea University Hospital
Umea SE-90185
Sweden

Colin L. Masters
Department of Pathology
The University of Melbourne
Parkville 3010
Australia

Ivar Mendez
Division of Neurosurgery
Dalhousie University
Halifax
NS
Canada

Hiroaki Miyajima
Edward Mallinckrodt Department of
Pediatrics
Washington University School of
Medicine
St Louis
MO
USA and
First Department of Medicine
Hamamatsu University School of
Medicine
Hamamatsu
Japan

Bruce L. Miller
Memory and Aging Center
Department of Neurology
University of California
350 Parnassus Ave
Suite 800, Box 1207
San Francisco
CA 94143-1207
USA

John H. Morrison
Department of Neuroscience
Mount Sinai School of Medicine
One Gustave Levy Place
New York
NY 10029
USA

Howard T. J. Mount
CRND
Department of Medicine
Division of Neurology
University of Toronto
Toronto
ON
Canada

Roger M. Nitsch
Division of Psychiatry Research
University of Zurich
August Forel Strasse 1
Zurich 8008
Switzerland

Frederick C. Nucifora
Division of Neurobiology
Department of Psychiatry
Johns Hopkins University School of
Medicine
Ross Research Building, Room 618
720 Rutland Avenue
Baltimore
MD 21205
USA

Matthew J. Parton
Department of Neurology
The Institute of Psychiatry and Guy's,
King's & St Thomas' School of Medicine
De Crespigny Park
London SE5 8AF
UK

Guilio Maria Pasinetti
Neuroinflammation Research
Laboratories
Department of Psychiatry
Mount Sinai School of Medicine
One Gustave Levy Place
New York
NY 10029
USA

Henry L. Paulson
Department of Neurology
University of Iowa Hospitals and Clinics
Iowa City
IA 52242
USA

Daniel Perl
Department of Neuropathology
Mount Sinai Medical Center
Box 1134
One Gustave Levy Place
New York
NY 10029-6500
USA

Susan Perlman
Department of Neurology
David Geffen School of Medicine at
UCLA
Los Angeles
CA
USA

Ronald C. Petersen
Mayo Alzheimer's Disease Research Center
Department of Neurology
Mayo Clinic
200 First Street
SW Rochester
MN 55905-0001
USA

Donald Price
Departments of Pathology, Neurology
and Neurosciences and Division of Neuropathology
The Johns Hopkins University School of Medicine
558 Ross Research Building
72 Rutland Avenue
Baltimore
MD 21205-2196
USA

Serge Przedborski
Departments of Neurology and Pathology, and
Center for Neurobiology and Behavior
BB-307 Columbia University
650 West 168th Street
New York
NY 10032
USA

Hélène Puccio
Institut de Génétique et de Biologie
Moléculaire et Cellulaire
1 rue Laurent Fries
BP 10142
674 Illkirch Cedex
France

Peter R. Rapp
Department of Neuroscience
Mount Sinai School of Medicine
One Gustave Levy Place
New York
NY 10029
USA

Normal Relkin
Weill Cornell Medical College
New York
NY
USA

Peter Riederer
Clinic and Poliklinik of Psychiatry and Psychotherapy
Department of Clinical Neurochemistry
University of Wurzburg
Fuchsleinstrasse 15
97080 Wurzburg Germany

Olaf Riess
Institute for Medical Genetics
Calwerstrasse 7
D-72076 Tübingen
Germany

Christopher A. Ross
Division of Neurobiology
Department of Psychiatry
Johns Hopkins University School of Medicine
Ross Research Building, Room 618
720 Rutland Avenue
Baltimore
MD 21205
USA

Sabine Rudnik-Schöneborn
Institute for Human Genetics
University of Technology
Pauwelsstr. 30
52074 Aachen
Germany

Michael Samuel
Department of Neurology
King's College Hospital
Denmark Hill
Camberwell
London SE5 9RS
UK

Rosario Sanchez-Pernaute
Udall Parkinson's Disease Research
Center of Excellence
Neuroregeneration Laboratories
McLean Hospital/Harvard Medical
School
115 Mill Street
Belmont
MA 02478
USA

Mary Sano
Alzheimer's Disease Research Center
Department of Psychiatry
Mount Sinai School of Medicine
New York
USA
and
Bronx VA Medical Center
139 W Kingsbridge Road
Code 151/Rm 1F01
Bronx
New York
NY 10468
USA

Chamsy Sarkis
Laboratoire de Génétique
Moleculaire de la Neurotransmission et
des Processus Neurodégeneratiffs
(LGN)
Centre National de la Recherche
Scientifique
UMR 7091
Paris
France

Anthony H. V. Schapira
Royal Free and University College
Medical School
University College London
Rowland Hill Street
London NW3 2PF
UK
and
Institute of Neurology
University College London
Queen Square
London WC1N 3BG
UK

Jorg B. Schulz
Department of Neurodegeneration and
Restorative Research
Center of Neurological Medicine
University of Göttingen
Waldweg 33
D-37073 Göttingen
Germany

Michael Sendtner
Institute for Clinical Neurobiology Josef-
Schneider-Str. 11
97080 Wurzburg
Germany

Pamela J. Shaw
Academic Neurology Unit
E Floor
Sheffield University Medical
School
Beech Hill Road
Sheffield S10 2RX
UK

Michael Y. Sherman
Department of Biochemistry
Bldg K323
Boston University Medical School
715 Albany Street
Boston
MA 02118
USA

Mika Shimoji
Department of Neurology
Johns Hopkins University School of Medicine
600 N Wolfe Street, Pathol 2-210

Baltimore
MD 21205
USA

Clifford W. Shults
Department of Neurosciences
University of California San Diego
Neurology Service
3350 La Jolla Village Drive
San Diego
CA 92101
USA

László Siklós
Department of Neurology
Baylor College of Medicine
Houston
TX
USA

Alexander Storch
Department of Neurology
Technical University of Dresden
Fetscherstrasse 74
01307 Dresden
Germany

David F. Tang-Wai
Division of Neurology
University Health Network
Toronto Western Hospital
Toronto
Ontario
Canada

Rudolph E. Tanzi
Genetics and Aging Research Unit
Department of Neurology
Massachusetts General Hospital
114 16th Street
Charlestown
MA 02129
USA

Patrick S. Thomas, Jr.
Department of Laboratory Medicine
and Center for Neurogenetics and Neurotherapeutics
University of Washington Medical Center
Seattle
WA
USA

Kim Tieu
Department of Environmental Medicine
and Center for Aging and Developmental Biology
University of Rochester
Rochester
NY 14642
USA

John Q. Trojanowski
Center for Neurodegenerative Disease
Research
Department of Pathology and
Laboratory Medicine
University of Pennsylvania School of
Medicine
3400 Spruce Street
Maloney Building, 3rd floor
Philadelphia
PA 19104
USA

Maja Trošt
Institute for Medical Research
Long Shore – Long Island
Jewish Health System
350 Community Drive
Manhasset
NY 11030
USA

Davide Trotti
Department of Neurology
Massachusetts General Hospital
Harvard Medical School
16th Street, Bldg 114
Charlestown
MA 02129
USA

Hayrettin Tumani
Department of Neurology
University of Ulm
Germany

Lechoslaw Turski
Solvay Pharmaceuticals Research
Laboratories
C J van Houtenlaan 36
1831 CP Weesp
The Netherlands

Craig van Horne
Udall Parkinson's Disease Research
Center of Excellence
Neuroregeneration Laboratories
McLean Hospital/Harvard Medical School
115 Mill Street
Belmont
MA 02478
USA

Gregor K. Wenning
Department of Neurology
University Hospital
A-6020 Innsbruck
Austria

Philip C. Wong
Department of Pathology and Division of
Neuropathology
The Johns Hopkins University School
of Medicine
558 Ross Research Building
72 Rutland Avenue
Baltimore
MD 21205-2196
USA

Jonathan D. Wood
The University of Sheffield
Academic Neurology Unit
E Floor, Medical School
Beech Hill Road
Sheffield S10 2RX
UK

Clare Wood-Allum
Academic Neurology Unit
E Floor
Sheffield University Medical School
Beech Hill Road
Sheffield S10 2RX
UK

Klaus Zerres
Institute for Human Genetics
University of Technology
Pauwelsstr. 30
52074 Aachen
Germany

Preface

Neurodegenerative diseases are becoming increasingly prevalent with the aging of the general population. The twentieth century witnessed a significant demographic change in the human population of the industrialized world that is currently followed by a similar shift of life expectancy to upper age ranges in Asia, Africa, and Middle and South America. Quality of life of the aging population of the world is, to a great extent, determined by the normal aging process of neurons in the central nervous system and especially by the occurrence of diseases characterized by accelerated neuronal loss: diseases which are traditionally designated as being neurodegenerative. They are presently amongst the major contributors to disability and disease in human populations.

Alzheimer's disease is the most prevalent of the neurodegenerative diseases followed by Parkinson's disease. Amyotrophic lateral sclerosis and Huntington's disease affect smaller numbers of patients but have devastating consequences. A large number of other rarer neurodegenerative diseases have similar profound effects on the patients and families who are afflicted by these illnesses. Research into the pathogenesis and treatment for these disorders is exploding exponentially. To a great extent this has been fostered by major advances in genetics, since we now know mutations that are associated with a large number of these illnesses. This includes familial forms of Alzheimer's disease, Parkinson's disease, fronto-temporal dementia, ALS, Huntington's disease and a variety of ataxias. Most of the sporadic cases of the common neurodegenerations such as Alzheimer's disease, Parkinson's disease, Amyotrophic lateral sclerosis appear to be polygenetic and are influenced by poorly characterized environmental factors.

The discovery of causative genetic mutations has led to the development of transgenic animal models of these disorders, which has enhanced our understanding of disease pathogenesis. Transgenic models are also useful for experimental therapeutics. Already, this is having a major impact on the development of novel therapeutic strategies for the treatment of these disorders. The ultimate goal is to either prevent these diseases in at-risk individuals before the onset of clinical manifestations or to develop effective neuroprotective therapies that slow down or halt disease progression in the earliest stages.

Given the pace of research and the burgeoning interest in the field, it appeared to be an auspicious time to put together a major textbook placing the neurodegenerative diseases into modern prospective. The objective of the present text is to present the latest research into the genetics, pathogenesis, biochemistry, animal models, clinical features, and treatment of neurodegenerative diseases. As such, we have been very fortunate to obtain the assistance of an internationally recognized group of authors who are amongst the foremost experts in neurodegenerative diseases.

In the first section we have compiled state-of-the-art chapters that reflect on basic aspects of neurodegeneration, including the roles of free radicals, mitochondria, excitotoxicity, calcium binding proteins, apoptosis, neurotrophins, protein aggregation, DNA repair systems, trace elements, nitric oxide/PARP, and inflammation. We have also obtained outstanding chapters on utilizing diagnostic and therapeutic tools in neurodegenerative diseases. This includes chapters on transgenic animal models, toxic animal models, strategies for molecular genetics, electrophysiological assessment, MRI, PET/SPECT, and MRI spectroscopy. Gene therapy, stem cells and transplantation are also covered.

The book then focuses on major aspects of neurodegenerative diseases, including normal aging of the nervous system. There are specific approaches to diseases dominated by dementia or behavioral disturbances, including Alzheimer's disease, Dementia with Lewy bodies, Pick's disease, fronto-temporal dementias, and fronto-temporal dementia with parkinsonism. There is also a chapter on prion diseases. The approach to the patient presenting with Parkinsonian symptoms is addressed, as well as more detailed chapters dealing with the clinical aspects, neuropathology and treatment of Parkinson's disease. There are also chapters on the so-called "atypical parkinsonisms" including multiple system atrophy, progressive supranuclear palsy and corticobasal degeneration. Subsequent sections deal with the neurodegenerative ataxias, motor neuron diseases, degenerative diseases with chorea (Huntington's disease, DRPLA, neurocanthocytosis), iron and copper disorders and finally mitochondria diseases. In each section we attempted to obtain chapters that detail the genetics and the clinical and neuropathologic features of these illnesses, as well as modern approaches to treatment.

Although the rapid pace of research in the field challenges the ability of any textbook to maintain its currency, we have conscripted a superlative group of contributors and compiled a text that we believe will be the most authoritative in the field for the forthcoming near future. We hope that this text will be useful to both neurologists and neuroscientists who are interested in the pathogenesis, clinical aspects, and treatment of these disorders. We also hope that this work will stimulate the further research necessary to relieve the human suffering caused by these tragic and devastating illnesses.

Flint Beal
Anthony Lang
Albert Ludolph

Basic aspects of neurodegeneration

Endogenous free radicals and antioxidants in the brain

Stefan L. Marklund

Department of Medical Biosciences, Clinical Chemistry, Umeå University Hospital, Sweden

The role of oxygen free radicals and antioxidants in Central Nervous System (CNS) pathology is of major interest for many reasons. While accounting for only 2% of the body weight, the brain uses 20% of the oxygen consumed by the resting body. Polyunsaturated lipids and catecholamines prone to autoxidize are abundant, and since the neurons are postmitotic, efficient protection against oxidants is vital. Accordingly, changes in most antioxidant and prooxidant factors result in phenotypes in the brain, which is exemplified in this chapter. Evidence for attack by oxygen free radicals on lipids, proteins and DNA has also been found in virtually every type of brain disease and in aging. The oxidants also exert signalling effects, but that aspect will not be covered in this chapter.

Formation of oxygen free radicals

Molecular oxygen is chemically a biradical with two unpaired electrons with equal spins in two antibonding $\Pi^{*}2p$ orbitals. This has the consequence that oxygen primarily is reduced one step at a time, since reactions with paired electrons are "forbidden." Reduction of oxygen to water may, in principle, be described in steps:

$$O_2 + e^- \rightarrow O_2 \cdot^-$$
$$O_2 \cdot^- + e^- + 2H^+ \rightarrow H_2O_2$$
$$H_2O_2 + e^- + H^+ \rightarrow OH \cdot + H_2O$$
$$OH \cdot + e^- + H^+ \rightarrow H_2O$$

The results are the intermediates: the superoxide anion radical, hydrogen peroxide and the hydroxyl radical. Hydrogen peroxide is not a free radical but is still reactive, and the intermediates are together often termed reactive oxygen species (ROS). Sometimes peroxyl (LOO·) and alkoxyl (LO·) radicals, e.g. formed in lipid peroxidation (below) are included among the ROS. The term is commonly used, because often the actual damaging species in the biological system under study is not well defined.

The bulk of oxygen in the body is reduced in four steps to water in the mitochondrial respiratory chain, without release of intermediates. A few percent of the oxygen consumed is estimated to be reduced stepwise under formation of ROS. With the exception of a few oxidase-catalyzed reactions, the reduction primarily proceeds via formation of superoxide radical.

Superoxide anion radical

Mitochondria

The major source of superoxide radicals in the body is the reaction of oxygen with electrons leaking from the mitochondrial respiratory chain. The major sites of superoxide formation are apparently FeS clusters or semiquinones in complex I and ubisemiquinone in complex III. Studies with depletion of Mn-SOD suggests that complex III superoxide formation may be directed vs. both the inner matrix and the intermembrane space (Raha et al., 2000). From the intermembrane space, the radicals may then enter the cytosol via the voltage-dependent anion channels (VDAC) (Han et al., 2003). Increased mitochondrial superoxide production apparently plays important roles in a variety of pathologies including glutamate-induced excitotoxicity (Nicholls et al., 1999), hyperglycemia (Du et al., 2000), TNF action (Hennet, Richter & Peterhans, 1993), some mitochondrial diseases (McEachern et al., 2000), and ischemia-reperfusion (Li & Jackson, 2002). (See also Chapter 3, Greenamyre and Chapter 62, Shapira.)

The NADPH oxidases

These are membrane-bound complexes that are major sources of superoxide radical in the body. Normally, the activity has useful purposes: in phagocytes for the defense against infections and in other cell types probably for signalling. However, activation of the oxidases may also exert toxic collateral effects. The catalytic subunit gp91phox and p22phox are membrane bound, while there are several cytosolic components that assemble with the membrane-bound components upon activation (Babior, Lambeth & Nauseef, 2002). There are at least five gp91phox homologs (NOX) (Bokoch & Knaus, 2003; Cheng *et al.*, 2001). The most extensively studied is the NOX2 of neutrophils, which also exists in macrophages/microglia. Oxidant production by activated microglia has been implicated in virtually every neurodegenerative disease, e.g. Gao *et al.* (2002). (See also Chapter 14, Pasinetti.) NOX isoforms are also expressed in vascular endothelial and smooth muscle cells (Sorescu *et al.*, 2002), and may be sources of superoxide in pathologies with vascular components, e.g. as induced by peptides derived from APP (Iadecola *et al.*, 1999). Furthermore, components of the NADPH oxidase complex have been demonstrated in cultured cortical neurons and astrocytes, and have been implicated in oxidant production induced by Zn (Noh & Koh, 2000), and neuronal apoptosis following NGF deprivation (Tammariello, Quinn & Estus, 2000).

Autoxidations

Autoxidations generally result in one-step reduction of oxygen to the superoxide radical. Multiple endogenous and exogenous drugs and toxins in the CNS are prone to autoxidation including dopamine, L-DOPA, adrenalin, noradrenalin, 6-OH-dopamine. Most reactions are relatively slow, but are promoted by transition metal ions. Such reactions are suspected to contribute to neurodegeneration, e.g. in Parkinson's disease (Jenner & Olanow, 1996). (See also Chapter 6, Przedborski.)

Xanthine oxidase

This is the final enzyme in the catabolism of purines in humans and catalyzes the stepwise formation of xanthine and urate from hypoxanthine under formation of both superoxide and hydrogen peroxide. Xanthine oxidase is proteolysed from its NADH-accepting form, e.g. following ischemia/reperfusion, which also will lead to increased formation of hypoxanthine. The enzyme has been demonstrated in the brain of some rodents (Patt *et al.*, 1988), but not with certainty in humans. The inhibitor allopurinol (Palmer *et al.*, 1993) or inhibition by pretreatment with tungsten (Patt *et al.*, 1988) has shown protective effects in some brain i/r models, for example, but many studies have failed to show effects (Nakashima *et al.*, 1999).

Nitric oxide synthase

Under suboptimal concentrations of arginine all nitric oxide synthase isoenzymes generate $O_2 \cdot^-$ under enzymic cycling (Pou *et al.*, 1992). This side reaction is also influenced by the cofactor tetrahydrobiopterin, which increases the rate of oxygen reduction, but also leads to some direct formation of hydrogen peroxide (Rosen *et al.*, 2002).

Prostanoid metabolism

Both PGH synthase and lipoxygenases release in the presence of NAD(P)H superoxide radical as a byproduct (Kukreja *et al.*, 1986). Such formation has been shown to contribute to microvascular abnormalities in the brain, e.g. induced by hypertension (Kontos *et al.*, 1981).

CYP450

The drug-metabolizing cytochrome P450s leak electrons to oxygen to form the superoxide radical. The 2E1 isoform is particularly prone to form superoxide and occurs in some parts of the brain (Tindberg & Ingelman-Sundberg, 1996). It is induced by ethanol and some xenobiotics, IL-1β, and ischemia/reperfusion (Tindberg *et al.*, 1996). Whether the activities in the brain are sufficient to exert toxic effects is not known, but 2E1 is strongly implicated in, e.g. liver pathology (Cederbaum *et al.*, 2001).

RAGE

Advanced glycation end products react with a cell surface receptor (RAGE) that transduces proinflammatory signals including formation of oxygen radicals, possibly via activation of NADPH oxidases (Wautier *et al.*, 2001). The receptor exists on microglia, astrocytes and hippocampal neurons and has been implicated in cellular activation, e.g. by Aβ peptides in Alzheimer's disease (Lue *et al.*, 2001; Sasaki *et al.*, 2001).

Reactions of the superoxide radical

The superoxide radical reacts very rapidly with NO to form peroxynitrite. This reaction is of great importance for the physiology and pathology of both molecules. (See Chapter 2, Crow and Chapter 12, Dawson.) There is also a rapid reaction with ascorbate (Nishikimi, 1975) and a slower complex reaction and interaction with reduced glutathione (Winterbourn & Metodiewa, 1994). The superoxide radical has, however, a low reactivity with most other biomolecules. The most important cellular targets are proteins with FeS clusters (Gardner & Fridovich, 1991), which occur particularly in mitochondria. The inactivation of the cytosolic and mitochondrial aconitases, which both contain FeS clusters, are useful markers for increased superoxide radical formation (Gardner & Fridovich, 1991; Huang *et al.*, 2002). Participation of superoxide radical in Haber Weiss chemistry may also be of importance, see below. The corresponding acid form, HOO·, is more reactive and may, e.g. initiate lipid peroxidation (Bielski, Arudi & Sutherland, 1983). The acid–base couple has a pK_a of 4.75, which is why such reactions will increase in importance with decreasing pH. It has been suggested that the superoxide radical can terminate lipid peroxidation chains and there is evidence for the existence of optimal superoxide concentrations in vivo (Nelson, Bose & McCord, 1994). The superoxide radical inhibits glutathione peroxidase (Blum & Fridovich, 1985) and catalase (Kono & Fridovich, 1982). On the other hand, the radical reactivates catalase inhibited by NO (Kim & Han, 2000). There are other in vivo effects of superoxide radical with more undefined mechanisms, but with a neurobiological interest. Thus superoxide activates mitochondrial uncoupling proteins (Echtay *et al.*, 2002), potentiates hippocampal synaptic transmission (Knapp & Klann, 2002) and inactivates a plasma membrane surface glutamate receptor-like complex (Agbas *et al.*, 2002).

Hydrogen peroxide

The major part of the hydrogen peroxide in the body is formed by superoxide dismutase-catalyzed or spontaneous dismutation of the superoxide radical. Some hydrogen peroxide is, however, formed directly by oxidases such as glycollate oxidase, urate oxidase (not in humans) and D-amino acid oxidase, which are localized to peroxisomes. Of particular importance in the CNS are the monoamine oxidases (MAO), situated in the outer membrane of mitochondria. MAO A primarily degrades serotonin and norepinephrine, and MAO B degrades phenylethylamine. Dopamine is metabolized by both (Shih, Chen & Ridd, 1999). Toxic effects may be caused by both the hydrogen peroxide formed upon the oxidative deamination of catecholamines as well as by some of the resulting metabolites. MAO effects have been suggested to contribute to, e.g. the loss of dopaminergic neurons in Parkinson's disease (Jenner & Olanow, 1996), where impairment of mitochondria may contribute (Gluck *et al.*, 2002).

Hydrogen peroxide generally has a low reactivity, but may oxidize some cysteines. Cysteine thiolate anions are readily oxidized to cysteine sulfenic acid, whereas (base) thiols are very resistant. The thiolate anions exist at physiological pH in cysteines with low pK_as caused by adjacent stabilizing positively charged amino acid residues. Protein tyrosine phosphatases can be inactivated by such cysteine oxidation, and this reaction is involved in some of the signaling effects of hydrogen peroxide (Meng, Fukada & Tonks, 2002). Another susceptible target is the active cysteine in glyceraldehyde-3-phosphate dehydrogenase (Brodie & Reed, 1987). This thiol is very susceptible overall for reactions with ROS. Most toxicity of hydrogen peroxide is caused apparently by the interaction with transition metal ions (below).

Hydroxyl radical

The hydroxyl radical reacts at close to diffusion limited rates with most biomolecules and is by far the most reactive of the ROS. It is mainly formed in vivo in the reaction of hydrogen peroxide with reduced forms of transition metal ions:

$$H_2O_2 + Me^+ \rightarrow OH\cdot + OH^- + Me^{2+}$$

The most important participating metals in vivo are Cu^+ and Fe^{2+}. The reaction with iron is called the Fenton reaction from its first description (Winterbourn, 1995). For the reactions to occur, the metal ions have to be reduced, e.g. by superoxide:

$$O_2\cdot^- + Fe^{3+} \rightarrow Fe^{2+} + O_2$$

The sum of the two reactions is called the Haber–Weiss reaction (Halliwell, 1978; McCord & Day, Jr., 1978). The transition metal ion reduction can, however, be accomplished by many other reductants, e.g. ascorbate. Fenton/Haber–Weiss chemistry probably underlies a major part of the toxicity of both hydrogen peroxide and the transition metal ions.

Hydroxyl radical may also be formed from peroxynitrite (Halliwell, Zhao & Whiteman, 1999) and by the reaction of superoxide with hypochlorite (Candeias *et al.*, 1993). HOCl can, for example, be formed from hydrogen peroxide and Cl^- catalysed by myeloperoxidase in neutrophil leukocytes.

$$HOCl + O_2\cdot^- \rightarrow OH\cdot + Cl^- + O_2$$

Singlet oxygen

An input of energy can transform ground state (triplet) molecular oxygen to singlet oxygen. The physiologically relevant form is called $^1\Delta_g$ singlet oxygen, which has the two antibonding electrons with opposite spins in one of the Π^*2p orbitals. Thereby, spin restrictions for reactions are removed and singlet oxygen reacts avidly with a wide variety of biomolecules, e.g. those containing double bonds. The reaction with unsaturated fatty acids results in the formation of lipid hydroperoxides, cf. below. Among amino acids residues, methionine and histidine are particularly susceptible, and in DNA the reaction primarily occurs with guanine residues (Sies & Menck, 1992). Singlet oxygen has a very short half-life in water, 3.8 µs. Protection can be achieved by quenching reactions where the energy is transferred to another molecule, which in turn dissipates it as heat. β-carotene and other carotenoids are efficient singlet oxygen quenchers.

Singlet oxygen can be formed by type II photosensitizing reactions, where molecules excited by light transfer the energy to (triplet) molecular oxygen. Porphyrins and many drugs, e.g. tetracyclins are efficient sensitizers, and singlet oxygen is a major cause of the light-induced skin reactions caused by these compounds. Singlet oxygen is also formed in the reaction between two lipid peroxyl radicals, cf. below, and slowly in a reaction between hydrogen peroxide and hypochlorite. Except for photosensitized reactions in the retina, singlet oxygen is probably not a major player in pathology of the nervous system.

Lipid peroxidation and vitamin E

The basis for lipid peroxidation is the labile *bis*-allylic hydrogens (LH below) bound to the methylene carbons between the double bonds in polyunsaturated fatty acids. The process can be initiated, for example, with the reaction of the hydrogen with a hydroxyl radical. Molecular oxygen rapidly adds to the resulting carbon-centred free radical, forming a lipid peroxyl radical. This, in turn, abstracts a *bis*-allylic hydrogen from a neighbor fatty acid forming a lipid hydroperoxide and again a carbon-centred free radical. Molecular oxygen adds to this radical resulting in a propagated chain reaction called lipid peroxidation.

$$LH + OH\cdot \rightarrow L\cdot + H_2O$$
$$L\cdot + O_2 \rightarrow LOO\cdot$$
$$LOO\cdot + LH \rightarrow LOOH + L\cdot$$

The reaction chain can be terminated by the radicals reacting with each other, e.g. the so-called Russel mechanism:

$$>LOO\cdot + >LOO\cdot \rightarrow >CHOH + >C = O + (singlet)O_2$$

The "phenolic" hydrogen (Toc-OH) on the chroman ring of the lipid-soluble vitamin E (α-tocopherol) efficiently competes with the *bis*-allylic hydrogens for donation to lipid peroxyl radicals.

$$LOO\cdot + Toc\text{-}OH \rightarrow LOOH + Toc\text{-}O\cdot$$

The resulting radical in vitamin E is delocalized and generally does not participate in propagation of lipid peroxidation. The result is termination of the lipid peroxidation chain. Following absorption, vitamin E is transported to the organs of the body via lipoproteins. Vitamin E enters the brain slowly, although this organ seems to be prioritized in vitamin E deficiency (Vatassery *et al.*, 1988). In a-β-lipoproteinemia there is a deficient absorption and transport of vitamin E, which results in neurological deficits that are ameliorated by vitamin E therapy. The secretion of vitamin E from the liver via VLDL is dependent on the α-tocopherol transfer protein. Loss of function mutations in this protein lead to very low plasma vitamin E levels and progressive spinocerebellar ataxia (Gotoda *et al.*, 1995) and retinitis pigmentosa (Yokota *et al.*, 1997).

The in vivo initiation mechanisms are not well understood, but commonly may involve reactions of transition metal ions with lipid hydroperoxides, which in turn can be preformed by several mechanisms in vivo:

$$LOOH + Fe^{2+} \rightarrow LO\cdot + OH^- + Fe^{3+}$$
$$LOOH + Fe^{3+} \rightarrow LOO\cdot + H^+ + Fe^{2+}$$

The resulting lipid alkoxyl and peroxyl radicals then abstract *bis*-allylic hydrogens initiating lipid peroxidation chains.

The lipid peroxidation results in detrimental structural changes of membranes and lipoproteins. The peroxidation-modified lipids degrade further to form a wide variety of toxic reactive compounds such as 4-OH-nonenal and malondialdehyde.

Transition metal ions

Transition metal ions are toxic, e.g. by participating in the Haber–Weiss reaction and in initiation of lipid peroxidation, and therefore have to be tightly controlled in vivo. In plasma, binding of Fe to transferrin prevents the reactivity, and normally less than 50% of the capacity is occupied. In the cytosol, storage in ferritin is protective. The form and mechanism of transit of Fe between intracellular pools and proteins, however, is not well defined, but there may be a 0.7–0.9 µM "labile" iron pool (Konijn *et al.*, 1999). Increased amounts of reactive iron may occur following release from ferritin by the superoxide radical (Biemond *et al.*, 1988) and some redox-cycling toxins (Winterbourn, Vile & Monteiro, 1991), disruption of FeS clusters, e.g. by superoxide radicals (Gardner & Fridovich, 1991), and degradation of heme from denatured hemoproteins. Heme itself is also prooxidant (Gutteridge & Smith, 1988).

The intracellular transit of Cu is better understood and involves different "Cu-chaperones" for different Cu protein targets (Huffman & O'Halloran, 2001). SOD1 is, for example, charged by a Cu-chaperone for SOD (Wong *et al.*, 2000). The intracellular concentration of "free" Cu has been estimated to be less than 1 molecule per cell (Rae *et al.*, 1999). Excess Cu (and Zn) in cells may be scavenged by metallothioneins (Hidalgo *et al.*, 2001). (See also Chapter 13, Bush, Chapter 60, Gitlin, and Chapter 61, Lewitt.)

Hemoprotein peroxidases and oxidants

Mammals contain at least four peroxidases with heme prosthetic groups; myeloperoxidase, eosinophil peroxidase, lactoperoxidase and thyroid peroxidase. Like the ubiquitous plant hemoperoxidases, they have the ability to catalyze the oxidation of a wide variety of phenolic and other substrates by hydrogen peroxide. In vivo, however, the mammalian peroxidases primarily oxidize halides.

Myeloperoxidase exists in granules of neutrophils, monocytes and can also be induced in tissue macrophages/microglia (Sugiyama *et al.*, 2001). Upon activation these cells produce hydrogen peroxide via NADPH oxidase, which myeloperoxidase uses to oxidize Cl^- to the strong oxidant hypochlorite.

$$H_2O_2 + Cl^- \rightarrow OCl^- + H_2O$$

The hypochlorite is not essential for, but contributes to, the killing of bacteria by the neutrophils (Hampton, Kettle & Winterbourn, 1996). Myeloperoxidase apparently can also catalyze the hydrogen peroxide-dependent oxidation nitrite to a nitrating species (Pfeiffer *et al.*, 2001). This leads to the formation protein-bound nitrotyrosine, previously thought to be a specific marker for the reaction product between superoxide radical and NO, peroxynitrite.

The peroxidase of eosinophil leukocytes can also produce hypochlorite, but seems primarily to oxidize bromide ions to hypobromite (Weiss *et al.*, 1986). The lactoperoxidase of tears, saliva and milk oxidizes thiocyanate to the bacteriostatic hypothiocyanate. The thyroid peroxidase iodinates and condensates tyrosine residues in thyroglobulin to form the thyroid hormones.

Myeloperoxidase has been demonstrated in microglia close to plaques in Alzheimer's disease and also in the β-amyloid, suggesting a potential involvement in the disease (Reynolds *et al.*, 1999). The enzyme may, however, also have a modulating effect on inflammatory reactions, since mice lacking myeloperoxidase are more susceptible to experimental autoimmune encephalitis (Brennan *et al.*, 2001a) and atherosclerosis (Brennan *et al.*, 2001b).

Low-molecular weight scavengers

Endogenous

GSH

The tripeptide glutathione, L-γ-glutamyl-L-cysteinyl-glycine (GSH) reaches cellular concentrations of several mmol/l, and is generally the most abundant low-molecular weight antioxidant in the body. GSH aids in metabolizing hydroperoxides by being the reducing substrate of the glutathione peroxidases (below), and of some of the peroxyredoxins (below). GSH can also directly reduce some free radical targets in biomolecules (Biaglow *et al.*, 1989). The reactions mostly result in formation of the disulfide oxidized glutathione (GSSG), which is in turn reduced back to GSH by glutathione reductase. The enzyme uses NADPH, derived from the glucose-6-phosphate dehydrogenase, the cytosolic (Jo *et al.*, 2002) and the mitochondrial (Jo *et al.*, 2001) NADP-dependent isocitrate dehydrogenase isoenzymes. These dehydrogenases thus form important parts of the antioxidant defence. GSH can also react with oxidized cysteines in proteins forming mixed disulfides. Increased concentrations of these are found in oxidant stress (Cotgreave & Gerdes, 1998). GSH is also used for conjugation of xenobiotics and other molecules catalyzed by glutathione transferases, and direct reaction with free radical intermediates, e.g. from dopamine and L-DOPA can also occur (Spencer *et al.*, 1998). These reactions can, however, also lead to depletion of GSH, causing toxic effects on tissues.

GSH is formed from its constituent amino acids in two steps synthesized by γ-glutamyl-cysteine-synthase and glutathione synthase. Cysteine may be limiting for the synthesis, and can experimentally and therapeutically be supplied by *N*-acetylcysteine or by 2-oxothiazolidine-4-carboxylate (Gwilt *et al.*, 1998). GSH can be exported over the plasma membrane and will then be hydrolyzed to γ-glutamine and cysteinyl-glycine by the ectoenzyme γ-glutamyltranspeptidase. The dipeptide is then hydrolyzed by dipeptidases. The constituent amino acids can then be taken up intracellularly for GSH resynthesis.

In the brain, the concentration of GSH appears to be higher in astrocytes (4 mmol/l) than in neurons (2.5 mmol/l) and other glial cells. Astrocytes can apparently protect neurons by degrading the diffusible hydrogen peroxide, and also supply neurons with the substrates for GSH synthesis by export of GSH (Dringen, Gutterer & Hirrlinger, 2000).

Bilirubin and heme oxygenases

Heme is degraded to biliverdin and the transmitter substance CO by the heme oxygenases (HO), the inducible HO-1 and the constitutive HO-2. HO-2 is the most abundant in the CNS. Biliverdin is then reduced by biliverdin reductase and NADPH to bilirubin. Since heme, that for example, can be released from denatured hemoproteins, is prooxidant (Gutteridge & Smith, 1988), the heme oxygenases may exert antioxidant roles, provided that the released iron is efficiently sequestered. Bilirubin, in addition, efficiently scavenges some reactive oxygen species such as singlet oxygen and peroxyl radicals, forming biliverdin again. Bilirubin has shown in vitro neuroprotective action (Dore et al., 1999), and a protective cycle involving biliverdin reductase can be envisioned. The β-amyloid precursor protein inhibits HO, and Alzheimer-linked mutant protein causes stronger inhibition. This effect has been suggested to contribute to the pathology in Alzheimer's disease (Takahashi et al., 2000).

Urate

This is the end product of purine catabolism in humans, who have an inactive urate oxidase. In most other species allantoin is formed by urate oxidase. The concentration of urate in humans furthermore is kept high by tubular reabsorption in the kidney. Urate can scavenge a variety of oxidants such as $ROO\cdot$, $ONOO^-$, NO_2 and O_3 (Becker et al., 1991) to form allantoin, parabanic acid and some other compounds. Urate at concentrations found in humans furthermore has been shown to protect the Cu-containing SOD1 and SOD3 in vivo against inactivation by (presumably) hydrogen peroxide (Hink et al., 2002). Administration of urate protects, for example, against experimental autoimmune encephalitis (Kastenbauer et al., 2001), and increased levels of the oxidized metabolites in CSF have, for example, been observed in humans with meningitis (Kastenbauer et al., 2002), suggesting a protective role of the compound in the CNS.

Exogenous

Ascorbate

This and vitamin E (see above) are the major dietary antioxidants in humans. Other mammals, with the exception of guinea pigs, synthesize ascorbate in the liver. Ascorbate occurs in 10–100-fold higher concentration in cells compared with blood plasma. In addition to participation in multiple metabolic reactions, ascorbate is an important antioxidant that reacts rapidly with superoxide radical, other free radicals and peroxynitrite and can also regenerate oxidized vitamin E (Chan, 1993). Ascorbate on the other hand can also reduce ferric iron and other oxidized transition metal ions and thereby promote Fenton-type reactions. Ascorbate easily autoxidizes, catalyzed by transition metal ions under oxygen radical formation (Buettner & Jurkiewicz, 1996). The importance of these prooxidant reactions may, however, be small in vivo where transition metal ions are mostly tightly controlled.

The reaction of ascorbate with oxygen free radicals primarily results in formation of semidehydroascorbate that disproportionates rapidly to dehydroascorbate and ascorbate. Semidehydro- and dehydroascorbate are reduced back rapidly to ascorbate by multiple mechanisms including GSH, thioredoxin reductase (Arrigoni & De Tullio, 2002; Nordberg & Arner, 2001), and a GSH-dependent dehydroascorbate reductase localized to the grey matter (Fornai et al., 1999).

Ascorbate reaches the brain primarily via the CSF. It is actively transported from blood plasma in the choroid plexus into the CSF via a Na-coupled transporter, SVCT2, to result in high extracellular concentrations in the brain, around 200–400 μmol/l (Rice, 2000). This concentration apparently is controlled, suggesting an extracellular antioxidant role. Neurons take up ascorbate via SVCT2 and contain around 10 mmol/l. Astrocytes contain much less, around 2 mmol/l. The mechanism of loss of ascorbate from neurons is not fully understood, but may include a heteroexchange mechanism with glutamate, and an export of dehydroascorbate via the glucose transporter Glut 3. It is suggested that astrocytes acquire dehydroascorbate by Glut 1, reduce it and secrete ascorbate again. This may serve as a supply mechanism for neurons (Rice, 2000). The presence in all cells of glucose transporters (Glut) that also allow transport of dehydroascorbate, coupled with efficient intracellular reduction, seems to account for a significant part of the cellular ascorbate uptake. Such uptake is enhanced by extracellular ascorbate oxidation via, for example, superoxide radicals (Nualart et al., 2003).

Flavonoids and other plant antioxidants

Dietary and intervention studies have indicated that fruit and vegetable consumption is important for neuronal health (Galli et al., 2002). Plants contain multiple potential active components, and mostly the actual active compounds are not identified with certainty. Many beneficial effects are presumed to be derived from a family of polyphenolic compounds called flavonoids, which occur abundantly in plants and are major constituents of many formulations, for example, from ginseng and *Ginkgo biloba*. Owing to their polyunsaturated substituted cyclic structures, the compounds function as reducing antioxidants, and have been shown to exert cytoprotective actions in a variety of experimental systems. The compounds may also reduce oxygen (autoxidize) under formation of oxygen radicals and thereby function as prooxidants. Many of the compounds show poor absorption and the extent of passage through the blood–brain barrier is little known. Their importance for the basal CNS integrity in humans is therefore not well established (Youdim *et al.*, 2002). Carotenoids, many of which are precursors of vitamin A, are efficient scavengers of singlet oxygen. Garlic extracts containing *S*-allycystein, *S*-allymercaptocysteine, allicin and diallosulfides have been shown to delay cognitive impairment in a senescent accelerated mouse model (Youdim & Joseph, 2001).

Antioxidant proteins and enzymes

Superoxide dismutases (SOD)
These dismute the superoxide radical under formation of molecular oxygen and hydrogen peroxide.

$$2O_2^- + 2H^+ \rightarrow O_2 + H_2O_2$$

Since this reaction occurs rapidly and spontaneously, the SODs generally do not alter the hydrogen peroxide formation, but rather reduce the steady-state concentration of the superoxide radical. When there are major competing reactions that reduce the radical (e.g. with ascorbate) SOD will decrease hydrogen peroxide formation and, if competing reactions oxidize the radical, SOD will tend to increase the hydrogen peroxide formation. If SOD competes with NO for reaction with the superoxide radical, hydrogen peroxide formation will also be increased by the enzyme (Gardner, Salvador & Moradas-Ferreira, 2002).

There are three different SODs with different locations and different roles in the body. The phenotypes of knockouts are very different (Carlsson *et al.*, 1995; Li *et al.*, 1995; Reaume *et al.*, 1996), and so far there is no evidence that the isoenzymes can complement each other (Copin, Gasche & Chan, 2000). One reason apparently is the poor penetration of the superoxide radical through biological membranes (Winterbourn & Stern, 1987).

The first discovered (McCord & Fridovich, 1969) and most extensively studied is CuZn–SOD (SOD1). It is a homodimeric enzyme with each 15 kDa subunit containing one Cu and one Zn atom. The Cu is liganded by 4 His and the Zn by 3 His and one Asp residue (Tainer *et al.*, 1982). SOD1 physically is a very stable protein. SOD1 is charged with Cu by the Cu-chaperone for superoxide dismutase (CCS) (Huffman & O'Halloran, 2001). Whereas CCS is essential in yeast, some residual SOD1 activity exists in mice lacking CCS (Wong *et al.*, 2000), suggesting additional ways of charging the enzyme with Cu in mammals. The major location of SOD1 is the cytosol, but the enzyme also occurs in the nucleus (Chang *et al.*, 1988) and in the intermembrane space of mitochondria (Weisiger & Fridovich, 1973). A location for peroxisomes has also been discussed (Keller *et al.*, 1991; Liou *et al.*, 1993). Whereas the other SOD isoenzymes are widely regulated, SOD1 is essentially a constitutive enzyme with tissue-specific differences in concentration (Marklund, 1984). All the cultured or isolated cell types studied so far have contained the enzyme and generally there are rather small differences between various cell types (Marklund, 1984, 1990). Overall the brain contains intermediate levels of SOD1 compared with other tissues, with slightly more in grey matter that in white (Marklund, 1984). SOD1 is an abundantly expressed enzyme and the level in grey matter corresponds to 0.3% of the soluble protein (Marklund, 1984). By immunohistochemistry, spinal motor neurons appear to contain more SOD1 than most other cells in the CNS (Shaw *et al.*, 1997), but a likely proposition is that all other cell types in the CNS also contain sizeable levels of SOD1. More than 100 different mutations in the SOD1 gene have been linked to heritable amyotrophic lateral sclerosis (ALS) (Andersen *et al.*, 2003; Rosen *et al.*, 1993). ALS is caused by the gain of a toxic property of mutant SOD1, and mice lacking SOD1 do not develop motor neuron degeneration or show any other obvious phenotype (Reaume *et al.*, 1996). Closer inspection, however, reveals axonopathy (Shefner *et al.*, 1999), and the mutant mice also show increased susceptibility to, e.g. the neurotoxin MPTP (Zhang *et al.*, 2000), and to ischemia/reperfusion of the CNS (Kondo *et al.*, 1997).

The mammalian Mn-SOD (SOD2) is homotetrameric, with each subunit liganding one Mn atom (Borgstahl *et al.*, 1992). The subunits are synthesized in the cytosol with a signal peptide with direct import into the mitochondrial matrix where the enzyme is matured by proteolysis and equipped with Mn atoms. The latter reaction may be accomplished by a specific Mn-transfer protein (Luk *et al.*, 2003). The severe phenotype of mice lacking SOD2 suggests that the enzyme is essential for mitochondrial integrity (Lebovitz *et al.*, 1996; Li *et al.*, 1995). Mitochondrial factors containing superoxide-susceptible FeS clusters are apparently major targets in SOD2 null mice. Brain grey matter contains high levels of Mn-SOD, whereas the level in white matter is threefold lower (Marklund, 1984).

Apparently, the high levels in the brain are important since CNS injury is a prominent feature of Mn-SOD null mice (Lebovitz *et al.*, 1996). Mice heterozygous for the SOD2 null allele show increased susceptibility to the neurotoxic mitochondrial toxins, malonate, 3-nitropropionic acid and MPTP (Andreassen *et al.*, 2001), and are more susceptible to ALS-linked mutant SOD1 (Andreassen *et al.*, 2000). SOD2 is widely regulated by a variety of inflammatory cytokines (Marklund, 1992; Wong & Goeddel, 1988) and somewhat less so by oxidant stress (Stralin & Marklund, 1994).

Extracellular-SOD (EC-SOD, SOD3) is a homotetrameric secreted glycoprotein (Marklund, 1982). The subunits are synthesized with a signal peptide, which is cleaved upon maturation. They ligand Cu and Zn and the sequence is similar to that of SOD1 in the part that defines the active site (Hjalmarsson *et al.*, 1987). SOD3 shows high affinity for heparin and heparan sulfate, conferred by the highly positively charged C-terminal end of the subunits. In vivo the enzyme is anchored primarily to heparan sulfate proteoglycans in the interstitial matrix of tissues (Karlsson *et al.*, 1994). In the vasculature, SOD3 forms an equilibrium between the plasma phase and the endothelial cell surfaces. The brain contains little SOD3, both in humans (Marklund, 1984) and in mice (Carlsson *et al.*, 1995). However, in the brain the enzyme is localized to neurons in a few discrete areas, and in addition is apparently mainly intracellular (Oury, Card & Klann, 1999). This intracellular location has also been observed in some other tissues and suggests that the enzyme may have an intracellular role or is stored for secretion under some circumstances. The enzyme may thus exert some specific roles in the CNS. SOD3 null mice do not show any spontaneous CNS or other phenotypes, but the lungs are highly susceptible to high oxygen tension (Carlsson, Jonsson, Edlund & Marklund, 1995). Impaired memory (Levin *et al.*, 1998), and enhanced injury in stroke models (Sheng *et al.*, 1999) has also been observed in SOD3 null mice. SOD3 is a highly regulated enzyme and the synthesis is influenced by inflammatory cytokines (Marklund, 1992), vasoactive factors and some sulphated glycosaminoglycans (Stralin & Marklund, 2001), but hardly by oxidant stress (Stralin & Marklund, 1994).

Catalase

The homotetrameric hemoprotein catalase catalyzes the dismutation of hydrogen peroxide.

$$2H_2O_2 \rightarrow O_2 + 2H_2O$$

The catalysed reaction is first order in hydrogen peroxide at all physiological concentrations, and unlike glutathione peroxidase catalase is equally efficient at all hydrogen peroxide concentrations. Except for erythrocytes, the enzyme is intracellularly localized to peroxisomes. Overall, the brain contains little catalase activity. Both grey and white matter of the human brain contains so little catalase that it is difficult to measure reliably due to contamination of the catalase-rich erythrocytes (Marklund *et al.*, 1982). In the rat brain catalase shows a widespread distribution, both to neurons and to glia (Moreno, Mugnaini & Ceru, 1995). Since hydrogen peroxide easily penetrates membranes (Winterbourn & Stern, 1987), the catalase-rich erythrocytes in the vasculature may degrade some of the hydrogen peroxide formed in the brain. In rats, an age-dependent decline in the catalase activity in various parts of the brain has been observed (Ciriolo *et al.*, 1997).

Glutathione peroxidases (GPX)

There are four GPX isoenzymes, all with selenocysteine in the active sites (Brigelius-Flohe, 1999). The highest activity is generally shown by the cytosolic GPX, which probably is expressed by all cells in the body. This cGPX also occurs in the mitochondria (Esworthy, Ho & Chu, 1997). The phospholipid hydroperoxide (PH) GPX also shows a wide distribution. There is an extracellular plasma GPX that is mainly secreted by the kidney, but which also is expressed in the CNS (Maser, Magenheimer & Calvet, 1994). The fourth isoenzyme is the gastrointestinal (GI) GPX. All GPXs reduce H_2O_2 and some organic hydroperoxides at the expense of reduced glutathione:

$$H_2O_2 + 2GSH \rightarrow 2H_2O + GSSG$$

In addition, PHGPX reduces a variety of complex lipidhydroperoxides and hydroperoxy groups on other biological compounds. Plasma GPX can also use thioredoxin as a reductant.

The human brain contains relatively low levels of GPX activity compared with other tissues (Marklund *et al.*, 1982), which, together with the low catalase activity, suggests that the organ may be vulnerable to increased formation of hydrogen peroxide. Note that the cGPX activity in the brain is, unlike in other organs, spared in selenium deficiency (Brigelius-Flohe, 1999). The enzyme appears to be mainly expressed in glial cells (Damier *et al.*, 1993). CGPX null mice do not show any spontaneous phenotype, but display an increased infarct size in a brain ischemia-reperfusion model (Crack *et al.*, 2001). They also show increased sensitivity to the neurotoxins: malonate, 3-nitropropionic acid and 1-methyl-4-phenyl-1,2,5,6-tetrahydropyridine (Klivenyi *et al.*, 2000; Zhang *et al.*, 2000).

Thioredoxin, glutaredoxin, and thioredoxin reductase

The major cytosolic thioredoxin (Trx-1) is a 12 kDA protein with a –Cys–Gly–Pro–Cys– active site motif, which is easily oxidized to a disulfide. Trx possesses potent protein disulfide oxidoreductase activity, and is involved in protein folding (Nordberg & Arner, 2001). Mitochondria contain another isoform, Trx-2. Reduced Trxs also serve as a substrate for the peroxyredoxin isoenzymes, see below. Trx-1 is widely expressed in neurons in the brain (Lippoldt et al., 1995), and overexpression has been shown to protect against, for example, brain ischemia-reperfusion damage (Takagi et al., 1999). Likewise, Trx-2 shows a wide distribution in the brain, apparently primarily to neurons (Rybnikova et al., 2000).

Glutaredoxin (thioltransferase) shows functions overlapping with the Trxs. Unlike these, glutaredoxin can be reduced by glutathione, and it can also reduce protein-GSH-mixed disulfides (Nordberg & Arner, 2001). This effect is, for example important in recovery of mitochondrial function following excitotoxic insult (Kenchappa et al., 2002).

Oxidized Trxs are reduced by thioredoxin reductases (TrxR) using NADPH as reductant (Nordberg & Arner, 2001). The TrxRs are flavoproteins containing active site selenocysteines, which occur in different isoforms in the cytosol and mitochondria (Nordberg & Arner, 2001). The TrxRs show wide substrate specificity and can, in addition to Trx, reduce GSH, dehydroascorbate and semidehydroascorbate, hydroperoxides including lipid hydroperoxides and protein disulfide isomerases (Nordberg & Arner, 2001). The main function of protein disulfide isomerases is to oxidize cysteines to form disulfide bonds during protein folding.

Methionine is easily oxidized by various oxidants to the sulfoxide form and is reduced back by methionine sulfoxide reductase. This enzyme uses the NADPH/Trx/TrxR system for reduction of its active site (Weissbach et al., 2002). Overexpression of methionine sulfoxide reductase predominantly in the brain of *Drosophila* prolongs the lifespan (Ruan et al., 2002). This suggests a role of methionine oxidation in aging.

Peroxyredoxins

In mammals the peroxyredoxins (Prx) comprise a family of six isoenzymes with structural and some functional similarities. The Prx isoenzymes are localized to different compartments with Prx1 and Prx2 in the cytosol, Prx3 in the mitochondria, Prx4 in the plasma membrane, Prx5 in mitochondria, peroxisomes and cytosol, while Prx6 has an extracellular location (Fujii & Ikeda, 2002). The Prx isoenzymes catalyze the reduction of hydrogen peroxide and organic hydroperoxides with all, except Prx6, using thioredoxin as the reductant. Prx1, 4 and 6 can also use GSH (Fujii & Ikeda, 2002). Notably, a bacterial peroxyredoxin has shown peroxynitrite reductase activity, which might be shared by the mammalian isoforms (Bryk, Griffin & Nathan, 2000). Unlike other enzymes that degrade hydroperoxides, the activities of Prx1 and 2 can be regulated (by phosphorylation), suggesting active involvement in cellular signaling by hydrogen peroxide (Chang et al., 2002). The Prx isoenzymes are generally highly expressed and show wide tissue distributions with comparatively high expression throughout the brain (Rhee et al., 2001). Given the low catalase and glutathione peroxidase activities, the Prx isoenzymes may conceivably exert particularly important roles in the CNS.

Markers of free radical damage

Chemical analysis

There are numerous relatively stable small molecules and protein and DNA modifications formed in reactions with oxygen free radicals, which can be used as markers for oxidant injury.

Peroxidative attack on polyunsaturated fatty acids results in the formation of various classes of isoprostanes, which are regarded as the most reliable markers of lipid peroxidation. The most widely studied is the F2 isoprostane 8-isoPGF2α, which derives from arachidonic acid. The isoprostanes are stable and have been determined, e.g. in brain extracts, cerebrospinal fluid, blood plasma and urine, and appear to parallel the peroxidation intensity (Greco, Minghetti & Levi, 2000; Janssen, 2001).

Malondialdehyde is a late breakdown product from peroxidized lipids and is generally detected as a reaction product with thiobarbituric acid (TBARS). The TBARS can be analysed by spectrophotometry, fluorimetry and by HPLC with increasing specificity (Moore & Roberts, 1998). A variety of other aldehydes and molecules can react with TBA, however, and MDA is also formed in prostanoid synthesis. The TBARS reaction therefore, has a very limited specificity and utility in complex matrices such as tissue extracts, plasma and CSF.

A major cytotoxic degradation product from peroxidized lipids is 4-hydroxynonenal. It easily forms thioether adducts and adducts with free amino groups in proteins. It is much less often analyzed than MDA (Moore & Roberts, 1998), but has a greater utility as a marker for immunohistochemical analysis.

Numerous oxidant-induced protein modifications are used as markers. The most commonly analyzed are carbonyls detected by the reaction with 2,4-dinitrophenylhydrazine. The carbonyls can be formed by OH-radical generated by the Fenton reaction, ionizing radiation, peroxynitrite, lipid peroxidation metabolites and glycoxidation (Berlett & Stadtman, 1997). The carbonyls are commonly detected by photometry in extracts and by histochemical analysis (Smith *et al.*, 1998), and should be considered as general markers of oxidant stress with limited information as to underlying oxidant mechanisms.

Oxidants are major endogenous mutagens and attack the bases in DNA under formation of a variety of modified forms. The most widely analysed is the mutagenic 8-OH-deoxyguanosine (Dizdaroglu *et al.*, 2002). The DNA is rapidly repaired by various excision mechanisms, and the concentration of modified bases thus represents a steady state between formation and excision. The rate of repair is induced in a variety of situations. On the other hand, the concentration of excised modified bases in extracellular fluids and the excretion in urine should be more proportional to the rate of oxidant injury. Increased levels have been found, for example, in CSF in ALS (Bogdanov *et al.*, 2000) and in various areas of the brain in Alzheimer's disease (Gabbita, Lovell & Markesbery, 1998). The results in different studies vary considerably, due to technical differences and the problem of artifactual base oxidation during sample preparation and analysis. (See also Chapter 10, Rolig.)

Modified low-molecular weight compounds are also analysed. In humans urate is oxidized to several different compounds (Becker *et al.*, 1991). The metabolites, allantoin and parabanic acid have been used as oxidant stress markers in humans, e.g. in brain microdialysis (Hillered & Persson, 1995; Marklund *et al.*, 2000) and in cerebrospinal fluid (Kastenbauer *et al.*, 2002).

Salicylate, which permeates tissues rapidly, is oxidized by hydroxyl radicals to 2,3- and 2,5-dihydroxybenzoic acid. The 2,3-compound is apparently specific for the hydroxyl radical, is easily extracted from tissues and can be analyzed by HPLC. Increases have, e.g. been shown in brain ischemia/reperfusion damage (Floyd, 1999).

Cellular and histochemical analyses

Histochemical analysis of oxidant stress markers has been widely employed and offers the advantage of cellular and subcellular location of the processes.

Vital staining for hydrogen peroxide formation can be accomplished via the reaction with Ce ions, which results in precipitation of electron-opaque cerium perhydroxides. Superoxide formation can be visualized with the Mn^{2+}/diaminobenzidine assay (Karnovsky, 1994). Another common vital stain is 2,7-dichlorofluorescein diacetate, which following intracellular hydrolysis of the acetate groups is oxidized to a fluorescent compound by "oxidants." The oxidation is caused primarily by hydrogen peroxide catalysed by hemoproteins. The fluorescent staining thus occurs at the location of the catalytic hemoproteins and not the site of formation of the diffusible hydrogen peroxide. Peroxynitrite, and possibly RO·, ROO· and HOCl will also oxidize DCF. Further complicating interpretation is the fact that DCF in the presence of peroxidases can engage in autoxidations artifactually generating hydrogen peroxide and fluorescence (Rota, Chignell & Mason, 1999).

Lipid peroxidation is most commonly studied with antibodies raised against malondialdehyde- and 4-hydroxynonenal-induced epitopes. These have been widely employed in studies of CNS pathology, e.g. Yoritaka *et al.* (1996). Advanced glycation end products are most commonly demonstrated with antibodies versus N–E-carboxymethyl-lysine adducts, a major end product of glycoxidation (Schleicher, Wagner & Nerlich, 1997). Oxidative damage to DNA and RNA has been demonstrated with antibodies vs., e.g. 8-OH-guanosine (Zhang *et al.*, 1999). Increased levels have, for example, been found in ALS (Shibata *et al.*, 2002).

REFERENCES

Agbas, A., Chen, X., Hong, O., Kumar, K. N. & Michaelis, E. K. (2002). Superoxide modification and inactivation of a neuronal receptor-like complex. *Free Radic. Biol. Med.*, **32** (6), 512–24.

Andersen, P. M., Sims, K. B., Xin, W. W. *et al.* (2003). Sixteen novel mutations in the Cu/Zn superoxide dismutase gene in amyotrophic lateral sclerosis: a decade of discoveries, defects and disputes. *Amyotroph. Lateral. Scler. Other Motor Neuron Disord.*, **4** (2), 62–73.

Andreassen, O. A., Ferrante, R. J., Klivenyi, P. *et al.* (2000). Partial deficiency of manganese superoxide dismutase exacerbates a transgenic mouse model of amyotrophic lateral sclerosis. *Ann. Neurol.*, **47** (4), 447–55.

Andreassen, O. A., Ferrante, R. J., Dedeoglu, A. *et al.* (2001). Mice with a partial deficiency of manganese superoxide dismutase show increased vulnerability to the mitochondrial toxins malonate, 3-nitropropionic acid, and MPTP. *Exp. Neurol.*, **167** (1), 189–95.

Arrigoni, O. & De Tullio, M. C. (2002). Ascorbic acid: much more than just an antioxidant. *Biochim. Biophys. Acta*, **1569** (1–3), 1–9.

Babior, B. M., Lambeth, J. D. & Nauseef, W. (2002). The neutrophil NADPH oxidase. *Arch. Biochem. Biophys.*, **397** (2), 342–4.

Becker, B. F., Reinholz, N., Leipert, B., Raschke, P., Permanetter, B. & Gerlach, E. (1991). Role of uric acid as an endogenous radical scavenger and antioxidant. *Chest*, **100** (3), Suppl, 176S–81S.

Berlett, B. S. & Stadtman, E. R. (1997). Protein oxidation in aging, disease, and oxidative stress. *J. Biol. Chem.*, **272** (33), 20313–16.

Biaglow, J. E., Varnes, M. E., Epp, E. R., Clark, E. P., Tuttle, S. W. & Held, K. D. (1989). Role of glutathione in the aerobic radiation response. *Int. J. Radiat. Oncol. Biol. Phys.*, **16** (5), pp. 1311–14.

Bielski, B. H., Arudi, R. L. & Sutherland, M. W. (1983). A study of the reactivity of HO_2/O^{2-} with unsaturated fatty acids. *J. Biol. Chem.*, **258** (8), 4759–61.

Biemond, P., Swaak, A. J., van Eijk, H. G. & Koster, J. F. (1988). Superoxide dependent iron release from ferritin in inflammatory diseases. *Free Radic. Biol. Med.*, **4** (3), 185–98.

Blum, J. & Fridovich, I. (1985). Inactivation of glutathione peroxidase by superoxide radical. *Arch. Biochem. Biophys.*, **240** (2), 500–8.

Bogdanov, M., Brown, R. H., Matson, W. *et al.* (2000). Increased oxidative damage to DNA in ALS patients. *Free Radic. Biol. Med.*, **29** (7), pp. 652–8.

Bokoch, G. M. & Knaus, U. G. (2003). NADPH oxidases: not just for leukocytes anymore! *Trends Biochem. Sci.*, **28** (9), 502–8.

Borgstahl, G. E., Parge, H. E., Hickey, M. J., Beyer, W. F., Jr., Hallewell, R. A. & Tainer, J. A. (1992). The structure of human mitochondrial manganese superoxide dismutase reveals a novel tetrameric interface of two 4-helix bundles. *Cell*, **71** (1), 107–18.

Brennan, M., Gaur, A., Pahuja, A., Lusis, A. J. & Reynolds, W. F. (2001a). Mice lacking myeloperoxidase are more susceptible to experimental autoimmune encephalomyelitis. *J. Neuroimmunol.*, **112** (1–2), 97–105.

Brennan, M. L., Anderson, M. M., Shih, D. M. *et al.* (2001b). Increased atherosclerosis in myeloperoxidase-deficient mice. *J. Clin. Invest.*, **107** (4), 419–30.

Brigelius-Flohe, R. (1999). Tissue-specific functions of individual glutathione peroxidases. *Free Radic. Biol. Med.*, **27** (9–10), 951–65.

Brodie, A. E. & Reed, D. J. (1987). Reversible oxidation of glyceraldehyde 3-phosphate dehydrogenase thiols in human lung carcinoma cells by hydrogen peroxide. *Biochem. Biophys. Res. Commun.*, **148** (1), 120–5.

Bryk, R., Griffin, P. & Nathan, C. (2000). Peroxynitrite reductase activity of bacterial peroxiredoxins. *Nature*, **407** (6801), 211–15.

Buettner, G. R. & Jurkiewicz, B. A. (1996). Catalytic metals, ascorbate and free radicals: combinations to avoid. *Radiat. Res.*, **145** (5), 532–41.

Candeias, L. P., Patel, K. B., Stratford, M. R. & Wardman, P. (1993). Free hydroxyl radicals are formed on reaction between the neutrophil derived species superoxide anion and hypochlorous acid. *FEBS Lett.*, **333** (1–2), 151–3.

Carlsson, L. M., Jonsson, J. Edlund, T. & Marklund, S. L. (1995). Mice lacking extracellular superoxide dismutase are more sensitive to hyperoxia. *Proc. Natl. Acad. Sci. USA*, **92** (14), 6264–8.

Cederbaum, A. I., Wu, D., Mari, M. & Bai, J. (2001). CYP2E1-dependent toxicity and oxidative stress in HepG2 cells. *Free Radic. Biol. Med.*, **31** (12), 1539–43.

Chan, A. C. (1993). Partners in defense, vitamin E and vitamin C. *Can. J. Physiol Pharmacol.*, **71** (9), 725–31.

Chang, L. Y., Slot, J. W., Geuze, H. J. & Crapo, J. D. (1988). Molecular immunocytochemistry of the CuZn superoxide dismutase in rat hepatocytes. *J. Cell Biol.*, **107** (6 Pt 1), 2169–79.

Chang, T. S., Jeong, W., Choi, S. Y., Yu, S., Kang, S. W. & Rhee, S. G. (2002). Regulation of peroxiredoxin I activity by Cdc2-mediated phosphorylation. *J. Biol. Chem.*, **277** (28), 25370–6.

Cheng, G., Cao, Z., Xu, X., van Meir, E. G. & Lambeth, J. D. (2001). Homologs of gp91phox: cloning and tissue expression of Nox3, Nox4, and Nox5. *Gene*, **269** (1–2), 131–40.

Ciriolo, M. R., Marasco, M. R., Iannone, M., Nistico, G. & Rotilio, G. (1997). Decrease of immunoreactive catalase protein in specific areas of ageing rat brain. *Neurosci. Lett.*, **228** (1), 21–4.

Copin, J. C., Gasche, Y. & Chan, P. H. (2000). Overexpression of copper/zinc superoxide dismutase does not prevent neonatal lethality in mutant mice that lack manganese superoxide dismutase. *Free Radic. Biol. Med.*, **28** (10), 1571–6.

Cotgreave, I. A. & Gerdes, R. G. (1998). Recent trends in glutathione biochemistry – glutathione–protein interactions: a molecular link between oxidative stress and cell proliferation?. *Biochem. Biophys. Res. Commun.*, **242** (1), 1–9.

Crack, P. J., Taylor, J. M., Flentjar, N. J. *et al.* (2001). Increased infarct size and exacerbated apoptosis in the glutathione peroxidase-1 (Gpx-1) knockout mouse brain in response to ischemia/reperfusion injury. *J. Neurochem.*, **78** (6), 1389–99.

Damier, P., Hirsch, E. C., Zhang, P., Agid, Y. & Javoy-Agid, F. (1993). Glutathione peroxidase, glial cells and Parkinson's disease. *Neuroscience*, **52** (1), 1–6.

Dizdaroglu, M., Jaruga, P., Birincioglu, M. & Rodriguez, H. (2002). Free radical-induced damage to DNA: mechanisms and measurement(1,2). *Free Radic. Biol. Med.*, **32** (11), 1102–15.

Dore, S., Takahashi, M., Ferris, C. D. *et al.* (1999). Bilirubin, formed by activation of heme oxygenase-2, protects neurons against oxidative stress injury. *Proc. Natl. Acad. Sci. USA*, **96** (5), 2445–50.

Dringen, R., Gutterer, J. M. & Hirrlinger, J. (2000). Glutathione metabolism in brain metabolic interaction between astrocytes and neurons in the defense against reactive oxygen species. *Eur. J. Biochem.*, **267** (16), 4912–16.

Du, X. L., Edelstein, D., Rossetti, L. *et al.* (2000). Hyperglycemia-induced mitochondrial superoxide overproduction activates the hexosamine pathway and induces plasminogen activator inhibitor-1 expression by increasing Sp1 glycosylation. *Proc. Natl. Acad. Sci. USA*, **97** (22), 12222–6.

Echtay, K. S., Roussel, D., St Pierre, J. *et al.* (2002). Superoxide activates mitochondrial uncoupling proteins. *Nature*, **415** (6867), 96–9.

Esworthy, R. S., Ho, Y. S. & Chu, F. F. (1997). The Gpx1 gene encodes mitochondrial glutathione peroxidase in the mouse liver. *Arch. Biochem. Biophys.*, **340** (1), 59–63.

Floyd, R. A. (1999). Antioxidants, oxidative stress, and degenerative neurological disorders. *Proc. Soc. Exp. Biol. Med.*, **222** (3), 236–45.

Fornai, F., Saviozzi, M., Piaggi, S. *et al.* (1999). Localization of a glutathione-dependent dehydroascorbate reductase within the central nervous system of the rat. *Neuroscience*, **94** (3), 937–48.

Fujii, J. & Ikeda, Y. (2002). Advances in our understanding of peroxiredoxin, a multifunctional, mammalian redox protein. *Redox. Rep.*, **7** (3), 123–30.

Gabbita, S. P., Lovell, M. A. & Markesbery, W. R. (1998). Increased nuclear DNA oxidation in the brain in Alzheimer's disease. *J. Neurochem.*, **71** (5), 2034–40.

Galli, R. L., Shukitt-Hale, B., Youdim, K. A. & Joseph, J. A. (2002). Fruit polyphenolics and brain aging: nutritional interventions targeting age-related neuronal and behavioral deficits. *Ann. NY Acad. Sci.*, **959**, 128–32.

Gao, H. M., Jiang, J., Wilson, B., Zhang, W., Hong, J. S. & Liu, B. (2002). Microglial activation-mediated delayed and progressive degeneration of rat nigral dopaminergic neurons: relevance to Parkinson's disease. *J. Neurochem.*, **81** (6), 1285–97.

Gardner, P. R. & Fridovich, I. (1991). Superoxide sensitivity of the *Escherichia* coli aconitase. *J. Biol. Chem.*, **266** (29), 19328–33.

Gardner, R., Salvador, A. & Moradas-Ferreira, P. (2002). Why does SOD overexpression sometimes enhance, sometimes decrease, hydrogen peroxide production? a minimalist explanation. *Free Radic. Biol. Med.*, **32** (12), 1351–7.

Gluck, M., Ehrhart, J., Jayatilleke, E. & Zeevalk, G. D. (2002). Inhibition of brain mitochondrial respiration by dopamine: involvement of H_2O_2 and hydroxyl radicals but not glutathione-protein-mixed disulfides. *J. Neurochem.*, **82** (1), 66–74.

Gotoda, T., Arita, M., Arai, H. *et al.* (1995). Adult-onset spinocerebellar dysfunction caused by a mutation in the gene for the alpha-tocopherol-transfer protein. *N. Engl. J. Med.*, **333** (20), 1313–18.

Greco, A., Minghetti, L. & Levi, G. (2000). Isoprostanes, novel markers of oxidative injury, help understanding the pathogenesis of neurodegenerative diseases. *Neurochem. Res.*, **25** (9–10), 1357–64.

Gutteridge, J. M. & Smith, A. (1988). Antioxidant protection by haemopexin of haem-stimulated lipid peroxidation. *Biochem. J.*, **256** (3), 861–5.

Gwilt, P. R., Radick, L. E., Li, X. Y., Whalen, J. J. & Leaf, C. D. (1998). Pharmacokinetics of 2-oxothiazolidine-4-carboxylate, a cysteine prodrug, and cysteine. *J. Clin. Pharmacol.*, **38** (10), 945–50.

Halliwell, B. (1978). Superoxide-dependent formation of hydroxyl radicals in the presence of iron salts. Its role in degradation of hyaluronic acid by a superoxide-generating system. *FEBS Lett.*, **96** (2), 238–42.

Halliwell, B., Zhao, K. & Whiteman, M. (1999). Nitric oxide and peroxynitrite. The ugly, the uglier and the not so good: a personal view of recent controversies. *Free Radic. Res.*, **31** (6), 651–69.

Hampton, M. B., Kettle, A. J. & Winterbourn, C. C. (1996). Involvement of superoxide and myeloperoxidase in oxygen-dependent killing of *Staphylococcus aureus* by neutrophils. *Infect. Immun.*, **64** (9), 3512–17.

Han, D., Antunes, F., Canali, R., Rettori, D. & Cadenas, E. (2003). Voltage-dependent anion channels control the release of the superoxide anion from mitochondria to cytosol. *J. Biol. Chem.*, **278** (8), 5557–63.

Hennet, T., Richter, C. & Peterhans, E. (1993). Tumour necrosis factor-alpha induces superoxide anion generation in mitochondria of L929 cells. *Biochem. J.*, **289** (2), 587–92.

Hidalgo, J., Aschner, M., Zatta, P. & Vasak, M. (2001). Roles of the metallothionein family of proteins in the central nervous system. *Brain Res. Bull.*, **55** (2), 133–45.

Hillered, L. & Persson, L. (1995). Parabanic acid for monitoring of oxygen radical activity in the injured human brain. *Neuroreport*, **6** (13), 1816–20.

Hink, H. U., Santanam, N., Dikalov, S. *et al.* (2002). Peroxidase properties of extracellular superoxide dismutase: role of uric acid in modulating in vivo activity. *Arterioscler. Thromb. Vasc. Biol.*, **22** (9), 1402–8.

Hjalmarsson, K., Marklund, S. L., Engstrom, A. & Edlund, T. (1987). Isolation and sequence of complementary DNA encoding human extracellular superoxide dismutase. *Proc. Natl. Acad. Sci. USA*, **84** (18), 6340–4.

Huang, T. T., Raineri, I., Eggerding, F. & Epstein, C. J. (2002). Transgenic and mutant mice for oxygen free radical studies. *Methods Enzymol.*, **349**, 191–213.

Huffman, D. L. & O'Halloran, T. V. (2001). Function, structure, and mechanism of intracellular copper trafficking proteins. *Annu. Rev. Biochem.*, **70**, 677–701.

Iadecola, C., Zhang, F., Niwa, K. *et al.* (1999). SOD1 rescues cerebral endothelial dysfunction in mice overexpressing amyloid precursor protein. *Nat. Neurosci.*, **2** (2), 157–61.

Janssen, L. J. (2001). Isoprostanes: an overview and putative roles in pulmonary pathophysiology. *Am. J. Physiol. Lung Cell Mol. Physiol.*, **280** (6), p. L1067–82.

Jenner, P. & Olanow, C. W. (1996). Oxidative stress and the pathogenesis of Parkinson's disease. *Neurology*, **47** (6, Suppl 3), S161–S70.

Jo, S. H., Son, M. K., Koh, H. J. *et al.* (2001). Control of mitochondrial redox balance and cellular defense against oxidative damage by mitochondrial NADP+-dependent isocitrate dehydrogenase. *J. Biol. Chem.*, **276** (19), 16168–76.

Jo, S. H., Lee, S. H., Chun, H. S. *et al.* (2002). Cellular defense against UVB-induced phototoxicity by cytosolic NADP(+)-dependent isocitrate dehydrogenase. *Biochem. Biophys. Res. Commun.*, **292** (2), 542–9.

Karlsson, K., Sandstrom, J., Edlund, A. & Marklund, S. L. (1994). Turnover of extracellular-superoxide dismutase in tissues. *Laborat. Invest.*, **70** (5), 705–10.

Karnovsky, M. J. (1994). Robert Feulgen Lecture 1994. Cytochemistry and reactive oxygen species: a retrospective. *Histochemistry*, **102** (1), 15–27.

Kastenbauer, S., Koedel, U., Becker, B. F. & Pfister, H. W. (2001). Experimental meningitis in the rat: protection by uric acid at human physiological blood concentrations. *Eur. J. Pharmacol.*, **425** (2), 149–52.

Kastenbauer, S., Koedel, U., Becker, B. F. & Pfister, H. W. (2002). Oxidative stress in bacterial meningitis in humans. *Neurology*, **58** (2), 186–91.

Keller, G. A., Warner, T. G., Steimer, K. S. & Hallewell, R. A. (1991). Cu,Zn superoxide dismutase is a peroxisomal enzyme in human fibroblasts and hepatoma cells. *Proc. Natl. Acad. Sci. USA*, **88** (16), 7381–5.

Kenchappa, R. S., Diwakar, L., Boyd, M. R. & Ravindranath, V. (2002). Thioltransferase (glutaredoxin) mediates recovery of motor neurons from excitotoxic mitochondrial injury. *J. Neurosci.*, **22** (19), 8402–10.

Kim, Y. S. & Han, S. (2000). Superoxide reactivates nitric oxide-inhibited catalase. *Biol. Chem.*, **381** (12), 1269–71.

Klivenyi, P., Andreassen, O. A., Ferrante, R. J. *et al.* (2000). Mice deficient in cellular glutathione peroxidase show increased vulnerability to malonate, 3-nitropropionic acid, and 1-methyl-4-phenyl 1,2,5,6-tetrahydropyridine. *J. Neurosci.*, **20** (1), 1–7.

Knapp, L. T. & Klann, E. (2002). Potentiation of hippocampal synaptic transmission by superoxide requires the oxidative activation of protein kinase C. *J. Neurosci.*, **22** (3), 674–83.

Kondo, T., Reaume, A. G., Huang, T. T. *et al.* (1997). Reduction of CuZn-superoxide dismutase activity exacerbates neuronal cell injury and edema formation after transient focal cerebral ischemia. *J. Neurosci.*, **17** (11), 4180–9.

Konijn, A. M., Glickstein, H., Vaisman, B., Meyron-Holtz, E. G., Slotki, I. N. & Cabantchik, Z. I. (1999). The cellular labile iron pool and intracellular ferritin in K562 cells. *Blood*, **94** (6), 2128–34.

Kono, Y. & Fridovich, I. (1982). Superoxide radical inhibits catalase. *J. Biol. Chem.*, **257** (10), 5751–4.

Kontos, H. A., Wei, E. P., Dietrich, W. D. *et al.* (1981). Mechanism of cerebral arteriolar abnormalities after acute hypertension. *Am. J. Physiol*, **240** (4), H511–27.

Kukreja, R. C., Kontos, H. A., Hess, M. L. & Ellis, E. F. (1986). PGH synthase and lipoxygenase generate superoxide in the presence of NADH or NADPH. *Circ. Res.*, **59** (6), 612–19.

Lebovitz, R. M., Zhang, H., Vogel, H. *et al.* (1996). Neurodegeneration, myocardial injury, and perinatal death in mitochondrial superoxide dismutase-deficient mice. *Proc. Natl. Acad. Sci. USA*, **93** (18), 9782–7.

Levin, E. D., Brady, T. C., Hochrein, E. C. *et al.* (1998). Molecular manipulations of extracellular superoxide dismutase: functional importance for learning. *Behav. Genet.*, **28** (5), 381–90.

Li, C. & Jackson, R. M. (2002). Reactive species mechanisms of cellular hypoxia-reoxygenation injury. *Am. J. Physiol Cell Physiol.*, **282** (2), C227–41.

Li, Y., Huang, T. T., Carlson, E. J. *et al.* (1995). Dilated cardiomyopathy and neonatal lethality in mutant mice lacking manganese superoxide dismutase. *Nat. Genet.*, **11** (4), 376–81.

Liou, W., Chang, L. Y., Geuze, H. J. *et al.* (1993). Distribution of CuZn superoxide dismutase in rat liver. *Free Radic. Biol. Med.*, **14** (2), 201–7.

Lippoldt, A., Padilla, C. A., Gerst, H. *et al.* (1995). Localization of thioredoxin in the rat brain and functional implications. *J. Neurosci.*, **15** (10), 6747–56.

Lue, L. F., Walker, D. G., Brachova, L. *et al.* (2001). Involvement of microglial receptor for advanced glycation end-products (RAGE) in Alzheimer's disease: identification of a cellular activation mechanism. *Exp. Neurol.*, **171** (1), 29–45.

Luk, E., Carroll, M., Baker, M. & Culotta, V. C. (2003). Manganese activation of superoxide dismutase 2 in Saccharomyces cerevisiae requires MTM1, a member of the mitochondrial carrier family. *Proc. Natl. Acad. Sci. USA*, **100** (18), 10353–7.

Marklund, N., Ostman, B., Nalmo, L., Persson, L. & Hillered, L. (2000). Hypoxanthine, uric acid and allantoin as indicators of in vivo free radical reactions. Description of a HPLC method and human brain microdialysis data. *Acta Neurochir. (Wien.)*, **142** (10), 1135–41.

Marklund, S. L. (1982). Human copper-containing superoxide dismutase of high molecular weight. *Proc. Natl. Acad. Sci. USA*, **79** (24), 7634–8.

  (1984). Extracellular superoxide dismutase in human tissues and human cell lines. *J. Clin. Invest.*, **74** (4), 1398–403.

  (1990). Expression of extracellular superoxide dismutase by human cell lines. *Biochem. J.*, **266** (1), 213–19.

  (1992). Regulation by cytokines of extracellular superoxide dismutase and other superoxide dismutase isoenzymes in fibroblasts. *J. Biol. Chem.*, **267** (10), 6696–701.

Marklund, S. L., Westman, N. G., Lundgren, E. & Roos, G. (1982). Copper- and zinc-containing superoxide dismutase, manganese-containing superoxide dismutase, catalase, and glutathione peroxidase in normal and neoplastic human cell lines and normal human tissues. *Cancer Res.*, **42** (5), 1955–61.

Maser, R. L., Magenheimer, B. S. & Calvet, J. P. (1994). Mouse plasma glutathione peroxidase. cDNA sequence analysis and renal proximal tubular expression and secretion. *J. Biol. Chem.*, **269** (43), 27066–73.

McCord, J. M. & Day, E. D., Jr. (1978). Superoxide-dependent production of hydroxyl radical catalyzed by iron-EDTA complex. *FEBS Lett.*, **86** (1), 139–42.

McCord, J. M. & Fridovich, I. (1969). Superoxide dismutase. An enzymic function for erythrocuprein (hemocuprein). *J. Biol. Chem.*, **244** (22), 6049–55.

McEachern, G., Kassovska-Bratinova, S. *et al.* (2000). Manganese superoxide dismutase levels are elevated in a proportion of amyotrophic lateral sclerosis patient cell lines. *Biochem. Biophys. Res. Commun.*, **273** (1), 359–63.

Meng, T. C., Fukada, T. & Tonks, N. K. (2002). Reversible oxidation and inactivation of protein tyrosine phosphatases in vivo. *Mol. Cell*, **9** (2), 387–99.

Moore, K. & Roberts, L. J. (1998). Measurement of lipid peroxidation. *Free Radic. Res.*, **28** (6), 659–71.

Moreno, S., Mugnaini, E. & Ceru, M. P. (1995). Immunocytochemical localization of catalase in the central nervous system of the rat. *J. Histochem. Cytochem.*, **43** (12), 1253–67.

Nakashima, M., Niwa, M., Iwai, T. & Uematsu, T. (1999). Involvement of free radicals in cerebral vascular reperfusion injury evaluated in a transient focal cerebral ischemia model of rat. *Free Radic.Biol.Med.*, **26** (5–6), 722–9.

Nelson, S. K., Bose, S. K. & McCord, J. M. (1994). The toxicity of high-dose superoxide dismutase suggests that superoxide can both initiate and terminate lipid peroxidation in the reperfused heart. *Free Radic. Biol. Med.*, **16** (2), 195–200.

Nicholls, D. G., Budd, S. L., Ward, M. W. & Castilho, R. F. (1999). Excitotoxicity and mitochondria. *Biochem. Soc. Symp.*, **66**, 55–67.

Nishikimi, M. (1975). Oxidation of ascorbic acid with superoxide anion generated by the xanthine-xanthine oxidase system. *Biochem. Biophys. Res.Commun.*, **63** (2), 463–8.

Noh, K. M. & Koh, J. Y. (2000). Induction and activation by zinc of NADPH oxidase in cultured cortical neurons and astrocytes. *J. Neurosci.*, **20** (23), RC111.

Nordberg, J. & Arner, E. S. (2001). Reactive oxygen species, antioxidants, and the mammalian thioredoxin system. *Free Radic. Biol. Med.*, **31** (11), 1287–312.

Nualart, F. J., Rivas, C. I. & Montecinos, V. P. (2003). Recycling of vitamin C by a bystander effect. *J. Biol. Chem.*, **278** (12), 10128–33.

Oury, T. D., Card, J. P. & Klann, E. (1999). Localization of extracellular superoxide dismutase in adult mouse brain. *Brain Res.*, **850** (1–2), 96–103.

Palmer, C., Towfighi, J., Roberts, R. L. & Heitjan, D. F. (1993). Allopurinol administered after inducing hypoxia–ischemia reduces brain injury in 7-day-old rats. *Pediatr. Res.*, **33** (4 Pt 1), 405–11.

Patt, A., Harken, A. H., Burton, L. K. *et al.* (1988). Xanthine oxidase-derived hydrogen peroxide contributes to ischemia reperfusion-induced edema in gerbil brains. *J. Clin. Invest.*, **81** (5), 1556–62.

Pfeiffer, S., Lass, A., Schmidt, K. & Mayer, B. (2001). Protein tyrosine nitration in cytokine-activated murine macrophages. Involvement of a peroxidase/nitrite pathway rather than peroxynitrite. *J. Biol. Chem.*, **276** (36), 34051–8.

Pou, S., Pou, W. S., Bredt, D. S., Snyder, S. H. & Rosen, G. M. (1992). Generation of superoxide by purified brain nitric oxide synthase. *J. Biol. Chem.*, **267** (34), 24173–6.

Rae, T. D., Schmidt, P. J., Pufahl, R. A., Culotta, V. C. & O'Halloran, T. V. (1999). Undetectable intracellular free copper: the requirement of a copper chaperone for superoxide dismutase. *Science*, **284** (5415), 805–8.

Raha, S., McEachern, G. E., Myint, A. T. & Robinson, B. H. (2000). Superoxides from mitochondrial complex III: the role of manganese superoxide dismutase. *Free Radic. Biol. Med.*, **29** (2), 170–80.

Reaume, A. G., Elliott, J. L., Hoffman, E. K. *et al.* (1996). Motor neurons in Cu/Zn superoxide dismutase-deficient mice develop normally but exhibit enhanced cell death after axonal injury. *Nat. Genet.*, **13** (1), 43–7.

Reynolds, W. F., Rhees, J., Maciejewski, D. *et al.* (1999). Myeloperoxidase polymorphism is associated with gender specific risk for Alzheimer's disease. *Exp. Neurol.*, **155** (1), 31–41.

Rhee, S. G., Kang, S. W., Chang, T. S., Jeong, W. & Kim, K. (2001). Peroxiredoxin, a novel family of peroxidases. *IUBMB.Life*, **52** (1–2), 35–41.

Rice, M. E. (2000). Ascorbate regulation and its neuroprotective role in the brain. *Trends Neurosci.*, **23** (5), 209–16.

Rosen, D. R., Siddique, T., Patterson, D. *et al.* (1993). Mutations in Cu/Zn superoxide dismutase gene are associated with familial amyotrophic lateral sclerosis. *Nature*, **362** (6415), 59–62.

Rosen, G. M., Tsai, P., Weaver, J. M. *et al.* (2002). Tetrahydrobiopterin: its role in the regulation of neuronal nitric oxide synthase-generated superoxide. *J.Biol.Chem.*

Rota, C., Chignell, C. F. & Mason, R. P. (1999). Evidence for free radical formation during the oxidation of 2′-7′-dichlorofluorescin to the fluorescent dye 2′-7′-dichlorofluorescein by horseradish peroxidase: possible implications for oxidative stress measurements. *Free Radic. Biol. Med.*, **27** (7–8), 873–81.

Ruan, H., Tang, X. D., Chen, M. L. *et al.* (2002). High-quality life extension by the enzyme peptide methionine sulfoxide reductase. *Proc. Natl. Acad. Sci. USA*, **99** (5), 2748–53.

Rybnikova, E., Damdimopoulos, A. E., Gustafsson, J. A., Spyrou, G. & Pelto-Huikko, M. (2000). Expression of novel antioxidant thioredoxin-2 in the rat brain. *Eur. J. Neurosci.*, **12** (5), 1669–78.

Sasaki, N., Toki, S., Chowei, H. *et al.* (2001). Immunohistochemical distribution of the receptor for advanced glycation end products in neurons and astrocytes in Alzheimer's disease. *Brain Res.*, **888** (2), 256–62.

Schleicher, E. D., Wagner, E. & Nerlich, A. G. (1997). Increased accumulation of the glycoxidation product N(epsilon)- (carboxymethyl)lysine in human tissues in diabetes and aging. *J. Clin. Invest*, **99** (3), 457–68.

Shaw, P. J., Chinnery, R. M., Thagesen, H., Borthwick, G. M. & Ince, P. G. (1997). Immunocytochemical study of the distribution of the free radical scavenging enzymes Cu/Zn superoxide dismutase (SOD1); MN superoxide dismutase (MN SOD) and catalase in the normal human spinal cord and in motor neuron disease. *J. Neurol. Sci.*, **147** (2), 115–25.

Shefner, J. M., Reaume, A. G., Flood, D. G. *et al.* (1999). Mice lacking cytosolic copper/zinc superoxide dismutase display a distinctive motor axonopathy. *Neurology*, **53** (6), 1239–46.

Sheng, H., Brady, T. C., Pearlstein, R. D., Crapo, J. D. & Warner, D. S. (1999). Extracellular superoxide dismutase deficiency worsens outcome from focal cerebral ischemia in the mouse. *Neurosci. Lett.*, **267** (1), 13–16.

Shibata, N., Hirano, A., Hedley-Whyte, E. T. *et al.* (2002). Selective formation of certain advanced glycation end products in spinal cord astrocytes of humans and mice with superoxide dismutase-1 mutation. *Acta Neuropathol. (Berl.)*, **104** (2), 171–8.

Shih, J. C., Chen, K. & Ridd, M. J. (1999). Monoamine oxidase: from genes to behavior. *Annu.Rev.Neurosci.*, **22**, 197–217.

Sies, H. & Menck, C. F. (1992). Singlet oxygen induced DNA damage. *Mutat. Res.*, **275** (3–6), 367–75.

Smith, M. A., Sayre, L. M., Anderson, V. E. *et al.* (1998). Cytochemical demonstration of oxidative damage in Alzheimer disease by immunochemical enhancement of the carbonyl reaction with 2,4 dinitrophenylhydrazine. *J. Histochem. Cytochem.*, **46** (6), 731–5.

Sorescu, D., Weiss, D., Lassegue, B. *et al.* (2002). Superoxide production and expression of nox family proteins in human atherosclerosis. *Circulation*, **105** (12), 1429–35.

Spencer, J. P., Jenner, P., Daniel, S. E. *et al.* (1998). Conjugates of catecholamines with cysteine and GSH in Parkinson's disease: possible mechanisms of formation involving reactive oxygen species. *J. Neurochem.*, **71** (5), 2112–22.

Stralin, P. & Marklund, S. L. (1994). Effects of oxidative stress on expression of extracellular superoxide dismutase, CuZn-superoxide dismutase and Mn-superoxide dismutase in human dermal fibroblasts. *Biochem. J.*, **298** (2), 347–52.

(2001). Vasoactive factors and growth factors alter vascular smooth muscle cell EC-SOD expression. *Am. J. Physiol. Heart Circ. Physiol.*, **281** (4), H1621–9.

Sugiyama, S., Okada, Y., Sukhova, G. K. *et al.* (2001). Macrophage myeloperoxidase regulation by granulocyte macrophage colony-stimulating factor in human atherosclerosis and implications in acute coronary syndromes. *Am. J. Pathol.*, **150** (3), 879–91.

Tainer, J. A., Getzoff, E. D., Beem, K. M. *et al.* (1982). Determination and analysis of the 2 A-structure of copper, zinc superoxide dismutase. *J. Mol. Biol.*, **160** (2), 181–217.

Takagi, Y., Mitsui, A., Nishiyama, A. *et al.* (1999). Overexpression of thioredoxin in transgenic mice attenuates focal ischemic brain damage. *Proc. Natl. Acad. Sci. USA*, **96** (7), 4131–6.

Takahashi, M., Dore, S., Ferris, C. D. *et al.* (2000). Amyloid precursor proteins inhibit heme oxygenase activity and augment neurotoxicity in Alzheimer's disease. *Neuron*, **28** (2), 461–73.

Tammariello, S. P., Quinn, M. T. & Estus, S. (2000). NADPH oxidase contributes directly to oxidative stress and apoptosis in nerve growth factor-deprived sympathetic neurons. *J. Neurosci.*, **20** (1), RC53.

Tindberg, N., Baldwin, H. A., Cross, A. J. & Ingelman-Sundberg, M. (1996). Induction of cytochrome P450 2E1 expression in rat and gerbil astrocytes by inflammatory factors and ischemic injury. *Mol. Pharmacol.*, **50** (5), 1065–72.

Tindberg, N. & Ingelman-Sundberg, M. (1996). Expression, catalytic activity, and inducibility of cytochrome P450 2E1 (CYP2E1) in the rat central nervous system. *J. Neurochem.*, **67** (5), 2066–73.

Vatassery, G. T., Brin, M. F., Fahn, S., Kayden, H. J. & Traber, M. G. (1988). Effect of high doses of dietary vitamin E on the concentrations of vitamin E in several brain regions, plasma, liver, and adipose tissue of rats. *J. Neurochem.*, **51** (2), 621–3.

Wautier, M. P., Chappey, O., Corda, S. *et al.* (2001). Activation of NADPH oxidase by AGE links oxidant stress to altered gene expression via RAGE. *Am. J. Physiol. Endocrinol. Metab.*, **280** (5), E685–94.

Weisiger, R. A. & Fridovich, I. (1973). Mitochondrial superoxide simutase. Site of synthesis and intramitochondrial localization. *J. Biol. Chem.*, **248** (13), 4793–6.

Weiss, S. J., Test, S. T., Eckmann, C. M. *et al.* (1986). Brominating oxidants generated by human eosinophils. *Science*, **234** (4773), 200–3.

Weissbach, H., Etienne, F. & Hoshi, T. (2002). Peptide methionine sulfoxide reductase: structure, mechanism of action, and biological function. *Arch. Biochem. Biophys.*, **397** (2), 172–8.

Winterbourn, C. C. (1995). Toxicity of iron and hydrogen peroxide: the Fenton reaction. *Toxicol. Lett.*, **82–83**, 969–74.

Winterbourn, C. C. & Metodiewa, D. (1994). The reaction of superoxide with reduced glutathione. *Arch. Biochem. Biophys.*, **314** (2), 284–90.

Winterbourn, C. C. & Stern, A. (1987). Human red cells scavenge extracellular hydrogen peroxide and inhibit formation of hypochlorous acid and hydroxyl radical. *J. Clin. Invest*, **80** (5), 1486–91.

Winterbourn, C. C., Vile, G. F. & Monteiro, H. P. (1991). Ferritin, lipid peroxidation and redox-cycling xenobiotics. *Free Radic. Res. Commun.*, **12–13** (1), 107–14.

Wong, G. H. & Goeddel, D. V. (1988). Induction of manganous superoxide dismutase by tumor necrosis factor: possible protective mechanism. *Science*, **242** (4880), 941–4.

Wong, P. C., Waggoner, D., Subramaniam, J. R. *et al.* (2000). Copper chaperone for superoxide dismutase is essential to activate mammalian Cu/Zn superoxide dismutase. *Proc. Natl. Acad. Sci. USA*, **97** (6), 2886–91.

Yokota, T., Shiojiri, T., Gotoda, T. *et al.* (1997). Friedreich-like ataxia with retinitis pigmentosa caused by the His101Gln mutation of the alpha-tocopherol transfer protein gene. *Ann. Neurol.*, **41** (6), 826–32.

Yoritaka, A., Hattori, N., Uchida, K. *et al.* (1996). Immunohistochemical detection of 4-hydroxynonenal protein adducts in Parkinson disease. *Proc. Natl. Acad. Sci. USA*, **93** (7), 2696–701.

Youdim, K. A. & Joseph, J. A. (2001). A possible emerging role of phytochemicals in improving age-related neurological dysfunctions: a multiplicity of effects. *Free Radic. Biol. Med.*, **30** (6), 583–94.

Youdim, K. A., Spencer, J. P., Schroeter, H. & Rice-Evans, C. (2002). Dietary flavonoids as potential neuroprotectants. *Biol. Chem.*, **383** (3–4), 503–19.

Zhang, J., Graham, D. G., Montine, T. J. & Ho, Y. S. (2000). Enhanced *N*-methyl-4-phenyl-1,2,3,6-tetrahydropyridine toxicity in mice deficient in CuZn-superoxide dismutase or glutathione peroxidase. *J. Neuropathol. Exp. Neurol.*, **59** (1), 53–61.

Zhang, J., Perry, G., Smith, M. A. *et al.* (1999). Parkinson's disease is associated with oxidative damage to cytoplasmic DNA and RNA in substantia nigra neurons. *Am. J. Pathol.*, **154** (5), 1423–9.

2

Biological oxidants and therapeutic antioxidants

John P. Crow

Department of Pharmacology and Toxicology, College of Medicine, University of Arkansas, Little Rock, AR, USA

Introduction

A book chapter represents a special type of literature overview, which offers the promise of covering topics and addressing issues which are relevant and topical but which will also stand the test of time. It is appealing to focus on topical issues, which will hopefully provide some immediate insight into problems and questions confronting investigators in the field. However, undue focus on topical issues predisposes the discussion to becoming dated prior to, or shortly after, appearing in print. Thus, the expressed purpose of this chapter will be to deal with broader concepts which will, hopefully, provide stable foundations to interpret results and permit better comprehension of both current and future topical issues relating to nitrogen oxide-derived oxidative injury relevant to neurodegenerative disease. The author's training and research background is in the chemistry and biochemistry of biologically produced oxidants, biochemical mechanisms of oxidative injury, and the pharmacology of endogenous and synthetic antioxidants. Thus, these perspectives will be emphasized, leaving the broader issues of neuroscience to the preeminent neuroscientists elsewhere in this volume. Also, because entire chapters could be devoted to many of the topics covered, citations for relevant literature reviews will be emphasized and the primary literature cited only when necessary.

Why is identification of reactive species and biomolecular targets so difficult?

For many decades, it has been understood that oxidative injury, both acute and chronic, plays a central role in numerous human disease processes and aging, yet major advances in identifying specific reactive species and/or the specific biomolecular targets responsible for cell injury and death have been few and far between. Reasons for the slow pace of progress abound, but the fundamental problem is rapid transmutation (spontaneous and/or enzymatic) of primary reactive species into secondary and even tertiary species, each with different reactivity profiles and targets. Since the seminal discovery of Cu,Zn superoxide dismutase by Joe McCord and Irwin Fridovich in 1969, overwhelming evidence has accumulated that scavenging of superoxide can, in many instances, prevent oxidative injury. However, superoxide itself is not a good oxidant and few direct reactions of superoxide (with biomolecular targets) have been identified that could readily account for oxidative injury. Logically, superoxide must, under some conditions, be transformed into something else. Besides rapid transmutations, reactive species are, by definition, short-lived and have defied direct measurement in most instances. Thus, it is necessary to rely on stable end-product analysis to infer both the species involved and the mechanisms by which they are formed – a process wrought with uncertainty. The notion that the devil is in the details certainly applies to the study of reactive species in biology. The discovery, some 15 years ago, that nitric oxide (NO) was formed in mammalian systems has opened new avenues of research into reactive species and oxidative injury and, while adding a host of heretofore unconsidered reactive nitrogen species to the fray, it may have, paradoxically, simplified many issues relating to superoxide-mediated toxicity.

The expressed purpose of this chapter is to discuss how, and under what conditions, NO is transformed from a benign second messenger to an aggressive neurotoxin and how pharmacological interventions may limit the latter effects of NO-derived species without altering the beneficial physiological effects of NO itself. To accomplish this goal, it will be necessary to examine some of the essential chemical and biophysical properties of NO, provide a rationale for the predominant species thought to mediate NO-derived toxicity, and characterize the broad classes of novel antioxidants that may act to prevent oxidative neuronal injury. Along the way, some fundamental principles of oxidant scavenging will be outlined, potential mechanisms of oxidative injury will be discussed, the relevance of some oxidative markers will be assessed, and the potential contribution of endogenous metalloproteins in oxidative injury will be examined. Mutant forms of Cu,Zn superoxide dismutase (SOD1) are known to cause some forms of familial amyotrophic lateral sclerosis (FALS), and recent evidence suggests that both beta amyloid peptide (Alzheimer's disease) and prion protein (bovine spongiform encephalopathy) bind the redox active metal copper. Recognition that these proteins can bind copper and potentially allow it to redox cycle, thereby producing oxidants that can injure neurons directly and/or modify proteins, may prove critical to solving the mysteries of how they are neurotoxic.

The good, the bad, and the unknown of NO

The fact that nitric oxide (NO) is produced enzymatically in mammalian systems and acts as a unique type of second messenger has been known for roughly 15 years. Almost from the beginning, it became clear that NO had a dark side: while it regulates numerous physiological processes, it can also contribute to oxidative injury. The simplest explanation for the duplicitous behavior of NO is that it can undergo chemical transformations and form reactive intermediates with very different properties. All NOS isoforms make at least some free NO, and free NO is what binds to the heme prosthetic group of guanylate cyclase (GC) and initiates cGMP production which, in turn, activates numerous physiological processes. What happens to NO in the interim – after its release from NOS and before it binds to GC – remains the subject of much debate, and intermediate chemical transformation is likely to be the primary determinant in whether or not NO participates in oxidative injury. In the beginning, most of what was known about NO chemistry came from work on atmospheric nitrogen oxides and their roles in air pollution. In recent years, that knowledge base has been extended to the solutional chemistry of NO; however, many of these studies have involved the use of relatively high concentrations of NO and the chemistry of NO changes dramatically as its concentration increases. Normal in vivo concentrations of NO are in the submicromolar range (GC is maximally stimulated by low nanomolar levels of NO) where the chemistry is less likely to be governed by reactions with itself or other NO-derived radicals, but where detection sensitivity limits the ability to

identify reactive intermediates in real time. Thus, like most reactive species, it is necessary to analyze the stable end products and attempt to deduce the mechanisms by which they were formed. The limited scope of this chapter dictates that we focus on those NO-derived species (i) that are most likely to form under physiological conditions, and (ii) that can account for the oxidative modifications and cellular injury seen. This "Occam's Razor" approach has the dual advantage of limiting the number of possibilities that must be considered and of focusing on those possibilities that are most likely to be pathologically relevant.

Interminable terminology

Prior to the introduction of NO, perhaps the most commonly used descriptor was "reactive oxygen species" or ROS. ROS has evolved to include "reactive nitrogen species" (RNS) as well as terms like "nitrative" and "nitrosative" stress to the previously used catchall phrase "oxidative stress." The introduction of NO into the field of free radical/oxidant-mediated cell injury and pathology has had the dual effect of providing alternative (and arguably more tenable) mechanistic explanations for such injury, while simultaneously complicating attempts to identify specific species and sources of reactive species. Adding NO to the fray also creates entirely new categories of terminology to an already bloated and confusing list. "Free radicals" refer to a specific type of reactive species that possess at least one unpaired electron and are, therefore, inherently unstable, although some free radicals – such as NO – are remarkably stable. Not all free radicals are oxidants and superoxide is a much better reductant than oxidant. Thus, it is imperative to provide some terms (and definitions) that encompass all biologically relevant reactive species in ways that the terms "free radical" or "reactive oxygen species" cannot do. Potent reductants such as glutathione (GSH) and ascorbic acid (vitamin C) can rightly be referred to as "reactive species," but in a different sense from that usually intended. Fortunately, the limited scope of this chapter allows/forces us to its focus on NO-derived reactive species and, for that, we will use the term "NO-derived oxidant" or "NODO." "NO" will refer specifically to the free radical nitric oxide (properly designated as $\cdot N=O$), and "peroxynitrite" (the product of NO and superoxide) will refer to either peroxynitrite anion or the more reactive protonated form, peroxynitrous acid. In addition, "oxidative stress" will be used to refer to cellular production of oxidants which does not exceed the threshold of acute repair. "Oxidative injury" will refer to oxidant production that exceeds the threshold of acute repair and produces discernable impairment of some critical cellular processes; if continued unabated, oxidative injury ultimately will lead to cell death.

Common oxidative pathways

Many exogenous compounds become toxicants by first being reduced enzymatically, and then spontaneously (i.e. non-enzymatically) reoxidizing to generate reactive oxygen species – initially superoxide.[1] Superoxide then becomes the starting material for the production of overtly injurious species. Thus, many different redox active toxicants may act via common pathways. By focusing on intercepting/ scavenging these common intermediates, it may be possible to design compounds which would be beneficial in a number of different disease conditions. For many reasons, the CNS is particularly susceptible to oxidative injury from exogenous toxicants as well from biologically produced oxidants. This is due, in part, to the relative inability of neurons to replenish injured cells and to the very high metabolic demand of neurons (Halliwell, 2001). It has been estimated that the brain accounts for 20% of total body oxygen consumption (Halliwell, 2001). Because oxygen consumption occurs in the mitochondria, high oxygen consumption reflects the second-to-second dependence of neurons on mitochondria. Many generic mitochondrial toxins (e.g. MPP^+ derived from MPTP, 3-nitroproprionic acid, barbiturates, rotentone, etc.) affect the CNS first, not so much because they are taken up specifically by neuronal mitochondria, but because the high energy demands of neurons make them more susceptible to even momentary decreases in electron transport and subsequent ATP production. Creatine may boost athletic performance and slow neurodegenerative processes by providing mitochondria with an alternate energy source (creatine phosphate) to buffer against momentary decreases in ATP.

Mitochondria as primary source of ROS

Given the oxygen handling by mitochondria, it is not surprising that they are the major source of reactive oxygen species in virtually all cell types. The mitochondrial electron transport chain is designed to store four electrons and pass them off to molecular oxygen to produce two molecules of water. However, this process is not 100% efficient and, even under normal physiological conditions, as much as 1% of total oxygen consumption results in incompletely reduced oxygen species including superoxide, hydrogen peroxide, and hydroxyl radical (the products of one, two, and three electron reductions of oxygen, respectively). A dizzying array of biochemical processes involving several multi-subunit copper- and iron-containing proteins as well as multiple redox active substrates must interact in a highly coordinated fashion to maintain proper electron flow through the system and avoid inadvertent transfer of single electrons to oxygen. Given this inherent complexity, the fact that the electron transport system functions with 99% efficiency is more incredible than a 1% misfire rate. Coincidentally, the fact that the proteins, enzymes, and substrates of the electron transport chain are redox active makes them more likely to be attacked by oxidants (electricians are more likely to get shocked than plumbers) and more likely to be inactivated by oxidants (e.g. electricians with weak hearts). Abnormal oxidative modifications frequently occur at several points along the chain and, in general, the more downstream the malfunction, the more likely that electron-charged enzymes and substrates upstream will accumulate and release single electrons prematurely. The fact that mitochondria require their own specific isoform of SOD (manganese superoxide dismutase, MnSOD, or SOD2) and that MnSOD is absolutely essential for life (Li *et al.*, 1995; Copin *et al.*, 2000), whereas the cytosolic form (Cu,Zn SOD or SOD1) is not (Reaume *et al.*, 1996), provide strong circumstantial evidence: (i) that superoxide is normally produced in mitochondria, (ii) that mitochondria are the principal source of ROS, and (iii) that critical targets susceptible to oxidative inactivation exist within mitochondria. The essential role of MnSOD and how its paradoxical susceptibility to oxidative inactivation may be pivotal to mitochondrial death will be discussed more fully later on.

How can superoxide be toxic?

Prior to the discovery that NO was produced enzymatically in vivo, free radical/oxidant-mediated injury was thought to involve primarily superoxide, hydrogen peroxide (H_2O_2), and hydroxyl radical. The fundamental problem was that, of these three species, hydroxyl radical was the only strong oxidant; superoxide and H_2O_2 are very weak oxidants and, in the absence of transition metals like copper, iron and manganese, relatively unreactive.[2] Yet it was clear from studies with superoxide dismutases, catalase and glutathione peroxidase (the primary H_2O_2 decomposing enzyme in mitochondria) that, not only could oxidative injury be largely prevented by scavenging superoxide and H_2O_2, but also that stable end-products associated with hydroxyl radical production (e.g. aromatic hydroxylation) could be measured in affected tissues. This led to the proposal of a three-tiered reaction cascade involving reduction of redox active Fe(III) to Fe(II) by superoxide, followed by reaction of Fe(II) with H_2O_2 (derived from the dismutation of superoxide) to produce hydroxyl radical. There are numerous problems with this mechanism, including relatively slow reaction rates and the need for simultaneous production and localization of all three reactants in biological systems containing redundant systems designed to keep all three reactants at extremely low concentrations (Kehrer, 2000; Koppenol, 2001). Equally important is the fact that hydroxyl radical is such a potent oxidant and so indiscriminately reactive that it can only diffuse a few angstroms before reacting with some molecular target. Thus, enthusiasm for hydroxyl radical as a predominant mediator of oxidative injury is dampened by the fact that (via the Fenton reaction) it is difficult to produce and any resulting damage is restricted to the site of production. In this context, the realization that peroxynitrite forms quite readily, possesses hydroxyl radical-like reactivity, and is capable of diffusing considerable distances before "detonating," becomes very significant (see below).

Reactive oxygen versus reactive nitrogen species

The seminal discoveries that NO is produced in vivo and that it reacts with superoxide extremely rapidly (rate constant $\sim10^{10}$ $M^{-1}s^{-1}$) (Kissner et al., 1997) to form a species – peroxynitrite – that has hydroxyl radical-like reactivity, have caused some serious rethinking of the original, fundamental in vivo mechanisms of oxidant production. If the NO/superoxide reaction had been known 30 years ago, the so-called Fenton Reaction (to produce hydroxyl radical) might never have gained such prominence in biology. That is not to say that reactive oxygen species cannot produce oxidative injury in the absence of NO; only that the species produced and mechanisms involved become more straightforward when NO is present, because the only two reactants required are superoxide and NO; redox active metals can interact with peroxynitrite and alter/exacerbate its reactivity, but are not required. It must be emphasized that many of the reactive species produced under biological conditions are too short-lived to be measured directly and that most of what we know about their production has been gleaned from analysis of products which may, or may not, be specific for any given reactive species. Because of the critical importance of product analysis (to assess production of reactive species), we will discuss this at greater length later on. First, it is necessary to examine some of the chemical and biophysical properties of NO, its reaction with superoxide, and the reactivity of peroxynitrite in order to understand how NODOs can account for many of the abnormal oxidative products measured in tissues as well as oxidative injury itself.

Why does "how" matter?

Considerable debate centers around the basic chemistry of NO and NO-derived species – debates which frequently generate considerably more heat than hight. Quite often, the biologists seek to avoid such issues and focus on "bottom line" issues related to the end result of NO-mediated toxicity, i.e. "just tell me what happens and don't bother me with the chemistry that underlies it." While this approach has some practical merit, the basic chemistry and biophysical properties of NO cannot be ignored if one seeks to successfully intervene pharmacologically. Many potent NOS inhibitors are currently available and it is a simple matter to inhibit all NO production with non-selective inhibitors. However, inhibiting all NO production to prevent oxidative injury is like disconnecting the water source to your house to stop a leaky faucet; the gain will be overwhelmed by the loss.

Physical/chemical properties of nitric oxide

NO is a unique second messenger molecule and an understanding of its biophysical and chemical properties is essential to an understanding of how it can be a benign physiological messenger under some conditions while giving rise to potent oxidizing, nitrating (addition of an – NO_2 group), and nitrosating (addition of an –NO group) species under other conditions. The singular biophysical property of NO that makes it truly unique is its diffusability; lipid membranes are no barrier to NO and it will diffuse through cell membranes virtually as fast as it diffuses through free aqueous solution (Liu et al., 1998).[3] This effectively means that NO produced by one cell will affect physiological and pathological processes in cells far removed from the site of production – a phenomenon that has important implications both in terms of probing biochemical mechanisms and in terms of inhibiting NO-related processes. The extremely efficient diffusability of NO means that selective inhibition (or genetic knockout) of one NOS isoform may or may not have any discernable effect; NO is NO regardless of whether it's made by nNOS, eNOS, or iNOS, and other isoforms can be up-regulated to compensate for the loss of one isoform. Thus, selective inhibition of a given NOS isoform may have short-term effects that are lost over a period of hours as other isoforms are biosynthesized de novo. To categorically rule out involvement of NO in any given physiological or pathological process, it is necessary non-specifically to inhibit all isoforms simultaneously. This may be accomplished successfully in cultured cells, but in whole animals inhibition of all NO production is inconsistent with life. Thus, it is not possible genetically to knock out all NOS isoforms, nor is it practical to attempt to prevent NO-mediated oxidative injury by chronically inhibiting all NO production with non-selective NOS inhibitors.

Nitric oxide does not react directly with thiols

One important chemical property of NO is its relative lack of reactivity with anything except other radicals[4] and with metalloproteins that retain some radical character. For example, the essential second messenger function of NO is a consequence of its binding to iron in the heme prosthetic group of guanylate cyclase which, in turn, is activated to produce cGMP. Likewise, NO binds to oxy-hemoglobin to yield innocuous nitrate; the high rate constant for this reaction and the enormous concentration of oxyhemoglobin in the blood argue that this is the primary pathway for normal physiological scavenging of NO that reaches the vasculature. We will provide a rationale for why the reaction of NO with the radical superoxide (to yield peroxynitrite) may be the predominant pathological reaction pathway for NO, but one thing that NO does not do is to react directly with thiols such as glutathione (GSH) or cysteine residues in proteins; this fact makes it difficult to reconcile the apparent production of nitrosothiol-containing compounds in vivo (Thomas *et al.*, 2001) without invoking an, as yet undiscovered, reaction pathway. Given sufficient time, NO will react with oxygen to form N_2O_3 and other species that can react directly with thiols, but, at physiological concentrations of NO and oxygen, this reaction is much too slow to be of much biological relevance.[5] The half-life of NO in biological systems ranges from 0.09 to 2 seconds (Thomas *et al.*, 2001). This short biological half-life places limits on which reactions NO can undergo and which species can be formed. One of the few known reactions of NO that is fast enough to occur within this half-life window is its reaction with superoxide to form peroxynitrite. It should be emphasized that the reaction between superoxide and NO is so fast ($\sim 10^{10}$ $M^{-1}s^{-1}$) (Kissner *et al.* 1997), that virtually every collision between these two radicals would result in covalent combination to form peroxynitrite; this reaction is roughly five times faster than superoxide can be scavenged by any superoxide dismutases (SODs). Thus, SODs can, at best, only limit peroxynitrite formation, but cannot eliminate it. We will explore the fundamental relationship between SODs, superoxide, H_2O_2, NO and peroxynitrite immediately after examining some of the properties of peroxynitrite that make it the ideal biological oxidant and nitrating agent.

Peroxynitrite – the predominant NO-derived oxidant (NODO)

Peroxynitrite was first described as a chemical entity in the early 1900s and characterized thoroughly as an oxidant and phenolic nitrating agent in the 1960s (Ray, 1962; Hughes & Nicklin, 1968). In the early 1990s, Dr Joseph Beckman suggested that peroxynitrite could be formed in vivo via the reaction of superoxide and NO (Beckman *et al.*, 1990). The first compelling measurement of the rate constant for this reaction was made by Huie and Padmaja in 1993 (Padmaja & Huie, 1993); their rate constant of 6.7×10^9 $M^{-1}s^{-1}$ has recently been revised upward to greater than 10^{10} $M^{-1}s^{-1}$ (Liu *et al.*, 1998). The reaction between superoxide and NO ranks among the fastest reactions known in biology and approaches the fastest rates that any two molecules can interact; hence the term "diffusion-limited" reaction. One does not need to be a physical chemist to appreciate that a reaction which occurs this rapidly is virtually assured to occur whenever NO and superoxide are produced simultaneously (the rate constant for oxidation of target molecules by hydroxyl radical – the most reactive species known in biology – is in the range of 10^{10} $M^{-1}s^{-1}$ to 10^{11} $M^{-1}s^{-1}$). To argue that peroxynitrite is not formed in vivo is to ignore the simple physical and chemical laws which govern bimolecular reactions in aqueous solution. Aside from the simple reality of a diffusion-limited rate constant, the very first descriptions of endothelium-derived relaxing factor (EDRF/NO) indicated that its biological half-life was enhanced by the addition of SODs – compelling evidence that NO is continuously reacting with superoxide to form peroxynitrite in biological systems (Gryglewski *et al.*, 1986; Rubanyi & Vanhoutte, 1986).

Peroxynitrite anion is the product formed initially from the radical/radical reaction of superoxide and NO; the anion becomes protonated at physiological pH (pK_a $\sim$7.0) and, in the absence of oxidizable targets, will rearrange spontaneously to nitrate (NO_3^-) with a half-life of $\sim$1 s at pH 7.4 and 37 °C (Beckman *et al.*, 1990). However, in the milieu of a cell, peroxynitrite anion will react with a wide array of functional groups on proteins, DNA, lipids, and various low molecular weight compounds such as glutathione (see Scheme 1). Peroxynitrite anion reacts directly with carbon dioxide to increase the yield of a nitrating species and this reaction (with CO_2) may largely govern its reactivity in vivo (Denicola *et al.*, 1996). At the very least, it means that scavengers of peroxynitrite will be effective only if they can out-compete the reaction (of peroxynitrite) with CO_2 and/or react with the peroxynitrite/CO_2 adduct that is formed. Oshima and coworkers (1990) were the first to measure nitrotyrosine (and its deaminated metabolite nitro-hydroxyphenylacetic acid) in the urine of smokers; however, the source of urinary nitrotyrosine was unknown at that time. Beckman and coworkers verified the in vivo formation of peroxynitrite by making an antibody to protein-bound nitrotyrosine and using that antibody to show that proteins in human ARDS lung contained tyrosyl residues that had been nitrated (Crow *et al.*, 1994). Since that time, nitrated proteins (as well as free nitrotyrosine and metabolites) have been shown to occur in many different human disease conditions including ALS, Alzheimer's disease, Parkinson's disease, and prion protein-related diseases as well as in experimental animals (for review, see Beckman, 2002). Whether nitration of proteins *per se* is fundamental to oxidative injury remains to be established. However, it should be emphasized that all work to date reveals a striking selectivity of nitration such that only a few proteins appear to be targets of nitration and that, as such, a high percentage of those specific protein target molecules may be nitrated even though the total cellular nitration, as a function of total protein-bound tyrosine, may be relatively low (0.01% to 1.0% of total tyrosine).

Nitrotyrosine as marker of NODOs

Nitrotyrosine is a stable modification, which is relatively specific for peroxynitrite. Nitrotyrosine has been measured with immunological techniques and by HPLC, validated via GC–MS and LC–MS (Beckman, 2002). However, it must be emphasized that peroxynitrite can modify a number of biomolecular targets in ways that may be more critical to oxidative cell injury and death, particularly within the CNS (see Scheme 1). Peroxynitrite can oxidize critical thiols of enzymes, metal centers in proteins, lipids, nucleic acids, as well as nitrate and hydroxylate phenolics like tyrosine, tryptophan (serotonin), and catecholamines such as dopamine (Daveu *et al.*, 1997; Riobo *et al.*, 2002).[6] Many of these modifications are irreversible under physiological conditions and can be readily measured; however, it is considerably more difficult to ascribe non-nitration modifications exclusively to peroxynitrite since other reactive species can produce some of these modifications, at least in vitro. Only when these modifications occur concomitantly with tyrosine nitration can they be attributed to peroxynitrite. The inability to assign specific reaction products to specific oxidants continues to confound attempts to identify precise reactive species and thereby design specific scavenger molecules as therapeutics. For this and many other reasons, the emphasis, in terms of therapeutic antioxidant drug design, is toward multifunctional agents and combination therapy which includes several compounds, each with specific scavenger profiles. It is important to point out that

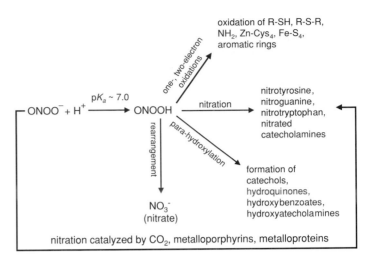

Scheme 1 Known reaction pathways for peroxynitrite.

peroxynitrite is capable of producing virtually all of the products previously ascribed to hydroxyl radical. This further illustrates how formation of NODOs – specifically peroxynitrite – may actually simplify efforts to define mechanisms of oxidant formation in vivo and simplify the search for the elusive endogenous oxidants most responsible for oxidative injury.

Other oxidative modifications by peroxynitrite

Oxidative modifications to biomolecules, whether by peroxynitrite, other NODOs, or other reactive oxygen species, almost always will be limited to a few particularly susceptible targets and then (with some notable exceptions), to only a small percentage of the total molecules making up that target. For example, activity measurements of enzymes known to be sensitive to oxidative inactivation may reveal that only a small percentage of the total enzyme activity is lost. Thus, questions naturally arise as to how modification of a small percentage of a few select targets can translate into significant oxidative injury. One example would be the oxidative *activation* of an enzyme; activation of even a very small fraction of an important tyrosine kinase (e.g. c-Src kinase (MacMillan-Crow *et al.*, 2000)) could trigger an inappropriate cascade of phosphorylation reactions leading to uncontrolled cell proliferation and tumorigenesis. A similar situation, of uncontrolled or inappropriately prolonged phosphorylation, could result from the inactivation of a phosphatase. Some of the fastest reactions yet described for peroxynitrite occur with the active site thiolates of the tyrosine phosphatases CD45, LAR, and PTP1B (Takakura *et al.*, 1999); because of their low cellular concentrations and extremely fast rate constants, a large fraction of the total tyrosine phosphatase activity may be lost in a short time. Physiological concentrations (nanomolar) of peroxynitrite irreversibly inactivate these three tyrosine phosphatases in vitro, and treatment of cells with peroxynitrite has been shown to produce a prolonged, hyperphosphorylation state (Mondoro et al., 1997; Mallozzi et al., 1997) – evidence suggesting that a large fraction of total tyrosine phosphatase activity was inhibited. Although other mechanisms have been proposed for hyperphosphorylation of tau protein in Alzheimer's and neurofilaments in amyotrophic lateral sclerosis (ALS), mechanisms involving oxidative activation of kinases and/or oxidative inactivation of thiol-dependent phosphatases in these diseases are possibilities which remain largely unexplored.

Hydroxylation of dopamine by peroxynitrite forms 6-hydroxydopamine (6-OHDA) – a well-characterized neurotoxin which readily kills neurons within the substantia nigra (Daveu et al., 1997; Riobo et al., 2002 and J. P. Crow, unpublished observations). Because neuronal lesions by 6-OHDA are irreversible, formation of even minute amounts of 6-OHDA over time could cause cumulative neuronal injury. The structural protein neurofilament L (NFL) is particularly susceptible to nitration by peroxynitrite and in vitro studies indicate that one nitrated tyrosyl residue on every tenth NFL molecule is sufficient to prevent self-assembly (Crow et al., 1997). Nitration of only a few subunits of actin or tubulin (Eiserich et al., 1999; Kalisz et al., 2000; Giannopoulou et al., 2002) could also disrupt assembly of these structural proteins via a process analogous to inserting a defective link into a chain. Unequivocal cause-and-effect relationships between these biochemical events and oxidative injury in vivo have not been established; they are used solely as examples of how low level modifications could, in theory, have dramatic effects either by inappropriate amplification of a signal (e.g. phosphorylation), by accumulation of damage (6-OHDA), or by interference with a sequential structural protein assembly process such as occurs with neurofilaments, actin, and tubulin. Considering that all of these biochemical insults could occur simultaneously, it is not difficult to envision how oxidative stress can overwhelm cellular repair mechanisms and escalate into oxidative injury.

MnSOD is a ubiquitous target of peroxynitrite in vivo

Nitration and inactivation of the mitochondrial form of manganese superoxide dismutase (MnSOD) represents one mechanism of oxidative injury where the consequences are more straightforward and quite profound. Studies with genetic knockouts for MnSOD reveal that it is essential for life (Li et al., 1995; Copin et al., 2000). Thus, it is possible to extrapolate that an acute loss of MnSOD activity (within a time frame which does not allow for compensation via de novo biosynthesis) could, in and of itself, lead to cell death. It stands to reason that loss of MnSOD activity per se would not be lethal but, instead, must be related to the increase in levels of reactive species secondary to loss of superoxide scavenging activity. MnSOD has been shown to be particularly susceptible to nitration/inactivation by peroxynitrite (MacMillan et al., 1996, 1998) in a number of human disease conditions including ALS (Aoyama et al., 2000). In vitro studies reveal that loss of MnSOD enzyme activity is a consequence of both nitration and other oxidative modifications including inter-subunit formation of dityrosine crosslinks (MacMillan et al., 1998). When MnSOD is found to be nitrated, it is possible to infer that it is also oxidatively inactivated and activity assays have confirmed this in many instances. Thus, this represents a classic example of where nitration may serve as a marker for a more pernicious modification that is less apparent but nonetheless significant in terms of loss of enzyme activity. The fact that MnSOD is inactivated so readily by the very oxidant that it acts to prevent is paradoxical and suggests that this process may serve as an oxidant sensing mechanism in mitochondria, i.e. to signal the cell that oxidative injury has crossed some critical threshold and perhaps to initiate active apoptosis. Because mitochondria in all cell types possess and require MnSOD, acute loss of MnSOD activity may serve as a generic cell death mechanism.

Protein nitration in neurodegenerative diseases

Nitrated proteins have been identified in affected tissues in Parkinson's Disease (Good et al., 1998; Giasson et al., 2000), in Alzheimer's dementia (Smith et al., 1997; Hensley et al., 1998; Tohgi et al., 1999; Williamson et al., 2002), in ALS (Aoyama et al., 2000; Abe et al., 1995; Beal et al., 1997; Strong et al., 1998; Cassina et al., 2002), and in prion protein-related diseases (Guentchev et al., 2000). Again, the presence of nitrated proteins simply may indicate that peroxynitrite was formed at some stage and modified other critical cellular targets in less discernible but functionally more important ways. Because the magnitude of modification via other pathways may greatly exceed the nitration pathways, the toxicological relevance of peroxynitrite formation may be grossly underestimated if one focuses solely on the extent of protein nitration. By the same token, a lack of clear correlation between the specific proteins which are nitrated and oxidative injury does not preclude peroxynitrite as the mediator of that injury. For example, the levels of peroxynitrite needed to nitrate 0.05% of the total protein-bound tyrosine in the cell may be sufficient to totally inactivate (via non-nitrative pathways) critical iron–sulfur proteins in the mitochondrial electron transport chain and effectively inhibit mitochondrial energy production. The mechanisms related to peroxynitrite-mediated cytotoxicity are only beginning to be understood and too narrow a focus on the functional consequences of protein nitration alone may be dangerously misleading.

Scavenging of reactive species: basic concepts

Before discussing some of the newer, novel antioxidants that are currently being developed and evaluated as potential human therapeutics, it is important to establish some basic concepts relating to oxidant scavenging (for review, see Crow, 2000). Misconceptions abound as to what constitutes a scavenger of free radicals and/or reactive species, how they work, and their limitations. Exogenously administered scavengers do not magically soak up all reactive species, they merely act as alternate targets. Their overall effectiveness in preventing oxidative injury is a function of several factors including: (i) which species they scavenge, (ii) how fast they react with various injurious species, (iii) their tissue and cellular concentration, and (iv) the mechanism by which they scavenge reactive species. There are few, if any, truly specific scavengers; this may be advantageous from the standpoint of therapeutic antioxidants, but it limits their utility as probes for identifying the specific reactive species responsible for oxidative injury.

With regard to scavenger specificity, it is important to point out that there is no such thing as a "hydroxyl radical scavenger" by virtue of the fact that essentially all biomolecules react with hydroxyl radical at near diffusion-limited rates. Hydroxyl radical is so reactive that it will diffuse only a few angstroms before reacting with any one of a host of target molecules (Kehrer, 2000; Koppenol, 2001). Also, hydroxyl radical production almost invariably requires the presence of redox active iron or copper. Thus, oxidative injury by hydroxyl radical is restricted to a very small radius near the site of production. For example, release of iron from safe storage depots such as ferritin can result in binding of free iron to the phosphate moieties of nucleic acids. Reduction of nucleic acid-bound iron by antioxidants such as acorbate, followed by diffusion of H_2O_2 to that site can result in hydroxyl radical production, which can oxidize a functional group on that, or an adjacent, nucleic acid, but not targets more than a few angstroms from the site of hydroxyl radical production. Several factors, including some discussed earlier, call into question the relevance of hydroxyl radical to oxidative injury. In any case, attempts to employ any compound as a specific "hydroxyl radical scavenger" call into question the comprehension of the investigator.

Direct-acting vs. indirect-acting scavengers

Oxidant and/or free radical scavengers can broadly be grouped as being either direct acting or indirect acting. Direct-acting scavengers, as the name implies, react directly with a reactive species in a bimolecular fashion. This means that, as the concentration of the scavenger is increased, a larger fraction of the reactive molecules will react with it rather than with other biomolecular targets. The fraction of reactive molecules scavenged will be a function of the scavenger concentration and the rate constant for its reaction with the given oxidant: the faster the rate constant, the lower the concentration of scavenger required to be effective. GSH is present in some cells at millimolar concentrations and reacts directly with peroxynitrite, but its effectiveness as an endogenous peroxynitrite scavenger is limited by the fact that the rate constant (for reaction with peroxynitrite) is low relative to other biomolecular targets. Indirect-acting scavengers typically provide electrons to "quench" secondary reactants formed when the primary oxidant attacks a biomolecular target. For example, attack of potent one-electron oxidants such as hydroxyl radical or nitrogen dioxide on tyrosine initially yields a tyrosyl radical, which can then be re-reduced quite effectively by ascorbic acid (vitamin C). By quenching the reactive intermediate (tyrosyl radical), further oxidation/modification of tyrosine is prevented. Ascorbate and tocopherol (vitamin E) are both, for the most part, indirect-acting scavengers which quench reactive intermediates in the cytosol and lipid membrane, respectively. Indirect-acting scavengers display a hyperbolic dose-response relationship (as opposed to a linear dose-response for direct-acting scavengers), meaning that they reach a saturating concentration above which no additional benefit is seen. This may be one reason why little or no additional benefit is seen with megadoses of ascorbate and tocopherol even in situations where oxidative stress is known to play a major role in cell injury.

Sacrificial vs. catalytic scavengers

Direct-acting scavengers can be categorized further as either sacrificial or catalytic. GSH is sacrificial, meaning that one mole of GSH is consumed for every mole of

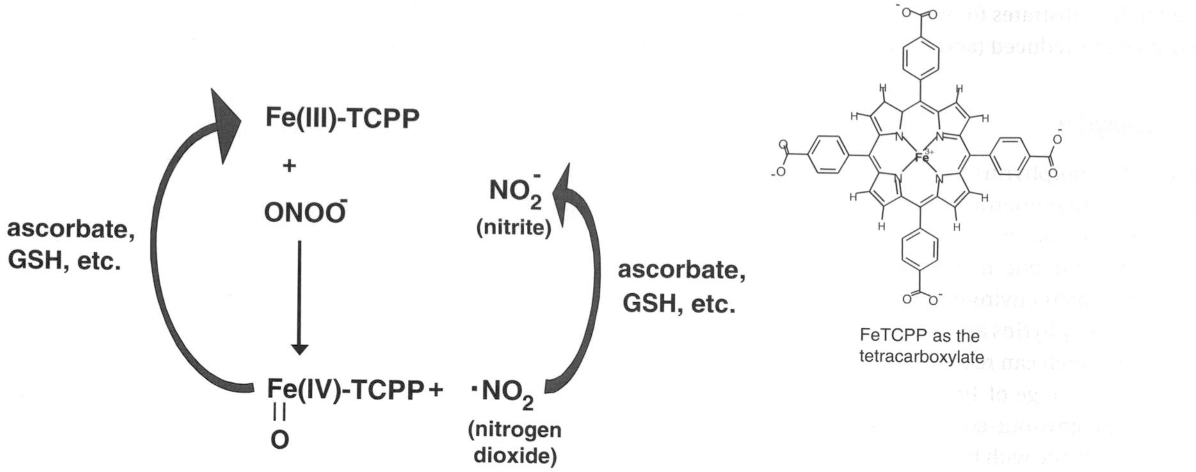

Based on its reactivity, peroxynitrite (or the protonated from, peroxynitrous acid) can be thought of as a hydroxyl radical bound to nitrogen dioxide (HO--ONO). The central Fe(III) ion of redox active metalloporphyrins like Fe TCPP donates one electron to reduce the "hydroxyl radical end" of peroxynitrite thereby yielding nitrogen dioxide and Fe(IV) prophyrin. Cellular antioxidants rapidly reduce the Fe(IV) back to Fe (III) and also reduce nitrogen dioxide to nitrite, thereby regenerating the reduced porphyrin and simultaneously quenching the secondary reactant. In vivo the Fe ion may be reduced to Fe(II) and thereby become capable of complete two-electron reduction of peroxynitrite, thereby bypassing production of nitrogen dioxide.

Scheme 2 Peroxynitrite scavenging by Fe porphyrins in vitro.

peroxynitrite scavenged. The primary reaction product – GSSG – can be recycled by the NADH-requiring enzyme glutathione reductase; however, this recycling cannot keep pace with GSH oxidation by peroxynitrite in real time, hence the designation sacrificial. Many low molecular weight Mn- and Fe-containing porphyrins are catalytic antioxidants. They can react with peroxynitrite to generate Mn(IV) or Fe(IV) species, which can be re-reduced to their respective +3 (or even +2) forms by ascorbate and GSH even faster than they are initially oxidized by peroxynitrite (for review, see Scheme 2 and Crow, 2000). Thus, they act catalytically in the sense that they are recycled back to their original reduced states in real time. As a general chemical class, many of the Mn and Fe porphyrins currently being investigated were first synthesized and introduced as low molecular weight SOD "mimics" or "mimetics." It is now clear that they are much more effective as peroxynitrite scavengers and that this may be the primary basis for their protective effect, but many are still referred to as SOD mimics and incorrectly used as probes for superoxide-dependent oxidative mechanisms.[7] Based on new findings of peroxynitrite decomposing activity, hydroperoxide reductase activity, and superoxide oxido-reductase activity of these metalloporphyrins, they have been termed collectively "catalytic antioxidants."

Scavengers based on pharmacophores in proteins

In terms of designing efficient low molecular weight scavengers for use as therapeutics, we can learn a lot from nature. Based on studies with thiol- and metal-containing proteins and enzymes, it is clear that thiol-based compounds hold the greatest promise for effective sacrificial scavengers whereas Mn and Fe porphyrins appear to be the best candidates for exogenously administered peroxynitrite decomposition catalysts. Studies with thiol-containing proteins and low molecular weight complexes indicate that the microenvironment of the thiol can be fine tuned to give reaction rates needed for effective scavenging. For example, the rate constant for GSH or N-acetyl cysteine (NAC) reacting with peroxynitrite is $\sim 10^3$ $M^{-1}s^{-1}$ (Radi et al., 1991). Zinc-thiolate complexes react ~ 100-fold faster than GSH and the active site thiolate of some tyrosine phosphatase enzymes (e.g. PTP1b, CD45, LAR phosphatases) reacts up to 10 000-fold faster than GSH (Takakura et al., 1999). Based on clinical experience with the thiol-containing compound NAC, it is reasonable to propose that tissue levels of 1–10 µM could be safely achieved. Thiol-based compounds designed to mimic the extraordinarily high reactivity of the active site thiolate of these tyrosine phosphatases effectively would scavenge a high percentage of peroxynitrite formed even at low micromolar concentrations. Such compounds could conceivably be designed to be substrates for various reductases such that they would be re-reduced (and hence recycled) in vivo.

Metalloporphyrins

The Mn and Fe porphyrins that have been shown to have broad antioxidant properties are, in effect, analogs of naturally occurring heme (iron protoporphyrin IX); the reactivities of the synthetic metalloporphyrins are not constrained by the microenvironment of protein-bound heme. These metalloporphyrins are planar molecules with a central metal ion which can react with peroxynitrite with rate constants in the range of 10^7 $M^{-1}s^{-1}$ (Ferrer-Sueta et al., 1999) – fast enough to out-compete most of the known reactions of peroxynitrite with biomolecular targets. Moreover, some metalloporphyrins appear to be capable of scavenging the CO_2 adduct of peroxynitrite as well (Ferrer-Sueta et al., 1999; Crow, 1999). Because these compounds are re-reduced by endogenous antioxidants like ascorbate and GSH in real time, their effective concentration would not be decreased by reaction with peroxynitrite; this is a key pharmacological advantage of the catalytic scavengers. The combination of fast rate constants for reaction with peroxynitrite and fast catalytic recycling means that these agents should be effective – and would continue to be effective – at low micromolar concentrations. Metalloporphyrins have been shown to be protective in a number of cell and animal models of oxidative injury, including ALS (Liu et al., 2002) and models of stroke (Mackensen et al., 2001). Evidence that these redox active porphyrins were working via peroxynitrite scavenging was provided by showing that protein nitration was prevented (Salvemini et al., 1999; Misko et al., 1998). (Prevention of protein nitration strongly suggests that other deleterious reactions of peroxynitrite were also prevented.) However, new evidence suggests that metalloporphyrins have protective effects independent of antioxidant activities, namely that they are potent inducers of heme oxygenases and other heat shock proteins – proteins which are known to enhance survivability to oxidative stress.

Selenium- and tellurium-based scavengers

Selenium and tellurium are in the same chemical family as sulfur and, with regard to reactions with biological oxidants, can be viewed as "hyperactive thiols." Ebselen is a selenium-containing compound introduced originally as a glutathione peroxidase (GPx) mimic. Much like the metalloporphyrins, ebselen was found to react even more efficiently with peroxynitrite (Sies & Masumoto, 1997). Problems with water solubility and with reactivity toward both low molecular weight thiols and protein thiols have limited the potential of ebselen as a clinically useful antioxidant. More soluble and less promiscuous compounds such as selenomethione have proved to be effective antioxidants, at least in cell culture models (Briviba et al., 1996) and may have potential as therapeutics in vivo. Compounds like selenium and tellurium which either exist in trace amounts in vivo or not at all, have a high potential for toxicity, particularly if they are released as free metals as a result of oxidation or enzymatic metabolism. New classes of selenium- and tellurium-containing compounds (Jacob et al., 2000) may overcome current limitations and prove to be clinically useful. Metalloporphyrins have the advantage of being remarkably stable toward metal release as the tetra-coordinate porphyrin backbone binds Mn and Fe with very high affinity while permitting the metals to redox cycle.

Superoxide, NO, H_2O_2, and peroxynitrite are inextricably intertwined with SODs

SODs can catalyze the interconversion between superoxide, NO, H_2O_2, and peroxynitrite; thus a fundamental relationship exists between these enzymes and the chemical entities that interact with them. This relationship has many important implications including: (i) why it is desirable to scavenge superoxide- and NODOs rather than the primary radicals, (ii) how H_2O_2-mediated toxicity may be SOD dependent, (iii) how and why SOD mutants cause ALS, (iv) how wild-type SOD may become toxic via the same mechanism as SOD mutants (and thereby cause sporadic ALS), and (v) how binding of copper by amyloid beta and prion protein (PrP) may contribute to Alzheimer's disease and prion-related diseases such as scrapie and bovine spongiform encephalopathies. This topic was reserved for the end because of the need to incorporate several concepts developed earlier.

Why do we need so much SOD activity?

As mentioned earlier, the fundamental problem with superoxide-dependent oxidative injury is that superoxide itself does not do much, i.e. despite its name, it is not a good oxidant and it simply does not react at all with most non-radical biomolecules.[8] Moreover, superoxide will undergo spontaneous dismutation (transfer an electron from one superoxide to another to yield molecular oxygen and H_2O_2) at a rate which is arguably fast enough to prevent superoxide-mediate modification of the few biomolecular targets that do exist (Gardner & Fridovich, 1992; Hausladen & Fridovich, 1994). So, why do we need superoxide dismutases – enzymes that simply increase the rate of a reaction that already occurs? Also, why do we need so much SOD (~1% of all soluble protein in the CNS is SOD1)? One possible reason could be the need to compete with NO for available superoxide and thereby prevent formation of peroxynitrite.[9] The reaction of superoxide with either SOD1 or SOD2 is 2×10^9 $M^{-1}s^{-1}$ (Forman & Fridovich, 1973). The reaction of superoxide with NO is ~five-fold faster than that; SODs are already as efficient as nature can make them and they simply cannot react any faster,[10] so biological systems compensate by making more of it and maintaining a very high cytosolic concentration of Cu,Zn SOD (~10 μM of Cu,Zn SOD exists in the cytosol of neurons and most other cell types). The steady-state concentration of superoxide in the cell has been estimated to be in the range of 10 picomolar, or 1 000 000 lower than the concentration of enzyme designed to scavenge it. This extremely high concentration ratio of enzyme to substrate is just the opposite of what exists with most enzymes and has important implications for physiology, pathology, and for the design of therapeutic antioxidants.

More SOD does not mean more H₂O₂

One obvious, yet often unappreciated implication of the 1 000 000:1 molar ratio of SOD1 to superoxide, is that further increasing the concentration of SOD1 will not increase the amount of H_2O_2 formed. The formation of H_2O_2 (via the dismutation of superoxide) is limited by the amount of superoxide formed, not by the rate at which it is converted to H_2O_2. Therefore, in the absence of an increase in superoxide production, merely increasing the concentration of SOD will have absolutely no effect on the amount of H_2O_2 formed. Despite this simple logic, toxicity associated with overexpressing SODs – and particularly SOD2 in the mitochondria – is quite often attributed to increased formation of H_2O_2 (Zhang et al., 2002). This conclusion seems reasonable, based on the fact that overexpression of catalase often abrogates the toxicity associated with SOD overexpression (Zhang et al., 2002). However, such results can also be explained on the basis of SODs catalyzing the reverse reaction whereby H_2O_2 is used as a substrate to produce superoxide (see below). The only conceivable circumstance where higher SOD concentration will lead to more H_2O_2 is when a significant fraction of superoxide is reacting with NO to make peroxynitrite. Under those conditions, increasing the concentration of SODs will "divert" more superoxide (from reacting with NO) to make H_2O_2. However, under these conditions, production of more H_2O_2 is very unlikely to be toxic since this would amount to substituting a very mild cytotoxin (H_2O_2) for a very potent one (peroxynitrite).

In the presence of NO, SODs can use H₂O₂ to run in reverse

Another consequence of overexpressing SODs will be to promote the reverse reaction whereby H_2O_2 becomes a substrate for SODs, resulting in the production of superoxide. SOD, like all enzymes, is capable of catalyzing reactions bidirectionally. The direction of the reaction is dictated by many factors including the relative energy states of substrates and products and by the relative concentrations of substrates and products. In the case of SODs, H_2O_2 would rarely build up to high concentrations because catalase, gluthathione peroxidase, and other peroxidases act to decompose H_2O_2 to water and oxygen. However, catalase is primarily localized to peroxisomes and GPx is localized to the mitochondria (Halliwell, 2001). Thus H_2O_2 may accumulate in the cytosol (or other subcellular compartment) to concentrations sufficient to drive the reverse reaction by SODs. Coincidentally, the normal substrate for SODs – superoxide – reacts with NO about five-fold faster than it reacts with SOD itself and NO is small enough to "invade" the active site of SODs. Thus, in the presence of NO, any superoxide produced by SODs can be quickly converted to peroxynitrite and the equilibrium can be "pulled" by NO in the reverse direction. The reverse reaction of SOD is more likely to be important in situations where H_2O_2 is added exogenously, e.g. when H_2O_2 is added to cultured cells. It is quite easy to demonstrate that SODs plus H_2O_2 and NO will yield peroxynitrite in vitro and McBride et al. have provided compelling evidence for this reaction occurring in cells where H_2O_2 has been added exogenously (McBride & Brown, 1997; McBride et al., 1999).

In the absence of enzyme-bound zinc, Cu,Zn SOD can be reduced to the Cu(I) form by other cellular reductants, thereby eliminating the need for H_2O_2 altogether. Thus, the Cu(I) form of zinc-deficient SOD1 can use ascorbate, GSH, NADH, etc. along with oxygen and NO to make peroxynitrite catalytically. This is the basis for one hypothesis regarding the gained function of SOD1 mutants in ALS and the reader is referred to a review of this mechanism (Beckman et al., 2001). One attractive aspect of this zinc deficiency hypothesis is that it provides a mechanism whereby wild-type SOD1 – via a failure to bind zinc – could become toxic in the same manner as ALS-associated mutants and thereby produce so-called sporadic ALS (Beckman et al., 2001).

The reverse dismutase reaction utilizing H_2O_2 should not be confused with so-called peroxidase activity of SODs. Peroxidase activity of SOD only occurs at extremely high (nonphysiological) concentrations of H_2O_2 and inactivates SOD after only a few turnovers (Hodgson & Fridovich, 1975;

Wiedan-Pazos *et al.*, 1996). The reverse reaction of SOD1 occurs at low micromolar concentrations of H_2O_2 and is enhanced in a concentration-dependent manner by NO (Crow *et al.*, unpublished observations).

Copper-binding proteins as a generic mechanism of toxicity in neurodegenerative disease

Much attention has been focused on abnormal aggregation of proteins as the basis for toxicity of beta amyloid peptide in Alzheimer's disease, Huntingtin protein in Huntington's disease, prion protein in Mad Cow disease (bovine spongiform encephalopathy and other prion-related diseases), and SOD1 mutants in ALS. There are many reasons to believe that these proteins are inherently unstable and have a greater tendency to aggregate, particularly in certain conformations or oxidatively modified forms. Binding of non-redox active metals such as zinc and aluminium by these proteins could stabilize abnormal conformations and thereby contribute to toxicity. However, a growing body of evidence suggests that copper binding may be critical to their toxicity, particularly with beta amyloid peptide, prion protein, and SOD1 mutants (Bush, 2000). Copper is inherently toxic due to its ability to steal electrons from cellular reductants such as ascorbate and GSH and hand them off to oxygen to generate superoxide. SOD1 "forces" copper to carry out the opposite reaction – namely to take electrons from superoxide, but abnormal conformations and/or abnormal copper binding by SOD1 mutants could "disinhibit" this inherent property of copper and allow it to become pro-oxidant. There is evidence that beta amyloid and prion protein bind copper in a redox active manner. Oxidants formed in this way could attack critical sites of energy production in mitochondria and/or oxidatively modify the copper binding protein itself, making it resistant to proteolytic degradation and more likely to accumulate and aggregate. Thus, abnormal generation of oxidants via redox cycling of bound copper may turn out to be a generic mechanism contributing to neurodegenerative disease.

ENDNOTES

1. Single, odd electrons could, in theory, be transferred to any molecule capable of accepting them. Odd electrons are transferred to molecular oxygen (to generate reactive species) because oxygen normally has two unpaired electrons and because it is the most abundant, diffusable, and proximal one electron acceptor present.

2. In the absence of redox metal catalysts, significant oxidation of thiols (-SH) such as glutathione by H_2O_2 requires many hours to occur. Superoxide is a much better reductant than oxidant and its ability to reduce Fe(III) cytochrome c serves as the basis for the most commonly used in vitro SOD assay.

3. NO, like oxygen, is lipid soluble and will partition into lipid bilayers. The fact that NO and oxygen accumulate to higher concentrations within lipid bilayers has important implications for NO/oxygen interactions and initiation of lipid peroxidation (Liu *et al.*, 1998).

4. Chemically speaking, the reaction of any radical with any non-radical is electronically unbalanced, thermodynamically unfavourable and, when it does occur, results in a new radical species. Thus, only radicals with very high oxidation potentials will react directly with neutral biological molecules and thereby abstract single electrons. Such electron abstraction neutralizes the oxidizing radical (e.g. hydroxyl radical gets reduced to hydroxide anion or $^-$OH) and simultaneously yields a new radical derived from the biomolecular target. The biomolecular radical may be quenched by one electron reductants such as ascorbate or tocopherol (so-called radical termination) or abstract an electron from another target, thereby propagating the radical reaction.

5. The exception to this rule is the reaction of NO with oxygen within a lipid bilayer as mentioned earlier. However, even under these conditions, the reactive species produced will most likely react with electron-rich unsaturated lipids in the bilayer and not escape to interact with soluble biomolecules.

6. Most of the peroxynitrite-mediated modifications that have been studied extensively in vitro are not reversed even by high concentrations of classic reductants such as dithiothreitol. Nitration and hydroxylation of aromatic amino acid residues or low molecular weight compounds represent covalent modifications which could only be reversed only by enzymes in vivo. However, no compelling evidence for reversal of these or other peroxynitrite-mediated modifications in vivo exists.

7. Simple calculations of specific dismutase activity per milligram of porphyrin – compared to true SOD enzyme activity already present in cells – reveals that millimolar concentrations of porphyrins would be needed to enhance total dismutase activity by even a small percentage. Thus, it is exceedingly unlikely that Mn and Fe porphyrins are exerting protective effects via dismutase activity.

8. The notable exception to this rule is iron–sulfur centers in many mitochondrial enzymes such as aconitase (Gardner & Fridovich, 1992; Hansladen & Fridovich, 1994). Iron-sulfur centers retain some degree of radical character and can be oxidized reversibly by superoxide.

9 The amino acid residues which comprise SOD1 support this teleological argument. Most enzymes that peroxynitrite has been shown to inactivate contain critical tyrosine, cysteine, or methionine residues. Human Cu,Zn SOD has only one methionine and two free cysteines – none of which is required for enzyme activity – and no tyrosines. Thus, human Cu,Zn SOD appears to have evolved to be highly resistant to oxidative modification/inactivation by peroxynitrite.

10 Many factors govern whether two molecules will react with each other, but the ultimate limit is imposed by how fast they can

diffuse and randomly collide with each other, i.e. no reaction can occur faster than the rate at which the two reactants can collide. A large protein like SOD cannot diffuse and collide as rapidly as a small molecule like NO. Under physiological conditions, $2 \times 10^9 \, M^{-1}s^{-1}$ (the rate constant for reaction of superoxide with SOD) is about as fast as a small molecule can collide with a large protein whereas two small molecules can collide from 10 to 100 times faster or 10^{10} to $10^{11} \, M^{-1}s^{-1}$. Thus, the reaction of superoxide with SOD represents a true diffusion-limited reaction for a protein and a small molecule, and the reaction of superoxide with NO ($\sim10^{10} \, M^{-1}s^{-1}$) approaches the diffusion limit for two small molecules.

REFERENCES

Abe, K., Pan, L. H., Watanabe, M., Kato, T. & Itoyama, Y. (1995). Induction of nitrotyrosine-like immunoreactivity in the lower motor neuron of amyotrophic lateral sclerosis. *Neurosci. Lett.*, **199** (2), 152–4.

Aoyama, K., Matsubara, K., Fujikawa, Y. *et al.* (2000). Nitration of manganese superoxide dismutase in cerebrospinal fluids is a marker for peroxynitrite-mediated oxidative stress in neurodegenerative diseases. *Ann. Neurol.*, **47** (4), 524–7.

Beal, M. F., Ferrante, R. J., Browne, S. E. Matthews, R. T., Kowall, N. W. & Brown, Jr., R. H. (1997). Increased 3-nitrotyrosine in both sporadic and familial amyotrophic lateral sclerosis. *Ann. Neurol.*, **42** (4), 644–54.

Beckman, J. S. (2002). Protein tyrosine nitration and peroxynitrite. *FASEB J.*, **16** (9), 1144.

Beckman, J. S., Beckman, T. W., Chen, J., Marshall, P. A. & Freeman, B. A. (1990). Apparent hydroxyl radical production by peroxynitrite: Implications for endothelial injury from nitric oxide and superoxide. *Proc. Natl Acad. Sci.* USA, **87**, 1620–4.

Beckman, J. S., Estevez, A. G. Crow, J. P. & Barbeito, L. (2001). Superoxide dismutase and the death of motoneurons in ALS. *Trends Neurosci.*, **24** (11 Suppl), S15–20.

Briviba, K., Roussyn, I., Sharov, V. S. & Sies, H. (1996). Attenuation of oxidation and nitration reactions of peroxynitrite by selenomethionine, selenocystine and ebselen. *Biochem. J.*, **319** (Pt 1), 13–15.

Bush, A. I. (2000). Metals and neuroscience. *Curr. Opin. Chem. Biol.*, **4** (2), 184–91.

Cassina, P., Peluffo, H., Pehar, M. *et al.* (2002). Peroxynitrite triggers a phenotypic transformation in spinal cord astrocytes that induces motor neuron apoptosis. *J. Neurosci. Res.*, **67** (1), 21–9.

Copin, J. C., Gasche, Y. & Chan, P. H. (2000). Overexpression of copper/zinc superoxide dismutase does not prevent neonatal lethality in mutant mice that lack manganese superoxide dismutase. *Free Radic. Biol. Med.*, **28** (10), 1571–6.

Crow, J. P. (1999). Manganese and iron porphyrins catalyze peroxynitrite decomposition and simultaneously increase nitration and oxidant yield: implications for their use as peroxynitrite scavengers in vivo. *Arch. Biochem. Biophys.*, **371** (1), 41–52.

(2000). Peroxynitrite scavenging by metalloporphyrins and thiolates. *Free Radic. Biol. Med.*, **28** (10), 1487–94.

Crow, J. P., Ye, Y., Royall, J., Kooy, N. & Beckman, J. S. (1994). Evidence of peroxynitrite formation *in vivo*: detection of nitrated proteins with an anti-nitrotyrosine antibody. In *Physiology of Nitric Oxide, 3rd edn.*

Crow, J. P., Ye, Y. Z., Strong, M., Kirk, M., Barnes, S. & Beckman, J. S. (1997). Superoxide dismutase catalyzes nitration of tyrosines by peroxynitrite in the rod and head domains of neurofilament-L. *J. Neurochem.*, **69** (5), 1945–53.

Daveu, C., Servy, C., Dendane, M., Marin, P. & Ducrocq, C. (1997). Oxidation and nitration of catecholamines by nitrogen oxides derived from nitric oxide. *Nitric Oxide.*, **1** (3), 234–43.

Denicola, A., Freeman, B. A., Trujillo, M. & Radi, R. (1996). Peroxynitrite reaction with carbon dioxide/bicarbonate: kinetics and influence on peroxynitrite-mediated oxidations. *Arch. Biochem. Biophys.*, **333** (1), 49–58.

Eiserich, J. P., Estevez, A. G., Bamberg, T. V. *et al.* (1999). Microtubule dysfunction by posttranslational nitrotyrosination of alpha-tubulin: a nitric oxide-dependent mechanism of cellular injury. *Proc. Natl Acad. Sci., USA*, **96** (11), 6365–70.

Ferrer-Sueta, G., Batinic-Haberle, I., Spasojevic, I., Fridovich, I. & Radi, R. (1999). Catalytic scavenging of peroxynitrite by isomeric Mn(III) *N*-methylpyridylporphyrins in the presence of reductants. *Chem. Res. Toxicol.*, **12** (5), 442–9.

Forman, H. J. & Fridovich, I. (1973). Superoxide dismutase: a comparison of rate constants. *Arch. Biochem. Biophys.*, **158** (1), 396–400.

Gardner, P. R. & Fridovich, I. (1992). Inactivation–reactivation of aconitase in *Escherichia coli*. A sensitive measure of superoxide radical. *J. Biol. Chem.*, **267** (13), 8757–63.

Giannopoulou, E., Katsoris, P., Polytarchou, C. & Papadimitriou, E. (2002). Nitration of cytoskeletal proteins in the chicken embryo chorioallantoic membrane. *Arch. Biochem. Biophys.*, **400** (2), 188–98.

Giasson, B. I., Duda, J. E., Murray, I. V. *et al.* (2000). Oxidative damage linked to neurodegeneration by selective alpha-synuclein nitration in synucleinopathy lesions. *Science*, **290** (5493), 985–9.

Good, P. F., Hsu, A., Werner, P., Perl, D. P. & Olanow, C. W. (1998). Protein nitration in Parkinson's disease. *J. Neuropathol. Exp. Neurol.*, **57** (4), 338–42.

Gryglewski, R. J., Palmer, R. M. & Moncada, S. (1986). Superoxide anion is involved in the breakdown of endothelium-derived vascular relaxing factor. *Nature*, **320** (6061), 454–6.

Guentchev, M., Voigtlander, T., Haberler, C., Groschup, M. H. & Budka, H. (2000). Evidence for oxidative stress in experimental prion disease. *Neurobiol. Dis.*, **7** (4), 270–3.

Halliwell, B. (2001). Role of free radicals in the neurodegenerative diseases: therapeutic implications for antioxidant treatment. *Drugs Aging*, **18** (9), 685–716.

Hausladen, A. & Fridovich, I. (1994). Superoxide and peroxynitrite inactivate aconitases, but nitric oxide does not. *J. Biol. Chem.*, **269** (47), 29405–8.

Hensley, K., Maidt, M. L., Yu, Z., Sang, H., Markesbery, W. R. & Floyd, R. A. (1998). Electrochemical analysis of protein nitrotyrosine and dityrosine in the Alzheimer brain indicates region-specific accumulation. *J. Neurosci.*, **18** (20), 8126–32.

Hodgson, E. K. & Fridovich, I. (1975). The interaction of bovine erythrocyte superoxide dismutase with hydrogen peroxide: inactivation of the enzyme. *Biochemistry*, **14** (24), 5294–9.

Hughes, M. N. & Nicklin, H. G. (1968). The chemistry of pernitrites. Part I. Kinetics of decomposition of pernitrous acid. *J. Chem. Soc.(A)*, 450–2.

Jacob, C., Arteel, G. E., Kanda, T., Engman, L. & Sies, H. (2000). Water-soluble organotellurium compounds: catalytic protection against peroxynitrite and release of zinc from metallothionein. *Chem. Res. Toxicol.*, **13** (1), 3–9.

Kalisz, H. M., Erck, C., Plessmann, U. & Wehland, J. (2000). Incorporation of nitrotyrosine into alpha-tubulin by recombinant mammalian tubulin-tyrosine ligase. *Biochim. Biophys. Acta*, **1481** (1), 131–8.

Kehrer, J. P. (2000). The Haber–Weiss reaction and mechanisms of toxicity. *Toxicology*, **149** (1), 43–50.

Kissner, R., Nauser, T., Bugnon, P., Lye, P. G. & Koppenol, W. H. (1997). Formation and properties of peroxynitrite as studied by laser flash photolysis, high-pressure stopped-flow technique, and pulse radiolysis. *Chem. Res. Toxicol.*, **10** (11), 1285–92.

Koppenol, W. H. (2001). The Haber–Weiss cycle: 70 years later. *Redox. Rep.*, **6** (4), 229–34.

Li, Y., Huang, T. T., Carlson, E. J. *et al.* (1995). Dilated cardiomyopathy and neonatal lethality in mutant mice lacking manganese superoxide dismutase. *Nat. Genet.*, **11** (4), 376–81.

Liu, X., Miller, M. J., Joshi, M. S., Thomas, D. D. & Lancaster, Jr., J. R. (1998). Accelerated reaction of nitric oxide with O_2 within the hydrophobic interior of biological membranes. *Proc. Natl Acad. Sci., USA*, **95** (5), 2175–9.

Lymar, S. V., Jiang, Q. & Hurst, J. K. (1996). Mechanism of carbon dioxide-catalyzed oxidation of tyrosine by peroxynitrite. *Biochemistry*, **35** (24), 7855–61.

McBride, A. G. & Brown, G. C. (1997). Production of peroxynitrite from nitric oxide, hydrogen peroxide and superoxide dismutase: pathological implications. *Biochem. Soc. Trans.*, **25** (3), 409S.

McBride, A. G., Borutaite, V. & Brown, G. C. (1999). Superoxide dismutase and hydrogen peroxide cause rapid nitric oxide breakdown, peroxynitrite production and subsequent cell death. *Biochim. Biophys. Acta*, **1454** (3), 275–88.

Mackensen, G. B., Patel, M., Sheng, H. *et al.* (2001). Neuroprotection from delayed postischemic administration of a metalloporphyrin catalytic antioxidant. *J. Neurosci.*, **21** (13), 4582–92.

MacMillan-Crow, L. A., Crow, J. P., Kerby, J. D., Beckman, J. S. & Thompson, J. A. (1996). Nitration and inactivation of manganese superoxide dismutase in chronic rejection of human renal allografts. *Proc. Natl. Acad. Sci. USA*, **93** (21), 11853–8.

MacMillan-Crow, L. A., Crow, J. P. & Thompson, J. A. (1998). Peroxynitrite-mediated inactivation of manganese superoxide dismutase involves nitration and oxidation of critical tyrosine residues. *Biochemistry*, **37** (6), 1613–22 .

MacMillan-Crow, L. A., Greendorfer, J. S., Vickers, S. M. & Thompson, J. A. (2000). Tyrosine nitration of c-SRC tyrosine kinase in human pancreatic ductal adenocarcinoma. *Arch. Biochem. Biophys.*, **377** (2), 350–6.

Mallozzi, C., Di Stasi, A. M. & Minetti, M. (1997). Peroxynitrite modulates tyrosine-dependent signal transduction pathway of human erythrocyte band 3. *FASEB J.*, **11** (14), 1281–90.

Misko, T. P., Highkin, M. K., Veenhuizen, A. W. *et al.* (1998). Characterization of the cytoprotective action of peroxynitrite decomposition catalysts. *J. Biol. Chem.*, **273** (25), 15646–53.

Mondoro, T. H., Shafer, B. C. & Vostal, J. G. (1997). Peroxynitrite-induced tyrosine nitration and phosphorylation in human platelets. *Free Radic. Biol. Med.*, **22** (6), 1055–63.

Ohshima, H., Friesen, M., Brouet, I. & Bartsch, H. (1990). Nitrotyrosine as a new marker for endogenous nitrosation and nitration of proteins. *Food Chem. Toxicol.*, **28** (9), 647–52.

Padmaja, S. & Huie, R. E. (1993). The reaction of nitric oxide with organic peroxyl radicals. *Biochem. Biophys. Res. Commun.*, **195** (2), 539–44.

Radi, R., Beckman, J. S., Bush, K. M. & Freeman, B. A. (1991). Peroxynitrite oxidation of sulfhydryls. The cytotoxic potential of superoxide and nitric oxide. *J. Biol. Chem.*, **266** (7), 4244–50.

Ray, J. D. (1962). Heat of isomerization of peroxynitrite to nitrate and kinetics of isomerization of peroxynitrous acid to nitric acid. *J. Inorg. Nucl. Chem.*, **24**, 1159–62.

Reaume. A. G., Elliott, J. L., Hoffman, E. K. *et al.* (1996). Motor neurons in Cu/Zn superoxide dismutase-deficient mice develop normally but exhibit enhanced cell death after axonal injury. *Nat. Genet.*, **13** (1), 43–7.

Riobo, N. A., Schopfer, F. J., Boveris, A. D., Cadenas, E. & Poderoso, J. J. (2002). The reaction of nitric oxide with 6-hydroxydopamine: implications for Parkinson's disease. *Free Radic. Biol. Med.*, **32** (2), 115–21.

Rubanyi, G. M. & Vanhoutte, P. M. (1986). Superoxide anions and hyperoxia inactivate endothelium-derived relaxing factor. *Am. J. Physiol.*, **250** (5 Pt 2), H822–7.

Salvemini, D., Riley, D. P., Lennon, P. J. *et al.* (1999). Protective effects of a superoxide dismutase mimetic and peroxynitrite decomposition catalysts in endotoxin-induced intestinal damage. *Br. J. Pharmacol.*, **127** (3), 685–92.

Sies, H. & Masumoto, H. (1997). Ebselen as a glutathione peroxidase mimic and as a scavenger of peroxynitrite. *Adv. Pharmacol.*, **38**, 229–46.

Smith, M. A., Richey Harris, P. L., Sayre, L. M., Beckman, J. S. & Perry, G. (1997). Widespread peroxynitrite-mediated damage in Alzheimer's disease. *J. Neurosci.*, **17** (8), 2653–7.

Strong, M. J., Sopper, M. M., Crow, J. P., Strong, W. L. & Beckman, J. S. (1998). Nitration of the low molecular weight neurofilament is equivalent in sporadic amyotrophic lateral sclerosis and control cervical spinal cord. *Biochem. Biophys. Res. Commun.*, **248** (1), 157–64 .

Strong, M. J., Strong, W. L., He, B. P. & Crow, J. P. (2002). High capacity, high affinity zinc binding by neurofilament proteins inhibits zinc incorporation into Cu,Zn superoxide dismutase (SOD1): implications for SOD1 mutant toxicity in ALS. (submitted 2002).

Takakura, K., Beckman, J. S., MacMillan-Crow, L. A. & Crow, J. P. (1999). Rapid and irreversible inactivation of protein tyrosine phosphatases PTP1B, CD45, and LAR by peroxynitrite. *Arch. Biochem. Biophys.*, **369** (2), 197–207.

Thomas, D. D., Liu, X., Kantrow, S. P. & Lancaster, Jr., J. R. (2001). The biological lifetime of nitric oxide: implications for the perivascular dynamics of NO and O2. *Proc. Natl Acad. Sci. USA*, **98** (1), 355–60.

Tohgi, H., Abe, T., Yamazaki, K., Murata, T., Ishizaki, E. & Isobe, C. (1999). Alterations of 3-nitrotyrosine concentration in the cerebrospinal fluid during aging and in patients with Alzheimer's disease. *Neurosci. Lett.*, **269** (1), 52–4.

Wiedau-Pazos, M., Goto, J. J., Rabizadeh, S. *et al.* (1996). Altered reactivity of superoxide dismutase in familial amyotrophic lateral sclerosis. *Science*, **271** (5248), 515–18.

Williamson, K. S., Gabbita, S. P., Mou, S. *et al.* (2002). The nitration product 5-nitro-gamma-tocopherol is increased in the Alzheimer brain. *Nitric Oxide*, **6** (2), 221–7.

Wu, A. S., Kiaei, M., Aguirre, N. *et al.* (2003). Iron porphyrin treatment extends survival in a transgenic animal model of amyotrophic lateral sclerosis. *J. Neurochem.*, **85** (1), 142–50.

Zhang, Y., Zhao, W., Zhang, H. J., Domann, F. E. & Oberley, L. W. (2002). Overexpression of copper zinc superoxide dismutase suppresses human glioma cell growth. *Cancer Res.*, **62** (4), 1205–12.

3

Mitochondria, metabolic inhibitors and neurodegeneration

James G. Greene[1] and J. Timothy Greenamyre[2]

[1]Center for Neurodegenerative Disease and Department of Neurology, Emory University, Atlanta, GA, USA
[2]Pittsburgh Institute for Neurodegenerative Diseases, University of Pittsburgh, PA, USA

The role of the mitochondrion in neurodegeneration is a paradox. On the one hand, vital mitochondrial tasks, such as energy production and calcium buffering, provide an important foundation for all neuronal functions. Yet, on the other, mitochondrial free radical production and involvement in cell-death cascades may lead to a neuron's untimely demise.

It is now clear that mitochondria are not merely neuronal "power plants", but are highly complex, integrated organelles whose function transcends that of simple energy production. In addition to providing the majority of neuronal energy via oxidative phosphorylation, mitochondria play a central role in intracellular ion homeostasis, free radical management, and gene and protein expression.

This chapter will focus on the biology of mitochondrial electron transport, oxidative phosphorylation and other mitochondrial functions, and will discuss the effects of mitochondrial toxins on mitochondrial function and neuronal viability. It will explore briefly one of the main consequences of oxidative metabolism, mitochondrial free radical production and how this and other mitochondrial factors potentially contribute to neuronal death.

Mitochondrial energy production and sites of action for metabolic inhibitors

Mitochondria efficiently convert the potential energy of glucose into a usable cellular energy currency, primarily ATP. Glucose is the primary basis for neuronal energy metabolism; ketone bodies can provide a limited energy source, but only in situations of chronic metabolic imbalance.

Glucose crosses the blood–brain barrier in an insulin-independent manner and is taken up by membrane transporters. It is phosphorylated almost immediately by hexokinase and enters glycolysis. Iodoacetate (IOA) is an inhibitor of glycolysis that acts by acetylating sulfhydryl groups on glucose-6-phosphate dehydrogenase and other proteins (Hochster & Quastel, 1963). Pyruvate, the end product of glycolysis, is transported through the double-layer mitochondrial membrane into the matrix where it is transformed into acetyl CoA by the pyruvate dehydrogenase complex (PDHC). Lactate, produced from glial metabolism of glucose, is also a significant source of neuronal pyruvate.

Acetyl CoA enters the tricarboxylic acid (TCA) cycle by combination with oxaloacetate to form citrate (Fig. 3.1). The TCA cycle is a sequence of nine reactions that results in the production of high-energy phosphates, reducing equivalents, and oxaloacetate for the next round of the cycle. One important reaction in this sequence is the transformation of succinate to fumarate by succinate dehydrogenase (SDH, complex II). This enzyme contains a flavin prosthetic group that is reduced from FAD^+ to $FADH_2$ in the process of succinate metabolism. Malonate is a reversible, competitive inhibitor of SDH (Hochster & Quastel, 1963); 3-nitropropionic acid (3-NP) is a suicide inhibitor of this enzyme (Alston et al., 1977). One mole of glucose produces a net gain of 2 moles each of ATP and NADH in the cytoplasm from glycolysis and 8 moles of NADH, 2 moles of $FADH_2$, and 2 moles of GTP in the mitochondrial matrix from the TCA cycle.

Since the inner mitochondrial membrane is impermeable to NADH, the reducing equivalents contained in cytosolic NADH are transferred to the mitochondrial matrix by two "shuttles." The glycerol-3-phosphate shuttle is irreversible and results in one mole of mitochondrial $FADH_2$ from one mole of cytoplasmic NADH; the malate–aspartate shuttle is reversible and results in one mole of mitochondrial NADH from one mole of cytoplasmic NADH. The

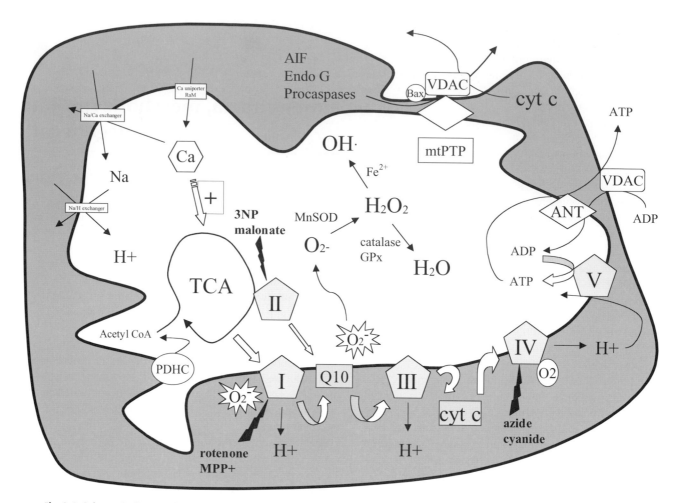

Fig. 3.1 Schematic diagram illustrating various aspects of mitochondrial metabolism. There is significant interaction between energy metabolism, calcium buffering, ROS production, and regulation of neuronal death.

malate–aspartate shuttle, because it requires no net energy expenditure, only operates if the NADH/NAD$^+$ ratio is higher in the cytoplasm than the mitochondrial matrix. Aminoxyacetic acid (AOAA) inhibits a variety of transamination reactions, including the transamination of oxaloacetate to aspartate in the mitochondrial matrix, which is a key step in the operation of the malate-aspartate shuttle (Kauppinen *et al.*, 1987).

Oxidative phosphorylation transforms the potential energy contained in NADH and FADH$_2$ into ATP. The electron transport chain (ETC) includes a series of enzymes in the inner mitochondrial membrane, two small electron carriers, and SDH (Fig. 3.1). Electrons from NADH enter the respiratory chain via complex I (NADH dehydrogenase; NADH: ubiquinone oxidoreductase). Rotenone and MPP$^+$ are inhibitors of this enzyme (Nicklas *et al.*, 1985; Ramsay *et al.*, 1991).

Electrons from complex I are passed to complex III (ubiquinol–cytochrome c oxidoreductase) via the small electron acceptor ubiquinone, also known as coenzyme Q10. Coenzyme Q10 is also the entry point for electrons derived from FADH$_2$. Most FADH$_2$ is generated via the TCA cycle by SDH (complex II; succinate: ubiquinone oxidoreductase), but some comes indirectly from glycolysis via the glycerol-3-phosphate shuttle.

Complex III, which can be inhibited by antimycin (Slater, 1973), donates electrons to a second small electron acceptor, cytochrome c, which passes them to complex IV (cytochrome oxidase). Complex IV transfers electrons to molecular oxygen, the final electron acceptor. Inhibitors of complex IV include cyanide (CN$^-$) and azide (N$_3^-$) (Hochster & Quastel, 1963).

Complexes I, III, and IV pump protons from the inner mitochondrial matrix to the outer mitochondrial matrix, creating potential energy stored in the form of an electro-chemical gradient. The establishment of this proton motive force (Δp) is vital to many mitochondrial functions, including ATP synthesis. Δp is a composite of mitochondrial membrane potential ($\Delta\psi$) and ΔpH, with $\Delta\psi$ being the larger contributor to Δp.

The potential energy in Δp is harnessed by complex V (ATP synthase), which produces ATP from ADP and inorganic phosphate when protons flow through the complex back into the mitochondrial matrix. Mitochondrial uncouplers, such as dinitrophenol and carbonyl cyanide trifluoromethoxyphenyl hydrazon (FCCP), disrupt the mitochondrial proton gradient and thereby uncouple electron transport from ATP synthesis (Hochster & Quastel, 1963).

The flow of two moles of electrons through complexes I, III, and IV provides energy for each enzyme complex to pump enough protons to make one mole of ATP. Metabolism of one mole of glucose through oxidative phosphorylation generates about 30 moles of ATP.

Under normal circumstances, glycolysis accounts for only about 5% of neuronal energy production, but it provides necessary precursors for the TCA cycle and oxidative phosphorylation. Under hypoxic conditions, NAD^+ may be regenerated via anaerobic mechanisms, such as lactate production, thereby increasing the energy production of anaerobic glycolysis, although the energy production capacity of this mechanism is limited. Regulation of neuronal energy metabolism is a subject beyond the scope of this review, but it is based on cellular energy charge, the need for anabolic precursors, the supply of glucose and oxygen, and second messenger signaling pathways, especially Ca^{2+} (Pulsinelli & Cooper, 1989; Stryer, 1988; Gunter et al., 1994).

Mitochondrial calcium homeostasis

As mentioned above, the potential energy represented by Δp is important for other mitochondrial functions besides ATP production, namely mitochondrial calcium uptake and homeostasis. The inner mitochondrial membrane contains two mechanisms that allow for passage of calcium ions into the mitochondrial matrix, the calcium uniporter and RaM. Calcium uptake is driven primarily by $\Delta\psi$. These uptake mechanisms have a low affinity for calcium, so they are only activated above a certain set-point calcium concentration (typically 500–1000 nM); however, mitochondria have an extremely high capacity for calcium uptake once that set point is reached (Gunter & Gunter, 2001).

Mitochondrial calcium is extruded by sodium-dependent and sodium-independent mechanisms. Sodium-dependent efflux is modulated by a Na^+/H^+ antiporter that extrudes sodium from the mitochondrial matrix at the expense of ΔpH. Sodium-independent efflux appears to depend on ΔpH as well, in the form of active Ca/H exchange. Thus, the proton-motive force mediates both mitochondrial uptake and release of calcium (Pfeiffer et al., 2001).

As might be imagined, due to their link through the proton motive force, not only does mitochondrial metabolism affect calcium flux, calcium flux modulates mitochondrial metabolism. Small increases in intramitochondrial calcium, such as would be seen with modest neuronal stimulation, act as an intracellular signal to produce increases in mitochondrial respiration. Higher levels of calcium sequestration are thought to induce Ca^{2+}-dependent Ca^{2+} release and propagation of further intracellular calcium signals (Ichas et al., 1997).

Under situations of extreme stress, large amounts of calcium can be sequestered in mitochondria. This serves as a valuable protective mechanism by maintaining cytosolic calcium in the physiologic range, but when overwhelmed, high levels of intramitochondrial calcium have deleterious effects. These include metabolic inhibition, dissipation of $\Delta\psi$, and increased ROS generation (Murphy et al., 1999; Ichas et al., 1997; Stout et al., 1998).

Mitochondrial free radical production

One of the inherent dangers in oxidative metabolism is ROS generation. Superoxide radical is produced by reduction of molecular oxygen by one electron. In mitochondria, this is most likely to occur when elements of the electron transport chain are in a highly-reduced state and, as such, more easily oxidizable. The physiological state during which this is most likely to occur is when matrix ADP concentration is low, resulting in a "bottleneck" at ATP synthase (state IV respiration). A similar highly-reduced state occurs when inhibitors of the electron transport chain are present, resulting in a "backup" of electrons. Under these circumstances oxygen accepts electrons from components other than complex IV. Furthermore, any event that enhances oxidative metabolism, thereby increasing electron flux, may cause an increased likelihood of superoxide generation. Conversely, mitochondrial ROS production is lowest during state III respiration, when ADP is plentiful and electrons proceed unimpeded through the chain (Boveris & Turrens, 1980; Boveris et al., 1972; Loschen et al., 1974). Superoxide production is most likely to occur at complex I and ubiquinone (Raha & Robinson, 2001).

Superoxide is converted to hydrogen peroxide (H_2O_2) by intramitochondrial manganese superoxide dismutase (Mn-SOD). H_2O_2 is reduced to water by glutathione peroxidase or catalase (Fridovitch, 1995). However, in the presence of reduced iron, such as that present in electron transport chain enzymes, H_2O_2 may be converted to the indiscriminate, highly reactive hydroxyl radical ($\cdot$OH) (Raha and Robinson, 2001) (Fig. 3.1). Accordingly, if mechanisms of superoxide detoxification are not functional or become overwhelmed, production of hydroxyl radical may increase. In addition, the iron–sulfur centers in electron transport chain enzymes are sensitive targets for ROS damage. This may, in turn, result in further mitochondrial inhibition and a vicious cycle of enhanced ROS production.

Mitochondrial permeability transition

One more aspect of mitochondrial physiology to discuss at this point is the mitochondrial permeability transition, which is characterized by sudden increased permeability of the inner membrane to ions and small molecules. This results in osmotic swelling of the mitochondrion and disruption of outer membrane integrity, leading to release of contents from the mitochondrial intermembrane space into the cytosol. This transition is mediated by a pore complex (mtPTP), the molecular composition of which is uncertain (Crompton, 1999). The probability of PTP opening is increased by many factors, including high ADP/ATP ratio, increased mitochondrial Ca^{2+}, and enhanced oxidative stress. This transition can be reversible, and it is inhibited by high mitochondrial membrane potential (Pfeiffer *et al.*, 2001). Several pharmacologic agents, including cyclosporin A, inhibit the mitochondrial permeability transition (Bernardi *et al.*, 1994).

It is worthwhile to note here that, although energy production, calcium buffering, ROS generation, and permeability transition are inextricably linked as aspects of mitochondrial function, mitochondrial deficits may be more pronounced in one aspect of function than another. For example, while a relatively severe complex I deficit may be required to produce noticeable effects on mitochondrial respiration and ATP production, much less intense inhibition of the same enzyme is sufficient to produce significant mitochondrial ROS generation and evidence of oxidative damage (Davey *et al.*, 1998; Betarbet *et al.*, 2000).

Mitochondria and cell death: necrosis

It is not surprising that malfunction of so central an organelle as the mitochondrion would result in cellular injury and possibly death. It is perhaps more intriguing to speculate that one of the functions of mitochondria in certain circumstances may be to induce cell death.

Historically, cellular death has been divided into two categories, and mitochondria may play a role in both types. Necrosis is typically described as a passive process that includes morphological features such as large-scale cellular swelling and rupture associated with inflammation. Apoptosis is an active, regulated form of "programmed" cell death that classically manifests cell shrinkage, chromatin condensation and fragmentation, and the formation of apoptotic bodies that are phagocytosed with little or no resultant inflammatory response (Kerr *et al.*, 1972).

The type of neuronal cell death that occurs in chronic neurodegenerative diseases is unclear. The focused death of individual neurons and neuronal subpopulations with minimal inflammatory response is suggestive of apoptosis, but necrosis on a neuron level cannot be ruled out. Study of this question is complicated in humans by the long duration of illness and poorly defined onset of neurodegenerative disease. It is also confounded by the relatively short time course of neurodegeneration in experimental models.

Necrosis can result from ATP depletion, calcium overload, and ROS generation, among other things, and as noted above, mitochondria are central to all three of those systems. A major fraction of ATP produced (approximately 40%) is consumed by the Na–K ATPase to maintain neuronal membrane potential during the resting state; this proportion increases during neuronal activation (Astrup *et al.*, 1981; Mata *et al.*, 1980). Preservation of sodium and potassium gradients is not only important to keep the neuron in the polarized state for neurotransmission, but the potential energy stored in that gradient is vital for calcium, pH and volume homeostasis.

During situations when mitochondrial capacity is overwhelmed by energy demand, either due to mitochondrial dysfunction or extreme neuronal stress, the ability of a neuron to maintain a polarized state might be compromised (Erecinska & Dagani, 1990). For example, mitochondrial complex II inhibition by 3-NP, markedly diminishes ATP levels in cultured striatal neurons. This diminished mitochondrial capacity is accompanied by depolarization of the resting neuronal membrane potential to 60% of its normal value (Greene *et al.*, 1998). Depolarization of the cellular membrane has a myriad of potential consequences, including excessive NMDA receptor activation ("indirect excitotoxicity") and activation of voltage-dependent calcium channels. Excessive NMDA receptor activation may be particularly devastating due to the apparent greater toxicity associated with NMDA receptor-dependent calcium loads, as opposed to other mechanisms of calcium influx (Kiedrowski & Costa, 1995; Peng & Greenamyre, 1998). This can result in dysregulation of neuronal calcium levels and potentially cause non-specific activation of calcium-dependent proteases and other enzymes, leading to rapid cell death in a necrotic manner.

Because the neuronal sodium gradient is dissipated by ATP depletion, secondary active transport via this gradient will stall. Since glutamate reuptake is a Na-dependent process, ATP depletion may result in massive increases in extracellular glutamate concentration and potential for excitotoxic damage (Cousin et al., 1995). Impaired Na/H exchange at the neuronal membrane may have significant effects on cytoplasmic pH, resulting in intraneuronal acidification and an accompanying rise in intraneuronal calcium (Koch & Barrish, 1994). Intraneuronal calcium levels may also increase dramatically due to impairment of Na/Ca exchange at the neuronal membrane. It is thought that this exchange is particularly important in the removal of calcium loads as opposed to the maintenance of resting calcium levels, similar to mitochondrial calcium buffering (Blaustein, 1988). Under circumstances when intraneuronal calcium load is increasing rapidly due to excess NMDA receptor activation, inhibition of Na/Ca exchange may be singularly damaging (Andreeva et al., 1991). The large sodium current associated with NMDA receptor activation only further short-circuits the neuronal sodium gradient and magnifies the effects of the NMDA calcium current (Kiedrowski et al., 1994).

Breakdown of the sodium gradient is essentially due to a large net influx of sodium ions from the extracellular space. This is a significant osmotic load that results in neuronal swelling which can cause, at the least, significant mechanical disturbance of cellular machinery and, at the worst, neuronal rupture.

In addition, ATP depletion will affect any energy-dependent neuronal process such as axonal transport, neurotransmitter uptake, release and reuptake, and ATP dependent calcium sequestration into ER. Furthermore, countless kinase-phosphatase reactions will be deranged, throwing the entire neuronal enzymatic machinery into disarray.

Since all mitochondrial functions are so intimately interrelated, it is difficult experimentally to separate individual mitochondrial functions to explore their specific contribution to cell survival and death. Be that as it may, strategies

that support neuronal ATP production have been shown to limit neuronal death in certain models. Support of brain ATP levels by administration of creatine or cyclocreatine produces significant neuroprotection from the damage resulting from multiple types of mitochondrial inhibition (Matthews et al., 1998a; Carter et al., 1995).

From the preceding discussion, it is apparent that ATP depletion leads to far-reaching neuronal effects that may contribute to neuronal necrosis. A central mediator in those pathways is calcium, which has long been thought to be a key mediator of necrosis. As such, overwhelming both mitochondrial energy production and calcium buffering may have a synergistic effect to damage neuronal calcium homeostasis resulting in accelerated neuronal death.

Mitochondria are important for buffering both physiologic and toxic calcium loads, and mitochondrial ETC dysfunction decreases mitochondrial calcium uptake capability by decreasing $\Delta\psi$ (Gunter & Gunter, 2001). This system has a high capacity for calcium uptake that is not easily exceeded, but calcium entering through NMDA receptors may have privileged access to mitochondria potentially resulting in impaired calcium homeostasis even with intact neuronal mitochondria (Peng & Greenamyre, 1998; Tymianski et al., 1993). Not only might this produce elevation in cytosolic calcium, but calcium-induced activation of the mtPTP (Pfeiffer et al., 2001). This may cause further rise in cytosolic calcium, and further impairment of mitochondrial function. In addition to nonspecific protease activation, calcium overload can induce ROS production via the arachadonic acid and nitric oxide pathways (Gunasekar et al., 1995).

Mitochondrial ROS production may also feed into this spiral toward neuronal necrosis. The most intuitive mechanism for this is non-specific oxidative damage to neuronal components, including nucleic acids, protein, and lipids. This damage can be additive or synergistic with that caused by destructive nonspecific enzyme activation associated with calcium overload.

In addition, since mitochondrial enzymes are ripe targets for ROS-induced damage, production of ROS may lead to further impairment of mitochondrial function (Flint et al., 1993; Yan et al., 1997; Zhang et al., 1990). This leads to ATP depletion, poor calcium handling, and yet more free radical production.

A free radical spin trap (N-tert-butyl-α-(2-sulfophenyl)-nitrone) has been shown to attenuate metabolic inhibitor-induced neurotoxicity without affecting ATP levels (Schulz et al., 1995). Free radical scavengers are also effective neuroprotectants in models of ischemic neuronal death, which is typically necrotic in the acute period (Yue et al., 1992;

Cao & Phillis, 1994). Additional evidence for the involvement of free radicals in the neurotoxicity induced by metabolic inhibition is the finding that 3-NP toxicity is attenuated in mice transgenic for human copper/zinc superoxide dismutase (Beal et al., 1995). Finally, antioxidants such as ubiquinone and lipoic acid derivatives are protective against acute mitochondrial inhibition in vivo (Matthews et al., 1998a; Greenamyre et al., 1994).

Mitochondrial and cell death: apoptosis

Because the neurodegeneration seen in human disease and animal models thereof typically does not fit cleanly into either the necrosis or apoptosis category, the separation of this discussion is somewhat artificial. However, there are some differences between massive mitochondrial dysfunction leading to nonspecific necrosis and more subtle abnormalities that may result in death that is more toward the apoptosis side of the continuum.

Apoptosis, as opposed to necrosis, is an active process. To a certain extent, this process is dependent on intracellular ATP levels, and it has been proposed that whether a cell undergoes necrosis or apoptosis depends on the intracellular ATP concentration (Ankarcrona et al., 1995; Leist et al., 1997; Volbracht et al., 1999). As such, in order for a neuron to undergo apoptosis, mitochondria must be at least partly, if not fully, functional. As mentioned earlier, partial mitochondrial inhibition may have dramatic effects on certain aspects of mitochondrial function with minimal effects on respiration (Davey et al., 1998). It follows that, while severe mitochondrial impairment may result in necrosis, more subtle defects may cause apoptosis.

The cell biology of apoptotic pathways is complicated, interrelated, and incompletely understood, but mitochondria are now recognized to be central mediators of apoptosis (Kroemer & Reed, 2000; Ravagnan et al., 2002). The majority of apoptotic pathways depend on release of mitochondrial intermembrane proteins that activate effectors of apoptotic cascades. Mitochondrial proteins described to be regulators of apoptosis include cytochrome c, AIF (apoptosis inducing factor), endonuclease G, Smac (second mitochondrial activator of caspases), DIABLO (direct IAp binding protein with low pI), HtrA2/Omi, and procaspases 2, 3, and 9 (Liu et al., 1996; Ravagnan et al., 2002).

A family of Bcl-2-like proteins modulates release of intermembrane proteins. This protein family includes both promoters (Bax, Bak, Bcl-x-s, Bad, Bim, Bid) and preemptors (Bcl-2, Bcl-x-l, Bcl-w) of apoptosis (Ravagnan et al., 2002).

Release of intermembrane space proteins is dependent on pore formation in the mitochondrial membrane. Two possible mechanisms have been described. The first involves oligomerization of Bax or Bak or formation of a Bax–VDAC complex that spans the inner and outer mitochondrial membrane (Antonsson et al., 2001). Antiapoptotic Bcl-2-like proteins may prevent formation of this pore by heterodimerization with Bax or Bak (Shimizu et al., 1999; Vander Heiden et al., 1999).

The second possible mechanism revolves around the mtPTP (Fig. 3.1). As discussed above, the mtPTP mediates the mitochondrial permeability transition, which may cause outer membrane rupture followed by release of intermembrane space proteins. As such, any stimulus that facilitates mtPTP opening (high ADP/ATP ratio, mitochondrial calcium, mitochondrial ROS) may cause induction of the apoptotic cascade. Binding of cyclophilin D to the ANT can also facilitate pore opening (Crompton et al., 1998; Woodfield et al., 1998). As further evidence of the interconnected nature of these pathways, it has recently been described that Bax translocation to mitochondria increases mitochondrial ROS production and that blocking ROS production prevents cell death (Kirkland et al., 2002, Narita et al., 1998).

The cellular signals that result in mitochondrial protein release are varied. Withdrawal of growth factors, UV damage, free radical production, and cytokine signals may all cause induction of p53, a key cell cycle regulator (Vogelstein et al., 2000). p53 can activate Bax and caspase 8 (Ding & Fisher, 1998). It can also activate a protein called PIG3, which, similar to Bax, can stimulate mitochondrial ROS production (Polyak et al., 1997).

Other cellular signals, including cytoskeletal disruption, TNF receptor activation, or elevated intracellular calcium may cause translocation of proapoptotic Bcl-2-like proteins to the mitochondria and facilitate protein release (Hengartner, 2000; Luo et al., 1998; Puthalakath et al., 1999).

In addition, anything that induces the mtPTP may result in release of mitochondrial proteins and activation of apoptotic cascades. This would include dysfunction of respiration and mitochondrial calcium overload, as well as mitochondrial inhibition and ROS production.

Mitochondrial protein release causes downstream activation of multiple apoptotic effecter molecules. Cytochrome c and procaspase 9 released from the intermembrane space combine with the cytosolic protein APAF-1 to form a complex termed the apoptosome (Ravagnan et al., 2002). Formation of the apoptosome results in activation of caspase 9 which cleaves procaspase 3 to activate caspase 3. Caspase 3 has been shown to be an important effecter of apoptosis and acts via CADNase (caspase-activated DNase) and ACINUS (apoptotic chromatin condensation inducer in the nucleus) to provoke chromatin condensation and DNA fragmentation (Hengartner, 2000; Ravagnan et al., 2002).

Smac/DIABLO, when released from the intermembrane space, bind to and inhibit several inhibitors of apoptosis proteins (IAPs) in the cytosol, including XIAP and cIAP1 and 2, thus promoting apoptosis (Du et al., 2000; Ekert et al., 2001). HtrA2/Omi also inhibits IAPs, and it further enhances apoptosis independent of its IAP inhibition through its serine protease activity (Verhagen et al., 2002).

AIF and Endonuclease G act in a caspase-independent manner to cleave nuclear DNA into high molecular weight fragments following mitochondrial release (Li et al., 2001; Zamzami et al., 1996).

There are many other proposed enzymatic pathways that contribute to the apoptotic cascade. The majority of them depend in some way on mitochondrial protein release for initiation or continuation. As such, functioning and malfunctioning mitochondria play a central role in cellular death by apoptotic mechanisms.

Mitochondrial inhibition and neurodegeneration

The previous sections have reviewed mitochondrial biology and the ways in which perturbation of this biology may cause neuronal death. The question as to whether or not mitochondria are involved in the pathogenesis and pathophysiology of human neurodegenerative disease has received extensive attention for more than a decade (Fiskum et al., 1999). It has now been convincingly described that there is impaired mitochondrial function in many neurodegenerative diseases not traditionally thought to be mitochondrial in nature (Orth & Schapira, 2001). Further exploration of the consequences of this decrease in ETC activity has involved extensive use of mitochondrial inhibitors in vitro and in vivo.

For example, decreased complex I activity has been described in substantia nigra and platelets from Parkinson's disease patients (Schapira et al., 1989, 1990; Parker et al., 1989). Cybrid cell lines made from Parkinson's disease mitochondria exhibit complex I deficiency, impaired calcium homeostasis, and increased ROS (Swerdlow et al., 1998; Sheehan et al., 1997b). The finding that led to investigation of complex I activity in Parkinson's disease patients was the discovery that MPP+, the active metabolite of MPTP, inhibits complex I (Nicklas et al., 1985; Ramsay et al., 1991).

Since MPP+ is taken up selectively into dopaminergic neurons, it is a poor model for a diffuse complex I defect.

Rotenone is a hydrophobic compound, used sometimes as a pesticide, which produces a generalized complex I inhibition when administered to rodents. This compound has been shown to mimic many of the behavioral and pathological hallmarks of Parkinson's disease, including symptomatic Parkinsonism, specific dopaminergic neuronal degeneration, protein aggregation, oxidative protein damage, and microglial activation. These effects occur in the presence of a rotenone concentration that produces complex I inhibition with minimal effect on mitochondrial respiration (Betarbet et al., 2000).

Rotenone has been shown to markedly enhance H_2O_2 production (Hensley et al., 1998). In addition, rotenone in vitro depletes neuronal glutathione, causes oxidative damage to protein and DNA, stimulates mitochondrial release of cytochrome c, and activates caspase 3 (Sherer et al., 2002). These data suggest that inhibition at complex I produces a behavioral and neuropathological model of Parkinson's disease and that mitochondrial dysfunction at complex I may play a significant role in the pathophysiology of Parkinson's disease.

In Huntington's disease, PET scanning has revealed decreased glucose utilization in cerebral cortex and basal ganglia in Huntington's disease patients and also in at-risk individuals (Mazziotta et al., 1987; Kuhl et al., 1982). In vivo magnetic resonance spectroscopy has revealed increased lactate in Huntington's disease basal ganglia and cortex, suggesting a shift toward anaerobic metabolism, and thus an oxidative defect (Jenkins et al., 1998). Several specific enzyme defects have been reported in Huntington's disease, including in complexes II, III, and IV (Beal, 1998 for review see). In addition, Huntington's disease mitochondria are less polarized (lower $\Delta\psi$) and handle calcium loads less efficiently than controls; it appears that this is a direct effect of polyglutaminated mutant huntingtin on the mitochondrion. This mitochondrial deficiency was observed in transgenic animals prior to clinical evidence for disease (Panov et al., 2002).

Local or systemic administration of complex II inhibitors (malonate or 3-NP) produces a behavioural and neuropathological syndrome similar to Huntington's disease in rodents and nonhuman primates. Hallmarks include chorea and bradykinesia, weight loss, specific degeneration of striatal projection neurons, sparing of striatal interneurons, and oxidative damage (Beal et al., 1993; Brouillet et al., 1995). Neurodegeneration is associated with perturbation of multiple mitochondrial functions, and it is prevented by manipulation of these functions, including support of neuronal ATP levels and free radical trapping (Matthews et al., 1998a,b; Schulz et al., 1995). Downstream modulation of effectors of neuronal death, such as membrane hyperpolarization or inhibition of the NMDA receptor is also an effective neuroprotective strategy (Greene & Greenamyre, 1995, 1996). Deficiency of MnSOD enhances and overexpression of Bcl-2 attenuates neurodegeneration seen in these models, consistent with an apoptotic process (Andreassen *et al.*, 2001; Bogdanov *et al.*, 1996). These data show that mitochondrial inhibition at complex II can replicate Huntington's disease pathology in animal models and suggest that mitochondrial dysfunction at complex II may play a significant role in the pathophysiology of Huntington's disease.

In Alzheimer's disease, several studies have revealed evidence of various energetic defects in autopsy and post-mortem tissue (Beal, 1998, for review). Experiments using cybrid cells constructed with Alzheimer's disease mitochondria have revealed complex IV defects, abnormal calcium homeostasis, and increased production of ROS, although the existence of a specific mitochondrial deficit in Alzheimer's disease is controversial (Swerdlow *et al.*, 1997; Sheehan *et al.*, 1997a).

Inhibition of complex IV in model systems by cyanide or azide also produces neuropathological sequelae, although this has been more extensively studied in vitro than in vivo. Complex IV inhibition has been shown to produce excitotoxic lesions in vivo and administration of complex IV inhibitors also produces deficits in learning and spatial memory (Bennett *et al.*, 1996; Brouillet *et al.*, 1994).

Azide and cyanide have also been used to replicate the mitochondrial dysfunction that occurs during hypoxic-ischemic events since the lack of oxygen occurring during these events represents *de facto* complex IV inhibition. Generalization from the acute neurodegeneration produced by hypoxia-ischemia to the chronic neuronal death seen in neurodegenerative disease is fraught with complication, but many of the mitochondrial mechanisms discussed above may be active (see Wieloch, 2001, for review).

Concluding remarks

Mitochondria are central neuronal organelles that play a vital role in neuronal life and death. Both mitochondrial dysfunction and proper function are essential components in neurodegeneration. Further elucidation of the mechanisms of interaction between mitochondria and neuronal death will allow better description of the pathogenesis of neurodegenerative diseases and provide potential targets for therapeutic intervention.

REFERENCES

Alston, T. A., Mela, L. & Bright, H. J. (1977). 3-nitropropionate, the toxic substance of Indigofera, is a suicide inactivator of succinate dehydrogenase. *Proc. Natl Acad. Sci., USA*, **74**, 3767–71.

Andreassen, O. A., Ferrante, R. J. & Dedeoglu, A. (2001). Mice with a partial deficiency of manganese superoxide dismutase show increased vulnerability to the mitochondrial toxins malonate, 3-nitropropionic acid, and MPTP. *Exp. Neurol.*, **167**, 189–95.

Andreeva, N., Khodorov, B., Stelmashook, E. *et al.* (1991). Inhibition of Na/Ca exchange enhances delayed neuronal deathelicited by glutamate in cerebellar granule cell cultures. *Brain Res.*, **548**, 322–5.

Ankarcrona, M., Dypbukt, J. M., Bonfoco, E. *et al.* (1995). Glutamate-induced neuronal death: a succession of necrosis or apoptosis depending on mitochondrial function. *Neuron*, **15**, 961–73.

Antonsson, B., Montessuit, S., Sanchez, B. & Martinou, J. C. (2001). Bax is present as a high molecular weight oligomer/complex in the mitochondrial membrane of apoptotic cells. *J. Biol. Chem.*, **276**, 11615–23.

Astrup, J., Sorensen, P. M. & Sorensen, H. R. (1981). Oxygen and glucose consumption related to Na-K transport in canine brain. *Stroke*, **12**, 726–30.

Beal, M. F. (1998). Mitochondrial dysfunction in neurodegenerative diseases. *Biochim. Biophys. Acta*, **1366**, 211–23.

Beal, M. F., Ferrante, R. J., Henshaw, R. *et al.* (1993). Neurochemical and histologic characterization of striatal excitotoxic lesions produced by the mitochondrial toxin 3-nitropropionic acid. *J. Neurosci.*, **13**, 4181–92.

Beal, M. F., Ferrante, R. J., Henshaw, R. *et al.* (1995). 3-Nitropropionic acid neurotoxicity is attenuated in copper/zinc superoxide dismutase transgenic mice. *J. Neurochem.*, **65**, 919–22.

Bennett, M. C., Mlady, G. W., Fleshner, M. & Rose, G. M. (1996). Synergy between chronic corticosterone and sodium azide treatments in producing a spatial learning deficit and inhibiting cytochrome oxidase activity. *Proc. Natl Acad, Sci., USA*, **93**, 1330–4.

Bernardi, P., Broekemeier, K. M. & Pfeiffer, D. R. (1994). Recent progress on regulation of the mitochondrial permeability transition pore: a cyclosperin-sensitive pore in the inner mitochondrial membrane. *J. Bioenerg. Biomembr.*, **26**, 509–17.

Betarbet, R., Sherer, T. B., Mackenzie, G., Garcia-Osuna, M., Panov, A. V. & Greenamyre, J. T. (2000). Chronic systemic pesticide exposure reproduces features of Parkinson's disease. *Nat. Neurosc.*, **3**, 1301–6.

Blaustein, M. P. (1988). Calcium transport and buffering in neurons. *Trends Neurosci.*, **10**, 438–43.

Bogdanov, M. B., Ferrante, R. J., Mueller, G., Ramos, L. E., Martinou, J. C. & Beal, M. F. (1999). Oxidative stress is attenuated in mice overexpressing BCL-2. *Neurosci. Lett.*, **262**, 33–6.

Boveris, A. & Turrens, J. F. (1980). Production of superoxide anion by the NADH-dehydrogenase of mammalian mitochondria. In *Aspects in Superoxide and Superoxide Dismutase.*

Developments in Biochemistry, ed. J. V. Bannister and H. A. O. Hill, Vol. 11A, pp. 84–91. New York: Elsevier-North Holland.

Boveris, A., Oshino, N. & Chance, B. (1972). The cellular production of hydrogen peroxide. *Biochem. J.*, **128**, 617–30.

Brouillet, E., Hyman, B. T., Jenkins, B. G. *et al.* (1994). Systemic or local administration of azide produces striatal lesions by an energy impairment-induced excitotoxic mechanism. *Exp. Neurol.*, **129**, 175–82.

Brouillet, E., Hantraye, P., Ferrante, R. J. *et al.* (1995). Chronic mitochondrial energy impairment produces selective striatal degeneration and abnormal choreiform movements in primates. *Proc. Natl Acad. Sci., USA*, **92**, 7105–9.

Cao, X. & Phillis, J. W. (1994). Alpha-phenyl-test-butyl nitrone reduces cortical infarct and edema in rats subjected to focal ischemia. *Brain Res.*, **644**, 267–72.

Carter, A. J., Muller, R. E., Pschorn, U. & Stransky, W. (1995). Preincubation with creatine enhances levels of creatine phosphate and prevents anoxic damage in rat hippocampal slices. *J. Neurochem.*, **64**, 2691–9.

Cousin, M. A., Nicholls, D. G. & Pocock, J. M. (1995). Modulation of ion gradients and glutamate release in cultured cerebellar granule cells by ouabain. *J. Neurochem.*, **64**, 2097–104.

Crompton, M. (1999). The mitochondrial permeability transition pore and its role in cell death. *Biochem. J.*, **341**, 233–49.

Crompton, M., Virji, S. & Ward, J. M. (1998). Cyclophilin-D binds strongly to complexes of the voltage-dependent anion channel and the adenine nucleotide translocase to form the permeability transition pore. *Eur. J. Biochem.*, **258**, 729–35.

Davey, G. P., Peuchen, S. & Clark, J. B. (1998). Energy thresholds in brain mitochondria. Potential involvement in neurodegeneration. *J. Biol. Chem.*, **273**, 12753–7.

Ding, H. F. & Fisher, D. E. (1998). Mechanisms of p53-mediated apoptosis. *Crit. Rev. Oncol.*, **9**, 83–98.

Du, C., Fang, M., Li, Y. & Wang, X. (2000). Smac, a mitochondrial protein that promotes cytochrome c-dependent caspase activation by eliminating IAP inhibition. *Cell*, **102**, 33–42.

Ekert, P. G., Silke, J., Hawkins, C. J., Verhagen, A. M. & Vaux, D. L. (2001). DIABLO promotes apoptosis by removing MIHA/XIAP from processed caspase 9. *J. Cell Biol.*, **152**, 483–90.

Erecinska, M. & Dagani, F. (1990) Relationships between the neuronal sodium/potassium pump and energy metabolism. *J. Gen. Physiol.*, **95**, 591–616.

Fiskum, G., Murphy, A. N. & Beal, M. F. (1999). Mitochondria in neurodegeneration: acute ischemia and chronic neurodegenerative diseases. *J. Cereb. Blood Flow Metab.*, **19**, 351–69.

Flint, D. H., Tuminello, J. F. & Emptage, M. H. (1993). The inactivation of Fe-S cluster containing hydro-lases by superoxide. *J. Biol. Chem.*, **268**, 22369–76.

Fridovitch, I. (1995). Superoxide radical and superoxide dismutases. *Ann. Rev. Biochem.*, **64**, 97–112.

Greenamyre, J. T., Garcia-Osuna, M. & Greene, J. G. (1994). The endogenous cofactors, thioctic acid and dihydrolipoic acid, are neuroprotective against NMDA and malonic acid lesions of striatum. *Neurosci. Lett.*, **171**, 17–20.

Greene, J. G. & Greenamyre, J. T. (1995). Characterization of the excitotoxic potential of the reversible succinate dehydrogenase inhibitor malonate. *J. Neurochem.*, **64**, 430–6.

(1996). Manipulation of membrane potential modulates malonate-induced striatal excitotoxicity. *J. Neurochem.*, **66**, 637–43.

Greene, J. G., Sheu, S. S., Gross, R. A. & Greenamyre, J. T. (1998). 3-nitropropionic acid exacerbates N-methyl-D-aspartate toxicity in striatal culture by multiple mechanisms. *Neuroscience*, **84**, 503–10.

Gunasekar, P. G., Kanthasamy, A. G., Borowitz, J. L. & Isom, G. (1995). NMDA receptor activation produces concurrent generation of nitric oxide and reactive oxygen species: implication for cell death. *J. Neurochem.*, **65**, 2016–21.

Gunter, T. E. & Gunter, K. K. (2001). Uptake of calcium by mitochondria: transport and possible function. *IUBMB Life*, **52**, 197–204.

Gunter, T. E., Gunter, K. K., Sheu, S.-S. & Gavin, C. E. (1994). Mitochondrial calcium transport. *Am. J. Physiol.*, **267**, C313–39.

Hengartner, M. O. (2000). The biochemistry of apoptosis. *Nature*, **407**, 770–6.

Hensley, K., Pye, Q. N., Maidt, M. *et al.* (1998). Interaction of alpha-phenyl-N-tert-butyl nitrone and alternative electron acceptors with complex I indicates a substrate reduction site upstream from the rotenone binding site. *J. Neurochem.*, **71**, 2549–57.

Hochster R. M. & Quastel J. H., eds. (1963). *Metabolic Inhibitors: A Comprehensive Treatise*. New York: Academic Press.

Ichas, F., Jouaville, L. S. & Mazat, J. P. (1997). Mitochondria are excitable organelles capable of generating and conveying electrical and calcium signals. *Cell*, **89**, 1145–53.

Jenkins, B. G., Rosas, H. D., Chen, Y. C. *et al.* (1998). 1H NMR spectroscopy studies of Huntington's disease: correlations with CAG repeat numbers. *Neurology*, **50**, 1357–65.

Kauppinen, R. A., Sihra, T. S. & Nicholls, D. G. (1987). Aminooxy-acetic acid inhibits the malate–aspartate shuttle in isolated nerve terminals and prevents the mitochondria from using glycolytic substrates. *Biochim. Biophys. Acta*, **930**, 173–8.

Kerr, J. F., Wyllie, A. H. & Currie, A. R. (1972). Apoptosis: a basic biological phenomenon with wide ranging implications in tissue kinetics. *Br. J. Cancer*, **26**, 239–47.

Kiedrowski, L. & Costa, E. (1995). Glutamate-induced destabilization of intracellular calcium concentration homeostasis in cultured cerebellar granul cells: role of mitochondria in calcium buffering. *Mol. Pharmacol.*, **53**, 974–80.

Kiedrowski, L., Brooker, G., Costa, E. & Wroblewski, J. T. (1994). Glutamate impairs neuronal calcium extrusion while reducing sodium gradient. *Neuron*, **12**, 295–300.

Kirkland, R. A., Windelborn, J. A., Kasprzak, J. M. & Franklin, J. L. (2002). A Bax-induced pro-oxidant state is critical for cytochrome c release during programmed neuronal death. *J. Neurosci.*, **22**, 6480–90.

Koch, R. A. & Barrish, M. E. (1994). Perturbation of intracellular calcium and hydrogen ion regulation in cultured mouse hippocamp-al neurons by reduction of the sodium ion concentration gradient. *J. Neurosci.*, **14**, 2585–93.

Kroemer, G. & Reed, J. C. (2000). Mitochondrial control of cell death. *Nat. Med.* **6**, 513–19.

Kuhl, D. E., Phelps, M. E., Markham, C. H., Metter, J., Riege, W. H. & Winter, J. (1982). Cerebral metabolism and atrophy in Huntington's disease determined by [18]FDG and computed tomographic scan. *Ann. Neurol.*, **12**, 425–34.

Leist, M., Single, B., Castoldi, A. F., Kuhnle, S. & Nicotera, P. (1997). Intracellular ATP concentration: a switch between apoptosis and necrosis. *J. Exp. Med.*, **185**, 1481–6.

Li, L. Y., Luo, X. & Wang, X. (2001). Endonuclease G is an apoptotic DNase when released from mitochondria. *Nature*, **412**, 95–9.

Liu, X., Kim, C. N., Yang, J., Jemmerson, R. & Wang, X. (1996). Induction of apoptotic program in cell-free extracts: requirement for dATP and cytochrome c. *Cell*, **86**, 147–57.

Loschen, G., Azzi, A., Richter, C. *et al.* (1974). Superoxide radicals as precursors of mitochondrial hydrogen peroxide. *FEBS Lett.*, **42**, 68–72.

Luo, X., Budihardjo, I., Zou, H., Slaughter, C. & Wang, X. (1998). Bid, a Bcl2 interacting protein, mediates cytochrome c release from mitochondria in response to activation of cell surface death receptors. *Cell*, **94**, 481–90.

Mata, M., Fink, D. J., Gainer, H. *et al.* (1980). Activity-dependent energy metabolism in rat posterior pituitary primarily reflects sodium pump activity. *J. Neurochem.*, **34**, 213–15.

Matthews, R. T., Yang, L., Browne, S., Baik, M. & Beal, M. F. (1998a). Coenzyme Q10 administration increases brain mitochondrial ATP concentrations and exerts neuroprotective effects. *Proc. Natl Acad. Sci., USA*, **95**, 8892–7.

Matthews, R. T., Yang, L., Jenkins, B. G. *et al.* (1998b). Neuroprotective effects of creatine and cyclocreatine in animal models of Huntington's disease. *J. Neurosci.*, **18**, 156–63.

Mazziotta, J. C., Phelps, M. E. & Pahl, J. I. (1987). Reduced cerebral glucose metabolism in asymptomatic subjects at risk for Huntington's disease. *N. Engl. J. Med.*, **316**, 356–62.

Murphy, A. N., Fiskum, G. & Beal, M. F. (1999). Mitochondria in neurodegeneration: bioenergetic function in cell life and death. *J. Cereb. Blood Flow Metab.*, **19**, 231–45.

Narita, M., Shimizu, S., Ito, T. *et al.* (1998). Bax interacts with the permeability transition pore to induce permeability transition and cytochrome c release in isolated mitochondria. *Proc. Natl Acad. Sci., USA*, **95**, 14681–6.

Nicklas, W. J., Vyas, I. & Heikkila, R. E. (1985). Inhibition of NADH-linked oxidation in brain mitochondria by 1-methyl-4-phenyl-pyridine, a metabolite of the neurotoxin, 1-methyl-4-phenyl-1,2,3,6-tetrahydropyridine. *Life Sci.*, **36**, 2503–8.

Orth, M. & Schapira, A. H. V. (2001). Mitochondria and degenerative disorders. *Am. J. Med. Genet. (Semin. Med. Genet.)*, **106**, 27–36.

Panov, A. V., Gutekunst, C-A., Leavitt, B. R. *et al.* (2002). Early mitochondrial calcium defects in Huntington's disease are a direct effect of polyglutamines. *Nat. Neurosci.*, **5**, 731–6.

Parker, W. D., Boyson, S. J. & Parks, J. K. (1989). Abnormalities of the electron transport chain in idiopathic Parkinson's disease. *Ann. Neurol.*, **26**, 719–23.

Peng, T. I. & Greenamyre, J. T. (1998). Privileged access to mitochondria of calcium influx through *N*-methyl-D-aspartate receptors. *Mol. Pharmacol.*, **53**, 974–80.

Pfeiffer, D. R., Gunter, T. E., Eliseev, R. *et al.* (2001). Release of Ca^{2+} from mitochondria via the saturable mechanisms and the permeability transition. *IUBMB Life*, **52**, 205–12.

Polyak, K., Xin, Y., Zweier, J. L., Kinzler, K. W. & Vogelstein, B. (1997). A model for p53-induced apoptosis. *Nature*, **289**, 300–4.

Pulsinelli, W. A. & Cooper, A. J. L. (1989). Metabolic encephalopathies and coma. In *Basic Neurochemistry*, ed. G. Siegel, B. Agranoff, R. W. Albers & P. Molinoff, pp. 765–81. New York: Raven Press.

Puthalakath, H., Huang, D. C., O'Reilly, L. A., King, S. M. & Strasser, A. (1999). The proapoptotic activity of the Bcl-2 family member Bim is regulated by interaction with the dynein motor complex. *Mol. Cell*, **3**, 287–96.

Raha, S. & Robinson, B. H. (2001). Mitochondria, oxygen free radicals, and apoptosis. *Am. J. Med. Genet. (Semin. Med. Genet.)*, **106**, 62–70.

Ramsay, R. R., Krueger, M. J. & Youngster, S. K. (1991). Interaction of 1-methyl-4-phenylpyridinium ion (MPP+) and its analogs with the rotenone/piericidin binding site of NADH dehydrogenase. *J. Neurochem.*, **56**, 1184–90.

Ravagnan, L., Roumier, T. & Kroemer, G. (2002). Mitochondria, the killer organells and their weapons. *J. Cell Physiol.*, **192**, 131–7.

Schapira, A. H. V., Cooper, J. M., Dexter, D., Jenner, P., Clark, J. B. & Marsden, C. D. (1989). Mitochondrial complex I deficiency in Parkinson's disease. *Lancet*, **i**, 1269.

Schapira, A. H. V., Mann, V. M. & Cooper, J. M. (1990). Anatomic and disease specificity of NADH CoQ1 reductase (complex I) deficiency in Parkinson's disease. *J. Neurochem.*, **55**, 2142–5.

Schulz, J. B., Henshaw, D. R., Siwek, D. *et al.* (1995) Involvement of free radicals in excitotoxicity in vivo. *J. Neurochem.*, **63**, 2239–47.

Sheehan, J. P., Swerdlow, R. H., Miller, S. W. *et al.* (1997a). Calcium homeostasis and reactive oxygen species production in cells transformed by mitochondria from individuals with sporadic Alzheimer's disease. *J. Neurosci.*, **17**, 4612–22.

Sheehan, J. P., Swerdlow, R. H., Parker, W. D., Miller, S. W., Davis, R. E. & Tuttle, J. B. (1997b). Altered calcium homeostasis in cells transformed by mitochondria from individuals with Parkinson's disease. *J. Neurochem.*, **68**, 1221–33.

Sherer, T. B., Betarbet, R., Stout, A. K. *et al.* (2002). An in vitro model of Parkinson's disease: linking mitochondrial impairment to altered alpha-synuclein metabolism and oxidative damage. *J. Neurosci.*, **22**, 7006–15.

Shimizu, S., Narita, M. & Tsujimoto, Y. (1999). Bcl-2 family proteins regulate the release of apoptogenic cytochrome c by the mitochondrial channel VDAC. *Nature*, **399**, 4833–7.

Slater, E. C. (1973). The mechanism of action of the respiratory inhibitor, antimycin. *Biochem. Biophys. Acta*, **301**, 129–54.

Stryer, L. (1988). In *Biochemistry*, pp. 349–426. New York: W. H. Freeman and Company.

Stout, A. K., Raphael, H. M., Kanterewicz, B. I. *et al.* (1998). Glutamate-induced neuron death requires mitochondrial calcium uptake. *Nat. Neurosci.*, **1**, 366–73.

Swerdlow, R. H., Parks, J. K., Cassarino, D. S. *et al.* (1997). Cybrids in Alzheimer's disease: a cellular model of the disease? *Neurology*, **49**, 918–25.

Swerdlow, R. H., Parks, J. K., Davis, J. N. *et al.* (1998). Matrilineal inheritance of complex I dysfunction I in a multigenerational Parkinson's disease family. *Ann. Neurol.*, **44**, 873–81.

Tymianski, M., Charlton, M. P., Carlen, P. L. & Tator, C. H. (1993). Source specificity of early calcium neurotoxicity in cultured embryonic spinal neurons. *J. Neurosci.*, **13**, 2085–104.

Vander Heiden, M. G., Chandel, N. S., Schumacker, P. T. & Thompson, C. B. (1999). Bcl-xl prevents cell death following growth factor withdrawal by facilitating mitochondrial ATP/ADP exchange. *Mol. Cell*, **3**, 159–67.

Verhagen, A. M., Silke, J., Ekert, P. G. *et al.* (2002). HtrA2 promotes cell death through its serine protease activity and its ability to antagonize inhibitor of apoptosis proteins. *J. Biol. Chem.*, **277**, 445–54.

Volbracht, C., Leist, M. & Nicotera, P. (1999). ATP controls neuronal apoptosis triggered by microtubule breakdown or potassium deprivation. *Mol. Med.* **5**, 477–89.

Vogelstein, B., Lane, D. & Levine, A. J. (2000). Surfing the p53 network. *Nature*, **408**, 307–10.

Wieloch, T. (2001). Mitochondrial involvement in acute neurodegeneration. *IUBMB Life*, **52**, 247–54.

Woodfield, K., Ruck, A., Brdiczka, D. & Halestrap, A. P. (1998). Direct demonstration of a specific interaction between cyclophilin-D and the adenine nucleotide translocase confirms their role in the mitochondrial permeability transition. *Biochem. J.* **336**, 287–90.

Yan, L. J., Levine, R. L. & Sohal, R. S. (1997). Oxidative damage during aging targets mitochondrial aconitase. *Proc. Natl Acad. Sci.*, *USA*, **94**, 11168–72.

Yue, T. L., Gou, J. L., Lysko, P. G., Cheng, H. Y., Barone, F. C. & Feuerstein, G. (1992). Neuroprotective effects of phenyl-t-butyl-nitrone in getbil global brain ischemia and in cultured rat cerebellar neurons. *Brain Res.*, **574**, 193–7.

Zamzami, N., Susin, S. A., Marchetti, P. *et al.* (1996). Mitochondrial control of nuclear apoptosis. *J. Exp. Med.*, **183**, 1661–72.

Zhang, Y., Marcillat, O., Giulivi, C., Ernster, L. & Davies, K. J. (1990). The oxidative inactivation of mitochondrial electron transport chain components and ATPase. *J. Biol. Chem.*, **265**, 16330–6.

4

Excitotoxicity and excitatory amino acid antagonists in chronic neurodegenerative diseases

Chrysanthy Ikonomidou[1] and Lechoslaw Turski[2]

[1]Department of Pediatric Neurology, Carl Gustav Carus University, Dresden, Germany
[2]Solvay Pharmaceuticals Research Laboratories, Weesp, the Netherlands

Introduction

In 1935 Krebs discovered that the amino acid glutamate increases metabolism in the isolated retina and that it is concentrated in the cerebral gray matter (Krebs, 1935). Hayashi (1952, 1958) first reported on excitatory properties of glutamate on neuronal tissue. Local administration of glutamate on the motor cortex of dogs and primates resulted in motor seizures. Curtis *et al.* (1959) subsequently demonstrated that glutamate and aspartate, when applied iontophoretically to the cat spinal cord, depolarized neurons. Since the 1960s there has been appreciation of the role of glutamate in the nervous system, and today it is considered the major excitatory neurotransmitter (Fonnum, 1984). It is essential for learning and memory, synaptic plasticity, neuronal survival and, in early development, for proliferation, migration and differentiation of neuronal progenitors and immature neurons (Guerrini *et al.*, 1995; Ikonomidou *et al.*, 1999; Komuro & Rakic, 1993).

Glutamate fulfils its various functions due to its compartmentalization (Fonnum, 1984). The largest pool of glutamate is the metabolic pool. The neuronal pool is located in nerve endings and represents the neurotransmission pool. A separate pool is located in glia and serves the recycling of transmitter glutamate. The smallest glutamate pool is involved in synthesis of the inhibitory neurotransmitter γ-aminobutyric acid (GABA). Glutamate is released from presynaptic terminals by a calcium-dependent mechanism, is removed subsequently by uptake into the surrounding glial cells and aminated to glutamine.

When released into the synaptic cleft, glutamate acts at the postsynaptic site on receptors (Hollmann & Heinemann, 1994; Nakanishi, 1992). These include the *N*-methyl-D-aspartate (NMDA), kainate, the α-amino-3-hydroxy-5-methylisoxazole-propionate (AMPA) and the metabotropic receptors. The first three are coupled to ion channels and are therefore called ionotropic glutamate receptors. Metabotropic glutamate receptors mediate their actions through G-proteins.

Receptor subtypes for both ionotropic and metabotropic glutamate receptors have been cloned and characterized (Hollmann & Heinemann, 1994).

Antagonists to these receptors were synthesized, enabling studies of the physiology of glutamate and opening perspectives pertaining to potential therapeutic applications of such compounds in human neurologic diseases.

NMDA receptors

NMDA receptors represent tetrameric heteromeric subunit assemblies whose physiological and pharmacological properties depend upon their subunit composition. Two major subunit families, NR1 and NR2 (A–D) have been cloned (Burnashev *et al.*, 1992; Monyer *et al.*, 1992). Recently NR3A and NR3B receptor subunits were characterized (Anderson *et al.*, 2001; Chatterton *et al.*, 2002; Das *et al.*, 1998; Matsuda *et al.*, 2002). Most NMDA receptors in the CNS are formed from NR1 and NR2 subunits. Alternative splicing results in 8 isoforms of NR1. The NR2 subunit family consists of four individual subunits termed NR2A–D (Hollmann & Heinemann, 1994; Monyer *et al.*, 1991; 1994). Different NR2 subunits result in different Ca^{2+}-permeability of the NMDA receptor channel, different gating properties and magnesium sensitivity (Monyer *et al.*, 1991, 1994).

Glycine is a coagonist at NMDA receptors and polyamines positive modulators (McBain and Mayer, 1994; Ozawa *et al.*, 1998). Physiological concentrations of glycine reduce the relatively rapid NMDA receptor desensitization. Another coagonist at NMDA receptors is D-serine.

Glycine shows different affinities at NMDA receptor sub-types. This affinity depends on the NR1 isoform and also the NR2 subunit composition of the receptor complex which allosterically influences the glycine recognition site located on the NR1 subunit (Monyer *et al.*, 1992; Woodward *et al.*, 1995).

Non-NMDA ionotropic glutamate receptors

AMPA receptors are composed of four subunits, GluR1–GluR4 (GluRA–GluRD). They are widely distributed throughout the mammalian central nervous system and mediate fast glutamatergic neurotransmission. The type of subunits within a tetrameric assembly determines biophysical and pharmacological profile of AMPA receptors. Two splice variants for GluR subunits have been described, *flip* and *flop*; these differ in their expression between brain regions and developmental stages. Other non-NMDA receptor subunits are designated GluR5, GluR6, GluR7, KA1 and KA2, and these form high affinity kainate receptors (Herb *et al.*, 1992, 1996; Hollmann & Heinemann, 1994).

The GluR2 subunit determines Ca^{2+} permeability of AMPA receptor channels. Receptors containing the GluR2 subunit show low Ca^{2+} permeability.

Metabotropic glutamate receptors

These are built from eight subunits, mGluR1–8. Within the mGluR-receptor family the sequence identity varies. Classification into three subclasses (I–III) has been proposed (Nakanishi, 1992; Pin & Duvoisin, 1995). Within each class the amino acid sequence identity is 70% and between classes 45%. mGluR1 and mGluR5 belong to Class I, mGluR2 and mGluR3 to class II, mGluR4 and mGluR6–8 to class III. Different transduction mechanisms are activated by each class. Class I activates phospholipase C, increases phosphoinositide turnover and Ca^{2+} release from internal stores and leads to formation of diacylglycerol which then might activate protein kinase C. Class II and III are coupled negatively to adenylate cyclase and reduce the intracellular amount of cAMP. Class II and III differ in their pharmacological profile against specific agonists (Pin & Duvoisin, 1995).

The neurotoxin glutamate

Excitotoxicity, a phenomenon originally discovered in the 1950s and extensively investigated and characterized in the 1970s and 1980s, describes a process in which an excess of the endogenous excitatory amino acid neurotransmitter glutamate causes overstimulation of glutamate receptors and destroys central neurons. Lucas and Newhouse (1957) first described that systemic administration of monosodium glutamate results in degeneration of retinal ganglion cells. Olney and colleagues (Olney, 1969, 1971; Olney & Ho, 1970; Olney *et al.*, 1972) subsequently observed that excitatory amino acids, when given to infant rodents and primates, cause neurodegeneration in brain areas that lack blood–brain barrier. The ability of acidic amino acids to destroy neurons correlates with their excitatory potencies (Olney, 1969, 1971; Olney & Ho, 1970; Olney *et al.*, 1972). This interaction was termed neuroexcitotoxicity. Both ionotropic and metabotropic glutamate receptors can mediate excitotoxicity (McDonald & Schoepp, 1992; Schoepp *et al.*, 1995).

The mechanisms that mediate excitotoxicity have been studied extensively since the 1960s. The acute component of glutamate toxicity is mediated through a massive influx of sodium and chloride ions into the cell (Choi *et al.*, 1987; Rothman, 1985). A second component of glutamate neurotoxicity is Ca^{2+}-dependent and mediated through activation of Ca^{2+}-sensitive proteases. (Choi, 1987; Frandsen & Shousboe, 1991, 1992; Tymianski *et al.*, 1993). Calpains and other proteases that degrade neurofilaments seem to be involved in the late phase of the calcium activated excitotoxic cascade (Bartus *et al.*, 1994; Lee *et al.*, 1991; Manev *et al.*, 1991). Another category of enzymes with potentially self-digesting properties are the phospholipase A2 and other lipases, also activated by elevations of intracellular calcium (Rordorf *et al.*, 1991; Rothman *et al.*, 1993). Agents which inhibit phospholipases can partially attenuate some forms of excitotoxic injury (Rothman *et al.*, 1993). Similarly, endonuclease and protease C inhibitors (Favaron *et al.*, 1990; Samples & Dubinski, 1993) have been shown to inhibit glutamate toxicity in cultures.

Nitric oxide is a potent second messenger implicated in pathogenesis of excitotoxic neuronal death (Dawson *et al.*, 1991). One mechanism that mediates the toxic effect of nitric oxide is the non-enzymatic reaction of nitric oxide with the superoxide anion and the formation of peroxynitrite ($ONOO^-$) (Beckman *et al.*, 1992; Ischiropoulos *et al.*, 1992). Peroxynitrite is a highly reactive molecule, which initiates lipid peroxidation in biologic membranes, hydroxylation and nitration of aromatic amino acid residues and sulfhydryl oxidation of proteins (Radi *et al.*, 1991a, b). These reactions can occur in vivo and are important in excitotoxic neuronal damage (Schulz *et al.*, 1995).

The second mechanism that mediates nitric oxide toxicity is via interaction with numerous cytosolic, mitochondrial and nuclear enzymes. Nitric oxide reacts with non-heme iron and causes inactivation of key mitochondrial enzymes such as mitochondrial aconitase and complex I and II of the mitochondrial electron transport chain

(Nathan, 1992; Pantopoulos & Hentze, 1995). It depletes intracellular glutathione levels (Clancy *et al.*, 1994), deaminates nucleotide bases and damages DNA, decreases intracellular levels of nicotinamide-adenine dinucleotide (NAD) and adenosine triphosphate (ATP) (Zhang *et al.*, 1994). Nitric oxide also inhibits the enzyme glyceraldehyde-3-phosphate dehydrogenase, which plays a key role during glycolysis and in the hexose monophosphate shunt and is involved in synthesis of the oxidized form of nicotinamide-adenine dinucleotide phosphate ($NADP^+$) and maintenance of glutathione levels (Brune & Lapetina, 1989).

Slow onset excitotoxicity

The concept of slow excitotoxicity arose from observations made by Novelli and coworkers showing that inhibitors of oxidative phosphorylation or of the Na^+/K^+ pump allow glutamate or NMDA to become neurotoxic (Novelli *et al.*, 1988). Subsequently, Zeevalk and Nicklas showed that cyanide triggers excitotoxic lesions sensitive to NMDA antagonists in the chick embryo retina (Zeevalk & Nicklas, 1991). Toxicity induced by metabolic inhibition can be mimicked by membrane depolarization with potassium or by relieving the Mg^{2+}-block of the NMDA receptor (Zeevalk & Nicklas, 1991). These observations were extended by findings in in vivo models showing that mitochondrial toxins (aminooxyacetic acid, an inhibitor of the maleate-aspartate shunt; 1-methyl-pyridine, a mitochondrial complex I toxin; 3-nitropropionic acid and malonic acid, inhibitors of mitochondrial complex II; the nicotinamide antagonist 3-acetylpyridine) produce axon sparing, excitotoxic lesions in the mammalian central nervous system, which can be blocked by NMDA and AMPA antagonists, glutamate release inhibitors and prior decortication (Beal *et al.*, 1991a, b; 1993a, b; Greene *et al.*, 1993; Henshaw *et al.*, 1994; McMaster *et al.*, 1991; Schulz *et al.*, 1994; Srivastava *et al.*, 1993; Urbanska *et al.*, 1991; Wüllner *et al.*, 1994). These observations led to the hypothesis that energy impairment at the postsynaptic site of glutamatergic synapse causes membrane depolarization, alleviation of the Mg^{2+}-block of the NMDA receptors and heightened neuronal vulnerability towards physiological concentrations of glutamate (Beal, 1992a; Ikonomidou & Turski, 1996).

Excitotoxicity and neurodegenerative diseases

Morphological changes produced by excitotoxic compounds in the brain and spinal cord in many aspects resemble those observed in the context of chronic neurodegenerative diseases, such as Parkinson's disease, Huntington's disease and amyotrophic lateral sclerosis. Therefore, it has been suggested that excitotoxic mechanisms may mediate these disorders (Beal, 1992b). Especially slow excitotoxicity, triggered by impairment of mitochondrial energy metabolism, has been implicated. It is conceivable that glutamate overactivity caused by exogenous or endogenous factors is an etiological factor for slow progressive death of vulnerable neuronal populations in chronic neurodegenerative diseases or contributes to their natural history and progression. Exogenous or endogenous compounds may activate glutamate receptors, may increase glutamate synthesis, release or reuptake, interfere with glutamate-linked ion channels or enhance glutamate-linked second messenger systems.

Although the genetic basis for some of these diseases has been defined in recent years, the actual mechanism(s) leading to neurodegeneration are still not understood. Slow excitotoxicity may constitute a contributing factor in pathogenesis of neuronal death that could be amenable to pharmacological treatment.

Excitotoxicity and Parkinson's disease

Parkinson's disease, one of the major neurodegenerative disorders of middle and old age, is associated with degeneration of dopaminergic neurons in the ventral mesencephalon. Clinical symptoms consist of tremor, rigidity, bradykinesia, postural deficits and impaired gait.

A gradual decline of dopaminergic neurons of the substantia nigra pars compacta and dopamine content with age is common in the general population. In Parkinson's disease there may be an accelerated rate of cell death, so that a critical level of dopaminergic cell loss (50–70% of neurons) is reached during normal lifespan and neurological symptoms of Parkinson's disease become obvious (Bernheimer *et al.*, 1973; Fearnley & Lees, 1991; McGeer *et al.*, 1989). It is also possible that an exogenous insult, such as an environmental toxin, may cause a partial loss of substantia nigra dopaminergic neurons which will be followed by further "physiological" decline with age (Calne & Langston, 1983). Careful neuropathological studies, serial positron emission tomography (PET) and single photon emission spectroscopy (SPECT) demonstrate a more rapid decline of dopaminergic neurons in the substantia nigra of Parkinson patients as compared to control aging subjects (Brooks, 1998; Fearnley & Lees, 1991; McGeer *et al.*, 1989). Such findings indicate that idiopathic Parkinson's disease is an active disease process in which nigral cell death is accelerated markedly.

The mechanisms by which these neurons degenerate are poorly understood but there is some evidence implicating excitotoxicity as one contributing mechanism to pathogenesis of Parkinson's disease. Initial observations linking excitotoxicity to Parkinson's disease were made by Spencer and colleagues (Spencer, 1987). They reported that the excitatory amino acid α-amino -β-methylaminopropionic acid (BMAA) is linked to Guam ALS-parkinsonism dementia syndrome. This observation became controversial because others found only low levels of BMAA in ingested cycad flour.

MPTP (1-methyl-4-phenyl-1,2,3,6-tetrahydropyridine) and its metabolite MPP$^+$ have been used to model Parkinson's disease, since it was discovered that MPTP can cause Parkinson's disease in man (Davis et al., 1979; Langston et al., 1983). The first report suggesting that excitotoxicity may play a role in the pathogenesis of MPTP-induced Parkinson's disease was made by Turski and colleagues (1991), who demonstrated that neurotoxicity of MPP$^+$, the active metabolite of MPTP, can be blocked in the substantia nigra with both competitive and non-competitive NMDA receptor antagonists. Such results could be reproduced by other groups (Brouillet & Beal, 1993; Chan et al., 1993; Jones-Humble et al., 1994; Santiago et al., 1992; Srivastava et al., 1993). Subsequent studies in primates confirmed that NMDA antagonists attenuated MPTP-induced depletion of substantia nigra dopaminergic neurons (Lange et al., 1993; Zuddas et al., 1992). In support of this hypothesis, both glutamate receptor blockers and neuronal NOS inhibitors have been reported to attenuate degeneration of dopamine neurons in MPTP-treated primates (Blum et al., 2001).

Considerable evidence exists implicating mitochondrial dysfunction in Parkinson's disease. Chronic systemic exposure to the lipophilic pesticide rotenone leads to inhibition of mitochondrial complex I and reproduces features of Parkinson's disease in rats, including accumulation of fibrillar cytoplasmic inclusions that contain ubiquitin and α-synuclein (Betarbet et al., 2000). Studies of the electron transport enzymes have been carried out in lymphocytes, platelets, muscle tissue and postmortem brain tissue from Parkinson's disease patients (DiDonato et al., 1993; Di Monte et al., 1991, 1993; Hattori et al., 1991; Janetzky et al., 1994; Mann et al., 1992; Nakagawa-Hattori et al., 1992; Schapira et al., 1990a, b). Decrease in complex I activity was found in brain, muscle tissue and platelets of Parkinson's disease patients compared to control subjects. Some studies also reported impaired acitivity of complexes II–IV in muscle tissue and complex II in lymphocytes of Parkinson's disease patients. A nuclear magnetic resonance spectroscopy study to measure occipital lobe lactate concentration revealed a highly significant increase of lactate concentrations in Parkinson's disease patients with the largest increases in Parkinson's disease patients with dementia (Bowen et al., 1994). Similar findings indicating increased lactate levels were reported for the striatum of Parkinson's disease patients (Chen et al., 1994; Taylor et al., 1994).

Impaired mitochondrial function may increase vulnerability of affected neurons towards physiological concentrations of glutamate (slow excitotoxicity). Given the fact that the substantia nigra receives rich glutamatergic inputs from neocortex and the subthalamic nucleus, contribution of slow excitotoxicity to the pathogenesis of this disease in the context of energy failure becomes a very attractive hypothesis.

There is evidence indicating that parkinsonian symptoms are caused by glutamatergic overactivity (corticostriatal pathway, subthalamopallidal pathway) (Schmidt & Kretschmer, 1997). Milacemide, a glycine prodrug, which enhances NMDA receptor function, worsens parkinsonian symptoms (Giuffra et al., 1993), whereas NMDA receptor antagonists elicit antiparkinsonian like activity in animal models in rodents and primates (Schmidt & Kretschmer, 1997, Uitti et al., 1996; Ossowska et al., 1994).

Antiparkinsonian activity was observed with the non-competitive NMDA antagonist dextromethorphan (Montastruc et al., 1994) and in initial trials with the glutamate release inhibitor lamotrigine (Zipp et al., 1993), but these findings could not be confirmed in subsequent studies (Montastruc et al., 1997; Zipp et al., 1995). So far, the only compounds with antiglutamatergic properties that are used for the treatment of patients with Parkinson's disease are amantadine, memantine and budipine (Adler et al., 1997; Schwab et al., 1969; Rabey et al., 1992). They are used to ameliorate clinical symptoms but there is no clinical evidence indicating that they influence the course of the disease due to neuroprotective properties. There is only one study by Uitti and coworkers who found that amantadine treatment is an independent predictor of improved survival in Parkinson's disease (Uitti et al., 1996). Studies with remacemide and budipine have demonstrated efficacy of these compounds alone and in combination with dopaminergic agents in relief of parkinsonian symptoms (Greenamyre et al., 1994; Malsch et al., 2001; Parkinson's Study Group, 2000, 2001; Parsons et al., 1998; Przuntek & Muller, 1999; Przuntek et al., 2002; Spieker et al., 1999; Verhagen et al., 1998). It should be noted though, that all NMDA antagonist drugs used in the therapy of Parkinson's disease have pharmacological functions in other neurotransmitter systems as well, thus the conclusion that their antiparkinsonian activities are due to NMDA antagonist properties is not necessarily correct.

There have been reports that the AMPA receptor antagonist NBQX improves symptoms and enhances the effect of L-DOPA in MPTP-treated monkeys (Klockgether et al., 1991; Wachtel et al., 1992) but these findings could not be replicated (Gossel et al., 1995; Luquin et al., 1993; Papa et al., 1993; Zadow & Schmidt, 1994). Owing to such inconsistencies, AMPA receptor antagonists have not made their way into the clinical treatment of Parkinson's disease.

Huntington's disease

Huntington's disease is inherited as an autosomal dominant disease that gives rise to progressive, selective (localized) neural cell death associated with choreic movements and dementia. The disease is associated with increases in the length of a CAG triplet repeat present in a gene called "huntingtin" located on chromosome 4p16.3. The classic signs of Huntington's disease are progressive chorea, rigidity and dementia, frequently associated with seizures. A characteristic atrophy of the caudate nucleus is seen radiographically. There is a prodromal phase of mild psychotic and behavioural symptoms, which precedes frank chorea by up to 10 years.

Initial efforts to model this disease before the genetic defect had been discovered were made by Schwarcz et al., who injected quinolinic acid (an NMDA agonist) into the striatum and produced loss of GABAergic output neurons sparing interneurons containing somatostatin-NPY (Schwarcz & Kohler, 1983; Schwarcz et al., 1983). This neuropathological pattern resembles that seen in Huntington's disease brains (Beal et al., 1986; Schwarcz & Kohler, 1983; Schwarcz et al., 1983). Based on these findings, an excitotoxicity hypothesis for the pathogenesis of Huntington's disease was formulated.

Administration of the mitochondrial toxin 3-NP to rodents produces pathology resembling Huntington's disease (Borlongan et al., 1997; Brouillet et al., 1995; Palfi et al., 1996). Striatal toxicity of 3-NP can be ameliorated by NMDA receptor antagonists, such as memantine (Wenk et al., 1996), and glutamate release inhibitors, such as riluzole (Guyot et al., 1997). Similarly, striatal toxicity of malonate, a complex II–III inhibitor, was prevented by NMDA receptor antagonists MK-801 and memantine and by the glutamate release inhibitor lamotrigine (Greene & Greenamyre, 1995). Thus, it has been postulated that mitochondrial dysfunction in Huntington's patients may be a trigger that constitutes striatal neurons prone to excitotoxicity. This hypothesis is supported by findings from Greenamyre's group, who reported increased apoptosis in Huntington's disease lymphoblasts associated with repeat length-dependent mitochondrial depolarization, which correlated with increased numbers of glutamine repeats (Sawa et al., 1999, Panov et al., 2002).

To gain insight into the pathogenesis of Huntington's disease, Schilling et al. (1999) generated transgenic mice that expressed a cDNA encoding an N-terminal fragment (171 amino acids) of huntingtin with 82, 44, or 18 glutamines. Mice expressing relatively low steady-state levels of N171 huntingtin with 82 glutamine repeats (N171–82Q) developed behavioural abnormalities, including loss of coordination, tremor, hypokinesia, and abnormal gait, before dying prematurely. In mice exhibiting these abnormalities, diffuse nuclear labeling, intranuclear inclusions, and neuritic aggregates, all immunoreactive with an antibody to the N-terminus (17 amino acids) of huntingtin, were found in multiple populations of neurons. None of these behavioural or pathologic phenotypes were seen in mice expressing N171–18Q. The authors considered these findings to be consistent with the idea that N-terminal fragments of huntingtin with a repeat expansion are toxic to neurons, and that N-terminal fragments are prone to form both intranuclear inclusions and neuritic aggregates.

The mechanism through which the widely expressed mutant Huntington's disease gene mediates a slowly progressing striatal neurotoxicity is unknown. Glutamate receptor-mediated excitotoxicity has been hypothesized to contribute to Huntington's disease pathogenesis. However, inconsistent with this hypothesis, Hansson et al. (1999) showed that transgenic Huntington's disease mice expressing exon 1 of the human Huntington's disease gene with an expanded number of CAG repeats are strongly protected from acute striatal excitotoxic lesions. Intrastriatal infusions of quinolinic acid, the agonist of the N-methyl-D-aspartate (NMDA) receptor, caused massive striatal neuronal death in wildtype mice, but no damage in transgenic Huntington's disease littermates. The remarkable neuroprotection in transgenic Huntington's disease mice occurred at the stage when they had not developed any neurologic symptoms caused by the mutant Huntington's disease gene. At this stage, there was no change in the number of striatal neurons and astrocytes in untreated transgenic mice, although the striatal volume was decreased by 17%. Hansson et al. (1999) proposed that the presence of exon 1 of the mutant Huntington's disease gene induces profound changes in striatal neurons that render these cells resistant to excessive NMDA receptor activation.

The antiglutamatergic compound remacemide, tested in a double-blind placebo controlled study in Huntington's disease patients showed only a trend towards symptomatological improvement (Kieburtz et al., 1996). Ketamine failed to show any symptomatological improvement (Murman et al., 1997). Thus, there is so far no evidence that symptomatological improvements should be expected by the use of antiglutamatergic compounds in Huntington's disease patients. Whether antiglutamatergic agents can be used as neuroprotectants remains controversial. As mentioned above, Hansson et al. demonstrated resistance of striatal neurons carrying exon 1 of the mutant Huntington's disease gene to NMDA receptor activation (Hansson et al., 1999). Worrisome are also experimental findings demonstrating that slow neurotoxicity of 3-NP can be enhanced by NMDA antagonists in rats (Ikonomidou et al., 2000).

Glutamate in Alzheimer's disease

Alzheimer's disease is by far the most common cause of dementia. Terry and Davies (1980) pointed out that the presenile form (with onset before age 65) is identical to the most common form of senile dementia. They recommended the term senile dementia of the Alzheimer type (SDAT). Senile (neuritic) plaques and neurofibrillary tangles comprise the major neuropathological lesions in Alzheimer's disease brains. Neuritic plaques are spherical lesions and are found in moderate or large numbers in limbic structures and association neocortex. They contain extracellular deposits of amyloid-β protein. Degenerating axons and dendrites are present within and around the amyloid deposits (Selkoe, 1999; Terry & Davies, 1980).

Neurofibrillary tangles are intraneuronal cytoplasmatic lesions consisting of paired, helically wound, 10 nm filaments. They occur in large numbers in Alzheimer's disease brains in limbic structures and association cortices of the parietal, frontal and temporal lobes. The subunit protein of neurofibrillary tangles is a hyperphosphorylated, insoluble form of the microtubule associated protein, tau. Insoluble tau accumulates in the tangles after conjugation to ubiquitin (Selkoe, 1999).

It has been known for decades that Alzheimer's disease can occur in a familial form that transmits in an autosomal dominant trait. As more and more mutations are identified, the idea that almost all cases of Alzheimer's disease have genetic determinants is being confirmed (Selkoe, 1999). There are, however, also indications that glutamate and the mechanism of excitotoxicity may be involved in pathogenesis and progression of Alzheimer's disease. Constituents of senile plaques stimulate production by microglia of an unknown NMDA agonist (Giulian et al., 1995) as well as production of nitric oxide (NO), known to enhance glutamate release and inhibit its uptake (Goodwin et al., 1995; Lees, 1993). β-Amyloid enhances glutamate toxicity (Brorson et al., 1995; Mattson and Goodman, 1995), enhances depolarization dependent glutamate release (Arias et al., 1995) and inhibits its glial uptake (Harris et al., 1996).

There is decrease in astroglial glutamate EAA2 carrier in the frontal cortex of Alzheimer's disease patients. Colocalization of glutamate neurons and neurofibrillary tangles was reported in Alzheimer's disease brain (Braak et al., 1993; Francis et al., 1992). Finally, intracerebroventricular administration of β-amyloid produced long-lasting depression of EPSP that was prevented by the NMDA antagonist CPP (Cullen et al., 1996), whereas subcutaneous administration of memantine prevented pathological alterations in the hippocampus produced by direct injection of β-amyloid.

Memantine has shown efficacy and has been approved for use in the treatment of dementia in Germany for over 10 years (Jain, 2000; Winblad & Poritis, 1999). Based on successful clinical trials, an application was filed to the EU Commission in 2002 to approve memantine for treatment of moderately-to-severe Alzheimer's disease (Kilpatrick & Tilbrook, 2002).

Another hypothesis describing a link between glutamate and Alzheimer's disease postulates that NMDA receptor hypofunction may be involved mechanistically. There is evidence that the NMDA receptor system becomes hypoactive with advancing age. Olney and colleagues demonstrated repeatedly that NMDA receptor hypofunction in the adult mammalian brain triggers a disinhibition syndrome in which low grade chronic excitotoxic activity (fuelled by acetylcholine and glutamate) causes a widespread pattern of neurodegeneration resembling that seen in Alzheimer's disease. The authors postulate that, in Alzheimer's disease brains, genetic and/or environmental factors may lead to much earlier and more profound NMDA receptor hypoactivity state than in "normal" aging brains, thus increasing the likelihood that widespread neurodegeneration will occur (Farber et al., 1998; Olney et al., 1997; Wozniak et al., 1998).

Amyotrophic lateral sclerosis

Amyotrophic lateral sclerosis (ALS) is the most common motor neuron disease in adults. It is characterized by selective degeneration of upper and lower motor neurons, progressive weakness and paralysis of all muscles and spasticity (Cleveland & Rothstein, 2001). Over 90% of cases occur sporadically, in 5–10% of cases the disease is inherited in a dominant mode (familial ALS).

ALS is a heterogeneous disorder and several pathogenetic mechanisms have been suggested. These include oxidative damage, neurofilament disorganization and subsequent axonal damage, toxicity from intracellular aggregates and excitotoxicity (Cleveland & Rothstein, 2001).

There is unquestionable and landmark evidence, that familial ALS and some forms of sporadic ALS are caused by mutations in the Cu/Zn superoxide dismutase (SOD1) gene (Andersen, 2001; Andersen et al., 2001; Gaudette et al., 2000). More than 90 mutations have been identified so far and almost all provoke a dominantly inherited disease. It appears that changes in activity level of the enzyme are not the key factor for the disease but rather that the mutated enzymes have acquired toxic properties, the nature of which still remains unresolved. The final event, however, has been shown to be activation of caspase 3, leading to active cell death (Li et al., 2000; Pasinelli et al., 2000; Vukosavic et al., 2000). Activation of caspase 3 is preceded by activation of caspase 1 (Pasinelli et al., 2000; Vukosavic et al., 2000).

One hypothesis to explain toxicity of SOD1 mutations is that such mutated forms release copper and allow it to catalyse oxidative reactions (Corson et al., 1998). Another one postulates that Zn-deficient SOD1 mutants facilitate conversion of oxygen to superoxide, which binds to nitric oxide and produces peroxynitrite.

Debate on involvement of excitotoxicity in ALS is based on studies suggesting that the metabolism of glutamate is abnormal in patients with ALS. Rothstein et al. (1992) postulated that the high-affinity glutamate transporter is the site of the defect at least in some forms of the disease. The primary mechanism for the inactivation of glutamate and aspartate is their removal from the extracellular space by a sodium-dependent transport system in astrocytes and neurons. This transport system has both high-affinity and low-affinity carriers for the two molecules. The low-affinity carrier subserves general metabolic activities. The high-affinity carrier is a component of the glutamate neurotransmitter system and is responsible for clearance of the neurotransmitter glutamate from the synaptic cleft. The inhibition of glutamate transport is toxic to neurons, due to persistent elevation of extracellular glutamate. A possible mechanism for the elevated cerebrospinal fluid concentrations of glutamate and aspartate in patients with ALS could be deficient transport into cells. Studying synaptosomes from neural tissue obtained from 13 patients with ALS as well as from controls, Rothstein et al. (1992) found that ALS patients showed a marked diminution in the maximal velocity of transport for high-affinity glutamate uptake in synaptosomes from spinal cord, motor cortex, and somatosensory cortex, but not in those from visual cortex, striatum, or hippocampus. This diminution was the result of a pronounced loss of the astroglial EAAT2 protein (Rothstein et al., 1995). Transport of other molecules (gamma-aminobutyric acid and phenylalanine) was normal in patients with ALS.

Fact is that in about one third of ALS patients glutamate concentrations are increased in the cerebrospinal fluid (Shaw et al., 1995), whereas intracellular glutamate concentrations are decreased (Ludolph et al., 1998; Perry et al., 1987; Young, 1990). Cerebrospinal fluid from ALS patients is toxic to hippocampal neurons via stimulation of AMPA receptors (Couratier et al., 1993). The glutamate release inhibitor riluzole attenuates damage induced by ALS CSF (Couratier et al., 1994; Terro et al., 1996). These findings, along with experimental evidence implicating selective vulnerability of spinal motoneurons to AMPA/kainate-receptor agonists (Hugon et al., 1989; Ikonomidou et al., 1996; Williams et al., 1997), implicate that glutamate, acting on AMPA/kainate receptors may be pathogenetically involved in motor neuron degeneration in ALS.

Excitotoxicity has been implicated in two other neurological disorders that resemble ALS, the Guam ALS-Parkinsonism dementia syndrome and a disease described in the Kii peninsula of Japan. These two disorders have been linked to food excitotoxins (Spencer et al., 1986, 1993).

Along with the finding that SOD1 mutants, when expressed in mice, lead to functional loss of EAAT2 (Nagano et al., 1996), it seems likely that deficient glutamate uptake may contribute to pathogenesis of some forms of ALS.

Several agents have been tested in ALS patients for potential neuroprotective properties, these include brain derived neurotrophic factors (The BDNF Study Group, 1999), ciliary neurotrophic factor (Akbar et al., 1997), insulin like growth factor (Borasio et al., 1998; Lai et al., 1997), various antioxidants, antiinflammatory agents, antibiotics, calcium regulators (Cleveland & Rothstein, 2001) and riluzole. Of all those agents, only riluzole, a glutamate-release inhibitor, achieved a modest effect at increasing survival in two independent trials (Bensimon et al., 1994; Lacomblez et al., 1996) and has been approved for the treatment of ALS, although patients do not experience slowing in disease progression.

Conclusions

There is evidence supporting the notion that excitotoxicity mediated by glutamate constitutes a contributing factor in the pathogenesis of chronic neurodegenerative diseases. Budipine, amantadine and memantine are in use for therapy of parkinsonism. Memantine is effective in therapy of Alzheimer's dementia and riluzole showed some efficacy in ALS. There is, however, evidence indicating that NMDA antagonists can be detrimental for neuronal survival in chronic models of neurodegeneration (Ikonomidou et al., 2000). Riepe et al. developed the paradigm of chemical preconditioning, in which they studied mechanisms of excitotoxicity hours to days after a conditioning excitotoxic stimulus (Riepe *et al.*, 1995, Riepe & Ludolph, 1997; Ludolph *et al.*, 1998). Chemical preconditioning is a neuroprotective strategy, which involves the activation of NMDA receptors (Kasischke *et al.*, 1996). If similar endogenous neuroprotective mechanisms become operant in the context of chronic neurodegenerative diseases, then perhaps blocking NMDA receptors may not be the right therapeutic strategy to pursue, despite the fact that these compounds are protective in acute models of neurodegeneration which we use to study these diseases in rodents and primates. Perhaps targeting non-NMDA receptor mediated excitotoxicity would be the better way to go and could better enable that these devastating diseases become amenable to neuroprotective treatment.

REFERENCES

Adler, C. H., Stern, M. B., Vernon, G. & Hurtig, H. I. (1997). Amantadine in advanced Parkinson's disease: good use of an old drug. *J. Neurol.*, **244**, 336–7.

Akbar, M. T., Torp, R., Danbolt, N. C., Levy, L. M., Meldrum, B. S. & Ottersen, O. P. (1997). Expression of glial glutamate transporters GLT-1 and GLAST is unchanged in the hippocampus in fully kindled rats. *Neuroscience*, **78**, 351–9.

Andersen, P. M. (2001). Genetics of sporadic ALS. *Amyotroph. Lateral Scler. Other Motor Neuron Disord.*, **2**, S37–41.

Andersen, P. M., Morita, M. & Brown, R. H. Jr. (2001). Nucleotide sequence, genomic organization, and chromosomal localization of genes encoding the human NMDA receptor subunits NR3A and NR3B. *Genomics*, **78**, 178–84.

Arias, C., Arrieta, I. & Tapia, R. (1995). beta-Amyloid peptide fragment 25–35 potentiates the calcium-dependent release of excitatory amino acids from depolarized hippocampal slices. *J. Neurosci. Res.*, **41**, 561–6.

Bartus, R. T., Baker, K. L., Heiser, A. D. *et al.* (1994). Postischemic administration of AK275, a calpain inhibitor, provides substantial protection against focal ischemic brain damage. *J. Cereb. Blood Flow Metab.*, **14**, 537–44.

Beal, M. F. (1992a). Does impairment of energy metabolism result in excitotoxic neuronal death in neurodegenerative illnesses? *Ann. Neurol.*, **31**, 119–30.

Beal, M. F. (1992b). Role of excitotoxicity in human neurological disease. *Curr. Opin. Neurol.*, **2**, 657–62.

Beal, M. F., Kowall, N. W., Ellison, D. W., Mazurek, M. F., Swartz, K. J. & Martin, J. B. (1986). Replication of the neurochemical characteristics of Huntington's disease by quinolinic acid. *Nature*, **321**, 168–71.

Beal, M. F., Ferrante, R. J., Swartz, K. J. & Kowall, N. W. (1991a). Chronic quinolinic acid lesions in rats closely resemble Huntington's disease. *J. Neurosci.*, **11**, 1649–59.

Beal, F., Swartz, K. J., Hyman, B. T., Storey, E., Finn, S. F. & Koroshetz, W. (1991b). Aminooxyacetic acid results in excitotoxic lesions by a novel indirect mechanism. *J. Neurochem.*, **57**, 1068–73.

Beal, M. F., Brouillet, E., Jenkins, B., Henshaw, R., Rosen, B. & Hyman, B. T. (1993a). Age-dependent striatal excitotoxic lesions produced by the endogenous mitochondrial inhibitor malonate. *J. Neurochem.*, **61**, 1147–50.

Beal, M. F., Brouillet, E., Jenkins, B. G. *et al.* (1993b). Neurochemical and histologic characterization of striatal excitotoxic lesions produced by the mitochondrial toxin 3- nitropropionic acid. *J. Neurosci.*, **13**, 4181–92.

Beckman, J. S., Ischiropoulos, H., Zhu, L. *et al.* (1992). Kinetics of superoxide-dismutase- and iron-catalyzed nitration of phenolics by peroxynitrite. *Arch. Biochem. Biophys.*, **298**, 438–45.

Bensimon, G., Lacomblez, L., Meininger, V. & The ALS/Riluzole Study Group. (1994). A controlled trial of riluzole in amyotrophic lateral sclerosis. *N. Engl. J. Med.*, **330**, 585–91.

Bernheimer, H., Birkmayer, W., Hornykiewicz, O., Jellinger K. & Seitelberger, F. (1973). Brain dopamine and the syndromes of Parkinson and Huntington. Clinical, morphological and neurochemical correlations. *J. Neurol. Sci.*, **20**, 415–55.

Betarbet, R., Sherer, T. B., MacKenzie, G., Garcia-Osuna, M., Panov, A. V. & Greenamyre, J. T. (2000). Chronic systemic pesticide exposure reproduces features of Parkinson's disease. *Nat. Neurosci.*, **3**, 1301–6.

Blum, D., Torch, S., Lambeng, N. *et al.* (2001). Molecular pathways involved in the neurotoxicity of 6-OHDA, dopamine and MPTP: contribution to the apoptotic theory in Parkinson's disease. *Prog. Neurobiol.*, **65**, 135–72.

Borasio, G. D., Robberecht, W., Leigh, P. N. *et al.* (1998). A placebo-controlled trial of insulin-like growth factor-I in amyotrophic lateral sclerosis. European ALS/IGF-I Study Group. *Neurology*, **51**, 583–6.

Borlongan, C. V., Koutouzis, T. K. & Sanberg, P. R. (1997). 3-Nitropropionic acid animal model and Huntington's disease. *Neurosci. Biobehav. Rev.*, **21**, 289–93.

Bowen, B. C., Block, R. E., Sanchez-Ramos, J. *et al.* (1994). Proton MR spectroscopy of the brain in 14 patients with Parkinson's disease. *Am. J. Neuroradiol.*, **16**, 61–8.

Braak, H., Braak, E. & Bohl, J. (1993). Staging of Alzheimer-related cortical destruction. *Eur. Neurol.*, **33**, 403–8.

Brooks, D. J. (1998). The early diagnosis of Parkinson's disease. *Ann. Neurol.*, **44** (Suppl), S10–18.

Brorson, J. R., Bindokas, V. P., Iwama, T., Marcuccilli, C. J., Chisholm, J. C. & Miller, R. J. (1995). The Ca^{2+} influx induced by beta-amyloid peptide 25–35 in cultured hippocampal neurons results from network excitation. *J. Neurobiol.*, **26**, 325–38.

Brouillet, E. & Beal, M. F. (1993). NMDA antagonists partially protect against MPTP induced neurotoxicity in mice. *NeuroReport*, **4**, 387–90.

Brouillet, E., Hantraye, P., Ferrante, R. J. *et al.* (1995). Chronic mitochondrial energy impairment produces selective striatal degeneration and abnormal choreiform movements in primates. *Proc. Natl. Acad. Sci., USA*, **92**, 7105–9.

Brune, B. & Lapetina, E. G. (1989). Activation of a cytosolic ADP-ribosyl transferase by nitric oxide generating agents. *J. Biol. Chem.*, **264**, 8455–8.

Burnashev, N., Schoepfer, R., Monyer, H. *et al.* (1992). Control by asparagine residues of calcium permeability and magnesium blockade in the NMDA receptors. *Science*, **257**, 1415–19.

Calne, D. B. & Langston, J. W. (1983). Aetiology of Parkinson's disease. *Lancet*, **ii**, 1457–9.

Chan, P., Langston, J. W. & Monte, D. A. (1993). MK-801 temporarily prevents MPTP-induced acute dopamine depletion and MPP⁺ elimination in the mouse striatum. *J. Pharmacol. Exp. Ther.*, **267**, 1515–20.

Chatterton, J. E., Awobuluyi, M., Premkumar, L. S. *et al.* (2002). Excitatory glycine receptors containing the NR3 family of NMDA receptor subunits. *Nature*, **415**, 793–8.

Chen, Y. I., Jenkins, B. G. & Rosen, B. R. (1994). Evidence for impairment of energy metabolism in Parkinson's disease using in vivo localized MR spectroscopy. *Proc. Soc. Magn. Res.*, **1**, 194.

Choi, D. W. (1987). Ionic dependence of glutamate neurotoxicity. *J. Neurosci.*, **7**, 369–79.

Choi, D. W., Maulucci-Gedde, M. & Kriegstein, A. R. (1987). Glutamate neurotoxicity in cortical cell culture. *J. Neurosci.*, **7**, 357–68.

Clancy, R. M., Levartovsky, D., Leszczynska-Piziak, J., Yegudin, J. & Abramson, S. B. (1994). Nitric oxide reacts with intracellular glutathione and activates the hexose monophosphate shunt in human neutrophils: Evidence for S-nitrosoglutathione as a biactive intermediary. *Proc. Natl Acad. Sci., USA*, **91**, 3680–4.

Cleveland, D. W. & Rothstein, J. D. (2001). From Charcot to Lou Gehrig: deciphering selective motor neuron death in ALS. *Nat. Rev. Neurosci.*, **2**, 806–19.

Corson, L. B., Strain, J. J., Culotta, V. C. & Cleveland, D. W. (1998). Chaperone-facilitated copper binding is a property common to several classes of familial amyotrophic lateral sclerosis-linked superoxide dismutase mutants. *Proc. Natl Acad. Sci., USA*, **95**, 6361–6.

Couratier, P., Hugon, J., Sindou, P., Vallat, J. M. & Dumas, M. (1993). Cell culture evidence for neuronal degeneration in amyotrophic lateral sclerosis being linked to glutamate AMPA/kainate receptors. *Lancet*, **341**, 265–8.

Couratier, P., Sindou, P., Esclaire, F. & Hugon, J. (1994). Neuroprotective effects of riluzole in ALS CSF toxicity. *Neuroreport*, **5**, 1012–14.

Cullen, W. K., Wu, J. Q., Anwyl, R. & Rowan, M. J. (1996). beta-Amyloid produces a delayed NMDA receptor-dependent reduction in synaptic transmission in rat hippocampus. *Neuroreport*, **8**, 87–92.

Curtis, D. R., Phillis, J. W. & Watkins, J. C. (1959). Chemical excitation of spinal neurones. *Nature*, **183**, 611–12.

Das, S., Sasaki, Y. F., Rothe, T. *et al.* (1998). Increased NMDA current and spine density in mice lacking the NMDA receptor subunit NR3A. *Nature*, **393**, 377–81.

Davis, G. C., Williams, A. C., Markey, S. P. *et al.* (1979). Chronic parkinsonism secondary to intravenous injection of meperidine analogues. *Psychiatry Res.*, **1**, 249–54.

Dawson, V. L., Dawson, T. M., London, E. D., Bredt, D. S. & Snyder, S. H. (1991). Nitric oxide mediates glutamate neurotoxicity in primary cortical culture. *Proc. Natl Acad. Sci., USA*, **88**, 6368–71.

DiDonato, S., Zeviani, M., Giovannini, P. *et al.* (1993). Respiratory chain and mitochondrial DNA in muscle and brain in Parkinson's disease patients. *Neurology*, **43**, 2262–8.

Di Monte, D., Tetrud, J. W. & Langston, J. W. (1991). Blood lactate in Parkinson's disease and senescence. *Biochem. Biophys. Res. Commun.*, **170**, 483–9.

Farber, N. B., Newcomer, J. W. & Olney, J. W. (1998). The glutamate synapse in neuropsychiatric disorders. Focus on schizophrenia and Alzheimer's disease. *Prog. Brain Res.*, **116**, 421–37.

Favaron, M., Manev, H., Siman, R. *et al.* (1990). Down regulation of protein kinase C protects cerebellar granule neurons in primary culture from glutamate-induced neuronal death. *Proc. Natl Acad. Sci., USA*, **87**, 1983–7.

Fearnley, J. & Lees, A. (1991). Parkinson's disease: neuropathology. *Brain*, **114**, 2283–301.

Fonnum, F. (1984). Glutamate: a neurotransmitter in mammalian brain. *J. Neurochem.*, **42**, 1–11.

Francis, P. T., Pangalos, M. N. & Bowen, D. M. (1992). Animal and drug modelling for Alzheimer synaptic pathology. *Prog. Neurobiol.*, **39**, 517–45.

Frandsen, A. & Schousboe, A. (1991). Dantrolene prevents glutamate cytotoxicity and Ca²⁺-release from intracellular stores in cultures cerebral cortical neurons. *J. Neurochem.*, **56**, 1075–8.

(1992). Mobilization of dantrolene-sensitive intracellular calcium pools is involved in the cytotoxicity induced by quisqualate and *N*-methyl-D-asparate but not 2-amino-3-(3-hydroxy-5-methylisoxazol-4-yl)propionate and kainate in cultured cerebral cortical neurons. *Proc. Natl Acad. Sci., USA*, **89**, 2590–4.

Gaudette, M., Hirano, M. & Siddique, T. (2000). Current status of SOD1 mutations in familial amyotrophic lateral sclerosis. *Amyotroph Lateral Scler. Other Motor Neuron Disord.*, **1**, 83–9.

Giuffra, M. E., Sethy, V. H., Davis, T. L., Mouradian, M. M. & Chase, T. N. (1993). Milacemide therapy for Parkinson's disease. *Movement Disord.*, **8**, 47–50.

Giulian, D., Haverkamp, L. J., Li, J. *et al.* (1995). Senile plaques stimulate microglia to release a neurotoxin found in Alzheimer brain. *Neurochem. Int.*, **27**, 119–37.

Goodwin, J. L., Uemura, E. & Cunnick, J. E. (1995). Microglial release of nitric oxide by the synergistic action of beta-amyloid and IFN-gamma. *Brain Res.*, **692**, 207–14.

Gossel, M., Schmidt, W. J., Loscher, W., Zajaczkowski, W. & Danysz, W. J. (1995). Effect of coadministration of glutamate receptor antagonists and dopaminergic agonists on locomotion in monoamine-depleted rats. *J. Neural Trans.*, **19**, 27–39.

Greenamyre, J. T., Eller, R. V., Zhang, Z., Ovadia, A., Kurlan, R. & Gash, D. M. (1994). Antiparkinsonian effects of remacemide hydrochloride, a glutamate antagonist, in rodent and primate models of Parkinson's disease. *Ann. Neurol.*, **35**, 655–61.

Greene, J. G. & Greenamyre, J. T. (1995). Manipulation of membrane potential modulates malonate-induced striatal excitotoxicity in vivo. *J. Neurochem.*, **64**, 2332–8.

Greene, J. G., Porter, R. H. P., Eller, R. V. & Greenamyre, J. T. (1993). Inhibition of succinate dehydrogenase by malonic acid produces an 'excitotoxic' lesion in rat striatum. *J. Neurochem.*, **61**, 1151–4.

Guerrini, L., Blasi, F. & Denis, D. (1995) Synaptic activation of NF-kappa B by glutamate in cerebellar granule neurons in vitro. *Proc. Natl Acad. Sci., USA*, **92**, 9077–81.

Guyot, M. C., Palfi, S., Stutzmann, J. M., Maziere, M., Hantraye, P. & Brouillet, E. (1997). Riluzole protects from motor deficits and striatal degeneration produced by systemic 3-nitropropionic acid intoxication in rats. *Neuroscience*, **81**, 141–9.

Hansson, O., Petersen, A., Leist, M., Nicotera, P., Castilho, R. F. & Brundin, P. (1999). Transgenic mice expressing a Huntington's disease mutation are resistant to quinolinic acid-induced striatal excitotoxicity. *Proc. Natl Acad. Sci., USA*, **96**, 8727–32.

Harris, M. E., Wang, Y., Pedigo, N. W. Jr., Hensley, K., Butterfield, D. A. & Carney, J. M. (1996). Amyloid beta peptide (25–35) inhibits Na$^+$-dependent glutamate uptake in rat hippocampal astrocyte cultures. *J. Neurochem.*, **67**, 277–86.

Hattori, N., Tanaka, M., Ozawa, T. & Mizuno, Y. (1991). Immunohistochemical studies on complexes I, II, III and IV of mitochondria in Parkinson's disease. *Ann. Neurol.*, **30**, 563–71.

Hayashi, T. (1952). A physiological study of epileptic seizures following cortical stimulation in animals and its application to human clinics. *Jpn J. Pharmacol.*, **3**, 46–64.

(1958). Inhibition and excitation due to γ-aminobutyric acid in the central nervous system. *Nature*, **182**, 1076–7.

Henshaw, R., Jenkins, B. G., Schulz, J. B. *et al.* (1994). Malonate produces striatal lesions by indirect NMDA receptor activation. *Brain Res.*, **647**, 161–6.

Herb, A., Burnashev, N., Werner, P., Sakmann, B., Wisden, W. & Seeburg, P. H. (1992). The KA-2 subunit of excitatory amino acid receptors shows widespread expression in brain and forms ion channels with distantly related subunits. *Neuron*, **8**, 775–85.

Herb, A., Higuchi, M., Sprengel, R. & Seeburg, P. H. (1996). Q/R site editing in kainate receptor GluR5 and GluR6 pre-mRNAs requires distant intronic sequences. *Proc. Natl Acad. Sci., USA*, **93**, 1875–80.

Hollmann, M. & Heinemann, S. (1994). Cloned glutamate receptors. *Annu. Rev. Neurosci.*, **17**, 31–108.

Hugon, J., Vallat, J. M., Spencer, P. S., Leboutet, M. J. & Barthe, D. (1989). Kainic acid induces early and delayed degenerative neuronal changes in rat spinal cord. *Neurosci. Lett.*, **104**, 258–62.

Ikonomidou, C. & Turski, L. (1996). Neurodegenerative disorders: clues from glutamate and energy metabolism. *Crit. Rev. Neurobiol.*, **10**, 239–63.

Ikonomidou, C., Bosch, F., Miksa, M. *et al.* (1999). Blockade of NMDA receptors and apoptotic neurodegeneration in the developing brain. *Science*, **283**, 70–4.

Ikonomidou, C., Stefovska, V. & Turski, L. (2000). Neuronal death enhanced by *N*-methyl-D-aspartate antagonists. *Proc. Natl Acad. Sci., USA*, **97**, 12885–90.

Ikonomidou, C., Qin, Y.-Q., Labruyere, J. & Olney, J. W. (1996). Motor neuron degeneration induced by excitotoxin agonists has features in common with those seen in the SOD-1 transgenic mouse model of amyotrophic lateral sclerosis. *J. Neuropathol. Exp. Neurol.*, **55**, 211–24.

Ischiropoulos, H., Zhu, L., Chen, J. *et al.* (1992). Peroxynitrite-mediated tyrosine nitration catalyzed by superoxide dismutase. *Arch. Biochem. Biophys.*, **298**, 431–7.

Jain, K. K. (2000). Evaluation of memantine for neuroprotection in dementia. *Expert Opin. Invest. Drugs*, **9**, 1397–406.

Janetzky, B., Hauck, S., Youdim, M. B. *et al.* (1994). Unaltered aconitase acitivity, but decreased complex I activity in substantia nigra pars compacta of patients with Parkinson's disease. *Neurosci. Lett.*, **169**, 126–8.

Jones-Humble, S. A., Morgan, P. F. & Cooper, B. R. (1994). The novel anticonvulsant lamotrigine prevents dopamine depletion in C57 black mice in the MPTP animal model of Parkinson's disease. *Life Sci.*, **54**, 245–52.

Kasischke, K., Ludolph, A. C. & Riepe, M. W. (1996). NMDA-antagonists reverse increased hypoxic tolerance by preceding chemical hypoxia. *Neurosci. Lett.*, **214**, 1–4.

Kieburtz, K., Feigin, A., McDermott, M. *et al.* (1996). A controlled trial of remacemide hydrochloride in Huntington's disease. *Movement Disord.*, **11**, 273–7.

Kilpatrick, G. J. & Tilbrook, G. S. (2002). Memantine. Merz. *Curr. Opin Investig Drugs*, **3**, 798–806.

Klockgether, T., Turski, L., Honore, T. *et al.* (1991). The AMPA receptor antagonist NBQX has antiparkinsonian effects in monoamine-depleted rats and MPTP-treated monkeys. *Ann. Neurol.*, **30**, 717–23.

Komuro, H. & Rakic, P. (1993). Modulation of neuronal migration by NMDA receptors. *Science*, **260**, 95–7.

Krebs, H. A. (1935). Metabolism of amino acids. III Deamination of amino acids. *Biochem. J.*, **29**, 1520–44.

Lacomblez, L., Bensimon, G., Leigh, P. N., Guillet, P. & Meininger, V. (1996). Dose-ranging study of riluzole in amyotrophic lateral sclerosis. Amyotrophic Lateral Sclerosis/Riluzole Study Group II. *Lancet*, **347**, 1425–31

Lai, E. C., Felice, K. J., Festoff, B. W. *et al.* (1997). Effect of recombinant human insulin-like growth factor-I on progression of ALS. A placebo-controlled study. The North America ALS/IGF-I Study Group. *Neurology*, **49**, 1621–30.

Lange, K. W., Loschmann, P. A., Sofic, E. *et al.* (1993). The competitive NMDA antagonists CPP protect substantia nigra neurons from MPTP-induced degeneration in primates. *Naunyn-Schmiedebergs Arch. Pharmacol.*, **348**, 586–92.

Langston, J. W., Ballard, P., Tetrud, J. W. & Irwin, I. (1983). Chronic Parkinsonism in humans due to a product of meperidine-analog synthesis. *Science*, **219**, 979–80.

Lee, K. S., Frank, S., Vanderklish, P., Arai, A. & Lynch, G. (1991). Inhibition of proteolysis protects hippocampal neurons from ischemia. *Proc. Natl Acad. Sci., USA*, **88**, 7233–7.

Lees, G. J. (1993). The possible contribution of microglia and macrophages to delayed neuronal death after ischemia. *J. Neurol. Sci.*, **114**, 119–22.

Li, M., Ona, V. O., Guegan, C. *et al.* (2000). Functional role of caspase-1 and caspase-3 in an ALS transgenic mouse model. *Science*, **288**, 335–9.

Lucas, D. R. & Newhouse, J. P. (1957). The toxic effect of sodium-L-glutamate on the inner layers of the retina. *Arch. Ophthalmol.*, **58**, 193–201.

Luquin, M. R., Obeso, J. A., Laguna, J., Guillen, J. & Martineslage, J. M. (1993). The AMPA receptor antagonist NBQX does not alter the motor response induced by selective dopamine agonists in MPTP-treated monkeys. *Eur. J. Pharmacol.*, **235**, 297–300.

Malsch, U, Bliesath, H., Bother, K., Ramm, H. & Luhmann, R. (2001). Monotherapy of Parkinson's disease with budipine. A double blind comparison with amantadine. *Fortsch. Neurol. Psychiatr.*, **69**, 56–9.

Manev, H., Favaron, M., Siman, R., Guidotti, A. & Costa, E. (1991). Glutamate neurotoxicity is independent of calpain I inhibition in primary cultures of cerebellar granule cells. *J. Neurochem.*, **57**, 1288–95.

Mann, V. M., Cooper, J. M., Krige, D., Daniel, S. E., Schapira, A. H. & Marsden, C. D. (1992). Brain, skeletal muscle and platelet homogenate mitochondrial function in Parkinson's disease. *Brain*, **115**, 333–42.

Matsuda, K., Kamiya, Y., Matsuda, S. & Yuzaki, M. (2002). Cloning and characterization of a novel NMDA receptor subunit NR3B: a dominant subunit that reduces calcium permeability. *Brain Res. Mol. Brain Res.*, **100**, 43–52.

Mattson, M. P. & Goodman, Y. (1995). Different amyloidogenic peptides share a similar mechanism of neurotoxicity involving reactive oxygen species and calcium. *Brain Res.*, **676**, 219–24.

McBain, C. J. & Mayer, M. L. (1994). *N*-methyl-D-aspartic acid receptor structure and function. *Physiol. Rev.*, **74**, 723–60.

McDonald, J. W. & Schoepp, D. D. (1992). The metabotropic excitatory amino acid receptors agonist 1S,3R-ACPD selectively potentiates *N*-methyl-D-asparate-induced brain injury. *Eur. J. Pharmacol.*, **215**, 353–4.

McGeer, P. L., Itagaki, S., Akiyama, H. & McGeer, E. G. (1989). Rate of cell death in parkinsonism indicates active neuropathological process. *Ann. Neurol.*, **24**, 574–6.

McMaster, O. G., Du, F., French, E. D. & Schwarcz, R. (1991). Focal injection of aminooxyacetic acid produces seizures and lesions in rat hippocampus: evidence for mediation by NMDA receptors. *Exp. Neurol.*, **113**, 378–85.

Montastruc, J. L., Fabre, N., Rascol, O., Senard, J. M. & Blin, O. (1994). *N*-methyl-D-aspartate (NMDA) antagonists and Parkinson's disease: a pilot study with dextromethorphan. *Mov. Disord.*, **9**, 242–3.

Montastruc, J. L., Rascol, O. & Senard, J. M. (1997). Glutamate antagonists and Parkinson's disease: a review of clinical data. *Neurosci. Biobehav. Rev.*, **21**, 477–80.

Monyer, H., Seeburg, P. H. & Wisden, W. (1991). Glutamate-operated channels: Developmentally early and mature forms arise by alternative splicing. *Neuron*, **6**, 799–810.

Monyer, H., Sprengel, R., Schoepfer, R. *et al.* (1992). Heteromeric NMDA receptors: molecular and functional distinction of subtypes. *Science*, **256**, 1217–21.

Monyer, H., Burnashev, N., Laurie, D. J., Sakmann, B. & Seeburg, P. H. (1994). Developmental and regional expression in the rat brain and functional properties of four NMDA receptors. *Neuron*, **12**, 529–40.

Murman, D. L., Giordani, B., Mellow, A. M. *et al.* (1997). Cognitive, behavioral, and motor effects of the NMDA antagonist ketamine in Huntington's disease. *Neurology*, **49**, 153–61.

Nakagawa-Hattori, Y., Yoshino, H., Kondo, T., Mizuno, Y. & Horai, S. (1992). Is Parkinson's disease a mitochondrial disorder? *J. Neurol. Sci.*, **107**, 29–33.

Nagano, I., Wong, P. C. & Rothstein, J. D. (1996). Nitration of glutamate transporters in transgenic mice with a familial amyotrophic lateral sclerosis-linked SOD1 mutation. *Ann. Neurol.*, **40**, 542.

Nakanishi, S. (1992). Molecular diversity of glutamate receptors and implications for brain function. *Science*, **258**, 597–603.

Nathan, C. (1992). Nitric oxide as a secretory product of mammalian cells. *FASEB J.*, **6**, 3051–64.

Novelli, A., Reilly, J. A., Lysko, P. G. & Henneberry, R. C. (1988). Glutamate becomes neurotoxic via the *N*-methyl-D-asparate receptors when intracellular energy levels are reduced. *Brain Res.*, **451**, 205–12.

Olney, J. W. (1969). Brain lesions, obesity and other disturbances in mice treated with monosodium glutamate. *Science*, **164**, 719–21.

(1971). Glutamate-induced neuronal necrosis in the infant mouse hypothalamus: an electron microscopic study. *J. Neuropathol. Exp. Neurol.*, **30**, 75–90.

Olney, J. W. & Ho, O. L. (1970). Brain damage in infant mice following oral intake of glutamate, aspartate or cysteine. *Nature*, **227**, 609–10.

Olney, J. W., Sharpe, L. G. & Feigin, R. D. (1972). Glutamate-induced brain damage in infant primates. *J. Neuropathol. Exp. Neurol.*, **31**, 464–88.

Olney, J. W., Wozniak, D. F. & Farber, N. B. (1997). Excitotoxic neurodegeneration in Alzheimer disease. New hypothesis and new therapeutic strategies. *Arch. Neurol.*, **54**, 1234–40.

Ossowska, K. (1994). The role of excitatory amino acids in experimental models of Parkinson's disease. *J. Neural Trans.*, **8**, 39–71.

Palfi, S. P., Ferrante, R. J., Brouillet, E. *et al.* (1996). Chronic 3-nitropropionic acid treatment in baboons replicates the cognitive and motor deficits of Huntington's disease. *J. Neurosci.*, **16**, 3019–25.

Panov, A. V., Gutenkunst, C. A., Leavitt, B. R. *et al.* (2002). Early mitochondrial calcium defects in Huntington's disease are a direct effect of polyglutamines. *Nat. Neurosci.*, **5**, 713–36.

Pantopoulos, H. & Hentze, M. W. (1995). Nitric oxide signaling to iron-regulatory protein: direct control of ferritin mRNA translation and transferrin receptor mRNA stability in transfected fibroblasts. *Proc. Natl Acad. Sci., USA*, **92**, 1267–71.

Papa, S. M., Engber, T. M., Boldry, R. C. & Chase, T. N. (1993). Opposite effects of NMDA and AMPA receptor blockade on catalepsy induced by dopamine receptor antagonists. *Eur. J. Pharmacol.*, **232**, 247–53.

Parkinson's Study Group (2000). A multicenter randomized controlled trial of remacemide hydrochloride as monotherapy for Parkinson's disease. *Neurology*, **54**, 1583–8.

(2001). Evaluation of dyskinesias in a pilot, randomized, placebo-controlled trial of remacemide in advanced Parkinson disease. *Arch. Neurol.*, **58**, 1660–8.

Parsons, C. G., Danysz, W. & Quack, G. (1998a). Glutamate in CNS disorders as a target for drug development: an update. *Drug News Perspect.*, **11**, 523–69.

Parsons, C. G., Hartmann, S. & Spielmanns, P. (1998b) Budipine is a low affinity, N-methyl-D-asparate receptor antagonist: patch clamp studies in cultured striatal, hippocampal, cortical and superior colliculus neurones. *Neuropharmacology*, **37**, 719–27.

Pasinelli, P., Houseweart, M. K., Brown, R. H. Jr & Cleveland, D. W. (2000). Caspase-1 and -3 are sequentially activated in motor neuron death in Cu,Zn superoxide dismutase-mediated familial amyotrophic lateral sclerosis. *Proc. Natl Acad. Sci., USA*, **97**, 13901–6.

Perry, T. L., Hansen, S. & Jones, K. (1987). Brain glutamate deficiency in amyotrophic lateral sclerosis. *Neurology*, **37**, 1845–8.

Pin, J. P. & Duvoisin, R. (1995). The metabotropic glutamate receptor: structure and function. *Neuropharmacology*, **34**, 1–26.

Przuntek, H. & Muller, T. (1999). Clinical efficacy of budipine in Parkinson's disease. *J. Neural Trans. Suppl*, **56**, 75–82.

Przuntek, H., Bittkau, S., Bliesaht, H. *et al.* (2002) Budipine provides additional benefit in patients with Parkinsons disease receiving a stable optimum dopaminergic drug regimen. *Arch Neurol.*, **59**, 803–6.

Radi, R., Beckman, J. S., Bush, K. M. & Freeman, B. A. (1991a). Peroxynitrite-induced membrane lipid peroxidation: the cytotoxic potential of superoxide and nitric oxide. *Arch. Biochem. Biophys.*, **288**, 484–7.

Radi, R., Beckman, J. S., Bush, K. M. & Freeman, B. A. (1991b). Peroxynitrite oxidation of sulfhydryls. *J. Biol. Chem.*, **266**, 4244–50.

Rabey, J. M., Nissipeanu, P. & Korczyn, A. D. (1992). Efficacy of memantine, an NMDA receptor antagonist, in the treatment of Parkinson's disease. *J. Neural Trans.*, **4**, 277–82.

Riepe, M. & Ludolph, A. C. (1997). Chemical preconditioning: a cytoprotective strategy. *Mol. Cell Biochem.*, **174**, 249–54.

Riepe, H. W., Hori, N., Ludolph, A. C. & Carpenter, D. O. (1995). Failure of neuronal ion exchange, not potentiated excitation, causes excitotoxicity after inhibition of oxidative phosphorylation. *Neuroscience*, **64**, 91–7.

Rordorf, G., Uemura, Y. & Bonventre, J. V. (1991) Characterization of phospholipase A2 (PLA2) activity in gerbil brain: enhanced activities of cytosolic, mitochondrial, and microsomal forms after ischemia and reperfusion. *J. Neurosci.*, **11**, 1829–36.

Rothman, S. M. (1985). The neurotoxicity of excitatory amino acids is produced by passive chloride influx. *J. Neurosci.*, **5**, 1483–9.

Rothman, S. M., Yamada, K. A. & Lancaster, N. L. (1993). Nordihydroguaiaretic acid attenuates NMDA neurotoxicity-action beyond the receptor. *Neuropharmacology*, **32**, 1279–88.

Rothstein, J. D., Martin, L. J. & Kuncl, R. W. (1992). Decreased glutamate transport by the brain and spinal cord in amyotrophic lateral sclerosis. *N. Engl. J. Med.*, **326**, 1464–8.

Rothstein, J. D., Van Kammen, M., Levey, A. I., Martin, L. J. & Kuncl, R. W. (1995). Selective loss of glial glutamate transporter GLT-1 in amyotrophic lateral sclerosis. *Ann. Neurol.*, **38**, 73–84.

Samples, S. D. & Dubinsky, J. M. (1993). Aurintricarboxylic acid protects hippocampal neurons from glutamate excitotoxicity in vitro. *J. Neurochem.*, **61**, 382–5.

Santiago, M., Venero, J. L., Machado, A. & Cano, J. (1992). In vivo protection of striatum from MPP$^+$ neurotoxicity by N-methyl-D-asparate antagonists. *Brain Res.*, **586**, 203–7.

Sawa, A., Wiegand, G. W., Cooper, J. *et al.* (1999). Increased apoptosis of Huntington disease lymphoblasts associated with repeat length-dependent mitochondrial depolarization. *Nat. Med.*, **5**, 1194–8.

Schapira, A. H., Cooper, J. M., Dexter, D., Clark, J. B., Jenner, P. & Marsden, C. D. (1990a). Mitochondrial complex I deficiency in Parkinson's disease. *J. Neurochem.*, **54**, 823–7.

Schapira, A. H., Mann, V. M., Cooper, J. M. *et al.* (1990b). Anatomic and disease specificity of NADH CoQ$_1$ reductase (complex I) deficiency in Parkinson's disease. *J. Neurochem.*, **55**, 2142–5.

Schilling, G., Becher, M. W., Sharp, A. H. *et al.* (1999). Intranuclear inclusions and neuritic aggregates in transgenic mice expressing a mutant N-terminal fragment of huntingtin. *Hum. Molec. Genet.*, **8**, 397–407.

Schmidt, W. J. & Kretschmer, B. D. (1997). Behavioural pharmacology of glutamate receptors in the basal ganglia. *Neurosci. Biobehav. Res.*, **21**, 381–92.

Schoepp, D. D., Tizzano, J. P., Wright, R. A. & Fix, A. S. (1995). Reversible and irreversible neuronal injury induced by intrahippocampal infusion of the mGluR agonist 1S,3R-ACPD in the rat. *Neurodegeneration*, **4**, 71–80.

Schulz, J. B., Henshaw, D. R., Jenkins, B. G. *et al.* (1994). 3-Acetylpyridine produces age-dependent neuronal lesions by an excitotoxic and free radical mediated mechanim. *J. Cereb. Blood Flow Metab.*, **14**, 1024–9.

Schulz, J. B., Matthews, R. T., Muqit, M. M., Browne, S. E. & Beal, M. F. (1995). Inhibition of neuronal nitric oxide synthase by 7-nitroindazole protects against MPTP induced neurotoxicity in mice. *J. Neurochem.*, **64**, 936–9.

Schwab, R. S., England, A. C., Poskranzer, D. C. & Young, R. R. (1969). Amantadine in the treatment of Parkinson's disease. *J. Ann. Med. Assn.*, **208**, 1168–70.

Schwarcz, R. & Kohler, C. (1983). Differential vulnerability of central neurons of the rat to quinolinic acid. *Neurosci. Lett.*, **38**, 85–90.

Schwarcz, R., Whetsell, W. O. & Mangano, R. M. (1983). Quinolinic acid: an endogenous metabolite that produces axon-sparing lesions in rat brain. *Science*, **219**, 316–18.

Schwarcz, R., Okuno, E., White, R. J., Bird, E. D. & Whetsell, W. O., Jr. (1988). 3-Hydroxyanthranilate oxygenase activity is increased in the brains of Huntington disease victims. *Proc. Natl Acad. Sci., USA*, **85**, 4079–81.

Selkoe, D. J. (1999). Translating cell biology into therapeutic advances in Alzheimer's disease. *Nature Suppl.*, **399**, A23–31.

Shaw, P. J., Forrest, V., Ince, P. G., Richardson, J. P. & Wastell, H. J. (1995). Studies on cellular free radical protection mechanisms in the anterior horn from patients with amyotrophic lateral sclerosis. *Neurodegeneration*, **4**, 209–16.

Spencer, P. S. (1987). Guam ALS/parkinsonism-dementia: a long-latency neurotoxic disorder caused by 'slow toxin(s)' in food? *Can. J. Neurol. Sci.*, **14** (3 Suppl), 347–57.

Spencer, P. S., Roy, D. N., Ludolph, A., Hugon, J., Dwivedi, M. P. & Schaumburg, H. H. (1986). Lathyrism: evidence for the role of the neuroexcitatory amino acid BOAA. *Lancet*, **ii**, 1066–7.

Spencer, P. S., Kisby, G. E., Ross, S. M. *et al.* (1993). Guam ALS-PDC: possible causes. *Science*, **262**, 825–6.

Spieker, S., Eisebitt, R., Breit, S. *et al.* (1999). Tremorlytic activity of budipine in Parkinson's disease. *Clin. Neuropharmacol.*, **22**, 115–19.

Srivastava, R., Brouillet, E., Beal, M. F., Storey, E. & Hyman, B. T. (1993). Blockade of 1-methyl-4-phenylpyridinium ion (MPP+) nigral toxicity in the rat by prior decortication or MK-801 treatment. *Neurobiol. Aging*, **14**, 295–301.

Taylor, D. J., Krige, D., Barnes, P. R. *et al.* (1994). A ^{31}P magnetic resonance spectroscopy study of mitochondrial function in skeletal muscle of patients with Parkinson's disease. *J. Neurol. Sci.*, **125**, 77–81.

Terro, F., Lasort, M., Vlader, F., Ludolph, A. & Hugon, J. (1996). Antioxidant drugs block in vitro the neurotoxicity of CSF from patients with amyotrophic lateral sclerosis. *Neuroreport*, **7**, 1970–2.

Terry, R. D. & Davies, P. (1980). Dementia of the Alzheimer type. *Ann. Rev. Neurosci.*, **3**, 77–95.

The BDNF Study Group. (1999). A controlled trial of recombinant methionyl human BDNF in ALS: (Phase III). *Neurology*, **52**, 1427–33.

Turski, L., Bressler, K., Rettig, K. J., Loschmann, P. A. & Wachtel, H. (1991). Protection of substantia nigra from MPP+ neurotoxicity by *N*-methyl-D-aspartate antagonists. *Nature*, **349**, 414–18.

Tymianski, M., Wallace, M. C., Spigelman, I. *et al.* (1993). Cell-permeant Ca^{2+}-chelators reduce early excitotoxic and ischemic neuronal injury in vitro and in vivo. *Neuron*, **11**, 221–35.

Uitti, R. J., Rajput, A. H., Ahlskog, J. E. *et al.* (1996). Amantadine treatment is an independent predictor of improved survival in Parkinson's disease. *Neurology*, **46**, 1551–6.

Urbanska, E., Ikonomidou, C., Sieklucka, M. & Turski, W. A. (1991). Aminooxyacetic acid produces excitotoxic lesions in the rat striatum. *Synapse*, **9**, 129–35.

Verhagen Metman, L., Del Dotto, P., Blanchet, P. J., van den Munckhof, P. & Chase, T. N. (1998) Blockade of glutamatergic transmission as treatment for dyskinesias and motor fluctuations in Parkinson's disease. *Amino Acids*, **14**, 75–82.

Vukosavic, S., Stefanis, L., Jackson-Lewis, V. *et al.* (2000). Delaying caspase activation by Bcl-2: a clue to disease retardation in a transgenic mouse model of amyotrophic lateral sclerosis. *J. Neurosci.*, **20**, 9119–25.

Wachtel, H., Kunow, M. & Loschmann, P. A. (1992). NBQX (6-nitro-sulfamoyl-benzo-quinoxaline-dione) and CPP (3-carboxy-piperazin-propyl phosphonic acid) potentiate dopamine agonist induced rotations in substantia nigra lesioned rats. *Neurosci. Lett.*, **142**, 179–82.

Williams, T. L., Day, N. C. Kamboj, R. K., Ince, P. G. & Shaw, P. J. (1997). Calcium-permeable alpha-amino-3-hydroxy-5-methyl-4-isoxazole propionic acid receptors: a molecular determinant of selective vulnerability in amyotrophic lateral sclerosis. *Ann. Neurol.*, **35**, 200–7.

Winblad, B. & Poritis, N. (1999) Memantine in severe dementia: results of the 9M-Best Study (Benefit and efficacy in severely demented patients during treatment with memantine). *Int. J. Geriatr. Psychiatry*, **14**, 135–46.

Wozniak, D. F., Dikranian, K., Ishimaru, M. J. *et al.* (1998). Disseminated corticolimbic neuronal degeneration induced in rat brain by MK-801: potential relevance to Alzheimer's disease. *Neurobiol. Dis.*, **5**, 305–22.

Wüllner, U., Young, A. B., Penney, J. B. & Beal, M. F. (1994). 3-Nitropropionic acid toxicity in the striatum. *J. Neurochem.*, **63**, 1772–81.

Young, A. B. (1990). What's the excitement about excitatory amino acids in amyotrophic lateral sclerosis? *Ann. Neurol.*, **28**, 9–11.

Zadow, B. & Schmidt, W. J. (1994). The AMPA antagonists NBQX and GYKI 52466 do not counteract neuroleptic-induced catalepsy. *Naunyn Schmied Arch. Pharmacol.*, **349**, 61–5.

Zeevalk, G. D. & Nicklas, W. J. (1991). Mechanisms underlying initiation of excitotoxicity associated with metabolic inhibition. *J. Pharmacol. Exp. Ther.*, **257**, 870–8.

Zhang, J., Dawson, V. L., Dawson, T. M. & Snyder, S. H. (1994). Nitric oxide activation of poly (ADP-ribose)synthetase in neurotoxicity. *Science*, **263**, 687–9.

Zipp, F., Baas, H. & Fischer, P. A. (1993). Lamotrigine – antiparkinsonian activity by blockade of glutamate release? *J. Neural Transm.*, **5**, 67–75.

Zipp, F., Burklin, F., Stecker, K., Baas, H. & Fischer, P. A. (1995). Lamotrigine in Parkinson's disease – a double blind study. *J. Neural Transm*, **10**, 199–206.

Zuddas, A., Oberto, G., Vaglini, F., Fascetti, F., Fornai, F. & Corsini, G. U. (1992). MK-801 prevents 1-methyl-4-phenyl-1,2,3,6-tetrahydropyridine-induced parkinsonism in primates. *J. Neurochem.*, **59**, 733–9.

Glutamate transporters

Davide Trotti and Stuart L. Gibb

Department of Neurology, Massachusetts General Hospital
Harvard Medical School, Charlestown, MS, USA

Introduction

In the central nervous system (CNS) of mammals, glutamate acts as a chemical transmitter of excitatory signals by binding to different glutamate receptors and activating a multitude of highly integrated molecular pathways. Termination of this excitatory neurotransmission occurs via re-uptake of glutamate by specialized high affinity transporters capable of maintaining glutamate at $\sim 1\,\mu M$ levels in the synaptic cleft. At higher concentrations, glutamate can also act as neurotoxin causing degeneration and death of neurons (Choi, 1992). This event is known as excitotoxicity and contributes to many chronic and acute neurodegenerative diseases. Therefore, glutamate homeostasis and the regulation of glutamate transporter abundance and function are a key element for the normal brain function.

High affinity, Na$^+$-dependent glutamate transporters: localization, functional properties and topology

Molecular cloning has identified five different subtypes of Na$^+$-dependent glutamate transporters, termed EAAT1–5 (excitatory amino acid transporters 1–5; nomenclature used for human subtypes). At present, two different nomenclatures are in use in the literature to indicate human and rodent isoforms (Table 5.1). However, the homologues show a high degree of interspecies conservation (>95%) and do not differ functionally. The gene names for the human transporter are as follows: EAAT3 or SLC1A1; EAAT2 or SLC1A2; EAAT1 or SLC1A3; EAAT4 or SLC1A4; EAAT5 or SLC1A5. The acronym SLC1 refers to 'Solute Carrier family' number 1 and A1 to family member number 1.

Localization

Immunohistochemistry studies revealed that the glutamate transporters EAAT1 and EAAT2 are localized to astroglial membranes that immediately oppose synaptic cleft regions of the neuropil. EAAT3–4 are expressed in neuronal membranes in a perisynaptic distribution with the highest concentration at the edge of postsynaptic densities, rather than within the synaptic cleft, and in general are expressed in a somatodendritic fashion on post-synaptic spines and somas. The glial transporter EAAT1 is highly expressed in the molecular layer of the cerebellum and less in the hippocampus, superior colliculus, and *substantia gelatinosa* of the spinal cord. In contrast, EAAT2 expression is generally high throughout all brain regions and the spinal cord but it is largely absent from the white matter tracts. EAAT3 is selectively enriched in neurons of the hippocampus, cerebellum, and basal ganglia, whereas EAAT4 is confined largely to the soma and dendrites of the Purkinje cells of the cerebellum. EAAT5 is located in retinal ganglion cells (for a detailed review, see Danbolt, 2001) (Table 5.1). Recent studies reported the cloning of a variant form of EAAT2 from rat forebrain neuronal cultures that localizes in the presynaptic terminals and dendritic shafts of neurons as well as in astrocytes (Chen *et al.*, 2002; Schmitt *et al.*, 2002).

Functional properties

Glutamate transporters are coupled to the inwardly directed electrochemical gradients of Na$^+$ and H$^+$, and to the outwardly directed gradient of K$^+$. This unique coupling stoichiometry allows efficient removal of glutamate from extracellular compartments. The coupling stoichiometry of EAAT2 and EAAT3 was examined in detail and the studies revealed that 3 Na$^+$ ions and 1 H$^+$ are co-transported with

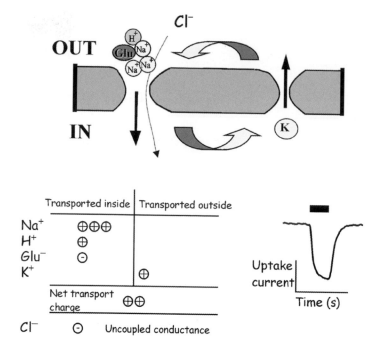

Fig. 5.1 Stoichiometry of the glutamate transporters. Glutamate transport involves loading of the empty carrier with glutamate $^-$/H$^+$ and 3 Na$^+$, following the translocation of the fully loaded carrier across the plasma membrane and release of the cotransported ions at the intracellular space. Thereafter, 1 K$^+$ binds to the carrier inside and promotes the relocation of the empty carrier. This implies that 2 positive net charges are moved inside the cell for each glutamate molecule taken up and the process can be monitored by electrophysiological techniques. The insert of the figure shows a representative recording of glutamate-mediated uptake current performed in a *Xenopus* oocyte expressing EAAT2. For net uptake of glutamate, the transporters must complete this cycle. If K$^+$ does not bind, the transporter does not enter the relocation step, binds Na$^+$ and glutamate$^-$ at the inside of the cell and translocates back in the reverse direction. In this case, the transporter behaves like an exchanger. The net uptake of glutamate is also accompanied by a chloride conductance, the extent of which varies among glutamate transporter subtypes.

each glutamate molecule, whereas 1 K$^+$ is transported in the opposite direction (Levy *et al.*, 1998a; Levy *et al.*, 1998b; Zerangue and Kavanaugh, 1996) (Fig. 5.1). This implies that two positive charges are translocated with each glutamate molecule. Functional analysis of EAAT4 has led to the identification of a substrate gated chloride conductance associated to the transport of glutamate. This feature is also displayed by other glutamate transporter family members, with the anion permeability decreasing in the order EAAT5–4 >> EAAT1 > EAAT3 >> EAAT2 (Seal & Amara, 1999).

Table 5.1. Distribution of glutamate transporters in the nervous system

Glutamate transporter	Rodent homologue	Cell type	Distribution
EAAT1	GLAST	Astrocyte	Highly expressed in cerebellum. Brain and spinal cord
EAAT2	GLT1	Astrocyte	All brain and spinal cord
EAAT3	EAAC1	Neuron	Hippocampus, cerebellum, basal ganglia
EAAT4	EAAT4	Neuron	Purkinje cells of cerebellum
EAAT5	EAAT5	Neuron	Retina

Topology

Recently, crystallographic studies have shed light on the molecular architecture of glutamate transporters. Yernool and colleagues (Yernool *et al.*, 2004) crystallized a glutamate transporter (Glt$_{ph}$) from the obligate anerobe, *Pyrococcus horikoshii*. Glt$_{ph}$ shares 37% homology with the eukaryotic EAAT2 glutamate transporter. Protomer structure contains eight transmembrane regions which are predominantly α-helical (regions 4 and 7 are segmented α-helices), a large extracellular loop connecting transmembrane regions 3 and 4, and two hairpin regions. A schematic representation is shown in Fig. 5.2. The Glt$_{ph}$ study also provided data on the residues mediating interactions between a homotrimeric functional complex. The first six transmembrane regions of Glt$_{ph}$ form a cylinder, the outer surface of which mediates intersubunit contact within the trimer complex. The remaining C-terminal residues form a structure within the cylinder that is implicated in substrate transport. Although there may be differences between this model and the structure of other glutamate transporter isomers, it is reasonable to expect that their structures will be similar. However, in models of three-dimentional topology, differences do exist. The crystal structure of Glt$_{ph}$ indicates that it exists as a trimer, stoichiometry which has previously been reported for other prokaryotic transporters. Furthermore, the study suggests that eukaryotic transporters such as EAAT2 also exist as a homotrimer. When EAAT2 was overexpressed in HEK cells and crossed linked with gluteraldehyde, a banding pattern consistent with trimer formation was observed. In a different study and using a variety of different approaches, Gendreau and colleagues, demonstrated that a bacterial glutamate transproter from *Escherichia coli* and the human glutamate transporter EAAT2 assemble as homotrimers,

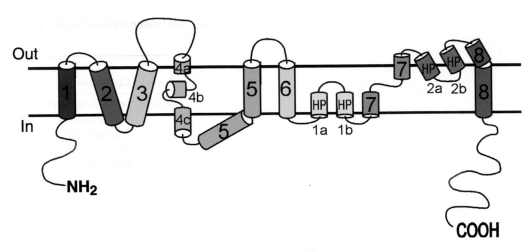

Fig. 5.2 Schematic representation of a glutamate transporter topology.

demonstrating an evolutionary conserved trimeric quaternary structure of glutamate transporter (Gendreau *et al.*, 2004). This is in contrast to data provided by freeze–fracture electron microscopy. Eskandari and colleagues reported that expressing EAAT3 in *Xenopus* oocytes revealed the presence of distinct 10 nm pentagonal particles, in which five well-defined domains could be identified. According to these observations, the functional EAAT3 complex was predicted to be a pentamer in the appearance of a penton-based pyramid (Eskandari *et al.*, 2000).

Regulation of glutamate transporters

Glutamate transporter levels and activity are subject to complex regulation by a variety of endogenous factors. There is evidence for neuronal and non-neuronal factors inducing upregulation of transporter levels as well as for substrate-mediated increase in transport activity (Poitry-Yamate *et al.*, 2002). Several hormones, growth and trophic factors, signaling molecules like reactive oxygen and nitrogen species, arachidonic acid and poly-unsaturated fatty acids or protein kinase C activity are capable of regulating expression, trafficking and activity of glutamate transporters (for review see Robinson, 2002). In addition, their associating proteins also regulate glutamate transporter activity. Two proteins, GTRAP41 and GTRAP48 specifically interact with the intracellular carboxy-terminal domain of EAAT4 and modulate its activity (Jackson *et al.*, 2001). The expression of either GTRAP41 or GTRAP48 resulted in the increase in the V_{max} of the transport without altering glutamate affinity. It is speculated that GTRAP41 couples EAAT4 to actin and GTRAP48 to a Rho GTPase signaling system. A completely different protein named GTRAP3-18 (Lin

et al., 2001) interacts with the intracellular carboxy-terminal domain of EAAT3. GTRAP3-18 is a predicted 188 amino acid hydrophobic protein with four possible trans-membrane domains, which possesses a sequence identity (95%) to F18, a protein encoded by a vitamin-A-responsive gene. In contrast to the effect exerted by GTRAP41 and GTRAP48 on EAAT4, GTRAP3-18 reduces the transport activity of EAAT3 by decreasing the affinity of glutamate to the transporter.

Excitatory neurotransmission and glutamate transporters

The concept that glutamate transporters control the termination of glutamatergic neurotransmission is based on the evidence that synaptically released glutamate is not inactivated by enzymatic degradation because of the lack of a specific enzyme in the synaptic cleft. Clements and colleagues empirically estimated the time course of decay of glutamate in the synaptic cleft and found that it is slower than that derived from theoretical calculation based on a simple diffusion model (Clements *et al.*, 1992). Consequently, these investigators proposed that neighboring structures restricted the diffusion of glutamate. This suggested that altering the location, density, and/or the function of glutamate transporters could influence the time course of the transmitter clearance in the synaptic cleft. The turnover rate of EAAT2 for a complete cycle of transport at −80 mV and 22 °C was found to be approximately 70 ms (Wadiche *et al.*, 1995) and 20 ms for EAAT1 (Wadiche & Kavanaugh, 1998). This is significantly slower than the estimated glutamate decay time constant in hippocampal synapses which is 1–2 ms (Clements *et al.*, 1992). This difference was predicted also to be true at physiological temperatures. Therefore, it can be argued as to whether glutamate transporters really constitute a major mechanism for removing released glutamate. Binding of glutamate to the transporters, however, exhibits fast kinetics. By applying glutamate with a time resolution of 100 microseconds using the laser-pulse photolysis technique of caged glutamate, the binding kinetics of the glutamate transporter EAAT3 occurred on a submillisecond time scale and preceded the subsequent slower glutamate translocation across the membrane by a few milliseconds after binding (Grewer et al., 2000). Thus, even though the turnover rate is low, the glutamate binding step itself is thought to be fast enough to participate in the removal of glutamate released in the synaptic cleft.

As suggested by experimental evidence (Lehre & Danbolt, 1998; Lehre & Rusakov, 2002), the geometry of the synapse is also an important determinant of the shaping of the glutamate-mediated neurotransmission (for review, see Rusakov & Lehre, 2002). The spatial confinement of glutamate in the synaptic cleft is not absolute as the cleft in which the neurotransmitter is released forms a continuum with the extracellular space. A glutamate molecule leaving the cleft is likely to be taken up by transporter proteins concentrated around the cleft on cell membranes of glia and neurons. However, experimental findings have suggested that glutamate molecules can exit the synaptic cleft, elude glutamate transporters and interact with glutamate receptors, such as metabotropic glutamate receptors (mGluRs) located perisynaptically (Brasnjo & Otis, 2001; Tempia et al., 1998).

Excitotoxicity and glutamate transporters

Based on the stoichiometry of glutamate transport and the prevailing ionic environment in which the transporters operate, it can be calculated that these proteins concentrate glutamate more than 10 000-fold across cell membranes (Levy et al., 1998b). Because of this high concentrating capacity, glutamate transporters are thought to play a major role in maintaining the extracellular glutamate concentration at low levels to protect neurons from excitotoxicity. This has been experimentally demonstrated both in vitro and in vivo. Protection of neurons by glutamate transporters from glutamate-mediated excitotoxicity was first demonstrated in vitro in organotypic rat spinal cord cultures using the glutamate transporter blockers. Treatment with these compounds generally resulted in elevated extracellular accumulation of glutamate that correlated with increased excitotoxic cell death (O'Shea et al., 2002;

Rothstein et al., 1993). In vivo, of particular note is the work of Rothstein and coworkers, who applied antisense oligonucleotides directed at glutamate transporters to the cerebroventricle of alert rats. Administration of antisense EAAT2 or EAAT1 oligonucleotides resulted in the degeneration of neurons whereas EAAT3 antisense oligonucleotides did not induce neurodegeneration, suggesting that the glial but not the neuronal glutamate transporters protect neurons from excitotoxicity. Complementary findings were obtained in EAAT1 and EAAT2 knockout mice which exhibited increased susceptibility to glutamate-mediated brain injury and suffered from lethal spontaneous seizures, whereas EAAT3 knockout mice did not show neurodegeneration (Peghini et al., 1997; Tanaka et al., 1997; Watanabe et al., 1999). The prevailing role of glial glutamate transporters in protecting neurons from excitotoxic insults stems from the different functional role that glial and neuronal glutamate transporters play in the CNS. In neurons, the intracellular glutamate concentration is ~ 10 mM. Considering the extracellular glutamate concentration of ~ 1 μM, this results in a steep gradient across neuronal cell membranes, which is essentially equal to the maximal concentration capacity of the high affinity glutamate transporters. Consequently, under normal conditions, neuronal glutamate transporters are almost at equilibrium and have little functional capacity. It is therefore not too surprising that the knockout of neuronal EAAT3 did not induce neurodegeneration. In glial cells, however, glutamate is taken up continuously and is then rapidly converted to glutamine by glutamine synthetase, a glial enzyme that maintains the concentration of glutamate as low as ~ 50 μM. Therefore, glial glutamate transporters are not at equilibrium and keep pumping glutamate into glial cells, generating a continuous stream of the neurotransmitter from glutamatergic synapse to glial cells.

Neurodegenerative diseases and glutamate transporters

Impairment in glutamate transporters has been reported in a number of acute and chronic neurodegenerative pathologies. However, in most cases it is not clear whether this impairment represents a primary defect, an event secondary to the primary insult, or both.

Amyotrophic lateral sclerosis (ALS)

Increased glutamate levels followed by excitotoxicity has been indicated as one possible pathogenic event occurring in ALS (Rothstein, 1995a, b), a neurodegenerative disorder of motor neurons in the spinal cord, motor cortex and brain stem. Reduced glutamate uptake and loss of the glutamate transporter EAAT2 has been observed in motor cortex from postmortem brains of ALS patients (Rothstein et al., 1992, 1995). Similarly, a reduction in EAAT2 was found in the spinal cord of transgenic mice models of ALS, as well as elevation of extracellular glutamate levels (Bruijn et al., 1997), suggesting that glutamate transport impairment is a common component in the pathway to motor neuron degeneration. The molecular mechanisms leading to EAAT2 loss in ALS are not yet understood. Levels of EAAT2 mRNA are unchanged (Bristol & Rothstein, 1996), suggesting that the reduction of EAAT2 is not due to decreased transcription of mRNA, but rather to an irresolute event at the translation or post-translation level. In a subset of sporadic ALS patients, abnormal EAAT2 mRNA editing and the presence of aberrant spliced forms with manifested dominant negative properties were found (Lin et al., 1998). However, other investigators failed to find a correlation between the presence of aberrant EAAT2 transcripts and ALS, as these transcripts were also detected in tissue specimens from control and Alzheimer's disease subjects (Flowers et al., 2001; Meyer et al., 1999). The case of ALS illustrates the involvement of glutamate transporters in a neurodegenerative pathology that is also characterized by oxidative stress. Studies by Rosen and colleagues (Rosen et al., 1993) showed that about 20% of familial ALS patients carry missense mutations in the gene encoding Cu^{2+}/Zn^{2+} superoxide dismutase (SOD1). Mutations in SOD1 catalyze the formation of deleterious oxidants, such as hydroxyl radical or peroxynitrite. Several lines of evidence suggested a link between SOD1 mutants and excitoxicity-mediated neuronal death. A loss of EAAT2 has been reported in the spinal cord of transgenic ALS mice and rats. In a Xenopus oocyte model, coexpression of some of the mutant forms of human SOD1 protein and EAAT2 caused inactivation of the transporter molecule (Trotti et al., 1999). Therefore, it is possible that the inactivation and loss of EAAT2 may be related to the properties of the SOD1 mutation.

Using single-strand conformation polymorphism analysis of genomic DNA, Brown and colleagues reported a mutation in the EAAT2 gene associated with sporadic ALS. This mutation substitutes an asparagine for a serine at position 206 (N206S) (Aoki et al., 1998) and avoided the glycosylation of the carrier at that site. It was also found that the EAAT2-N206S mutant had a pronounced reduction in the transport rate and a substantial dominant negative impact on the wild-type activity. The decreased rate of transport was because of decreased trafficking of the mutated carrier to the plasma membrane. Moreover, the EAAT2-N206S exhibited an increased reverse transport capability (Trotti et al., 2000). These combined effects significantly impair the ability of EAAT2 to clear glutamate at the synaptic cleft of neurons.

Alzheimer's disease

Alzheimer's disease is a chronic degenerative neurological disorder. Hallmarks of the disease are accumulation of β-amyloid peptide, a major constituent of the amyloid plaques characteristic of the disease, as well as widespread oxidative injury. The role of β-amyloid peptide in the neuropathology of Alzheimer's disease, including free radical injury and excitotoxicity is well documented. Treatment of neuron/astrocyte co-cultures with high concentrations of β-amyloid peptide increases the vulnerability of neurons to glutamate-induced cell death, probably due to the inhibition of astrocytic glutamate transporters (Harris et al., 1996). Two recent studies showed that, at concentrations compatible to those found in Alzheimer's disease brains, the β-amyloid peptide causes instead a substantial increase in glutamate uptake in astrocytes and attenuates synaptic efficacy (Abe & Misawa, 2003; Ikegaya et al., 2002). These findings are also supported by an electrophysiological study done in cultured microglia in which chronic treatment with low concentrations of β-amyloid peptide enhanced glutamate transport currents (Noda et al., 1999). An excessive removal of glutamate may cause depressed glutamatergic neurotransmission which is at the basis of the amnesia in Alzheimer's disease. A different study based on antibodies reported reduced levels of EAAT2 protein in frontal cortex of Alzheimer's patients but normal levels of EAAT2 mRNA as well as of EAAT1 and EAAT3 (Li et al., 1997). Note that trangenic mice expressing mutant amyloid precursor protein appear to have reduced EAAT2 and EAAT1 protein levels (Masliah et al., 2000).

Huntington's disease

Huntington's disease is a late-onset neurodegenerative disease for which the mutation is CAG/polyglutamine repeat expansion. The R6 mice expressing an N-terminal fragment of mutant huntingtin develop a movement disorder that is preceded by the formation of neuronal polyglutamine aggregates. The phenotype is probably caused by a widespread neuronal dysfunction, whereas neuronal cell death occurs late and is very selective. Decreased mRNA and protein levels of the major astroglial glutamate transporter EAAT2 in the striatum and cortex of these mice is accompanied by a concomitant decrease in glutamate uptake (Behrens et al., 2002; Lievens et al., 2001).

In contrast, the expression of the glutamate transporters EAAT1 and EAAT3 remained unchanged. These changes in expression and function occurred prior to any evidence of neurodegeneration and suggest that a defect in astrocytic glutamate uptake may contribute to the phenotype and neuronal cell death in Huntington's disease.

Parkinson's disease

Indirect observations suggested a possible malfunctioning of glutamate transporters in the pathogenesis of Parkinson's disease. 1-methyl-4-phenyl-1,2,3,6-tetrahydropyridine (MPTP), a neurotoxin known to target dopaminergic neurons in Parkinson's disease, reversibly inhibits astroglial glutamate uptake in cultured astrocytes (Hazell et al., 1997).

Ischemia

Reversed operation of glutamate transporters appears to contribute to the rise in extracellular glutamate and the excitotoxicity that occurs during an ischemic insult (Rossi et al., 2000). Because glutamate uptake is driven by the energy stored in the form of electrochemical gradients across the plasma membranes, the impairment of the ionic gradients caused by insufficient energy supply, which occurs during brain ischemia, results in a decrease in concentrating capacity of glutamate transporters and favors their reversed operation. Neurons have a much higher content of glutamate than glial cells; therefore neuronal glutamate transporters are more likely to run in reverse in ischemia and to contribute to the extracellular rise in glutamate to excitotoxic levels (Hamann et al., 2002; Rossi et al., 2000). During ischemia, glutamate transporter expression is also altered (An et al., 2002; Rao et al., 2001) and their activity can be further downregulated by polyunsaturated fatty acids, particularly by arachidonic acid, and reactive oxygen species (ROS), both of which are produced in response to excessive glutamate receptor activation (Volterra et al., 1994).

Glutamate transporters and mercury neurotoxicity

Sensory disturbance and ataxia were described in a number of neurological cases attributed to the ingestion of fish contaminated with methylmercury (MeHg) (Harada, 1995; Malm et al., 1995). Poisoning with elementary mercury (Hg^0) vapours was also shown to produce similar neurological symptoms. Several lines of evidence indicate that glutamate-mediated excitotoxicity is probably involved. For example, glutamate receptor (NMDA type)

antagonists effectively blocked the neurotoxic action of mercury in cerebral neuronal cultures (Park et al., 1996). MeHg and Hg^0 would act, at least in part, through the common oxidation product mercuric mercury (Hg^{2+}). Submicromolar concentrations of Hg^{2+} were found to inhibit selectively the uptake of excitatory amino acids in cultured astrocytes. MeHg mimicked this effect but not other divalent cations (Aschner, 1996; Aschner, 2001; Aschner et al., 2000). It was also shown that mercuric chloride uncouples glutamate uptake from the co-transport of 1 H$^+$ (Nagaraja & Brookes, 1996), and that micromolar concentrations of it is sufficient to induce a dramatic inhibition of the glutamate transporters EAAT1-T3 (Trotti et al., 1997).

Concluding remarks

Regulation of glutamate transporter abundance and function is a very important element in the normal brain function as impairment in glutamate uptake is associated with many neurodegenerative diseases. This has also led to the identification of the glutamate transport system as a desirable therapeutic target. In recent years, important advances have been made in understanding basic molecular and cellular mechanisms governing the expression and regulation of glutamate transporters. These achievements are expected to facilitate further studies on the roles of individual transporter subtypes and to develop new strategies for the diagnosis and treatment of diseases associated with the malfunctioning of glutamate transporters.

REFERENCES

Abe, K. & Misawa, M. (2003). Amyloid beta protein enhances the clearance of extracellular L-glutamate by cultured rat cortical astrocytes. Neurosci. Res., 45, 25–31.

An, S. J., Kang, T. C., Park, S. K. et al. (2002). Oxidative DNA damage and alteration of glutamate transporter expressions in the hippocampal Ca1 area immediately after ischemic insult. Mol. Cells, 13, 476–80.

Aoki, M., Lin, C. L., Rothstein, J. D. et al. (1998). Mutations in the glutamate transporter EAAT2 gene do not cause abnormal EAAT2 transcripts in amyotrophic lateral sclerosis. Ann. Neurol., 43, 645–53.

Aschner, M. (1996). Astrocytes as modulators of mercury-induced neurotoxicity. Neurotoxicology, 17, 663–9.

Aschner, M. (2001). Mercury toxicity. J. Pediatr., 138, 450–1.

Aschner, M., Yao, C. P., Allen, J. W. & Tan, K. H. (2000). Methylmercury alters glutamate transport in astrocytes. Neurochem. Int., 37, 199–206.

Behrens, P. F., Franz, P., Woodman, B., Lindenberg, K. S. & Landwehrmeyer, G. B. (2002). Impaired glutamate transport and glutamate-glutamine cycling: downstream effects of the Huntington mutation. *Brain*, **125**, 1908–22.

Brasnjo, G. & Otis, T. S. (2001). Neuronal glutamate transporters control activation of postsynaptic metabotropic glutamate receptors and influence cerebellar long-term depression. *Neuron*, **31**, 607–16.

Bristol, L. A. & Rothstein, J. D. (1996). Glutamate transporter gene expression in amyotrophic lateral sclerosis motor cortex. *Ann. Neurol.*, **39**, 676–9.

Bruijn, L. I., Becher, M. W., Lee, M. K. *et al.* (1997). ALS-linked SOD1 mutant G85R mediates damage to astrocytes and promotes rapidly progressive disease with SOD1-containing inclusions. *Neuron*, **18**, 327–38.

Chen, W., Aoki, C., Mahadomrongkul, V. *et al.* (2002). Expression of a variant form of the glutamate transporter GLT1 in neuronal cultures and in neurons and astrocytes in the rat brain. *J. Neurosci.*, **22**, 2142–52.

Choi, D. W. (1992). Excitotoxic cell death. *J. Neurobiol.*, **23**, 1261–76.

Clements, J. D., Lester, R. A., Tong, G., Jahr, C. E. & Westbrook, G. L. (1992). The time course of glutamate in the synaptic cleft. *Science*, **258**, 1498–501.

Danbolt, N. C. (2001). Glutamate uptake. *Prog. Neurobiol.*, **65**, 1–105.

Eskandari, S., Kreman, M., Kavanaugh, M. P., Wright, E. M. & Zampighi, G. A. (2000). Pentameric assembly of a neuronal glutamate transporter. *Proc. Natl Acad. Sci., USA*, **97**, 8641–6.

Flowers, J. M., Powell, J. F., Leigh, P. N., Andersen, P. & Shaw, C. E. (2001). Intron 7 retention and exon 9 skipping EAAT2 mRNA variants are not associated with amyotrophic lateral sclerosis. *Ann. Neurol.*, **49**, 643–9.

Gendreau, S., Voswinkel, S., Torres-Salazar, D. *et al.* (2004). A trimeric quaternary structure is conserved in bacterial and human glutamate transporters. *J. Biol. Chem.*, **279**, 39505–12.

Grewer, C., Watzke, N., Wiessner, M. & Rauen, T. (2000). Glutamate translocation of the neuronal glutamate transporter EAAC1 occurs within milliseconds. *Proc. Natl Acad. Sci., USA* **97**, 9706–11.

Hamann, M., Rossi, D. J., Marie, H. & Attwell, D. (2002). Knocking out the glial glutamate transporter GLT-1 reduces glutamate uptake but does not affect hippocampal glutamate dynamics in early simulated ischaemia. *Eur. J. Neurosci.*, **15**, 308–14.

Harada, M. (1995). Minamata disease: methylmercury poisoning in Japan caused by environmental pollution. *Crit. Rev. Toxicol.*, **25**, 1–24.

Harris, M. E., Wang, Y., Pedigo, N. W., Jr., Hensley, K., Butterfield, D. A. & Carney, J. M. (1996). Amyloid beta peptide (25–35) inhibits Na$^+$-dependent glutamate uptake in rat hippocampal astrocyte cultures. *J. Neurochem.*, **67**, 277–86.

Hazell, A. S., Itzhak, Y., Liu, H. & Norenberg, M. D. (1997). 1-Methyl-4-phenyl-1,2,3,6-tetrahydropyridine (MPTP) decreases glutamate uptake in cultured astrocytes. *J. Neurochem.*, **68**, 2216–19.

Ikegaya, Y., Matsuura, S., Ueno, S. *et al.* (2002). Beta-amyloid enhances glial glutamate uptake activity and attenuates synaptic efficacy. *J. Biol. Chem.*, **277**, 32180–6.

Jackson, M., Song, W., Liu, M. Y. *et al.* (2001). Modulation of the neuronal glutamate transporter EAAT4 by two interacting proteins. *Nature*, **410**, 89–93.

Lehre, K. P. & Danbolt, N. C. (1998). The number of glutamate transporter subtype molecules at glutamatergic synapses: chemical and stereological quantification in young adult rat brain. *J. Neurosci.*, **18**, 8751–7.

Lehre, K. P. & Rusakov, D. A. (2002). Asymmetry of glia near central synapses favors presynaptically directed glutamate escape. *Biophys. J.* **83**, 125–34.

Levy, L. M., Attwell, D., Hoover, F., Ash, J. F., Bjoras, M. & Danbolt, N. C. (1998a). Inducible expression of the GLT-1 glutamate transporter in a CHO cell line selected for low endogenous glutamate uptake [published erratum appears in *FEBS Lett.* 1998 May 1;427(1):152]. *FEBS Lett.*, **422**, 339–42.

Levy, L. M., Warr, O. & Attwell, D. (1998b). Stoichiometry of the glial glutamate transporter GLT-1 expressed inducibly in a Chinese hamster ovary cell line selected for low endogenous Na$^+$-dependent glutamate uptake. *J. Neurosci.*, **18**, 9620–8.

Li, S., Mallory, M., Alford, M., Tanaka, S. & Masliah, E. (1997). Glutamate transporter alterations in Alzheimer disease are possibly associated with abnormal APP expression. *J. Neuropathol. Exp. Neurol.*, **56**, 901–11.

Lievens, J. C., Woodman, B., Mahal, A. *et al.* (2001). Impaired glutamate uptake in the R6 Huntington's disease transgenic mice. *Neurobiol. Dis.*, **8**, 807–21.

Lin, C. I., Orlov, I., Ruggiero, A. M. *et al.* (2001). Modulation of the neuronal glutamate transporter EAAC1 by the interacting protein GTRAP3–18. *Nature*, **410**, 84–8.

Lin, C.-L. G., Bristol, L. A., Jin, L. *et al.* (1998). Aberrant RNA processing in a neurodegenerative disease: the cause for absent EAAT2, a glutamate transporter, in amyotrophic lateral sclerosis. *Neuron*, **20**, 589–602.

Malm, O., Branches, F. J., Akagi, H. *et al.* (1995). Mercury and methylmercury in fish and human hair from the Tapajos river basin. *Brazil. Sci. Total Environ.*, **175**, 141–50.

Masliah, E., Alford, M., Mallory, M., Rockenstein, E., Moechars, D. & Van Leuven, F. (2000). Abnormal glutamate transport function in mutant amyloid precursor protein transgenic mice. *Exp. Neurol.*, **163**, 381–7.

Meyer, T., Fromm, A., Munch, C. *et al.* (1999). The RNA of the glutamate transporter EAAT2 is variably spliced in amyotrophic lateral sclerosis and normal individuals. *J. Neurol. Sci.*, **170**, 45–50.

Nagaraja, T. N. & Brookes, N. (1996). Mercuric chloride uncouples glutamate uptake from the countertransport of hydroxyl equivalents. *Am. J. Physiol.*, **271**, C1487–93.

Noda, M., Nakanishi, H. & Akaike, N. (1999). Glutamate release from microglia via glutamate transporter is enhanced by amyloid-beta peptide. *Neuroscience*, **92**, 1465–74.

O'Shea, R. D., Fodera, M. V., Aprico, K. *et al.* (2002). Evaluation of drugs acting at glutamate transporters in organotypic hippocampal cultures: new evidence on substrates and blockers in excitotoxicity. *Neurochem. Res.*, **27**, 5–13.

Park, S. T., Lim, K. T., Chung, Y. T. & Kim, S. U. (1996). Methylmercury-induced neurotoxicity in cerebral neuron

culture is blocked by antioxidants and NMDA receptor antagonists. *Neurotoxicology*, **17**, 37–45.

Peghini, P., Janzen, J. & Stoffel, W. (1997). Glutamate transporter
EAAC-1-deficient mice develop dicarboxylic aminoaciduria
and behavioral abnormalities but no neurodegeneration.
EMBO J., **16**, 3822–32.

Poitry-Yamate, C. L., Vutskits, L. & Rauen, T. (2002). Neuronal-
induced and glutamate-dependent activation of glial glutamate transporter function. *J. Neurochem.*, **82**, 987–97.

Rao, V. L., Bowen, K. K. & Dempsey, R. J. (2001). Transient focal cerebral ischemia down-regulates glutamate transporters GLT-1
and EAAC1 expression in rat brain. *Neurochem. Res.*, **26**, 497–
502.

Robinson, M. B. (2002). Regulated trafficking of neurotransmitter
transporters: common notes but different melodies. *J. Neurochem.*, **80**, 1–11.

Rosen, D. R., Siddique, T., Patterson, D. *et al.* (1993). Mutations in
Cu/Zn superoxide dismutase gene are associated with familial
amyotrophic lateral sclerosis. *Nature*, **362**, 59–62.

Rossi, D. J., Oshima, T. & Attwell, D. (2000). Glutamate release in
severe brain ischaemia is mainly by reversed uptake. *Nature*,
403, 316–21.

Rothstein, J. D. (1995a). Excitotoxic mechanisms in the pathogenesis of amyotrophic lateral sclerosis. *Adv. Neurol.*, **68**, 7–20.

(1995b). Excitotoxicity and neurodegeneration in amyotrophic
lateral sclerosis. *Clin. Neurosci.*, **3**, 348–59.

Rothstein, J. D., Martin, L. J. & Kuncl, R. W. (1992). Decreased glutamate transport by the brain and spinal cord in amyotrophic
lateral sclerosis [see comments]. *N. Engl. J. Med.*, **326**, 1464–8.

Rothstein, J. D., Jin, L., Dykes-Hoberg, M. & Kuncl, R. W. (1993).
Chronic inhibition of glutamate uptake produces a model of
slow neurotoxicity. *Proc. Natl Acad. Sci., USA*, **90**, 6591–5.

Rothstein, J. D., Van Kammen, M., Levey, A. I., Martin, L. J. & Kuncl,
R. W. (1995). Selective loss of glial glutamate transporter GLT-1
in amyotrophic lateral sclerosis. *Ann. Neurol.*, **38**, 73–84.

Rothstein, J. D., Dykes-Hoberg, M., Pardo, C. A. *et al.* (1996). Knockout of glutamate transporters reveals a major role for astroglial
transport in excitotoxicity and clearance of glutamate. *Neuron*,
16, 675–86.

Rusakov, D. A. & Lehre, K. P. (2002). Perisynaptic asymmetry of glia:
new insights into glutamate signalling. *Trends Neurosci.*, **25**,
492–4.

Schmitt, A., Asan, E., Lesch, K. P. & Kugler, P. (2002). A splice variant
of glutamate transporter GLT1/EAAT2 expressed in neurons:

cloning and localization in rat nervous system. *Neuroscience*,
109, 45–61.

Seal, R. P. & Amara, S. G. (1999). Excitatory amino acid transporters:
a family in flux. *Annu. Rev. Pharmacol. Toxicol.*, **39**, 431–56.

Slotboom, D. J., Konings, W. N. & Lolkema, J. S. (2001). Glutamate
transporters combine transporter- and channel-like features.
Trends Biochem. Sci., **26**, 534–9.

Tanaka, K., Watase, K., Manabe, T. *et al.* (1997). Epilepsy and exacerbation of brain injury in mice lacking the glutamate transporter
GLT-1. *Science*, **276**, 1699–702.

Tempia, F., Miniaci, M. C., Anchisi, D. & Strata, P. (1998). Postsynaptic current mediated by metabotropic glutamate receptors in
cerebellar Purkinje cells. *J. Neurophysiol.*, **80**, 520–8.

Trotti, D., Nussberger, S., Volterra, A. & Hediger, M. A. (1997). Differential modulation of the uptake currents by redox interconversion of cysteine residues in the human neuronal glutamate
transporter EAAC1. *Eur. J. Neurosci.*, **9**, 2207–12.

Trotti, D., Rolfs, A., Danbolt, N. C., Brown, R. H., Jr. & Hediger, M. A.
(1999). SOD1 mutants linked to amyotrophic lateral sclerosis
selectively inactivate a glial glutamate transporter [published
erratum appears in *Nat. Neurosci.* 1999 Sep;2(9):848]. *Nat. Neurosci.*, **2**, 427–33.

Trotti, D., Aoki, M., Pasinelli, P. *et al.* (2000). Amyotrophic lateral
sclerosis-linked glutamate transporter mutant has impaired
glutamate clearance capacity. *J. Biol. Chem.*, **276**, 576–82.

Volterra, A., Trotti, D. & Racagni, G. (1994). Glutamate uptake
is inhibited by arachidonic acid and oxygen radicals via
two distinct and additive mechanisms. *Mol. Pharmacol.*, **46**,
986–92.

Wadiche, J. I., Arriza, J. L., Amara, S. G. & Kavanaugh, M. P. (1995).
Kinetics of a human glutamate transporter. *Neuron*, **14**, 1019–
27.

Wadiche, J. I. & Kavanaugh, M. P. (1998). Macroscopic and microscopic properties of a cloned glutamate transporter/chloride
channel. *J. Neurosci.*, **18**, 7650–61.

Watanabe, T., Morimoto, K., Hirao, T., Suwaki, H., Watase, K. &
Tanaka, K. (1999). Amygdala-kindled and pentylenetetrazole-
induced seizures in glutamate transporter GLAST-deficient
mice. *Brain Res.*, **845**, 92–6.

Yernool, D., Boudker, O., Jin, Y. & Gouaux, E. (2004). Structure of a
glutamate transporter homologue from *Pyrococcus horikoshii*.
Nature, **431**, 811–18.

Zerangue, N. & Kavanaugh, M. P. (1996). Flux coupling in a neuronal
glutamate transporter. *Nature*, **383**, 634–7.

6

Calcium binding proteins in selective vulnerability of motor neurons

László Siklós[1] and Stanley H. Appel[2]

[1]Institute of Biophysics, Biological Research Center, Szeged, Hungary
[2]Department of Neurology, Baylor College of Medicine, Houston, TX, USA

Introduction

Since the mid-1990s, the specific etiologies and mechanisms leading to dysfunction and loss of motor neurons in ALS have been under intensive investigation. No single mechanism appears to explain the devastating and inexorable injury to motor neurons. What appears far more likely is a convergence of a number of different mechanisms that collectively or sequentially impair motor neuron structure and function. Among the various proposals implicated, increased free radicals and oxidative stress, increased glutamate excitotoxicity, increased cellular aggregates and increased intracellular calcium have received the most attention (Rothstein, 1995; Cleveland, 1999; Shaw & Eggett, 2000; Rowland, 2000; Julien, 2001; Rowland & Shneider, 2001; Cleveland & Rothstein, 2001). None of these mechanisms is mutually exclusive and altered calcium homeostasis, free radicals, and glutamate excitotoxicity may all participate in the cell injury cascade leading to motor neuron death. Alterations in one parameter can lead to alterations in other parameters, and each can enhance and propagate the injury cascade. Such perturbations could critically impair motor neuron mitochondria and neurofilaments, compromise energy production and axoplasmic flow, and impair synaptic function. However, these alterations would be expected to adversely affect most neurons, and the critical question is why motor neurons are uniquely sensitive to injury in ALS, and why some motor neurons are relatively resistant to injury. Our own hypothesis focuses on the critical role of intracellular calcium and the inability of vulnerable motor neurons to handle an increased intracellular calcium load, possibly related to the relative paucity of the calcium binding proteins, calbindin D_{28k} and parvalbumin. With this hypothesis, impaired calcium homeostasis is considered a "final common pathway" leading to motor neuron injury through a calcium-dependent positive feedback loop (Appel et al., 2001).

Intracellular ionized calcium $[Ca^{2+}]_i$ is a ubiquitous second messenger, which plays an important role in a variety of neuronal functions in physiological as well as pathological states (Berridge et al., 1998; Berridge et al., 2000). Unlike other second messengers, ionic calcium cannot be metabolized, thus numerous mechanisms have evolved to regulate $[Ca^{2+}]_i$ and prevent toxicity (Clapham, 1995). Calcium can enter the cell from the extracellular space through various Ca channels including voltage-gated and ligand-gated channels, and can be actively extruded from the cell by calcium pumps and Na/Ca-exchangers (Carafoli & Stauffer, 1994). Calcium can also be released from high affinity intracellular stores through inositol triphosphate or ryanodine receptors, and can be taken up into these stores by Ca pumps (Pozzan et al., 1994). Mitochondria also accumulate calcium through a passive low-affinity uniporter and release calcium through Na-dependent and Na-independent pathways (Gunter et al., 1998). Perturbations in calcium homeostasis can have significant untoward effects on cell function, which could lead to irreversible cell injury. However, it is also possible that increased intracellular calcium is a marker of motor neuron degeneration rather than the cause of motor neuron degeneration. In the discussion that follows, we marshal the evidence that increased intracellular calcium within motor neurons may contribute to motor neuron injury as well as act as a secondary marker of motor neuron injury.

Increased calcium in motor neurons in ALS

The first direct demonstration of altered intracellular calcium in ALS came from ultrastructural studies of muscle biopsy samples from patients with sporadic ALS

(Siklós *et al.*, 1996). Using oxalate-pyroantimonate fixation to visualize tissue calcium as electron dense deposits, we demonstrated an increased number of calcium precipitates in synaptic vesicles and mitochondria of ALS motor axon terminals, accompanied by an increased number of vesicles and swelling of mitochondria (Siklós *et al.*, 1996). Since many of these biopsies were from patients in early stages of disease, it is unlikely that such findings were a late marker of motor neuron degeneration. Furthermore, the increased calcium in ALS motor axon terminals paralleled the increased intracellular calcium and increased number of synaptic vesicles demonstrated in motor nerve terminals of mice injected intraperitoneally with immunoglobulin G (IgG) from ALS patients (Engelhardt *et al.*, 1995; Pullen & Humphreys, 2000; Pullen *et al.*, 2004). Increased calcium with degenerative changes in the endoplasmic reticulum and Golgi complex was also demonstrated in motor neuron cell bodies in the spinal cord following passive transfer with ALS IgG. In SOD1 transgenic mice with the $G^{93}A$ mutation, a model of the familial form of ALS (Gurney *et al.*, 1994), a robust increase of intracellular calcium was demonstrated in cell bodies of spinal motor neurons and proportional disintegration of the corresponding motor axon terminals was also documented (Siklós *et al.*, 1998).

In cell cultures, glutamate neurotoxicity is mediated by the entry of calcium (Choi *et al.*, 1987; Tymianski *et al.*, 1993). Given the important potential role of glutamate excitotoxicity in motor neuron injury in ALS (Rothstein, 1995), we investigated alterations in calcium distribution in spinal motor neurons following in vivo application of D,L homocysteic acid, a non-specific glutamate agonist (Adalbert *et al.*, 2002). We noted increased accumulation of calcium in the cytoplasm, followed by gradual increases in calcium in degenerating intracellular organelles (endoplasmic reticulum, Golgi complex and mitochondria). Thus calcium is increased in degenerating spinal motor neurons in several different models of both sporadic and familial ALS.

Cellular calcium homeostasis and calcium binding proteins

Since ionic calcium plays a universal second messenger role, its concentration and intracellular distribution require tight regulation (Brini & Carafoli, 2000). A steep concentration gradient of Ca^{2+} can develop across the plasma membrane of neurons, spanning four orders of magnitude. This gradient guarantees fast signal transduction in physiological conditions, but could easily lead to large increases in $[Ca^{2+}]_i$ and cellular degeneration, if control mechanisms are compromised (Nicotera & Orrenius, 1998; Sattler & Tymianski, 2000). In the past several years

much has been learned about these control mechanisms, especially the major calcium sequestering organelles: the rapidly exchanging endoplasmic reticulum (Berridge, 1998; Paschen & Doutheil, 1999) and the high buffering capacity of mitochondria (Gunter *et al.*, 1998), and their possible cooperation in regulating calcium signals in health and disease (Meldolesi, 2001; Siesjö *et al.*, 1999).

Within the cell, calcium can interact with numerous proteins. However, the possible geometrical formations of the binding sites are quite limited. The most common calcium binding domain of proteins is the EF-hand motif, which is a helix–loop–helix structure of usually 12 residues with a special sequence, forming a loop that can accommodate calcium ions (Marsden *et al.*, 1990; Lewit-Bentley & Réty, 2000). To date, over 200 proteins are known to be capable of binding Ca^{2+} in one or more EF-hand motifs (Yap *et al.*, 1999). The EF-hand proteins are members of 45 distinct subfamilies, originally identified by functional and/or chemical characteristics of the first known representatives (Kawasaki *et al.*, 1998). Through their Ca^{2+}-binding EF-hand motifs, these proteins do influence local concentrations of $[Ca^{2+}]$. For many of the EF-hand proteins such as calmodulin or troponin C, their buffering capacity is far less significant than the regulatory function triggered by calcium-induced conformational changes (Miller, 1995; Yap *et al.*, 1999). Additional studies are necessary to define the actual coordinating function of the majority of EF-hand proteins and how they mediate intracellular calcium signalling. At present, this information is lacking, and most explanations attempt to understand the unique aspects of calcium homeostasis in different cell types based upon the buffering capacity of CaBPs. The limitation of this approach is exemplified by the approximately 10 μM intracellular concentration of calmodulin, which is equipped with four calcium binding motifs and theoretically might possess significant buffering capacity (Brini & Carafoli, 2000). Yet calmodulin appears to function more as a regulatory molecule (Cheung, 1980; Means *et al.*, 1982) than a passive buffer.

The strategic localization of CaBPs in the cytosol appears to be extremely important for influencing calcium homeostasis. For example, distribution of CaBPs in the vicinity of plasmalemmal calcium pumps and channels, as well as around mitochondria and endoplasmic reticulum, might indicate their relevance in calcium-mediated cellular death/life issues (Miller, 1998). In contrast to earlier concepts of active calcium accumulation, it is now clear that mitochondria are equipped with a uniporter for the passive uptake of Ca^{2+} from the cytosol (Gunter & Pfeiffer, 1990; Bernardi, 1999). The rapid flow of Ca^{2+} from the cytoplasm to the mitochondrial matrix ensures that changes in $[Ca^{2+}]_i$, assumed to be proportional to cellular

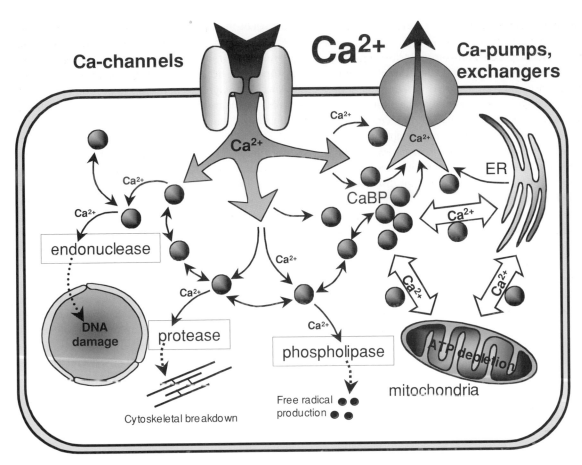

Fig. 6.1 An overload of intracellular Ca^{2+} may induce injury directly, by activating destructive enzymes (endonucleases, proteases), or indirectly, by activating phospholipases, which generate toxic intermediates. Furthermore, if the capacity of the sequestering organelles, particularly mitochondria, were exceeded, mitochondrial dysfunction would result in energy depletion and increased free radicals. The decreased levels of ATP could impair active defense processes (Ca-extruding mechanisms) and ultimately, collapse the mitochondrial membrane potential, and induce release of apoptotic factors. With high amount of mobile CaBP-s in the cytosol, however, the amplitude of $[Ca^{2+}]_i$ would be attenuated. The presence of CaBP-s might shortcut Ca^{2+} to the extrusion pumps, or recycle Ca^{2+} to the high affinity ER store before final extrusion, thus prevent or delay the overload of mitochondria.

activity, are quickly copied into corresponding intramitochondrial changes (Werth & Thayer, 1994). The calcium dependence of the activity of certain intramitochondrial enzymes involved in energy metabolism has been implicated in adjusting energy production to the actual demand of the cell under physiological conditions (Cox & Matlib, 1993; Robb-Gaspers *et al.*, 1998). If the system is overwhelmed by large increases in $[Ca^{2+}]_i$, the special mitochondrial defense system is activated by opening the mitochondrial megachannel (permeability transition pore), leading to the release of substances such as cytochrome c and initiating cell injury (Kroemer *et al.*, 1998; Murphy *et al.*, 1999). This mechanism has been implicated in acute lesions as well as chronic degenerative disorders (Schapira, 1998). One role for CaBPs might be to attenuate the amplitude of $[Ca^{2+}]_i$, and either facilitate the extrusion

of Ca^{2+} or recycle it to the fast exchanging endoplasmic reticulum store. The presence of CaBPs could help keep the relevant cytosolic $[Ca^{2+}]_i$ in the normal range while the elevation of the total calcium level remains hidden. This phenomenon might provide the basis of the findings of Brini *et al.* (2000), and Mogami *et al.* (1997), without assuming the presence of special intracellular tunnels for Ca^{2+} (Mogami *et al.*, 1997), who reported that, either lowering the calcium level in the endoplasmic reticulum (ER), or replenishing ER stores could occur without detectable changes in the cytosolic calcium level. Thereby, besides decreasing the activation of destructive enzymes by lowering $[Ca^{2+}]_i$, CaBPs reduce the likelihood of mitochondrial calcium overload, thus decrease the likelihood of megachannel openings and the release of apoptosis-inducing factors (Fig. 6.1) [Brustovetsky *et al.*, 2002].

Calcium binding proteins in motor neurons

One of the unique aspects of amyotrophic lateral sclerosis is that motor neuron pools are affected to differing extents (Swash & Schwartz, 1995). This selectivity, particularly the relative preservation of some motor neuron functions (e.g. voluntary sphincter and oculomotor) has prompted a search for constituents which could provide such protection. The variable content of parvalbumin and/or calbindin-D_{28k} in different motor neuron populations offers one potential explanation. The discovery of calmodulin, the isolation of an increasing number of other calcium binding proteins (CaBPs) (e.g. Waisman et al., 1983) and the first detailed description of the distribution of calbindin-D_{28K} and parvalbumin in the brain and spinal cord of the rat (Celio, 1990), have increased our understanding of the potential functions of CaBPs in the nervous system (Baimbridge et al., 1992). Reports that followed the studies of Celio confirmed the different composition of CaBPs in different populations of motor neurons in the spinal cord of rats (Ren & Ruda, 1994), as well as in the brainstem of primates (Reiner et al., 1995). In rodents, the presence of parvalbumin mRNA was documented to be a marker of ALS-resistant motor neurons (Elliott & Snider, 1995). The most pertinent studies were the demonstrations in human CNS that motor neurons most vulnerable in ALS are relatively deficient in the CaPBs calbindin-D_{28k} and/or parvalbumin, and those motor neurons most resistant in ALS have relatively abundant concentrations in either or both of these CaBPs (Ince et al., 1993; Alexianu et al., 1994).

Not all of the published reports of CaBPs in motor neurons of adult mammalian models agree that the paucity of parvalbumin and/or calbindin-D_{28k} in spinal motor neurons best explains vulnerability in ALS (Laslo et al., 2000). Part of the misleading interpretations may relate to the immunocytochemical techniques used, including differences in the source and type of (monoclonal or polyclonal) primary antibodies and, particularly, the degree of the calcium-binding status of CaBPs, which cannot be always and/or easily controlled (Winsky & Kuznicki, 1996). However, to date, no studies of human CNS (including ALS specimens) have refuted the hypothesis that motor neuron parvalbumin and/or calbindin-D_{28k} play a significant role in resistance or vulnerability to injury in ALS.

AMPA/kainate receptors and selective vulnerability

An alternative approach to explain the calcium-dependent vulnerability of motor neurons in ALS might be based on the details of the composition of their surface receptors. AMPA/kainate receptors are the major glutamate receptors present on motor neurons, and activation of these receptors would be expected to promote the entry of extracellular calcium and thereby contribute to selective vulnerability (Williams et al., 1997). However, under normal circumstances, the mRNA for the GluR2 subunit of the AMPA/kainate receptor is edited with high efficiency resulting in an arginine in place of a glutamine, and rendering the receptor impermeable to calcium (Puchalski et al., 1994). No differences in GluR2 subunits have been demonstrated in vulnerable compared to resistant motor neurons in vivo. In G86R mSOD1 transgenic mice, the distribution and intensity of GluR2 immunoreactivity was not altered between transgenic and control mice, and was equivalent in vulnerable motor neurons and resistant sensory neurons, although editing of the GluR2 was not examined (Morrison et al., 1998). Vandenberghe et al. [2000] demonstrated that rat spinal motor neurons were more vulnerable to AMPA and kainate than dorsal horn neurons, despite edited GluR2 being expressed equivalently in both spinal and dorsal horn neurons. Further, whole cell calcium permeability was similar in both neuronal populations. Nevertheless, in tissue culture, both Ca-permeable and Ca-impermeable AMPA receptors have been demonstrated in motor neurons that express GluR2 (Van Den Bosch et al., 2000). However, it is not clear whether the Ca-permeable AMPA receptors in such preparations have absent GluR2, or unedited GluR2. Short exposures of kainate did not affect dorsal horn neurons but did kill motor neurons through Ca-permeable AMPA receptors. Furthermore, both GluR2-containing and GluR2-lacking AMPA receptors coexist in clusters at synapses in motor neurons (Vandenberghe et al., 2001). The key question is whether the Ca-permeable AMPA receptors present in motor neurons in vitro are also present in adult human motor neurons in vivo.

In human ALS, Takuma et al. (1999) demonstrated specific alterations in the AMPA/kainate receptors. They documented reduced efficiency of GluR2 RNA editing, and decreased expression of the GluR2 subunit in the ventral gray of ALS tissue compared to controls. Both of these changes would be anticipated to increase permeability to calcium. However, these results could be the consequence and not the cause of motor neuron injury or selective vulnerability. At present, it is still unclear whether Ca-permeable AMPA/kainate receptors contribute to selective vulnerability and selective resistance in ALS. Are specific Ca-permeable AMPA/kainate receptors present in adult human spinal motor neurons (to explain their vulnerability), and are such receptors relatively absent in eye muscle motor neurons (to explain their resistance)? Recent studies in rat suggest no differences in the mRNA and protein for the GluR2 subunit of AMPA/kainate receptors in vulnerable hypoglossal motor neurons and resistant oculomotor motor neurons (Laslo et al., 2001). Such studies would suggest that differences in AMPA/kainate R may not be the best explanation for selective vulnerability.

Mechanism of protection of motor neurons by calcium binding proteins: axon terminals

Evidence for the potential importance of CaBPs in selective vulnerability is revealed in the calcium distribution of different motor neurons of SOD1 mutant mice and rats regularly injected with ALS IgG (Siklós et al., 1999). For this comparative analysis of models of sporadic and familial ALS, we selected spinal motoneurons and oculomotor neurons, since their CaBP composition was clearly different (Alexianu et al., 1994; Siklós et al., 1998). In light of earlier data from passive transfer experiments (Engelhardt et al., 1995) we expected major changes at the neuromuscular junction and focused on motor axon terminals in the interosseus and external eye muscles.

The analysis of motor axon terminals of the interosseus muscle in both models of ALS revealed mitochondrial degeneration and extensive calcium accumulation in mitochondria. These results were in agreement with previous findings obtained by examination of the same muscle after acute IgG treatment of animals (Engelhardt et al., 1995), or by analysis of muscle biopsy samples of sporadic ALS patients (Siklós et al., 1996).

Microscopic examination of the neuromuscular junctions in the external eye muscles also revealed changes different from those seen in the interosseus muscle. The major finding in the neuromuscular junctions in the external eye muscles was the appearance of large vacuolar structures (endosomes) accumulating the majority of intraterminal calcium. Such changes were not noted in neuromuscular junctions of interosseous muscles. The development of calcium filled endosomes was seen in motor nerve terminals of the superior rectus muscle of SOD1 transgenic mice (Siklós et al., 1998), and following injection of IgG from patients with sporadic ALS. Such endosomes were in contact with the extracellular space via a narrow channel. Thus, oculomotor neurons with ample levels of parvalbumin could resist the applied stress conditions, probably by specialized management of intracellular calcium.

The exact origin or identity of endosomes could not be determined. However, their development was probably connected to the peculiar modification of synaptic transmission in the oculomotor synapses. Stimulation of

nerve terminals has been reported to lead to a transient increase of endosome-like organelles, because of the different kinetics of exo- and endocytosis (Takei et al., 1996). Such vacuoles could possess very narrow channels communicating with the extracellular space (Gad et al., 1998), similar to the endosomes documented in our study. Since increased intracellular calcium has been demonstrated to hinder vesicle membrane retrieval in a graded fashion (von Gersdorff & Matthews, 1994; Brodin et al., 1997), differential formation of endosomes in vulnerable and resistant motoneurons could result from different ways of handling intracellular calcium possibly influenced by the calcium binding protein content. Indeed, in a recent study, Burrone and colleagues (2002) demonstrated that intracellular (endogenous) calcium buffers could decrease the release of vesicles towards the active zone, thus decreasing the size of the rapidly releasable pool of vesicles. The consequent saturation of the reserve pool of vesicles may favour a decreased rate of endocytosis and formation of a non-pinched off membrane-enclosed structure, i.e. endosome (Fig. 6.2). Alternatively, endosome-like structures may develop after prolonged stimulation (Leenders et al., 2002). Such stimulation could increase intracellular calcium triggered by increased glutamate excitotoxicity, increased oxidative stress, or ALS IgG (Smith et al., 1992). Thus endosomes may constitute an alternative route for vesicle recycling, probably to compensate for the exhaustion of the releasable pool of vesicles. If calcium binding proteins (i.e. endogenous calcium buffers) were present, the releasable pool would be exhausted faster (Burrone et al., 2002), and endosomes might develop preferentially at those axon terminals with larger calcium buffering capacity. If the membrane of such structures is constituted from that of synaptic vesicles, the incorporated ATP-ase in these structures (Michaelson et al., 1980) would facilitate the removal of the increased calcium load from the intracellular space. Accordingly, the presence of CaBPs could explain the ex vivo resistance of extraocular terminals to physiological effects of amyotrophic lateral sclerosis sera, i.e. differences in the frequency of spontaneous transmitter release, compared to motor axon terminals of spinal motor neurons (Mosier et al., 2000). These observations suggest that axon terminals with high CaBP content may develop a specialized mechanism against calcium load, which might be particularly important for motor neurons where axon terminals and cell bodies could be at large distances. However, so far, no direct evidence demonstrates that the presence of parvalbumin (or any other calcium binding protein) in oculomotor neurons is the sole factor responsible for the selective resistance of these motor neurons or their ability to handle an increased intracellular calcium load.

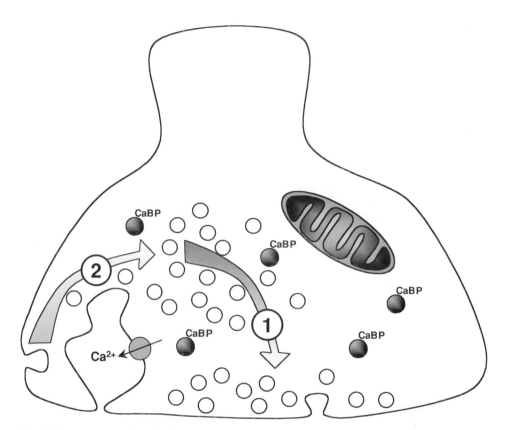

Fig. 6.2 Endogenous calcium buffers (CaBP) in axon terminals could retard vesicle mobilization to the active zone (1). The consequent saturation of the reserve pool of vesicles provides a negative feedback for recycling (2), which, in parallel with the exhaustion of the readily releasable pool of vesicles, facilitate the development of an alternative route of membrane retrieval. The calcium pump of endosomes would help to keep cytoplasmic calcium low.

Mechanism of protection of motor neurons by calcium binding proteins: cell bodies

The basic principles of the protection of motor neurons from calcium-mediated degeneration are summarized in Fig. 6.1, which models the potential neuroprotective effects of CaBPs. Such a model is supported by the differential survival of motor neurons and the parallel levels and distribution of intracellular calcium in the oculomotor nucleus and the spinal motor neurons of mutant SOD1 transgenic mice (Siklós et al., 1998). Although the exact mechanism of mutant SOD1 toxicity is still undefined (Cleveland & Liu, 2000; Cleveland & Rothstein, 2001), the interaction of altered calcium- and free radical homeostasis (Mattson, 1998) suggest that the presence of CaBP could be neuroprotective.

Direct electrophysiological evidence for differences in vulnerable and resistant motor neurons was provided by using the "added buffer" approach of Neher and Augustine (1992). With this technique to monitor "calcium buffering" Keller's laboratory was able to document that calcium binding ratios were five- to sixfold greater in oculomotor neurons than in spinal motor neurons (Vanselow & Keller, 2000). Prolonged Ca recovery times were noted in oculomotor neurons, in contrast to spinal motor neurons that had more rapid recovery times.

The proposed synergetic effect of free radical and calcium homeostasis (Mattson, 1998) prompted us to study the calcium distribution in SOD1 knockout animals, which, though, more prone to injury, develop normally (Reaume et al., 1996). We noted a selective age-dependent increase of calcium levels of spinal motoneurons compared with oculomotor neurons in wild-type animals (Siklós et al., 2000), supporting the notion of altered calcium homeostasis with aging (Kirischuk & Verkhratsky, 1996; Verkhratsky & Toescu, 1998). Lack of such changes in oculomotor neurons suggests that stabilization of calcium homeostasis during aging, associated with the presence of calcium binding proteins, might enhance neuroprotection (Clementi et al., 1996).

An unexpected finding of the present experiments was the relative decrease of calcium from the ER stores and the cytoplasm of spinal motor neurons of SOD1 knockout animals compared to age-matched controls. No such changes were noted in oculomotor neurons. These data suggest that decrements in the free-radical defense system could selectively impair calcium homeostasis in neurons with presumably lower calcium buffer capacity. Recent physiological and anatomical characterization of SOD1 knockout mice revealed a slow development of a mild, chronic peripheral hindlimb axonopathy and a moderate decline in motor unit number, suggesting impaired sprouting (D. Flood & J. Shefner, personal communication). This finding is in accord with the reduction of calcium in spinal motor neurons, since suitable intracellular calcium levels and intact intracellular stores are known to be necessary for synapse remodeling and neurite elongation (Kocsis et al., 1993; Mattson & Kater, 1987; Suarez-Isla et al., 1984). The protection of oculomotor neurons, particularly their internal stores from such a decrease of intracellular calcium could be explained on the basis of their higher CaBP content, as proposed by Hofer et al. (1998), assuming that Ca^{2+} released from the stores can be captured immediately and recycled into the stores by CaBPs (see Fig. 6.1).

In vitro transfection study

To test the protective effects of CaBP directly, we used our motor neuron cell line (VSC 4.1 cell line) and studied the effects of purified IgG from sporadic ALS patients on cellular viability and physiological properties (Smith et al., 1994). Cytotoxicity of ALS IgG in these cells was associated with increased calcium currents through voltage-gated calcium channels (Mosier et al., 1995). Furthermore, with direct calcium imaging by laser scanning confocal microscopy, it was demonstrated that ALS IgG could induce transient increases in the intracellular calcium level, with amplitudes proportional to the cytotoxic potential of the actual IgG preparation (Colom et al., 1997). The initial transient increase in calcium was clearly different from the later sustained increases in calcium, which appeared to accompany actual cell degeneration. This initial signaling of subsequent cell injury is also a hallmark of glutamate-induced cell degeneration (Tymianski, et al. 1993). The cytotoxicity of VSC 4.1 cells with ALS IgG was only noted in differentiated cells with low calbindin-D_{28k} content. When calbindin-D_{28k} expression was increased following retroviral infection of VSC 4.1 cells, the ALS IgG was no longer toxic. When calbindin-D_{28k} antisense oligonucleotides were injected into the cells, the calbindin-D_{28k}

content was decreased markedly, and the toxic effects of ALS IgG were restored (Ho et al., 1996). Similar neuroprotective effects of calbindin-D_{28k} in cell culture were documented by Roy et al. (1998). More recently, Van Den Bosch et al. (2002) have documented that the application of kainic acid results in marked increases in intracellular calcium leading to subsequent motor neuron death, which can be relatively protected by overexpression of parvalbumin.

In vivo studies

To study the effects of CaBP in vivo, transgenic animals were developed with increased expression of parvalbumin in their motor neurons (Beers et al., 2001). A rat calmodulin II (CaMII) promoter was employed because it has been shown to promote β-galactosidase expression in embryonic and adult mouse neurons. Transgenic lines (two altogether) were bred to homozygosity and determined to contain eight to ten integrated copies of the CaMII/parvalbumin construct. Presence of parvalbumin was confirmed by in situ hybridization and immunocytochemistry in ventral horn neurons of the lumbar section of the spinal cord. None of the parvalbumin transgenic mice exhibited ALS-like signs of weakness or paralysis, or died prematurely. When homozygous PV+ mice (eight to ten copies of parvalbumin construct) were injected intraperitoneally with immunoglobulins from ALS patients, neither elevation of the calcium content of the motor neurons, nor increase in the frequency of the spontaneous trasmitter release were noted. Similar treatments increased calcium in wild-type animals. Thus the increased parvalbumin expression in spinal motor neurons completely prevented the increased intracellular calcium noted in motor axon terminals.

When mice with mutant SOD1 (mSOD1) transgenic mice with the $G^{93}A$ mutation were bred to the parvalbumin transgenic mice (PV+ × mSOD1), we noted increased preservation of spinal neurons (by approximately 33%), a delayed disease onset (by 17%) and a prolonged survival (by 11%), compared to mSOD1 mice. These modest effects were in marked contrast to the complete blockade of increased calcium following injection of ALS IgG. One potential explanation for the discrepancy may relate to the fact that homozygous PV transgenic mice with high integrated PV copy number were used for the IgG experiments, while hemizygous mice with low integrated PV copy number were studied in the PV/mSOD1 transgenic mice. The moderate protective effect of the upregulation of PV on motoneuron survival in the familial ALS model suggests that a focus on motor neurons alone is insufficient. We must also consider the maintenance of calcium homeostasis in cells such as neighboring glia which can certainly contribute significantly to motor neuron viability.

Stress-related changes of CaBPs in motoneurons and glial cells

The traditional tool to study physiological and cellular reactions during degeneration – axotomy (Koliatsos & Price, 1996) – revealed that a certain number of the surviving motor neurons in the hypoglossal nucleus (Krebs et al., 1997; Dassesse et al., 1998) and in the spinal cord of the operated rats (Fallah & Clowry, 1999) respond to stress with increased levels of CaBPs. The upregulation of CaBP expression was explained as a self-protective mechanism to facilitate the survival of injured motoneurons by maintaining Ca^{2+} homeostasis. This concept was supported by axotomy experiments in mice (Obál, 2002) correlating changes of calcium- and CaBP levels in the oculomotor neurons (prototype of resistant neurons in ALS) and hypoglossal neurons (representing vulnerable cells in ALS). In the oculomotor nucleus, CaBP-staining was significantly increased in the perikarya, in contrast to the hypoglossal nucleus, in which the elevated staining intensity was localized primarily to the neuropil, with no, or only occasional, staining of the cell bodies. Accordingly, by electron microscopy changes in intracellular calcium in oculomotor neurons were small, demonstrating only a fast transient increase, while in hypoglossal neurons, calcium levels were markedly increased and lasted considerably longer.

There is increasing evidence in ALS that motor neurons do not die by themselves but require other cells: the process is non-cell autonomous (Clement et al., 2003). In mutant SOD1 transgenic mice, which are models of familial ALS, neither the neuron-specific expression of the mutant SOD1 (Lino et al., 2002; Pramatarova et al., 2001), nor astrocyte-specific expression of mSOD1 (Gong et al., 2000) induced the degeneration of motor neurons. Furthermore, studies of chimeric mice confirm the non-cell autonomy of motor neuron cell death, and support the potential participation of glia in motor neuron degeneration (Clement et al., 2003).

Indeed, as demonstrated in the model of fALS, astrocytes are exposed to oxidative stress, leading to their injury and manifested in the loss/inactivation of the (EAAT2) glutamate transporter (Trotti et al., 1999; Howland et al., 2002), which increases the likelihood of further excitotoxicity. The phenotypic transformation of spinal cord astrocytes, triggered either directly by oxidative stress (Cassina et al., 2002), or by excess calcium influx (Du et al., 1999), may lead to a loss of astrocytic functions including buffering potassium and glutamate, as well as inhibiting feedback control of microglial NO release, and thereby aggravating neuronal damage (Schubert et al., 2001). The importance of calcium influx in altering astrocytic function is highlighted by the findings that astrocytic transformation/reactive gliosis could be minimized by the L-type Ca^{2+} channel blocker, nifedipine (Du et al., 1999). Furthermore, under certain experimental conditions (3-nitropropionic acid stress), astrocytes proved to be even more sensitive to calcium overload than neurons (Fukuda et al., 1998).

S100 is a family of CaBPs which are localized mainly to glial cells in the nervous system. They have a wide range of effects, which are still not completely understood (Rothermundt et al., 2003). It is possible that under conditions of stress, astrocytes utilize a similar defense tool as neurons, i.e. they overexpress their available (naturally occurring) CaBPs to attenuate the effect of the calcium overload. Accordingly, upregulation of S100β was documented in astrocytes in the spinal cord of ALS patients (Migheli et al., 1999). Furthermore, in parallel studies on ALS patients and SOD1 transgenic mice S100A overexpression was also documented (Hoyaux et al., 2000, 2002). In wobbler mice, another model of motor neuron degeneration, the distribution of S100β overexpressing astrocytes paralleled the presence of neurons showing oxidative damage (Corvino et al., 2003).

Although the contribution of elevated glial Ca^{2+} in the degenerative process has not been proven definitely, these findings highlight the potential contribution of calcium-mediated damage of astrocytes in the pathogenesis of motor neuron injury in ALS. Such data also highlights the protective effects of astrocytes, and the need to guard the guardians. The combination of interventions aiming to improve the defense mechanisms against calcium-mediated injury in astrocytes as well as in motor neurons might yield more effective overall neuroprotection.

Neuroprotective role of CaBPs in other systems

Diverse studies have suggested that CaBPs may exert a general neuroprotective effect in neurodegenerative diseases. The concept was supported by the observation of age-dependent decline of expression of calcium binding proteins, particularly calbindin-D_{28k} (Iacopino & Christakos, 1990; Potier et al., 1994; Villa et al., 1994; Amenta et al., 1994; Kishimoto et al., 1998), and by recognizing that calbindin-D_{28k} could protect cells from excitotoxicity in a wide variety of in vitro systems (Mattson et al., 1991; Lledo et al., 1992; Clementi et al., 1996; McMahon et al., 1998). Other supportive in vivo studies demonstrated increased survival

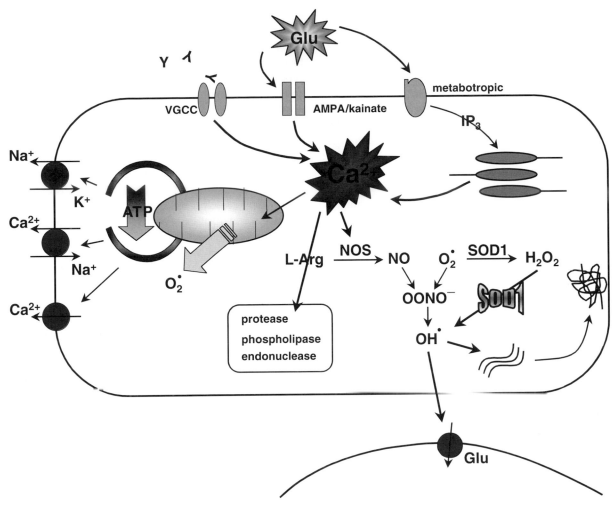

Fig. 6.3 Calcium-dependent mechanisms of motoneuronal degeneration integrating different models of ALS. If intracellular calcium is increased, several direct (proteases, phopholipases, endonucleases) and indirect destructive mechanisms (production of free radicals) are initiated. Normally, free radicals are neutralized by appropriate components of the cellular defense system. However, the presence of mutant SOD1 results in a series of toxic reactions, which damage cytoskeletal components, as well as pumps/transport molecules (e.g. glutamate transporters) on neighboring glia. Impaired glutamate glial uptake could lead to increased glutamate available to stimulate AMPA/kainate receptors, and further increase intracellular calcium. The mechanism might be amplified by calcium influx through voltage-gated calcium channels due to IgG, and release of calcium from intracellular stores as a consequence of activation of metabotropic receptors. If the calcium increase endures, it might overwhelm extrusion pumps and intracellular organelles, particularly mitochondria. Such increased calcium might impair mitochondrial function, leading to overproduction of free radicals, and depletion of ATP. Finally, if not interrupted, the process may culminate in the opening of the mitochondrial megachannel leading to apoptotic or necrotic cell death, depending on the energy actually available.

of neurons containing calbindin-D_{28k} (Rami *et al.*, 1992), or parvalbumin (Tortosa & Ferrer, 1993) after ischemia, or deafferentation (Beck *et al.*, 1994).

Studies aiming to correlate calcium binding protein content of neurons in affected brain regions and the degree of degeneration revealed positive correlations in Parkinson's and Alzheimer's disease. Calretinin-containing neurons were resistant to intrastriatal 6-hydroxydopamine

lesions (Tsuboi *et al.*, 2000), and calbindin-D_{28k} containing substantia nigra dopamine neurons are relatively spared in Parkinson's disease (Yamada *et al.*, 1990). Similarly, parvalbumin immunoreactive neurons in the neocortex of patients with Alzheimer's disease were relatively resistant to degeneration (Ferrer *et al.*, 1991; Hof *et al.*, 1991). Further indirect evidence for the protective role of PV or calbindin-D_{28k} is derived from studies on transgenic animals expressing the spinocerebellar ataxia-1 gene, which demonstrate that the reduced immunoreactivity to CaBPs in Purkinje cells precedes the onset of ataxia and loss of Purkinje cells (Vig *et al.*, 1998). Not all studies support the protective role of CaBPs. For example, it was claimed that the presence of calbindin-D_{28k} may not be relevant to the pathogenesis of Parkinson's disease (McRitchie & Halliday, 1995). Freund *et al.* (1990) reported the lack of a consistent and systematic relationship between neuronal calbindin-D_{28k} or parvalbumin content and ischemic vulnerability in different brain regions. Hartley *et al.* (1996) reported that increased expression of parvalbumin in cultured cortical neurons using a HSV-1 vector system actually enhanced NMDA neurotoxicity. Furthermore, Klapstein *et al.* (1998) demonstrated that hippocampal neurons in calbindin-D_{28k} knockout mice with reduced calcium buffering capacity were relatively protected against calcium-mediated damage. Thus, the relative protective role of calbindin-D_{28k} and parvalbumin in motor neurons does not necessarily extend to other neuronal systems. The neuroprotective effects of CaBP may depend on the nature of the insult, and the unique intrinsic, e.g. particular CaBP compositions/content (Parvizi *et al.*, 2003) or network properties of the affected neurons. To clarify these discrepancies, the specific modulatory effects of CaBP must be defined in each class of neurons, and determinations made as to whether CaBP specifically modify voltage-gated channels, ligand-gated channels (such as the AMPA/kainate receptor), Ca ATPases, or other structural and functional properties.

Conclusions: calcium-mediated degeneration of motor neurons

Increased intracellular calcium appears to be the key factor in coupling different pathways to cell destruction in models of ALS. Thus, stabilization of motoneuronal calcium homeostasis could be a potential tool to increase motor neuron resistance to stress. The summary of our present concept is illustrated in Fig. 6.3.

The proposed model addresses an increasing number of literature data documenting the interplay of some of the individual mechanisms, assuming a calcium-dependent link (see e.g. La Bella *et al.*, 1997; Roy *et al.*, 1998). Furthermore, the data suggest that degeneration of motor neurons could be attenuated by increasing the levels of calcium binding proteins in vulnerable motor neurons. It is important, however, that these neurons could not be ultimately rescued, which is in accord with the observation that certain motor functions such as eye muscles and voluntary

sphincter functions are only relatively spared (Bergmann *et al.*, 1995). This failure to completely prevent ultimate motor neuron injury could be the consequence of failing to address all of the cellular participants of the destructive process during the in vivo attempts of neuroprotection, or it could be the consequence of the role of the calcium binding proteins as calcium buffers. By definition, all buffers would be saturated sooner or later, if the stress signal endures. Nevertheless, CaBPs, considered as "buffers," could minimize the calcium-mediated pathological mechanisms and slow progression, but the loop could not be broken, or the mechanism halted. To be effective, therapy must be initiated at early stages prior to the start of irreversible changes in the cells and organelles. The goal then would be to delay injury in spinal motor neurons and provide the same relative neuroprotection that is present in relatively resistant motor neurons. Even achieving that goal would be worthwhile.

Acknowledgements

We acknowledge the support from the Muscular Dystrophy Association, the National Scientific Research Fund of Hungary (T 034314) and the Hungarian Ministry of Health (T04/001/2000).

REFERENCES

Adalbert, R. J., Engelhardt, J. I. & Siklós, L. (2002). DL-homocysteic acid application disrupts calcium homeostasis and induces degeneration of spinal motoneurons *in vivo*. *Acta Neuropathol.*, **103**, 428–36.

Alexianu, M. E., Ho, B. K., Mohamed, H., La Bella, V., Smith, R. G. & Appel, S. H. (1994). The role of calcium-binding proteins in selective motoneuron vulnerability in amyotrophic lateral sclerosis. *Ann. Neurol.*, **36**, 846–58.

Amenta, F., Cavalotta, D., Del Valle, M. E. *et al.* (1994). Calbindin D-28k immunoreactivity in the rat cerebellar cortex: age-related changes. *Neurosci. Lett.*, **178**, 131–4.

Appel, S. H., Beers, D., Siklós, L., Engelhardt J. I. & Mosier, D. R. (2001). Calcium: the Darth Vader of ALS. *ALS Other Motor Neuron Disord.*, **2**, S47–54.

Baimbridge, K. G., Celio, M. R. & Rogers, J. H. (1992). Calcium-binding proteins in the nervous system. *Trends Neurosci.*, **15**, 303–8.

Beck, K. D., Hefti, F. & Widmer, H. R. (1994). Deafferentation removes calretinin immunopositive terminals, but does not induce degeneration of calbindin D-28k and parvalbumin expressing neurons in the hippocampus of adult rats. *J. Neurosci. Res.*, **39**, 298–304.

Beers, D. R., Ho, B. K., Siklós, L. *et al.* (2001). Parvalbumin over-expression alters immune-mediated increases in intracellular calcium, and delays disease onset in a transgenic model of familial amyotrophic lateral sclerosis. *J. Neurochem.*, **79**, 499–509.

Bergmann, M., Volpel, M. & Kuchelmeister, K. (1995). Onuf's nucleus is frequently involved in motor neuron disease/ amyotrophic lateral sclerosis. *J. Neurol. Sci.*, **129**, 141–6.

Bernardi, P. (1999). Mitochondrial transport of cations: channels, exchangers, and permeability transition. *Physiol. Rev.*, **79**, 1127–55.

Berridge, M. J. (1998). Neuronal calcium signaling. *Neuron*, **21**, 13–26.

Berridge, M. J., Bootman, M. D. & Lipp, P. (1998). Calcium – a life and death signal. *Nature*, **395**, 645–8.

Berridge, M. J., Lipp, P. & Bootman, M. D. (2000). The versatility and universality of calcium signalling. *Nat. Rev.*, **1**, 11–21.

Brini, M. & Carafoli, E. (2000). Calcium signalling: a historical account, recent developments and future perspectives. *Cell Mol. Life. Sci.*, **57**, 354–70.

Brini, M., Bano, D., Manni, S., Rizzuto, R. & Carafoli, E. (2000). Effects of PMCA and SERCA pump overexpression on the kinetics of cell Ca^{2+} signalling. *EMBO J.*, **19**, 4926–35.

Brodin, L., Löw, P., Gad, H., Gustaffson, J., Pieribone, V. A. & Shupliakov, O. (1997). Sustained neurotransmitter release: new molecular clues. *Eur. J. Neurosci.*, **9**, 2503–11.

Brustovetsky, N., Brustovetsky, T., Jemmerson, R. & Dubinsky, J. M. (2002). Calcium-induced cytochrome C release from CNS mitochondria is associated with the permeability transition and rupture of the outer membrane. *J. Neurochem.*, **80**, 207–18.

Burrone, J., Guilherme, N., Gomis, A., Cooke, A. & Lagnado, L. (2002). Endogenous calcium buffers regulate fast exocytosis in the synaptic terminal of retinal bipolar cells. *Neuron.*, **33**, 101–12.

Carafoli, E. & Stauffer, T. (1994). The plasma membrane calcium pump: functional domains, regulation of the activity, and tissue specificity of isoform expression. *J. Neurobiol.*, **25**, 312–24.

Cassina, P., Peluffo, H., Pehar, M. *et al.* (2002). Peroxynitrite triggers a phenotypic transformation in spinal cord astrocytes that induces motor neuron apoptosis. *J. Neurosci. Res.*, **67**, 21–9.

Celio, M. (1990). Calbindin D-28k and parvalbumin in the rat nervous system. *Neuroscience*, **35**, 375–475.

Cheung, W. Y. (1980). Calmodulin plays a pivotal role in cellular regulation. *Science*, **207**, 19–27.

Choi, D. W., Maulucci-Gedde, M. & Kriegstein, A. R. (1987). Glutamate neurotoxicity in cortical cell ulture. *J. Neurosci.*, **7**, 357–68.

Clapham, D. E. (1995). Calcium signaling. *Cell*, **80**, 259–68.

Clement, A. M., Nguyen, M. D., Roberts, E. A. *et al.* (2003). Wild-type nonneural cells extend survival of SOD1 mutant motor neurons in ALS mice. *Science*, **302**, 113–17.

Clementi, E., Racchetti, G., Melino, G. & Meldolesi, J. (1996). Cytosolic Ca^{2+} buffering, a cell property that in some

neurons markedly decreases during aging, has a protective effect against NMDA/nitric oxide-induced excitotoxicity. *Life Sci.*, **59**, 389–97.

Cleveland, D. W. (1999). From Charcot to SOD1: mechanisms of selective motor neuron death in ALS. *Neuron*, **24**, 515–20.

Cleveland, D. W. & Liu, J. (2000). Oxidation versus aggregation – how do SOD1 mutants cause ALS? *Nat. Med.*, **6**, 1320–1.

Cleveland, D. W. & Rothstein, J. D. (2001). From Charcot to Lou Gehrig: deciphering selective motor neuron death in ALS. *Nat. Rev. Neurosci.*, **2**, 806–19.

Colom, L. V., Alexianu, M. E., Mosier, D. R., Smith, R. G. & Appel, S. H. (1997). Amyotrophic lateral sclerosis immunoglobulins increase intracellular calcium in a motoneuron cell line. *Exp. Neurol.*, **146**, 354–60.

Corvino, V., Businaro, R., Geloso, M. C. *et al.* (2003). S100B protein and 4-hydroxynonenal in the spinal cord of wobbler mice. *Neurochem. Res.*, **28**, 341–5.

Cox, D. A. & Matlib, M. A. (1993). Modulation of intramitochondrial free Ca^{2+} concentration by antagonists of Na^{+}–Ca^{2+} exchange. *Trends Pharm. Sci.*, **14**, 408–13.

Dassesse, D., Cuvelier, L., Krebs, C. *et al.* (1998). Differential expression of calbindin and calmodulin in motoneurons after hypoglossal axotomy. *Brain Res.*, **786**, 181–8.

Du, S., Rubin, A., Klepper, S. *et al.* (1999). Calcium influx and activation of calpain I mediate acute reactive gliosis in injured spinal cord. *Exp. Neurol.*, **157**, 96–105.

Engelhardt, J. I., Siklós, L., Kőműves, L., Smith, R. G. & Appel, S. H. (1995). Antibodies to calcium channels from ALS patients passively transferred to mice selectively increase intracellular calcium and induce ultrastructural changes in motor neurons. *Synapse*, **20**, 185–99.

Elliott, J. L. & Snider, W. D. (1995). Parvalbumin is a marker of ALS-resistant motor neurons. *NeuroReport*, **6**, 449–52.

Fallah, Z. & Clowry, G. J. (1999). The effect of a peripheral nerve lesion on calbindin D28k immunoreactivity in the cervical ventral horn of developing and adult rats. *Exp. Neurol.*, **156**, 111–20.

Ferrer, I., Soriano, E., Tunon, T., Fonseca, M. & Guionnet, N. (1991). Parvalbumin immunoreactive neurons in normal human temporal neocortex and in patients with Alzheimer's disease. *J. Neurol. Sci.*, **106**, 135–41.

Freund, T. F., Buzsáki, G., Leon, A., Baimbridge, K. G. & Somogyi, P. (1990). Relationship of neural vulnerability and calcium binding protein immunoreactivity in ischemia. *Exp. Brain. Res.*, **83**, 55–66.

Fukuda, A., Deshpande, S. B., Shimano, Y. & Nishino, H. (1998). Astrocytes are more vulnerable than neurons to cellular Ca^{2+} overload induced by a mitochondrial toxin, 3-nitropropionic acid. *Neuroscience*, **87**, 497–507.

Gad, H., Löw, P., Zotova, E., Brodin, L. & Shupliakov, O. (1998). Dissociation between Ca^{2+}-triggered synaptic vesicle exocytosis and clathrin-mediated endocytosis at a central synapse. *Neuron*, **21**, 607–16.

Gong, Y. H., Parsadanian, A. S., Andreeva, A., Snider, W. D. & Elliott, J. S. (2000). Restricted expression of G86R Cu/Zn superoxide dismutase in astrocytes results in astrocytosis but does not cause motoneuron degeneration. *J. Neurosci.*, **20**, 660–5.

Gunter, T. E. & Pfeiffer, D. R. (1990). Mechanisms by which mitochondria transport calcium. *Am. J. Physiol.*, **27**, C755–86.

Gunter, T. E., Buntinas, L., Sparagne, G. C. & Gunter, K. K. (1998). The Ca^{2+} transport mechanism of mitochondria and Ca^{2+} uptake from physiological-type Ca^{2+} transients. *Biochim. Biophys. Acta*, **1366**, 5–15.

Gurney, M. E., Pu, H., Chiu, A. Y. *et al.* (1994). Motor neuron degeneration in mice that express a human Cu, Zn superoxide dismutase mutation. *Science*, **164**, 1772–5.

Hartley, D. M., Neve, R. L., Bryan, J. *et al.* (1996). Expression of the calcium-binding protein, parvalbumin, in cultured cortical neurons using a HSV-1 vector system enhances NMDA neurotoxicity. *Brain Res. Mol. Brain Res.*, **40**, 285–96.

Ho, B. K., Alexianu, M. E., Colom, L. V., Mohamed, A. H., Serrano, F. & Appel, S. H. (1996). Expression of calbindin-D_{28K} in motoneuron hybrid cells after retroviral infection with calbindin-D_{28K} cDNA prevents amyotrophic lateral sclerosis IgG-mediated cytotoxicity. *Proc. Natl Acad. Sci., USA*, **93**, 6796–801.

Hof, P. R., Cox, K., Young, W. G., Celio, M. R., Rogers, J. & Morrison, J. H. (1991). Parvalbumin-immunoreactive neurons in the neocortex are resistant to degeneration in Alzheimer's disease. *J. Neuropathol. Exp. Neurol.*, **50**, 451–62.

Hofer, A. M., Landolfi, B., Debellis, L., Pozzan, T. & Curci, S. (1998). Free $[Ca^{2+}]$ dynamics measured in agonist-sensitive strores of single living intact cells: a new look at the refilling process. *EMBO J.*, **17**, 1986–95.

Howland, D. S., Liu, J., She, Y. *et al.* (2002). Focal loss of the glutamate transporter EAAT2 in a transgenic rat model of SOD1 mutant-mediated amyotrophic lateral sclerosis (ALS). *Proc. Natl Acad. Sci. USA*, **99**, 1604–9.

Hoyaux, D., Alao, J., Fuchs, J. *et al.* (2000). S100A6, a calcium- and zinc-binding protein, is overexpressed in SOD1 mutant mice, a model for amyotrophic lateral sclerosis. *Biochim. Biophys. Acta*, **1498**, 264–72.

Hoyaux, D., Boom, A., Van den Bosch, L. *et al.* (2002). S100A6 overexpression within astrocytes associated with impaired axons from both ALS mouse model and human patients. *J. Neuropathol. Exp. Neurol.*, **61**, 736–44.

Iacopino, A. M. & Christakos, S. (1990). Specific reduction of calcium-binding protein (28-kilodalton calbindin-D) gene expression in aging and neurodegenerative diseases. *Proc. Natl Acad. Sci., USA*, **87**, 4078–82.

Ince, P., Stout, N., Shaw, P. *et al.* (1993). Parvalbumin and calbindin D-28k in the human motor system and in motor neuron disease. *Neuropathol. Appl. Neurobiol.*, **19**, 291–9.

Julien, J. P. (2001). Amyotrophic lateral sclerosis: unfolding the toxicity of the misfolded. *Cell*, **104**, 581–91.

Kawasaki, H., Nakayama, S. & Kretsinger, R. H. (1998). Classification and evolution of EF-hand proteins. *BioMetals*, **11**, 277–95.

Kirischuk, S. & Verkhratsky, A. (1996). Calcium homostasis in aged neurons. *Life Sci.*, **59**, 451–9.

Kishimoto, J., Tsuchiya, T., Cox, H., Emson, P. C. & Nakayama, Y. (1998). Age-related changes of calbindin-D28k, calretinin, and parvalbumin mRNAs in the hamster brain. *Neurobiol. Aging*, **19**, 77–82.

Klapstein, G. J., Vietla, S., Lieberman, D. N. *et al.* (1998). Calbindin-D28k fails to protect hippocampal neurons against ischemia in spite of its cytoplasmic calcium buffering properties: evidence from calbindin-D28k knockout mice. *Neuroscience*, **85**, 361–73.

Kocsis, J. D., Rand, M. N., Lankford, K. L. & Waxman, S. G. (1993). Intracellular calcium mobilization and neurite outgrowth in mammalian neurons. *J. Neurobiol.*, **25**, 252–64.

Koliatsos, V. E. & Price, D. L. (1996). Axotomy as an experimental model of neuronal injury and cell death. *Brain Pathol.*, **6**, 447–65.

Krebs, C., Neiss, W. F., Streppel, M. *et al.* (1997). Axotomy induces transient calbindin D28K immunoreactivity in hypoglossal motoneurons in vivo. *Cell Calcium*, **22**, 367–72.

Kroemer, G., Dallaporta, B. & Resche-Rigon, M. (1998). The mitochondrial death/life regulator in apoptosis and necrosis. *Ann. Rev. Physiol.*, **60**, 619–42.

La Bella, V., Goodman, J. C. & Appel, S. H. (1997). Increased CSF glutamate following injection of ALS immunoglobulins. *Neurology*, **48**, 1270–2.

Laslo, P., Lipski, J., Nicholson, L. F. B., Miles, G. B. & Funk, G. D. (2000). Calcium binding proteins in motoneurons at low and high risk for degeneration in ALS. *NeuroReport*, **11**, 3305–8.

(2001). GluR2 AMPA receptor subunit expression in motoneurons at low and high risk for degeneration in amyotrophic lateral sclerosis. *Exp. Neurol.*, **169**, 461–71.

Leenders, A. G. M., Scholten, G., De Lange, R. P. J., Lopes da Silva, F. H. & Ghijsen, W. E. J. M. (2002). Sequential changes in synaptic vesicle pools and endosome-like organelles during depolarization near the active zone of central nerve terminals. *Neuroscience*, **109**, 195–206.

Lewit-Bentley, A. & Réty, S. (2000). EF-hand calcium-binding proteins. *Curr. Opin. Struct. Biol.*, **10**, 637–43.

Lino. M. M., Schneider, C. & Caroni, P. (2002). Accumulation of SOD1 mutants in postnatal motoneurons does not cause motoneuron pathology or motoneuron disease. *J. Neurosci.*, **22**, 4825–32.

Lledo, P. M., Somasundaram, B., Morton, A. J., Emson, P. C. & Mason, W. T. (1992). Stable transfection of calbindin-D_{28k} into the GH_3 cell line alters calcium currents and intracellular calcium homeostasis. *Neuron*, **9**, 943–54.

Marsden, B. J., Shaw, G. S. & Sykes, B. D. (1990). Calcium binding proteins. Elucidating the contributions to calcium affinity from an analysis of species variants and peptide fragments. *Biochem. Cell. Biol.*, **68**, 587–601.

Mattson, M. P. (1998). Free radicals, calcium, and the synaptic plasticity – cell death continuum: emerging role of the transcription factor NFκB. *Int. Rev. Neurobiol.*, **49**, 103–68.

Mattson, M. P. & Kater, S. B. (1987). Calcium regulation of neurite elongation and growth cone mobility. *J. Neurosci.*, **7**, 4034–43.

Mattson, M. P., Rychlik, B., Chu, C. & Christakos, S. (1991). Evidence for calcium-reducing and excito-protective roles for the calcium-binding protein calbindin-D_{28k} in cultured hippocampal neurons. *Neuron*, **6**, 41–51.

McMahon, A., Wong, B. S., Iacopino, A. M., Ng, M. C., Chi, S. & German, D. C. (1998). Calbindin-D_{28k} buffers intracellular calcium and promotes resistance to degeneration in PC12 cells. *Mol. Brain Res.*, **54**, 56–63.

McRitchie, D. A. & Halliday, G. M. (1995). Calbindin D_{28k}-containing neurons are restricted to the medial substantia nigra in humans. *Neuroscience*, **65**, 87–91.

Means, A. R., Tash, J. S. & Chafouleas, J. G. (1982). Physiological implications of the presence, distribution and regulation of calmodulin in eukaryotic cells. *Physiol. Rev.*, **62**, 1–39.

Meldolesi, J. (2001). Rapidly exchanging Ca^{2+} stores in neurons: molecular, structural and functional properties. *Prog. Neurobiol.*, **65**, 309–38.

Michaelson, D. M., Ophir, I. & Angel, I. (1980). ATP-stimulated Ca^{2+} transport into cholinergic *Torpedo* synaptic vesicles. *J. Neurochem.*, **35**, 116–24.

Migheli, A., Cordera, S., Bendotti, C., Atzori, C., Piva, R. & Schiffer, D. (1999). S-100B protein is upregulated in astrocytes and motor neurons in the spinal cord of patients with amyotrophic lateral sclerosis. *Neurosci. Lett.*, **261**, 25–8.

Miller, R. J. (1995). Regulation of calcium homeostasis in neurons: the role of calcium-binding proteins. *Biochem. Soc. Trans.*, **23**, 629–32.

(1998). Mitochondria – the Kraken wakes! *Trends Neurosci.*, **21**, 95–7.

Mogami, H., Nakano, K., Tepikin, A. V. & Petersen, O. H. (1997). Ca^{2+} flow via tunnels in polarized cells: recharging of apical Ca^{2+} stores by focal Ca^{2+} entry through basal membrane patch. *Cell*, **88**, 49–55.

Morrison, B. M., Janssen, W. G., Gordon, J. W. & Morrison, J. H. (1998). Light and electron microscopic distribution of the AMPA receptor subunit GluR2 in the spinal cord of control and G86R mutant superoxide dismutase transgenic mice. *J. Comp. Neurol.*, **395**, 523–34.

Mosier, D. R., Baldelli, P., Delbono, O. *et al.* (1995). Amyotrophic lateral sclerosis immunoglobulins increase Ca^{2+} currents in a motoneuron cell line. *Ann. Neurol.*, **37**, 102–9.

Mosier, D. R., Siklós, L. & Appel, S. H. (2000). Resistance of extraocular motoneuron terminals to effects of amyotrophic lateral sclerosis sera. *Neurology*, **54**, 252–5.

Murphy, A. N., Fiskum, G. & Beal, M. F. (1999). Mitochondria in neurodegeneration: Bioenergetic function in cell life and death. *J. Cereb. Blood Flow Metab.*, **19**, 231–45.

Neher, E. & Augustine, G. J. (1992). Calcium gradients and buffers in bovine chromaffin cells. *J. Physiol.*, **450**, 273–301.

Nicotera, P. & Orrenius, S. (1998). The role of calcium in apoptosis. *Cell Calcium*, **23**, 173–80.

Obál, I. (2002). Immune-mediated damages and the role of intracellular calcium homeostasis in the degeneration of neurons. PhD Thesis, University of Szeged, Hungary.

Parvizi, J. & Damasio, A. R. (2003). Differential distribution of calbindin D28k and parvalbumin among functionally distinctive sets of structures in the macaque brainstem. *J. Comp. Neurol.*, **462**, 153–67.

Paschen, W. & Doutheil, J. (1999). Disturbances of the functioning of endoplasmic reticulum: a key mechanism underlying neuronal cell injury? *J. Cereb. B F Metab.*, **19**, 1–18.

Potier, B., Krzywkowski, P., Lamour, Y. & Dutar, P. (1994). Loss of calbindin-immunoreactivity in CA1 hippocampal stratum radiatum and lacunosum-moleculare interneurons in the aged rat. *Brain Res.*, **661**, 181–8.

Pozzan, T., Rizzuto, R., Volpe, P. & Meldolesi, J. (1994). Molecular and cellular physiology of intracellular calcium stores. *Physiol. Rev.*, **74**, 595–636.

Pramatarova, A., Laganiere, J., Roussel, J., Brisebois, K. & Rouleau, G. A. (2001). Neuron-specific expression of mutant superoxide dismutase 1 in transgenic mice does not lead to motor impairment. *J. Neurosci.*, **21**, 3369–74.

Puchalski, R. B., Louis, J. C., Brose, N. *et al.* (1994). Selective RNA editing and subunit assembly of native glutamate receptor. *Neuron*, **13**, 131–47.

Pullen, A. H., Demestre, M., Howard, R. S. & Orrell, R. W. (2004). Passive transfer of purified IgG from patients with amyotrophic lateral sclerosis to mice results in degeneration of motor neurons accompamied by Ca^{2+} enhancement. *Acta Neuropathol.*, **107**, 35–46.

Pullen, A. H. & Humphreys, P. (2000). Ultrastructural analysis of spinal motoneurons from mice treated with IgG from ALS patients, healthy individuals, or disease controls. *J. Neurol. Sci.*, **180**, 35–45.

Rami, A., Rabié, A., Thomasset, M. & Krieglstein, J. (1992). Calbindin-D_{28K} and ischemic damage of pyramidal cells in rat hippocampus. *J. Neurosci. Res.*, **31**, 89–95.

Reaume, A. G., Elliott, J. L., Hoffman, E. K., *et al.* (1996). Motor neurons in Cu/Zn superoxide dismutase-deficient mice develop normally but exhibit enhanced cell death after axonal injury. *Nat. Genet.*, **13**, 43–7.

Reiner, A., Medina, L., Figueredo-Cardenas, G. & Anfinson, S. (1995). Brainstem motoneuron pools that are selectively resistant in amyotrophic lateral sclerosis are preferentially enriched in parvalbumin: Evidence from monkey brainstem for a calcium-mediated mechanism in sporadic ALS. *Exp. Neurol.*, **131**, 239–50.

Ren, K. & Ruda, M. A. (1994). A comparative study of the calcium-binding proteins calbindin-D28K, calretinin, calmodulin and parvalbumin in the rat spinal cord. *Brain Res. Rev.*, **19**, 163–79.

Robb-Gaspers, L. D., Rutter, G. A., Burnett, P., Hajnóczky, G., Denton, R. M. & Thomas, A. P. (1998). Coupling between cytosolic and mitochondrial calcium oscillations: role in the regulation of hepatic metabolism. *Biochim. Biophys. Acta*, **1366**, 17–32.

Rothermundt, M., Peters, M., Prehn, J. H. & Arolt, V. (2003). S100B in brain damage and neuro-degeneration. *Microsc. Res. Tech.*, **60**, 614–32.

Rothstein, J. D. (1995). Excitotoxic mechanisms in the pathogenesis of amyotrophic lateral sclerosis. *Adv. Neurol.*, **68**, 7–20.

Rowland, L. P. (2000). Six important themes in amyotrophic lateral sclerosis (ALS) research, 1999. *J. Neurol. Sci.*, **180**, 2–6.

Rowland, L. P. & Shneider, N. A. (2001). Amyotrophic lateral sclerosis. *N. Engl. J. Med.*, **344**, 1688–700.

Roy, J., Minotti, S., Dong, L., Figlewicz, D. A. & Durham, H. D. (1998). Glutamate potentiates the toxicity of mutant Cu/Zn-superoxide dismutase in motor neurons by post-synaptic calcium-dependent mechanisms. *J. Neurosci.*, **18**, 9673–84.

Sattler, R. & Tymianski, M. (2000). Molecular mechanisms of calcium-dependent excitotoxicity. *J. Mol. Med.*, **78**, 3–13.

Schapira, A. H. V. (1998). Mitochondrial dysfunction in neurodegenerative disorders. *Biochim. Biophys. Acta*, **1366**, 225–33.

Schubert, P., Ogata, T., Marchini, C. & Ferroni, S. (2001). Glia-related pathomechanisms in Alzheimer's disease: a therapeutic target? *Mech. Ageing Dev.*, **123**, 47–57.

Shaw, P. J. & Eggett, C. J. (2000). Molecular factors underlying selective vulnerability of motor neurons to degeneration in amyotrophic lateral sclerosis. *J. Neurol.*, **247** (suppl 1), 17–27.

Siesjö, B. K., Hu, B. & Kristián, T. (1999). Is the cell death pathway triggered by the mitochondrion or the endoplasmic reticulum? *J. Cereb. Blood Flow Metab.*, **19**, 19–26.

Siklós, L., Engelhardt, J., Harati, Y., Smith, R. G., Joó, F. & Appel, S. H. (1996). Ultrastructural evidence for altered calcium in motor nerve terminals in amyotrophic lateral sclerosis. *Ann. Neurol.*, **39**, 203–16.

Siklós, L., Engelhardt, J. I., Alexianu, M. E., Gurney, M. E., Siddique, T. & Appel, S. H. (1998). Intracellular calcium parallels motor neuron degeneration in SOD-1 mutant mice. *J. Neuropathol. Exp. Neurol.*, **57**, 571–87.

Siklós, L., Engelhardt, J. I., Adalbert, R. & Appel, S. H. (1999). Calcium-containing endosomes at oculomotor terminals in animal models of ALS. *NeuroReport*, **10**, 2539–45.

Siklós, L., Engelhardt, J. I., Reaume, A. G. *et al.* (2000). Altered calcium homeostasis in spinal motoneurons but not in oculomotor neurons of SOD-1 knockout mice. *Acta Neuropathol.*, **99**, 517–24.

Smith, R. G., Hamilton, S., Hofmann, F. *et al.* (1992). Serum antibodies to L-type calcium channels in patients with amyotrophic lateral sclerosis. *N. Engl. J. Med.*, **327**, 1721–8.

Smith, R. G., Alexianu, M. E., Crawford, G., Nyormoi, O., Stefani, E. & Appel, S. H. (1994). The cytotoxicity of immunoglobulins from amyotrophic lateral sclerosis patients on an hybrid motoneuron cell line. *Proc. Natl Acad. Sci., USA*, **91**, 3393–7.

Suarez-Isla, B. A., Pelto, D. J., Thompson, J. M. & Rapoport, S. I. (1984). Blockers of calcium permeability inhibit neurite extension and formation of neuromuscular synapses in cell culture. *Dev. Brain Res.*, **14**, 263–70.

Swash, M. & Schwartz, M. S. (1995). Motor neuron disease: the clinical syndrome. In *Motor Neuron Disease. Biology and Management*, ed. P. N. Leigh & M. Swash. London, Berlin, Heidelberg, New York, Paris, Tokyo, Hong Kong, Barcelona, Budapest: Springer-Verlag. pp. 1–17.

Takei, K., Mundigl, O., Daniell, L. & De Camilli, P. (1996). The synaptic vesicle cycle: A single vesicle budding step involving clathrin and dynamin. *J. Cell. Biol.*, **133**, 1237–50.

Takuma, H., Kwak, S., Yoshizawa, T. & Kanazawa, I. (1999). Reduction of GluR2 RNA editing, a molecular change that increases calcium influx through AMPA receptors, selective in the spinal ventral gray of patients with amyotrophic lateral sclerosis. *Ann. Neurol.*, **46**, 806–15.

Trotti, D., Rolfs, A., Danbolt, N. C., Brown, Jr R. H. & Hediger, M. A. (1999). SOD1 mutant linked amyotrophic lateral sclerosis selectively inactivate a glial glutamate transporter. *Nat. Neurosci.*, **2**, 427–33.

Tortosa, A. & Ferrer, I. (1993). Parvalbumin immunoreactivity in the hippocampus of the gerbil after transient forebrain ischaemia: a qualitative and quantitative sequential study. *Neuroscience*, **55**, 33–43.

Tsuboi, K., Kimber, T. A. & Shults, C. W. (2000). Calretinin-containing axons and neurons are resistant to an intrastriatal 6-hydroxydopamine lesion. *Brain Res.*, **866**, 55–64.

Tymianski, M., Charlton, M. P., Carlen, P. L. & Tator, C. H. (1993). Source specificity of early calcium neurotoxicity in cultured embryonic spinal neurons. *J. Neurosci.*, **13**, 2085–114.

Vandenberghe, W., Robberecht, W. & Brorson, J. R. (2000). AMPA receptor calcium permeability, GluR2 expression, and selective motoneuron vulnerability. *J. Neurosci.*, **20**, 123–32.

Vandenberghe, W., Bindokas, V. P., Miller, R. J. *et al.* (2001). Subcellular localization of calcium permeable AMPA receptors in spinal motor neurons. *Eur. J. Neurosci.*, **14**, 305–14.

Van Den Bosch, L., Vandenberghe, W., Klaassen, H. *et al.* (2000). Ca^{2+}-permeable AMPA receptors and selective vulnerability of motor neurons. *J. Neurol. Sci.*, **180**, 29–34.

Van Den Bosch, L., Schwaller, B., Vleminckx, V. *et al.* (2002). Protective effect of parvalbumin on excitotoxic motor neuron death. *Exp. Neurol.*, **174**, 150–61.

Vanselow, B. K. & Keller, B. U. (2000). Calcium dynamics and buffering in oculomotor neurones from mouse that are particularly resistant during amyotrophic lateral sclerosis (ALS)-related motoneurone disease. *J. Physiol.*, **525**, 433–45.

Verkhratsky, A. & Toescu, E. C. (1998). Calcium and neuronal ageing. *Trends Neurosci.*, **21**, 2–7.

Vig, P. J. S., Subramony, S. H., Burright, E. N. *et al.* (1998). Reduced immunoreactivity to calcium binding proteins in Purkinje cells precedes onset of ataxia in spinocerebellar ataxia-1 transgenic mice. *Neurology*, **50**, 106–13.

Villa, A., Podini, P., Panzeri, M. C., Racchetti, G. & Meldolesi, J. (1994). Cytosolic Ca^{2+} binding proteins during rat brain ageing: Loss of calbindin and calretinin in the hippocampus, with no change in the cerebellum. *Eur. J. Neurosci.*, **6**, 1491–9.

Von Gersdorff, H. & Matthews, G. (1994). Inhibition of endocytosis by elevated internal calcium in synaptic terminal. *Nature*, **370**, 652–5.

Waisman, D. M., Smallwood, J. I., Lafreniere, D. & Rasmussen, H. (1983). Identification of novel calcium-binding proteins of heart and brain 1000,000 x G supernatant. *Biochem. Biophys. Res. Commun.*, **116**, 435–41.

Werth, J. L. & Thayer, S. A. (1994). Mitochondria buffer physiological calcium loads in cultured rat dorsal root ganglion neurons. *J. Neurosci.*, **14**, 348–56.

Williams, T. L., Day, N. C., Ince, P. G. *et al.* (1997). Calcium-permeable alpha-amino-3-hydroxy-5-methyl-4-isoxazole proprionic acid receptors: a molecular determinant of selective vulnerability in amyotrophic lateral sclerosis. *Ann. Neurol.*, **42**, 200–7.

Winsky, L. & Kuznicki, J. (1996). Antibody recognition of calcium-binding proteins depends on their calcium-binding status. *J. Neurochem.*, **66**, 764–71.

Yamada, T., McGeer, P. L., Baimbridge, K. G. & McGeer, E. G. (1990). Relative sparing in Parkinson's disease of substantia nigra dopamine neurons containing calbindin-D_{28k}. *Brain Res.*, **526**, 303–7.

Yap, K. L., Ames, J. B., Swindells, M. B. & Ikura, M. (1999). Diversity of conformational states and changes within the EF-hand protein superfamily. *Proteins*, **37**, 499–507.

7

Apoptosis in neurodegenerative diseases

Jörg B. Schulz

Department of Neurodegeneration and Restorative Research, University of Göttingen, Germany

Introduction

Although reports on the morphological characteristics of apoptosis in neurodegenerative diseases remain controversial, accumulating evidence suggests that the molecular and biochemical pathways of apoptosis are involved in neuronal death of various neurodegenerative disorders and in related cellular and animal models. This includes stroke, head trauma, Huntington's (HD), Parkinson's (PD), Alzheimer's disease (AD and amyotrophic lateral sclerosis (ALS)). This evidence includes the activation of the mitogen activated protein (MAP) kinase pathway, the induction of Bax, prostate apoptosis response-4 (Par-4) and glyceraldehyde-3-phosphate dehydrogenase (GAPDH), evidence of aberrant activation of the cell cycle machinery, and the activation of caspases. Caspases are the mammalian cell-death-effector proteins. They may have an important role in acute and chronic neurodegenerative diseases. They execute cell death but may also be linked to the initiation of chronic neurodegenerative diseases. Peptide or protein inhibitors of caspases protect neurons in vitro or in animal models of neurological disorders. Although preclinical results are promising, clinical studies have not been performed because of the lack of synthetic caspase inhibitors that cross the blood–brain barrier. Such agents are a major focus in current programs of drug development and will hopefully become available soon. However, in some cell culture and animal models caspase inhibitors block cell death but may result in survival of a dysfunctional neuron. In contrast, therapeutic interference with the signaling phase of apoptosis, e.g. inhibition of the MAP kinase pathway, or the combination of caspase inhibitors with neurotrophins may provide morphological and functional protection.

Apoptosis

Apoptosis is an important form of cell death characterized by a series of distinct morphological and biochemical alterations, suggesting the presence of a common execution machinery in different cells. Condensation and fragmentation of nuclear chromatin, compaction of cytoplasmic organelles, a decrease in cell volume and alterations to the plasma membrane are classically observed resulting in the recognition and phagocytosis of apoptotic cells. The nuclear alterations are often associated with internucleosomal cleavage of DNA, recognized as DNA laddering on conventional agarose gel electrophoresis. Internucleosomal cleavage of DNA is a relatively late event in the apoptotic process, which in some models of neuronal cell death may be dissociated from early critical steps (Yakovlev et al., 1997; Namura et al., 1998; Springer et al., 1999). Apoptosis is not restricted to nucleated cells (Kroemer, 1997). Nevertheless, detecting DNA fragmentation is simple and often used as a criterion to determine whether or not a cell is dying by apoptosis. Unfortunately, it is often overinterpreted and not without shortcomings. In addition, it has become clear that there is no clear-cut difference between necrosis and apoptosis. In addition, several forms of non-caspase-mediated forms of programmed cell death have been reported. Based on morphological grounds, one may differentiate (Leist & Jaattela, 2001) among

(i) classical apoptosis,
(ii) apoptosis-like programmed cell death, in which the chromatin condensation characteristically is less compact and complete than in apoptosis (the typical feature found in non-caspase mediated forms of programmed cell death),

(iii) necrosis-like programmed cell death, in which chromatin condensation is lacking (the initiation of this cell death may be dependent on caspase activation; however the execution is independent of caspases and

(iv) accidental necrosis and cell lysis.

Caspases

Caspases are the major executioners of apoptosis but some caspases are also involved in cytokine processing and inflammation. A family of at least 14 related cysteine proteases are known, named caspase-1 to caspase-14, depending upon their sequence of discovery. The family includes two murine homologues (caspase-11 and -12) that have no known human counterparts yet. Caspases are synthesized and stored as inactive proenzymes. They contain an N-terminal prodomain together with one large (p17 to p20) and one small (p10 to p12) subunit. The activation of caspases requires cleavage (usually by other caspases) to liberate one large and one small subunit, which associate into a heterotetramer, containing two small and two large subunits (Nicholson, 1999). Owing to their differential substrate specificities, they may be divided into three major groups, which also provides insight into their biological roles in inflammation and apoptosis (Rano *et al.*, 1997; Thornberry *et al.*, 1997). The three groups can be largely distinguished by their P4 preferences, a crucial determinant in caspase specificity. Group-I enzymes (caspases-1, -4, -5 and -13) prefer hydrophobic residues at P4 and are involved in the maturation of multiple pro-inflammatory cytokines. Group II enzymes (caspases-2, -3, and -7 and) have a strict requirement for Asp at P4 and will cleave DxxD apoptotic substrates. The cleaved substrates will disable cellular repair, halt cell cycle progression, inactivate inhibitors of DNA fragmentation, dismantle structural elements and mark dying cells for engulfment (Fischer *et al.*, 2003). Group III enzymes (caspases-6, -8, -9, -10) prefer branched-chain aliphatic amino acids in the position P4 and will activate group II caspases and other group III caspases.

Death receptor, exogenous pathway of apoptosis

The exogenous pathway of apoptosis is recruited following the activation of cell-surface death receptors such as Fas/CD95 and the tumour necrosis factor receptor 1 (TNFR1). These receptors are activated by specific ligands like Fas/CD95 and TNFα. On binding, the intracellular death domains (DD) of these receptors associate with adaptor proteins that contain the death effector domains,

e.g. FADD (Fig. 7.1). Adaptor proteins recruit procaspase-8, leading to its activation. Activated caspase-8 then activates other caspases, either directly or indirectly, by cleaving Bid. The exogenous pathway plays a major role in cancer cells and in immunity. However, its role in neuronal death is discussed controversially. Although caspase-8 is activated in several pathological conditions, including stroke, Huntington's disease and Parkinson's disease (Sanchez *et al.*, 1999; Velier *et al.*, 1999; Hartmann *et al.*, 2001b) and caspase-8 is activated in neurons in experimental paradigms of apoptosis, neurons in many models appear to be resistant to the activation of the cell death receptors that trigger the exogenous cell death pathway even in the presence of these receptors at the cell surface (Gerhardt *et al.*, 2001; Putcha *et al.*, 2002). Certain inhibitory mechanisms that interfere with Fas/CD95-mediated signaling including the expression of inhibitory proteins like c-Flip (Raoul *et al.*, 1999) and Lifeguard (Somia *et al.*, 1999), appear to silence the death receptors.

Mitochondrial, endogenous pathway of apoptosis

In mature, postmitotic and differentiated neurons apoptosis in most instances is induced through the mitochondrial, endogenous cell death pathway (Gerhardt *et al.*, 2001; Putcha *et al.*, 2002). Mitochondria are life-essential organelles for the production of metabolic energy in the form of ATP. Paradoxically mitochondria also play a key role in pathways leading to cell death (van Loo *et al.*, 2002). This role of mitochondria is not just a loss of function resulting in an energy deficit but is an active process involving different mitochondrial proteins. Cytochrome c was the first characterized mitochondrial factor shown to be released from the mitochondrial intermembrane space and to be actively implicated in apoptotic cell death. Since then, other mitochondrial proteins, such as the apoptosis-inducing factor (AIF), the second mitochondria-derived activator of caspase (Smac)/direct inhibitor of Apoptosis (AIT)-binding protein with low pI (DIABLO), endonuclease G and Omi/high temperature requirement A2 (HtrA2), were found to undergo release during apoptosis and have been implicated in various aspects of the cell death process. Pro- (Bid, Bax, Bak, Bok, Bik, Bnip3, Bad, Bim, Bmf, Noxa, Puma) and antiapoptotic (Bcl-2, Bcl-x$_L$, Bcl-w, Mcl-1, Boo, Bcl-B) members of the Bcl-2 protein family control the integrity and response of mitochondria to apoptotic signals. The precise molecular mechanisms by which Bcl-2 family proteins protect from or induce mitochondrial damage are still controversial (Martinou & Green, 2001).

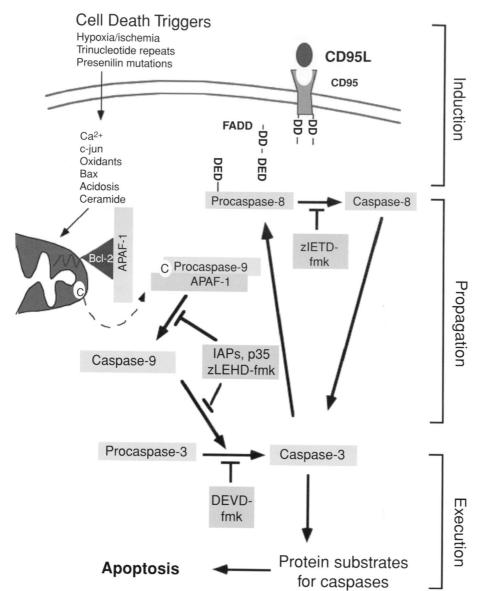

Fig. 7.1 Cascade of apoptotic events in acute and chronic neurodegenerative diseases. The panel depicts our current understanding of intracellular events leading to the activation of effector caspases, e.g. caspase-3. Different apoptosis-triggering pathways employ distinct signal transduction pathways that culminate in the release of cytochrome c from mitochondria. Alternatively, caspase-8 which contains two death effector domain-like molecules (DED), reacts with FADD (Fas-associating protein with death domain), and is recruited for activation at either the CD95 death-inducing signaling complex (DISC) or the tumor necrosis factor-α receptor-1 (TNF-R). However this mechanism has not clearly been shown to occur in mature, differentiated neurons (**Induction phase**). Two general mechanisms for release of cytochrome c (or other caspase-activating proteins) have been proposed: one involves osmotic disequilibrium leading to an expansion of the matrix space, organellar swelling, and subsequent rupture of the outer membrane; the other envisions opening of channels in the outer membrane, thus releasing cytochrome c from the intermembrane space of mitochondria into the cytosol. Members of the Bcl-2 family may perform double duty, controlling cytochrome c release from mitochondria and also possibly binding Apaf-1. Cytochrome c activates caspases by binding to Apaf-1 causing it to associate with initiator procaspases (e.g. procaspase-9). Apaf-1 shares sequence similarity with the prodomain of Ced-3 and other initiator caspases with long prodomains including caspase-1, -2, -8, -9 and -10. This domain may serve as a <u>c</u>aspase <u>r</u>ecruitment <u>d</u>omain (CARD complex) by binding to caspases that have similar CARDs at their NH$_2$ termini. Upon reception of a death stimulus, the complex might dissociate, freeing Apaf-1 and thereby triggering the activation of initiator caspases (**Propagation phase**). Active initiator caspases may activate effector caspases (e.g. caspase-3), initiating the proteolytic cascade that culminates in apoptosis (**Execution phase**). Potential sides for peptide (zIETD-fmk, caspase-8 inhibitor; zLEHD-fmk, caspase-9 inhibitor; DEVD-fmk, caspase-3 inhibitor) and protein inhibitors (IAP, p35) of caspases to interfere with this pathway are noted.

Following release from mitochondria, cytochrome c, together with the apoptosis protease-activating factor (Apaf-1), dATP and the cytosolic procaspase-9, forms a high molecular weight caspase-activating complex, termed apoptosome (Fig. 7.1). Once assembled, the apoptosome activates procaspase-9 as the initiator caspase, which in turn proteolytically activates the executioner procaspase-3 (Fig. 7.1) (Li *et al.*, 1997). A proteolytic cascade is then initiated in which caspase-3 activates procaspase-2, -6, -8 and -10, resulting in a feedback amplification of the apoptotic signal (Slee *et al.*, 1999).

AIF was originally discovered as a mitochondrial protein that, like cytochrome c, is released into the cytoplasm during cell death. Following an apoptotic stimulus AIF translocates to the nucleus in response to apoptogenic stimuli to induce apoptosis characterized by large-scale (~50 kb) DNA fragmentation instead of oligonucleosomal DNA laddering. The molecular mechanisms of cell death induced by AIF are only poorly understood; they are independent of caspases (Cande *et al.*, 2002). Overexpression of the heat shock protein (HSP)70 antagonizes AIF (Ravagnan *et al.*, 2001). New evidence suggests, however, that a redox-active enzymatic region of AIF may be antiapoptotic while the DNA binding region is proapoptotic (Klein *et al.*, 2002; Lipton & Bossy-Wetzel, 2002).

The Apaf-1/cytochrome c apoptosome complex contains the X-chromosome-linked IAP (XIAP), which binds and inhibits caspase-3 and caspase-9 (Bratton *et al.*, 2001; Srinivasula *et al.*, 2001). Smac/DIABLO, a 29 kDa mitochondrial protein, is a mitochondrial XIAP antagonist. It is processed to a 23 kDa mature protein and translocates to the cytosol after an apoptotic trigger. Besides its interaction with XIAP, Smac/DIABLO also binds other IAP proteins including c-IAP1, c-IAP2, surviving and baculoviral OpIAP. Whether Smac/DIABLO is an essential factor in the apoptotic process is still unclear. Smac/DIABLO-deficient mice are completely viable and do not show any abnormality. Further, all types of Smac/DIABLO-deficient primary cells respond normally to a broad range of apoptotic stimuli (Okada *et al.*, 2002). These observations suggest the existence of redundant factors compensating for the loss of Smac/DIABLO, e.g. Omi/HtrA2, or that Smac/DIABLO has no essential and general role in apoptosis during development.

The serine protease Omi/Htra2 shares functional properties with Smac/DIABLO. Upon induction of apoptosis, the protease is released from the mitochondrial intermembrane space and interacts with cytosolic IAP proteins with an IAP binding motif. In contrast to Smac/DIABLO, which shows a differential expression pattern with abundant expression in skeletal muscle, lung,

thymus and brain, Omi/HtrA is expressed ubiquitously. Besides its IAP-interacting property, Omi/HtrA is also an inducer/accelerator of cell death through its serine protease catalytic domain. When the mature protein, without its mitochondrial presequence, is overexpressed in the cytoplasm, it induces cell death independent of caspase activation or IAP interaction. The catalytic domain is essential for its cytotoxic, caspase-independent activity, whereas the IAP binding domain is necessary for caspase-dependent mechanisms (Hegde *et al.*, 2002). Mutations in Omi/HtrA have been linked to the mouse mutant *motor neuron degeneration* 2 (mnd 2) (Jones *et al.*, 2003). This mutant mouse does not only show a neuromuscular disorder but also striatal damage and a Parkinsonian phenotype (Rathke-Hartlieb *et al.*, 2002).

Evidence for apoptosis and caspase activation in human diseases

The development of therapeutic targets for acute and chronic neurodegenerative diseases depends in part upon identifying specific mechanisms of cell death in humans and animal models. In sporadic and inherited neurodegenerative disorders like Huntington's disease (Portera-Cailliau *et al.*, 1995), Alzheimer's disease (Anderson *et al.*, 1996) and ALS (Martin, 1999), the presence of chromatin condensation and DNA fragmentation suggests that cells are dying by an apoptotic-like mechanism. The results are more controversial for Parkinson's disease: two studies reported that 5–8% of neurons in the *substantia nigra pars compacta* (SNpc) of Parkinson's disease patients show DNA-end labeling, a third study reported 6% of the melanin-containing neurons with chromatin changes upon electron microscopy (Mochizuki *et al.*, 1996; Anglade *et al.*, 1997; Tompkins *et al.*, 1997). On the other hand, others have failed to detect apoptotic changes in the SNpc (Kosel *et al.*, 1997; Banati *et al.*, 1998; Wüllner *et al.*, 1999), possibly because apoptotic DNA fragments have a relatively short half-life. While the significance of morphologic features suggestive of apoptosis remains controversial in human postmortem tissue, the detection of molecular apoptotic markers in human brain tissue and in animal models supports the pathological evidence. In Parkinson's disease (Hartmann *et al.*, 2000; 2001b), Huntington's disease (Ona *et al.*, 1999; Sanchez *et al.*, 1999), Alzheimer's disease (Gervais *et al.*, 1999), and ALS (Guegan *et al.*, 2001) translocation of cytochrome c from mitochondria to cytosol, activation of caspases, or appearance of substrate cleavage products support the hypothesis that apoptosis and processed caspases are important mediators of neuronal cell death in neurodegenerative diseases.

In brain tissue taken during surgical decompression for acute intracranial hypertension following trauma, cleavage of caspase-1, upregulation and cleavage of caspase-3 were found along with DNA fragmentation with both apoptotic and necrotic morphologies (Clark et al., 1999).

Evidence for apoptotic cell death in human stroke is scant at the present time. In two autopsy cases, a significant number of TUNEL-positive granule cells were found in the cerebellum after global ischemia (Hara et al., 1995); the importance of such changes to postmortem interval was not clarified. Unlike rodents, human cerebral neurons reportedly exhibit little or no caspase-3 immunoreactivity under normal conditions (Krajewska et al., 1997). However, during ischemic degeneration, caspase-3 protein expression increases.

T-cell mediated inflammation may play a key role in the pathogenic mechanism sustaining multiple sclerosis. At nearly all stages of multiple sclerosis, apoptotic cells bearing myelin markers, presumably oligodendrocytes, are present in brain (Ozawa et al., 1994; Dowling et al., 1996). Multiple sclerosis plaques show a pronounced expression of Fas/Apo-1/CD95 and Fas ligand death signaling molecules on glia cells, including oligodendrocytes, suggesting that the Fas signaling pathway may be pathogenetically relevant to multiple sclerosis (D'Souza et al., 1996; Dowling et al., 1996).

Studies in animal models

Because postmortem brains often contain artifacts due to autopsy delay, and typically show end stage disease rather than an evolving disease process, the best clues to mechanisms underlying neurodegenerative diseases come from animal studies.

Stroke

Morphological and biochemical characterization of central neurons following global or focal ischemia suggest that apoptosis contributes to ischemic death of neurons (MacManus et al., 1993; MacManus et al., 1994). Two lines of evidence indicate that caspase-3 activation plays a key role following transient forebrain ischemia. First, immunohistochemical and biochemical studies show that caspase-3 activation occurs in susceptible cortical and hippocampal neurons following temporary (2 h) middle cerebral artery occlusion produced by filament insertion into the carotid artery or four vessel occlusion for 12 min and global ischemia, respectively (Namura et al., 1998; Xu et al., 1999).

Second, intracerebral administration of selective caspase peptide inhibitors reduce cellular and behavioral deficits following transient focal (30 min to 2 h filament insertion into the carotid artery) or global ischemia (bilateral carotid artery occlusion for 5 min) (Hara et al., 1997b; Endres et al., 1998; Himi et al., 1998). Moreover, neuroprotection can still be achieved when intracerebral administration of a caspase-3-specific (DEVD-cmk) or a pan-specific (zVAD-fmk)-caspase inhibitor was delayed by 6–9 h after mild transient (30 min) focal ischemia (Endres et al., 1998; Fink et al., 1998) or after chemically induced hypoxia (Schulz et al., 1998). In both models the N-methyl-D-aspartic acid receptor antagonist dizolcipine (MK-801) is only efficacious when administered less than 1 hour after the initial insult. The prolonged therapeutic window makes caspase inhibitors particularly attractive for the treatment of stroke.

The observation that distinct mechanisms of cell protection reduce neuronal injury in ischemia suggests the possibility that, when combined, these treatments may act in synergy. Pretreatment with subthreshold doses of MK-801, and delayed treatment with subthreshold doses of zVAD-fmk, provide synergistic protection compared with either treatment alone. Moreover, both treatments extend the therapeutic window for caspase inhibition for an additional 2 to 3 hours (Ma et al., 1998; Schulz et al., 1998). The data suggest the potential value of combining treatment strategies to reduce potential side effects and to extend the treatment window in cerebral ischemia.

Inhibitors of apoptosis proteins (IAPs) are a family of proteins which confer resistance to neuronal apoptosis (Simons et al., 1999) by caspase inhibition (Deveraux et al., 1998; Robertson et al., 2000). Adenovirally mediated overexpression of neuronal apoptosis inhibitory protein (NAIP) and of X-chromosomal IAP (XIAP) attenuates ischemic damage in the hippocampus after global ischemia induced by four vessel occlusion for 12 min and behavioral deficits(Xu et al., 1997, 1999).

Spinal cord ischemia activates caspases-8 and -3, which colocalize in neurons with cells showing DNA fragmentation. The Fas receptor expressed in neurons coexpressing caspase-8, may provide one upstream mechanism for caspase activation (Matsushita et al., 2000).

Trauma

The inhibition of caspases may offer therapeutic potential in the treatment of traumatic brain or spinal cord injury. Caspases-1 and -3 are cleaved and activated after fluid percussion-, impact- or cold injury-induced brain trauma (Yakovlev et al., 1997; Fink et al., 1999; Morita-Fujimura *et al.*, 1999) and impact spinal trauma (Springer *et al.*, 1999) in neurons and oligodendrocytes. Intracerebroventricular injection of zVAD-fmk, a panspecific caspase inhibitor, zDEVD-fmk, a caspase-3 specific inhibitor, or YVAD-fmk, a caspase-1 specific inhibitor, markedly reduces posttraumatic apoptotic cell death and significantly enhances neurological recovery (Yakovlev *et al.*, 1997; Fink *et al.*, 1999; Morita-Fujimura *et al.*, 1999). Intraocular application of caspase inhibitors reduces delayed cell death of retinal ganglion cells caused by transection of the optical nerve (Kermer *et al.*, 1998).

Multiple sclerosis

Inhibition of oligodendrocyte apoptosis in autoimmune demyelinating diseases may block or attenuate the neurological manifestations of the disorder. Experimental autoimmune encephalomyelitis (EAE) is a rodent model of multiple sclerosis. Oligodendrocytes from transgenic mice that express the baculovirus anti-apoptotic protein p35 (inhibits multiple caspases), were resistant to cell death induced by TNF-α, agonistic anti-Fas antibody and INF-γ. Further, cre/p35 transgenic mice were resistant to EAE induction by immunization with the myelin oligodendrocyte glycoprotein. The numbers of infiltrating T cells and macrophages/microglia in the EAE lesions were significantly reduced, as were the numbers of apoptotic oligodendrocytes expressing the activated form of caspase-3 (Hisahara *et al.*, 2000).

Huntington's disease

This disease is characterized by the presence of mutated Huntingtin protein containing extended repeats of the amino acid glutamine; this mutated protein appears to be neurotoxic, but proteolytic cleavage may be needed to generate a neurotoxic fragment from the full-length, mutated huntingtin protein. Caspase-3 cleaves huntingtin in vitro and in apoptotic cells (Goldberg *et al.*, 1996; Wellington *et al.*, 1998). Recently, caspase-cleaved huntingtin fragments were identified in postmortem brains of Parkinson's disease patients, but also in controls, indicating that caspase-mediated cleavage of huntingtin may occur as a normal physiological event (Wellington *et al.*, 2002). However it was thought that the cleavage of mutant huntingtin would release fragments with the potential for increased toxicity and accumulation, due to the presence of the expanded polyglutamine tract (Wellington *et al.*, 2002). According to conventional theories, procaspases are not active; recently, however, several groups have shown that procaspases may also have catalytic activity, albeit at a level

much lower than that of active caspases (Stennicke *et al.*, 1999). Mutant, full-length huntingtin with extended polyglutamine tracts may provide a suitable substrate for basal procaspase activity in the absence of apoptosis generating neurotoxic huntingtin fragments.

Ona and colleagues have shown that a dominant-negative mutant of interleukin-1β-converting enzyme (caspase-1), delays the onset and progression of pathology in a transgenic model of Huntington's disease expressing a mutant human Huntingtin exon 1 encoding an expanded polyglutamine repeat (Ona *et al.*, 1999). Further, intracerebroventricular administration of the panspecific caspase inhibitor zVAD-fmk (Ona *et al.*, 1999) and minocycline (Chen *et al.*, 2000), which indirectly inhibits caspase-1 and -3, delays mortality in this model.

Caspase-8 is another caspase that might be involved in the pathogenesis of Huntington's disease. More evidence points to an endogenous activation of caspase-8 than an activation through death receptors. The caspase is recruited to intracellular aggregates and is subsequently activated in neuronal cells that express an expanded polyglutamine repeat (Sanchez *et al.*, 1999). In a cellular system, caspase inhibition prevents cell death but not inclusion formation (Saudou *et al.*, 1998). Activated caspase-8 has been detected in the insoluble fraction of brains of Huntington's disease patients but not of controls (Sanchez *et al.*, 1999). Caspase-8 may also be activated by the formation of proapoptotic heterodimers consisting of huntingtin interacting protein 1 (Hip1) and Hip1 protein interactor (Hippi), which is favored by the disease-associated polyglutamine expansion (Gervais *et al.*, 2002).

Parkinson's disease

1-Methyl-4-phenyl-1,2,3,6-tetrahydropyridine (MPTP) produces clinical, biochemical and neuropathologic changes reminiscent of those occurring in idiopathic Parkinson's disease (PD). The toxicity of its active metabolite MPP$^+$ involves the activation of caspases in vitro (Dodel *et al.*, 1998; von Coelln *et al.*, 2001) and in vivo (Yang *et al.*, 1998; Eberhardt *et al.*, 2000; Hartmann *et al.*, 2000). In mice chronic administration of MPTP induces apoptotic cell death in dopaminergic *substantia nigra* neurons. Transgenic mice expressing a dominant-negative mutant of interleukin-1β converting enzyme are relatively resistant to MPTP toxicity (Klevenyi *et al.*, 1999). Further, the overexpression of the antiapoptic protein, Bcl-2, prevents activation of caspases and provides protection against MPTP toxicity (Yang *et al.*, 1998).

The mitochondrial activation pathway requires the release of cytochrome c from mitochondria in connection with the opening of the mitochondrial transition pore. Cytochrome c then forms a ternary complex with Apaf-1 and caspase-9 in the cytosol. MPP$^+$ has been reported to be able to induce the opening of the mitochondrial transition pore (Cassarino et al., 1999). Adeno-associated virus mediated expression of a dominant negative form of Apaf-1, consisting of the wild-type caspase recruitment domain, provides protection against dopaminergic cell loss and striatal catecholamine depletion in the mouse MPTP model (Mochizuki et al., 2001). Consequently, nigral neurons showing activated caspase-3 were only found on the non-injected side.

Neurons expressing non-activated caspase-3 seem to be particularly prone to early degeneration as their number is low in parkinsonian SNpc compared with controls, whereas a higher number of cells with activated caspase-3 (6.5% vs. 3.9%) than in non-affected controls was observed (Hartmann et al., 2000); and, as MPP$^+$-induced cell loss proceeds in culture, the number of neurons expressing activated caspase-3 declines rapidly.

Caspase inhibition is achieved by tri- or tetrapeptide inhibitors or viral proteins and their mammalian homologues (IAPs) with different substrate specificity (Deveraux & Reed, 1999; Robertson et al., 2000). Some of the peptide inhibitors are not entirely specific in that they also block cathepsins. Peptide caspase inhibitors (zVAD-fmk or selective caspase-3 inhibitors) protect primary mesencephalic cultures against MPP$^+$ (Dodel et al., 1998; Eberhardt et al., 2000; Bilsland et al., 2002). However, the loss of [^{3}H]dopamine uptake as a marker for dendritic function is not reversed (Eberhardt et al., 2000). Recently, more detailed analysis provided evidence that, although caspase inhibitors are protective against MPP$^+$ toxicity in primary dopaminergic neurons or dopaminergic cell lines in culture, this rescue may be temporary, may cause a switch from apoptosis to necrosis or may not result in functional benefit (Choi et al., 1999; Eberhardt et al., 2000; Hartmann et al., 2001b). An inhibitor of caspase-1 like enzymes was not effective against MPP$^+$ in primary mesencephalic or cerebellar granule cells (Du et al., 1997; Bilsland et al., 2002).

Inhibitors of apoptosis proteins (IAP) were first discovered as viral proteins and were shown to suppress the defensive apoptotic host response to viral infection. Ectopic expression in mammalian cells blocks apoptosis (Deveraux & Reed, 1999). They share one or several baculoviral IAP repeat (BIR) domains. Many of them also have a RING domain (dispensable for antiapoptotic effect) and some of them possess a caspase recruitment domain (CARD). They block caspase activity by direct binding to specific pro-caspases or active caspases (Deveraux et al., 1998). The baculoviral protein p35, for example, is a broad inhibitor of caspase function, while cowpox virus product CrmA inhibits primarily caspase-1 and -8. In humans, at least six homologous proteins were discovered: NAIP, cIAP1/HIAP-2, cIAP2/HIAP-1, Survivin, Bruce and X-linked inhibitor of apoptosis protein (XIAP).

In cellular models we compared the efficacy of different adenoviral constructs (AdV-XIAP, AdV-HIAP1, AdV-HIAP2, AdV-NAIP, AdV-p35, AdV-crmA) against apoptotic stimuli and found XIAP expression to be most effective (Simons et al., 1999; Kugler et al., 2000; Gerhardt et al., 2001). XIAP preferably blocks activation of pro-caspase-3, -6 and -7 by inhibiting the processing of procaspase-9. The XIAP protein contains a RING finger domain and three BIR domains, of which BIR-3 assumed to associate with caspase-9, and BIR-1/2 with caspase-3 and -7 (Robertson et al., 2000). It is expressed ubiquitously in human tissues, but is sequestered from caspases by the Smac/Diablo protein under normal circumstances. In some instances, an intact JNK1 signalling pathway seems to be required for its antiapoptotic function (Sanna et al., 1998, 2002). Interestingly, XIAP has been identified as a ubiquitin ligase, providing possible cross-talk to the ubiquitin-proteasome system.

Transfection of the nigrostriatal pathway with an Ad-XIAP led to a strong expression of XIAP protein in the striatum and in dopaminergic neurons of the SNpc (Eberhardt et al., 2000). Expression of XIAP provided protection against the MPTP-induced loss of tyrosine hydroxylase-positive neurons but not against the reduction of striatal catecholamine concentrations, suggesting a dissociation between neuronal survival and the loss of neuritic function. Additional studies in primary mesencephalic cultures provided evidence that caspase inhibition by zVAD-fmk rescued the tyrosine hydroxylase-positive somata, but not their neurites and synapses from MPP$^+$- and 6-hydroxydopamine-induced toxicity (Eberhardt et al., 2000; von Coelln et al., 2001). In contrast, the adenovirus-mediated expression of GDNF resulted in higher striatal catecholamine concentrations but did not protect against the MPTP-induced loss of dopaminergic neurons. The combination of adenoviral gene transfer of XIAP and GDNF provided synergistic effects: the MPTP-induced loss of tyrosine hydroxylase-positive neurons was almost completely blocked and the dopamine concentrations in the striatum were fully restored (Eberhardt et al., 2000).

In transgenic mice expressing p35, a broad-spectrum viral caspase inhibitor, cell loss after MPTP treatment was reduced and striatal catecholamines were preserved partially (Viswanath et al., 2000). In these mice, activation of caspase-3, -8 and -9, release of cytochrome c and cleavage of Bid (a proapoptotic Bcl-2 family member) after MPTP injections was reduced compared with wild-type mice (Viswanath *et al.*, 2001). Studying the effects of MPP$^+$ in PC12 cells and primary mesencephalic culture, a temporal sequence of activation after cytochrome c release from caspase-9 to caspase-3 and finally caspase-8 was established, all of which could be abrogated by a caspase-9 inhibitor (LEHD-CHO). A caspase-8 inhibitor (IETD-CHO) decreased caspase-3 or -9 activation only slightly (Viswanath *et al.*, 2001). Bid was cleaved by caspase-8 and promoted cytochrome c release, providing integration between the mitochondrial and the death-receptor pathway of caspase activation (Hengartner, 2000). The activation of caspase-8 occurs in a minority of neurons and glial cells in parkinsonian SNpc and in nigral neurons after MPTP treatment of mice (Hartmann *et al.*, 2001b). These data would be compatible with a model of cytochrome c-induced caspase-9 activation leading to caspase-3 activation that mediates the effector phase of apoptosis, and with an amplification loop involving caspase-8 (Fig. 7.1). The induction of CD 95 Fas could provide another source of caspase-8 activation, but has been denied at least in cell culture experiments with MPP$^+$ (Gomez *et al.*, 2001). Minocycline, a clinically approved tetracycline derivative that inhibits microglial activation and presumably also inhibits caspase-1 and caspase-3, mitigates MPTP-induced neurodegeneration (Du *et al.*, 2001; Wu *et al.*, 2002). However, these protective effects of minocycline in MPP+/MPTP toxicity have been disputed by others (Yang *et al.*, 2003, Cornet *et al.*, 2004, Diguet *et al.*, 2004). Taken together, this would suggest that caspase inhibition is effective in preventing MPTP-induced death of dopaminergic neurons; however, an additional neurorestorative treatment may be required to fully restore their functional activity.

Mitochondrial dysfunction plays a central role in the pathogenesis of Parkinson's disease and MPTP toxicity. Several mechanisms have been proposed in models of neuronal apoptosis and MPTP/MPP$^+$ toxicity, by which pro-apoptotic factors may be released from mitochondria to activate the caspase cascade. Prostate apoptosis response-4 (Par-4) was identified as being upregulated in prostate tumour cells undergoing apoptosis, but is now known to be essential in developmental and pathological neuronal death (Guo *et al.*, 1997; Mattson, 2000). Levels of Par-4 increase rapidly in response to various apoptotic stimuli through enhanced translation of Par-4 mRNA. A leucine zipper domain in the carboxy-terminus of Par-4 is essential for its pro-apoptotic function, and interactions of Par-4 with other proteins, including protein kinase C · and Bcl-2, through this zipper may be central to the mechanisms by which Par-4 induces mitochondrial dysfunction. Levels of Par-4 are increased selectively before death in dopaminergic neurons of SNpc in

Parkinson's disease brain and in mice and monkeys following MPTP treatment (Duan *et al.*, 1999). In culture a block of Par-4 induction by antisense treatment provides protection.

Bax may have a central role in mediating mitochondria-dependent apoptosis in neurons (Deckwerth *et al.*, 1996). Models of Bax activation indicate that its oligomerization may result in a homomultimeric pore (Saito *et al.*, 2000), a VDAC-containing pore (Shimizu *et al.*, 1999), or a permeabilization of mitochondrial outer membrane (Kluck *et al.*, 1999) to release cytochrome c. Following MPTP treatment there is an upregulation of Bax in the SNpc (Hartmann *et al.*, 2001a). Bax upregulation appears to be of functional relevance since mutant mice lacking Bax are significantly more resistant to MPTP toxicity than their wild-type littermates (Vila *et al.*, 2001). Collectively, the results indicate that Bax plays a pivotal role in SNpc dopaminergic neuronal death in the MPTP mouse model likely by acting in injured neurons before the onset of irreversible cell death events.

One way by which the new transcription of death inducing genes, including Bax, Par-4, or Bim (Putcha *et al.*, 2001; Whitfield *et al.*, 2001) that lead to the translocation of cytochrome c from mitochondria may occur is activation of the mitogen activated protein (MAP) kinase pathway. Saporito and colleagues were the first to show that in the MPTP model the JNK pathway is activated and that the pharmacological inhibition of this pathway with CEP1347 leads to neuroprotection (Saporito *et al.*, 1999, 2000). Recently we investigated the role of the pro-apoptotic c-Jun NH$_2$-terminal kinase (JNK) signaling cascade in SH-SY5Y human neuroblastoma cells in vitro and in mice in vivo (Xia *et al.*, 2001). MPTP/MPP$^+$ led to the sequential phosphorylation and activation of JNK kinase (MKK4), JNK and c-Jun, the activation of caspases and apoptosis. In mice, adenoviral gene transfer of the JNK binding domain of JNK-interacting protein-1 (a scaffold protein and inhibitor of JNK) inhibited this cascade downstream of MKK4 phosphorylation, blocked JNK, c-Jun and caspase activation, death of dopaminergic neurons and the loss of catecholamines in the striatum. Furthermore, the gene transfer resulted in behavioral benefit. Therefore, inhibition of the JNK pathway offers a new treatment strategy for Parkinson's disease which blocks the death signaling pathway upstream of the execution of apoptosis in dopaminergic neurons, providing a therapeutic advantage over the direct inhibition of caspases.

Glyceraldehyde-3-phosphate dehydrogenase (GAPDH) has been shown to play a role in apoptosis in some cellular models. Age- and cytosine arabinoside-induced apoptosis in cerebellar granule cells and age-induced apoptosis in cerebral cortical cultures are associated with an increased expression of GAPDH and prevented by treatment with GAPDH antisense oligonucleotides (Ishitani & Chuang, 1996; Ishitani et al., 1996a, b). Cell death associated with nuclear translocation of GAPDH and antisense protection occurs in several neuronal and non-neuronal systems (Ishitani et al., 1997; Saunders et al., 1999; Shashidharan et al., 1999). Downregulation of GAPDH expression by antisense oligonucleotides protected mesencephalic dopaminergic neurons from MPP$^+$ toxicity (Fukuhara et al., 2001). CGP 3466 (dibenzo[b,f]oxepin-10-ylmethyl-methyl-prop-2-ynyl-amine) is structurally related to R-(−)-deprenyl and shares its ability to bind to GAPDH and rescue neurons in several in vitro and in vivo paradigms (Kragten et al., 1998; Carlile et al., 2000). CGP3466 was shown to protect against MPTP- and 6-hydroxydopamine-induced toxicity and behavioral deficits in vivo without affecting monoamine oxidase B activity (Andringa & Cools, 2000; Andringa et al., 2000; Waldmeier et al., 2000). However, crucial experiments including the proof of GAPDH upregulation and nuclear translocation and the effects of CGP 3446 on these changes have not been done yet in dopaminergic neurons. A phase II clinical trial for Parkinson's disease was initiated.

Amyotrophic lateral sclerosis

Whereas 90% of human cases with ALS are sporadic, about 10% are inherited. Of these, about 10 to 20% carry a dominant mutation in the superoxide dismutase 1 (SOD1) gene. Expression of these mutations in mice replicate the clinical and pathological hallmarks of ALS. In mice transgenic for mutant SOD1, there are clear apoptotic cells in the spinal cord, though they are rare (Vukosavic et al., 2000). In the spinal cord of human ALS patients and in affected transgenic SOD1 mice, Bax is not only upregulated but it is also expressed mainly in its deleterious homodimeric conformation. In mice, Bax is translocated from the cytosol to the mitochondria (Vukosavic et al., 1999). Overexpression of Bcl-2 prolongs survival of transgenic SOD1 mice (Kostic et al., 1997). Evidence for a prominent recruitment of the mitochondrial pathways of apoptosis has been found in the spinal cord of patients and transgenic SOD1 mice (Guegan et al., 2001). Pharmacological inhibition of cytochrome c release delays disease onset and extends the survival of transgenic SOD1 mice (Zhu et al., 2002). A functional role for caspases has been implicated by studies showing that the panspecific caspase inhibitor, zVAD-fmk, attenuates mutant SOD1-mediated cell death in transfected PC12 cells and in transgenic SOD1 mice (Ghadge et al., 1997; Li et al., 2000). Motor neurons isolated from transgenic mice that overexpress different ALS-

linked SOD1 mutants showed increased susceptibility to activation of the Fas-triggered death pathway (Raoul et al., 2002). However, in general differentiated motor neurons are more resistant to FasL/CD95L than immature motor neurons, This resistance that has been linked to an increased expression of c-Flip (Raoul et al., 1999). In mice transgenic of mutant SOD1 activation of caspase-8, like induction of TNF α (Nguyen et al., 2001), occurs in the spinal cord only near end-stages of the cell death process (Guegan et al., 2002). This observation indicates that the extrinsic pathway of apoptosis in this model – if at all – only makes a late contribution to cell death.

Caspase inhibition and inflammation

Until recently, the brain was considered immunologically priviledged and unable to develop inflammation unless the blood–brain barrier was disrupted. We now know that the brain is capable of sustaining its own endogenous inflammatory reaction, and the evidence in Alzheimer's disease is particularly strong (McGeer et al., 1988), but information occurs in other neurodegenerative diseases as well. It has been hypothesized that this reaction contributes heavily to progressive neuronal death.

Non-specific caspase inhibitors block group II and III caspases involved in apoptosis, and caspase-1, the enzyme that cleaves pro-interleukin-1β to mature interleukin-1β. Since interleukin-1 receptor antagonists prevent damage after focal ischemia induced by permanent middle cerebral artery occlusion (Loddick & Rothwell, 1996), the first study using pan-caspase inhibitors was intended to show that blocking ICE activity prevents ischemic damage in the same model (Loddick et al., 1996). Transgenic mice expressing a dominant negative caspase-1 are protected in animal models of stroke induced by 3 h of cerebral artery occlusion followed by 24 h of reperfusion (Hara et al., 1997a), impact-induced head trauma (Fink et al., 1999), Parkinson's disease (Klevenyi et al., 1999), amyotrophic lateral sclerosis (Friedlander et al., 1997) and Huntington's disease (Ona et al., 1999). It remains to be elucidated whether both inhibition of inflammation and inhibition of caspase-mediated neuronal apoptosis contribute to the protective effects of caspase inhibitors. Of note, murine caspase-11, with homology to human caspase-4, promotes both caspase-1 and caspase-3 processing, thereby enhancing both apoptosis and cytokine maturation (Kang et al., 2000).

Limitations and cautions

Caspases and related proteins are emerging as important therapeutic targets in a variety of acute and chronic CNS diseases. Preclinical evidence in stroke supports the need to investigate anti-apoptotic treatment strategies, particularly because caspase inhibitors reduce tissue injury when administered many hours after mild ischemia. In the clinical setting, anti-apoptotic strategies might become useful to treat brief episodes of brain ischemia or be given in advance of risky surgical procedures (e.g. cardiopulmonary by-pass) or combined with thrombolytics or agents in which synergy has been documented (e.g. glutamate receptor antagonists). Furthermore, caspase inhibitors may provide promising opportunities for other neurological conditions in which cell death is prominent. Although the results of treatment in animals with caspase inhibitors are promising, clinical studies have not yet been performed because of the lack of synthetic caspase inhibitors that cross the blood–brain barrier. Such agents are a major focus in current programs of drug development and hopefully will become available soon. In addition, therapies that lead to the increased expression of IAPs are a potential avenue for treatment of chronic neurodegenerative disorders.

REFERENCES

Anderson, A. J., Su, J. H. & Cotman, C. W. (1996). DNA damage and apoptosis in Alzheimer's disease: colocalization with c-Jun immunoreactivity, relationship to brain area, and effect of postmortem delay. *J. Neurosci.*, **16**, 1710–19.

Andringa, G. & Cools, A. R. (2000). The neuroprotective effects of CGP 3466B in the best in vivo model of Parkinson's disease, the bilaterally MPTP-treated rhesus monkey. *J. Neural Transm. Suppl.*, 215–25.

Andringa, G., van Oosten, R. V., Unger, W. *et al.* (2000). Systemic administration of the propargylamine CGP 3466B prevents behavioural and morphological deficits in rats with 6-hydroxydopamine-induced lesions in the substantia nigra. *Eur. J. Neurosci.*, **12**, 3033–43.

Anglade, P., Vyas, S., Javoy-Agid, F. *et al.* (1997). Apoptosis and autophagy in nigral neurons of patients with Parkinson's disease. *Histol. Histopathol.*, **12**, 25–31.

Banati, R. B., Daniel, S. E. & Blunt, S. B. (1998). Glial pathology but absence of apoptotic nigral neurons in long-standing Parkinson's disease. *Mov. Disord.*, **13**, 221–7.

Bilsland, J., Roy, S., Xanthoudakis, S. *et al.* (2002). Caspase inhibitors attenuate 1-methyl-4-phenylpyridinium toxicity in primary cultures of mesencephalic dopaminergic neurons. *J. Neurosci.*, **22**, 2637–49.

Bratton, S. B., Walker, G., Srinivasula, S. M. *et al.* (2001). Recruitment, activation and retention of caspases-9 and -3 by Apaf-1 apoptosome and associated XIAP complexes. *EMBO J*, **20**, 998–1009.

Cande, C., Cohen, I., Daugas, E. *et al.* (2002). Apoptosis-inducing factor (AIF): a novel caspase-independent death effector released from mitochondria. *Biochimie*, **84**, 215–22.

Carlile, G. W., Chalmers-Redman, R. M., Tatton, N. A. *et al.* (2000). Reduced apoptosis after nerve growth factor and serum withdrawal: conversion of tetrameric glyceraldehyde-3-phosphate dehydrogenase to a dimer. *Mol. Pharmacol.*, **57**, 2–12.

Cassarino, D. S., Parks, J. K., Parker, W. D., Jr. & Bennett, J. P., Jr. (1999). The parkinsonian neurotoxin MPP+ opens the mitochondrial permeability transition pore and releases cytochrome c in isolated mitochondria via an oxidative mechanism. *Biochim. Biophys. Acta*, **1453**, 49–62.

Chen, M., Ona, V. O., Li, M. *et al.* (2000). Minocycline inhibits caspase-1 and caspase-3 expression and delays mortality in a transgenic mouse model of Huntington disease. *Nat. Med.*, **6**, 797–801.

Choi, W. S., Yoon, S. Y., Oh, T. H. *et al.* (1999). Two distinct mechanisms are involved in 6-hydroxydopamine- and MPP+-induced dopaminergic neuronal cell death: role of caspases, ROS, and JNK. *J. Neurosci. Res.*, **57**, 86–94.

Clark, R. S., Kochanek, P. M., Chen, M. *et al.* (1999). Increases in Bcl-2 and cleavage of caspase-1 and caspase-3 in human brain after head injury. *FASEB J.*, **13**, 813–21.

Cornet, S., Spinnewyn, B., Delaflotte, S. *et al.* (2004). Lack of evidence of direct mitochondrial involvement in the neuroprotective effect of minocycline. *Eur. J. Pharmacol.*, **505**, 111–19.

D'Souza, S. D., Bonetti, B., Balasingam, V. *et al.* (1996). Multiple sclerosis: Fas signaling in oligodendrocyte cell death. *J. Exp. Med.*, **184**, 2361–70.

Deckwerth, T. L., Elliott, J. L., Knudson, C. M., Johnson, E. M., Snider, W. D. & Korsmeyer, S. J. (1996). Bax is required for neuronal death after trophic factor deprivation and during development. *Neuron*, **17**, 401–11.

Deveraux, Q. L. & Reed, J. C. (1999). IAP family proteins – suppressors of apoptosis. *Genes Dev.*, **13**, 239–52.

Deveraux, Q. L., Roy, N., Stennicke, H. R. *et al.* (1998). IAPs block apoptotic events induced by caspase-8 and cytochrome c by direct inhibition of distinct caspases. *EMBO J.*, **17**, 2215–23.

Diguet, E., Fernagut, P. O., Wel, X. *et al.* (2004). Deleterious effects of minocycline in animal models of Parkinson's disease and Huntington's disease. *Eur. J. Neurosci.*, **19**, 3266–76.

Dodel, R. C., Du, Y., Bales, K. R., Ling, Z. D., Carvey, P. M. & Paul, S. M. (1998). Peptide inhibitors of caspase-3-like proteases attenuate 1-methyl-4-phenylpyridinum-induced toxicity of cultured fetal rat mesencephalic dopamine neurons. *Neuroscience*, **86**, 701–7.

Dowling, P., Shang, G., Raval, S., Menonna, J., Cook, S. & Husar, W. (1996). Involvement of the CD95 (APO-1/Fas) receptor/ligand system in multiple sclerosis brain. *J. Exp. Med.*, **184**, 1513–18.

Du, Y., Dodel, R. C., Bales, K. R., Jemmerson, R., Hamilton-Byrd, E. & Paul, S. M. (1997). Involvement of caspase-3-like cysteine protease in 1-methyl-4-phenylpyridinium-mediated apoptosis of cultured cerebellar granule neurons. *J. Neurochem.*, **69**, 1382–8.

Du, Y., Ma, Z., Lin, S. *et al.* (2001). Minocycline prevents nigrostriatal dopaminergic neurodegeneration in the MPTP model of Parkinson's disease. *Proc. Natl Acad. Sci., USA*, **98**, 14669–74.

Duan, W., Zhang, Z., Gash, D. M. & Mattson, M. P. (1999). Participation of prostate apoptosis response-4 in degeneration of dopaminergic neurons in models of Parkinson's disease. *Ann. Neurol.*, **46**, 587–97.

Eberhardt, O., Coelln, R. V., Kugler, S. *et al.* (2000). Protection by synergistic effects of adenovirus-mediated X-chromosome-linked inhibitor of apoptosis and glial cell line-derived neurotrophic factor gene transfer in the 1-methyl-4-phenyl-1,2,3,6-tetrahydropyridine model of Parkinson's disease. *J. Neurosci.*, **20**, 9126–34.

Endres, M., Namura, S., Shimizu-Sasamata, M. *et al.* (1998). Attenuation of delayed neuronal death after mild focal ischemia in mice by inhibition of the caspase family. *J. Cereb. Blood Flow Metab.*, **18**, 238–47.

Fink, K., Zhu, J., Namura, S. *et al.* (1998). Prolonged therapuetic window for ischemic brain damage caused by delayed caspase activation. *J. Cereb. Blood. Flow Metab.*, **18**, 1071–6.

Fink, K. B., Andrews, L. J., Butler, W. E. *et al.* (1999). Reduction of post-traumatic brain injury and free radical production by inhibition of the caspase-1 cascade. *Neuroscience*, **94**, 1213–18.

Fischer, U., Janicke, R. U. & Schulze-Osthoff, K. (2003). Many cuts to ruin: a comprehensive update of caspase substrates. *Cell Death Differ.*, **10**, 76–100.

Friedlander, R. M., Brown, R. H., Gagliardini, V., Wang, J. & Yuan, J. (1997). Inhibition of ICE slows ALS in mice [letter]. *Nature*, **388**, 31.

Fukuhara, Y., Takeshima, T., Kashiwaya, Y., Shimoda, K., Ishitani, R. & Nakashima, K. (2001). GAPDH knockdown rescues mesencephalic dopaminergic neurons from MPP+ -induced apoptosis. *NeuroReport*, **12**, 2049–52.

Gerhardt, E., Kügler, S., Leist, M. *et al.* (2001). Cascade of caspase-activation in potassium-deprived cerebellar granule neurons: targets for treatment with peptide and protein inhibitors of apoptosis. *Mol. Cell Neurosci.*, **17**, 717–31.

Gervais, F. G., Singaraja, R., Xanthoudakis, S. *et al.* (2002). Recruitment and activation of caspase-8 by the Huntingtin-interacting protein Hip-1 and a novel partner Hippi. *Nat. Cell Biol.*, **4**, 95–105.

Gervais, F. G., Xu, D., Robertson, G. S. *et al.* (1999). Involvement of caspases in proteolytic cleavage of Alzheimer's amyloid-beta precursor protein and amyloidogenic A beta peptide formation. *Cell*, **97**, 395–406.

Ghadge, G. D., Lee, J. P., Bindokas, V. P. *et al.* (1997). Mutant superoxide dismutase-1-linked familial amyotrophic lateral sclerosis: molecular mechanisms of neuronal death and protection. *J. Neurosci.*, **17**, 8756–66.

Goldberg, Y. P., Nicholson, D. W., Rasper, D. M. *et al.* (1996). Cleavage of huntingtin by apopain, a proapoptotic cysteine protease, is modulated by the polyglutamine tract. *Nat. Genet.*, **13**, 442–9.

Gomez, C., Reiriz, J., Pique, M., Gil, J., Ferrer, I. & Ambrosio, S. (2001). Low concentrations of 1-methyl-4-phenylpyridinium ion induce caspase-mediated apoptosis in human SH-SY5Y neuroblastoma cells. *J. Neurosci. Res.*, **63**, 421–8.

Guegan, C., Vila, M., Rosoklija, G., Hays, A. P. & Przedborski, S. (2001). Recruitment of the mitochondrial-dependent apoptotic pathway in amyotrophic lateral sclerosis. *J. Neurosci.*, **21**, 6569–76.

Guegan, C., Vila, M., Teissman, P. *et al.* (2002). Instrumental activation of bid by caspase-1 in a transgenic mouse model of ALS. *Mol. Cell Neurosci.*, **20**, 553–62.

Guo, N., Krutzsch, H. C., Inman, J. K. & Roberts, D. D. (1997). Thrombospondin 1 and type I repeat peptides of thrombospondin 1 specifically induce apoptosis of endothelial cells. *Cancer Res.*, **57**, 1735–42.

Hara, A., Yoshimi, N., Hirose, Y., Ino, N., Tanaka, T. & Mori, H. (1995). DNA fragmentation in granular cells of human cerebellum following global ischemia. *Brain Res.*, **697**, 247–50.

Hara, H., Fink, K., Endres, M. *et al.* (1997a). Attenuation of transient focal cerebral ischemia injury in transgenic mice expressing a mutant ICE inhibitory protein. *J. Cereb. Blood Flow Metab.*, **17**, 370–5.

Hara, H., Friedlander, R. M., Gagliardini, V. *et al.* (1997b). Inhibition of interleukin 1β converting enzyme family proteases reduces ischemic and excitotoxic neuronal damage. *Proc. Natl Acad. Sci., USA*, **94**, 2007–12.

Hartmann, A., Hunot, S., Michel, P. P. *et al.* (2000). Caspase-3: A vulnerability factor and final effector in apoptotic death of dopaminergic neurons in Parkinson's disease. *Proc. Natl Acad. Sci., USA*, **97**, 2875–80.

Hartmann, A., Michel, P. P., Troadec, J. D. *et al.* (2001a). Is Bax a mitochondrial mediator in apoptotic death of dopaminergic neurons in Parkinson's disease? *J. Neurochem.*, **76**, 1785–93.

Hartmann, A., Troadec, J. D., Hunot, S. *et al.* (2001b). Caspase-8 is an effector in apoptotic death of dopaminergic neurons in Parkinson's disease, but pathway inhibition results in neuronal necrosis. *J. Neurosci.*, **21**, 2247–55.

Hegde, R., Srinivasula, S. M., Zhang, Z. *et al.* (2002). Identification of Omi/HtrA2 as a mitochondrial apoptotic serine protease that disrupts inhibitor of apoptosis protein-caspase interaction. *J. Biol. Chem.*, **277**, 432–8.

Hengartner, M. O. (2000). The biochemistry of apoptosis. *Nature*, **407**, 770–6.

Himi, T., Ishizaki, Y. & Murota, S. (1998). A caspase inhibitor blocks ischaemia-induced delayed neuronal death in the gerbil. *Eur. J. Neurosci.*, **10**, 777–81.

Hisahara, S., Araki, T., Sugiyama, F. *et al.* (2000). Targeted expression of baculovirus p35 caspase inhibitor in oligodendrocytes protects mice against autoimmune-mediated demyelination. *EMBO J.*, **19**, 341–8.

Ishitani, R. & Chuang, D. M. (1996). Glyceraldehyde-3-phosphate dehydrogenase antisense oligodeoxynucleotides protect against cytosine arabinonucleoside-induced apoptosis in cultured cerebellar neurons. *Proc. Natl Acad. Sci., USA*, **93**, 9937–41.

Ishitani, R., Kimura, M., Sunaga, K., Katsube, N., Tanaka, M. & Chuang, D. M. (1996a). An antisense oligodeoxynucleotide to glyceraldehyde-3-phosphate dehydrogenase blocks age-induced apoptosis of mature cerebrocortical neurons in culture. *J. Pharmacol. Exp. Ther.*, **278**, 447–54.

Ishitani, R., Sunaga, K., Hirano, A., Saunders, P., Katsube, N. & Chuang, D. M. (1996b). Evidence that glyceraldehyde-3-phosphate dehydrogenase is involved in age-induced apoptosis in mature cerebellar neurons in culture. *J. Neurochem.*, **66**, 928–35.

Ishitani, R., Sunaga, K., Tanaka, M., Aishita, H. & Chuang, D. M. (1997). Overexpression of glyceraldehyde-3-phosphate dehydrogenase is involved in low K⁺-induced apoptosis but not necrosis of cultured cerebellar granule cells. *Mol. Pharmacol.*, **51**, 542–50.

Jones, J. M., Datla, P., Srinivasula, S. M. *et al.* (2003). Loss of Ori mitochondrial protease activity causes the neuromuscular disorder of mnd2 mutant mice. *Nature, ***425**, 721–7.

Kang, S. J., Wang, S., Hara, H. *et al.* (2000). Dual role of caspase-11 in mediating activation of caspase-1 and caspase-3 under pathological conditions. *J. Cell Biol.*, **149**, 613–22.

Kermer, P., Klöcker, N., Labes, M. & Bähr, M. (1998). Inhibition of CPP32-like proteases rescues axotomized retinal ganglion cells from secondary cell death *in vivo*. *J. Neurosci.*, **15**, 4656–62.

Klein, J. A., Longo-Guess, C. M., Rossmann, M. P. *et al.* (2002). The harlequin mouse mutation downregulates apoptosis-inducing factor. *Nature*, **419**, 367–74.

Klevenyi, P., Andreassen, O., Ferrante, R. J., Schleicher, J. R., Jr., Friedlander, R. M. & Beal, M. F. (1999). Transgenic mice expressing a dominant negative mutant interleukin-1beta converting enzyme show resistance to MPTP neurotoxicity. *NeuroReport*, **10**, 635–8.

Kluck, R. M., Esposti, M. D., Perkins, G. *et al.* (1999). The pro-apoptotic proteins, Bid and Bax, cause a limited permeabilization of the mitochondrial outer membrane that is enhanced by cytosol. *J. Cell Biol.*, **147**, 809–22.

Kosel, S., Egensperger, R., Voneitzen, U., Mehraein, P. & Graeber, M. B. (1997). On the question of apoptosis in the parkinsonian substantia nigra. *Acta Neuropathol.*, **93**, 105–8.

Kostic, V., Jackson-Lewis, V., de Bilbao, F., Dubois-Dauphin, M. & Przedborski, S. (1997). Bcl-2: prolonging life in a transgenic mouse model of familial amyotrophic lateral sclerosis. *Science*, **277**, 559–62.

Kragten, E., Lalande, I., Zimmermann, K. *et al.* (1998). Glyceraldehyde-3-phosphate dehydrogenase, the putative target of the antiapoptotic compounds CGP 3466 and R-(−)-deprenyl. *J. Biol. Chem.*, **273**, 5821–8.

Krajewska, M., Wang, H.-G., Krajewski, S. *et al.* (1997). Immunohistochemical analysis of *in vivo* patterns of expression of CPP32 (Caspase-3), a cell death protease. *Cancer Res.*, **57**, 1605–13.

Kroemer, G. (1997). Mitochondrial implication in apoptosis. Towards an endosymbiont hypothesis of apoptosis evolution. *Cell Death Differ.*, **4**, 443–56.

Kugler, S., Straten, G., Kreppel, F., Isenmann, S., Liston, P. & Bahr, M. (2000). The X-linked inhibitor of apoptosis (XIAP) prevents cell death in axotomized CNS neurons in vivo. *Cell Death Differ.*, **7**, 815–24.

Leist, M. & Jaattela, M. (2001). Four deaths and a funeral: from caspases to alternative mechanisms. *Nat. Rev. Mol. Cell Biol.*, **2**, 589–98.

Li, P., Nijhawan, D., Budihardjo, I. *et al.* (1997). Cytochrome c and dATP-dependent formation of Apaf-1/caspase-9 complex initiates an apoptotic protease cascade. *Cell*, **91**, 479–89.

Li, M., Ona, V. O., Guegan, C. *et al.* (2000). Functional role of caspase-1 and caspase-3 in an ALS transgenic mouse model. *Science*, **288**, 335–9.

Lipton, S. A. & Bossy-Wetzel, E. (2002). Dueling activities of AIF in cell death versus survival: DNA binding and redox activity. *Cell*, **111**, 147–50.

Loddick, S. A. & Rothwell, N. J. (1996). Neuroprotective effects of human recombinant interleukin-1 receptor antagonist in focal cerebral ischemia in the rat. *J. Cereb. Blood Flow Metab.*, **16**, 932–40.

Loddick, S. A., MacKenzie, A. & Rothwell, N. J. (1996). An ICE inhibitor, z-VAD-DCB attenuates ischaemic brain damage in the rat. *NeuroReport*, **7**, 1465–8.

Ma, J., Endres, M. & Moskowitz, M. A. (1998). Synergistic effects of caspase inhibitors and MK-801 in brain injury after transient focal cerebral ischemia in mice. *Br. J. Pharmacol.*, **124**, 756–62.

MacManus, J. P., Buchan, A. M., Hill, I. E., Rasquinha, I. & Preston, E. (1993). Global ischemia can cause DNA fragmentation indicative of apoptosis in rat brain. *Neurosci. Lett.*, **164**, 89–92.

MacManus, J. P., Hill, I. E., Huang, Z. G., Rasquinha, I., Xue, D. & Buchan, A. M. (1994). DNA damage consistent with apoptosis in transient focal ischaemic neocortex. *NeuroReport*, **5**, 493–6.

Martin, L. J. (1999). Neuronal death in amyotrophic lateral sclerosis is apoptosis: possible contribution of a programmed cell death mechanism. *J. Neuropathol. Exp. Neurol.*, **58**, 459–71.

Martinou, J. C. & Green, D. R. (2001). Breaking the mitochondrial barrier. *Nat. Rev. Mol. Cell. Biol.*, **2**, 63–7.

Matsushita, K., Wu, Y., Qiu J. *et al.* (2000). Fas receptor and neuronal cell death after spinal cord ischemia. *J. Neurosci.*, **20**, 6879–87.

Mattson, M. P. (2000). Apoptosis in neurodegenerative disorders. *Nat. Rev. Mol. Cell Biol.*, **1**, 120–9.

McGeer, P. L., Itagaki, S., Akiyama, H. & McGeer, E. G. (1988). Rate of cell death in parkinsonism indicates active neuropathological process. *Ann. Neurol.*, **24**, 574–6.

Mochizuki, H., Goto, K., Mori, H. & Mizuno, Y. (1996). Histochemical detection of apoptosis in Parkinson's disease. *J. Neurol. Sci.*, **137**, 120–3.

Mochizuki, H., Hayakawa, H., Migita, M. *et al.* (2001). An AAV-derived Apaf-1 dominant negative inhibitor prevents MPTP toxicity as antiapoptotic gene therapy for Parkinson's disease. *Proc. Natl Acad. Sci., USA*, **98**, 10918–23.

Morita-Fujimura, Y., Fujimura, M., Kawase, M., Murakami, K., Kim, G. W. & Chan, P. H. (1999). Inhibition of interleukin-1 beta converting enzyme family proteases (caspases) reduces cold injury-induced brain trauma and DNA fragmentation in mice. *J. Cereb. Blood Flow Metab.*, **19**, 634–42.

Namura, S., Zhu, J., Fink, K. *et al.* (1998). Activation and cleavage of caspase-3 in apoptosis induced by experimental cerebral ischemia. *J. Neurosci.*, **18**, 3659–68.

Nguyen, M. D., Julien, J. P. & Rivest, S. (2001). Induction of proinflammatory molecules in mice with amyotrophic lateral sclerosis: no requirement for proapoptotic interleukin-1beta in neurodegeneration. *Ann. Neurol.*, **50**, 630–9.

Nicholson, D. W. (1999). Caspase structure, proteolytic substrates, and function during apoptotic cell death. *Cell Death Differ.*, **6**, 1028–42.

Okada, H., Suh, W. K., Jin, J. *et al.* (2002). Generation and characterization of Smac/DIABLO-deficient mice. *Mol. Cell Biol.*, **22**, 3509–17.

Ona, V. O., Li, M., Vonsattel, J. P. *et al.* (1999). Inhibition of caspase-1 slows disease progression in a mouse model of Huntington's disease. *Nature*, **399**, 263–7.

Ozawa, K., Suchanek, G., Breitschopf, H. *et al.* (1994). Patterns of oligodendroglia pathology in multiple sclerosis. *Brain*, **117**, 1311–22.

Portera-Cailliau, C., Hedreen, J. C., Price, D. L. & Koliatsos, V. E. (1995). Evidence for apoptotic cell death in Huntington disease and excitotoxic animal models. *J. Neurosci.*, **15**, 3775–87.

Putcha, G. V., Moulder, K. L., Golden, J. P. *et al.* (2001). Induction of BIM, a proapoptotic BH3-only BCL-2 family member, is critical for neuronal apoptosis. *Neuron*, **29**, 615–28.

Putcha, G. V., Harris, C. A., Moulder, K. L., Easton, R. M., Thompson, C. B. & Johnson, E. M., Jr. (2002). Intrinsic and extrinsic pathway signaling during neuronal apoptosis: lessons from the analysis of mutant mice. *J. Cell Biol.*, **157**, 441–53.

Rano, T. A., Timkey, T., Peterson, E. P. *et al.* (1997). A combinatorial approach for determining protease specificities: application to interleukin-1beta converting enzyme (ICE). *Chem. Biol.*, **4**, 149–55.

Raoul, C., Henderson, C. E. & Pettmann, B. (1999). Programmed cell death of embryonic motoneurons triggered through the Fas death receptor. *J. Cell Biol.*, **147**, 1049–62.

Raoul, C., Estevez, A. G., Nishimune, H. *et al.* (2002). Motoneuron death triggered by a specific pathway downstream of Fas potentiation by ALS-linked SOD1 mutations. *Neuron*, **35**, 1067–83.

Rathke-Hartlieb, S., Schlomann, U., Heirnann, P., Meisler, M. H., Jackusch, H. & Bartsch, J. W. (2002). Progressive loss of striatal neurons causes motor dysfunction in MND2 mutant mice and is not prevented by Bcl-2. *Exp. Neurol.*, **175**, 87–97.

Ravagnan, L., Gurbuxani, S., Susin, S. A. *et al.* (2001). Heat-shock protein 70 antagonizes apoptosis-inducing factor. *Nat. Cell Biol.*, **3**, 839–43.

Robertson, G. S., Crocker, S. J., Nicholson, D. W. & Schulz, J. B. (2000). Neuroprotection by the inhibition of apoptosis. *Brain Pathol.*, **10**, 283–92.

Saito, M., Korsmeyer, S. J. & Schlesinger, P. H. (2000). BAX-dependent transport of cytochrome c reconstituted in pure liposomes. *Nat. Cell Biol.*, **2**, 553–5.

Sanchez, I., Xu, C. J., Juo, P., Kakizaka, A., Blenis, J. & Yuan, J. (1999). Caspase-8 is required for cell death induced by expanded polyglutamine repeats. *Neuron*, **22**, 623–33.

Sanna, M. G., Duckett, C. S., Richter, B. W., Thompson, C. B. & Ulevitch, R. J. (1998). Selective activation of JNK1 is necessary for the anti-apoptotic activity of hILP. *Proc. Natl Acad. Sci., USA*, **95**, 6015–20.

Sanna, M. G., da Silva Correia, J., Ducrey, O. *et al.* (2002). IAP suppression of apoptosis involves distinct mechanisms: the TAK1/JNK1 signaling cascade and caspase inhibition. *Mol. Cell Biol.*, **22**, 1754–66.

Saporito, M. S., Brown, E. M., Miller, M. S. & Carswell, S. (1999). CEP-1347/KT-7515, an inhibitor of c-jun N-terminal kinase activation, attenuates the 1-methyl-4-phenyl tetrahydropyridine-mediated loss of nigrostriatal dopaminergic neurons in vivo. *J. Pharmacol. Exp. Ther.*, **288**, 421–7.

Saporito, M. S., Thomas, B. A. & Scott, R. W. (2000). MPTP activates c-Jun NH(2)-terminal kinase (JNK) and its upstream regulatory kinase MKK4 in nigrostriatal neurons in vivo. *J. Neurochem.*, **75**, 1200–8.

Saudou, F., Finkbeiner, S., Devys, D. & Greenberg, M. E. (1998). Huntingtin acts in the nucleus to induce apoptosis but death does not correlate with the formation of intranuclear inclusions. *Cell*, **95**, 55–66.

Saunders, P. A., Chen, R. W. & Chuang, D. M. (1999). Nuclear translocation of glyceraldehyde-3-phosphate dehydrogenase isoforms during neuronal apoptosis. *J. Neurochem.*, **72**, 925–32.

Schulz, J. B., Weller, M., Matthews, R. T. *et al.* (1998). Extended therapeutic window for caspase inhibition and synergy with MK-801 in the treatment of cerebral histotoxic hypoxia. *Cell Death Differ.*, **5**, 847–57.

Shashidharan, P., Chalmers-Redman, R. M., Carlile, G. W. *et al.* (1999). Nuclear translocation of GAPDH-GFP fusion protein during apoptosis. *NeuroReport*, **10**, 1149–53.

Shimizu, S., Narita, M. & Tsujimoto, Y. (1999). Bcl-2 family proteins regulate the release of apoptogenic cytochrome c by the mitochondrial channel VDAC. *Nature*, **399**, 483–7.

Simons, M., Beinroth, S., Gleichmann, M. *et al.* (1999). Adenovirus-mediated gene transfer of IAPs delays apoptosis of cerebellar granule neurons. *J. Neurochem.*, **72**, 292–301.

Slee, E. A., Harte, M. T., Kluck, R. M. *et al.* (1999). Ordering the cytochrome c-initiated caspase cascade: hierarchical activation of caspases-2, -3, -6, -7, -8, and -10 in a caspase-9-dependent manner. *J. Cell Biol.*, **144**, 281–92.

Somia, N. V., Schmitt, M. J., Vetter, D. E., Van Antwerp, D., Heinemann, S. F. & Verma, I. M. (1999). LFG: An anti-apoptotic gene that provides protection from fas-mediated cell death. *Proc. Natl Acad. Sci., USA*, **96**, 12667–72.

Springer, J. E., Azbill, R. D. & Knapp, P. E. (1999). Activation of the caspase-3 apoptotic cascade in traumatic spinal cord injury. *Nat. Med.*, **5**, 943–6.

Srinivasula, S. M., Hegde, R., Saleh, A. *et al.* (2001). A conserved XIAP-interaction motif in caspase-9 and Smac/DIABLO regulates caspase activity and apoptosis. *Nature*, **410**, 112–16.

Stennicke, H. R., Deveraux, Q. L., Humke, E. W., Reed, J. C., Dixit, V. M. (1999). Caspase-9 can be activated without proteolytic processing. *J. Biol. Chem.*, **274**, 8359–62.

Thornberry, N. A., Rano, T. A., Peterson, E. P. *et al.* (1997). A combinatorial approach defines specificities of members of the caspase family and granzyme B. Functional relationships established for key mediators of apoptosis. *J. Biol. Chem.*, **272**, 17907–11.

Tompkins, M., Basgall, E., Zamrini, E. & Hill, W. (1997). Apoptotic-like changes in Lewy-body-associated disorders and normal aging in substantia nigral neurons. *Am. J. Pathol.*, **150**, 119–31.

van Loo, G., Saelens, X., van Gurp, M., MacFarlane, M., Martin, S. J. & Vandenabeele, P. (2002). The role of mitochondrial factors in apoptosis: a Russian roulette with more than one bullet. *Cell Death Differ.*, **9**, 1031–42.

Velier, J. J., Ellison, J. A., Kikly, K. K., Spera, P. A., Barone, F. C. & Feuerstein, G. Z. (1999). Caspase-8 and caspase-3 are expressed by different populations of cortical neurons undergoing delayed cell death after focal stroke in the rat. *J. Neurosci.*, **19**, 5932–41.

Vila, M., Jackson-Lewis, V. V., Vukosavic, S. *et al.* (2001). Bax ablation prevents dopaminergic neurodegeneration in the 1-methyl-4-phenyl-1,2,3,6-tetrahydropyridine mouse model of Parkinson's disease. *Proc. Natl Acad. Sci., USA*, **98**, 2837–42.

Viswanath, V., Wu, Z., Fonck, C., Wei, Q., Boonplueang, R. & Andersen, J. K. (2000). Transgenic mice neuronally expressing baculoviral p35 are resistant to diverse types of induced apoptosis, including seizure-associated neurodegeneration. *Proc. Natl Acad. Sci., USA*, **97**, 2270–5.

Viswanath, V., Wu, Y., Boonplueang, R. *et al.* (2001). Caspase-9 activation results in downstream caspase-8 activation and bid cleavage in 1-methyl-4-phenyl-1,2,3,6-tetrahydropyridine-induced Parkinson's disease. *J. Neurosci.*, **21**, 9519–28.

von Coelln, R., Kugler, S., Bahr, M., Weller, M., Dichgans, J. & Schulz, J. B. (2001). Rescue from death but not from functional impairment: caspase inhibition protects dopaminergic cells against 6-hydroxydopamine-induced apoptosis but not against the loss of their terminals. *J. Neurochem.*, **77**, 263–73.

Vukosavic, S., Dubois-Dauphin, M., Romero, N. & Przedborski, S. (1999). Bax and Bcl-2 interaction in a transgenic mouse model of familial amyotrophic lateral sclerosis. *J. Neurochem.*, **73**, 2460–8.

Vukosavic, S., Stefanis, L., Jackson-Lewis, V. *et al.* (2000). Delaying caspase activation by Bcl-2: a clue to disease retardation in a transgenic mouse model of amyotrophic lateral sclerosis. *J. Neurosci.*, **20**, 9119–25.

Waldmeier, P. C., Spooren, W. P. & Hengerer, B. (2000). CGP 3466 protects dopaminergic neurons in lesion models of Parkinson's disease. *Naunyn Schmiedebergs Arch. Pharmacol.*, **362**, 526–37.

Wellington, C. L., Ellerby, L. M., Hackam, A. S. *et al.* (1998). Caspase cleavage of gene products associated with triplet expansion disorders generates truncated fragments containing the polyglutamine tract. *J. Biol. Chem.*, **273**, 9158–67.

Wellington, C. L., Ellerby, L. M., Gutekunst, C. A. *et al.* (2002). Caspase cleavage of mutant huntingtin precedes neurodegeneration in Huntington's disease. *J. Neurosci.*, **22**, 7862–72.

Whitfield, J., Neame, S. J., Paquet, L., Bernard, O. & Ham, J. (2001). Dominant-negative c-Jun promotes neuronal survival by reducing BIM expression and inhibiting mitochondrial cytochrome c release. *Neuron*, **29**, 629–43.

Wu, D. C., Jackson-Lewis, V., Vila, M. *et al.* (2002). Blockade of microglial activation is neuroprotective in the 1-methyl-4-phenyl-1,2,3,6-tetrahydropyridine mouse model of Parkinson disease. *J. Neurosci.*, **22**, 1763–71.

Wüllner, U., Kornhuber, J., Weller, M. *et al.* (1999). Cell death and apoptosis regulating proteins in Parkinson's disease – a cautionary note. *Acta Neuropathol.*, **97**, 408–12.

Xia, X. G., Harding, T., Weller, M., Bieneman, A., Uney, J. B. & Schulz, J. B. (2001). Gene transfer of the JNK interacting protein-1 protects dopaminergic neurons in the MPTP model of Parkinson's disease. *Proc. Natl Acad. Sci., USA*, **98**, 10433–8.

Xu, D. G., Crocker, S. J., Doucet, J.-P. *et al.* (1997). Elevation of neuronal expression of NAIP reduces ischemic damage in the rat hippocampus. *Nat. Med.*, **3**, 997–1004.

Xu, D., Bureau, Y., McIntyre, D. C. *et al.* (1999). Attenuation of ischemia-induced cellular and behavioral deficits by X chromosome-linked inhibitor of apoptosis protein overexpression in the rat hippocampus. *J. Neurosci.*, **19**, 5026–33.

Yakovlev, A. G., Knoblach, S. M., Fan, L., Fox, G. B., Goodnight, R. & Faden, A. I. (1997). Activation of CPP32-like caspases contributes to neuronal apoptosis and neurological dysfunction after traumatic brain injury. *J. Neurosci.*, **17**, 7415–24.

Yang, L., Matthews, R. T., Schulz, J. B. *et al.* (1998). MPTP neurotoxicity is attenuated in mice overexpressing Bcl-2. *J. Neurosci.*, **18**, 8145–52.

Yang, L., Sugama, S., Chirichigno, J. W. *et al.* (2003). Minocycline enhances MPTP toxicity to dopaminergic neurons, *J. Neurosci. Res.*, **74**, 278–85.

Zhu, S., Stavrovskaya, I. G., Drozda, M. *et al.* (2002). Minocycline inhibits cytochrome c release and delays progression of amyotrophic lateral sclerosis in mice. *Nature*, **417**, 74–8.

8

Neurotrophic factors

Michael Sendtner

Institute for Clinical Neurobiology, Würzburg, Germany

Introduction

During development of higher vertebrates, many types of neurons including spinal and bulbar motoneurons are generated in excess. When developing motoneurons become postmitotic, they grow out axons and make contact with their target tissue, the skeletal muscle. Subsequently, about 50% of the motoneurons are lost during a critical process, which is called physiological motoneuron cell death. This phenomenon has been the focus of research for about a century and has led to the identification of neurotrophic factors that regulate survival of motoneurons during this developmental period. Motoneuron cell death is also observed in vitro when these neurons are isolated from the embryonic avian or rodent spinal cord. These cultured motoneurons have been a useful tool for studying basic mechanisms underlying neuronal degeneration. Such studies have revealed insights into signaling pathways that modulate survival during development and that might be disturbed under pathophysiological conditions in neurodegenerative disorders such as amyotrophic lateral sclerosis (ALS). However, specific differences in mechanisms that regulate survival of developing and postnatal motoneurons have also been identified. These findings could help to develop new therapeutic strategies that could counteract the pathophysiological processes underlying ALS.

Developmental motoneuron cell death

Viktor Hamburger and other pioneer researchers have shown during the first part of the twentieth century that the developmental cell death of motoneurons is guided by influences provided from the target tissue (Hamburger, 1934, 1958). Removal of limb buds in developing chick embryos enhances massively developmental motoneuron death, and transplantation of an additional limb reduces the number of dying motoneurons. This kind of plasticity allows the individual organism to react to deviations from genetically determined developmental programs, and thus might have contributed during evolution to the generation of a highly complex nervous system in higher vertebrates. On the other hand, this high complexity also implies possibilities for disturbances by gene mutations and dysregulation of gene expression, which then could lead to specific diseases.

The concept that factors from skeletal muscle play a major role in regulating motoneuron survival during development has been challenged recently by the observation that mice deficient for erb-B3, the receptor for glial growth factor (GGF), show a severe deficit of developing Schwann cells, and then, as a consequence, a significant reduction (79%) in motoneurons (Riethmacher *et al.*, 1997). Thus, developing Schwann cells appear to be at least as important for motoneurons as skeletal muscle. However, these findings are not necessarily contradictory. These data could also indicate that motoneurons first become dependent on muscle-derived neurotrophic support and then, subsequently, on Schwann cell-derived factors. When skeletal muscle is destroyed (Grieshammer *et al.*, 1998), motoneuron survival in the lumbar spinal cord is reduced highly during embryonic development, thus confirming earlier data obtained from experiments in chick when limb buds are removed (Oppenheim, 1985). In conclusion, neurotrophic factors provided from various cell types apparently play together in regulating survival and functional integrity of motoneurons both during development and in the adult.

This scenario appears even more complex with respect to early findings that motoneuron cell death in vertebrates can also occur in a target-independent manner. Rita Levi-Montalcini and others have shown (Levi-Montalcini,

1950; O'Connor & Wyttenbach, 1974; Oppenheim *et al.*, 1989) that, during early development of the chick embryo around day 4, massive cell death can be observed in a specific population of motoneurons in the ventral cervical spinal cord. This type of cell death is highly synchronized, in contrast to motoneuron cell death observed in this and other regions of the developing chick spinal cord between embryonic day 6 and 10, which roughly corresponds to embryonic day 14 and postnatal day 3 in the mouse or rat. A recent study (Yaginuma *et al.*, 1996) has shown that this type of early motoneuron cell death occurs in a target-independent manner and may be determined by a cell-autonomous program. Taken together, these data suggest that cell death programs in motoneurons probably change during development, and at least some of the motoneurons pass through an early phase when cell-autonomous and/or target-independent processes regulate cell death and then undergo a phase when signals from skeletal muscle play a major role. Subsequently, signals from Schwann cells such as CNTF and other survival factors acting through signaling pathways that involve Stat-3 contribute to the maintenance of motoneurons, and evidence from experiments with various mouse mutants suggests that postnatal survival of motoneurons becomes increasingly dependent again on cell autonomous processes such as sufficient expression of the "survival of motoneuron" (SMN) protein (Jablonka *et al.*, 2000; Monani *et al.*, 2000) and protection from glutamate-mediated toxicity (Rothstein, 1995). Further research has to show how these signals and the intracellular signaling pathways play together and how the motoneurons react to disturbances of individual signals. The availability of mouse mutants, in which individual signals are disrupted either by classical homologous recombination or in a cell type-specific or otherwise inducible manner by use of the Cre/loxP and other recombination techniques, will help to understand such processes and thus could provide a basis for rational design of therapeutic strategies for treatment of various forms of motoneuron disease.

Neurotrophic factors for motoneurons

Nerve growth factor (NGF) was the first neurotrophic factor to be discovered. It is a prototypic target-derived neurotrophic molecule that regulates survival of subpopulations of sensory and sympathetic neurons. Since 1989, more than ten neurotrophic factors have been identified and characterized on a molecular level. This list includes factors called neurotrophins, which are related to NGF. At least three neurotrophins, brain-derived neurotrophic

Table 8.1. Neurotrophic factors for motoneurons and their receptors

	Receptor on motoneurons
1. Neurotrophins	
Brain-derived neurotrophic factor (BDNF)	p75^{NTR}, trk-B
Neurotrophin-3 (NT-3)	p75^{NTR}, trk-C
Neurotrophin-4/5 (NT-4/5)	p75^{NTR}, trk-B
2. CNTF/LIF family	
Ciliary neurotrophic factor (CNTF)	CNTFRα, LIFRß, gp130
Leukemia inhibitory factor (LIF)	LIFRß, gp130
Cardiotrophin-1 (CT-1)	?, LIFRß, gp130
Cardiotrophin-1 like cytokine (CLC)	CNTFRα, LIFRß, gp130
3. Hepatocyte growth factor/scatter factor (HGF/SF)	c-met
4. Insulin-like growth factors	
IGF-I	IGFR-1
IGF-II	IGFR-1, Mannose-6P receptor
5. Glial-derived neurotrophic factor and related factors	
Glial-derived neurotrophic factor (GDNF)	GFRα1, c-ret
Neurturin (NTR)	GFRα2, c-ret
Persephin	GFRα4, c-ret
Artemin	GFRα3, c-ret

factor, neurotrophin-4 and neurotrophin-3, but not NGF, support motoneuron survival (Henderson *et al.*, 1993; Hughes *et al.*, 1993; Sendtner *et al.*, 1992a). Motoneurons are also supported by other neurotrophic molecules, indicating that motoneuron survival and function is a highly complex process, which is influenced by a cooperative function of these molecules so far not fully understood. Some of these molecules are expressed only postnatally. Thus the requirement for neurotrophic factors seems to change from developmental periods to postnatal life. Moreover, neurotrophic factors do not only act on motoneuron survival but also on functional parameters such as the regulation of transmitter synthesis and release, axon outgrowth and synaptic stability (for review, see Sendtner, 1998).

The CNTF family supports motoneuron survival through the activation of complex membrane receptors involving gp130 and LIFR-β (Nakashima & Taga, 1998). Factors that bind to such complexes are the ciliary neurotrophic factor (Arakawa *et al.*, 1990), the leukemia-inhibitory factor (Hughes *et al.*, 1993), cardiotrophin-1 (Pennica *et al.*, 1995) and the recently identified cardiotrophin-like cytokine (CLC) (Pennica *et al.*, 1995; Senaldi *et al.*, 1999; Shi *et al.*, 1999), which also can bind to the CNTF receptor complex (Elson *et al.*, 2000).

Survival of cultured motoneurons is also supported by members of the glial-derived neurotrophic factor (GDNF) gene family of transforming growth factor-β-related survival factors (Henderson *et al.*, 1994; Zurn *et al.*, 1994). Factors that support motoneuron survival include GDNF (Henderson *et al.*, 1994), neurturin (Klein *et al.*, 1997), persephin (Milbrandt *et al.*, 1998), and artemin (Baloh *et al.*, 1998). These molecules act through receptors involving the c-ret tyrosine kinase, and specific α-receptors (Baloh *et al.*, 1997).

HGF is a heterodimeric protein with similarities to plasminogen. However, it lacks enzymatic activity (Weidner *et al.*, 1991). Only lumbar motoneurons from 5-day old chick embryos survive with HGF, but not motoneurons from thoracic or cervical spinal cord (Novak *et al.*, 2000). In chick embryos, the c-met tyrosine kinase is expressed in lumbar but not in thoracic motoneurons between embryonic day 5 and 10 during the period of physiological motoneuron cell death. However, the expression of c-met in lumbar motoneurons seems to be regulated by target tissue-derived factors other than HGF. This conclusion is based on the observation that the massive cell death of motoneurons that occurs in the lumbar spinal cord after limb-bud removal cannot be reduced by treatment with HGF, probably because the c-met receptor is downregulated by limb-bud removal and signals that lead to expression of this receptor are thus removed. Thus, HGF is another example of a neurotrophic factor (Wong *et al.*, 1997) that influences survival of specific subpopulations of motoneurons, and needs cooperation with other signals in order to exert its survival-promoting effect. The list of molecules that support motoneuron survival is still growing, and it is expected that it will become even longer in the future.

Motoneurons are also supported by insulin-like growth factor-1 and IGF-2 (Arakawa *et al.*, 1990; Ebens *et al.*, 1996; Yamamoto *et al.*, 1997). In cultures of isolated embryonic chick spinal motoneurons, the survival-promoting effects of IGFs are relatively low, in contrast to cultures of embryonic rat motoneurons, which can be maintained in serum-free medium (Hughes *et al.*, 1993). However, when IGFs are combined with other neurotrophic factors such as CNTF, this leads to supraadditive survival effects (Arakawa *et al.*, 1990). Thus neurotrophic factors potentate each other, suggesting that survival of motoneurons in vivo depends on a complex cooperation of more than one factor. Similarly, when BDNF was administered for prolonged

periods to lesioned facial motoneurons via a gene therapeutic approach, it supported survival but could not prevent atrophy of the motoneuron cell bodies (Gravel *et al.*, 1997). Only when BDNF and CNTF were added together was a significant anti-atrophic effect observed.

This observation is important for designing therapies with neurotrophic factors. The administration of a single factor does not meet the physiological requirements of motoneurons, in particular when these cells suffer from a chronic degenerative process, and combinations of factors might be necessary to influence the course of the disease in ALS.

Identification of cellular signaling pathways responsible for neurotrophic factor mediated survival of motoneurons

A major focus of molecular neurobiology is signaling pathways, which mediate the various functions of neurotrophic factors. These pathways could serve as targets for rational drug design and thus for development of therapeutics to treat symptoms such as axon degeneration and cell death of motoneurons, the hallmarks of ALS (Chou, 1992). Neurotrophins have served as a prototypic gene family for investigation of such signaling pathways in primary neurons (Segal & Greenberg, 1996). Signaling through high affinity neurotrophin receptors that include members of the trk gene family involves several pathways. Initiation of these pathways depends on the cytosolic adapter protein Shc, the activation of PLC-γ and the activation of the PI-3-kinase/AKT-pathways directly at the level of the trk transmembrane tyrosine kinases.

The Shc adapter proteins have been the focus of research, as they can couple trk-signaling to the Ras/MAP-kinase pathway. This pathway is involved in promoting neuronal survival and neurite outgrowth. Experiments with PC-12 cells (Bar-Sagi & Feramisco, 1985), with primary sympathetic neurons (Borasio *et al.*, 1993) and with mice in which the Shc binding site in trk receptors is altered demonstrate that activated Ras supports differentiation and survival of neuronal cells. At least in PC-12 cells, sustained activation of the MAPK pathway (Aletta, 1994; Traverse *et al.*, 1992; Wixler *et al.*, 1996) supports differentiation vs mitogenic effects of NGF in comparison to epidermal growth factor (EGF), and sustained activation of the MAPK pathway also appears necessary for neurotrophin-mediated survival of motoneurons. Moreover, a second Ras-independent pathway for activation of the MAPK pathway has been found to be involved in mediating the differentiation effects of NGF (York *et al.*, 1998). This redirects the focus of interest on activation mechanisms upstream from Ras and other small GTP-binding proteins, which transduce the signal from receptor molecules to the MAPK and other intracellular signaling pathways.

In neurons, several forms of Shc exist, which are named ShcA, ShcB, and ShcC/N-shc (Cattaneo & Pelicci, 1998). The expression of these Shc isoforms is under strict control during development. The ratio of ShcA and ShcC/N-Shc expression deserves particular attention. ShcC/N-Shc has been detected as a neuron-specific Shc isoform (Nakamura et al., 1996), which mediates the coupling of trk signaling to Ras activation. Whereas ShcA is expressed ubiquitously, ShcC expression is only found in the nervous system. The upregulation of ShcC corresponds to downregulation of ShcA expression in the brain at a developmental stage when neuronal cells become postmitotic (Conti et al., 1997) and at least some populations of neurons including the motoneurons become dependent on neurotrophic factors for their survival. It is tempting to speculate that this switch from ShcA to ShcC expression is responsible for a switch in response to neurotrophic factors from a differentiation signal to a survival signal (Segal & Greenberg, 1996). This could be of importance for understanding how developing motoneurons become responsible to neurotrophic factors for their survival.

Recent evidence from mice in which the Shc binding site in trkB was mutated (Minichiello et al., 1998) suggests that differences between various neurotrophic factors exist in the utilization of this pathway for survival and neurite outgrowth. Mice in which the Shc binding site of trkB is mutated show that NT-4-mediated survival effects were reduced more dramatically than BDNF-dependent differentiation or survival. These mice display a complete loss of the NT-4-dependent D-hair sensory cells but no change in BDNF-dependent, slowly adapting mechanotransducing sensory neurons. However, survival of motoneurons has not been investigated in such mice so far, and it remains to be demonstrated whether survival or functional properties in subpopulations of motoneurons are altered when the Shc binding site is mutated in the trkB receptor. Nevertheless, this report showed that significant differences exist between various ligands in the activation of downstream pathways, even if shared receptor components such as trkB in the case of BDNF and NT-4 are involved.

Besides the Ras/MAPK pathway, a second pathway involving activation of PI-3K is highly important for neuronal survival (Dudek et al., 1997). PI-3K can associate directly with trk receptors under various experimental conditions (Obermeier et al., 1993). However, it is now accepted widely that Shc signaling plays a major role for activation of PI-3K downstream of trks in neuronal cells (Baxter et al., 1995; Datta et al., 1997; Greene & Kaplan, 1995). The PI-3-kinase in turn activates Akt, a serine/threonine kinase with a broad spectrum of substrates including the proapoptotic Bad (Datta et al., 1997), caspase-9 (Cardone et al., 1998), the forkhead transcription factor FKHRL1 (Brunet et al., 1999) and IKKα kinase (Ozes et al., 1999; Romashkova & Makarov, 1999). Future studies will show which of these downstream pathways could modulate motoneuron survival under pathophysiological conditions such as ALS.

A third important pathway, which could be of importance in particular for motoneurons is the activation of PLCγ1 (Obermeier et al., 1994; Segal & Greenberg, 1996; Tinhofer et al., 1996). Activation of PLCγ1 leads to increased release of free Ca^{2+} from intracellular stores, which in turn activates cyclic AMP response-element-binding protein (CREB) (Finkbeiner et al., 1997). In addition, elevated intracellular Ca^{2+} levels have also been described to activate the small GTP-binding protein Rap1 but not Ras (Grewal et al., 2000). Rap1 activates B-Raf but not Raf-1. In developing motoneurons, B-Raf is expressed at relatively high levels during the period of physiological cell death (Wiese et al., 2001). Thus increased levels of Ca^{2+} could contribute to activation of Rafs, which seem to play a central role both in activation of the MAPK pathway and also as effector kinases for bcl-2, which phosphorylates BAD and thus inhibits its proapoptotic activity (Wang et al., 1994, 1996).

Dysregulation of these processes might also contribute to the pathophysiology of motoneuron disease, and future studies have to show which members of the Shc family are expressed in motoneurons in ALS patients, and whether changes in expression levels could alter signals from target tissues, glial cells and possibly also from pharmacologically applied neurotrophic factors.

The role of neuronal activity and glutamate for motoneuron survival

Removal of afferent synpase activity leads to increased cell death in vivo (Okado & Oppenheim, 1984) in various neuronal cell types. This finding corresponds to observations in cell culture that neurons can be maintained under conditions that mimic depolarization, such as elevated potassium concentration (Wakade et al., 1983) or even addition of glutamate receptor agonists at optimal concentrations (Meyer Franke et al., 1995). However, various types of neurons differ in their capacity to survive in culture in the presence of increased levels of potassium or glutamate. Whereas 35 mM K^+ in the culture medium supports survival of sympathetic neurons from 10-day-old chick embryos (Wakade *et al.*, 1983), motoneurons from 5- or 6-day old chick embryos cannot survive for periods longer than 3 days under the same conditions. In this respect, motoneurons resemble retinal ganglion cells, which cannot survive for prolonged periods with elevated potassium concentration in the culture medium (Meyer Franke *et al.*, 1995). On the other side, BDNF-mediated survival was enhanced strongly in isolated retinal ganglion cells when the cells were depolarized or when NMDA or kainic acid were added to these cultures. The effect appears to be mediated by elevation of cAMP, as inhibitors of protein kinase A inhibit the potentiation of the BDNF survival effect by increased potassium or glutamate agonists. These data also suggest that intracellular Ca^{2+} elevation is involved in potentiating survival effects of neurotrophic factors.

Glutamate toxicity is considered as a major pathomechanism in amyotrophic lateral sclerosis (Choi, 1992). Although first clinical trials with specific glutamate receptor inhibitors failed (Gredal *et al.*, 1997), Riluzole is thought to delay progression of the disease by interfering with excitotoxic mechanisms (Bensimon *et al.*, 1994). However, it is not clear whether the effect occurs at the presynaptic or postsynaptic site, or even by interference with pathogenic mechanisms other than glutamatergic signaling such as presynaptic potassium channels.

Embryonic motoneurons express NMDA receptors (Kalb *et al.*, 1992) and AMPA receptors including subtypes of AMPA receptors that mediate Ca^{2+} influx in response to glutamate (Metzger *et al.*, 2000). When these motoneurons are exposed to enhanced concentrations of glutamate or NMDA in vitro, motoneuron cell death is not enhanced (Metzger *et al.*, 1998). This seems surprising with respect to the observation that massive cell death occurs under the same conditions in other types of neurons, for example in cultures of cortical neurons (M.S., unpublished observations). Even when the motoneurons are depolarized in order to remove the Mg^{2+}-block in NMDA receptors, this does not influence the survival of motoneurons in cell culture. On the other hand, NMDA or glutamate exposure does not potentiate the survival effect of BDNF or other neurotrophic factors, as observed with isolated retinal ganglion cells (Meyer Franke *et al.*, 1995). Despite this negative effect, motoneurons show specific responses to enhanced glutamate levels in the culture medium. Glutamate treatment leads to specific inhibition of dendrite growth in a fully reversible manner. Axon outgrowth was not affected under the same culture conditions by glutamate exposure, suggesting that glutamate could play an important role in plasticity of dendrite growth and synapse formation between motoneurons and other types of neurons within the spinal cord.

An active role of NGF signaling in motoneuron cell death?

Genetic determination of cell death plays an important role during development of non-vertebrates such as *Caenorhabditis elegans*. The ces-2 gene apparently acts cell-autonomously to trigger programmed cell death (Metzstein *et al.*, 1996). Ces-2 is expressed specifically in two distinct pharyngeal motoneurons in the worm and initiates death in these specific cells. Such cell-autonomous cell death genes have not been identified so far in motoneurons from higher vertebrates, although it is likely that they could play a role, for example during an early phase of development when motoneuron cell death apparently occurs in a target-independent manner. The cell death receptor Fas and the corresponding Fas ligand are expressed in early motoneurons, and Fas has been found to transmit a cell death signal in cultured motoneurons from 12.5-day-old mouse embryos (Raoul *et al.*, 1999). Fas and Fas-ligand are expressed early during development in motoneurons, and coexpression of these two molecules is expected to confer cell-autonomous cell death programs. When embryonic motoneurons are cultured for 3 days with neurotrophic factors, they become resistant to Fas-induced cell death, either by interference with downstream-effectors such as activated caspase-8 and caspase-3, or by promoting motoneuron maturation to a stage when they are resistant to other mediators of cell-autonomous cell death programs, or by both mechanisms. Thus, Fas and Fas-ligand could play a role during early stages of motoneuron cell death when these cells do not yet depend, or even cannot react, to neurotrophic factors, and further studies for example involving Bid-deficient mice, which are resistant to Fas-induced cell death, could be of great help in understanding the physiological role of Fas-mediated cell death for motoneurons.

The p75 neurotrophin receptor (p75[NTR]) shares structural and functional similarities with other transmembrane molecules of the Fas/Apo-1/CD95 and tumor necrosis factor receptor – 1 family (for review see Nagata, 1997). In a variety of cellular contexts in vitro and in vivo, p75[NTR] mediates cell death after the binding of NGF, in particular when trkA is not expressed (Chao *et al.*, 1998; Friedman & Greene, 1999). Injection of neutralizing antibodies into the eye of early chick embryos has shown that NGF and p75[NTR] are involved in early developmental cell death of retinal ganglion cells that have just been formed and are starting to grow axons (Frade *et al.*, 1996; Frades Barde, 1998). This early phase of cell death is not regulated by the target tissue. In the specific case, the source of NGF were microglial cells that had invaded the retina during these early developmental stages (Frade *et al.*, 1996).

The role of p75^{NTR} as a mediator of cell death has also been shown in basal forebrain cholinergic neurons (Yeo *et al.*, 1997). Overexpression of the cytoplasmic part of the p75^{NTR} in mice (Majdan *et al.*, 1997) leads to significant loss of several populations of neurons, including motoneurons in the facial nucleus. Thus, it appears intriguing that p75^{NTR} could have similar functions in motoneurons, in particular when this receptor is expressed at high levels after axotomy. When the expression of this receptor was abolished in adult p75^{NTR} $-/-$ mice, survival and regeneration of axotomized motoneurons were improved in comparison to control animals (Ferri *et al.*, 1998), and overexpression of the cytoplasmic part of p75^{NTR} enhances lesion-induced cell death of facial motoneurons in adult mice (Majdan *et al.*, 1997). Moreover, application of NGF to axotomized sciatic (Miyata *et al.*, 1986) or facial (Sendtner *et al.*, 1992a) motoneurons significantly increases the rate of cell death (Wiese *et al.*, 1999b). These results are compatible with the assumption that p75^{NTR} is a cell death receptor in developing motoneurons. On the other side, and in contrast to other neuronal populations (Bamji *et al.*, 1998; Van der Zee *et al.*, 1996, 1998; Yeo *et al.*, 1997), the number of motoneurons in 6–9 week old p75^{NTR} $-/-$ mice is reduced in comparison to wild-type mice, as revealed by quantification of facial motoneuron numbers and axon profiles in brainstem and peripheral nerves (Ferri *et al.*, 1998; Wiese *et al.*, 1999b). However, in the case of basal forebrain cholinergic neurons, contradictory results have been obtained in the meantime so that at least one of the originally published reports apparently is not reproducible, and the findings thus do not support a proapoptotic function through the p75 neurotrophin receptor as has been reported originally for postnatal basal forebrain cholinergic neurons (Van der Zee *et al.*, 1996).

Motoneurons do not only express high levels of p75^{NTR} in neurodegenerative disease including ALS (Kerkhoff *et al.*, 1991) or after axotomy, but also under physiological conditions during early development. Expression of this receptor molecule occurs before the motoneurons contact skeletal muscle and before they become responsive to neurotrophins for their survival. In order to test the possibility that NGF and p75^{NTR} are mediators of the early phase of motoneuron cell death in brachial spinal cord, cell death in the spinal cord of p75^{NTR} $-/-$ and NGF $-/-$ mice has been investigated. Between E10.5 and 12.5, before the period of classical target-dependent cell death starts (Frade & Barde, 1999), an increase in the thickness of the mantle zone was observed. However, the number of ISLET-1 positive motoneurons was not increased in the ventral portion of the spinal cord of these mutant mice.

The role of p75^{NTR} in motoneuron cell death is different at later developmental stages (Wiese *et al.*, 1999b). NGF reduces the survival effects of BDNF and NT-3 in wild-type but not in p75^{NTR} $-/-$ motoneurons. These data thus favor a model of p75^{NTR} functioning as a cell death receptor in motoneurons. However, the quantities of NGF that interfere with the survival responses of BDNF and NT-3 are very low (7×10^{-13} M) (Fig. 8.1). They do not reach the levels necessary for saturating those low-affinity binding sites on primary neurons that are thought to correspond to p75^{NTR} receptors (Meakin & Shooter, 1992; Rodriguez-Tébar *et al.*, 1990). It has been described that p75^{NTR} can be expressed in neuronal cells in a conformation conferring high-affinity binding of NT-3 (Dechant *et al.*, 1997). However, under the same experimental conditions, NGF did not bind to p75^{NTR} when added at 10^{-12} M.

Observations that very low quantities of NGF interfere with BDNF and NT-3 effects in neurons could be explained by a model in which the p75^{NTR} is part of the high-affinity receptors for BDNF and NT-3. Previous observations that NGF enhances motoneuron survival at later developmental stages in chick (Qin-Wei *et al.*, 1994) when p75^{NTR} expression is low (Ernfors *et al.*, 1988) suggest that the presence of p75^{NTR} increases the specificity of BDNF and NT-3 binding to their receptors. Reduction of NT-3- and BDNF-mediated survival by NGF is not seen in p75^{NTR} $-/-$ motoneurons. This observation supports the model that p75^{NTR} receptors are components of the high-affinity binding sites for NT-3 and BDNF on E14 lumbar motoneurons and do not constitute separate NGF receptors. The BDNF dose necessary for half-maximal survival is shifted from 1.2×10^{-12} M in wild-type motoneurons to 5.4×10^{-12} M in p75^{NTR} $-/-$ motoneurons. This supports previous data that trk homodimers are not equivalent to high-affinity neurotrophin receptors in primary neurons (Mahadeo *et al.*, 1994; Wolf *et al.*, 1995). Thus p75^{NTR} appears as part of the high-affinity receptor complex for BDNF and possibly also NT-3 on motoneurons. Only part, if any, of the p75^{NTR} transmembrane molecule receptors should exist separately and function independently as cell death receptors on these cells. In the latter case, one would expect that NGF signaling through p75^{NTR} should also reduce the survival response mediated through CNTF or GDNF receptors. However, even high quantities of NGF (20 ng/ml) known to saturate low-affinity receptors on neuronal cells (Rodriguez-Tébar *et al.*, 1990) did not reduce CNTF- and GDNF-mediated survival of motoneurons. This was surprising insofar as the CNTF-mediated survival response of embryonic chick mesencephalic trigeminal neurons was

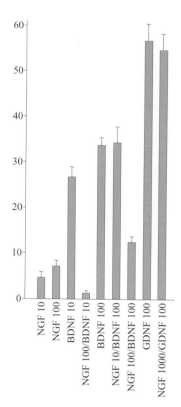

Fig. 8.1 NGF antagonizes BDNF-mediated survival of mouse motoneurons in culture. Motoneurons were isolated from lumbar spinal cord of 14-day-old mouse embryos (Wiese *et al.*, 1999b). Survival of motoneurons was determined by counting surviving motoneurons after 3 days in culture. Values shown are a percentage of initially plated neurons in the culture dish. BDNF and NGF were added at concentrations indicated at 10 or 100 pg/ml. The survival effect of BDNF is significantly reduced in the presence of NGF at equimolar concentrations, and completely abolished when NGF is given at doses 10 times higher than BDNF. Note that maximal concentration of NGF in this experiment was 100 pg/ml, which is below the concentration thought to saturate low-affinity neurotrophin receptors. NGF could not reduce the survival response initiated by GDNF, even when the concentration was increased to a level of 1000 pg/ml, thus suggesting that NGF acts as a specific antagonist, probably at the receptor level, rather than acting as an independent cell death effector on these cultured motoneurons.

Downstream signals which mediate the neuronal survival response to neurotrophins and CNTF: the role of members of the IAP family

Not very much is known about the downstream signals involved in execution of motoneuron cell death and neurotrophic factor-mediated survival. Research on the role of bcl-2 has guided the way to our present knowledge. Overexpression of bcl-2 significantly reduces the extent of motoneuron cell death during development (Dubois-Dauphin *et al.*, 1994; Martinou *et al.*, 1994). However, mice in which bcl-2 expression is abolished by homologous recombination show only a small reduction of motoneuron numbers at birth (Michaelidis *et al.*, 1996), indicating either that bcl-2-related molecules can substitute for this deficiency or that bcl-2 and related molecules are not necessary physiologically for motoneuron survival during development. Motoneuron cell death in bcl-2 $-/-$ mice is enhanced only during the postnatal period, leading to loss of 40% of facial motoneurons in 6-week-old mice. This suggests that bcl-2 becomes important for postnatal survival at least of subpopulations of motoneurons. However, bcl-2 deficient motoneurons do not lose their responsiveness to neurotrophic factors. BDNF and CNTF are still capable of rescuing motoneurons from lesion-induced cell death after facial nerve transection in newborn animals. Nevertheless, survival in response to these neurotrophic factors was lower in bcl-2 deficient mice, indicating that subpopulations depend on bcl-2 for survival after nerve lesion, and/or that compensation by other antiapoptotic members of the bcl-2 family is only incomplete in these cells.

Observations that neurons from BAX-deficient mice (Deckwerth *et al.*, 1998; Knudson *et al.*, 1995) are resistant against cell death after neurotrophic factor deprivation provide a second indication that members of the bcl-2 family are involved, and that mitochondria play a role in motoneuron cell death. Recently, it has been shown that BAX-dependent release of cytochrome c from mitochondria plays an essential role in the initiation of cell death in NGF-deprived sympathetic neurons (Deshmukh & Johnson, Jr., 1998). However, microinjection of cytochrome c into the cytoplasm could not initiate cell death when the primary sympathetic neurons were grown in the presence of NGF. Based on these observations, it was speculated that NGF leads to a rapid production of an intracellular protein, which protects cells from proapoptotic actions of cytochrome c (Newmeyer & Green, 1998). Furthermore, it was concluded that such protective molecules are expressed at low basal levels and upregulated within a short time after NGF exposure.

reduced by NGF (Davey & Davies, 1998). Thus, the role of p75^{NTR} differs depending on cell type and developmental stage. Whether such differences are caused by the presence or absence of downstream-effectors of trk and p75^{NTR} signaling, or simply by the fact that apoptosis through p75^{NTR} requires higher expression levels than those found in motoneurons from E14 mouse spinal cord, remains to be seen.

Members of the IAP/ITA family are candidates for such protective proteins. They inhibit the activation of procaspase-9 (Deveraux *et al.*, 1998), which is initiated by cytochrome c and Apaf-1 (Slee *et al.*, 1999; Stennicke *et al.*, 1999). Furthermore, they inhibit the function of activated caspase-3, -6 and -7, and thus interfere at at least two levels with cellular programs for apoptosis (Devereaux *et al.*, 1997; Roy *et al.*, 1997). The identification and cloning of the chick *ita* gene (Digby *et al.*, 1996), which encodes a protein of 611 amino acids with highest homology to human cIAP-2, allowed investigation on the role of this protein in NGF-mediated survival of developing chick neurons. ITA expression is induced rapidly by neurotrophic factors (Fig. 8.2). This upregulation of ITA mRNA and protein levels involves the PI-3K pathway. Overexpression of ITA in primary sensory and sympathetic neurons can promote neuronal survival in the absence of NGF, and antisense expression of ITA abolishes NGF-mediated survival in sensory and sympathetic neurons. These actions involve the baculovirus IAP repeat (BIR) domains of the ITA protein, as expression of a BIR-deleted form of ITA was without any effect on neuronal survival.

These data suggest that members of the IAP family, which include the mammalian IAP-2 and XIAP, are key regulators in the signaling machinery for neurotrophic factor-mediated neuronal survival. The expression of inhibitors for caspases could be an essential mechanism, which contributes to motoneuron survival once these caspases are activated (Fig. 8.3), and they probably could be of high importance in protecting motoneurons against any kind of proapoptotic signaling that occurs during postnatal life.

Animal models for human motoneuron disease

Despite significant progress in the understanding of survival and cell death signaling for developing motoneurons, little is known about how these mechanisms relate to pathological cell death in human motoneuron disease. A subtype of autosomal dominant familial amyotrophic lateral sclerosis is caused by mutations of the superoxide-dismutase gene (Rosen *et al.*, 1993; Deng *et al.*, 1993). Overexpression of mutated SOD-1 in motoneurons causes cytoplasmic aggregation of the enzyme, and neurons with such aggregates subsequently undergo apoptotic cell death (Durham *et al.*, 1997). Mice in which mutated SOD-1 (G93A) is overexpressed exhibit postnatal degeneration of motoneurons (Gurney *et al.*, 1994). When these mice are crossbred with bcl-2 overexpressing mice, onset of disease is delayed (Kostic *et al.*, 1997), suggesting that

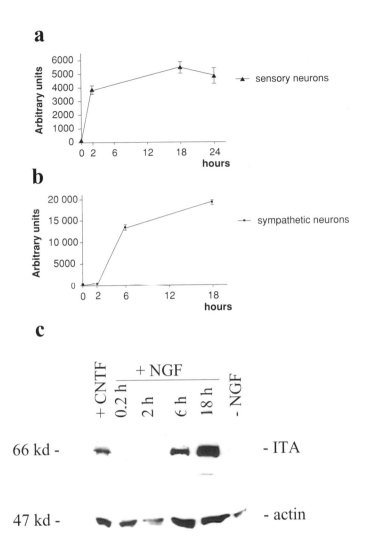

Fig. 8.2 NGF and CNTF promote rapid upregulation of the IAPs in cultured neurons. IAPs are potent inhibitors of caspases, and thus could participate in the survival response of neurons to neurotrophic factors. See Wiese *et al.* (1999a) for details. Reproduced with permission from this publication.

bcl-2 protects the motoneurons from pathogenic processes caused by mutated SOD-1. Therefore, whatever the pathogenic process in patients with mutations of SOD-1 or in transgenic mice overexpressing mutated SOD-1 is, it seems to interfere with classical cell death programs.

Similar findings have also been made with other mutant mice in which the underlying gene mutation is not known so far. Treatment with neurotrophic factors can interfere with motoneuron degeneration in mouse mutants, such as progressive motoneuronopathy (pmn) (Sendtner *et al.*, 1992b) and wobbler (Mitsumoto *et al.*, 1994) mice, and it is not clear whether the underlying gene defects are involved

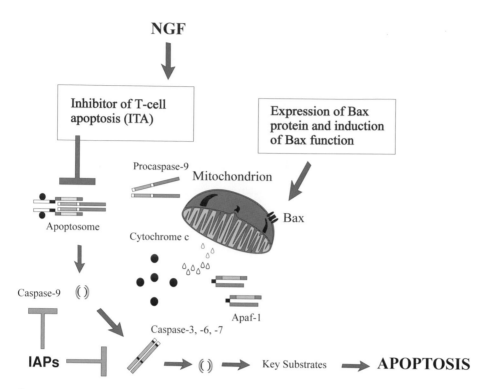

Fig. 8.3 Signaling pathways for neurotrophic factor-mediated survival of motoneurons. Recent studies (Deshmukh & Johnson, Jr., 1998) have shown that injection of cytochrome-C into the cytoplasm of cultured neurons can induce apoptosis only when nerve growth factor is absent or added after the injection of cytochrome-C. This has led to the conclusion that nerve growth factor and other neurotrophic factors lead to upregulation of an activity, which directly interferes with the activation of apoptosome activity and downstream caspases. In the absence of neurotrophic factors, cytochrome-C is released from mitochondria by a process in which Bax is involved. This leads to the formation of apoptosomes by a process also requiring Apaf-1 and ATP. By this means, procaspase-9 is cleaved and activated. Caspase-9 in turn can cleave procaspase-3, -6 and/or -7, which then activate downstream substrates, among them ICAD (inhibitor of caspase-activated Dnase (CAD)) and finally leads to apoptosis of the neuron. Members of the IAP-family (inhibitor of apoptosis protein) can block activated caspases and inhibit these regulatory steps in the execution of apoptosis. In cultured sensory and sympathetic neurons, NGF and CNTF upregulate ITA expression at least 20-fold. This upregulation takes place within less than 6 hours. Thus, ITA and mammalian homologues of this protein could be essential mediators in the downstream signaling machinery for neurotrophic factor-mediated survival of primary neurons.

in cell death or survival signaling pathways. Overexpression of bcl-2 in pmn mice does not delay the onset of the disease or prolong survival of pmn mice, although it inhibits the degeneration and cell death of motoneurons cell bodies in these mutant mice (Ikeda *et al.*, 1995). Similar observations have also been made when pmn mice were treated with GDNF (Sagot *et al.*, 1996). However, in contrast to CNTF, GDNF treatment does not lead to prolonged survival of the pmn mice. Although this neurotrophic factor reduces the extent of degeneration of motoneuron cell bodies, the degeneration of axons was not prevented, indicating that various families of neurotrophic factors differ in their potential to influence specific parameters of motoneurons such as axon maintenance or axon regeneration, at least in pmn mice.

During recent years accumulating evidence suggests that nitric oxide (NO) also plays a role in motoneuron cell death (Estevez *et al.*, 1998b; Estevez *et al.*, 1998a). Deprivation of embryonic motoneurons in culture from neurotrophic factors leads to enhanced production of neuronal nitric acid synthetase. Moreover, enhanced nitrotyrosine immunoreactivity could be observed in these motoneurons. NOS inhibitors could prevent apoptosis of cultured motoneurons, at least for short periods up to 3 days. Similar findings were made when a cell-permeable scavenger of superoxide was added to neurotrophic factor deprived motoneurons in culture. Thus enhanced superoxide and NO production, possibly also the production of peroxinitrite, could play a role as proapoptotic signals, which represent a first step in the execution of cell death in motoneurons. Recently, it was demonstrated that NO mediates the cell death of motoneurons when the superoxide-dismutase protein lacks a zinc ion, a scenario which could underlie familial ALS (Estevez *et al.*, 1999). Nevertheless, very little is known so far about how these pathways are connected with activation of caspases in motoneurons, or whether these mechanisms represent an independent proapoptotic stimulus, which acts in a caspase-independent fashion.

First evidence for interaction between these proapoptotic stimuli was shown by crossbreeding mice carrying the G93A mutation in the SOD gene with mice overexpressing a dominant-negative ICE isoform, which prevents caspases from activation of cell death pathways (Friedlander *et al.*, 1997). Thus, it will be interesting to know how neurotrophic factors interfere with such proapoptotic pathways. This could be at the transcriptional level, preventing the upregulation of proapoptotic genes such as NOS, or by upregulation of members of the IAP family, which block caspase activity. Future research has to show how pro- and antiapoptotic signaling in motoneurons is regulated in individual motoneurons, and how individual cell-specific genetic programmes at specific developmental stages, and signals from contacting cells such as muscle, glial cells and neurons, play together in these regulatory processes.

REFERENCES

Aletta, J. M. (1994). Differential effect of NGF and EGF on ERK in neuronally differentiated PC12 cells. *NeuroReport*, **5**, 2090–2.

Arakawa, Y., Sendtner, M. & Thoenen, H. (1990). Survival effect of ciliary neurotrophic factor (CNTF) on chick embryonic motoneurons in culture: comparison with other neurotrophic factors and cytokines. *J. Neurosci.*, **10**, 3507–15.

Baloh, R. H., Tansey, M. G., Golden, J. P. *et al.* (1997). TrnR2, a novel receptor that mediates neurturin and GDNF signaling through Ret. *Neuron*, **18**, 793–802.

Baloh, R. H., Tansey, M. G., Lampe, P. A. *et al.* (1998). Artemin, a novel member of the GDNF ligand family, supports peripheral and central neurons and signals through the GFRalpha3–RET receptor complex. *Neuron*, **21**, 1291–302.

Bamji, S. X., Majdan, M. & Pozniak, C. D. (1998). The p75 neurotrophin receptor mediates neuronal apoptosis and is essential for naturally occurring sympathetic neuron death. *J. Cell Biol.*, **140**, 911–23.

Bar-Sagi, D. & Feramisco, J. R. (1985). Microinjection of the ras oncogene protein into PC12 cells induces morphological differentiation. *Cell*, **42**, 841–8.

Baxter, R. M., Cohen, P., Obermeier, A., Ullrich, A., Downes, C. P. & Doza, Y. N. (1995). Phosphotyrosine residues in the nerve-growth-factor receptor (Trk-A). Their role in the activation of inositolphospholipid metabolism and protein kinase cascades in phaeochromocytoma (PC12) cells. *Eur. J. Biochem.*, **234**, 84–91.

Bensimon, G., Lacomblez, L., Meininger, V. & ALS-Riluzole Study Group (1994). A controlled trial of riluzole in amyotrophic lateral sclerosis. *N. Engl. J. Med.*, **330**, 585–91.

Borasio, G. D., Markus, A., Wittinghofer, A., Barde, Y. A. & Heumann, R. (1993). Involvement of ras p21 in neurotrophin-induced response of sensory, but not sympathetic neurons. *J. Cell Biol.*, **121**, 665–72.

Brunet, A., Bonni, A., Zigmond, M. J. *et al.* (1999). Akt promotes cell survival by phosphorylating and inhibiting a Forkhead transcription factor. *Cell*, **96**, 857–68.

Cardone, M. H., Roy, N., Stennicke, H. R. *et al.* (1998). Regulation of cell death protease caspase-9 by phosphorylation. *Science*, **282**, 1318–21.

Cattaneo, E. & Pelicci, P. G. (1998). Emerging roles for SH2/PTB-containing Shc adaptor proteins in the developing mammalian brain. *Trends Neurosci.*, **21**, 476–81.

Chao, M., Casaccia-Bonnefil, P., Carter, B., Chittka, A., Kong, H. & Yoon, S. O. (1998). Neurotrophin receptors: mediators of life and death. *Brain Res. Rev.*, **26**, 295–301.

Choi, D. W. (1992). Amyotrophic lateral sclerosis and glutamate – too much of a good thing. *N. Engl. J. Med.*, **326**, 1493–5.

Chou, S. M. (1992). Pathology-light microscopy of amyotrophic lateral sclerosis. In *Handbook of Amyotrophic Lateral sclerosis*, ed. R. A. Smith, New York: Marcel Dekker, Inc., pp. 133–82.

Conti, L., De Fraja, C., Gulisano, M., Migliaccio, E., Govoni, S. & Cattaneo, E. (1997). Expression and activation of SH2/PTB-containing ShcA adaptor protein reflects the pattern of neurogenesis in the mammalian brain. *Proc. Natl Acad. Sci. USA*, **94**, 8185–90.

Datta, S. R., Dudek, H., Tao, X. *et al.* (1997). Akt phosphorylation of BAD couples survival signals to the cell-intrinsic death machinery. *Cell*, **91**, 231–41.

Davey, F. & Davies, A. M. (1998). TrkB signaling inhibits p75-mediated apoptosis induced by nerve growth factor in embryonic proprioceptive neurons. *Curr. Biol.*, **8**, 915–18.

Dechant, G., Tsoulfas, P., Parada, L. F. & Barde, Y. A. (1997). The neurotrophin receptor p75 binds neurotrophin-3 on sympathetic neurons with high affinity and specificity. *J. Neurosci.*, **17**, 5281–7.

Deckwerth, T. L., Easton, R. M., Knudson, C. M., Korsmeyer, S. J. & Johnson, E. M., Jr. (1998). Placement of the BCL2 family member BAX in the death pathway of sympathetic neurons activated by trophic factor deprivation. *Exp. Neurol.*, **152**, 150–62.

Deng, H.-X., Hentati, A., Tainer, J. A. *et al.* (1993). Amyotrophic lateral sclerosis and structural defects in Cu,Zn superoxide dismutase. *Science*, **261**, 1047–51.

Deshmukh, M. & Johnson, E. M., Jr. (1998). Evidence of a novel event during neuronal death: development of competence-to-die in response to cytoplasmic cytochrome c [see comments]. *Neuron*, **21**, 695–705.

Devereaux, Q. L., Takahashi, R., Salvesen, G. S. & Reed, J. C. (1997). X-linked IAP is a direct inhibitor of cell-death proteases. *Nature*, **388**, 300–4.

Devereaux, Q. L., Roy, N., Stennicke, H. R. *et al.* (1998). IAPs block apoptotic events induced by caspase-8 and cytochrome c by direct inhibition of distinct caspases. *EMBO J.*, **17**, 2215–23.

Digby, M. R., Kimpton, W. G., York, J. J., Connick, T. E. & Lowenthal, J. W. (1996). ITA, a vertebrate homologue of IAP that is expressed in T lymphocytes. *DNA Cell Biol.*, **15**, 981–8.

Dubois-Dauphin, M., Frankowski, H., Tsujimoto, Y., Huarte, J. & Martinou, J.-C. (1994). Neonatal motoneurons overexpressing the *bcl-2* protooncogene in transgenic mice are protected from axotomy-induced cell death. *Proc. Natl Acad. Sciences, USA*, **91**, 3309–13.

Dudek, H., Datta, S. R., Franke, T. F. *et al.* (1997). Regulation of neuronal survival by the serine-threonine protein kinase Akt [see comments]. *Science*, **275**, 661–5.

Durham, H. D., Roy, J., Dong, L. & Figlewicz, D. A. (1997). Aggregation of mutant Cu/Zn superoxide dismutase proteins in a culture model of ALS. *J. Neuropathol. Exp. Neurol.*, **56**, 523–30.

Ebens, A., Brose, K., Leonardo, E. D. *et al.* (1996). Hepatocyte growth factor/scatter factor is an axonal chemoattractant and a neurotrophic factor for spinal motor neurons. *Neuron*, **17**, 1157–72.

Elson, G. C., Lelievre, E., Guillet, C. *et al.* (2000). CLF associates with CLC to form a functional heteromeric ligand for the CNTF receptor complex. *Nat. Neurosci.*, **3**, 867–72.

Ernfors, P., Hallböök, F., Ebendal, T. *et al.* (1988). Developmental and regional expression of β-nerve growth factor receptor mRNA in the chick and rat. *Neuron*, **1**, 983–96.

Estevez, A. G., Spear, N., Manuel, S. M., Barbeito, L., Radi, R. & Beckman, J. S. (1998a). Role of endogenous nitric oxide and peroxynitrite formation in the survival and death of motor neurons in culture. *Prog. Brain Res.*, **118**, 269–80.

Estevez, A. G., Spear, N., Manuel, S. M. *et al.* (1998b). Nitric oxide and superoxide contribute to motor neuron apoptosis induced by trophic factor deprivation. *J. Neurosci.*, **18**, 923–31.

Estevez, A. G., Crow, J. P., Sampson, J. B. *et al.* (1999). Induction of nitric oxide-dependent apoptosis in motor neurons by zinc-deficient superoxide dismutase. *Science*, **286**, 2498–500.

Ferri, C. C., Moore, F. A. & Bisby, M. A. (1998). Effects of facial nerve injury on mouse motoneurons lacking the p75 low-affinity neurotrophin receptor. *J. Neurobiol.*, **34**, 1–9.

Finkbeiner, S., Tavazoie, S. F., Maloratsky, A., Jacobs, K. M., Harris, K. M. & Greenberg, M. E. (1997). CREB: a major mediator of neuronal neurotrophin responses. *Neuron*, **19**, 1031–47.

Frade, J. M. & Barde, Y. A. (1998). Microglia-derived nerve growth factor causes cell death in the developing retina. *Neuron*, **20**, 35–42.

Frade, J. M. & Barde, Y. A. (1999). Genetic evidence for cell death mediated by nerve growth factor and the neurotrophin receptor p75 in the developing mouse retina and spinal cord. *Development*, **126**, 683–90.

Frade, J. M., Rodriguez Tebar, A. & Barde, Y. A. (1996). Induction of cell death by endogenous nerve growth factor through its p75 receptor. *Nature*, **383**, 166–8.

Friedlander, R. M., Brown, R. H., Gagliardini, V., Wang, J. & Yuan, J. (1997). Inhibition of ICE slows ALS in mice [letter] [published erratum appears in *Nature* 1998 Apr 9;392(6676):560]. *Nature*, **388**, 31.

Friedman, W. J. & Greene, L. A. (1999). Neurotrophin signaling via Trks and p75. *Exp. Cell Res.*, **253**, 131–42.

Gravel, C., Götz, R., Lorrain, A. & Sendtner, M. (1997). Adenoviral gene transfer of ciliary neurotrophic factor and brain-derived neurotrophic factor leads to longterm survival of axotomized motoneurons. *Nat. Med.*, **3**, 765–70.

Gredal, O., Werdelin, L., Bak, S. *et al.* (1997). A clinical trial of dextromethorphan in amyotrophic lateral sclerosis. *Acta Neurol. Scand.*, **96**, 8–13.

Greene, L. A. & Kaplan, D. R. (1995). Early events in neurotrophin signaling via Trk and p75 receptors. *Curr. Opin. Neurobiol.*, **5**, 579–87.

Grewal, S. S., Horgan, A. M., York, R. D., Withers, G. S., Banker, G. A. & Stork, P. J. (2000). Neuronal calcium activates a rap1 and b-raf signaling pathway via the cyclic adenosine monophosphate-dependent protein kinase. *J. Biol. Chem.*, **275**, 3722–8.

Grieshammer, U., Lewandoski, M., Prevette, D. *et al.* (1998). Muscle-specific cell ablation conditional upon Cre-mediated DNA recombination in transgenic mice leads to massive spinal and cranial motoneuron loss neuronal cell death. *Neuron*, **20**, 633–47.

Gurney, M. E., Pu, H., Chiu, A. Y. *et al.* (1994). Motor neuron degeneration in mice that express a human Cu,Zn superoxide dismutase mutation. *Science*, **264**, 1772–5.

Hamburger, V. (1934). The effects of wing bud extirpation on the development of the central nervous system in chick embryos. *J. Exp. Zool.*, **68**, 449–94.

(1958). Regression versus peripheral control of differentiation in motor hyperplasia. *Am. J. Anat.*, **102**, 365–10.

Henderson, C. E., Camu, W., Mettling, C. *et al.* (1993). Neurotrophins promote motor neuron survival and are present in embryonic limb bud. *Nature*, **363**, 266–70.

Henderson, C. E., Phillips, H. S., Pollock, R. A. *et al.* (1994). GDNF: a potent survival factor for motoneurons present in peripheral nerve and muscle. *Science*, **266**, 1062–4.

Hughes, R. A., Sendtner, M. & Thoenen, H. (1993). Members of several gene families influence survival of rat motoneurons in vitro and in vivo. *J. Neurosci. Res.*, **36** (6), 663–71.

Ikeda, K., Klinkosz, B., Greene, T. *et al.* (1995). Effects of brain-derived neurotrophic factor on motor dysfunction in wobbler mouse motor neuron disease. *Ann. Neurol.*, **37**, 505–11.

Jablonka, S., Schrank, B., Kralewski, M., Rossoll, W. & Sendtner, M. (2000). Reduced survival motor neuron (Smn) gene dose in mice leads to motor neuron degeneration: an animal model for spinal muscular atrophy type III. *Hum. Mol. Genet.*, **9**, 341–6.

Kalb, R. G., Lidow, M. S., Halsted, M. & Hockfield, S. (1992). N-Methyl-D-aspartate receptors are transiently expressed in the developing spinal cord ventral horn. *Proc. Natl Acad. Sci. USA*, **89**, 8502–6.

Kerkhoff, H., Jennekens, F. G. I., Troost, D. & Veldman, H. (1991). Nerve growth factor receptor immunostaining in the spinal cord and peripheral nerves in amyotrophic lateral sclerosis. *Acta Neuropathol.(Berl.)*, **81**, 649–56.

Klein, R. D., Sherman, D., Ho, W. H. *et al.* (1997). A GPI-linked protein that interacts with Ret to form a candidate neurturin receptor. *Nature*, **387**, 717–21.

Knudson, C. M., Tung, K. S., Tourtellotte, W. G., Brown, G. A. & Korsmeyer, S. J. (1995). Bax-deficient mice with lymphoid hyperplasia and male germ cell death. *Science*, **270**, 96–9.

Kostic, V., Jackson-Lewis, V., De Bilbao, F., Dubois-Dauphin, M. & Przedborski, S. (1997). Bcl-2: prolonging life in a transgenic mouse model of familial amyotrophic lateral sclerosis. *Science*, **277**, 559–62.

Levi-Montalcini, R. (1950). The origin and development of the visceral system in the spinal cord of the chick embryo. *J. Morphol.*, 253–84.

Mahadeo, D., Kaplan, L., Chao, M. V. & Hempstead, B. L. (1994). High affinity nerve growth factor binding displays a faster rate of association than p140^{trk} binding. Implications for multisubunit polypeptide receptors. *J. Biol. Chem.*, **269**, 6884–91.

Majdan, M., Lachance, C., Gloster, A. *et al.* (1997). Transgenic mice expressing the intracellular domain of the p75 neurotrophin receptor undergo neuronal apoptosis. *J. Neurosci.*, **17**, 6988–98.

Martinou, J.-C., Dubois-Dauphin, M., Staple, J. K. *et al.* (1994). Overexpression of BCL-2 in transgenic mice protects neurons from naturally occurring cell death and experimental ischemia. *Neuron*, **13**, 1017–30.

Meakin, S. O. & Shooter, E. M. (1992). The nerve growth factor family of receptors. *Trends Neurosci.*, **15**, 323–31.

Metzger, F., Wiese, S. & Sendtner, M. (1998). Effect of glutamate on dendritic growth in embryonic rat motoneurons. *J. Neurosci.*, **18**, 1735–42.

Metzger, F., Kulik, A., Sendtner, M. & Ballanyi, K. (2000). Contribution of Ca^{2+}-permeable AMPA/KA receptors to glutamate-induced Ca^{2+} rise in embryonic lumbar motoneurons *in situ*. *J. Neurophysiol.*, **83**, 50–9.

Metzstein, M. M., Hengartner, M. O., Tsung, N., Ellis, R. E. & Horvitz, H. R. (1996). Transcriptional regulator of programmed cell death encoded by *Caenorhabditis elegans* gene ces-2. *Nature*, **382**, 545–7.

Meyer Franke, A., Kaplan, M. R., Pfrieger, F. W. & Barres, B. A. (1995). Characterization of the signaling interactions that promote the survival and growth of developing retinal ganglion cells in culture. *Neuron*, **15**, 805–19.

Michaelidis, T. M., Sendtner, M., Cooper, J. D. *et al.* (1996). Inactivation of the bcl-2 gene results in progressive degeneration of motoneurons, sensory and sypathetic neurons during early postnatal development. *Neuron*, **17**, 75–89.

Milbrandt, J., de Sauvage, F. J., Fahrner, T. J. *et al.* (1998). Persephin, a novel neurotrophic factor related to GDNF and neurturin. *Neuron*, **20**, 245–53.

Minichiello, L., Casagranda, F., Tatche, R. S. *et al.* (1998). Point mutation in trkB causes loss of NT4-dependent neurons without major effects on diverse BDNF responses. *Neuron*, **21**, 335–45.

Mitsumoto, H., Ikeda, K., Klinkosz, B., Cedarbaum, J. M., Wong, V. & Lindsay, R. M. (1994). Arrest of motor neuron disease in *wobbler* mice cotreated with CNTF and BDNF. *Science*, **265**, 1107–10.

Miyata, Y., Kashihara, Y., Homma, S. & Kuno, M. (1986). Effects of nerve growth factor on the survival and synaptic function of Ia sensory neurons axotomized in neonatal rats. *J. Neurosci.*, **6**, 2012–18.

Monani, U. R., Sendtner, M., Coovert, D. D. *et al.* (2000). The human centromeric survival motor neuron gene (SMN2) rescues embryonic lethality in Smn(−/−) mice and results in a mouse with spinal muscular atrophy [In Process Citation]. *Hum. Mol. Genet.*, **9**, 333–9.

Nagata, S. (1997). Apoptosis by death factor. *Cell*, **88**, 355–65.

Nakamura, T., Sanokawa, R., Sasaki, Y., Ayusawa, D., Oishi, M. & Mori, N. (1996). N-Shc: a neural-specific adapter molecule that mediates signaling from neurotrophin/Trk to Ras/Mapk pathway. *Oncogene*, **13**, 1111–21.

Nakashima, K. & Taga, T. (1998). gp130 and the IL-6 family of cytokines: signaling mechanisms and thrombopoietic activities. *Semin. Hematol.*, **35**, 210–21.

Newmeyer, D. D. and Green, D. R. (1998). Surviving the cytochrome seas [comment]. *Neuron*, **21**, 653–5.

Novak, K. D., Prevette, D., Wang, S., Gould, T. W. & Oppenheim, R. W. (2000). Hepatocyte growth factor/scatter factor is a neurotrophic survival factor for lumbar but not for other somatic motoneurons in the chick embryo. *J. Neurosci.*, **20**, 326–37.

O'Connor, T. M. & Wyttenbach, C. R. (1974). Cell death of the embryonic chick spinal cord. *J. Cell Biol.*, **60**, 448–59.

Obermeier, A., Lammers, R., Wiesmuller, K. H., Jung, G., Schlessinger, J. & Ullrich, A. (1993). Identification of Trk binding sites for SHC and phosphatidylinositol 3′-kinase and formation of a multimeric signaling complex. *J. Biol. Chem.*, **268**, 22963–6.

Obermeier, A., Bradshaw, R. A., Seedorf, K., Choidas, A., Schlessinger, J. & Ullrich, A. (1994). Neuronal differentiation signals are controlled by nerve growth factor receptor/Trk binding sites for SHC and PLCgamma. *EMBO J.*, **13**, 1585–90.

Okado, N. & Oppenheim, R. W. (1984). Cell death of motoneurons in the chick embryo spinal cord. IX. The loss of motoneurons following removal of afferent inputs. *J. Neurosci.*, **4**, 1639–52.

Oppenheim, R. W. (1985). Naturally occurring cell death during neural development. *Trends Neurosci.*, **8**, 487–93.

Oppenheim, R. W., Cole, T. & Prevette, D. (1989). Early regional variations in motoneuron numbers arise by differential proliferation in the chick embryo spinal cord. *Dev. Biol.*, **133**, 468–74.

Ozes, O. N., Mayo, L. D., Gustin, J. A., Pfeffer, S. R., Pfeffer, L. M. & Donner, D. B. (1999). NF-kappaB activation by tumour necrosis factor requires the Akt serine- threonine kinase. *Nature*, **401**, 82–5.

Pennica, D., Shaw, K. J., Swanson, T. A. *et al.* (1995). Cardiotrophin-1. Biological activities and binding to the leukemia inhibitory factor receptor/gp130 signaling complex. *J. Biol. Chem.*, **270**, 10915–22.

Qin-Wei, Y., Johnson, J., Prevette, D. & Oppenheim, R. W. (1994). Cell death of spinal motoneurons in the chick embryo following deafferentiation: rescue effects of tissue extracts, soluble proteins, and neurotrophic agents. *J. Neurosci.*, **14**, 7629–40.

Raoul, C., Henderson, C. E. & Pettmann, B. (1999). Programmed cell death of embryonic motoneurons triggered through the Fas death receptor. *J. Cell Biol.*, **147**, 1049–62.

Riethmacher, D., Sonnenberg-Riethmacher, E., Brinkmann, V., Vamaai, T., Lewin, G. R. & Birchmeier, C. (1997). Severe neuropathies in mice with targeted mutations in the ErbB3 receptor. *Nature*, **389**, 725–30.

Rodriguez-Tébar, A., Dechant, G. & Barde, Y.-A. (1990). Binding of brain-derived neurotrophic factor to the nerve growth factor receptor. *Neuron*, **4**, 487–92.

Romashkova, J. A. & Makarov, S. S. (1999). NF-kappaB is a target of AKT in anti-apoptotic PDGF signaling. *Nature*, **401**, 86–90.

Rosen, D. R., Siddique, T., Patterson, D. *et al.* (1993). Mutation in Cu/Zn superoxide dismutase gene are associated with familial amyotrophic lateral sclerosis. *Nature*, **362**, 59–62.

Rothstein, J. D. (1995). Excitotoxic mechanisms in the pathogenesis of amyotrophic lateral sclerosis. *Adv. Neurol.*, **68**, 7–20.

Roy, N., Deveraux, Q. L., Takahashi, R., Salvesen, G. S. & Reed, J. C. (1997). The c-IAP-1 and c-IAP-2 proteins are direct inhibitors of specific caspases. *EMBO J.*, **16**, 6914–25.

Sagot, Y., Tan, S. A., Hammang, J. P., Aebischer, P. & Kato, A. C. (1996). GDNF slows loss of motoneurons but not axonal degeneration or premature death of pmn/pmn mice. *J. Neurosci.*, **16**, 2335–41.

Segal, R. A. & Greenberg, M. E. (1996). Intracellular signaling pathways activated by neurotrophic factors. *Annu. Rev. Neurosci.*, **19**, 463–89.

Senaldi, G., Varnum, B. C., Sarmiento, U. *et al.* (1999). Novel neurotrophin-1/B cell-stimulating factor-3: a cytokine of the IL-6 family. *Proc. Natl Acad. Sci. USA*, **96**, 11458–63.

Sendtner, M. (1998). Neurotrophic factors: effects in modulating properties of the neuromuscular endplate. *Cytokine Growth Factor Rev.*, **9**, 1–7.

Sendtner, M., Holtmann, B., Kolbeck, R., Thoenen, H. & Barde, Y.-A. (1992a). Brain-derived neurotrophic factor prevents the death of motoneurons in newborn rats after nerve section. *Nature*, **360**, 757–8.

Sendtner, M., Schmalbruch, H., Stöckli, K. A., Carroll, P., Kreutzberg, G. W. & Thoenen, H. (1992b). Ciliary neurotrophic factor prevents degeneration of motor neurons in mouse mutant progressive motor neuronopathy. *Nature*, **358**, 502–4.

Shi, Y., Wang, W., Yourey, P. A. *et al.* (1999). Computational EST database analysis identifies a novel member of the neuropoietic cytokine family. *Biochem. Biophys. Res. Commun.*, **262**, 132–8.

Slee, E. A., Harte, M. T., Kluck, R. M. *et al.* (1999). Ordering the cytochrome c-initiated caspase cascade: hierarchical activation of caspases-2, -3, -6, -7, -8, and -10 in a caspase-9- dependent manner. *J. Cell Biol.*, **144**, 281–92.

Stennicke, H. R., Deveraux, Q. L., Humke, E. W., Reed, J. C., Dixit, V. M. & Salvesen, G. S. (1999). Caspase-9 can be activated without proteolytic processing. *J. Biol. Chem.*, **274**, 8359–62.

Tinhofer, I., Maly, K., Dietl, P. *et al.* (1996). Differential Ca^{2+} signaling induced by activation of the epidermal growth factor and nerve growth factor receptors. *J. Biol. Chem.*, **271**, 30505–9.

Traverse, S., Gomez, N., Paterson, H., Marshall, C. & Cohen, P. (1992). Sustained activation of the mitogen-activated protein (MAP) kinase cascade may be required for differentiation of PC12 cells. Comparison of the effects of nerve growth factor and epidermal growth factor. *Biochem. J.*, **288** (2), 351–5.

Van der Zee, C. E., Ross, G. M., Riopelle, R. J., and Hagg, T. (1996). Survival of cholinergic forebrain neurons in developing p75NGFR-deficient mice [see comments] [retracted by Hagg T. In: *Science* 1999 Jul 16;285(5426):340]. *Science*, **274**, 1729–32.

van der Zee, C. E. E. M., Ross, G. M., Riopelle, R. J. & Hagg, T. (1998). Survival of cholinergic forebrain neurons in developing p75 NGFR-deficient mice. *Science*, 1729–32.

Wakade, A. R., Edgar, D. & Thoenen H (1983). Both nerve growth factor and high K concentration support the survival of chick embryo sympathetic neurons. *Exp. Cell Res.*, **144**, 377–84.

Wang, H.-G., Miyashita, T., Takayama, S. *et al.* (1994). Apoptosis regulation by interaction of Bcl-2 protein and Raf-1 kinase. *Oncogene*, **9**, 2751–6.

Wang, H.-G., Rapp, U. R. & Reed, J. C. (1996). Bcl-2 targets the protein kinase Raf-1 to mitochondria. *Cell*, **87**, 629–38.

Weidner, K. M., Arakaki, N., Hartmann, G. *et al.* (1991). Evidence for the identity of human scatter factor and human hepatocyte growth factor. *Proc. Natl Acad. Sci. USA*, **88**, 7001–5.

Wiese, S., Digby, M. R., Gunnersen, J. M. *et al.* (1999a). The anti-apoptotic protein ITA is essential for NGF-mediated survival of embryonic chick neurons. *Nat. Neurosci.*, **2**, 978–83.

Wiese, S., Metzger, F., Holtmann, B. & Sendtner, M. (1999b). The role of p75NTR in modulating neurotrophin survival effects in developing motoneurons. *Eur. J. Neurosci.*, **11**, 1668–76.

Wiese, S., Pei, G., Karch, C. *et al.* (2001). Specific function of B-Raf in mediating survival of embryonic motoneurons and sensory neurons. *Nat. Neurosci.*, **4**, 137–42.

Wixler, V., Smola, U., Schuler, M. & Rapp, U. (1996). Differential regulation of Raf isozymes by growth versus differentiation inducing factors in PC12 pheochromocytoma cells. *FEBS Lett.*, **385**, 131–7.

Wolf, D. E., McKinnon, C. A., Daou, M. C., Stephens, R. M., Kaplan, D. R. & Ross, A. H. (1995). Interaction with TrkA immobilizes gp75 in the high affinity nerve growth factor receptor complex. *J. Biol. Chem.*, **270**, 2133–8.

Wong, V., Glass, D. J., Arriga, R., Yancopoulos, G. D., Lindsay, R. M. & Conn, G. (1997). Hepatocyte growth factor promotes motor neuron survival and synergizes with ciliary neurotrophic factor. *J. Biol. Chem.*, **272**, 5187–91.

Yaginuma, H., Tomita, M., Takashita, N. *et al.* (1996). A novel type of programmed neuronal death in the cervical spinal cord of the chick embryo. *J. Neurosci.*, **16**, 3685–703.

Yamamoto, Y., Livet, J., Polock, R. *et al.* (1997). Hepatocyte growth factor (HGF/SF) is a muscle-derived survival factor for a sub-population of embryonic motoneurons. *Development (Suppl)*, **124**, 2903–13.

Yeo, T. T., Chua-Couzens, J., Butcher, L. L. *et al.* (1997). Absence of p75NTR causes increased basal forebrain cholinergic neuron size, choline acetyltransferase activity, and target innervation. *J. Neurosci.*, **17**, 7594–605.

York, R. D., Yao, H., Dillon, T. *et al.* (1998). Rap1 mediates sustained MAP kinase activation induced by nerve growth factor. *Nature*, **392**, 622–6.

Zurn, A. D., Baetge, E. E., Hammang, J. P., Tan, S. A. & Aebischer, P. (1994). Glial cell line-derived neurotrophic factor (GDNF), a new neurotrophic factor for motoneurones. *NeuroReport*, **6**, 113–18.

9

Protein misfolding and cellular defense mechanisms in neurodegenerative diseases

Michael Y. Sherman[1] and Alfred L. Goldberg[2]

[1] Department of Biochemistry, Boston University Medical School, MA, USA
[2] Department of Cell Biology, Harvard Medical School, Boston, MA, USA

Introduction

In many major neurodegenerative diseases, including amyotrophic lateral sclerosis (ALS), Alzheimer's disease, Parkinson's disease, and several hereditary diseases caused by expansions of polyglutamine (PolyQ) tracts (e.g. Huntington's disease and the spinocerebellar ataxias) (Table 9.1), the pathology and the eventual death of specific neuronal populations occur due to the accumulation of specific abnormal polypeptides, which form insoluble intracellular inclusions. Many observations suggest that these various types of inclusions arise through common mechanisms and elicit similar host responses. For example, all these inclusions contain components of the ubiquitin-proteasome degradation pathway and also molecular chaperones, which represent the two main systems that eukaryotic cells use to protect themselves against the buildup of unfolded polypeptides. The accumulation of abnormal polypeptides in the form of inclusions in various neurological disorders must result from an inability of neurons to either refold or degrade these abnormal species. Because these neurological diseases are of late onset, and the very same mutant proteins are expressed without causing obvious pathology in younger individuals, it seems likely that the failure to adequately deal with these abnormal molecules progresses with aging.

Because the continued accumulation of unfolded, non-functional polypeptides is likely to cause cell toxicity, it is not surprising that defense mechanisms emerged early in evolution that enable cells to withstand the appearance of large amounts of unfolded proteins, as may result from mutations, errors in protein synthesis, or inefficient folding of nascent polypeptides. These mechanisms are activated upon various experimental conditions that cause widespread damage to cell proteins and massive accumulation of abnormal polypeptides, such as exposure to high temperatures, oxygen radicals, heavy metals, certain antibiotics that reduce the fidelity of translation, or genetic diseases. It seems very likely that these defense mechanisms also function during the slower accumulation of mutant or damaged proteins in neurodegenerative disease. The major adaptation is the induction of a set of highly conserved heat-shock proteins (Hsps), which function as the major cellular defense against the buildup of unfolded proteins. Among the Hsps in eukaryotic cells are molecular chaperones (Feldman & Frydman, 2000; Frydman, 2001), which reduce protein denaturation and aggregation and promote refolding of denatured polypeptides, several antioxidant enzymes (Hass & Massaro, 1988; Xi et al., 2001; Yamashita et al., 1998), which reduce oxidative damage to cell proteins, and components of the ubiquitin-proteasome pathway (Seufert & Jentsch, 1990; Sommer & Seufert, 1992; Watt & Piper, 1997), which catalyse the selective degradation of unfolded polypeptides (Glickman & Ciechanover, 2002; Hershko & Ciechanover, 1998; Schwartz & Ciechanover, 1999) (Table 9.2).

The trigger for induction of the heat shock proteins is the accumulation of unfolded polypeptides in the cytosol or nucleus (Ananthan et al., 1986; Goff & Goldberg, 1985). For example, the heat-shock response can be induced by treatments that cause the production of large amounts of abnormal polypeptides, such as incorporation of amino acid analogs (which prevent normal folding) or puromycin (which leads to premature termination of nascent polypeptides) (Goff & Goldberg, 1985). Furthermore, direct microinjection into cells of unfolded polypeptides or the expression of recombinant abnormal polypeptides, but not the corresponding native proteins, induces this response (Ananthan et al., 1986; Goff & Goldberg, 1985). Presumably, the ability of unfolded proteins to stimulate the expression of heat-shock genes may play an important role in protection from

Table 9.1. Neurodegenerative diseases with inclusion bodies associated with ubiquitin and proteasome

Disease	Inclusion	Major Constituent
Alzheimer's	Neurofibrilatory tangles	Tau
Parkinson's	Lewy body	α-synuclein, crystallins
Lewy body dementia	Lewy body	α-synuclein
Amyotrophic lateral Sclerosis	Skein, Bunina bodies	SOD, neurofilaments
Polyglutamine extension disorders		
Huntington's	Nuclear, cytosolic	huntingtin
Spinocerebellar Ataxias 1, 2 and 3	Nuclear, cytosolic	ataxins 1, 2 and 3
Spinobulbar muscular Atrophy (Kennedy's)	Nuclear, cytosolic	Androgen receptor

Table 9.2. Functions of cytosolic and ER chaperones probably important for protection against neurodegenerative diseases

- Prevent aggregation of mutant and damaged proteins
- Catalyze protein folding and multimer assembly
- Solubilize aggregated proteins in cells
- Promote ubiquitination and degradation of abnormal proteins
- In ER, promote proper folding and glycosylation of membrane and secreted proteins
- Suppress protein kinases (e.g. JNK) and thus inhibit apoptotic program
- Regulate their own expression in cytosol (heat shock response) and ER ("unfolded protein response")

Ubiquitin conjugation to protein substrates

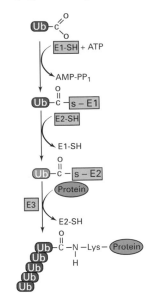

THE UBIQUITIN - PROTEASOME PATHWAY

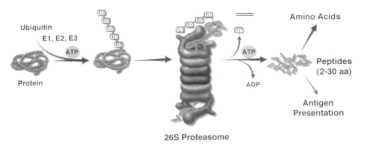

Fig. 9.1 Ubiquitin-proteasome pathway.

neuronal loss in neurological disorders associated with accumulation of damaged and mutant proteins and their aggregation.

Cells also contain efficient mechanisms to prevent accumulation of mutant or misfolded proteins in the endoplasmic reticulum (ER). Such abnormal secreted or membrane molecules are transported from the ER back into the cytosol where they are rapidly degraded (da Costa *et al.*, 1999; Fewell *et al.*, 2001; Honda *et al.*, 1999; Kopito, 1999; Steiner *et al.*, 1998; Tsai *et al.*, 2002; Xiong *et al.*, 1999). This degradative process is important in various inherited diseases (e.g. cystic fibrosis), but the retrograde transport system may also account for the generation of the self-perpetuating forms of prion protein in neurons (Ma *et al.*, 2002). If this degradative mechanism is insufficient to prevent the accumulation of the abnormal proteins in the ER, cells respond by activation of the "unfolded protein response". This transcriptional program is analogous to the heat shock response in the cytosol and is triggered by the buildup of unfolded proteins within the ER. This adaptive response increases production of a group of molecular chaperones in the ER (often termed Grps), many of which are homologous to the cytosolic Hsps (Chapman *et al.*, 1998; Welihinda *et al.*, 1999). This adaptation further enhances the ER's capacity to generate properly folded membrane and secreted proteins and to translocate such unfolded molecules back into the cytosol for degradation by the ubiquitin-proteasome pathway (Fig. 9.1). Interestingly, defects in the "unfolded protein response" have been observed in cells that express the mutant Presenilin 1 (Imaizumi *et al.*, 2001; Katayama *et al.*, 2001; Katayama *et al.*, 1999), which predisposes to Alzheimer's disease (see below).

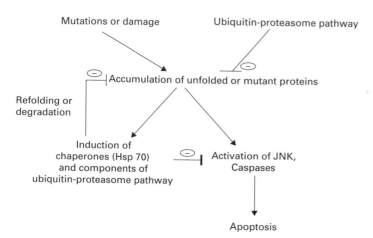

Fig. 9.2 Induction of protective and apoptotic programs by abnormal proteins.

Protective functions of heat shock proteins

Molecular chaperones, i.e. members of the Hsp70, Hsp90, Hsp104, Hsp40, and small Hsp (Hsp27, α-crystallins) families, bind selectively to denatured or partially unfolded domains in polypeptides (Feder & Hofmann, 1999; Johnson & Craig, 1997; Samali & Orrenius, 1998). Most of these chaperones are major cell constituents under normal conditions, where they are essential to ensure the proper folding and intracellular localization of newly synthesized polypeptides (Table 9.2). Surprisingly, in spite of the function of molecular chaperones, a significant fraction (perhaps up to 30%) of newly synthesized polypeptides normally fails to achieve the correct conformation and is rapidly digested (Schubert et al., 2000). Under conditions that cause protein damage (e.g. heat shock) or upon accumulation of mutant proteins (e.g. huntingtin with expanded polyQ sequences), the cell's need for the chaperones increases, and their expression is stimulated (Fig. 9.2). Cells also utilize the capacity of chaperones to bind selectively unfolded polypeptides to monitor the intracellular levels of such abnormal, potentially toxic molecules. In unstressed cells, the expression of heat shock genes normally is inhibited by the presence of molecular chaperones (Baler et al., 1996; Liberek et al., 1992; Voellmy, 1996). Increased transcription of the heat shock genes is triggered when the abnormal proteins accumulate and bind preferentially to Hsp 90 (Zou et al., 1998) and Hsp70 (Shi et al., 1998), thus preventing these chaperones from inhibiting the expression of heat shock genes.

Damage from oxygen radicals has been associated with several neurodegenerative diseases and accompanies acti-

vation of inflammatory responses. A specific group of heat shock proteins serves to protect cells against oxygen free radicals. For example, superoxide dismutase, heme oxygenase, and catalase can all be induced as part of the heat shock response and help protect against oxidative damage to cell proteins, DNA, and lipids (Amrani et al., 1993; Massa et al., 1996). If any of these enzymes is overproduced in transgenic animals or in cultured cells, it can protect cells from ischemia-reperfusion injury (Chan, 1996), which is associated with extensive production of reactive oxygen species (ROS) and oxidative protein damage. Another enzyme that appears to play an important role in maintaining the proper redox potential in the cytosol is gamma-glutamylcysteine synthetase, a rate-limiting enzyme in the synthesis of glutathione (Soltaninassab et al., 2000). Gamma-glutamylcysteine synthetase is strongly induced in response to oxidative stress and other stressful treatments that lead to protein damage, and this enzyme therefore is likely to be important for cell protection (Sekhar et al., 2000; Soltaninassab et al., 2000). The amino acid in proteins most susceptible to oxidative damage is methionine, and many tissues, especially the brain and retina, contain the enzyme methionine sulfoxide reductase (Kuschel et al., 1999); (Moskovitz et al., 1996), which specifically repairs this type of damage to proteins. Decreased levels of this enzyme have been reported in brains of Alzheimer's disease patients (Gabbita et al., 1999), while overexpression of this enzyme helps protect cells from oxidative stress (Moskovitz et al., 1998). Enzymes that protect from oxidative damage may be particularly important in defense against Parkinson's and perhaps Alzheimer's diseases, where oxidative stress seems to be a critical aspect of the disease process.

Selective degradation of abnormal proteins

The ubiquitin-proteasome degradation system rapidly eliminates certain proteins, including mutant and damaged polypeptides, without causing non-specific destruction of other cell proteins. To achieve this selectivity, proteins to be degraded are first marked by covalent linkage to the small polypeptide cofactor ubiquitin (Fig. 9.1). The linkage of a chain of four or more ubiquitins to a lysine on the substrate marks it for rapid breakdown by the very large proteolytic complex, the 26S proteasome (Coux et al., 1996; Glickman & Ciechanover, 2002; Hershko & Ciechanover, 1998; Rock et al., 1994). The 26S proteasome consists of two 19S regulatory complexes situated at either end of the 20S core proteasome, a hollow, barrel-shaped structure, within which proteins are degraded. Substrates first bind via their ubiquitin chains to the 19S regulatory complex (Fig. 9.1). This structure contains a ring of six homologous ATPase molecules, which have many of the properties of molecular chaperones; for example, they can unfold globular proteins and translocate them into the 20S proteasome for degradation (Benaroudj & Goldberg, 2000; Navon & Goldberg, 2001). Concomitantly, the regulatory complex releases the chain of ubiquitin molecules, which are then recycled for use in the degradation of other proteins.

The ubiquitin requirement for degradation and the isolation of proteolysis within a microcompartment of the cell, to which substrate entry is highly restricted, all help ensure that degradation occurs in a highly selective and efficient manner. Proteolysis occurs within the central chamber of the 20S proteasome, which contains six proteolytic sites, two of which preferentially cleave after hydrophobic residues, two after basic ones, and two after acidic residues (Coux et al., 1996; Kisselev et al., 1999a). Thus the proteasome, unlike typical proteases, does not simply cut a protein into two pieces, but instead these six sites function together to degrade proteins processively to small peptides ranging from three to 25 residues long (Kisselev et al., 1999b). These products once released from the proteasome are hydrolyzed rapidly to amino acids by cytosolic peptidases. Thus, the proteasome has the capacity to cleave a large variety of peptide bonds within proteins, but it lacks the capacity to hydrolyze within repeated sequences of glutamine, which may be an important factor in the ability of extended polyglutamine sequences to cause neurodegenerative diseases (Ventrakaman & Goldberg, unpublished data).

The exquisite specificity of the degradative process results from the properties of enzymes for ubiquitin conjugation (Fig. 9.1). In this process, the ubiquitin molecule is activated first by the enzyme, E1, which transfers the ubiquitin to one of the cell's approximately 20 distinct ubiquitin-carrier proteins (E2s), which then, together with a specific ubiquitin-protein ligase (E3), transfers the activated ubiquitin molecule to lysine residues on the protein substrate. The selectivity in this pathway comes primarily from the E3. Mammalian cells typically contain hundreds of different E3s, which function with a specific E2 in the ubiquitination of different types of protein. Although much has been learned recently about E3 function (Fig. 9.1), it is still unclear exactly how most unfolded or damaged proteins are recognized and degraded selectively. Amongst the genes induced as part of the heat-shock response are certain ubiquitin-carrier proteins (E2s) and the polyubiquitin gene, which encodes multiple ubiquitin molecules in

a linear polymer (Glickman & Ciechanover, 2002; Hershko & Ciechanover, 1998; Watt & Piper, 1997). Its expression and subsequent cleavage represent a special mechanism that enables the cell to generate large amounts of ubiquitin quickly when the overall rate of proteolysis rises (Mitch & Goldberg, 1996) (Finley et al., 1987).

The two main protective strategies, the repair of damaged proteins and their selective degradation, are complementary mechanisms to eliminate unfolded polypeptides, which may perturb cell function and initiate cell death programs (see below). However, refolding and degradation are not independent processes involving distinct cellular components, but rather appear to be linked at several levels. The ATPases within the 26S proteasome, in addition to promoting proteolysis, have chaperone-like activities and can block protein aggregation and even promote the refolding of denatured proteins (Braun et al., 1999; Strickland et al., 2000), at least in model experiments. In addition, the chaperones Hsp70 and Hsp40, not only play an important role in preventing aggregation and refolding, but are also essential for the ubiquitination and rapid degradation of many abnormal species (Bercovich et al., 1997; Lee et al., 1996a; Meacham et al., 2001; Ohba, 1997; Sherman & Goldberg, 1996; Zhang et al., 2001). Apparently, the capacity of these chaperones to associate selectively with unfolded polypeptides facilitates substrate recognition by E3s and perhaps degradation by proteasomes. One such E3, termed CHIP, seems to function together with Hsp70 and Hsp40 or with Hsp90 in the ubiquitination of various unfolded proteins (Meacham et al., 2001; Murata et al., 2001). It remains to be seen whether this system is important in degrading the abnormal proteins that cause these various neurodegenerative disorders. An interesting finding was that CHIP enhances the activity of Parkin, another E3 ligase, mutations which cause the majority of familial Parkinson's disease cases (Imai et al., 2002).

The dual roles of the chaperones in refolding and degradation of unfolded proteins appear highly advantageous to the organism in dealing with damaged polypeptides (Table 9.2). Since it must be impossible for the chaperones to refold many types of abnormal proteins (e.g. certain mutant proteins or ones covalently damaged by oxygen radicals), the ability of the chaperones to also facilitate the destruction of these proteins appears quite important, since it should reduce the concentration of these toxic species in a cell. In many neurodegenerative disorders and upon aging, the capacity of both chaperone and degradation systems appear to be reduced (see below), which may result in the inability of certain populations of neurons to cope with mutant or damaged proteins, leading to neuronal toxicity.

Protein inclusions and aggresome formation

If a eukaryotic or prokaryotic cell's ability to degrade or refold abnormal polypeptides is exceeded, as occurs experimentally when a mutant protein is expressed at high levels or when the proteasome is inhibited, the denatured or partially unfolded molecules accumulate and tend to aggregate (Cotner & Pious, 1995; Dubois *et al.*, 1991; Gragerov *et al.*, 1991; Johnston *et al.*, 1998; Kampinga *et al.*, 1995; Klemes *et al.*, 1981; Prouty *et al.*, 1975; Wigley *et al.*, 1999) eventually forming large inclusion bodies. Because these structures have not been isolated and characterized rigorously biochemically in the various human diseases or animal models, their precise composition and the forces holding them together in these various conditions are largely unknown.

It had been assumed initially that the formation of inclusion bodies results solely from the inherent tendency of denatured protein molecules to associate with one other to form insoluble aggregates. However, recent findings indicate that inclusion body formation in mammalian cells is a more complex process, in which cellular machinery appears to be actively involved. Generally, these structures are found in the cytoplasm at the microtubular organization center (MTOK or centrosome) (Anton *et al.*, 1999; Fabunmi *et al.*, 2000; Garcia-Mata *et al.*, 1999; Vidair *et al.*, 1999; Wigley *et al.*, 1999; Wojcik *et al.*, 1996), while in the nucleus, these bodies tend to be found in discrete structures that had been termed "promyelocytic leukemia oncogenic domains" (PODS) (Anton *et al.*, 1999). Several recent publications indicate that the formation of these inclusions is a multistep process, which involves transport of smaller aggregates from the cell's periphery towards the MTOK along the microtubuli (Garcia-Mata *et al.*, 1999; Johnston *et al.*, 1998, 2002). Hsps, ubiquitinated proteins, ubiquitin-conjugating enzymes, and 26S proteasomes associate with the inclusion bodies (Anton *et al.*, 1999; Fabunmi *et al.*, 2000; Garcia-Mata *et al.*, 1999; Vidair *et al.*, 1999; Wigley *et al.*, 1999) and form a large structure, recently termed the aggresome (Johnston *et al.*, 1998). Aggregates of mutated membrane proteins, such as the CFTR variants in cystic fibrosis and the presenilin-1 mutant associated with Alzheimer's disease (Johnston *et al.*, 1998; Wigley *et al.*, 1999), as well as cytosolic abnormal proteins (Garcia-Mata *et al.*, 1999), can all be found in aggresomes. It is noteworthy that aggresome formation is accelerated when proteasome inhibitors are added to block the degradation of the abnormal polypeptides (Garcia-Mata *et al.*, 1999; Johnston *et al.*, 1998). The process of aggresome formation is very rapid, and the first indications of this process (e.g. the

relocalization of Hsp25 to the centrosome) can be seen 10 min after addition of a proteasome inhibitor (M. Borreli, personal communication). It appears likely that reducing proteolysis generally exposes a process that occurs in patients during the slow progression of many neurodegenerative diseases.

In the neurodegenerative diseases associated with polyQ repeats, such as Huntington's disease and the spinocerebellar ataxias, as well as in Alzheimer's disease, and the prion disorders, the inclusions appear to involve protein–protein interaction that are especially stable due to extensive formation of β-sheet structures, which are held together by multiple hydrogen bonds (Bates *et al.*, 1998; Lathrop *et al.*, 1998). In addition, in the polyQ disorders some aggregated polypeptides may be covalently crosslinked by transglutaminase (Cooper *et al.*, 1997; Igarashi *et al.*, 1998; Kahlem *et al.*, 1998). Inclusion bodies formed by the polyQ-containing proteins are strikingly similar to aggresomes. When expressed in cultured cells, the polyQ-containing proteins form several inclusion bodies in the nucleus or one per cell in the cytosol. Results from several groups indicate that huntingtin fragments with an expanded polyQ tract form inclusions at the centrosome in the cytosol (Hoffner *et al.*, 2002; Meriin *et al.*, 2001; Sathasivam *et al.*, 2001; Waelter *et al.*, 2001), while ataxin 1-containing inclusions colocalize with promyelocytic leukemia bodies in the nucleus (Chai *et al.*, 1999b; Takahashi *et al.*, 2002). Like the formation of aggresomes, the generation of inclusion bodies requires transport of small aggregates to the centrosome along microtubuli, at least in some models of polyQ-expansion diseases (Muchowski *et al.*, 2002; Shimohata *et al.*, 2002).

Despite their chemical stability, protein aggregates composed of β-sheets, once formed are not necessarily permanent cellular components, and can disappear with time, due to protein refolding or degradation. In experimental models, the proteins in the inclusions appear to be in a dynamic state, continually turning over and being replaced by other unfolded molecules. For example, in transgenic mice, induction of huntingtin with an expanded polyQ repeat leads to the formation of inclusion bodies and neurodegeneration, but, if subsequently huntingtin expression is prevented, the inclusion bodies can disappear (Yamamoto *et al.*, 2000), apparently via a proteasome-dependent mechanism, since this process is blocked by proteasome inhibitors (Martin-Aparicio *et al.*, 2001). Moreover, the behavioral symptoms associated with the disease are reversed. Even when a large fraction of the cytosol of bacteria (Prouty *et al.*, 1975) or reticulocytes (Klemes

POSSIBLE INTERRELATION BETWEEN SOLUBLE ABNORMAL
PROTEINS AND LARGE INCLUSIONS

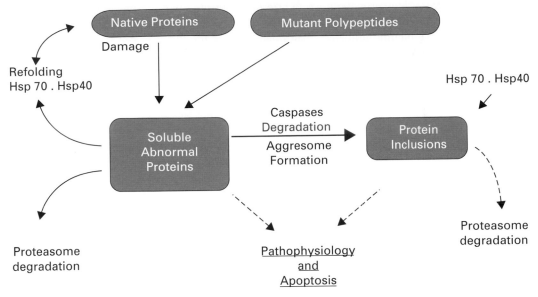

Fig. 9.3 Possible interrelation between soluble abnormal proteins and aggregated proteins. This model summarizes the different possible fates of a mutant or damaged protein in neurons and the factors that can influence these alternative paths. Once synthesized, the abnormal protein may be partially or completely unfolded and tend to form microaggregates with itself and with other cell constituents. Eventually, these structures can be transported into microscopically visible inclusions (resembling "aggresomes"). Opposing these developments are the molecular chaperones, which functioning in teams may refold or solubilize the abnormal polypeptides, and the Ub-proteasome pathway, which may degrade them. On the other hand, ubiqutin-conjugation or cleavage by caspases may also reduce the protein's solubility, thus favoring formation of large inclusion bodies. There is also clear evidence that even after inclusion formation, the mutant polypeptides within these bodies can be degraded or solubilized. In addition, the soluble abnormal proteins, by interacting with other cell components may disturb neuronal function or by soaking up proteasomes or chaperones (especially Hsp70) can and trigger neurodegeneration and apoptosis. It remains unclear whether the insoluble inclusions also contribute to the neurodegeneration or if by sequestering the potentially damaging polypeptides, their formation may help reduce the cytotoxic effects. This summary also emphasizes how the apparent failure of abnormal proteins in aged organisms to activate the heat-shock response may reduce these protective mechanisms that help defend against these deleterious consequences.

et al., 1981) is occupied by such inclusions, the cells can completely eliminate these inclusions by proteolysis, if the production of the denatured proteins ceases. Similarly, in cells treated with a proteasome inhibitor, short-lived forms of the influenza virus nucleoprotein accumulated in the aggresome but then were lost rapidly from these structures after the inhibitor was removed (Anton *et al.*, 1999). Either the insoluble ubiquitinated proteins are digested directly by proteasomes (e.g. those present in the inclusions), or they undergo chaperone-mediated solubilization followed by proteasome-dependent hydrolysis. In either case, the aggresome may function as a storage compartment that protects the cell by temporarily isolating the denatured, potentially damaging polypeptides until they can be refolded or digested (Fig. 9.3).

The formation of inclusion bodies by mutant proteins in polyQ expansion diseases, like the formation of aggresomes in general, appears to be a highly regulated process. For example, treatment of cells with glucocorticoids was found to strongly suppress the aggregation and nuclear localization of both the androgen receptor and huntingtin fragments containing expanded polyQ sequences (Diamond *et al.*, 2000). This steroid hormone appears to be acting through its receptor to cause the transcription of a still-unidentified factor that inhibits the aggregation of these mutant proteins. Other components of cellular signaling pathways were also found to regulate the formation of inclusion bodies. When the protein kinase MEKK1, which catalyzes an early step in the JNK signaling pathway, is activated, it stimulates the formation of the inclusion bodies (Meriin *et al.*, 2001). A similar enhancement of inclusion formation was seen upon expression of arfaptin 2, a guanine nucleotide exchange factor for small GTP-binding proteins (Peters *et al.*, 2002). Moreover, both MEKK1 and arfaptin 2 were found to be colocalized with the inclusion bodies. Since small GTP-binding proteins can regulate MEKK1, it is possible that both components are acting through the same signaling pathway, and may even be related to the glucocorticoid effect. Importantly, MEKK1 appears to promote an early nucleation step(s) in the formation of small seeds of polyQ aggregates, and it was hypothesized that this kinase activates a putative cellular factor that catalyzes the nucleation of polyQ aggregates (Meriin *et al.*, 2001).

In a *C. elegans* model of human Spinocerebellar Ataxia type 1, formation of inclusion bodies was regulated by the PI3-kinase pathway, which also involves AKT kinase and the transcription factor Forkhead (encoded by daf-16 gene of *C. elegans*) (Morley *et al.*, 2002). This signalling pathway controls aging of the worms. Mutations in any of these signaling proteins reduced the formation of inclusion bodies and delayed the age of onset of cell abnormalities (Morley *et al.*, 2002). At present, it is not clear whether these effects are associated directly with alterations in this signaling pathway or related to a general delay in aging in the mutant worms. In any case, this finding is especially intriguing, since it establishes a link between signaling pathways that regulate formation of inclusion bodies and aging. Taken together, these observations further indicate that inclusion body formation represents a complex, regulated cellular response, even though the inherent tendency of unfolded proteins to aggregate and leave solution must play a key role. Further understanding of this process is of importance, since such information could have therapeutic implications.

The finding that a large fraction of the cell's chaperones and proteasomes are found in aggresomes (Fabunmi *et al.*, 2000), indicates that either inclusion bodies are sites specialized for protein refolding and proteolysis or, alternatively, that the aggregated polypeptides in the inclusion bodies resist degradation and may even trap proteasomes in nonfunctional degradative complexes. The trapping of proteasomes in inclusion bodies may contribute to a reduction in the total capacity of the cells for protein breakdown in neurological diseases (Bence *et al.*, 2001; Helmuth, 2001). Therefore, when the cell's protective machinery is overwhelmed with abnormal proteins, the stressed cells appear to localize them, together with the chaperones and degradative apparatus, in a special compartment in which the potentially toxic polypeptides can be resolubilized or refolded or undergo degradation. By contrast, in non-stressed cells, where chaperones and the proteasome are dispersed throughout the cytosol and the nucleus, degradation of the majority of proteins appears to take place outside the aggresome. This segregation of the unfolded molecules within the aggresome probably also helps reduce the threat to cell homeostasis by limiting the capacity of these unfolded proteins to associate with other cell constituents (e.g. nascent polypeptides, cell membranes, etc.), which potentially could disrupt various cellular functions. On the other hand, in many models of neurodegenerative diseases inclusion bodies certainly cause toxicity, although the mechanisms of the toxicity associated with formation of inclusion bodies have not been dissected yet.

Like aggresomes, inclusion bodies containing proteins with polyQ domains (Chai *et al.*, 1999a; Cummings *et al.*, 1998; Wyttenbach *et al.*, 2000) and other abnormal polypeptides involved in neurological pathology associate in the cytosol with molecular chaperones, in this instance Hsc70 and Hsp40 (Fig. 9.3). Overexpression of these chaperones leads to an inhibition of the inclusion body formation in various disease models (Carmichael *et al.*, 2000; Chan *et al.*, 2000; Jana *et al.*, 2000; Zhou *et al.*, 2001), which is consistent with the well-established role of molecular chaperones in prevention of protein aggregation. Furthermore, reduction of Hsps levels by downregulation of the transcription factor HSF1 in *C. elegans* expressing ataxin-1 led to an increase in the formation of inclusion bodies and increased toxicity (Morley *et al.*, 2002). On the other hand, experiments with yeast models of polyQ expansion disease showed that the relationship between chaperones and inclusion body formation is more complex. There are two steps that can be distinguished genetically in inclusion body formation – seeding and growth of small aggregates. Mutations in chaperones Hsp104 and the Hsp40 homolog, Sis1, prevented seeding of the polyQ aggregates, while mutations in Hsp70 and another Hsp40 homolog, Ydj1, slowed down the growth of aggregates (Meriin *et al.*, 2002). Overexpression of either Hsp104 or Hsp70 also suppressed polyQ aggregation in these models (Muchowski *et al.*, 2000). Although the mechanisms of these effects are not understood, it appears that some optimal levels of chaperones are necessary for inclusion body formation, and over- or underexpression of various chaperones reduces the efficiency of aggregation.

Recent study in yeast models of polyQ expansion disease demonstrated that another factor that controls aggregation and toxicity of polyQ-containing polypeptides is the yeast prion Rnq1. Like other prions, this glutamine- and asparagine-rich protein (Sondheimer & Lindquist, 2000; Sondheimer *et al.*, 2001; Wickner *et al.*, 2001) can be present in cells in either a normal (soluble) or prion (insoluble) conformation. The presence of molecules in the prion conformation forces soluble Rnq1 molecules to change their conformation and to join the aggregates. These aggregates can somehow propagate and be transferred into daughter cells. In a *rnq1* deletion strain, in spite of very high expression levels of polyQ, its aggregation was suppressed, and there was no toxicity. Furthermore, Rnq1 could promote aggregation of polyQ-containing polypeptides only when present in the prion conformation (Meriin *et al.*, 2002). The dependence on Rnq1 was specific for polyQ aggregation and was not seen with other polypeptides that form inclusions (e.g. a mutant form of SOD that can cause Amyotrophic Lateral Sclerosis) (Meriin *et al.*, 2002). The obvious question raised by these findings is whether the aggregation of proteins with expanded polyQ domains in neurons also requires an unknown prion-like protein.

Proteasomal hydrolysis of polyQ-containing proteins

It is unclear whether the presence within the inclusions of a high concentration of ubiquitinated proteins and proteasomes indicates that proteolysis is occurring at high rates in such structures or that there has been an unsuccessful attempt of the proteasomal apparatus to efficiently eliminate the abnormal insoluble molecules. The β-sheets formed by extended polyQ sequences and other fibril-forming polypeptides present in various types of inclusion bodies are likely to represent a major challenge for the proteasomal ATPases, which unfold and translocate substrates into the 20S particle (Navon & Goldberg, 2001). It is presently unknown how the proteasome digests a ubiquitinated polypeptide containing an extended polyQ domain, but it must do so successfully most of the time. For example, in Huntington's disease patients, the abnormal form of huntingtin accumulates in inclusions only in specific regions of the brain, even though this gene is also expressed in other neurons and non-neuronal cells. In these cells, the mutant huntingtin must be continually degraded without the formation of toxic aggregates or large inclusion bodies. Indeed, recent data indicate that in non-neuronal cells in culture, huntingtin with extended polyQ is degraded with a half-life of several hours by a proteasomal mechanism (Martin-Aparicio *et al.*, 2001). Recent data indicate that in none of the 20S proteasome's peptidase sites, which are trypsin-like, chymotrypsin-like, or caspase-like in their substrate specificity, can cleave within a polyQ stretch (Venkatraman & Goldberg, unpublished data). Therefore, when the proteasome digests a protein containing a normal or extended polyQ tract, it probably

releases long polyQ sequences, and one or more of the cytosolic peptidases that complete the hydrolysis of proteasome products must be able to digest peptides containing only glutamine residues. Otherwise, these relatively insoluble polyQ sequences would aggregate and form inclusion bodies.

In principle, each of these steps in the degradative pathway could on occasion fail, leading to the accumulation of the abnormal polypeptides. There is evidence that the mutant form of ataxin-1 with an extended polyQ sequence is degraded by proteasomes inefficiently, despite normal rates of ubiquitination (Cummings *et al.*, 1999). Perhaps the extended polyQ sequence interferes with complete degradation by the 26S proteasome by causing tight associations with other molecules and preventing protein entry into the 20S particle. In such a case, either the 26S proteasome may release a polyQ-containing fragment, which could be more toxic than huntingtin itself, or the aggregated polyQ sequence may stay attached to the 19S particle and prevent degradation of other proteins (Navon & Goldberg, 2001). In cultured cell models, caspase 3 seems to serve such a pathogenic role by cleaving the extended forms of huntingtin, ataxin, and the androgen receptor to smaller fragments that contain the deleterious polyQ domains (Ellerby *et al.*, 1999; Martindale *et al.*, 1998; Wellington *et al.*, 1997, 1998). However, it remains uncertain what step actually fails in the affected neurons of patients, leading to an accumulation of these abnormal species.

There is growing evidence that the failure of proteasomes to degrade efficiently polyQ-containing polypeptides and other abnormal proteins (e.g., alpha-synuclein, mutant SOD) and their accumulation can result in an inhibition of proteasome function and a general reduction in protein degradation by the ubiquitin-proteasome pathway (Bence *et al.*, 2001; Helmuth, 2001; Jana *et al.*, 2001). An inhibition of this pathway has been observed in various cellular and animal models of Huntington's and Parkinson's diseases and amyotrophic lateral sclerosis (Chung *et al.*, 2001a; McNaught & Jenner, 2001; McNaught *et al.*, 2002; McNaught *et al.*, 2001; Tanaka *et al.*, 2001; Urushitani *et al.*, 2002). The proteasome-associated peptidase activities were suppressed in these conditions, suggesting a general defect in proteasome function in these diseases. In addition, the ubiquitination step of this pathway is also affected in at least some disorders, most clearly in inherited Parkinson's disease (see below) (Chung *et al.*, 2001b; Shimura *et al.*, 2000, 2001). In cell culture, only neurons with inclusion bodies have general defects in protein degradation, while cells that express the same abnormal proteins in soluble form do not demonstrate the defect (Bence *et al.*, 2001). These data argue that inhibition of protein degradation in these neurodegenerative disorders is associated with the emergence of inclusion bodies. One potential mechanism of such an inhibition is the trapping of the proteasomes in the inclusions, which may make these particles inaccessible to their normal substrates. Another possibility is that mutations that retard the degradation of certain domains in normally unstable proteins (e.g. expanded polyglutamine domains) may lead to a tight association of the mutant polypeptide within the proteasome and an inhibition of its activity towards other substrates. Model experiments with a protein substrate which was chemically linked to a large globular protein so that it could not be translocated through the ATPase ring to the 20S core particle showed that such a modified polypeptide can become tightly associated with the ATPase and acts like a dominant inhibitor of protein breakdown (Navon & Goldberg, 2001). Independently of the specific mechanism, the non-translocated protein complex causes failure of proteasomes to remove abnormal proteins, which in vivo would cause their further accumulation in an autocatalytic process (Table 9.2).

One of the great mysteries concerning these neurodegenerative diseases is their tendency to specifically affect only certain neuronal populations (e.g. basal ganglia in Huntington's disease or motor neurons in ALS). In these susceptible cell populations, the defenses against these specific abnormal proteins must be different or defective. When the abnormal genes responsible for Huntington's (Saudou et al., 1998) or Parkinson's (Masliah et al., 2000) diseases are expressed in cultured neurons or in the brain, the neuropathology is evident in those cell types affected by the human disease. An alternative possibility, for which there is some evidence in Huntington's disease, is that these susceptible neurons are the sites of somatic mutations, such that their DNA contains a huntingtin with exceptionally long polyQ sequences. In other words, these neurons may be expressing an even more abnormal gene product than the rest of the brain (Aronin et al., 1995; Telenius et al., 1994).

Protein damage can induce apoptosis

If a cell's protective systems are unable to handle the buildup of abnormal polypeptides, and if the induction of Hsps is insufficient to prevent their continued accumulation, a program for cell suicide (apoptosis) is initiated (Gabai et al., 1998). In other words, when the cell's mechanisms for repair, segregation, and digestion of the unfolded proteins are inadequate, this situation is sufficiently threatening to the organism to trigger programmed cell death.

For example, apoptosis occurs in response to a variety of highly stressful treatments that are damaging to cell proteins (e.g. exposure to high temperatures). Cell death apparently occurs before the cells have sufficient time to induce the Hsps to achieve enhanced protection (Gabai et al., 1997; Mosser et al., 1997; Mosser & Martin, 1992). Similarly, apoptosis can be triggered by incubation with amino acid analogues or low doses of puromycin (Sugita et al., 1995), which causes the production of improperly folded or incomplete proteins. If shorter fragments of proteins are generated, they appear less toxic than longer ones, perhaps because they are more readily degraded or less likely to associate with other cell components (Chow et al., 1995).

Recently, important insights have been obtained as to how abnormal proteins can trigger apoptosis. When mammalian cells are subjected to a variety of stressful conditions, a number of protein kinases are activated. One of these stress-activated kinases, called JNK, plays a key role in the activation of apoptosis triggered by unfolded proteins (for review, see Gabai et al., 1998). Inhibition of the JNK signaling pathway reduces the ability of protein-damaging conditions, such as high temperatures, to induce programmed cell death. JNK activates apoptosis by multiple mechanisms. It increases the phosphorylation of the major anti-apoptotic proteins Bcl-2 and Bcl-x, thus reducing their anti-apoptotic activity (Kharbanda et al., 2000; Srivastava et al., 1999). JNK can also somehow promote cleavage and activation of the pro-apoptotic protein Bid (Gabai et al., 2002). These effects of JNK control the major mitochondria-dependent apoptotic pathway (Gabai et al., 2002). The two major isoforms, JNK1 and JNK2, play an essential role in apoptosis induced by DNA damage (Tournier et al., 2000) and in neuronal apoptosis during brain development (Kuan et al., 1999). JNK can also activate apoptosis through the induction of the FAS ligand (Faris et al., 1998a; Faris et al., 1998b). In the brain, there is a specific JNK isoform, JNK3, which is essential for the neuronal apoptosis induced by excitotoxic agents (e.g. kainic acid), and perhaps other stimuli (Yang et al., 1997). It remains unclear which of the JNK isoforms is critical in cell death caused by the accumulation of mutant polypeptides in neuronal cells. Inhibition of proteasomes by lactacystin or other specific inhibitors activates JNK, and this activation leads to induction of apoptosis in both neuronal and non-neuronal cell lines (Hideshima et al., 2002; Masaki et al., 2000; Meriin et al., 1998). This activation of the JNK-dependent apoptotic pathway by the proteasome inhibitors is likely to lead to a stabilization and accumulation of pro-apoptotic proteins (e.g. p53 or Bax). A similar accumulation of the pro-apoptotic proteins was seen in cellular models of Huntington's disease (Jana et al., 2001). These findings are also consistent with results from proposed models in which neuronal loss in these neurodegenerative disorders results from an inhibition of the ubiquitin-proteasome pathway.

It is noteworthy that the expression of proteins with extended polyQ sequences can activate signaling pathways and induce apoptosis in similar ways as other types of unfolded polypeptides. Cell death induced by overexpression of mutant huntingtin has been reported to depend on the activation of JNK (Liu, 1998; Yasuda *et al.*, 1999). However, other apoptotic pathways, perhaps independent of JNK, may also be involved in Huntington's disease. For example, there is evidence that caspase 8 can be activated by association with inclusion bodies, and this activation may also contribute to huntingtin-induced dysfunction and apoptosis (Sanchez *et al.*, 1999; Urushitani *et al.*, 2001).

The major heat shock protein Hsp70 plays a key role in the regulation of JNK. Specific inhibition of Hsp72 induction with anti-sense RNA enhances JNK activation by protein-damaging insults (Gabai *et al.*, 2000), while increased expression of Hsp72 dramatically reduces the capacity of protein damage to activate JNK (Gabai *et al.*, 1997) (Fig. 9.2). This crosstalk between the chaperone machinery and the apoptotic signaling pathway may play an important role in reducing the toxicity of abnormal polypeptides in neurological disorders. Direct inhibition of the apoptotic pathway by Hsp70 can explain the findings in *Drosophila* and in certain cellular models of polyQ-expansion diseases that overexpression of Hsp70 did not reduce the number of inclusion bodies but dramatically suppressed apoptosis (Warrick *et al.*, 1999; Zhou *et al.*, 2001). These data indicate that Hsp70 probably also protects cells at a step that follows inclusion body formation.

Key unresolved issues

There are several closely related fundamental questions that have to be resolved if we are fully to understand the pathogenesis of the polyQ-expansion disorders: (a) Is neuronal death critical in the disease process? (b) Is it a soluble form of the abnormal proteins or the inclusion bodies that cause cell toxicity? (c) What are the molecular pathways that lead to neuronal dysfunction and/or death in these disorders?

(a) In Huntington's disease patients, there is extensive neuronal loss in the striatum and cerebral cortex, leading to a marked reduction in brain size at later stages of the disease. On the other hand, in transgenic mouse models that express fragments of huntingtin containing the expanded

polyQ, there are behavioral abnormalities similar to those in Huntington's disease, but massive neuronal death was not found (Davies *et al.*, 1997; Yamamoto *et al.*, 2000). Neurons that express the mutant huntingtin differ from ones expressing the normal forms in several respects, including a reduced number of dendrites and reduced transport of dyes along the neuron (Young, 1998). Furthermore, an altered expression of NMDA receptors, which led to enhanced sensitivity of neurons to excitotoxic stimuli, was seen in animal models of Huntington's disease (Cepeda *et al.*, 2001; Zeron *et al.*, 2001, 2002). At present, it is not clear which of these alterations (if any) causes the neurological symptoms, cellular loss, and eventually disease progression. In *C. elegans* transfected with the mutant huntingtin, the expressing neurons do not undergo apoptosis, but show symptoms of neurodegeneration that could be suppressed by inhibitors of caspases, the key proteolytic enzymes in the apoptotic pathway (Faber *et al.*, 1999). Thus, activation of certain components of the cell death program seems to play a role in the neurodegeneration, even without causing classic apoptosis. In case of huntingtin-caused cell death, caspases may be involved not in the execution step of the apoptosis, but rather in production of toxic huntingtin fragments. Several observations on transfected cells in culture suggest that the truncated forms of huntingtin and ataxins that are found in inclusions may be generated by caspase-mediated cleavages (Ellerby *et al.*, 1999; Kobayashi *et al.*, 1998; Martindale *et al.*, 1998; Wellington *et al.*, 1998). The inclusions themselves may also bind and further activate caspase, thus perhaps inducing programmed cell death or promoting neurodegeneration (Miyashita *et al.*, 1999; Ona *et al.*, 1999; Sanchez *et al.*, 1999; Wang *et al.*, 1999). In striatal cells transfected with huntingtin, there is a dramatic enhancement of autophagy, i.e. the incorporation of large regions of the cytoplasm into vacuoles followed by their digestion in lysosomes (Kegel *et al.*, 2000; Petersen *et al.*, 2001). A similar activation of autophagy was seen with PC-12 cells expressing the mutant form of alpha-synuclein, which is responsible for an inherited form of Parkinson's disease (Anglade *et al.*, 1997; Stefanis *et al.*, 2001). Autophagy is activated in most cell types deprived of essential growth factors. In several cell types, including neurons, enhanced autophagy may lead to cell dysfunction and eventually death and may thus represent an alternative to the classical apoptotic mechanism of programmed cell death (Stefanis *et al.*, 2001). It is possible that the enhanced autophagy may contribute to neurodegeneration in polyQ expansion disorders. On the other hand, autophagy may also contribute to the elimination of the mutant huntingtin molecules (Ravikumar *et al.*, 2002).

Table 9.3. Consequences of accumulation of unfolded proteins demonstrated in model systems

1. Proteasomes form aggresome-like inclusions
2. Non-translocatable aggregated proteins may bind to ATPases in 26S proteasome, block its function, and cause further accumulation of abnormal proteins
3. Trapping of proteasomes and chaperones in inclusions may cause further accumulation of abnormal proteins
4. Binding of normal polyQ-containing proteins to aggregates of mutant polyQ proteins may interfere with normal cell function (e.g. trapping of histone acetylase in inclusions may block transcription of many genes)

(b) The formation of inclusion bodies generally precedes neurodegeneration in all models, and in instances where cell death has been documented, the formation of large inclusions precedes it as well. Such observations initially led to the widely held assumption that aggregate formation is the critical event triggering neuropathology in Huntington's disease and related diseases. On the other hand, there is appreciable evidence that soluble polyQ-containing polypeptides cause neuronal toxicity. This apparent contradiction probably indicates that there are multiple mechanisms of neuronal toxicity, which may be initiated by either soluble or aggregated abnormal polypeptides.

There are several hypotheses on the mechanisms of toxicity of polypeptides with expanded polyQ domains related to inclusion body formation (Table 9.3). All these hypotheses consider that various types of essential proteins are recruited into inclusion bodies, leading to the cessation of critical cellular functions. Toxicity due to the trapping of proteasomes in inclusion bodies and related inhibition of the ubiquitin-proteasome degradation pathway is discussed above. Another hypothesis stipulates that the trapping of Hsp70 and Hsp40 in inclusion bodies may deplete the pool of free chaperones, thus leading to cessation of protein-folding activity and eventually to neurodegeneration. This idea is consistent with the fact that overexpression of Hsp70 or Hsp40 strongly suppresses the polyQ-induced toxicity in *Drosophila* and in cellular models (Warrick *et al.*, 1999; Zhou *et al.*, 2001) (although there are other explanations of these data, as discussed above). Furthermore, inhibition of Hsp70 function by expression of a dominant-negative Hsp70 mutant in Drosophila led to neurodegeneration similar to that seen upon expression of ataxin-1 with an expanded polyQ domain (Chan *et al.*, 2000).

Another hypothesized pathogenic mechanism is that the mutant polypeptides with expanded polyQ domains co-aggregate with normal essential proteins with polyQ or glutamine/asparagine-rich domains, leading to neuronal

dysfunction (Table 9.3). Although the human genome has not been analyzed extensively for the presence of such proteins, in *Drosophila* and yeast, there are hundreds of such polypeptides, and some of them are essential for cell growth and survival. In model experiments, a polypeptide with short polyQ (25Q) co-aggregated with a polypeptide with long polyQ (103Q) (Kazantsev *et al.*, 1999; Preisinger *et al.*, 1999). Furthermore, some of the normal critical polyQ-containing proteins were found to be present in inclusion bodies, including CBP, a transcription co-activator CREB-binding protein (Nucifora *et al.*, 2001; Steffan *et al.*, 2000), and nucleolin (Preisinger *et al.*, 1999). Recruitment to inclusion bodies of CBP also leads to the inhibition of its histone acetyltransferase activity and a reduction of histone acetylation in a cellular model of Huntington's disease (Nucifora *et al.*, 2001). Accordingly, inhibition of histone deacetylase, which leads to a net increase in the level of acetylated histones and thus opposes the inhibition of histone acetyltransferase, increased cell survival and partially suppressed neurodegeneration in the *Drosophila* model (Steffan *et al.*, 2001). Therefore, recruitment of CBP, and perhaps other transcriptional regulators, to inclusion bodies represents at least one of the mechanisms of neurodegeneration in the polyQ expansion diseases.

(c) Although apoptosis is often associated with the formation of inclusion bodies in cells expressing proteins with extended polyQ, soluble forms of the polypeptides may also cause cell death. For example, deletion of the C-terminal portion of huntingtin enhances formation of inclusions but does not increase the fraction of apoptotic cells (Saudou *et al.*, 1998). Furthermore, deletion of the self-association regions of ataxin 1 blocks aggregation but does not suppress apoptosis (Klement *et al.*, 1998). Moreover, in transgenic mice lacking the ubiquitin-protein ligase E6-AP, formation of ataxin-1 inclusion bodies is reduced, while toxicity is more prominent (Cummings *et al.*, 1999). In another example, when the dominant negative form of the ubiquitin-conjugating enzyme Cdc34 was transfected into such cells, it suppressed the formation of inclusions, but actually led to increased apoptosis (Saudou *et al.*, 1998). These observations all suggest that a soluble form of these abnormal molecules could be the primary trigger of apoptosis in these systems. Among potential mechanisms of induction of cell death by soluble polyQ-containing proteins are direct interaction of these proteins with various pro- or anti-apoptotic factors. One of these putative mechanisms is the interaction of soluble huntingtin with normal polyQ with a pro-apoptotic protein Hip1 (Kalchman *et al.*, 1997), leading to its inhibition and cell survival. Huntingtin with an expanded polyQ domain cannot interact with Hip1 and can no longer inhibit it, leading to interaction of Hip1 with another pro-apoptotic protein

Hippi, which can activate caspase 8 and cause cell death (Gervais *et al.*, 2002).

It should be emphasized that activation of cell malfunction and death by polyQ polypeptides need not involve a single molecular mechanism; in fact, as discussed above, strong evidence has been obtained for multiple mechanisms, all of which may function synergistically in causing cell damage and death. Moreover, additional mechanisms of toxicity may also be discovered as these models are studied in further depth. In any case, as discussed above, the activation of JNK, cytochrome C release, and the activation of caspases are probably the downstream events initiated independently of the particular mechanism triggering apoptosis. Finally, while many aspects of neuronal function are clearly altered in these neurodegenerative diseases (e.g. the number of dendrites, transport of molecules along the neuron, expression of receptors for excitotoxic transmitters), it is quite unclear whether the inclusions or the soluble species may cause such changes, since only their relationship to apoptosis has been studied.

Neuronal protection by molecular chaperones

Based on findings in non-neuronal cells expressing various mutant proteins, it seems very likely that chaperones, especially Hsp70 and Hsp40, also serve important protective roles in neurons that express mutant proteins, including those with polyQ expansions. As mentioned above, in Drosophila models of human polyQ diseases, overproduction of Hsp70 and Hsp40 strongly protected neurons that expressed mutant forms of human huntingtin (Fernandez-Funez *et al.*, 2000; Kazemi-Esfarjani & Benzer, 2000; Warrick *et al.*, 1999). In neuronal cultures, expression of Hsp70 and Hsp40 protected cells from apoptosis induced by the mutant androgen receptor (Kobayashi *et al.*, 2000). Similarly, overexpression of the inducible isoform of Hsp70 reduced neuronal degeneration in mice caused by an extended form of ataxin-1 (Cummings *et al.*, 2001). Also, overproduction of another chaperone Hsp104 in *C. elegans* dramatically reduced neurotoxicity of the mutant huntingtin (Satyal *et al.*, 2000).

There are several possible mechanisms by which these chaperones might help protect the neurons. (a) The Hsps may help combat the tendencies of huntingtin and ataxin to unfold and aggregate. In yeast cells, these chaperones can reduce the formation of inclusion bodies by a huntingtin fragment with expanded polyQ, and in vitro decrease aggregation of this fragment (Muchowski *et al.*, 2000). The huntingtin fragment tends to form two types of aggregates, either amyloid-like fibrils that are unusual in resisting solubilization by the ionic detergent SDS, or amorphous structures that can be solubilized with detergents. Hsp70 and its cofactor Hsp40 can bind to the soluble molecules, and facilitate the formation of the amorphous aggregates, while suppressing formation of the fibrillar structures (Muchowski *et al.*, 2000). It seems very likely, although it remains to be proven, that chaperones have similar effects in neurons. (b) The abnormal species, whether soluble or aggregated, probably serve as seeds to which other partially unfolded proteins associate, and thus may inhibit the successful folding of newly synthesized polypeptides. By binding to the abnormal species, the Hsps may reduce the harmful consequences of this accumulation. (c) In addition to associating with aggregated species and perhaps promoting their resolubilization, the chaperones may bind preferentially to the soluble polyQ-extended molecules and reduce their toxicity by preventing them from interacting with proteins that trigger apoptosis and neurodegeneration. (d) The Hsps may also facilitate the ubiquitination and degradation of huntingtin and ataxins, as Hsp70 and Hsp40 do for certain other abnormal proteins (Bercovich *et al.*, 1997; Lee *et al.*, 1996a; Sherman & Goldberg, 1996). Other chaperones may also contribute to these effects; for example, in yeast a distinct chaperone, Hsp104 (but not Hsp70 or Hsp40), is essential for the degradation of ataxin-1 (Lee *et al.*, in press).

(e) Finally, Hsp72, by inhibiting the activation of JNK, should directly inhibit the ability of these mutant polypeptides to cause apoptosis. It therefore appears likely that at some stages of the disease, the heat shock response is activated as part of the standard cellular response to a buildup of abnormal proteins. However, reliable information on the levels of Hsp expression in neurons during progression of these diseases is unfortunately not available (see below). This question is of appreciable importance, since, in principle, treatments that cause induction of Hsps could be a very useful approach for therapy of these neurodegenerative diseases.

Abnormal protein inclusions in Parkinson's disease

In addition to the polyQ diseases, several other major neurodegenerative diseases are also associated with an accumulation of proteinaceous inclusions and neuronal apoptosis (Table 9.1, Fig. 9.2). For example, in the substantia nigra of patients with Parkinson's disease, α-synuclein, a very abundant pre-synaptic protein of unknown function, accumulates in inclusions, termed Lewy bodies, in cell bodies and neurites (Mezey *et al.*, 1998) of dopaminergic neurons. α-synuclein was first implicated in the pathogenesis of Parkinson's disease through the identification of mutated forms of this protein in families having the rare inherited forms of this disease (Polymeropoulos *et al.*, 1997). In more recent studies, Lewy bodies, the characteristic inclusions in non-inherited forms of these and other neurodegenerative diseases (e.g. multiple systems atrophy) have been shown to contain an abnormal form of α-synuclein, which contains nitrated tyrosine residues (Giasson *et al.*, 2000). This covalent modification results from oxidative damage to the protein, and there had been appreciable evidence implicating oxidative injury in the pathogenesis of this disease (Giasson *et al.*, 2000). By reacting with nitric oxide, oxygen free radicals (especially superoxide) generate the highly reactive species, peroxynitrite, which modifies tyrosines in proteins, and presumably the resulting abnormal form of α-synuclein is particularly prone to aggregate in cells. Nitrative insult of cells that caused generation of peroxynitrite led to aggregation of α-synuclein (Paxinou *et al.*, 2001). A similar aggregation of α-synuclein was seen upon exposure of cells to mitochondrial inhibitors (Lee *et al.*, 2002) that cause oxidative stress and produce Parkinson's-like symptoms in an animal model. Similar inclusions containing ubiquitin and α-synuclein are also seen in patients with Dementia with Lewy Bodies (DLB) (Baba *et al.*, 1998; Spillantini *et al.*, 1998; Takeda *et al.*, 1998).

Like the inclusions containing huntingtin and the ataxins, the α-synuclein inclusions contain large amounts of ubiquitin and proteasomes (Bennett *et al.*, 1999; Ii *et al.*, 1997). Importantly, the major hereditary form of Parkinson's disease results from mutations in the protein parkin (Kitada *et al.*, 1998; Tanaka *et al.*, 1998), which was shown to be a ubiquitin-protein ligase (E3). In the patients with this form of the disease, this enzymatic activity is lost. The question of what the natural substrates for parkin are is presently highly controversial. It appears that normal α-synuclein cannot bind to parkin and cannot be ubiquitinated by parkin (Shimura *et al.*, 2001). However, parkin can associate with an α-synuclein-interacting protein, synphilin-1, and ubiquitinate it (Chung *et al.*, 2001b). Importantly, in transfected cells the presence of all three components, α-synuclein, synphilin-1, and parkin, was essential for the appearance of Lewy body-like inclusions (Chung *et al.*, 2001b), and all three components are found in these inclusions. Furthermore, mutations in parkin that inactivate the E3 ubiquitin ligase activity and cause familial forms of Parkinson's disease prevented the interaction of parkin with synphilin-1 and prevented inclusion body formation (Chung *et al.*, 2001b). Accordingly, in cases of familial Parkinson's disease associated with mutations in parkin (Mizuno *et al.*, 2001), there is a lack of Lewy bodies, which are characteristic of other forms of this disease. These data

suggest that ubiquitination of synphilin-1, or other proteins, is essential for formation of inclusion bodies. This idea is in accord with observations that formation of inclusion bodies in models of polyQ expansion diseases was suppressed upon inactivation of the ubiquitin-conjugating enzymes Cdc34 and E6-AP (Cummings *et al.*, 1999; Saudou *et al.*, 1998).

Other hereditary forms of Parkinson's disease are also associated with distinct mutations affecting the ubiquitination system. In one form, the mutation inactivates the ubiquitin carboxy-terminal hydrolase L1 (Leroy *et al.*, 1998). This enzyme is one of the cell's many isopeptidases, or enzymes capable of removing ubiquitin from peptide conjugates, but recent findings indicate that under certain in vitro, and possibly in vivo, conditions, it can also promote ubiquitin conjugation (Liu *et al.*, 2002). For unknown reasons, this enzyme is one of the most abundant proteins in the brain, and it is rapidly induced in aplysia during post-synaptic facilitation (Hegde *et al.*, 1997). Curiously, mutations in a distinct deubiquitinating enzyme are associated with a distinct neurodegenerative disease, gracile axonal dystrophy (Saigoh *et al.*, 1999). However, the precise role of these deubiquitinating enzymes in overall ubiquitin metabolism and in protein degradation is uncertain. Most likely, such mutations lead to a general disorder in ubiquitin recycling, but it is quite unclear why such a defect would lead in Parkinson's disease to a specific accumulation of α-synuclein and not other abnormal brain proteins. If ubiquitination is, in fact, critical for Lewy body formation, one would expect that mutations in ubiquitin carboxy-terminal hydrolase L1 would increase the levels of ubiquitin-conjugated proteins, thus increasing the formation of inclusion bodies. In any case, it is conceivable that the α-synuclein mutation, free radical damage to this protein, or a failure to ubiquitinate α-synuclein leads to an accumulation of abnormal species, which interfere with normal cell function and eventually trigger apoptosis of the dopaminergic neurons. If so, Hsps would be anticipated to play a role in retarding the development of Parkinson's disease, by reducing α-synuclein aggregation, promoting its solubilization or degradation, or inhibiting the events leading to apoptosis.

Apoptosis and inclusions in other neurodegenerative diseases

Another late-onset neurodegenerative disease that appears to involve some similar cellular mechanisms is amyotrophic lateral sclerosis (ALS), a rapidly progressive disease characterized by death of motor neurons (Brown,

1998). Some of the hereditary forms of ALS are due to mutations in superoxide dismutase, including ones that cause a loss-of-function or a gain-of-function (Brown, 1998; Cleveland, 1999). Initially, oxidative stress associated with dysfunction of SOD was suggested to be the primary cause of ALS (Cleveland & Rothstein, 2001), but subsequent experiments have ruled out this possibility and indicated instead that accumulation of misfolded SOD is the cause of the disease. Briefly, it was shown that the progression of the disease does not correlate with SOD activity and production of reactive oxygen species, and symptoms develop even in individuals with mutations in SOD that completely lack enzyme activity (Brown, 1998; Cleveland, 1999). Furthermore, a specific "copper chaperone" is necessary for loading of Cu^{2+} onto SOD, and deletion of this gene, while dramatically reducing SOD activity, did not change the course of the disease in animal models (Subramaniam *et al.*, 2002). Thus, ALS appears to represent another "abnormal protein disorder". In transgenic animals expressing the mutant SODs, apoptosis is evident and can be retarded by central administration of caspase inhibitors (Li *et al.*, 2000) or by mutations affecting certain caspases (Friedlander & Yuan, 1998). ALS, in both its hereditary and acquired versions, is associated with the presence in affected motor neurons of proteinaceous inclusions that contain mutant forms of SOD, stain with anti-ubiquitin antibodies (Ii *et al.*, 1997; Kawashima *et al.*, 1998; Mayer *et al.*, 1996; Shibata *et al.*, 1999; Tu *et al.*, 1997), and contain excess neurofilaments. The development of these inclusions containing SOD closely resembles the formation of aggresomes (Johnston *et al.*, 2000). Although rigorous demonstration of abnormal polypeptides is lacking in the common nonhereditary form of ALS, there is evidence for oxidative or heavy-metal-mediated damage to neuronal proteins. Importantly, in culture the viability of neurons expressing the mutant SOD can be improved by increasing the content of Hsp72 (Bruening *et al.*, 1999).

Alzheimer's disease, the most common cause of senile dementia, appears (at least) superficially to be very different from these other diseases. This condition is associated with extracellular amyloid plaques, but Alzheimer's-affected brains are also characterized by intracellular accumulation of ubiquitin conjugate of the cytoskeletal protein tau, which also accumulates in neurons in the much rarer disease, progressive supranuclear palsy. The molecular basis for these inclusions and their relationship to the extracellular amyloid-related damage is quite unclear, especially since in transgenic mouse models of Alzheimer's disease, extracellular plaques are seen without the intracellular inclusions. One intriguing observation is the finding in the brains of some Alzheimer's disease patients

an anomalous form of ubiquitin (UBB⁺) (van Leewen *et al.*, 1998), resulting from transcriptional misreading of the stress-induced polyubiquitin gene (see below). As a result, some ubiquitin molecules are generated with aberrant C-terminal extensions and therefore cannot be conjugated to substrates. Such an extended version, however, can become linked to other ubiquitin molecules and, in principle, such ubiquitin chains might competitively inhibit proteasomal function. Recent experiments demonstrated that UBB⁺ can be incorporated in ubiquitin trees, and overexpression of UBB⁺ in cells can dramatically inhibit protein degradation by the ubiquitin-proteasome pathway (Lindsten *et al.*, 2002; van Leeuwen *et al.*, 2002). Such an inhibition could significantly contribute to the toxicity of various types of abnormal polypeptides involved in neurodegenerative disorders, especially since production of UBB⁺ increases in aged organisms (van Leeuwen *et al.*, 1998, 2002).

Because of these striking similarities, it is attractive to hypothesize that diverse neurodegenerative diseases develop through a common mechanism, in which the accumulation of abnormal proteins in the affected neurons is recognized as evidence of massive and probably irreparable damage to cell constituents, leading to neuronal dysfunction and the activation of the apoptotic program. Although such a unifying mechanism remains unproven and largely untested, these various observations emphasize that, in very long-lived non-dividing cells, such as neurons, any rare event favoring production of an aberrant protein (e.g. free radical damage) can lead to its slow accumulation, with toxic consequences. Because structural defects in any of a variety of neuronal proteins can generate pathology, the proper functioning of the molecular chaperones and the ubiquitin-proteasome pathway must be particularly important in host defenses against neuronal degeneration.

Aging, Hsps, and susceptibility to neurodegenerative diseases

An important common feature of many of these neurological diseases that has long puzzled investigators is their late onset. In most cases, the marked neurodegeneration (e.g. in Huntington's disease or ALS) occurs in middle age or later (Brown, 1998; Young, 1998). The mechanisms proposed here for cell protection and pathology in these various conditions also suggest a possible explanation for their late onset. The onset of an inherited disease in middle age or later implies that the affected neurons can deal successfully with the mutant proteins for many years. During this time the potentially toxic polypeptides must be continually synthesized and degraded without causing disease symptoms or cell death, until, with aging, abnormal molecules accumulate in certain neurons and eventually reach toxic levels. In other words, with aging, the cell's capacity to handle the aberrant polypeptides becomes insufficient to prevent their accumulation and toxic consequences. It is noteworthy that earlier onset of disease is seen in Huntington's disease and related polyQ disease as the extent of the abnormality in protein structure becomes greater (i.e. as the length of the polyQ repeat increases) (Young, 1998). Similarly, in transgenic mouse models of ALS, earlier onset occurs if the extent of the expression of the abnormal gene product is increased (i.e. they show a gene dosage effect) (Cleveland, 1999).

We suggest that one important factor contributing to the enhanced sensitivity of aged organisms to these disorders is a reduced capacity of cells from older individuals to cope with abnormal proteins. Of particular interest in this regard are various observations indicating that aged organisms and senescent cultures of mammalian cells are less able to induce Hsps in response to protein-damaging conditions (Heydari et al., 1994; Rattan & Derventzi, 1991), due to the defect in activation of transcription factor HSF1 (Heydari et al., 2000; Lee et al., 1996b). For example, in rodents, the magnitude of the increase in Hsp expression in various tissues, including brain, after a mild heat shock is much smaller in aged animals than in young ones (Heydari et al., 1994). A similar reduction with aging in the ability of rat and human tissues to induce Hsps has been observed upon exposure to oxidative stress and amino acid analogs (Locke & Tanguay, 1996; Muramatsu et al., 1996). In agreement with this suggestion, inhibition of HSF1 in the *C. elegans* model of polyQ expansion disease leads to significantly earlier onset of the disease (Morley et al., 2002).

Since these Hsps can promote refolding, solubilization and degradation of damaged polypeptides, the loss of this protective response should seriously compromise the cell's capacity to cope with the mutant or damaged proteins, which could have been handled successfully at younger ages. These considerations predict that neurons from aged humans should be defective in inducing Hsps when mutant huntingtin, ataxins, α-synuclein, and other abnormal proteins tend to accumulate. As a consequence of decreased Hsp inducibility, the mutant polypeptides should build up in cells of aged individuals to higher levels and result in a greater tendency to form inclusions, to cause neurodegeneration, and to trigger apoptosis. Decreased expression or inducibility of chaperones may account for the large number of observations suggesting the presence in

aged organisms and senescent cultures of various types of abnormal polypeptides (Grune et al., 1997; Sastre et al., 1996), including oxidatively damaged polypeptides, ones containing isomerized residues and inactive proteins due to altered conformations (Chiu & Liu, 1997; Mrak et al., 1997; Sastre et al., 1996; Tarcsa et al., 2000). It is also interesting that cells infected with the mutant prion protein (Tatzelt et al., 1995) also show diminished capacity to induce Hsps, which may increase their vulnerability to prion-induced apoptosis. Furthermore, mutations in Presenilin 1, which cause early onset of Alzheimer's disease, reduce the neuron's capacity to induce chaperones in the ER (Katayama et al., 1999). This defect could contribute to the enhanced production of Aβ peptide in these cells and to the greater susceptibility of such cells to apoptosis and neurodegeneration. Also, it was recently reported that brains of aged individuals have a specific mechanism that causes frame-shift mutations at the RNA level and thus generation of nonsense polypeptides (van Leewen et al., 1998).

With aging, cells also seem to have a reduced capacity for protein degradation, although this issue has not been rigorously examined. One proteolytic pathway affected by aging is the lysosomal pathway (Cuervo & Dice, 1998b), which catalyzes the breakdown of endocytosed components, including most surface membrane proteins. The breakdown of proteins that are specifically targeted to lysosomes for degradation is dramatically reduced in senescent cultures and in cells isolated from aged organisms (Cuervo & Dice, 1998a; Dice, 1993). This defect seems to be due to a reduced capacity to translocate polypeptides into lysosomes for degradation (Cuervo & Dice, 1996, 1998a; Hayes and Dice, 1996). These observations would also suggest a reduced capacity for proteolysis by autophagic vacuole formation, which has been reported in certain cellular models of polyQ disease. The capacity of the ubiquitin-proteasome pathway also seems to be reduced with aging, although the data on age-dependent alteration of the pathway are sometimes contradictory (Carrard et al., 2002; Shringarpure & Davies, 2002; Szweda et al., 2002). It should be noted, however, that in some tissues and cell types, a clear decline of the ubiquitin-proteasome-dependent degradation of certain proteins and of proteasome activity was demonstrated (Shang et al., 1997). Also, in aged mouse muscles, expression of mRNA for multiple components of this pathway is reduced (Shang et al., 1997). Another potentially important age-related alteration is the recently described mutant form of ubiquitin, UBB+, resulting from a frame shift at the RNA level (van Leewen et al., 1998), which, as noted above, may reduce the cell's capacity to degrade aberrant molecules. Production of UBB+ has been seen not only in aging, but especially in several neurological disorders (Bardag-Gorce *et al.*, 2002; De Vrij *et al.*, 2001; van Leeuwen *et al.*, 2000), and was suggested to play a major role in reducing the capability of neurons to degrade abnormal polypeptides (van Leeuwen *et al.*, 2002).

Whatever the molecular basis for these intriguing observations, such changes in the cell's proteolytic capacity, and the general increase in unfolded molecules, should further limit the capacity of the aged organism to cope with a mutant protein or other abnormal polypeptides and may thus indirectly contribute to the development of neurodegenerative diseases.

Acknowledgements

This work was made possible by grants from the Hereditary Disease Foundation to MS and from the Hereditary Disease Foundation, ALS foundation, and NIGMS to ALG. We are grateful to Ms. Sarah Trombley for expert assistance in the preparation of this manuscript.

REFERENCES

Amrani, M., Allen, N. J., O'Shea, J. *et al.* (1993). Role of catalase and heat shock protein on recovery of cardiac endothelial and mechanical function after ischemia. *Cardioscience*, **4**, 193–8.

Ananthan, J., Goldberg, A. L. & Voellmy, R. (1986). Abnormal proteins serve as eukaryotic stress signals and trigger the activation of heat shock genes. *Science*, **232**, 522–4.

Anglade, P., Vyas, S., Javoy-Agid, F. *et al.* (1997). Apoptosis and autophagy in nigral neurons of patients with Parkinson's disease. *Histol. Histopathol.*, **12**, 25–31.

Anton, L. C., Schubert, U., Bacik, I. *et al.* (1999). Intracellular localization of proteasomal degradation of a viral antigen. *J. Cell Biol.*, **146**, 113–24.

Aronin, N., Chase, K., Young, C. *et al.* (1995). Cag expansion affects the expression of mutant huntingtin in the huntington's disease brain. *Neuron*, **15**, 1193–201.

Baba, M., Nakajo, S., Tu, P. H. *et al.* (1998). Aggregation of alpha-synuclein in Lewy bodies of sporadic Parkinson's disease and dementia with Lewy bodies. *Am. J. Pathol.*, **152**, 879–84.

Baler, R., Zou, J. & Voellmy, R. (1996). Evidence for a role of Hsp70 in the regulation of the heat shock response in mammalian cells. *Cell Stress Chaperones*, **1**, 33–9.

Bardag-Gorce, F., van Leeuwen, F. W., Nguyen, V. *et al.* (2002). The role of the ubiquitin-proteasome pathway in the formation of mallory bodies. *Exp. Mol. Pathol.*, **73**, 75–83.

Bates, G. P., Mangiarini, L. & Davies, S. W. (1998). Transgenic mice in the study of polyglutamine repeat expansion diseases. *Brain Pathol.*, **8**, 699–714.

Benaroudj, N. & Goldberg, A. L. (2000). PAN, the proteasome-activating nucleotidase from archaebacteria, is a protein-unfolding molecular chaperone. *Nat. Cell Biol.*, **2**, 833–9.

Bence, N. F., Sampat, R. M. & Kopito, R. R. (2001). Impairment of the ubiquitin-proteasome system by protein aggregation. *Science*, **292**, 1552–5.

Bennett, M. C., Bishop, J. F., Leng, Y., Chock, P. B., Chase, T. N. & Mouradian, M. M. (1999). Degradation of alpha-synuclein by proteasome. *J. Biol. Chem.*, **274**, 33855–8.

Bercovich, B., Stancovski, I. & Mayer, A. (1997). Ubiquitin-dependent degradation of certain protein substrates in vitro requires the molecular chaperone Hsc70. *J. Biol. Chem.*, **272**, 9002–10.

Braun, B. C., Glickman, M., Kraft, R. *et al.* (1999). The base of the proteasome regulatory particle exhibits chaperone-like activity. *Nat. Cell Biol.*, **1**, 221–6.

Brown, R. (1998). *Amyotrophic Lateral Sclerosis and the Inherited Motor Neuron Diseases*. New York: Scientific American, Inc.

Bruening, W., Roy, J., Giasson, B., Figlewicz, D. A., Mushynski, W. E. & Durham, H. D. (1999). Up-regulation of protein chaperones preserves viability of cells expressing toxic Cu/Zn-superoxide dismutase mutants associated with amyotrophic lateral sclerosis. *J. Neurochem.*, **72**, 693–9.

Carmichael, J., Chatellier, J., Woolfson, A., Milstein, C., Fersht, A. R. & Rubinsztein, D. C. (2000). Bacterial and yeast chaperones reduce both aggregate formation and cell death in mammalian cell models of Huntington's disease. *Proc. Natl Acad. Sci., USA*, **97**, 9701–5.

Carrard, G., Bulteau, A. L., Petropoulos, I. & Friguet, B. (2002). Impairment of proteasome structure and function in aging. *Int. J. Biochem. Cell Biol.*, **34**, 1461–74.

Cepeda, C., Ariano, M. A., Calvert, C. R. *et al.* (2001). NMDA receptor function in mouse models of Huntington disease. *J. Neurosci. Res.*, **66**, 525–39.

Chai, Y., Koppenhafer, S. L., Bonini, N. M. & Paulson, H. L. (1999a). Analysis of the role of heat shock protein (Hsp) molecular chaperones in polyglutamine disease. *J. Neurosci.*, **19**, 10338–47.

Chai, Y. H., Koppenhafer, S. L., Shoesmith, S. J., Perez, M. K. & Paulson, H. L. (1999b). Evidence for proteasome involvement in polyglutamine disease: localization to nuclear inclusions in SCA3/MJD and suppression of polyglutamine aggregation in vitro. *Hum. Mol. Genet.*, **8**, 673–82.

Chan, H. Y., Warrick, J. M., Gray-Board, G. L., Paulson, H. L. & Bonini, N. M. (2000). Mechanisms of chaperone suppression of polyglutamine disease: selectivity, synergy and modulation of protein solubility in Drosophila. *Hum. Mol. Genet.*, **9**, 2811–20.

Chan, P. H. (1996). Role of oxidants in ischemic brain damage. *Stroke*, **27**, 1124–9.

Chapman, R., Sidrauski, C. & Walter, P. (1998). Intracellular signaling from the endoplasmic reticulum to the nucleus. *Ann. Rev. Cell Dev. Biol.*, **14**, 459–85.

Chiu, D. T. Y. & Liu, T. Z. (1997). Free radical and oxidative damage in human blood cells. *J. Biomedi. Sci.*, **4**, 256–9.

Chow, S. C., Peters, I. & Orrenius, S. (1995). Reevaluation of the role of de novo protein synthesis in rat thymocyte apoptosis. *Exp. Cell Res.*, **216**, 149–59.

Chung, K. K., Dawson, V. L. & Dawson, T. M. (2001a). The role of the ubiquitin-proteasomal pathway in Parkinson's disease and other neurodegenerative disorders. *Trends Neurosci.*, **24**, S7–S14.

Chung, K. K., Zhang, Y., Lim, K. L. *et al.* (2001b). Parkin ubiquitinates the alpha-synuclein-interacting protein, synphilin-1: implications for Lewy-body formation in Parkinson disease. *Nat. Med.*, **7**, 1144–50.

Cleveland, D. W. (1999). From Charcot to SOD1: mechanisms of selective motor neuron death in ALS. *Neuron*, **24**, 515–20.

Cleveland, D. W. & Rothstein, J. D. (2001). From Charcot to Lou Gehrig: deciphering selective motor neuron death in ALS. *Nat. Rev. Neurosci.*, **2**, 806–19.

Cooper, A. J., Sheu, K. F., Burke, J. R. *et al.* (1997). Polyglutamine domains are substrates of tissue transglutaminase: does transglutaminase play a role in expanded CAG/poly-Q neurodegenerative diseases? *J. Neurochem.*, **69**, 431–4.

Cotner, T. & Pious, D. (1995). HLA-DR beta chains enter into an aggregated complex containing GRP-78/BiP prior to their degradation by the pre-Golgi degradative pathway. *J. Biol. Chem.*, **270**, 2379–86.

Coux, O., Tanaka, K. & Goldberg, A. L. (1996). Structure and functions of the 20S and 26S proteasomes. *Ann. Rev. Biochem.*, **65**, 801–47.

Cuervo, A. M. & Dice, J. F. (1996). A receptor for the selective uptake and degradation of proteins by lysosomes. *Science*, **273**, 501–3.

(1998a). How do intracellular proteolytic systems change with age? *Frontiers Biosci.*, **3**, 25–43.

(1998b). Lysosomes, a meeting point of proteins, chaperones, and proteases. *J. Mol. Med.*, **76**, 6–12.

Cummings, C. J., Mancini, M. A., Antalffy, B. DeFranco, D. B., Orr, H. T. & Zoghbi, H. Y. (1998). Chaperone suppression of aggregation and altered subcellular proteasome localization imply protein misfolding in SCA1. *Nat. Genet.*, **19**, 148–54.

Cummings, C. J., Reinstein, E., Sun, Y. *et al.* (1999). Mutation of the E6-AP ubiquitin ligase reduces nuclear inclusion frequency while accelerating polyglutamine-induced pathology in SCA1 mice. *Neuron*, **24**, 879–92.

Cummings, C. J., Sun, Y., Opal, P. *et al.* (2001). Over-expression of inducible HSP70 chaperone suppresses neuropathology and improves motor function in SCA1 mice. *Hum. Mol. Genet.*, **10**, 1511–18.

da Costa, C. A., Ancolio, K. & Checler, F. (1999). C-terminal maturation fragments of presenilin 1 and 2 control secretion of APP alpha and A beta by human cells and are degraded by proteasome. *Mol. Med.*, **5**, 160–8.

Davies, S. W., Turmaine, M., Cozens, B. A. *et al.* (1997). Formation of neuronal intranuclear inclusions underlies the neurological dysfunction in mice transgenic for the Hd mutation. *Cell*, **90**, 537–48.

De Vrij, F. M., Sluijs, J. A., Gregori, L. *et al.* (2001). Mutant ubiquitin expressed in Alzheimer's disease causes neuronal death. *FASEB J.*, **15**, 2680–8.

Diamond, M. I., Robinson, M. R. & Yamamoto, K. R. (2000). Regulation of expanded polyglutamine protein aggregation and nuclear localization by the glucocorticoid receptor. *Proc. Natl Acad. Sci. USA*, **97**, 657–61.

Dice, J. F. (1993). Cellular and molecular mechanisms of aging. *Physiol. Rev.*, **73**, 149–59.

Dubois, M. F., Hovanessian, A. G. & Bensaude, O. (1991). Heat-shock-induced denaturation of proteins. Characterization of the insolubilization of the interferon-induced p68 kinase. *J. Biol. Chem.*, **266**, 9707–11.

Ellerby, L. M., Andrusiak, R. L., Wellington, C. L. *et al.* (1999). Cleavage of atrophin-1 at caspase site aspartic acid 109 modulates cytotoxicity. *J. Biol. Chem.*, **274**, 8730–6.

Faber, P. W., Alter, J. R., MacDonald, M. E. & Hart, A. C. (1999). Polyglutamine-mediated dysfunction and apoptotic death of a *Caenorhabditis elegans* sensory neuron. *Proc. Natl Acad. Sci. USA*, **96**, 179–84.

Fabunmi, R. P., Wigley, W. C., Thomas, P. J. & DeMartino, G. N. (2000). Activity and regulation of the centrosome-associated proteasome. *J. Biol. Chem.*, **275**, 409–13.

Faris, M., Kokot, N., Latinis, K. *et al.* (1998a). The c-jun N-terminal kinase cascade plays a role in stress-induced apoptosis in Jurkat cells by up-regulating fas ligand expression. *J. Immunol.*, **160**, 134–44.

Faris, M., Latinis, K. M., Kempiak, S. J., Koretzky, G. A. & Nel, A. (1998b). Stress-induced fas ligand expression in T cells is mediated through a mek kinase 1-regulated response element in the fas ligand promoter. *Mol. Cell. Biol.*, **18**, 5414–24.

Feder, M. E. & Hofmann, G. E. (1999). Heat-shock proteins, molecular chaperones, and the stress response: evolutionary and ecological physiology. *Ann. Rev. Physiol.*, **61**, 243–82.

Feldman, D. E. & Frydman, J. (2000). Protein folding in vivo: the importance of molecular chaperones. *Curr. Opin. Struct. Biol.*, **10**, 26–33.

Fernandez-Funez, P., Nino-Rosales, M. L., de Gouyon, B. *et al.* (2000). Identification of genes that modify ataxin-1-induced neurodegeneration. *Nature*, **408**, 101–6.

Fewell, S. W., Travers, K. J., Weissman, J. S. & Brodsky, J. L. (2001). The action of molecular chaperones in the early secretory pathway. *Annu. Rev. Genet.*, **35**, 149–91.

Finley, D., Ozkaynak, E. & Varshavsky, A. (1987). The yeast polyubiquitin gene is essential for resistance to high temperatures, starvation, and other stresses. *Cell*, **48**, 1035–46.

Friedlander, R. M. & Yuan, J. Y. (1998). ICE, neuronal apoptosis and neurodegeneration. *Cell Death Differ.*, **5**, 823–31.

Frydman, J. (2001). Folding of newly translated proteins in vivo: the role of molecular chaperones. *Annu. Rev. Biochem.*, **70**, 603–47.

Gabai, V. L., Meriin, A. B., Mosser, D. D., Caron, A. W., Rits, S. Shifrin, V. I. & Sherman, M. Y. (1997). HSP70 prevent activation of stress kinases: a novel pathway of cellular thermotolerance, **272**, 18033–7.

Gabai, V. L., Meriin, A. B., Yaglom, J. A., Volloch, V. Z. & Sherman, M. Y. (1998). Role of Hsp70 in regulation of stress-kinase JNK: implication in apoptosis and aging. *FEBS Lett.*, **438**, 1–4.

Gabai, V. L., Yaglom, J. A., Volloch, V. *et al.* (2000). Hsp72-mediated suppression of c-Jun N-terminal kinase is implicated in development of tolerance to caspase-independent cell death. *Mol. Cell. Biol.*, **20**, 6826–36.

Gabai, V. L., Mabuchi, K., Mosser, D. D. & Sherman, M. Y. (2002). Hsp72 and stress kinase c-jun N-terminal kinase regulate the bid-dependent pathway in tumor necrosis factor-induced apoptosis. *Mol. Cell. Biol.*, **22**, 3415–24.

Gabbita, S. P., Aksenov, M. Y., Lovell, M. A. & Markesbery, W. R. (1999). Decrease in peptide methionine sulfoxide reductase in Alzheimer's disease brain. *J. Neurochem.*, **73**, 1660–6.

Garcia-Mata, R., Bebok, Z., Sorscher, E. J. & Sztul, E. S. (1999). Characterization and dynamics of aggresome formation by a cytosolic GFP-chimera. *J. Cell. Biol.*, **146**, 1239–54.

Gervais, F. G., Singaraja, R., Xanthoudakis, S. *et al.* (2002). Recruitment and activation of caspase-8 by the Huntingtin-interacting protein Hip-1 and a novel partner Hippi. *Nat. Cell. Biol.*, **4**, 95–105.

Giasson, B. I., Duda, J. I., Murray, I. V. *et al.* (2000). Oxidative damage linked to neurodegeneration by selective α-synuclein nitration in syncleinopathy lesions. *Science*, **290**, 285–9.

Glickman, M. H. & Ciechanover, A. (2002). The ubiquitin-proteasome proteolytic pathway: destruction for the sake of construction. *Physiol. Rev.*, **82**, 373–428.

Goff, S. A. & Goldberg, A. L. (1985). Production of abnormal proteins in *E. coli* stimulates transcription of lon and other heat shock genes. *Cell*, **41**, 587–95.

Gragerov, A. I., Martin, E. S., Krupenko, M. A., Kashlev, M. V. & Nikiforov, V. G. (1991). Protein aggregation and inclusion body formation in *Escherichia coli* rpoH mutant defective in heat shock protein induction. *FEBS Lett.*, **291**, 222–4.

Grune, T., Reinheckel, T. & Davies, K. J. (1997). Degradation of oxidized proteins in mammalian cells. *FASEB J.*, **11**, 526–34.

Hass, M. A. & Massaro, D. (1988). Regulation of the synthesis of superoxide dismutases in rat lungs during oxidant and hyperthermic stresses. *J. Biol. Chem.*, **263**, 776–81.

Hayes, S. A. & Dice, J. F. (1996). Roles of molecular chaperones in protein degradation. *J. Cell Biol.*, **132**, 255–8.

Hegde, A. N., Inokuchi, K., Pei, W. *et al.* (1997). Ubiquitin C-terminal hydrolase is an immediate-early gene essential for long-term facilitation in Aplysia. *Cell*, **89**, 115–26.

Helmuth, L. (2001). Cell biology. Protein clumps hijack cell's clearance system. *Science*, **292**, 1467–8.

Hershko, A. & Ciechanover, A. (1998). The ubiquitin system. *Ann. Rev. Biochem.*, **67**, 425–79.

Heydari, A. R., Takahashi, R., Gutsmann, A., You, S. & Richardson, A. (1994). Hsp70 and aging. *Experientia*, **50**, 1092–8.

Heydari, A. R., You, S., Takahashi, R., Gutsmann-Conrad, A., Sarge, K. D. & Richardson, A. (2000). Age-related alterations in the activation of heat shock transcription factor 1 in rat hepatocytes. *Exp. Cell Res.*, **256**, 83–93.

Hideshima, T., Mitsiades, C., Akiyama, M. *et al.* (2002). Molecular mechanisms mediating anti-myeloma activity of proteasome inhibitor PS-341. *Blood*, **26**, 26.

Hoffner, G., Kahlem, P. & Djian, P. (2002). Perinuclear localization of huntingtin as a consequence of its binding to microtubules through an interaction with beta-tubulin: relevance to Huntington's disease. *J. Cell. Sci.*, **115**, 941–8.

Honda, T., Yasutake, K., Nihonmatsu, N. *et al.* (1999). Dual roles of proteasome in the metabolism of presenilin 1. *J. Neurochem.*, **72**, 255–61.

Igarashi, S., Koide, R., Shimohata, T. *et al.* (1998). Suppression of aggregate formation and apoptosis by transglutaminase inhibitors in cells expressing truncated DRPLA protein with an expanded polyglutamine stretch. *Nat. Genet.*, **18**, 111–17.

Ii, K., Ito, H., Tanaka, K. & Hirano, A. (1997). Immunocytochemical co-localization of the proteasome in ubiquitinated structures in neurodegenerative diseases and the elderly. *J. Neuropath. Exp. Neurol.*, **56**, 125–31.

Imai, Y., Soda, M., Hatakeyama, S. *et al.* (2002). CHIP is associated with Parkin, a gene responsible for familial Parkinson's disease, and enhances its ubiquitin ligase activity. *Mol. Cell*, **10**, 55–67.

Imaizumi, K., Katayama, T. & Tohyama, M. (2001). Presenilin and the UPR. *Nat. Cell. Biol.*, **3**, E104.

Jana, N. R., Tanaka, M., Wang, G. & Nukina, N. (2000). Polyglutamine length-dependent interaction of Hsp40 and Hsp70 family chaperones with truncated N-terminal huntingtin: their role in suppression of aggregation and cellular toxicity. *Hum. Mol. Genet.*, **9**, 2009–18.

Jana, N. R., Zemskov, E. A., Wang, G. & Nukina, N. (2001). Altered proteasomal function due to the expression of polyglutamine-expanded truncated N-terminal huntingtin induces apoptosis by caspase activation through mitochondrial cytochrome c release. *Hum. Mol. Genet.*, **10**, 1049–59.

Johnson, J. L. & Craig, E. A. (1997). Protein folding in vivo: unraveling complex pathways. *Cell*, **90**, 201–4.

Johnston, J. A., Ward, C. L. & Kopito, R. R. (1998). Aggresomes: a cellular response to misfolded proteins. *J. Cell Biol.*, **143**, 1883–98.

Johnston, J. A., Dalton, M. J., Gurney, M. E. & Kopito, R. R. (2000). Formation of high molecular weight complexes of mutant cu, Zn-superoxide dismutase in a mouse model for familial amyotrophic lateral sclerosis. *Proc. Natl Acad. Sci. USA*, **97**, 12571–6.

Johnston, J. A., Illing, M. E. & Kopito, R. R. (2002). Cytoplasmic dynein/dynactin mediates the assembly of aggresomes. *Cell Motil. Cytoskeleton*, **53**, 26–38.

Kahlem, P., Green, H. & Djian, P. (1998). Transglutaminase as the agent of neurodegenerative diseases due to polyglutamine expansion. *Pathol. Biol.*, **46**, 681–2.

Kalchman, M. A., Koide, H. B., McCutcheon, K. *et al.* (1997). HIP1, a human homologue of *S. cerevisiae* Sla2p, interacts with membrane-associated huntingtin in the brain. *Nat. Genet.*, **16**, 44–53.

Kampinga, H. H., Brunsting, J. F., Stege, G. J., Burgman, P. W. & Konings, A. W. (1995). Thermal protein denaturation and protein aggregation in cells made thermotolerant by various chemicals: role of heat shock proteins. *Exp. Cell Res.*, **219**, 536–46.

Katayama, T., Imaizumi, K., Sato, N. *et al.* (1999). Presenilin-1 mutations downregulate the signalling pathway of the unfolded-protein response. *Nat. Cell Biol.*, **1**, 479–85.

Katayama, T., Imaizumi, K., Honda, A. *et al.* (2001). Disturbed activation of endoplasmic reticulum stress transducers by familial Alzheimer's disease-linked presenilin-1 mutations. *J. Biol. Chem.*, **276**, 43446–54.

Kawashima, T., Kikuchi, H., Takita, M. *et al.* (1998). Skein-like inclusions in the neostriatum from a case of amyotrophic lateral sclerosis with dementia. *Acta Neuropath.*, **96**, 541–5.

Kazantsev, A., Preisinger, E., Dranovsky, A., Goldgaber, D. & Housman, D. (1999). Insoluble detergent-resistant aggregates form between pathological and nonpathological lengths of polyglutamine in mammalian cells. *Proc. Natl Acad. Sci. USA*, **96**, 11404–9.

Kazemi-Esfarjani, P. & Benzer, S. (2000). Genetic suppression of polyglutamine toxicity in *Drosophila*. *Science*, **287**, 1837–40.

Kegel, K. B., Kim, M., Sapp, E. *et al.* (2000). Huntingtin expression stimulates endosomal-lysosomal activity, endosome tubulation, and autophagy. *J. Neurosci.*, **20**, 7268–78.

Kharbanda, S., Saxena, S., Yoshida, K. *et al.* (2000). Translocation of SAPK/JNK to mitochondria and interaction with Bcl-x(L) in response to DNA damage. *J. Biol. Chem.*, **275**, 322–7.

Kisselev, A. F., Akopian, T. N., Castillo, V. & Goldberg, A. L. (1999a). Proteasome active sites allosterically regulate each other, suggesting a cyclical bite-chew mechanism for protein breakdown. *Mol. Cell*, **4**, 395–402.

Kisselev, A. F., Akopian, T. N., Woo, K. M. & Goldberg, A. L. (1999b). The sizes of peptides generated from protein by mammalian 26 and 20 S proteasomes. Implications for understanding the degradative mechanism and antigen presentation. *J. Biol. Chem.*, **274**, 3363–71.

Kitada, T., Asakawa, S., Hattori, N. *et al.* (1998). Mutations in the parkin gene cause autosomal recessive juvenile parkinsonism [see comments]. *Nature*, **392**, 605–8.

Klement, I. A., Skinner, P. J., Kaytor, M. D. *et al.* (1998). Ataxin-1 nuclear localization and aggregation: role in polyglutamine-induced disease in SCA1 transgenic mice [see comments]. *Cell*, **95**, 41–53.

Klemes, Y., Etlinger, J. D. & Goldberg, A. L. (1981). Properties of abnormal proteins degraded rapidly in reticulocytes. Intracellular aggregation of the globin molecules prior to hydrolysis. *J. Biol. Chem.*, **256**, 8436–44.

Kobayashi, Y., Miwa, S., Merry, D. E. *et al.* (1998). Caspase-3 cleaves the expanded androgen receptor protein of spinal and bulbar muscular atrophy in a polyglutamine repeat length-dependent manner. *Biochem. Biophys. Res. Commun.*, **252**, 145–50.

Kobayashi, Y., Kume, A., Li, M. *et al.* (2000). Chaperones Hsp70 and Hsp40 suppress aggregate formation and apoptosis in cultured neuronal cells expressing truncated androgen receptor protein with expanded polyglutamine tract. *J. Biol. Chem.*, **275**, 8772–8.

Kopito, R. R. (1999). Biosynthesis and degradation of CFTR. *Physiol. Rev.*, **79**, S167–73.

Kuan, C. Y., Yang, D. D., Roy, D. R. S., Davis, R. J., Rakic, P. & Flavell, R. A. (1999). The Jnk1 and Jnk2 protein kinases are required for regional specific apoptosis during early brain development. *Neuron*, **22**, 667–76.

Kuschel, L., Hansel, A., Schoherr, R. *et al.* (1999). Molecular cloning and functional expression of a human peptide methionine sulfoxide reductase (hMsrA). *FEBS Lett.*, **456**, 17–21.

Lathrop, R. H., Casale, M., Tobias, D. J., Marsh, J. L. & Thompson, L. M. (1998). Modeling protein homopolymeric repeats: possible polyglutamine structural motifs for Huntington's disease. *Proc. Int. Conf. Intell. Syst. Mol. Biol.*, **6**, 105–14.

Lee, D. H., Sherman, M. Y. & Goldberg, A. L. (1996a). Involvement of the molecular chaperone Ydj1 in the ubiquitin-dependent degradation of short-lived and abnormal proteins in *Saccharomyces cerevisiae*. *Mol. Cell. Biol.*, **16**, 4773–81.

Lee, H. J., Shin, S. Y., Choi, C., Lee, Y. H. & Lee, S. J. (2002). Formation and removal of alpha-synuclein aggregates in cells exposed to mitochondrial inhibitors. *J. Biol. Chem.*, **277**, 5411–17.

Lee, Y. K., Manalo, D. & Liu, A. Y. (1996b). Heat shock response, heat shock transcription factor and cell aging. *Biol. Signals*, **5**, 180–91.

Leroy, E., Boyer, R., Auburger, G. *et al.* (1998). The ubiquitin pathway in Parkinson's disease [letter]. *Nature*, **395**, 451–2.

Li, M. W., Ona, V. O., Guegan, C. *et al.* (2000). Functional role of caspase-1 and caspase-3 in an ALS transgenic mouse model. *Science*, **288**, 335–9.

Liberek, K., Galitski, T. P., Zylicz, M. & Georgopoulos, C. (1992). The DnaK chaperone modulates the heat shock response of *Escherichia coli* by binding to the sigma 32 transcription factor. *Proc. Natl Acad. Sci., USA*, **89**, 3516–20.

Lindsten, K., de Vrij, F. M., Verhoef, L. G. *et al.* (2002). Mutant ubiquitin found in neurodegenerative disorders is a ubiquitin fusion degradation substrate that blocks proteasomal degradation. *J. Cell Biol.*, **157**, 417–27.

Liu, Y., Fallon, L., Lashuel, H. A., Liu, Z. & Lansbury, P. T., Jr. (2002). The UCH-L1 gene encodes two opposing enzymatic activities that affect alpha-synuclein degradation and Parkinson's disease susceptibility. *Cell*, **111**, 209–18.

Liu, Y. F. (1998). Expression of polyglutamine-expanded Huntingtin activates the SEK1-JNK pathway and induces apoptosis in a hippocampal neuronal cell line. *J. Biol. Chem.*, **273**, 28873–7.

Locke, M. & Tanguay, R. M. (1996). Diminished heat shock response in the aged myocardium. *Cell Stress Chaperones*, **1**, 251–60.

Ma, J., Wollmann, R. & Lindquist, S. (2002). Neurotoxicity and neurodegeneration when PrP accumulates in the cytosol. *Science*, **298**, 1781–5.

Martin-Aparicio, E., Yamamoto, A., Hernandez, F., Hen, R., Avila, J. & Lucas, J. J. (2001). Proteasomal-dependent aggregate reversal and absence of cell death in a conditional mouse model of Huntington's disease. *J. Neurosci.*, **21**, 8772–81.

Martindale, D., Hackam, A., Wieczorek, A. *et al.* (1998). Length of huntingtin and its polyglutamine tract influences localization and frequency of intracellular aggregates. *Nat. Genet.*, **18**, 150–4.

Masaki, R., Saito, T., Yamada, K. & Ohtani-Kaneko, R. (2000). Accumulation of phosphorylated neurofilaments and increase in apoptosis-specific protein and phosphorylated c-Jun induced by proteasome inhibitors. *J. Neurosci. Res.*, **62**, 75–83.

Masliah, E., Rockenstein, E., Veinbergs, I. *et al.* (2000). Dopaminergic loss and inclusion body formation in alpha-synuclein mice: implications for neurodegenerative disorders. *Science*, **287**, 1265–9.

Massa, S. M., Swanson, R. A. & Sharp, F. R. (1996). The stress gene response in brain. *Cerebrovasc. Brain Metab. Rev.*, **8**, 95–158.

Mayer, R. J., Tipler, C., Arnold, J. *et al.* (1996). Endosome-lysosomes, ubiquitin and neurodegeneration. *Adv. Exp. Medi. Biol.*, **389**, 261–9.

McNaught, K. S. & Jenner, P. (2001). Proteasomal function is impaired in substantia nigra in Parkinson's disease. *Neurosci. Lett.*, **297**, 191–4.

McNaught, K. S., Olanow, C. W., Halliwell, B., Isacson, O. & Jenner, P. (2001). Failure of the ubiquitin-proteasome system in Parkinson's disease. *Nat. Rev. Neurosci.*, **2**, 589–94.

McNaught, K. S., Mytilineou, C., Jnobaptiste, R. *et al.* (2002). Impairment of the ubiquitin-proteasome system causes dopaminergic cell death and inclusion body formation in ventral mesencephalic cultures. *J. Neurochem.*, **81**, 301–6.

Meacham, G. C., Patterson, C., Zhang, W., Younger, J. M. & Cyr, D. M. (2001). The Hsc70 co-chaperone CHIP targets immature CFTR for proteasomal degradation. *Nat. Cell Biol.*, **3**, 100–5.

Meriin, A., Gabai, V., Yaglom, J., Shifrin, V. & Sherman, M. (1998). Proteasome inhibitors activate stress-kinases and induce Hsp72: diverse effects on apoptosis. *J. Biol. Chem.*, **273**, 6373–9.

Meriin, A. B., Mabuchi, K., Gabai, V. L., Yaglom, J. A., Kazantsev, A. & Sherman, M. Y. (2001). Intracellular aggregation of polypeptides with expanded polyglutamine domain is stimulated by stress-activated kinase MEKK1. *J. Cell Biol.*, **153**, 851–64.

Meriin, A. B., Zhang, X., He, X., Newnam, G. P., Chernoff, Y. O. & Sherman, M. Y. (2002). Huntington toxicity in yeast model depends on polyglutamine aggregation mediated by a prion-like protein Rnq1. *J. Cell Biol.*, **157**, 997–1004.

Mezey, E., Dehejia, A., Harta, G., Papp, M. I., Polymeropoulos, M. H. & Brownstein, M. J. (1998). Alpha synuclein in neurodegenerative disorders – murderer or accomplice. *Nat. Med.*, **4**, 755–7.

Mitch, W. E. & Goldberg, A. L. (1996). Mechanisms of muscle wasting. The role of the ubiquitin-proteasome pathway. *N. Engl. J. Med.*, **335**, 1897–905.

Miyashita, T., Matsui, J., Ohtsuka, Y. *et al.* (1999). Expression of extended polyglutamine sequentially activates initiator and effector caspases. *Biochem. Biophys. Res. Commun.*, **257**, 724–30.

Mizuno, Y., Hattori, N., Mori, H., Suzuki, T. & Tanaka, K. (2001). Parkin and Parkinson's disease. *Curr. Opin. Neurol.*, **14**, 477–82.

Morley, J. F., Brignull, H. R., Weyers, J. J. & Morimoto, R. I. (2002). The threshold for polyglutamine-expansion protein aggregation and cellular toxicity is dynamic and influenced by aging in

Caenorhabditis elegans. Proc. Natl Acad. Sci. USA, **99**, 10417–22.

Moskovitz, J., Flescher, E., Berlett, B. S., Azare, J., Poston, J. M. & Stadtman, E. R. (1998). Overexpression of peptide-methionine sulfoxide reductase in *saccharomyces cerevisiae* and human T cells provides them with high resistance to oxidative stress. *Proc. Natl Acad. Sci. USA*, **95**, 14071–5.

Moskovitz, J., Jenkins, N. A., Gilbert, D. J. *et al.* (1996). Chromosomal localization of the mammalian peptide-methionine sulfoxide reductase gene and its differential expression in various tissues. *Proc. Natl Acad. Sci. USA*, **93**, 3205–8.

Mosser, D. D. & Martin, L. H. (1992). Induced thermotolerance to apoptosis in a human T lymphocyte cell line. *J. Cell. Physiol.*, **151**, 561–70.

Mosser, D. D., Caron, A. W., Bourget, L., Denis-Larose, C. & Massie, B. (1997). Role of the human heat shock protein hsp70 in protection against stress-induced apoptosis. *Mol. Cell. Biol.*, **17**, 5317–27.

Mrak, R. E., Griffin, W. S. T. & Graham, D. I. (1997). Aging-associated changes in human brain. *J. Neuropath. Exp. Neurol.*, **56**, 1269–75.

Muchowski, P. J., Schaffar, G., Sittler, A. Wanker, E. E., Hayer-Hartl, M. K. & Hartl, F. U. (2000). Hsp70 and Hsp40 chaperones can inhibit self-assembly of polyglutamine proteins into amyloid-like fibrils. *Proc. Natl Acad. Sci. USA*, **97**, 7841–6.

Muchowski, P. J., Ning, K., D'Souza-Schorey, C. & Fields, S. (2002). Requirement of an intact microtubule cytoskeleton for aggregation and inclusion body formation by a mutant huntingtin fragment. *Proc. Natl Acad. Sci. USA*, **99**, 727–32.

Muramatsu, T., Hatoko, M., Tada, H., Shirai, T. & Ohnishi, T. (1996). Age-related decrease in the inductability of heat shock protein 72 in normal human skin. *Br. J. Dermatol.*, **134**, 1035–8.

Murata, S., Minami, Y., Minami, M., Chiba, T. & Tanaka, K. (2001). CHIP is a chaperone-dependent E3 ligase that ubiquitylates unfolded protein. *EMBO Rep*, **2**, 1133–8.

Navon, A. & Goldberg, A. L. (2001). Proteins are unfolded on the surface of the ATPase ring before transport into the proteasome. *Mol. Cell*, **8**, 1339–49.

Nucifora, F. C., Jr., Sasaki, M., Peters, M. F. *et al.* (2001). Interference by huntingtin and atrophin-1 with cbp-mediated transcription leading to cellular toxicity. *Science*, **291**, 2423–8.

Ohba, M. (1997). Modulation of intracellular protein degradation by SSB1-SIS1 chaperon system in yeast *S. cerevisiae. FEBS Lett.*, **409**, 307–11.

Ona, V. O., Li, M., Vonsattel, J. P. *et al.* (1999). Inhibition of caspase-1 slows disease progression in a mouse model of Huntington's disease [see comments]. *Nature*, **399**, 263–7.

Paxinou, E., Chen, Q., Weisse, M. *et al.* (2001). Induction of alpha-synuclein aggregation by intracellular nitrative insult. *J. Neurosci.*, **21**, 8053–61.

Peters, P. J., Ning, K., Palacios, F. *et al.* (2002). Arfaptin 2 regulates the aggregation of mutant huntingtin protein. *Nat. Cell Biol.*, **4**, 240–5.

Petersen, A., Larsen, K. E., Behr, G. G. *et al.* (2001). Expanded CAG repeats in exon 1 of the Huntington's disease gene stimulate dopamine-mediated striatal neuron autophagy and degeneration. *Hum. Mol. Genet.*, **10**, 1243–54.

Polymeropoulos, M. H., Lavedan, C., Leroy, E. *et al.* (1997). Mutation in the alpha-synuclein gene identified in families with Parkinson's disease [see comments]. *Science*, **276**, 2045–7.

Preisinger, E., Jordan, B. M., Kazantsev, A. & Housman, D. (1999). Evidence for a recruitment and sequestration mechanism in Huntington's disease. *Phil. Trans. Roy. Soc. Lond. B. Biol. Sci.*, **354**, 1029–34.

Prouty, W. F., Karnovsky, M. J. & Goldberg, A. L. (1975). Degradation of abnormal proteins in *Escherichia coli*. Formation of protein inclusions in cells exposed to amino acid analogs. *J. Biol. Chem.*, **250**, 1112–22.

Rattan, S. I. & Derventzi, A. (1991). Altered cellular responsiveness during ageing. *Bioessays*, **13**, 601–6.

Ravikumar, B., Duden, R. & Rubinsztein, D. C. (2002). Aggregate-prone proteins with polyglutamine and polyalanine expansions are degraded by autophagy. *Hum. Mol. Genet.*, **11**, 1107–17.

Rock, K. L., Gramm, C., Rothstein, L. *et al.* (1994). Inhibitors of the proteasome block the degradation of most cell proteins and the generation of peptides presented on MHC class I molecules. *Cell*, **78**, 761–71.

Saigoh, K., Wang, Y. L., Suh, T. G. *et al.* (1999). Intragenic deletion in the gene encoding ubiquitin carboxy-terminal hydrolase in gad mice. *Nat. Genet.*, **23**, 47–51.

Samali, A. & Orrenius, S. (1998). Heat shock proteins: regulators of stress response and apoptosis. *Cell Stress Chaperones*, **3**, 228–36.

Sanchez, I., Xu, C. J., Juo, P., Kakizaka, A., Blenis, J. & Yuan, J. (1999). Caspase-8 is required for cell death induced by expanded polyglutamine repeats [see comments]. *Neuron*, **22**, 623–33.

Sastre, J., Pallardo, F. V. & Vina, J. (1996). Glutathione, oxidative stress and aging. *Age*, **19**, 129–39.

Sathasivam, K., Woodman, B., Mahal, A. *et al.* (2001). Centrosome disorganization in fibroblast cultures derived from R6/2 Huntington's disease (HD) transgenic mice and HD patients. *Hum. Mol. Genet.*, **10**, 2425–35.

Satyal, S. H., Schmidt, E., Kitagawa, K. *et al.* (2000). Polyglutamine aggregates alter protein folding homeostasis in *Caenorhabditis elegans*. *Proc. Natl Acad. Sci. USA*, **97**, 5750–5.

Saudou, F., Finkbeiner, S., Devys, D. & Greenberg, M. E. (1998). Huntingtin acts in the nucleus to induce apoptosis but death does not correlate with the formation of intranuclear inclusions. *Cell*, **95**, 55–66.

Schubert, U., Anton, L. C., Gibbs, J., Norbury, C. C., Yewdell, J. W. & Bennink, J. R. (2000). Rapid degradation of a large fraction of newly synthesized proteins by proteasomes. *Nature*, **404**, 770–4.

Schwartz, A. L. & Ciechanover, A. (1999). The ubiquitin-proteasome pathway and pathogenesis of human diseases. *Annu. Rev. Med.*, **50**, 57–74.

Sekhar, K. R., Soltaninassab, S. R., Borrelli, M. J. *et al.* (2000). Inhibition of the 26S proteasome induces expression of GLCLC,

the catalytic subunit for gamma-glutamylcysteine synthetase. *Biochem. Biophys. Res. Commun.*, **270**, 311–17.

Seufert, W. & Jentsch, S. (1990). Ubiquitin-conjugating enzymes UBC4 and UBC5 mediate selective degradation of short-lived and abnormal proteins. *EMBO J.*, **9**, 543–50.

Shang, F., Gong, X., Palmer, H. J., Nowell, T. R., Jr. & Taylor, A. (1997). Age-related decline in ubiquitin conjugation in response to oxidative stress in the lens. *Exp. Eye Res.*, **64**, 21–30.

Sherman, M. & Goldberg, A. L. (1996). Involvement of molecular chaperones in intracellular protein breakdown. In *Stress-inducible Cellular Responses*, ed. U. Feige, R. I. Morimoto, I. Yahara, B. S. Polla, Basel: Birkhauser Verlag, pp. 57–78.

Shi, Y., Mosser, D. D. & Morimoto, R. I. (1998). Molecular chaperones as HSF1-specific transcriptional repressors. *Genes Dev.*, **12**, 654–66.

Shibata, N., Hirano, A., Kato, S. *et al.* (1999). Advanced glycation endproducts are deposited in neuronal hyaline inclusions: a study on familial amyotrophic lateral sclerosis with superoxide dismutase-1 mutation. *Acta Neuropath.*, **97**, 240–6.

Shimohata, T., Sato, A., Burke, J. R., Strittmatter, W. J., Tsuji, S. & Onodera, O. (2002). Expanded polyglutamine stretches form an 'aggresome'. *Neurosci. Lett.*, **323**, 215–18.

Shimura, H., Hattori, N., Kubo, S. *et al.* (2000). Familial Parkinson disease gene product, parkin, is a ubiquitin-protein ligase. *Nat. Genet.*, **25**, 302–5.

Shimura, H., Schlossmacher, M. G., Hattori, N. *et al.* (2001). Ubiquitination of a new form of alpha-synuclein by parkin from human brain: implications for Parkinson's disease. *Science*, **293**, 263–9.

Shringarpure, R. & Davies, K. J. (2002). Protein turnover by the proteasome in aging and disease. *Free Radic. Biol. Med.*, **32**, 1084–9.

Soltaninassab, S. R., Sekhar, K. R., Meredith, M. J. & Freeman, M. L. (2000). Multi-faceted regulation of gamma-glutamylcysteine synthetase. *J. Cell Physiol.*, **182**, 163–70.

Sommer, T. & Seufert, W. (1992). Genetic analysis of ubiquitin-dependent protein degradation. *Experientia*, **48**, 172–8.

Sondheimer, N. & Lindquist, S. (2000). Rnq1: an epigenetic modifier of protein function in yeast. *Mol. Cell*, **5**, 163–72.

Sondheimer, N., Lopez, N., Craig, E. A. & Lindquist, S. (2001). The role of Sis1 in the maintenance of the [RNQ+] prion. *EMBO J.*, **20**, 2435–42.

Spillantini, M. G., Crowther, R. A., Jakes, R., Hasegawa, M. & Goedert, M. (1998). alpha-Synuclein in filamentous inclusions of Lewy bodies from Parkinson's disease and dementia with lewy bodies. *Proc. Natl Acad. Sci. USA*, **95**, 6469–73.

Srivastava, R. K., Mi, Q.-S., Hardwick, J. M. & Longo, D. L. (1999). Deletion of the loop region of Bcl-2 completely blocks paclitaxel-induced apoptosis. *Proc. Natl Acad. Sci. USA*, **96**, 3775–80.

Stefanis, L., Larsen, K. E., Rideout, H. J., Sulzer, D. & Greene, L. A. (2001). Expression of A53T mutant but not wild-type alpha-synuclein in PC12 cells induces alterations of the ubiquitin-dependent degradation system, loss of dopamine release, and autophagic cell death. *J. Neurosci.*, **21**, 9549–60.

Steffan, J. S., Kazantsev, A., Spasic-Boskovic, O. *et al.* (2000). The Huntington's disease protein interacts with p53 and CREB-binding protein and represses transcription. *Proc. Natl Acad. Sci. USA*, **97**, 6763–8.

Steffan, J. S., Bodai, L., Pallos, J. *et al.* (2001). Histone deacetylase inhibitors arrest polyglutamine-dependent neurodegeneration in *Drosophila. Nature*, **413**, 739–43.

Steiner, H., Capell, A., Pesold, B. *et al.* (1998). Expression of Alzheimer's disease-associated presenilin-1 is controlled by proteolytic degradation and complex formation. *J. Biol. Chem.*, **273**, 32322–31.

Strickland, E., Hakala, K., Thomas, P. J. & DeMartino, G. N. (2000). Recognition of misfolding proteins by PA700, the regulatory subcomplex of the 26 S proteasome. *J. Biol. Chem.*, **275**, 5565–72.

Subramaniam, J. R., Lyons, W. E., Liu, J. *et al.* (2002). Mutant SOD1 causes motor neuron disease independent of copper chaperone-mediated copper loading. *Nat. Neurosci.*, **5**, 301–7.

Sugita, M., Morita, T. & Yonesaki, T. (1995). Puromycin induces apoptosis of developing chick sympathetic neurons in a similar manner to NGF-deprivation. *Zool. Sci.*, **12**, 419–25.

Szweda, P. A., Friguet, B. & Szweda, L. I. (2002). Proteolysis, free radicals, and aging. *Free Radic. Biol. Med.*, **33**, 29–36.

Takahashi, J., Fujigasaki, H., Zander, C. *et al.* (2002). Two populations of neuronal intranuclear inclusions in SCA7 differ in size and promyelocytic leukaemia protein content. *Brain*, **125**, 1534–43.

Takeda, A., Mallory, M., Sundsmo, M., Honer, W., Hansen, L. & Masliah, E. (1998). Abnormal accumulation of NACP/alpha-synuclein in neurodegenerative disorders. *Am. J. Path.*, **152**, 367–72.

Tanaka, K., Suzuki, T. & Chiba, T. (1998). The ligation systems for ubiquitin and ubiquitin-like proteins. *Mol. Cell*, **8**, 503–12.

Tanaka, Y., Engelender, S., Igarashi, S. *et al.* (2001). Inducible expression of mutant alpha-synuclein decreases proteasome activity and increases sensitivity to mitochondria-dependent apoptosis. *Hum. Mol. Genet.*, **10**, 919–26.

Tarcsa, E., Szymanska, G., Lecker, S., O'Connor, C. M. & Goldberg, A. L. (2000). Ca^{2+}-free calmodulin and calmodulin damaged by in vitro aging are selectively degraded by 26 S proteasomes without ubiquitination. *J. Biol. Chem.*, **275**, 20295–301.

Tatzelt, J., Zuo, J. R., Voellmy, R. *et al.* (1995). Scrapie prions selectively modify the stress response in neuroblastoma cells. *Proc. Natl Acad. Sci. USA*, **92**, 2944–8.

Telenius, H., Kremer, B. & Goldberg, Y. P. (1994). Somatic and gonadal mosaicism of the huntington disease gene cag repeat in brain and sperm. *Nat. Genet.*, **6**, 409–14.

Tournier, C., Hess, P., Yang, D. D. *et al.* (2000). Requirement of JNK for stress-induced activation of the cytochrome c-mediated death pathway. *Science*, **288**, 870–4.

Tsai, B., Ye, Y. & Rapoport, T. A. (2002). Retro-translocation of proteins from the endoplasmic reticulum into the cytosol. *Nat. Rev. Mol. Cell. Biol.*, **3**, 246–55.

Tu, P. H., Gurney, M. E., Julien, J. P., Lee, V. M. & Trojanowski, J. Q. (1997). Oxidative stress, mutant SOD1, and neurofilament pathology in transgenic mouse models of human motor neuron disease [published erratum appears in *Lab. Invest.* 1997 Jun;76(6): following table of contents]. *Lab. Invest.*, **76**, 441–56.

Urushitani, M., Miyashita, T., Ohtsuka, Y., Okamura-Oho, Y., Shikama, Y. & Yamada, M. (2001). Extended polyglutamine selectively interacts with caspase-8 and -10 in nuclear aggregates. *Cell Death Differ.*, **8**, 377–86.

Urushitani, M., Kurisu, J., Tsukita, K. & Takahashi, R. (2002). Proteasomal inhibition by misfolded mutant superoxide dismutase 1 induces selective motor neuron death in familial amyotrophic lateral sclerosis. *J. Neurochem.*, **83**, 1030–42.

van Leewen, F. W., de Kleijn, D. P., van den Hurk, H. H. *et al.* (1998). Frameshift mutants of beta amyloid precursor protein and ubiquitin-B in Alzheimer's and Down patients. *Science*, **279**, 242–7.

van Leeuwen, F. W., Fischer, D. F., Benne, R. & Hol, E. M. (2000). Molecular misreading. A new type of transcript mutation in gerontology. *Ann. NY Acad. Sci.*, **908**, 267–81.

van Leeuwen, F. W., Gerez, L., Benne, R. & Hol, E. M. (2002). +1 Proteins and aging. *Int. J. Biochem. Cell Biol.*, **34**, 1502–5.

Vidair, C. A., Huang, R. N. & Doxsey, S. J. (1999). Heat shock causes protein aggregation and reduced protein solubility at the centrosome and other cytoplasmic locations. *Int. J. Hyperthermia*, **12**, 681–95.

Voellmy, R. (1996). Sensing stress and responding to stress. In *stress-inducible Cellular Responses*, ed. U. Feige, I. Morimoto, I. Yahara & B. Polla. Basel: Birkhauser Verlag, pp. 121–37.

Waelter, S., Boeddrich, A., Lurz, R. *et al.* (2001). Accumulation of mutant huntingtin fragments in aggresome-like inclusion bodies as a result of insufficient protein degradation. *Mol. Biol. Cell.*, **12**, 1393–407.

Wang, G. H., Mitsui, K., Kotliarova, S. *et al.* (1999). Caspase activation during apoptotic cell death induced by expanded polyglutamine in N2a cells. *NeuroReport*, **10**, 2435–8.

Warrick, J. M., Chan, H. Y., Gray-Board, G. L., Chai, Y., Paulson, H. L. & Bonini, N. M. (1999). Suppression of polyglutamine-mediated neurodegeneration in *Drosophila* by the molecular chaperone HSP70. *Nat. Genet.*, **23**, 425–8.

Watt, R. & Piper, P. W. (1997). UBI4, the polyubiquitin gene of *Saccharomyces cerevisiae*, is a heat shock gene that is also subject to catabolite derepression control. *Mol. Gen. Genet.*, **253**, 439–47.

Welihinda, A. A., Tirasophon, W. & Kaufman, R. J. (1999). The cellular response to protein misfolding in the endoplasmic reticulum. *Gene Expression*, **7**, 293–300.

Wellington, C. L., Brinkman, R. R., Okusky, J. R. & Hayden, M. R. (1997). Toward understanding the molecular pathology of huntingtons disease. *Brain Path.*, **7**, 979–1002.

Wellington, C. L., Ellerby, L. M., Hackam, A. S. *et al.* (1998). Caspase cleavage of gene products associated with triplet expansion disorders generates truncated fragments containing the polyglutamine tract. *J. Biol. Chem.*, **273**, 9158–67.

Wickner, R. B., Edskes, H. K., Roberts, B. T., Pierce, M. M., Baxa, U. & Ross, E. (2001). Prions beget prions: the [PIN+] mystery! *Trends Biochem. Sci.*, **26**, 697–9.

Wigley, W. C., Fabunmi, R. P., Lee, M. G. *et al.* (1999). Dynamic association of proteasomal machinery with the centrosome. *J. Cell Biol.*, **145**, 481–90.

Wojcik, C., Schroeter, D., Wilk, S., Lamprecht, J. & Paweletz, N. (1996). Ubiquitin-mediated proteolysis centers in hela cells – indication from studies of an inhibitor of the chymotrypsin-like activity of the proteasome. *Euro. J. Cell Biol.*, **71**, 311–18.

Wyttenbach, A., Carmichael, J., Swartz, J. *et al.* (2000). Effects of heat shock, heat shock protein 40 (HDJ-2), and proteasome inhibition on protein aggregation in cellular models of Huntington's disease. *Proc. Natl Acad. Sci. USA*, **97**, 2898–903.

Xi, L., Tekin, D., Bhargava, P. & Kukreja, R. C. (2001). Whole body hyperthermia and preconditioning of the heart: basic concepts, complexity, and potential mechanisms. *Int. J. Hyperthermia*, **17**, 439–55.

Xiong, X., Chong, E. & Skach, W. R. (1999). Evidence that endoplasmic reticulum (ER)-associated degradation of cystic fibrosis transmembrane conductance regulator is linked to retrograde translocation from the ER membrane. *J. Biol. Chem.*, **274**, 2616–24.

Yamamoto, A., Lucas, J. J. & Hen, R. (2000). Reversal of neuropathology and motor dysfunction in a conditional model of Huntington's disease. *Cell*, **101**, 57–66.

Yamashita, N., Hoshida, S., Taniguchi, N., Kuzuya, T. & Hori, M. (1998). Whole-body hyperthermia provides biphasic cardioprotection against ischemia/reperfusion injury in the rat. *Circulation*, **98**, 1414–21.

Yang, D. D., Kuan, C. Y., Whitmarsh, A. J. *et al.* (1997). Absence of excitotoxicity-induced apoptosis in the hippocampus of mice lacking the Jnk3 gene. *Nature*, **389**, 865–70.

Yasuda, S., Inoue, K., Hirabayashi, M. *et al.* (1999). Triggering of neuronal cell death by accumulation of activated SEK1 on nuclear polyglutamine aggregations in PML bodies. *Genes to Cells*, **4**, 743–56.

Young, A. (1998). *Huntington's Disease and other Trinucleotide Repeat Disorders.* New York: Scientific American, Inc.

Zeron, M. M., Chen, N., Moshaver, A. *et al.* (2001). Mutant huntingtin enhances excitotoxic cell death. *Mol. Cell. Neurosci.*, **17**, 41–53.

Zeron, M. M., Hansson, O., Chen, N. *et al.* (2002). Increased sensitivity to *N*-methyl-D-aspartate receptor-mediated excitotoxicity in a mouse model of Huntington's disease. *Neuron*, **33**, 849–60.

Zhang, Y., Nijbroek, G., Sullivan, M. L. *et al.* (2001). Hsp70 molecular chaperone facilitates endoplasmic reticulum-associated protein degradation of cystic fibrosis transmembrane conductance regulator in yeast. *Mol. Biol. Cell*, **12**, 1303–14.

Zhou, H., Li, S. H. & Li, X. J. (2001). Chaperone suppression of cellular toxicity of huntingtin is independent of polyglutamine aggregation. *J. Biol. Chem.*, **276**, 48417–24.

Zou, J. Y., Guo, Y. L., Guettouche, T., Smith, D. F. & Voellmy, R. (1998). Repression of heat shock transcription factor Hsf1 activation by Hsp90 (Hsp90 complex) that forms a stress-sensitive complex with Hsf1. *Cell*, **94**, 471–80.

10

Neurodegenerative disease and the repair of oxidatively damaged DNA

Marcus S. Cooke

Departments of Cancer Studies and Genetics
University of Leicester, Leicester Royal Infirmary, UK

Free radicals and oxidative damage to DNA

In addition to endogenous sources of free radicals, such as those derived from normal metabolism (see Chapter 1), pathophysiological or environmental events may also generate free radicals. Cellular biomolecules, including nucleic acids, proteins and lipids are all targets for these damaging species. Reactive oxygen species (ROS) are of particular interest. Enzymic and non-enzymic antioxidants (discussed in Chapter 2) contribute to the limit on the extent to which ROS are produced, and hence their interaction with cellular components. If the balance between the anti- and pro-oxidant factors is altered in favour of the latter, a condition of oxidative stress arises, with a concomitant increase in biomolecule modification. Given its central role in cellular events, modification of DNA, for example 8-hydroxyguanine (8-OH-Gua), and thymine glycol (Tg), has been the subject of intense study. Such lesions may have a plethora of effects, most notably mutation, but also replicative block, deletions, microsatellite instability and loss of heterozygosity, as well as various epigenetic effects (for review see Cooke et al., 2003). Furthermore, a great deal of literature exists that describes elevated levels of lesions in a variety of diseases, suggesting that the induction of damage is an important event in pathogenesis (for review, see Cooke et al., 2003). Unlike oxidatively modified lipids and proteins, which may be removed and replaced as part of normal turnover, DNA needs to be repaired, and intense study has revealed much about the processes that maintain genome integrity.

Maintenance of genome integrity

In terms of repair, it may be viewed that genome integrity is maintained via two approaches: (i) the prevention of incorporation of oxidatively modified deoxynucleotide triphosphates into nuclear and mitochondrial genomes, and (ii) removal of oxidative lesions, formed in situ, from nuclear and mitochondrial DNA. By far the most studied oxidative DNA lesion is 8-OH-Gua, and consequently the remainder of the chapter will focus principally upon this lesion. It may be implied, although not taken for granted, that similar principles apply for other lesions.

Prevention of incorporation

Free deoxynucleotides have a greater propensity for oxidation compared with base-paired deoxynucleotides in DNA (Mo et al., 1992). Furthermore, mitochondrial sources of deoxynucleotides are larger than nuclear sources (mitochondria: 18.0 pmol dGTP/μg DNA vs nuclear: 8.0 pmol dGTP/μg DNA; Bestwick et al., 1982). Taken together, these would suggest an imperative for preventing modified DNA precursors being incorporated into the genome. The best characterized enzyme which performs such a role is 8-hydroxy-2′-deoxyguanosine triphosphatase (8-oxodGTPase; Bialkowski & Kasprzak, 1998), hydrolysing 8-oxodGTP to 8-oxodGMP (Fig. 10.1). Further processing, perhaps by 5′(3′)-nucleotidases, may give rise to the deoxynucleoside form of this lesion, 8-hydroxy-2′-deoxyguanosine (8-OH-dG), which can be excreted (Cooke et al., 2000).

Removal of oxidative lesions from DNA

Numerous repair systems, with overlapping substrate specificities, ensure that a failure in one enzyme does not render a lesion irreparable. Broadly speaking, these multiple pathways can be divided into base excision repair (BER) and nucleotide excision repair (NER) and are targeted towards global genome repair (GGR) and repair

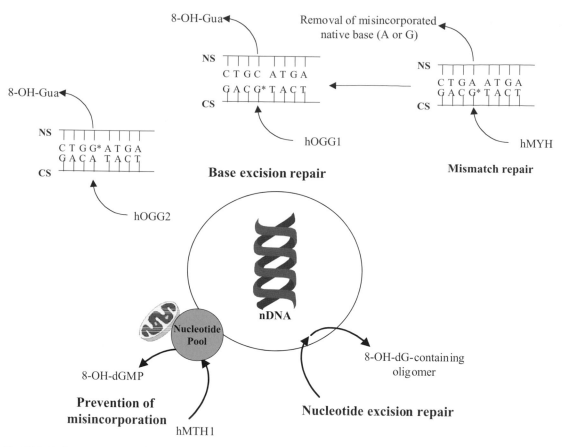

Fig. 10.1 Pathways to prevent the persistence of oxidatively damaged DNA, using 8-hydroxyguanine (8-OH-Gua) as a representative lesion. CS, coding strand; NS, nascent strand.

of actively transcribed regions (via transcription-coupled repair, TCR).

Base excision repair

The prevailing understanding is that, quantitatively, BER is by far the most important route for the removal of the majority of oxidative lesions. At its simplest, this process involves a specific enzyme, with a defined repertoire of substrate, removing the modified base, leaving an apurinic-apyrimidinic (AP) site. The subsequent fate of this AP site is proposed to be dependent upon whether the glycosylase also possesses an AP lyase activity, and may involve simply the removal of one nucleotide (short patch repair), or 2–6 nucleotides (long patch repair; Fortini *et al.*, 1999), followed by gap filling and ligation.

The glycosylase considered to have the primary responsibility for the removal of 8-OH-Gua in human cells, is the human 8-OH-Gua glycosylase (hOGG1; Arai *et al.*, 1997, Rosenquist *et al.*, 1997). This enzyme acts via short patch repair, and has a specificity for 8-OH-Gua: C pairs present in double-stranded DNA, i.e. formed *in situ* (Fig. 10.1). The hOGG1 characterisation studies revealed two isoforms, designated α- and β-hOGG1, which exhibited specificity for subcellular localization to the nucleus and mitochondrial inner membrane, respectively (Croteau *et al.*, 1997, Nishioka *et al.*, 1999). The activity of hOGG1 is complemented by another enzyme, denoted hOGG2, which removes the 8-OH-Gua from the nascent strand in 8-OH-Gua: A or 8-OH-Gua: G pairs, arising from misincorporation of 8-OH-dGTP (Nishioka *et al.*, 1999; Fig. 10.1). Similarly, 8-OH-Gua: A and 8-OH-Gua: G mispairs may arise from misincorporation of A or G opposite 8-OH-Gua in the coding strand. In this case, the unmodified base in the nascent strand is removed by mismatch repair, involving the human homologue of *Escherichia coli* MutY protein, hMYH (McGoldrick *et al.*, 1995, Slupska *et al.*, 1996; Fig. 10.1). Repair synthesis, after removal of the mismatched native base is more likely to insert a C opposite 8-OH-Gua, and hence become a target for hOGG1.

Nucleotide excision repair

Despite appearing to be directed principally towards bulky lesions, such as cyclobutane thymine dimers (T<>T), there is evidence that NER (Figs. 10.1 and 10.2) may act upon non-bulky lesions such as 8-OH-Gua and Tg (Cooper *et al.*, 1997, Reardon *et al.*, 1997). The rate of 8-OH-Gua removal appears comparable to that for T<>T, generating a lesion-containing oligomer, approximately 24–32 nucleotides long (Reardon *et al.*, 1997). In the case of T<>T, at least, these oligomers are then subject to 5′–3′ exonucleolytic attack (Galloway *et al.*, 1994), whether this is the case for 8-oxoGua, and ultimately generates the 8-OH-dG moiety so often measured extracellularly (for review, see Cooke *et al.*, 2002), remains uninvestigated.

NER of oxidative DNA damage may be a backup for BER, being dependent upon cell type, and under specific conditions, e.g. when BER is compromised. Despite this, evidence from studies examining the significance of oxidative DNA damage in xeroderma pigmentosum (XP), implies that the NER of such damage, although not necessarily 8-OH-Gua specifically, has some functional significance.

Transcription coupled repair

The purpose of TCR is to remove lesions from actively transcribed genes. In general, lesions that block the processivity of RNA polymerase (RNAP) are subject to TCR (Tornaletti & Hanawalt, 1999). Whilst some proteins of the NER pathway are also involved in TCR, this does not necessarily make TCR a sub-pathway of NER, as the function of these proteins can be clearly separated between the two pathways (Evans *et al.*, 2004). Some studies exist which suggest that non-bulky lesions, such as 8-OH-Gua and Tg, may also be substrates for TCR (Le Page *et al.*, 2000, Cooper *et al.*, 1997), implying the recruitment of glycosylases to this role. TCR is vital to cell metabolism as it removes the stalled RNAP, allowing the recruited repair proteins to act upon the lesion.

DNA repair abnormalities and neurological symptoms

Oxidative stress, and concomitant elevated levels of oxidative DNA damage, has been proposed to be important in a number of neurodegenerative conditions, such as Alzheimer's disease (for review, see Evans *et al.*, 2004), a role supported by promising results from antioxidant supplementation studies (Mattson *et al.*, 2002). Whilst numerous factors may affect levels of damage, it is becoming increasingly clear that DNA repair, in particular, may have a crucial role.

The association between DNA repair and the neurological deficits in neurodegenerative diseases is perhaps most evident in the (rare) human hereditary diseases caused by mutations in DNA repair genes, as discussed below.

Xeroderma pigmentosum

Xeroderma pigmentosum is a rare, autosomal recessive condition, displaying acute photosensitivity and an associated strong predisposition to skin cancer. The condition arises from mutations in the key genes (complementation groups) associated with NER (Sancar, 1995). Of the seven complementation groups with NER defects (A–G), A, B, D and G display varying degrees of neurological deficiency (Table 10.1). This deficiency manifests in early infancy, arising from the progressive loss of neurones from the cerebral cortex (Sarasin, 1991), reportedly due to the failure to repair DNA damage (Robbins, 1988, Robbins *et al.*, 1991, 1993). More specifically, it is the failure of NER to remove a class of oxidative DNA damage, which appears associated with neurological symptoms in the affected complementation groups (Chopp *et al.*, 1996). Exactly which lesions are responsible is not clear. XPA has received perhaps the most attention, due to the most severe symptoms, and almost total loss of NER activity (2%; Table 10.1). Indeed, XPA cells have been shown to be deficient in the removal of 8-OH-Gua, Tg (Reardon *et al.*, 1997), 5-hydroxycytosine, 2,6-diamino-4-hydroxy-5-formamidopyrimidine, 4,6-diamino-5-formamidopyrimidine (Lipinski *et al.*, 1999), and 8,5′-cyclo-2′-deoxyadenosine (Brooks *et al.*, 2000). In contrast XPD, for example, demonstrates efficient 8-OH-Gua repair (Cappelli *et al.*, 2000). Whilst further work is still required, these findings strongly implicate ROS, and the resulting oxidative DNA damage, in the pathogenesis of the neurological symptoms in XP, with implications for other neurodegenerative diseases.

Cockayne's syndrome

Unlike XP, this recessive, progeroid disease is not associated with an increased cancer incidence, although patients are photosensitive. Patients have short stature, progressive neurological degeneration and mental retardation. Whilst levels of global genome NER are normal, accounting for the absence of cancer predisposition, TCR is defective (van Hoffen *et al.*, 1993, Leadon & Cooper, 1993). This condition can be divided into two complementation groups (CS–A and CS–B), and again the defective repair of oxidative DNA damage has been proposed to contribute to the CS phenotype (Hanawalt, 1994, Dianov *et al.*, 1997), and neurological abnormalities, specifically. CSB cells have been shown to possess downregulated *hOGG1* expression, resulting in a deficiency in GGR of 8-OH-Gua specifically, uracil and

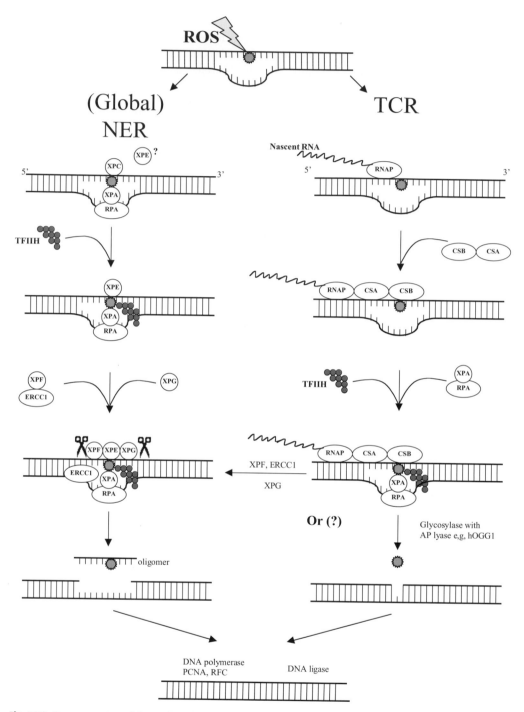

Fig. 10.2 Representation of the nucleotide excision repair (NER) and transcription-coupled repair pathways. (i) NER: lesion recognition by XPC and possibly XPE, perhaps aided XPA in conjunction with replication protein A (RPA, a.k.a human single strand binding protein). Recruitment of other proteins; TFIIH (containing the helicase sub-units XPB and XPD), and the XPF/ERCC1 complex. The 5' incision is made by the XPF/ERCC1 complex and 3' by XPG. The oligomer is removed, and the gap filled and sealed by DNA polymerases δ or ε, proliferating cell nuclear antigen (PCNA), replication factor C (RFC) and DNA ligase. (ii) TCR: RNA polymerase II (RNAPII) stalls at the lesion, at which point CSA and CSB proteins are recruited. The following steps are as for NER, although there is a suggestion that glycosylases may also be recruited to perform a TCR function at the lesion excision stage.

Table 10.1. Summary of major disorders associated with nucleotide excision repair/transcription-coupled repair deficiency[1].

Mutated gene	Gene function in NER/TCR	Residual NER activity (% of wild type)	Neurological symptoms	Clinical symptoms				
				XP	CS	XP + CS	TTD	UV -sensitive COFS syndrome
XPA	DNA damage recognition	< 2	Severe	X				
XPB	DNA unwinding, subunit (helicase) of TFIIH	< 10	Severe			X	X	
XPC	Repair of non-transcribed DNA	+/− 20	Absent	X				
XPD	DNA unwinding, subunit (helicase) of TFIIH	+/− 30	Variable			X	X	X
XPE	DNA damage recognition?	+/− 45	Absent	X				
XPF	Incision 5′ to DNA damage	+/− 20	Absent	X				
XPG	Incision 3′ to DNA damage	+/− 10	Variable	X		X		X
CSA	TCR	100	Severe		X			X
CSB	Transcription-coupling factor	100	Severe		X			
TTD-A	Unidentified subunit of TFIIH	+/− 10	Severe				X	

[1] Table derived from de Vries and van Steeg (1996), and Graham *et al.* (2001).

Tg being unaffected (Dianov *et al.*, 1997). For other oxidative lesions, the impact of mutated *CSB* in TCR may jeopardize their removal from actively transcribed genes, even their GGR is unaffected. It appears to be defects in TCR that are responsible for the CS phenotype. For example, the rare mutations in *XPB*, *XPD* and *XPG* all give rise to a combined XP/CS phenotype, at least in part due to the impact they have on TCR (Cooper *et al.*, 1997, Le Page *et al.*, 2000) and, as noted above, are all associated with severe neurological abnormalities (de Vries & van Steeg, 1996). The basis for this relationship has been proposed. Given the brain's high requirement for oxygen, the generation of ROS, and hence DNA damage, is likely to be equally high. Therefore, to maintain cell activity and neurological function, repair of actively transcribed genes is of great importance. As long as TCR is present, cells can function when global levels of lesions would normally be lethal. However, in the case of CS, not only is TCR absent, but lesions in transcribed strands are inaccessible to GGR due to the stalled RNAP, leading to an accumulation of lesions which block transcription. Protein synthesis ceases as mRNA levels decline, postulated to account for the symptoms of neurological deterioration and wasting (Le Page *et al.*, 2000).

Trichothiodystrophy

Patients with TTD have sulfur-deficient, brittle hair and nails, are of short stature, and are mentally retarded. Of the TTD patients, only those who are photosensitive have a repair defect, associated with the *XPB* or *XPD* genes.

Another class of TTD exists that cannot be associated with XP. Neurological symptoms are present, as well as defective DNA repair, seemingly associated with the transcription initiation complex, TFIIH, designated TTD-A (Vermeulen *et al.*, 1994; Table 10.1; Fig. 10.2).

Repair of mitochondrial DNA damage and neurodegenerative disease

Increasingly, mitochondria are being proposed an important role in neurodegenerative diseases, such as Alzheimer's disease, Parkinson's disease, amyotrophic lateral sclerosis and multiple sclerosis (Calabrese *et al.*, 2001). There is evidence that oxidative damage to mitochondrial DNA (mtDNA), and its repair, may be important, not only for neurodegenerative disease, but also other conditions, as a small number of mtDNA mutations have been associated with a significant number of mitochondrial myopathy disorders and aging (Wallace, 1992, 1994).

Certainly, mtDNA contains more damage than its nuclear counterpart (Yakes & Van Houten, 1997), not least because mitochondria produce 90% of the free radicals in a cell (Berdanier & Everts, 2001), but also mtDNA possesses little of the structural features that serve to protect nuclear DNA. Another factor is repair. As mentioned above, β-hOGG1 is targeted towards mitochondria, as are other repair proteins, such as hMTH1 (Kang *et al.*, 1995), hMYH, and hNTH1 (Takao *et al.*, 1998).

Table 10.2. Evidence for elevated levels of oxidatively damaged DNA in human neurodegenerative disease.

Disease	Damage increased?	Observations
Parkinson's disease (PD)	↑	• DNA levels of 8-OH-dG significantly elevated ($P=0.0002$) in substantia nigra of PD brains (Alam et al., 1997)
	↑	• Levels of 8-OH-dG and 8-OH-Gua in cytoplasmic DNA and RNA, respectively, are elevated in substantia nigra neurons of Parkinson's disease patients and, although to a lesser extent, in multiple system atrophy-Parkinsonian type and dementia with Lewy bodies (Zhang et al., 1999).
	↑	• Serum and CSF levels of 8-OH-dG significantly higher in PD and multiple system atrophy, compared to matched controls (Kikuchi et al., 2002).
Alzheimer's disease (AD)	→	• DNA levels of 8-OH-dG in Alzheimer's disease brain, not associated with disease (Koppele et al., 1996).
	↑	• Higher levels of 8-OH-dG in cortex and cerebellum of AD patients vs. controls (Lezza et al., 1999).
	↑	• Ventricular cerebrospinal fluid (CSF) DNA levels of 8-OH-dG significantly ($P<0.05$) elevated and CSF levels of free 8-OH-dG significantly reduced ($P<0.05$) compared to controls (Lovell et al., 1999).
	↑	• Significantly higher levels ($P<0.001$) of 8-OH-dG in lymphocytes from AD patients compared to controls (Mecocci et al., 1998).
	↑	• Significant increase in 8-OH-Guo[2] levels in CSF of AD patients, compared to controls, which decreased with duration of illness, and progression of cognitive dysfunction (Abe et al., 2002). Consistent with the observation that oxidative damage to nucleic acids is an early event in pathogenesis of AD (Nunomura et al., 2001).
	↑	• Significant increase in nuclear DNA 8-OH-dG levels and highly significant, threefold increase in mitochondrial DNA levels of 8-OH-dG in parietal cortex of AD patients compared with controls (Mecocci et al., 1994).
Huntington's disease (HD)	→	• No difference between the levels of 8-OH-Gua, FapyAde[3], 8-OH-Ade, FapyGua, 2-OH-Ade, xanthine and hypoxanthine in caudate, putamen and frontal cortex from HD brains, compared to controls (Alam et al., 2000).
	↑	• Nuclear levels of 8-OH-dG significantly elevated in HD caudate (Browne et al., 1997)
	↑	• Significantly increased mitochondrial 8-OH-dG levels in parietal cortex of HD patients, compared to controls. No significant differences in lesion levels in frontal cortex or cerebellum of HD patients, compared to controls (Polidori et al., 1999).
Dementia with Lewy Bodies (DLB)	↑	• Increased levels of 8-OH-Gua, FapyGua, 5-OHCyt, 5-OHUra, 5-OHMUra and xanthine in cortical region of brain in DLB patients compared to control tissue (Lyras et al., 1998).
Multiple sclerosis	↑	Significantly elevated levels of 8-OH-dG in plaques, compared to normal-appearing white matter in multiple sclerosis-affected cerebella (Vladimirova et al., 1998).
Amyotrophic lateral sclerosis (ALS)	↑	• Levels of 8-OH-dG significantly increased in plasma, urine and CSF, compared to controls; levels of urinary 8-OH-dG increased over a nine month period and correlated with disease severity (Bogdanov et al., 2000)
Down syndrome (DS) and AD	→	No difference in levels of 8-OH-dG in either cerebral cortex, or cerebellum in DS or AD brains, compared to controls Seidl et al., 1997).

[1] 8-OH-Guo; 8-hydroxyguanosine.

[2] FapyAde (4,6-diamino-5-formamidopyrimidine); 8-OH-Ade (8-hydroxyadenine); FapyGua (2,6-diamino-4-hydroxy-5-formamidopyrimidine); 2-OH-Ade (2-hydroxyadenine); 5-OHCyt (5-hydroxycytosine); 5-OHUra (5-hydroxyuracil); 5-OHMUra (5-hydroxymethyluracil).

It appears that mtDNA is only subject to GGR (Anson *et al.*, 1998). This situation is exacerbated in CSB where hOGG1 activity is deficient, eliminating 8-OH-Gua repair, although other lesions (uracil, hypoxanthine and Tg) do not appear affected (Stevnsner *et al.*, 2002). Whilst there are suggestions that NER might be involved in the repair of damage to mtDNA (for review see Croteau *et al.*, 1999), the inability to remove T<>T casts doubt upon this (Clayton *et al.*, 1974), emphasizing the importance of BER.

Inefficient repair of damage to mtDNA has a potential involvement in neurodegenerative disease, and yet, apart from the diseases arising from hereditary repair defects, there appear to be few studies directly linking repair deficiency and major neurodegenerative diseases. However, given the central role of repair in damage limitation, the numerous reports of elevated lesion levels in a variety of neurodegenerative diseases (see Table 10.2), and in corresponding mouse models (Bogdanov *et al.*, 2001; Aguirre *et al.*, unpublished data, 2004), might suggest defective DNA repair to be a common factor. Supportive of this hypothesis are a number of emerging reports which have considered repair. Of these, there are indications of impaired repair of oxidatively damaged mtDNA in Down syndrome (Druzhyna *et al.*, 1998), although repair of nuclear DNA was not considered. In contrast, an increased expression of poly(ADP)-ribose polymerase, involved in the repair of strand breaks, has been reported in the brains of ALS patients, albeit suggested to be simply response to widespread oxidative stress (Kim *et al.*, 2004).

Marginally, more appears to be known about DNA repair and AD, with the suggestion that a repair defect may be present (Parshad *et al.*, 1996), although this does not appear to be TCR, given findings with T←→T (Link *et al.*, 1995). A more recent report notes that hOGG1 activity and helicase activity is significantly reduced in specific regions of AD brain (Lovell *et al.*, 2000). Consistent with this is the finding that lymphocytes from AD patients have a diminished repair of hydrogen peroxide-induced oxidized purines (Morocz *et al.*, 2002), which also implies that the repair defect is not restricted to neuronal tissue. A study with amyloid precursor protein mutant mice demonstrated that folic acid deficiency reduced the repair of amyloid β-peptide induced oxidative modification of DNA bases (Kruman *et al.*, 2002). This would suggest that environmental conditions, e.g. diet, may be responsible for the reduction in DNA repair capacity, rather than a genetic defect, perhaps explaining the reduced repair capacity in both neuronal cells and lymphocytes, described above.

Defects in the DNA damage response and neurological symptoms

The BRCA1-associated genome surveillance complex (BASC) is a large multiprotein complex, which comprises many proteins involved in the maintenance of genome stability, including: ATM (ataxia telangiectasia, AT), BLM (Bloom's syndrome, BS), and FANCD2 (Fanconi anemia, FA; (Watters, 2003) proteins. Whilst not involved in the repair of DNA *per se*, these proteins are worth mentioning, for when defective, they give rise to clinical symptoms with some similarity to those arising from DNA repair defects. For example, amongst the symptoms of AT is sensitivity to ionizing radiation, susceptibility to cancer, progressive neurodegeneration and premature aging (Watters, 2003). Similarly, symptoms of BS include cancer predisposition and mental retardation; FA, cancer predisposition, ventricular defects and micropthalmia (Rolig & McKinnon, 2000). Like XPB and XPD, FA and BLM are helicases, as are RECQL4 and WRN. Whilst not part of BASC, patients with defects in RECQL4 and WRN develop the cancer prone syndromes, Rothmund–Thomson syndrome and Werner syndrome (premature aging), with progressive neurodegeneration and mental retardation, respectively (Rolig & McKinnon, 2000).

Concluding remarks

Evidence for elevated levels of oxidative DNA damage has been reported in many of the major neurodegenerative diseases. Whether this arises from an overwhelming oxidant production, defects in repair, or a combination of the two, appears unclear. More certain is that, in general, diseases associated with DNA repair deficiencies, and TCR specifically, do exhibit neurological problems. In a broader context, defects in the response to DNA damage, may also result in neurological symptoms, particularly where helicases are involved. Therefore, a link between DNA repair deficiencies and neurological impairment does exist. Whilst there is some tantalizing evidence that this same mechanism may contribute to the pathogenesis of at least one of the major neurodegenerative diseases, further studies need to be performed, with the subsequent potential for intervention.

Acknowledgements

The author would like to thank the UK Food Standards Agency, Arthritis Research Campaign and Leicester

Dermatology Research Funds for research support, and Dr. Mark D. Evans for his comments on the manuscript.

REFERENCES

Abe, T., Tohgi, H., Isobe, C., Murata, T. & Sato, C. (2002). Remarkable increase in the concentration of 8-hydroxyguanosine in cerebrospinal fluid from patients with Alzheimer's disease. *J. Neurosci., Res.*, **70**, 447–50.

Alam, Z. I., Jenner, A., Daniel, S. E. *et al.* (1997). Oxidative DNA damage in the Parkinsonian brain: an apparent selective increase in 8-hydroxyguanine levels in substantia nigra. *J. Neurochem.*, **69**, 1196–203.

Alam, Z. I., Halliwell, B. & Jenner, P. (2000). No evidence for increased oxidative damage to lipids, proteins, or DNA in Huntington's disease. *J. Neurochem*, **75**, 840–6.

Anson, R. M., Croteau, D. L., Stierum, R. H., Filburn, C., Parsell, R. & Bohr, V. A. (1998). Homogenous repair of singlet oxygen-induced DNA damage in differentially transcribed regions and strands of human mitochondrial DNA. *Nucl. Acids Res.*, **26**, 662–8.

Arai, K., Morishita, K., Shinmura, K. *et al.* (1997). Cloning of a human homolog of the yeast OGG1 gene that is involved in the repair of oxidative DNA damage. *Oncogene*, **14**, 2857–61.

Berdanier, C. D. & Everts, H. B. (2001). Mitochondrial DNA in aging and degenerative disease. *Mutat. Res.*, **475**, 169–83.

Bestwick, R. K., Moffett, G. L. & Mathews, C. K. (1982). Selective expansion of mitochondrial nucleoside triphosphate pools in antimetabolite-treated HeLa cells. *J. Biol. Chem.*, **257**, 9300–4.

Bialkowski, K. & Kasprzak, K. S. (1998). A novel assay of 8-oxo-2′-deoxyguanosine 5′-triphosphate pyrophosphohydrolase (8-oxo-dGTPase) activity in cultured cells and its use for evaluation of cadmium(II) inhibition of this activity. *Nucl. Acids Res.*, **26**, 3194–201.

Bogdanov, M., Brown, R. H., Matson, W. *et al.* (2000). Increased oxidative damage to DNA in ALS patients. *Free Radical Biol. Med.*, **29**, 652–8.

Bogdanov, M. B., Andreassen, O. A., Dedeoglu, A., Ferrante, R. J. & Beal, M. F. (2001). Increased oxidative damage to DNA in a transgenic mouse model of Huntington's disease. *J. Neurochem.*, **79**, 1246–9.

Brooks, P. J., Wise, D. S., Berry, D. A. *et al.* (2000). The oxidative DNA lesion 8,5′-(S)-cyclo-2′-deoxyadenosine is repaired by the nucleotide excision repair pathway and blocks gene expression in mammalian cells. *J. Biol. Chem.*, **275**, 22355–62.

Browne, S. E., Bowling, A. C., MacGarvey, U. *et al.* (999). Oxidative damage and metabolic dysfunction in Huntington's disease: selective vulnerability of the basal ganglia. *Ann. Neurol.*, **41**, 646–53.

Calabrese, V., Scapagnini, G., Giuffrida Stella, A. M., Bates, T. E. & Clark, J. B. (2001). Mitochondrial involvement in brain function and dysfunction: relevance to aging, neurodegenerative disorders and longevity. *Neurochem. Res.*, **26**, 739–64.

Cappelli, E., Degan, P., Thompson, L. H. & Frosina, G. (2000). Efficient repair of 8-oxo-7,8-dihydrodeoxyguanosine in human and hamster xeroderma pigmentosum D cells. *Biochemistry*, **39**, 10408–12.

Chopp, M., Chan, P. H., Hsu, C. Y., Cheung, M. E. & Jacobs, T. P. (1996). DNA damage and repair in central nervous system injury: National Institute of Neurological Disorders and Stroke Workshop Summary. *Stroke*, **27**, 363–9.

Clayton, D. A., Doda, J. N. & Friedberg, E. C. (1974). The absence of a pyrimidine dimer repair mechanism in mammalian mitochondria. *Proc. Natl Acad. Sci., USA*, **71**, 2777–81.

Cooke, M. S., Evans, M. D., Herbert, K. E. & Lunec, J. (2000). Urinary 8-oxo-2′-deoxyguanosine-source, significance and supplements. *Free Rad. Res.*, **32**, 381–97.

Cooke, M. S., Lunec, J. & Evans, M. D. (2002). Progress in the analysis of urinary oxidative DNA damage. *Free Rad. Biol. Med.*, **33**, 1601–14.

Cooke, M. S., Evans, M. D., Dizdaroglu, M. & Lunec, J. (2003). Oxidative DNA damage: mechanisms, mutation, and disease. *FASEB. J.*, **17**, 1195–214.

Cooper, P. K., Nouspikel, T., Clarkson, S. G. & Leadon, S. A. (1997). Defective transcription-coupled repair of oxidative base damage in Cockayne syndrome patients from XP group G. *Science*, **275**, 990–3.

Croteau, D. L., Rhys, C. M., Hudson, E. K., Dianov, G. L., Hansford, R. G. & Bohr, V. A. (1997). An oxidative damage-specific endonuclease from rat liver mitochondria. *J. Biol. Chem.*, **272**, 27338–44.

Croteau, D. L., Stierum, R. H. & Bohr, V. A. (1999). Mitochondrial DNA repair pathways. *Mutat. Res.*, **434**, 137–48.

de Vries, A. & van Steeg, H. (1996). Xpa knockout mice. *Semin. Cancer Biol.*, **7**, 229–40.

Dianov, G. L., Houle, J. F., Iyer, N., Bohr, V. A. & Friedberg, E. C. (1997). Reduced RNA polymerase II transcription in extracts of cockayne syndrome and xeroderma pigmentosum/Cockayne syndrome cells. *Nucl. Acids Res.*, **25**, 3636–42.

Druzhyna, N., Nair, R. G., LeDoux, S. P. & Wilson, G. L. (1998). Defective repair of oxidative damage in mitochondrial DNA in Down's syndrome. *Mutat. Res.*, **409**, 81–9.

Evans, M. D., Dizdaroglu, M. & Cooke, M. S. (2004). Oxidative DNA damage and disease: induction, repair and significance. *Mutat. Res. Rev.*, **567**, 1–61.

Fortini, P., Parlanti, E., Sidorkina, O. M., Laval, J. & Dogliotti, E. (1999). The type of DNA glycosylase determines the base excision repair pathway in mammalian cells. *J. Biol. Chem.*, **274**, 15230–6.

Galloway, A. M., Liuzzi, M. & Paterson, M. C. (1994). Metabolic processing of cyclobutyl pyrimidine dimers and (6–4) photoproducts in UV-treated human cells. Evidence for distinct excision-repair pathways. *J. Biol. Chem.*, **269**, 974–80.

Graham, J. M., Anyane-Yeboa, K., Raams, A. *et al.* (2001). Cerebro-oculo-facio-skeletal syndrome with a nucleotide excision-repair defect and a mutated XPD gene, with prenatal diagnosis in a triplet pregnancy. *Am. J. Hum. Genet.*, **69**, 291–300.

Hanawalt, P. C. (1994). Transcription-coupled repair and human disease. *Science*, **266**, 1957–8.

Kang, D., Nishida, J., Iyama, A. *et al*. (1995). Intracellular localization of 8-oxo-dGTPase in human cells, with special reference to the role of the enzyme in mitochondria. *J. Biol. Chem.*, **270**, 14659–65.

Kikuchi, A., Takeda, A., Onodera, H. *et al*. (2002). Systemic increase of oxidative nucleic acid damage in Parkinson's disease and multiple system atrophy. *Neurobiol. Dis.*, **9**, 244–8.

Kim, S. H., Engelhardt, J. I., Henkel, J. S. *et al*. (2004). Widespread increased expression of the DNA repair enzyme PARP in brain in ALS. *Neurology*, **62**, 319–22.

Koppele, J., Lucassen, P. J., Sakkee, A. N. *et al*. (1996). 8-OHdG levels in brain do not indicate oxidative DNA damage in Alzheimer's disease. *Neurobiol. Aging*, **17**, 819–26.

Kruman, I. I., Kumaravel, T. S., Lohani, A. *et al*. (2002). Folic acid deficiency and homocysteine impair DNA repair in hippocampal neurons and sensitize them to amyloid toxicity in experimental models of Alzheimer's disease. *J. Neurosci.*, **22**, 1752–62.

Le Page, F., Kwoh, E. E., Avrutskaya, A. *et al*. (2000). Transcription-coupled repair of 8-oxoguanine: requirement for XPG, TFIIH, and CSB and implications for Cockayne syndrome. *Cell*, **101**, 159–71.

Leadon, S. A. & Cooper, P. K. (1993). Preferential repair of ionizing radiation-induced damage in the transcribed strand of an active human gene is defective in Cockayne syndrome. *Proc. Natl Acad. Sci., USA*, **90**, 10499–503.

Lezza, A., Mecocci, P., Cormio, A. *et al*. (1999). Area-specific differences in OH8dG and mtDNA4977 levels in Alzheimer disease patients and aged controls. *J. Anti-Aging Med.*, **2**, 209–15.

Link, C. J., Robbins, J. H. & Bohr, V. A. (1995). Gene specific DNA repair of damage induced in familial Alzheimer disease cells by ultraviolet irradiation or by nitrogen mustard. *Mutat. Res.*, **336**, 115–21.

Lipinski, L. J., Hoehr, N., Mazur, S. J. *et al*. (1999). Repair of oxidative DNA base lesions induced by fluorescent light is defective in xeroderma pigmentosum group A cells. *Nucl. Acids Res.*, **27**, 3153–8.

Lovell, M. A., Xie, C. & Markesbery, W. R. (2000). Decreased base excision repair and increased helicase activity in Alzheimer's disease brain. *Brain Res.*, **855**, 116–23.

Lyras, L., Perry, R. H., Perry, E. K. *et al*. (1998). Oxidative damage to proteins, lipids, and DNA in cortical brain regions from patients with dementia with Lewy bodies. *J. Neurochem.*, **71**, 302–12.

Mattson, M. P., Chan, S. L. & Duan, W. (2002). Modification of brain aging and neurodegenerative disorders by genes, diet, and behaviour. *Physiol. Rev.*, **82**, 637–72.

McGoldrick, J. P., Yeh, Y. C., Solomon, M., Essigmann, J. M. & Lu, A. L. (1995). Characterization of a mammalian homolog of the *Escherichia coli* MutY mismatch repair protein. *Mol. Cell Biol.*, **15**, 989–96.

Mecocci, P., MacGarvey, U. & Beal, M. F. (1994). Oxidative damage to mitochondrial DNA is increased in Alzheimer's disease. *Ann. Neurol.*, **36**, 747–51.

Mecocci, P., Polidori, M. C., Ingegni, T. *et al*. (1998). Oxidative damage to DNA in lymphocytes from Alzheimer's disease patients. *Neurology*, **51**, 1014–17.

Mo, J. Y., Maki, H. & Sekiguchi, M. (1992). Hydrolytic elimination of a mutagenic nucleotide, 8-oxodGTP, by human 18-kilodalton protein: sanitization of nucleotide pool. *Proc. Natl Acad. Sci., USA*, **89**, 11021–5.

Morocz, M., Kalman, J., Juhasz, A. *et al*. (2002). Elevated levels of oxidative DNA damage in lymphocytes from patients with Alzheimer's disease. *Neurobiol. Aging*, **23**, 47–53.

Nishioka, K., Ohtsubo, T., Oda, H. *et al*. (1999). Expression and differential intracellular localization of two major forms of human 8-oxoguanine DNA glycosylase encoded by alternatively spliced OGG1 mRNAs. *Mol. Biol. Cell*, **10**, 1637–52.

Nunomura, A., Perry, G., Aliev, K. *et al*. (2001). Oxidative damage is the earliest event in Alzheimer disease. *J. Neuropath. Exp. Neurol.*, **60**, 759–67.

Parshad, R. P., Sanford, K. K., Price, F. M. *et al*. (1996). Fluorescent light-induced chromatid breaks distinguish Alzheimer disease cells from normal cells in tissue culture. *Proc. Natl Acad. Sci., USA*, **93**, 5146–50.

Polidori, M. C., Mecocci, P., Browne, S. E., Senin, U. & Beal, M. F. (1999). Oxidative damage to mitochondrial DNA in Huntington's disease parietal cortex. *Neurosci. Lett.*, **272**, 53–6.

Reardon, J. T., Bessho, T., Kung, H. C., Bolton, P. H. & Sancar, A. (1997). In vitro repair of oxidative DNA damage by human nucleotide excision repair system: possible explanation for neurodegeneration in xeroderma pigmentosum patients. *Proc. Natl Acad. Sci., USA*, **94**, 9463–8.

Robbins, J. H. (1988). Xeroderma pigmentosum. Defective DNA repair causes skin cancer and neurodegeneration. *J. Am. Med. Acad.*, **260**, 384–8.

Robbins, J. H., Brumback, R. A., Mendiones, M. *et al*. (1991). Neurological disease in xeroderma pigmentosum. Documentation of a late onset type of the juvenile onset form. *Brain*, **114 (3)**, 1335–61.

Robbins, J. H., Brumback, R. A. & Moshell, A. N. (1993). Clinically asymptomatic xeroderma pigmentosum neurological disease in an adult: evidence for a neurodegeneration in later life caused by defective DNA repair. *Eur. Neurol.*, **33**, 188–90.

Rolig, R. L. & McKinnon, P. J. (2000). Linking DNA damage and neurodegeneration. *Trends Neurosci.*, **23**, 417–24.

Rosenquist, T. A., Zharkov, D. O. & Grollman, A. P. (1997). Cloning and characterization of a mammalian 8-oxoguanine DNA glycosylase. *Proc. Natl Acad. Sci., USA*, **94**, 7429–34.

Sancar, A. (1995). DNA repair in humans. *Ann. Rev. Genet.*, **29**, 69–105.

Sarasin, A. (1991). The paradox of DNA repair-deficient disease. *Cancer J.*, **4**, 233–7.

Seidl, R., Greber, S., Schuller, E., Bernert, G., Cairns, N. & Lubec, G. (1997). Evidence against increased oxidative DNA damage in Down syndrome. *Neurosci. Lett.*, **235**, 137–40.

Slupska, M. M., Baikalov, C., Luther, W. M., Chiang, J. H., Wei, Y. F. & Miller, J. H. (1996). Cloning and sequencing a human homolog (hMYH) of the *Escherichia coli* mutY gene whose function is required for the repair of oxidative DNA damage. *J. Bacteriol.*, **178**, 3885–92.

Stevnsner, T., Nyaga, S., de Souza-Pinto, N. C. *et al.* (2002). Mitochondrial repair of 8-oxoguanine is deficient in Cockayne syndrome group B. *Oncogene*, **21**, 8675–82.

Takao, M., Aburatani, H., Kobayashi, K. & Yasui, A. (1998). Mitochondrial targeting of human DNA glycosylases for repair of oxidative DNA damage. *Nucl. Acids Res.*, **26**, 2917–22.

Tornaletti, S. & Hanawalt, P. C. (1999). Effect of DNA lesions on transcription elongation. *Biochimie*, **81**, 139–46.

van Hoffen, A., Natarajan, A. T., Mayne, L. V., van Zeeland, A. A., Mullenders, L. H. & Venema, J. (1993). Deficient repair of the transcribed strand of active genes in Cockayne's syndrome cells. *Nucl. Acids Res.*, **21**, 5890–5.

Vermeulen, W., van Vuuren, A. J., Chipoulet, M. *et al.* (1994). Three unusual repair deficiencies associated with transcription factor BTF2(TFIIH): evidence for the existence of a transcription syndrome. *Cold Spring Harbour Symp. Quant. Biol.*, **59**, 317–29.

Vladimirova, O., O'Connor, J., Cahill, A., Alder, H., Butunoi, C. & Kalman, B. (1998). Oxidative damage to DNA in plaques of MS brains, *Multiple Sclerosis*, **4**, 413–18.

Wallace, D. C. (1992). Mitochondrial genetics: a paradigm for aging and degenerative diseases? *Science*, **256**, 628–32.

Wallace, D. C. (1994). Mitochondrial DNA Mutations in diseases of energy metabolism. *J. Bioenerg. Biomemb.*, **26**, 241–50.

Watters, D. J. (2003). Oxidative stress in ataxia telangiectasia. *Redox Rep.*, **8**, 23–9.

Yakes, F. M. & Van Houten, B. (1997). Mitochondrial DNA damage is more extensive and persists longer than nuclear DNA damage in human cells following oxidative stress. *Proc. Natl Acad. Sci., USA*, **94**, 514–19.

Zhang, J., Perry, G., Smith, M. A. *et al.* (1999). Parkinson's disease is associated with oxidative damage to cytoplasmic DNA and RNA in substantia nigra neurons, *Am. J. Path.*, **154**, 1423–9.

11

Compounds acting on ion channels

Holger Lerche and Frank Lehmann-Horn

Departments of Neurology and Applied Physiology, University of Ulm, Germany

Important factors of neuronal death in various diseases ranging from acute illness such as head trauma or stroke to rapidly or slowly progressive disorders such as amyotrophic lateral sclerosis or idiopathic parkinsonism are energy deficit and membrane depolarization. The communication of nerve cells via action potentials and synaptic transmission needs a highly negative resting membrane potential as well as strong transmembrane ionic gradients, which guarantee a regulated ion flow across the membrane. A large part of the energy demand of neurons is therefore required for active ionic pumps such as the Na/K ATPase. A reduction of membrane excitability preventing membrane depolarization and decreasing the transmembrane ionic flow therefore diminishes the energy demand of neurons considerably. The pharmacological modification of the gating of voltage- or ligand-activated ion channels thus provides potentially powerful strategies for neuroprotection. The block of voltage-gated sodium or calcium channels directly reduces the influx of respective ions and decreases excitability, whereas the activation of potassium channels leads to a membrane hyperpolarization reducing excitability and secondarily influx of sodium and calcium through voltage-gated channels and other mechanisms. These neuroprotective strategies, the targets and compounds used for pharmacotherapy and available studies in animal models and humans are discussed in this chapter. The concept of excitoxicity and neuroprotection by its antagonism by a block of glutamate receptors belonging to the group of ligand-gated ion channels is discussed in Chapter 4 of this book.

Sodium channel blockers

Voltage-gated sodium channels provide the basis for the generation and conduction of action potentials in nerve and muscle cells. They open briefly upon depolarization and then close to a fast inactivated state, which limits the duration of an action potential and initiates its repolarizing phase. Upon repolarization they recover from inactivation and will be available for another action potential after a certain refractory period. Brain sodium channels consist of a main α- and two auxiliary β-subunits. The α-subunit is built of four homologous repeats with six transmembrane segments each. It constitutes both the gating and permeation machinery of the sodium channel as well as all known drug binding sites (Catterall, 2000a).

Sodium channel blockers can be divided into several different groups. The two most important categories are blockers of the outer pore such as Tetrodotoxin (TTX), and so-called use-dependent blockers binding to the inner pore, which are in clinical use as local anesthetics, antiarrhythmics or anticonvulsants. Whereas TTX is not suited for clinical use because of its toxicity due to a high-affinity block even in the resting state of the channel, use-dependent blockers bind predominantly to the inactivated state of the channel, which occurs only upon depolarization. These agents suppress series of action potentials increasingly with their frequency (therefore called "use dependence") but do not considerably disturb activation, thus excitation, from the resting state (Urenjak & Obrenovitch, 1996).

The influx of sodium into neurons seems to have an intrinsic neurotoxicity as could be shown by experiments using the sodium channel opener veratridine or ischemia models in brain preparations or cell cultures. Whereas removing extracellular calcium had relatively small beneficial effects in these models and did not prevent cell death, replacing extracellular sodium in various of such experiments prevented neuronal death presumably due to failure of depolarization and subsequent influx of NaCl with excessive osmotic load, cell swelling and bleb formation.

Moreover, excessive sodium influx leads to an increase of calcium influx via a reversal of the Na/Ca exchanger, which under resting conditions extrudes calcium driven by the large transmembrane sodium gradient. Sodium channel blockers thus should have several different potentially neuroprotective mechanisms such as (i) a direct reduction of sodium influx, (ii) an indirect reduction of calcium entry, (iii) a direct reduction of membrane excitability and (iv) an indirect reduction of transmitter release via a decrease of presynaptic membrane excitability. The latter two mechanisms reduce the energy demand of nerve cells as well as the excitotoxicity by glutamate. Therefore, the block of sodium channels should be a very effective neuroprotective strategy, which has been demonstrated in a large number of animal studies (for review see Urenjak & Obrenovitch, 1996; Taylor & Meldrum, 1995).

The high affinity pore blocker tetrodotoxin as well as local anesthetics (e.g. lidocaine), anticonvulsants (e.g. phenytoin) and more unspecific drugs with action on sodium channels like flunarizine or vinpocetine showed neuroprotective effects in numerous anoxic in vitro and in vivo animal models such as cell cultures, the optic nerve, hippocampal and neocortical slice preparations or transient global and focal ischemia. Measurable effects were an improved recovery of population spikes in the hippocampus or of compound action potentials in the optic nerve, as well as a reduction of infarct volume and the extent of cell death. Cellular and molecular mechanisms, which might have been involved in these neuroprotective effects, included a delay of extracellular acidosis and anoxic depolarization, block of sodium and calcium entry as well as potassium efflux, reduction of ATP depletion and of the brain metabolic rate (comprehensive overview: Urenjak & Obrenovitch, 1996). Clinical trials with different sodium channel blockers in early therapy of ischemic stroke are under way or planned, but results have not been published until now. Since most of the described neuroprotective effects in animal studies were observed with early application of the drugs, sometimes before the injury, it might be difficult to obtain a measurable benefit in clinical trials of acute stroke therapy.

Riluzole is the only drug that has been shown to have a neuroprotective effect in a chronic neurodegenerative disease, amyotrophic lateral sclerosis (Bensimon et al., 1994), besides its well-documented effect in numerous animal models ranging from brain ischemia to spinal cord injury (Obrenovitch & Urenjak, 1997). The drug also blocks sodium channels in a use-dependent manner with a high affinity for the inactivated state similar to local anesthetics and anticonvulsants. This might be one of the main mechanisms of action in neuroprotection of riluzole as

derived from in vitro investigations (Doble, 1997). However, other pharmacological properties of this drug might be even more important for its neuroprotective effects as will be outlined further below (see potassium channel activators).

Potassium channel openers

There is a huge variety of potassium channels expressed in excitable and non-excitable tissues (comprehensive and detailed overview: Hille, 2001). Voltage-gated potassium channels (K_v) activate upon membrane depolarization and contribute to the repolarizing phase of the action potential. They can be inactivating or not. The inactivating channels yield the transient A current, whereas the non-inactivating ones the so-called delayed rectifier potassium current characterized by sustained activation increasing with depolarization. K_v channels are structurally similar to sodium and calcium channels with six transmembrane regions but are built of four identical domains. Large-conductance calcium-activated potassium channels (BK_{Ca}) have a similar structure but a much weaker voltage dependence and are opened by elevated intracellular calcium concentrations. Inward rectifier potassium channels (K_{ir}) may be important for the resting membrane potential since they open at negative potentials and close with depolarization. They are tetramers of only two transmembrane domains, which are structurally conserved among potassium channels and form the pore region with the selectivity filter as was first demonstrated for the crystallized bacterial potassium channel KcsA (Doyle et al., 1998). ATP-dependent potassium channels (K_{ATP}) are derived from K_{ir} and have an octameric structure with another subunit yielding the ADP/ATP-sensitivity, the sulfonylurea receptor. K_{ATP} channels are closed when enough ATP is present intracellularly. They open with falling ATP and increasing ADP levels, thus when cells are energetically exhausted. Recently, a different class of potassium channels with four transmembrane segments has been identified, called 'two P domain potassium channels' (K_{2P}), due to their two pore regions. They are responsible for background or 'leak' potassium currents and are regulated by several different mechanisms such as membrane stretching, pH, lipids, second messengers and drugs (for review see Patel & Honore, 2001).

As a potassium outward current hyperpolarizes the cell membrane until the potassium equilibrium potential of about -85 mV is reached, an activation of potassium channels is needed for a neuroprotective effect based on a reduction of membrane excitability and secondarily of the neuronal energy demand. However, a lot of potassium channels for which activators have been developed are more or less expressed ubiquitously in mammalian cells which makes their use as therapeutic targets for a neuroprotective therapy difficult, due to systemic, mainly cardiovascular side effects.

The first potassium channel activators were available for K_{ATP} channels and a neuroprotective effect, for example, in ischemic models of rat hippocampus could be shown for several different types of these drugs (Heurteaux *et al.*, 1993). The neuroprotective mechanism seems to be related to an endogenous form of neuroprotection. During neuronal hypoxia, an initial hyperpolarization is followed by the final and lethal depolarization (Hansen, 1985). The hyperpolarization is caused by an activation of K_{ATP} channels (Riepe *et al.*, 1992). Activation of K_{ATP} channels might play an important role in ischemic and chemical preconditioning as the neuroprotective effect of chemical preconditioning could be partly antagonized by glibenclamide, a classical blocker of K_{ATP} channels (Riepe *et al.*, 1997). An endogenous neuroprotective role of these channels is also suggested by experiments showing that differential expression of the sulfonylurea receptor correlates to the expression of functional K_{ATP} channels and might contribute to the selective vulnerability in dopaminergic midbrain neurons (Liss *et al.*, 1999). Owing to cardiovascular side effects, K_{ATP} channel openers have not been used in clinical trials. New compounds with direct or indirect action on these channels dissociating vasorelaxation from protective effects in the heart and/or the brain might be key to a clinical use of these drugs (Yoo *et al.*, 2001).

Another newly developed potassium channel opener, BMS-204352, with neuroprotective effects acts on BK_{Ca} channels and a type of slow delayed rectifier potassium channels, so-called KCNQ channels. This compound was effective in rodent stroke models (Gribkoff *et al.*, 2001). It was well tolerated in patients but failed to be efficient in therapy of acute stroke in a Phase III trial (Jensen, 2002).

As already mentioned above, the neuroprotective mechanism of action of riluzole in amyotrophic lateral sclerosis as well as in various models of ischemia and trauma is not completely understood. Recently, it was demonstrated that two types of K_{2P} channels (TREK-1 and TRAAK), both activated by arachidonic acid and stretching, are activated directly by riluzole (Duprat *et al.*, 2000). Similar to the block of sodium channels by riluzole, this different mechanism of action would stabilize the resting membrane potential and decrease membrane excitability which first has a direct neuroprotective effect and second could also explain the known reduction of glutamate release. While TREK-1 is expressed in many tissues, TRAAK is found only in brain, spinal cord and retina. Therefore, in particular, TRAAK may

be a very attractive target for future selective neuroprotective agents.

Calcum channel antagonists

Voltage-gated calcium channels were first divided physiologically in low-voltage activated, fast inactivating ("transient," T-type) channels and high-voltage activated, slowly inactivating ("long-lasting," L-type) channels. Both channel types are mainly found in muscle and nerve cells. L-type channels are key players of electromechanical coupling transferring an action potential into a muscle contraction. They are blocked by three classes of drugs, dihydropyridines (e.g. nifedipine), phenylalkylamines (e.g. verapamil) and benzothiazepines (e.g. diltiazem). In neurons, several additional types of calcium channels were found, which are similar in their electrophysiological properties with activation by large depolarizations (high-voltage activated) and a slow inactivation. They could be differentiated by their response to peptide toxins from cone snails and spiders. N-type channels (*neuronal*) are sensitive to ω-conotoxin GVIA and P/Q-type channels (*purkinje*) to ω-Aga IVA, whereas R-type channels are resistant to these toxins. These neuronal channels are dominant at presynaptic nerve terminals and important for transferring an action potential into the secretion of neurotransmitters into the synaptic cleft. Calcium channels are all structurally very similar to sodium channels and built of several subunits, a main α_1-subunit containing the pore, gating machinery and drug binding sites, and different auxiliary subunits called β, $\alpha_2\delta$ and γ (Hille, 2001; Catterall, 2000b).

Since a calcium overload is thought to be one of the crucial steps in neurodegeneration (see Chapters 4 and 6) and since calcium enters the cell upon depolarization through ion channels, a block of voltage-gated calcium channels should be a promising strategy for neuroprotection. Various L-type calcium channel antagonists are in clinical use as antihypertensive and antiarrhythmic drugs. They have been investigated for many years for their neuroprotective effects in in vitro and in vivo models of ischemia and many clinical trials have been performed with acute stroke patients. While beneficial effects in animal models seemed first to be convincing, the clinical trials could only partly reveal positive effects. In two recent meta-analyses, Horn and colleagues evaluated both animal studies and clinical trials with L-type calcium channel antagonists designed for the treatment of stroke (Horn *et al.*, 2001; Horn & Limburg, 2001). The overall results were not promoting a neuroprotective effect of these drugs (mainly nifedipine or flunarizine, isradipine or nicardipine in one trial each) in stroke patients. The authors even concluded that the animal studies did not reveal a clear neuroprotective effect of nifedipine and discussed whether clinical trials should have been performed at all with regard to these poor experimental results. Furthermore, there are also reports that L-type calcium channel antagonists or low extracellular calcium or potassium concentrations may induce apoptotic cell death via a permanently reduced calcium influx or a reduced intracellular calcium concentration (Koh & Cotman, 1992; Galli *et al.*, 1995). Altogether, the hints for a possible neuroprotective effect of L-type calcium channel antagonists are weak and these drugs seem not to be suited for clinical use, at least in acute stroke therapy.

However, compounds blocking neuronal calcium channels (N-type, P/Q-type) might be more effective (Kobayashi & Mori, 1998), but they have yet not been investigated in clinical trials. For example, the imidazoline compound, antazoline, which protects against hypoxia and NMDA toxicity in neuronal cell cultures, was shown to block P/Q- and N-type calcium channels (Milhaud *et al.*, 2002). The N-type calcium channel antagonist, SNX-111, a synthetic product of the naturally occurring ω-conotoxin MVIIA, also seems to have a neuroprotective potential (Perez-Pinzon *et al.*, 1997; Bowersox & Luther, 1998).

Concluding remarks

In summary, many different drugs acting on ion channels have proved to be neuroprotective in various animal and cell culture models. The clinical benefit of such drugs, however, remains questionable as long as only for a single compound – riluzole, for which the mechanism of action is still not fully understood – a neuroprotective effect could be shown in a single disease, amyotrophic lateral sclerosis. A major problem of all clinical trials, in particular those for acute stroke therapy, might be that therapy starts always too late. We can only hope that earlier diagnosis and treatment in both stroke and neurodegenerative disorders will be possible in the future and that trials starting therapy as early as possible will be able to transfer the positive laboratory results into a clinical benefit for our patients.

REFERENCES

Bensimon, G., Lacomblez, L. & Meininger, V. (1994). A controlled trial of riluzole in amyotrophic lateral sclerosis. ALS/Riluzole Study Group. *N. Engl. J. Med.*, **330**, 585–91.

Bowersox, S. S. & Luther, R. (1998). Pharmacotherapeutic potential of ω-conotoxin MVIIA (SNX-111), an N-type neuronal calcium channel blocker found in the venom of *Conus magus. Toxicon*, **36**, 1651–8.

Catterall, W. A. (2000a). From ionic currents to molecular mechanisms: the structure and function of voltage-gated sodium channels. *Neuron*, **26**, 13–25.

(2000b). Structure and regulation of voltage-gated calcium channels. *Annu. Rev. Cell. Dev. Biol.*, **16**, 521–55.

Doble, A. (1997). Effects of riluzole on glutamatergic neurotransmission in the mammalian central nervous system, and other pharmacological effects. *Rev. Contemp. Pharmacother.*, **8**, 213–25.

Doyle, D. A., Morais Cabral, J., Pfuetzner, R. A. *et al.* (1998). The structure of the K+ channel: molecular basis of K+ conduction and selectivity. *Science*, **280**, 69–77.

Duprat, F., Lesage, F., Patel, A. J., Fink, M., Romey, G. & Lazdunski, M. (2000). The neuroprotective agent riluzole activates the two P domain K+ channels TREK-1 and TRAAK. *Mol. Pharmacol.*, **57**, 906–12.

Galli, C., Meucci, O., Scorziello, A., Werge, T. M., Calissano, P. & Schettini, G. (1995). Apoptosis in cerebellar granule cells is blocked by high KCl, forskolin, and IGF-1 through distinct mechanisms of action: the involvement of intracellular calcium and RNA synthesis. *J. Neurosci.*, **15**, 1172–9.

Gribkoff, V. K., Starrett, J. E. Jr., Dworetzky, S. I. *et al.* (2001). Targeting acute ischemic stroke with a calcium-sensitive opener of maxi-K potassium channels. *Nat. Med.*, **7**, 471–7.

Hansen, A. J. (1985). Effects of anoxia on ion distribution in the brain. *Physiol. Rev.*, **65**, 101–48.

Heurteaux, C., Bertaina, V., Widmann, C. & Lazdunski, M. (1993). K+ channel openers prevent global ischemia-induced expression of c-fos, c-jun, heat shock protein, and amyloid beta-protein precursor genes and neuronal death in rat hippocampus. *Proc. Natl Acad. Sci., USA*, **90**, 9431–5.

Hille, B. (2001). *Ion Channels of Excitable Membranes*. Sunderland, Massachusetts, USA: Sinauer Associates Inc.

Horn, J. & Limburg, M. (2001). Calcium antagonists for ischemic stroke: a systematic review. *Stroke*, **32**, 570–6.

Horn, J., de Haan, R. J., Vermeulen, M., Luiten, P. G. & Limburg, M. (2001). Nimodipine in animal model experiments of focal cerebral ischemia: a systematic review. *Stroke*, **32**, 2433–8.

Jensen, B. S. (2002). BMS-204352: a potassium channel opener developed for the treatment of stroke. *CNS Drug Rev.*, **8**, 353–60.

Kobayashi, T. & Mori, Y. (1998). Ca2+ channel antagonists and neuroprotection from cerebral ischemia. *Eur. J. Pharmacol.*, **363**, 1–15.

Koh, J.-Y. & Cotman, C. W. (1992). Programmed cell death: its possible contribution to neurotoxicity mediated by calcium channel antagonists. *Brain Res.*, **587**, 233–40.

Liss, B., Bruns, R. & Roeper, J. (1999). Alternative sulfonylurea receptor expression defines metabolic sensitivity of K-ATP channels in dopaminergic midbrain neurons. *EMBO J.*, **18**, 833–46.

Milhaud, D., Fagni, L., Bockaert, J. & Lafon-Cazal, M. (2002). Inhibition of voltage-gated Ca2+ channels by antazoline. *NeuroReport*, **13**, 1711–14.

Obrenovitch, T. P. & Urenjak, J. (1997). Actions of riluzole in animal models of CNS ischemia and trauma. *Rev. Contemp. Pharmacother.*, **8**, 227–35.

Patel, A. J. & Honore, E. (2001). Properties and modulation of mammalian 2P domain K$^+$ channels. *Trends Neurosci.*, **24**, 339–46.

Perez-Pinzon, M. A., Yenari, M. A., Sun, G. H., Kunis, D. M. & Steinberg, G. K. (1997). SNX-111, a novel, presynaptic N-type calcium channel antagonist, is neuroprotective against focal cerebral ischemia in rabbits. *J. Neurol. Sci.*, **153**, 25–31.

Riepe, M., Hori, N., Ludolph, A. C., Carpenter, D. O., Spencer, P. S. & Allen, C. N. (1992). Inhibition of energy metabolism by 3-nitropropionic acid activates ATP-sensitive potassium channels. *Brain Res.*, **586**, 61–6.

Riepe, M. W., Esclaire, F., Kasischke, K. *et al.* (1997). Increased hypoxic tolerance by chemical inhibition of oxidative phosphorylation: 'chemical preconditioning'. *J. Cereb. Blood Flow Metab.*, **17**, 257–64.

Taylor, C. P. & Meldrum, B. S. (1995). Na$^+$ channels as targets for neuroprotective drugs. *Trends Pharmacol. Sci.*, **16**, 309–16.

Urenjak, J. & Obrenovitch, T. P. (1996). Pharmacological modulation of voltage-gated Na$^+$ channels: a rational and effective strategy against ischemic brain damage. *Pharmacol. Rev.*, **48**, 21–67.

Yoo, S. E., Yi, K. Y., Lee, S. *et al.* (2001). A novel anti-ischemic ATP-sensitive potassium channel (K(ATP)) opener without vasorelaxation: *N*-(6-aminobenzopyranyl)-*N*'-benzyl-*N*''-cyanoguanidine analogue. *J. Med. Chem.*, **44**, 4207–15.

12

The role of nitric oxide and PARP in neuronal cell death

Mika Shimoji, Valina L. Dawson and Ted M. Dawson

Department of Neurology, Johns Hopkins University School of Medicine, Baltimore, MD, USA

Nitric oxide

Nitric oxide (NO) is a novel neuronal messenger molecule that is not confined to the synaptic cleft and can mediate rapid signaling by diffusing freely in three dimensions to act throughout local regions of neural tissue (Dawson & Dawson, 1998). NO can be generated in most tissues in the body and was first identified as endothelium-derived relaxing factor (EDRF) in blood vessels where it is the major regulator of vascular tone (Furchgott & Zawadzki, 1980; Palmer *et al.*, 1987; Kilbourn & Belloni, 1990; Ignarro, 1991). NO is produced by the enzymatic conversion of L-arginine to L-citrulline by nitric oxide synthase (NOS). In the NO biosynthetic scheme, L-arginine is first oxygenated to the intermediate N^G-hydroxy-L-arginine, which is then oxygenated to produce NO and L-citrulline. NO has a short half-life due to the pervasive action of superoxide (Palmer *et al.*, 1987). There are three isoforms of NOS. Two isoforms are expressed constitutively (neuronal; nNOS, endothelial; eNOS) and one that expressed only after induction (inducible; iNOS) (Fujisawa *et al.*, 1994; Chartrain *et al.*, 1994; Marsden *et al.*, 1993). Both the constitutive and inducible forms are tetrahydrobiopterin (BH_4) dependent (Tayeh & Marletta, 1989; Kwon *et al.*, 1989). The constitutive isoforms, nNOS and eNOS are Ca^{2+}/calmodulin regulated and thus NO generation is dependent on calcium signaling events. However, iNOS is Ca^{2+}/calmodulin independent and therefore NO is generated from iNOS upon protein expression. NO generation from iNOS is regulated by the duration of mRNA expression for iNOS (Dawson & Dawson, 1998). Regulation of iNOS occurs primarily at the transcriptional and translational level, once the transcriptional signal has been eliminated, iNOS message and protein are rapidly degraded (Lowenstein *et al.*, 1993).

NO can elicit such diverse cellular signaling due to a wide variety of molecular targets including soluble guanylylate cyclase, other heme-containing enzymes including cyclooxygenase, thiol moieties and tyrosine residues on proteins, iron–sulfur-containing proteins and superoxide anion. Although NO is a free radical, it is not widely reactive and has a limited chemistry restricting the potential target molecules it can modify. Signaling is thought to occur largely through nitrosylation and nitration reactions (Stamler *et al.*, 2001; Marshall *et al.*, 2000). While NO is important in normal neuronal signaling, when NO production is unregulated or excessive, NO can mediate neuronal degeneration. Many of the toxic actions of NO have been linked to the generation of peroxynitrite following the reaction with superoxide anion. NO has been implicated in the neuropathology of stroke, trauma, AIDS dementia, Alzheimer's disease, Parkinson's disease, multiple sclerosis, as well as bacterial and viral encephalitis (Dawson & Dawson, 1998).

Poly(ADP-ribose) polymerase-1

Poly(ADP-ribose) polymerase-1 (PARP-1; EC 2.4.2.30) is a nuclear zinc-finger DNA binding enzyme that facilitates DNA repair upon activation by DNA damage (Shall & de Murcia, 2000; Lautier *et al.*, 1993). DNA strand breaks, generated either directly by endogenous free radicals (i.e. oxygen radicals), exogenous DNA damaging agents (i.e. ionizing radiation, mono-functional alkylating agents) or indirectly following enzymatic incision of DNA, can trigger an acute cellular response accompanied by the synthesis of poly(ADP-ribose) by PARP-1. At the site of DNA breakage, PARP-1 catalyzes the successive transfer of ADP-ribose moiety units from its substrate, β-nicotinamide adenine dinucleotide (NAD^+), to a variety of proteins (Chambon *et al.*, 1963) including PARP-1 itself. Poly(ADP-ribose) polymers are negatively charged, therefore proteins that are poly(ADP-ribosy)lated such as those involved in chromatin structure including histones H1, H2B, high mobility group (HMG) proteins and lamin B or proteins involved in DNA metabolism lose their affinity for DNA. PARP enzyme activity has been documented in many different classes of organisms from lower eukaryotes such as *Dictyostelium discoideum* and *Crypthecodinium cohnii* (Rickwood & Osman, 1979; Werner *et al.*, 1984), to higher eukaryotes from snail, *Helix pomatia* to man (Burtscher *et al.*, 1986, 1987; Ushiro *et al.*, 1987). The nucleotide and amino acid sequence comparison among different organisms reveals 61 to 88% homology and structural conservation of functional elements (two zinc fingers, nuclear localization signal, leucine-zipper motif and NAD-binding structure) among *Drosophila melanogaster*, *Xenopus laevis*, chick, mouse, bovine and human PARP-1 (Uchida & Miwa, 1994).

PARP-1 is a very abundant enzyme with up to one PARP-1 molecule for each 1000 bp of DNA (Lautier *et al.*, 1993) or one million molecules per cell (Ludwig *et al.*, 1988; Yamanaka *et al.*, 1988) and it has a long half-life. PARP-1 is the isoform of PARP family that produces the large, branched chain polymers. It is a 113 kDa protein localized to the nucleus of all cells. PARP-1 is composed of three major domains: the NH_2-terminal region, the central auto-modification domain, and COOH-terminal region. The 42 kDa NH_2 terminal is the DNA binding domain containing two zinc fingers for DNA strand break recognition (Cherney *et al.*, 1987; Mazen *et al.*, 1989) and it contains the nuclear localization signal for targeting PARP-1 to the cell nucleus (Uchida *et al.*, 1987). The 16 kDa internal region of PARP-1 includes the auto-modification domain (Alkhatib *et al.*, 1987; Kurosaki *et al.*, 1987) containing 15 conserved glutamic acids that are presumed targets for poly(ADP-ribose) (Cherney *et al.*, 1987; Uchida *et al.*, 1987) and a BRCT (BRCA1 C terminus) domain at amino acids 384–479 (Zhang *et al.*, 1998). BRCT domains are suggested to be protein–protein interaction modules, allowing strong and specific associations with other BRCT-motif containing proteins. The 55 kDa COOH-terminal region of PARP-1 contains the NAD^+ binding site and catalytic domain, which synthesizes the poly(ADP-ribose), and is the most conserved region of the protein in all species (Ruf *et al.*, 1996; Uchida & Miwa, 1994).

PARP-1 is inactive in the absence of DNA damage or fragmentation; however, its enzymatic activity can increase 500-fold on binding to DNA fragments. PARP-1 ribosy-lates histones (Krupitza & Cerutti, 1989), topoisomereases I and II (Krupitza & Cerutti, 1989; Scovassi *et al.*, 1993), DNA-dependent protein kinase (Ruscetti *et al.*, 1998), DNA polymerase a and b (Ohashi *et al.*, 1986; Yoshihara *et al.*,

1985), DNA ligase I and II (Yoshihara *et al.*, 1985), HMG proteins (Tanuma *et al.*, 1985; Tsai *et al.*, 1992), p53 (Wesierska-Gadek *et al.*, 1996a; Wesierska-Gadek *et al.*, 1996b), and PARP-1 itself (Lautier *et al.*, 1993). PARP-1 activation following DNA damage/fragmentation is an early event and is elicited by very small amounts of DNA damage. Poly(ADP-ribosyl)ation of histones results in chromatin relaxation (Frechette *et al.*, 1985; Niedergang *et al.*, 1985). The chromatin de-condensation is restored when poly(ADP-ribose) is degraded (de Murcia *et al.*, 1986). The de-condensation of chromatin is believed to facilitate the DNA repair at sites of DNA damage and affects DNA transcription at transcription initiation sites. Auto-poly(ADP-ribosyl)ation inhibits PARP-1 activity by separating PARP-1 from DNA. The release of PARP-1 from DNA permits DNA repair enzymes access to the break points (de Murcia & Menissier de Murcia, 1994). The timing of PARP-1 attachment to and release from DNA helps to synchronize the repair process. Binding of PARP-1 to DNA may also prevent inappropriate DNA recombination by repelling other DNA molecules (Chatterjee *et al.*, 1999, de Murcia *et al.*, 1997; Morrison *et al.*, 1997; Wang *et al.*, 1997).

Activation of PARP-1 is energetically expensive, for every mole of ADP-ribose transferred from NAD^+, one mole of NAD^+ is consumed and four free energy equivalents of ATP are required to regenerate NAD^+ to normal cellular levels (Shall & de Murcia, 2000; Lautier *et al.*, 1993). Intense activation of PARP-1 can result in a rapid depletion of cellular NAD^+ and ATP (Berger, 1985; Carson *et al.*, 1986). During PARP-1 activation, it consumes up to 200 molecules of NAD^+ at each catalytic step and leads to cellular depletion of NAD^+ and ATP, decreased DNA, RNA, and protein synthesis (Berger, 1985; Carson *et al.*, 1986; Oleinick & Evans, 1985). Additionally, excessive PARP-1 activation often occurs in a setting of impaired cellular respiration and metabolism, which combined with the loss of NAD^+ and ATP may contribute to eventual cell death. This process, however, can be prevented by chemical inhibition of PARP-1 activity or PARP-1 gene deletion in mice (Pieper *et al.*, 1999b; Szabo & Dawson, 1998; Pieper *et al.*, 1999a).

PARP-1 mediated neurotoxicity is executed by apoptosis inducing factor

Studies from different laboratories link production of NO and other free radical species to PARP-1 activation and to the cell death and tissue damage after excitotoxic or immunologic insults (Smith, 2001). However, it is still uncertain how activation of PARP triggers the cell death cascade. Recent investigations indicate that excitotoxicity followed by PARP-1 activation is likely mediated via apoptosis inducing factor (AIF) and its translocation from mitochondria to the nucleus (Yu *et al.*, 2002).

AIF is a mitochondrial flavoprotein that mediates caspase-independent cell death (Ferri & Kroemer, 2001). In response to toxic stimuli, AIF initiates cell death by translocation from mitochondria to the nucleus to induce nuclear condensation and DNA fragmentation (Susin *et al.*, 1999; Joza *et al.*, 2001; Daugas *et al.*, 2000). Excitotoxic concentrations of NMDA triggers neurotoxicity that is caspase independent and PARP-1 dependent (Yu *et al.*, 2002). Following PARP-1 activation AIF translocates from mitochondria to the nucleus, preceding cytochrome c release and activation of the major execution caspase, caspase 3. The time course of AIF translocation is coincident with changes in nuclear morphology (nuclear condensation) and DNA damage (Yu *et al.*, 2002). Accompanying AIF translocation is mitochondrial membrane depolarization and phosphatidylserine exposure on the cell surface. Overexpression of Bcl-2, an anti-apoptotic protein, can delay or prevent AIF translocation and protect against PARP-1 dependent cell death (Yu *et al.*, 2002). Furthermore, neutralizing antibodies to AIF provides substantial cytoprotection against PARP-1 dependent cell death (Yu *et al.*, 2002). Taken together, these data suggest a key role for AIF in affecting caspase-independent forms of cell death in the nervous system.

Excitotoxicity and experimental stroke

NO is an important signaling molecule; however, in the presence of superoxide anion the potent neurotoxin, peroxynitrite is produced (Dawson *et al.*, 1993a). The reaction of NO with superoxide anion results in peroxynitrite that can oxidize proteins, lipids, RNA, and DNA (Beckman *et al.*, 1994a, b; Koppenol *et al.*, 1992). In particular, peroxynitrite oxidizes DNA leading to single strand breaks that trigger PARP-1 activation. There is an important link between NO formation and neurotoxic PARP-1 activation (Zhang *et al.*, 1994). Brain extracts treated with NO results in ADP-ribosylation of PARP-1 (Zhang *et al.*, 1994).

In cerebral cortical cultures and primary brain cultures excess stimulation of glutamate receptors results in excitotoxicity. NO-mediated excitotoxicity occurs primarily through activation of the *N*-methyl-D-aspartate (NMDA) subtype of glutamate receptors. nNOS is physically coupled to the NMDA receptor via postsynaptic density 95 protein (PSD95) (Christopherson *et al.*, 1999). Disruption of this interaction results in loss of NO production and rescue from excitotoxic and ischemic cell death (Sattler *et al.*, 1999; Aarts *et al.*, 2002). Pharmacological inhibition of nNOS or genetic deletion of nNOS provides neuroprotection. Exposure of cerebral cortical cultures to chemical donors of NO also results in neurotoxicity (Dawson *et al.*, 1991, 1993a). Exposure to superoxide dismutase (SOD) reduced NMDA and NO neurotoxicity implicating superoxide anion and peroxynitrite formation in excitotoxicity. These findings in cell culture have been extended into whole animals. In the nNOS knockout mice experimental stroke damage is diminished in male mice (Huang *et al.*, 1994), and NOS inhibitors reduce stroke damage to a similar extent as glutamate antagonists (Samdani *et al.*, 1997). Although nNOS knockout mice are very resistant to focal and global ischemia (Hara *et al.*, 1996; Panahian *et al.*, 1996), the resistance to ischemia diminishes with non-specific NOS inhibitors treatment (Dalkara & Moskowitz, 1997). In part this is due to non-specific inhibition of eNOS. Regulation of cerebral blood flow is critically dependent on NO generated by eNOS. Infarct volume is increased in eNOS knockout mice, and this injury is reduced following treatment with NOS inhibitors (Huang *et al.*, 1996). Thus, NO derived from nNOS mediates neurotoxicity following focal ischemia, while NO derived from eNOS is important in maintaining cerebral blood flow and has a protective role in focal ischemia (Moskowitz & Dalkara, 1996).

Although peroxynitrite can oxidize most cellular constituents including proteins, lipids, RNA and DNA, it is its actions on damaging DNA and activating PARP-1 that appears to be the primary mechanism of triggering neurotoxicity. Primary cortical cultures treated with pharmacologic antagonists of PARP are resistant to exposure to neurotoxic concentrations of NMDA, NO or oxygen-glucose deprivation (Eliasson *et al.*, 1997; Zhang *et al.*, 1994). Similarly, cultures generated from PARP-1 null mice are also resistant to these toxic insults (Eliasson *et al.*, 1997). In the transient middle cerebral artery occlusion experimental mouse model of stroke, PARP-1 knockout mice show 78% decrease and PARP-1 heterozygous mice show 65% decrease in ischemic tissue damage as compared to wild-type mice (Eliasson *et al.*, 1997). Similarly, the potent PARP inhibitor, 3,4-dihydro-5-[4-(1-piperidinyl)butox]-1(2H)-isoquinolinone (DPQ), protects against experimental stroke damage in rats (Takahashi *et al.*, 1999). A role for PARP activation in human stroke is suggested by the observation of elevated levels of poly(ADP-ribose) in patients who suffered global cerebral ischemia after cardiac arrest when compared with matched controls (Love *et al.*, 1999b).

Parkinson's disease

Some of the neuropathology of Parkinson's disease can be elicited by selective destruction of dopamine (DA) neurons of substantia nigra (SN) following administration of the neurotoxin, 1-methyl-4-penyl-1,2,3,6-tetrahydropyridine (MPTP) in primates and rodent animal models (Burns et al., 1983; Lau et al., 1990; Petroske et al., 2001). The neurotoxic effect of MPTP that results in the parkinsonian syndrome was first discovered in the intravenous drug user community in early 1980s (Langston et al., 1983). MPTP is a highly lipophilic chemical that can easily cross the blood–brain barrier; however, MPTP itself is not toxic in the brain. Once MPTP is inside the brain, it is taken up by astrocytes and metabolized to MPDP$^+$ by monoamine oxidase B (MAO-B) (Chiba et al., 1984; Markey et al., 1984) then oxidized to MPP$^+$. MPP$^+$ is then released to the extracellular space and taken up selectively and actively by the high affinity DA transporter and accumulated in DA neurons (Chiba et al., 1985; Javitch et al., 1985). In DA neurons MPP$^+$ accumulates in mitochondria via energy driven uptake (Singer et al., 1987), where it binds to complex I (Nicklas et al., 1985; Ramsay et al., 1991) and disrupts the NAD-linked mitochondrial respiratory chain. This disturbance in mitochondrial respiration results in a decrease in ATP production and an increase in superoxide anion formation in DA neurons (Ramsay & Singer, 1992). The increase in superoxide anion formation can lead to formation of peroxynitrite, further inhibition of mitochondrial function by damaging MnSOD activity (MacMillan-Crow et al., 1996), and more superoxide formation, starting a self-destructive cycle of events. Peroxynitrite can also damage DNA leading to PARP activation (Zhang et al., 1994, 1995), loss of energy and possibly AIF translocation. Preliminary data suggest that AIF translocates following MPTP intoxication. Consistent with the hypothesis that DA neurons dies via this pathway following MPTP intoxication are the findings that nNOS, iNOS and PARP-1 knockout mice are resistant to MPTP neurotoxicity (Przedborski et al., 1996; Liberatore et al., 1999; Mandir et al., 1999).

Aggregated alpha-synuclein is a major component of Lewy bodies, which are the histochemical hallmarks of Parkinson's disease. In vitro, exposure of human recombinant alpha-synuclein to peroxynitrite induces formation of highly stable nitrated alpha-synuclein oligomers and nitrated pre-assembled alpha-synuclein filaments leads to the formation of high molecular mass aggregates (Souza et al., 2000). Nitration of alpha-synuclein also occurs in the mouse striatum and ventral midbrain following intoxication with MPTP (Przedborski et al., 2001). In human postmortem tissue nitrated alpha-synuclein is present in Lewy bodies from patients with Parkinson's disease (Giasson et al., 2000). Taken together, these findings support the hypothesis that NO plays a major role in the neurodegeneration and neurotoxicity of Parkinson's disease.

Inflammatory neurodegenerative diseases

Acquired immunodeficiency syndrome patients often present with neurological symptoms and cognitive impairment that is sometimes associated with pronounced cortical atrophy (Navia et al., 1986; Atwood et al., 1993; Power & Johnson, 1995). However, the localization of the HIV virus in the CNS is almost exclusively in macrophages, microglia and multi-nucleated giant cells (Takahashi et al., 1996; Wiley et al., 1986). First, it was suggested that this atrophy was caused indirectly by toxic effects of HIV coat protein, gp120 (Lipton, 1992) activating glutamate excitotoxicity through a NMDA receptor/nNOS pathway (Dawson et al., 1993b). However, local inflammatory responses including expression of cytokines and iNOS are a consistent observation in human tissue. In HIV-associated dementia, the HIV coat protein gp41 may be the molecule that significantly contributes to the induction of iNOS and other inflammatory molecules leading to the production of NO and subsequent neuronal cell death/tissue atrophy (Adamson et al., 1996). There is evidence of increased iNOS mRNA expression and protein level in cortical brain tissues of HIV patients with severe HIV-1 dementia that correlates with the levels of HIV-1 coat protein gp41, but not gp120 (Adamson et al., 1996). Gp41 can induce iNOS in mixed neural cultures to trigger neuronal cell death in a NO-dependent manner. Neuronal cultures from iNOS knockout mice are resistant to gp41 neurotoxicity (Adamson et al., 1999). The actions of gp41 are specific to the N-terminal region of gp41, which induces iNOS protein activity and iNOS-dependent neurotoxicity at picomolar concentrations in a manner similar to recombinant gp41 (Adamson et al., 1999).

Alzheimer's disease is a progressive dementing neurologic disorder, and the most frequent cause of dementia in the elderly. Pathologically, Alzheimer's disease is characterized by excessive deposition of the protein beta-amyloid and the formation of neuritic plaques and tangles. A striking feature of neuritic plaques is the presence of activated microglia, cytokines, and complement components, suggestive of "inflammatory foci" within Alzheimer's disease brain (Butterfield et al., 2002). Included in these inflammatory foci is the expression of iNOS and markers of increased oxidation (Luth et al., 2001; Heneka et al., 2001; Floyd, 1999) implicating expression of iNOS and NO as a contributory factor in the pathogenesis of Alzheimer's disease. Although it is not clear by which mechanism PARP-1 might play a role in Alzheimer's disease, study of postmortem tissue reveals increased poly(ADP-ribose) levels in brains of Alzheimer's disease patients implicating PARP activation in neuronal cell loss in this disorder (Love *et al.*, 1999a).

Nitric oxide (NO) has been implicated as a pathogenic mediator in central nervous system demylinating disease states, including multiple sclerosis and the animal model of experimental allergic encephalomyelitis. Induction of iNOS occurs in active demyelinating regions in brains of patients with multiple sclerosis (Liu *et al.*, 2001; Bo *et al.*, 1994; Bagasra *et al.*, 1995; De Groot *et al.*, 1997). Induction of iNOS is observed in experimental allergic encephalomyelitis (Lin *et al.*, 1993; Parkinson *et al.*, 1997; Gold *et al.*, 1997; Cross *et al.*, 1997; Sun *et al.*, 1998). Experimental induction of iNOS is toxic to neurons (Dawson *et al.*, 1994) and to the myelin producing oligodendrocytes (Merrill *et al.*, 1993). NO generated from iNOS may contribute significantly to the cytotoxicity of oligodendrocytes and destruction of myelin in brain and spinal cord in patients suffering from multiple sclerosis.

Inhibitors of nitric oxide synthase

Although there are three structurally distinct isoforms of NOS: neuronal (nNOS), endothelial (eNOS) and inducible (iNOS), the catalytic domains of these proteins are similar which has hampered development of selective agents. Since overactivation of nNOS and iNOS are injurious to the nervous system but eNOS is critical for the maintenance of cerebral blood flow, the development of selective agents is critical for the successful therapeutic use of NOS inhibitors for the treatment of neurologic disease. However, information on the enzyme structure at all levels from the primary to quaternary structure may facilitate the development of selective therapeutic tools (Alderton *et al.*, 2001). The NOS enzymes are dimers in their active form, although they require calmodulin at each subunit and therefore could be considered tetramers (two NOS monomers associated with two calmodulins). They contain tightly bound cofactors including: (6R)-5,6,7,8-tetrahydrobiopterin, FAD, FMN and iron protoporphyrin IX (heme). *In situ*, NOSs are regulated by cofactor binding or expression, phosphorylation, localization, protein–protein interactions, myristoylation, and palmitoylation. Most pharmacologic development, however, has focused on generating agents active towards the catalytic domain. Unfortunately, a comparison of human eNOS and iNOS oxygenase structures reveals them to be very similar in overall molecular shape, relative orientation of cofactors

and stereochemistry within the catalytic center and so it is not obvious from a structural starting point how selective inhibitors may be designed. There are numerous NOS inhibitors described in the literature and used as pharmacological tools. The most widely used have been L-NMMA, L-NNA, NG-nitro-L-arginine methyl ester (L-NAME) and aminoguanidine. These agents are commercially available and have good tissue penetration, however, they are generally non-specific and so experimental data must be interpreted with caution. There is currently no consideration for the use of these agents in the clinic. The general classes of inhibitors are arginine analogs, thiocitrullines, indazoles, substituted guanidoamines, thioureas and noncompetitive agents. Specificity has been assigned by small differences in potency for inhibiting one isoform over another, apparent in vivo selectivity due to bioavailability (such as the case for 7-nitroindazol), or differences in the time course to inhibit the difference enzymes. Unfortunately, most inhibitors are relatively non-selective to NOS isoform. The identification of selective inhibitors of iNOS and nNOS has been a goal of both academic and pharmaceutical scientists. The observation of very high structural homology between the catalytic and regulatory domains of the three isoforms has led to concern about whether selective inhibition is feasible. Recently, there have been reports of agents that are selective for iNOS/nNOS over eNOS and some agents that are highly selective for iNOS. These sulfur-substituted acetamidine amino acids (GW273629 and GW274150) are an advance over previously reported iNOS selective inhibitors in that they have tissue penetration and are not acutely toxic (Alderton *et al.*, 2001). There are still many questions regarding the biology of NOS isoforms that may shed light on the development of selective agents. Are there post-translational modifications that are significantly different in the regulation of the three isoforms that can be capitalized on? What is the significance and basis of the subcellular localization of the NOSs? Where are splice variants of the NOS isoforms expressed and do they have biologic significance in disease states? What is the molecular and structural basis of the high isoform selectivity of some NOS inhibitors? If selective iNOS, nNOS or dual iNOS/nNOS inhibitors can be identified, it is expected that they will prove to be of value in the treatment of human diseases.

PARP inhibitors

Development of neuroprotective PARP inhibitors faces additional challenges because activation of PARP has dual effects on the survival or death of cells. Comprehending the complex role of PARP in the cell death process is important to understanding how PARP inhibition can protect from or enhance cytotoxicity depending on the nature and severity of DNA damage. The exact mechanism of how PARP activation promotes cell death in certain systems or protects from cytotoxicity in others requires further investigation. The nature of genotoxic stimuli (oxidative stress, alkylating agents, ionizing radiation, etc.) and cellular metabolism are usually considered to be key factors in determining the role of poly(ADP-ribosylation) in the cell death process. Depending on the intensity of the stimulus, genotoxic agents can trigger three different pathways. In the case of mild DNA damage, poly(ADP-ribosylation) facilitates DNA repair and thus survival. Increasing DNA damage may activate the p53-dependent (or possibly independent) apoptotic pathway(s). The most severe DNA damage may cause excessive PARP activation, depleting cellular NAD^+/ATP stores and resulting in necrotic-like cell death. Inhibiting PARP in cells that are attempting DNA repair will send the cells into apoptosis however, inhibiting PARP in cells that are undergoing cell death may facilitate their survival.

The prototype PARP inhibitors include nicotinamide, benzamide and 3-aminobenzamide that have long served as experimental agents suitable for laboratory investigations. These compounds inhibit the enzyme with a low potency, have limited cell uptake and have a short half-life. Additionally, these agents are non-specific to PARP isoform as well as exhibiting other non-specific effects, including acting as antioxidants. Recently, several other classes of more potent and selective PARP inhibitors have been synthesized. Most PARP inhibitors fall into the categories of monoaryl amides and bi-, tri-, or tetracyclic lactams. Most PARP inhibitors are designed as competitive inhibitors blocking the NAD^+ binding site in the catalytic domain. 3,4-dihydro-5-methyl-isoquinolin-1(2H)-one, benzoxazole-4-carboxamide, dihydroisoquinolin-1(2H)-nones, 1,6-naphthyridine-5(6H)-ones, quinazolin-4(3H)-ones, thieno[3,4-c]pyridin-4(5H)ones and thieno[3,4-d]pyrimidin-4(3H)ones, 1,5-dihydroxyisoquinoline, and 2-methyl-quinazolin-4[3H]-one are potent and relatively selective inhibitors of PARP. Their isoform selectivity is not yet known. 1,8-Naphthalimide derivatives and (5H)-phenanthridin-6-ones are new PARP inhibitors represented by PJ34 and GPI 6150. These agents have been shown to be effective in limiting injury in experimental rodent models of focal cerebral ischemia, traumatic brain injury, 1-methyl-4-phenyl-1,2,3,6-tetrahydropyridine (MPTP)-induced damage to dopaminergic neurons, regional myocardial ischemia, streptozotocin-induced diabetes, septic shock, and arthritis. PARP inhibitors have been shown not only to block early neuronal injury elicited in large part by excitotoxic cascades but to also limit inflammatory reactions. This secondary effect of PARP inhibitors may prevent the secondary injury seen in many neurological diseases due to activation of local inflammation around the site of injury. Inhibition of PARP will be most important in disease states where inflammatory activation is augmented in systems by MAP kinase activation and NF-kB translocation resulting from free-radical and oxidant formation. In the nervous system PARP inhibitors have the potential to protect against two different types of insult triggered by a single disease trigger thus eliciting a greater overall protection than anti-excitotoxic or anti-inflammatory approaches alone. The marked protection achieved with various PARP inhibitors in animal models of many different diseases suggests that PARP inhibitors can be developed to treat human diseases. However, before PARP inhibitors can be used in humans, certain safety issues should be addressed to determine under what conditions PARP inhibition should be advised. Because PARP has been implicated in DNA repair and maintenance of genomic integrity, one possible risk associated with long-term PARP inhibition might be increased mutation rate and cancer formation. While this will not be a concern for the treatment of acute neurological injuries such as stroke, for chronic neurodegenerative disorders such as Parkinson's disease, this might be a serious consideration. The risk–benefit ratios associated with the development of PARP inhibitors for therapeutic purposes is not yet known, yet this class of therapeutic agents holds promise for the treatment of neurologic diseases.

In the initiation phase of neurotoxicity, activation of NMDA glutamate receptors leads to increased intracellular calcium that activates neuronal nitric oxide synthase (nNOS) producing nitric oxide (NO) (Fig. 12.1). Neuronal activation will also result in increased oxidative phosphorylation and subsequently increased superoxide anion production. Superoxide anion production can also be elevated by complex 1 inhibition with chemicals such as MPTP, rotenone or paraquat and decrements in complex 1 are observed in Parkinson's patients. Superoxide is not membrane permeable and resides largely in the mitochondria where it is generated. NO and superoxide anion react to form the potent oxidant, peroxynitrite. Peroxynitrite generation can trigger an amplification phase of neurotoxicity by attacking mitochondrial proteins in the electron transport chain including complex I and IV as well as the superoxide scavenging enzyme, manganese superoxide

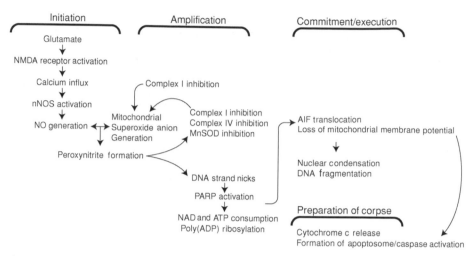

Fig. 12.1 Model of nitric oxide, poly (ADP-ribose) polymerase mediated neuronal cell death.

dismutase (MnSOD). This initiates a viscous cycle of per-oxynitrite generation through sustained superoxide anion generation. Peroxynitrite is membrane permeable and can move to the nucleus triggering DNA strand breaks. Damaged DNA activates poly (ADP-Ribose) polymerase (PARP) resulting in the synthesis of PAR polymers, ribosylation of proteins and consumption of NAD and ATP. These PARP dependent events signal to the mitochondria to release apoptosis inducing factor (AIF) that translocate to the nucleus. In the nucleus AIF triggers large-scale DNA fragmentation and nuclear condensation. These nuclear changes in neurons are likely to be the final commitment and execution point in the neurotoxic cascade. Subsequent to these events Cytochrome c is released and caspases are activated. Blocking these events does not prevent NO/PARP dependent neurotoxicity but may be important in preparation of the corpse and the degradation of the cell.

REFERENCES

Aarts, M., Liu, Y., Liu, L. *et al.* (2002). Treatment of ischemic brain damage by perturbing NMDA receptor– PSD-95 protein interactions. *Science*, **298**, 846–50.

Adamson, D. C., Wildemann, B., Sasaki, M. *et al.* (1996). Immunologic NO synthase: elevation in severe AIDS dementia and induction by HIV-1 gp41. *Science*, **274**, 1917–21.

Adamson, D. C., McArthur, J. C., Dawson, T. M. & Dawson, V. L. (1999a). Course of HIV-Associated Dementia: Correlation's with gp41, iNOS and Macrophage/Microglial Activation. *Mol. Med.*, **5**, 98–109.

Adamson, D. C., Kopnisky, K. L., Dawson, T. M. & Dawson, V. L. (1999b). Mechanisms and structural determinants of HIV-1

coat protein, gp41-induced neurotoxicity. *J. Neurosci.*, **19**, 64–71.

Alderton, W. K., Cooper, C. E. & Knowles, R. G. (2001). Nitric oxide synthases: structure, function and inhibition. *Biochem. J.*, **357**, 593–615.

Alkhatib, H. M., Chen, D. F., Cherney, B. *et al.* (1987). Cloning and expression of cDNA for human poly(ADP-ribose) polymerase. *Proc. Nat. Acad. Sci., USA*, **84**, 1224–8.

Atwood, W. J., Berger, J. R., Kaderman, R., Tornatore, C. S. & Major, E. O. (1993). Human immunodeficiency virus type 1 infection of the brain. *Clin. Microbiol. Rev.*, **6**, 339–66.

Bagasra, O., Michaels, F. H., Zheng *et al.* (1995). Activation of the inducible form of nitric oxide synthase in the brains of patients with multiple sclerosis. *Proc. Natl Acad. Sci., USA*, **92**, 12041–5.

Beckman, J. S., Chen, J., Crow, J. P. & Ye, Y. Z. (1994a). Reactions of nitric oxide, superoxide and peroxynitrite with superoxide dismutase in neurodegeneration. *Prog. Brain. Res.*, **103**, 371–80.

Beckman, J. S., Chen, J., Ischiropoulos, H. & Crow, J. P. (1994b). Oxidative chemistry of peroxynitrite. *Methods Enzymol.*, **233**, 229–40.

Berger, N. A. (1985). Poly(ADP-ribose) in the cellular response to DNA damage. *Radiat. Res.*, **101**, 4–15.

Bo, L., Dawson, T. M., Wesselingh, S. *et al.* (1994). Induction of nitric oxide synthase in demyelinating regions of multiple sclerosis brains. *Ann. Neurol.*, **36**, 778–86.

Burns, R. S., Chiueh, C. C., Markey, S. R., Ebert, M. H., Jacobowitz, D. M., & Kopin, I. J. (1983). A primate model of parkinsonism: selective destruction of dopaminergic neurons in the pars compacta of the substantia nigra by *N*-methyl-4-phenyl-1, 2, 3, 6-tetrahydropyridine. *Proc. Natl Acad. Sci. USA*, **80** (14), 4546–50.

Burtscher, H. J., Auer, B., Klocker, H., Schweiger, M. & Hirsch-Kauffmann, M. (1986). Isolation of ADP-ribosyltransferase by affinity chromatography. *Anal. Biochem.*, **152**, 285–90.

Burtscher, H. J., Klocker, H., Schneider, R., Auer, B., Hirsch-Kauffmann, M. & Schweiger, M. (1987). ADP-ribosyltransferase from Helix pomatia. Purification and characterization. *Biochem. J.*, **248**, 859–64.

Butterfield, D. A., Griffin, S., Munch, G. & Pasinetti, G. M. (2002). Amyloid beta-peptide and amyloid pathology are central to the oxidative stress and inflammatory cascades under which Alzheimer's disease brain exists. *J. Alzheimers Dis.*, **4**, 193–201.

Carson, D. A., Seto, S., Wasson, D. B. & Carrera, C. J. (1986). DNA strand breaks, NAD metabolism, and programmed cell death. *Exp. Cell. Res.*, **164**, 273–81.

Chambon, P., Weill, J. D. & Mandel, P. (1963). Nicotinamide mononucleotide activation of new DNA-dependent polyadenylic acid synthesizing nuclear enzyme. *Biochem. Biophys. Res. Commun.*, **11**, 39–43.

Chartrain, N. A., Geller, D. A., Koty, P. P. et al. (1994). Molecular cloning, structure, and chromosomal localization of the human inducible nitric oxide synthase gene. *J. Biol. Chem.*, **269**, 6765–72.

Chatterjee, S., Berger, S. J. & Berger, N. A. (1999). Poly(ADP-ribose) polymerase: a guardian of the genome that facilitates DNA repair by protecting against DNA recombination. *Mol. Cell. Biochem.*, **193**, 23–30.

Cherney, B. W., McBride, O. W., Chen, D. F. et al. (1987). cDNA sequence, protein structure, and chromosomal location of the human gene for poly(ADP-ribose) polymerase. *Proc. Natl Acad. Sci., USA*, **84**, 8370–4.

Chiba, K., Trevor, A. & Castagnoli, N., Jr. (1984). Metabolism of the neurotoxic tertiary amine, MPTP, by brain monoamine oxidase. *Biochem. Biophys. Res. Commun.*, **120**, 574–8.

Chiba, K., Trevor, A. J. & Castagnoli, N., Jr. (1985). Active uptake of MPP⁺, a metabolite of MPTP, by brain synaptosomes. *Biochem. Biophys. Res. Commun.*, **128**, 1228–32.

Christopherson, K. S., Hillier, B. J., Lim, W. A. & Bredt, D. S. (1999). PSD-95 assembles a ternary complex with the *N*-methyl-D-aspartic acid receptor and a bivalent neuronal NO synthase PDZ domain. *J. Biol. Chem.*, **274**, 27467–73.

Cross, A. H., Manning, P. T., Stern, M. K. & Misko, T. P. (1997). Evidence for the production of peroxynitrite in inflammatory CNS demyelination. *J. Neuroimmunol.*, **80**, 121–30.

Dalkara, T. & Moskowitz, M. A. (1997). Neurotoxic and neuroprotective roles of nitric oxide in cerebral ischaemia. *Int. Rev. Neurobiol.*, **40**, 319–36.

Daugas, E., Susin, S. A., Zamzami, N. et al. (2000). Mitochondrio-nuclear translocation of AIF in apoptosis and necrosis. *FASEB J.*, **14**, 729–39.

Dawson, V. L. & Dawson, T. M. (1998). Nitric oxide in neurodegeneration. *Prog. Brain Res.*, **118**, 215–29.

Dawson, V. L., Dawson, T. M., London, E. D., Bredt, D. S. & Snyder, S. H. (1991). Nitric oxide mediates glutamate neurotoxicity in primary cortical cultures. *Proc. Natl Acad. Sci., USA*, **88**, 6368–71.

Dawson, V. L., Dawson, T. M., Bartley, D. A., Uhl, G. R. & Snyder, S. H. (1993a). Mechanisms of nitric oxide-mediated neurotoxicity in primary brain cultures. *J. Neurosci.*, **13**, 2651–61.

Dawson, V. L., Dawson, T. M., Uhl, G. R. & Snyder, S. H. (1993b). Human immunodeficiency virus type 1 coat protein neurotoxicity mediated by nitric oxide in primary cortical cultures. *Proc. Natl Acad. Sci., USA*, **90**, 3256–9.

Dawson, V. L., Brahmbhatt, H. P., Mong, J. A. & Dawson, T. M. (1994). Expression of inducible nitric oxide synthase causes delayed neurotoxicity in primary mixed neuronal-glial cortical cultures. *Neuropharmacology*, **33**, 1425–30.

De Groot, C. J., Ruuls, S. R., Theeuwes, J. W., Dijkstra, C. D. & Van der Valk, P. (1997). Immunocytochemical characterization of the expression of inducible and constitutive isoforms of nitric oxide synthase in demyelinating multiple sclerosis lesions. *J. Neuropathol. Exp. Neurol.*, **56**, 10–20.

de Murcia, G., Huletsky, A., Lamarre, D. et al. (1986). Modulation of chromatin superstructure induced by poly(ADP-ribose) synthesis and degradation. *J. Biol. Chem.*, **261**, 7011–7.

de Murcia, G. & Menissier de Murcia, J. (1994). Poly(ADP-ribose) polymerase: a molecular nick-sensor. *Trends Biochem. Sci.*, **19**, 172–6.

de Murcia, J. M., Niedergang, C. Trucco, C. et al. (1997). Requirement of poly(ADP-ribose) polymerase in recovery from DNA damage in mice and in cells. *Proc. Natl Acad. Sci., USA*, **94**, 7303–7.

Eliasson, M. J., Sampei, K., Mandir, A. S. et al. (1997). Poly(ADP-ribose) polymerase gene disruption renders mice resistant to cerebral ischemia. *Nat. Med.*, **3**, 1089–95.

Ferri, K. F. & Kroemer, G. (2001). Organelle-specific initiation of cell death pathways. *Nat. Cell. Biol.*, **3**, E255–63.

Floyd, R. A. (1999). Antioxidants, oxidative stress, and degenerative neurological disorders. *Proc. Soc. Exp. Biol. Med.*, **222**, 236–45.

Frechette, A., Huletsky, A., Aubin, R. J. et al. (1985). Poly(ADP-ribosyl)ation of chromatin: kinetics of relaxation and its effect on chromatin solubility. *Can. J. Biochem. Cell. Biol.*, **63**, 764–73.

Fujisawa, H., Ogura, T., Kurashima, Y., Yokoyama, T., Yamashita, J. & Esumi, H. (1994). Expression of two types of nitric oxide synthase mRNA in human neuroblastoma cell lines. *J. Neurochem.*, **63**, 140–5.

Furchgott, R. F. & Zawadzki, J. V. (1980). The obligatory role of endothelial cells in the relaxation of arterial smooth muscle by acetylcholine. *Nature*, **288**, 373–6.

Giasson, B. I., Duda, J. E., Murray, I. V. et al. (2000). Oxidative damage linked to neurodegeneration by selective alpha-synuclein nitration in synucleinopathy lesions. *Science*, **290**, 985–9.

Gold, D. P., Schroder, K., Powell, H. C. & Kelly, C. J. (1997). Nitric oxide and the immunomodulation of experimental allergic encephalomyelitis. *Eur. J. Immunol.*, **27**, 2863–9.

Hara, H., Huang, P. L., Panahian, N., Fishman, M. C. & Moskowitz, M. A. (1996). Reduced brain edema and infarction volume in mice lacking the neuronal isoform of nitric oxide synthase after transient MCA occlusion. *J. Cereb. Blood Flow Metab.*, **16** (4), 605–11.

Heneka, M. T., Wiesinger, H., Dumitrescu-Ozimek, L., Riederer, P., Feinstein, D. L. & Klockgether, T. (2001). Neuronal and glial coexpression of argininosuccinate synthetase and inducible nitric oxide synthase in Alzheimer disease. *J. Neuropathol. Exp. Neurol.*, **60**, 906–16.

Huang, Z., Huang, P. L., Panahian, N., Dalkara, T., Fishman, M. C. & Moskowitz, M. A. (1994). Effects of cerebral ischemia in mice deficient in neuronal nitric oxide synthase. *Science*, **265**, 1883–5.

Huang, Z., Huang, P. L., Ma, J. *et al.* (1996). Enlarged infarcts in endothelial nitric oxide synthase knockout mice are attenuated by nitro-L-arginine. *J. Cereb. Blood Flow Metab.*, **16**, 981–7.

Ignarro, L. J. (1991). Signal transduction mechanisms involving nitric oxide. *Biochem. Pharmacol.*, **41**, 485–90.

Javitch, J. A., D'Amato, R. J., Strittmatter, S. M. & Snyder, S. H. (1985). Parkinsonism-inducing neurotoxin, *N*-methyl-4-phenyl-1, 2, 3, 6-tetrahydropyridine: uptake of the metabolite *N*-methyl-4-phenylpyridine by dopamine neurons explains selective toxicity. *Proc. Natl Acad. Sci., USA*, **82**, 2173–7.

Joza, N., Susin, S. A., Daugas, E. *et al.* (2001). Essential role of the mitochondrial apoptosis-inducing factor in programmed cell death. *Nature*, **410**, 549–54.

Kilbourn, R. G. & Belloni, P. (1990). Endothelial cell production of nitrogen oxides in response to interferon gamma in combination with tumor necrosis factor, interleukin-1, or endotoxin. *J. Natl Cancer Inst.*, **82**, 772–6.

Koppenol, W. H., Moreno, J. J., Pryor, W. A., Ischiropoulos, H. & Beckman, J. S. (1992). Peroxynitrite, a cloaked oxidant formed by nitric oxide and superoxide. *Chem. Res. Toxicol.*, **5**, 834–42.

Krupitza, G. & Cerutti, P. (1989). Poly(ADP-ribosylation) of histones in intact human keratinocytes. *Biochemistry*, **28**, 4054–60.

Kurosaki, T., Ushiro, H., Mitsuuchi, Y. *et al.* (1987). Primary structure of human poly(ADP-ribose) synthetase as deduced from cDNA sequence. *J. Biol. Chem.*, **262**, 15990–7.

Kwon, N. S., Nathan, C. F. & Stuehr, D. J. (1989). Reduced biopterin as a cofactor in the generation of nitrogen oxides by murine macrophages. *J. Biol. Chem.*, **264**, 20496–501.

Langston, J. W., Ballard, P. A., Tetrud, J. W. & Irwin, I. (1983). Chronic Parkinsonism in humans due to a product of meperidine-analog synthesis. *Science*, **219**, 979–80.

Lau, Y. S., Trobough, K. L., Crampton, J. M. & Wilson, J. A. (1990). Effects of probenecid on striatal dopamine depletion in acute and long-term 1-methyl-4-phenyl-1, 2, 3, 6-tetrahydropyridine (MPTP)-treated mice. *Gen. Pharmacol.*, **21** (2), 181–7.

Lautier, D., Lagueux, J., Thibodeau, J., Menard, L. & Poirier, G. G. (1993). Molecular and biochemical features of poly (ADP-ribose) metabolism. *Mol. Cell. Biochem.*, **122**, 171–93.

Liberatore, G. T., Jackson-Lewis, V., Vukosavic, S. *et al.* (1999). Inducible nitric oxide synthase stimulates dopaminergic neurodegeneration in the MPTP model of Parkinson disease. *Nat. Med.*, **5**, 1403–9.

Lin, R. F., Lin, T. S., Tilton, R. G. & Cross, A. H. (1993). Nitric oxide localized to spinal cords of mice with experimental allergic encephalomyelitis: an electron paramagnetic resonance study. *J. Exp. Med.*, **178**, 643–8.

Lipton, S. A. (1992). Memantine prevents HIV coat protein-induced neuronal injury in vitro. *Neurology*, **42**, 1403–5.

Liu, J. S., Zhao, M. L., Brosnan, C. F. & Lee, S. C. (2001). Expression of inducible nitric oxide synthase and nitrotyrosine in multiple sclerosis lesions. *Am. J. Pathol.*, **158**, 2057–66.

Love, S., Barber, R. & Wilcock, G. K. (1999a). Increased poly(ADP-ribosyl)ation of nuclear proteins in Alzheimer's disease. *Brain*, **122** (2), 247–53.

Love, S., Barber, R. & Wilcock, G. K. (1999b). Neuronal accumulation of poly(ADP-ribose) after brain ischaemia. *Neuropathol. Appl. Neurobiol.*, **25**, 98–103.

Lowenstein, C. J., Alley, E. W., Raval, P. *et al.* (1993). Macrophage nitric oxide synthase gene: two upstream regions mediate induction by interferon gamma and lipopolysaccharide. *Proc. Natl Acad. Sci., USA*, **90**, 9730–4.

Ludwig, A., Behnke, B., Holtlund, J. & Hilz, H. (1988). Immunoquantitation and size determination of intrinsic poly(ADP-ribose) polymerase from acid precipitates. An analysis of the in vivo status in mammalian species and in lower eukaryotes. *J. Biol. Chem.*, **263**, 6993–9.

Luth, H. J., Holzer, M., Gartner, U., Staufenbiel, M. & Arendt, T. (2001). Expression of endothelial and inducible NOS-isoforms is increased in Alzheimer's disease, in APP23 transgenic mice and after experimental brain lesion in rat: evidence for an induction by amyloid pathology. *Brain Res.*, **913**, 57–67.

MacMillan-Crow, L. A., Crow, J. P., Kerby, J. D., Beckman, J. S. & Thompson, J. A. (1996). Nitration and inactivation of manganese superoxide dismutase in chronic rejection of human renal allografts. *Proc. Natl Acad. Sci., USA*, **93**, 11853–8.

Mandir, A. S., Przedborski, S., Jackson-Lewis, V. *et al.* (1999). Poly(ADP-ribose) polymerase activation mediates 1-methyl-4-phenyl-1,2,3,6-tetrahydropyridine (MPTP)-induced parkinsonism. *Proc. Natl Acad. Sci., USA*, **96**, 5774–9.

Markey, S. P., Johannessen, J. N., Chiueh, C. C., Burns, R. S. & Herkenham, M. A. (1984). Intraneuronal generation of a pyridinium metabolite may cause drug-induced parkinsonism. *Nature*, **311**, 464–7.

Marsden, P. A., Heng, H. H., Scherer, S. W. *et al.* (1993). Structure and chromosomal localization of the human constitutive endothelial nitric oxide synthase gene. *J. Biol. Chem.*, **268**, 17478–88.

Marshall, H. E., Merchant, K. & Stamler, J. S. (2000). Nitrosation and oxidation in the regulation of gene expression. *FASEB J.*, **14**, 1889–900.

Mazen, A., Menissier-de Murcia, J., Molinete, M. *et al.* (1989). Poly(ADP-ribose)polymerase: a novel finger protein. *Nucl. Acids Res.*, **17**, 4689–98.

Merrill, J. E., Ignarro, L. J., Sherman, M. P., Melinek, J. & Lane, T. E. (1993). Microglial cell cytotoxicity of oligodendrocytes is mediated through nitric oxide. *J. Immunol.*, **151**, 2132–41.

Morrison, C., Smith, G. C., Stingl, L., Jackson, S. P., Wagner, E. F. & Wang, Z. Q. (1997). Genetic interaction between PARP and DNA-PK in V(D)J recombination and tumorigenesis. *Nat. Genet.*, **17**, 479–82.

Moskowitz, M. A. & Dalkara, T. (1996). Nitric oxide and cerebral ischemia. *Adv. Neurol.*, **71**, 365–7; discussion 367–9.

Navia, B. A., Jordan, B. D. & Price, R. W. (1986). The AIDS dementia complex: I. Clinical features. *Ann. Neurol.*, **19**, 517–24.

Nicklas, W. J., Vyas, I. & Heikkila, R. E. (1985). Inhibition of NADH-linked oxidation in brain mitochondria by 1-methyl-4-phenyl-pyridine, a metabolite of the neurotoxin, 1-methyl-4-phenyl-1,2,5,6-tetrahydropyridine. *Life Sci.*, **36**, 2503–8.

Niedergang, C. P., de Murcia, G., Ittel, M. E., Pouyet, J. & Mandel, P. (1985). Time course of polynucleosome relaxation and ADP-ribosylation. Correlation between relaxation and histone H1 hyper-ADP-ribosylation. *Eur. J. Biochem.*, **146**, 185–91.

Ohashi, Y., Itaya, A., Tanaka, Y., Yoshihara, K., Kamiya, T. & Matsukage, A. (1986). Poly(ADP-ribosyl)ation of DNA polymerase beta in vitro. *Biochem. Biophys. Res. Commun.*, **140**, 666–73.

Oleinick, N. L. & Evans, H. H. (1985). Poly(ADP-ribose) and the response of cells to ionizing radiation. *Radiat. Res.*, **101**, 29–46.

Palmer, R. M., Ferrige, A. G. & Moncada, S. (1987). Nitric oxide release accounts for the biological activity of endothelium-derived relaxing factor. *Nature*, **327**, 524–6.

Panahian, N., Yoshida, T., Huang, P. L. *et al.* (1996). Attenuated hippocampal damage after global cerebral ischemia in mice mutant in neuronal nitric oxide synthase. *Neuroscience*, **72** (2), 343–54.

Parkinson, J. F., Mitrovic, B. & Merrill, J. E. (1997). The role of nitric oxide in multiple sclerosis. *J. Mol. Med.*, **75**, 174–86.

Petroske, E., Meredith, G. E., Callen, S., Totterdell, S. & Lau, Y. S. (2001). Mouse model of Parkinsonism: a comparison between subacute MPTP and chronic MPTP; probenecid treatment. *Neuroscience*, **106** (3), 589–601.

Pieper, A. A., Brat, D. J., Krug, D. K. *et al.* (1999a). Poly(ADP-ribose) polymerase-deficient mice are protected from streptozotocin-induced diabetes. *Proc. Natl Acad. Sci., USA*, **96**, 3059–64.

Pieper, A. A., Verma, A., Zhang, J. & Snyder, S. H. (1999b). Poly(ADP-ribose) polymerase, nitric oxide and cell death. *Trends Pharmacol. Sci.*, **20**, 171–81.

Power, C. & Johnson, R. T. (1995). HIV-1 associated dementia: clinical features and pathogenesis. *Can. J. Neurol. Sci.*, **22**, 92–100.

Przedborski, S., Jackson-Lewis, V., Yokoyama, R., Shibata, T., Dawson, V. L. & Dawson, T. M. (1996). Role of neuronal nitric oxide in 1-methyl-4-phenyl-1,2,3,6-tetrahydropyridine (MPTP)-induced dopaminergic neurotoxicity. *Proc. Natl Acad. Sci., USA*, **93**, 4565–71.

Przedborski, S., Chen, Q., Vila, M. *et al.* (2001). Oxidative post-translational modifications of alpha-synuclein in the 1-methyl-4-phenyl-1,2,3,6-tetrahydropyridine (MPTP) mouse model of Parkinson's disease. *J. Neurochem.*, **76**, 637–40.

Ramsay, R. R., Krueger, M. J., Youngster, S. K., Gluck, M. R., Casida, J. E. & Singer, T. P. (1991). Interaction of 1-methyl-4-phenylpyridinium ion (MPP$^+$) and its analogs with the rotenone/piericidin binding site of NADH dehydrogenase. *J. Neurochem.*, **56**, 1184–90.

Ramsay, R. R. & Singer, T. P. (1992). Relation of superoxide generation and lipid peroxidation to the inhibition of NADH-Q oxidoreductase by rotenone, piericidin A, and MPP$^+$. *Biochem. Biophys. Res. Commun.*, **189**, 47–52.

Rickwood, D. & Osman, M. S. (1979). Characterisation of poly(ADP-Rib) polymerase activity in nuclei from the slime mould Dictyostelium discoideum. *Mol. Cell. Biochem.*, **27**, 79–84.

Ruf, A., Mennissier de Murcia, J., de Murcia, G. & Schulz, G. E. (1996). Structure of the catalytic fragment of poly(AD-ribose) polymerase from chicken. *Proc. Natl Acad. Sci., USA*, **93**, 7481–5.

Ruscetti, T., Lehnert, B. E., Halbrook, J. *et al.* (1998). Stimulation of the DNA-dependent protein kinase by poly(ADP-ribose) polymerase. *J. Biol. Chem.*, **273**, 14461–7.

Samdani, A. F., Dawson, T. M. & Dawson, V. L. (1997). Nitric oxide synthase in models of focal ischemia. *Stroke*, **28**, 1283–8.

Sattler, R., Xiong, Z., Lu, W. Y., Hafner, M., MacDonald, J. F. & Tymianski, M. (1999). Specific coupling of NMDA receptor activation to nitric oxide neurotoxicity by PSD-95 protein. *Science*, **284**, 1845–8.

Scovassi, A. I., Mariani, C., Negroni, M., Negri, C. & Bertazzoni, U. (1993). ADP-ribosylation of nonhistone proteins in HeLa cells: modification of DNA topoisomerase II. *Exp. Cell. Res.*, **206**, 177–81.

Shall, S. & de Murcia, G. (2000). Poly(ADP-ribose) polymerase-1: what have we learned from the deficient mouse model? *Mutat. Res.*, **460**, 1–15.

Singer, T. P., Castagnoli, N., Jr., Ramsay, R. R. & Trevor, A. J. (1987). Biochemical events in the development of parkinsonism induced by 1-methyl-4-phenyl-1,2,3,6-tetrahydropyridine. *J. Neurochem.*, **49**, 1–8.

Smith, S. (2001). The world according to PARP. *Trends Biochem. Sci.*, **26**, 174–9.

Souza, J. M., Giasson, B. I., Chen, Q., Lee, V. M. & Ischiropoulos, H. (2000). Dityrosine cross-linking promotes formation of stable alpha-synuclein polymers. Implication of nitrative and oxidative stress in the pathogenesis of neurodegenerative synucleinopathies. *J. Biol. Chem.*, **275**, 18344–9.

Stamler, J. S., Lamas, S. & Fang, F. C. (2001). Nitrosylation. the prototypic redox-based signaling mechanism. *Cell*, **106**, 675–83.

Sun, D., Coleclough, C., Cao, L., Hu, X., Sun, S. & Whitaker, J. N. (1998). Reciprocal stimulation between TNF-alpha and nitric oxide may exacerbate CNS inflammation in experimental autoimmune encephalomyelitis. *J. Neuroimmunol.*, **89**, 122–30.

Susin, S. A., Lorenzo, H. K., Zamzami, N. *et al.* (1999). Molecular characterization of mitochondrial apoptosis-inducing factor. *Nature*, **397**, 441–6.

Szabo, C. & Dawson, V. L. (1998). Role of poly(ADP-ribose) synthetase in inflammation and ischaemia-reperfusion. *Trends Pharmacol. Sci.*, **19**, 287–98.

Takahashi, K., Wesselingh, S. L., Griffin, D. E., McArthur, J. C., Johnson, R. T. & Glass, J. D. (1996). Localization of HIV-1 in human brain using polymerase chain reaction/in situ hybridization and immunocytochemistry. *Ann. Neurol.*, **39**, 705–11.

Takahashi, K., Pieper, A. A., Croul, S. E., Zhang, J., Snyder, S. H. & Greenberg, J. H. (1999). Post-treatment with an inhibitor of poly(ADP-ribose) polymerase attenuates cerebral damage in focal ischemia. *Brain Res.*, **829**, 46–54.

Tanuma, S., Yagi, T. & Johnson, G. S. (1985). Endogenous ADP ribo-sylation of high mobility group proteins 1 and 2 and histone H1 following DNA damage in intact cells. *Arch. Biochem. Biophys.*, **237**, 38–42.

Tayeh, M. A. & Marletta, M. A. (1989). Macrophage oxidation of L-arginine to nitric oxide, nitrite, and nitrate. Tetrahydro-biopterin is required as a cofactor. *J. Biol. Chem.*, **264**, 19654–8.

Tsai, Y. J., Aoki, T., Maruta, H. *et al.* (1992). Mouse mammary tumor virus gene expression is suppressed by oligomeric ellag-itannins, novel inhibitors of poly(ADP-ribose) glycohydrolase. *J. Biol. Chem.*, **267**, 14436–42.

Uchida, K. & Miwa, M. (1994). Poly(ADP-ribose) polymerase: struc-tural conservation among different classes of animals and its implications. *Mol. Cell. Biochem.*, **138**, 25–32.

Uchida, K., Morita, T., Sato, T. *et al.* (1987). Nucleotide sequence of a full-length cDNA for human fibroblast poly(ADP-ribose) polymerase. *Biochem. Biophys. Res. Commun.*, **148**, 617–22.

Ushiro, H., Yokoyama, Y. & Shizuta, Y. (1987). Purification and characterization of poly (ADP-ribose) synthetase from human placenta. *J. Biol. Chem.*, **262**, 2352–7.

Wang, Z. Q., Stingl, L., Morrison, C. *et al.* (1997). PARP is important for genomic stability but dispensable in apoptosis. *Genes Dev.*, **11**, 2347–58.

Werner, E., Sohst, S., Gropp, F., Simon, D., Wagner, H. & Kroger, H. (1984). Presence of poly (ADP-ribose) polymerase and poly (ADP-ribose) glycohydrolase in the dinoflagellate *Cryptheco-dinium cohnii*. *Eur. J. Biochem.*, **139**, 81–6.

Wesierska-Gadek, J., Bugajska-Schretter, A. & Cerni, C. (1996a). ADP-ribosylation of p53 tumor suppressor protein: mutant but not wild-type p53 is modified. *J. Cell. Biochem.*, **62**, 90–101.

Wesierska-Gadek, J., Schmid, G. & Cerni, C. (1996b). ADP-ribosylation of wild-type p53 in vitro: binding of p53 protein to specific p53 consensus sequence prevents its modification. *Biochem. Biophys. Res. Commun.*, **224**, 96–102.

Wiley, C. A., Schrier, R. D., Nelson, J. A., Lampert, P. W. & Old-stone, M. B. (1986). Cellular localization of human immunod-eficiency virus infection within the brains of acquired immune deficiency syndrome patients. *Proc. Natl Acad. Sci., USA*, **83**, 7089–93.

Yamanaka, H., Penning, C. A., Willis, E. H., Wasson, D. B. & Carson, D. A. (1988). Characterization of human poly(ADP-ribose) polymerase with autoantibodies. *J. Biol. Chem.*, **263**, 3879–83.

Yoshihara, K., Itaya, A., Tanaka, Y. *et al.* (1985). Inhibition of DNA polymerase alpha, DNA polymerase beta, terminal deoxynucleotidyl transferase, and DNA ligase II by poly(ADP-ribosyl)ation reaction in vitro. *Biochem. Biophys. Res. Com-mun.*, **128**, 61–7.

Yu, S. W., Wang, H., Poitras, M. F. *et al.* (2002). Mediation of poly(ADP-ribose) polymerase-1-dependent cell death by apoptosis-inducing factor. *Science*, **297**, 259–63.

Zhang, J., Dawson, V. L., Dawson, T. M. & Snyder, S. H. (1994). Nitric oxide activation of poly(ADP-ribose) synthetase in neurotoxi-city. *Science*, **263**, 687–9.

Zhang, J., Pieper, A. & Snyder, S. H. (1995). Poly(ADP-ribose) synthetase activation: an early indicator of neurotoxic DNA damage. *J. Neurochem.*, **65**, 1411–14.

Zhang, X., Morera, S., Bates, P. A. *et al.* (1998). Structure of an XRCC1 BRCT domain: a new protein-protein interaction module. *EMBO J.*, **17**, 6404–11.

13

Copper and zinc in Alzheimer's disease and amyotrophic lateral sclerosis

Avi L. Friedlich[1] and Ashley I. Bush[2]

[1,2]Laboratory for Oxidation Biology, Genetics and Aging Research Unit, Massachusetts General Hospital, Charlestown, MA, USA and Mental Health Research Institute of Victoria, and Department of Pathology, University of Melbourne, Australia

Introduction

The non-infectious neurodegenerative disorders, Alzheimer's disease, and amyotrophic lateral sclerosis are heterogeneous with respect to etiology, neuropathology and clinical presentation. Yet, these disorders share a number of features in common to suggest some common pathogenic events. Each disorder is age related and is characterized by progressive and symmetric degeneration of discrete populations of neurons. Each disorder is associated with biochemical markers of oxidative attack, and each is associated with deposition of a CuZn metalloprotein in affected tissue.

Molecular genetic analysis has linked autosomal dominant forms of AD, PD, and amyotrophic lateral sclerosis, respectively, to mutations in ß-amyloid precursor protein, α-synuclein, and superoxide dismutase 1. Each of these proteins or its proteolytic products may aggregate in affected tissue during the course of disease.

In this chapter we summarize current knowledge of CNS Cu and Zn metabolism in normal physiology. Then, focusing on AD and ALS, we review evidence for pathophysiologic Cu and Zn metabolism and evidence linking Cu and Zn to the physiologic and toxic activities of ß-amyloid protein and superoxide dismutase 1.

Protein interactions in brain copper and zinc metabolism

At the active site of many enzymes, Cu participates in one-electron transfer reactions. Zn, which is electrochemically inert, maintains structural stability of many proteins. In addition to these essential and ubiquitous roles for Cu and Zn, brain-specific functions exist for these metals. The brain contains high concentrations of Cu and Zn in the neocortex and spinal cord (reviewed in Bush, 2000), the functions of which are poorly understood but may relate to the specialized metabolism of neurotransmission.

Zn^{2+} is sequestered into pre-synaptic vesicles in a subset of corticofugal glutamatergic fibers by the zinc transporter 3 protein (Palmiter et al., 1996; Frederickson et al., 2000). Its release on depolarization may raise the concentration of Zn^{2+} in the synaptic cleft to 300 μM (Assaf & Chung, 1984; Howell et al., 1984). Cu^{2+} may also have a role in neurotransmission, as extracellular Cu^{2+} concentrations have been observed to rise transiently to 15 μM during neuronal depolarization (Hartter & Barnea, 1988a,b).

Because free Cu and Zn are potentially neurotoxic (for review see Atwood et al., 1999) stringent homeostatic mechanisms exist to regulate extracellular and intracellular concentrations, and the blood–brain barrier is relatively impermeable to transient changes in plasma Cu and Zn levels, such as those which occur prandially and post-prandially. The concentrations of Cu and Zn in neocortex are >1 order of magnitude higher than that in plasma, and the concentrations in plasma are 10 to 20 orders of magnitude higher than those in cerebrospinal fluid (CSF). These large metal concentration gradients suggest that energy-dependent pathways exist to transport Cu and Zn from plasma or CSF to neocortex and that passive transport mechanisms may exist for their clearance into CSF or plasma. Zn^{2+} in some regions of the brain is in rapid exchange with the plasma, but these are still poorly understood (Pullen et al., 1990).

Zn^{2+} released during neurotransmission is in an ionic, dissociable form. Less is known about the chemical form of Cu^{2+} that is released during neurotransmission into the synapse. The mechanisms for transport, storage, and release of Cu and Zn are currently being elaborated. Knowledge of Cu transport mechanisms has been augmented by elucidating the mechanisms of Mendelian genetic diseases of Cu and Zn metabolism associated with neurodegeneration. Wilson's disease and Menkes disease, two disorders of systemic Cu metabolism associated with pronounced neurodegeneration, are associated with different genes from the same family. These genes encode cation transporting P-type ATPases localizing to the trans-Golgi network (Chelly *et al.*, 1993; Tanzi *et al.*, 1993; Mercer, 2001). The major Cu binding protein in serum is ceruloplasmin, and aceruloplasminemia is associated with basal ganglia degeneration (Morita *et al.*, 1995). Other Cu transport and loading proteins have also been identified. Ctr1 is a transmembrane protein involved in Cu uptake at the plasma membrane (Zhou & Thiele, 2001; Lee *et al.*, 2001). Ctr1 knockout mice have decreased Cu levels in brain (Kuo *et al.*, 2001; Lee *et al.*, 2001).

For Zn^{2+} sequestration and transport, several families of proteins are now known. Intestinal absorption of Zn and cellular zinc uptake are largely mediated by the zip family of transport proteins (Wang *et al.*, 2002). Transendothelial zinc transport at the blood–brain barrier is probably mediated by receptors for Zn-histidine or Zn-albumin. Intracellular sequestration and transport of Zn^{2+} is largely mediated by the metallothionein (MT) family of proteins (Vallee, 1995; Jacob *et al.*, 1998), with MTII and MTIII being the most significant in brain. The zinc transporter (ZnT) family is involved in sub-cellular zinc compartmentation. ZnT3 mediates the vesicular sequestration of synaptic zinc (Masters *et al.*, 1994; Palmiter & Findley, 1995; Palmiter *et al.*, 1996). ZnT3 seems generally to stimulate zinc migration through the blood–brain cerebral spinal fluid system, as targeted disruption of ZnT3 decreases cerebral zinc levels (Cole *et al.*, 1999). Even with elaborate mechanism for Cu and Zn homeostasis, a steady rise in brain Cu and Fe levels is observed as a function of age in post-reproductive life (Maynard *et al.*, 2002). The reasons for this are unclear. Elevated levels of Cu or Fe may increase oxidative stress and render the brain more susceptible to neurodegenerative disorders such as AD and ALS.

Alzheimer's disease

A consensus has yet to emerge about the levels of total Zn and Cu in plasma and CSF in AD. Zn and Cu are largely bound in an ionic form to ligands such as proteins and amino acids in these fluids. Fasting serum Zn 1 year prior to death has been reported to correlate negatively with amyloid plaque density in seven brain regions (Tully *et al.*, 1995) Two reports have indicated that that serum Cu is elevated in Alzheimer compared to age-matched control patients (Kapaki *et al.*, 1993; Squitti *et al.*, 2002). It remains to be

determined whether there are specific biochemical fractions associated with Zn^{2+} and Cu^{2+} within the blood that are altered in AD.

In AD CSF, one study has reported an increase in Cu (Basun *et al.*, 1991), two studies have reported an increase in Zn (Hershey *et al.*, 1983; Rulon *et al.*, 2000), and two studies have reported a decrease in Zn (Kapaki *et al.*, 1993; Molina *et al.*, 1998). Other reports have found no differences between AD and control CSF, with respect to Cu and Zn (Hershey *et al.*, 1983; Sahu *et al.*, 1988).

While a consensus has emerged that Cu and Zn are elevated in amyloid, reports of alterations in bulk metal levels in AD have not shown consistency. Cu and Zn accumulation in AD amyloid deposits has been demonstrated by micro particle X-ray emission (PIXE; Lovell *et al.*, 1998). Cu was localized predominantly to the senile plaque rim, while Zn was elevated in the senile plaque rim and core. Additionally, Zn was elevated in the AD neuropil, compared to age-matched control. Histochemically reactive Zn has also been localized to amyloid plaques and amyloid angiopathy in AD tissue (Suh *et al.*, 2000), and APP2576 transgenic mouse brain (Lee *et al.*, 1999). Another PIXE study demonstrated increased Zn levels in the Alzheimer hippocampus and amygdala in unstained cryostat sections, though no correlation with plaques was made (Danscher *et al.*, 1997). Raman microscopy from purified plaque cores suggests that Cu and Zn present in senile plaques are coordinated to histidine residues and the only metals ion coordinating Aß (Dong *et al.*, 2003).

Numerous studies have quantified metal levels in gross brain specimens or homogenates using instrumental neutron activating analysis (INAA) and inductively coupled plasma mass spectroscopy (ICP–MS), with conflicting results. The ICP–MS studies have demonstrated decreased Zn in the AD hippocampus, thalamus and gyri (Panayi *et al.*, 2002) and also in the frontal, occipital and temporal cortices (Corrigan *et al.*, 1993). An INAA study found decreased Cu and increased Zn in AD hippocampus and amygdala (Deibel *et al.*, 1996). An INAA sub-cellular fractionation study found decreased nuclear Zn in the temporal lobe (Wenstrup *et al.*, 1990).

Investigations of the expression and distribution of Cu and Zn transport and sequestration proteins in AD provide additional evidence for disrupted Cu and Zn metabolism in AD. Expression of ceruloplasmin (Castellani *et al.*, 1999), MT-III (Yu *et al.*, 2001), MMP-1 (Leake *et al.*, 2000), MMP2 (Backstrom *et al.*, 1992), and MMP-9 (Asahina *et al.*, 2001) have all been reported to be altered in the Alzheimer brain.

MTIII is deficient in AD brain tissue (Uchida *et al.*, 1988; Uchida *et al.*, 1991; Yu *et al.*, 2001), which may impair the buffering capacity of the cortical tissue, and contribute to the extracellular pooling of Zn and Cu that occurs in AD.

Whereas abnormal Cu^{2+} elevation may drive the toxicity of Aß (Huang *et al.*, 1999b), interstitial Zn^{2+} elevation may reflect a homeostatic antioxidant response. Mechanistically, this could be due to Zn^{2+} release from the metallothionein (MT) pool upon glial activation (Penkowa *et al.*, 1999) or due to MT thiols being oxidized by H_2O_2 (Maret & Vallee, 1998), perhaps produced by Aß (Huang *et al.*, 1999a,b; Opazo *et al.*, 2002). The hypothesis that Zn^{2+} elevation forms amyloid is supported by the distribution of exchangeable Zn^{2+} in the synaptic vesicles of the glutamatergic corticofugal system (Frederickson, 1989), paralleling the anatomical sites most prone to amyloid deposition.

Other Aß-associated proteins may also modulate the precipitation of Aß in the presence of Zn^{2+}, and so play a role in amyloid formation. The Zn^{2+} binding properties of alpha-2-macroglobulin, a genetic risk factor for AD (Blacker *et al.*, 1998) modulate its binding to Aß (Du *et al.*, 1997). Also, apolipoprotein E preserves Aß solubility in the presence of Zn^{2+}, and the ApoE4 isoform, a risk factor for amyloid deposition and AD, is the poorest solubility chaperone under these conditions (Moir *et al.*, 1999). Therefore, in ApoE4 carriers, Aß is more likely to be precipitated by Zn^{2+}.

Beta amyloid protein

The ~4 kDa ß amyloid protein (Aß) deposits as amyloid in the neuropil and cerebrovasculature in Alzheimer disease. Strong genetic evidence links Aß and its precursor the ß-amyloid precursor protein (APP) to Alzheimer's disease pathogenesis. Although much progress has been made over the past few years towards understanding the biology and pathobiology of Aß and APP, consensus on the biologic and pathogenic functions of each protein has not been reached. The ß-amyloid protein (Aß) possesses high and low affinity binding sites for Cu and Zn (Bush *et al.*, 1994; Atwood *et al.*, 1998; Miura *et al.*, 2000). The affinity of the Zn^{2+} binding sites on Aß1-40 are 100 nM and 5 μM (Table 13.1), indicating that they might be occupied under physiological conditions (Atwood *et al.*, 1998, 2000). The highest affinity Cu^{2+} binding site on Aß1–42 has a measured $K_a \approx 10^{-18}$ M, much greater than the highest affinity Cu^{2+} binding site on Aß1-40 ($K_a \approx 10^{-10}$ M) (Atwood *et al.*, 1998, 2000).

The differential affinity of $Aß_{42}$ and $Aß_{40}$ for Cu^{2+} (Atwood *et al.*, 2000) may account for the differential redox behaviour and toxicity of these two species (Huang *et al.*, 1999). The Cu^{2+}–Aß1–42 complex has a strong reduction

Table 13.1. Copper and zinc binding affinities of the 40 and 42 residue beta amyloid protein. Data are from Atwood *et al.* (2000).

K_d (M)	High affinity	Low affinity
Aß1-40/Zn	1.0×10^{-7}	1.3×10^{-6}
Aß1-42/Zn	1.0×10^{-7}	1.3×10^{-6}
Aß1-40/Cu	4.6×10^{-11}	1.3×10^{-6}
Aß1-42/Cu	7.0×10^{-18}	5.0×10^{-9}

potential (+550 mM vs Ag/AgCl) compared with the blue copper proteins. Such strong electrochemical potential probably denotes a biological significance, and because Aß binds Cu^{2+} and Zn^{2+} to form a superoxide dismutase like structure (Curtain *et al.*, 2001), we hypothesized that metal binding to Aß in health may subserve a physiological function, such as metal clearance. A role for Aß or the Aß precursor protein (AßPP) in metal ion homeostasis is consistent with the observed reduction of brain Cu and Fe levels in mutant AßPP expressing (Tg2576 and C100-V717F) transgenic mice (Maynard *et al.*, 2002). The presence of an iron responsive element on the 5^1 untranslated region of the AßPP mRNA is also consistent with a role for Aß or AßPP in metal ion homeostasis (Rogers *et al.*, 2002). The oxidative damage induced by Aß may be mechanistically related to the oxidative stress induced by mutant SOD1 (Atwood *et al.*, 1998, 2000). Hydrogen peroxide (H_2O_2), implicated in AD pathogenesis, is produced by Cu Aß (Huang *et al.*, 1999b). Among Aß species, Cu $Aß_{42}$ produces H_2O_2 at a faster rate that Cu $Aß_{40}$, while mouse Cu Aß produces much less H_2O_2 (Huang *et al.*, 1999a). The redox activities of these Cu Aß species correlate with their respective neurotoxicity in culture, which is largely mediated by H_2O_2 formed by Cu Aß (Huang *et al.*, 1999b). H_2O_2 formation by Cu Aß and CuZn Aß can also be inhibited by chelation (Huang *et al.*, 1999b), and the H_2O_2 mediated toxicity of Aß in culture can be exaggerated by Cu^{2+} and ameliorated by Zn^{2+} (Cuajungco *et al.*, 2000).

It is now well established that Aß is rapidly precipitated by physiological concentrations of Zn^{2+}, a redox inert cation. Under mildly acidic conditions (pH 6.8 to 7.0), the redox-active metals Cu^{2+} and Fe^{3+} induce greater Aß aggregation than does Zn (Atwood *et al.*, 1998). Significantly, the turbidity of rodent Aß1-40 (with substitutions of Arg→Gly, Tyr→Phe and His→Arg at positions 5, 10 and 13, respectively) is unaffected by Zn^{2+} or Cu^{2+} at low micromolar concentrations (Atwood *et al.*, 1998).

CuZn selective chelators markedly enhance the resolubilization of Aß deposits from post-mortem AD brain samples (Cherny *et al.*, 1999) supporting the possibility that

Cu and Zn ions play a significant role in assembling these deposits. The metallochemistry of Aß links oxidative damage and amyloidosis in AD. In vitro precipitation of Aß by Cu^{2+} or Zn^{2+} can be completely reversed by chelation (Huang et al., 1997). In postmortem AD brain, selective Cu or Zn chelators can induce the resolubilization of Aß from plaques (Cherny et al., 1999). Oxidative damage may be the earliest pathological event in AD (Nunomura et al., 2001), and a negative correlation exists between amyloid burden and levels of 8-hydroxyguanosine, a marker of hydroxyl radical activity (Cuajungco et al., 2000). This is possibly because Zn supresses H_2O_2 formation from Aß. Thus, the mature plaque in AD may form through a compensatory mechanism where Zn^{2+} is sequestered into accumulations of Aß.

Pre-clinical and clinical data now support Cu and Zn metabolism as a valid therapeutic target in AD. Clioquinol (CQ), a retired antibiotic with a 0.5 billion patient day history, was evaluated by Cherny et al. (2001) for efficacy in 21 month old APP2576 transgenic mice. Administration by gavage of 30 mg/kg for 9 weeks resulted in a 49% decrease in brain Aß load, a decrease in serum Aß, with no evidence of drug-induced toxicity or systemic loss of metals. General health and body weight parameters were significantly improved in the treated animals after only 16 days of treatment. Treatment of APP2576 mice with CQ induced a $\approx$15% *increase* in brain Cu and Zn, indicating that the therapeutic mechanism of CQ is not simply chelation and clearance. A phase II double-blinded clinical trial of CQ in Alzheimer patients has recently been completed. CQ decreased plasma Aß levels and, in more advanced AD patients, slowed the rate of cognitive decline (Colin L. Masters et al., personal communication). Continued investigation into Cu and Zn metabolism, the metallobiology of Aß and APP, and the mechanism of action of CQ seems likely to increase understanding of AD pathogenesis and lead to new treatments for the millions of patients suffering from the disorder.

Amyotrophic lateral sclerosis

In frontal and occipital gray matter, Zn levels have been reported to be decreased by INAA (Yasui et al., 1993). Decreased serum and CSF Cu but not Zn has been reported in ALS (Kapaki et al., 1997). Metallothionein immunoreactivity is increased in the spinal cord in ALS, and liver and kidney metallothionein levels are also elevated in ALS (Sillevis-Smitt et al., 1992; Sillevis-Smitt et al., 1994). The same pattern of elevated metallothionein immunoreactivity occurs in a transgenic model of ALS. SOD1-G93A

transgenic mice demonstrate increased MT1 and MTII, and MTIII expression in astrocytes in both white and gray matter. Neuronal MT-III expression is also elevated (Gong & Elliott, 2000). Metalothionein elevation is likely compensatory and protective. In the G93A mutant SOD1 transgenic model of ALS, deficiency of MTI, MTII or MTIII exacerbates the ALS phenotype (Nagano et al., 2001; Puttaparthi et al., 2002). Total body and cerebral Cu and Zn metabolism in ALS may be altered, though the pathophysiological metabolism remains to be characterized.

Superoxide dismutase 1

Over 100 mutations in CuZn superoxide dismutase (SOD1) are associated with autosomal dominant ALS (Rosen, 1993; Brown & Robberecht, 2001). SOD1 represents a major biochemical pool of Cu^{2+} and Zn^{2+} in all tissues. That toxicity of mutant SOD1 (mSOD1) is independent of wild type activity has been established. The ALS associated mSOD1 species possess varying amounts of wild-type enzymatic activity, ranging from 0% (e.g. H46R and G85R) to 100% (e.g. G37R) of wild-type activity. SOD1 knockout mice do not develop the ALS phenotype (Reaume et al., 1996), and the age of onset and duration of disease in ALS transgenic mice is unaffected by levels of wild-type SOD1 activity (Bruijn et al., 1998). Thus, the toxicity of mSOD1 is a gain-of-function.

Several gain-of-function redox reactions have been proposed for mSOD1, and at least two currently appear plausible. Increased peroxidase activity has been reported in vitro (Wiedau-Pazos et al., 1996; Liochev et al., 1997) in the H48Q, A4V, and G93A variants, although not consistently (Singh et al., 1998). Increased peroxidase activity in vivo has been reported in the A4V and G93A (Roe et al., 2002) species.

Also, peroxynitrite formation from nitric oxide and dioxygen has been proposed as a toxic gain-of function for mSOD1:

Reaction 1: $X + Cu^{2+} \longrightarrow X^+ + Cu^+$
Reaction 2: $NO^- + O_2 + Cu^+ \longrightarrow ONOO^- + Cu^{2+}$

Cu replete, Zn deficient SOD1 has been reported to confer toxicity by producing peroxynitrite according to these reactions (Estevez et al., 1999), and loss of Zn from mSOD1 has been proposed as a primary pathogenic event (Crow et al., 1997).

Pathological findings in mSOD1-associated ALS and in transgenic models are consistent with the redox hypotheses for mSOD1 pathogenicity. Elevated levels of nitrotyrosine and its major metabolite 3-nitro-4-hydroxyphenylacetic acid have been demonstrated in the lumbar and thoracic spinal cord in familial ALS (Beal *et al.*, 1997). Motor neuron immunopositivity for 3-nitrotyrosine, malondialdehyde, and heme oxygenase have been reported as well (Beal *et al.*, 1997). Similar patterns of immunoreactive oxidative adducts have been reported in the G93A and G37R transgenic mice (Ferrante *et al.*, 1997; Bruijn *et al.*, 1997), and protein carbonyl levels have been found to be elevated in the G93A mice as early as 30 days of age (Andrus *et al.*, 1998). Further, mitochondrial vacuolation is a prominent feature in the ALS transgenic mice (Wong *et al.*, 1995; Gurney *et al.*, 1998), and impairment of respiratory transport chain function has been confirmed in the G93A model (Mattiazzi *et al.*, 2002). The copper chelators trientine (Nagano *et al.*, 1999) and D-penicillamine (Hottinger *et al.*, 1997) have shown efficacy in the transgenic models.

The possibility of copper involvement in mSOD1 pathogenicity must now be carefully reassessed in light of work by Subramaniam *et al.* (2002) demonstrating that CCS dependent Cu transport does not contribute to mSOD1 toxicity. Those authors crossed the G37R, G85R, and G93A transgenic mice with CCS-knockouts and found no modification of disease phenotype with the CCS−/−background. They confirmed in the CCS knockouts that wild type SOD1 activity was reduced by 80% and that ^{64}Cu incorporation into SOD1 was markedly decreased 24 hours after intraperitoneal ^{64}Cu injections.

A pathogenic role for Cu properly inserted into the mSOD1 active site cannot be ruled out on the basis of data reported by Subramaniam *et al.* (2002). The CCS knockout mice do retain 20% of wild-type SOD1 activity, and the results of Subramaniam *et al.* (2002) would still be consistent with toxic Cu reactivity at the mSOD1 catalytic site if (a) the pathogenic mSOD1 species were compartmentalized (e.g. localized to mitochondria or other subcellular compartment) throughout the course of disease and (b) the compartmentalized SOD1 pool conferring pathogenicity were activated with copper loading through a mechanism independent of CCS.

In addition, Cu mediated mSOD1 pathogenicity from Cu coordinated at sites other than the catalytic site (Bush, 2002) cannot be ruled out on the basis of data reported by Subramaniam *et al.* (2002). Cu can be coordinated by mSOD1 at several locations, including the wild type Zn binding site (Goto *et al.*, 2000) and the surface residue C111 (Liu *et al.*, 2000). Such metallated species would not be expected to possess significant wild type SOD1 activity. The ^{64}Cu experiments of Subramaniam *et al.* (2002) demonstrate a decrease in the rate of Cu incorporation into SOD1 but do not demonstrate a decrease in the amount of Cu incorporated at all metal binding sites: SOD1 : Zn : Cu

stoichiometry was not measured in that report. Total Cu levels in brain are elevated in the CCS knockouts (Subramaniam *et al.*, 2002). The evidence favoring a Cu mediated pathogenic mechanism for mSOD1 therefore remains fundamentally unchallenged.

Future prospects

Growing evidence exists to support pathophysiological Cu and Zn metabolism in AD and ALS. Moreover, pre-clinical data in ALS and pre-clinical and clinical trials data in AD now support a pathogenic role for Cu and Zn. Increased understanding of the pathogenic mechanism of Cu and Zn in AD and ALS will identify new targets for drug discovery, which can then be tested for efficacy in transgenic animal models of AD and ALS, as well as other neurodegenerative disorders such as Parkinson's disease. Thus, for AD, ALS and other neurodegenerative disorders, clinical trials with agents that interdict pathogenic Cu and Zn metabolism may be rapidly approaching. Demonstrating therapeutic efficacy of drugs attenuating pathogenic Cu and Zn metabolism will be required to establish a role for these metals in the non-infectious degenerative disorders of the central nervous system.

Acknowledgements

Supported by funds from the Alzheimer Association, ALS Association, NIA, NINDS, and NHMRC.

REFERENCES

Andrus, P. K., Fleck, T. J., Gurney, M. E. & Hall, E. D. (1998). Protein oxidative damage in a transgenic mouse model of familial amyotrophic lateral sclerosis. *J. Neurochem.*, **71**(5), 2041–8.

Asahina, M., Yoshiyama, Y. & Hattori, T. (2001). Expression of matrix metalloproteinase-9 and urinary-type plasminogen activator in Alzheimer's disease brain. *Clin. Neuropathol.*, **20**(2): 60–3.

Assaf, S. Y. & Chung, S.-H. (1984). Release of endogenous Zn^{2+} from brain tissue during activity. *Nature*, **308**, 734–6.

Atwood, C. S., Moir, R. D., Huang, X. *et al.* (1998). Dramatic aggregation of Alzheimer Aß by Cu(II) is induced by conditions representing physiological acidosis. *J. Biol. Chem.*, **273**, 12817–26.

Atwood, C. S., Huang, X., Moir, R. D., Tanzi, R. E. & Bush, A. I. (1999). Role of free radicals and metal ions in the pathogenesis of Alzheimer's disease. *Met. Ions Biol. Syst.*, **36**, 309–64.

Atwood, C. S., Scarpa, R. C., Huang, X. *et al.* (2000). Characterization of copper interactions with Alzheimer Aß peptides – identification of an attomolar affinity copper binding site on Aß1-42. *J. Neurochem.*, **75**, 1219–33.

Backstrom, J. R., Miller, C. A. & Tokes, Z. A. (1992). Characterization of neutral proteinases from Alzheimer-affected and control brain specimens: identification of calcium-dependent metalloproteinases from the hippocampus. *J. Neurochem.*, **58**(3), 983–92.

Basun, H., Forssell, L. G., Wetterberg, L. & Winblad, B. (1991). Metals and trace elements in plasma and cerebrospinal fluid in normal aging and Alzheimer's disease. *J. Neural. Transm. Park. Dis. Dement. Sect.*, **3**(4), 231–58.

Beal, M. F., Ferrante, R. J., Browne, S. E., Matthews, R. T., Kowall, N. W. & Brown R. H., Jr. (1997). Increased 3-nitrotyrosine in both sporadic and familial amyotrophic lateral sclerosis. *Ann. Neurol.*, **42**(4), 644–54.

Blacker, D., Wilcox, M. A., Laird, N. M. *et al.* (1998). Alpha-2 macroglobulin is genetically associated with Alzheimer disease. *Nat. Genet.*, **19**(4), 357–60.

Brown, R. H., Jr. & Robberecht, W. (2001). Amyotrophic lateral sclerosis: pathogenesis. *Semin. Neurol.*, **21**(2), 131–9.

Bruijn, L. I., Beal, M. F., Becher, M. W. *et al.* (1997). Elevated free nitrotyrosine levels, but not protein-bound nitrotyrosine or hydroxyl radicals, throughout amyotrophic lateral sclerosis (ALS)-like disease implicate tyrosine nitration as an aberrant in vivo property of one familial ALS-linked superoxide dismutase 1 mutant. *Proc. Natl. Acad. Sci., USA*, **94**(14), 7606–11.

Bruijn, L. I., Houseweart, M. K., Kato, S. *et al.* (1998). Aggregation and motor neuron toxicity of an ALS-linked SOD1 mutant independent from wild-type SOD1. *Science*, **281**(5384), 1851–4.

Bush, A. I. (2000). Metals and neuroscience. *Curr. Opin. Chem. Biol.*, **4**(2), 184–91.

Bush, A. I. (2002). Is ALS caused by an altered oxidative activity of mutant superoxide dismutase? *Nat. Neurosci.*, **5**(10), 919; author reply 919–20.

Bush, A. I., Pettingell, W. H., Multhaup, G. *et al.* (1994). Rapid induction of Alzheimer Aß amyloid formation by zinc. *Science*, **265**, 1464–7.

Castellani, R. J., Smith, M. A., Nunomura, A., Harris, P. L. & Perry, G. (1999). Is increased redox-active iron in Alzheimer disease a failure of the copper-binding protein ceruloplasmin? *Free Radic. Biol. Med.*, **26**(11–12), 1508–12.

Chelly, J., Tumer, Z., Tonnesen, T. *et al.* (1993). Isolation of a candidate gene for Menkes disease that encodes a potential heavy metal binding protein. *Nat. Genet.*, **3**(1), 14–19.

Cherny, R. A., Legg, J. T., McLean, C. A. *et al.* (1999). Aqueous dissolution of Alzheimer's disease Aß amyloid deposits by biometal depletion. *J. Biol. Chem.*, **274**, 23223–8.

Cherny, R. A., Atwood, C. S., Xilinas, M. E. *et al.* (2001). Treatment with a copper–zinc chelator markedly and rapidly inhibits beta-amyloid accumulation in Alzheimer's disease transgenic mice. *Neuron*, **30**(3), 665–76.

Cole, T. B., Wenzel, H. J., Kafer, K. E., Schwartzkroin, P. A. & Palmiter, R. D. (1999). Elimination of zinc from synaptic vesicles in the intact mouse brain by disruption of the ZnT3 gene. *Proc. Natl Acad. Sci., USA*, **96**, 1716–21.

Corrigan, F. M., Reynolds, G. P. & Ward, N. I. (1993). Hippocampal tin, aluminum and zinc in Alzheimer's disease. *Biometals*, **6**, 149–54.

Crow, J. P., Sampson, J. B., Zhuang, Y., Thompson, J. A. & Beckman, J. S. (1997). Decreased zinc affinity of amyotrophic lateral sclerosis-associated superoxide dismutase mutants leads to enhanced catalysis of tyrosine nitration by peroxynitrite. *J. Neurochem.*, **69**(5), 1936–44.

Cuajungco, M. P., Goldstein, L. E., Nunomura, A. *et al.* (2000). Evidence that the beta-amyloid plaques of Alzheimer's disease represent the redox-silencing and entombment of abeta by zinc. *J. Biol. Chem.*, **275**(26), 19439–42.

Curtain, C. C., Ali, F., Volitakis, I. *et al.* (2001). Alzheimer's disease amyloid- binds Cu and Zn to generate an allosterically-ordered membrane-penetrating structure containing SOD-like subunits. *J. Biol. Chem.*, **276**(23), 20466–73.

Danscher, G., Jensen, K. B., Frederickson, C. J. *et al.* (1997). Increased amount of zinc in the hippocampus and amygdala of Alzheimer's diseased brains: a proton-induced X-ray emission spectroscopic analysis of cryostat sections from autopsy material. *J. Neurosci. Methods*, **76**(1), 53–9.

Deibel, M. A., Ehmann, W. D. & Markesbery, W. R. (1996). Copper, iron, and zinc imbalances in severely degenerated brain regions in Alzheimer's disease: possible relation to oxidative stress. *J. Neurol. Sci.*, **143**, 137–42.

Dong, J., Atwood, C. S., Anderson, V. E. *et al.* (2003). Metal binding and oxidation of amyloid-beta within isolated senile plaque cores: Raman microscopic evidence. *Biochemistry*, **42**(10), 2768–73.

Du, Y., Ni, B., Glinn, M. *et al.* (1997). alpha2-Macroglobulin as Aß-amyloid peptide-binding plasma protein. *J. Neurochem.*, **69**(1), 299–305.

Estevez, A. G., Crow, J. P., Sampson, J. B. *et al.* (1999). Induction of nitric oxide-dependent apoptosis in motor neurons by zinc-deficient superoxide dismutase. Science, **286**(5449), 2498–500.

Ferrante, R. J., Shinobu, L. A. Schulz, J. B. *et al.* (1997). Increased 3-nitrotyrosine and oxidative damage in mice with a human copper/zinc superoxide dismutase mutation. *Ann. Neurol.*, **42**(3), 326–34.

Frederickson, C. J. (1989). Neurobiology of zinc and zinc-containing neurons. *Int. Rev. Neurobiol.*, **31**, 145–328.

Frederickson, C. J., Suh, S. W., Silva, D. & Thompson, R. B. (2000). Importance of zinc in the central nervous system: the zinc-containing neuron. *J. Nutr.*, **130**(5S Suppl), 1471S–83S.

Glenner, G. G. & Wong, C. W. (1984). Alzheimer's disease: initial report of the purification and characterization of a novel cerebrovascular amyloid protein. *Biochem. Biophys Res. Commun.*, **120**, 885–90.

Gong, Y. H. & Elliott J. L. (2000). Metallothionein expression is altered in a transgenic murine model of familial amyotrophic lateral sclerosis. *Exp. Neurol.*, **162**(1), 27–36.

Goto, J. J., Zhu, H., Sanchez, R. J. *et al.* (2000). Loss of in vitro metal ion binding specificity in mutant copper-zinc superoxide dismutases associated with familial amyotrophic lateral sclerosis. *J. Biol. Chem.*, **275**(2), 1007–14.

Gurney, M. E., Liu, R., Althaus, J. S., Hall E. D. & Becker, D. A. (1998). Mutant CuZn superoxide dismutase in motor neuron disease. *J. Inherit. Metab. Dis.*, **21**(5), 587–97.

Hambidge, M. & Krebs, N. F. (2001). Interrelationships of key variables of human zinc homeostasis: relevance to dietary zinc requirements. *Annu. Rev. Nutr.*, **21**, 429–52.

Hartter, D. E. & Barnea, A. (1988a). Brain tissue accumulates 67copper by two ligand-dependent saturable processes. *J. Biol. Chem.*, **263**, 799–805.

(1988b). Evidence for release of copper in the brain: depolarization-induced release of newly taken-up 67copper. *Synapse*, **2**(4), 412–15.

Hershey, C. O., Hershey, L. A., Varnes, A., Vibhakar, S. D., Lavin, P. & Strain, W. H. (1983). Cerebrospinal fluid trace element content in dementia: clinical, radiologic, and pathologic correlations. *Neurology*, **33**, 1350–3.

Howell, G. A., Welch, M. G. & Frederickson, C. J. (1984). Stimulation-induced uptake and release of zinc in hippocampal slices. *Nature*, **308**, 736–8.

Hottinger, A. F., Fine, E. G., Gurney, M. E., Zurn, A. D. & Aebischer, P. (1997). The copper chelator d-penicillamine delays onset of disease and extends survival in a transgenic mouse model of familial amyotrophic lateral sclerosis. *Eur. J. Neurosci.*, **9**(7), 1548–51.

Huang, X., Atwood, C. S., Moir, R. D. *et al.* (1997). Zinc-induced Alzheimer's Aß1-40 aggregation is mediated by conformational factors. *J. Biol. Chem.*, **272**, 26464–70.

Huang, X., Atwood, C. S., Hartshorn, M. A. *et al.* (1999a). The Aß peptide of Alzheimer's Disease directly produces hydrogen peroxide through metal ion reduction. *Biochemistry*, **38**, 7609–16.

Huang, X., Cuajungco, M. P., Atwood, C. S. *et al.* (1999b). Cu(II) potentiation of Alzheimer Aß neurotoxicity: correlation with cell-free hydrogen peroxide production and metal reduction. *J. Biol. Chem.*, **274**, 37111–16.

Jacob, C., Maret, W. & Vallee, B. L. (1998). Control of zinc transfer between thionein, metallothionein, and zinc proteins. *Proc. Natl Acad. Sci., USA*, **95**(7), 3489–94.

Kang, J., Lemaire, H. G., Unterbeck, A. *et al.* (1987). The precursor of Alzheimer's disease amyloid A4 protein resembles a cell-surface receptor. *Nature*, **325**, 733–6.

Kapaki, E. N., Zournas, C. P., Segdistsa, I. T., Xenos, D. S. & Papageorgiou, C. T. (1993). Cerebrospinal fluid aluminum levels in Alzheimer's disease. *Biol. Psychiatry*, **33**(8–9): 679–81.

Kapaki, E., Zournas, C., Kanias, G., Zambelis, T., Kakami, A. & Papageorgiou, C. (1997). Essential trace element alterations in amyotrophic lateral sclerosis. *J. Neurol. Sci.*, **147**(2), 171–5.

King, J. C., Shames, D. M. & Woodhouse, L. R. (2000). Zinc homeostasis in humans. *J. Nutr.*, **130**(5S Suppl), 1360S–6S.

Krebs, N. F. (2000). Overview of zinc absorption and excretion in the human gastrointestinal tract. *J. Nutr.*, **130**(5S Suppl), 1374S–7S.

Kuo, Y. M., Zhou, B., Cosco, D. & Gitschier, J. (2001). The copper transporter CTR1 provides an essential function in mammalian embryonic development. *Proc. Natl Acad. Sci., USA*, **98**(12), 6836–41.

Leake, A., Morris, C. M. & Whateley, J. (2000). Brain matrix metalloproteinase 1 levels are elevated in Alzheimer's disease. *Neurosci. Lett.*, **291**(3), 201–3.

Lee, D. Y., Prasad, A. S., Hydrick-Adair, C., Brewer, G. & Johnson, P. E. (1993). Homeostasis of zinc in marginal human zinc deficiency: role of absorption and endogenous excretion of zinc. *J. Lab. Clin. Med.*, **122**(5), 549–56.

Lee, J.-Y., Mook-Jung, I. & Koh, J.-Y. (1999). Histochemically reactive zinc in plaques of the Swedish mutant beta-amyloid precursor protein transgenic mice. *J. Neurosci.*, **19**, RC10, 1–5.

Lee, J., Prohaska, J. R. & Thiele, D. J. (2001). Essential role for mammalian copper transporter Ctr1 in copper homeostasis and embryonic development. *Proc. Natl Acad. Sci., USA*, **98**(12), 6842–7.

Liochev, S. I., Chen, L. L., Hallewell, R. A. & Fridovich, I. (1997). Superoxide-dependent peroxidase activity of H48Q: a superoxide dismutase variant associated with familial amyotrophic lateral sclerosis. *Arch. Biochem. Biophys.*, **346**(2), 263–8.

Liu, H., Zhu, H., Eggers, D. K. *et al.* (2000). Copper(2+) binding to the surface residue cysteine 111 of His46Arg human copper-zinc superoxide dismutase, a familial amyotrophic lateral sclerosis mutant. *Biochemistry*, **39**(28), 8125–32.

Lovell, M. A., Robertson, J. D., Teesdale, W. J., Campbell, J. L. & Markesbery, W. R. (1998). Copper, iron and zinc in Alzheimer's disease senile plaques. *J. Neurol. Sci.*, **158**(1), 47–52.

Maret, W. & Vallee, B. L. (1998). Thiolate ligands in metallothionein confer redox activity on zinc clusters. *Proc. Natl Acad. Sci., USA*, **95**(7), 3478–82.

Masters, B. A., Quaife, C. J., Erickson, J. C. *et al.* (1994). Metallothionein III is expressed in neurons that sequester zinc in synaptic vesicles. *J. Neurosci.*, **14**, 5844–57.

Mattiazzi, M., D' Aurelio, M., Gajewski, C. D. *et al.* (2002). Mutated human SOD1 causes dysfunction of oxidative phosphorylation in mitochondria of transgenic mice. *J. Biol. Chem.*, **277**(33), 29626–33.

Maynard, C. J., Cappai, R., Volitakis, I. *et al.* (2002). Overexpression of Alzheimer's disease amyloid-beta opposes the age-dependent elevations of brain copper and iron. *J. Biol. Chem.*, **277**, 44670–6.

Mercer, J. F. (2001). The molecular basis of copper-transport diseases. *Trends Mol. Med.*, **7**(2), 64–9.

Miura, T., Suzuki, K., Kohata, N. & Takeuchi, H. (2000). Metal binding modes of Alzheimer's amyloid ß-peptide in insoluble aggregates and soluble complexes. *Biochemistry*, **39**(23), 7024–31.

Moir, R. D., Atwood, C. S., Romano, D. M. *et al.* (1999). Differential effects of apolipoprotein E isoforms on metal-induced aggregation of Aß using physiological concentrations. *Biochemistry*, **38**(14), 4595–603.

Molina, J. A., Jimenez-Jimenez, F. J., Aguilar, M. V. *et al.* (1998). Cerebrospinal fluid levels of transition metals in patients with Alzheimer's disease. *J. Neural Transm.*, **105**(4–5), 479–88.

Morita, H., Ikeda, S., Yamamoto, K. *et al.* (1995). Hereditary ceruloplasmin deficiency with hemosiderosis: a clinicopathological study of a Japanese family. *Ann. Neurol.*, **37**(5), 646–56.

Nagano, S., Ogawa, Y., Yanagihara, T. & Sakoda, S. (1999). Benefit of a combined treatment with trientine and ascorbate in familial amyotrophic lateral sclerosis model mice. *Neurosci. Lett.*, **265**(3), 159–62.

Nagano, S., Satoh, M., Sumi, H. *et al.* (2001). Reduction of metallothioneins promotes the disease expression of familial amyotrophic lateral sclerosis mice in a dose-dependent manner. *Eur. J. Neurosci.*, **13**(7), 1363–70.

Nunomura, A., Perry, G., Aliev, G. *et al.* (2001). Oxidative damage is the earliest event in Alzheimer disease. *J. Neuropathol. Exp. Neurol.*, **60**(8), 759–67.

Opazo, C., Huang, X. & Cherny, R. (2002). Metalloenzyme-like activity of Alzheimer's disease ß-amyloid: Cu-dependent catalytic conversion of dopamine, cholesterol and biological, reducing agents to neurotoxic H_2O_2. *J. Biol. Chem.*, **277**, 40302–8.

Palmiter, R. D. & Findley, S. D. (1995). Cloning and functional characterization of a mammalian zinc transporter that confers resistance to zinc. *EMBO J.*, **14**(4), 639–49.

Palmiter, R. D., Cole, T. B. & Findley, S. D. (1996a). ZnT-2, a mammalian protein that confers resistance to zinc by facilitating vesicular sequestration. *EMBO J.*, **15**(8), 1784–91.

Palmiter, R. D., Cole, T. B., Quaife, C. J. & Findley, S. D. (1996b). ZnT-3, a putative transporter of zinc into synaptic vesicles. *Proc. Natl Acad. Sci., USA*, **93**(25), 14934–9.

Panayi, A. E., Spyrou, N. M., Iversen, B. S., White, M. A. & Part, P. (2002). Determination of cadmium and zinc in Alzheimer's brain tissue using Inductively Coupled Plasma Mass Spectrometry. *J. Neurol. Sci.*, **195**(1), 1–10.

Penkowa, M., Giralt, M., Moos, T., Thomsen, P. S., Hernandez, J. & Hidalgo, J. (1999). Impaired inflammatory response to glial cell death in genetically metallothionein-I- and -II-deficient mice. *Exp. Neurol.*, **156**(1), 149–64.

Pullen, R. G., Franklin, P. A. & Hall, G. H. (1990). ^{65}Zinc uptake from blood into brain and other tissues in the rat. *Neurochem. Res.*, **15**(10), 1003–8.

Puttaparthi, K., Gitomer, W. L., Krishnan, U., Son, M., Rajendran, B. & Elliott, J. L. (2002). Disease progression in a transgenic model of familial amyotrophic lateral sclerosis is dependent on both neuronal and non-neuronal zinc binding proteins. *J. Neurosci.*, **22**(20), 8790–6.

Reaume, A. G., Elliott, J. L., Hoffman, E. K. *et al.* (1996). Motor neurons in Cu/Zn superoxide dismutase-deficient mice develop normally but exhibit enhanced cell death after axonal injury. *Nat. Genet.*, **13**(1), 43–7.

Roe, J. A., Wiedau-Pazos, M., Moy, V. N., Goto, J. J., Gralla, E. B. & Valentine, J. S. (2002). In vivo peroxidative activity of FALS-mutant human CuZnSODs expressed in yeast. *Free Radic. Biol. Med.*, **32**(2), 169–74.

Rogers, J. T., Randall, J. D. Cahill, C. M. *et al.* (2002). An iron-responsive element type II in the 5′-untranslated region of the Alzheimer's amyloid precursor protein transcript. *J. Biol. Chem.*, **277**(47), 45518–28.

Rosen, D. R. (1993). Mutations in Cu/Zn superoxide dismutase gene are associated with familial amyotrophic lateral sclerosis. *Nature*, **364**(6435), 362.

Rulon, L. L., Robertson, J. D., Lovell, M. A., Deibel, M. A., Ehmann, W. D. & Markesber, W. R. (2000). Serum zinc levels and Alzheimer's disease. *Biol. Trace Elem. Res.*, **75**(1–3), 79–85.

Sahu, R. N., Pandey, R. S., Subhash, M. N., Arya, B. Y., Padmashree, T. S. & Srinivas, K. N. (1988). CSF zinc in Alzheimer's type dementia. *Biol. Psychiatry*, **24**(4), 480–2.

Sandstead, H. H. (2000). Causes of iron and zinc deficiencies and their effects on brain. *J. Nutr.*, **130**(2S Suppl), 347S–9S.

Sillevis-Smitt, P. A., Blaauwgeers, H. G., Troost, D. & de Jong, J. M. (1992). Metallothionein immunoreactivity is increased in the spinal cord of patients with amyotrophic lateral sclerosis. *Neurosci. Lett.*, **144**(1–2), 107–10.

Sillevis-Smitt, P. A., Mulder, T. P., Verspaget, H. W., Blaauwgeers, H. G., Troost, D. & de Jong, J. M. (1994). Metallothionein in amyotrophic lateral sclerosis. *Biol. Signals*, **3**(4), 193–7.

Singh, R. J., Karoui, H., Gunther, M. R., Beckman, J. S., Mason, R. P. & Kalyanaraman, B. (1998). Reexamination of the mechanism of hydroxyl radical adducts formed from the reaction between familial amyotrophic lateral sclerosis-associated Cu, Zn superoxide dismutase mutants and H_2O_2. *Proc. Natl Acad. Sci., USA*, **95**(12), 6675–80.

Squitti, R., Rossini, P. M., Cassetta, E. *et al.* (2002). d-penicillamine reduces serum oxidative stress in Alzheimer's disease patients. *Eur. J. Clin. Invest.*, **32**(1), 51–9.

Strausak, D., Mercer, J. F., Dieter, H. H., Stremmel, W. & Multhaup, G. (2001). Copper in disorders with neurological symptoms: Alzheimer's, Menkes, and Wilson diseases. *Brain Res. Bull.*, **55**(2), 175–85.

Subramaniam, J. R., Lyons, W. E., Liu, J. *et al.* (2002). Mutant SOD1 causes motor neuron disease independent of copper chaperone-mediated copper loading. *Nat. Neurosci.*, **5**(4), 301–7.

Suh, S. W., Jensen, K. B., Jensen, M. S. *et al.* (2000). Histochemically-reactive zinc in amyloid plaques, angiopathy, and degenerating neurons of Alzheimer's diseased brains. *Brain Res.*, **852**(2), 274–8.

Szerdahelyi, P. & Kasa, P. (1984). Histochemistry of zinc and copper. *Int. Rev. Cytol.*, **89**, 1–29.

Tanzi, R. E., Petrukhin, K., Chernov, I. *et al.* (1993). Identification of the Wilson's disease gene; a copper transporting ATPase with homology to the Menkes' disease gene. *Nat. Genet.*, **3**(4), 344–50.

Tully, C. L., Snowdon, D. A. & Markesbery, W. R. (1995). Serum zinc, senile plaques, and neurofibrillary tangles: findings from the Nun Study. *NeuroReport*, **6**, 2105–8.

Uchida, Y., Ihara, Y. & Tomonaga, M. (1988). Alzheimer's disease brain extract stimulates the survival of cerebral cortical neurons from neonatal rats. *Biochem. Biophys. Res. Commun.*, **150**(3), 1263–7.

Uchida, Y., Takio, K., Titani, K., Ihara, Y. & Tomonaga, M. (1991). The growth-inhibitory factor that is deficient in the Alzheimer's disease brain is a 68-amino acid metallothionein-like protein. *Neuron*, **7**, 337–47.

Vallee, B. L. (1995). The function of metallothionein. *Neurochem. Int.*, **27**(1), 23–33.

Wang, K., Zhou, B., Kuo, Y. M., Zemansky, J. & Gitschier, J. (2002). A novel member of a zinc transporter family is defective in acrodermatitis enteropathica. *Am. J. Hum. Genet.*, **71**(1), 66–73.

Wenstrup, D., Ehmann, W. D. & Markesbery, W. R. (1990). Trace element imbalances in isolated subcellular fractions of Alzheimer's disease brains. *Brain Res.*, **533**(1), 125–31.

Wiedau-Pazos, M., Goto, J. J., Rabizadeh, S. *et al.* (1996). Altered reactivity of superoxide dismutase in familial amyotrophic lateral sclerosis. *Science*, **271**(5248), 515–18.

Wong, P. C., Pardo, C. A., Borchelt, D. R. *et al.* (1995). An adverse property of a familial ALS-linked SOD1 mutation causes motor neuron disease characterized by vacuolar degeneration of mitochondria. *Neuron*, **14**(6), 1105–16.

Wong, P. C., Waggoner, D., Subramaniam, J. R. *et al.* (2000). Copper chaperone for superoxide dismutase is essential to activate mammalian Cu/Zn superoxide dismutase. *Proc. Natl Acad. Sci., USA*, **97**(6), 2886–91.

Yasui, M., Ota, K. & Garruto, R. M. (1993). Concentrations of zinc and iron in the brains of Guamanian patients with amyotrophic lateral sclerosis and parkinsonism-dementia. *Neurotoxicology*, **14**(4), 445–50.

Yu, W. H., Lukiw, W. J., Bergeron, C., Niznik, H. B. & Fraser, P. E. (2001). Metallothionein III is reduced in Alzheimer's disease. *Brain Res.*, **894**(1), 37–45.

Zhou, H. & Thiele, D. J. (2001). Identification of a novel high affinity copper transport complex in the fission yeast *Schizosaccharomyces pombe*. *J. Biol. Chem.*, **276**(23), 20529–35.

14

The role of inflammation in Alzheimer's disease neuropathology and clinical dementia. From epidemiology to treatment

Giulio Maria Pasinetti

Neuroinflammation Research Laboratories, Mount Sinai, School of Medicine, New York, USA

Several epidemiological studies have demonstrated a significantly lower incidence of Alzheimer's disease in individuals who regularly consume non-steroidal anti-inflammatory drugs (NSAIDs) compared with the general population. Despite this evidence, therapeutic studies investigating NSAIDs, including inhibitors of cyclooxygenase (COX)-1 and COX-2 and steroids, do not support this hypothesis. This discrepancy might be due to the fact that the bulk of epidemiological evidence has examined the likely incidence of AD prior to the onset of clinical symptoms of the disease. This inconsistency has led to the hypothesis that NSAIDs may be optimally effective as a preventive therapy prior to the onset of clinical symptoms or in individuals at high risk for AD, such as cases with mild cognitive impairment. This review will discuss recent findings from experimental models of AD neuropathology describing novel mechanisms involved in the potential beneficial role of NSAIDs. It will then examine the importance of evidence for the potential role of inflammation in amyloidosis in the AD brain. The implications of this evidence will be considered in the context of the potential negative role of inflammation in the brain during amyloid vaccination therapy in AD trials. On the basis of this information, this review will attempt to formulate a possible scenario in which optimal NSAIDs might be tested in the most favorable clinical therapeutic conditions in order to determine whether NSAIDs can provide beneficial treatment for the clinical progression of AD dementia. Alzheimer's disease is a chronic, progressive, irreversible neurodegenerative disorder associated with the process of ageing (McGeer *et al.*, 1996; In't Veld *et al.*, 2001; Stewart *et al.*, 1997). Presently, there are four million patients afflicted with AD in the USA, and the incidence is expected to increase exponentially over the next 10 years (Hebert *et al.*, 2003). Neuropathologically, AD is characterized by abnormal deposition of amyloid plaques in the brain parenchyma. The abnormal deposition appears to be the consequence of an elevation in amyloid peptides caused by altered processing of the amyloid precursor protein (APP) (Selkoe 2001). Abnormal phosphorylation of the microtubule-binding protein, tau (τ), also appears to play an important role in AD neuropathology and leads to neurofibrillary degeneration (Mandelkow & Mandelkow, 1998).

At present, there is no cure for AD. However, in the past year, research on AD has brought us closer to realizing the fundamental goal of sparing future generations the ravages of AD. A large body of evidence indicates progress in understanding the biological mechanisms of the disease, improving treatment options, and providing quality care. In the realm of therapeutics, we have gained new insights into the promising class of drugs known as non-steroidal anti-inflammatory drugs. Although it is not presently known whether inflammatory mechanisms (e.g. elevation of amyloid content and neurodegeneration) are responsible for AD neuropathology, or whether neurodegenerative events actually lead to inflammation (Pasinetti 1998), much of the epidemiological data support a protective effect for NSAIDs against AD (McGeer *et al.*, 1996; In't Veld *et al.*, 2001; Stewart *et al.*, 1997). Recent studies have further reinforced this evidence by suggesting that, in addition to beneficial anti-inflammatory actions, NSAIDs might also target AD amyloid pathology and possibly mediate neuroprotection. Ongoing investigations on the role of NSAIDs in AD dementia presently focus on preventive initiatives to slow the progression and possibly onset of AD dementia rather than exploring NSAIDs as a potential therapeutic agent in AD.

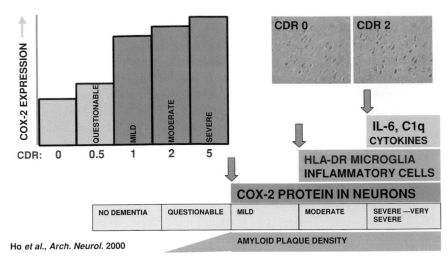

Fig. 14.1 Hippocampal COX-2 protein content correlates linearly with clinical progression of Early AD dementia.

Inflammation as a function of clinical progression of AD dementia

Recent studies suggest that select segments of inflammatory cascades are elevated in the AD brain as a function of the progression of clinical dementia in AD. The Clinical Dementia Rating (CDR) (Morris, 1993; Luterman *et al.*, 2000; Haroutunian *et al.*, 1998) measures stages of AD from early to late onset. The CDR scale ranges from mild cognitive impairment (MCI; CDR 0.5) through mild (CDR 1), moderate (CDR 2) and severe dementia (CDR 5). Pro-inflammatory activities have been found as early as the CDR 1 stage and become increasingly evident as the disease progresses. For example, as will be discussed below, recent evidence indicates that cyclooxygenase (COX)-2, an enzyme responsible for converting arachidonic acid to prostaglandin, is upregulated in the brain of AD cases, and increases between cases of CDR 0.5 to CDR 1.0 (Ho *et al.*, 2001) (Fig. 14.1). Other classical markers of inflammation such as cytokine expression and major histocompatibility complex (MHC) HLA-DR immunoreactive microglia are also apparent in AD, but occur in later, more-severe phases of the disease, such as in cases with CDR 5 (Fig. 14.1). Extensive oxidative damage and widespread activation of caspase pathways involved in apoptotic brain cell death are also found but, again, predominantly in severe cases of AD dementia (CDR 5) (Pompl *et al.*, 2003). Consequently, anti-inflammatory treatments designed to target inflammatory cascades specific to each stage of AD might optimize efficacy.

Implications for the potential beneficial role of NSAIDs in cases with MCI

As mentioned earlier, several epidemiological studies support the hypothesis that anti-inflammatory drugs delay the onset and possibly the progression of AD (McGeer *et al.*, 1996). In a meta-analysis review of 17 epidemiological studies (McGeer *et al.*, 1996), it was suggested that anti-inflammatory treatment such as NSAIDs and steroids might decrease the risk for AD by as much as 50%. Moreover, a prospective study found that relative risk (RR) for AD fell with increasing duration of NSAID use (In't Veld *et al.*, 2001). The same study showed that two or more years of NSAID treatment resulted in a 40% decrease in RR (In't Veld *et al.*, 2001).

However, epidemiological and therapeutic studies are inconsistent. For example, in a 6-month study of the NSAID Indomethacin (100–150 mg day^{-1}), patients showed some improvement on a battery of cognitive tests (Rogers *et al.*, 1993), yet this finding could not be reproduced in a study using other NSAID compounds such as Diclofenac-Misoprostol (although a high drop-out rate prevented statistically significant results) (Scharf *et al.*, 1999) or Prednisone (Aisen *et al.*, 2000) (among others). Although these data appear discouraging, it is likely that subclasses of NSAIDs have varying levels of efficacy for AD treatment. Furthermore, the epidemiological evidence was based on studies of patients prior to the apparent clinical manifestation of AD, in contrast with therapeutic studies conducted on patients with illnesses severe enough to exceed the clinical detection threshold (e.g. ≥CDR 1). Thus, patients at high risk for AD, such as cases affected by MCI, might represent a better population for testing the potential preventive role of anti-inflammatory activities in AD.

MCI is a term used to describe memory decline or other specific cognitive impairment in individuals who do not yet have AD dementia or significant impairment of other cognitive functions beyond that expected for their age or education (Petersen *et al.*, 1999). However, despite the high conversion rate to early AD dementia, MCI cannot be used synonymously with early or mild AD, as patients with AD are impaired not only in memory performance but in other cognitive domains as well, and meet diagnostic criteria for dementia (Shah *et al.*, 2000; Sramek *et al.*, 2001). Furthermore, there is heterogeneity among MCI cases with regard to the likelihood of conversion to early AD. Thus, it might be expected that inflammatory activities in the brain may ultimately affect the progression from MCI to early AD. We hypothesize that anti-inflammatory therapeutic approaches administered in cases with CDR exceeding MCI (CDR 0.5), such as CDR 1, might not be optimally effective, possibly explaining the discrepancy between epidemiological and therapeutic evidence for the role of NSAIDs in AD.

AD anti-inflammatory prevention trial (ADAPT)

A large body of epidemiological evidence supports a protective role for NSAIDs in AD; however, several attempts to translate these findings into successful treatment strategies for AD have largely failed. NSAIDs may impart neuroprotective effects that slow the progression of AD pathology, but we need to keep in mind that, most probably, these compounds will not yield short-term improvement in clinical symptoms. A further consideration is that the trials with NSAIDs have been conducted in diagnosed (clinically progressed) AD patients, and it may be the case that these drugs prove effective only when administered prior to the development of significant AD pathology. Thus, traditional clinical trial designs and clinical outcome measures (e.g. as have been employed in clinical efficacy trials of the classic cholinesterase inhibitors and other symptomatic drugs) are unlikely to be useful for testing anti-inflammatory compounds. For example, the ongoing AD Anti-inflammatory Prevention Trial (ADAPT) may prove that the "penultimate" test of NSAID efficacy may be primary prevention trials, wherein thousands of subjects at high risk for AD are treated for a number of years prior to clinical symptoms of AD. The significant sample size and high cost necessitated by such trials is a significant barrier to the effective demonstrating of primary prevention. For these reasons, current research

is focusing on developing more efficient assessment methods for use in AD primary prevention trials, and focusing on the development of biomarkers to help steer future prevention measures.

In part because of these considerations, the Alzheimer's Disease Anti-Inflammatory Prevention Trial (ADAPT) currently in progress was designed to test the hypothesis that NSAIDs might delay or prevent the onset of AD and age-related cognitive decline (Breitner, personal communication, 2003, Pompl *et al.*, 2003). This ongoing 5–7-year randomized clinical study at Johns Hopkins (sponsored by the National Institute of Aging) is testing the NSAID medications Naproxen and Celecoxib (a non-selective and a selective COX-2 inhibitor, respectively, see below) in patients who have not been diagnosed with AD. Adapting more-refined criteria for stages of AD in clinical trials should increase our understanding of NSAID treatment efficacy, and hopefully should resolve the inconsistency between epidemiological and therapeutic studies.

COX: a target for NSAIDs in AD

While the mechanism of action of NSAIDs is not entirely clear, it is generally believed that their effects are attributable to a competitive inhibition of COX catalytic activity, and a subsequent reduction of inflammatory PG production. COX exists in two isoforms, COX-1 and COX-2, that are encoded by distinct genes on different chromosomes (Kujubu *et al.*, 1991; Cao *et al.*, 1995; O'Banion *et al.*, 1992). There is an approximate 50% homology between these enzymes, as well as similar catalytic activity (Kujubu *et al.*, 1991; Cao *et al.*, 1995; O'Banion *et al.*, 1992). However, the isoforms are physiologically distinct. COX-2 is inducible in response to inflammatory signals such as cytokines and lipopolysaccharide, and is downregulated by glucocorticoids. By contrast, COX-1 is generally constitutive. Thus, it would appear that the COX-2 isoform is responsible for the normal mediation of inflammatory activity, while COX-1 maintains housekeeping functions (including gastric cytoprotection and platelet aggregation.

Traditional NSAIDs are non-selective COX inhibitors, effecting both COX-1 and COX-2 at varying levels. However, the effects of these compounds on inflammation are believed to derive from inhibition of COX-2 activity. COX-1 inhibition, on the other hand, has previously been implicated in gastrointestinal, renal and platelet toxicity associated with some non-selective COX inhibitors. Thus, the use of newly developed highly selective COX-2 inhibitors in AD treatment hold promise for anti-inflammatory action and reduced toxicity (Vane & Botting, 1995; Warner *et al.*, 1999).

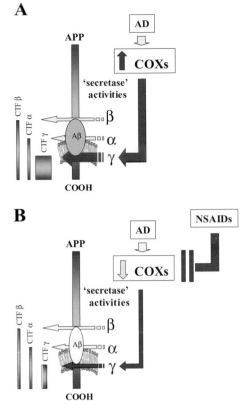

Fig. 14.2 Hypothetical mechanism through which COX-2 may influence amyloidosis.

As discussed, major efforts are under way to determine whether COX inhibitors can help control the progression of AD dementia. However, given the growing number of candidate NSAIDs and their widely divergent activities, it is vital that drug selection and study design are optimized. As discussed, proper characterization of NSAID activities, and administration of these compounds in a fashion that is specific to the phase of the disease, is essential. Better understanding of the influence of inflammatory activity in AD, and identification of specific mechanisms that play an early role in the progression of the disease, will vastly improve the likelihood of assessing the potential value of NSAID treatment strategies.

Novel evidence for the beneficial role of NSAIDs in AD neuropathology

Though the preponderance of research on NSAIDs in AD supports the theory that the anti-inflammatory "COX-inhibiting" properties of these drugs are responsible for their prophylaxis (Aisen 1997), recent in vitro studies offer alternative/additional explanations (Weggen et al., 2001; Lim et al., 2000). For example, there is evidence that non-selective COX inhibitors, rather than selective COX-2 (the inducible form of COX) inhibitors may inhibit the production of the fibril forming β-amyloid $(A\beta)_{1-42}$ (the major component of $A\beta$ plaques) at mM concentrations; and in some instances, in cellular systems devoid of COX activity. While this new evidence is of extreme interest, it is unclear these data will impact clinical studies in humans due the toxic doses studied. For example, it has been calculated that the in vitro efficacious dose for $A\beta$ inhibition would be the equivalent of approximately 10 g a day of NSAIDs (e.g. ibuprofen). However, it is without question that these mechanisms deserve continued exploration, so that we can eventually define the mechanisms by which certain NSAIDs, and other compounds, preferentially reduce $A\beta_{1-42}$ production. Addressing these questions will help determine the utility of this approach in reducing $A\beta$ deposition and other AD-associated pathology in vivo. Future studies in AD-like disease mice should prove to be useful tools for determining the relative merits of NSAIDs on selective $A\beta$ lowering activities and for altering $A\beta$ deposition and other AD like pathology in transgenic mice. Moreover, it is extremely important to consider that although certain NSAIDs may prevent $A\beta$ production in COX deficient cells in vitro systems, this evidence does not preclude involvement of COX in the onset/propagation of AD neuropathology in the brain. Indeed these studies do in no way disprove the relevance of COX to AD neuropatholgy, nor indicate that the COX inhibiting actions of NSAIDS are dispensable. For example, COX-2 and also COX-1 is significantly elevated in AD (Ho et al., 1999; Pasinetti & Aisen, 1998; Oka & Takashima, 1997; Yasojima et al., 1999), and the predominance of epidemiological evidence supporting a protective role for NSAIDs, exclusively find COX inhibitors to be effective. Thus, although alternative/additional mechanisms for NSAIDs are being explored (e.g. anti-amyloidogenic, peroxisome proliferator activated receptor-γ activation), it remains possible that the COX inhibiting properties of these drugs are what imparts their protection against AD. This hypothesis is further supported by the fact that previous studies (including Weggen) show that ibuprofen potently diminishes amyloid pathology as does that potently inhibiting COX activity in the brain, and recent findings from our laboratory demonstrate that COX overexpression in a mouse model of AD type neuropathology significantly exacerbates amyloid pathology (Xiang et al., 2002), possibly through a mechanism involving prostaglandin mediated induction of γ-secretase activity (Qin et al., 2003). This is schematized in Fig. 14.2.

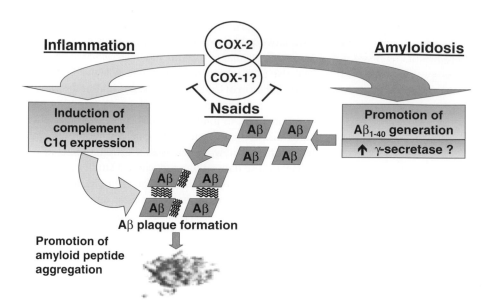

Fig. 14.3 Hypothesized roles of COX's in the creation of Aβ plaques and NSAIDs' blocking roles.

Hypothesis for the role of COX-2 in Aβ-amyloid plaques

On the basis of the above findings, we hypothesize that an additional factor that might promote Aβ fibril formation in AD is through COX-2-mediated pro-inflammatory activities in the brain (e.g. the induction of pro-inflammatory complement components) (Fig. 14.3). Evidence has recently been found that COX-2 might promote the expression of the complement component C1qB (Spielman *et al.*, 2002), which is known for its role in promoting Aβ aggregation (Webster *et al.*, 1994). In the light of the Weggen *et al.*, 2001 study showing that non-selective COX inhibitors, rather than selective COX-2-specific inhibitors, prevent Aβ peptide production and our data showing that COX-2 expression in the brain may potentiate AD-type amyloidogenesis and Aβ peptide generation in the brain (Xiang *et al.*, 2002), add a new layer of complexity to understanding the relationship between inflammation and AD neuropathology. For example, while COX-2 may be an important promoter of amyloidogenic activities in the AD brain, non-selective, rather than selective, COX inhibitors could preferentially influence APP processing and result in decreased Aβ production in vitro (Lim *et al.*, 2000).

Thus, a preferential COX-2 inhibitor with tolerable (i.e. minimal) COX-1 inhibitory activity (e.g. without gastrointestinal toxicity) may be an "ideal" NSAID with respect to anti-amyloidogenic activity for chronic treatment in cases at high risk of developing AD (MCI 0.5) (Fig. 14.1).

Future studies investigating the pharmacological relevance of NSAIDs in amyloidosis, and the role of COX, will help clarify the potential efficacy of COX-inhibiting drugs as therapeutic treatment in AD. The following sections will discuss recent evidence suggesting that COX-2 might also influence cell-cycle activities implicated in AD neuropathology.

Paradoxical role of inflammatory mediators in the brain. Implications for AD dementia

Although current data indicate that inflammation is closely correlated with AD neuropathology, the role of inflammatory mediators in the brain and AD may demand more complex measures than mere suppression of inflammation. For example, there is evidence that the complement derived pro-inflammatory anaphylatoxin C5a may exert neuroprotective properties in the brain (as demonstrated in C5 knock-out mice), possibly through activation of MAP kinase pathways (Mukherjee & Pasinetti, 2001). This evidence is consistent with the demonstration that activation of the complement system in the brain can protect against Aβ-induced neurotoxicity, and reduces amyloidosis (either by blocking deposition or promoting the clearance of amyloid) in mouse models of AD neuropathology. These results indicate that complement activation products can protect against brain injury, including Aβ, and possibly influence amyloidosis. Collectively, these findings support the concept that certain inflammatory defense mechanisms in the brain may be beneficial in neurodegenerative disease.

Thus, therapeutic designs aimed at non-specifically suppressing segments of inflammatory cascades may inhibit select neuroprotective actions of the complement system (among others), and possibly exacerbate neurodegenerative mechanisms. It is certain that future elucidation of the role of target inflammatory mediators will lead to the development of more successful therapeutic strategies that are specific for each (progressive) stage of AD dementia/neuropathology.

The role of COX derived prostaglandin in the cell cycle

Four phases comprise the cell division cycle: G1 (growth), S (DNA synthesis and replication), G2 (growth for cell division) and M (mitosis). The main regulators of the progression of the cell cycle are the cyclin/cyclin-dependent kinase (CDK) complexes. The sequential expression/activation of these proteins not only orchestrates the transition from one phase to the next, but can also serve as markers of different stages of the cell cycle (Grana & Reddy, 1995). The transition of resting cells from the G0 to G1 phase is controlled by the cyclinD–CDK4/6 complexes. Activation of these complexes is triggered by mitogenic growth factors and inhibited by the CDK4/6 inhibitor protein (p)18 (see below).

Little is known about the role of CDK4/6 inhibitors in the brain, including p18. Using a high-throughput microarray DNA technique, it was found that overexpression of hCOX-2 in neurons coincided with decreased mRNA expression of CDK4/6 inhibitor p18 in the brains of hCOX-2 transgenic mice (Mirjany et al., 2002). Conversely, the hCOX-2-mediated inhibition of p18 expression was reversed by treatment of mice with the preferential COX-2 inhibitor Nimesulide. Similarly, hippocampal expression of CDK4 and COX-2 in hippocampal neurons appears to be coregulated during the clinical progression of AD dementia, which is consistent with evidence that COX-2 may facilitate the re-entry of neurons into the cell cycle (G. M. Pasinetti, unpublished observations). Generally, it is thought that the CDK4/6 and cyclinD complex regulate the G0 to G1 transition.

One important target substrate for this complex is the retinoblastoma protein (Rb), a tumour suppressor that is phosphorylated by activated cyclinD–CDK4/6. Recent evidence shows that RB can also be phosphorylated during the cell response to Aβ-mediated neurotoxicity (Giovanni et al., 2000). Hyperphosphorylated Rb is released from the transcription factor complex E2F, which then activates genes required for S phase transition. COX-2 is induced in neurons following glutamate excitotoxic injury (Kelley

et al., 1999), and aggregated Aβ peptides (Pasinetti & Aisen, 1998) may promote cell-cycle activities by decreasing the expression of the CDK4/6 inhibitor p18 (Mirjany et al., 2002). Thus, it might be possible that COX leads neurons to attempt (prostaglandin mediated) unsuccessfully to re-enter the cell cycle, and eventually to die. We suggest that prostaglandin-responsive cell-cycle activities could facilitate transition of resting neurons from the G0 into G1 phase, representing an important target for neuroprotection by NSAIDs.

Cell cycle, COX-2 and AD neuropathology

The search for factors responsible for the formation of neurofibrillary and neuritic plaque pathology has yielded several clues to the hypothesis that the cell cycle may play an important role in AD neurodegeneration. For example, the accumulation of potentially mitogenic growth factors (e.g. epidermal growth factor) in AD amyloid plaques could represent a trigger that initiates the re-entry of neurons into the cell cycle. COX-2, whose expression is also regulated by growth factors and tumour promoters (Fletcher et al., 1991), might represent an important link between amyloid pathology and the cell cycle. Another factor associated with amyloid pathology, also known to influence cell-cycle pathways is oxidative stress (Raina et al., 2000). Thus, it is possible that, if neuronal COX-2 expression leads to increased oxidative stress in brain (for review, see Pasinetti 1998), this might influence susceptibility of neurons to injury through control of cell-cycle activities. This hypothesis is consistent with evidence showing that COX inhibitors can also arrest the progression of cell division (Shiff et al., 1996).

An important step towards understanding AD-related neuritic pathology was the identification of protein kinases involved in τ phosphorylation. For example, there is evidence showing that, in vitro, CDK5 can phosphorylate τ into AD-type NFTs (Baumann et al., 1993). The importance of this finding is that it might explain intracellular changes and increased phosphorylation of cytoskeletal proteins, such as τ neurofilaments, seen in AD. While destabilization of microtubules and coincidental activation of different kinases that are able to phosphorylate τ are features of the cell division cycle, COX-2 expression is preferentially elevated in NFT[+] neurons of the hippocampal formation (Oka & Takashima, 1997).

Thus, inappropriate re-entry into the cell cycle and interrupted mitotic processes might be significant factors not only in the neuronal degeneration but also in the cytoskeleton that characterizes the pathology of AD. In addition to its potential role on amyloidosis, it could still be possible that

COX-2, by promoting cell-cycle activities, might also participate in abnormal τ phosphorylation, further influencing AD neuropathology and possibly the clinical progression of AD dementia.

Inflammation and Aβ vaccination therapy in AD

Recent studies have found that highly specific immune responses may yield clinical benefits for AD. Investigators at Elan Pharmaceuticals studying neuropathological changes in a murine model of AD found that immunization with Aβ peptides can evoke an antibody response that is capable of preventing amyloidosis in pre-treated animals, and can significantly mitigate existing pathology in already affected subjects. These results have been replicated in numerous laboratories (Bard *et al.*, 2000; Janus *et al.*, 2000; Morgan *et al.*, 2000; Schenk *et al.*, 1999), and preliminary studies have already begun with human AD patients. On the basis of observations from animal models, investigators have found that either passive (intraperitoneal (IP) injection of pre-derived Aβ antibodies) or active (IP injection of Aβ peptides) immunization with Aβ can activate pro-inflammatory microglial cells through immunoglobulin receptor signaling, which facilitates clearance and degradation of Aβ plaques (Bard *et al.*, 2000; Schenk *et al.*, 1999); this presents a potentially beneficial role for features of inflammation in AD. These studies are undoubtedly the most significant leap in understanding the role of Aβ in AD neuropathology in the past decade.

However, the induction of pro-inflammatory cascades, such as inducing microglial cytokine synthesis and generation of free radicals (Levi *et al.*, 1998), are little understood and have been implicated in neuronal injury (Ulvestad *et al.*, 1994). As already discussed in this chapter, these underlying phenomenon are characteristic of AD, and raise significant concern about potential pro-inflammatory consequences of Aβ immunization (Mukherjee & Pasinetti, 2001; Pasinetti *et al.*, 2002). Furthermore, these data offer new challenges for the development of anti-inflammatory strategies to be used as therapeutic treatment in conjunction with vaccination therapy. For example, if the induction of specific cytokines or other unknown microglial pro-inflammatory factors are integral to microglial scavenging of Aβ plaques, the use of anti-inflammatory drugs that interfere with microglial cytokine activity may aberrantly affect immunization-based Aβ plaque clearance. If Aβ immunization induces/intensifies inflammation in patients with early-stage AD dementia, this treatment could potentially promote neurodegeneration and lead to acceleration of dementia.

Thus, it is early to speculate on the outcome of this therapy, either in conjunction with NSAIDs or alone, particularly as the trials have been discontinued owing to cerebral inflammation in a small subset of cases. Without question, vaccination is the most promising therapeutic treatment known so far. However, I believe this therapy is in the very early stages of development and requires much more investigation before it can safely be used for AD.

Research in progress and outstanding research questions: is there a "better" NSAID for AD?

Toxicity remains a major roadblock for studying dosages of traditional NSAIDs. One way to reduce NSAID toxicity is to add a cytoprotective agent to the treatment regimen. However, it is unlikely that a study of a treatment regimen that is tolerated (over the course of a year) by a minority of subjects will yield definitive results. The Alzheimer's Disease Cooperative Study (ADCS; http://antimony.ucsd.edu/) has opted to study two NSAID-type regimens that are expected to have substantially less toxicity than the Indomethacin and Diclofenac regimens reported (see above).

The first drug chosen by the ADCS is a new selective COX-2 inhibitor called Rofecoxib. As discussed, COX-2 may be the target of action of NSAIDs in the AD brain, and since COX-2 inhibitors appear to carry much reduced risk of serious gastrointestinal toxicity, Rofecoxib may be effective in preventive but not therapeutic trials.

The second active drug regimen in the new ADCS trial is low-dose Naproxen. Naproxen is a non-selective COX inhibitor, and therefore carries the risk of toxicity at full dose, similar to Indomethacin and Diclofenac. However, if in fact COX-1 is an important target for NSAID action in AD amyloidosis, Naproxen could be more effective than a selective COX-2 inhibitor. It is important to note that 200 mg is the over-the-counter analgesic dose, which is substantially less than a full anti-inflammatory dose. Nevertheless, studies suggest that this regimen is reasonably well tolerated in the elderly (DeArmond *et al.*, 1995; Geczy *et al.*, 1987), although there is little data on long-term treatment. In rodents, it has been found that systemic administration of Naproxen suppresses COX activity in the brain (Abdel-Halim *et al.*, 1978; Ferrari *et al.*, 1990), indicating effective brain penetration. But will the low dose tested in the ADCS trial be sufficient to alter the AD process? The epidemiological studies suggest that casual use of NSAIDs obtained over-the-counter may be neuroprotective, supporting further study of a low-dose regimen.

Collectively, the studies discussed above demonstrate significant support for the use of NSAIDs in the treatment of cases at high risk of developing AD dementia such as those with MCI. Specifically, studies on the role of COX inhibitors in amyloidogenesis indicate that non-selective COX inhibitors might be more favorable candidates for such therapies. These compounds should be proven highly tolerable both in experimental and in clinical studies, and demonstrate beneficial effects on AD-type neuropathology at lower concentration, possibly through their potential high penetrability of the blood–brain barrier. Thus, the optimal COX inhibitor needs superior tolerability relative to other COX inhibitors and should promote (directly or indirectly) anti-amyloidogenic activities, and possibly exert neuroprotective functions (as previously demonstrated for some categories of COX inhibitors) (Mirjany *et al.*, 2002).

In conclusion, elucidating the role of inflammatory processes provides an impetus for further development of anti-inflammatory therapies for AD. However, it remains critical that diagnosis of patients in the very earliest stages of AD is improved. Continued research is necessary to identify very early neurobiological inflammatory abnormalities clearly so that effective treatments can be developed.

Acknowledgements

I thank Ms. Isabela Diaconescu and Ms. Rainy Horvath for the outstanding editorial role in the preparation of this manuscript.

REFERENCES

Abdel-Halim, M. S., Sjoquist, B. & Anggard, E. (1978). Inhibition of prostaglandin synthesis in rat brain. *Acta Pharmacol. Toxicol.(Copenh)*, **43**, 266–72.

Aisen, P. S. (1997). Inflammation and Alzheimer's disease: mechanisms and therapeutic strategies. *Gerontology*, **43**, 143–9.

Aisen, P. S., Davis, K. L., Berg, J. D., Schafer, K., Campbell, K. & Thomas, R. G. (2000). A randomized controlled trial of prednisone in Alzheimer's disease. Alzheimer's Disease Cooperative Study. *Neurology*, **54**, 588–93.

Bard, F., Cannon, C., Barbour, R., Burke, R. L., Games, D. & Grajeda, H. (2000). Peripherally administered antibodies against amyloid beta-peptide enter the central nervous system and reduce pathology in a mouse model of Alzheimer disease. *Nat. Med.*, **6**, 916–19.

Baumann, K., Mandelkow, E. M., Biernat, J., Piwnica-Worms, H. & Mandelkow, E. (1993). Abnormal Alzheimer-like phosphorylation of tau-protein by cyclin-dependent kinases cdk2 and cdk5. *FEBS Lett.*, **336**, 417–24.

Cao, C., Matsumura, K., Yamagata, K. & Watanabe, Y. (1995). Induction by lipopolysaccharide of cyclooxygenase-2 mRNA in rat brain; its possible role in the febrile response. *Brain Res.*, **697**, 187–96.

DeArmond, B., Francisco, C. A., Lin, J. S., Huang, F. Y., Halladay, S. & Bartziek, R. D. (1995). Safety profile of over-the-counter naproxen sodium. *Clin. Ther.*, **17**, 587–601.

Ferrari, R. A., Ward, S. J., Zobre, C. M., Van Liew, D. K., Perrone, M. H. & Connell, M. J. (1990). Estimation of the in vivo effect of cyclooxygenase inhibitors on prostaglandin E2 levels in mouse brain. *Eur. J. Pharmacol.*, **179**, 25–34.

Fletcher, B. S., Lim, R. W., Varnum, B. C., Kujubu, D. A., Koski, R. A. & Herschman, H. R. (1991). Structure and expression of TIS21, a primary response gene induced by growth factors and tumor promoters. *J. Biol. Chem.*, **266**, 14511–18.

Geczy, M., Peltier, L. & Wolbach, R. (1987). Naproxen tolerability in the elderly: a summary report. *J. Rheumatol.*, **14**, 348–54.

Giovanni, A., Keramaris, E., Morris, E. J., Hou, S. T., O'Hare, M. & Dyson, N. (2000). E2F1 mediates death of B-amyloid-treated cortical neurons in a manner independent of p53 and dependent on Bax and caspase 3. *J. Biol. Chem.*, **275**, 11553–60.

Grana, X. & Reddy, E. P. (1995). Cell cycle control in mammalian cells: role of cyclins, cyclin dependent kinases (CDKs), growth suppressor genes and cyclin-dependent kinase inhibitors (CKIs). *Oncogene*, **11**, 211–19.

Haroutunian, V., Perl, D. P., Purohit, D. P., Marin, D., Khan, K. & Lantz, M. (1998). Regional distribution of neuritic plaques in the nondemented elderly and subjects with very mild Alzheimer disease. *Arch. Neurol.*, **55**, 1185–91.

Hebert, L. E., Scherr, P.A, Bienias, J. L., Bennett, D. A. & Evans D. A. (2003). Alzheimer disease in the US population. *Arch. Neurol.*, **60**, 1119–22.

Ho, L., Pieroni, C., Winger, D., Purohit, D. P., Aisen, P. S. & Pasinetti, G. M. (1999). Regional distribution of cyclooxygenase-2 in the hippocampal formation in Alzheimer's disease. *J. Neurosci. Res.*, **57**, 295–303.

Ho, L., Purohit, D., Haroutunian, V., Luterman, J. D., Willis, F. & Naslund, J. (2001). Neuronal cyclooxygenase 2 expression in the hippocampal formation as a function of the clinical progression of Alzheimer disease. *Arch. Neurol.*, **58**, 487–92.

In't Veld, B. A., Ruitenberg, A., Hofman, A., Launer, L. J., van Duijn, C. M. & Stijnen, T. (2001). Nonsteroidal antiinflammatory drugs and the risk of Alzheimer's disease. *N. Engl. J. Med.*, **345**, 1515–21.

Janus, C., Pearson, J., McLaurin, J., Mathews, P. M., Jiang, Y. & Schmidt, S. D. (2000). A beta peptide immunization reduces behavioural impairment and plaques in a model of Alzheimer's disease. *Nature*, **408**, 979–82.

Kelley, K. A., Ho, L., Winger, D., Freire-Moar, J., Borelli, C. B. & Aisen, P. S. (1999). Potentiation of excitotoxicity in transgenic mice overexpressing neuronal cyclooxygenase-2. *Am. J. Pathol.*, **155**, 995–1004.

Kujubu, D. A., Fletcher, B. S., Varnum, B. C., Lim, R. W. & Herschman, H. R. (1991). TIS10, a phorbol ester tumor promoter-inducible mRNA from Swiss 3T3 cells, encodes a novel prostaglandin synthase/cyclooxygenase homologue. *J. Biol. Chem.*, **266**, 12866–72.

Levi, G., Minghetti, L. & Aloisi, F. (1998). Regulation of prostanoid synthesis in microglial cells and effects of prostaglandin E2 on microglial functions. *Biochimie*, **80**, 899–904.

Lim, G. P., Yang, F., Chu, T., Chen, P., Beech, W. & Teter, B. (2000). Ibuprofen suppresses plaque pathology and inflammation in a mouse model for Alzheimer's disease. *J. Neurosci.*, **20**, 5709–14.

Luterman, J. D., Haroutunian, V., Yemul, S., Ho, L., Purohit, D. & Aisen, P. S. (2000). Cytokine gene expression as a function of the clinical progression of Alzheimer disease dementia. *Arch. Neurol.*, **57**, 1153–60.

Mandelkow, E. M. & Mandelkow, E. (1998). Tau in Alzheimer's disease. *Trends Cell Biol.*, **8**, 425–7.

McGeer, P. L., Schulzer, M. & McGeer, E. G. (1996). Arthritis and anti-inflammatory agents as possible protective factors for Alzheimer's disease: a review of 17 epidemiologic studies. *Neurology*, **47**, 425–32.

Mirjany, M., Ho, L. & Pasinetti, G. M. (2002). Role of cyclooxygenase-2 in neuronal cell cycle activity and glutamate-mediated excitotoxicity. *J. Pharmacol. Exp. Ther.*, **301**, 494–500.

Morgan, D., Diamond, D. M., Gottschall, P. E., Ugen, K. E., Dickey, C. & Hardy, J. (2000). A beta peptide vaccination prevents memory loss in an animal model of Alzheimer's disease. *Nature*, **408**, 982–5.

Morris, J. C. (1993). The Clinical Dementia Rating (CDR): current version and scoring rules. *Neurology*, **43**, 2412–14.

Mukherjee, P. & Pasinetti, G. M. (2001). Complement anaphylatoxin C5a neuroprotects through mitogen activated protein kinase dependent inhibition of caspase 3. *J. Neurochem.*, **76**, 1–8

O'Banion, M. K., Winn, V. D. & Young, D. A. (1992). cDNA cloning and functional activity of a glucocorticoid-regulated inflammatory cyclooxygenase. *Proc. Natl Acad. Sci. USA*, **89**, 4888–92.

Oka, A. & Takashima, S. (1997). Induction of cyclo-oxygenase 2 in brains of patients with Down's syndrome and dementia of Alzheimer type: specific localization in affected neurones and axons. *NeuroReport*, **8**, 1161–4.

Pasinetti, G. M. (1998). Cyclooxygenase and inflammation in Alzheimer's disease: experimental approaches and clinical interventions. *J. Neurosci. Res.*, **54**, 1–6.

Pasinetti, G. M. & Aisen, P. S. (1998). Cyclooxygenase-2 expression is increased in frontal cortex of Alzheimer's disease brain. *Neuroscience*, **87**, 319–24.

Pasinetti, G. M. & Pompl, P. (2002). Inflammation and Alzheimer's disease: are we well-ADAPTed? *Lancet Neurol.*, **1**, 403–4.

Pasinetti, G. M., Ho, L. & Pompl, P. (2002a). Amyloid immunization in Alzheimer's disease: do we promote amyloid scavenging at the cost of inflammatory degeneration? *Neurobiol. Aging*, **23**, 665–6.

Pasinetti, G. M., Ho, L. & Pompl, P. (2002b). AN1792 vaccination immunotherapy in Alzheimer's disease: the case of a therapy before its time. *Neurobiol Aging*, **23**, 683–4.

Petersen, R. C., Smith, G. E., Waring, S. C., Ivnik, R. J., Tangalos, E. G. & Kokmen, E. (1999). Mild cognitive impairment: clinical characterization and outcome. *Arch. Neurol.*, **56**, 303–8.

Pompl, P. N., Yemul, S., Xiang, Z. *et al.* (2003). Caspase gene expression in the brain as a function of the clinical progression of Alzheimer's disease. *Arch. Neurol.*, **60**, 369–76.

Qin, W., Ho, L., Pompl, P. N. *et al.* (2003). Cyclooxygenase (COX)-2 and COX-1 potentiate beta-amyloid peptide generation through mechanisms that involve gamma secretase activity. *J. Biol. Chem.*, **278**, 50970–7.

Raina, A. K., Zhu, X., Rottkamp, C. A., Monteiro, M., Takeda, A. & Smith, M. A. (2000). Cyclin' toward dementia: cell cycle abnormalities and abortive oncogenesis in Alzheimer disease. *J. Neurosci. Res.*, **61**, 128–33.

Rogers, J., Kirby, L. C., Hempelman, S. R., Berry, D. L., McGeer, P. L. & Kaszniak, A. W. (1993). Clinical trial of indomethacin in Alzheimer's disease. *Neurology*, **43**, 1609–11.

Scharf, S., Mander, A., Ugoni, A., Vajda, F. & Christophidis, N. (1993). A double-blind, placebo-controlled trial of diclofenac/misoprostol in Alzheimer's disease. *Neurology*, **53**, 197–201.

Schenk, D., Barbour, R., Dunn, W., Gordon, G., Grajeda, H. & Guido, T. (1999). Immunization with amyloid-beta attenuates Alzheimer-disease-like pathology in the PDAPP mouse. *Nature*, **400**, 173–7.

Selkoe, D. J. (2001). Alzheimer's disease: genes, proteins, and therapy. *Physiol Rev.*, **81**, 741–66.

Shah, Y., Tangalos, E. G. & Petersen, R. C. (2000). Mild cognitive impairment. When is it a precursor to Alzheimer's disease? *Geriatrics*, **55**, 62, 65–8.

Shiff, S. J., Koutsos, M. I., Qiao, L. & Rigas, B. (1996). Nonsteroidal antiinflammatory drugs inhibit the proliferation of colon adenocarcinoma cells: effects on cell cycle and apoptosis. *Exp. Cell Res.*, **222**, 179–88.

Spielman, L., Winger, D., Ho, L., Aisen, P. S., Shohami, E. & Pasinetti, G. M. (2002). Induction of the complement component C1qB in brain of transgenic mice with neuronal overexpression of human cyclooxygenase-2. *Acta Neuropathol. (Berl.)*, **103**, 157–62.

Sramek, J. J., Veroff, A. E. & Cutler, N. R. (2001). The status of ongoing trials for mild cognitive impairment. *Expert. Opin. Investig. Drugs*, **10**, 741–52.

Stewart, W. F., Kawas, C., Corrada, M. & Metter, E. J. (1997). Risk of Alzheimer's disease and duration of NSAID use. *Neurology*, **48**, 626–32.

Ulvestad, E., Williams, K., Matre, R., Nyland, H., Olivier, A. & Antel, J. (1994). Fc receptors for IgG on cultured human microglia mediate cytotoxicity and phagocytosis of antibody-coated targets. *J. Neuropathol. Exp. Neurol.*, **53**, 27–36.

Vane, J. R. & Botting, R. M. (1995). New insights into the mode of action of anti-inflammatory drugs. *Inflamm. Res.*, **44**, 1–10.

Warner, T. D., Giuliano, F., Vojnovic, I., Bukasa, A., Mitchell, J. A. & Vane, J. R. (1999). Nonsteroid drug selectivities for cyclo-oxygenase-1 rather than cyclo-oxygenase-2 are associated with human gastrointestinal toxicity: a full in vitro analysis. *Proc. Natl. Acad. Sci., USA*, **96**, 7563–8.

Webster, S., O'Barr, S. & Rogers, J. (1994). Enhanced aggregation and beta structure of amyloid beta peptide after coincubation with C1q. *J. Neurosci. Res.*, **39**, 448–56.

Weggen, S., Eriksen, J. L., Das, P., Sagi, S. A., Wang, R. & Pietrzik, C. U. (2001). A subset of NSAIDs lower amyloidogenic Abeta42 independently of cyclooxygenase activity. *Nature*, **414**, 212–16.

Xiang, Z., Ho, L., Yemul, S. *et al.* (2002). Cyclooxygenase-2 promotes amyloid plaque deposition in a mouse model of Alzheimer's disease neuropathology. *Gene Expression*, **10**, 271–8.

Yasojima, K., Schwab, C., McGeer, E. G. & McGeer, P. L. (1999). Distribution of cyclooxygenase-1 and cyclooxygenase-2 mRNAs and proteins in human brain and peripheral organs. *Brain Res.*, **830**, 226–36.

15

Selected genetically engineered models relevant to human neurodegenerative disease

Donald L. Price[1], David R. Borchelt[2], Michael K. Lee[3] and Philip C. Wong[4]

[1,2,3,4]Departments of Pathology, [1]Neurology, and [1]Neuroscience, and the [1,2,3,4]Division of Neuropathology,
The Johns Hopkins University School of Medicine, Baltimore, MD, USA

Introduction

This review on selected neurodegenerative diseases, including Alzheimer's disease, amyotrophic lateral sclerosis (ALS), and Parkinson's disease, and frontotemporal dementia with Parkinsonism (FTD-P), focuses on the ways by which genetically engineered models have clarified the mechanisms of these disorders and have identified new targets for therapy, and been used to test new treatment strategies. These neurodegenerative diseases are some of the most challenging diseases in medicine because of their general prevalence, cost, lack of mechanism-based treatments, and impact on individuals and caregivers (Lipp & Wolfer, 1998; Wong et al., 2002). The classical clinical phenotypes are, for the most part, quite distinct and reflect the dysfunction and death of specific populations of neurons. These brain lesions are characterized by the presence of intracellular or extracellular peptides/aggregates, which appear to be critical contributors to neurotoxicity, partially damaging to synapses. Genetic risk factors influence these age-associated, chronic illnesses. In rare instances, cases are inherited in Mendelian fashion (usually as autosomal dominants). Susceptibility genes, environmental risk factors, or other influences remain to be defined. Information from genetics has allowed investigators to express or to target genes in efforts to model these diseases and to study the (Armstrong et al., 1996) molecular participants critical in pathogenic pathways. This body of research is the principal topic of this review.

In this review, we emphasize the value of genetically engineered mouse models for studies of mechanisms and for experimental therapeutics, but we also briefly describe the extraordinary utility of non-mammalian genetic models. The identification of mutations in specific genes causing each of these illnesses has provided new opportunities for scientists to investigate the molecular participants in pathological processes and to explore disease mechanisms using transgenic approaches. In these autosomal dominant disorders, the mutant proteins often do not exhibit reductions in normal functions, but instead, malfolded mutant peptides acquire toxic properties that directly or indirectly impact on the structures, functions and viabilities of neural cells. Introducing mutant genes into mice reproduces some features of these diseases. Moreover, targeting of the genes that influence pathogenic pathways has provided new insights into disease mechanisms and has led to identification of potential therapeutic targets. Over the next several years, we anticipate that additional targets will be identified and novel treatments will be tested in these model systems and eventually will be examined in clinical trials. Because of limitations on citations, our references are predominantly reviews (Cleveland & Rothstein, 2001; Dawson et al., 2002; Dunnett & Bjorklund, 1999; Goedert, 2001a,b; Julien, 2001; Kopan & Goate, 2002; Lee-Price, 2001; Lee & Trojanowski, 1999; Lin et al., 1999; Lipp & Wolfer, 1998; Olanow & Tatton, 1999; Price et al., 1998; Selkoe, 2001; Sherman & Goldberg, 2001; Sisodia & George-Hyslop, 2002; Tanzi & Bertram, 2001; Vassar & Citron, 2000; Wichmann & DeLong, 1996; Wong et al., 2002; Wong et al., 1998; Cleveland & Rothstein, 2001).

Alzheimer's disease

Clinical features, pathology and genetics

Affected individuals usually develop clinical manifestations (difficulty in memory and cognitive functions followed by progressive dementia) during the seventh decade (earlier in familial cases) (Lipp & Wolfer, 1998; Price et al., 1998; Selkoe, 2001; Sisodia & George-Hyslop, 2002; Wong *et al.*, 2002). Alzheimer's disease is the most common cause of senile dementia, a term that refers to a syndrome, occurring in elderly people, resulting in memory loss and cognitive impairments of sufficient severity to interfere with social, occupational, and personal functions. This type of dementia affects more than 4 million people. Because of increased life expectancy and the postwar baby boom, the elderly are the fastest growing segment of our society. During the next 25 years, the number of people with Alzheimer's disease in the United States will triple, as will the cost. Thus, Alzheimer's disease is one of society's major public health problems.

Most individuals with sporadic Alzheimer's disease exhibit the first clinical signs during their seventh decade. However, some cases develop in mid-life; in these cases, it is more likely that there is a family history of the disease. In both the sporadic and familial forms of Alzheimer's disease, affected individuals show abnormalities of memory, problem solving, language, calculation, visuospatial perceptions, judgment, and behavior. Some patients develop psychotic symptoms, such as hallucinations and delusions. In these patients, mental functions and activities of daily living are increasingly impaired. In the late stages, these individuals are mute, incontinent, and bedridden and usually die of intercurrent medical illnesses. To make a diagnosis, clinicians rely on histories from patients and informants as well as physical, neurological, and psychiatric examinations, neuropsychological testing, laboratory studies, and a variety of diagnostic tests including neuroimaging studies. The clinical profile, in concert with a variety of laboratory assessments, allows the clinician to make a diagnosis of possible or probable Alzheimer's disease. Alterations in levels of specific proteins in the serum or cerebrospinal fluid, such as the Aβ peptide and tau, may eventually prove useful in diagnosis, but values may vary between individuals, and single measures are not of great diagnostic value. The presence of the ApoE-4 allele confers risk in late-onset disease (see below) and ApoE genotyping is a useful research tool but is not helpful for routine diagnostic purposes. Computerized tomography (CT) or magnetic resonance imaging (MRI), performed on the majority of patients with this syndrome, can identify other potentially treatable diseases and may detect abnormalities, particularly in the medial temporal lobe (atrophy of hippocampus and entorhinal cortex), that may have predictive value for establishing a diagnosis of Alzheimer's disease. In Alzheimer's disease, positron emission tomography (PET) and single photon emission computerized tomography (SPECT) usually show decreased regional blood flow in the parietal and temporal lobes with involvement of other cortical areas at later stages. At present, except for brain biopsy,

there are no tests that definitively establish the diagnosis of Alzheimer's disease in living subjects. It is extremely important for the physician to exclude other causes of dementia because some other types of dementia respond to specific treatments. However, Alzheimer's disease is a disorder for which there are no mechanism-based therapies. Only symptomatic treatments are available at present.

There are five principal risk factors for Alzheimer's disease: age; mutations in the *presenilin 1* (*PS1*) gene on chromosome 14; mutations in the *presenilin 2* (*PS2*) gene on chromosome 1; mutations in the *APP* gene on chromosome 21; and ApoE alleles positioned on the proximal long arm of chromosome 19. The presence of any of the mutations in the genes encoding *APP*, *PS1*, or *PS2* causes the disorder to occur earlier in the third through sixth decades. Specific A*poE* alleles appear to predispose to later onset Alzheimer's disease and some cases of late-onset familial Alzheimer's disease. Thus approximately 10% of cases of Alzheimer's disease exhibit clinical syndromes in mid life (early onset) and are inherited in an autosomal dominant manner.

In a small fraction of early-onset families, missense mutations have been identified in the APP gene on chromosome 21. In all cases, mutations invariably occur within, or immediately proximal to, the Aβ region. In several families, the normally occurring valine residue at position 717 (of APP-770) is replaced with Ile, Gly, or Phe. Cells that express APP with mutations at position 717 secrete increased levels of Aβ1-42,43. These longer Aβ forms have a propensity to nucleate rapidly into amyloid fibrils. In two large, related, early-onset Alzheimer's disease families from Sweden, a double mutation at codons 670 and 671 results in a substitution of the normal Lys–Met dipeptide to Asn–Leu; cells that express this mutant polypeptide secrete approximately 6–8-fold higher levels of Aβ. In a hereditary disease associated with Aβ deposition around blood vessels and cerebral hemorrhage, an APP mutation at position 693 leads to a Glu–Gln substitution (corresponding to amino acid 22 of Aβ). This mutation is associated with the Aβ peptide species that are more prone to aggregate into fibrils. Thus, some of the mutations linked to Alzheimer's disease can change the processing of APP and influence the biology of Aβ by increasing the production of Aβ peptides or the amounts of the longer, more toxic Aβ42, or by promoting fibril formation. In those pedigrees in which missense mutations in either *APP* or *PS* genes promote the formation of the more toxic form of Aβ, it is highly likely that Aβ is central to the pathogenesis of disease.

Nearly 50% of cases of early-onset familial Alzheimer's disease are linked to the *PS1* gene (chromosome 14), which encodes a 467-amino acid polypeptide containing between seven and nine transmembrane domains. Two mutations in the *PS2* gene, which encodes a protein homologous to PS1, cause autosomal dominant Alzheimer's disease in two familial Alzheimer's disease pedigrees. Approximately 50% of *PS1* mutations occur within, or immediately adjacent to, predicted transmembrane domains. Mutant PS1 and PS2 influence APP processing in a fashion that results in the elevated production of $A\beta 1$–42/43. In cultured cells and brains (human, monkey, and mouse), PS1 accumulates as an N-terminal ~28 kDa fragment, and a C-terminal ~18 kDa fragment, providing strong support for the idea that PS1 is subject to endoproteolytic processing in vivo. In view of the paucity of accumulated full-length PS, it has been suggested that PS fragments may be functional units. As indicated above, it is believed that PS are critical components of the γ-secretase complex. PS are highly homologous to sel-12, a gene product that plays a role in the determination of cell fates during development, suggesting roles for PS in these processes. Recent work indicates that γ-secretase cleaves APP and Notch-1, generating intracellular domains that traffic to the nucleus where they are involved in transcriptional activation. The results of studies of PS1 and Nct studies are consistent with the concept that they are components of γ-secretase and the phenotype of knockout mouse embryos are the result of failed Notch1 signaling. Mutant PS1 and PS2 influence APP processing in a fashion that results in the elevated production of $A\beta 1$–42/43.

An allele of ApoE, a glycoprotein that carries cholesterol and other lipids in the blood, has been implicated as a risk factor for the disease in Alzheimer's disease. At the single ApoE locus, three alleles are expressed: apoE2, apoE3, and apoE4. The apoE3 allele is most common in the general population (frequency of 0.78), whereas the allelic frequency of apoE4 is 0.14. However, in clinic-based studies, patients with late-onset disease (>65 years of age) have an apoE4 allelic frequency of 0.50; thus, the risk for Alzheimer's disease is increased by the presence of apoE4. The mechanisms whereby the apoE allele type elevates the risk for late-onset disease are not known but may reflect differences in the abilities of apoE isoforms to bind $A\beta$ and possibly influence aggregation, deposition and/or clearance.

In some individuals with autosomal dominant Alzheimer's disease, mutations have been identified in three different genes: *Amyloid Precursor Protein* (*APP*); *Presenilin1* (*PS1*); *and Presenilin2* (*PS2*). APP, a type I transmembrane protein existing as several isoforms, is expressed in many different cell types. Significantly, APP is particularly abundant in neurons, is synthesized in cell bodies, and is transported rapidly anterograde in axons, by interacting with a kinesin motor, possibly serving as a cargo receptor (Goldstein & Yang, 2000). Cleavages of APP generates $A\beta$ peptides via the activities of BACE1 (β-site APP cleaving enzyme 1) and the γ-secretase complex (Cai *et al.*, 2001; Sisodia & George-Hyslop, 2002; Vassar *et al.*, 1999; Vassar & Citron, 2000), which generate the N- and C-termini of $A\beta$ peptides, respectively. The γ-secretase cleavage liberates the APP intracellular domain (AICD), which, upon translocation to the nucleus, appears to play a role in transcription. (Cao & Südhof, 2001; Sisodia & George-Hyslop, 2002). The levels and distributions of APP and the neuronal pro-amyloidogenic cleavage enzymes, particularly BACE1, are hypothesized to be the principal determinants of high levels of $A\beta$ in the brain (Cai *et al.*, 2001; Wong *et al.*, 2001). In contrast, formation of $A\beta$ is precluded by cleavage of APP within the $A\beta$ domain by α-secretase and by BACE2, which are either expressed at low or non-detectable levels, respectively, in the brain, but at variably higher levels in other organs (Lipp & Wolfer, 1998).

Several FAD linked *APP* mutations are located in proximity to the pro-amyloidogenic cleavage sites (Sisodia & George-Hyslop, 2002; Tanzi & Bertram, 2001). For example, the *APPswe* mutation, a double mutation at the N-terminus of $A\beta$, enhances BACE1 cleavage many-fold and is associated with elevated levels of all $A\beta$ peptides, including $A\beta 42$, the *APP 717* mutation, located near the C-terminus of $A\beta$, promotes γ-secretase activity, leading to increased secretion of $A\beta 42$, the longer and more toxic $A\beta$ peptide.

PS1 and *PS2*, which encode two highly homologous 43 to 50 kD multipass transmembrane proteins that are processed to stable N-terminal and C-terminal fragments, are conserved from invertebrates to humans and are involved in Notch 1 signaling critical for cell fate decisions (Kopan & Goate, 2002; Sisodia & George-Hyslop, 2002). They are widely expressed at low abundance in the CNS. PS influence APP processing and are recognized as components of the γ-secretase complex along with Nicastrin, a type I transmembrane glycoprotein (Kopan & Goate, 2002; Sisodia & George-Hyslop, 2002), as well as Aph1 and Pen2, two multipass transmembrane proteins (Francis *et al.*, 2002). The *PS1* gene has been reported to harbor more than 80 different FAD mutations, whereas only a small number of mutations have been found in *PS2*-linked families (Sherrington *et al.*, 1995; Sisodia & George-Hyslop, 2002; Tanzi & Bertram, 2001). The majority of abnormalities in *PS* genes are missense mutations that result in single amino acid substitutions, which enhance γ-secretase activity and increase the levels of the $A\beta 42$ peptides. See below for discussion of the results of gene targeting studies, which have begun to clarify some of the properties of APP, BACE1, and components of γ-secretase complex.

BACE1 and BACE2, encoded by genes on chromosomes 11 and 21, respectively, have been shown to be transmembrane aspartyl proteases that are directly involved in the cleavage of APP. BACE1 mRNA is present in a variety of tissues, and BACE1 mRNA levels are high in many regions of brain. Intriguingly, BACE1 protein is only abundant in the brain while it is undetectable in other non-neural tissues, such as the pancreas, where the mRNA is alternatively spliced to a smaller protein incapable of cleaving APP. BACE2 mRNA is very low in neural tissues, except for scattered nuclei in the hypothalamus and brainstem. The functions of BACE1 processed peptides generated from APP are unknown, but it has been suggested that Aβ may influence synaptic activity. Interestingly, BACE1, along with APP and components of γ-secretase complex, is transported in axons and enriched at some synapses in several highly plastic structures of brain (i.e. the mossy fiber pathway originating from hippocampal granule cells and the glomeruli of olfactory bulb, observations consistent with the idea that Aβ released in synaptic fields may influence synaptic plasticity.

BACE1 preferentially cleaves APP at the +1 and +11 sites of Aβ in APP and is critical for the generation of Aβ. *BACE1* deficient mice show no overt developmental phenotype. In cultures of BACE1−/−neurons, the secretion of Aβ1-40/42 as well as Aβ11-40/42 is abolished. Thus, BACE1 is the principal neuronal β-secretase and makes proamyloidogenic cleavages. In contrast, BACE2 makes antiamyloidogenic cleavages at +19/+20 of Aβ. Thus, BACE2 acts more like a α-secretase. While BACE1 is critical for amyloidogenesis in brain, BACE2 does not appear to play a significant role in APP processing in neurons. In contrast to the ubiquitous expression of BACE1 mRNA in a variety of tissues, BACE1 protein is abundantly expressed in the brain while it is undetectable in other non-neural tissues, such as the pancreas. Although BACE1 protein is expressed at comparable levels in most brain regions, BACE1-specific immunoreactivities are particularly localized in the hippocampus.

γ-Secretase activity is essential for the regulated intramembraneous proteolysis of a variety of transmembrane proteins dependent upon a multiprotein catalytic complex, including PS and several other transmembrane proteins. It is not clear whether PS1 itself acts as an aspartyl protease, functions as a co-factor critical for the activity of γ-secretase, or exerts its influence by playing a role in trafficking of APP or other essential protein critical for enzyme activity, to the proper compartment for γ-secretase cleavage. The concept that PS1 may act as an aspartyl protease or may be a critical co-factor essential for the activity of γ-secretase is suggested by several observations: PS1 is isolated with γ-secretase under specific detergent soluble conditions; PS1 is selectively cross-linked or photoaffinity labeled by transition state inhibitors; substitutions of aspartate residues at D257 in TM6 (although controversial) and at D385 in TM7 have been reported to reduce secretion of A and ultimately cleavage of Notch1 in vitro; cells in which *PS1* has been targeted show decreased levels of secretion of A. Recent work is focused on roles of different proteins in the multiprotein catalytic complex, including Nicastrin (NCT), Aph-1, and Pen-2 domain. *NCT* null (*NCT*/−) mice and *NCT*/− fibroblasts have shown that *NCT* is an integral member of the γ-secretase complex. Partial decreases in the level of NCT significantly reduce the secretion of Aβ and NCT may be a valuable therapeutic target for Alzheimer's disease. Aph-1 and Pen-2 are novel transmembrane proteins: Aph1 has seven predicted transmembrane domain; while Pen-2 has two predicted transmembrane regions. These proteins interact with sel-12/PS and aph-1/nicastrin and their inactivation with RNAi methods in *Drosophila* cells decreases γ-sectetase of APP and Notch and reduces levels of processed PS. For these reasons, Aph-1 and Pen-2 are now believed to be critical components of γ-secretase complex.

Models of Aβ amyloidosis

Both spontaneously occurring and genetically produced diseases in animals have now been used to model features of Alzheimer's disease. Rhesus monkeys, *Macaca mulatta*, with an estimated lifespan of >35 years, show cognitive and memory deficits that appear at the end of the second and the beginning of the third decades of life. These animals develop virtually all of the brain abnormalities observed in older humans and, to a lesser degree, patients with Alzheimer's disease.

In mice, expression of APPswe or APP717 minigenes encoding FAD-linked mutations (with or without mutant *PS1*) leads to an Aβ amyloidosis in the CNS. Levels of Aβ, are elevated, and diffuse Aβ deposits and neuritic plaques appear in the hippocampus and cortex (Benoist & Mathis, 1997; Lipp & Wolfer, 1998; Price et al., 1998; Wong et al., 2002). Classical neurofibrillary tangles are not present in a region of the brain. The pathology evolves in stages: elevated levels of Aβ; synaptic alterations; formation of neurites, axon degeneration; and diffuse amyloid evolving to plaques. The nature and levels of the expressed transgene and the specific mutation influence the severity of the pathology. Mice expressing both mutant *PS1* and mutant *APP* develop accelerated disease (Benoist & Mathis, 1997). Learning deficits, problems in object recognition memory, and difficulties performing tasks assessing spatial reference and working memory have been identified in some of the lines of mutant mice (Chen *et al.*, 2000). Thus, these animals have an Aβ amyloidosis in the CNS, although the mutant mice do not fully recapitulate the full phenotypes of Alzheimer's disease; they are very useful subjects for research designed to examine mechanisms and to test therapies for this type of disease.

In attempts to obtain mice with both plaques and tangles, mutant *APP* transgenic mice have been mated to mice expressing the *P301L tau* mutant, a mutation linked to familial frontotemporal dementia with parkinsonism (FTDP). These mice appear to have a greater number of tangles and an apparent shift in distribution of NFT (Lewis *et al.*, 2001). Moreover, tau pathology appears to be induced by introducing Aβ fibrils into the brains of *P301L tau* mutant mice. However, mice bearing both mutant *tau* and *APP* or mutant *tau* mice injected with Aβ are problematic as models of FAD because the FTDP mutation alone is associated with the presence of tangles. A more appropriate model of Alzheimer's disease might be achieved by co-expression of mutant *FAD* linked genes and all six isoforms of wild type human *tau*.

Gene targeting relevant to Alzheimer's disease

In an effort to understand the functions of some of the genes thought to play roles in Alzheimer's disease, investigators have targeted a variety of genes including: *APP*; *APLPs*; *BACE1*; and *PS1*.

Homozygous $APP^{-/-}$ mice are viable and fertile, but appear to have subtle decreases in locomotor activity and forelimb grip strength (Zheng *et al.*, 1995). The absence of substantial phenotypes in $APP^{-/-}$ mice is thought to be related to functional redundancy of two amyloid precursor-like proteins, APLP1 and APLP2, homologous to APP. Consistent with this idea, $APLP2^{-/-}$ mice appear normal, but *APP* and *APLP2* null mice and *APLP1* and *APLP2* null mice do not survive the perinatal period (Heber *et al.*, 2000).

BACE1, a type 1 transmembrane aspartyl protease, is relatively abundant in brain, and is transported by axons to terminals. *BACE1* null mice are viable and healthy, have no obvious phenotype or pathology, and can mate successfully (Cai *et al.*, 2001; Luo *et al.*, 2001; Vassar & Citron, 2000). Importantly, cortical neurons cultured from *BACE1−/−* embryos, do not show cleavages at the +1 and +11 sites of Aβ, and the secretion of Aβ peptides is abolished even in the presence of elevated levels of exogenous weight or mutant APP (Cai *et al.*, 2001). In brains of *BACE1* null mice, Aβ peptides are not produced. These results establish that BACE1 is the neuronal β-secretase required to cleave APP to generate the N-termini of Aβ (Cai *et al.*, 2001). At present, there

is no consensus on other substrates cleaved by BACE1. Behavioral studies of the null mice, in vitro and in vivo challenges of *BACE1* neural cells, and two-dimensional gels of organs from BACE1 +/+, +/−, −/− mice will be critical in determining the consequences of the absence of BACE1 on behavior, susceptibility to challenge, and other substrates that may be cleaved by the enzyme. Results thus far indicate that BACE1 is an excellent therapeutic target for development of an anti-amyloidogenic drug.

In contrast to BACE1 null mice, $PS1^{-/-}$ mice do not survive beyond the early postnatal period and show severe developmental abnormalities of the axial skeleton, ribs and spinal ganglia, features resembling a partial Notch 1−/− phenotype (Wong *et al.*, 1997). These abnormalities occur because PS1 along with Nicastrin, APH1 and PEN2 and perhaps other proteins are components of the γ-*secretase* complex that carries out the S3 intramembranous cleavage of Notch1, a receptor protein involved in critical cell-fate decisions during development. Without this cleavage, the Notch1 intracellular domain (NICD) is not released from the plasma membrane and does not reach the nucleus to initiate transcriptional processes essential for cell fate decisions. In cell culture, absence of *PS1* or substitution of particular aspartate residues leads to reduced levels of γ-secretase cleavage products and levels of Aβ. *PS2* null mice are viable and fertile, though they develop age-associated mild pulmonary fibrosis and hemorrhage. Mice lacking *PS1* and heterozygous for *PS2* die midway through gestation with full *Notch1* null-like phenotype. To study the role of PS1 in vivo in adult mice, two groups generated conditional *PS1*-targeted mice lacking PS1 expression in the forebrain after embryonic development. As expected, the absence of PS1 resulted in decreased generation of Aβ; further establishing that PS1 is critical for γ-secretase activity in the brain. As indicated above, more recent work has established that Nicastrin, APH1 and PEN2 are also components of the γ-secretase complex and are critical for stabilizing PS and for generation of Aβ (Francis *et al.*, 2002). In concert, these findings suggest that γ-secretase inhibitors may be useful as therapeutic agents for Aβ amyloidosis.

Alzeimer's disease, a neuronal disease

The source of APP giving rise to Aβ has been debated (Wong *et al.*, 2001). Significantly, key participants in Aβ amyloidosis (APP, PS1 and BACE1) are synthesized by neurons, transported to terminals, and are colocalized with neurites in immediate proximity to sites of Aβ deposition in brain, providing circumstantial evidence consistent with a neuronal origin for Aβ. Moreover, APP is cleaved by BACE1 in distal axon terminal to generate C-terminal amyloidogenic peptides. More compelling is the demonstration that lesions of specific neuronal populations or their axonal projections (i.e. entorhinal cortex or perforant pathway) reduces the levels of Aβ and the numbers of plaques in terminal fields of these neurons (Sheng *et al.*, 2002).

Because BACE1 is the principal β-secretase in neurons and BACE2 and α-secretase may serve to limit the secretion of Aβ peptides in other organs, we have hypothesized that the relative levels of BACE1 and BACE2 activities, in conjunction with high levels of APP in neurons, are major determinants of Aβ amyloidosis in the CNS (Cai *et al.*, 2001; Wong *et al.*, 2001). This hypothesis predicts that the secretion of Aβ peptides will be the highest in neurons and brain as compared to other cell types or tissues because neurons express high levels of APP and BACE1 coupled with low level expression of BACE2 and α-secretase. Seemingly inconsistent with this hypothesis is a study showing high levels of BACE1 mRNA in the pancreas. BACE1 is critical for Aβ amyloidosis and both BACE1 and APP are expressed in β cells of the pancreas. Why do Alzheimer's disease and diabetes mellitus not occur together? It now appears that BACE1 mRNAs in the pancreas are alternatively spliced to generate a BACE1 isoform that is incapable of cleaving APP. Taken together with the observations that pancreas possesses low levels of normal BACE1 protein and activity, these results are consistent with the view that a high ratio of BACE1 to BACE2 activity leads to the selective vulnerability of neurons to Aβ amyloidosis, whereas the cells of the pancreas are spared.

One important member of the γ-secretase complex is nicastrin (NCT), a type I transmembrane glycoprotein, which forms high molecular weight complexes with presenilins (Yu *et al.*, 2000) and binds to the membrane-tethered form of Notch1 (Chen *et al.*, 2001). Recent studies have indicated that nicastrin is required for Notch signaling and APP processing (Chung & Struhl, 2001; Edbauer *et al.*, 2002; Hu *et al.*, 2002; Lopez-Schier & St Johnston, 2002; Yu *et al.*, 2000). Studies in *Drosophila* have shown that nicastrin may function to stabilize PSs and appears to be critical for the trafficking of PSs to the cell surface. Likewise, PS is required for the maturation and cell surface accumulation of nicastrin (Edbauer *et al.*, 2002; Kaether *et al.*, 2002; Leem *et al.*, 2002). These results have suggested that nicastrin and PSs form functional components of a multimeric complex required for the intramembraneous proteolysis of both Notch and APP.

To determine whether nicastrin is required for proteolytic processing of Notch and APP in mammals and the role of nicastrin in presenilin/γ-secretase complex assembly, we generated nicastrin-deficient ($NCT^{-/-}$) mice and derived fibroblasts from $NCT^{-/-}$ embryos. Nicastrin-null embryos died by embryonic day 10.5 and exhibited several patterning defects, including abnormal somite segmentation, phenotypes that are reminiscent of embryos lacking Notch1 or both presenilins. Importantly, secretion of Aβ peptides is abolished in $NCT^{-/-}$ fibroblasts, whereas it is reduced by ~50% in $NCT^{+/-}$ cells; the failure to generate Aβ peptides in $NCT^{-/-}$ cells is accompanied by destabilization of the presenilin/γ-secretase complex and accumulation of APP-C-terminal fragments. Moreover, APP trafficking analysis in $NCT^{-/-}$ fibroblasts revealed a significant delay in the rate of APP reinternalization compared with that of control cells. Together, these results establish that nicastrin is an essential component of the multimeric γ-secretase complex in mammals required for both γ-secretase activity and APP trafficking and suggest that nicastrin may be a valuable therapeutic target for Alzheimer's disease.

Among the most challenging mysteries of Alzheimer's disease is the identification of factors that render the brain particularly susceptible to the extracellular deposition of b-amyloid (Aβ). Aβ peptides are thought to be toxic and are the central component of neuritic plaques, which are preferentially localized to brain regions that are critical for memory, cognition, emotional state, and personality.

Recent research has begun to provide new clues concerning the biological basis for the vulnerability of the brain to these abnormalities, and this information has relevance to developing therapies for Alzheimer's. Aβ is generated from cleavages of the b-amyloid precursor protein (APP) by b site APP-cleaving enzyme 1 (BACE1) and by an enzyme activity termed g-secretase. In vivo, BACE1 has been found to be the principal b-secretase necessary to cleave APP to generate Aβ. In contrast, APP can also be cleaved within the Aβ sequence by putative "α-secretases" or by BACE2 to release the ectodomain (the amino-terminal soluble fragment) of APP; these cleavages within the Aβ domain of APP preclude the formation of Aβ. In Alzheimer's, why is the brain but not any other organ (such as the pancreas, for example) particularly vulnerable to Aβ deposition?

BACE1 and BACE2 are expressed ubiquitously, but levels of BACE1 messenger RNA (mRNA) are particularly high in brain and pancreas, whereas the levels of BACE2 mRNA are relatively low in all tissues, except in the brain, where it is nearly undetectable. Because BACE1 is the principal b-secretase in neurons and BACE2 limits the secretion of Aβ peptides, we propose that BACE1 is a pro-amyloidogenic enzyme, whereas BACE2 is an anti-amyloidogenic enzyme.

In this scenario, the relative levels of BACE1 and BACE2, in concert with the abundance of APP in neurons, are major determinants of Aβ formation. Under this model, the secretion of Aβ peptides would be expected to be highest in neurons and brain, as compared with other cell types or organs, because neurons express high levels of BACE1 coupled with low expression of BACE2. If the ratio of the level of BACE1 to BACE2 is a critical factor that selectively predisposes the brain to the formation of Aβ, Alzheimer's disease would be predicted to involve the brain rather than heart or pancreas.

Seemingly inconsistent with this hypothesis is the observation that there are very high levels of BACE1 mRNA in the pancreas. It appears that some of this mRNA is alternatively spliced to generate a BACE1 isoform that is incapable of cleaving APP; thus, Aβ is not deposited in the pancreas. Taken together with the observations that the pancreas has low levels of BACE1 protein, as well as low BACE1 enzymatic activity, these results are consistent with the view that a high ratio of BACE1 to BACE2 activity is a major determinant of selective vulnerability of the brain to formation of Aβ plaques.

Potential therapeutics for Alzheimer's disease

Although these mutant transgenic mice do not recapitulate the full phenotype of Alzheimer's disease, they represent excellent models of Aβ amyloidosis and are highly suitable for identification of therapeutic targets and for testing new treatments. Although both β- and γ-secretase activities represent therapeutic targets for the development of novel protease inhibitors for Alzheimer's disease, the demonstration that BACE1 is the principal β-secretase in cultured neurons and that, in contrast to $PS1^{-/-}$ mice, the $BACE1^{-/-}$ mice seem to be normal, provides an excellent rationale for focusing on the design of novel therapeutics to inhibit BACE1 activity in brain. Significantly, BACE1-deficient neurons fail to secrete Aβ even when co-expressing the *APP-swe* and mutant *PS1* genes, and these *BACE-1* coexpressing mutant *APP/PS* gene mice lacking BACE1 do not exhibit Aβ plaques in the brain (H.Cai, D.L.P. and P.C.W., unpublished data). PS, Nicastrin, APH1, and PEN2 are necessary for γ-secretase activity. With the latter, these proteins stabilize PS. Recent work suggests that PS1 is essential for activity, but it is not the protease performing γ cleavage (at least for Notch1) (Taniguchi *et al.*, 2002). Because of the role of the γ-secretase complex in Notch processing, it may be valuable to try to design therapeutics that inhibit selectively the γ-secretase activity, with regard to APP, without allowing the activity involved in Notch1 processing. This approach is being pursued because several populations of cells, hematopoetic stem cells in particular, use Notch 1 signaling for cell-fate decisions even in adults.

A variety of other treatments have been tested in mouse models, but space constraints limit discussion. However, to illustrate the challenges of extrapolating outcomes in mice to trials with humans, it is useful to briefly discuss recent problems with Aβ immunotherapy. In both prevention and treatment trials, both Aβ immunization (with Freund's adjuvant) and passive transfer of Aβ antibodies reduce levels of Aβ and plaque burden in mutant APP transgenic mice. Efficacy seems to be related to antibody titer. The mechanisms of enhanced clearance are not certain, but two not mutually exclusive hypotheses have been suggested: (i) a small amount of Aβ antibody reaches the brain, binds to Aβ peptides, promotes the disassembly of fibrils, and via the Fc antibody domain, attracts activated microglia that remove Aβ (Schenk *et al.*, 1999); and (ii) serum antibodies serve as a sink to draw the amyloid peptides from the brain into the circulation, thus changing the equilibrium of Aβ in different compartments and promoting removal from the brain (DeMattos *et al.*, 2001). Immunotherapy in transgenic mice was successful in clearing Aβ and attenuates learning and behavioral deficits in at least two cohorts of mutant *APP* mice. Although phase 1 trials with Aβ peptide and adjuvant were not associated with any adverse events, phase 2 trials of this strategy have been suspended because of severe adverse reactions (encephalomyelitis) in a subset of patients.

One of these patients arrived in autopsy in comparison with unimmunized cases of Alzheimer's disease, several unusual features were identified in the immunized case. Specifically, there were areas of cortex with very few plaques, yet they contained a relatively high density of tangles in neuropil and vascular amyloid deposits but lack plaque associated dystrophic neurites and astrocytic clusters; Aβ immunoreactivity was associated with microglia; and a T-cell predominant meningoencephalitis was identified (Nicoll *et al.*, 2003). Investigators have continued to pursue the passive immunization approach, experimental systems using passive immunization and attempting to make antigens that do not stimulate T-cell mediated immunologic attacks.

It is clear that amyloid burden can be significantly reduced by a variety of approaches. As indicated above, lesions of the entorhinal cortex or the perforant pathway reduced the levels of Aβ and the number of plaques in the terminal fields (molecular dentate gyrus). This work clearly shows that APP is a major source of the Aβ peptide in the brain (Lazarov *et al.*, 2002; Sheng *et al.*, 2002).

Another approach to reduce the amyloid burden is to use the Lentiviral vector system to express human neprilysin, a putative Aβ degrading enzyme, into the brain of transgenic mice with amyloid deposits. Unilateral intercerebral injections of lentivirus expressing neprilysin reduce Aβ deposits and may attenuate neurodegenerative processes. Another strategy is the use of non-steroidal anti-inflammatory drugs (NSAIDS) as a therapeutic approach. Retrospective studies had suggested that the prevalence of Alzheimer's disease was reduced in individuals who had (used NSAIDS. Lim *et al.* (2000) demonstrated that Ibuprofen suppresses plaque pathology and inflammation in a transgenic model of Aβ amyloidosis. Initially, this outcome was thought to be attributable to the impact of NSAIDS on CNS inflammation. However, more recent results suggest that ibuprofen (Weggen *et al.*, 2001) may lower Aβ42 independent of inhibition of cyclo oxygenase activity. Experiments by Weggen *et al.* (2001) show that several, but not all, NSAIDS decrease the levels of Aβ42 and increase the levels of Aβ1–38, a less toxic isoform. These studies suggest that NSAIDS can impact on the pathology in the brain by reducing levels of Aβ42 independent of COX activity and lead to the suggestion that other types of NSAIDS may do this with a greater degree of specificity. Another approach has been to target copper and zinc, which are enriched in Aβ deposits in the brains of individuals with Alzheimer's disease. It has been suggested that these metals play a role in aggregation of Aβ and local H_2O_2 production and thus, their removal might attenuate the deposition of Aβ and its consequences. In one study (Cherny *et al.*, 2001) they used clioquinol, a brain penetrate antibiotic that binds zinc and copper to reduce the levels of these metals in the brain. Nine-week therapy was associated with a modest increase in soluble Aβ and a reduction in Aβ deposition in the brain.

Amyotrophic lateral sclerosis

Clinical features, pathology and genetics

Individuals with this motor neuron disease have muscle weakness and atrophy, as well as spastic paralysis (Cleveland & Rothstein, 2001; Julien, 2001; Wong *et al.*, 1998). These signs result from selective degeneration of spinal and corticospinal motor neurons, respectively. In motor neurons, proximal axonal segments are swollen with accumulations of neurofilaments and cell bodies show ubiquitin-positive protein aggregates. Distal motor axons degenerate and terminals become disconnected from the denervated muscles, and, presumably, as trophic support is compromised, cell bodies shrink and then dendrites are attenuated. Clinical signs appear to be most closely linked to the disconnection of the motor terminals from their targets. Ultimately, neurons degenerate, exhibiting several features

consistent with oxidative damage, and programmed cell death. Ultimately, the numbers of motor neurons in the spinal cord and brainstem nuclei are reduced.

Approximately 10% of cases of ALS are familial, and, in most of these individuals, the disease is inherited in an autosomal dominant pattern. Approximately 15–20% of patients with autosomal dominant FALS (up to 2% of all ALS cases) have mutations in the gene that encodes cytosolic Cu/Zn superoxide dismutase (SOD1), a widely expressed and abundant antioxidant enzyme that catalyzes the conversion of $_-O^-_2$ to O_2 and H_2O_2. To date, at least 90 different missense mutations have been identified in the *SOD1* gene. Although some FALS *SOD1* mutants show reduced enzymatic activities, many variants retain full activity as occurs with the G37R *SOD1* mutation (Borchelt *et al.*, 1995). These mutations are scattered throughout the protein and are not preferentially localized near the active site or the dimer interface. It is puzzling how these mutations lead to a common phenotype. Thus, it is hypothesized that the mutant enzyme causes selective neuronal degeneration through a gain of toxic property, a concept consistent with autosomal dominant inheritance (Wong *et al.*, 1995). It has been suggested that the misfolded mutant SOD1 could catalyze aberrant reactions, including enhanced peroxidase activity, increased reactions with peroxinitrite, and mutation-induced conformational changes that result in aberrant activity catalyzed by Cu bound to mutant SOD1 (see below for discussion of potential aberrant copper chemistry in mutant SOD mediated disease) (Wong *et al.*, 1995). The presence of ubiquitin aggregates containing mutant SOD1 protein raises the possibility that aggregated mutant proteins, which may exhibit conformational changes, are toxic, that the protein aggregates sequester molecules which are critical for cell viability, or the malfolded mutant proteins damage proteosomal degradative machinery (Cleveland & Rothstein, 2001).

Several chronic experimental and clinical axonopathies are associated with the accumulation of cytoskeletal pathology, particularly accumulation of NF. The experimental toxin β,β'-iminodipropionitrile (IDPN), the prototype for this type of disorder, selectively blocks NF transport, perhaps by altering interactions of NF with microtubules or with anterograde motors. The transport of other cytoskeletal proteins, including actin and tubulin, is relatively unaffected, and fast anterograde and retrograde transport appear to be relatively normal. NF synthesis is unaltered, and newly synthesized NF proteins continue to enter the axon normally after systemic intoxication with IDPN. However, the transport of these proteins along the axon is markedly impaired, resulting in the accumulation of NF and distension of the proximal axon. Similar kinds of NF axonal pathology occur in other experimental models: aluminum intoxication; the overexpression of a species of wild-type NF proteins (altering their stoichometry); and the expression of mutant NF proteins, which fail to interact properly for accurate assembly; a dominant disorder that occurs in Brittany spaniels (hereditary canine spinal muscular atrophy); *PMN* mice; and mutant *SOD1* mice. Similar pathology occurs in human amyotrophic lateral sclerosis (Lou Gehrig's disease). These diseases are characterized by the abnormal accumulation of NF in the neuronal cell bodies and proximal axons. This form of pathology, which is a distinct form of pathology seen in ALS and several other models, appears to reflect the impaired transfer of newly synthesized NF proteins from the cell body to the axon, is associated with axonal degeneration and neuronal death, which raises the possibility that the accumulation of NF in the cell body may reflect a more general derangement of the entire axonal transport mechanism, including the transport of membranous organelles. As mentioned above, NF pathology also occurs in the distal portions of axons in a number of clinical and experimental disorders, including giant axonal neuropathy and intoxication with n-hexane, and acrylamide, and BPAU. The mechanisms that lead to distal NF swellings have not been clarified, but these changes may also reflect a general impairment of both the fast and slow transport systems because they are also associated with the distal accumulation of membranous organelles and distal axonal degeneration. The distal accumulation of membranous organelles in these settings occurs in axons devoid of NF (i.e. in the quiverer quail, where NF assembly is prevented by a mutation that blocks the transcription of NF-L) (Brown, 2000; Bruijn *et al.*, 1998; Terada & Hirokawa, 2000).

Pathology indicative of altered transport occurs in several genetic diseases in rodents and humans, including: Charcot Marie Tooth type 2A (*KIFIB* β mutations); in a form of autosomal recessive motor neuron disease (mutant *dynactin*); and in a mouse model of *dynamitin* overexpression (a situation where there is interference with the dynein/dynatcin complex). Moreover, it is likely that disorders associated with tau abnormalities (i.e. Alzheimer's disease and tauopathies, including Frontotemporal Dementia) are associated with alterations of transport. In these disorders, pathological filaments (comprised of tau) accumulate in cells.

Although distal axons show Wallerian degeneration after transaction (and following other insults), the degeneration of these axons and nerve terminals can be prevented by the presence of an unusual gene. In the slow Wallerian degeneration mutant mouse (C57BL/WLd^s), transected distal axons survive several weeks after transac-

tion. The protective gene encodes an N-terminal fragment of ubiquitination factor E4B (Ube4b) fused to a nicatinimide mononucleotide adenyl transferase. The mechanism of this autosomal semi-dominant protection is unknown, but is suspected to be related to altered ubiquitination or changed purine nucleotide metabolism. This unique genetic model provides an opportunity to discover new pathways of degeneration and protection.

Other forms of motor neuron degeneration or motor axonopathies have been linked to mutations

Als 2 is associated with mutations in the alsin gene. Charcot Marie Tooth disease is associated with microtubule motor Kif 1B β, a mutation associated with dynactin. Although motor neuron disease has been linked to a mutation in dynactin, this single base pair change results in a substitution that is predicted to alter the folding of dynactin's microtubule binding domain leading to motor neuron disease in humans (Puls *et al.*, 2003).

A disruption of dynein dynactin inhibits transported motor neurons and causes a late onset progressive neurodegeneration in transgenic mice. In this study, mice overexpressing dynamytin demonstrate a late onset slowly progressive motor neuron disease associated with muscle weakness, trembling, altered posture and gait, and weakness. Neurofilament accumulations and evidence of degeneration of motor neurons and denervation atrophy of muscle described in this mouse model with disrupted axonal transport (LaMonte *et al.*, 2002).

Other disease models of motor neuron disease are in progress. In addition to models of spinal muscular atrophy created by manipulations of the survivor motor neuron disease, mutations in dinine result in progressive motor neuron degeneration in heterozygous mice (Jan *et al.*, 2003; Kriz *et al.*, 2003; Rothstein, 2003).

SOD1 mutant mice

Although there are a variety of other extraordinarily interesting models of motor neuron disease (Cleveland & Rothstein, 2001; Julien, 2001), this review focuses on mice expressing FALS-linked mutant *SOD1*. The mice harboring mutations develop progressive weakness and muscle atrophy, and cellular pathology closely resembling that occurring in ALS. For example, the *G37R SOD1* mice accumulate to 3–12 times the endogenous levels in the spinal cord, and the levels of the mutant protein influence the age of onset (Wong *et al.*, 1995). High molecular weight complexes of mutant SOD1 accumulate in neural tissues but not in non-nervous system organs (Bruijn *et al.*, 1997). Some neuronal cell bodies show SOD1, ubiquitin, and phosphorylated NF–H immunoreactive inclusions (Wang *et al.*, 2002); in some lines of mutant mice, vacuolization and swelling of mitochondria appear early in some motor neurons. Toxic SOD1 is transported anterograde in axons, and early on, SOD1 accumulates in axons, where it is associated with structural pathology, occurring approximately 2–3 months before the appearance of clinical signs. Thus, SOD1, neurofilaments and degenerating mitochondria appear in irregular, swollen, intraparenchymal portions of motor axons, and axonal transport is abnormal. Wallerian degeneration of axons occurs, and the mice become weak (Bruijn *et al.*, 1997; Li *et al.*, 2000; Lipp & Wolfer, 1998; Wong *et al.*, 1995). In mutant mice (and in cases of ALS), it has been reported that caspsase 1 and 3 activities increase (early and late, respectively), followed by evidence of action of caspase 9 (Bruijn *et al.*, 1998; Cleveland & Rothstein, 2001). Eventually, the number of motor neurons is decreased and glial proliferation is present in the anterior horns.

Potential therapies for ALS

Mutant *SOD1* mice have been used to test pharmacological and gene-based therapies (Cleveland & Rothstein, 2001). Several potential treatments, including administration of vitamin E, selenium, riluzole, gabapentin, and d-penicillamine (a copper chelator), have been tested with unencouraging results. Treatments with creatine, caspase inhibitors, mincycline (which inhibits release of cytochrome C from mitchondria 138 have had modest influences on onset of disease and survival.

Treatment strategies would be more effectively targeted if the molecular mechanisms whereby mutant *SOD1* causes selective degeneration of motor neurons were better understood. Although it was initially speculated that loss of enzyme activity might be a factor in disease, this idea is not compatible with the following observations: some mutants show full activity; SOD1 null mice do not develop motor neuron phenotypes; and elevations or reductions in mutant SOD1 by mating to *SOD1* overexpressors of *SOD1* null mice, respectively to animals with mutations, does not influence phenotype (Cleveland & Rothstein, 2001; Subramaniam *et al.*, 2002). It has been proposed that the toxic property of mutant *SOD1* involves mutation-induced conformational changes in SOD1 that result in aberrant oxidative activities. In this scenario, cell dysfunction and death could be initiated by chemistries catalyzed by Cu bound in the active site of mutant SOD1 (Wong *et al.*, 2000). To test this hypothesis, we took advantage of the discovery in yeast of Lys7 and its mammalian homologue Cu chaperone

for SOD1 (CCS), and generated mice lacking *CCS*. Inactivation of the *CCS* gene in mice demonstrates that CCS is required for efficient Cu incorporation into SOD1 in mammals, and the phenotypes of the *CCS* null mice resemble those of the *SOD1* null mice. These mice were crossed with multiple lines of mutant SOD1 mice. Metabolic Cu labeling studies in mutant *SOD1* mice lacking CCS show that copper incorporation into wild-type and mutant SOD1 is significantly diminished. Thus, CCS is necessary for efficient copper incorporation into SOD1 of motor neurons. However, although the absence of the CCS results in a significant reduction in the level of Cu-loaded mutant SOD1, the CCS−/− genotype has no effect on the onset, progression or pathology of the motor neuron disease occurring in mutant *SOD1* mice (Wong *et al.*, 2000), a result which is inconsistent with the concept that aberrant, Cu-dependent activity of mutant SOD1 is involved in the pathogenesis of FALS (Finney & O'Halloran, 2003; Subramaniam *et al.*, 2002).

A pathological hallmark of ALS is the accumulation of neurofilaments in swollen proximal axons (and cell bodies) of motor neurons, whether primary or secondary, these abnormalities are associated with axonal transport, a process important for the long-term viability of neurons (Cleveland & Rothstein, 2001; Julien, 2001; Wong *et al.*, 1998). To test the role of neurofilaments in mutant *SOD1*-induced motor neuron disease, mutant *SOD1* mice were cross-bred to several lines of mice with altered levels/distributions of neurofilament proteins. When mice expressing an *NF-H-β-galactosidase* fusion protein (NF-H-lacZ), which cross-links neurofilaments and prevents their export into axons, are crossed with mutant *SOD1* mice, the progeny show no changes in progression of disease. Mutant *SOD1* mice lacking *NF-L* (neurofilament light chain) have a moderate increase in lifespan, while mutant *SOD1* mice overexpressing wild-type *NF-*L exhibit attenuation of disease progression and an increased lifespan. A more significant protection of motor neurons was achieved by introducing the *NF-H gene* into lines of mutant *SOD1* mice. However, it is possible that some of the influences on phenotype described with genetic mutations may be related to the introduction of new strain backgrounds into mutant mice rather than the presence or absence of specific genes.

Although the molecular mechanisms underlying mutant *SOD1*-linked familial ALS remain unclear, several pathogenic mechanisms (Cleveland & Rothstein, 2001; Higuchi *et al.*, 1998; Wong *et al.*, 2002) other than the copper hypothesis have been proposed, including roles for: toxicity or sequestration of mutant SOD1-containing aggregates; excitotoxicity related to reduction in levels of GLT1 or activity of this glial transporter important in glutamate uptake in the spinal cord; reduced chaperone activity; damage to the proteosomal degradative machinery by malfolded or aggregated mutant SOD1 and activation of caspases. These hypotheses are being explored. For example, overexpression of *Bcl2* in mutant *SOD1* mice has a modest impact on onset and survival.

At present, Riluzole is the only drug approved for therapy in human ALS, but the benefits are modest. Investigators are examining other ways to ameliorate excitotoxicity, possibly by influencing the levels or activity of the glial glutamate transporter. Trials with growth factors were stopped because of complications. To date, there have been no trials of inhibitors of apoptosis nor have engineered cells or stem cells been implanted, although these areas of research are promising for the future.

A variety of therapies have utilized mouse models. Minocycline inhibits the activity of caspase-1, caspase-3, inducible nitric oxide synthase (iNOS), and p38 mytogen activated protein kinase (MAPK). Several of these enzymes have been implicated in motor neuron disease; Zhu *et al.* (2002) have shown that minocycline delays disease onset; and extends survival in mutant SOD1 mice. Perhaps by inhibiting mitochondrial permeability transition mediated cytochrome release (Zhu *et al.*, 2002).

In another study, creatine was administered orally to G93A SOD mice. The disease onset was delayed and the survival of the mice was prolonged, though the effects were very modest. Recent clinical trials of creatine in patients with ALS did not find beneficial evidence of survival or disease progression (Growlenvelt, page 437 *Annals of Neurology*). Combination of creatine and minocycline showed enhanced survival, which extended beyond the effects of creatine. More recently, a combination of minocycline, creatine, and riluzole showed an additive effect on survival (Rothstein paper, *Annals of Neurology* and Criz paper, *Annals of Neurology* – same as Growlenvelt).

Parkinson's disease

Clinical features, pathology and genetics

Usually appearing in the sixth or seventh decade, classical parkinsonism, is characterized by resting tremor, rigidity, slowness of voluntary movement (bradykinesia), stooped posture, impaired postural stability, and shuffling gate (Baron *et al.*, 1996; Dunnett & Bjorklund, 1999; Edbauer *et al.*, 2002; Foix, 1921; Goedert, 2001b; Lozano *et al.*, 1998; Markham & Diamond, 1993; Olanow & Tatton, 1999; Vazques *et al.*, 1996; Wichmann & DeLong, 1996). PD

is the second most common neurodegenerative disease (to Alzheimer's disease) and affects ~1% of individuals >65 years of age, both sexes are equally affected. The motor deficits are related to degeneration of pigmented dopaminergic neurons in the substantia nigra, pars compacta (SNpc) (Forno, 1966; Forno *et al.*, 1986; Greenfield & Bosanquet, 1953; Hassler, 1938; Oppenheimer & Esiri, 1992; Sima *et al.*, 1996). These neurons often exhibit: Lewy bodies (LB), spherical, intracytoplasmic, usually ubiquitin–immunoreactive inclusions with a filamentous core often surrounded by clear halo; and Lewy neurites (LN), which are LB-like, smaller inclusions in processes of nigral neurons and several other affected neuronal populations (Braak *et al.*, 1999, 2000; Forno, 1966; Oppenheimer & Esiri, 1992; Spillantini *et al.*, 1997). A major fibrillar component of these two types of inclusions is α-synuclein (α-syn) (Chung *et al.*, 2001) (see Genetics Section below), but other proteins, including synphilin (Lozano *et al.*, 1998) are associated with these inclusions. The abnormalities in the nigral neurons are associated with reductions (80–95%) in dopaminergic markers are the number of dopamine receptors in striatum (Lozano *et al.*, 1998). In the basal ganglia, the loss of dopaminergic influences on striatal cells (Lee *et al.*, 2001; Lozano *et al.*, 1998; Wichmann & DeLong, 1996) leads to overactivity of the indirect pathway and decreased activity of the direct pathway. Because of different actions of D1 and 2 receptors in these two pathways, the result of dopaminergic deafferentation of the striatum leads to increased activity of nerve cells in the globus pallidus interna, leading to enhanced inhibition of thalamocortical neurons; the clinical outcome is bradykinesia.

The disease may be familial in ~10% of cases, and mutations have been identified in *α-syn*, *Ubiquitin Carboxy Terminal Hydrolase L1 (UCH-L1)* and *Parkin* (Armstrong *et al.*, 1996; Dawson *et al.*, 2002; Goedert, 2001b; Kitada *et al.*, 1998; Kruger *et al.*, 1998). The first disease-specific mutation (A53Tα) was located within the exon 4 of *γ-syn* (chromosome 4aq21–q23) (Polymeropoulos, 1998; Polymeropoulos *et al.*, 1997) a sequence is normally present in α-syn (of rodents) and in synelfin, an avian α-syn homologue (zebra finch) (Ueda *et al.*, 1993). The same mutation was found in several Greek kindreds. More recently, a second *α-syn* mutation (i.e. A30P) was discovered in two affected members of a small German pedigree (Kruger *et al.*, 1998; Polymeropoulos, 1998; Polymeropoulos *et al.*, 1997). α-syn, comprised 140 amino acids, is highly conserved protein found in mammals, fish, and birds (95% to 86% identity) (George *et al.*, 1995; Irizarry *et al.*, 1996; Maroteaux *et al.*, 1988; Südhof, 1995). In mammals, *α-syn* is a member of a multigene family consisting of at least two other *synuclein* genes (β-*Syn* and γ-*Syn*) (Goedert, 1997;

Lucking *et al.*, 2000). The synucleins, small cytosolic proteins of unknown function enriched at the synaptic terminals of neurons, show a conserved N-terminal repeat region (100 amino acids) consisting of seven imperfect repeats of 11 amino acid residues (KTKEGV), a hydrophobic sequence in the middle of the protein, and a less well conserved, negatively charged C-terminal domain.

Mutations (l93M) in the *UCH-L1* gene have been identified in two members of kindred with autosomal dominant PD. However, it is not certain that this mutation is truly causative of disease.

An autosomal recessive form of juvenile Parkinsonism (AR-JP) has been linked to truncations, frame shifts, and missense/nonsense mutations in *parkin* (chromosome 6q27) (Armstrong *et al.*, 1996; Kitada *et al.*, 1998; Kruger *et al.*, 1998; Zhang *et al.*, 2000). Parkin, a protein that shows some features common with ubiquitin at the amino terminus and has a cysteine ring finger motive at the carboxy-terminus, acts as (Zhang *et al.*, 2000) an E3-ubiquitin ligase, and, as such, provides for substrate specificity of ubiquitination (Dawson *et al.*, 2002; Imai *et al.*, 2000; Laptook *et al.*, 1994; Zhang *et al.*, 2000). Parkin may participate in ubiquitination and metabolism of α-syn and synphilin, α-syn-interacting protein implicated in α-syn aggregation. It is generally believed that *parkin* mutations lead to Parkinson's disease without LBs and that other substrates of parkin, such as Pae 1 receptor, may be toxic to neurons if not degraded. It has been suggested that reduced parkin activity may result in the accumulation of proteins/peptides (α-syn and Pae 1 receptor) that are toxic to dopaminergic neurons leading to parkinsonian phenotype in vivo (Dawson *et al.*, 2002).

α-syn transgenic mice

To understand the mechanisms whereby mutant *α-syn* leads to motoric abnormalities and neurodegeneration, investigators have produced multiple lines of transgenic mice (Abediovich *et al.*, 2000; Giasson *et al.*, 2002; Masliah *et al.*, 2000; Van der Putten *et al.*, 2000). For example, we expressed high levels of either wild-type or FPD-linked A30P or A53T human *α-syn* in mice (Masliah *et al.*, 2000). To achieve high levels of transgene expression in mice, the transgene expression (cDNAs encoding human *wild type, A30P,* or *A53T α-syn*) was controlled by the murine prion promotor (MoPrP-*Hu α-syn;*). Analysis of transgene-derived mRNA and protein shows high levels of *Hu α-syn* expression in the brains of these mice. The levels of total α-syn protein (human and mouse combined) in the brains of MoPrP-*Hu α-syn* mice are 4–15 times higher than in the non-transgenic mice. *In situ* hybridization discloses widespread expression of transgene-derived Hu α-syn mRNA in all brain regions, particularly the brainstem. The *A53T Hu α-syn* mice, but not mice with wild-type or the *A30P* variants, develop adult-onset, progressive motoric dysfunction leading to death. Affected mice accumulate α-syn and ubiquitin in neuronal perikarya and neurites, and brain regions with pathology show detergent-insoluble α-syn and α-syn aggregates. Immunoblot analyses of total SDS-soluble proteins disclose three α-syn polypeptides and peptide fragments corresponding to the full-length α-syn polypeptide (α-syn 16) and two truncated α-syn polypeptides (α-syn 12 and α-syn 10). The majority of α-syn fractionates with the S1 fraction, an observation consistent with α-syn being a cytosolic protein. However, α-syn in the P2 fractions from the brainstems of clinically affected A53T *Hu α-syn* mice is different quantitatively and qualitatively from α-syn polypeptides in the other P2 fractions. Specifically, the brainstem P2 fraction from the affected *A53T* Hu α-syn mice contains significantly more detergent-insoluble full-length ($\approx$16-kDa) α-syn. Moreover, the P2 fraction is also enriched for α-syn species with a lower molecular mass α-syn (α-syn 10 and 12) and a series of higher molecular mass aggregates of α-syn. Parallel analysis of (wt) Hu α-syn and A30P Hu α-syn mice shows that the α-syn species enriched in the P2 fraction is specific of A53T Hu α-syn or the expression. These results suggest that mutant α-syn can be cleaved (by "synucleinases") in both the N- and C-terminal regions, generating peptides that aggregate, gain a toxic property, and track with the disease. Moreover, the A53T α-syn and derived peptides are associated with significantly greater in vivo neurotoxicity as compared with other α-syn variants, and α-syn-dependent neurodegeneration is associated with abnormal accumulation of detergent-insoluble α-syn. In a similar study (Van der Putten *et al.*, 2000), mice were generated expressing either wild-type or *A53T Hu α-syn*; only the mice expressing the mutant protein developed motor impairments, paralysis, premature death, and age-dependent intracytoplasmic α-syn fibrillary inclusions in neurons. α-Syn was present in the detergent insoluble fraction, but α-syn peptide fragments were not commented upon. A major research question in this field is whether these α-syn fragments are present in FPD and in sporadic Parkinson's disease. If such is the case, it will be critical to identify the enzymes carrying out these cleavages, which may be targets for therapy.

Thus, although the expression of wild-type or mutant *α-syn* has been associated with neuropathology in several lines of transgenic mice and in flies, these studies of A53T α-syn document that the expression of this mutant gene leads to formation of truncated α-syn peptide high molecular aggregates in vivo neurotoxicity compared with either the A30P or WT Huα-*syn* variants associated with progressive neurodegeneration and death (but not classical PD). Although increase in vivo toxicity of the A53T mutation is consistent with this mutation being associated with a more aggressive disease course in humans than the A30P mutation, the lack of significant neuropathology in mice expressing A30P Huα-*Syn* is unexpected. Although the A30P mutation is found in a small pedigree with only two affected members, the potential for toxicity was assumed to be greater than with A53T mutation because A30P is a highly non-conservative substitution, whereas the A53T mutation is actually a normal sequence in rodents. It remains possible that the two mutations in *Huα-syn* initiate disease in different ways, or that the A30P variant could be a rare polymorphism.

α-Syn gene targeted mice

Initial studies of α-syn$^{-/-}$ mice indicate that α-syn is not essential for the viability of the mice. Knockout mice are viable and fertile; neural development appears normal; the complement of dopaminergic cell bodies, fibers, and synapses is normal; and the pattern of dopamine discharge and reuptake in response to electric stimulation is unremarkable. However, dopaminergic terminals in α-syn$^{-/-}$ mice exhibit faster recovery from paired pulse stimuli (Feany, 2000). Shortened recovery from the prepulse can be mimicked in the wild-type mice by elevations of extracellular calcium. Significantly, *α-syn*$^{-/-}$ mice exhibit reductions in total striatal dopamine levels and in the dopamine-dependent locomotor response to amphetamines. These results are consistent with the concept that α-syn is a presynaptic, activity-dependent, negative regulator of dopaminergic neurotransmission. It is possible that both β- and γ-syn can compensate for the loss of α-synuclein expression, and it will be useful to study mice that display other syn isotypes to determine the importance of various syn proteins with regards to normal synaptic activity.

The tauopathies

Clinical features, pathology and genetics

The tauopathies are a group of disorders that include frontotemporal dementia with parkinsonism linked to chromosone 17 (FTD-P 17) (Edbauer *et al.*, 2002; Hutton *et al.*, 1998; Lee *et al.*, 2001; Lee & Trojanowski, 1999; Munoz *et al.*, 2003), progressive supranuclear palsy (PSP), and corticobasal degeneration (CBD). The clinical phenotypes reflect the involvement of populations of neurons that exhibit fibrillar tau immunoreactive inclusions (Edbauer *et al.*, 2002; Lee *et al.*, 2001; Lee & Trojanowski, 1999; Munoz *et al.*, 2003) and degeneration of subsets of neural cells. These diseases are less common than classical Alzheimer's disease and Parkinson's disease. Alzheimer's disease is also a tauopathy, in that the neurofibrillary tangles, neuropil threads, and swollen neurites in plaques are enriched in filamentous aggregates of hyperphosphorylated tau (Lee *et al.*, 2001) (See section on Alzheimer's disease).

In this section, we focus principally on FTD-P 17, usually occurring in mid to late life, manifest as two principal phenotypes: an illness in which dementia is conspicuous; and a less common phenotype in which the movement disorder is a major feature (Edbauer *et al.*, 2002). In addition to dementia and parkinsonism, affected individuals may show other clinical signs reflecting abnormalities of the cortico-spinal pathways, and of circuits controlling eye movements and speech. Magnetic resonance imaging (MRI) (Pasquier *et al.*, 2003) discloses frontotemporal atrophy, and [^{18}F]-deoxy-glucose positron emission tomography (PET) shows hypometabolism, usually marked in the frontal and temporal regions (Pasquier *et al.*, 2003).

Neuropathological exams confirm that atrophy of the frontal and temporal lobes is accompanied by dilation of the third ventricles. Evidence of neuronal degeneration exists in the substantia nigra, hippocampus, and neocortex. Surviving neurons in these areas often contain intracellular aggregates of phosphorylated tau; similar inclusions may also be seen in oligodendroglial cells, and there may be evidence of white matter pathology.

Several other tauopathies manifest somewhat different clinical and pathological phenotypes. For example, PSP is characterized by progressive axial rigidity, slowed movements, vertical gaze palsy, IPS, dysarthia, and dementia. In PSP, globose neurofibrillary tangles, reactive astrocytosis, and evidence of neuronal loss are observed particularly in brainstem nuclei (Edbauer *et al.*, 2002). CBD also manifests as a movement disorder (rigidity and apraxia) with frontal type dementia. PET scans of these patients show alterations in glucose metabolism in parts of the cortex and thalamus regions; neuropathological analyses disclose regional atrophy (usually frontal), ballooned tau immunoreactive neurons, and glial pathology (Edbauer *et al.*, 2002).

As indicated above, the tauopathies share a disease-defining neuropathological feature: affected cells contain inclusions enriched in tau, a low molecular weight microtubule-associated protein (MAP) (Cleveland *et al.*, 1997a,b; Johnson & Hartigan, 1999). Normally, tau, a protein transported anterograde in axons (Mercken *et al.*, 1995), acts to stabilize tubulin polymers critical for microtubule assembly and stability (Caceres & Kosik, 1990). In mature human brains, the six isoforms of tau are derived by alternative splicing from a single gene on chromosome 17, and all six isoforms contain repeat regions, which interact with tubulin (Bird *et al.*, 2003; Edbauer *et al.*, 2002; Lee *et al.*, 2001; Munoz *et al.*, 2003). The isoforms consist of three isoforms of three repeat tau (3-R tau) and three isoforms of four repeat (4-R) tau encoded by exon 10 (Bird *et al.*, 2003; Lee *et al.*, 2001; Munoz *et al.*, 2003). The poorly soluble post-translationally modified tau underlying the cellular pathology differs somewhat in the different tauopathies: the six isoforms of tau are present in Alzheimer's disease; 4-R tau characterize the inclusions of PSP and CBD; 3-R tau is enriched in PiD (Munoz *et al.*, 2003). In contrast, in Alzheimer's disease, paired helical filaments of tangles are composed primarily of six isoforms of tau.

In FTD-P 17, *tau* mutations can be divided into three classes: mutations in exons; mutations in alternatively spliced exon 10; and mutations at the exon 10 5′ splice site (Bird *et al.*, 2003; Dumanchin *et al.*, 1998; Hong *et al.*, 1998; Hutton *et al.*, 1998; Kitada *et al.*, 1998; Lee *et al.*, 2001; Spillantini *et al.*, 1998). The most commonly encountered *tau* mutation is P301L. The effects of some of the intronic mutations have come from knowledge of the importance of a stem–loop structure that begins with the final codons of exon 10 and continues into intron 10. The stem–loop decreases the efficiency inclusion of exon 10; when the mutations destabilize this loop, there is increased inclusion of exon 10 in sequences in the protein leading to an increase in 4-R tau in the soluble and insoluble pools of tau. The P301L *tau* mutation is absorbed predominantly with aggregates of 4-R tau. Mutations that influence tau mRNA splicing, 4-R, are enriched in filamentous lesions. In contrast, mutations that alter the 4-R/3-R tau ratios result in twisted ribbons essentially composed of 4-R tau; these filaments accumulate in both neurons and glia. Individuals with PSP or CSB share the H1 tau haplotype, which appears to be a risk factor linked to the accumulation of 4-R tau in aggregates.

Gene targeting of *tau*

Tau was isolated initially as a stabilizer of microtubules (Hong *et al.*, 1998). In cultures, antisense strategies showed that downregulation of tau adversely influenced neurite outgrowth (Caceres & Kosik, 1990). However, when the *tau* gene was targeted, the only phenotype was mild differences in the organization of microtubules in small caliber axons (Harada *et al.*, 1994). MAPs exist and the lack of phenotype in tau −/− mice presumably reflects some redundancy in MAPs. Consistent with this idea is the observation that

mating of tau −/− and MAP1B −/− mice leads to a lethal postnatal phenotype (Takai *et al.*, 1999, 2000).

Models of tauopathies

In examining the outcomes of a variety of transgenic approaches in mice, it is important to remember that mice express three copies of the murine variant of 4-R tau, while humans express three copies of both 3-R tau and 4-R tau. The early efforts to produce mice expressing mutant *tau* transgenes did not lead to striking clinical phenotypes or pathology (Duff *et al.*, 2000). However, subsequent studies were more successful in producing disease (Probst *et al.*, 2000; Spittaels *et al.*, 1999). Thus overexpression of human tau can lead to weakness and hypophosphorylated insoluble tau immunoreactivity in neurons in the spinal cord, brainstem, and cortex; motor axons showed degeneration (Ishihara *et al.*, 1999; Lee *et al.*, 2001; Lee & Trojanowski, 1991). Tau immunoreactive lesions occur in some human *tau* mice (Hinguchi *et al.*, 2002).

Efforts have been made to overexpress wild-type tau to produce NFT of the Alzheimer's disease type (Lee *et al.*, 1999). More striking are the mice overexpressing *tau P301L* (Lewis *et al.*, 2000). When the prion or Thy1 promoter was used to drive *P301L tau*, neurofibrillary tangles occurred In neurons of the brain and spinal cord (Gotz *et al.*, 2001; Ishihara *et al.*, 1999; Lewis *et al.*, 2000). Moreover, when Aβ42 fibrils were injected into P301L mice, there was an increase in the number of tangles at injection sites.

Mice expressing wt human *tau* transgene do not develop pathology. However, when similar strategies are used to introduce human *tau* into tau −/− mice, the animals show accumulations of tau immunoreactivity in neurons, including the presence of certain phosphorylated and conformational epitopes seen in human disease (Peter Davies, personal communication). These observations have been interpreted to suggest that, in mice, endogenous mouse tau may interfere with the formation of tangles by human tau.

Investigators have created genetic models of tau-related neurodegeneration in invertebrates (Feany, 2000). For example, when wild-type or mutant *tau* are expressed in *Drosophila melanogaster*, transgenic flies develop a variety of clinical abnormalities; adult onset progressive disease; early lethality; greater toxicity with mutant tau; and accumulation of abnormal tau in nerve cells (Feany, 2000; Wittmann *et al.*, 2001).

Experimental therapeutics

The human tauopathies and genetically engineered animal models of these disorders are under active investigation, but it is clear that introduction of mutant *tau* and changes in the ratios of 3-R and 4-R tau lead to clinical disease and to accumulation of hypophosphorylated tau filamentous inclusions. It is likely that these biochemical abnormalities impact on the stability of tubulin and on microtubules, and thus might be expected to perturb axonal transport. It seems likely that the nature of tau iosforms, their ratios, and the balance of protein kinases/phosphatses activities acting on tau play roles in the pathogenesis of tauopathies. Understanding these issues is very important in that selected inhibitors of the appropriate kinases or phosphatases could be the basis for design of novel strategies to ameliorate abnormalities associated with alterations in this disease. Moreover, it is increasingly apparent that tau pathology can be associated with other abnormalities of protein aggregation. For example, in cases of Alzheimer's disease, the accumulation of Aβ42 peptide is in some way, as yet uncertain, linked to the appearance of tau pathology manifest by tangles, threads, and neuritis (in plaques). Similarly, the presence of α-synuclein, possibly specific peptide fragments of α-synuclein (Lee *et al.*, 2002) as occurs in Parkinson's disease and mouse models of synucleinopathies, is often associated with tau pathology in some of the neurodegenerative diseases (Giasson *et al.*, 2003; Trojanowski, 2002). The interactions of these conformationally altered pathological peptides are very active exciting areas of research, and understanding the abnormalities of biology of their proteins is critical for developing new mechanism-based therapies for these disorders.

Conclusions

The identification of genes mutated or deleted in the inherited forms of many neurodegenerative diseases has allowed investigators to create in vivo and in vitro model systems relevant to a wide variety of human neurological disorders.

In this review, we emphasized the value of transgenic and gene targeted models and the lessons they provided for understanding mechanisms of their neurodegenerative diseases. For example, the study of *BACE1*$^{-/-}$ mice and mutant *APP/PS1* transgenic models has provided extraordinary new insights into the mechanisms of Aβ amyloidogenesis, the reasons why Alzheimer's disease is a brain amyloidosis, and into potential therapeutic targets. In contrast, our studies of mutant *SOD1* mice lacking *CCS* demonstrate that aberrant activities dependent on copper-loaded SOD1 are unlikely to be involved with pathogenic mechanisms, and that other mechanisms/targets should be explored. Finally, with regard to mutant α-*syn* linked FPD, results from studies of mouse models suggest that α-syn may

undergo C- and N-terminal cleavages, generating toxic peptides. Strategies designed to delineate the participants in these cleavage processes, discover separate synucleinases, the consequence of deleting or inhibiting these enzymes will need to be explored. If these cleavages occur in humans with Parkinson's disease, it will be essential to understand the mechanisms of cell injury and to design inhibitors that block cleavages of α-syn.

Invertebrate organisms, like *C. elegans* or *Drosophila melanogaster*, provide excellent genetically manipulatable model systems for examining many aspects of neurodegenerative diseases (Kamal *et al.*, 2001; Lin *et al.*, 1999; Warrick *et al.*, 1998, 1999; Wittmann *et al.*, 2001). Invertebrates harboring mutant transgenes can be generated rapidly and their nervous systems are relatively simple. Moreover, behavior can be scored, with flies having the ability to carry out more complex behaviors and having a longer lifespan than worms. Significant new information has come from transgenic technologies, which have allowed mutant genes to be introduced into, or ablated in, flies and worms. For example, when wild-type or mutant human α-*syn* is expressed in the nervous system of flies, dopaminergic neurons degenerate in adult life, nerve cells show accumulations of γ-syn and filamentous inclusions, and animals develop progressive motor dysfunction (Warrick *et al.*, 1999). Similar experiments have been carried out in models of the CAG repeat diseases that encode expansions of polyglutamine (Kamal *et al.*, 2001; Warrick *et al.*, 1998; Wittmann *et al.*, 2001). When expanded *ataxin-3* is expressed in the retina of *Drosophila*, the retina degenerates, but the disease can be attenuated by manipulations of p35 or Hsp70. Similarly, introductions of wild-type or mutant human *tau* into flies, models tau-related neurodegenerative disease. Flies carrying these transgenes exhibit adult onset progressive neurodegeneration, evidence of enhanced toxicity of mutant tau, accumulations of abnormal tau in cells (but without neurofibrillary tangles), and early lethality (Kamal *et al.*, 2001). Because these invertebrate models reproduce aspects of pathologies occurring in human neurodegenerative diseases, studies of these systems should prove very useful in delineating disease pathways, identifying suppressors and enhancers of these processes, and in testing the influences of drugs on phenotypes in flies and worms.

These new models allow investigators to examine the molecular mechanisms by which mutant proteins cause selective dysfunction and death of neurons and to determine possible pathogenic pathways that can be tested by crossing animals with either mutated or deleted alleles of other molecular players in the pathogenic process. The use of RNA methods will accelerate the validation of molecules involved in pathogenic pathways. The results of these approaches will provide us with a better understanding of the mechanisms leading to diseases.

In summary, investigations of genetically engineered (transgenic or gene targeted) mice have disclosed participants in pathogenic pathways, have reproduced some of the features of human neurodegenerative disorders, have provided important new information about the disease mechanisms, and allow identification of new therapeutic targets. Moreover, the models can be used for testing novel treatments. These lines of research have made spectacular progress over the past few years, and we anticipate that discoveries will lead to the design of more promising therapies that can be tested in models of these devastating diseases.

REFERENCES

Abeliovich, A., Schmitz, Y., Farinas, I. *et al.* (2000). Mice lacking alpha-synuclein display functional deficits in the nigrostriatal dopamine system. *Neuron*, **25**, 239–52.

Armstrong, R. A., Cairns, N. J., Myers, D., Smith, C. U. M., Lantos, P. L. & Rossor, M. N. (1996). A comparison of β-amyloid deposition in the medial temporal lobe in sporadic Alzheimer's disease, Down's syndrome and normal elderly brains. *Neurodegeneration*, **5**, 35–41.

Baron, M. S., Vitek, J. L., Bakay, R. A. E. *et al.* (1996). Treatment of advanced Parkinson's disease by posterior GPi pallidotomy: 1-year results of a pilot study. *Ann. Neurol.*, **40**, 355–66.

Benoist, C. & Mathis, D. (1997). Cell death mediators in autoimmune diabetes – no shortage of suspects. *Cell*, **89**, 1–3.

Bird, T., Knopman, D., VanSwieten, J. *et al.* (2003). Epidemiology and genetics of frontotemporal dementia / Pick's disease. *Ann. Neurol.*, **54** Suppl 5, S29–31.

Borchelt, D. R., Guarnieri, M., Wong, P. C. *et al.* (1995). Superoxide dismutase 1 subunits with mutations linked to familial amyotrophic lateral sclerosis do not affect wild-type subunit function. *J. Biol. Chem.*, **270**, 3234–8.

Braak, H., Sandmann-Keil, D., Gai, W. & Braak, E. (1999). Extensive axonal Lewy neurites in Parkinson's disease: a novel pathological feature revealed by alpha-synuclein immunocytochemistry. *Neurosci. Lett.*, **265**, 67–9.

Braak, H., Rub, U., Sandmann-Keil, D. *et al.* (2000). Parkinson's disease: affection of brain stem nuclei controlling premotor and motor neurons of the somatomotor system. *Acta Neuropathol. (Berl.)*, **99**, 489–95.

Brown, A. (2000). Slow axonal transport: stop and go traffic in the axon. *Nat. Rev. Molec. Cell Biol.*, **1**, 153–6.

Bruijn, L. I., Becher, M. W., Lee, M. K. *et al.* (1997). ALS-linked SOD1 mutant G85R mediates damage to astrocytes and promotes rapidly progressive disease with SOD1-containing inclusions. *Neuron*, **18**, 327–8.

Bruijn, L. I., Houseweart, M. K., Kato, S. *et al.* (1998). Aggregation and motor neuron toxicity of an ALS-linked SOD1 mutant independent from wild-type SOD1. *Science*, **281**, 1851–4.

Caceres, A. & Kosik, K. J. (1990). Inhibition of neurite polarity by tau antisense oligonucleotides in primary cerebellar neurons. *Nature*, **343**, 461–3.

Cai, H., Wang, Y., McCarthy, D. *et al.* (2001). BACE1 is the major beta-secretase for generation of Abeta peptides by neurons. *Nat. Neurosci.*, **4**, 233–4.

Cao, X. & Südhof, T. C. (2001). A transcriptively active complex of APP with Fe65 and histone acetyltransferase Tip60. *Science*, **293**, 115–20.

Chen, G., Chen, K. S., Knox, J. *et al.* (2000). A learning deficit related to age and β-amyloid plaques in a mouse model of Alzheimer's disease. *Nature*, **408**, 975–9.

Chen, F., Yu, G., Arawaka, S. *et al.* (2001). Nicastrin binds to membrane-tethered Notch. *Nat. Cell Biol.*, **3**, 751–4.

Cherny, R. A., Atwood, C. S., Xilinas, M. E. *et al.* (2001). Treatment with a copper–zinc chelator markedly and rapidly inhibits β-amyloid accumulation in Alzheimer's disease transgenic mice. *Neuron*, **30**, 665–76.

Chung, H. M. & Struhl, G. (2001). Nicastrin is required for Presenilin-mediated transmembrane cleavage in *Drosophila*. *Nat. Cell Biol.*, **3**, 1129–32.

Chung, K. K., Zhang, Y., Lim, K. L. *et al.* (2001). Parkin ubiquitinates the alpha-synuclein-interacting protein, synphilin-1: implications for Lewy-body formation in Parkinson disease. *Nat. Med.*, **7**, 1144–50.

Cleveland, D. W., Hwo, S.-Y. & Kirschner, M. W. (1977a). Physical and chemical properties of purified tau factor and the role of tau in microtubule assembly. *J. Mol. Biol.*, **116**, 227–47.

(1977b). Purification of tau, a microtubule-associated protein that induces assembly of microtubules from purified tubulin. *J. Mol. Biol.*, **116**, 207–25.

Cleveland, D. W. & Rothstein, J. D. (2001). From Charcot to Lou Gehrig: deciphering selective motor neuron death in ALS. *Nat. Rev. Neurosci.*, **2**, 806–19.

Dawson, T., Mandir, A. & Lee, M. (2002). Animal models of PD: pieces of the same puzzle? *Neuron*, **35**, 219–22.

DeMattos, R. B., Bales, K. R., Cummins, D. J., Dodart, J. C., Paul, S. M. & Holtzman, D. M. (2001). Peripheral anti-Aβ antibody alters CNS and plasma Aβ clearance and decreases brain Aβ burden in a mouse model of Alzheimer's disease. *Proc. Natl Acad. Sci. USA*, **98**, 8850–5.

Duff, K., Knight, H., Refolo, L. M. *et al.* (2000). Characterization of pathology in transgenic mice over-expressing human genomic and cDNA tau transgenes. *Neurobiol. Dis.*, **7**, 87–98.

Dumanchin, C., Camuzat, A., Campion, D. *et al.* (1998). Segregation of a missense mutation in the microtubule-associated protein tau gene with familial frontotemporal dementia and parkinsonism. *Hum. Mol. Genet.*, **7**, 1825–9.

Dunnett, S. B. & Bjorklund, A. (1999). Prospects for new restorative and neuroprotective treatments in Parkinson's Disease. *Nature*, **399**, A32–9.

Edbauer, D., Winkler, E., Haass, C. & Steiner, H. (2002). Presenilin and nicastrin regulate each other and determine amyloid beta-peptide production via complex formation. *Proc. Natl Acad. Sci., USA*, **99**, 8666–71.

Feany, M. B. (2000). Studying human neurodegenerative diseases in flies and worms. *J. Neuropath. Exp. Neurol.*, **59**, 847–56.

Finney, L. A. & O'Halloran, T. V. (2003). Transition metal speciation in the cell: insights from the chemistry of metal ion receptors. *Science*, **300**, 931–6.

Foix, M. C. (1921). Les lesions anatomiques de la maladie de Parkinson. *Rev. Neurol.*, **28**, 595–600.

Forno, L. S. (1966). Pathology of parkinsonism. A preliminary report of 24 cases. *J. Neurosurg.*, **24**, 266–71.

Forno, L. S., Langston, J. W., DeLanney, L. E., Irwin, I. & Ricaurte, G. A. (1986). Locus ceruleus lesions and eosinophilic inclusions in MPTP-treated monkeys. *Ann. Neurol.*, **20**, 449–55.

Francis R., McGrath G., Zhang J. *et al.* (2002). aph-1 and pen-2 are required for notch pathway signaling, gamma-secretase cleavage of betaAPP, and presenilin protein accumulation. *Dev. Cell*, **3**, 85–97.

George, J. M., Jin, H., Woods, W. S. & Clayton, D. F. (1995). Characterization of a novel protein regulated during the critical period for song learning in the zebra finch. *Neuron*, **15**, 361–72.

Giasson, B. I., Duda, J. E., Quinn, S. M., Zhang, B., Trojanowski, J. Q. & Lee, V. M. (2002). Neuronal alpha-synucleinopathy with severe movement disorder in mice expressing A53T human alpha-synuclein. *Neuron*, **34**, 521–33.

Giasson, B. I., Forman, M. S., Higuchi, M. *et al.* (2003). Initiation and synergistic fibrillization of tau and alpha-synuclein. *Science*, **300**, 636–40.

Goedert, M. (1997). The awakening of α-synuclein. *Nature*, **388**, 232–3.

(2001a). Alpha-synuclein and neurodegenerative diseases. *Nature*, **2**, 492.

(2001b). The significance of tau and α-synuclein inclusions in neurodegenerative diseases. *Curr. Opin. Genet. Dev.*, **11**, 343–51.

Goldstein, L. S. B. & Yang, Z. (2000). Microtubule-based transport systems in neurons: the roles of kinesins and dyneins. *Annu. Rev. Neurosci.*, **23**, 39–71.

Gotz, J., Chen, F., Van Dorpe, J. & Nitsch, R. M. (2001). Formation of neurofibrillary tangles in P301l tau transgenic mice induced by Abeta fibrils. *Science*, **293**, 1491–5.

Greenfield, J. G. & Bosanquet, F. D. (1953). The brain-stem lesions in parkinsonism. *J. Neurol. Neurosurg. Psychiatry*, **16**, 213–26.

Harada, A., Oguchi, K., Okabe, S. *et al.* (1994). Altered microtubule organization in small-calibre axons of mice lacking *tau* protein. *Nature*, **369**, 488–91.

Hassler, R. (1938). Zur Pathologie der Paralysis agitans und des postencephalitischen Parkinsonismus. *J. Psychol. Neurol. (Lpz.)*, **48**, 367–476.

Heber, S., Herms, J., Gajic, V. *et al.* (2000). Mice with combined gene knock-outs reveal essential and partially redundant functions of amyloid precursor protein family members. *J. Neurosci.*, **20**, 7951–63.

Higuchi, M., Ishihara, T., Zhang, B. *et al.* (2002). Transgenic mouse model of tauopathies with glial pathology and nervous system degeneration. *Neuron*, **35**, 433–46.

Higuchi, S., Arai, H. & Matsushita, S. (1998). Mutation in the alpha-synuclein gene and sporadic Parkinson's disease, Alzheimer's disease, and dementia with lewy bodies. *Exp. Neurol.*, **153**, 164–6.

Hong, M., Zhukareva, V., Vogelsberg-Ragaglia, V. *et al.* (1998). Mutation-specific functional impairments in distinct tau isoforms of hereditary FTDP-17. *Science*, **282**, 1914–17.

Hu, Y., Ye, Y. & Fortini, M. E. (2002). Nicastrin is required for gamma-secretase cleavage of the *Drosophila* Notch receptor. *Dev. Cell*, **2**, 69–78.

Hutton, M., Lendon, C. L., Rizzu, P. *et al.* (1998). Association of missense and 5-splice-site mutations in tau with the inherited dementia FTDP-17. *Nature*, **393**, 702–5.

Imai, Y., Soda, M. & Takahashi, R. (2000). Parkin suppresses unfolded protein stress-induced cell death through its E3 ubiquitin-protein ligase activity. *J. Biol. Chem.*, **275**, 35661–4.

Irizarry, M. C., Kim, T. W., McNamara, M. *et al.* (1996). Characterization of the precursor protein of the non-A beta component of senile plaques (NACP) in the human central nervous system. *J. Neuropathol. Exp. Neurol.*, **55**, 889–95.

Ishihara, T., Hong, M., Zhang, B. *et al.* (1999). Age-dependent emergence and progression of a taupathy in transgenic mice overexpressing the shortest human tau isoform. *Neuron*, **24**, 751–62.

Jan, G. G., Veldink, J. H., van, d.T., I. *et al.* (2003). A randomized sequential trial of creatine in amyotrophic lateral sclerosis. *Ann. Neurol.*, **53**, 437–45.

Johnson, G. V. & Hartigan, J. A. (1999). Tau protein in normal and Alzheimer's disease brain: an update. *J. Alzheimers Dis.*, **1**, 329–51.

Julien, J.-P. (2001). Amyotrophic lateral sclerosis: unfolding the toxicity of the misfolded. *Cell*, **104**, 581–91.

Kaether, C., Lammich, S., Edbauer, D. *et al.* (2002). Presenilin-1 affects trafficking and processing of betaAPP and is targeted in a complex with nicastrin to the plasma membrane. *J. Cell Biol.*, **158**, 551–61.

Kamal, A., Almenar-Queralt, A., LeBlanc, J. F., Roberts, E. A. & Goldstein, L. S. (2001). Kinesin-mediated axonal transport of a membrane compartment containing beta-secretase and presenilin-1 requires APP. *Nature*, **414**, 643–8.

Kitada, T., Asakawa, S., Hattori, N. *et al.* (1998). Mutations in the *parkin* gene cause autosomal recessive juvenile parkinsonism. *Nature*, **392**, 605–8.

Kopan, R. & Goate, A. (2002). Aph-2/Nicastrin: an essential component of gamma-secretase and regulator of notch signaling and presenilin localization. *Neuron*, **33**, 321–4.

Kriz, J., Gowing, G. & Julien, J. P. (2003). Efficient three-drug cocktail for disease induced by mutant superoxide dismutase. *Ann. Neurol*, **53**, 429–36.

Kruger R., Kuhn W., Muller T. *et al.* (1998). Ala30Pro mutation in the gene encoding alpha-synuclein in Parkinson's disease. *Nat. Genet.*, **18**, 106–8.

LaMonte, B. H., Wallace, K. E., Holloway, B. A. *et al.* (2002). Disruption of dynein/dynactin inhibits axonal transport in motor neurons causing late-onset progressive degeneration. *Neuron*, **34**, 715–27.

Laptook, A. R., Corbett, R. J. T., Arencibia-Mireles, O., Ruley, J. & Garcia, D. (1994). The effects of systemic glucose concentration on brain metabolism following repeated brain ischemia. *Brain Res.*, **638**, 78–84.

Lazarov, O., Lee, M., Peterson, D. A. & Sisodia, S. S. (2002). Evidence that synaptically released beta-amyloid accumulates as extracellular deposits in the hippocampus of transgenic mice. *J. Neurosci.*, **22**, 9785–93.

Lee M. K. & Price, D. L. (2001). Advances in genetic models of Parkinson's diseases. *Clin. Neurosci. Res.*, **1**, 456–66.

Lee, M. K., Stirling, W. & Xu, Y. (2002). Human alpha-synuclein-harboring familial Parkinson's disease-linked Ala-53 → Thr mutation causes neurodegenerative disease with alpha-synuclein aggregation in transgenic mice. *Proc. Natl Acad. Sci., USA*, **99**, 8968–73.

Lee, V. M. Y. & Trojanowski, J. Q. (1999). Neurodegenerative taupathies: human disease and transgenic mouse models. *Neuron*, **24**, 507–10.

Lee, V. M., Goedert, M. & Trojanowski, J. Q. (2001). Neurodegenerative tauopathies. *Annu. Rev. Neurosci.*, **24**, 1121–59.

Leem, J. Y., Vijayan, S., Han, P. *et al.* (2002). Presenilin 1 is required for maturation and cell surface accumulation of nicstrin. *J. Biol. Chem.*, **277**, 19236–40.

Lewis, J., McGowan, E., Rockwood, J. *et al.* (2000). Neurofibrillary tangles, amyotrophy and progressive disturbance in mice expressing mutant (P301L) tau protein. *Nat. Genet.*, **25**, 402–5.

Lewis, J., Dickson, D. W., Lin, W.-L. *et al.* (2001). Enhanced neurofibrillary degeneration in transgenic mice expressing mutant tau and APP. *Science*, **293**, 1487–91.

Li, M., Ona, V. O., Gugan, C. *et al.* (2000). Functional role of caspase-1 and caspase-3 in an ALS transgenic mouse model. *Science*, **288**, 335–9.

Lim, G. P., Yang, F., Chu, T. *et al.* (2000). Ibuprofen suppresses plaque pathology and inflammation in a mouse model for Alzheimer's disease. *J. Neurosci.*, **20**, 5709–14.

Lin, X., Cummings, C. J. & Zoghbi, H. Y. (1999). Expanding our understanding of polyglutamine diseases through mouse models. *Neuron*, **24**, 499–502.

Lipp, H. P. & Wolfer, D. P. (1998). Genetically modified mice and cognition. *Curr. Opin. Neurobiol.*, **8**, 272–80.

Lopez-Schier, H. & St Johnston, D. (2002). *Drosophila* nicastrin is essential for the intramembranous cleavage of notch. *Dev. Cell*, **2**, 79–89.

Lozano, A. M., Lang, A. E., Hutchison, W. D. & Dostrovsky, J. O. (1998). New developments in understanding the etiology of Parkinson's Disease and in its treatments. *Curr. Opin. Neurobiol.*, **8**, 783–90.

Lozano, A. M., Lang, A. E., Hutchison, W. D. & Dostrovsky, J. O. (1998). New developments in understanding the etiology of Parkinson's disease and in its treatment. *Curr. Opin. Neurobiol.*, **8**, 783–90.

Lucking, C. B., Durr, A., Bonifati, V. *et al.* (2000). Association between early-onset Parkinson's disease and mutations in the parkin gene. *N. Engl. J. Med.*, **342**, 1560–7.

Luo, Y., Bolon, B. & Kahn, S. (2001). Mice deficient in BACE1, the Alzheimer's β-secretase, have normal phenotype and abolished β-amyloid generation. *Nature*, **4**, 231–2.

Markham, C. H. & Diamond, S. G. (1993). Clinical overview of Parkinson's disease. *Clin. Neurosci.*, **1**, 5–11.

Maroteaux, L., Campanelli, J. T. & Scheller, R. H. (1988). Synuclein: a neuron-specific protein localized to the nucleus and presynaptic nerve terminal. *J. Neurosci.*, **8**, 2804–15.

Masliah, E., Rockenstein, E. & Veinbergs, I. (2000). Dopaminergic loss and inclusion body formation in alpha-synuclein mice: implications for neurodegenerative disorders. *Science*, **287**, 1265–9.

Mercken, M., Fischer, I., Kosik, K. S. & Nixon, R. A. (1995). Three distinct axonal transport rates for tau, tubulin, and other microtubule-associated proteins: evidence for dynamic interactions of tau with microtubules *in vivo*. *J. Neurosci.*, **15**, 8259–67.

Munoz, D. G., Dickson, D. W., Bergeron, C., Mackenzie, I. R., Delacourte, A. & Zhukareva, V. (2003). The neuropathology and biochemistry of frontotemporal dementia. *Ann. Neurol.*, **54** Suppl 5, S24–8.

Nicoll, J. A., Wilkinson, D., Holmes, C., Steart, P., Markham, H. & Weller, R. O. (2003). Neuropathology of human Alzheimer disease after immunization with amyloid-beta peptide: a case report. *Nat. Med.*, **9**, 448–52.

Olanow, C. W. & Tatton, W. G. (1999). Etiology and pathogenesis of Parkinson's disease. *Annu. Rev. Neurosci.*, **22**, 123–44.

Oppenheimer, D. R. & Esiri, M. M. (1992). Diseases of the basal ganglia, cerebellum and motor neurons. In *Greenfield's Neuropathology*, ed. J. H. Adams & L. W. Duchen, pp. 988–1045. New York: Oxford University Press.

Pasquier, F., Fukui, T., Sarazin, M. *et al.* (2003). Laboratory investigations and treatment in frontotemporal dementia. *Ann. Neurol.*, **54** Suppl 5, S32–5.

Polymeropoulos, M. H. (1998). Autosomal dominant Parkinson's disease and alpha-synuclein. *Ann. Neurol.*, **44**, S63–4.

Polymeropoulos, M. H., Lavedan, C., Leroy, E. *et al.* (1997). Mutation in the alphasynuclein gene identified in families with Parkinson's disease. *Science*, **276**, 2045–7.

Price D. L., Tanzi R. E., Borchelt D. R. & Sisodia S. S. (1998). Alzheimer's disease: genetic studies and transgenic models. *Annu. Rev. Genet.*, **32**, 461–93.

Probst, A., Götz, J., Wiederhold, K. H. *et al.* (2000). Axonopathy and amyotrophy in mice transgenic for human four-repeat tau protein. *Acta Neuropathol.*, **99**, 469–81.

Puls, I., Jonnakuty, C., LaMonte, B. H. *et al.* (2003). Mutant dynactin in motor neuron disease. *Nat. Genet.*, **33**, 455–6.

Rothstein, J. D. (2003). Of mice and men: reconciling preclinical ALS mouse studies and human clinical trials. *Ann. Neurol.*, **53**, 423–6.

Schenk, D., Barbour, R., Dunn, W. *et al.* (1999). Immunization with amyloid-beta attenuates Alzheimer disease-like pathology in the PDAPP mouse. *Nature*, **400**, 173–7.

Selkoe, D. J. (2001a). Alzheimer's disease: genes, proteins, and therapy. *Physiol. Rev.*, **81**, 741–66.

(2001b). Clearing the brain's amyloid cobwebs. *Neuron*, **32**, 177–80.

Sheng, J. G., Price, D. L. & Koliatsos, V. E. (2002). Disruption of corticocortical connections ameliorates amyloid burden in terminal fields in a transgenic model of Abeta amyloidosis. *J. Neurosci.*, **22**, 9794–9.

Sherman, M. Y. & Goldberg, A. L. (2001). Cellular defenses against unfolded proteins: a cell biologist thinks about neurodegenerative diseases. *Neuron*, **29**, 15–32.

Sherrington, R., Rogaev, E. I., Liang, Y. *et al.* (1995). Cloning of gene bearing missense mutations in early-onset familial Alzheimer's disease. *Nature*, **375**, 754–60.

Sima, A. A. F., Defendini, R., Keohane, C. *et al.* (1996). The neuropathology of chromosome 17-linked dementia. *Ann. Neurol.*, **39**, 734–43.

Sisodia, S. S. & George-Hyslop, P. H. (2002). gamma-Secretase, Notch, Abeta and Alzheimer's disease: where do the presenilins fit in? *Nat. Rev. Neurosci.*, **3**, 281–90.

Spillantini, M. G., Schmidt, V. M. L., Trojanowski, J. Q., Jakes, R. & Goedert, M. (1997). Alpha-synuclein in lewy bodies [letter]. 839–40.

Spillantini, M. G., Murrell, J. R., Goedert, M., Farlow, M. R., Klug, A. & Ghetti, B. (1998). Mutation in the tau gene in familial multiple system tauopathy with presenile dementia. *Proc. Natl Acad. Sci., USA*, **95**, 7737–41.

Spittaels, K., Van den Haute, C., Van Dorpe, J. *et al.* (1999). Prominent axonopathy in the brain and spinal cord of transgenic mice overexpressing four-repeat human tau protein. *Am. J. Pathol.*, **155**, 2153–65.

Subramaniam, J. R., Lyons, W. E. & Liu, J. (2002). Mutant SOD1 causes motor neuron disease independent of copper chaperone-mediated copper loading. *Nat. Neurosci.*, **5**, 301–7.

Südhof, T. C. (1995). The synaptic vesicle cycle: a cascade of protein-protein interactions. *Nature*, **375**, 645–53.

Takei, Y., Kondo, S., Harada, A., Inomata, S., Noda, T. & Hirokawa, N. (1997). Delayed development of nervous system in mice homozygous for disrupted microtubule-associated protein 1B (MAP1B) gene. *J. Cell Biol.*, **137**, 1615–26.

Takei, Y., Teng, J., Harada, A. & Hirokawa, N. (2000). Defects in axonal elongation and neuronal migration in mice with disrupted tau and map 1b genes. *J. Cell Biol.*, **150**, 989–1000.

Taniguchi, Y., Karlstrom, H., Lundkvist, J. *et al.* (2002). Notch receptor cleavage depends on but is not directly executed by presenilins. *Proc. Natl Acad. Sci., USA*, **99**, 4014–19.

Tanzi, R. E. & Bertram, L. (2001). New frontiers in Alzheimer's disease genetics. *Neuron*, **32**, 181–4.

Terada, S. & Hirokawa, K. (2000). Moving on to the cargo problem of microtubule-dependent motors in neurons. *Curr. Opin. Neurobiol.*, **10**, 566–73.

Trojanowski, J. Q. (2002). Tauists, baptists, syners, apostates, and new data. *Ann. Neurol.*, **52**, 263–5.

Ueda, K., Fukushima, H., Masliah, E. *et al.* (1993). Molecular cloning of cDNA encoding an unrecognized component of amyloid in Alzheimer disease. *Proc. Natl Acad. Sci. USA*, **90**, 11282–6.

Van der Putten, H., Wiederhold, K. H., Probst, A., *et al.* (2000). Neuropathology in mice expressing human alpha-synuclein. *J. Neurosci.*, **20**, 6021–9.

Vassar, R., Bennett, B. D., Babu-Khan, S. *et al.* (1999). β-secretase cleavage of Alzheimer's amyloid precursor protein by the transmembrane aspartic protease BACE. *Science*, **286**, 735–41.

Vassar, R. & Citron, M. (2000). Aβ-generating enzymes: recent advances in β- and γ-secretase research. *Neuron*, **27**, 419–22.

Vázques, J., Fernández-Shaw, C., Marina, A., Haas, C., Cacabelos, R. & Valdivieso, F. (1996). Antibodies to human brain spectrin in Alzheimer's disease. *J. Neuroimmunol.*, **68**, 39–44.

Wang, J., Xu, G. & Borchelt, D. R. (2002). High molecular weight complexes of mutant superoxide dismutase 1: age-dependent and tissue-specific accumulation. *Neurobiol. Dis.*, **9**, 139–48.

Warrick, J. M., Paulson, H. L., Gray-Board Y. E. *et al.* (1998). Expanded polyglutamine protein forms nuclear inclusions and causes neural degeneration in *Drosophila*. *Cell*, **93**, 939–49.

Warrick, J. M., Chan, H., Gray-Board, Y. E., Chai, Y., Paulson, H. L. & Bonini, N. M. (1999). Suppression of polyglutamine-mediated neurodegeneration in *Drosophila* by the molecular chaperone HSP70. *Nat. Genet.*, **23**, 425–8.

Weggen, S., Eriksen, J. L., Das, P. *et al.* (2001). A subset of NSAIDs lower amyloidogenic Aβ42 independently of cyclooxygenase activity. *Nature*, **414**, 212–16.

Wichmann, T. & DeLong, M. R. (1996). Functional and pathophysiological models of the basal ganglia. *Curr. Opin. Neurobiol.*, **6**, 752–8.

Wittmann, C. W., Wszolek, M. F., Shulman, J. M. *et al.* (2001). Tauopathy in *Drosophila:* neurodegeneration without neurofibrillary tangles. *Science*, **293**, 711–14.

Wong, P. C., Pardo, C. A., Borchelt, D. R. *et al.* (1995). An adverse property of a familial ALS-linked SOD1 mutation causes motor neuron disease characterized by vacuolar degeneration of mitochondria. *Neuron*, **14**, 1105–16.

Wong, P. C., Zheng, H., Chen, H. *et al.* (1997). Presenilin 1 is required for Notch 1 and DII1 expression in the paraxial mesoderm. *Nature*, **387**, 288–92.

Wong, P. C., Rothstein, J. D. & Price, D. L. (1998). The genetic and molecular mechanisms of motor neuron disease. *Curr. Opin. Neurobiol.*, **8**, 791–9.

Wong, P. C., Waggoner, D., Subramaniam, J. R. *et al.* (2000). Copper chaperone for superoxide dismutase is essential to activate mammalian Cu/Zn superoxide dismutase. *Proc. Natl Acad. Sci., USA*, **97**, 2886–91.

Wong, P. C., Price, D. L. & Cai, H. (2001). The brain's susceptibility to amyloid plaques. *Science*, **293**, 1434–5.

Wong, P. C., Cai, H., Borchelt, D. R. & Price, D. L. (2002). Genetically engineered mouse models of neurodegenerative diseases. *Nat. Neurosci.*, **5**, 633–9.

Yu, G., Nishimura, M., Arawaka, S. *et al.* (2000). Nicastrin modulates presenilin-mediated notch/glp-1 signal transduction and betaAPP processing. *Nature*, **407**, 48–54.

Zhang, Y., Gao, J., Chung, K. K. *et al.* (2000). Parkin functions as an E2-dependent ubiquitin-protein ligase and promotes the degradation of the synaptuc vesicle-associated protein, CDCrel-1. *Proc. Natl Acad. Sci., USA*, **97**, 13354–9.

Zheng, H., Jiang, M.-H., Trumbauer, M. E. *et al.* (1995). β-amyloid precursor protein-deficient mice show reactive gliosis and decreased locomotor activity. *Cell*, **81**, 525–31.

Zhu, S., Stavrovskaya, I. G., Drozda, M. *et al.* (2002). Minocycline inhibits cytochrome c release and delays progression of amyotrophic lateral sclerosis in mice. *Nature*, **417**, 74– 8.

16

Toxic animal models

Serge Przedborski[1] and Kim Tieu[2]

[1]Departments of Neurology and Pathology, and Center for Neurobiology and Behavior, Columbia University, NY, USA
[2]Department of Environmental Medicine and Center for Aging and Developmental Biology, University of Rochester, NY, USA

Introduction

As discussed elsewhere (Przedborski *et al.*, 2003), the term "neurodegenerative disease" refers to a group of neurological disorders with heterogeneous clinical and pathological expressions. These diseases are all characterized by a loss of specific subpopulations of neurons confined to functional anatomic systems, arising in most cases for unknown reasons and progressing in a relentless manner. Among the variety of neurodegenerative disorders, the lion's share of attention has been given only to a handful, including Alzheimer's disease, Parkinson's disease, Huntington's disease, and amyotrophic lateral sclerosis (ALS). So far, the most consistent risk factor for developing a neurodegenerative disorder, especially AD and PD, is increasing age. Over the past century the growth rate of the population age 65 and beyond in the industrialized countries has far exceeded that of the population as a whole. Thus it can be anticipated that, over the next generations, the proportion of elderly citizens will double and, with this, the number of individuals suffering from a neurodegenerative disorder. This prediction is at the centre of the growing concerns from the medical community and from legislators, as one can easily foresee a dramatic increase in the emotional, physical, and financial burden on patients, caregivers, and society related to these disabling illnesses. The problem is made worse by the fact that, although to date several approved drugs do, to some extent, alleviate symptoms of several neurodegenerative diseases, their chronic use is often associated with debilitating side effects, and none seems to stop the progression of the degenerative processes. It is now clear that the development of effective preventive or protective therapies has been thus far impeded by our limited knowledge of the causes and mechanisms by which neurons die in neurodegenerative diseases. Thanks to the development of experimental models, several neurobiological

breakthroughs have brought closer than ever the day that the secrets of several neurodegenerative disorders will be unlocked and effective therapeutic strategies will become available. So far, among the various accepted experimental models, neurotoxins have been the most popular means employed to produce selective neuronal death in both in vitro and in vivo systems. In this chapter, we will thus review the key neurotoxic models of neurodegeneration, which will be categorized based on their main molecular targets as we currently know them. For each of the selected neurotoxins, attention will be paid to providing the reader with information regarding their respective mechanisms of action and the kinds of diseases that they model. Although in vitro data will be mentioned whenever necessary, this chapter will focus on in vivo studies.

1-Methy-4-phenyl-1,2,3,6-tetrahydropyridine

1-Methy-4-phenyl-1,2,3,6-tetrahydropyridine (MPTP) is a byproduct of the chemical synthesis of a meperidine analogue with potent heroin-like effects. MPTP can induce a parkinsonian syndrome in humans almost indistinguishable from PD (Langston & Irwin, 1986). Recognition of MPTP as a neurotoxin occurred early in 1982, when several young drug addicts mysteriously developed a profound parkinsonian syndrome after the intravenous use of street preparations of meperidine analogs which, unknown to anyone, were contaminated with MPTP (Langston *et al.*, 1983). In humans and non-human primates, depending on the regimen used, MPTP can produce an irreversible and severe parkinsonian syndrome that replicates almost all of the features of PD; in non-human primates, a resting tremor characteristic of PD has only been demonstrated convincingly in the African green monkey (Tetrud *et al.*, 1986). It is believed that, in PD, the neurodegenerative process occurs over several years, while the most active phase of neurodegeneration is completed within a few days following MPTP administration (Langston, 1987; Jackson-Lewis et al., 1995). However, recent data suggest that, following the main phase of neuronal death, MPTP-induced neurodegeneration may continue to progress "silently" over several decades, at least in humans intoxicated with MPTP (Vingerhoets et al., 1994; Langston et al., 1999). Except for four cases (Davis et al., 1979; Langston et al., 1999), no human pathological material has been available for study, and thus the comparison between PD and the MPTP model is mainly based on non-human primates (Forno et al., 1993). Neuropathological data show that MPTP administration causes damage to the nigrostriatal dopaminergic pathway identical to that seen in PD (Dauer & Przedborski, 2003), yet there is a resemblance that goes beyond the loss of SNpc dopaminergic neurons. Like PD, MPTP causes a greater loss of dopaminergic neurons in the SNpc than in the ventral tegmental area (Seniuk et al., 1990; Muthane et al., 1994) and, in monkeys treated with low doses of MPTP (but not in humans), a greater degeneration of dopaminergic nerve terminals in the putamen than in the caudate nucleus (Moratalla et al., 1992; Snow et al., 2000). However, two typical neuropathologic features of PD have, until now, been lacking in the MPTP model. First, except for the SNpc, pigmented nuclei such as the locus coeruleus have been inconsistently affected, according to most published reports. Second, the eosinophilic intraneuronal inclusions, called "Lewy bodies," so characteristic of PD, thus far, have not been convincingly observed in MPTP-induced parkinsonism (Forno et al., 1993); although, in MPTP-injected monkeys, intraneuronal inclusions reminiscent of Lewy bodies have been described (Forno et al., 1986). Despite these imperfections, MPTP continues to be regarded as the best animal model of PD, and it is believed that studying MPTP toxic mechanisms will shed light on the molecular basis of PD.

Over the years, MPTP has been used in a large variety of animal species, ranging from worms to mammals. To date, the most frequently used animals for MPTP studies are monkeys, mice and rats. The administration of MPTP through a number of different routes using different dosing regimens has led to the development of several distinct models, each characterized by some unique behavioral and biochemical features. The manner in which these models were developed is based on the concept of delivering MPTP in a fashion that creates the most severe and stable form of nigrostriatal damage with the least number of undesirable side effects such as acute death, dehydration and malnutrition. Although MPTP can be given by a number of different routes, including gavage and stereotaxic injection into the brain, the most common, reliable, and reproducible lesion is provided by its systemic administration (i.e. subcutaneous, intravenous, intraperitoneal or intramuscular). The most commonly used regimens in monkeys are the multiple intraperitoneal or intramuscular injections and the intracarotid infusion of MPTP (Petzinger & Langston, 1998). The former is easy to perform and produces a bilateral parkinsonian syndrome. However, often the monkey exhibits a generalized parkinsonian syndrome so severe that chronic administration of drugs such as L-DOPA is required to enable the animal to eat and drink adequately (Petzinger & Langston, 1998). Although unilateral intracarotid infusion is technically more difficult, this regimen causes symptoms mainly on one side (Bankiewicz et al., 1986; Przedborski et al., 1991), so it has the advantage of allowing the monkey to maintain normal nutrition and hydration without the use of L-DOPA. For many years monkeys were mainly, if not exclusively, treated with harsh regimens of MPTP to produce an acute and severe dopaminergic neurodegeneration (Petzinger and Langston, 1998). More recently, several investigators have treated monkeys with low doses of MPTP (e.g. 0.05 mg/kg 2–3 times per week) for a prolonged period of time (i.e. weeks to months) in an attempt to better model the slow neurodegenerative process of PD (Schneider & Roeltgen, 1993; Bezard et al., 1997; Schneider et al., 1999). While both the acute and the chronic MPTP-monkey models are appropriate for the testing of experimental therapies aimed at alleviating PD symptoms, the chronic model is presumably the most suitable for testing neuroprotective strategies. Among the numerous mammalian species susceptible to MPTP (Kopin & Markey, 1988; Heikkila et al., 1989; Przedborski et al., 2000), in addition to monkeys, mice have become the animals most commonly used. However, several problems need to be emphasized. First, mice are much less sensitive to MPTP than monkeys; thus, much higher doses are required to produce significant SNpc damage in this animal species. Higher doses present a far greater hazard, requiring tighter safety precautions (Przedborski et al., 2001b). Second, unlike monkeys, mice treated with MPTP do not develop parkinsonism. Third, the magnitude of striatal dopamine nigrostriatal damage depends on the dose and dosing schedule (Sonsalla & Heikkila, 1986). The use of MPTP in rats presents an interesting situation (Kopin & Markey, 1988). For instance, rats injected with mg/kg doses of MPTP comparable to those used in mice do not exhibit any significant dopaminergic neurodegeneration (Giovanni et al., 1994a,b). Conversely, rats injected with much higher doses of MPTP do exhibit significant dopaminergic neurodegeneration (Giovanni et al., 1994a,b) although, at these high doses, rats have

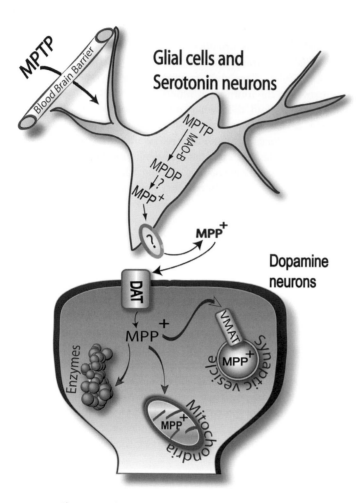

Fig. 16.1 Schematic representation of MPTP metabolism. After its systemic administration, MPTP crosses the blood-brain barrier. Once in the brain, MPTP is converted to MPDP$^+$ by MAO-B within non-dopaminergic cells, and then to MPP$^+$ by an unknown mechanism (?). Thereafter, MPP$^+$ is released, again by an unknown mechanism (?), into the extracellular space. From there, MPP$^+$ is taken up by the DAT and thus enters dopaminergic neurons. Inside dopaminergic neurons, MPP$^+$ can (i) bind to the vesicular monoamine transporters (VMAT) and translocate into synaptosomal vesicles, (ii) accumulate into the mitochondria by an active process, and (iii) remain in the cytosol and interact with different cytosolic enzymes.

to be pretreated with guanethidine to prevent dramatic peripheral catecholamine release and extensive mortality (Giovanni et al., 1994a). These findings indicate that rats are relatively insensitive to MPTP, but regardless of this drawback, rats continue to be used quite often in MPTP studies (Storey et al., 1992; Giovanni et al., 1994a,b; Staal & Sonsalla, 2000; Staal et al., 2000). In rats, however, the systemic administration of MPTP is rarely

used and the vast majority of studies involve the stereo-taxic infusion of 1-methyl-4-phenylpyridinium (MPP$^+$), a toxic metabolite of MPTP (Storey et al., 1992; Giovanni et al., 1994a,b; Staal & Sonsalla, 2000; Staal et al., 2000).

Prior to using the MPTP model it is crucial to remember that several factors influence the reproducibility of the lesion in monkeys, rats and mice. However, to our knowledge, an extensive and systematic assessment of these factors has only been done in mice (Heikkila et al., 1989; Giovanni et al., 1991, 1994a,b; Miller et al., 1998; Hamre et al., 1999; Staal & Sonsalla, 2000) and the results can be summarized as follows: different strains of mice (and even within a given strain, mice from different vendors) can exhibit strikingly distinct sensitivity to MPTP. This differential seems to be inherited as an autosomal dominant trait (Hamre et al., 1999). As discussed in greater detail in (Przedborski & Vila, 2001), gender, age and body weight are also factors that modulate MPTP sensitivity and reproducibility of the lesion.

MPTP mode of action

As illustrated in Fig. 16.1, the metabolism of MPTP is a complex, multistep process (Przedborski & Vila, 2003; Dauer & Przedborski, 2003). After its systemic administration, MPTP, which is highly lypophilic, rapidly crosses the blood–brain barrier (BBB). Once in the brain, the pro-toxin MPTP is metabolized to 1-methyl-4-phenyl-2,3-dihydropyridinium (MPDP$^+$) by the enzyme monoamine oxidase B (MAO-B) within non-dopaminergic cells such as glial cells, and then (probably by spontaneous oxidation) to 1-methyl-4-phenylpyridinium (MPP$^+$), the active toxic compound. Thereafter, MPP$^+$ is released (by an unknown mechanism) into the extracellular space. Since MPP$^+$ is a polar molecule, unlike its precursor MPTP, it cannot freely exit cells within which it has been produced or enter cells within which it will cause toxicity. It is thus likely that the translocation of MPP$^+$ from its site of production to its site of cytotoxicity depends on the plasma membrane carriers. Consistent with this view is the fact that MPP$^+$ has a high affinity for plasma membrane dopamine transporter (DAT) (Mayer et al., 1986), as well as for norepinephrine and serotonin transporters, enabling it to gain access to monoaminergic neurons and more particularly dopaminergic neurons. The obligatory character of this step in the MPTP neurotoxic process is demonstrated by the fact that blockade of DAT by specific antagonists such as mazindol (Javitch et al., 1985) or ablation of the DAT gene in mutant mice (Bezard et al., 1999) completely prevents

MPTP-induced toxicity. Conversely, transgenic mice with increased brain DAT expression are more sensitive to MPTP (Donovan *et al.*, 1999).

Once inside dopaminergic neurons, MPP[+] can follow at least three routes (Fig. 16.1): (i) it can bind to the vesicular monoamine transporters (VMAT) which will translocate MPP[+] into synaptosomal vesicles (Liu *et al.*, 1992), (ii) it can be concentrated within the mitochondria (Ramsay & Singer, 1986), and (iii) it can remain in the cytosol and interact with different cytosolic enzymes (Klaidman *et al.*, 1993). The fraction of MPP[+] destined to each of these routes is probably a function of MPP[+] intracellular concentration and affinity for VMAT, mitochondrial membrane potential, and cytosolic enzymes. The importance of the vesicular sequestration of MPP[+] is demonstrated by the fact that cells transfected to express greater density of VMAT are converted from MPP[+]-sensitive to MPP[+]-resistant cells (Liu *et al.*, 1992). Conversely, we demonstrated that mutant mice with 50% lower VMAT expression are significantly more sensitive to MPTP-induced dopaminergic neurotoxicity compared to their wild-type littermates (Takahashi *et al.*, 1997). These findings indicate that there is a clear inverse relationship between the capacity of MPP[+] sequestration (i.e. VMAT density) and the magnitude of MPTP neurotoxicity. Inside dopaminergic neurons, MPP[+] can also be concentrated within the mitochondria (Fig. 16.1) (Ramsay & Singer, 1986), where it impairs mitochondrial respiration by inhibiting complex I of the electron transport chain (Nicklas *et al.*, 1985; Mizuno *et al.*, 1987) through its binding at or near the site of the mitochondrial poison rotenone (Ramsay *et al.*, 1991; Higgins, Jr. & Greenamyre, 1996; Schuler & Casida, 2001).

MPTP mechanism of action

Currently, it is believed that the neurotoxic process of MPTP is made up of a cascade of multiple deleterious events, which can be divided into early and late neuronal perturbations and secondary non-neuronal alterations. All of these, to a variable degree and at different stages of the degenerative process, participate in the ultimate demise of dopaminergic neurons.

Early events
Soon after its entry into dopaminergic neurons, MPP[+] binds to complex I and, by interrupting the flow of electrons, leads to an acute deficit in ATP formation (Chan *et al.*, 1992). It appears, however, that complex I activity should be reduced >70% to cause severe ATP depletion in non-synaptic mitochondria (Davey & Clark, 1996) and that, in contrast to in vitro, in vivo MPTP causes only a

transient 20% reduction in mouse striatal and midbrain ATP levels (Chan *et al.*, 1991), raising the question as to whether MPP[+]-related ATP deficit can be the sole factor underlying MPTP-induced dopaminergic neuronal death.

Another consequence of complex I inhibition by MPP[+] is an increased production of reactive oxygen species (ROS), especially of superoxide (Rossetti *et al.*, 1988; Hasegawa *et al.*, 1990; Cleeter *et al.*, 1992). Early ROS production can also occur in this model from the auto-oxidation of dopamine resulting from an MPP[+]-induced massive release of vesicular dopamine to the cytosol (Lotharius & O'Malley, 2000). Dopamine can also be oxidized to the highly reactive dopamine-quinone by cyclooxygenase-2, an enzyme which is upregulated in SNpc dopaminergic neurons in MPTP-intoxicated mice and PD postmortem samples (Teismann *et al.*, 2003). The importance of MPP[+]-related ROS production in the dopaminergic toxicity process in vivo is demonstrated by the fact that transgenic mice with increased brain activity of copper/zinc superoxide dismutase (SOD1), a key ROS scavenging enzyme, are significantly more resistant to MPTP-induced dopaminergic toxicity than their non-transgenic littermates (Przedborski *et al.*, 1992). However, several lines of evidence support the concept that ROS exert many or most of their toxic effects in the MPTP model in conjunction with other reactive species such as nitric oxide (NO) (Schulz *et al.*, 1995b; Ara *et al.*, 1998; Pennathur *et al.*, 1999; Przedborski *et al.*, 2001a) produced in the brain by both the neuronal and the inducible isoforms of the enzyme NO synthase (Przedborski *et al.*, 1996; Liberatore *et al.*, 1999). A comprehensive review of the source and the role of NO in the MPTP model can be found in the following references (Przedborski & Vila, 2001; Przedborski & Dawson, 2001; Tieu *et al.*, 2003).

Late events
In response to the variety of functional perturbations caused by the depletion in ATP and the production of ROS, death signals, which can activate the molecular pathways of apoptosis, arise within intoxicated dopaminergic neurons. Although at this time we cannot exclude with certainty the possibility that apoptotic factors are not consistently recruited regardless of MPTP regimen, only prolonged administration of low to moderate doses of MPTP is associated with definite morphologically defined apoptotic neurons (Jackson-Lewis *et al.*, 1995; Tatton & Kish, 1997). Supporting the implication of apoptotic molecular factors in the demise of dopaminergic neurons after MPTP administration is the demonstration that the pro-apoptotic protein Bax is instrumental in this toxic model (Vila *et al.*, 2001a). Overexpression of the anti-apoptotic Bcl-2 also protects dopaminergic cells against MPTP-induced

neurodegeneration (Offen *et al.*, 1998; Yang *et al.*, 1998). Similarly, adenovirus-mediated transgene expression of the X-chromosome-linked inhibitor of apoptosis protein (XIAP), an inhibitor of executioner caspases such as caspase-3, also blocks the death of dopaminergic neurons in the SNpc following the administration of MPTP (Eberhardt *et al.*, 2000). Other caspases are also activated in MPTP-intoxicated mice such as caspase-8, which is a proximal effector of the tumor necrosis factor receptor family death pathway (Hartmann *et al.*, 2001). Other observations supporting a role of apoptosis in the MPTP neurotoxic process include the demonstration of the resistance to MPTP of mutant mice deficient in p53 (Trimmer *et al.*, 1996), a cell cycle control gene involved in programmed cell death, or the resistance of mice treated with inhibitors of c-Jun N-terminal kinases (Saporito *et al.*, 1999, 2000). Collectively, these data show that, during the degenerative process, the apoptotic pathways are activated and contribute to the actual death of intoxicated neurons in the MPTP model.

Secondary events

The loss of dopaminergic neurons in the MPTP mouse model is associated with a glial response composed mainly of activated microglial cells and, to a lesser extent, of reactive astrocytes (Vila *et al.*, 2001b). From a neuropathological standpoint, microglial activation is indicative of an active, ongoing process of cell death. The presence of activated microglia in postmortem samples from MPTP-intoxicated individuals who came to autopsy several decades after being exposed to the toxin (Langston *et al.*, 1999) suggests an ongoing degenerative process and thus challenges the notion that MPTP produces a "hit-and-run" kind of damage. Therefore, this important observation (Langston *et al.*, 1999) suggests that a single acute insult to the SNpc by MPTP could set in motion a self-sustained cascade of events with long-lasting deleterious effects. Looking at mice injected with MPTP and killed at different time points thereafter, it appears that the time course of reactive astrocyte formation parallels that of dopaminergic structure destruction in both the striatum and the SNpc, and that GFAP expression remains upregulated even after the main wave of neuronal death has passed (Czlonkowska *et al.*, 1996; Kohutnicka *et al.*, 1998; Liberatore *et al.*, 1999). These findings suggest that, in the MPTP mouse model (Przedborski *et al.*, 2000), the astrocytic reaction is secondary to the death of neurons and not the reverse. This conclusion is supported by the demonstration that blockade of MPP^+ uptake into dopaminergic neurons completely prevents not only SNpc dopaminergic neuronal death but also GFAP up-regulation (O'Callaghan *et al.*, 1990). Remarkably, activation of microglial cells, which is also quite strong

in the MPTP mouse model (Czlonkowska *et al.*, 1996; Kohutnicka *et al.*, 1998; Liberatore *et al.*, 1999; Dehmer *et al.*, 2000), occurs much earlier than that of astrocytes and, more importantly, reaches a maximum before the peak of dopaminergic neurodegeneration (Liberatore *et al.*, 1999). In the light of the MPTP data presented above, it can be surmised that the response of both astrocytes and microglial cells in the SNpc occurs within a timeframe allowing these glial cells to participate in the demise of dopaminergic neurons in the MPTP mouse model and possibly in PD. Activated microglial cells can produce a variety of noxious compounds including ROS and reactive nitrogen species (RNS) via NADPH-oxidase (Wu *et al.*, 2003) and inducible NOS (Liberatore *et al.*, 1999) as well as proinflammatory cytokines and prostaglandins. Observations showing that blockade of microglial activation mitigates nigrostriatal damage caused by MPTP supports the notion that microglia participate in MPTP-induced neurodegeneration (Wu *et al.*, 2002).

Reactive oxygen species-producing neurotoxins

Reactive oxygen species, such as superoxide radicals, are produced constantly during normal cellular metabolism, primarily as byproducts of the mitochondrial respiratory chain and, when it applies, catecholamine metabolism. Defense mechanisms, however, exist to limit the levels of ROS and the damage they inflict on cellular components such as lipids, proteins, and DNA. It has been hypothesized that the finely tuned balance between the production and destruction of ROS is skewed in a number of pathological conditions including neurodegenerative disorders such as Parkinson's disease, resulting in oxidative stress that leads to severe cellular dysfunction and, ultimately, to cell death. For this reason, ROS-generating neurotoxins such as 6-hydroxydopamine (6-OHDA) and paraquat have been extensively used to model neurodegeneration.

6-Hydroxydopamine and related compounds

Since the introduction of 6-OHDA more than 30 years ago, several related compounds have been synthesized and tested both in vitro and in vivo. So far, however, none of them have been found to be superior to 6-OHDA as a monoamine neurotoxin. Among the 6-OHDA analogues, only 6-OH-DOPA and 6-aminodopamine have been used to a certain extent, especially to damage noradrenergic pathways. Yet, the much greater body of information available on the use of 6-OHDA over any other of its derivatives (Jonsson, 1980) may also explain why 6-OHDA is the preferred compound of its group for producing catecholaminergic lesions. With respect to the mode and mechanism of action, it is well established that 6-OHDA accumulates specifically in catecholaminergic neurons, causes depletion of norepinephrine and dopamine and, ultimately, inflicts structural damage to these neurons (Jonsson, 1983). The specificity of 6-OHDA's action on catecholaminergic neurons is explained by the high affinity of the toxin for the plasma membrane catecholamine transporter, allowing 6-OHDA to be rapidly and efficiently taken up by norepinephrine and dopamine neurons. Given this fact, it is not surprising that pre-treatment of animals with a norepinephrine uptake (Herve *et al.*, 1986; Luthman *et al.*, 1989) or dopamine uptake blocker (Luthman *et al.*, 1987, 1989), by preventing the entry of the toxin in these neurons, mitigates 6-OHDA cytotoxicity. Once inside of the neurons, 6-OHDA accumulates in the cytosol where it produces quinones, which inactivate some biological macromolecules by binding to their nucleophilic groups (Saner & Thoenen, 1971), as well as a variety of ROS (Cohen & Werner, 1994). Although quinone-based and ROS-based mechanisms are probably both operative in 6-OHDA cytotoxicity, available evidence favors the notion that ROS play the dominant neurotoxic role (Graham, 1978; Cohen & Werner, 1994). Of note, since 6-OHDA forms the *para*-quinone it does not react as well with external nucleophiles as the dopamine *ortho*-quinone does. ROS generated by the metabolism of 6-OHDA emanate from its autooxidation and from its oxidative deamination mediated by the MAO. However, the finding that pretreatment with MAO inhibitor such as pargyline, rather than mitigating 6-OHDA toxicity, instead enhances it (Jonsson, 1980), suggests that auto-oxidation and not oxidative deamination is instrumental in 6-OHDA-induced neuronal death. Because auto-oxidation of 6-OHDA can occur both intra- and extraneuronally, this neurotoxin is prone to causing specific and nonspecific effects. Consistent with this view is the demonstration that, in mesencephalic cultures, 6-OHDA toxicity is not restricted to dopaminergic neurons (Lotharius *et al.*, 1999), and that several cell types devoid of catecholaminergic transporters including C6 glioma, NIH-3T3, and CHO cells can be damaged by the toxin (Blum *et al.*, 2001). It is thus important to use as low a dose of 6-OHDA as possible and to prevent auto-oxidation of 6-OHDA from occurring extraneuronally by, for example, administering a reducing agent such as ascorbic acid with 6-OHDA. Under experimental conditions devoid of non-specific toxicity, 6-OHDA affects primarily dopaminergic and noradrenergic neurons, much less peripheral adrenergic neurons, and, according to most reports, not at all central adrenergic and serotoninergic neurons (at least in rodents). Among

the various central catecholaminergic pathways, the locus coeruleus noradrenergic system (nerve terminals) appears to be the one most sensitive to 6-OHDA, whereas the adrenergic neuron systems are most resistant (Jonsson *et al.*, 1976). The dopaminergic systems range from being relatively sensitive (e.g. the nigrostriatal pathway) to almost completely resistant (e.g. the tubero-infundibular pathway) to 6-OHDA (Jonsson, 1980). In general, it has been observed that the nerve terminals appear to be the most sensitive, that the axons are less so, and that the cell body structures are least sensitive to the neurotoxic action of 6-OHDA (Jonsson, 1983). These differences can at least partly be related to differences in surface–volume relationships. Since the 6-OHDA dose, injection volume, time and route of administration, and the injection technique are the crucial factors, one may find it worthwhile to refer to Jonsson (1980) to optimize lesioning conditions.

In adult animals, 6-OHDA has been used most commonly in rats and to a lesser extent in mice, cats, dogs, and monkeys (Jonsson, 1983), but no one species has a real scientific advantage over the other. Since 6-OHDA does not easily cross the BBB it has to be injected intraventricularly, intracisternally, or intracerebrally to damage the central catecholaminergic systems (Jonsson, 1983). Intraventricular and intracisternal administration of 6-OHDA calls for high doses (500–1000 μg/kg in 25–50 μl) and produces a bilateral catecholaminergic lesion, observed within a few hours of the injection of the toxin, with generally limited regrowth of affected nerve fibers (Jonsson, 1983). Unexpectedly, these routes of administration produce a very heterogenous pattern of denervation with profound reductions in norepinephrine in the cerebral cortex and cerebellum and only mild reductions in the hypothalamus and brainstem (Jonsson, 1983). Similarly, reductions in dopamine are maximal at the level of the nigrostriatal pathway and minimal at the level of other dopaminergic pathways (Jonsson, 1983). Within the ventral midbrain dopaminergic neuronal groups, the highest loss is found in the substantia nigra, followed by the retrorubral field, and ventral tegmental area (Rodriguez *et al.*, 2001). When a bilateral 6-OHDA lesion is severe, rats will often die primarily due to the occurrence of marked aphagia, adipsia, and seizures (Ungerstedt, 1971a; Bourn *et al.*, 1972). However, the few rats which survive and recover normal ingestion and weight show interesting behavioral abnormalities including hypokinesia, purposeless chewing, and catalepsia which can, at least partially, be reversed by the administration of dopaminergic agonists (Rodriguez *et al.*, 2001). In contrast to this widespread mode of lesioning, local intracerebral injection of 6-OHDA is often used to target a specific catecholaminergic pathway of the brain (Ungerstedt,

1968, 1971c). This kind of lesion is achieved by stereotaxic administration usually of 1–10 μg of toxin infused in 1–10 μl at a rate of 1 to 5 μl/min. To avoid non-specific damage the solution injected should not contain more than 2.5 μg/μl of 6-OHDA (Przedborski et al., 1995). Also it is important to keep in mind the fact that the size of the lesioned areas and the magnitude of the lesion (specific and non-specific) are dependent on the volume of 6-OHDA solution infused as well as its concentration and the rate at which it is infused (Agid et al., 1973). To specifically target the nigrostriatal dopaminergic pathway, 6-OHDA must be injected stereotaxically into the substantia nigra, the nigrostriatal tract or the striatum (Javoy et al., 1976; Jonsson, 1983). Following 6-OHDA injections into substantia nigra or the nigrostriatal tract, dopaminergic neurons start degenerating within 24 hours and die by non-apoptotic morphology (Jeon et al., 1995). Maximal reduction of striatal dopamine is reached within 3 to 4 days post-lesion (Faull & Laverty, 1969) and, in most studies, residual striatal dopamine content is less than 20% of controls. When injected into the striatum, 6-OHDA produces a more protracted retrograde degeneration of the nigrostriatal system which can last from 1 to 3 weeks post-lesion (Sauer & Oertel, 1994; Przedborski et al., 1995). Here, the death of nigral dopaminergic neurons occurs by retrograde degeneration and dying neurons exhibit a mixed morphology (Marti et al., 1997), which is quite distinct from that seen following the injection of the toxin directly into the nigra (Jeon et al., 1995). Regardless of the site of 6-OHDA injection along the nigrostriatal pathway, a number of pre- and postsynaptic changes occur, even with only moderate damage (Joyce et al., 1996). These include increased dopaminergic turnover within the remaining dopaminergic terminals (Zigmond et al., 1990) and upregulation of striatal dopamine D2 receptors (Ungerstedt, 1971b); the latter is only seen for a dopamine depletion greater than 90% and is maximal within 2–3 weeks postlesion (Marshall et al., 1989). Usually, 6-OHDA is injected into one hemisphere while the other hemisphere serves as an internal control. Unilateral injections lead to asymmetric circling motor behavior whose magnitude depends on the degree of nigrostriatal lesion (Ungerstedt & Arbuthnott, 1970; Hefti et al., 1980; Przedborski et al., 1995) and is best observed after administration of direct (rotation away from the lesion) or indirect (rotation toward the lesion) dopamine agonists, due to physiological imbalance between the lesioned and the unlesioned striatum. Over the years, this turning behavior, which can be quantified, has been widely used to assess the antiparkinsonian properties of new drugs, as illustrated in (Jiang et al., 1993), or the success of transplantation and gene therapies in repairing the lesioned pathways (Kirik et al., 2002; Bjorklund et al., 2002). The 6-OHDA model does not mimic all the clinical and pathological features characteristic of PD nor does it result in formation of the cytoplasmic inclusions (Lewy bodies) so typical of PD. Furthermore, the acute nature of the nigrostriatal neurodegeneration seen after the injection of 6-OHDA differs from the more progressive time course of PD.

Studies in rodents have demonstrated that developing monoaminergic neurons respond differently to 6-OHDA than their mature counterparts (Jonsson, 1983). In neonatal rats 6-OHDA has been mainly administered systemically, which can only be done during the first postnatal week, due to the development of the BBB around 7–10 days of life, and intracisternally to produce widespread lesion of the nervous system. Both routes of administration induce profound alterations of the norepinephrine systems, particularly in the nucleus ceruleus and cerebral cortex as well as of the dopaminergic systems (Jonsson, 1983; Breese et al., 1984). Upon reaching adulthood, in contrast to the noradrenergic denervation in the nucleus ceruleus and cerebral cortex, neonatally lesioned rats exhibit noradreneric and serotonergic hyperinnervation in other brain regions, such as the brainstem (Jonsson, 1983; Joyce et al., 1996). Of note, some serotonergic sprouting in the striatum also occurs after 6-OHDA in adult animals, too. They also show increased serotonin receptor density and functional dopamine D1 receptor supersensitivity (Joyce et al., 1996). The latter can be elicited by challenging neonatally lesioned rats with dopamine D1 receptor agonists, which results in behavioral abnormalities such as increased locomotion and self-mutilation (Breese et al., 1990). The association of the aforementioned biochemical and behavioral alterations has led experts to propose neonatal 6-OHDA-lesioned rats as an experimental model of Lesch–Nyhan syndrome, a rare genetic disorder characterized by chorea, spasticity, and compulsive auto-mutilation (Moy et al., 1997). Neonatal rats have also been lesioned with 6-OHDA by intra-striatal infusion to study the mode of cell death of injured developing nigrostriatal dopaminergic neurons (Marti et al., 1997). In this study the authors demonstrate that the lesion results in an induction of apoptotic cell death in phenotypically defined dopaminergic neurons; this appears on the third postlesion day and persists until the tenth and is most marked when the lesion is performed before postnatal day 14 (Marti et al., 1997).

Finally, 6-OHDA can be utilized to produce a chemical sympathectomy, which is preferentially achieved by intravenous injection of the toxin at a dose of 50 to 500 mg/kg either once or twice at 16-hour intervals (Jonsson, 1983). Of note, while 50 mg/kg, which is well tolerated, reduces norepinephrine content by 90% in most peripheral organs such as the iris and heart, higher doses (e.g. 250–500 mg/kg), which cause high lethality, are needed to damage cell bodies in the sympathetic ganglia (Jonsson, 1983). Although 6-OHDA-induced sympathectomy is permanent in neonatal animals, it is transient in adults and, with time, there is regeneration of noradrenergic fibers (Jonsson, 1983). Over the years, 6-OHDA-induced sympathectomy has proved to be a useful model for studying the role of sympathetic innervation in a large variety of symptoms such as pain, and in physiologic functions such as immune, cardiovascular, bone, and glucose metabolisms (Khalil & Helme, 1989; Kaul, 1999; Sherman & Chole, 2000; Cao et al., 2002).

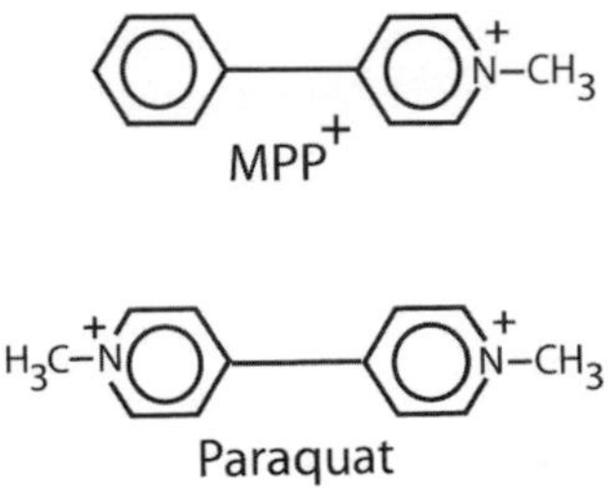

Paraquat

The potent herbicide paraquat (*N,N'*-dimethyl-4-4'-bipiridinium) is another prototypic toxin known to exert deleterious effects through oxidative stress. It is now well established that paraquat toxicity is mediated by redox cycling with cellular diaphorase such as nitric oxide synthase (Day et al., 1999), thereby elevating intracellular levels of the ROS superoxide. Since its introduction in agriculture, there have been several cases of lethal poisoning resulting from ingestion or even from dermal exposure (Smith, 1988). Until recently, most experimental studies of paraquat were related to its effects on lung, liver and kidney probably because the toxicity induced by this herbicide in these organs is responsible for death after acute exposure. However, the structural similarity of paraquat to the neurotoxin MPP$^+$ (Fig. 16.2) has sparked major interest in this herbicide as a potential environmental parkinsonian toxin. In support of this view are the published observations that significant damage to the brain is seen in individuals who died from paraquat intoxication (Grant et al., 1980; Hughes, 1988) despite the fact that paraquat poorly crosses the BBB (Shimizu et al., 2001). Furthermore, epidemiological studies have suggested an increased risk for PD due to paraquat exposure (Liou et al., 1997). Yet, paraquat accumulation in the brain appears not to follow any known enzymatic or neurotransmitter distribution (Widdowson et al., 1996a,b). While oral administration of paraquat to rats appears ineffective in lesioning the central nervous system (Widdowson et al., 1996b), its intraventricular or intracerebral injection produces unequivocal neurodegeneration which, however, does not seem restricted to any specific neuronal groups (De Gori et al., 1988; Liou et al., 1996). When injected systemically into mice, conflicting results are obtained. Some authors have reported reduced motor activity and dose-dependent losses of striatal dopaminergic nerve fibers and

Fig. 16.2 Structural similarity between paraquat and MPP$^+$. The only difference between these two compounds is the second *N*-methyl-pyridium group that paraquat has instead of the phenyl group as seen in MPP$^+$.

substantia nigra neuronal cell bodies in paraquat-treated mice (Brooks et al., 1999). Conversely, others have failed to see any behavioral abnormality or nigrostriatal dopaminergic pathway damage in similarly treated mice (Thiruchelvam et al., 2000a,b). This discrepancy may be explained by the fact that the propensity of paraquat to damage the nigrostriatal pathway in mice is not only dose-, but also age-dependent (McCormack et al., 2002; Thiruchelvam et al., 2003). The use of stereology to assess cell loss in some, but not all, studies may also be a reason for the previous inconsistent results. Aside from killing dopaminergic neurons, paraquat induces α-synuclein upregulation and aggregation (Manning-Bog et al., 2002). This suggests that the paraquat model could be quite valuable to recapitulate some of the key neuropathological features of PD such as SNpc neuronal loss and α-synuclein-positive inclusions.

It is worth mentioning that manganese ethylenebis-dithiocarbamate, or "Maneb," which is used in overlapping geographical areas with paraquat, has been shown to decrease locomotor activity and potentiate paraquat effects on the nigrostriatal pathway in mice (Thiruchelvam et al., 2000a,b). In these studies, combined paraquat and Maneb exposures produce greater loss of dopaminergic neurons than either of the chemicals alone (Thiruchelvam et al., 2000a,b). However, none of these studies has found meaningful reductions in striatal dopamine levels after paraquat injection, even when combined with Maneb. This paradoxical finding may be due to some kind of compensation mechanism that makes up for the modest loss of neurons caused by these toxins. In light of this, the biochemical basis for the reported behavioural abnormalities found in these animals cannot be attributed to a deficit in brain dopamine as in PD; thus, based on our current knowledge of this model, those motoric perturbations cannot be used to mimic PD symptoms.

In contrast to SNpc dopaminergic neurons, GABAergic elements in the substantia nigra and the striatum are not

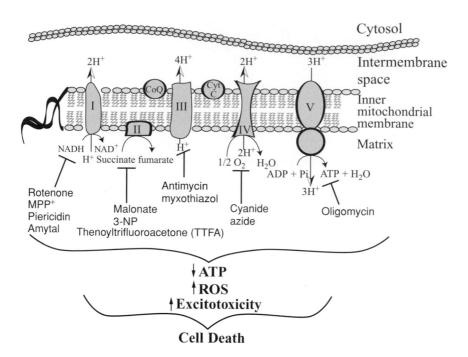

Fig. 16.3 Inhibitors of electron transport chain (ETC). Under normal physiological conditions, electrons donated from NADH to Complex I (NADH: ubiquinone oxidoreductase) or from succinate to Complex II (succinate: ubiquinone oxidoreductase) are passed to coenzyme Q (ubiquinone), ubisemiquinone, ubiquinol, Complex III (ubiquinol: cytochrome c oxidoreductase), cytochrome c, Complex IV (cytochrome c oxidase) and finally to O_2 to produce H_2O. The energy released from this ETC is used to pump the protons out of the inner mitochondrial membrane into intermembrane space creating a membrane potential gradient. This potential energy then drives the flow of protons back into the mitochondrial matrix via Complex V (ATP synthase) and thereby producing ATP. The specific sites of action of various inhibitors are illustrated here.

affected by paraquat as evidenced by Western blot and immunohistochemical studies of glutamic acid decarboxylase (GAD) (McCormack *et al.*, 2002; Thiruchelvam *et al.*, 2003). Beyond these two neuronal populations, none of the studies cited above has systematically assessed the status of other neuronal types such as cholinergic, serotonergic or adrenergic in the brain. At this point, therefore, it remains unclear whether the observed paraquat/Maneb cytotoxicity is really specific to the dopaminergic systems and could thus be regarded as a reliable experimental model of PD.

Mitochondrial neurotoxins

Mitochondrion is a small organelle, which assures by itself a large number of vital cellular metabolic pathways such as the tricarboxylic acid cycle, the fatty acid beta-oxidation, and the electron transport chain (ETC), to cite only a few. Despite the multiplicity of potential mitochondrial metabolic targets, so far, investigators interested in producing toxic experimental models of neurodegeneration essentially have used natural or synthetic compounds capable of inhibiting various enzymatic components of the

ETC to achieve their goals (Fig. 16.3). Presumably the main reason for this intense research effort is that defects in mitochondrial ETC function have been identified in several prominent neurodegenerative disorders in which they are believed to play a pathogenic role. Although a long list of ETC inhibitors has been tested, especially in rodents, only a handful, which include rotenone, malonate, and 3-nitropropionic acid (3-NP) have been used more than anecdotally and will be discussed here. Although these toxins will also be discussed by Timothy Greenamyre elsewhere in this book, here we will focus our review on the use of rotenone, malonate, and 3-NP in the production of experimental models of neurological diseases. Of note, MPTP and isoquinoline, which are known to affect the ETC, but whose cytotoxic mechanisms may involve additional cellular targets, will not be discussed in this section.

Rotenone

Rotenone is the most potent member of the rotenoids, a family of natural cytotoxic compounds extracted from *Leguminosa* plants, used as insect and fish poison and more recently also regarded as a potential parkinsonian environmental toxin. Rotenone is highly lipophylic and can thus readily gain access to all organs with an apparent fast pharamacokinetic. For instance, after a single intravenous injection, rotenone reaches maximal concentration in the brain within 15 min and decays to about half of this level in approximately 100 min (Talpade *et al.*, 2000). Although it accumulates throughout the CNS, the distribution of rotenone in the brain is heterogeneous (Talpade *et al.*, 2000), apparently not because of regional variations in cerebral blood flow (Kilbourn *et al.*, 1997), but rather regional differences in oxidative metabolism (Talpade *et al.*, 2000). By virtue of its lipophilicity, rotenone freely enters all cells and, once inside, it probably diffuses into all organelles including mitochondria, where it blocks complex I of the ETC. The effect of rotenone on mitochondrial respiration is time and dose dependent and results from its insertion in a large binding pocket in the hydrophobic part of complex I (Okun *et al.*, 1999), probably made of the ND1 subunit. While rotenone has been used extensively as a prototypic mitochondrial poison in vitro, only a limited number of studies used rotenone to specifically kill dopaminergic neurons or to model PD. Treatment of embryonic ventral midbrain cultures with rotenone has been shown to cause major neurotoxicity (Marey-Semper *et al.*, 1995), especially in the presence of glial cells (Gao *et al.*, 2002). In both studies dopamine uptake was significantly more affected than GABA uptake, thus supporting the hypothesis of selective vulnerability of dopaminergic cells. In vivo, rotenone has been administered to animals by different routes. Oral administration of rotenone appears to cause little neurotoxicity (Betarbet *et al.*, 2000). By contrast, stereotaxic injection of rotenone into the median forebrain bundle causes substantial depletion of striatal dopamine and serotonin (Heikkila *et al.*, 1985), findings consistent with the notion that rotenone lesions the median forebrain bundle, which carries dopaminergic and serotoninergic fibers into the striatum. In rats treated for 7–9 days with high doses of rotenone (10–18 mg/kg/d) as a continuous intravenous infusion, there were major lesions in both the striatum and the globus pallidus, characterized by neuronal loss and gliosis (Ferrante *et al.*, 1997). The nigrostriatal pathway, however, appeared intact (Ferrante *et al.*, 1997). This latter finding is consistent with the demonstration that the systemic acute administration of high doses of rotenone (15 mg/kg), while causing high lethality, failed to affect striatal dopamine contents (Thiffault *et al.*, 2000). The possibility that nigrostriatal injury may be induced by rotenone under less severe experimental conditions and different paradigms of administration has also been evaluated. In one such study (Thiffault *et al.*, 2000), the effect of multiple subcutaneous injections of rotenone (1.5 mg/kg three times per week for 3 weeks) failed to

cause any significant neurochemical signs of dopaminergic damage in rats. However, when rotenone was intravenously infused (2–3 mg/kg/day) for 1–3 weeks, treated rats developed no apparent striatal lesion, but exhibited the specific nigrostriatal pathway neurodegeneration associated with nigral intraneuronal proteinaceous inclusions (Betarbet *et al.*, 2000) reminiscent of Lewy bodies, a neuropathological hallmark of PD. However, in this study only 50% of the treated rats exhibited clear nigrostriatal damage and only Lewis rats showed a consistent lesion (Betarbet *et al.*, 2000), indicative of a significant inter-individual and inter-strain variability in the observed effect of rotenone. Although this toxic model of PD appears quite promising, it is also quite challenging. A review of the current problems and limitations that surround this model can be found in Perier *et al.* (2003). Moreover, subsequent studies have challenged the notion that rotenone infusion would cause a selective lesion of the nigrostriatal pathway (Lapointe *et al.*, 2004; Hoglinger *et al.*, 2003).

Malonate and 3-nitropropionic acid

Malonate and 3-NP share similar mechanisms of action and both have been used to model the same type of neurological disorder; therefore, these two toxins will be discussed together. Although malonate and 3-NP can be readily synthesized, both are natural molecules in that the former is a product of animal fatty acid metabolism and the latter is a secondary metabolite of the fungus *Arthrinium*, considered to cause a form of acute food poisoning called "moldy sugarcane poisoning." It is now well established that malonate and 3-NP inhibit, in a competitive reversible and irreversible manner respectively, the binding of succinate to the enzyme succinate dehydrogenase (SDH) (Alston *et al.*, 1977; Cooper & Clark, 1994). Because SDH is a main enzymatic component of both the tricarboxylic acid cycle and the ETC complex II, its blockade impairs tricarboxylic acid metabolism and mitochondrial respiration. Not surprisingly, therefore, the administration of malonate and 3-NP is associated with impaired ATP synthesis (Beal *et al.*, 1993b; Zeevalk *et al.*, 1995; Kaal *et al.*, 2000) and increased local lactate production (Beal *et al.*, 1993a), metabolic alterations which, upon equimolar intrastrial injections, are less pronounced and short lasting with the reversible inhibitor malonate than with the irreversible inhibitor 3-NP. It is believed that the interference of electron flow in ETC by 3-NP and malonate leads to membrane depolarization which, in turn, activates the voltage-dependent NMDA receptors (Greene & Greenamyre, 1996). According to this scenario, once NMDA receptors are activated, a massive influx of calcium occurs, thus triggering numerous cell death pathways and stimulating ROS production which ultimately cause cell demise (Albin & Greenamyre, 1992; Dugan & Choi, 1994). Consistent with a role for NMDA receptors in this deleterious cascade are the autoradiographic and electrophysiologic demonstrations that malonate- and 3-NP-induced SDH inhibition does activate NMDA receptors (Wullner *et al.*, 1994; Calabresi *et al.*, 2001) and that NMDA antagonists such as MK-801 can attenuate malonate- and 3-NP-induced neurotoxicity (Greene & Greenamyre, 1996; Massieu *et al.*, 2001). In addition, after exposure to these toxins, NMDA-dependent increased intracellular calcium (Calabresi *et al.*, 2001; Lee *et al.*, 2002), activation of proteases such as caspases (Schulz *et al.*, 1998; Lee *et al.*, 2002), and rise in ROS (Schulz *et al.*, 1996; Ferger *et al.*, 1999) were all documented. While most steps of the outlined sequence of events have been studied in great detail, there is a surprising lack of information about the process by which 3-NP and malonate actually enter the central nervous system and subsequently the neurons and mitochondria. Because these two toxins share structural similarity with succinate it may be surmised that malonate and 3-NP entry into the mitochondria may be facilitated by one of the succinate carriers (Kakhniashvili *et al.*, 1997). It should be mentioned that several variants of the mitochondrial succinate carriers are expressed at the level of the BBB and the plasma membrane of neurons (Pajor *et al.*, 2001). It is thus possible that these transporter variants participate in the translocation of 3-NP and malonate into the brain and neurons. If correct, it would appear that 3-NP benefits more from this mechanism than malonate since only 3-NP, and not malonate, can cause neurodegenerative changes after systemic administration. It would also suggest that the reported protective effects of large doses of succinate against malonate may be due, not to a rescue of SDH function as speculated by the authors (Greene *et al.*, 1993), but simply to the excess of succinate impeding malonate cellular and mitochondrial entry.

From the very beginning, the rat has emerged as the preferred species to study malonate and 3-NP neurotoxicity, although occasionally mice and monkeys have also been used (Brouillet *et al.*, 1999). Thus, most available data regarding the use of these toxins emanates primarily from investigations in rats and, as far as 3-NP is concerned, this toxin has been effectively administered systemically or intracerebrally to rats using very different regimens to cause very different behavioral and neuropathological alterations and death rates (Brouillet *et al.*, 1999). Higher doses of 3-NP have also been used in mice (Klivenyi *et al.*, 2000; Fernagut *et al.*, 2002) to induce striatal lesions; however, under these harsh regimens, death rate is as high as 50% in these animals. Surprisingly, while 3-NP is known to cause neurotoxicity following its ingestion, we did not come across any studies in which this toxin was administered orally. Among the different regimens used, it appears that conspicuous brain neuropathology with low lethality can be obtained in rats by intraperitoneal injections or subcutaneous infusion of 10 to 20 mg/kg/day of 3-NP for 5 to 30 days (Brouillet *et al.*, 1999). As depicted in (Brouillet *et al.*, 1999), after a prolonged low dose regimen, lesions are small and restricted consistently to the dorsolateral part of the anterior striatum, whereas after a brief high dose regimen, lesions are larger, invading the entire lateral striatum and involving, in several cases, the most caudal part of the striatum. In addition, while chronic 3-NP-treatment is not associated with extrastriatal lesions, acute and subacute 3-NP treatment is frequently associated with significant pallidal and hippocampal damage. These data indicate that the consistency and extent of the damage to the brain produced by 3-NP depends on the dose and rate of administration. In keeping with this, it should be emphasized that the chronic delivery of a low dose of 3-NP (e.g. 12 mg/kg/day) induces motor abnormalities and selective neuropathology in less than half of the treated animals (Beal *et al.*, 1993b). Other factors known to influence 3-NP neurotoxicity are the age and the genetic background of the rats (Brouillet *et al.*, 1993; Ouary *et al.*, 2000). As for malonate, because of its inability to cross the BBB, 2 to 4 μmol of the toxin is usually injected stereotaxically into the striatum. As with 3-NP, malonate neurotoxicity is age dependent as, after intrastriatal injections, 4- and 12-month-old rats show greater extent of striatal lesions than do 1-month-old animals (Beal *et al.*, 1993a). However, there is no difference in the extent of neuronal loss between 6- and 27-month-old rats (Meldrum *et al.*, 2000).

Microscopically, 3-NP injected systemically or intrastriatally produces tissue damage similar to that produced by stereotaxic injection of malonate in the striatum, consisting of a necrotic core at the centre of the lesion surrounded by an intermediate zone between the core and the normal striatal tissue in which there is gliosis and a loss of only certain subtypes of neurons. However, in the case of 3-NP, only with chronic low dosage are the size of the intermediate zone substantial and the pattern of neuronal loss similar to that produced by malonate. For instance, harsh 3-NP treatment appears to affect all striatal subpopulations of neurons (Beal *et al.*, 1993b), whereas more gentle 3-NP treatment, like intrastriatal injection of 2 μmol of malonate, affects medium-sized GABAergic spiny neurons and spares the medium-sized aspiny NADPH-diaphorase in rodents and monkeys (Beal *et al.*, 1993a,b; Brouillet *et al.*, 1995). In addition, malonate, but apparently not 3-NP, also affects striatal dopaminergic structures and causes some degree of nigral dopaminergic loss through a retrograde degeneration process (Sonsalla *et al.*, 1997; Zeevalk *et al.*, 1997); why there should be no retrograde degeneration after 3-NP treatment is an enigma. Although not identical (Borlongan *et al.*, 1995; Sun *et al.*, 2002), this pattern of neuronal loss is reminiscent of that seen in Huntington's disease, thus supporting the usefulness of both 3-NP and malonate in modeling HD. However, while malonate and 3-NP recapitulate rather faithfully HD's chemical neuropathology, neither in rats nor in monkeys do they reproduce well HD's motor abnormalities. From the 3-NP perspective, both in rats and monkeys a harsh treatment produces mostly hypokinesia and limb weakness, and occasionally dystonia, uncoordination, and even somnolence (Brouillet *et al.*, 1995; Borlongan *et al.*, 1997; Sun *et al.*, 2002). In rats, the more chronic regimen was associated with hyperkinesia initially, followed by hypokinesia (Borlongan *et al.*, 1997) or subtle motor abnormalities only observable using sophisticated motor testing (Guyot *et al.*, 1997). In monkeys, the situation appears even more deceiving in that no spontaneous motor abnormalities were detected in three animals treated for 3–6 weeks with 8 mg/kg/day of 3-NP, and only foot dyskinesia and dystonia were seen in two others treated for an even longer period with a slightly higher dose (Brouillet *et al.*, 1995). Although the significance of this is unclear, these authors also show that a variety of abnormal movements, including chorea, could be induced in otherwise asymptomatic 3-NP-treated monkeys by the administration of a dopamine agonist such as apomorphine. Regardless of the type of abnormal movements observed in these animals, it was found that the degree of neurological impairment correlates with the severity of striatal lesions, consistent with the view that most of the observed motor symptoms directly result from striatal cell loss (Guyot *et al.*, 1997).

The reason that 3-NP and possibly malonate cause preferential damage to the striatum despite widespread brain SDH inhibition (Brouillet *et al.*, 1998) is unknown. To date, two hypotheses, which are not mutually exclusive, prevail. First, as discussed above, several in vitro and in vivo studies have demonstrated the importance of excitotoxicity in 3-NP's and malonate's deleterious effects (Brouillet *et al.*, 1999). Therefore, since the striatum receives prominent glutamatergic input from the cerebral cortex and the thalamus, it may be hypothesized that the rich striatal glutamatergic innervation is a key factor in 3-NP striatal selectivity. In favor of this view is the finding that the ablation of the cortical glutamatergic afferences to the striatum mitigates 3-NP striatal neurotoxicity (Beal *et al.*, 1993b). However, the fact that there is no evidence of increased striatal extracellular glutamate concentrations after systemic administration of 3-NP and that several brain areas not affected by 3-NP possess even greater glutamatergic

innervation than the striatum represent strong arguments against this idea. Second, mounting evidence indicates that dopamine is instrumental in 3-NP and malonate's deleterious actions (Reynolds *et al.*, 1998; Maragos *et al.*, 1998; Moy *et al.*, 2000; Calabresi *et al.*, 2001; Xia *et al.*, 2001), which fits well with the fact that the striatum contains a conspicuous dopaminergic innervation and that virtually all striatal neurons are dopaminoceptive. It has been found consistently that striatal dopamine depletion, produced either by 6-OHDA lesion or by pharmacological inhibition of dopamine synthesis, attenuates the effects of malonate and 3-NP (Reynolds *et al.*, 1998; Maragos *et al.*, 1998; Moy *et al.*, 2000; Calabresi *et al.*, 2001; Xia *et al.*, 2001). So far, however, the molecular basis of the role of dopamine in the malonate and 3-NP models may be mediated by oxidative stress (mainly due to autooxidation of dopamine), dopamine receptor activation, or both. Relevant to both mechanisms are the demonstrations that antioxidant strategies protect from malonate- and 3-NP-induced toxicity (Schulz *et al.*, 1995a; Schulz *et al.*, 1996) and that dopamine D2 receptor agonists can restore the effect of malonate or of 3-NP in 6-OHDA-lesioned animals, whereas D2 receptor antagonists attenuate the effects of both neurotoxins (Calabresi *et al.*, 2001; Xia *et al.*, 2001). In conclusion, from all of the above evidence it appears quite obvious that, except for moldy sugarcane poisoning, both 3-NP and malonate do not represent perfect models of HD or any other neurodegenerative disorder of the basal ganglia. This fact should not undermine, however, the critical importance of these two neurotoxins as tools to further dissect the functional chemical neuroanatomy of the basal ganglia and the role of excitotoxicity and dopamine in the striatal neurodegenerative process.

Other ETC mitochondrial toxins

For each mitochondrial enzymatic complex of the ETC, numerous reasonably specific inhibitors are available (Cooper & Clark, 1994). Some of these, namely MPP^+, rotenone, malonate, and 3-NP, have already been discussed. Others such as piericidin (complex I), antimycin A (complex III), and cyanide and azide (complex IV), while extensively used in vitro, have rarely been used in vivo to model neurological disorders. Because the rare surviving victims from cyanide suicide or homicidal attempts may develop parkinsonism and dementia or delayed onset dystonia combined with a severe parkinsonism (Sanchez-Ramos, 1993), animals have been treated with cyanide to elucidate the chemical neuroanatomy underlying the emergence of the movement disorders. In keeping with this, it has been reported that a third of the mice injected subcutaneously with potassium cyanide (6 mg/kg) twice daily for 7 days exhibited reduced locomotor activity, which could be reversed by L-DOPA, as well as catalepsy, which could not be reversed by L-DOPA (Kanthasamy *et al.*, 1994). Although behavioral abnormalities were only seen in a fraction of the treated mice, all had significant dopaminergic loss at the level of the basal ganglia (Kanthasamy *et al.*, 1994); since the authors only studied the dopaminergic system in these mice, it is unknown whether or not cyanide affects these neurons preferentially. While there is no in vivo evidence that any specific neurotransmitter pathway would be more sensitive to cyanide than any other, note that, following infusion of cyanide to cats, severe lesions were only seen in the corpus callosum, pallidus and substantia nigra (Funata *et al.*, 1984). More surprisingly and in contrast to neuropathological reports from human autopsy, the treated cats did not show significant lesions in the cerebral cortex and the hippocampus (Funata *et al.*, 1984). Except for the lack of the cortical and hippocampal damage, the topography of neuropathological changes resembles that reported in carbon monoxide intoxication, thus suggesting that cyanide may be a useful model of chemical brain hypoxia. Alternatively, given the prominent pallidal lesion, the administration of cyanide to animals may produce a unique means to explore the pathophysiology of akinetic-rigid syndromes.

Neurotoxic amphetamines

Amphetamines are potent, highly addictive and widely abused psychostimulants. Among the amphetamine derivatives, four have been shown to have neurotoxic effects on the nervous system, namely *p*-chloroamphetamine (PCA), methamphetamine (METH), 3,4-methylenedioxymethamphetamine (MDMA) and fenfluramine. These four compounds have been extensively used in various mammals to study the basis and the lasting consequences of amphetamine addiction on the brain. The neurotoxic profile of these four analogues, however, is not identical in that PCA and fenfluramine, when used in moderate doses, tend to affect serotoninergic neurons specifically, while methamphetamine and MDMA are toxic to both dopaminergic and serotoninergic neurons.

While neurotoxic amphetamines can be administered effectively to animals through a variety of routes, systemic injection is by far the most popular. From these animal studies we learned that, almost immediately after amphetamine administration, there is a massive release of monoamines from their storage sites in the nerve terminals from both the central and peripheral nervous system (Segal & Kuczenski, 1994); compared with the other amphetamines' analogues, methamphetamine causes more pronounced central effects and fewer peripheral ones. In the brain, the release of dopamine begins soon after the injection of amphetamines and peaks within 1 hour (Clausing & Bowyer, 1999; Kita *et al.*, 2000). This time course coincides with the brain levels of amphetamine following its systemic injection (Clausing & Bowyer, 1999). As in humans, during this early phase, animals such as rats and monkeys injected with low doses of amphetamines exhibit a range of acute behavioral changes such as increased locomotor activity (Segal & Kuczenski, 1994). However, as the doses increase, the motor activity becomes more stereotyped (e.g. sniffing) (Segal & Kuczenski, 1994), and increased salivation and self-injurious behaviors occur (Kita *et al.*, 2000). In addition, animals develop a dose-dependent hyperthermia (potentially exceeding 41°C) whose magnitude correlates with the levels of brain amphetamine and released dopamine and whose time course is delayed by about 30 minutes compared to that of brain amphetamine and released dopamine (Clausing & Bowyer, 1999). Although our knowledge of the pathophysiology underlying amphetamine-induced hyperthermia remains incomplete, it is well known that it correlates with lethality and neurotoxicity (Ali *et al.*, 1994; Albers & Sonsalla, 1995; Malberg & Seiden, 1998).

Following the acute phase, it is now well accepted that neurotoxic amphetamine analogues not only cause functional deficits, such as profound monoamine depletion, but also structural alterations. Amphetamine-induced neurotoxicity depends on the regimen used since only high dosage and repeated injections will produce significant and consistent neurodegeneration (Davidson *et al.*, 2001). As reviewed in Axt *et al.* (1994), neurotoxic regimens of amphetamine and analogs cause selective loss of dopaminergic and serotonergic nerve terminals with relatively little effects on the corresponding cell bodies. Furthermore, data obtained from rats and non-human primates show that the destruction of the serotonergic and dopaminergic nerve terminal is not even throughout the various regions of the brains. Amphetamines consistently destroy the fine serotonergic terminals that originate from the dorsal raphe nucleus but spare the beaded ones that originate from the median raphe nucleus (Axt *et al.*, 1994). Similarly, amphetamines selectively destroy dopaminergic nerve terminals in the striatum, nucleus accumbens and frontal cortex but spare dopaminergic cell bodies in the ventral tegmental area and substantia nigra (Axt *et al.*, 1994). Although this represents the prevalent view, some studies have reported significant neuronal loss especially in the substantia nigra of rodents following very high levels of methamphetamine administration (Trulson *et al.*, 1985; Sonsalla *et al.*, 1996). Among the affected dopaminergic brain areas, the dorsal aspect of the striatum appears to be the most susceptible to the neurotoxic amphetamines, whereas the ventral aspect of the striatum and the shell of the nucleus accumbens are much less sensitive, and the olfactory tubercle and the septum are rather resistant (Axt *et al.*, 1994). Moreover, within the striatum it would appear that dopaminergic projections to the matrix are affected, while those to the patches are resistant (Axt *et al.*, 1994). Surprisingly, despite these dramatic biochemical and structural changes, there is still no consensus regarding the nature of their spontaneous behavioral correlates, neither in monkeys nor in rodents (Ricaurte *et al.*, 1994). However, several studies have reported strikingly abnormal responses to pharmacological challenges in amphetamine-treated animals (Ricaurte *et al.*, 1994), thus suggesting that such an approach may represent an effective and reliable means to reveal lasting behavioral alterations in these lesioned animals.

Several studies have shown that, after the administration of neurotoxic amphetamines to monkeys and rodents, monoaminergic innervation, especially in the forebrain, exhibits signs of recovery (Axt *et al.*, 1994). It appears that the milder the lesion the more extensive the re-innervation, but with the current regimens, recovery is moderate at best. Because this process is slow by nature, it is important to remember that it may take anywhere from several months to several years before re-innervation is completed and conclusions about the extent of the recovery can be drawn. For example, in non-human primates injected with MDMA (5mg/kg twice daily for 4 days, SC), the recovery of serotonin axon density in frontal cortex is only about 60% after 7 years (Hatzidimitriou *et al.*, 1999). Rostral neocortex and ventral forebrain are reinnervated sooner and more completely than the caudal neocortex and dorsal forebrain, which is a pattern of axonal re-growth reminiscent of that of axonal growth during development.

Major disagreements still persist about the mechanisms by which neurotoxic amphetamines destroy nerve terminals. All neurotoxic amphetamines cited above are quite lipophilic and can thus readily gain access to all organs including the brain. While amphetamine analogs may, to a certain extent, enter cells such as neurons by diffusion, their accumulation within dopaminergic neurons, for example, is facilitated by DAT (Zaczek *et al.*, 1991a,b). It is thus not surprising that mutant mice deficient in DAT are more resistant to methamphetamine (Fumagalli *et al.*, 1998). Once inside monoaminergic neurons, amphetamines inhibit MAO (Scorza *et al.*, 1997), promote flux reversal by plasma membrane monoamine trans-

porters (Sulzer *et al.*, 1993), and induce monoamine efflux from vesicles (Sulzer *et al.*, 1995). The latter redistribution of monoamines from vesicles to cytosol is believed to be a pivotal event in amphetamine analog neurotoxicity as it gives rise to massive intracellular production of ROS (Cubells *et al.*, 1994; Fumagalli *et al.*, 1999). Although the evidence summarized above suggests that endogenous monoamines and monoamine-derived ROS play a critical role in amphetamine analog neurotoxicity, recent in vivo data indicate that at least some of the results implicating monoamines such as dopamine in the neurotoxic process may have been confounded by secondary drug effects on core temperature. The neuroprotective effects of several pharmacologic agents on MDMA and methamphetamine neurotoxicity appear to be related to their thermoregulatory actions, rather than to their primary pharmacologic actions (Miller & O'Callaghan, 1994; Albers & Sonsalla, 1995; Callahan & Ricaurte, 1998). One of the most damaging findings against the actual role of dopamine in the neurotoxic process is the demonstration that hypothermia rather than catecholamine depletion contributes to the neuroprotective effects of reserpine and α-methyl-p-tyrosine in MDMA and methamphetamine-treated animals, since prevention of drug-induced hypothermia abolishes the neuroprotection of reserpine and α-methyl-p-tyrosine, alone or in combination (Yuan *et al.*, 2001, 2002). In contrast to the above findings in animals, however, in vitro data obtained from cell cultures question whether change in body temperature is related to methamphetamine toxicity. Using postnatally derived ventral midbrain mouse cultures, it is shown that the specific loss of neurites in dopaminergic neurons induced by methamphetamine is a consequence of its upregulation of TH activity, leading to elevated levels of cytosolic dopamine and consequently increased production of toxic cytosolic ROS (Larsen *et al.*, 2002). This study also demonstrates that, in the absence of vesicular sequestration of dopamine as seen in cultures derived from VMAT-deficient mice, the toxicity of methamphetamine is exacerbated, further supporting the deleterious role of dopamine. Since all cultures are maintained at constant temperature, the authors argue that, in their system, temperature is not involved in the toxicity of methamphetamine. From all these studies, the issue of core temperature and toxicity of amphetamine and its analogs warrants further investigation. At the moment, at least in the animal models, hyperthermia is likely involved but itself *per se* may not be solely responsible for toxicity (Albers & Sonsalla, 1995). Caution should be exercised especially when these compounds are to be used in animals. The above discussion shows that administration of neurotoxic amphetamines to animals provides a powerful model to explore the molecular basis of acute and chronic amphetamine exposure on the brain. Aside from this, it also provides a unique model to elucidate the mechanisms governing regeneration in the adult brain, which is a topic of major importance in the field of neurorepair.

Isoquinolines derivatives

As reviewed in McNaught *et al.* (1998), isoquinoline derivatives refer to isoquinoline itself, substituted congeners such as 6-methoxyisoquinoline, and the various reduced species 1,2- or 3,4-dihydroisoquinolines, and 1,2,3,4-tetrahydroisoquinolines (TIQ), all of which may occur in their neutral or charged form, i.e. the isoquinolinium ion. These compounds are heterocycles in which a benzene ring and a pyridine ring are fused through carbon, and are formed from Pictet-Spengler non-enzymatic condensation of catecholamines (e.g. dopamine and L-DOPA) with aldehydes (Deitrich & Erwin, 1980). Among the isoquinoline derivatives, TIQ, 1-benzyl-TIQ and (R)-1,2-dimethyl-5,6-dihydroxy-TIQ ((R)-*N*-methyl-salsolinol) have the most potent toxicity (Nagatsu, 1997); of note, contrary to the other derivatives mentioned above, (R)salsolinol is formed enzymatically from dopamine and acetaldehyde by (R)salsolinol synthase (Naoi *et al.*, 1996). Many isoquinoline derivatives are found naturally in the environment and in foodstuffs as well as in human body fluids and brain tissues (McNaught *et al.*, 1998).

All available data support the notion that the mode and mechanism of action of isoquinolines is very close to that of MPTP and will thus not be discussed here. However, readers may find a comprehensive review on these topics in (Nagatsu, 1997; McNaught *et al.*, 1998). Isoquinolines have been used as neurotoxins both in vitro and in vivo, but, so far, they have produced much more consistent cytotoxicity in cell cultures than in animals (McNaught *et al.*, 1998). For instance, the administration of both TIQ and 1-benzyl-TIQ to monkeys produced behavioral and neuroanatomical abnormalities consistent with a lesion of the nigrostriatal dopaminergic pathway (Nagatsu & Yoshida, 1988; Yoshida *et al.*, 1990; Kotake *et al.*, 1996). In contrast, administration of *N*-methyl-TIQ, *N*-methylisoquinolinium, or *N*-methylnorsalsolinol to monkeys failed to produce any pathological change in the substantia nigra (Yoshida *et al.*, 1993). A similar confusing situation exists in rodents where both lesion (Yoshida *et al.*, 1993; Antkiewicz-Michaluk *et al.*, 2000; Lorenc-Koci *et al.*, 2000; Abe *et al.*, 2001) and no lesion of the nigrostriatal pathway has been reported following the systemic administration of various TIQ analogues (Perry *et al.*, 1988). More disturbing is the lack of dopaminergic

neurotoxicity found following the stereotaxic injection of *N*-methyl-norsalsolinol into the medial forebrain bundle of rats (Yoshida *et al.*, 1993; Moser *et al.*, 1996). These discrepancies may relate to technical differences among the cited studies or to distinct physicochemical properties among the various analogues used, such as lipophilicity, making the particular isoquinoline derivatives differ in the degree to which they enter the brain. Regardless of the reason for this inconsistency, at this point the available data raise serious doubts about the ability of this group of toxins to produce a reliable experimental model of PD.

Glutamate and analogues

As discussed by Ikonomidou and Turski in this book, the amino acid glutamate is the main excitatory neurotransmitter in the brain implicated in a large array of physiological actions mediated through the activation of the glutamate receptors. These authors also remind us that, aside from its role in numerous normal functions of the brain, glutamate and its analogues have emerged as potent neurotoxins. The concept of glutamate and analogues as neurotoxins is quite interesting and emanates primarily from the demonstration that excitatory properties of various glutamate analogues correlate with their ability to cause neurotoxic damage (Olney *et al.*, 1971). Yet, while the list of identified neurotoxic excitatory amino acids, or "excitotoxins," is long, up to now only glutamate and a few of its analogues have been extensively utilized to lesion the nervous system, especially in vivo. By far the most popular excitotoxins include kainic acid (KA) and ibotenic acid (IA), which are isolated from the marine algae *Diginea simplex* off the coast of Japan and the mushroom *Amanita muscara*, respectively, and quinolinic acid (QA) which is formed endogenously from tryptophan through kynurenine pathways. Like other amino acids, neither glutamate nor KA, IA or QA efficiently cross the BBB, thus requiring their stereotaxic injection in the brain or CSF to produce significant excitotoxic lesions of the central nervous system. So far, excitotoxins have been regarded as unique chemical tools for killing intrinsic neurons while sparing passing axons, nerve terminals and glial cells in discrete regions of the brain. Although this mode of lesioning may appear straightforward at first, accurate injury often requires laborious pilot studies to determine the appropriate coordinates, toxin concentrations, and injection volumes to produce a specific axon-sparing neuronal lesion with minimal necrosis confined within the boundary of the nucleus of interest. However, once those conditions are set, the lesion is quite reproducible, whether it is performed in rodents or in monkeys, in adult or immature animals, or to target large or small brain areas. Although all of the different excitotoxins mentioned above are effective in producing axon-sparing lesions, it may be important for certain investigators to remember that the actual morphology of the degenerating neurons (e.g. apoptosis or necrosis) is quite different depending on the excitotoxin used and the age of the animals (Portera-Cailliau *et al.*, 1997a,b). Beyond these technical considerations, it must be emphasized that, over the past decades excitotoxins, through their ability to produce axon-sparing lesions, have contributed tremendously in our understanding of the role of specific neuronal systems in both normal and pathological situations. This fact is particularly well illustrated in the context of the MPTP monkey, where the use of IA stereotaxic injection has led to the demonstration of the pivotal role of the subthalamic nucleus in the pathophysiology of parkinsonism (Bergman *et al.*, 1990).

In addition, excitotoxins are thought to be implicated in the pathogenesis of a variety of acute and chronic neurological diseases and have thus been tested with more or less success in various animal species in attempts to model these pathological conditions. For instance, it has been well established that the systemic, intracerebroventricular, or intraparenchymal injection of KA produces an excellent experimental model of epilepsy (Ben Ari & Cossart, 2000). KA, IA and QA have also been proposed as suitable neurotoxins to generate an animal model of HD given the fact that their intrastriatal injections replicate many of the biochemical, neuropathological and even behavioral hallmarks of this neurodegenerative disorder. Using choline acetyltransferase (CAT), GAD and TH as markers, intrastriatal injections of glutamate, KA and IA produce significant reduction in cholinergic and GABAergic markers with normal or even increased dopaminergic markers on the site of injection (McGeer & McGeer, 1976; Coyle & Schwarcz, 1976; Schwarcz *et al.*, 1978, 1979). These alterations occur as early as 6 h after injection, with maximal effect observed at 48 h and lasting up to 21 days after KA injection (Schwarcz & Coyle, 1977). Consistent with the known chemical neuroanatomy of the striatal projections, the excitotoxic lesion of the striatum is accompanied with a reduction of GAD activity (McGeer & McGeer, 1976) and substance P content (Hong *et al.*, 1977) in the ipsilateral substantia nigra. KA has also been demonstrated to induce other biochemical changes that parallel those found in HD such as reduced levels of the angiotensin converting enzyme as well as receptors for serotonin, dopamine, acetylcholine, and GABA (McGeer & McGeer, 1982). Despite these striking similarities to HD, the enthusiasm for the intrastriatal KA model was dampened after it became clear

that KA fails to spare striatal somatostatin-containing neurons (Araki *et al.*, 1985) as seen in HD, and, even more troublesome, that KA causes remote neurodegeneration in, for example, the hippocampus, following its intrastriatal injection (Zaczek *et al.*, 1980). Unfortunately, intrastriatal injection of IA has not been proven to be more selective than KA in killing neurons and has thus been usually regarded as not particularly suitable to model HD either (Kohler & Schwarcz, 1983; Beal *et al.*, 1986). In contrast to KA and IB, QA has been proposed as a more suitable agent to model HD, since intrastriatal injections of QA (240 nmol), unlike the other two, result in marked depletions of both GABA and substance P, with selective sparing of somatostatin and neuropeptide Y neurons (Beal *et al.*, 1986, 1991). Likewise, quantitative assessment of QA-induced striatal lesion in rats using radioligand binding assays has also shown the selectivity of the damage (Levivier *et al.*, 1994). However, other laboratories have failed to observe similar selective effects from QA (Davies & Roberts, 1987; Boegman *et al.*, 1987). Although technical differences may underlie the discrepancy, to date, the actual reason remains obscure.

From a behavioral point of view, rats receiving bilateral striatal injection of KA (1 μg) exhibit locomotor changes such as increased swing time and decreased stance time (Hruska & Silbergeld, 1979). These animals spend more time swinging their feet in the air than on the ground, movements that are somewhat reminiscent of chorea (Hruska & Silbergeld, 1979). Rats with this kind of lesion also show enhanced locomotor response to amphetamine but not to apomorphine (Mason *et al.*, 1978), a type of dissociate response that has been reported in HD patients. In addition to motor abnormalities, KA-lesioned rats also show impairments in learning (Dunnett & Iversen, 1981). Although, as with other animal models, the behavioral changes induced by KA are difficult to extrapolate to the abnormalities seen in humans, KA appears to mimic at least some behavioral features of HD. The abnormal behavioral profiles of IA and QA have not been as well characterized as those of KA. In one study different doses of QA ranging from 75 to 300 nmol were injected in to rats and behavioral testings were performed 2 and 4 weeks afterward (Sanberg *et al.*, 1989). The animals receiving 150 and 225 nmol were hyperactive and lost weight, whereas those that received 75 nmol behaved similar to controls and those that received 300 nmol died. Abnormal movements closer to HD have been induced in monkeys with excitotoxic lesion of the striatum (Kanazawa *et al.*, 1986, 1990; Hantraye *et al.*, 1990; Burns *et al.*, 1995). However, as seen with 3-NP, typical chorea in these animals was only elicited after administration of dopaminergic agonists (Kanazawa *et al.*, 1986, 1990; Hantraye *et al.*,

1990; Burns *et al.*, 1995) and, more importantly, only in animals with lesions encompassing the posterior putamen (Kanazawa *et al.*, 1986; Burns *et al.*, 1995).

When using KA, IA and QA as a model for HD, there are several variables to consider (McGeer & McGeer, 1978; Coyle & Schwarcz, 1983). Dose-response studies (0.5–5 μg) of KA show a steep curve and toxicity is not linear with increasing doses (Coyle & Schwarcz, 1976; Coyle *et al.*, 1978). For example, an injection of 0.5 μg reduces by 20% the activity of GAD but 2 μg causes a near maximal GAD loss (80%) (Coyle & Schwarcz, 1976). Similarly, a histological study from Nissl-stained sections shows that at a dose of 0.5 μg, KA produces a discrete spherical lesion with a radius of 0.3 mm, but at 1 μg, the lesion increases to 1.4 mm (Coyle *et al.*, 1978). Also, due to differing sensitivity to excitotoxins among cell types, the dose of glutamate or analogues selected is dependent on the type of targeted cells and the desired magnitude of lesion. However, as a rule of thumb, to avoid non-specific damage due to pressure, excitotoxins should be delivered in the smallest possible volume slowly over a prolonged period of time. Furthermore, variation in response to excitotoxins has been linked to differences in strains (Sanberg *et al.*, 1979) and age of animals (Gaddy *et al.*, 1979). When given unilateral intrastriatal injections of either 2.5 or 5 nmol of KA, Wistar are more sensitive than Sprague–Dawley rats (Sanberg *et al.*, 1979). Similar types of injections produce a greater magnitude of damage in older (69–172 days) than in younger (48–49 days) Sprague–Dawley rats (Gaddy *et al.*, 1979). Sex and hormones have also been shown to influence the effect of excitotoxins. Bilateral striatal injections of QA produces higher locomotor activity (Emerich *et al.*, 1991) but less weight loss (Zubrycki *et al.*, 1990) in female than in male or overiectomized female rats. Since KA induces seizures, if the animals were to be pretreated with anticonvulsants one should bear in mind that pharmacological agents such as diazepam and carbamazepine attenuate the excitotoxic effect of KA (Zaczek *et al.*, 1978). The type of anesthetics used has also been shown to influence the effect of excitotoxins. Anesthetics with a short half-life such as ether or hexobarbital potentiate the action of KA whereas those with a long half-life such as chloral hydrate or pentobarbital attenuate it (Zaczek *et al.*, 1978). When IA is used, one should be aware that the injected animals may sleep for a long time (up to 8h) even at a low dose (5 μg) (Coyle & Schwarcz, 1983). This might present a drawback for the behavioral assessment of the animals. Finally, care should also be taken to avoid non-enzymatic decomposition of IA since this chemical is thermolabile and photosensitive.

Acknowledgements

The authors wish to thank Drs Donato A. Di Monte, Jim Greene, J Timothy Greenamyre, Theresa Hasting, Jörg Schultz, and David Sulzer for their insightful comments on the manuscript, and Ms Pat White, Mr Brian Jones, and Mr Matthew Lucas for their help in its preparation. This study is supported by NIH/NINDS Grants RO1 NS38586 and NS42269, P50 NS38370, and P01 NS11766-27A1, the US Department of Defense Grant (DAMD 17-99-1-9471 and DAMD 17-03-1), the Lowenstein Foundation, the Lillian Goldman Charitable Trust, and the Parkinson's Disease Foundation.

REFERENCES

Abe, K., Taguchi, K., Wasai, T. *et al.* (2001). Stereoselective effect of (R)- and (S)-1-methyl-1,2,3,4-tetrahydroisoquinolines on a mouse model of Parkinson's disease. *Brain Res. Bull.*, **56**, 55–60.

Agid, Y., Javoy, F., Glowinski, J., Bouvet, D. & Sotelo, C. (1973). Injection of 6-hydroxydopamine into the substantia nigra of the rat. II. Diffusion and specificity. *Brain Res.*, **58**, 291–301.

Albers, D. S. & Sonsalla, P. K. (1995). Methamphetamine-induced hyperthermia and dopaminergic neurotoxicity in mice: pharmacological profile of protective and nonprotective agents. *J. Pharmacol. Exp. Ther.*, **275**, 1104–14.

Albin, R. L. & Greenamyre, J. T. (1992). Alternative excitotoxic hypotheses. *Neurology*, **42**, 733–8.

Ali, S. F., Newport, G. D., Holson, R. R., Slikker, W., Jr. & Bowyer, J. F. (1994). Low environmental temperatures or pharmacologic agents that produce hypothermia decrease methamphetamine neurotoxicity in mice. *Brain Res.*, **658**, 33–8.

Alston, T. A., Mela, L. & Bright, H. J. (1977). 3-Nitropropionate, the toxic substance of Indigofera, is a suicide inactivator of succinate dehydrogenase. *Proc. Natl Acad. Sci., USA*, **74**, 3767–71.

Antkiewicz-Michaluk, L., Romanska, I. Papla, I. *et al.* (2000). Neurochemical changes induced by acute and chronic administration of 1,2,3,4-tetrahydroisoquinoline and salsolinol in dopaminergic structures of rat brain. *Neuroscience*, **96**, 59–64.

Ara, J., Przedborski, S., Naini, A. B. *et al.* (1998). Inactivation of tyrosine hydroxylase by nitration following exposure to peroxynitrite and 1-methyl-4-phenyl-1,2,3,6-tetrahydropyridine (MPTP). *Proc. Natl Acad. Sci., USA*, **95**, 7659–63.

Araki, M., McGeer, P. L. & McGeer, E. G. (1985). Differential effect of kainic acid on somatostatin, GABAergic and cholinergic neurons in the rat striatum. *Neurosci. Lett.*, **53**, 197–202.

Axt, K. J., Mamounas, L. A. & Molliver, M. E. (1994). Structural features of amphetamine neurotoxicity in the brain. In *Amphetamine and its Analogs. Psychopharmacology,*

Toxicology, and Abuse, ed. A. K. Cho & D. S. Segal, pp. 315–367. New York: Academic Press.

Bankiewicz, K. S., Oldfield, E. H., Chiueh, C. C., Doppman, J. L., Jacobowitz, D. M. & Kopin, I. J. (1986). Hemiparkinsonism in monkeys after unilateral internal carotid artery infusion of 1-methyl-4-phenyl-1,2,3,6-tetrahydropyridine (MPTP). *Life Sci.*, **39**, 7–16.

Beal, M. F., Kowall, N. W., Ellison, D. W., Mazurek, M. F., Swartz, K. J. & Martin, J. B. (1986). Replication of the neurochemical characteristics of Huntington's disease by quinolinic acid. *Nature*, **321**, 168–71.

Beal, M. F., Ferrante, R. J., Swartz, K. J. & Kowall, N. W. (1991). Chronic quinolinic acid lesions in rats closely resemble Huntington's disease. *J. Neurosci*, **11**, 1649–59.

Beal, M. F., Brouillet, E., Jenkins, B., Henshaw, R., Rosen, B. & Hyman, B. T. (1993a). Age-dependent striatal excitotoxic lesions produced by the endogenous mitochondrial inhibitor malonate. *J. Neurochem.*, **61**, 1147–50.

Beal, M. F., Brouillet, E., Jenkins, B. G. *et al.* (1993b). Neurochemical and histologic characterization of striatal excitotoxic lesions produced by the mitochondrial toxin 3-nitropropionic acid. *J. Neurosci.*, **13**, 4181–92.

Ben Ari, Y. & Cossart, R. (2000). Kainate, a double agent that generates seizures: two decades of progress. *Trends Neurosci.*, **23**, 580–7.

Bergman, H., Wichmann, T. & DeLong, M. R. (1990). Reversal of experimental parkinsonism by lesions of the subthalamic nucleus. *Science*, **249**, 1436–8.

Betarbet, R., Sherer, T. B., MacKenzie, G., Garcia-Osuna, M., Panov, A. V. & Greenamyre, J. T. (2000). Chronic systemic pesticide exposure reproduces features of Parkinson's disease. *Nat. Neurosci.*, **3**, 1301–6.

Bezard, E., Imbert, C., Deloire, X., Bioulac, B. & Gross, C. E. (1997). A chronic MPTP model reproducing the slow evolution of Parkinson's disease: evolution of motor symptoms in the monkey. *Brain Res.*, **766**, 107–12.

Bezard, E., Gross, C. E., Fournier, M. C., Dovero, S., Bloch, B. & Jaber, M. (1999). Absence of MPTP-induced neuronal death in mice lacking the dopamine transporter. *Exp. Neurol.*, **155**, 268–73.

Bjorklund, L. M., Sanchez-Pernaute, R., Chung, S. *et al.* (2002). Embryonic stem cells develop into functional dopaminergic neurons after transplantation in a Parkinson rat model. *Proc. Natl Acad. Sci., USA*, **99**, 2344–9.

Blum, D., Torch, S., Lambeng, N. *et al.* (2001). Molecular pathways involved in the neurotoxicity of 6-OHDA, dopamine and MPTP: contribution to the apoptotic theory in Parkinson's disease. *Prog. Neurobiol.*, **65**, 135–72.

Boegman, R. J., Smith, Y. & Parent, A. (1987). Quinolinic acid does not spare striatal neuropeptide Y-immunoreactive neurons. *Brain Res.*, **415**, 178–82.

Borlongan, C. V., Koutouzis, T. K., Freeman, T. B., Cahill, D. W. & Sanberg, P. R. (1995). Behavioral pathology induced by repeated systemic injections of 3-nitropropionic acid mimics the motoric symptoms of Huntington's disease. *Brain Res.*, **697**, 254–7.

Borlongan, C. V., Koutouzis, T. K. & Sanberg, P. R. (1997). 3-Nitropropionic acid animal model and Huntington's disease. *Neurosci. Biobehav. Rev.*, **21**, 289–93.

Bourn, W. M., Chin, L. & Picchioni, A. L. (1972). Enhancement of audiogenic seizure by 6-hydroxydopamine. *J. Pharm. Pharmacol.*, **24**, 913–14.

Breese, G. R., Baumeister, A. A., McCown, T. J., Emerick, S. G., Frye, G. D. & Mueller, R. A. (1984). Neonatal-6-hydroxydopamine treatment: model of susceptibility for self-mutilation in the Lesch–Nyhan syndrome. *Pharmacol. Biochem. Behav.*, **21**, 459–61.

Breese, G. R., Criswell, H. E., Duncan, G. E. & Mueller, R. A. (1990). A dopamine deficiency model of Lesch–Nyhan disease – the neonatal-6-OHDA-lesioned rat. *Brain Res. Bull.*, **25**, 477–84.

Brooks, A. I., Chadwick, C. A., Gelbard, H. A., Cory-Slechta, D. A. & Federoff, H. J. (1999). Paraquat elicited neurobehavioral syndrome caused by dopaminergic neuron loss. *Brain Res.*, **823**, 1–10.

Brouillet, E., Jenkins, B. G., Hyman, B. T. *et al.* (1993). Age-dependent vulnerability of the striatum to the mitochondrial toxin 3-nitropropionic acid. *J. Neurochem.*, **60**, 356–9.

Brouillet, E., Hantraye, P., Ferrante, R. J. *et al.* (1995). Chronic mitochondrial energy impairment produces selective striatal degeneration and abnormal choreiform movements in primates. *Proc. Natl Acad. Sci., USA*, **92**, 7105–9.

Brouillet, E., Guyot, M. C., Mittoux, V. *et al.* (1998). Partial inhibition of brain succinate dehydrogenase by 3-nitropropionic acid is sufficient to initiate striatal degeneration in rat. *J. Neurochem.*, **70**, 794–805.

Brouillet, E., Conde, F., Beal, M. F. & Hantraye, P. (1999). Replicating Huntington's disease phenotype in experimental animals. *Prog. Neurobiol.*, **59**, 427–68.

Burns, L. H., Pakzaban, P., Deacon, T. W. *et al.* (1995). Selective putaminal excitotoxic lesions in non-human primates model the movement disorder of Huntington disease. *Neuroscience*, **64**, 1007–17.

Calabresi, P., Gubellini, P., Picconi, B. *et al.* (2001). Inhibition of mitochondrial complex II induces a long-term potentiation of NMDA-mediated synaptic excitation in the striatum requiring endogenous dopamine. *J. Neurosci.*, **21**, 5110–20.

Callahan, B. T. & Ricaurte, G. A. (1998). Effect of 7-nitroindazole on body temperature and methamphetamine-induced dopamine toxicity. *NeuroReport*, **9**, 2691–5.

Cao, L., Filipov, N. M. & Lawrence, D. A. (2002). Sympathetic nervous system plays a major role in acute cold/restraint stress inhibition of host resistance to *Listeria monocytogenes*. *J. Neuroimmunol.*, **125**, 94–102.

Chan, P., DeLanney, L. E., Irwin, I., Langston, J. W. & Di Monte, D. (1991). Rapid ATP loss caused by 1-methyl-4-phenyl-1,2,3,6-tetrahydropyridine in mouse brain. *J. Neurochem.*, **57**, 348–51.

Chan, P., DeLanney, L. E., Irwin, I., Langston, J. W. & Di Monte, D. (1992). MPTP-induced ATP loss in mouse brain. *Ann. NY Acad. Sci.*, **648**, 306–8.

Clausing, P. & Bowyer, J. F. (1999). Time course of brain temperature and caudate/putamen microdialysate levels of amphetamine and dopamine in rats after multiple doses of d-amphetamine. *Ann. NY Acad. Sci.*, **890**, 495–504.

Cleeter, M. W., Cooper, J. M. & Schapira, A. H. (1992). Irreversible inhibition of mitochondrial complex I by 1-methyl-4-phenylpyridinium: evidence for free radical involvement. *J. Neurochem.*, **58**, 786–9.

Cohen, G. & Werner, P. (1994). Free radicals, oxidative stress, and neurodegeneration. In *Neurodegenerative Diseases*, ed. D. B. Calne, pp. 139–161. Philadelphia: W. B. Saunders.

Cooper, J. M. & Clark, J. B. (1994). The structural organization of the mitochondrial respiration chain. In *Mitochondrial Disorders in Neurology*, ed. A. H. Schapira & S. DiMauro, pp. 1–30. Boston: Butterworth-Heinemann Ltd.

Coyle, J. T. & Schwarcz, R. (1976). Lesion of striatal neurones with kainic acid provides a model for Huntington's chorea. *Nature*, **263**, 244–6.

Coyle, J. T. & Schwarcz, R. (1983). The use of excitatory amino acids as selective neurotoxins. In *Handbook of Chemical Neuroanatomy. Method in Chemical Neuroanatomy*, ed. A. Björklund & T. Hökfelt, pp. 508–27. New York: Elsevier.

Coyle, J. T., Molliver, M. E. & Kuhar, M. J. (1978). *In situ* injection of kainic acid: a new method for selectively lesioning neuronal cell bodies while sparing axons of passage. *J. Comp. Neurol.*, **180**, 301–24.

Cubells, J. F., Rayport, S., Rajendran, G. & Sulzer, D. (1994). Methamphetamine neurotoxicity involves vacuolation of endocytic organelles and dopamine-dependent intracellular oxidative stress. *J. Neurosci.*, **14**, 2260–71.

Czlonkowska, A., Kohutnicka, M., Kurkowska-Jastrzebska, I. & Czlonkowski, A. (1996). Microglial reaction in MPTP (1-methyl-4-phenyl-1,2,3,6-tetrahydropyridine) induced Parkinson's disease mice model. *Neurodegeneration*, **5**, 137–43.

Dauer, W. & Przedborski, S. (2003). Parkinson's disease: mechanisms and models. *Neuron*, **39**, 889–909.

Davey, G. P. & Clark, J. B. (1996). Threshold effects and control of oxidative phosphorylation in nonsynaptic rat brain mitochondria. *J. Neurochem.*, **66**, 1617–24.

Davidson, C., Gow, A. J., Lee, T. H. & Ellinwood, E. H. (2001). Methamphetamine neurotoxicity: necrotic and apoptotic mechanisms and relevance to human abuse and treatment. *Brain Res. Rev.*, **36**, 1–22.

Davies, S. W. & Roberts, P. J. (1987). No evidence for preservation of somatostatin-containing neurons after intrastriatal injections of quinolinic acid. *Nature*, **327**, 326–9.

Davis, G. C., Williams, A. C., Markey, S. P. *et al.* (1979). Chronic parkinsonism secondary to intravenous injection of meperidine analogs. *Psychiatry Res.*, **1**, 249–54.

Day, B. J., Patel, M., Calavetta, L., Chang, L. Y. & Stamler, J. S. (1999). A mechanism of paraquat toxicity involving nitric oxide synthase. *Proc. Natl. Acad. Sci., USA*, **96**, 12760–5.

De Gori, N., Froio, F., Strongoli, M. C., De Francesco, A., Calo, M. & Nistico, G. (1988). Behavioural and electrocortical changes induced by paraquat after injection in specific areas of the brain of the rat. *Neuropharmacology*, **27**, 201–7.

Dehmer, T., Lindenau, J., Haid, S., Dichgans, J. & Schulz, J. B. (2000). Deficiency of inducible nitric oxide synthase protects against MPTP toxicity in vivo. *J. Neurochem.*, **74**, 2213–16.

Deitrich, R. & Erwin, V. (1980). Biogenic amine-aldehyde condensation products: tetrahydroisoquinolines and tryptolines (beta-carbolines). *Annu. Rev. Pharmacol. Toxicol.*, **20**, 55–80.

Donovan, D. M., Miner, L. L., Perry, M. P. *et al.* (1999). Cocaine reward and MPTP toxicity: alteration by regional variant dopamine transporter overexpression. *Mol. Brain Res.*, **73**, 37–49.

Dugan, L. L. & Choi, D. W. (1994). Excitotoxicity, free radicals, and cell membrane changes. *Ann. Neurol.*, **35 Suppl.**, S17–S21.

Dunnett, S. B. & Iversen, S. D. (1981). Learning impairments following selective kainic acid-induced lesions within the neostriatum of rats. *Behav. Brain Res.*, **2**, 189–209.

Eberhardt, O., Coelln, R. V., Kugler, S. *et al.* (2000). Protection by synergistic effects of adenovirus-mediated X-chromosome-linked inhibitor of apoptosis and glial cell line-derived neurotrophic factor gene transfer in the 1-methyl-4-phenyl-1,2,3,6-tetrahydropyridine model of Parkinson's disease. *J. Neurosci.*, **20**, 9126–34.

Emerich, D. F., Zubricki, E. M., Shipley, M. T., Norman, A. B. & Sanberg, P. R. (1991). Female rats are more sensitive to the locomotor alterations following quinolinic acid-induced striatal lesions: effects of striatal transplants. *Exp. Neurol.*, **111**, 369–78.

Faull, R. L. & Laverty, R. (1969). Changes in dopamine levels in the corpus striatum following lesions in the substantia nigra. *Exp. Neurol.*, **23**, 332–40.

Ferger, B., Eberhardt, O., Teismann, P., de Groote, C. & Schulz, J. B. (1999). Malonate-induced generation of reactive oxygen species in rat striatum depends on dopamine release but not on NMDA receptor activation. *J. Neurochem.*, **73**, 1329–32.

Fernagut, P. O., Diguet, E., Stefanova, N. *et al.* (2002). Subacute systemic 3-nitropropionic acid intoxication induces a distinct motor disorder in adult C57Bl/6 mice: behavioural and histopathological characterisation. *Neuroscience*, **114**, 1005–17.

Ferrante, R. J., Schulz, J. B., Kowall, N. W. & Beal, M. F. (1997). Systemic administration of rotenone produces selective damage in the striatum and globus pallidus, but not in the substantia nigra. *Brain Res.*, **753**, 157–62.

Forno, L. S., Langston, J. W., DeLanney, L. E., Irwin, I. & Ricaurte, G. A. (1986). Locus ceruleus lesions and eosinophilic inclusions in MPTP- treated monkeys. *Ann. Neurol.*, **20**, 449–55.

Forno, L. S., DeLanney, L. E., Irwin, I. & Langston, J. W. (1993). Similarities and differences between MPTP-induced parkinsonism and Parkinson's disease: Neuropathologic considerations. *Adv. Neurol.*, **60**, 600–8.

Fumagalli, F., Gainetdinov, R. R., Valenzano, K. J. & Caron, M. G. (1998). Role of dopamine transporter in methamphetamine-induced neurotoxicity: evidence from mice lacking the transporter. *J. Neurosci.*, **18**, 4861–9.

Fumagalli, F., Gainetdinov, R. R., Wang, Y. M., Valenzano, K. J., Miller, G. W. & Caron, M. G. (1999). Increased methamphetamine neurotoxicity in heterozygous vesicular monoamine transporter 2 knock-out mice. *J. Neurosci.*, **19**, 2424–31.

Funata, N., Song, S. Y., Okeda, R., Funata, M. & Higashino, F. (1984). A study of experimental cyanide encephalopathy in the acute phase – physiological and neuropathological correlation. *Acta Neuropathol. (Berl)*, **64**, 99–107.

Gaddy, J. R., Britt, M. D., Neill, D. B. & Haigler, H. J. (1979). Susceptibility of rat neostriatum to damage by kainic acid: age dependence. *Brain Res.*, **176**, 192–6.

Gao, H. M., Hong, J. S., Zhang, W. & Liu, B. (2002). Distinct role for microglia in rotenone-induced degeneration of dopaminergic neurons. *J. Neurosci.*, **22**, 782–90.

Giovanni, A., Sieber, B.-A., Heikkila, R. E. & Sonsalla, P. K. (1994a). Studies on species sensitivity to the dopaminergic neurotoxin 1-methyl-4-phenyl-1,2,3,6-tetrahydropyridine. Part 1: Systemic administration. *J. Pharmacol. Exp. Ther.*, **270**, 1000–7.

Giovanni, A., Sieber, B. A., Heikkila, R. E. & Sonsalla, P. K. (1991). Correlation between the neostriatal content of the 1-methyl-4- phenylpyridinium species and dopaminergic neurotoxicity following 1-methyl-4-phenyl-1,2,3,6-tetrahydropyridine administration to several strains of mice. *J. Pharmacol. Exp. Ther.*, **257**, 691–7.

Giovanni, A., Sonsalla, P. K. & Heikkila, R. E. (1994b). Studies on species sensitivity to the dopaminergic neurotoxin 1-methyl-4-phenyl- 1,2,3,6-tetrahydropyridine. Part 2: Central administration of 1-methyl-4-phenylpyridinium. *J. Pharmacol. Exp. Ther.*, **270**, 1008–14.

Graham, D. G. (1978). Oxidative pathways for catecholamines in the genesis of neuromelanin and cytotoxic quinones. *Mol. Pharmacol.*, **14**, 633–43.

Grant, H., Lantos, P. L. & Parkinson, C. (1980). Cerebral damage in paraquat poisoning. *Histopathology*, **4**, 185–95.

Greene, J. G. & Greenamyre, J. T. (1996). Manipulation of membrane potential modulates malonate-induced striatal excitotoxicity in vivo. *J. Neurochem.*, **66**, 637–43.

Greene, J. G., Porter, R. H. P., Eller, R. V. & Greenamyre, J. T. (1993). Inhibition of succinate dehydrogenase by malonic acid produces an 'excitotoxic' lesion in rat striatum. *J. Neurochem.*, **61**, 1151–4.

Guyot, M. C. & Hantraye, P., Dolan, R., Palfi, S., Maziere, M. & Brouillet, E. (1997). Quantifiable bradykinesia, gait abnormalities and Huntington's disease-like striatal lesions in rats chronically treated with 3-nitropropionic acid. *Neuroscience*, **79**, 45–56.

Hamre, K., Tharp, R., Poon, K., Xiong, X. & Smeyne, R. J. (1999). Differential strain susceptibility following 1-methyl-4-phenyl-1,2,3,6-tetrahydropyridine (MPTP) administration acts in an autosomal dominant fashion: quantitative analysis in seven strains of *Mus musculus*. *Brain Res.*, **828**, 91–103.

Hantraye, P., Riche, D., Maziere, M. & Isacson, O. (1990). A primate model of Huntington's disease: behavioral and anatomical studies of unilateral excitotoxic lesions of the caudate-putamen in the baboon. *Exp. Neurol.*, **108**, 91–104.

Hartmann, A., Troadec, J. D., Hunot, S. *et al.* (2001). Caspase-8 is an effector in apoptotic death of dopaminergic neurons in

Parkinson's disease, but pathway inhibition results in neuronal necrosis. *J. Neurosci.*, **21**, 2247–55.

Hasegawa, E., Takeshige, K., Oishi, T., Murai, Y. & Minakami, S. (1990). 1-Methyl-4-phenylpyridinium (MPP+) induces NADH-dependent superoxide formation and enhances NADH-dependent lipid peroxidation in bovine heart submitochondrial particles. *Biochem. Biophys. Res. Commun.*, **170**, 1049–55.

Hatzidimitriou, G., McCann, U. D. & Ricaurte, G. A. (1999). Altered serotonin innervation patterns in the forebrain of monkeys treated with (+/−)3,4-methylenedioxymethamphetamine seven years previously: factors influencing abnormal recovery. *J. Neurosci.*, **19**, 5096–107.

Hefti, F., Melamed, E. & Wurtman, R. J. (1980). Partial lesions of the dopaminergic nigrostriatal system in rat brain: biochemical characterization. *Brain Res.*, **195**, 123–37.

Heikkila, R. E., Nicklas, W. J., Vyas, I. & Duvoisin, R. C. (1985). Dopaminergic toxicity of rotenone and the 1-methyl-4-phenylpyridinium ion after their stereotaxic administration to rats: implication for the mechanism of 1-methyl-4-phenyl-1,2,3,6-tetrahydropyridine toxicity. *Neurosci. Lett.*, **62**, 389–94.

Heikkila, R. E., Sieber, B. A., Manzino, L. & Sonsalla, P. K. (1989). Some features of the nigrostriatal dopaminergic neurotoxin 1-methyl-4-phenyl-1,2,3,6-tetrahydropyridine (MPTP) in the mouse. *Mol. Chem. Neuropathol.*, **10**, 171–83.

Herve, D., Studler, J. M., Blanc, G., Glowinski, J. & Tassin, J. P. (1986). Partial protection by desmethylimipramine of the mesocortical dopamine neurones from the neurotoxic effect of 6-hydroxydopamine injected in ventral mesencephalic tegmentum. The role of noradrenergic innervation. *Brain Res.*, **383**, 47–53.

Higgins, D. S., Jr. & Greenamyre, J. T. (1996). [^{3}H]dihydrorotenone binding to NADH: ubiquinone reductase (Complex I) of the electron transport chain: An autoradiographic study. *J. Neurosci.*, **16**, 3807–16.

Hoglinger, G. U., Feger, J., Annick, P. *et al.* (2003). Chronic systemic complex I inhibition induces a hypokinetic multisystem degeneration in rats. *J. Neurochem.*, **84**, 1–12.

Hong, J. S., Yang, H. Y., Racagni, G. & Costa, E. (1977). Projections of substance P containing neurons from neostriatum to substantia nigra. *Brain Res*, **122**, 541–4.

Hruska, R. E. & Silbergeld, E. K. (1979). Abnormal locomotion in rats after bilateral intrastriatal injection of kainic acid. *Life Sci.*, **25**, 181–93.

Hughes, J. T. (1988). Brain damage due to paraquat poisoning: a fatal case with neuropathological examination of the brain. *Neurotoxicology*, **9**, 243–8.

Jackson-Lewis, V., Jakowec, M., Burke, R. E. & Przedborski, S. (1995). Time course and morphology of dopaminergic neuronal death caused by the neurotoxin 1-methyl-4-phenyl-1,2,3,6-tetrahydropyridine. *Neurodegeneration*, **4**, 257–69.

Javitch, J. A., D'Amato, R. J., Strittmatter, S. M. & Snyder, S. H. (1985). Parkinsonism-inducing neurotoxin, *N*-methyl-4-phenyl-1,2,3,6-tetrahydropyridine: uptake of the metabolite

N-methyl-4-phenylpyridinium by dopamine neurons explain selective toxicity. *Proc. Natl Acad. Sci., USA*, **82**, 2173–7.

Javoy, F., Sotelo, C., Herbert, A. & Agid, Y. (1976). Specificity of dopaminergic neuronal degeneration induced by intracerebral injection of 6-hydroxydopamine in the nigrostriatal dopamine system. *Brain Res.*, **102**, 210–15.

Jeon, B. S., Jackson-Lewis, V. & Burke, R. E. (1995). 6-hydroxydopamine lesion of the rat substantia nigra: time course and morphology of cell death. *Neurodegeneration*, **4**, 131–7.

Jiang, H., Jackson-Lewis, V., Muthane, U. *et al.* (1993). Adenosine receptor antagonists potentiate dopamine receptor agonist-induced rotational behavior in 6-hydroxydopamine-lesioned rats. *Brain Res.*, **613**, 347–51.

Jonsson, G. (1980). Chemical neurotoxins as denervation tools in neurobiology. *Annu. Rev. Neurosci.*, **3**, 169–87.

Jonsson, G. (1983). Chemical lesioning techniques: monoamine neurotoxins. In *Handbook of Chemical Neuroanatomy. Vol. 1: Methods in Chemical Neuroanatomy*, ed. A. Björklund & T. Hökfelt, pp. 463–507. Amsterdam: Elsevier Science Publishers B. V.

Jonsson, G., Fuxe, K., Hokfelt, T. & Goldstein, M. (1976). Resistance of central phenylethanolamine-n-methyl transferase containing neurons to 6-hydroxydopamine. *Med. Biol.*, **54**, 421–6.

Joyce, J. N., Frohna, P. A. & Neal-Beliveau, B. S. (1996). Functional and molecular differentiation of the dopamine system induced by neonatal denervation. *Neurosci. Biobehav. Rev.*, **20**, 453–86.

Kaal, E. C., Vlug, A. S., Versleijen, M. W., Kuilman, M., Joosten, E. A. & Bar, P. R. (2000). Chronic mitochondrial inhibition induces selective motoneuron death in vitro: a new model for amyotrophic lateral sclerosis. *J. Neurochem.*, **74**, 1158–65.

Kakhniashvili, D., Mayor, J. A., Gremse, D. A., Xu, Y. & Kaplan, R. S. (1997). Identification of a novel gene encoding the yeast mitochondrial dicarboxylate transport protein via overexpression, purification, and characterization of its protein product. *J. Biol. Chem.*, **272**, 4516–21.

Kanazawa, I., Kimura, M., Murata, M., Tanaka, Y. & Cho, F. (1990). Choreic movements in the macaque monkey induced by kainic acid lesions of the striatum combined with L-dopa. Pharmacological, biochemical and physiological studies on neural mechanisms. *Brain*, **113**, 509–35.

Kanazawa, I., Tanaka, Y. & Cho, F. (1986). 'Choreic' movement induced by unilateral kainate lesion of the striatum and L-DOPA administration in monkey. *Neurosci. Lett.*, **71**, 241–6.

Kanthasamy, A. G., Borowitz, J. L., Pavlakovic, G. & Isom, G. E. (1994). Dopaminergic neurotoxicity of cyanide: neurochemical, histological, and behavioral characterization. *Toxicol. Appl. Pharmacol.*, **126**, 156–63.

Kaul, C. L. (1999). Role of sympathetic nervous system in experimental hypertension and diabetes mellitus. *Clin. Exp. Hypertens.*, **21**, 95–112.

Khalil, Z. & Helme, R. D. (1989). Sympathetic neurons modulate plasma extravasation in the rat through a non-adrenergic mechanism. *Clin. Exp. Neurol.*, **26**, 45–50.

Kilbourn, M. R., Charalambous, A., Frey, K. A., Sherman, P., Higgins, D. S., Jr. & Greenamyre, J. T. (1997). Intrastriatal neuro-toxin injections reduce in vitro and in vivo binding of radiolabeled rotenoids to mitochondrial complex I. *J. Cereb. Blood Flow Metab.*, **17**, 265–72.

Kirik, D., Georgievska, B., Burger, C. *et al.* (2002). Reversal of motor impairments in parkinsonian rats by continuous intrastriatal delivery of L-dopa using rAAV-mediated gene transfer. *Proc. Natl Acad. Sci., USA*, **99**, 4708–13.

Kita, T., Matsunari, Y., Saraya, T. *et al.* (2000). Methamphetamine-induced striatal dopamine release, behavior changes and neurotoxicity in BALB/c mice. *Int. J. Dev. Neurosci.*, **18**, 521–30.

Klaidman, L. K., Adams, J. D., Jr., Leung, A. C., Kim, S. S. & Cadenas, E. (1993). Redox cycling of MPP+: evidence for a new mechanism involving hydride transfer with xanthine oxidase, aldehyde dehydrogenase, and lipoamide dehydrogenase. *Free Radic. Biol. Med.*, **15**, 169–79.

Klivenyi, P., Andreassen, O. A., Ferrante, R. J. *et al.* (2000). Mice deficient in cellular glutathione peroxidase show increased vulnerability to malonate, 3-nitropropionic acid, and 1-methyl-4-phenyl-1,2,5,6-tetrahydropyridine. *J. Neurosci.*, **20**, 1–7.

Kohler, C. & Schwarcz, R. (1983). Comparison of ibotenate and kainate neurotoxicity in rat brain: a histological study. *Neuroscience*, **8**, 819–35.

Kohutnicka, M., Lewandowska, E., Kurkowska-Jastrzebska, I., Czlonkowski, A. & Czlonkowska, A. (1998). Microglial and astrocytic involvement in a murine model of Parkinson's disease induced by 1-methyl-4-phenyl-1,2,3,6-tetrahydropyridine (MPTP). *Immunopharmacology*, **39**, 167–80.

Kopin, I. J. & Markey, S. P. (1988). MPTP toxicity: implication for research in Parkinson's disease. *Annu. Rev. Neurosci.*, **11**, 81–96.

Kotake, Y., Yoshida, M., Ogawa, M., Tasaki, Y., Hirobe, M. & Ohta, S. (1996). Chronic administration of 1-benzyl-1,2,3,4-tetrahydroisoquinoline, an endogenous amine in the brain, induces parkinsonism in a primate. *Neurosci. Lett.*, **217**, 69–71.

Langston, J. W. (1987). MPTP: the promise of a new neurotoxin. In *Movement Disorders 2*, ed. C. D. Marsden & S. Fahn, pp. 73–90. London: Butterworths.

Langston, J. W. & Irwin, I. (1986). MPTP: current concepts and controversies. *Clin. Neuropharmacol.*, **9**, 485–507.

Langston, J. W., Ballard, P. & Irwin, I. (1983). Chronic parkinsonism in humans due to a product of meperidine-analog synthesis. *Science*, **219**, 979–80.

Langston, J. W., Forno, L. S., Tetrud, J., Reeves, A. G., Kaplan, J. A. & Karluk, D. (1999). Evidence of active nerve cell degeneration in the substantia nigra of humans years after 1-methyl-4-phenyl- 1,2,3,6-tetrahydropyridine exposure. *Ann. Neurol.*, **46**, 598–605.

Lapointe, N., St-Hilaire, M., Martinoli, M. G. *et al.* (2004). Rotenone induces non-specific central nervous system and systemic toxicity. *FASEB J.*, **18**, 717–19.

Larsen, K. E., Fon, E. A., Hastings, T. G., Edwards, R. H. & Sulzer, D. (2002). Methamphetamine-induced degeneration of dopaminergic neurons involves autophagy and upregulation of dopamine synthesis. *J. Neurosci.*, **22**, 8951–60.

Lee, W. T., Yin, H. S. & Shen, Y. Z. (2002). The mechanisms of neuronal death produced by mitochondrial toxin 3-nitropropionic acid: the roles of *N*-methyl-D-aspartate glutamate receptors and mitochondrial calcium overload. *Neuroscience*, **112**, 707–16.

Levivier, M., Holemans, S., Togasaki, D. M., Maloteaux, J.-M., Brotchi, J. & Przedborski, S. (1994). Quantitative assessment of quinolinic acid-induced striatal toxicity in rats using radioligand binding assays. *Neurol. Res.*, **16**, 194–200.

Liberatore, G., Jackson-Lewis, V., Vukosavic, S. *et al.* (1999). Inducible nitric oxide synthase stimulates dopaminergic neurodegeneration in the MPTP model of Parkinson's disease. *Nat. Med.*, **5**, 1403–9.

Liou, H. H., Chen, R. C., Tsai, Y. F., Chen, W. P., Chang, Y. C. & Tsai, M. C. (1996). Effects of paraquat on the substantia nigra of the wistar rats: neurochemical, histological, and behavioral studies. *Toxicol. Appl. Pharmacol.*, **137**, 34–41.

Liou, H. H., Tsai, M. C., Chen, C. J. *et al.* (1997). Environmental risk factors and Parkinson's disease: a case-control study in Taiwan. *Neurology*, **48**, 1583–8.

Liu, Y., Roghani, A. & Edwards, R. H. (1992). Gene transfer of a reserpine-sensitive mechanism of resistance to *N*-methyl-4-phenylpyridinium. *Proc. Natl Acad. Sci., USA*, **89**, 9074–8.

Lorenc-Koci, E., Smialowska, M., Antkiewicz-Michaluk, L., Golembiowska, K., Bajkowska, M. & Wolfarth, S. (2000). Effect of acute and chronic administration of 1,2,3,4-tetrahydroisoquinoline on muscle tone, metabolism of dopamine in the striatum and tyrosine hydroxylase immunocytochemistry in the substantia nigra, in rats. *Neuroscience*, **95**, 1049–59.

Lotharius, J. & O'Malley, K. L. (2000). The parkinsonism-inducing drug 1-methyl-4-phenylpyridinium triggers intracellular dopamine oxidation. A novel mechanism of toxicity. *J. Biol. Chem.*, **275**, 38581–8.

Lotharius, J., Dugan, L. L. & O'Malley, K. L. (1999). Distinct mechanisms underlie neurotoxin-mediated cell death in cultured dopaminergic neurons. *J. Neurosci.*, **19**, 1284–93.

Luthman, J., Bolioli, B., Tsutsumi, T., Verhofstad, A. & Jonsson, G. (1987). Sprouting of striatal serotonin nerve terminals following selective lesions of nigro-striatal dopamine neurons in neonatal rat. *Brain Res. Bull.*, **19**, 269–74.

Luthman, J., Fredriksson, A., Sundstrom, E., Jonsson, G. & Archer, T. (1989). Selective lesion of central dopamine or noradrenaline neuron systems in the neonatal rat: motor behavior and monoamine alterations at adult stage. *Behav. Brain Res.*, **33**, 267–77.

Malberg, J. E. & Seiden, L. S. (1998). Small changes in ambient temperature cause large changes in 3,4-methylenedioxymethamphetamine (MDMA)-induced serotonin neurotoxicity and core body temperature in the rat. *J. Neurosci.*, **18**, 5086–94.

Manning-Bog, A. B., McCormack, A. L., Li, J., Uversky, V. N., Fink, A. L. & Di Monte, D. A. (2002). The herbicide paraquat causes up-regulation and aggregation of alpha-synuclein in mice: paraquat and alpha-synuclein. *J. Biol. Chem.*, **277**, 1641–4.

Maragos, W. F., Jakel, R. J., Pang, Z. & Geddes, J. W. (1998). 6-Hydroxydopamine injections into the nigrostriatal pathway attenuate striatal malonate and 3-nitropropionic acid lesions. *Exp. Neurol.*, **154**, 637–44.

Marey-Semper, I., Gelman, M. & Lévi-Strauss, M. (1995). A selective toxicity toward cultured mesencephalic dopaminergic neurons is induced by the synergistic effects of energetic metabolism impairment and NMDA receptor activation. *J. Neurosci.*, **15**, 5912–18.

Marshall, J. F., Navarrete, R. & Joyce, J. N. (1989). Decreased striatal D1 binding density following mesotelencephalic 6-hydroxydopamine injections: an autoradiographic analysis. *Brain Res.*, **493**, 247–57.

Marti, M. J., James, C. J., Oo, T. F., Kelly, W. J. & Burke, R. E. (1997). Early developmental destruction of terminals in the striatal target induces apoptosis in dopamine neurons of the substantia nigra. *J. Neurosci.*, **17**, 2030–9.

Mason, S. T., Sanberg, P. R. & Fibiger, H. C. (1978). Kainic acid lesions of the striatum dissociate amphetamine and apomorphine stereotypy: similarities to Huntington's chorea. *Science*, **201**, 352–5.

Massieu, L., Del Rio, P. & Montiel, T. (2001). Neurotoxicity of glutamate uptake inhibition in vivo: correlation with succinate dehydrogenase activity and prevention by energy substrates. *Neuroscience*, **106**, 669–77.

Mayer, R. A., Kindt, M. V. & Heikkila, R. E. (1986). Prevention of the nigrostriatal toxicity of 1-methyl-4-phenyl-1, 2,3,6-tetrahydropyridine by inhibitors of 3,4-dihydroxyphenylethylamine transport. *J. Neurochem.*, **47**, 1073–9.

McCormack, A. L., Thiruchelvam, M., Manning-Bog, A. B., Thiffault, C., Langston, J. W., Cory-Slechta, D. A. & Di Monte, D. A. (2002). Environmental risk factors and Parkinson's disease: selective degeneration of nigral dopaminergic neurons caused by the herbicide paraquat. *Neurobiol. Dis.*, **10**, 119–27.

McGeer, E. G. & McGeer, P. L. (1976). Duplication of biochemical changes of Huntington's chorea by intrastriatal injections of glutamic and kainic acids. *Nature*, **263**, 517–19.

McGeer, E. G. & McGeer, P. L. (1978). Some factors influencing the neurotoxicity of intrastriatal injections of kainic acid. *Neurochem. Res.*, **3**, 501–17.

(1982). Kainic acid: the neurotoxic breakthrough. *Crit. Rev. Toxicol.*, **10**, 1–26.

McNaught, K. S., Carrupt, P. A., Altomare, C. *et al.* (1998). Isoquinoline derivatives as endogenous neurotoxins in the aetiology of Parkinson's disease. *Biochem. Pharmacol.*, **56**, 921–33.

Meldrum, A., Page, K. J., Everitt, B. J. & Dunnett, S. B. (2000). Age-dependence of malonate-induced striatal toxicity. *Exp. Brain Res.*, **134**, 335–43.

Miller, D. B., O'Callaghan, J. P. (1994). Environment-, drug- and stress-induced alterations in body temperature affect the neurotoxicity of substituted amphetamines in the C57BL/6J mouse. *J. Pharmacol. Exp. Ther.*, **270**, 752–60.

Miller, D. B., Ali, S. F., O'Callaghan, J. P. & Laws, S. C. (1998). The impact of gender and estrogen on striatal dopaminergic neurotoxicity. *Ann. NY Acad. Sci.*, **844**, 153–65.

Mizuno, Y., Sone, N. & Saitoh, T. (1987). Effects of 1-methyl-4-phenyl- 1,2,3,6-tetrahydropyridine and 1-methyl-4-phenylpyridinium ion on activities of the enzymes in the electron transport system in mouse brain. *J. Neurochem.*, **48**, 1787–93.

Moratalla, R., Quinn, B., DeLanney, L. E., Irwin, I., Langston, J. W. & Graybiel, A. M. (1992). Differential vulnerability of primate caudate-putamen and striosome-matrix dopamine systems to the neurotoxic effects of 1-methyl-4-phenyl-1,2,3,6-tetrahydropyridine. *Proc. Natl Acad. Sci., USA*, **89**, 3859–63.

Moser, A., Siebecker, F., Nobbe, F. & Bohme, V. (1996). Rotational behaviour and neurochemical changes in unilateral *N*-methyl-norsalsolinol and 6-hydroxydopamine lesioned rats. *Exp. Brain Res.*, **112**, 89–95.

Moy, S. S., Criswell, H. E. & Breese, G. R. (1997). Differential effects of bilateral dopamine depletion in neonatal and adult rats. *Neurosci. Biobehav. Rev.*, **21**, 425–35.

Moy, L. Y., Zeevalk, G. D. & Sonsalla, P. K. (2000). Role for dopamine in malonate-induced damage in vivo in striatum and in vitro in mesencephalic cultures. *J. Neurochem.*, **74**, 1656–65.

Muthane, U., Ramsay, K. A., Jiang, H. *et al.* (1994). Differences in nigral neuron number and sensitivity to 1-methyl-4-phenyl-1,2,3,6-tetrahydropyridine in C57/bl and CD-1 mice. *Exp. Neurol.*, **126**, 195–204.

Nagatsu, T. (1997). Isoquinoline neurotoxins in the brain and Parkinson's disease. *Neurosci. Res.*, **29**, 99–111.

Nagatsu, T. & Yoshida, M. (1988). An endogenous substance of the brain, tetrahydroisoquinoline, produces parkinsonism in primates with decreased dopamine, tyrosine hydroxylase and biopterin in the nigrostriatal regions. *Neurosci. Lett.*, **87**, 178–82.

Naoi, M., Maruyama, W., Dostert, P. *et al.* (1996). Dopamine-derived endogenous 1(R),2(N)-dimethyl-6,7-dihydroxy-1,2,3,4-tetrahydroisoquinoline, *N*-methyl-(R)-salsolinol, induced parkinsonism in rat: biochemical, pathological and behavioral studies. *Brain Res.*, **709**, 285–95.

Nicklas, W. J., Vyas, I. & Heikkila, R. E. (1985). Inhibition of NADH-linked oxidation in brain mitochondria by MPP$^+$, a metabolite of the neurotoxin MPTP. *Life Sci.*, **36**, 2503–8.

O'Callaghan, J. P., Miller, D. B. & Reinhard, J. F. (1990). Characterization of the origins of astrocyte response to injury using the dopaminergic neurotoxicant, 1-methyl-4-phenyl-1,2,3,6-tetrahydropyridine. *Brain Res.*, **521**, 73–80.

Offen, D., Beart, P. M., Cheung, N. S. *et al.* (1998). Transgenic mice expressing human Bcl-2 in their neurons are resistant to 6-hydroxydopamine and 1-methyl-4-phenyl-1,2,3,6-tetrahydropyridine neurotoxicity. *Proc. Natl Acad. Sci., USA*, **95**, 5789–94.

Okun, J. G., Lummen, P. & Brandt, U. (1999). Three classes of inhibitors share a common binding domain in mitochondrial complex I (NADH: ubiquinone oxidoreductase). *J. Biol. Chem.*, **274**, 2625–30.

Olney, J. W., Ho, O. L. & Rhee, V. (1971). Cytotoxic effects of acidic and sulphur containing amino acids on the infant mouse central nervous system. *Exp. Brain Res.*, **14**, 61–76.

Ouary, S., Bizat, N., Altairac, S. *et al.* (2000). Major strain differences in response to chronic systemic administration of the mitochondrial toxin 3-nitropropionic acid in rats: implications for neuroprotection studies. *Neuroscience*, **97**, 521–30.

Pajor, A. M., Gangula, R. & Yao, X. (2001). Cloning and functional characterization of a high-affinity Na(+)/dicarboxylate cotransporter from mouse brain. *Am. J. Physiol. Cell Physiol.*, **280**, C1215–23.

Pennathur, S., Jackson-Lewis, V., Przedborski, S. & Heinecke, J. W. (1999). Mass spectrometric quantification of 3-nitrotyrosine, ortho-tyrosine, and o,o′-dityrosine in brain tissue of 1-methyl-4-phenyl-1,2,3,6-tetrahydropyridine-treated mice, a model of oxidative stress in Parkinson's disease. *J. Biol. Chem.*, **274**, 34621–8.

Perier, C., Bove, J., Vila, M. & Przedborski, S. (2003). The rotenone model of Parkinson's disease. *Trends Neurosci.*, **26**, 345–6.

Perry, T. L., Jones, K. & Hansen, S. (1988). Tetrahydroisoquinoline lacks dopaminergic nigrostriatal neurotoxicity in mice. *Neurosci. Lett.*, **85**, 101–4.

Petzinger, G. M. & Langston, J. W. (1998). The MPTP-lesioned non-human primate: a model for Parkinson's disease. In *Advances in Neurodegenerative Disorders. Parkinson's Disease*, ed. J. Marwah, H. Teiltelbaum, pp. 113–48. Scottsdale: Prominent Press.

Portera-Cailliau, C., Price, D. L. & Martin, L. J. (1997a). Excitotoxic neuronal death in the immature brain is an apoptosis–necrosis morphological continuum. *J. Comp. Neurol.*, **378**, 70–87.

Portera-Cailliau, C., Price, D. L. & Martin, L. J. (1997b). Non-NMDA and NMDA receptor-mediated excitotoxic neuronal deaths in adult brain are morphologically distinct: further evidence for an apoptosis-necrosis continuum. *J. Comp. Neurol.*, **378**, 88–104.

Przedborski, S. & Dawson, T. M. (2001). The role of nitric oxide in Parkinson's disease. In *Parkinson's Disease. Methods and Protocols*, ed. M. M. Mouradian, pp. 113–36. New Jersey: Humana Press.

Przedborski, S. & Vila, M. (2003). The 1-methyl-4-phenyl 1-1, 2, 3, 6-tetrahydropyridine mouse model: a tool to explore the pathogenesis of Parkinson's disease. *Ann. N. Y. Acad. Sci.*, **991**, 189–98.

Przedborski, S., Jackson-Lewis, V., Popilskis, S. *et al.* (1991). Unilateral MPTP-induced parkinsonism in monkeys: a quantitative autoradiographic study of dopamine D1 and D2 receptors and re-uptake sites. *Neurochirurgie*, **37**, 377–82.

Przedborski, S., Kostic, V., Jackson-Lewis, V. *et al.* (1992). Transgenic mice with increased Cu/Zn-superoxide dismutase activity are resistant to *N*-methyl-4-phenyl-1,2,3,6-tetrahydropyridine-induced neurotoxicity. *J. Neurosci.*, **12**, 1658–67.

Przedborski, S., Levivier, M., Jiang, H. *et al.* (1995). Dose-dependent lesions of the dopaminergic nigrostriatal pathway induced by intrastriatal injection of 6-hydroxydopamine. *Neuroscience*, **67**, 631–47.

Przedborski, S., Jackson-Lewis, V., Yokoyama, R., Shibata, T., Dawson, V. L. & Dawson, T. M. (1996). Role of neuronal nitric oxide in MPTP (1-methyl-4-phenyl-1,2,3,6-tetrahydropyridine)-induced dopaminergic neurotoxicity. *Proc. Natl Acad. Sci., USA*, **93**, 4565–71.

Przedborski, S., Jackson-Lewis, V., Djaldetti, R. *et al.* (2000). The parkinsonian toxin MPTP: action and mechanism. *Restor Neurol. Neurosci*, **16**, 135–42.

Przedborski, S., Chen, Q., Vila, M. *et al.* (2001a). Oxidative post-translational modifications of alpha-synuclein in the 1-methyl-4-phenyl-1,2,3,6-tetrahydropyridine (MPTP) mouse model of Parkinson's disease. *J. Neurochem.*, **76**, 637–40.

Przedborski, S., Jackson-Lewis, V., Naini, A. *et al.* (2001b). The parkinsonian toxin 1-methyl-4-phenyl-1,2,3,6-tetrahydropyridine (MPTP): a technical review of its utility and safety. *J. Neurochem.*, **76**, 1265–74.

Przedborski, S. & Vila, M. (2001). MPTP: A review of its mechanisms of neurotoxicity. *Clin. Neurosci. Res.*, **1**, 407–18.

Przedborski, S., Vila, M. & Jackson-Lewis, V. (2003). Series Introduction: Neurodegeneration: What is it and where are we? *J. Clin. Invest.*, **111**, 3–10.

Ramsay, R. R. & Singer, T. P. (1986). Energy-dependent uptake of *N*-methyl-4-phenylpyridinium, the neurotoxic metabolite of 1-methyl-4-phenyl-1,2,3,6-tetrahydropyridine, by mitochondria. *J. Biol. Chem.*, **261**, 7585–7.

Ramsay, R. R., Krueger, M. J., Youngster, S. K., Gluck, M. R., Casida, J. E. & Singer, T. P. (1991). Interaction of 1-methyl-4-phenylpyridinium ion (MPP$^+$) and its analogs with the rotenone/piericidin binding site of NADH dehydrogenase. *J. Neurochem.*, **56**, 1184–90.

Reynolds, D. S., Carter, R. J. & Morton, A. J. (1998). Dopamine modulates the susceptibility of striatal neurons to 3-nitropropionic acid in the rat model of Huntington's disease. *J. Neurosci.*, **18**, 10116–27.

Ricaurte, G. A., Sabol, K. E. & Seiden, L. S. (1994). Functional consequences of neurotoxic amphetamine exposure. In *Amphetamine and its Analogs. Psychopharmacology, Toxicology, and Abuse*, ed. A. K. Cho & D. S. Segal, pp. 297–313. New York: Academic Press.

Rodriguez, D. M., Abdala, P., Barroso-Chinea, P., Obeso, J. & Gonzalez-Hernandez, T. (2001). Motor behavioural changes after intracerebroventricular injection of 6-hydroxydopamine in the rat: an animal model of Parkinson's disease. *Behav. Brain Res.*, **122**, 79–92.

Rossetti, Z. L., Sotgiu, A., Sharp, D. E., Hadjiconstantinou, M. & Neff, M. (1988). 1-Methyl-4-phenyl-1,2,3,6-tetrahydropyridine (MPTP) and free radicals in vitro. *Biochem. Pharmacol.*, **37**, 4573–4.

Sanberg, P. R., Pisa, M. & McGeer, E. G. (1979). Strain differences and kainic acid neurotoxicity. *Brain Res.*, **166**, 431–5.

Sanberg, P. R., Calderon, S. F., Giordano, M., Tew, J. M. & Norman, A. B. (1989). The quinolinic acid model of Huntington's disease: locomotor abnormalities. *Exp. Neurol.*, **105**, 45–53.

Sanchez-Ramos, J. R. (1993). Toxin-induced parkinsonism. In *Parkinsonian Syndromes*, ed. M. B. Stern & W. C. Koller, pp. 155–71. New York: Marcel Dekker, Inc.

Saner, A. & Thoenen, H. (1971). Model experiments on the molecular mechanism of action of 6-hydroxydopamine. *Mol. Pharmacol.*, **7**, 147–54.

Saporito, M. S., Brown, E. M., Miller, M. S. & Carswell, S. (1999). CEP-1347/KT-7515, an inhibitor of c-jun N-terminal kinase activation, attenuates the 1-methyl-4-phenyl tetrahydropyridine-mediated loss of nigrostriatal dopaminergic neurons in vivo. *J. Pharmacol. Exp. Ther.*, **288**, 421–7.

Saporito, M. S., Thomas, B. A. & Scott, R. W. (2000). MPTP activates c-Jun NH(2)-terminal kinase (JNK) and its upstream regulatory kinase MKK4 in nigrostriatal neurons in vivo. *J. Neurochem.*, **75**, 1200–8.

Sauer, H. & Oertel, W. H. (1994). Progressive degeneration of nigrostriatal dopamine neurons following intrastriatal terminal lesions with 6-hydroxydopamine: a combined retrograde tracing and immunocytochemical study in the rat. *Neuroscience*, **59**, 401–15.

Schneider, J. S. & Roeltgen, D. P. (1993). Delayed matching-to-sample, object retrieval, and discrimination reversal deficits in chronic low dose MPTP-treated monkeys. *Brain Res.*, **615**, 351–4.

Schneider, J. S., Tinker, J. P., Van Velson, M., Menzaghi, F. & Lloyd, G. K. (1999). Nicotinic acetylcholine receptor agonist SIB-1508Y improves cognitive functioning in chronic low-dose MPTP-treated monkeys. *J. Pharmacol. Exp. Ther.*, **290**, 731–9.

Schuler, F. & Casida, J. E. (2001). Functional coupling of PSST and ND1 subunits in NADH: ubiquinone oxidoreductase established by photoaffinity labeling. *Biochim. Biophys. Acta*, **1506**, 79–87.

Schulz, J. B., Matthews, R. T., Jenkins, B. G., Brar, P. & Beal, M. F. (1995a). Improved therapeutic window for treatment of histotoxic hypoxia with a free radical spin trap. *J. Cereb. Blood Flow Metab.*, **15**, 948–52.

Schulz, J. B., Matthews, R. T., Muqit, M. M. K., Browne, S. E. & Beal, M. F. (1995b). Inhibition of neuronal nitric oxide synthase by 7-nitroindazole protects against MPTP-induced neurotoxicity in mice. *J. Neurochem.*, **64**, 936–9.

Schulz, J. B., Henshaw, D. R., MacGarvey, U. & Beal, M. F. (1996). Involvement of oxidative stress in 3-nitropropionic acid neurotoxicity. *Neurochem. Int.*, **29**, 167–71.

Schulz, J. B., Weller, M., Matthews, R. T. *et al.* (1998). Extended therapeutic window for caspase inhibition and synergy with MK-801 in the treatment of cerebral histotoxic hypoxia. *Cell Death Differ.*, **5**, 847–57.

Schwarcz, R. & Coyle, J. T. (1977). Striatal lesions with kainic acid: neurochemical characteristics. *Brain Res.*, **127**, 235–49.

Schwarcz, R., Scholz, D. & Coyle, J. T. (1978). Structure-activity relations for the neurotoxicity of kainic acid derivatives and glutamate analogues. *Neuropharmacology*, **17**, 145–51.

Schwarcz, R., Hokfelt, T., Fuxe, K., Jonsson, G., Goldstein, M. & Terenius, L. (1979). Ibotenic acid-induced neuronal degeneration:

a morphological and neurochemical study. *Exp. Brain Res.*, **37**, 199–216.

Scorza, M. C., Carrau, C., Silveira, R., Zapata-Torres, G., Cassels, B. K. & Reyes-Parada, M. (1997). Monoamine oxidase inhibitory properties of some methoxylated and alkylthio amphetamine derivatives: structure-activity relationships. *Biochem. Pharmacol.*, **54**, 1361–9.

Segal, D. S. & Kuczenski, R. (1994). Behavioral pharmacology of amphetamine. In *Amphetamine and its Analogs. Psychopharmacology, Toxicology, and Abuse*, ed. A. K. Cho & D. S. Segal, pp. 115–50. New York: Academic Press.

Seniuk, N. A., Tatton, W. G. & Greenwood, C. E. (1990). Dose-dependent destruction of the coeruleus-cortical and nigral-striatal projections by MPTP. *Brain Res.*, **527**, 7–20.

Sherman, B. E. & Chole, R. A. (2000). Sympathectomy, which induces membranous bone remodeling, has no effect on endochondral long bone remodeling in vivo. *J. Bone. Miner. Res.*, **15**, 1354–60.

Shimizu, K., Ohtaki, K., Matsubara, K. *et al.* (2001). Carrier-mediated processes in blood–brain barrier penetration and neural uptake of paraquat. *Brain Res.*, **906**, 135–42.

Smith, J. G. (1988). Paraquat poisoning by skin absorption: a review. *Hum. Toxicol.*, **7**, 15–19.

Snow, B. J., Vingerhoets, F. J., Langston, J. W., Tetrud, J. W., Sossi, V. & Calne, D. B. (2000). Pattern of dopaminergic loss in the striatum of humans with MPTP induced parkinsonism. *J. Neurol. Neurosurg. Psychiatry*, **68**, 313–16.

Sonsalla, P. K. & Heikkila, R. E. (1986). The influence of dose and dosing interval on MPTP-induced dopaminergic neurotoxicity in mice. *Eur. J. Pharmacol.*, **129**, 339–45.

Sonsalla, P. K., Jochnowitz, N. D., Zeevalk, G. D., Oostveen, J. A. & Hall, E. D. (1996). Treatment of mice with methamphetamine produces cell loss in the substantia nigra. *Brain Res.*, **738**, 172–5.

Sonsalla, P. K., Manzino, L., Sinton, C. M., Liang, C. L., German, D. C. & Zeevalk, G. D. (1997). Inhibition of striatal energy metabolism produces cell loss in the ipsilateral substantia nigra. *Brain Res.*, **773**, 223–6.

Staal, R. G. & Sonsalla, P. K. (2000). Inhibition of brain vesicular monoamine transporter (VMAT2) enhances 1-methyl-4-phenylpyridinium neurotoxicity in vivo in rat striata. *J. Pharmacol. Exp. Ther.*, **293**, 336–42.

Staal, R. G., Hogan, K. A., Liang, C. L., German, D. C. & Sonsalla, P. K. (2000). In vitro studies of striatal vesicles containing the vesicular monoamine transporter (VMAT2): rat versus mouse differences in sequestration of 1-methyl-4-phenylpyridinium. *J. Pharmacol. Exp. Ther.*, **293**, 329–35.

Storey, E., Hyman, B. T., Jenkins, B. *et al.* (1992). 1-Methyl-4-phenylpyridinium produces excitotoxic lesions in rat striatum as a result of impairment of oxidative metabolism. *J. Neurochem.*, **58**, 1975–8.

Sulzer, D., Maidment, N. T. & Rayport, S. (1993). Amphetamine and other weak bases act to promote reverse transport of dopamine in ventral midbrain neurons. *J. Neurochem.*, **60**, 527–35.

Sulzer, D., Chen, T.-K., Lau, Y. Y., Kristensen, H., Rayport, S. & Ewing, A. (1995). Amphetamine redistributes dopamine from synaptic vesicles to the cytosol and promotes reverse transport. *J. Neurosci.*, **15**, 4102–8.

Sun, Z., Xie, J. & Reiner, A. (2002). The differential vulnerability of striatal projection neurons in 3-nitropropionic acid-treated rats does not match that typical of adult-onset Huntington's disease. *Exp. Neurol.*, **176**, 55–65.

Takahashi, N., Miner, L. L., Sora, I. *et al.* (1997). VMAT2 knockout mice: heterozygotes display reduced amphetamine-conditioned reward, enhanced amphetamine locomotion, and enhanced MPTP toxicity. *Proc. Natl Acad. Sci., USA*, **94**, 9938–43.

Talpade, D. J., Greene, J. G., Higgins, D. S., Jr. & Greenamyre, J. T. (2000). In vivo labeling of mitochondrial complex I (NADH: ubiquinone oxidoreductase) in rat brain using [(3)H]dihydrorotenone. *J. Neurochem.*, **75**, 2611–21.

Tatton, N. A. & Kish, S. J. (1997). *In situ* detection of apoptotic nuclei in the substantia nigra compacta of 1-methyl-4-phenyl-1,2,3,6-tetrahydropyridine-treated mice using terminal deoxynucleotidyl transferase labelling and acridine orange staining. *Neuroscience*, **77**, 1037–48.

Teismann, P., Tieu, K., Choi, D. K. *et al.* (2003). Cyclooxygenase-2 is instrumental in Parkinson's disease neurodegeneration. *Proc. Natl Acad. Sci., USA*, **100**, 5473–8.

Tetrud, J. W., Langston, J. W., Redmond, D. E., Jr., Roth, R. H., Sladek, J. R. & Angel, R. W. (1986). MPTP-induced tremor in human and non-human primates. *Neurology*, **36 (suppl 1)**, 308.

Thiffault, C., Langston, J. W. & Di Monte, D. A. (2000). Increased striatal dopamine turnover following acute administration of rotenone to mice. *Brain Res.*, **885**, 283–8.

Thiruchelvam, M., Brockel, B. J., Richfield, E. K., Baggs, R. B. & Cory-Slechta, D. A. (2000a). Potentiated and preferential effects of combined paraquat and maneb on nigrostriatal dopamine systems: environmental risk factors for Parkinson's disease? *Brain Res.*, **873**, 225–34.

Thiruchelvam, M., Richfield, E. K., Baggs, R. B., Tank, A. W. & Cory-Slechta, D. A. (2000b). The nigrostriatal dopaminergic system as a preferential target of repeated exposures to combined paraquat and maneb: implications for Parkinson's disease. *J. Neurosci.*, **20**, 9207–14.

Thiruchelvam, M., McCormack, A., Richfield, E. K. *et al.* (2003). Age-related irreversible progressive nigrostriatal dopaminergic neurotoxicity in the paraquat and maneb model of the Parkinson's disease phenotype. *Eur. J. Neurosci.*, **18**, 589–600.

Tieu, K., Ischiropoulos, H. & Przedborski, S. (2003). Nitric oxide and reactive oxygen species in Parkinson's disease. *IUBMB Life*, **55**, 329–35.

Trimmer, P. A., Smith, T. S., Jung, A. B. & Bennett, J. P., Jr. (1996). Dopamine neurons from transgenic mice with a knockout of the p53 gene resist MPTP neurotoxicity. *Neurodegeneration*, **5**, 233–9.

Trulson, M. E., Cannon, M. S., Faegg, T. S. & Raese, J. D. (1985). Effects of chronic methamphetamine on the nigral-striatal dopamine system in rat brain: tyrosine hydroxylase immunochemistry and quantitative light microscopic studies. *Brain Res. Bull.*, **15**, 569–77.

Ungerstedt, U. (1968). 6-Hydroxydopamine induced degeneration of central monoamine neurons. *Eur. J. Pharmacol.*, **5**, 107–10.

(1971a). Adipsia and aphagia after 6-hydroxydopamine induced degeneration of the nigro-striatal dopamine system. *Acta Physiol. Scand. Suppl*, **367**, 95–122.

(1971b). Postsynaptique supersensitivity after 6-hydroxydopamine induced degeneration of the nigro-striatal system in the rat brain. *Acta Physiol. Scand.*, **Suppl**. 367, 69–93.

(1971c). Stereotaxic mapping of the monoamine pathways in the rat brain. *Acta Physiol. Scand.*, **Suppl**. 367, 1–48.

Ungerstedt, U. & Arbuthnott, G. (1970). Quantitative recording of rotational behaviour in rats after 6-hydroxydopamine lesions of the nigrostriatal dopamine system. *Brain Res.*, **24**, 485–93.

Vila, M., Jackson-Lewis, V., Vukosavic, S. *et al.* (2001a). Bax ablation prevents dopaminergic neurodegeneration in the 1-methyl-4-phenyl-1,2,3,6-tetrahydropyridine mouse model of Parkinson's disease. *Proc. Natl Acad. Sci., USA*, **98**, 2837–42.

Vila, M., Jackson Lewis, V., Guégan, C. *et al.* (2001b). The role of glial cells in Parkinson's disease. *Curr. Opin. Neurol.*, **14**, 483–9.

Vingerhoets, F. J., Snow, B. J., Tetrud, J. W., Langston, J. W., Schulzer, M. & Calne, D. B. (1994). Positron emission tomographic evidence for progression of human MPTP-induced dopaminergic lesions. *Ann. Neurol.*, **36**, 765–70.

Widdowson, P. S., Farnworth, M. J., Simpson, M. G. & Lock, E. A. (1996a). Influence of age on the passage of paraquat through the blood–brain barrier in rats: a distribution and pathological examination. *Hum. Exp. Toxicol.*, **15**, 231–6.

Widdowson, P. S., Farnworth, M. J., Upton, R. & Simpson, M. G. (1996b). No changes in behaviour, nigro-striatal system neurochemistry or neuronal cell death following toxic multiple oral paraquat administration to rats. *Hum. Exp. Toxicol.*, **15**, 583–91.

Wu, D. C., Jackson-Lewis, V., Vila, M. *et al.* (2002). Blockade of microglial activation is neuroprotective in the 1-methyl-4-phenyl-1,2,3,6-tetrahydropyridine mouse model of Parkinson disease. *J. Neurosci.*, **22**, 1763–71.

Wu, D. C., Teismann, P., Tieu, K. *et al.* (2003). NADPH oxidase mediates oxidative stress in the 1-methyl-4-phenyl-1,2,3,6-tetrahydropyridine model of Parkinson's disease. *Proc. Natl Acad. Sci., USA*, **100**, 6145–50.

Wullner, U., Young, A. B., Penney, J. B. & Beal, M. F. (1994). 3-Nitropropionic acid toxicity in the striatum. *J. Neurochem.*, **63**, 1772–81.

Xia, X. G., Schmidt, N., Teismann, P., Ferger, B. & Schulz, J. B. (2001). Dopamine mediates striatal malonate toxicity via dopamine

transporter-dependent generation of reactive oxygen species and D2 but not D1 receptor activation. *J. Neurochem.*, **79**, 63–70.

Yang, L., Matthews, R. T., Schulz, J. B. *et al.* (1998). 1-Methyl-4-phenyl-1,2,3,6-tetrahydropyride neurotoxicity is attenuated in mice overexpressing Bcl-2. *J. Neurosci.*, **18**, 8145–52.

Yoshida, M., Niwa, T. & Nagatsu, T. (1990). Parkinsonism in monkeys produced by chronic administration of an endogenous substance of the brain, tetrahydroisoquinoline: the behavioral and biochemical changes. *Neurosci. Lett.*, **119**, 109–13.

Yoshida, M., Ogawa, M., Suzuki, K. & Nagatsu, T. (1993). Parkinsonism produced by tetrahydroisoquinoline (TIQ) or the analogues. *Adv. Neurol.*, **60**, 207–11.

Yuan, J., Callahan, B. T., McCann, U. D. & Ricaurte, G. A. (2001). Evidence against an essential role of endogenous brain dopamine in methamphetamine-induced dopaminergic neurotoxicity. *J. Neurochem.*, **77**, 1338–47.

Yuan, J., Cord, B. J., McCann, U. D., Callahan, B. T. & Ricaurte, G. A. (2002). Effect of depleting vesicular and cytoplasmic dopamine on methylenedioxymethamphetamine neurotoxicity. *J. Neurochem.*, **80**, 960–9.

Zaczek, R., Nelson, M. F. & Coyle, J. T. (1978). Effects of anaesthetics and anticonvulsants on the action of kainic acid in the rat hippocampus. *Eur. J. Pharmacol.*, **52**, 323–7.

Zaczek, R., Simonton, S. & Coyle, J. T. (1980). Local and distant neuronal degeneration following intrastriatal injection of kainic acid. *J. Neuropathol. Exp. Neurol.*, **39**, 245–64.

Zaczek, R., Culp, S. & De Souza, E. B. (1991a). Interactions of [3H]amphetamine with rat brain synaptosomes. II. Active transport. *J. Pharmacol. Exp. Ther.*, **257**, 830–5.

Zaczek, R., Culp, S., Goldberg, H., Mccann, D. J. & De Souza, E. B. (1991b). Interactions of [3H]amphetamine with rat brain synaptosomes. I. Saturable sequestration. *J. Pharmacol. Exp. Ther.*, **257**, 820–9.

Zeevalk, G. D., Derr-Yellin, E. & Nicklas, W. J. (1995). NMDA receptor involvement in toxicity to dopamine neurons in vitro caused by the succinate dehydrogenase inhibitor 3-nitropropionic acid. *J. Neurochem.*, **64**, 455–8.

Zeevalk, G. D., Manzino, L., Hoppe, J. & Sonsalla, P. (1997). In vivo vulnerability of dopamine neurons to inhibition of energy metabolism. *Eur. J. Pharmacol.*, **320**, 111–19.

Zigmond, M. J., Abercrombie, E. D., Berger, T. W., Grace, A. A. & Stricker, E. M. (1990). Compensations after lesions of the central dopaminergic neurons: some clinical and basic implications. *Trends Neurosci.*, **13**, 290–6.

Zubrycki, E. M., Emerich, D. F. & Sanberg, P. R. (1990). Sex differences in regulatory changes following quinolinic acid-induced striatal lesions. *Brain Res. Bull.*, **25**, 633–7.

17

A genetic outline of the pathways to cell death in Alzheimer's disease, Parkinson's disease, frontal dementias and related disorders

John Hardy

Laboratory of Neurogenetics, National Institute on Aging, National Institutes of Health, Bethesda, MD, USA

Over the last 10 years, genetic and pathological analysis has allowed the dissection of the major pathways to cell death in Alzheimer's disease, Pick's disease and Lewy body disease. The central findings are these.

First, the pathology of Alzheimer's disease consists of plaques, made of the Aβ peptide, derived from the APP protein, and neurofibrillary tangles made of the tau protein: Lewy bodies, made of the synuclein protein, are a frequent, but not invariant pathology of Alzheimer's disease (Hansen & Samuel, 1997).

Second, all pathogenic mutations in the APP and presenilin genes alter APP metabolism such that more of the peptide, Aβ42, is produced (Hardy & Selkoe, 2002). These data suggest that Aβ is the primary molecule in the pathogenic cascade for Alzheimer's disease and that tau dysfunction and tangle formation are a necessary downstream event in disease pathogenesis and that α-synuclein dysfunction and Lewy body formation are an occasional downstream event in disease pathogenesis.

Third, mutations in the tau gene causes some frontal temporal dementias and other entities in which tau is deposited (Hutton et al., 1998). In some sporadic tangle disorders, the tau haplotype is a risk factor for disease (Baker et al., 1999). These data suggest that cell death and dementia are a consequence of tau dysfunction and tangle formation (Hardy et al., 1998).

Fourth, mutations in the α-synuclein gene cause Parkinson's disease and other entities in which α-synuclein is deposited (Polymeropoulos et al., 1997). In sporadic Lewy body disorders, the α-synuclein haplotype is a risk factor for disease (Farrer et al., 2001a). These data suggest that cell death and dementia are a consequence of synuclein dysfunction and Lewy body formation.

Fifth, transgenic mice in which only Aβ levels are manipulated show plaque deposition, but only marginal cell loss (Irizarry et al., 1997) and a subtle behavioral phenotype

(Morgan et al., 2000): however, mice which have been primed for either tangle formation through a mutant tau transgene (Lewis et al., 2000), or primed for α-synuclein pathology with an α-synuclein transgene (Masliah et al., 2000), show much more fulminant pathology and cell loss (Lewis et al., 2001; Masliah et al., 2001), which, certainly in the case of the tau transgene, closely resembles the full pathology of Alzheimer's disease including the cell loss.

All of these genetic data, pathological data and data derived from mouse models can be incorporated into a remarkably simple scheme shown in Fig. 17.1, or represented by two alternate pathways for cell death shown in Figs. 17.2 and 17.3.

These skeletal pathways of pathogenesis are useful because they suggest points at which therapy might be aimed; however, they also provide a framework within which to discuss the many gaps in our knowledge.

Gaps in our knowledge

There are many gaps in our knowledge. It is most convenient to organize these gaps in a hierarchical fashion.

First, to what extent do the entities represent single pathogenic processes?

For Alzheimer's disease, the answer seems clear; the disease process seems to be similar in all cases since, with few exceptions, the final pathology is the same. For frontal dementias, the relationship between clinical phenotypes and pathogenesis is much less clear: some frontal dementias appear to have different pathologies and may therefore have either completely different, or may have overlapping pathogeneses. Conversely, some tangle disorders show no tau association or mutations suggesting that there are other

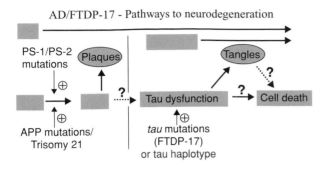

AD/FTDP-17 - Pathways to neurodegeneration

Fig. 17.1 Diagram showing the hierarchical relationship between APP/Aβ/plaques, tau/tangles and cell death based on observations in families with hereditary disease and on transgenic mouse models.

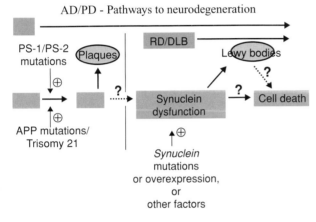

AD/PD - Pathways to neurodegeneration

Fig. 17.2 Diagram showing the hierarchical relationship between APP/Aβ/plaques, α-synuclein/Lewy bodies and cell death based on observations in families with hereditary disease and on transgenic mouse models.

routes to this final pathway. Finally, for Parkinson's disease, the answer is extremely unclear: while some mutations in the parkin gene lead to disease with Lewy body pathology (suggesting a common pathogenesis: Farrer *et al.*, 2001b), the majority do not: thus, determining whether all cases of Parkinson's disease share a single pathogenic process is not yet possible.

Second: what other genes are involved in disease pathogeneses?

The answer to this question is dependent on the answers to the issues of whether the entities are single pathogenic entities, or multiple entities. Since the evidence is that Alzheimer's disease is indeed a single pathogenic entity, the strong suggestion is that any genetic loci which contribute to the familial clustering of late onset Alzheimer's

disease should be involved in Aβ production or clearance, as apolipoprotein E appears to be (Bales *et al.*, 1999). For frontal dementias, there are at least two extant linkages to chromosomes 9 and 3 (Hosler *et al.*, 2000; Brown *et al.*, 1995) but the pathology does not seem to involve tau, and thus the question as to whether identification of this gene will directly aid in developing an understanding of the tau pathway to cell death remains open. For Parkinson's disease, there are seven extant genetic linkages (Gwinn-Hardy *et al.*, 2002): in the absence of detailed neuropathological descriptions of the characteristics of these forms of Parkinson's disease, the pathogeneses of these forms of disease, relative to the synuclein pathway outlined above, remains uncertain.

Third, what are the relationships between the molecules involved in these pathogenic processes?

The outlined pathogenic pathways shown in Figs. 17.1 and 17.2 show clearly the deficits in our knowledge: perhaps most clearly, we do not know the nature of the interaction between Aβ or either tau or α-synuclein. However, at least we now have animal models in which these important issues can be probed.

Fourth, what are the toxic species of these pathogenic molecules?

The plaque, the tangle, and the Lewy body are the pathological hallmarks of these prevalent diseases and these lesions certainly mark damaged and dying neurons. It is not clear, however, whether these lesions are themselves damaging or merely relatively harmless space filling accumulations of material. While most recent data suggests that Aβ oligomers, rather than plaques, may be the primary pathogenic species, it is difficult to believe that the disruption to neuronal circuitry evident in a neuritic plaque is benign: perhaps, the Aβ deposited within the plaque acts as a reservoir for the toxic species. Similarly, it is not clear the extent to which tangles and Lewy bodies are damaging species or whether they too are "just" space-filling inert lesions and reflect dysfunction of the cognate protein. However, when one sees electron micrographs of neurons with tangles in them, it is difficult to imagine that they are benign since they can fill up one-third of the cells volume and apparently block off the axon hillock (Sumpter *et al.*, 1986). With respect to Lewy bodies, while one might previously have hypothesized that their formation reflects a disruption of normal α-synuclein function, the fact that individuals with a triplication of the α-synuclein locus develop severe Parkinson's disease with extensive Lewy body formation (Singleton *et al.*, 2003) does not easily fit with the notion that the problem is caused by a lack of normal α-synuclein function. In both these cases it would seem likely that the visible pathological lesions contribute to the problem, although the possibility that pathologic oligomers contribute to the cellular dysfunction cannot be ruled out.

Experimental therapies based on the amyloid cascade hypothesis

The disease schemes outlined in Figs. 17.1 and 17.2 lead directly to suggestions concerning potential points of intervention. For Alzheimer's disease, if disease initiation represents the effects of a chronic imbalance between Aβ production and Aß clearance, there are several ways in which the disease may be treated. Five broad strategies have been proposed with this idea in mind.

First, one could attempt to partially inhibit either of the two proteases, ß- and γ-secretase, that generate Aß from APP. In the case of the former enzyme, compound screening and medicinal chemistry are being vigorously pursued to identify potent small molecule inhibitors that can fit the large active site of this aspartyl protease and still penetrate the blood brain barrier. In the case of the latter, potent membrane-permeable inhibitors are already in hand, but their testing in humans has barely been attempted, in light of the theoretical concern that most such compounds might interfere importantly with signaling by Notch proteins and other cell surface receptors which would likely lead to serious disorders in turn (Haass & DeStrooper, 1999).

Second, one could attempt to prevent the oligomerization of Aß or enhance its clearance from the cortex. This approach is exemplified by the use of active or passive Aß immunization, in which antibodies to Aß decrease cerebral levels of the peptide by promoting microglial clearance (Schenk *et al.*, 1999; Bard *et al.*, 2000) and/or by redistributing the peptide from the brain to the systemic circulation (DeMattos *et al.*, 2002). Although active immunization with synthetic Aß1–42 peptide produces robust benefits in APP transgenic mice without detectable toxicity, the recent extension of this approach to AD patients resulted in a small but unacceptable fraction of the study subjects developing a usually transient CNS inflammatory reaction which, in a few cases, was fatal (Nicoll *et al.*, 2003), precluding further testing with this preparation. Of note, those who were enrolled in the clinical trial surely had a significant plaque and tangle burden: it is possible that if this treatment were possible very early, even presymptomatically in the course, this unacceptable adverse effect could be

avoidable. Analysis of a subset of Aß immunized patients suggested that the treatment may have slowed disease progression (Hock *et al.*, 2003) although definitive conclusions on this await the report of the analysis of the whole trial (Winblad & Blum, 2003). Several alternative preparations intended to provide Aß antibodies by either active or passive routes have been formulated (e.g. Weiner *et al.*, 2000), and one or more of these is likely to reach clinical testing before long.

The third broad approach to the treatment of Alzheimer's disease is anti-inflammatory. This strategy was initiated based on evidence that a cellular inflammatory response in the cortex is elicited by the progressive accumulation of Aß (Rogers *et al.*, 2002). Additionally, it has recently been shown that some anti-inflammatory drugs may have direct effects on the cleavage of APP by γ-secretase, independent of their inhibition of cyclo-oxygenase 2 and other inflammatory mediators (Weggen *et al.*, 2003). Some such drugs have been shown to reduce cytopathology in APP transgenic mice (Lim *et al.*, 2001; Jantzen *et al.*, 2002).

The fourth approach is based on modulating cholesterol homeostasis (Burns & Duff, 2003). Chronic use of cholesterol-lowering drugs has recently been associated with a lower incidence of AD (Wolozin *et al.*, 2000; Jick *et al.*, 2000). Concurrently, high cholesterol diets have been shown to increase Aβ pathology in animals (Sparks *et al.*, 2000; Refolo *et al.*, 2001), and cholesterol-lowering drugs have been shown to reduce pathology in APP transgenic mice (Refolo *et al.*, 2000). These effects seem to be caused by a direct (though poorly understood) effect of cholesterol on APP processing (Fassbender *et al.*, 2001; Wahrle *et al.*, 2002). A particular advantage of this approach is that statin drugs are generally well tolerated and have already been widely prescribed. Again, clinical trials are under way.

The fifth approach is based on the surprising observation that Aß aggregation is, in part, dependent on Cu^{2+} and Zn^{2+} ions (Bush *et al.*, 1994). This has led to the suggestion that chelation of these ions may have therapeutic potential and clinical trials of such a chelating agent, clioquinol, which has been used "successfully" in the transgenic model (Cherny *et al.*, 2001), are currently under way.

Another approach would be to try and break the link between Aß and tangle formation: this approach has only been amenable to experimental attack since the development of mice in which both pathologies occur (Lewis *et al.*, 2001). One approach which may have merit is to inhibit glycogen synthase kinase-3β as this seems to be one of the key enzymes involved in tau phosphorylation and this seems to be a key initiator of tangle formation (Takashima *et al.*, 1998). While inhibiting tangle formation would have the potential merit of being a useful therapeutic approach for other diseases such as progressive supranuclear palsy as well as for Alzheimer's disease, it has the potential drawback of allowing other routes to cell death, such as the α-synuclein pathway, come into operation.

Conclusions

We are at a pivotal point in research into neurodegenerative diseases: currently, all the therapies for these diseases are based are transmitter replacement approaches and not at dealing with underlying pathogenic mechanisms. Now, especially for Alzheimer's disease, but increasingly for the other diseases reviewed above, we are beginning to understand the mechanisms underlying cell death and to believe that we can alter these underlying mechanisms: over the next few years, it is to be hoped that this apparent understanding does indeed lead to a radically different, and more mechanistic approach to therapy for these devastating and prevalent disorders.

REFERENCES

Baker, M., Litvan, I., Houlden, H. *et al.* (1999). Association of an extended haplotype in the tau gene with progressive supranuclear palsy. *Hum. Mol. Genet.*, **8**(4), 711–15.

Bales, K. R., Verina, T., Cummins, D. J. *et al.* (1999). Apolipoprotein E is essential for amyloid deposition in the APP (V717F) transgenic mouse model of Alzheimer's disease. *Proc. Natl Acad. Sci., USA*, **96**, 15233–8.

Bard, F., Cannon, C., Barbour, R. *et al.* (2000). Peripherally administered antibodies against amyloid beta-peptide enter the central nervous system and reduce pathology in a mouse model of Alzheimer disease. *Nat. Med.*, **6**, 916–19.

Brown, J., Ashworth, A., Gydesen, S. *et al.* (1995). Familial nonspecific dementia maps to chromosome 3. *Hum. Mol. Genet.*, **4**, 1625–8.

Burns, M. & Duff, K. (2003). Use of in vivo models to study the role of cholesterol in the etiology of Alzheimer's disease. *Neurochem. Res.*, **28**(7), 979–86.

Bush, A. I., Pettingell, W. H., Multhaup, G. *et al.* (1994). Rapid induction of Alzheimer A beta amyloid formation by zinc. *Science*, **265**, 1464–7.

Cherny, R. A., Atwood, C. S., Xilinas, M. E. *et al.* (2001). Treatment with a copper–zinc chelator markedly and rapidly inhibits beta-amyloid accumulation in Alzheimer's disease transgenic mice. *Neuron*, **30**, 665–76.

DeMattos, R. B., Bales, K. R., Cummins, D. J., Paul, S. M. & Holtzman, D. M. (2002). Brain to plasma amyloid-beta efflux: a measure of brain amyloid burden in a mouse model of Alzheimer's disease. *Science*, **295**, 2264–7.

Farrer, M., Maraganore, D. M., Lockhart, P. *et al.* (2001a). Alpha-synuclein gene haplotypes are associated with Parkinson's disease. *Hum. Mol. Genet.*, **10**, 1847–51.

Farrer, M., Chan, P., Chen, R. *et al.* (2001b). Lewy bodies and parkinsonism in families with parkin mutations. *Ann. Neurol.*, **50**(3), 293–300.

Fassbender, K., Simons, M., Bergmann, C. *et al.* (2001). Simvastatin strongly reduces levels of Alzheimer's disease beta-amyloid peptides Abeta 42 and Abeta 40 in vitro and in vivo. *Proc. Natl Acad. Sci., USA*, **98**, 5856–61.

Gwinn-Hardy, K. (2002). Genetics of parkinsonism. *Mov. Disord.*, **17**(4), 645–56.

Haass, C. & De Strooper, B. (1999). The presenilins in Alzheimer's disease – proteolysis holds the key. *Science*, **286**, 916–19.

Hansen, L. A. & Samuel, W. (1997). Criteria for Alzheimer's disease and the nosology of dementia with Lewy bodies. *Neurology*, **48**(1), 126–32.

Hardy, J. & Selkoe, D. J. (2002). The amyloid hypothesis of Alzheimer's disease: progress and problems on the road to therapeutics. *Science*, **297**, 353–6.

Hardy, J. & Duff, K., Gwinn-Hardy, K., Pérez-Tur, J. & Hutton, M. (1998). Genetic dissection of Alzheimer's disease and related dementias: amyloid and its relationship to tau. *Nat. Neurosci.*, **1**, 95–9.

Hock, C., Konietzko, U., Streffer, J. R. *et al.* (2003). Antibodies against beta-amyloid slow cognitive decline in Alzheimer's disease. *Neuron*, **38**, 547–54.

Hosler, B. A., Siddique, T., Sapp, P. C. *et al.* (2000). Linkage of familial amyotrophic lateral sclerosis with frontotemporal dementia to chromosome 9q21–q22. *J. Am. Med. Assoc.*, **284**(13), 1664–9.

Hutton, M., Lendon, C. L., Rizzu, P. *et al.* (1998). Association of missense and 5′-splice-site mutations in tau with the inherited dementia FTDP-17. *Nature*, **393**(6686), 702–5.

Irizarry, M. C., Soriano, F., McNamara, M. *et al.* (1997). Abeta deposition is associated with neuropil changes, but not with overt neuronal loss in the human amyloid precursor protein V717F (PDAPP) transgenic mouse. *J. Neurosci.*, **17**, 7053–9.

Jick, H., Zornberg, G. L., Jick, S. S., Seshadri, S. & Drachman, D. A. (2000). Statins and the risk of dementia. *Lancet*, **356**, 1627–31.

Lewis, J., McGowan, E., Rockwood, J. *et al.* (2000). Neurofibrillary tangles, amyotrophy and progressive motor disturbance in mice expressing mutant (P301L) tau protein. *Nat. Genet.*, **25**, 402–5.

Lewis, J., Dickson, D. W., Lin, W. L. *et al.* (2001). Enhanced neurofibrillary degeneration in transgenic mice expressing mutant tau and APP. *Science*, **293**, 1487–91.

Lim, G. P., Yang, F., Chu, T. *et al.* (2001). Ibuprofen effects on Alzheimer pathology and open field activity in APPsw transgenic mice. *Neurobiol. Aging*, **22**, 983–91.

Masliah, E., Rockenstein, E., Veinbergs, I. *et al.* (2000). Dopaminergic loss and inclusion body formation in alpha-synuclein mice: implications for neurodegenerative disorders. *Science*, **287**, 1265–9.

Masliah, E., Rockenstein, E., Veinbergs, I. *et al.* (2001). Beta-amyloid peptides enhance alpha-synuclein accumulation and neuronal deficits in a transgenic mouse model linking Alzheimer's disease and Parkinson's disease. *Proc. Natl Acad. Sci. USA.*, **98**, 12245–50.

Morgan, D., Diamond, D. M., Gottschall, P. *et al.* (2000). Vaccination with Aß peptide prevents memory deficits in an animal model of Alzheimer's disease. *Nature*, **408**, 982–5.

Nicoll, J. A., Wilkinson, D., Holmes, C., Steart, P., Markham, H. & Weller, R. O. (2003). Neuropathology of human Alzheimer disease after immunization with amyloid-beta peptide: a case report. *Nat Med.*, **9**, 448–52.

Polymeropoulos, M. H., Lavedan, C., Leroy, E. *et al.* (1997). Mutation in the alpha-synuclein gene identified in families with Parkinson's disease. *Science*, **276**, 2045–7.

Refolo, L. M., Malester, B., LaFrancois, J. *et al.* (2000). Hypercholesterolemia accelerates the Alzheimer's amyloid pathology in a transgenic mouse model. *Neurobiol Dis.*, **7**, 321–31.

Refolo, L. M., Pappolla, M. A., LaFrancois, J. *et al.* (2001). A cholesterol-lowering drug reduces beta-amyloid pathology in a transgenic mouse model of Alzheimer's disease. *Neurobiol. Dis.*, **8**(5), 890–9.

Rogers, J., Strohmeyer, R., Kovelowski, C. J. & Li, R. (2002). Microglia and inflammatory mechanisms in the clearance of amyloid beta peptide. *Glia*, **40**(2), 260–9.

Schenk, D., Barbour, R., Dunn, W. *et al.* (1999). Immunization with amyloid-beta attenuates Alzheimer-disease-like pathology in the PDAPP mouse. *Nature*, **400**, 173–7.

Singleton, A. B., Farrer, M., Johnson, J. *et al.* (2003). α-Synuclein locus triplication causes Parkinson's disease. *Science*, **302**, 841.

Sparks, D. L., Martin, T. A., Gross, D. R. & Hunsaker, J. C. 3rd. (2000). Link between heart disease, cholesterol, and Alzheimer's disease: a review. *Microsi. Res. Tech.*, **50**, 287–90.

Sumpter, P. Q., Mann, D. M., Davies, C. A., Yates, P. O., Snowden, J. S. & Neary, D. (1986). An ultrastructural analysis of the effects of accumulation of neurofibrillary tangle in pyramidal neurons of the cerebral cortex in Alzheimer's disease. *Neuropathol. Appl. Neurobiol.*, **12**(3), 305–19.

Takashima, A., Honda, T., Yasutake, K. *et al.* (1998). Activation of tau protein kinase I/glycogen synthase kinase-3β by amyloid beta peptide (25–35) enhances phosphorylation of tau in hippocampal neurons. *Neurosci. Res.*, **31**(4), 317–23.

Wahrle, S., Das, P., Nyborg, A. C. *et al.* (2002). Cholesterol-dependent gamma-secretase activity in buoyant cholesterol-rich membrane microdomains. *Neurobiol. Dis.*, **9**, 11–23.

Weggen, S., Eriksen, J. L., Sagi, S. A. *et al.* (2003). Evidence that nonsteroidal anti-inflammatory drugs decrease Abeta 42 production by direct modulation of gamma – secretase activity. *J. Biol. Chem.*, **278**(34), 31831–7.

Weiner, H. L., Lemere, C. A., Maron, R. *et al.* (2000). Nasal administration of amyloid-beta peptide decreases cerebral amyloid burden in a mouse model of Alzheimer's disease. *Ann. Neurol.*, **48**, 567–79.

Winblad, B. & Blum, K. I. (2003). Hints of a therapeutic vaccine for Alzheimer's? *Neuron*, **38**, 517–18.

Wolozin, B., Kellman, W., Ruosseau, P., Celesia, G. G. & Siegel, G. (2000). Decreased prevalence of Alzheimer disease associated with 3-hydroxy-3-methyglutaryl coenzyme A reductase inhibitors. *Arch. Neurol.*, **57**, 1439–43.

18

Neurophysiology of Parkinson's disease, levodopa-induced dyskinesias, dystonia, Huntington's disease and myoclonus

Antonio Currà, Rocco Agostino and Alfredo Berardelli

Department of Neurological Sciences and I.N.M. Neuromed IRCCS, University of Rome "La Sapienza", Italy

Introduction

Movement disorders are a disease group related to functional or structural abnormalities of the basal ganglia.

The term "basal ganglia" refers to the following structures: the striatum (caudate and putamen), globus pallidus (internal and external segments, GPi and GPe), subthalamic nucleus, and substantia nigra (SN) (SN pars compacta, SNpc, and SN pars reticulata, SNpr). The striatum receives connections from specific cortical areas and from the SNpc; the basal ganglia output nuclei, the GPi and SNpr, exert an inhibitory effect on the thalamus. Diminished phasic activity in the GPi/SNpr disinhibits the thalamus thus facilitating cortical motor areas, whereas increased phasic activity in the GPi/SNpr causes the opposite effect. The GPi–SNpr inhibition of the thalamus is modulated through two parallel pathways. According to the classical model of basal ganglia functioning (Albin *et al.*, 1989; Alexander & Crutcher, 1990; Alexander *et al.*, 1990; De Long, 1990; Parent & Hazarati, 1995; Wichmann & De Long, 1996) the first is an inhibitory "direct" pathway that originates in the striatum and projects directly onto the GPi/SNr; the second is an "indirect" inhibitory pathway that crosses the GPe and subthalamic nucleus to project indirectly onto the GPi/SNpr. Activation of the direct pathway tends to disinhibit the thalamus. Activation of the indirect pathway disinhibits the subthalamic nucleus thereby increasing GPi/SNpr excitation thus resulting in increased thalamic inhibition: the two parallel circuits have an opposing action on the GPi/SNr and hence on the thalamus. The direct pathway plays a positive feedback role on central motor areas and facilitates movement; the indirect pathway plays a negative feedback role and suppresses unwanted motor activity (Fig. 18.1).

Because movement disorders present with distinct clinical features, they can usually be differentiated on clinical grounds alone. The role of neurophysiological techniques in the clinical setting is chiefly to provide supplementary information in atypical cases and in patients in whom clinical features alone fail to specify the precise movement disorder.

The most prominent role of neurophysiological techniques is to increase our understanding of the mechanisms and pathophysiology underlying these diseases. A review of all neurophysiological studies in neurodegenerative diseases is beyond the scope of a single chapter, and certain specifics are covered in chapters discussing individual diseases in detail. In this chapter we therefore chose to review the neurophysiological findings and the results obtained from neurosurgical interventions in patients with Parkinson's disease (and levodopa-induced dyskinesias), dystonia, Huntington's disease, and myoclonus. Readers will find additional information in the tables summarizing the currently available neurophysiological tests (Table 18.1) and their use in neurodegenerative disorders (Table 18.2).

We based our selection of the topics to review on the two criteria. First, the importance and the greater understanding of the disease; second, the conditions we have chosen serve as examples of the use of some electrophysiological techniques and the insights that they provide.

Parkinson's disease (PD)

Parkinson's disease is a neurodegenerative disease primarily due to the progressive loss of neurons in the pars compacta of the substantia nigra. The main motor symptoms of PD are bradykinesia, rigidity and tremor.

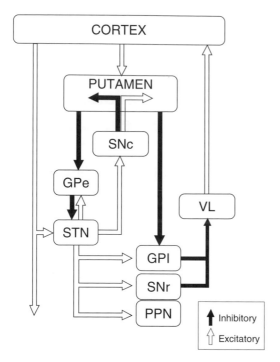

Fig. 18.1 Physiological model of the basal ganglia thalamo-cortical motor circuit under normal conditions. Indirect and direct pathways from the striatum are labeled. GPe and GPi, external and internal segments, respectively, of the globus pallidus; PPN pedunculopontine nucleus; SNc, substantia nigra pars compacta; SNr, substantia nigra pars reticulata; STN, subthalamic nucleus; VL ventrolateral thalamus.

Neurophysiological findings obtained in experimental parkinsonism and in patients undergoing surgery

In patients with PD an abnormal output from the basal ganglia generates error signals. Recordings from GPi and STN cells show hyperactivity in patients off-medication and reduced rates after dopaminergic activation by apomorphine injection. Conversely, GPe cells fire at low rates in the off-medication period, and the rates increase when patients are on-medication (Hutchison *et al.*, 1997, 1998; Stephani *et al.*, 1997). Increased output from the GPi neurons modifies the activity in the thalamo-cortical neurons and consequently in the cortical motor areas (Berardelli *et al.*, 2001; Marsden & Obeso, 1994).

Important physiological measures of basal ganglia function include not only the absolute level of discharges but also the temporal and spatial pattern of output from GPi and SNpr (Berardelli *et al.*, 1998). A normal discharge pattern might help focus cortical activation so that appropriate muscles are activated and others suppressed during performance of a task. In Parkinson's disease, the temporal variability of pallidal discharges increases, and discharges tend to be more synchronized between distant cells in parkinsonian patients than in the healthy state.

Bradykinesia: EMG, movement studies, sensorimotor integration studies, movement-related potentials, transcranial magnetic stimulation

To investigate the causes of bradykinesia, EMG and kinematic recording techniques (trajectories, velocity, and acceleration) have been used to study patients with PD during voluntary movement tasks (Berardelli & Currà, 2002; Berardelli *et al.*, 2001). The movements studied are classically of two types: simple movements (performed under isometric or isotonic conditions and by activating a single joint) and complex movements (combination of several simple movements executed sequentially or simultaneously).

In normal subjects performing rapid simple voluntary movements, EMG recordings from agonist and antagonists muscles show three successive phases of activity forming a "triphasic pattern": the first "burst" of activity in the agonist muscles (AG1) produces the force required to move the limb, the second antagonist (ANT) muscle burst stops the movement at the desired point, and the third antagonist muscle burst (AG2) serves mainly to stabilize the limb when it approaches the target point. This triphasic pattern originates in the central nervous system and is modulated by inputs of various origins. Parkinsonian patients perform "simple" rapid movements with cycles of multiple EMG "bursts" and are slower than normal subjects in initiating and performing movements (Berardelli *et al.*, 2001; Hallett & Khoshbin, 1980). The AG1 "burst" is insufficient not because the production mechanism saturates but because patients are unable to adapt activation to movement amplitude ("scaling" defect) (Berardelli *et al.*, 1986b). Patients with PD tend to compensate the defective activation of AG1 with multiple EMG activations (Fig. 18.2).

Simple clinical observation of parkinsonian patients suggests as a key feature of their motor disorder abnormal performance of "complex" movements (Agostino *et al.*, 1998). Defects have been reported in simultaneous isotonic elbow flexion and isometric thumb and finger oppositions. Unlike normal subjects, patients with PD accomplish single movements executed separately faster than the same single movements executed simultaneously (Benecke *et al.*, 1986, 1987). Baseline hypometria also worsens when patients are distracted by a second simultaneous non-motor task (for example a lexical decision). Hence the difficulty in executing simultaneous movements is not simply due to

Table 18.1. Neurophysiological investigations for neurodegenerative disorders

Neurophysiological test	Description
Accelerometry and EMG analysis of tremor	Frequency and amplitude recordings of tremor by devices applied to the trembling body parts; surface EMG recording of the activity evoked in at least two antagonistic muscles involved in the tremor
Resetting of tremor rhythm	Resetting of tremor rhythm at accelerometry and EMG following various perturbing events (muscle stretch, mechanical perturbation, electrical stimulation of peripheral nerves, transcranial electric or magnetic stimulation)
EMG analysis of fast single joint movements	Surface recording of agonist and antagonist muscles acting at the joint
EMG analysis of involuntary movements	Surface EMG recording of the activity evoked in the muscle involved in the involuntary movement
EMG analysis of external anal sphincter	Needle recording of motor unit potentials in the external anal sphincter
Blink reflex excitability	Surface recording of the R2 component of the blink reflex from the orbicularis oculi muscles following paired electrical stimuli at various interstimulus intervals (ISI) or electrical repetitive single stimuli delivered at fixed rate
Facial reflexes to upper limb stimulation	Simultaneous EMG recording in upper and lower facial muscles of the activity evoked by electrical stimulation of the median nerve at the wrist
Auditory startle responses	Surface EMG recording in various cranial and limb muscles of the responses evoked by high-intensity auditory stimuli which differ randomly in tonal frequency and intensity, and delivered at very long ISIs (minutes)
Reciprocal inhibition	EMG recording of the H reflex in forearm flexor muscles conditioned by a radial nerve stimulus delivered at various ISIs
Stretch reflexes and long-latency reflexes	EMG recording in limb muscle of the activity evoked by muscle stretching or electrical stimulation of a mixed/cutaneous nerve
Motor potential (MEP) evoked by transcranial magnetic stimulation (TMS)	EMG recording of the compound motor action potential evoked by TMS of the motor cortex
TMS-induced silent period	Period of inactivity in the EMG recordings during voluntary contraction induced by single pulse TMS of the motor cortex
Intracortical inhibition to paired-pulse TMS	MEP size reduction following paired pulse TMS at short (1–5 ms) or long (100–150 ms) ISIs
Premotor potentials	Slow rising negative EEG waves recorded from the scalp before the onset of a self-paced voluntary movement (Bereitshaftpotential), or between the warning and the go signal in a reaction time paradigm (Contingent Negative Variation)
EEG analysis of myoclonus with or without back-averaging	Scalp recording of the EEG activity simultaneous or preceding the myoclonus detected by polygraphic EMG
Somatosensory, visual and auditory evoked potentials	Averaged scalp recordings of cortical and subcortical activity evoked by peripheral multimodal sensory stimuli
Autonomic nervous system testing	Specific tests designed to investigate the autonomic function in the cardiovascular, genito-urinary, gastrointestinal, cutaneous, and ocular districts

altered planning of two simultaneous movements. Similar abnormalities are seen for sequential movements (Benecke *et al.*, 1987; Berardelli *et al.*, 1986a). When patients with PD perform short motor sequences of various types, movement times are longer for each movement in the sequence than for the same movement performed separately. An abnormally long interval also elapses between the end of one movement and the beginning of the next, showing a defect in assembling two sequential motor programs. The difficulty in producing sequential movements (improved by dopaminergic treatment) becomes increasingly evident as the motor sequence progresses (sequence effect) and involves passing from one movement to the next (Agostino *et al.*, 1992, 1994).

Studies of sequential finger oppositions in patients with PD show that bradykinesia impairs individual more than non-individual finger movements (Agostino *et al.*, 2003). Patients perform these movements slowly and with

Table 18.2. Neurophysiological investigations in neurodegenerative movement disorders

Disease	Neurophysiological test	Expected finding
Parkinson's disease	Tremor accelerometry	Measure of tremor frequency
	EMG analysis of tremor	Alternating, co-contracting pattern
	Postural tremor resetting	By mechanical, peripheral electric, transcranial electric and magnetic stimulation
	EMG analysis of fast single joint movement	Defective scaling of the first agonist burst
	EMG analysis of external anal sphincter	May be neurogenic in longstanding patients
	Blink reflex excitability	Enhanced
	Auditory startle responses	Delayed
	Reciprocal inhibition	Abnormally modulated before movement
	Long-latency and stretch reflexes	Enhanced amplitude
	Premotor potentials	Reduced amplitude
	Central motor conduction time to TMS	Normal
	TMS-induced silent period	Shortened
	Intracortical inhibition to paired-pulse TMS	
	Autonomic nervous system testing	Abnormal
Corticobasal degeneration	EMG analysis of external anal sphincter	Neurogenic
	Blink reflex excitability	Normal
	Somatosensory evoked potentials	Abnormal or absent frontal component
	Central motor conduction time to TMS	May be prolonged
	MEP to TMS	May be increased
	Paired-pulse TMS (inhibition, facilitation)	Increased size of conditioned MEP
Progressive supranuclear palsy	EMG analysis of external anal sphincter	Neurogenic
	Facial reflexes to median nerve stimulation	Absent responses in upper facial muscles
	Blink reflex excitability	Enhanced
	Auditory startle responses	Strongly delayed or absent
	Central motor conduction time to TMS	May be prolonged
	MEP to TMS	May be abnormal
Multiple system atrophy	EMG analysis of external anal sphincter	Neurogenic in almost all patients
	Blink reflex excitability	Enhanced
	Auditory startle responses	Enhanced and exaggerated
	Central motor conduction time to TMS	May be prolonged
		May be abnormal
	Multimodal sensory evoked potentials	May be abnormal
	Autonomic nervous system testing	Abnormal
Dystonia	EMG analysis of fast single joint movement	Increased duration of EMG bursts; co-contraction; overflow
	EMG analysis of involuntary movements	Very long bursts; co-contraction; exacerbation during voluntary movement
	Blink reflex excitability	Enhanced
	Reciprocal inhibition	Abnormal early and late phase
	Long latency reflexes	LLR-1 amplitude may be enhanced; LLR2 may be decreased in amplitude or absent
	Premotor potentials	Reduced amplitude
	Central motor conduction time to TMS	Normal
	TMS-induced silent period	Shortened
	Intracortical inhibition to paired-pulse TMS	Reduced
	Somatosensory evoked potentials	Abnormal spatial and temporal summation; abnormal premovement gating

Table 18.2. (*cont.*)

Disease	Neurophysiological test	Expected finding
Huntington's disease	EMG analysis of fast single joint movement	Disorganised triphasic pattern, variable duration of EMG bursts
	EMG analysis of involuntary movements	Variable and random patterns of muscle activation
	Blink reflex excitability	Reduced
	Long-latency and stretch reflexes	Reduced or absent M2; delayed LLRs in leg muscles
	Central motor conduction time to TMS	Normal
	TMS-induced silent period	Often prolonged; may be reduced in rigid patients
	Premotor potentials	Absent before choreic movement
	Somatosensory evoked potentials	Reduced amplitude of early cortical components
Myoclonus	EMG analysis of involuntary movements	Short-duration EMG bursts in cortical jerks
	Long latency reflexes	Increased amplitude
	EEG analysis (back-averaging technique)	Positive EEG transient before muscle jerk in cortical myoclonus
	Somatosensory evoked potentials	Often giant potentials in cortical myoclonus
	Central motor conduction time to TMS	Normal
	TMS-induced silent period	May be shortened
	Intracortical inhibition to paired-pulse TMS	Reduced
Essential tremor	Accelerometry	Frequency, amplitude and power spectrum
	EMG analysis of two antagonist muscles	Co-contracting, alternating pattern
	Tremor resetting	By mechanical, peripheral electric, transcranial electric and magnetic stimulation
	Long latency reflexes	LLR1 may be increased

reduced amplitude, but their slowness worsens as finger oppositions progress predominantly when patients have to move fingers individually. This finding suggests that finer cortical control is needed to promote and sustain the highly fractionated motor output responsible for individual finger movements.

Kinematic defects in producing sequential movements have been described also in motor tasks requiring bimanual simultaneous movements or reaching a target in space, normal activities of daily life such as drinking from a cup, or grasping a small object and placing it on top of a larger one (Bennett *et al.*, 1995). The conclusions of these studies is that bradykinesia originates mainly from abnormalities in movement execution.

Patients with PD are abnormally dependent on sensory information for motor performance, especially on visual information available during the task. Various studies have shown that the difficulty in executing movements diminishes when patients are allowed visual control (Georgiou *et al.*, 1993, 1994). In a series of experiments involving the sequential pressing of ten illuminated or non-illuminated buttons, the PD group's slow motor performance in sequential motor tasks worsened without illumination and improved when they received acoustic stimuli. In various motor tasks, such as walking, writing and daily activities, patients with PD can at least partly reduce their bradykinesia by using external visual and non-visual stimuli to improve their degree of attention.

Sensorimotor integration refers to those cerebral processes that link sensory input to motor output to produce appropriate voluntary movements (Abbruzzese & Berardelli, 2003). Many studies have been designed to investigate whether, and to what extent, abnormal sensorimotor integration is responsible for bradykinesia in parkinsonian patients. Among tasks studied is precision gripping of an object between the thumb and index finger and raising the index finger, or maintaining the index finger at a fixed height above a table, applying various load perturbations under the two conditions (Fellows *et al.*, 1998). Another study investigating discrimination between two points and the positional sense of patients with PD reported diminished precision (Demirci *et al.*, 1997). A study of limb movements that tested the effects of visual and kinesthetic information reported altered peripheral feedback (Klockgether

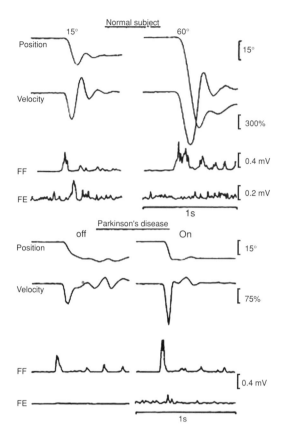

Fig. 18.2 Rapid movements performed at a single joint (15° and 60° of movement amplitude) in a normal subject and a patient with Parkinson's disease (off and on therapy). The normal subject performed the movement with a single triphasic pattern in the agonist and antagonist muscles, whereas the patient performed the movement with multiple EMG bursts. EMG activity was recorded from forearm flexors (FF) and extensors (FE) muscles. (From Berardelli *et al.*, 1986, with permission.)

et al., 1995). Last, when parkinsonian patients use kinesthetic information to approach a visual target they perceive distances as shorter than they really are. All these observations imply that altered sensorimotor integration is among the causes of hypometria or bradykinesia and that kinesthesia may have a role in the pathophysiology of PD. What remains unclear is whether the motor deficit originates from changes in peripheral cutaneous receptors or from abnormal central processing of this afferent input due to basal ganglia dysfunction.

Bradykinesia: cortical function (reaction times, movement-related potentials, magnetic stimulation)

Studies of reaction times (RT) and premotor potentials have provided information on abnormal motor

programming in PD (Evarts *et al.*, 1981; Jahanshahi *et al.*, 1992, 1993, 1995). The term RT refers to the interval elapsing between the stimulus to move and movement initiation. In simple RT (sRT) experiments subjects receive a complete advance description of the required movement so that they can preprogram it. In choice RT (cRT) experiments they receive only a partial description of the movement so that the movement can be only partially preprogrammed. Numerous studies have provided evidence of increased RTs in parkinsonian patients whereas the results for cRTs are controversial. Among the various mechanisms held responsible for increased RTs are difficulty in incorporating advance information into the motor plan, in retaining the appropriate motor programs in memory and in enacting them. Regardless of the precise mechanisms responsible, increased RT implies that preparation for voluntary movement is in some way abnormal in PD.

In normal subjects, preparation for movement can also be studied by recording the slow-rising negative EEG potentials generated before the onset of a voluntary movement (premotor potentials). The premotor potential (bereitschaftspotential, BP) begins during the 2 seconds that precede the onset of self-initiated movements and can be recorded from the scalp. The BP comprises two components: the early component (BP1) is a bilateral, symmetric negative potential that precedes the onset of movement by 1–2 seconds and increases to reach maximum amplitude at the vertex. The late component (BP2) precedes the onset of movement-related EEG activity by 650–50 ms. Recordings from subdural electrodes have shown that the BP1 component predominantly reflects the activation of the primary motor area and supplementary motor area (SMA), whereas BP2 originates exclusively from the primary motor area (Ikeda *et al.*, 1992). In patients with PD in the "off" condition the amplitude of the BP1 is reduced whereas the amplitude of BP2 is increased. The reduction of the early BP component has been attributed to reduced SMA activation, compensated during the preparation for movement by hyperactivity in the lateral motor areas (Cunnington *et al.*, 1995; Dick *et al.*, 1989).

In normal subjects, transcranial magnetic stimulation (TMS) primarily activates the motor cortex and elicits recordable EMG responses in limb muscles contralateral to the stimulated hemisphere (motor evoked potentials, MEP), due to activation of the corticospinal system (Hallett, 2000). Most investigators also report that these patients have normal motor threshold, defined as the minimum stimulation intensity required to evoke a MEP (Dick *et al.*, 1984). Experiments investigating changes in MEP amplitudes as a function of stimulus intensity and degree of voluntary contraction have shown that stimuli of equal intensity delivered at rest induce abnormally large-amplitude MEPs in patients with PD. Conversely, stimuli of similar intensity delivered during a muscle contraction elicit abnormally small-amplitude MEPs (Valls-Solè *et al.*, 1994).

As well as inducing an MEP, magnetic stimuli delivered during a voluntary contraction induce a period of EMG inactivity termed the silent period (SP) that lasts about 200 ms. Consensus is that the interruption of voluntary EMG activity originates from the cortex possibly through the activation of inhibitory interneurons that project onto pyramidal cells in the motor cortex. Patients with PD have an abnormally short-lasting SP (Cantello *et al.*, 1991; Priori *et al.*, 1994a). This reduction may depend on a loss of striatal dopamine that, by increasing GPi/SNr inhibition on the thalamus in turn, results in reduced cortical facilitation. Besides improving patients' clinical conditions, dopaminergic therapy lengthens the SP (Priori *et al.*, 1994a), whereas surgical therapy lengthens or shortens the SP duration according to the lesion/stimulation site and the pre-surgery clinical condition (Chen *et al.*, 2001; Cunic *et al.*, 2002; Strafella *et al.*, 1997; Young *et al.*, 1997).

Another application of TMS consists of delivering paired pulse in a conditioning–test paradigm at various interstimulus intervals (ISIs). This experimental technique is used to study the intracortical inhibitory and excitatory circuits. Patients with PD tested at rest with short ISIs have reduced intracortical inhibition, thought to reflect altered basal ganglia input (Ridding *et al.*, 1995a). When suprathreshold conditioning-test stimuli are delivered at long ISIs, inhibition increases at ISIs of 100 and 150 ms. The reduced thalamic excitatory action on cortical motor areas could therefore flatten the excitability curve of the motoneuronal pool thereby facilitating tonic activity thus inhibiting the final increase in excitability needed for rapid motor tasks (Berardelli *et al.*, 1996b).

This interpretation is in line with findings reported in studies using repetitive TMS. Modern magnetic stimulating devices allow stimuli to be delivered in trains (rTMS) at various frequencies and intensities. In normal subjects, during rTMS trains at 5 Hz the MEP to each stimulus progressively increases in size. This effect is absent in parkinsonian patients in the "off" state and is partially restored with dopaminergic medications. Reduced MEP facilitation together with normal SP lengthening during rTMS in patients with PD reflects a decreased facilitation of the excitatory cells in the cortical motor areas (Gilio *et al.*, 2002).

A recent application of TMS techniques is to investigate how cortical excitability changes during the transition from rest to voluntary movement, by delivering single or paired-pulse during the reaction time. In patients with PD, the period of increasing excitability before EMG onset is prolonged and the rate of rise slower than normal (Pascual-Leone *et al.*, 1994; Chen *et al.*, 2001b). The period of increased excitability following EMG offset is also prolonged (Chen *et al.*, 2001b). Thus, both activation and deactivation of the corticospinal system associated with simple movements is slower in PD.

Conclusions on bradykinesia

The data reviewed suggest that the main deficit underlying bradykinesia is an insufficient recruitment of muscle force during the initiation of movement. Important features are the underscaling of muscle force and increased dependence on external cues. Bradykinesia seems to result primarily from the underscaling of movement commands in internally generated movements (Currà *et al.*, 1997; Klockgether *et al.*, 1995). This defect reflects the role of the basal ganglia in selecting and reinforcing the pattern of cortical activity during movement preparation and performance. Finally, other regions of the CNS can adapt to the primary basal ganglia deficit of PD (Berardelli & Currà, 2002; Berardelli *et al.*, 2001).

Tremor: neuroimaging and TMS studies

In patients with PD, tremor typically has a frequency of 4–5 Hz and manifests on the EMG with the alternating activation of agonist and antagonist muscles. Some patients also have action tremor (postural and kinetic), at a frequency ranging from 6 to 12 Hz. Tremor at rest can be reproduced in experimental animals with lesions of the ventromedial tegment of the mesencephalon that involve the nigro-striatal, cerebello-rubral, cerebellar-thalamic and rubro-olivary pathways. To produce tremor, the association between lesions of the nigrostriatal dopaminergic pathways and the cerebellar pathways seems to be important. Recent experimental observations in monkeys with MPTP-induced parkinsonisms have shown periodic discharges in the pallidal cells of the pars interna (GPi) and subthalamic nucleus at frequencies similar to those of tremor. An important role in producing tremor is played also by the thalamus and cerebral cortex. Accordingly, tremor can be reduced or abolished by lesions of these structures. The thalamic lesioning site that yields the greatest reduction in limb oscillations is the ventral intermediate nucleus (VIM). This small area contains large cells, is well developed in superior primates and humans and lies between the pars oralis of the posterior lateroventral nucleus (VPLo) and the

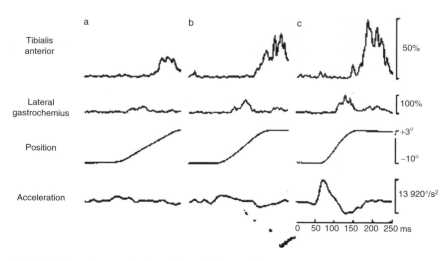

Fig. 18.3 Shortening reaction in Parkinson's disease. Electromyographic responses in tibialis anterior (shortening reaction) and lateral gastrocnemius (stretch reflex) produced by dorsiflexion stretch at three different acceleration levels (a,b,c) in a patient who was exerting a slight voluntary plantar flexion background force. (From Berardelli & Hallett, 1984, with permission.)

ventrolateral nucleus. Investigating the role of the motor cortex in tremor, Britton *et al.* (1992) noted that the tremor phase in patients with PD can be modulated by TMS most probably through the activation of cortical motor areas. Imaging studies using positron emission tomography (PET) have indicated a cerebellar role in tremor related to PD (Deiber *et al.*, 1993). In patients undergoing thalamic stimulation a reduction in tremor was associated with reduced regional blood flow to the median and paramedian rostral cerebellar areas. This reduction, mediated by the rubro-olivo-cerebellar circuit and activated by the cerebellar nuclei, is thought to represent the final inhibitory outcome of a central oscillator that passes through the VIM nucleus of the thalamus.

Cross-spectral analysis (including coherence and phase) of the electromyographic tremor activity in the arm, leg and neck muscles showed that multiple oscillators are responsible for the tremor in the different extremities (Raethyen *et al.*, 2000).

Rigidity: spinal and long loop reflexes, spinal inhibitory mechanisms

Although the increased muscle tone is thought to reflect patients' difficulty in maintaining muscles completely at rest, it is also secondary to the increased stretch reflex.

Numerous studies have shown that the monosynaptic spinal component of the stretch reflex is normal whereas the long-latency stretch reflex has an abnormally increased amplitude. Rigidity may therefore be caused by an increased long-latency stretch reflex (Rothwell *et al.*, 1983; Tatton & Lee, 1975). Long-latency reflexes (LLRs)

may be elicited also by electrical stimulation of the median nerve and recorded from thenar muscles under isometric contraction. These responses are thought to be mediated by transcortical anatomic circuits (thalamus, sensorimotor cortex, and spinal cord) and by functional changes in basal ganglia caused by hyperactivity in these circuits. In particular, the reduced SMA activation (present in parkinsonian patients) could reduce tonic inhibition of the long-latency reflexes. An alternative explanation is that the increased LLR depends on the increased activity in group II fibers (owing to their low conduction velocity these fibers result in long-latency muscle responses) (Berardelli *et al.*, 1983).

A recent study investigating the early and late facilitation of the quadriceps H reflex deriving from non-monosynaptic group I and group II excitations showed that group II facilitation was enhanced in the rigid lower limb of unilaterally affected PD patients (Simonetta Moreau *et al.*, 2002). Facilitation of the transmission in the interneuronal pathway activated by group II afferents in rigid lower limb is thought to result from a change in their descending monoaminergic inhibitory control.

Another possibility is that rigidity is caused by an increased shortening reaction to passive movements generated by joint and tendon organ afferents (Fig. 18.3) (Berardelli & Hallett, 1984).

Last, other possible pathophysiological mechanisms to explain rigidity in patients with PD are increased reciprocal inhibition between agonist and antagonist muscles, and reduced Ib tendon inhibition (Delwaide *et al.*, 1991). Reciprocal inhibition (RI) between agonist and antagonist muscles in the forearm consists of an initial short-lasting disynaptic Ia inhibitory phase followed by a long-lasting, presynaptic, phase of inhibition of the large proprioceptive afferent fibers. Disynaptic Ia reciprocal inhibition acts, at the spinal level, by actively inhibiting antagonist motor neurons and reducing the inhibition of agonist motor neurons. Changes in these spinal circuits probably reflect the increased activity in the dorsal reticulospinal system. A recent study investigated the short-lasting inhibitory phase of RI at rest and at the onset of a voluntary wrist flexion (Meunier et al., 2000). At rest, patients had normal RI. In contrast, before voluntary movements patients lacked the descending supraspinal modulation seen in normal subjects. On the less affected side, the descending modulation was present but less intense than in controls; on the more affected side, the modulation was almost absent. Recent studies also suggest that changes in the activity of the pedunculopontine nucleus – partly involving the ventral tegmental segment – contribute to changes in muscular tone.

EMG of the external anal sphincter for the differential diagnosis of parkinsonism

External anal sphincter electromyography (Sph-EMG) is a helpful test to disclose Onuf's nucleus degeneration. Quantitative Sph-EMG in normal controls showed a trend for increased motor unit potential (MUP) amplitude, duration, area, and polyphasicity with advancing age (Giladi et al., 2001). Pathological studies show that various neurodegenerative disorders including PD, multiple system atrophy (MSA), progressive supranuclear palsy (PSP), may reduce the neuronal population of this spinal nucleus far more than normal aging.

Multiple system atrophy (MSA) is a degenerative disease manifesting a combination of parkinsonism, cerebellar, pyramidal, and autonomic (including urinary, sexual, and anorectal) dysfunction. Compared with normal subjects patients with MSA almost invariably exhibit neurogenic abnormalities (Pramstaller et al., 1995). A more recent study also showed MUP size and fiber density similar to normal subjects, but a reduced recruitment pattern and number of active MUPs at rest (Giladi et al., 2001). Abnormal Sph-EMG has been found also in patients with MSA without clinical urological or anorectal problems (Giladi et al., 2001), and may reflect either the decreased number of motor cells in Onuf's nucleus without significant consequential reinnervation, or upper motor neuron involvement affecting the anal sphincter in MSA.

In a recent study investigating Sph-EMG in patients with PD, patients with probable MSA of parkinsonian type (MSA-p), and patients with probable MSA of cerebellar type (MSA-c) abnormal, denervated Sph-EMG was observed in 95.7% of patients with MSA-p, 86.4% of those with MSA-c,

and 33.3% of those with PD. These results did not correlate with the severity of parkinsonism (Lee et al., 2002). Previous papers showed that abnormalities in Sph-EMG were present early in patients with MSA, whereas similar abnormalities appeared only later (after 5 years or more) in patients with PD (Stocchi et al., 1997). Because patients with early PD do not show severe Sph-EMG abnormalities (Pramstaller et al., 1995) Sph-EMG helps to distinguish patients with PD from patients with other forms of parkinsonism in the first 5 years after the onset of symptoms and signs. Sph-EMG also distinguishes MSA from pure autonomic failure, as well as from cerebellar ataxias (if other causes of sphincter denervation have been ruled out) but not from progressive supranuclear palsy and corticobasal degeneration (Vodusek, 2001).

Levodopa-induced dyskinesias (LIDs)

Dyskinesias are one of the major problems in the long-term management of patients with PD. Patients manifest an array of motor symptoms that differ also in their time of onset after levodopa intake (Fahn, 2000).

Neurophysiological findings in experimental dyskinesias and during surgery

Early studies suggested that dyskinesias were due to reduced firing of neurons in the GPi, resulting in the loss of its inhibitory function on the thalamus and consequently in increased thalamo-cortical drive (Merello et al., 1999; Wichmann & De Long, 1996). Evidence that lesions in the GPe did alleviate LIDs (Blanchet et al., 1994), however, suggested that changes in the indirect pathway alone were not enough to generate LIDs. A recent neurophysiological study suggested that stimulation of the ventral pallidum controls dyskinesias by activating the large GPe axons responsible for inhibiting GPi neurons (Wu et al., 2001). Not only abnormal firing rates but also changes in the quality of signaling, i.e. the pattern, synchronization, and somatosensory responsiveness, are responsible for the emergence of dyskinesias. Changes in the quality of signaling in the GPi neurons provoke corresponding changes in the activity of the thalamus that interfere with thalamo-cortical signal transmission. Disruption of the normal spatio-temporal pattern of cortical neuronal activity leads to disordered cortical output and altered motor control (Berardelli et al., 2001). In patients with LIDs, most STN neurons have a high mean firing rate and an irregular firing pattern (Hutchison et al., 1998). Krack et al. (1999) found that off-period dystonia was associated with cellular hyperactivity, that diphasic dystonia reflected an altered pattern of STN activity with alternating periods of hyperactivity, and that decreased activity in cells responsible for specific dyskinetic muscles and peak-dose dyskinesias were accompanied by STN hypoactivity.

EMG recordings

On surface EMG studies LIDs typically consist of synchronous or asynchronous irregular antagonist muscle bursts that last up to 500–800 ms (Hallett, 2000; Yanagisawa & Nezu, 1987). The most typical LID pattern is that of chorea associated with synchronous EMG activity. When LIDs manifest as repetitive alternating movements, the EMG pattern consists of asynchronous, alternating and pseudo-rhythmic bursts at about 1 Hz (Luquin *et al.*, 1992).

Blinking and brainstem function in patients with LIDs

Blinking is a function subserved by the brainstem trigeminal-facial circuitry that is sensitive to changes in brain dopamine concentrations. Spontaneous blinking is reduced in patients with PD and increases with dopamine replacement (Agostino *et al.*, 1987; Karson, 1983). The blink rate is faster in patients with LIDs (Karson, 1983).

The function of trigeminal–facial pathways in the brainstem may be studied by testing the blink reflex and masseter inhibitory reflex. In normal subjects, the blink reflex consists of an early unilateral response (R1), followed by a late bilateral response (R2). Excitability of the brainstem circuitry is commonly studied by investigating the blink reflex recovery curve. In parkinsonian patients the inhibition of the R2 component is reduced during the off state and increases during the on state (Agostino *et al.*, 1987). R2 inhibition is more intense in dyskinetic than in non-dyskinetic patients (Iriarte *et al.*, 1989). In conclusion, in off-therapy parkinsonian patients the deficiency of dopamine leads to decreased spontaneous blinking but increased blink reflex excitability. Excessively high dopamine plasma levels are necessary to reverse these abnormalities, because they disappear during peak-dose dyskinesias, but do not disappear with optimal treatment.

Primary dystonia

Dystonia is defined as a syndrome of sustained muscle contractions frequently causing twisting or repetitive movements or abnormal postures. Primary dystonia is the commonest form of dystonia and the term refers to patients who have no signs of structural abnormality in the CNS. Primary dystonia can be manifested as focal (writer's cramp,

torticollis or blepharospasm), segmental or generalized dystonia. Segmental dystonia affects two contiguous body parts, whereas generalized dystonia is more widespread and involves at least one lower limb plus another body segment. Focal dystonias affect only a single part of the body. These forms of dystonia include blepharospasm, cervical dystonia, and writer's cramp. An important feature in focal dystonia is that it is often task specific.

Neurophysiological findings in experimental dystonia and during surgery

The pathogenesis of dystonia depends partly on changes in the activity of the basal ganglia (GPi and STN) and thalamus (VOP/VIM). Animal studies suggested a lowered GPi output. Numerous studies in patients with dystonia have described a decreased mean discharge rate with a change in the pattern and somatosensory responsiveness of neurons in the internal and external pallidum (Krack *et al.*, 1999; Lenz *et al.*, 1998; Lozano *et al.*, 1999; Vitek *et al.*, 1998, 1999).

These findings suggest that hyperkinetic disorders results from underactive basal ganglia output (Krack *et al.*, 1999; Lenz *et al.*, 1998; Lozano *et al.*, 1999; Vitek *et al.*, 1998, 1999). Recent microelectrode exploration of the GPi in patients with segmental and generalized dystonia undergoing stereotactic surgery under local or generalized anesthesia showed that GPi firing rates and pattern change according to the type of anesthesia used. In patients who underwent surgery under local anesthesia, the mean GPi firing rate was similar to that observed in patients with PD, whereas in dystonic patients under propofol anesthesia, the mean GPi firing rate was substantially reduced, and the firing pattern characterized by long pauses in activity. These findings indicate that pathophysiology of dystonia does not rely on abnormally low basal ganglia output, and suggest that the widely accepted pathophysiological models of dystonia need to be reconsidered (Hutchison *et al.*, 2003).

EMG recordings

Dystonic movements are characterized by prolonged EMG bursts in agonist and antagonist muscles and by overflow activity in other distant muscles.

Brainstem reflexes

In patients with cranial dystonia, the recovery cycle of the late bilateral R2 component of the blink reflex, conditioned by electrical and photic stimuli, is enhanced (Berardelli *et al.*, 1985; Katayama *et al.*, 1996) (Fig. 18.4). The recovery cycle of the R2 component is abnormal also in patients

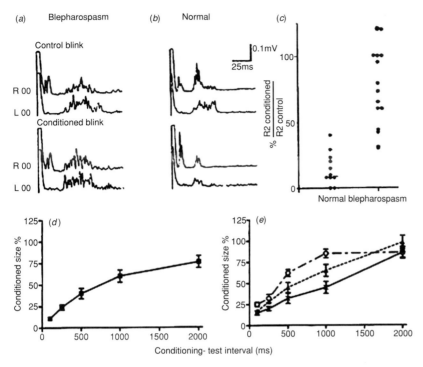

Fig. 18.4 Averaged data of the blink reflex from a representative patient with blepharospasm (*a*) and (*b*) a normal subject. Please note the increased duration and amplitude of the control and conditioned (interstimulus interval, ISI 500 ms) R2 responses. (*c*) Ratio between the amplitude of the conditioned and control R2 response in patients and controls at ISI 500 ms. (*d*), (*e*) The blink reflex recovery curve, i.e. the curve relating the amplitude of R2 response to the ISI. (*d*) controls; (*e*) crosses represent patients with arm dystonia; triangles represent patients with torticollis; circles represent patients with segmental dystonia. (Modified from Berardelli *et al.*, 1985, with permission.)

with dystonia without blepharospasm (Pauletti *et al.*, 1993). Prepulse inhibition was found to be abnormal in patients with blepharospasm: the R2 response of the blink reflex was abnormally gated by sensory stimulation, particularly in those patients who did not use a sensory trick (Gromez-Wong *et al.*, 1998).

Another way to investigate the function of trigeminal-facial pathways in the brainstem is to test the masseter inhibitory reflex. This response consists of an early phase (SP1), followed by a late phase (SP2) of inhibition in the ongoing EMG activity. The recovery cycle of the late phase of the masseter inhibitory reflex is enhanced in patients with cranial dystonia, even in those without jaw closing dystonia (Cruccu *et al.*, 1991).

Spinal reflexes and spinal inhibitory circuits

Vibration over the muscle tendon is an effective means for stimulating muscle spindle afferents (group Ia). After a short latency, in normal subjects vibration evokes a tonic contraction of the stimulated muscle, known as the tonic vibration reflex. This response is mediated by spinal and supraspinal circuitry, and is abnormal in patients with hand dystonia. In patients with dystonia, after a short delay, vibration evokes dystonic contractions also in other muscles (Kaji *et al.*, 1995a). Despite having normal positional sense, patients with hand dystonia have severely impaired vibration-induced kinesthetic sense (Grunewald *et al.*, 1997), a finding that strengthens the notion of an abnormal sensory–motor link in dystonia.

In patients with writer's cramp, the late phase of reciprocal inhibition (RI), and sometimes both the early and late phases, are reduced (Nakashima *et al.*, 1989). Abnormalities in the presynaptic phase usually return to normal after botulinum toxin injection (Priori *et al.*, 1995). RI is also abnormal in the unaffected arms of patients with writer's cramp as well as in patients with cervical dystonia. Abnormal RI reflects altered processing of Ia input to the spinal cord in dystonia. The normalization of presynaptic inhibition after botulinum toxin is thought to be mediated by changes in the activity of intrafusal fibers that decrease the muscle spindle input to the spinal cord.

The technique of tendon stimulation allows one to study group III-elicited presynaptic inhibition of group I afferents (Priori *et al.*, 1998). In patients with dystonia, group III fibers exert an abnormal presynaptic inhibition on Ia fibers (Lorenzano *et al.*, 2000). Abnormalities in presynaptic inhibition could originate from abnormal supraspinal control of the interneurons that mediate presynaptic inhibition or from altered spinal input.

Movement studies

Besides abnormal movements, clinical observation also shows that patients with dystonia produce abnormal voluntary movement (Berardelli & Currà, 2002). In patients with dystonia the RT is normal during simple arm reaching movements (Inzelberg *et al.*, 1995), head rotation and finger extension (Kaji *et al.*, 1995b), and single pointing movements (Currà *et al.*, 2000b). Conversely, during tasks requiring consecutive motor responses, patients with generalized dystonia have slow RTs whereas patients with focal dystonia do not (Currà *et al.*, 2000b).

Patients with dystonia perform rapid elbow movements slowly and with variable amplitude, and the EMG activity shows longer agonist muscle bursts, co-contraction activity between agonist and antagonist muscles, and activity in remote muscles (van der Kamp *et al.*, 1989). EMG recordings during distal movements of isolated fingers in patients with hand cramps show a spread of EMG activity in muscles not directly involved in the desired movement (Cohen & Hallett, 1988).

Studies of arm reaching movements have also shown slowness, increased variability of movement, and a prolonged deceleration phase (Inzelberg *et al.*, 1995). During sequential movements patients with dystonia are slower than controls and take longer than controls to switch from one sub-movement to the next (Agostino *et al.*, 1992). In addition to this general impairment in the execution of sequential movements patients with generalized dystonia (but not patients with focal dystonia) are slower in executing self-initiated than externally triggered movements (Currà *et al.*, 2000b).

Sensory function and sensorimotor integration

Several studies have reported clinically detectable sensory abnormalities in dystonia. Discomfort, pain or kinesthetic sensations are frequently reported at various times before dystonia develops (i.e. patients with blepharospasm often complain of irritation or dry eyes) (Defazio *et al.*, 1998). Risk factors for the development of focal dystonia include preceding loco-regional traumas and overuse of muscle groups.

Even though patients with dystonia have no abnormality in a single-touch, gross localization task, they perform worse than healthy subjects on somatosensory discrimination tasks. The abnormality correlates with the severity of dystonia (Bara-Jimenez *et al.*, 2000). Patients with generalized dystonia not only present with difficulties in timing functions but they also fail in cross-modal processing of visual–tactile stimuli (Aglioti *et al.*, 2003). Patients with hand dystonia are substantially worse also on graphesthesia and manual form perception (Byl *et al.*, 1996a). Functional MRI studies investigating the response in the primary sensory cortex to simultaneous tactile stimulation of the index and middle finger, and stimulation of each finger alone disclosed a non-linear interaction between the sensory cortical response to individual finger stimulation in patients with dystonia (Sanger *et al.*, 2002). These findings can be easily explained by observations from electrophysiology studies in a monkey model of focal dystonia disclosing noteworthy de-differentiation of sensory maps and the existence of single cells in hand regions of area 3b with enlarged receptive fields that extend to the surfaces of more than one digit (Byl *et al.*, 1996a). These changes may lead to abnormal processing of simultaneous sensory inputs and would explain clinical sensory deficits in human dystonia.

An important clinical feature of focal dystonia is the sensory trick (geste antagonistique), namely a tactile or proprioceptive sensory input to a nearby body part. This sensory input dramatically improves abnormal posture or movement. For example, in patients with blepharospasm, wearing sunglasses to avoid bright light effectively reduces contractions in the orbicularis oculi muscles.

The effectiveness of sensory tricks in improving dystonia suggests an abnormal link between muscle afferents and efferents in dystonia. Although traditional opinion considered the "sensory trick" as a sort of psychogenic maneuvre for distracting patients' attention, later physiological studies showed that it can actually modify EMG recruitment (Wissel *et al.*, 1999), and selectively affect dystonic tremor but not other forms of tremor (Masuhr *et al.*, 2000). In patients with cervical dystonia, PET scans showed that sensory tricks induce a perceptual dysbalance reducing the activation of the supplementary motor area and of the primary sensorimotor cortex (Naumann *et al.*, 2000). The additional sensory stimulus represented by the trick apparently acts by re-adjusting the abnormal link between afferent sensory input and movement output. Overall, current findings from neurophysiological investigations suggest a

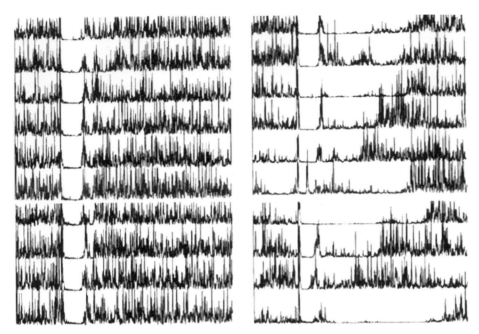

Fig. 18.7 On the left, raw data from consecutive unselected traces of the silent period evoked by suprathreshold transcranial magnetic stimuli in a normal subject. Note the constant duration of the silent period. On the right, raw data from consecutive unselected traces in a patient with Huntington's disease. Note the variable duration of the cortical silent period. Recordings are from the first dorsal interosseous muscle during slight voluntary contraction. Horizontal calibration = 200 ms, vertical calibration = 500 mV. (From Modugno *et al.*, 2001, with permission.)

Conclusions

Patients with HD have abnormalities of spinal inhibitory circuits probably due to a loss of supraspinal control on spinal mechanisms. In addition, neurophysiological findings show that the cortical motor areas are not globally hyperexcitable, implying that the model of hyperkinetic movement disorders need to be reappraised (Priori *et al.*, 2000). Besides chorea, bradykinesia is one of the cardinal manifestations of disordered movement in HD (Berardelli & Currà, 2002; Berardelli *et al.*, 1999). Patients with HD therefore have a generalized deficit in movement execution. HD disturbs external as well as internal cueing mechanisms. Yet, like other movement disorders originating from basal ganglia abnormalities, it predominantly affects the mechanisms controlling the internal cueing of sub-movements (Currà *et al.*, 2000a).

Myoclonus

Myoclonus refers to sudden shock-like muscular movements. These movements may be caused by the contraction of a group of muscles lasting less than 300 ms (positive myoclonus) or they may be caused by the sudden relaxation of a group of muscles (negative myoclonus or asterixis).

Myoclonus may be observed in a variety of conditions including certain seizure disorders and hereditary, metabolic, infectious, vascular, neoplastic, mitochondrial, toxic, or neuro-degenerative disease processes. Myoclonus should be distinguished from other movement disorders such as tics, some forms of tremor, chorea, and dystonia, but – not rarely – myoclonus and other movement disorders coexist in the same patient. Indeed, myoclonus is observed in PD and Lewy body related disorders, MSA, cortical basal degeneration, progressive supranuclear palsy, HD, dentato-rubro-pallido-luysian atrophy, in frontotemporal dementia and parkinsonism linked to chromosome 17 (Berardelli *et al.*, 1998; Thompson *et al.*, 1994; Chen *et al.*, 1992).

Myoclonus may be classified according to anatomic distribution (focal, segmental, multifocal, generalized), triggering factors (spontaneous, reflex-, action-myclonus), pattern of muscle contractions (rhythmic or irregular), etiology (physiological, essential, and secondary myoclonus), and finally pathophysiology. This classification best fits in with the scope of this chapter and therefore will be emphasized. It is based on the evidence that myoclonus results

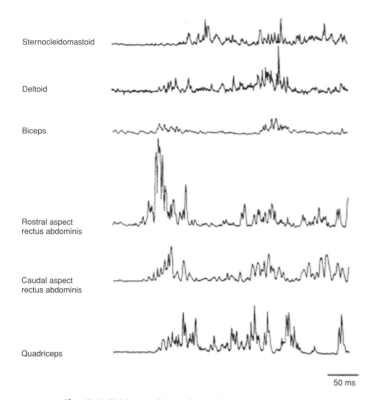

Sternocleidomastoid

Deltoid

Biceps

Rostral aspect
rectus abdominis

Caudal aspect
rectus abdominis

Quadriceps

50 ms

Fig. 18.8 EMG recordings of a single spontaneous jerk in different axial and limb muscles in a patient with propriospinal myoclonus. The leading muscle in the axial jerk is the rectus abdominis followed at various intervals by activation of the quadriceps and sternocleidomastoid muscles. This suggests propagation from a site within the thoracic spinal cord. Vertical calibration: top three channels 100 μV, bottom three channels 200 μV. (From Brown *et al.*, 1991, with permission.)

from abnormal electrical discharges originating in the nervous system.

According to the site of origin of the abnormal neuronal discharge myoclonus is categorized as cortical, subcortical, spinal, or peripheral (Marsden *et al.*, 1981). Cortical myoclonus arises from areas of the cerebral cortex, is considered "epileptic," and is often associated with other types of seizures. Subcortical myoclonus arises within the brainstem, and spinal myoclonus arises within the spinal cord. Myoclonic jerks generated by nerve fibers are recognised as peripheral myoclonus (for example hemifacial spasm, stump myoclonus).

Cortical types of myoclonus appear spontaneously, or in response to voluntary movement or somatosensory stimulation. The EMG bursts of myoclonus are of short duration, 10 to 30 ms. The EEG recording may show simultaneous spike or spike-and-wave discharges. The technique of back-averaging shows that the jerks are preceded by a

positive EEG transient over the contralateral sensorimotor cortex, 20 ms before for the arm and 35 ms for the legs. Cortical somatosensory evoked potentials are enlarged in many of these patients (Shibasaki *et al.*, 1978).

Subcortical myoclonus is typically generalized and occurs in response to auditory stimulation or sensory stimulation to the head and neck area. It activates the sternocleidomastoid muscles first, then the facial, masseter, cranial and trunk and limb muscles. The order of activation is therefore up the brainstem and down the spinal cord (Marsden *et al.*, 1981). EMG recordings show bursts of muscle activity 100 ms in duration. The EEG may show generalized spike discharges though these are not time-locked to the myoclonus. Back-averaging the EEG activity before the jerks fails to demonstrate a preceding cortical event.

Spinal myoclonus arises from an abnormal discharge of spinal motoneurones. In spinal segmental myoclonus, muscle jerking is rhythmic and repetitive; it is confined to adjacent spinal segments and persists at a frequency of 0.5–2 Hz during sleep. In propriospinal myoclonus, an abnormal spinal generator recruits predominantly axial muscles over many segments of the spinal cord through a propriospinal network (Brown *et al.*, 1991). These result in brisk trunkal flexion or less commonly extension movements. The order of muscle activation in each jerk spreads slowly from an axial focus upwards and down the spinal cord (Fig. 18.8). The accompanying EMG bursts often have long duration. These jerks are arrhythmic and stimulus sensitivity is uncommon and variable.

A widely accepted mechanism for myoclonus of peripheral nerve origin is ephatic transmission from peripheral ectopically generated potentials (ectopic generator) as suggested by abolition of the abnormal movement by local nerve anesthesia (Assal *et al.*, 1998). Peripheral myoclonus is common in the facial district (hemifacial spasm), but has been also described in limb muscles (Evidente and Caviness, 1998). Central structures contribute to maintain or reinforce peripheral myoclonus, as supported by the evidence of secondary central reorganization after peripheral nerve lesion, and by the cases in which the innervation between the efferent motor activity responsible for myoclonus differs from that of the sensory afference able to modulate it (Assal *et al.*, 1998).

Diagnosis of myoclonus is centered on clinical assessment (careful patient and family history, and clinical examination). Neurophysiological testing (EEG, EMG, SEP, reflex studies) helps to evaluate the pathophysiological mechanism of the myoclonus, the possible factors able to induce the symptoms, and to determine the site of origin of the abnormal neuronal discharge within the nervous system.

REFERENCES

Abbruzzese, G. & Berardelli, A. (2003). Sensorimotor integration in movement disorders. *Mov. Disord.*, **18**, 231–40.

Abbruzzese, G., Dall'Agata, D., Morena, M., Reni, L. & Favale, E. (1990). Abnormalities of parietal and prerolandic somatosensory evoked potentials in Huntington's disease. *Electroencephalogr. Clin. Neurophysiol.*, **77**, 340–6.

Abbruzzese, G., Buccolieri, A., Marchese, R., Trompetto, C., Mandich, P. & Schieppati, M. (1997). Intracortical inhibition and facilitation are abnormal in Huntington's disease: a paired magnetic stimulation study. *Neurosci. Lett.*, **228**, 87–90.

Abbruzzese, G., Marchese, R., Buccolieri, A., Gasparetto, B. & Trompetto, C. (2001). Abnormalities of sensorimotor integration in focal distonia. A transcranial magnetic stimulation study. *Brain*, **124**, 537–45.

Aglioti, S. M., Fiori, M., Forster, B. & Tinazzi, M. (2003). Temporal discrimination of cross-modal and unimodal stimuli in generalized dystonia. *Neurology*, **60**, 782–5.

Agostino, R., Berardelli, A., Cruccu, G. *et al.* (1987). Corneal and blink reflexes in Parkinson's disease with 'on–off' fluctuations. *Mov. Disord.*, **2**, 227–35.

Agostino, R., Berardelli, A., Cruccu, G., Pauletti, G., Stocchi, F. & Manfredi, M. (1988). Correlation between facial involuntary movements and abnormalities of blink and corneal reflexes in Huntington's chorea. *Mov. Disord.*, **3**, 281–9.

Agostino, R., Berardelli, A., Formica, A., Accornero, N. & Manfredi, M. (1992). Sequential arm movements in patients with Parkinson's disease, Huntington's disease and dystonia. *Brain*, **115**, 1481–95.

Agostino, R., Berardelli, A., Currà, A., Accornero, N. & Manfredi, M. (1998). Clinical impairment of sequential finger movements in Parkinson's disease. *Mov. Disord.*, **13**, 418–21.

Agostino, R., Berardelli, A., Formica, A., Stocchi, F., Accornero, N. & Manfredi, M. (1994). Analysis of repetitive and non repetitive sequential arm movements in patients with Parkinson's disease. *Mov. Disord.*, **57**, 368–70.

Agostino, R., Currà, A., Giovannelli, M., Modugno, N., Manfredi, M. & Berardelli, A. (2003). Impairment of individual finger movements in Parkinson's disease. *Mov. Disord.*, **18**, 560–5.

Albin, R. L., Young, A. B. & Penney, J. B. (1989). The functional anatomy of basal ganglia disorders. [Review]. *Trends. Neurosci.*, **12**, 366–75.

Albin, R. L., Reiner, A., Anderson, K. D., *et al.* (1992). Preferential loss of striato-external pallidal projection neurons in presymptomatic Huntington's disease. *Ann. Neurol.*, **31**, 425–30.

Alexander, G. E. & Crutcher, M. D. (1990). Functional architecture of basal ganglia circuits. Neural substrates of parallel processing. *Trends Neurosci.*, **13**, 266–71.

Alexander, G. E., Crutcher, M. D. & Delong, M. R. (1990). Basal ganglia-thalamocortical circuits – parallel substrates for motor, oculomotor, prefrontal and limbic functions. *Progr. Brain. Res.*, **85**, 119–46.

Assal, F., Magistris, M. R. & Vingerhoets, F. J. (1998). Post-traumatic stimulus suppressible myoclonus of peripheral origin. *J. Neurol. Neurosurg. Psychiatry*, **64**(5), 673–5.

Bara-Jimenez, W., Shelton, P., Sanger, T. D. & Hallett, M. (2000). Sensory discrimination capabilities in patients with focal hand dystonia. *Ann. Neurol.*, **47**, 377–80.

Benecke, R. Rothwell, J. C., Dick, J. P. R. *et al.* (1986). Performance of simultaneous movements in patients with Parkinson's disease. *Brain*, **109**, 739–57.

(1987). Disturbance of sequential movements in patients with Parkinson's disease. *Brain*, **110**, 361–79.

Bennett, K. M., Marchetti, M., Iovine, R. & Castiello, U. (1995). The drinking action of Parkinson's disease subjects. *Brain*, **118**, 959–70.

Berardelli, A. & Currà, A. (2002). Voluntary movement disorders. In *Clinical Neurophysiology and Neuromuscular Diseases*, ed. W. F. Brown, Ch. F. Bolton & M. Aminoff, pp. 1727–48. Philadelphia: W. B. Saunders.

Berardelli, A. & Hallett, M. (1984). Shortening reaction of human tibialis anterior. *Neurology*, **34**, 242–5.

Berardelli, A., Sabra, A. F. & Hallett, M. (1983). Physiological mechanisms of rigidity in Parkinson's disease. *J. Neurol. Neurosurg. Psychiatry*, **46**, 45–53.

Berardelli, A., Rothwell, J. C., Day, B. L. & Marsden, C. D. (1985). Pathophysiology of blepharospasm and oromandibular dystonia. *Brain*, **108**, 593–608.

Berardelli, A., Accornero, N., Argenta, M. *et al.* (1986a). Fast complex arm movements in Parkinson's disease. *J. Neurol. Neurosurg. Psychiatry*, **49**, 1146–9.

Berardelli, A., Dick, J. P. R., Rothwell, J. C., Day, B. L. & Marsden, C. D. (1986b). Scaling of the size of the first agonist EMG burst during rapid wrist movements in patients with Parkinson's disease. *J. Neurol. Neurosurg. Psychiatry*, **49**, 1273–9.

Berardelli, A., Rona, S., Inghilleri, M. & Manfredi, M. (1996b). Cortical inhibition in Parkinson's disease. A study with paired magnetic stimuli. *Brain*, **119**, 71–7.

Berardelli, A., Rothwell, J. C., Hallett, M., Thompson, P. D., Manfredi, M. & Marsden, C. D. (1998). The pathophysiology of primary dystonia. *Brain*, **121**, 1195–212.

Berardelli, A., Noth, J., Thompson, P. D. *et al.* (1999). Pathophysiology of chorea and bradykinesia in Huntington's disease. *Mov. Disord.*, **14**, 398–403.

Berardelli, A., Rothwell, J. C., Thompson, P. D. & Hallett, M. (2001). Pathophysiology of bradykinesia in Parkinson's disease. *Brain*, **124**, 2131–46.

Berardelli, A., Thompson, P. D. & Priori, A. (1998). *Myoclonus*. In Tolosa, E., Koller. W. C., Gershanik, O. S. (Eds). *Differential diagnosis and treatment of movement disorders*. Butterworth-Heinemann, Boston, 89–97.

Blanchet, P. J., Boucher, R. & Bédard, P. J. (1994). Excitotoxic lateral pallidotomy does not relieve L-dopa-induced dyskinesia in MPTP parkinsonian monkeys. *Brain Res.*, **650**, 32–9.

Bradshaw, J. L., Phillips, J. G., Dennis, C., *et al.* (1992). Initiation and execution of movement sequences in those suffering from and at-risk of developing Huntington's disease. *J. Clin. Exp. Neuropsychol.*, **14**, 179–92.

Britton, T. C., Thompson, P. D., Day, B. L., Rothwell, J. C., Findley, L. J. & Marsden, C. D. (1992). 'Resetting' of postural tremors at the wrist with mechanical stretches in Parkinson's disease, essential tremor, and normal subjects mimicking tremor. *Ann. Neurol.*, **31**, 507–14.

Brown, P., Thompson, P. D., Rothwell, J. C., Day, B. L. & Marsden, C. D. (1991). Axial myoclonus of propriospinal origin. *Brain*, **114**, 197–214.

Byl, N., Wilson, F., Merzenich, M. *et al.* (1996a). Sensory dysfunction associated with repetitive strain injuries of tendonitis and focal hand dystonia: a comparative study. *J. Orthop. Sports Phys. Ther.*, **23**, 234–44.

Byl, N. N., Merzenich, M. M. & Jenkins, W. M. (1996b). A primate genesis model of focal dystonia and repetitive strain injury: I. Learning-induced dedifferentiation of the representation of the hand in the primary somatosensory cortex in adult monkeys. *Neurology*, **47**, 508–20.

Byrnes, M. L., Thickbroom, G. W., Wilson, S. A. *et al* (1998). The corticomotor representation of upper limb muscles in writer's cramp and changes following botulinum toxin injection. *Brain*, **121**, 977–88.

Cantello, R., Gianelli., M., Bettucci, D., Civardi, C., De Angelis, M. S. & Mutani, R. (1991). Parkinson's disease rigidity: magnetic motor evoked potentials in a small hand muscle. *Neurology*, **41**, 1449–56.

Caraceni, T., Avanzini, G., Spreafico, R., Negri, S., Broggi, G. & Girotti, F. (1976). Study of the excitability of the blink reflex in Huntington's chorea. *Eur. Neurol.*, **14**, 465–72.

Caviness, J. N. (2003). Myoclonus and neurodegenerative disease – what's in a name? *Parkinsonism and Related Disorders*, **9**, 185–92.

Chen, R., Ashby, P. & Lang, A. E. (1992). Stimulus-sensitive myoclonus in akinetic-rigid syndromes. *Brain*, **115**, 1875–88.

Chen, R., Wassermann, E. M. Canos, M., & Hallett, M. (1997). Impaired inhibition in writer's cramp during voluntary muscle activation. *Neurology*, **49**, 1054–9.

Chen, R., Garg, R. R., Lozano, A. M. & Lang, A. E. (2001a). Effects of internal globus pallidus stimulation on motor cortex excitability. *Neurology*, **56**, 716–23.

Chen, R., Kumar, S., Garg, R. R. & Lang, A. E. (2001b). Impairment of motor cortex activation and deactivation in Parkinson's Disease. *Clin. Neurophysiol.*, **112**, 600–7.

Churchyard, A. J., Morris, M. E., Georgiou, N., Chiu, E., Cooper, R. & Iansek, R. (2001). Gait dysfunction in Huntington's disease: parkinsonism and a disorder of timing. Implications for movement rehabilitation. *Adv. Neurol.*, **87**, 375–85.

Cohen, L. G. & Hallett, M. (1988). Hand cramps: clinical features and electromyographic patterns in a focal dystonia. *Neurology*, **38**, 1005–12.

Crossman, A. R., Mitchell, I. J., Sambrook, M. A. & Jackson, A. (1988). Chorea and myoclonus in the monkey induced by gamma-aminobutyric acid antagonism in the lentiform complex. *Brain*, **111**, 1211–33.

Cruccu, G., Pauletti, G., Agostino, R., Berardelli, A. & Manfredi, M. (1991). Masseter inhibitory reflex in movement disorders, Huntington's chorea, Parkinson's disease, dystonia, and unilateral masticatory spasm. *Electroencephalogr. Clin. Neurophysiol.*, **81**, 24–30.

Cunic, D., Roshan, L., Khan. F. I., Lozano, A. M., Lang, A. E. & Chen, R. (2002). Effects of subthalamic nucleus stimulation on motor cortex excitability in Parkinson's disease. *Neurology*, **58**, 1665–72.

Cunnington, R., Iansek, R., Bradshaw, J. L. & Philips, J. G. (1995). Movement related potentials in Parkinson's disease: presence and predictability of temporal and spatial cues. *Brain*, **118**, 935–50.

Currà, A., Berardelli, A., Agostino, R., *et al.* (1997). Performance of sequential arm movement with and without advance knowledge of motor pathways in Parkinson's disease. *Mov. Disord.*, **12**, 646–54.

Currà, A., Agostino, R., Galizia, P., Fittipaldi, F., Manfredi, M. & Berardelli, A. (2000a). Sub-movement cueing and motor sequence execution in patients with Huntington's disease. *Clin. Neurophysiol.*, **111**, 1184–90.

Currà, A., Berardelli, A., Agostino, R., Giovannelli, M., Koch, G. & Manfredi, M. (2000b). Movement cueing and motor execution in dystonia. *Mov. Disord.*, **15**, 103–12.

Currà, A., Romaniello, A., Berardelli, A., Cruccu, G. & Manfredi, M. (2000c). Shortened cortical silent period in facial muscles of patients with cranial dystonia. *Neurology*, **54**, 130–5.

De Long, M. R. (1990). Primate models of movement disorders of basal ganglia origin. *Trends Neurosci.*, **13**, 281–5.

Defazio, G., Berardelli, A., Abbruzzese, G. *et al.* (1998). Possible risk factors for primary adult onset dystonia: a case control investigation by the Italian Movement Disorders Study Group. *J. Neurol. Neurosurg. Psychiatry*, **64**, 25–32.

Deiber, M. P., Pollak, P., Passingham, R. *et al.* (1993). Thalamic stimulation and suppression of parkinsonian tremor. Evidence of a cerebellar deactivation using positron emission tomography, *Brain*, **116**, 267–79.

Delwaide, P. J., Pepin, J. L. & Maertens de Noordhout, A. (1991). Short-latency autogenic inhibition in patients with Parkinsonian rigidity. *Ann. Neurol.*, **30**, 83–9.

Demirci, M., Grill, S., McShane, L. *et al.* (1997). A mismatch between kinesthetic and visual perception in Parkinson's disease. *Ann. Neurol.*, **41**, 781–8.

Deuschl, G., Toro, C., Matsumoto, J. & Hallett, M. (1995). Movement related cortical potential in writer's cramp. *Ann. Neurol.*, **38**, 862–8.

Dick, J. P. R., Cowan, J. M. A., Day, B. L. *et al.* (1984). Corticomotoneurone connection is normal in Parkinson's disease. *Nature*, **310**, 407–9.

Dick, J. P. R., Rothwell, J. C., Day, B. L. *et al.* (1989). The Bereitschaftspotential is abnormal in Parkinson's disease. *Brain*, **112**, 233–44.

Evarts, E. V., Teravainem, H. & Calne, D. B. (1981). Reaction time in Parkinson's disease. *Brain*, **104**, 167–86.

Evidente, V. G. & Caviness, J. N. (1999). Myoclonus of peripheral origin. *J. Neurol. Neurosurg. Psychiatry*, **66**(1), 123–4.

Fahn, S. (2000). The spectrum of levodopa-induced dyskinesias. *Ann. Neurol.*, **47**, suppl.1, S2–S11.

Fellows, S. J., Noth, J. & Schartz, M. (1998). Precision grip and Parkinson's disease. *Brain*, **12**, 1771–84.

Féve, A., Bathien, N. & Rondot, P. (1984). Abnormal movements related potentials in patients with lesions of the basal ganglia and anterior thalamus. *J. Neurol. Neurosurg. Psychiatry*, **57**, 100–4.

Filipovic, S. R., Ljubisavljevic, M., Svetel, M., Milanovic, S., Kacar, A. & Kostic, V. S. (1997). Impairment of cortical inhibition in writer's cramp as revealed by changes in electromyographic silent period after transcranial magnetic stimulation. *Neurosci. Lett.*, **222**, 167–70.

Georgiou, N., Iansek, R., Bradshaw, J. L. *et al.* (1993). An evaluation of the role of internal cues in the pathogenesis of parkinsonian hypokinesia. *Brain*, **116**, 1575–87.

Georgiou, N., Bradshaw, J. L., Iansek, R. *et al.* (1994). Reduction in external cues and movement sequencing in Parkinson's disease. *J. Neurol. Neurosurg. Psychiatry*, **57**, 368–70.

Georgiou, N., Bradshaw, J. L., Philips, J. G., Chiou, E. & Bradshaw, J. A. (1995). Reliance on advance information and movement sequencing in Huntington's disease. *Mov. Disord.*, **10**, 477–81.

Georgiou, N., Phillips, J. G., Bradshaw, J. L. *et al.* (1997). Impairments of movement kinematics in patients with Huntington's disease: a comparison with and without a concurrent task. *Mov. Disord.*, **12**, 386–96.

Gilad, R., Giladi, N., Korczyn, A. D., Gurevich, T. & Sadeh, M. (2001). Quantitative anal sphincter EMG in multisystem atrophy and 100 controls. *J. Neurol. Neurosurg. Psychiatry*, **71**(5), 596–9.

Gilio, F., Currà, A., Lorenzano, C., Modugno, N., Manfredi, M. & Berardelli, A. (2000). Effects of botulinum toxin type A on intracortical inhibition in patients with dystonia. *Ann. Neurol.*, **48**, 20–6.

Gilio, F., Currà, A., Inghilleri, M., Lorenzo, C., Manfredi, M. & Berardelli, A. (2002). Repetitive magnetic stimulation of cortical motor areas in Parkinson's disease: implications for the pathophysiology of cortical function. *Mov. Disord.*, **17**, 467–73.

Gilio, F., Currà, A., Inghilleri, M., Lorenzano, C., Suppa, A., Manfredi, M. & Berardelli, A. (2003). Abnormalities of motor cortex excitability preceding movement in patients with distonia. *Brain, in press.*

Gomez-Wong, E., Marti, M. J., Tolosa, E. & Valls-Sole, J. (1998). Sensory modulation of the blink reflex in patients with blepharospasm. *Arch. Neurol.*, **55**, 1233–7.

Grissom, J. R., Lackland, A. F. B., Toro, C., Trerrau, J. & Hallett, M. (1995). The N30 and N140–P190 median somatosensory evoked potential waveforms in dystonia involving the upper extremity. *Neurology*, **45**(Suppl 4), A458.

Grunewald, R. A., Yoneda, Y., Shipman, J. M. & Sagar, H. J. (1997). Idiopathic focal dystonia: a disorder of muscle spindle afferent processing? *Brain*, **120**, 2179–85.

Hallett, M. (1995). Is dystonia a sensory disorder? [editorial] *Ann. Neurol.*, **38**, 139–40.

(2000a). Clinical physiology of dopa-induced dyskinesia. *Ann. Neurol.*, **47**, S147–53.

(2000b). Transcranial magnetic stimulation and the human brain. *Nature*, **406**, 147–50.

Hallett, M. & Khoshbin, S. (1980). Physiological mechanisms of bradykinesia. *Brain*, **103**, 301–14.

Hanajima, R., Ugawa, Y., Terao, Y., Ugata, K. & Kanazawa, I. (1996). Ipsilateral cortico-cortical inhibition of the motor cortex in various neurological disorders. *J. Neurol. Sci.*, **140**, 109–16.

Hefter, H., Homberg, V., Lange, H. W. & Freund, H. J. (1987). Impairment of rapid movement in Huntington's disease. *Brain*, **110**, 585–612.

Hutchison, W. D., Levy, R., Dostrovsky, J. O., Lozano, A. M. & Lang, A. E. (1997). Effects of apomorphine on globus pallidus neurons in parkinsonian patients. *Ann. Neurol.*, **42**, 767–75.

Hutchison, W. D., Allan, R. I., Opitz, H. *et al.* (1998). Neurophysiological identification of the subthalamic nucleus in surgery for Parkinson's disease. *Ann. Neurol.*, **44**, 622–8.

Hutchison, W. D., Lang, A. E., Dostrovsky, J. O. & Lozano, A. M. (2003). Pallidal neuronal activity: implications for models of dystonia. *Ann. Neurol.*, **53**(4), 480–8.

Ikeda, A., Luders, H. O., Burgess, R. C. & Shibasaki, H. (1992). Movement-related potentials recorded from supplementary motor area and primary motor area: role of supplementary motor area in voluntary movements. *Brain*, **115**, 1017–43.

Ikeda, A., Shibasaki, H., Kaji, R. *et al.* (1996b). Abnormal sensorimotor integration in writer's cramp: study of contingent negative variation. *Mov. Disord.*, **11**, 638–90.

Ikoma, K., Samii, A., Mercuri, B., Wassermann, E. M. & Hallett, M. (1996a). Abnormal cortical motor excitability in dystonia. *Neurology*, **46**, 1371–6.

Inzelberg, R., Flash, T., Schechtman, E. *et al.* (1995). Kinematic properties of upper limb trajectories in idiopathic torsion dystonia. *J. Neurol. Neurosurg. Psychiatry*, **58**, 312–19.

Iriarte, L. M., Chacon, J., Madrazo, J. *et al.* (1989). Blink reflex in dyskinetic and nondyskinetic patients with Parkinson's disease. *Eur. Neurol.*, **29**, 67–70.

Jahanshahi, M., Brown, R. G. & Marsden, C. D. (1992). Simple and choice reaction time and the use of advance information for motor preparation in Parkinson's disease. *Brain*, **115**, 539–64.

Jahanshahi, M., Brown, R. G. & Marsden, C. D. (1993). A comparative study of simple and choice reaction time in Parkinson's, Huntington's and cerebellar disease. *J. Neurol. Neurosurg. Psychiatry*, **56**, 1169–77.

Jahanshahi, M., Jenkins, I. H., Brown, R. G., Marsden, C. D., Passingham, R. E. & Brooks, D. J. (1995). Self-initiated versus externally triggered movements. I. An investigation using measurement of regional cerebral blood flow with PET and movement-related potentials in normal and Parkinson's disease subjects. *Brain*, **118**, 913–33.

Johnson, K. A., Bennett, J. E., Georgiou, N. *et al.* (2000). Bimanual co-ordination in Huntington's disease. *Exp. Brain Res.*, **134**, 483–9.

Johnson, K. A., Cunnington, R., Iansek, R., Bradshaw, J. L., Georgiou, N. & Chiu, E. (2001). Movement-related potentials in Huntington's disease: movement preparation and execution. *Exp. Brain Res.*, **138**, 492–9.

Johnson, K.A., Cunnington, R., Bradshaw, J. L., Chiu, E. & Iansek, R. (2002). Effect of an attentional strategy on movement-related potentials recorded from subjects with Huntington's disease. *Mov. Disord.*, **17**, 998–1003.

Kaji, R., Ikeda, A., Ikeda, T. *et al.* (1995a). Physiological study of cervical dystonia. Task-specific abnormality in contingent negative variation. *Brain*, **118**, 511–22.

Kaji, R., Murase, N. (2001). Sensory function of basal ganglia. *Mov. Disord.*, **16**, 593–4.

Kaji, R., Rothwell, J. C., Katayama, M. *et al.* (1995b). Tonic vibration reflex and muscle afferent block in writer's cramp. *Ann. Neurol.*, **38**, 155–62.

Kanovsky, P., Streitova, H., Dufek, J. *et al.* (1998). Change in lateralization of the P22/N30 cortical component of median nerve somatosensory evoked potentials in patients with cervical dystonia after successful treatment with botulinum toxin A. *Mov. Disord.*, **13**, 108–17.

Karson, C. N. (1983). Spontaneous eye blink rates and dopaminergic systems. *Brain*, **106**, 643–53.

Katayama, M., Kohara, N., Kaji, R., Kojima, Y., Shibasaki, H. & Kimura, J. (1996). Effect of photic conditioning on blink reflex recovery function in blepharospasm. *Electroencephalogr. Clin. Neurophysiol.*, **101**, 446–52.

Klockgether, T., Borutta, M., Spieker, S. & Dichgans, J. (1995). A defect of kinesthesia in parkinson's disease. *Mov. Disord.*, **10**, 460–5.

Krack, P., Pollak, P., Limousin, P., Benazzouz, A., Deuschl, G. & Benabid, A. L. (1999). From off-period dystonia to chorea: the clinical spectrum of varying subthalamic nucleus activity. *Brain*, **122**, 1133–46.

Lee, E. A., Kim, B. J. & Lee, W. Y. (2002). Diagnosing multiple system atrophy with greater accuracy: combined analysis of the clonidine-growth hormone test and external anal sphincter electromyography. *Mov. Disord.*, **17**(6), 1242–7.

Lenz, F. A., Suarez, J. I., Verhagen Metman, L. *et al.* (1998). Pallidal activity during dystonia: somatosensory reorganisation and changes with severity. *J. Neurol. Neurosurg. Psychiatry*, **65**, 767–70.

Lorenzano, C., Priori, A., Currà, A. *et al.* (2000). Impaired EMG inhibition elicited by tendon stimulation in dystonia. *Neurology*, **26**, 1789–93.

Lozano, A. M., Kumar, R., Gross, R. E. *et al.* (1999). Globus pallidus internus pallidotomy for generalized dystonia. *Mov. Disord.*, **14**, 481–3.

Luquin, M. R., Scipioni, O., Vaamonde, J. *et al.* (1992) Levodopa-induced dyskinesias in Parkinson's disease: clinical and pharmacological classification. *Mov. Disord.*, **7**, 117–24.

Marsden, C. D. & Obeso, O. (1994). The functions of the basal ganglia and the paradox of stereotactic surgery in Parkinson's disease. *Brain*, **117**, 856–76.

Marsden, C. D., Hallett, M. & Fahn, S. (1981). The nosology and pathophysiology of myoclonus. In Marsden, C. D., Fahn, S. (Eds). *Movement Disorders 2*. Butterworth, London, 196.

Martinez, M. S., Fontoira, M., Celester, G., Castro del Rio, M., Permuy, J. & Iglesias, A. (2001). Myoclonus of peripheral origin: case secondary to a digital nerve lesion. *Mov. Disord.*, **16**, 970–4.

Masuhr, F., Wissel, J., Muller, J., Scholz, U. & Poewe, W. (2000). Quantification of sensory trick impact on tremor amplitude and frequency in 60 patients with head tremor. *Mov. Disord.*, **15**, 960–4.

Mavroudakis, N., Caroyer, J. M., Brunko, E. & Zegers de Beyl, D. (1995). Abnormal motor evoked responses to transcranial magnetic stimulation in focal dystonia. *Neurology*, **45**, 1671–7.

Mazzini, L., Zaccala, M. & Balzarini, C. (1994). Abnormalities of somatosensory evoked potentials in spasmodic torticollis. *Mov. Disord.*, **9**, 426–30.

Merello, M., Lees, A. J., Balej, J., Cammarota, A. & Leiguarda, R. (1999). GPi firing rate modification during beginning-of-dose motor deterioration following acute administration of apomorphine. *Mov. Disord.*, **14**, 481–3.

Meunier, S., Pol, S., Houeto, J. L. & Vidailhet, M. (2000). Abnormal reciprocal inhibition between antagonist muscles in Parkinson's disease. *Brain*, **123** (5), 1017–26.

Mitchell, J., Jackson, A., Sambrook, M. A. & Crossman, A. R. (1989). The role of the subthalamic nucleus in experimental chorea. Evidence from 2-deoxyglucose metabolic mapping and horseradish peroxidase tracing studies. *Brain*, **112**, 1533–48.

Modugno, N., Currà, A., Giovannelli, M. *et al.* (2001). The prolonged cortical silent period in patients with Huntington's disease. *Clin. Neurophysiol.*, **112**, 1470–4.

Murase, N., Kaji, R., Shimazu, H. *et al.* (2000). Abnormal premovement gating of somatosensory input in writer's cramp. *Brain*, **123**, 1813–29.

Nakashima, K., Rothwell, J. C., Day, B. L., Thompson, P. D. & Marsden, C. D. (1989). Reciprocal inhibition between forearm muscles in patients with writer's cramp and other occupational cramps, symptomatic hemidystonia and hemiparesis due to stroke. *Brain*, **112**, 681–97.

Nardone, A., Mazzini, L. & Zaccala, M. (1992). Changes in EMG response to perturbations and SEPs in a group of patients with idiopathic spasmodic torticollis. *Mov. Disord.*, **7**(Suppl 1), 25.

Naumann, M. & Reiners, K. (1997). Long-latency reflexes of hand muscles in idiopathic focal dystonia and their modification by botulinum toxin. *Brain*, **120**, 409–16.

Naumann, M., Magyar-Lehmann, S., Reiners, K., Erbguth, F. & Leenders, K. L. (2000). Sensory tricks in cervical dystonia: perceptual dysbalance of parietal cortex modulates frontal motor programming. *Ann. Neurol.*, **47**, 322–8.

Noth, J., Engel, L., Friedemann, H. H. & Lange, H. W. (1984). Evoked potentials in patients with Huntington's disease and their offspring. *Electroencephalogr. Clin. Neurophysiol.*, **32**, 134–41.

Noth, J., Podoll, K. & Friedemann, H. H. (1985). Long loop reflexes in small hand muscles studied in normal subjects and in patients with Huntington's disease. *Brain*, **108**, 65–80.

Parent, A. & Hazrati, L. N. (1995). Functional anatomy of the basal ganglia. I. The cortico-basal ganglia-thalamo-cortical loop. *Brain Res. Rev.*, **20**, 91–127.

Pascual-Leone, A., Valls-Solé, J., Brasil-Neto, J. P., Cohen, L. G. & Hallett, M. (1994). Akinesia in Parkinson's disease. I. Shortening of simple reaction time with focal, single-pulse transcranial magnetic stimulation. *Neurology*, **44**, 884–91.

Pauletti, G., Berardelli, A., Cruccu, G., Agostino, R. & Manfredi, M. (1993). Blink reflex and the masseter inhibitory reflex in patients with dystonia. *Mov. Disord.*, **8**, 495–500.

Pramstaller, P. P., Wenning, G. K., Smith, S. J., Beck, R. O., Quinn, N. P. & Fowler, C. J. (1995). Nerve conduction studies, skeletal muscle EMG, and sphincter EMG in multiple system atrophy. *J. Neurol. Neurosurg. Psychiatry*, **58**, 618–21.

Priori, A., Berardelli, A., Inghilleri, I., Accornero, N. & Manfredi, M. (1994a). Motor cortical inhibition and the dopaminergic system. *Brain*, **117**, 317–23.

Priori, A., Berardelli, A., Inghilleri, M., Polidori, L. & Manfredi, M. (1994b). Electromyographic silent period after transcranial brain stimulation in Huntington's disease. *Mov. Disord.*, **9**, 178–82.

Priori, A., Berardelli, A., Mercuri, B. & Manfredi, M. (1995). Physiological effects produced by BoNT treatment of upper limb dystonia. Changes in reciprocal inhibition between forearm muscles. *Brain*, **118**, 801–7.

Priori, A., Berardelli, A., Inghilleri, M., Pedace, F., Giovannelli, M. & Manfredi, M. (1998). Electrical stimulation over muscle tendons in humans. Evidence favouring presynaptic inhibition of Ia fibres due to the activation of group III tendon afferents. *Brain*, **121**, 373–80.

Priori, A., Polidori, L., Rona, S., Manfredi, M. & Berardelli, A. (2000). Spinal and cortical inhibition in Huntington's disease. *Mov. Disord.*, **15**, 938–46.

Raethjen, J., Lindemann, M., Schmaljohann, H., Wenzelburger, R., Pfister G. & Deuschl, G. (2000). Multiple oscillators are causing parkinsonian and essential tremor. *Mov. Disord.*, **15**, 84–94.

Reilly, J. A., Hallett, M., Cohen, L. G., Tarkka, I. M. & Dang, N. (1992). The N30 component of somatosensory evoked potentials in patients with dystonia. *Electroencephalogr. Clin. Neurophysiol.*, **84**, 243–7.

Ridding, M. C., Inzelberg, R. & Rothwell, J. C. (1995a). Changes in excitability of motor circuitry in patients with Parkinson's disease. *Ann. Neurol.*, **37**, 181–8.

Ridding, M. C., Sheean, G., Rothwell, J. C., Inzelberg, R. & Kujirai, T. (1995b). Changes in the balance between motor cortical excitation and inhibition in focal, task specific dystonia. *J. Neurol. Neurosurg. Psychiatry*, **53**, 493–8.

Rona, S., Berardelli, A., Vacca, L., Inghilleri, M. & Manfredi, M. (1998). Alterations of motor cortical inhibition in patients with dystonia. *Mov. Disord.*, **13**, 118–24.

Rothwell, J. C., Obeso, J. A., Traub, M. M. & Marsden, C. D. (1983). The behaviour of the long-latency stretch reflex in patients with Parkinson's disease. *J. Neurol. Neurosurg. Psychiatry*, **46**, 35–44.

Sanger, T. D., Pascual-Leone, A., Tarsy, D. & Schlaug, G. (2002). Non-linear sensory cortex response to simultaneous tactile stimuli in writer's cramp. *Mov. Disord.*, **17**, 105–11

Shibasaki, H., Yamashita, Y. & Kuroiwa, Y. (1978). Electroencephalographic studies myoclonus. *Brain*, **101**, 447–60.

Simonetta Moreau, M., Meunier, S., Vidailhet, M., Pol, S., Galitzky, M. & Rascol, O. (2002). Transmission of group II heteronymous pathways is enhanced in rigid lower limb of de novo patients with Parkinson's disease. *Brain*, **125**, 2125–33.

Stefani, A., Stanzione, P., Bassi, A., Mazzone, P., Vangelista, T. & Bernardi, G. (1997). Effects of increasing doses of apomorphine during stereotaxic neurosurgery in Parkinson's disease: clinical score and internal globus pallidus activity. *J. Neural. Transm.*, **104**, 895–904.

Stocchi, F., Carbone, A., Inghilleri, M., Monge, A., Ruggieri, S., Berardelli, A. & Manfredi, M. (1997). Urodynamic and neurophysiological evaluation in Parkinson's disease and multiple system atrophy. *J. Neurol. Neurosurg. Psychiatry.*, **62**, 507–11.

Storey, E. & Beal, M. F. (1993). Neurochemical substrates of rigidity and chorea in Huntington's disease. *Brain*, **116**, 1201–22.

Strafella, A., Ashby, P., Lozano, A. & Lang, A. E. (1997). Pallidotomy increases cortical inhibition in Parkinson's disease. *Can. J. Neurol. Sci.*, **24**, 133–6.

Tamburin, S., Manganotti, P., Marzi, C. A., Fiaschi, A. & Zanette, G. (2002). Abnormal somatotopic arrangement of sensorimotor interactions in dystonic patients. *Brain*, **125**, 2719–30.

Tatton, W. G. & Lee, R. G. (1975). Evidence for abnormal long-loop reflexes in rigid parkinsonian patients. *Brain Res.*, **100**, 671–6.

Tegenthoff, M., Vorgerd, M., Juskowiak, F., Roos, V. & Malin, J. P. (1996). Postexcitatory inhibition after transcranial magnetic single and double brain stimulation in Huntington's disease. *Electroencephalogr. Clin. Neurophysiol.* **101**, 298–303.

Thickbroom, G. W., Byrnes, M. L., Stell, R. & Mastaglia, F. L. (2003). Reversible reorganisation of the motor cortical representation of the hand in cervical dystonia. *Mov. Disord.*, **18**, 395–402.

Thompson, P. D., Dick, J. P., Day, B. L. *et al.* (1986). Electrophysiology of the corticomotoneurone pathways in patients with movement disorders. *Mov. Disord.*, **1**, 113–17.

Thompson, P. D., Berardelli, A., Rothwell, J. C. *et al.* (1988). The coexistence of bradykinesia and chorea in Huntington's disease and its implications for theories of basal ganglia control of movement. *Brain*, **111**, 223–44.

Thompson, P. D., Day, B. L., Rothwell, J. C., Brown, P., Britton, T. C. & Marsden, C. D. (1994). The myoclonus in corticobasal degeneration. Evidence for two forms of cortical reflex myoclonus. *Brain*, **117**, 1197–207.

Tinazzi, M., Priori, A., Bertolasi, L., Frasson, E., Mauguiere, F. & Fiaschi, A. (2000). Abnormal central integration of a dual somatosensory input in dystonia. Evidence for sensory overflow. *Brain*, **123**, 42–50.

Valls-Solè, J., Pascual-Leone, A., Brasil-Neto, J. P., Cammarota, A., McShane, L. & Hallett, M. (1994). Abnormal facilitation of the response to transcranial magnetic stimulation in patients with Parkinson's disease. *Neurology*, **44**, 735–41.

van der Kamp, W., Berardelli, A., Rothwell, J. C., Thompson, P. D., Day, B. L. & Marsden, C. D. (1989). Rapid elbow movements in patients with torsion dystonia. *J. Neurol. Neurosurg. Psychiatry*, **52**, 1043–9.

van der Kamp, W., Rothwell, J. C., Thompson, P. D., Day, B. L. & Marsden, C. D. (1995). The movement related cortical potential is abnormal in patients with idiopathic torsion dystonia. *Mov. Disord.*, **5**, 630–3.

Vitek, J. L., Zhang, J., Evatt, M. *et al.* (1998). GPi pallidotomy for dystonia: clinical outcome and neuronal activity. *Adv. Neurol.*, **78**, 211–19.

Vitek, J. L., Chockkan, V., Zhang, J. *et al.* (1999). Neuronal activity in the basal ganglia in patients with generalized dystonia and hemiballism. *Ann. Neurol.*, **46**, 22–35.

Vodusek, D. B. (2001). Sphincter EMG and differential diagnosis of multiple system atrophy. *Mov. Disord.*, **16**, 600–7.

Weeks, R. A., Ceballos-Baumann, A., Piccini, P., Boecker, H., Harding, A. E. & Brooks, D. J. (1997). Cortical control of movement in Huntington's disease. A PET activation study. *Brain*, **120**, 1569–78.

Wichmann, T. & De Long, R. R. (1996). Functional and pathophysiological models of basal ganglia. *Curr. Opin. Neurobiol.*, **6**, 751–8.

Wissel, J., Muller, J., Ebersbach, G. & Poewe, W. (1999). Trick maneuvers in cervical dystonia: investigation of movement- and touch-related changes in polymyographic activity. *Mov. Disord.*, **14**, 994–9.

Wu, Y. R., Levy, R., Ashby, P., Tasker, R. R. & Dostrovsky, J. O. (2001). Does stimulation of the GPi control dyskinesia by activating inhibitory axons? *Mov. Disord.*, **16**, 208–16.

Yanagisawa, N. & Nezu, A. (1987). Pathophysiology of involuntary movements in Parkinson's disease. *Eur. Neurol.*, **26**, 30–40.

Young, M. S., Triggs, W. J., Bowers, D., Greer, M. & Friedman, W. A. (1997). Stereotactic pallidotomy lengthens the transcranial magnetic cortical stimulation silent period in Parkinson's disease. *Neurology*, **49**, 1278–83.

Part II

Neuroimaging in neurodegeneration

19

Structural and functional magnetic resonance imaging in neurodegenerative diseases

Michael Samuel[1,2] and Alan Colchester[1,3]

[1]Department of Neurology, William Harvey Hospital, Ashford, Kent, UK
[2]Department of Neurology, King's College Hospital, London, UK
[3]Kent Institute of Medicine and Health Sciences, Canterbury, UK

Introduction

A full account of structural and functional MRI in neurodegenerative diseases would require an extensive volume. There are many neuroradiology texts which describe the common structural MRI abnormalities. MRI acquisition and processing techniques continue to develop apace and this chapter focuses on non-routine structural MRI and functional MRI (fMRI).

We define neurodegenerative diseases as having a distinct clinical picture, progressive natural history, focal or global pathology, and characteristic histopathology. This chapter describes diseases where neurodegeneration occurs intracranially, rather than in the spinal cord or peripheral nervous system. We do not include diseases where neurodegeneration occurs secondary to vascular or inflammatory processes, so we exclude diseases such as cerebral autosomal dominant arteriopathy with subcortical infarcts and leukoencephalopathy, multiple sclerosis or complex biochemical disorders (e.g. leukodystrophies), but we do include some disorders of copper, iron and calcium metabolism as well as prion diseases. Accepting our limitations, we limit our discussion to five categories of neurodegenerative disorders: [i] dementias, [ii] extrapyramidal disorders, [iii] motor system disorders, [iv] ataxias and [v] prion diseases. Of these, the application of non-routine MRI and fMRI to dementia and movement disorders has seen the largest expansion so far.

Structural MRI in neurodegenerative disorders

Structural MRI acquisition and postprocessing techniques

Typical routine clinical sequences, such as T_1 and T_2-weighted, fluid attenuated inversion recovery (FLAIR) and Short Tau Inversion Recovery (STIR) are effective at showing the location of pathological changes, but are seldom specific for the type of pathology. For this reason newer MRI techniques are being developed. A notable exception is the "eye of the tiger" appearance on T_2-weighted MRI in the pallidum in Neurodegeneration with Brain Iron Accumulation-1 (NBIA-1) (Hallervorden–Spatz syndrome) (Sethi et al., 1988; Guillerman, 2000). The low signal on T_2, in the absence of calcification determined by CT, indicates deposition of iron compounds, while the non-specific high signal reflects vacuolation, gliosis, demyelinated fibers and swelling of axons (Savoiardo et al., 1993) (Fig. 19.1). Although not specific to NBAI1 (Davie et al., 1997; Molinuevo et al., 1999; Guillerman, 2000), this sign in an appropriate clinical context is highly suggestive of this syndrome.

Very high spatial resolution can be achieved using small bore magnets having high magnetic field strengths of up to 7.1 tesla. This method, called "magnetic resonance microscopy," has been applied to postmortem in vitro specimens (Huesgen et al., 1993) and has recently been used to visualize neuritic plaques of Alzheimer's disease (Benveniste et al., 1999) (Fig. 19.2). It is yet to be determined whether this method can be developed further for in vivo use to show other pathological structures, e.g. Lewy bodies in Parkinson's disease or glial intracytoplasmic inclusions in multiple systems atrophy (MSA).

Visual judgment of abnormalities of size, shape and intensity of structures is the basis of routine clinical approaches. More objective computer-assisted methods are being developed, in principle to provide more accurate and reproducible measures of abnormality, which may be important for understanding disease processes, improving diagnosis, evaluating therapy, recruiting patients for treatment and survival studies and reducing the time needed for manual measurements. Here we review some of the more important of these methods.

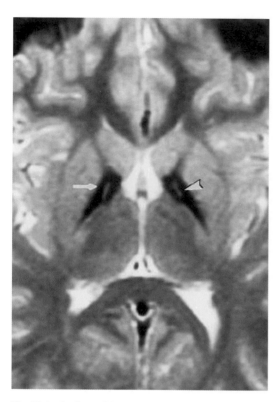

Fig. 19.1 The "eye of the tiger" sign of Neurodegeneration with Brain Iron Accumulation 1 (Hallervorden-Spatz syndrome). Transverse T_2-weighted MR image depicts a low signal intensity ring (arrow) surrounding a central high signal intensity region (arrowhead) in the medial aspect of the globus pallidus. (Modified with permission Guillerman, 2000.)

Manual segmentation

The usual approach assumes that the user has made a prior decision about the location of the region or volume of interest (ROI or VOI), as opposed to methods where the goal is to identify regions as a result of computer processing. An interactive computer program is used to outline the relevant structures. Area, volume, shape and intensity measures are computed. Such methods have been particularly important in the quantification of atrophy (see section on dementias). An alternative to outlining boundaries is a tool where a matrix of regularly spaced points is superimposed on the image, so-called "stereology." The user marks all points that are perceived to be inside the ROI. The spacing between the points is pre-determined, so an estimate of the area or volume is simply calculated from the number of points so marked.

Automated segmentation by analysis of image intensities

Methods for segmenting a large field of view using statistical analysis of the distribution of intensity values have been widely used. It is assumed that gray matter, white matter and CSF can be separated into different intensity classes using one or more MRI sequences but in practice there is significant overlap between the tissue classes. One method of successful implementation depends on non-rigid coregistration of the subject's MRI to a standard MRI from a probabilistic atlas in which gray and white matter and CSF voxels[1] have already been labeled (Van Leemput *et al.*, 1998). This labeling is copied to the subject's MRI to initialize the processing. The intensity values from the subject are used to revise the intial labeling, to compute the probability of a voxel belonging to a particular tissue class. The likelihood of assigning a particular voxel to one class is increased if its neighbors have already been assigned to that class. A correction for inhomogeneities may be included (Wells *et al.*, 1996) and additional specific tissue classes may be allowed, e.g. for multiple sclerosis lesions (Van Leemput *et al.*, 2001). Similar methods may in future be particularly useful for segmentation of regions of altered signal in neurodegenerative diseases.

This approach has a number of difficulties but also advantages. The intensity classes overlap significantly and vary widely between scanners. Even on one scanner, repeat scan–scan variability is evident. However, the fact that each voxel is assigned a probability of being, for example gray matter has been used to advantage. Many voxels will only be partially occupied by gray matter (particularly at boundaries), and the probability of belonging to the gray matter tissue class is taken to represent the fractional occupancy of the voxel by gray matter, i.e gray matter concentration (Ashburner & Friston, 1997). Statistical approaches to comparing group differences on a voxel-by-voxel basis can be directly applied to estimate volume. Measures of whole brain, total gray or white matter or subregional volumes – "volumetry" – are important outcome variables in many studies, and automated intensity-based segmentation is increasingly used in such studies. These are also the basis of voxel-based morphometry (VBM) (Ashburner & Friston, 2000). The advantage of these methods is that they can be applied to the whole brain and are not restricted to areas of pathology visible by inspection.

Automated measurement of volume differences using deformation analysis

An approach to measuring change is to quantify the shifts needed to bring a boundary from one image into alignment with another. This depends on prior coarse coregistration of the images to bring the majority of structures into

---

[1] A voxel is a 3-D volume element. A pixel is a 2-D picture element.

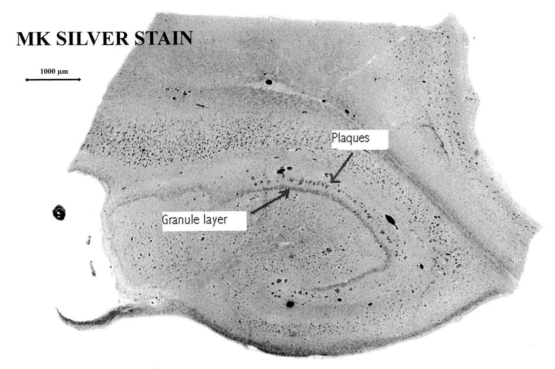

MK SILVER STAIN

1000 μm

Plaques

Granule layer

Fig. 19.2 (*a*) A silver stained pathological hippocampal section from a patient with Alzheimer's disease showing a row of plaques in parallel with the granule cell layer.

approximate correspondence, so that residual differences in position represent a biologically meaningful measure – such as the rate of atrophy. The term "deformation-based morphometry" tends to be applied to approaches which use a global non-rigid coregistration method. As with VBM, these methods allow identification of regions of significant change to be localized. For example, the boundary shift integral method of Freeborough and Fox (1997) has proved a sensitive method for detecting volume loss at the cortical surface in AD (Fox & Freeborough, 1997) (see below).

Diffusion-weighted imaging (DWI)

This method probes cerebral structures to provide clues to microscopic geometry (Bammer, 2003). The MR signal is sensitized to the diffusion of water molecules. Diffusion normally occurs randomly by Brownian motion and when unrestricted, water molecules move distances of around 10 μm in 50 ms. Their motion can be restricted by cell membranes, tortuous structures and other molecules (Pierpaoli *et al.*, 1996; Le Bihan *et al.*, 2001). Diffusion characteristics of separate components of the brain differ. Axons are notable because of the lack of restriction to diffusion along their length but their transverse restriction is highly consistent. Basic diffusion weighted images show signal intensity in a voxel when the diffusion-sensitizing gradient is applied in a single direction. Three images of the same slice are

typically displayed, each acquired with gradients in three directions, one orthogonal to the slice and the other two in the plane of the slice. Signal is attenuated (dark) in voxels where the diffusion gradient is aligned with fiber bundles running in the same direction. The images are influenced by the T_2 value of the tissue, so a limitation is that areas with increased T_2 cannot be distinguished from areas with impeded diffusion. By varying the strength ("b value") of the diffusion gradient, an apparent diffusion coefficient (ADC) in the direction of the gradient can be calculated for each voxel. ADC maps are displayed so that voxels of high diffusion are bright, i.e. the opposite of basic diffusion weighted images. So far, the most practical use has been the early detection of areas of acute ischemia (Warach *et al.*, 1992), but since DWI can be performed on conventional scanners and scanning time is short, its use in neurodegenerative disorders is increasing.

Diffusion tensor imaging (DTI): quantitative analysis of DWI

Information provided by DWI and ADC maps is limited by the directions of the applied field gradients. A more general approach is to apply gradients in at least six directions and to fit a function (the tensor) that allows several quantities, independent of the directions of the applied gradients, to be derived (Pierpaoli *et al.*, 1996; Le Bihan *et al.*, 2001). Scalar

1000 μm

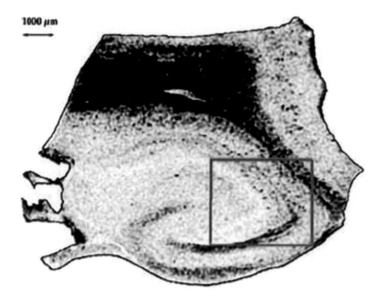

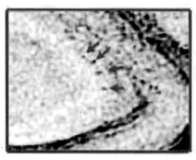

Fig. 19.2 (*b*) Corresponding T_2^* proton stain "magnetic resonance microscopy" with voxel size of $5.9 \times 10^{-5} \text{mm}^3$. A row of black rounded elements (arrowheads) can be located above the brighter band representing the granule layer. (Modified with permission from Benveniste *et al.*, 1999. Copyright 1999 National Academy of Sciences, USA.)

measures (non-directional) include mean diffusivity (MD) and fractional anisotropy (FA) (isotropy means equal in all directions). MD is the average of the ADCs estimated along any three orthogonal directions. This is also reported as the trace which is the sum rather than the average of the three values. FA expresses the extent to which diffusion varies in different directions and shows good contrast between gray and white matter. If disruption occurs in an organized fiber path, water will diffuse more along fiber tracts than across it and FA will decrease.

Directional measures provide information about the orientation of locally anisotropic structures. Many large fiber tracts form bundles several millimetres wide. Voxels within such bundles have a very clear direction of minimally restricted diffusion. However, other voxels may contain fibers running in more than one direction. The diffusion

tensor has six parameters which expresses the magnitude of the directional components in three orthogonal directions: (*a*) in the direction of the strongest component, (*b*) within the plane orthogonal to this in the direction with the strongest component, and (*c*) in the remaining direction orthogonal to these two. The function can be interpreted as an ellipsoid (Westin *et al.*, 1999). The width of the ellipsoid represents the strength of the component. Where there is only one predominant orientation of structures, the ellipsoid is needle-like. Where there are two strong components, the ellipsoid becomes like a two-dimensional disk. Where diffusion is equal in all directions, the ellipsoid is like a sphere (isotropy).

Fiber tracking (tractography) using DTI

Adjacent voxels within large fiber bundles have similar principal directions. The main direction of diffusivity can be mapped as a voxel-wise colour coded scale and superimposed on a structural MRI (Basser *et al.*, 2000; Jones *et al.*, 2002; Bammer *et al.*, 2003). The course of tracts can be followed by computing "streamlines," that is chains of voxels in which one voxel is linked to its neighbor in the direction of principal diffusion (Conturo *et al.*, 1999; Jones *et al.*, 1999). For example, "streamlines" can be initiated in the optic radiation, which lead to the calcarine cortex. This method has an important potential application in interpreting functional imaging data to show how activated foci are anatomically connected.

However, away from major fiber bundles, little is known of human white matter anatomy. Many assumptions come from extrapolation from animal studies and small human tracts remain to be defined; some of these will be important for our understanding of neurodegenerative diseases. Tracking small bundles through areas of crossing fibers is difficult and several approaches are under investigation (Basser *et al.*, 2000; Poupon *et al.*, 2000; Parker *et al.*, 2001). For in vivo tractography in patients with neurodegenerative diseases, it will be important to validate methods by correlation with post-mortem studies on the same patient. Appropriate validation methods are under development (Bardinet *et al.*, 2001; Kenwright *et al.*, 2003).

Structural MRI in neurodegenerative diseases

Here, initially we give representative examples of some routine clinical structural MRI abnormalities seen in our five categories of neurodegenerative disorders (Fig. 19.3, parts 1–23). So far, non-routine structural MRI has been predominantly applied to normal subjects, stroke (Warach *et al.*, 1992; Chabriat *et al.*, 1999), disconnection syndromes (Molko *et al.*, 2002) and psychiatric disorders (Foong *et al.*,

2000). The newer applications have not been applied to the spectrum of neurodegenerative disorders. Below, we focus on specific examples where publications exist and, for clarity, we compare these to routine structural MRI. Figure 19.3 (parts 1–23) shows characteristic abnormalities of some common neurodegenerative diseases. For a more complete discussion on each disease, the reader is referred to relevant chapters in this volume.

Dementias

Alzheimer's disease

MRI in AD is used to exclude treatable disorders, to establish the extent of vascular white matter abnormalities and to assess focal atrophy. Medial temporal lobe atrophy (MTA) is an important feature of AD and is best seen on coronal sections orientated perpendicular to the inferior (temporal) horn of the lateral ventricle (Fig. 19.3(1)). Enlargement of the CSF spaces is seen early as an increased height of the choroid fissure superomedial to the hippocampus. Enlargement of the temporal horn of the lateral ventricle and reduction of the height of the hippocampus generally become visible later (Scheltens *et al.*, 1992), but the correlation with the degree of atrophy is poor. Visual impression of atrophy can be made more robust by grading specific features (Scheltens *et al.*, 1992). A series of studies have assessed the sensitivity and specificity of medial temporal atrophy using visual rating schemes in the diagnosis of AD (Scheltens *et al.*, 1992; Erkinjuntti *et al.*, 1993; Desmond *et al.*, 1994; de Leon *et al.*, 1996; Frisoni *et al.*, 1996; O'Brien *et al.*, 1997; Scheltens *et al.*, 1997; Pucci *et al.*, 1998; Barber *et al.*, 1999a; Wahlund *et al.*, 2000). The diagnosis of AD was based on clinical criteria in these studies, but the correlation between clinical and pathological classifications is known to be poor. Despite the limitations of using clinical diagnostic criteria as the standard by which to judge the accuracy of MR criteria, sensitivity was surprisingly high in most of the studies, ranging from 70–100% (Scheltens *et al.*, 1992; Desmond *et al.*, 1994; de Leon *et al.*, 1996; Frisoni *et al.*, 1996; O'Brien *et al.*, 1997; Scheltens *et al.*, 1997; Pucci *et al.*, 1998; Barber *et al.*, 1999a; Wahlund *et al.*, 2000), although one study showed only 41% sensitivity (Erkinjuntti *et al.*, 1993). Specificity ranged from 67–96%. The control groups were mostly normals, but similar high specificities were obtained against other dementias (O'Brien *et al.*, 1997; Pucci *et al.*, 1998) or patients with minimal cognitive impairment (de Leon *et al.*, 1996). The results of these small studies (mostly <50 patients) have been corroborated by two larger studies with 130 and 77 AD patients, respectively (de Leon *et al.*, 1996; O'Brien *et al.*, 1997). It is

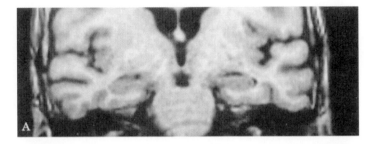
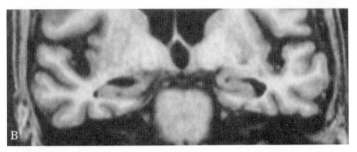
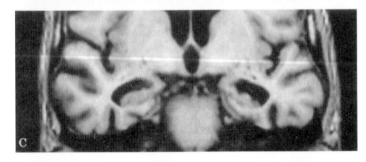
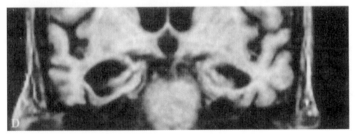

Fig. 19.3(1) Alzheimer's disease. T_1-weighted MR images orientated perpendicular to the long axis of the hippocampus showing progressive medial temporal lobe atrophy (MTA). (Modified with permission from Barber *et al.*, 1999a). Figure supplied by Drs Barber and O'Brian, Newcastle University, England, UK.)

now well established that assessing MTA by these methods is sensitive for AD and also specific within the context of the dementia subtypes included in the studies.

Most volumetry studies of medial temporal structures in dementia have used interactive segmentation methods. These allow volume measurement of the hippocampus, parahippocampal gyrus and other temporal substructures.

Comparing volumes of MTA with clinical diagnosis, sensitivity ranged from 0.80–0.94 for AD (Jack *et al.*, 1992, 1997; Ikeda *et al.*, 1994; Laakso *et al.*, 1995; Convit *et al.*, 1997; Pantel *et al.*, 1997, 1998; Krasuski *et al.*, 1998; Laakso *et al.*, 1998; Lehericy *et al.*, 1998; Frisoni *et al.*, 1999; Juottonen *et al.*, 1999), against normal controls specificities were 0.8–1.0 (Jack *et al.*, 1992, 1997; Ikeda *et al.*, 1994; Laakso *et al.*, 1995, 1998; Pantel *et al.*, 1997, 1998; Krasuski *et al.*, 1998; Lehericy *et al.*, 1998; Juottonen *et al.*, 1999). Against patients with minimal cognitive impairment or frontotemporal dementia (FTD), two small studies found similarly high specificity (Convit *et al.*, 1997; Frisoni *et al.*, 1999) of 0.86 and 0.90, respectively.

Limitations of volumetric quantification are evident even with structures which are primarily defined by their anatomy (Colchester *et al.*, 2001), e.g. the fusiform gyrus, inferior, medial and superior temporal gyri. The difficulties are compounded when assessing the perirhinal and entorhinal cortex, the definitions of which draw on animal data and cytoarchitectonic studies. Progress has been made in defining operational criteria for defining the boundaries of these structures (Insausti *et al.*, 1995; Insausti *et al.*, 1998) but substantial inter-subject variations cause significant difficulties. Juotonnen (Juottonen *et al.*, 1999) estimated entorhinal cortex volumes and reported improved sensitivity and specificity (0.90 and 0.94). Patients with minimal cognitive impairment, as well as those with AD, have reduced entorhinal cortex volumes, but the hippocampus was significantly atrophied only in patients with AD (Dickerson *et al.*, 2001). Progression of minimal cognitive impairment to AD was best predicted by "partial entorhinal volume" (Killany *et al.*, 2000). While such detailed subdivision of the temporal cortex is important for functional localization, subdivisions of the medial temporal lobe into hippocampus and parahippocampal gyrus is probably sufficient for diagnosis. The value of volumetry or semi-quantitative rating scales in the diagnosis of AD remains controversial, which is understandable noting the methodological difficulties described above. Some groups conclude that there is little or no value (Knopman *et al.*, 2001) while others suggest that the diagnostic value of hippocampal volumetry probably surpasses, and is at least equal to, clinical accuracy (Laakso, 2002).

For whole brain studies, Fox *et al.* used a technique in which the shift of boundaries was measured over time in a coregistered series of MR scans (Fox & Freeborough, 1997; Freeborough & Fox, 1997). By studying autosomal dominant AD, they followed the change in rate of atrophy associated with symptom onset and could predict the onset of clinical dementia (Fig. 19.4) (Fox *et al.*, 1997; Chan *et al.*, 2003). The use of voxel-based morphometry has allowed the main areas of atrophy to be investigated without depending on prior definition of the region of interest (Baron *et al.*, 2001; Ohnishi *et al.*, 2001). As expected, these studies confirmed that the medial temporal lobe was the most severely affected region, but Baron *et al.* (2001) identified several other areas outside the medial temporal lobe which were also affected.

Dementia with Lewy bodies (DLB)

This is the second most common dementia in the elderly and importantly differs from AD in its good response to cholinesterase inhibitors and greater sensitivity to neuroleptics (Barber *et al.*, 2001b). Thus differentiation from AD has clear therapeutic goals. Early studies using volumetry showed that although patients with DLB have more MTA than controls (Barber *et al.*, 1999a), they have relative preservation of the hippocampus compared with AD (Fig. 19.3(2)) (Hashimoto *et al.*, 1998). These differences are present across the entire length of the hippocampus (Barber *et al.*, 2001a). There were no differences in amygdala (Hashimoto *et al.*, 1998), lateral temporal lobes (Barber *et al.*, 2001a), frontal lobes (Barber *et al.*, 2000a), occipital lobes (Middelkoop *et al.*, 2001) or whole brain volumes, and the rate of focal atrophy did not differ between AD and DLB (O'Brien *et al.*, 2001). The absence of MTA had a specificity of 100% and 88% for separating DLB from AD and vascular dementia respectively, and a sensitivity of 88% (Barber *et al.*, 1999a). Despite the fact that MTA correlated with memory decline in all dementia groups (Barber *et al.*, 1999a), these findings led some groups to suggest that the preservation of the medial temporal lobe on MRI volumetry should be incorporated into the consensus criteria for diagnosis of DLB (Barber *et al.*, 1999a).

White matter changes are common to normal aging, DLB, AD and vascular dementia. The relationship to cortical atrophy has been studied by semi-quantitative volumetric MRI and correlated to whole brain and ventricular volume. White matter changes are best visualized on T_2 or proton density images. Periventricular hyperintensity is positively correlated with age and ventricular dilatation and is more severe in all dementia groups than controls. Deep white matter hyperintensity correlates with a history of hypertension, does not correlate with age, atrophy or ventricular dilatation, is also significantly greater in all dementia groups but is highest in patients with vascular dementia (Barber *et al.*, 1999b, 2000b). These findings suggest that volumetric MRI can distinguish two pathological processes, which lead to periventricular or deep white matter changes and which may have a different impact on the clinical presentation of cognitive decline.

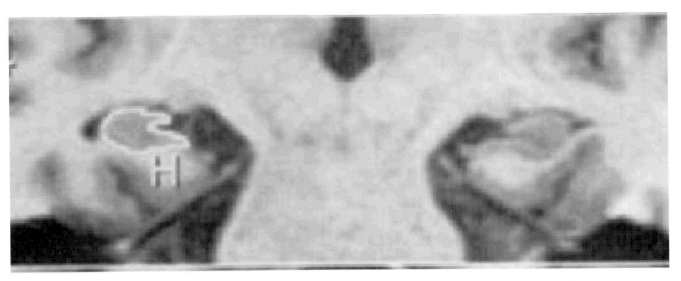

Fig. 19.3(2) Dementia with Lewy bodies. Selected T_1-weighted MRI slice from a 71-year-old female patient with dementia with Lewy bodies illustrating boundaries of the hippocampal formation (H = hippocampal formation). In contrast to Alzheimer's disease, there is sparing of the hippocampus. (Modified with permission from Hashimoto *et al.*, 1998.)

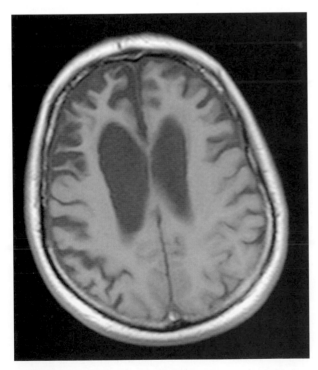

Fig. 19.3(3) Frontotemporal lobar degeneration. Striking frontal atrophy in a patient with frontotemporal dementia. T_1-weighted MRI.

Subcortical structures have also been investigated in DLB, AD and vascular dementia since they are implicated by the common presence of parkinsonism. Normalized volumetric measurements of the caudate from T_1-weighted MR images showed no significant differences between the patient groups although the left caudate volume was reduced significantly in AD and DLB compared with controls (Barber *et al.*, 2002). This finding was not found in the first whole brain VBM study comparing AD, DLB and controls, although thalamic atrophy was found in AD (Burton *et al.*, 2002). The results of subcortical imaging are at an early stage and their significance is currently uncertain.

Fronto-temporal dementia (FTD)

The dementias associated with focal atrophy of the frontal and temporal lobes form a heterogeneous group for which nomenclature is evolving and often confusing (Fig. 19.3(3)). The term Pick's disease is best reserved as a neuropathological diagnosis, where marked frontal atrophy is associated with swollen tau- and ubiquitin-positive neurones with Pick body inclusions. "Dementia lacking distinctive histopathology" is another neuropathological category; cases show significant neuronal loss and gliosis and may have spongiform changes in the superficial layers, but (as the name implies) do not have Pick bodies or other distinctive features. No specific neuroimaging features have been identified to distinguish between these categories of FTD. The main emphasis is on distinction from cases of AD, with variable results. The rate of atrophy may be even higher than in AD (Chan *et al.*, 2001). In primary progressive aphasia, atrophy is as expected most marked in the left temporal lobe (Radanovic et al., 2001).

Extrapyramidal disorders

Huntington's disease

MRI is a sensitive marker for bi-caudate atrophy (Fig. 19.3(4)) and striatal high signal change (Oliva et al., 1993). Striatal iron is increased in caudate, putamen and pallidum (Bartzokis & Tishler, 2000) and striatal atrophy is correlated with CAG repeat number (Rosas et al., 2001). High-resolution MR and cortical surface reconstruction allows measurement of cortical thickness. Thinning of the cortex was detected early in HD, progressed from a posterior to anterior direction and correlated with disease progression (Rosas et al., 2002). Affected regions included white matter, cerebral cortex, brainstem and cerebellum (Rosas et al., 2003) suggesting that some of the clinical spectrum of HD may occur as a result of extra-striatal degeneration. In dentatorubropallidoluysian atrophy, there are more extensive thalamic, midbrain and pontine high signal abnormalities (Fig. 19.3(5)) (Tomiyasu et al., 1998).

Parkinson's Disease

High-resolution MRI is not normal and can show cortical atrophy. Subtle changes in the substantia nigra have been identified specifically by thin section T_2-weighted images. Hutchinson and Raff used two inversion recovery sequences (white matter suppressed and grey matter suppressed) to calculate images of the ratio of these, which were color scaled. The ratio images show the width of the hyperintense substantia nigra band to decrease in PD, even in early cases (Fig. 19.5) (Hutchinson & Raff, 1999). This is not demonstrable on routine images (Adachi et al., 1999; Oikawa et al., 2002). It is possible that early (or even subclinical PD) might be detectable with refinement of this technique.

The subthalamic nucleus is of central importance in the pathophysiology and treatment of PD. High resolution MRI, specifically tailored with long TR, can visualize the subthalamic nucleus for neurosurgical interventions such as deep brain stimulation (Fig. 19.3(6)).

Atypical forms of parkinsonism and their differentiation from PD

The presence of high signal in white matter on T_2-weighted MRI and the clinical presentation of is usually sufficient to diagnose vascular pseudoparkinsonism. Midbrain atrophy (Fig. 19.3(7)) and enlargement of the third ventricle on mid-sagittal MRI suggests progressive supranuclear palsy (PSP), the so called "hummingbird sign" (Kato et al., 2003) (Fig. 19.3(8)). Superior cerebellar peduncle signal dropout occurred in 4/9 patients with PSP on proton-density images and may represent focal gliosis or demyelination (Oka et al., 2001).

Putaminal atrophy correlates with contralateral parkinsonism in the parkinsonian form of multiple system atrophy (MSA-P). On 0.5 tesla T_2 and proton density-weighted images, this is seen as a high signal in the posterolateral putamen. In contrast, using a higher field on 1.5 tesla images, the posterior putamen appears markedly hypointense on T_2-weighted images because of the deposition of iron. Putaminal high signal intensity may be evident as a rim lateral to the low signal in the posterolateral putamen (Fig. 19.3(9)). Cerebellar, pontine and middle cerebellar peduncle high signal or atrophy suggests the cerebellar form of MSA (MSA-C) (Fig. 19.3(10)), although there is an overlap with other types of MSA (Naka et al., 2002). Sparing of some pontine fibers and pyramidal tracts gives the "hot cross bun" sign in the pons but this is not specific to MSA and can also be seen in spinocerebellar ataxia. High signal changes around the dentate nuclei may be seen in the fragile X pre-mutation syndrome (Fig. 19.3(11)) (Brunberg et al., 2002).

In corticobasal degeneration (CBD), MRI reveals asymmetrical frontal or parietal atrophy, especially affecting the perirolandic region and parasagittal regions (Fig. 19.3(12)). T_2-weighted images show further low signal in putamen and globus pallidus and ventricular enlargement (Tokumaru et al., 1996; Hauser et al., 1996; Soliveri et al., 1999; Kitagaki et al., 2000). One patient is described with T_2-weighted hyperintensity of white matter adjacent to bilateral frontal cortex atrophy (Doi et al., 1999). These signal changes might reflect focal demyelination secondary to neuronal loss.

The degree of cortical grey matter volume loss has been studied in parkinsonian disorders. Whole brain 3D volumetry (Cordato et al., 2002) with manually discerned cortical and ventricular ROIs was used to compare PD and PSP groups and showed an 8% whole brain volume loss in PSP with 77% increase in whole ventricular size. The frontal lobe (particularly the posterior frontal cortex) showed more atrophy in PSP (19% compared with PD) and this regional atrophy correlated with clinical measures of frontal behavioral changes (Fig. 19.6).

One early 3-D volumetry study of subcortical structures showed normal striatal, cerebellar, and brainstem volumes in PD, whereas brainstem and striatal atrophy were detected in atypical parkinsonism (MSA-C, MSA-P and PSP) (Schulz et al., 1999). MSA patients showed additional cerebellar atrophy. With the exception of brainstem

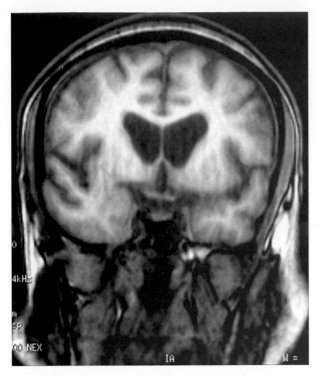

Fig. 19.3(4) Huntington's disease. Coronal T_1-weighted MRI showing caudate atrophy. (Courtesy of Dr J. Jarosz, King's College Hospital, London, UK.)

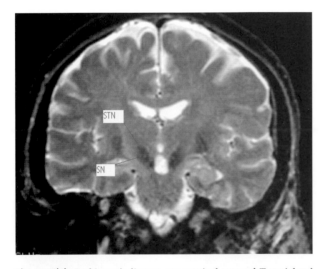

Fig. 19.3(6) Parkinson's disease, pre surgical coronal T_2-weighted MRI showing location of subthalamic nucleus (STN) and substantia nigra (SN). (Courtesy of Dr J. Jarosz, King's College, Hospital, London, UK.)

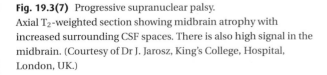

Fig. 19.3(7) Progressive supranuclear palsy. Axial T_2-weighted section showing midbrain atrophy with increased surrounding CSF spaces. There is also high signal in the midbrain. (Courtesy of Dr J. Jarosz, King's College, Hospital, London, UK.)

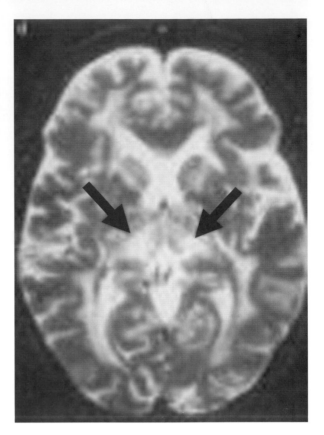

Fig. 19.3(5) DRPLA. T_2-weighted MRI showing high signal in the thalamus bilaterally. Signal changes are also seen in the pons, and midbrain. (Modified with permission from Tomiyasu *et al.*, 1998.)

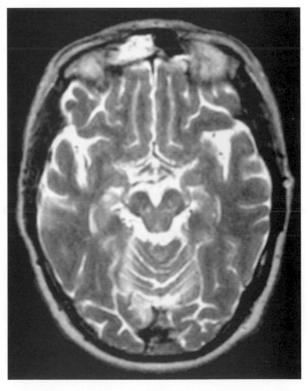

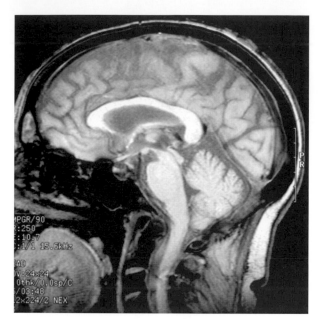

Fig. 19.3(8) Progressive supranuclear palsy. Mid-sagittal T_1-weighted section showing the beaked rostral midbrain, tegmentum and pontine base – the "hummingbird" sign (Courtesy of Dr J. Jarosz, King's College, Hospital, London, UK.)

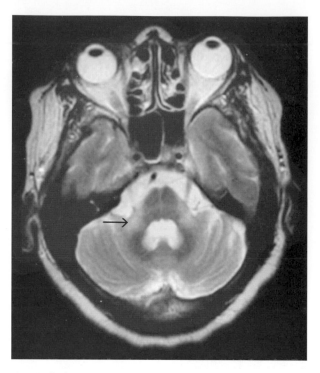

Fig. 19.3(10) Multiple system atrophy. 1.5 T T_2-weighted axial MRI showing pontine signal change, representing sparing of the pontine white matter tracts – the "hot cross bun" sign (courtesy of Dr J. Jarosz, King's College, Hospital, London, UK). There is also high signal of the middle cerebellar peduncle at arrow. High signal of the middle cerebellar peduncle may also seen in Fragile X premutation syndrome (Brunberg *et al.*, 2002).

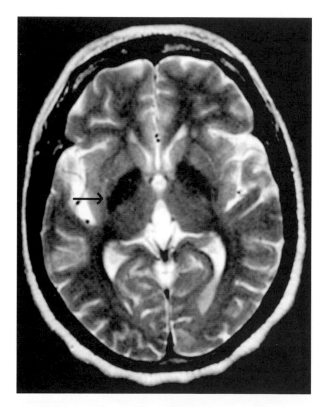

Fig. 19.3(9) Multiple systems atrophy (MSA). 1.5 T T_2-weighted axial MRI of low signal of the postero-lateral putamen with adjacent lateral rim of high signal (arrow) (Courtesy of Dr J. Jarosz, King's College, Hospital, London, UK.)

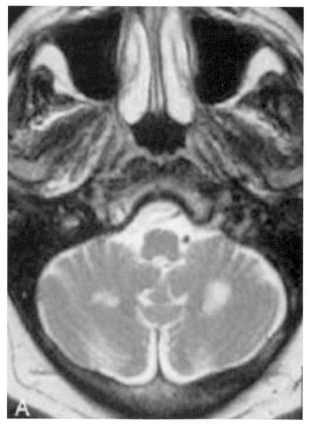

Fig. 19.3(11) Fragile X permutation syndrome. T_2-weighted MRI showing high signal intensity in white matter inferior and lateral to the deep cerebellar nuclei. (Modified with permission from Brunberg *et al.*, 2002. © American Society of Neuroradiology.)

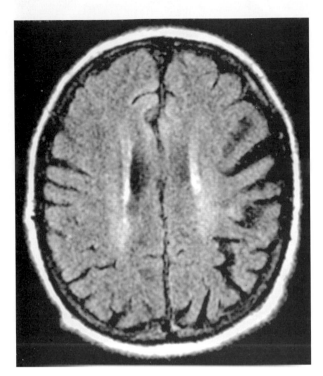

Fig. 19.3(12) Corticobasal ganglionic degeneration. FLAIR MRI showing asymmetrical left focal atrophy of the posterior frontal and parietal cortex (Courtesy of Dr J. Jarosz, King's College, Hospital, London, UK.)

atrophy in MSA-C, individuals and groups could not be differentiated on the basis of regional volumetry, unless a stepwise discriminant analysis was employed. The technique is, however, still considered insensitive in that typical PD could not be distinguished from controls, while MSA-P could not be distinguished from PSP. Another recent study showed similar patterns of midbrain volumes in both MSA-P and PD but that there was 50% greater putaminal atrophy in MSA-P (Ghaemi *et al.*, 2002).

A single study of subcortical structures using VBM found an increase in grey matter density in the nucleus ventralis intermedius (VIM) of thalamus contralateral to resting tremor in PD (Fig. 19.7) (Kassubek *et al.*, 2002). This is the first study to describe a structural difference in thalamus in PD. Whereas a loss of grey matter intensity might represent neuronal loss and could be straightforward to interpret, the nature of an *increase* in grey matter intensity is unclear, but could speculatively represent neuronal hypertyrophy or a higher neuronal density secondary to reduced local inhibitory input.

Using DWI, Schocke *et al.* demonstrated that MSA-P could be differentiated from idiopathic PD (Schocke *et al.*,

2002) based on an increase in diffusion of water molecules in the putamen in atypical parkinsonism, implying disruption of striatal architecture. This study extended previous work on increased ADC in frontal and precentral white matter in patients with PSP compared with normals (Ohshita *et al.*, 2000). Most recently, regional ADC values in putamen and caudate were shown to be significantly increased in PSP and MSA-P compared with PD, reflecting neurodegeneration and gliosis (Seppi *et al.*, 2003). There was only one patient with PD whose putaminal ADC value was greater than the lowest value of the MSA-P group. No significant differences were found in thalamus, substantia nigra, pons, periventricular white matter or grey matter. This may reflect reduced sensitivity of DWI in these areas where a variable orientation of fiber tracts may hinder detection of differences. To date, only one DTI study has reported a significant finding in PD, that of a decrease of FA in the region between the substantia nigra and inferior basal ganglia when compared with controls (Yoshikawa *et al.*, 2004).

Disorders of copper, iron and calcium (Figs. 19.3(16))

In these conditions, there is usually extensive but non-specific signal change in the basal ganglia. Examples of routine MRI abnormalities in Wilson's disease, acquired hepatolenticular degeneration (Ueki *et al.*, 2002), idiopathic calcification and neuroferritinopathy (Wills *et al.*, 2002) are shown in Figs. 19.3(13)–19.3(16).

Motor system disorders

MRI is undertaken in motor neuron disease (MND) to exclude differential diagnoses. The diagnosis of MND rests upon the clinical detection of predominantly lower motor neuron signs combined with upper motor neuron signs. The former are difficult to identify with MRI because of the small structure of the spinal cord and brainstem, and the latter are more variable (Leigh *et al.*, 2002). The use of MRI has focused on the detection and interpretation of upper motor neuron signs. Recently, high signal of the corticospinal tracts and low signal of the motor cortex have been described in T_2-weighted images of amyotropic lateral sclerosis (ALS) (Figs. 19.3(17) and 19.3(18)) (Carella *et al.*, 1995; Ellis *et al.*, 1999a).

MND is not solely a disorder of the motor system and imaging has been used to study both motor and non-motor cortical regions. Quantification of grey matter intensity by whole brain automated VBM has revealed deficits in grey

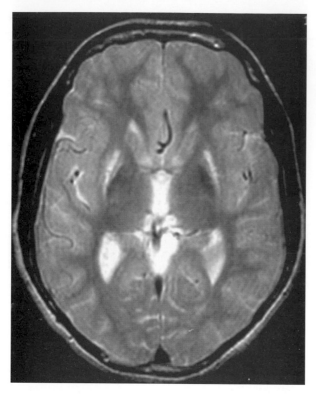

Fig. 19.3(13) Wilson's disease showing low density in the pallidum and high density lesions in caudate and putamen bilaterally. (Courtesy of Dr J. Jarosz, King's College Hospital, London, UK.)

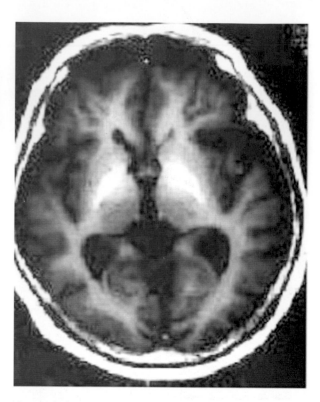

Fig. 19.3(14) Acquired hepatolenticular degeneration. Symmetrical high signal on T_1-weighted MRI in pallidum. (Modified with permission from Ueki *et al.*, 2002. Acknowledgement to Blackwell Publishing Ltd.)

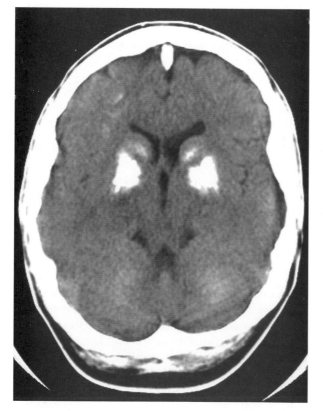

Fig. 19.3(15a) Idiopathic calcification of the brain. CT showing marked high signal in the basal ganglia.

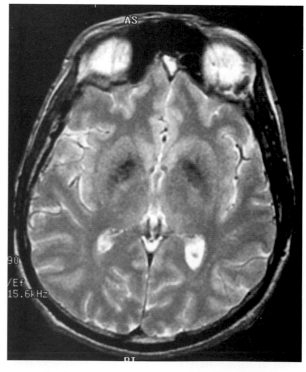

Fig. 19.3(15b) Idiopathic calcification of the brain. In contrast, T_2 axial MRI shows modest dark signal in the analogous areas.

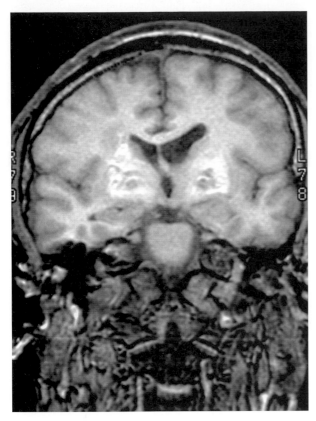

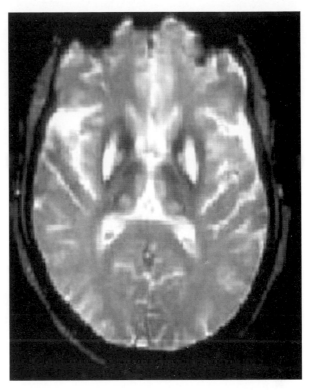

Fig. 19.3(15c) Idiopathic calcification of the brain. T_1 coronal MRI depicts the calcium deposition as a combination of high and low signal. (Courtesy of Dr J. Jarosz, King's College Hospital, London, UK.)

Fig. 19.3(16) Neuroferritinopathy. T_2-weighted MRI of central hyperintensity surrounded by hypointensity in pallidum, putamen and thalamus. (Modified with permission from Wills *et al.*, 2002, and with permission from BMJ Publishing Group.)

matter volume in Brodmann areas 8, 9, and 10 bilaterally (Ellis *et al.*, 2001). Patients with bulbar-onset ALS also have deficits in the white matter volume extending from the precentral gyrus to the internal capsule and brainstem, consistent with the course of the corticospinal tract, but without grey matter volume loss in the motor cortex. Combining these two findings suggests that ALS is a multisystem disease in which grey matter volume loss may occur at sites distinct from sites of white matter abnormalities (Ellis *et al.*, 2001).

Preliminary results on DTI in ALS (Ellis *et al.*, 1999b; Sach *et al.*, 2004) show increased mean diffusivity and decreased fractional anisotropy along the internal capsule in bulbar-onset disease, indicating disruption of water diffusion along the corticospinal tracts. Mapping such results to a whole brain volume may herald a new method to detect functional disruption. Although fractional anisotropy correlated with disease severity and mean diffusivity correlated with disease duration, the results overlapped considerably with normals. A decrease in FA can also be detected despite the absence of clinical upper motor neuron signs (Sach *et al.*, 2004). It is possible that development of VBM and DTI will provide further in vivo evidence to corroborate the extensive nature of pathological changes of MND.

Ataxias

Ataxic disorders have not generally been studied with nonroutine MRI. Routine T_1-weighted MRI, may show nonspecific cerebellar and brainstem atrophy (Fig. 19.3(19)). In the context of palatal tremor, this may be combined with hyperintensity and hypertrophy of the olivary nucleus (Fig. 19.3(20)) to suggest the diagnosis of the progressive ataxia and palatal tremor syndrome (Sperling & Herrmann, Jr., 1985; Phanthumchinda, 1999; Samuel *et al.*, 2004).

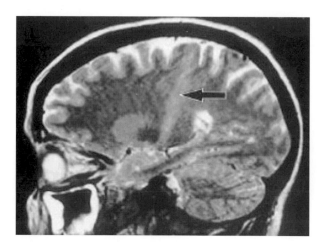

Fig. 19.3(17) Amyotrophic lateral sclerosis.
T_2-weighted sagittal MRI showing high signal intensity along pyramidal tracts. (Modified with permission from Ellis *et al.*, 1999a.)

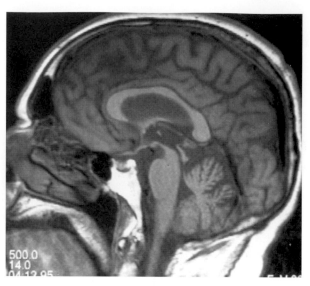

Fig. 19.3(19) Cerebellar degeneration.
Spinocerebellar ataxia. Sagittal T_1-weighted MRI showing cerebellar atrophy. (Courtesy of Dr J. Jarosz, King's College Hospital, London, UK.)

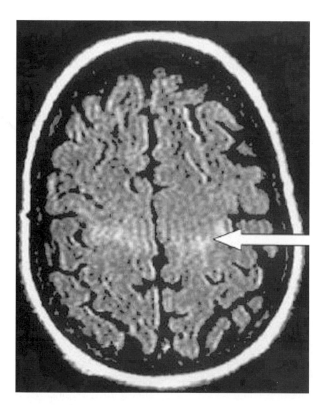

Fig. 19.3(18) Amyotropic lateral stenosis.
Axial FLAIR MRI showing high signal beneath primary motor cortex. (Modified with permission from Ellis *et al.*, 1999a.)

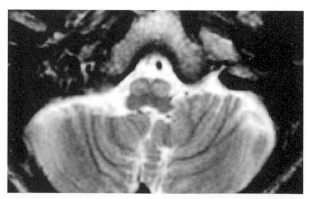

Fig. 19.3(20) Progressive ataxia and palatal tremor. T_2-weighted MRI showing high signal and hypertrophy of the olivary region bilaterally. (Courtesy of Dr AE Lang, Toronto Western Hospital, Toronto, Ontario, Canada).

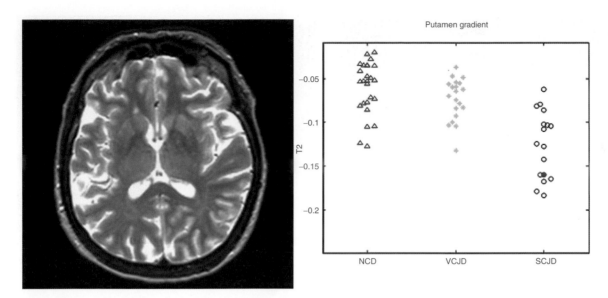

Putamen gradient

Fig. 19.3(21) Prion disease.

T_2-weighted MRI in a patient with confirmed sporadic CJD showing hyperintensity of the head of the caudate and anterior part of the putamen, although this can be difficult to judge by eye. The graph shows quantitative data of the "putamen gradient" (rate of change of intensity from front to back along the putamen) in three groups of patients: non-CJD dementia NCD (left), confirmed vCJD (centre); and confirmed sCJD (right). The blue-filled circle in the sCJD group is from the patient whose MRI is shown, demonstrating that the "putamen gradient" for this patient falls outside the complete range of values for the two comparison groups ($p < 0.01$).

Prion diseases

Sporadic CJD (sCJD)

The earliest reports of MRI described only generalized atrophy (Kovanen *et al.*, 1985). Subsequently, there were reports of increased intensity, usually symmetrical, in the basal ganglia (Gertz *et al.*, 1988; Pearl & Anderson 1989; Kruger *et al.*, 1990; Milton *et al.*, 1991; Uchino *et al.*, 1991; Falcone *et al.*, 1992; Di Rocco *et al.*, 1993; Barboriak *et al.*, 1994; Garcia-Santos *et al.*, 1996) on T_2 and proton density MRI. In the first substantial series (Finkenstaedt *et al.*, 1996), high signal in the putamen and caudate head were observed in 79% of sCJD patients (14 definite and 15 probable), but this study lacked controls (Fig. 19.3(21)). The same patients were included in a review of a larger group of 157 sCJD patients (Poser *et al.*, 1999; Schroter *et al.*, 2000) where 67% of 29 sCJD patients had basal ganglia hyperintensity (sensitivity), while 52 of 56 non-CJD dementia controls did not show such changes (92% specificity). A less consistent finding is high signal in the cerebral cortex, which is often asymmetrical (Gertz *et al.*, 1988; Esmonde & Will, 1992; Falcone *et al.*, 1992, 1996; Garcia-Santos *et al.*, 1996; Tzeng *et al.*, 1997; Urbach *et al.*, 1998; Samman *et al.*, 1999; Collie *et al.*, 2001).

Signal changes have also been seen in periaqueductal grey matter (Collie *et al.*, 2001), thalamus (Gertz *et al.*, 1988), hippocampus (Sellar *et al.*, 2002), cerebellum (Tzeng *et al.*, 1997) and occasionally in the white matter of the hemispheres (Falcone *et al.*, 1992; Collie *et al.*, 2001) (Fig. 19.3(22)). Abnormal signal intensities in the deep grey matter are less conspicuous in sCJD than variant CJD. In a recent multi-centre quantitative study (Hojjat *et al.*, 2002), 34 digital MR scans were analyzed (12 sCJD, 11 variant CJD and 10 non-CJD dementia patients). Absolute intensities in the putamen and caudate head were generally increased but varied widely, and no simple reference structures for normalization could be identified that allowed confident discrimination of sCJD patients. However, intensity abnormalities of the caudate and putamen relative to frontal white matter were predictive of variant CJD (although with less sensitivity and specificity than the pulvinar), while sCJD could not be distinguished from non-CJD dementia controls. The most significant finding was that the normal gradient of intensity within the putamen (reducing signal from front to back on long TR MRI) was significantly greater in sCJD than either variant CJD or non-CJD dementia (Hojjat *et al.*, 2002). Using the optimum threshold, the sensitivity and specificity for

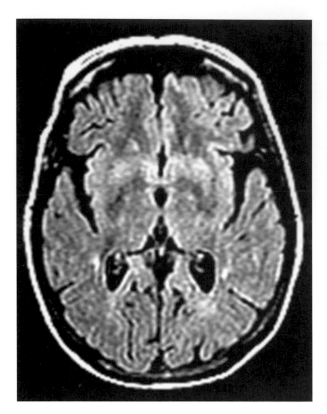

Fig. 19.3(22) FLAIR MRI of confirmed sporadic CJD showing marked hyperintensity in the caudate head and putamen, which is easier to detect visually on FLAIR than on T_2-weighted images. There is also some hyperintensity of the insular cortex.

sCJD diagnosis using the "putamen gradient" were both 89%, comparable to any other non-invasive test for sCJD (Fig. 19.3(21)). Further evaluation of this test in a larger group is required.

FLAIR sequences improve the detection of grey and white matter hyperintensities and will almost certainly improve the sensitivity of visual analysis of MRI in sCJD (Fig. 19.3(22)). DWI has been described in sCJD in a number of case reports and small series (Demaerel *et al.*, 1997, 1999; Bahn *et al.*, 1997a; Bahn & Parchi, 1999; Na *et al.*, 1999; Samman *et al.*, 1999; Yee *et al.*, 1999; Kropp *et al.*, 2000; Oppenheim *et al.*, 2000; Kim, 2001; Matoba, 2001; Mao-Draayer *et al.*, 2002; Mittal *et al.*, 2002; Murata *et al.*, 2002; Rabinstein *et al.*, 2002; Martindale *et al.*, 2003; Mendez *et al.*, 2003) showing striking altered diffusion in the basal ganglia and cerebral cortex (Collie *et al.*, 2001; Mao-Draayer *et al.*, 2002; Murata *et al.*, 2002) (Fig. 19.8).

Variant CJD (vCJD)

MRI is very important for the diagnosis of vCJD. Following the first description of vCJD (Will *et al.*, 1996), two case

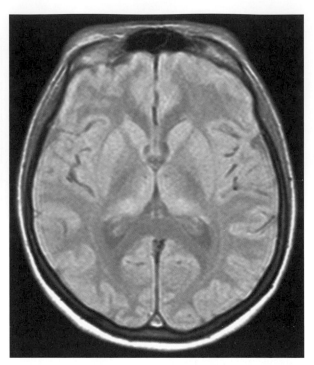

Fig. 19.3(23) Confirmed vCJD. Proton density axial MRI. There is striking hyperintensity of the posterior thalamus ("pulvinar sign") with less hyperintensity of the medial thalamus. This combination has been referred to as the "hockey-stick" sign.

reports described high signal in the posterior thalamus (pulvinar) on proton density and T_2-weighted MRI (Chazot *et al.*, 1996; Howard, 1996). In 12 of the first 14 cases, the initial MRI reports were unremarkable or showed non-specific atrophy (Zeidler *et al.*, 1997), but with re-examination, symmetrical high signal was seen in the posterior and medial thalamus in a majority of cases (Sellar *et al.*, 1997; Zeidler *et al.*, 2000). Zeidler *et al.* (2000) analysed scans from 36 patients with vCJD obtained between 1 and 23 months after symptom onset (ranging from 7 to 38 months from presentation to death) and compared them with two groups of patient controls: (*a*) 17 patients referred with suspected CJD but in whom CJD was subsequently ruled out, and (*b*) 40 patients with other types of CJD. Clear hyperintensity of the pulvinar was termed the 'pulvinar sign' (Fig. 19.3(23)) and was present in 78% of the vCJD cases (sensitivity). The sign was seen in 5–29% of the controls giving specificities of 71–95% (Zeidler *et al.*, 1997). Hyperintensity can be seen in vCJD in other grey matter areas: in about 2/3 of cases in dorsomedial thalamic nuclei (Sellar *et al.*, 2002), putamen (in 33%), head of caudate nucleus (in about 25%), and periaqueductal grey matter and / or tectal plate (Coulthard *et al.*, 1999; Oppenheim *et al.*, 2000; Zeidler *et al.*, 2000).

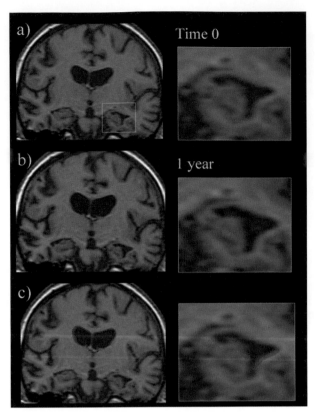

Fig. 19.4 Progression of atrophy in a 55-year-old subject with Alzheimer's disease. Enlarged regions show the left hippocampus. (*a*) Coronal slice taken from the baseline T_1-weighted image. (*b*) Coronal slice taken from the repeat (approximately 1 year later) T_1-weighted image. (*c*) Repeat image registered to the baseline image. Areas shaded red represent areas of change, based on voxels with significantly (greater than 20% of mean brain) lower intensity on the repeat image. (Courtesy of Dr N. Fox, Dementia Research Group, Institute of Neurology, London, UK.)

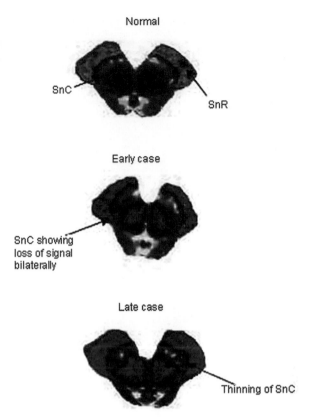

Fig. 19.5 Substantia nigra imaging in Parkinson's disease. Ratio images of normal, early and late PD (see text) presented as a coloured scaled figure (from 0–255). The substantia nigra compacta (SnC) reaches the cerebral peduncles in the normal but is thinner and smaller in the early and late cases. (Modified with permission from Hutchinson & Raff, 1999, and with permission BMJ Publishing Group.)

Hyperintensity may occasionally also be seen diffusely in the white matter of the centrum semiovale (Collie *et al.*, 2001).

Quantification of changes in three cases of vCJD (Coulthard *et al.*, 1999) confirmed the "pulvinar sign" when compared with a group of normal subjects. In a larger UK multi-centre study, 11 confirmed vCJD cases were compared with 28 controls (12 sCJD, 16 non-CJD dementia cases) (Colchester *et al.*, 2002). This study evaluated several different structures for normalizing intensities across subjects. The pulvinar-to-frontal white matter T_2 intensity ratio was an excellent discriminator between vCJD and non-CJD dementia and also between vCJD and sCJD (specificity 89% with sensitivity 100% when a T_2 intensity

ratio of 1.51. was used). Such a ratio cannot be readily judged by eye. The pulvinar-to-putamen proton density ratio was also found to be a good discriminator (91% sensitivity and 89% specificity) (Colchester *et al.*, 2002) using a ratio of 1.0. This is more appropriate for visual reporting because the required discrimination is whether the pulvinar is brighter than the putamen. Confirmation of these findings is needed in a larger study but there is no doubt of the diagnostic importance of pulvinar hyperintensity in distinguishing vCJD from non-CJD dementias and sCJD.

With only small numbers of vCJD patients, there is a shortage of information about other MRI sequences. FLAIR shows changes in the deep nuclei clearly but the numbers of patients examined is very small, 3 of 36 patients in one study (Zeidler *et al.*, 2000). DWI was only carried out in 4/100 vCJD cases in the UK (Sellar *et al.*, 2002). Estimation

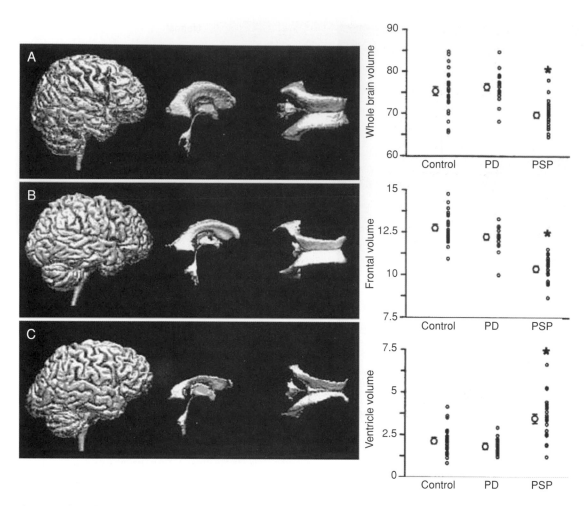

Fig. 19.6 Three-dimensional volumetry in extrapyramidal disorders. Volume rendered 3-D MRI reconstructions of the whole brain and ventricular system in PSP (A), PD (B), and a normal control (C). Left images: cortical atrophy, particularly is apparent in PSP. Middle images: lateral view of the ventricular system showing dilation in PSP compared with PD and controls. Right images: superior view of the ventricular images again shows dilation in PSP compared with PD and controls. The graphs on the right show the measured volumes as a percentage of the total intracranial volume. (Modified with permission from Cordato *et al.*, 2002. Also by permission of Oxford University Press.)

of the ADC was reported in one French vCJD case (Oppenheim *et al.*, 2000) where reduced striatal ADC was found in contrast to increased ADC in the pulvinar. These changes probably reflect different regional pathologies in vCJD: in the striatum, spongiosis predominates, while in the pulvinar, gliosis and neuronal loss are more prominent (Zeidler *et al.*, 2000).

Iatrogenic and familial CJD

There is much less information about the iatrogenic (iCJD) and familial (fCJD) forms. Iatrogenic CJD has arisen as a result of the use of contaminated neurosurgical instruments or EEG electrodes, grafts of dura mater or cornea,

and injection of human-derived pituitary growth hormone and gonadotrophin. It is notable that MRI signal abnormalities have not been observed in these cases (Thadani *et al.*, 1988; Pocchiari *et al.*, 1992; Lane *et al.*, 1994; Billette de Villemeur *et al.*, 1996; Rabinstein *et al.*, 2002). About 15% of all human CJD patients have a genetic basis, and more than 30 genotypes have been identified including various subtypes of the Gerstmann–Straussler–Scheinker syndrome and fatal familial insomnia. The phenotypes vary considerably. MRI findings of atrophy and basal ganglia signal hyperintensity in a small number of patients have been described (Windl *et al.*, 1996). In a time series study of 4 fCJD patients (Murata *et al.*, 2002), abnormalities

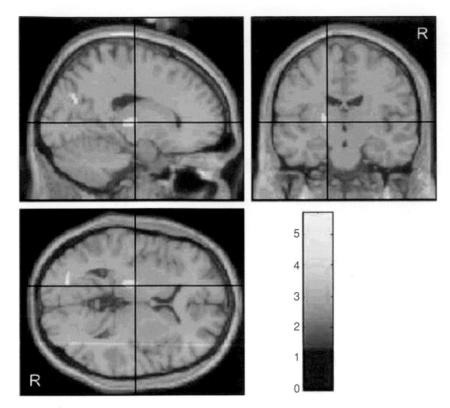

Fig. 19.7 Voxel-based morphometry in tremulous Parkinson's disease. Grouped analysis showing the areas of significantly increased grey matter density rendered on to three orthogonal slices of a stereotaxically normalized brain. Significance is denoted by the color code which represents Z scores. The cross hairs represent the thalamic area with the highest significance. This was located in the ventralis intermedius nucleus. (Modified with permission from Kassubek *et al.*, 2002. Reprinted from *Neurosci.Lett.*, Copyright 2002 with permission from Elsevier.)

on DWI appeared earlier in the caudate than in the putamen.

Functional MRI (fMRI) in neurodegenerative diseases

Introduction

Functional MRI is perhaps the most complex of the current MRI techniques. It is used as an index of regional cerebral blood flow (rCBF). FMRI measures a relative signal change between two states – active and baseline. This is a marker for a change in rCBF that is interpreted as a marker of neuronal metabolic activity. The result is correlated to performance of a specific task that was performed during scanning (Belliveau *et al.*, 1991; Rao *et al.*, 1993; Turner *et al.*, 1998). Advantages over radiotracer-based techniques (PET and SPECT) include the wider availability of imaging systems, independence of tracers, avoidance of ionizing radi-

ation and a relatively short scanning time. The use of fMRI in clinical practice is currently limited to case reports of planning of neurosurgical interventions, e.g. localizing the motor strip (Puce *et al.*, 1995; Atlas *et al.*, 1996) or language areas prior to resection of vascular malformations or tumours (Binder *et al.*, 1996; Bahn *et al.*, 1997b; Pouratian *et al.*, 2002; Baciu *et al.*, 2003) (Fig. 19.9). It is probable that its use in neurodegenerative disorders will increase in a similar manner.

For fMRI, the pattern of rCBF in an individual, or in a group of subjects, is compared with a control group who are scanned under identical conditions to make inferences concerning the activation. Questions which may be answered by fMRI can include the following.

Does a structurally abnormal area of cerebral tissue activate normally?
A structurally abnormal area would be hypothesized to have impaired activation. A structurally normal area may

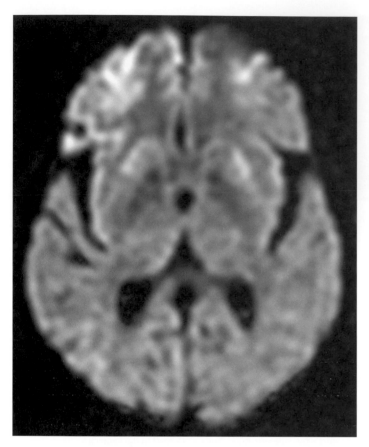

Fig. 19.8 Diffusion-weighted image of confirmed sporadic CJD showing high signal in the anterior basal ganglia, and striking high signal in the right frontal lobe, with less marked cortical hyperintensity in the right insular and left frontal lobe.

however activate abnormally, providing pathophysiological information which is not detectable by routine structural imaging. Studies can also determine if activation is modulated by drugs (Loubinoux *et al.*, 1999; Pariente *et al.*, 2001).

Can fMRI detect subclinical or preclinical states?
One may be able to identify which members of an at-risk group have abnormal activation, e.g. the hippocampal activation in subjects with a family history of AD (Smith *et al.*, 1999). This could potentially lead to early enrolment of at-risk individuals in presymptomatic drug trials when neuroprotective therapies become available.

Does a cerebral region overactivate during task performance?
Regional overactivation may be a compensatory mechanism by which the diseased brain attempts to improve performance by recruiting cerebral regions which are less

affected by the disease. This method lends itself particularly to the study of developmental and learning disorders, e.g. dyslexia, but also applies to degenerative disorders, e.g. overactivation of lateral premotor cortex in PD during performance of sequential finger movements (Sabatini *et al.*, 2000). Over-activation should be cautiously interpreted since overactivation of an inhibitory nucleus may impair clinical function.

What is the time scale of the rCBF changes?
PET and SPECT have temporal resolutions of minutes, but changes in rCBF occur over seconds (Kleinschmidt *et al.*, 1996). The temporal resolution of fMRI allows for detection of haemodynamic changes which occur over approximately 1–3 seconds (Turner *et al.*, 1998; Samuel *et al.*, 1998).

Are discrete regions functionally related?
The spatial and temporal patterns of a set of activated regions allows inferences to be made on connectivity within a known neural network (Rowe *et al.*, 2002).

Method of fMRI

Basic principles
Some methods and pitfalls relevant to fMRI are similar to those of non-routine structural MRI, but others are specific to fMRI. To appreciate these, some knowledge of terminology is required and a brief account of fMRI will be given below.

Signal changes increase in proportion to the magnetic field strength: at 1.5 tesla, signal changes may be 2–4% (Kwong *et al.*, 1992), but at 4 tesla up to 28% signal change may be detected (Turner *et al.*, 1993). However, the safety of high field strength is not as well determined in humans, especially when combined with use of electrical equipment and most fMRI is currently performed on commercially available 1.5 tesla scanners. The abundance of hydrogen (^{1}H) nuclei and its large magnetic moment make it ideal for fMRI. As ^{1}H nuclei are excited by an applied radiofrequency (RF) pulse, some gain enough energy to flip (through a flip angle) to align anti-parallel to the magnetic field. A RF pulse sequence that involves application of a 90° followed by a 180° refocusing pulse is called a spin echo sequence. Relatively long TE (60 ms) and TR times (up to 2.5 s) are typically required[2]. MRI data are encoded in a system called

---

[2] TE is the time from application of one RF pulse to the detection of the signal in the receiving coil (i.e. an echo) and determines the amount of decay. TR is the time from application of one RF pulse to the application of the next RF pulse (i.e. repetition) and determines the amount of recovery.

k-space (conceptually similar to a two-dimensional grid). Data are mathematically modelled along the rows of *k*-space, usually filling one row at a time. An image of voxels is generated after deconvolution. In conventional MRI, one line of *k*-space is filled every TR (i.e. during 1 echo, 1 line of voxels is filled). For a matrix of 256 voxels in one dimension and a TR of 0.5 s, filling 256 lines takes $256 \times 0.5 = 128$ seconds.

The two major advances which led to the development of fMRI from structural MRI were the ability to acquire MRI data very rapidly and the discovery of endogenous contrast.

Methods to acquire ultra-fast MRI

Involuntary head motion (even millimeters) from lengthy scanning protocols can seriously distort MR images (Weisskoff & Cohen, 1997). Cyclical motion artefact from heartbeat or respiration can be reduced by cardiorespiratory-gating but this adds to scanning time. Hemodynamic responses in vivo occur over 6–9 seconds (Frahm *et al.*, 1992) but can habituate over seconds (Samuel *et al.*, 1998). FMRI data are acquired in a slice-by-slice fashion and since the whole brain volume needs to be scanned in seconds, this means that each slice must be acquired in milliseconds.

A RF pulse sequence that varies as it is applied is called a gradient echo sequence. This requires additional coils within the bore of the magnet, leading to small inhomogeneities in the magnetic field. This causes additional loss of signal, called T_2^* decay. Gradient echo sequences are particularly susceptible to inhomogeneities and these were originally considered a nuisance in structural MRI, but it is the T_2^* signal which is used in fMRI. Hence, fMRI images are termed T_2^* weighted. By reducing flip angles and using gradient echo sequences, both TE and TR can be reduced (to about 5 and 50 milliseconds, respectively), enabling image acquisition in seconds. Fast MRI using gradient echo hardware has been achieved with different systems which have names depending on the manufacturer, e.g. FLASH (fast low angled shot) with Siemens. Using FLASH, visual cortex activation was detected during photic stimulation with a scanning time of 1.5 seconds (Frahm *et al.*, 1992). These conventional methods typically yield low signals and are sensitive to inflow phenomena and have now largely been superseded by the more advanced techniques described below.

Another method to reduce scanning time is to reduce encoding time. In the early 1980s, Mansfield's group were studying fast cardiac imaging and succeeded in acquiring whole body transverse human images in 57 ms (Chapman *et al.*, 1987) by filling *k*-space continually rather than sequentially. This encoding system fills a 2D plane of *k*-space for each TR (i.e. during 1 echo, 1 plane was filled) and has become known as echo planar imaging (EPI). This approach generates more image distortion, especially near bony structures, such as sinuses. Technical advances have improved the signal/noise ratio and gradient echo EPI is now the basis for most fMRI studies (Kwong, 1995).

fMRI contrast

Exogenous contrast

This is analogous to the radiotracer method of PET. When Gadolinium diethylene triamine pentaacetic acid (Gd-DTPA) is injected during task performance, it accumulates in metabolically active areas. However, bolus injections render fMRI invasive and has now been replaced by methods relying on endogenous contrast.

Endogenous contrast

The BOLD (blood oxygenation level dependent) technique is the most commonly used method (Ogawa *et al.*, 1990). During activation, a mismatch occurs between the delivery of oxygenated blood and oxygen extraction (Fox & Raichle, 1986; Fox *et al.*, 1988; Frostig *et al.*, 1990), leading to a reduced concentration of deoxyhaemoglobin (dxHb) in venous capillaries of the activated region. Since dxHb is paramagnetic and decreases MR signal, a fall in the concentration of dxHb leads to an increase in T_2^*-weighted signal. In vivo, using 7 tesla gradient echo sequences, veins in rat cortex became brighter as blood flow through them increased (i.e. the veins received more oxygenated blood) (Ogawa *et al.*, 1990). Subsequently, in humans in vivo using a 1.5 tesla system, a 1.8% increase in signal was confirmed in primary visual cortex during photic stimulation (Kwong *et al.*, 1992). The decrease in dxHb concentration during activation has now been also shown by near infrared spectroscopy (NIRS). Motor cortex was identified by FLASH fMRI during finger movement and NIRS demonstrated a delay of <10 s from task performance to the fall in dxHb signal in the same region, demonstrating too the existence of the hemodynamic lag from neuronal activation to measured response (Kleinschmidt *et al.*, 1996).

Image pre-processing and analysis

This includes co-registration with emphasis on reduction of artefactual motion and removal of high and low frequency noise (Friston *et al.*, 1995a, c, 1996). For between-group comparisons in multi-subject studies, each individual's images can be spatially transformed into a standard stereotaxic space (Talairach & Tournoux, 1988). Spatial and temporal smoothing are applied to increase the signal to noise ratio. In the simplest form of analysis, each voxel

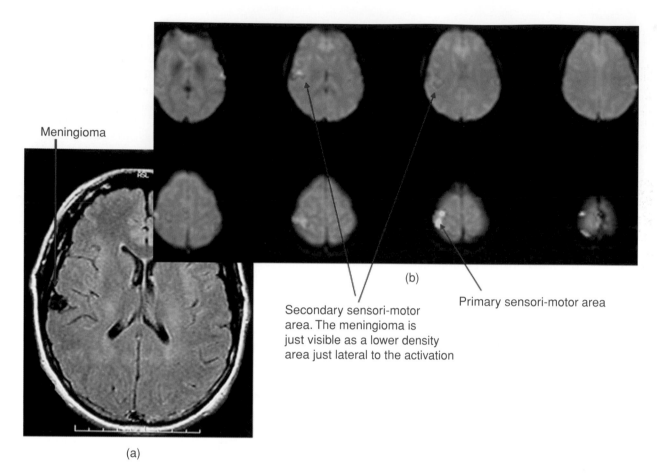

Meningioma

(b)

Secondary sensori-motor
area. The meningioma is
just visible as a lower density
area just lateral to the activation

Primary sensori-motor area

(a)

Fig. 19.9 The clinical application of fMRI in neurosurgical planning. (*a*) Structural axial FLAIR MRI of patient with a right superficial meningioma lying adjacent to the right secondary sensorimotor area. (*b*) FMRI activation associated with stimulation (using a brush) of the patient's left hand showing activation of right primary and secondary sensorimotor cortex. The activation is rendered directly on to T_2^*-weighted functional images in which the meningioma is visible as a low intensity area adjacent to the second sensorimotor area. The meningioma was successfully resected without sensorimotor compromise. (Personal communication, Courtesy of Mr R. Selway, King's College Hospital, London and Dr V. Ng, Maudsley Hospital, London.)

will display a time series, that is with a signal which alternates from lower intensity (during the baseline tasks) to a higher intensity (during the activated state). The task, hemodynamic response and BOLD effect can be modeled as a box–car function, i.e. alternating periods of "high" and "low" periods (e.g. see Fig. 19.10B), with the haemodynamic response typically lagged by 6–9 seconds after task performance. Alternatively, the hemodynamic response can be modelled as a sine wave or half-sine wave. Typically 60–100 T_2^*-weighted multi-slice data sets are acquired. Averaged "low" periods, (baseline state) are compared with averaged "high" periods (activated state) to determine activated voxels – so-called blocked-design subtraction studies.

Another method of fMRI analysis examines the hemodynamic responses but does not depend on prior assump-

tions of the shape or delay of the hemodynamic response, so called event-related fMRI. Voxels that are activated by a task are hypothesized to have a stereotyped hemodynamic response, irrespective of the shape of the response. Single cognitive or motor tasks are performed repeatedly every few seconds and fMRI signal is averaged in a manner similar to the back-averaging used in electrophysiological studies (Buckner *et al.*, 1996; Humberstone *et al.*, 1997b; Friston *et al.*, 1998; Clare *et al.*, 1999; Watanabe *et al.*, 2002). The variance of activated voxels would be expected to be lower than the variance of voxels depicting random noise. The magnitude of signal changes in event-related fMRI is generally smaller than in blocked-design subtraction studies and higher magnetic fields strengths (3 and 4 tesla) are usually required (Richter *et al.*, 1997; Humberstone *et al.*, 1997b; Clare *et al.*, 1999), although results have been reported using conventional scanners (Toma *et al.*, 1999).

Presentation of results

FMRI comparisons involve the analysis of tens of thousands of voxels by using automated statistical programs. Differences surviving a predetermined threshold are considered physiologically significant. Results are presented as color-coded maps rendered on to a structural MRI for gyral localization, giving a spatial resolution of 1–3 mm (Turner *et al.*, 1998) (e.g Fig. 19.11). An alternative method is to present black and white 3-D maximum intensity projections (e.g. Fig. 19.12) with the spatially normalized stereotaxic coordinates of the voxel with peak statistical significance, representing the center of a cluster. One can determine the number of voxels in a cluster and the magnitude of the difference, usually 0.5–5% with conventional strength MRI scanners. The time course of the change can also be inspected (e.g. Fig. 19.10B).

Pitfalls in fMRI for neurodegenerative disorders

Experimental design

During fMRI, subjects are isolated from examiners and direct visual assessment is not possible. Claustrophobia can be a problem in normal subjects but more so in subjects with degenerative disorders. Cueing and stimulation equipment should be outside the scanner and signals delivered to the subjects via VDU projection systems or headphones. Assessment of task performance is by repetition of the task outside the scanner or by use of specifically designed, non-ferromagnetic equipment which can be safely introduced into the magnet. Long coiled cables can induce heating and can be dangerous if in contact with a subject.

Inter-subject variability

Early fMRI studies in normal humans reported results of several, single-subject analyses. Generally these were in agreement with PET results but some individual variability existed (Tyszka *et al.*, 1994; Richter *et al.*, 1997; Humberstone *et al.*, 1997a; Toma *et al.*, 1999). Possible explanations include motion artifact, task strategies, gyral anatomy and vessel architecture. These different activation patterns during performance of identical tasks in healthy controls will cause difficulty in the interpretation of patient studies, e.g. how should one interpret the results of a study in which a patient with PD, who fails to activate mesial frontal cortex, is compared with a control volunteer who also fails to

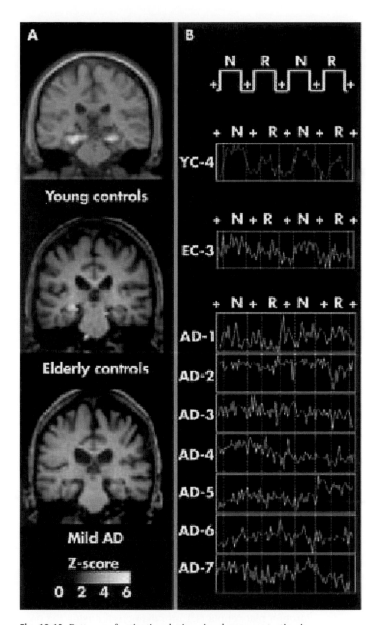

Fig. 19.10 Patterns of activation during visual memory testing in controls and AD. (A) Within-group activation in young controls, elderly controls and mild AD during presentation of novel and repeated face-name pairs. There is much less activation in the elderly controls and no activation in the AD group at the hippocampus. (B) The box car function of the paradigm of presentation of novel (N) and repeated (R) face-name pairs (upper tracing) shows a clear similarity to the fMRI signal in the hippocampal region from a young-control subject (YC-4), less similarity in an elderly control (EC-3) and little similarity in the seven AD subjects (AD-1 to 7). (Modified with permission from Sperling *et al.*, 2003 and with permission of BMJ Publishing Group.)

activate this region? It is anticipated that fMRI will evolve sufficiently to allow interpretation of individual studies.

Spatial normalization of brains with degenerative diseases
For multi-subject grouped studies, spatial normalization is required. This has the disadvantage of loss of spatial resolution but gives the advantage of less variability when making inferences about a disease process. While this may seem appropriate for normal scans, it may be less meaningful in studies of degenerative diseases with regional atrophy, because spatial normalization of an atrophic region may be inappropriate. Hence the stringency of spatial transformations should be considered.

Differing analytical software
The field of data analysis has seen an explosion of methods over the last decade (Gold *et al.*, 1998), each method developed by an institution with expertise in imaging (e.g. statistical parametric mapping (Friston *et al.*, 1995b), AFNI (Cox, 1996), STIMULATE (Strupp, 1996), Generic brain activation mapping (Brammer *et al.*, 1997)). One group showed that event-related fMRI detects activation which may not be detected by blocked-design subtraction methods (Mechelli *et al.*, 2003). Currently, there is no standard analysis method. This hinders the uniform interpretation of results form different centres. Also, high field strength scanners are more sensitive to small changes in signal and so the possibility of false negatives results on lower field scanners with high statistical thresholds should be recognized.

The brain–vein issue
In an early motor study of the precentral cortex, fMRI signal increased by 2–32% during finger–thumb oppositions. One individual who underwent a magnetic resonance angiogram (MRA) showed a correlation between the location of the activated fMRI focus and the location of a pial venule (<1 mm diameter), raising the possibility that BOLD signal might originate form draining venules (Lai *et al.*, 1993). Similarly, when primary visual cortex was directly viewed through cranial windows in lightly anesthetized monkeys during optical stimulation (Turner & Grinvald, 1994), the delayed decrease in dxHB concentration occurred 2–3 seconds following stimulus onset as expected but was predominantly detected in subpial venules up to 2 mm distant from the cortical parenchyma. These findings suggest that BOLD signal may have 2 components: one from parenchymal capillaries; the other from venules draining an area larger than the focus of activity. Flow components can be minimized by applying tailored RF pulses (Frahm *et al.*, 1987) and some groups compare fMRI activations with MRA (Frahm *et al.*, 1992; Lai *et al.*, 1993). However, it would be surprising to see changes far downstream in a venule since effects of oxygenation and inflow in a small cortical domain are likely to be diluted rapidly. In multi-subject studies, it is unlikely that the location of individual venules is sufficiently similar to allow signal to persist after inter-subject averaging. Nonetheless, it should be remembered that BOLD signal may not originate solely from activated capillaries (Cannestra *et al.*, 2001).

Having described the methods and pitfalls of fMRI, we shall now review its current use in the investigation of neurodegenerative disorders.

Dementias

Alzheimer's disease
The majority of current literature relates to AD. Activation studies have interrogated the hippocampus and entorhinal cortex, where pathological studies, volumetric MRI and neuropsychological studies have demonstrated early changes in AD. Significant activation at these loci using auditory and visual encoding paradigms initially had to be demonstrated in young normal individuals (Kato *et al.*, 1998, 2000; Stark & Squire, 2000). In one study, no differences were found between younger and older nondemented individuals (Kato *et al.*, 2001) during visual encoding, whereas another study showed a decline of right hippocampal activation in the elderly during encoding of novel faces who also showed less prefrontal and greater bi-parietal activation than the younger individuals (Sperling *et al.*, 2003). Elderly individuals with age-related memory decline (Small *et al.*, 2002) showed a variable loss of entorhinal activation and less activation of the subiculum and dentate gyrus (Small *et al.*, 1999).

In contrast, patients with AD show a marked lack of activation in the entire hippocampal formation and the entorhinal cortex (Small *et al.*, 1999) (Fig. 19.10) (Small *et al.*, 2000; Kato *et al.*, 2001; Sperling *et al.*, 2003) and less activation in left temporal lobe, right prefrontal cortex and right supramarginal gyrus during visual encoding (Fig. 19.13). Another study employed a visuospatial angle estimation paradigm to specifically engage visual association cortex and showed less activity in superior parietal lobule but more activity in oculotemporal cortex in AD (Prvulovic *et al.*, 2002). A study of visually-guided saccadic tracking found impaired activation of the right intraparietal sulcus in 2/3 of patients, while the remaining 1/3 had normal patterns (Thulborn *et al.*, 2000). The reasons for these differences are currently unclear.

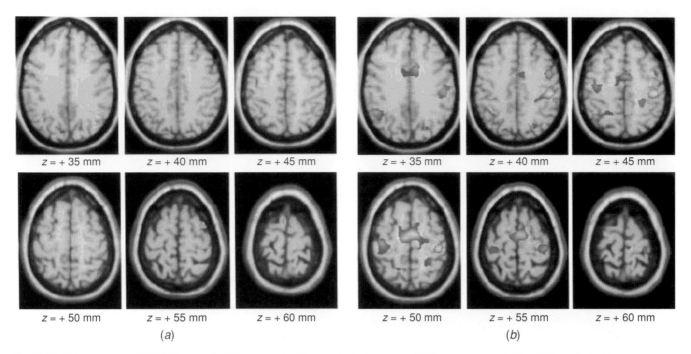

Fig. 19.11 Between group fMRI differences in PD compared with controls during sequential finger movements ($P < 0.01$, z = height in mm from commissural plane in spatially normalized images). (*a*) Areas of relative underactivity in PD compared with controls. (*b*) Areas of relative overactivity in PD compared with controls. (Modified with permission from Sabatini *et al.*, 2000. Also by permission of Oxford University Press.)

One multi-subject, between-group study showed no correlation between activation and atrophy in non-demented elderly individuals. In contrast, patients with AD showed a positive correlation between activation and atrophy in left inferior frontal gyrus, i.e. more activation in an area with more atrophy. This suggests a possible specific compensatory mechanism in left inferior frontal gyrus in AD (Johnson *et al.*, 2000). Additional regions of overactivation in AD have been described in bilateral frontal and cingulate cortex during match–mismatch verbal tasks requiring decision making (Saykin *et al.*, 1999). Treatment with rivastigmine enhances activation in fusiform and frontal cortex during visual encoding but simultaneously decreases activation in frontal cortex (Rombouts *et al.*, 2002), suggesting that the mechanism of action of anticholinesterases may not be uniform throughout the cortex.

In summary, the failure of activation of the entorhinal cortex appears to be a consistent feature of AD but the differences of activation of the other cortical sites is more variable and should always be interpreted in relation to the nature of the performed task. The variable results raise awareness that fMRI in neurodegenerative disorders should generally be considered preliminary and highlight the difficulties with interpretation as outlined earlier.

Individuals at risk of AD

Studies of subjects at risk of developing AD have attempted to detect early abnormalities which are undetectable by structural imaging or neuropsychological testing. In these studies, patients were considered at risk if they had a positive family history and the presence of at least one ApoEe4 allele. At risk individuals showed reduced activation in the mid- and posterior inferotemporal regions bilaterally during naming and letter fluency tasks despite identical performance to controls (Smith *et al.*, 1999). However, in other studies of at-risk individuals, hippocampal overactivation was detected along with a greater number of activated regions generally, including inferior frontal, prefrontal and temporal cortex, suggesting that at-risk individuals may need early recruitment of preserved cortical areas to maintain normal function (Bookheimer *et al.*, 2000; Burggren *et al.*, 2002). These studies require further corroboration as they hold a potential to identify at risk individuals who may benefit from disease-modifying therapies when these become available.

Other dementias

An early study on a single patient with DLB showed less primary visual cortex activation during a period with hallucinations compared with a period on treatment with

(a)   (b)   (c)

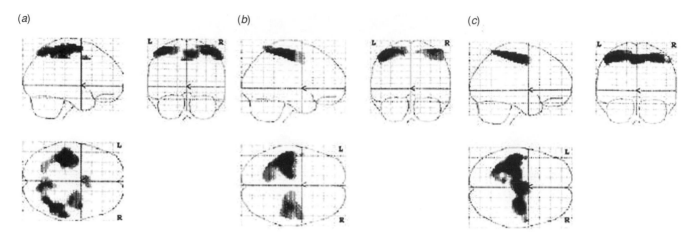

Fig. 19.12 Within-group maximum intensity projection maps of fMRI activation associated with joystick movements for controls, PD off and on treatment ($P < 0.01$ uncorrected, extent threshold 10 voxels). (*a*) Control group. (*b*) PD group off treatment. (*c*) PD group on levodopa. (Modified with permission from Haslinger *et al.*, 2001). Also by permission from Oxford University Press.)

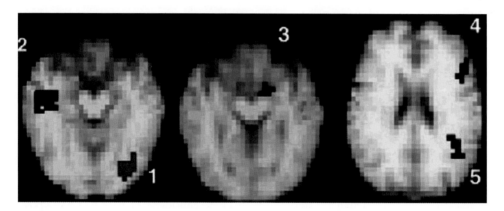

Fig. 19.13 Grouped differences between young controls, elderly non-demented controls and AD during visual stimulation. The area depicted in red is the right visual association area (1), where activation occurred in all three groups. The areas in blue are left anterior–inferior temporal lobe (2), the right entorhinal cortex (3), the right lateral prefrontal regions (4) and the right supramarginal gyrus (5), where there was activation in all non-demented subjects but no activation in AD subjects ($p < 0.0005$). (Modified with permission from Kato *et al.*, 2001.)

risperidone without hallucinations (Howard *et al.*, 1997). There have been no reported studies in other dementias. Undoubtedly, study of these will be rewarding since the presence of early associated features (e.g. aphasia, myoclonus, parkinsonism, hallucinations, apraxia, incontinence) offers new opportunities to study functional correlates of these less common symptoms and signs.

Extrapyramidal disorders

Parkinson's Disease
The majority of studies relate to PD. It is generally easier to study PD than other extrapyramidal syndromes because the MR images do not have discrete regions of altered signal,

which distorts MRI, (e.g. MSA Fig. 19.3(9), Wilson's disease Fig. 19.3(13)) and atrophy is usually not extensive early in the course of the illness. Many PET studies on PD also provide a standard with which to corroborate fMRI. One drawback of studying PD is motion artefact since most patients have tremor and those who do not may not represent typical idiopathic PD.

An early fMRI study comparing PD with controls confirmed that activation in dorsolateral prefrontal cortex (DLPFC) and rostral supplementary motor area (SMA) was reduced, while activation in caudal SMA, lateral premotor, primary motor and inferior parietal cortex was enhanced, during performance of complex finger movements (Sabatini *et al.*, 2000) (Fig. 19.11). These results replicate previous PET studies (Playford *et al.*, 1992; Samuel *et al.*, 1997), although overactivation of primary motor cortex was not detected by PET. Similarly, primary motor cortex overactivation, associated with a diffuse hemispheric overactivation, has now also been demonstrated in vivo (Haslinger *et al.*, 2001) (Fig. 19.12) and in a rat model of parkinsonism during electrical stimulation of a forepaw (Pelled *et al.*, 2002). In contrast, primary motor cortex hypo-activation was detected in another recent study during finger movements and this hypo-activation reversed with levodopa treatment, in a manner analogous to the levodopa- and apomorphine-induced reversal of hypoactive SMA detected with PET (Jenkins *et al.*, 1992; Rascol *et al.*, 1994). Taken together, fMRI studies of PD are in broad agreement with PET studies, although the nature of primary motor cortex abnormality – or compensation – is more variable and needs clarification.

Studies of cognitive function using a sentence comprehension task in PD have shown a similar phenomenon (Grossman *et al.*, 2003). While a control group of seniors showed activation in temporal, ventral and inferior frontal regions of the left hemisphere and striatum, patients with PD showed under-activity of striatal, prefrontal, and right temporal regions but over-activity in right inferior frontal and left temporal-parietal areas. This study extends the concept of compensatory cortical overactivation for cognitive function in PD, in a manner similar to the proposed overactivation of premotor–parietal–cerebellar circuits to compensate for impaired motor performance (Samuel *et al.*, 1997; Sabatini *et al.*, 2000).

More complex analyses of cognitive processes in PD can be studied with fMRI. Rowe *et al.* studied effective connectivity (the influence of one brain region on another) by measuring fMRI signal during sequential finger movement tasks when subjects had either no additional cognitive load, or they were asked to "think about the next move" (i.e. attention to action), or during presentation of colored lights (a distractor task) (Rowe *et al.*, 2002). Comparing all motor tasks with rest, an atypical overactivation in SMA was detected in PD. This had previously been demonstrated only under specific conditions of additional cognitive load with PET (Catalan *et al.*, 1999; Samuel *et al.*, 2001). Normal subjects showed an increase in coupling between prefrontal cortex and SMA during attention to action, which did not occur with the distractor task. Patients with PD failed to show an increase in coupling during attention to action. This supports the view that in PD, there is a functional disconnection of SMA from prefrontal cortex during attention to action and implies that the typical underactivity of mesial frontal cortex is task dependent, rather than a fixed deficit.

Treatment of PD includes deep brain stimulation (DBS) of the thalamus, subthalamic nucleus, and globus pallidus. The safety of fMRI during DBS with external stimulation (i.e. before implantation of the pulse generator) was shown in patients with chronic pain and essential tremor (Rezai *et al.*, 1999). At the point of stimulation, the electrode tip causes an artefact which hinders analysis, but at sites distant to DBS, fMRI can assess metabolic responses. Patients with PD with DBS (of subthalamic nucleus or ventral intermedius nucleus of the thalamus) showed increased activation in subcortical nuclei ipsilateral to stimulation (thalamus, globus pallidus, substantia nigra, superior colliculus) and in prefrontal cortex and lateral premotor cortex (Jech *et al.*, 2001, 2003). There was, however, considerable individual variability and these results are considered preliminary.

In contrast to cortical signals, there is limited and variable information on subcortical activation. The subcortical nuclei, in particular dorsal striatum, are believed to be dysfunctional in PD and theoretically, fMRI would be an ideal tool with which to demonstrate abnormal metabolic activity here. Analysis methods may have to be tailored to specifically detect activation in the basal ganglia, for example the spatial smoothing applied to enhance cortical signal may be suboptimal for detection of a small number of voxels with low amplitude signal change. Some groups have detected basal ganglia activation in normal volunteers (Bucher *et al.*, 1995) and in patients with a variety of focal pallidal lesions, although results have been subtle and variable (Bucher *et al.*, 1996). In 15 normal volunteers studied by double slice (4 mm) FLASH fMRI, the mean number of activated voxels within pallidum was 7 ± 1, contralateral to a limb during very rapid pronation-supination movements. Putaminal activation was more variable. Patients with pallidal lesions had generally less pallidal activation (mean = 5 ± 1 voxels). Only recently has striatal activation been detected in normal subjects with grouped studies (McClure *et al.*, 2003). Grouped studies may provide one manner with which to increase the signal/noise ratio in the basal ganglia. Detection of robust signals in basal ganglia is therefore at an early stage. FMRI of subcortical structures in neurodegenerative disorders is further hampered by the combination of atrophy, gliosis, and the local deposition of metallic compounds.

Other extra-pyramidal syndromes

There have been few studies of fMRI in Huntington's disease. During performance of a maze task, reduced fMRI signal was observed in caudate nucleus and sensorimotor, occipital, parietal cortex while increased activation was found in left postcentral and right middle frontal gyri (Clark

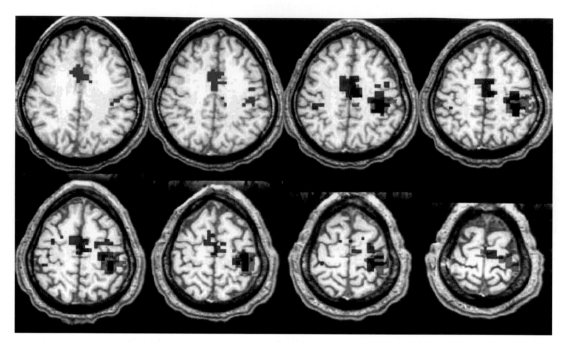

Fig. 19.14 Between-group fMRI differences in ALS compared with controls during right hand movements, showing the re-organization of the motor network in ALS. ALS (red) controls (blue). (Modified with permission from Springer–Verlag Journal; Konrad *et al.*, 2002.)

et al., 2002). The significance of these changes is undetermined and has not been correlated to focal regions of cortical atrophy. Cognitive and motor symptoms in HD have been suggested to result from a failure of central inhibitory mechanisms in basal ganglia–thalamo–cortical circuits. The presence of inhibitory central processing is postulated to prevent involuntary reactions from interfering with normal behavior. This phenomenon has been studied with fMRI with a "masked prime" task, in which visible left- or right-pointing arrows are presented, preceded by briefly presented and subsequently masked prime arrows (Aron *et al.*, 2003). Subjects performed key-presses to each target in either the same (a compatible response) or opposite direction (an incompatible response). Normally, there is a faster reaction time for incompatible responses. Choreic HD subjects showed an absence of this effect while non-choreic subjects showed an excessive inhibition compared with controls. These results suggest that dysfunction of basal ganglia-thalamo-cortical circuits can lead to either lack of motor inhibition or excessive inhibition but does not further distinguish the site of these mechanisms.

To date, there have been no reported fMRI studies of other extrapyramidal syndromes.

Motor system disorders
Currently available publications relate to upper motor neuron dysfunction in amyotrophic lateral sclerosis (ALS),

whereas the brunt of pathological change occurs in the anterior horn cells and in the giant Betz cells of the motor cortex. One early study investigated cortical reorganization in ALS by studying performance of simple finger flexions with a force generation of only 10% of the maximum in order to avoid the confounding effects of recruitment of additional muscles as patients attempt to overcome their motor impairment (Konrad *et al.*, 2002). This grouped study showed activation of primary motor, lateral premotor, mesial frontal and inferior parietal cortex, but in the ALS group the center of mass of activation of primary motor cortex was shifted anteriorly by 4–7 mm in stereotaxic space to encroach on the posterior aspect of lateral premotor cortex. This corroborates previous PET studies in ALS (Kew *et al.*, 1993). In addition, enhanced ipsilateral primary motor cortex activation was present. Premotor cortex has a direct projection to spinal cord (Dum & Strick, 1991) and the expansion of activation of motor areas in ALS may represent cortical reorganization in response to corticospinal tract disruption and Betz cell loss (Fig. 19.14).

It is, however, also possible that expansion of cortical motor areas during movement in ALS represents impaired cortico-cortical inhibition (Ziemann *et al.*, 1997) as a result of glutamate excitotoxicity. In direct contrast to motor studies, passively stroking the palm of ALS patients during a pure sensory paradigm consistently showed reduced activation of sensorimotor cortex without significant differences in thalamic or cerebellar activation, indicating that the sensory system appears intact at least up to, but not including, the cortical level (Brooks *et al.*, 2000). The impaired cortical activation following passive sensory stimulation may simply be a result of loss of cortical neurons, detected subclinically. If reproducible, it raises the possibility that passive fMRI sensory studies can be performed in severely motorically impaired ALS patients for a potentially useful diagnostic test. Further studies of passive and cognitive tasks in motor neuron disease are eagerly awaited. There are no fMRI reports on the other forms of motor neuron diseases.

Ataxias

To date, there have been no reported studies of fMRI in degenerative sporadic or hereditary ataxias, such as SCA syndromes, Friedreich's ataxia, ataxia telangiectasia, ataxia with oculomotor apraxia or other idiopathic disorders. Cerebellar activation can, however, be studied with fMRI in cerebellar degeneration. One early study demonstrated cerebellar somatotopy (Wessel & Nitschke, 1997). It is likely that cerebellar studies will become more widespread in future.

Prion diseases

To date, there are no published reports of fMRI in prion diseases.

Acknowledgement

We are very grateful to Dr J. Jarosz, Professor SCR Williams and Dr C Bain for their helpful contribution to this chapter. MS is supported by the Peel Medical Research Trust, London.

REFERENCES

Adachi, M., Hosoya, T., Haku, T., Yamaguchi, K. & Kawanami, T. (1999). Evaluation of the substantia nigra in patients with Parkinsonian syndrome accomplished using multishot diffusion-weighted MR imaging. *Am. J. Neuroradiol.*, **20**, 1500–6.

Aron, A. R., Schlaghecken, F., Fletcher, P. C. *et al.* (2003). Inhibition of subliminally primed responses is mediated by the caudate and thalamus: evidence from functional MRI and Huntington's disease. *Brain*, **126**, 713–23.

Ashburner, J. & Friston, K. J. (1997). Multimodal image coregistration and partitioning – a unified framework. *Neuroimage*, **6**, 209–17.

(2000). Voxel-based morphometry – the methods. *Neuroimage*, **11**, 805–21.

Atlas, S. W., Howard, R. S., Maldjian, J. *et al.* (1996). Functional magnetic resonance imaging of regional brain activity in patients with intracerebral gliomas: findings and implications for clinical management. *Neurosurgery*, **38**, 329–38.

Baciu, M., Le Bas, J. F., Segebarth, C. & Benabid, A. L. (2003). Presurgical fMRI evaluation of cerebral reorganization and motor deficit in patients with tumors and vascular malformations. *Eur. J. Radiol.*, **46**, 139–46.

Bahn, M. M., Kido, D. K., Lin, W. & Pearlman, A. L. (1997a). Brain magnetic resonance diffusion abnormalities in Creutzfeldt–Jakob disease. *Arch. Neurol.*, **54**, 1411–15.

Bahn, M. M., Lin, W., Silbergeld, D. L. *et al.* (1997b). Localization of language cortices by functional MR imaging compared with intracarotid amobarbital hemispheric sedation. *Am. J. Roentgenol.*, **169**, 575–9.

Bahn, M. M. & Parchi, P. (1999). Abnormal diffusion-weighted magnetic resonance images in Creutzfeldt–Jakob disease. *Arch. Neurol.*, **56**, 577–83.

Bammer, R. (2003). Basic principles of diffusion-weighted imaging. *Eur. J. Radiol.*, **45**, 169–84.

Bammer, R., Acar, B. & Moseley, M. E. (2003). In vivo MR tractography using diffusion imaging. *Eur. J. Radiol.*, **45**, 223–34.

Barber, R., Gholkar, A., Scheltens, P., Ballard, C., McKeith, I. G. & O'Brien, J. T. (1999a). Medial temporal lobe atrophy on MRI in dementia with Lewy bodies. *Neurology*, **52**, 1153–8.

Barber, R., Scheltens, P., Gholkar, A. *et al.* (1999b). White matter lesions on magnetic resonance imaging in dementia with Lewy bodies, Alzheimer's disease, vascular dementia, and normal aging. *J. Neurol. Neurosurg. Psychiatry*, **67**, 66–72.

Barber, R., Ballard, C., McKeith, I. G., Gholkar, A. & O'Brien, J. T. (2000a). MRI volumetric study of dementia with Lewy bodies: a comparison with AD and vascular dementia. *Neurology*, **54**, 1304–9.

Barber, R., Gholkar, A., Scheltens, P., Ballard, C., McKeith, I. G. & O'Brien, J. T. (2000b). MRI volumetric correlates of white matter lesions in dementia with Lewy bodies and Alzheimer's disease. *Int. J. Geriatr. Psychiatry*, **15**, 911–16.

Barber, R., McKeith, I. G., Ballard, C., Gholkar, A. & O'Brien, J. T. (2001a). A comparison of medial and lateral temporal lobe atrophy in dementia with Lewy bodies and Alzheimer's disease: magnetic resonance imaging volumetric study. *Dement. Geriatr. Cogn Disord.*, **12**, 198–205.

Barber, R., Panikkar, A. & McKeith, I. G. (2001b). Dementia with Lewy bodies: diagnosis and management. *Int. J. Geriatr. Psychiatry*, **16** Suppl 1, S12–18.

Barber, R., McKeith, I., Ballard, C. & O'Brien, J. (2002). Volumetric MRI study of the caudate nucleus in patients with dementia with Lewy bodies, Alzheimer's disease, and vascular dementia. *J. Neurol. Neurosurg. Psychiatry*, **72**, 406–7.

Barboriak, D. P., Provenzale, J. M. & Boyko, O. B. (1994). MR diagnosis of Creutzfeld–Jakob disease: significance of high signal intensity of the basal ganglia. *Am. J. Radiol.*, **162**, 137–40.

Bardinet, E., Colchester, A. C. F., Roche, A. *et al.* (2001). Registration of reconstructed post-mortem optical data with MR scans of the same patient. In *Medical Image Computing and Computer-Assisted Intervention, Lecture Notes in Computer Science 2208.* ed. W. J. Niessen & M. A. Viergever, pp. 957–965 Berlin: Springer.

Baron, J.-C., Chetalat, G., Desgranges, B. *et al.* (2001). In vivo mapping of grey matter loss with voxel-based morphometry in mild Alzheimer's disease. *Neuroimage*, **14**, 298–309.

Bartzokis, G. & Tishler, T. A. (2000). MRI evaluation of basal ganglia ferritin iron and neurotoxicity in Alzheimer's and Huntington's disease. *Cell Mol. Biol.*, (Noisy.-le-grand) **46**, 821–33.

Basser, P. J., Pajevic, S., Pierpaoli, C., Duda, J. & Aldroubi, A. (2000). In vivo fiber tractography using DT-MRI data. *Magn. Reson. Med.*, **44**, 625–32.

Belliveau, J. W., Kennedy, D. N. J., McKinstry, R. C. *et al.* (1991). Functional mapping of the human visual cortex by magnetic resonance imaging. *Science*, **254**, 716–19.

Benveniste, H., Einstein, G., Kim, K. R., Hulette, C. & Johnson, G. A. (1999). Detection of neuritic plaques in Alzheimer's disease by magnetic resonance microscopy. *Proc. Natl Acad. Sci. USA*, **96**, 14079–84.

Billette de Villemeur, T., Deslys, J. P. & Gelot, A. (1996). Clinical and pathological aspects of iatrogenic Cruetzfeldt–Jakob disease. In *Transmissable Subacute Spongiform Encephalopathies: Prion Diseases*, ed. L. Court & B. Dodet, pp. 451–7. Paris: Elsevier.

Binder, J. R., Swanson, S. J., Hammeke, T. A. *et al.* (1996). Determination of language dominance using functional MRI: a comparison with the Wada test. *Neurology*, **46**, 978–84.

Bookheimer, S. Y., Strojwas, M. H., Cohen, M. S. *et al.* (2000). Patterns of brain activation in people at risk for Alzheimer's disease. *N. Engl. J. Med.*, **343**, 450–6.

Brammer, M. J., Bullmore, E. T., Simmons, A. *et al.* (1997). Generic brain activation mapping in functional magnetic resonance imaging: a nonparametric approach. *Magn. Reson. Imaging*, **15**, 763–70.

Brooks, B. R., Bushara, K., Khan, A. *et al.* (2000). Functional magnetic resonance imaging (fMRI) clinical studies in ALS – paradigms, problems and promises. *Amyotroph. Lateral. Scler. Other Motor Neuron Disord.*, **1** Suppl 2, S23–32.

Brunberg, J. A., Jacquemont, S., Hagerman, R. J. *et al.* (2002). Fragile X premutation carriers: characteristic MR imaging findings of adult male patients with progressive cerebellar and cognitive dysfunction. *Am. J. Neuroradiol.*, **23**, 1757–66.

Bucher, S. F., Seelos, K. C., Stehling, M., Oertel, W. H., Paulus, W. & Reiser, M. (1995). High-resolution activation mapping of basal ganglia with functional magnetic resonance imaging. *Neurology*, **45**, 180.

Bucher, S. F., Seelos, K. C., Dodel, R. C., Paulus, W., Reiser, M. & Oertel, W. H. (1996). Pallidal lesions. Structural and functional magnetic resonance imaging. *Arch. Neurol.*, **53**, 682–6.

Buckner, R. L., Bandettini, P. A., O'Craven, K. M. *et al.* (1996). Detection of cortical activation during averaged single trials of a cognitive task using functional magnetic resonance imaging. *Am. J. Neuroradiol. USA*, **93**, 14878–83.

Burggren, A. C., Small, G. W., Sabb, F. W. & Bookheimer, S. Y. (2002). Specificity of brain activation patterns in people at genetic risk for Alzheimer disease. *Am. J. Geriatr. Psychiatry*, **10**, 44–51.

Burton, E. J., Karas, G., Paling, S. M. *et al.* (2002). Patterns of cerebral atrophy in dementia with Lewy bodies using voxel-based morphometry. *Neuroimage*, **17**, 618–30.

Cannestra, A. F., Pouratian, N., Bookheimer, S. Y., Martin, N. A., Beckerand, D. P. & Toga, A. W. (2001). Temporal spatial differences observed by functional MRI and human intraoperative optical imaging. *Cereb. Cortex*, **11**, 773–82.

Carella, F., Grisoli, M., Savoiardo, M. & Testa, D. (1995). Magnetic resonance signal abnormalities along the pyramidal tracts in amyotrophic lateral sclerosis. *Ital. J. Neurol. Sci.*, **16**, 511–15.

Catalan, M. J., Ishii, K., Honda, M., Samii, A. & Hallett, M. (1999). A PET study of sequential finger movements of varying length in patients with Parkinson's disease. *Brain*, **122**, 483–95.

Chabriat, H., Pappata, S., Poupon, C. *et al.* (1999). Clinical severity in CADASIL related to ultrastructural damage in white matter: in vivo study with diffusion tensor MRI. *Stroke*, **30**, 2637–43.

Chan, D., Fox, N. C., Scahill, R. I. *et al.* (2001). Patterns of temporal lobe atrophy in semantic dementia and Alzheimer's disease. *Ann. Neurol.*, **49**, 433–42.

Chan, D., Janssen, J. C., Whitwell, J. L. *et al.* (2003). Change in rates of cerebral atrophy over time in early-onset alzheimer's disease: longitudinal MRI study. *Lancet*, **362**, 1121–2.

Chapman, B., Turner, R., Ordidge, R. J. *et al.* (1987). Real-time movie imaging from a single cardiac cycle by NMR. *Magn. Reson. Med.*, **5**, 246–54.

Chazot, G., Brousolle, E., Lapras, C., Blatter, T. & Aguzzi, A. (1996). New variant of Creutzfeld–Jakob disease in a 26-year old French man. *Lancet*, **347**, 1181.

Clare, S., Humberstone, M., Hykin, J., Blumhardt, L. D., Botwell, R. & Morris, P. (1999). Detecting activations in event–related fMRI using analysis of variance. *Magn. Reson. Med.*, **42**, 1117–22.

Clark, V. P., Lai, S. & Deckel, A. W. (2002). Altered functional MRI responses in Huntington's disease. *Neuroreport*, **13**, 703–6.

Colchester, A. C. F., Hojjatoleslami, S. A., Will, R. G. & Collie, D. A. (2002). Quantitative validation of MR intensity of abnormalities in variant CJD. *J. Neurol. Neurosurg. Psychiatry*, **73**(2), 216.

Colchester, A. C. F., Kingsley, D., Lasserson, D. *et al.* (2001). Structural MRI volumetric analysis in patients with organic amnesia, 1: methods and comparative findings across diagnostic groups. *J. Neurol. Neurosurg. Psychiatry*, **71**, 13–22.

Collie, D. A., Sellar, R. J., Zeidler, M., Colchester, A. C. F., Knight, R. & Will, R. G. (2001). MRI of Creutzfeldt–Jakob disease: imaging features and recommended MRI protocol. *Clin. Radiol.*, **56**, 726–39.

Conturo, T. E., Lori, N. F., Cull, T. S. *et al.* (1999). Tracking neuronal fibre pathways in the living human brain. *Proc. Natl Acad. Sci.*, USA, **96**, 10422–7.

Convit, A., de Leon, M. J., Tarshish, C. *et al.* (1997). Specific hippocampal volume reductions in individuals at risk for Alzheimer's disease. *Neurobiol. Aging*, **18**, 131–8.

Cordato, N. J., Pantelis, C., Halliday, G. M. *et al.* (2002). Frontal atrophy correlates with behavioural changes in progressive supranuclear palsy. *Brain*, **125**, 789–800.

Coulthard, A., Hall, K., English, P. T. *et al.* (1999). Quantitative analysis of MRI signal intensity in new variant Creutzfeldt–Jakob disease. *Br. J. Radiol.*, **72**, 742–8.

Cox, R. W. (1996). AFNI: software for analysis and visualization of functional magnetic resonance neuroimages. *Comput. Biomed. Res.*, **29**, 162–73.

Davie, C. A., Barker, G. J., Machado, C., Miller, D. H. & Lees, A. J. (1997). Proton magnetic resonance spectroscopy in Steele–Richardson–Olszewski syndrome. *Mov. Disord.*, **12**, 767–71.

de Leon, M. J., Convit, A., George, A. E. *et al.* (1996). In vivo structural studies of the hippocampus in normal aging and in incipient Alzheimer's disease. *Ann. NY Acad. Sci.*, **17**, 1–13.

Demaerel, P., Baert, A. L., Vanopdensboch, W. & Robberecht, R. (1997). Diffusion-weighted magnetic resonance imaging in Creutzfeldt–Jakob disease. *Lancet*, **349**, 847–8.

Demaerel, P., Heiner, L., Robberecht, W., Sciot, R. & Wilms, G. (1999). Diffusion-weighted MRI in sporadic Creutzfeldt–Jakob disease. *Neurology*, **52**, 205–8.

Desmond, P. M., O'Brien, J. T., Tress, B. M. *et al.* (1994). Volumetric and visual assessment of the mesial temporal structures in Alzheimer's disease. *Austr. N. Z. J. Med.*, **24**, 547–53.

Di Rocco, A., Molinari, S., Stollman, A. L., Decker, A. & Yahr, M. D. (1993). MRI abnormalities in Creutzfeldt–Jakob disease. *Neuroradiology*, **35**, 584–5.

Dickerson, B. C., Goncharova, II., Sullivan, M. P. *et al.* (2001). MRI-derived entorhinal and hippocampal atrophy in incipient and very mild Alzheimer's disease. *Neurobiol. Aging*, **22**, 747–54.

Doi, T., Iwasa, K., Makifuchi, T. & Takamori, M. (1999). White matter hyperintensities on MRI in a patient with corticobasal degeneration. *Acta Neurol. Scand.*, **99**, 199–201.

Dum, R. P. & Strick, P. L. (1991). The origin of corticospinal projections from the premotor areas in the frontal lobe. *J. Neurosci.*, **11**, 667–89.

Ellis, C. M., Simmons, A., Dawson, J. M., Williams, S. C. & Leigh, P. N. (1999a). Distinct hyperintense MRI signal changes in the corticospinal tracts of a patient with motor neuron disease. *Amyotroph. Lateral. Scler. Other Motor Neuron Disord.*, **1**, 41–4.

Ellis, C. M., Simmons, A., Jones, D. K. *et al.* (1999b). Diffusion tensor MRI assesses corticospinal tract damage in ALS. *Neurology*, **53**, 1051–8.

Ellis, C. M., Suckling, J., Amaro, E. Jr. *et al.* (2001). Volumetric analysis reveals corticospinal tract degeneration and extramotor involvement in ALS. *Neurology*, **57**, 1571–8.

Erkinjuntti, T., Leee, D. H., Gao, F. Q. *et al.* (1993). Temporal lobe atrophy on magnetic resonance imaging in the diagnosis of early Alzheimer's disease. *Arch. Neurol.*, **50**, 305–10.

Esmonde, T. F. G. & Will, R. G. (1992). Magnetic resonance imaging in Creutzfeldt–Jakob disease. *Ann. Neurol.*, **31**, 230–1.

Falcone, S., Quencer, R. M., Bowen, B. *et al.* (1992). Creutzfeldt–Jakob disease: focal symmetrical cortical involvement demonstrated by MR imaging. *Am. J. Neuroradiol.*, **13**, 403–6.

Finkenstaedt, M., Szudra, A., Zerr, I. *et al.* (1996). MR imaging of Creutzfeldt–Jakob disease. *Radiology*, **199**, 793–8.

Foong, J., Maier, M., Clark, C. A., Barker, G. J., Miller, D. H. & Ron, M. A. (2000). Neuropathological abnormalities of the corpus callosum in schizophrenia: a diffusion tensor imaging study. *J. Neurol. Neurosurg. Psychiatry*, **68**, 242–4.

Fox, N. C. & Freeborough, P. A. (1997). Brain atrophy progression measured from serial MRI: validation and application to Alzheimer's disease. *J. Magn. Reson. Imaging*, **7**, 1069–75.

Fox, N. C., Freeborough, P. A., Mekkaoui, K. F., Stevens, J. M. & Rossor, M. N. (1997). Cerebral and cerebellar atrophy on serial magnetic resonance imaging in an initially symptom free subject at risk of familial prion disease. *Br. Med. J.*, **315**, 856–7.

Fox, P. T. & Raichle, M. E. (1986). Focal physiological uncoupling of cerebral blood flow and oxidative metabolism during somatosensory stimulation in human subjects. *Proc. Natl Acad. Sci., USA*, **83**, 1140–4.

Fox, P. T., Raichle, M. E., Mintun, M. A. & Dence, C. (1988). Nonoxidative glucose consumption during focal physiologic neural activity. *Science*, **241**, 462–4.

Frahm, J., Bruhn, H., Merboldt, K.-D. & Hänicke, W. (1992). Dynamic MR imaging of human brain oxygenation during rest and photic stimulation. *J. Magn. Reson. Imaging*, **2**, 501–5.

Frahm, J., Merboldt, K. D., Hanicke, W. & Haase A. (1987). Flow suppression in rapid FLASH NMR images. *Magn. Reson. Med.*, **4**, 372–7.

Freeborough, P. A. & Fox, N. C. (1997). The boundary shift integral: an accurate and robust measure of cerebral volume changes from registered repeat MRI. *IEEE Trans. Med. Imaging*, **16**, 623–9.

Frisoni, G. B., Beltramello, A., Weiss, C., Geroldi, C., Bianchetti, A. & Trabucchi, M. (1996). Linear measures of atrophy in mild Alzheimer's disease. *Neuroradiology*, **17**, 913–23.

Frisoni, G. B., Laakso, M. P., Beltramello, A. *et al.* (1999). Hippocampal and entorhinal cortex atrophy in frontotemporal dementia and Alzheimer's disease. *Neurology*, **52**, 91–100.

Friston, K. J., Ashburner, J., Poline, J.-P., Frith, C. D., Heather, J. D. & Frackowiak, R. S. J. (1995a). Spatial registration and normalization of images. *Hum. Brain Mapp.*, **2**, 165–89.

Friston, K. J., Fletcher, P., Josephs, O., Holmes, A., Rugg, M. D. & Turner, R. (1998). Event-related fMRI: characterizing differential responses. *Neuroimage*, **7**, 30–40.

Friston, K. J., Holmes, A. P., Worsley, K. J., Poline, J.-P., Frith, C. D. & Frackowiak, R. S. J. (1995b). Statistical parametric maps in functional imaging: a general linear approach. *Hum. Brain Mapp.*, **2**, 189–210.

Friston, K. J., Holmes, A. P., Poline, J.-B. *et al.* (1995c). Analysis of fMRI time-series revisited. *Neuroimage*, **2**, 45–53.

Friston, K. J., Williams, S. C., Howard, R., Frackowiak, R. S. J. & Turner, R. (1996). Movement related effects on fMRI time-series. *Magn. Reson. Med.*, **35**, 346–55.

Frostig, R. D., Lieke, E. E., T'so, D. Y. & Grinvald, A. (1990). Cortical functional architecture and local coupling between neuronal activity and the microcirculation revealed by in vivo high-resolution imaging of intrinsic signals. *Proc. Natl Acad. Sci., USA*, **87**, 6082–6.

Garcia-Santos, J. M., Lopez-Corbalan, J. A., Martinez-Lage, J. F. & Sicilia-Guillen, J. (1996). CT and MRI in iatrogenic and sporadic Creutzfeld–Jakob disease: as far as imaging perceives. *Neuroradiology*, **38**, 226–31.

Gertz, H.-J., Henkes, H. & Cervos-Navarro, J. (1988). Creutzfeldt–Jakob disease: correlation of MRI and neuropathological findings. *Neurology*, **38**, 1481–2.

Ghaemi, M., Hilker, R., Rudolf, J., Sobesky, J. & Heiss, W. D. (2002). Differentiating multiple system atrophy from Parkinson's disease: contribution of striatal and midbrain MRI volumetry and multi-tracer PET imaging. *J. Neurol. Neurosurg. Psychiatry*, **73**, 517–23.

Gold, S., Christian, B., Arndt, S. *et al.* (1998). Functional MRI statistical software packages: a comparative analysis. *Hum. Brain Mapp.*, **6**, 73–84.

Grossman, M., Cooke, A., DeVita, C. *et al.* (2003). Grammatical and resource components of sentence processing in Parkinson's disease: an fMRI study. *Neurology*, **60**, 775–81.

Guillerman, R. P. (2000). The eye-of-the-tiger sign. *Radiology*, **217**, 895–6.

Hashimoto, M., Kitagaki, H., Imamura, T. *et al.* (1998). Medial temporal and whole-brain atrophy in dementia with Lewy bodies: a volumetric MRI study. *Neurology*, **51**, 357–62.

Haslinger, B., Erhard, P., Kampfe, N. *et al.* (2001). Event-related functional magnetic resonance imaging in Parkinson's disease before and after levodopa. *Brain*, **124**, 558–70.

Hauser, R. A., Murtaugh, F. R., Akhter, K., Gold, M. & Olanow, C. W. (1996). Magnetic resonance imaging of corticobasal degeneration. *J. Neuroimaging*, **6**, 222–6.

Hojjat, S. A., Collie, D. A. & Colchester, A. C. F. (2002). The putamen intensity gradient in CJD diagnosis. In *Medical Image Computing and Computer-Assisted Intervention*, Lecture Notes in Computer Science, ed. T. Dohi & R. Kikinis, pp. 524–32. Berlin: Springer.

Howard, R., David, A., Woodruff, P. *et al.* (1997). Seeing visual hallucinations with functional magnetic resonance imaging. *Dement. Geriatr. Cogn. Disord.*, **8**, 73–7.

Howard, R. S. (1996). Creutzfeldt–Jakob disease in a young woman. *Lancet*, **347**, 945–8.

Huesgen, C. T., Burger, P. C., Crain, B. J. & Johnson, G. A. (1993). In vitro MR microscopy of the hippocampus in Alzheimer's disease. *Neurology*, **43**, 145–52.

Humberstone, M., Clare, S., Hykin, J., Morris, P. G. & Sawle, G. V. (1997a). Measuring single cognitive events with whole brain functional magnetic resonance imaging. *J. Neurol. Neurosurg. Psychiatry*, **62**, 204.

Humberstone, M., Sawle, G.V., Clare, S. *et al.* (1997b). Functional magnetic resonance imaging of single motor events reveals human presupplementary motor area. *Ann. Neurol.*, **42**, 632–7.

Hutchinson, M. & Raff, U. (1999). Parkinson's disease: a novel MRI method for determining structural changes in the substantia nigra. *J. Neurol. Neurosurg. Psychiatry*, **67**, 815–18.

Ikeda, M., Tanabe, H., Nakagawa, Y. *et al.* (1994). MRI-based quantitative assessment of the hippocampal region in very mild to moderate Alzheimer's disease. *Neuroradiology*, **36**, 7–10.

Insausti, R., Juottonen, K., Soininen, H. *et al.* (1998). MR volumetric analysis of the human entorhinal, perirhinal, and temporopolar cortices. *Am. J. Neuroradiol.*, **19**, 659–71.

Insausti, R., Tunon, T., Sobreviela, T. *et al.* (1995). The human entorhinal cortex: a cytoarchitectonic atlas. *J. Compar. Neurol.*, **335**, 171–98.

Jack, C. R., Petersen, R. C., O'Brien, P. C. & Tangalos, E. G. (1992). MR-based hippocampal volumetry in the diagnosis of Alzheimer's disease. *Neurology*, **42**, 183–8.

Jack, C. R., Petersen, R. C., Zu, Y. C. *et al.* (1997). Medial temporal atrophy on MRI in normal aging and very mild Alzheimer's disease. *Neurology*, **49**, 786–94.

Jech, R., Urgosik, D., Tintera, J. *et al.* (2001). Functional magnetic resonance imaging during deep brain stimulation: a pilot study in four patients with Parkinson's disease. *Mov. Disord.*, **16**, 1126–32.

Jech, R., Ruzicka, E., Tintera, J. & Urgosik, D. (2003). Reply: fMRI during deep brain stimulation. *Mov Disord.*, **18**, 461–2.

Jenkins, I. H., Fernandez, W., Playford, E. D. *et al.* (1992). Impaired activation of the supplementary motor area in Parkinson's disease is reversed when akinesia is treated with apomorphine. *Ann. Neurol.*, **32**, 749–57.

Johnson, S. C., Saykin, A. J., Baxter, L. C. *et al.* (2000). The relationship between fMRI activation and cerebral atrophy: comparison of normal aging and alzheimer disease. *Neuroimage.*, **11**, 179–87.

Jones, D. K., Simmons, A., Williams, S. C. R. & Horsfield, M. A. (1999). Non-invasive assessment of axonal fibre connectivity in the human brain via diffusion tensor MRI. *Magn. Reson. Med.*, **42**, 37–41.

Jones, D. K., Griffin, L. D., Alexander, D. C. *et al.* (2002). Spatial normalization and averaging of diffusion tensor MRI data sets. *Neuroimage*, **17**, 592–617.

Juottonen, K., Laakso, M. P., Partanen, K. & Soininen, H. (1999). Comparative MR analysis of the entorhinal cortex and hippocampus in diagnosing Alzheimer's disease. *Am. J. Neuroradiol.*, **20**, 139–44.

Kassubek, J., Juengling, F. D., Hellwig, B., Spreer, J. & Lucking, C. H. (2002). Thalamic gray matter changes in unilateral Parkinsonian resting tremor: a voxel-based morphometric analysis of 3-dimensional magnetic resonance imaging. *Neurosci. Lett.*, **323**, 29–32.

Kato, N., Arai, K. & Hattori, T. (2003). Study of the rostral midbrain atrophy in progressive supranuclear palsy. *J. Neurol. Sci.*, **210**, 57–60.

Kato, T., Erhard, P., Takayama, Y. *et al.* (1998). Human hippocampal long-term sustained response during word memory processing. *Neuroreport*, **9**, 1041–7.

Kato, T., Ogawa, S. & Ugurbil, K. (2000). Functional suppression of long-term sustained response in the human hippocampal formation due to memory distraction. *Neurosci. Lett.*, **291**, 33–6.

Kato, T., Knopman, D. & Liu, H. (2001). Dissociation of regional activation in mild AD during visual encoding: a functional MRI study. *Neurology*, **57**, 812–16.

Kenwright, C., Bardinet, E., Hojjat, S. A., Malandain, G., Ayache, N. & Colchester, A. C. F. (2003). 2-D to 3-D refinement of post-mortem optical and MRI co-registration. In *Medical Image Computing and Computer-Assisted Intervention*, ed. R. E. Ellis & T. M. Peters, pp. 935–44. Berlin: Springer.

Kew, J. J., Leigh, P. N., Playford, E. D. *et al.* (1993). Cortical function in amyotrophic lateral sclerosis. A positron emission tomography study. *Brain*, **116**, 655–80.

Killany, R. J., Gomez-Isla, T., Moss, M. *et al.* (2000). Use of structural magnetic resonance to predict who will get alzheimer's disease. *Ann. Neurol.*, **47**, 430–9.

Kim, H. C. (2001). Diffusion-weighted MR imaging in biopsy-proven Creutzfeldt–Jakob disease. *Korean J. Radiol.*, **2**, 192–6.

Kitagaki, H., Hirono, N., Ishii, K. & Mori, E. (2000). Corticobasal degeneration: evaluation of cortical atrophy by means of hemispheric surface display generated with MR images. *Radiology*, **216**, 31–8.

Kleinschmidt, A., Orbig, H., Requardt, M. *et al.* (1996). Simultaneous recording of cerebral blood oxygenation changes during human brain activation by magnetic resonance imaging and near – infrared spectroscopy. *J. Cereb. Blood Flow Metab.*, **16**, 817–26.

Knopman, D. S., DeKosky, S. T., Cummings, J. L. *et al.* (2001). Practice parameter: diagnosis of dementia (an evidence-based review). *Neurology*, **56**, 1143–53.

Konrad, C., Henningsen, H., Bremer, J. *et al.* (2002). Pattern of cortical reorganization in amyotrophic lateral sclerosis: a functional magnetic resonance imaging study. *Exp. Brain Res.*, **143**, 51–6.

Kovanen, J., Erkinjuntii, T., Livanainen, M. *et al.* (1985). Cerebral MR and CT imaging in Creutzfeldt–Jakob disease. *J. Comput. Assist. Tomogr.*, **9**, 125–8.

Krasuski, J. S., Alexander, G. E., Horwitz, B. *et al.* (1998). Volumes of medial temporal lobe structures in patients with Alzheimer's disease and mild cognitive impairment. *Biol. Psychiatry*, **43**, 60–8.

Kropp, S., Finkenstaedt, M., Zerr, I., Schroeter, A. & Poser, S. (2000). Diffusion-weighted MRI in patients with Creutzfeldt–Jakob disease. *Nervenarzt*, **71**, 91–5.

Kruger, H., Meesmann, C., Rohrbach, E., Muller, J. & Mertens, H. G. (1990). Panencephalopathic type of Creutzfeldt–Jakob disease with primary extensive involvement of white matter. *Eur. Neurol.*, **30**, 115–19.

Kwong, K. K. (1995). Functional magnetic resonance imaging with echo planar imaging. *Magn. Reson. Quart.*, **11**, 1–20.

Kwong, K. K., Belliveau, J. W., Chesler, D. A. *et al.* (1992). Dynamic magnetic resonance imaging of human brain activity during primary sensory stimulation. *Proc. Natl Acad. Sci., USA*, **89**, 5675–9.

Laakso, M. P. (2002). Structural imaging in cognitive impairment and the dementias. *Curr. Opin. Neurol.*, **15**, 415–21.

Laakso, M. P., Soininen, H., Partanen, K. *et al.* (1995). Volumes of hippocampus, amygdala and frontal lobes in the MRI-based diagnosis of early Alzheimer's disease: correlation with memory functions. *J. Neural Transm., Parkinson's. Dis. Demen.*, **9**, 73–86.

Laakso, M. P., Soininen, H., Partanen, K. *et al.* (1998). MRI of the hippocampus in Alzheimer's disease: sensitivity, specificity, and analysis of the incorrectly classified subjects. *Neurobiol. Aging*, **19**, 23–31.

Lai, S., Hopkins, A. L., Haacke, E. M. *et al.* (1993). Identification of vascular structures as a major source of signal contrast in high resolution 2D and 3D functional activation imaging of the motor cortex at 1.5 Tesla: preliminary results. *Magn. Reson. Med.*, **30**, 387–92.

Lane, K. L., Brown, P., Howel, D. N. *et al.* (1994). Creutzfeldt–Jakob disease in a pregnant woman with an implanted dura mater graft. *Neurosurgery*, **34**, 737–40.

Le Bihan, D., Mangin, J. F., Poupon, C. *et al.* (2001). Diffusion tensor imaging: concepts and applications. *J. Magn. Reson. Imaging*, **13**, 534–46.

Lehericy, S., Baulac, M., Chiras, J. *et al.* (1998). Amygdalohippocampal MR volume measurements in the early stages of Alzheimer disease. *Am. J. Neuroradiol.*, **15**, 929–37.

Leigh, P. N., Simmons, A., Williams, S., Williams, V., Turner, M. & Brooks, D. (2002). Imaging: MRS/MRI/PET/SPECT: summary. *Amyotroph. Lateral. Scler. Other Motor Neuron Disord.*, **3** Suppl 1, S75–S80.

Loubinoux, I., Boulanouar, K., Ranjeva, J. P. *et al.* (1999). Cerebral functional magnetic resonance imaging activation modulated by a single dose of the monoamine neurotransmission enhancers fluoxetine and fenozolone during hand sensorimotor tasks. *J. Cereb. Blood Flow Metab.*, **19**, 1365–75.

Mao-Draayer, Y., Braff, S. P., Nagle, K. J., Pendlebury, W., Penar, P. L. & Shapiro, R. E. (2002). Emerging patterns of diffusion-weighted MR imaging in Creutzfeld–Jakob disease: case report and review of the literature. *Am. J. Neuroradiol.*, **23**, 550–6.

Martindale, J. L., Geschwind, M. D. & Miller, B. L. (2003). Psychiatric and neuroimaging findings in Creutzfeldt–Jakob disease. *Geriat. Disord.*, **5**, 43–6.

Matoba, M. (2001). Creutzfeldt-Jakob disease: serial changes on diffusion-weighted MRI. *J. Comput. Assist. Tomogr.*, **25**, 274–7.

McClure, S. M., Berns, G. S. & Montague, P. R. (2003). Temporal prediction errors in a passive learning task activate human striatum. *Neuron*, **38**, 339–46.

Mechelli, A., Henson, R. N., Price, C. J. & Friston, K. J. (2003). Comparing event-related and epoch analysis in blocked design fMRI. *Neuroimage*, **18**, 806–10.

Mendez, O. E., Shang, J., Jungreis, C. A. & Kaufer, D. I. (2003). Diffusion-weighted MRI in Creutzfeldt–Jakob disease: a better diagnostic marker than CSF protein 14-3-3? *J. Neuroimaging*, **13**, 147–51.

Middelkoop, H. A., van der Flier, W. M., Burton, E. J. *et al.* (2001). Dementia with Lewy bodies and AD are not associated with occipital lobe atrophy on MRI. *Neurology*, **57**, 2117–20.

Milton, W. J., Atlas, S. W., Lavi, E. & Mollman, J. E. (1991). Magnetic resonance imaging of Creutzfeldt–Jakob disease. *Ann. Neurol.*, **29**, 438–40.

Mittal, S., Farmer, P., Kalina, P., Kingsley, P. B. & Halperin, J. (2002). Correlation of diffusion-weighted magnetic resonance imaging with neuropathology in Creutzfeld–Jakob Disease. *Arch. Neurol.*, **59**, 128–34.

Molinuevo, J. L., Munoz, E., Valldeoriola, F. & Tolosa, E. (1999). The eye of the tiger sign in cortical-basal ganglionic degeneration. *Mov. Disord.*, **14**, 169–71.

Molko, N., Cohen, L., Mangin, J. F. *et al.* (2002). Visualizing the neural bases of a disconnection syndrome with diffusion tensor imaging. *J. Cogn. Neurosci.*, **14**, 629–36.

Murata, T., Shiga, Y., Higano, S., Takahashi, S. & Mugikura, S. (2002). Conspicuity and evolution of lesions in Creutzfeldt–Jakob disease at diffusion-weighted imaging. *Am. J. Neuroradiol.*, **23**, 1164–72.

Na, D. L., Suh, C. K., Choi, S. H., *et al.* (1999). Diffusion-weighted magnetic resonance imaging in probable Creutzfeldt–Jakob disease. *Arch. Neurol.*, **56**, 951–7.

Naka, H., Ohshita, T., Murata, Y., Imon, Y., Mimori, Y. & Nakamura, S. (2002). Characteristic MRI findings in multiple system atrophy: comparison of the three subtypes. *Neuroradiology*, **44**, 204–9.

O'Brien, J. T., Desmond, P. M., Ames, D., Schweitzer, I., Chiu, E. & Tress, B. M. (1997). Temporal lobe magnetic resonance imaging can differentiate Alzheimer's disease from normal ageing, depression, vascular dementia and other causes of cognitive impairment. *Psychol. Med.*, **27**, 1267–75.

O'Brien, J. T., Paling, S., Barber, R. *et al.* (2001). Progressive brain atrophy on serial MRI in dementia with Lewy bodies, AD, and vascular dementia. *Neurology*, **56**, 1386–8.

Ogawa, S., Lee, T. M., Kay, A. R. & Tank, D. W. (1990). Brain magnetic resonance imaging with contrast dependent on blood oxygenation. *Proc. Natl Acad. Sci., USA*, **3**, 9868–72.

Ohshita, T., Oka, M., Imon, Y., Yamaguchi, S., Mimori, Y. & Nakamura, S. (2000). Apparent diffusion coefficient measurements in progressive supranuclear palsy. *Neuroradiology*, **42**, 643–7.

Ohnishi, T., Matsuda, H., Tabira, T. *et al.* (2001). Changes in brain morphology in Alzheimer disease and normal aging: is Alzheimer disease an exaggerated aging process? *Am. J. Neuroradiol.*, **22**, 1680–5.

Oikawa, H., Sasaki, M., Tamakawa, Y., Ehara, S. & Tohyama, K. (2002). The substantia nigra in Parkinson disease: proton density-weighted spin-echo and fast short inversion time inversion-recovery MR findings. *Am. J. Neuroradiol.*, **23**, 1747–56.

Oka, M., Katayama, S., Imon, Y., Ohshita, T., Mimori, Y. & Nakamura, S. (2001). Abnormal signals on proton density-weighted MRI of the superior cerebellar peduncle in progressive supranuclear palsy. *Acta Neurol. Scand.*, **104**, 1–5.

Oliva, D., Carella, F., Savoiardo, M. *et al.* (1993). Clinical and magnetic resonance features of the classic and akinetic-rigid variants of Huntington's disease. *Arch. Neurol.*, **50**, 17–19.

Oppenheim, C., Brandel, J.-P., Hauw, J.-J., Deslys, J.-P. & Fontaine, B. (2000). MRI and the second French case of vCJD. *Lancet*, **356**, 253–4.

Pantel, J., Schroder, J., Schad, L. R. *et al.* (1997). Quantitative magnetic resonance imaging and neuropsychological functions in dementia of the Alzheimer type. *Psychol. Med.*, **27**, 221–9.

Pantel, J., Schroder, J., Essig, M. *et al.* (1998). In vivo quantification of brain volumes in subcortical vascular dementia and Alzheimer's disease. An MRI-based study. *Demen, Geriatr. Cogn. Disord.*, **9**, 316.

Pariente, J., Loubinoux, I., Carel, C. *et al.* (2001). Fluoxetine modulates motor performance and cerebral activation of patients recovering from stroke. *Ann. Neurol.*, **50**, 718–29.

Parker, G. J. M., Wheeler-Kingshott, C. A. M. & Barker, G. J. (2001). Distributed anatomical brain connectivity derived from diffusion tensor imaging. In *Information Processing in Medical Imaging*, ed. M. F. Sana, pp. 106–120. Berlin: Springer.

Pearl, G. S. & Anderson, R. E. (1989). Creutzfeldt–Jakob disease: high caudate signal on magnetic resonance imaging. *South. Med. J.*, **82**, 1177–80.

Pelled, G., Bergman, H. & Goelman, G. (2002). Bilateral overactivation of the sensorimotor cortex in the unilateral rodent model of Parkinson's disease – a functional magnetic resonance imaging study. *Eur. J. Neurosci.*, **15**, 389–94.

Phanthumchinda, K. (1999). Syndrome of progressive ataxia and palatal myoclonus: a case report. *J. Med. Assoc. Thai.*, **82**, 1154–7.

Pierpaoli, C., Jezzard, P., Basser, P. J., Barnett, A. & Di Chiro, G. (1996). Diffusion tensor MR imaging of the human brain. *Radiology*, **201**, 637–48.

Playford, E. D., Jenkins, I. H., Passingham, R. E., Nutt, J., Frackowiak, R. S. & Brooks, D. J. (1992). Impaired mesial frontal and putamen activation in Parkinson's disease: a positron emission tomography study. *Ann. Neurol.*, **32**, 151–61.

Pocchiari, M., Masullo, C., Salvatore, M., Genuardi, M. & Galgani, S. (1992). Creutzfeldt–Jakob disease after non-commercial dura mater graft. *Lancet*, **340**, 614–15.

Poser, S., Mollenhauer, B., Kraubeta, A. *et al.* (1999). How to improve the clinical diagnosis of Creutzfeldt–Jakob disease. *Brain*, **122**, 2345–51.

Poupon, C., Clark, C. A., Frouin, V. *et al.* (2000). Regularisation of diffusion-based maps for the tracking of brain white matter fascicles. *Neuroimage*, **12**, 184–95.

Pouratian, N., Bookheimer, S. Y., Rex, D. E., Martin, N. A. & Toga, A. W. (2002). Utility of preoperative functional magnetic resonance imaging for identifying language cortices in patients with vascular malformations. *J. Neurosurg.*, **97**, 21–32.

Prvulovic, D., Hubl, D., Sack, A. T. *et al.* (2002). Functional imaging of visuospatial processing in Alzheimer's disease. *Neuroimage*, **17**, 1403–14.

Pucci, E., Belardinelli, N., Regnicolo, L. *et al.* (1998). Hippocampus and parahippocampal gyrus linear measurements based on magnetic resonance in Alzheimer's disease. *Eur. Neurol.*, **39**, 16–25.

Puce, A., Constable, R. T., Luby, M. L. *et al.* (1995). Functional magnetic resonance imaging of sensory and motor cortex: comparison with electrophysiological localization. *J. Neurosurg.*, **83**, 262–70.

Rabinstein, A. A., Whiteman, M. L. & Shebert, R. T. (2002). Abnormal diffusion-weighted magnetic resonance imaging in Creutzfeldt–Jakob disease following corneal transplantations. *Arch. Neurol.*, **59**, 637–9.

Radanovic, M., Senaha, M. L. H., Mansur, L. L. *et al.* (2001). Primary progressive aphasia: analysis of 16 cases. *Arch. Neuropsychiat.*, **59**, 512–20.

Rao, S. M., Binder, J. R., Bandettini, P. A. *et al.* (1993). Functional magnetic resonance imaging of complex human movements. *Neurology*, **43**, 2311–18.

Rascol, O., Sabatini, U., Chollet, F. *et al.* (1994). Normal activation of the supplementary motor area in patients with Parkinson's disease undergoing long-term treatment with levodopa. *J. Neurol. Neurosurg. Psychiatry*, **57**, 567–71.

Rezai, A. R., Lozano, A. M., Crawley, A. P. *et al.* (1999). Thalamic stimulation and functional magnetic resonance imaging: localization of cortical and subcortical activation with implanted electrodes. Technical note. *J. Neurosurg.*, **90**, 583–90.

Richter, W., Andersen, P. M., Georgopoulos, A. P. & Kim, S.-G. (1997). Sequential activity in human motor areas during a delayed cued finger movement task studied by time – resolved fMRI. *Neuroreport*, **8**, 1257–61.

Rombouts, S. A., Barkhof, F., Van Meel, C. S. & Scheltens, P. (2002). Alterations in brain activation during cholinergic enhancement with rivastigmine in Alzheimer's disease. *J. Neurol. Neurosurg. Psychiatry*, **73**, 665–71.

Rosas, H. D., Goodman, J., Chen, Y. I. *et al.* (2001). Striatal volume loss in HD as measured by MRI and the influence of CAG repeat. *Neurology*, **57**, 1025–8.

Rosas, H. D., Liu, A. K., Hersch, S. *et al.* (2002). Regional and progressive thinning of the cortical ribbon in Huntington's disease. *Neurology*, **58**, 695–701.

Rosas, H. D., Koroshetz, W. J., Chen, Y. I. *et al.* (2003). Evidence for more widespread cerebral pathology in early HD: an MRI-based morphometric analysis. *Neurology*, **60**, 1615–20.

Rowe, J., Stephan, K. E., Friston, K., Frackowiak, R., Lees, A. & Passingham, R. (2002). Attention to action in Parkinson's disease: impaired effective connectivity among frontal cortical regions. *Brain*, **125**, 276–89.

Sabatini, U., Boulanouar, K., Fabre, N. *et al.* (2000). Cortical motor reorganization in akinetic patients with Parkinson's disease: a functional MRI study. *Brain*, **123** (Pt 2), 394–403.

Sach, M., Winkler, G., Glauche, V. *et al.* (2004). Diffusion tensor MRI of early upper motor neuron involvement in amyotrophic lateral sclerosis. *Brain*, **127**, 340–50.

Samman, I., Wöhrle, J. C., Sommer, A., Hennerici, M., Schulz-Schaeffer, W. J. & Kretzschmar, H. A. (1999). Clinical range and MRI in Creutzfeldt–Jakob disease with heterozygosity at codon 129 and prion protein type 2. *J. Neurol. Neurosurg., Psychiatry*, **67**, 678–81.

Samuel, M., Ceballos-Baumann, A. O., Blin, J. *et al.* (1997). Evidence for lateral premotor and parietal overactivity in Parkinson's disease during sequential and bimanual movements. A PET study. *Brain*, **120**, 963–76.

Samuel, M., Williams, S. C., Leigh, P. N. *et al.* (1998). Exploring the temporal nature of hemodynamic responses of cortical motor areas using functional MRI. *Neurology*, **51**, 1567–75.

Samuel, M., Ceballos-Baumann, A. O., Boecker, H. & Brooks, D. J. (2001). Motor imagery in normal subjects and Parkinson's disease patients: an H215O PET study. *Neuroreport*, **12**, 821–8.

Samuel, M., Tuite, P., Torus, N., Sharpe, J. & Lang, A. E. (2004). Progressive ataxia and palatal tremor (PAPT): clinical, ocular, motility and MRI assessment with review of palatal tremors. *Brain*, **127**, 1252–68.

Savoiardo, M., Halliday, W. C., Nardocci, N. *et al.* (1993). Hallervorden-Spatz disease: MR and pathologic findings. *Am. J. Neuroradiol.*, **14**, 155–62.

Saykin, A. J., Flashman, L. A., Frutiger, S. A. *et al.* (1999). Neuroanatomic substrates of semantic memory impairment in Alzheimer's disease: patterns of functional MRI activation. *J. Int. Neuropsychol. Soc.*, **5**, 377–92.

Scheltens, P., Launer, L. J., Barkhof, F., Weinstein, H. C. & Jonker, G. (1997). The diagnostic value of magnetic resonance imaging and technetium 99m-HMPAO single-photo-emission-computed-tomography for the diagnosis of Alzheimer disease in a community-dwelling elderly population. *Alzheimer Dis. Assoc. Disord.*, **11**, 63–70.

Scheltens, P., Leys, D., Barkhol, F. *et al.* (1992). Atrophy of medial temporal lobes on MRI in probable Alzheimer's disease and normal aging: diagnostic value and neuropsychological correlates. *J. Neurol. Neurosurg. Psychiatry*, **55**, 967–72.

Schocke, M. F., Seppi, K., Esterhammer, R. *et al.* (2002). Diffusion-weighted MRI differentiates the Parkinson variant of multiple system atrophy from PD. *Neurology*, **58**, 575–80.

Schroter, A., Zerr, I., Henkel, K., Tschampa, H. J., Finkenstaedt, M. & Poser, S. (2000). Magnetic resonance imaging in the clinical diagnosis of Creutzfeldt–Jakob disease. *Arch. Neurol.*, **57**, 1751–7.

Schulz, J. B., Skalej, M., Wedekind, D. *et al.* (1999). Magnetic resonance imaging-based volumetry differentiates idiopathic Parkinson's syndrome from multiple system atrophy and progressive supranuclear palsy. *Ann. Neurol.*, **45**, 65–74.

Sellar, R. J. Will, W. & Zeidler, M. (1997). MR Imaging of new variant Creutzfeldt–Jakob disease: the pulvinar sign. *Neuroradiology*, **39**, S53.

Sellar, R. J. , Collie, D. A. & Will, R. G. (2002). Progress in understanding Creutzfeldt–Jakob disease. *Am. J. Neuroradiol.*, **23**, 1070–2.

Seppi, K., Schocke, M. F., Esterhammer, R. *et al.* (2003). Diffusion-weighted imaging discriminates progressive supranuclear palsy from PD, but not from the parkinson variant of multiple system atrophy. *Neurology*, **60**, 922–7.

Sethi, K. D., Adams, R. J., Loring, D. W. & el Gammal, T. (1988). Hallervorden-Spatz syndrome: clinical and magnetic resonance imaging correlations. *Ann. Neurol.*, **24**, 692–4.

Small, S. A., Perera, G. M., DeLaPaz, R., Mayeux, R. & Stern, Y. (1999). Differential regional dysfunction of the hippocampal formation among elderly with memory decline and Alzheimer's disease. *Ann. Neurol.*, **45**, 466–72.

Small, S. A., Nava, A. S., Perera, G. M., DeLaPaz, R. & Stern, Y. (2000). Evaluating the function of hippocampal subregions with high-resolution MRI in Alzheimer's disease and aging. *Microsc. Res. Tech.*, **51**, 101–8.

Small, S. A., Tsai, W. Y., DeLaPaz, R., Mayeux, R. & Stern, Y. (2002). Imaging hippocampal function across the human life span: is memory decline normal or not? *Ann. Neurol.*, **51**, 290–5.

Smith, C. D., Andersen, A. H., Kryscio, R. J. *et al.* (1999). Altered brain activation in cognitively intact individuals at high risk for Alzheimer's disease. *Neurology*, **53**, 1391–6.

Soliveri, P., Monza, D., Paridi, D. *et al.* (1999). Cognitive and magnetic resonance imaging aspects of corticobasal degeneration and progressive supranuclear palsy. *Neurology*, **53**, 502–7.

Sperling, M. R. & Herrmann C, Jr. (1985). Syndrome of palatal myoclonus and progressive ataxia: two cases with magnetic resonance imaging. *Neurology*, **35**, 1212–14.

Sperling, R. A., Bates, J. F., Chua, E. F. *et al.* (2003). fMRI studies of associative encoding in young and elderly controls and mild Alzheimer's disease. *J. Neurol. Neurosurg. Psychiatry*, **74**, 44–50.

Stark, C. E. & Squire, L. R. (2000). Functional magnetic resonance imaging (fMRI) activity in the hippocampal region during recognition memory. *J. Neurosci.*, **20**, 7776–81.

Strupp, J. (1996). Stimulate. A GUI based fMRI analysis software package. *Neuroimage*, **3**, 306.

Talairach, J. & Tournoux, P. (1988). A Co-planar Stereotaxic Atlas of a Human *Brain*. Stuttgart: *Thieme*.

Thadani, V., Penar, P. L., Partington, J. *et al.* (1988). Creutzfeldt–Jakob disease probably acquired from a cadaveric dura mater graft. *J. Neurosurg.*, **69**, 766–9.

Thulborn, K. R., Martin, C. & Voyvodic, J. T. (2000). Functional MR imaging using a visually guided saccade paradigm for comparing activation patterns in patients with probable Alzheimer's disease and in cognitively able elderly volunteers. *Am. J. Neuroradiol.*, **21**, 524–31.

Tokumaru, A. M., O'uchi, T., Kuru, Y., Maki, T., Murayama, S. & Horichi, Y. (1996). Corticobasal degeneration: MR with histopathologic comparison. *Am. J. Neuroradiol.*, **17**, 1849–52.

Toma, K., Honda, M., Hanakawa, T. *et al.* (1999). Activities of the primary and supplementary motor areas increase in preparation and execution of voluntary muscle relaxation: An event – related fMRI study. *J. Neurosci.*, **19**, 3527–34.

Tomiyasu, H., Yoshii, F., Ohnuki, Y., Ikeda, J. E. & Shinohara, Y. (1998). The brainstem and thalamic lesions in dentatorubral-pallidoluysian atrophy: an MRI study. *Neurology*, **50**, 1887–90.

Turner, R. & Grinvald, A. (1994). Direct visualization of patterns of deoxygenation and reoxygenation in monkey cortical vasculature during functional brain activation. *Proc. Soc. Magn. Reson. Med.*, **2**, 430.

Turner, R., Howseman, A., Rees, G. E., Josephs, O. & Friston, K. (1998). Functional magnetic resonance imaging of the human brain: data acquisition and analysis. *Exp. Brain Res.*, **123**, 5–12.

Turner, R., Jezzard, P., Wen, H. *et al.* (1993). Functional mapping of the human visual cortex at 4 and 1.5 tesla using deoxygenation contrast EPI. *Magn. Reson. Med.*, **29**, 277–9.

Tyszka, J. M., Grafton, S. T., Chew, W., Woods, R. P. & Colletti, P. M. (1994). Parceling of mesial frontal motor areas during ideation and movement using functional magnetic resonance imaging at 1.5 tesla [see comments]. *Ann. Neurol.*, **35**, 746–9.

Tzeng, B.-C., Chen, C.-Y., Lee, C.-C., Chen, F.-H., Chou, T.-Y. & Zimmerman, R. A. (1997). Rapid spongiform degeneration of the cerebrum and cerebellum in Creutzfeldt–Jakob disease. *Am. J. Neuroradiol.*, **18**(3), 583–6.

Uchino, A., Yoshinaga, M., Shiokawa, O., Hata, H. & Ohno, M. (1991). Serial MR imaging in Creutzfeldt–Jakob disease. *Neuroradiology*, **33**, 364–7.

Ueki, Y., Isozaki, E., Miyazaki, Y. *et al.* (2002). Clinical and neuroradiological improvement in chronic acquired hepatocerebral degeneration after branched-chain amino acid therapy. *Acta Neurol. Scand.*, **106**, 113–16.

Urbach, H., Klisch, J., Wolf, H. K., Brechtelsbauer, D., Gass, S. & Solymosi, L. (1998). MRI in sporadic Creutfeld–Jakob disease: correlation with clinical and neuropathological data. *Neuroradiology*, **40**, 65–70.

Van Leemput, K., Maes, F., Vandermeulen, D. & Suetens, P. (1998). Automatic segmentation of brain tissues and MR bias field correction using a digital brain atlas. In *Medical Image Computing and Computer-Assisted Intervention – MICCAI'98*, ed. W. M. Wells III, A. C. F. Colchester & S. Delp, pp. 1222–9. Berlin: Springer.

Van Leemput, K., Maes, F., Vandermeulen, D., Colchester, A. C. F. & Suetens, P. (2001). Automated segmentation of multiple sclerosis lesions by model outlier detection. *IEEE Trans. Med. Imaging*, **20**, 677–88.

Wahlund, L. O., Julin, P., Johansson, S. E. & Scheltens, P. (2000). Visual rating and volumetry of the medial temporal lobe on magnetic resonance imaging in dementia. A comparative study. *J. Neurol. Neurosurg. Psychiatry*, **69**, 630–5.

Warach, S., Chien, D., Li, W., Ronthal, M. & Edelman, R. R. (1992). Fast magnetic resonance diffusion-weighted imaging of acute human stroke. *Neurology*, **42**, 1717–23.

Watanabe, J., Sugiura, M., Sato, K. *et al.* (2002). The human prefrontal and parietal association cortices are involved in NO-GO performances: an event-related fMRI study. *Neuroimage*, **17**, 1207–16.

Weisskoff, R. M. & Cohen, M. S. (1997). Echo planar imaging: technology and techniques. In *Advancd MR Imaging Techniques*, ed. W. G., Bradley & G. M. Bydder, pp. 63–98. London: Martin Dunitz Ltd.

Wells, W. M., Grimson, W. E. L., Kikinis, R. & Jolesz, F. A. (1996). Adaptive segmentation of MRI data. *IEEE Trans. Med. Imaging*, **15**, 429–42.

Wessel, K. & Nitschke, M. F. (1997). Cerebellar somatotopic representation and cerebro-cerebellar interconnections in ataxic patients. *Prog. Brain Res.*, **114**, 577–88.

Westin, C.-F., Maier, S. E., Khidir, B., Everett, P., Jolesz, F. A. & Kikinis, R. (1999). Image processing for diffusion tensor magnetic resonance imaging. In *Medical Image Computing and*

Computer-Assisted Intervention, ed. C. J. Tayler & A. C. F. Colchester, pp. 441–52. Berlin: Springer.

Will, R. G., Ironside, J. W., Zeidler, M. *et al.* (1996). A new variant of Creutzfeldt–Jakob disease in the UK. *Lancet*, **347**, 921–6.

Wills, A. J., Sawle, G. V., Guilbert, P. R. & Curtis, A. R. (2002). Palatal tremor and cognitive decline in neuroferritinopathy. *J. Neurol. Neurosurg. Psychiatry*, **73**, 91–2.

Windl, O., Dempster, M., Estibiero, J. P. *et al.* (1996). Genetic basis of Creutzfeldt–Jakob disease in the United Kingdom: a systematic analysis of predisposing mutations and allelic variations in the PRNP gene. *Hum. Genet.*, **98**, 259–64.

Yee, A. S., Simon, J. H., Anderson, C. A., Sze, C.-I. & Filley, C. M. (1999). Diffusion-weighted MRI of right hemisphere dysfunction in Creutzfeldt–Jakob disease. *Neurology*, **52**, 1514–15.

Yoshikawa, K., Nakata, Y., Yamada, K. & Nakagawa, M. (2004). Early pathological changes in the parkinsonian brain demonstrated by diffusion tensor MRI. *J. Neurol. Neurosurg. Psychiatry*, **75**, 481–4.

Zeidler, M., Sellar, R. J., Collie, D. A. *et al.* (2000). The pulvinar sign on magnetic resonance imaging in variant Creutzfeldt–Jakob disease. *Lancet*, **355**, 1412–18.

Zeidler, M., Stewart, G. E., Barraclough, C. R. *et al.* (1997). New variant Creutzfeldt–Jakob disease: neurological features and diagnostic tests. *Lancet*, **350**, 903–7.

Ziemann, U., Winter, M., Reimers, C. gD, Reimers, K., Tergau, F. & Paulus, W. (1997). Impaired motor cortex inhibition in patients with amyotrophic lateral sclerosis. Evidence from paired transcranial magnetic stimulation. *Neurology*, **49**, 1292–8.

20

PET/SPECT

Maja Trošt, Vijay Dhawan, Andrew Feigin, and David Eidelberg

Institute for Medical Research, North Shore – Long Island
Jewish Health System, Manhasset, USA

Introduction

Neurodegenerative diseases, particularly those affecting the basal ganglia and related pathways, are often associated with abnormal activity of nigrostriatal dopaminergic projections. The integrity of this system can be assessed by neuroimaging methods utilizing radioligands that bind to pre or postsynaptic components. By contrast, the functional organization of the basal ganglia and its projections can be assessed by imaging regional cerebral blood flow and metabolism as measures of neural activity. Single photon and positron emission tomographic imaging (SPECT and PET) have been applied in studies of network activity. While these studies have relied mainly upon PET imaging in the resting state and during brain activation, SPECT and magnetic resonance techniques have also been used for this purpose. In this chapter, we will review the development of PET and SPECT techniques as markers of neurodegenerative processes specifically to assess rates of disease progression and the effects of novel therapeutic interventions.

Presynaptic dopaminergic function

Dopamine transporter imaging

The dopamine transporter (DAT) enables the release and reabsorption of dopamine in the nigrostriatal intersynaptic cleft. Different radiotracers, mostly cocaine analogues, have been developed to quantify striatal DAT binding as an objective marker of the integrity of presynaptic nigrostriatal dopamine terminals (Wilson *et al.*, 1996; Ma *et al.*, 2002) (Fig. 20.1). DAT imaging can be implemented with a variety of radiotracers using either SPECT or PET techniques. The major SPECT compounds in current

use include [123I]-2β-carbomethyl-3β-(4-iodophenyl) tropane (βCIT) and its fluoropropyl derivative [123I] FPCIT, [123I]-Altropane, [123I]-(N)-(3-iodopropen-2-yl)-2β-carbomethoxy-3β-(4-chlorophenyl) tropane (IPT), and [99mTc]-2β-((N, N'-bis(2-mercaptoethyl)ethylene diamino)methyl), 3β-(4-chlorophenyl)tropane) (TRODAT). DAT binding can be assessed with a variety of PET ligands including [18F]-FPCIT, [76Br]-(fluorethyl-methyl-2β-carboxymethoxy-3β-4-bromophenyl-tropane) (FE-CBT), to name only a few (Dhawan & Eidelberg, 2001; Ribeiro *et al.*, 2002). Striatal DAT binding can be quantified by any of these methods, which differ primarily in the time of attained equilibrium and the duration of the scanning procedure.

The major application of DAT binding imaging procedures has been to assess the rate of decline in presynaptic dopaminergic function in patients with Parkinson's disease (Fig. 20.1). In SPECT studies with [123I]-βCIT (Pirker *et al.*, 2002), striatal DAT binding declined by 7.1% per year in short duration PD, and 14.9% in short duration atypical parkinsonian syndromes. The rate of decline in PD appears to slow markedly with evolving disease (Pirker *et al.*, 2002). In another [123I]-βCIT study, 32 PD patients and 24 healthy controls underwent longitudinal SPECT imaging over a 1–4 year period. PD subjects demonstrated a decline in striatal DAT binding of approximately 11.2% per year from baseline as compared to 0.8% per year in control subjects (Marek *et al.*, 2001).

Given that the rate of disease progression is likely to differ in typical and atypical parkinsonism, differential diagnosis may be an important attribute of imaging in the study of neuroprotective interventions for PD. A number of DAT binding studies have been performed to assess the use of this method in differentiating parkinsonian syndromes. Booij and colleagues (2001) used [123I]-FPCIT to differentiate idiopathic PD patients

FPCIT/PET Images

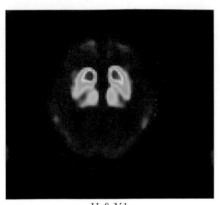
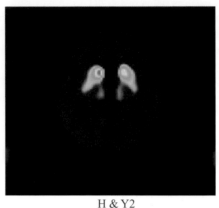

H & Y1   H & Y2
Baseline   3 Years

Fig. 20.1 FPCIT PET images (see text) showing continued losses of dopamine transporters in the striatum of a patient with early stage Parkinson's disease scanned over a 3-year period. Annual declines in DAT binding of approximately 5% were present in the caudate and putatmen of this subject. (Courtesy of Dr Yilong Ma.)

from those with other forms of parkinsonism (Booij *et al.*, 2001). [^{123}I]-βCIT has also been used to distinguish PD from vascular parkinsonism, in which striatal DAT binding was retained (Gerschlager *et al.*, 2002). In Wilson's disease, striatal DAT binding with [^{123}I]-βCIT was shown to be normal in asymptomatic patients and in patients with hepatic disease. By contrast, DAT binding was reduced in patients with neurological disease; the severity of neurological signs correlated with this measure (Barthel *et al.*, 2001). Another study revealed that patients with essential tremor do not exhibit abnormal reductions in striatal DAT binding (Antonini *et al.*, 2001). Striatal DAT binding is also normal in dopa responsive dystonia (DRD) (Jeon *et al.*, 1998), which differentiates these patients from those with young onset PD.

In a recent study, 157 PD and 26 multiple systems atrophy (MSA) patients were studied with [^{123}I]-βCIT/SPECT. Striatal uptake was markedly reduced in both the PD and MSA groups. However, the MSA subjects displayed more symmetric DAT loss compared with the PD patients, in accord with their clinical manifestations. Comparison of the relative loss of DAT binding in the caudate and putamen did not improve diagnostic accuracy in distinguishing between PD and MSA (Varrone *et al.*, 2001). SPECT can also detect decreased striatal DAT binding in asymptomatic relatives of PD patients, who are proposed to be at greater risk to develop PD (Maraganore *et al.*, 1999).

The assessment of striatal DAT binding with [^{123}I]-βCIT/SPECT has good test–retest reproducibility (Seibyl *et al.*, 1997); treatment with pergilide and L-selegiline has

no effect on imaging results (Ahlskog *et al.*, 1999; Innis *et al.*, 1999). Thus, patients may remain on these medications during scanning, although imaging parameters may be affected by concurrent levodopa administration (Guttman *et al.*, 2001). It has been shown that striatal DAT binding decreases with age in healthy volunteers and PD patients (Tissingh *et al.*, 1997; Kazumata *et al.*, 1998; Dhawan & Eidelberg, 2001). Therefore, age correction is generally needed when comparing subjects of different age groups or when conducting longitudinal progression studies (Sawle *et al.*, 1990; Eidelberg *et al.*, 1993; Kish *et al.*, 1995; van Dyck *et al.*, 1995; Ishikawa *et al.*, 1996; Volkow *et al.*, 1996; Kazumata *et al.*, 1998).

Dopa decarboxylase activity

Presynaptic nigrostriatal dopaminergic dysfunction has also been assessed extensively with [^{18}F]-FDOPA/PET. This imaging technique estimates the rate of decarboxylation of FDOPA to [^{18}F]-fluorodopamine, a function of dopa decarboxylase (DDC) activity, as well as its storage in dopaminergic nerve terminals. FDOPA/PET scans have routinely been analyzed by a multiple time graphical approach incorporating plasma or brain input functions (Brooks *et al.*, 1990; Ishikawa *et al.*, 1996; Eidelberg *et al.*, 2000), or by formal compartmental models to estimate specific kinetic rate constants for striatal DDC activity (Gjedde *et al.*, 1991; Dhawan *et al.*, 1996; Eidelberg *et al.*, 2000). The results of recent studies using this tracer suggest that the striato-occipital FDOPA uptake ratio determined from a single 10 min 3-D PET scan can be as accurate as the more complex measures (Ishikawa *et al.*, 1996; Nakamura *et al.*, 2001; Dhawan *et al.*, 2002). Those PET approaches have been used to obtain objective correlates of disease severity and to discriminate early stage PD patients from normal volunteers (Eidelberg *et al.*, 2000; Dhawan & Eidelberg, 2001). Striatal FDOPA measurements were found to correlate with dopamine cell counts measured in postmortem specimens (Pate *et al.*, 1993; Snow *et al.*, 1993).

The progression of PD has also been widely studied with FDOPA/PET (Morrish *et al.*, 1996). In a 5-year follow-up study, it was estimated that the annual decline in FDOPA uptake is 10.3% in the posterior putamen, 8.3% in the anterior putamen, and 5.9% in the caudate (Nurmi *et al.*, 2001). According to these findings, the preclinical period was calculated to be 6.5 years for the posterior putamen, while caudate FDOPA uptake was likely to be normal at disease onset.

Additionally, FDOPA/PET has been used to differentiate among parkinsonian syndromes (Eidelberg *et al.*, 2000). For example, in early idiopathic PD, FDOPA uptake is diminished primarily in posterior putamen and relatively preserved in anterior putamen and caudate; this gradient is not present in MSA (Brooks *et al.*, 1990). Nonetheless, subsequent studies have shown that caudate/putamen differences are not always sufficiently precise to categorize individual cases (Eidelberg *et al.*, 1995, 2000). In a subsequent study, striatal FDOPA separated healthy subjects from patients with parkinsonism, but did not differentiate PD from MSA patients (Antonini *et al.*, 1997).

This method may, however, differentiate corticobasal ganglionic degeneration (CBGD) from PD (Laureys *et al.*, 1999). Mild nigrostriatal presynaptic dopaminergic hypofunction, with equally affected caudate and putamen, has also been described in periodic limb movements and restless legs syndrome (Ruottinen *et al.*, 2000), although FDOPA/PET was found to be normal in a prior study (Trenkwalder *et al.*, 1999).

The pathophysiology of hereditary PD has also been studied with FDOPA/PET. This technique was used to assess dopaminergic function in adult-onset parkinsonism of pseudo-dominant inheritance associated with parkin mutations (Hilker *et al.*, 2001, 2002). Striatal FDOPA uptake was reduced in patients with compound heterozygous parkin mutations, most prominently in the posterior putamen. In asymptomatic carriers of a single parkin mutation with an apparently normal allele, a mild but significant decrease in uptake was present in both caudate and putamen. The reduction in striatal FDOPA uptake increased in magnitude with the number of mutated alleles.

The dopaminergic innovation of extrastriatal brain regions have also has been studied using FDOPA/PET. In one study, frontal mesocortical monoamine projections were imaged in unmedicated early PD patients and found to have increased activity (Rakshi *et al.*, 1999). A gender difference in this dopamine projection system has also been described in early stage disease (Kaasinen *et al.*, 2001).

Nigrostriatal dopaminergic function has been assessed in PD patients undergoing embryonic dopamine cell implantation. Transplant recipients rescanned one year following surgery demonstrated a 40.3% increase in putamen FDOPA uptake while placebo operated patients demonstrated a minimal decrement (Nakamura *et al.*, 2001). FDOPA/PET was also used to study the pathogenesis of the transplantation procedure. Caudate and putamen FDOPA uptake was compared between dyskinetic and non-dyskinetic transplant recipients. In the dyskinesia group, putamen FDOPA uptake was greater than in the non-dyskinetic group. The relative increases were localized to posterodorsal and ventral areas of the left putamen (Ma *et al.*, 2002) (Fig. 20.2).

Vesicular monoamine transporter

The presynaptic vesicular monoamine transporter (VMAT) is involved in the packaging and transport of monoamines to storage vesicles located in nerve terminals. Radioligands that bind to VMAT have been used to measure nerve terminal density (Frey *et al.*, 1996). These compounds may be especially valuable as markers of presynaptic dopaminergic function in PD patients because of the high level of VMAT2 in striatal terminals and the insensitivity of protein expression to antiparkinsonian therapeutic agents. Precise and specific in vivo measures of VMAT2 are possible with [^{11}C]-dihydrotetrabenazine (DTBZ) and PET imaging. This approach appears to be well suited to assess nigrostriatal dysfunction and disease progression (Frey *et al.*, 2001).

Postsynaptic dopaminergic function

In an earlier review, we summarized imaging studies of D1 and D2 neuroreceptor binding in PD (Eidelberg *et al.*, 2000). Subsequently, this approach has been used to differentiate between parkinsonian syndromes. A SPECT study was performed using [^{123}I]-(S)-5-iodo-7-N-[(1-ethyl-2-pyrrolidinyl)methyl] carboxamido-2,3-dihydrobenzofuran (IBF) to assess D2 receptor binding in patients with PD, MSA, and progressive supranuclear palsy (PSP) (Kim *et al.*, 2002). D2 binding in posterior putamen was abnormally elevated in the untreated PD cohort, and significantly reduced in the MSA group. The

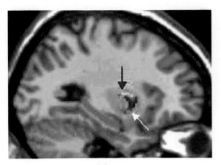

$x = -28$ mm

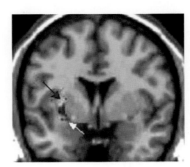
$y = 2$ mm

Fig. 20.2 Striatal FDOPA uptake in dopamine cell transplant recipients with and without postoperative dyskinesia (DYS+ and DYS −, respectively). In the DYS + group, post-transplantation FDOPA uptake was significantly elevated ($p < 0.001$, corrected) in a crescent-shaped cluster of voxels within the left putamen. Group differences in engraftment were greatest in the dorsal aspect of this structure ($Z_{max} = 3.58$; $x = -32$, $y = -2$, $z = 6$ mm, *red arrows*). A second focal area of increased uptake in DYS+ subjects was localized ventrally and more anteriorly ($Z_{max} = 3.39$; $x = -28$, $y = 2$, $z = -8$ mm, *white arrows*). No significant group differences were present in the right putamen. [The color stripe represents Z scores thresholded at 3.27 ($p = 0.001$). Representative sagittal (*left*) and coronal (*right*) MRI sections are displayed with reference to the anterior–posterior commissure line].

ratio of posterior putamen to caudate D2 binding revealed the caudate to be greater in 16 of 18 PD patients and in all PSP patients; the caudate was lower in 5 of 7 MSA patients. These findings suggest that SPECT quantification of striatal D2 receptor binding can be helpful in discriminating MSA from other forms of parkinsonism. Similarly, [123I]-iodolisuride was used with SPECT to discriminate PD from parkinson-plus syndromes (PPS) (Prunier *et al.*, 2001). The striato-occipital ratio was different statistically between PD and PPS.

D2 receptor function in early stage PD has been assessed utilizing two PET ligands: [11C]-raclopride (RAC) and [11C]-N-methylspiperone (NMSP) (Kaasinen *et al.*, 2000). With both methods, receptor binding was increased in the putamen contralateral to the predominant symptoms as compared with the ipsilateral side. Because this increase was seen with both the reversible (RAC) and the irreversible ligand (NMSP), this phenomenon is not likely to be a consequence of altered endogenous dopamine levels.

RAC was used to measure synaptic dopamine release from embryonic nigral transplants in the striatum of a patient with advanced PD. In this patient, who had received a transplant in the right putamen 10 years previously, the grafts had restored both basal and drug-induced dopamine release to normal levels (Piccini *et al.*, 1999). PET scanning was also performed with the high-affinity D2/D3 receptor radioligand [11C]-FLB 457 (Kaasinen *et al.*, 2000). The results suggest that extrastriatal (prefrontal, anterior cingulate, and thalamic) D2/D3 receptor binding is reduced in advanced PD but not in the early stages of the disease. The relationship of these findings to cognitive functioning in advanced PD is unknown.

The progressive loss of striatal D2 receptor binding was assessed in extrapyramidal movement disorders using [123I]-(S)-2-hydroxy-3-iodo-6-methoxy-[(1-ethyl-2-pyrrolidinyl)methyl] benzamide (IBZM) and SPECT. Results from a 4-year follow-up study of nine PD patients showed constant D2 receptor binding. In contrast, patients with PPS revealed a decline of the binding of the D2 receptor (Hierholzer *et al.*, 1998). In another SPECT study with IBZM, decreased striatal D2 receptor densities in advanced PD reduced the "safety factor" for synaptic transmission and contributed to the development of motor fluctuation (Hwang *et al.*, 2002).

Functional brain imaging

Besides quantifying dopaminergic function in neurodegenerative disorders, functional brain imaging can also be used to measure regional cerebral perfusion and glucose utilization as indices of local synaptic activity. In PET, regional cerebral blood flow is routinely measured with [15O]-H_2O. PET can also provide unique information on resting glucose metabolism with [18F]-fluorodeoxyglucose (FDG). In SPECT, cerebral perfusion can be assessed with [133Xe], [99mTc]-D,L-hexamethyl-propylene amine oxime (HMPAO), [123I]-iodoamphetamine (IMP) and [99mTc]-ethylcysteinate dimer (ECD).

It is well appreciated that, although the primary pathology of PD lies in dopaminergic substantia nigra, the overall clinical picture reflects system-wide abnormalities of regional cerebral functioning involving the basal ganglia and cortico-striato-pallido-thalamo-cortical loops

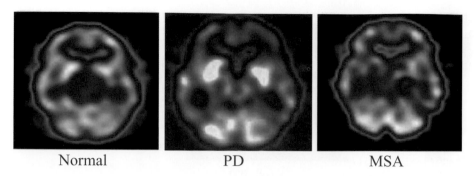

Normal   PD   MSA

Fig. 20.3 Typical axial ECD/SPECT images of cerebral perfusion from a normal volunteer, a PD subject, and an MSA subject. Lentiform hyperperfusion is evident in the PD subject; relative lentiform hypoperfusion is evident in the MSA subject. (Courtesy of Dr Angelo Antonini.)

(CSPTC) (Wichmann & DeLong, 1996). PET and other forms of functional brain imaging can be used to assess the impact of nigrostriatal degeneration on the functioning of these related motor pathways (Carbon & Eidelberg, 2002).

In this review, we will discuss the use of resting regional metabolism and blood flow as surrogate measures of neural function in movement disorders patients.

A recent FDG/PET study performed in 11 nondemented PD patients with advanced disease and 10 age-matched controls revealed significant regional reductions of glucose uptake in the parietal, frontal, temporal cortex, and in the caudate nucleus (Berding *et al.*, 2001). Local reductions in the frontal and temporal cortex correlated with parkinsonian disability.

Of particular clinical interest are studies employing this method to differentiate parkinsonian syndromes. In one such study, PD patients did not differ from controls in local glucose metabolism, whereas patients with striatonigral degeneration (SND) and PSP displayed relative hypometabolism in the basal ganglia (Arahata *et al.*, 1997). In a subsequent large retrospective study, 48 parkinsonian patients suspected as having possible atypical parkinsonism (APD) and a group of 56 patients with likely idiopathic PD were scanned with FDG/PET. A linear combination of caudate, lentiform, and thalamic values accurately discriminated APD from PD patients (Antonini *et al.*, 1998). A similar approach to differential diagnosis has been reported using ECD/SPECT for cerebral perfusion (Feigin *et al.*, 2002) (Fig. 20.3).

Statistical parametric mapping (SPM) analysis of FDG / PET data comparing CBGD to controls revealed metabolic decreases in premotor, primary motor, supplementary motor, primary sensory, prefrontal, and parietal associative cortices, as well as in the caudate and thalamus contralateral to the worse affected limbs (Laureys *et al.*, 1999). Except for the prefrontal regions, a similar metabolic pattern was observed when CBGD was compared to PD. In a similar PET study, PD patients with autonomic failure displayed metabolic reductions in parietal and occipital regions, as compared to their counterparts without this manifestation (Arahata *et al.*, 1999).

In a recent study, FDG/PET was performed on 17 nondemented patients with uncomplicated PD undergoing a stable therapeutic regimen and correlational analysis was performed to determine the metabolic substrates of bradykinesia and tremor. Bradykinesia scores were positively correlated with putamen and globus pallidus metabolism, while tremor scores were correlated negatively with metabolism in the putamen and cerebellar vermis. There was a large overlap between areas of the putamen correlating with both extrapyramidal figures (Lozza *et al.*, 2002).

In order to identify specific metabolic brain networks associated with PD and other movement disorders, we have used PET imaging with FDG in conjunction with a multivariate analysis of regional data (Carbon & Eidelberg, 2002). This technique is based upon principal component analysis (PCA), which allows for the identification of disease–related patterns of regional metabolic covariation (i.e. brain networks) and the quantification of pattern expression (i.e. network activity) in individual subjects.

Utilizing this mathematical approach, we identified a specific regional metabolic network in PD patients scanned in the resting state (Eidelberg *et al.*, 1990, 1994). The PD-related covariance pattern (PDRP) is characterized by pallidal and thalamic hypermetabolism associated with metabolic decrements in the lateral premotor cortex (PMC), the supplementary motor area (SMA), the dorsolateral prefrontal cortex (DLPFC) and the parieto-occipital association regions. This abnormal topography has since been validated in different ways: (i) PDRP activity reproducibility discriminates PD patients from controls in subsequent populations scanned with FDG/PET (Wichmann

& DeLong 1996), as well as ECD/SPECT perfusion methods (Feigin *et al.*, 2002); (ii) network activity correlates with nigrostriatal dopamine deficiency as determined by FDOPA/PET (Eidelberg *et al.*, 1990) and is modulated by exogenous dopamine (Feigin *et al.*, 2001); (iii) network activity in individual patients correlates consistently with motor disability (Eidelberg *et al.*, 1994, 1995); (iv) the PDRP is detectable early in the course of PD (Eidelberg *et al.*, 1995) and its expression increases with disease progression (Moeller & Eidelberg, 1997; Trošt *et al.*, 2002); (v) PDRP activity correlates with internal pallidal (GPi) single unit activity recorded during surgery (Eidelberg *et al.*, 1997). These data relate the PDRP network to the motoric features of parkinsonism. It is of interest that recent analyses of FDG/PET data have revealed additional metabolic topographies associated with the cognitive and affective manifestations of this disorder (Lozza *et al.*, 2001; Mentis *et al.*, 2002).

Interventional modulation of brain glucose metabolism in PD

Having established the PDRP as a functional imaging marker of parkinsonism, we examined the hypothesis that effective antiparkinsonian therapy is associated with modulation of abnormal network activity. We proposed that interventions at individual nodes of the motor CSPTC loop (Alexander *et al.*, 1990; Wichmann & DeLong, 1996) lead to significant reductions in PDRP expression. Additionally, we expected that the degree of network modulation would correlate with clinical improvement. To assess changes in network activity with therapy, we applied an automated computational procedure to quantify pattern expression in individual scans obtained in different treatment conditions (Eidelberg *et al.*, 1995; Moeller *et al.*, 1996). This algorithm is blind to intervention (drug, deep brain stimulation) and treatment status (ON, OFF).

In an FDG/PET study of GPi deep brain stimulation (DBS), we assessed seven patients off medication, comparing brain glucose metabolism ON and OFF stimulation (Fukuda *et al.*, 2001). GPi stimulation led to significant suppression of PDRP network activity. The degree to which the network was reduced by stimulation correlated with improvement in standardized motor ratings. Voxel analysis localized stimulation-induced increases within the network to the ipsilateral PMC and both cerebellar hemispheres. The metabolic increase in the PMC correlated significantly with clinical improvement, indicating the importance of functional modulation of neural activity at this CSPTC node for therapeutic efficacy.

Modulation of the PDRP is not unique to DBS, but is also present in other antiparkinsonian interventions in

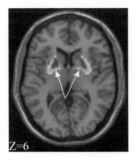
Caudate/putamen

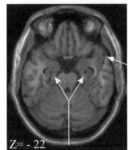
Right Superior temporal
gyrus (BA 38)

Hippocampus/hippocampus gyrus (BA 28)

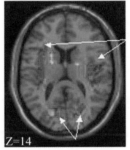
Insula

Cuneus (BA 18)

Fig. 20.4 Display of the regional metabolic covariance pattern associated with preclinical Huntington's disease overlaid on standardized MRI sections. This network topography was identified in a voxel analysis of FDG/PET scans from a combined group of 10 presymptomatic HD gene carriers and 20 gene negative controls. The HD-related pattern (HDRP) discriminated carriers from controls ($P < 0.0001$) and was characterized by relative metabolic decreases (*blue*) in the striatum associated with increases (*red*) in the temporal cortex, insula, and occipital association cortex. Region weights on this pattern correlated with those of the original HDRP that we identified in an independent population of preclinical HD gene carriers (Feigin *et al.*, 2001).

PD (Eidelberg *et al.*, 1996; Feigin *et al.*, 2001; Su *et al.*, 2001). In a cohort of eight patients undergoing unilateral pallidotomy, clinical outcome following surgery correlated with a reversal of the PDRP features, i.e. decreases in the glucose metabolism in the lentiform nucleus and the thalamus, parallel to an increase in glucose metabolism in the SMA (Eidelberg *et al.*, 1996). Furthermore, in a cohort of six patients undergoing unilateral subthalamic nucleus ablation, a highly significant reduction in PDRP expression was present in all operated hemispheres, correlating with improvement in off-medication motor ratings (Su *et al.*, 2001). These subjects exhibited marked postoperative metabolic decrements within the network in the ipsilateral GPi, substantia nigra pars reticularis (SNr), and in the ventrolateral and anterior thalamic nuclei.

PDRP modulation is also a feature of dopamine replacement. We used FDG/PET to study seven patients during intravenous levodopa infusion titrated to maximal clinical benefit (Feigin *et al.*, 2001). PDRP expression declined with therapy in all subjects. This treatment-induced change correlated with the degree of motor improvement as measured by serial clinical ratings. Voxel analysis localized the treatment-mediated metabolic reductions within the network to the putamen, ventral thalamus, and cerebellar hemispheres.

In summary, these studies suggest a common mechanism of intervention in successful antiparkinsonian therapy. Both stereotaxic surgical and medical treatments reduce PDRP activity, although different nodes within the motor CSPTC loop and cerebellar pathways may be preferentially modulated by different interventions. Moreover, our findings suggest that despite comparable clinical benefit, the degree of metabolic network modulation during treatment can differ across interventions. Additionally, studies of novel therapeutic strategies such as gene therapy (During *et al.*, 2001) are being performed with network imaging to quantify the effects of treatment on neural systems as well as behavior.

Huntington's disease

Imaging markers of disease progression may be helpful in assessing the efficacy of potential neuroprotective interventions to retard the onset of symptoms in individuals at risk for Huntington's disease. PET has been used to identify functional abnormalities in the brains of HD gene carriers both preclinically and following the onset of symptoms. FDG/PET studies in symptomatic HD patients have consistently demonstrated reduced striatal metabolic rates (Kuhl *et al.*, 1982; Hayden *et al.*, 1986; Young *et al.*, 1986; Kuwert *et al.*, 1990). By contrast, regional metabolic data in presymptomatic individuals at risk have been inconsistent, with some studies demonstrating normal metabolic rates (Young *et al.*, 1987) and others demonstrating reduced levels of striatal glucose

metabolism (Hayden *et al.*, 1987; Mazziotta *et al.*, 1987; Kuwert *et al.*, 1992; Antonini *et al.*, 1996). Similarly, RAC/PET studies of postsynaptic D_2 dopamine neuroreceptor binding in HD have disclosed a reduction in striatal receptor binding in symptomatic patients (Turjanski *et al.*, 1995; Antonini *et al.*, 1996), but not consistently in the presymptomatic phase of the illness (Antonini *et al.*, 1996; Weeks *et al.*, 1996). In a recent PET investigation of preclinical and early stage HD, a brain metabolic pattern relating to gene carrier status and independent of symptoms was identified through the network analysis of FDG/PET data from preclinical gene carriers (with normal RAC binding) and gene-negative control subjects (Feigin *et al.*, 2001). This HD-related pattern (HDRP) of regional brain metabolism was characterized by relative hypometabolism in the caudate, putamen, and temporal cortex, that covaried with metabolic increases in the occipital lobe. In a cross-sectional study, HDRP expression was found to be elevated in presymptomatic subjects with abnormal reductions in RAC binding and further increased in symptomatic HD patients (Feigin *et al.*, 2001), suggesting that this may be a useful marker for following both presymptomatic and symptomatic HD. This study has now been reproduced and validated in a new cohort of presymptomatic HD gene carriers analyzed using a voxel-based network analytical approach (Feigin *et al.*, 2001) (Fig. 20.4).

Recently, the same investigators measured the change in expression of the HDRP over 18 months in seven presymptomatic HD gene carriers, and correlated these changes with declines in dopamine D_2 receptor binding (Feigin *et al.*, 2003). They found that RAC binding declined by 3.9% per year in caudate and by 4.1% per year in putamen, and that HDRP subject scores increased by a mean of 4.1 points over the period of follow-up. Baseline HDRP subject scores correlated with baseline striatal RAC binding. It remains unknown whether striatal atrophy is the primary determinant of these PET measures. In this regard, volumetric measures with magnetic resonance imaging also hold great promise for providing an objective measure of neurodegeneration in both presymptomatic and symptomatic HD (Aylward *et al.*, 2000; Rosas *et al.*, 2001).

Conclusions

Functional neuroimaging with both SPECT and PET can provide valuable information in assessing *in vivo* neurochemical abnormalities, especially involving the dopamine system. In Parkinson's disease, these methods are being used to quantify presynaptic nigrostriatal function at the time of diagnosis as a means of assessing the integrity of dopaminergic projections from the substantia nigra. These imaging approaches may prove valuable in determining rates of neurodegeneration as part of the natural history of the disease and may facilitate the validation of potential neuroprotective agents. Similarly, postsynaptic measurements of dopamine neuroreceptors may be of great value in the study of hyperkinetic movement disorders such as Huntington's disease. Additional information concerning neurodegenerative processes can also be provided through network analytical strategies applied to images of brain blood flow and metabolism. This approach has recently yielded unique data concerning the modulation of neural systems during successful antiparkinsonian interventions. Multiregional network analysis has also been used to identify abnormal metabolic topographies in a variety of other neurological conditions and may be valuable in assessing rates of neurodegeneration, especially in the absence of other markers of disease progression.

Acknowledgements

This work was supported by NIH RO1 NS 35069, 37564, and P50 NS 38370. Dr Trošt was supported by the Veola T. Kerr Fellowship of the Parkinson Disease Foundation. Dr Feigin was supported by NIH KO8 NS 02011. Dr Eidelberg was supported by NIH K24 NS 02101.

REFERENCES

Ahlskog, J. E., Uitti, R. J., O'Connor, M. K. *et al.* (1999). The effect of dopamine agonist therapy on dopamine transporter imaging in Parkinson's disease. *Mov. Disord.*, **14**(6), 940–6.

Alexander, G. E., Crutcher, M. D. & DeLong, M. R. (1990). Basal ganglia-thalamocortical circuits: parallel substrates for motor, oculomotor, 'prefrontal' and 'limbic' functions. *Prog. Brain Res.*, **85**, 119–46.

Antonini, A., Leenders, K. L., Spiegel, R. *et al.* (1996). Striatal glucose metabolism and dopamine D2 receptor binding in asymptomatic gene carriers and patients with Huntington's disease. *Brain*, **119**(Pt 6), 2085–95.

Antonini, A., Leenders, K. L., Vontobel, P. *et al.* (1997). Complementary PET studies of striatal neuronal function in the differential diagnosis between multiple system atrophy and Parkinson's disease. *Brain*, **120**(12), 2187–95.

Antonini, A., Kazumata, K., Feigin, A. *et al.* (1998). Differential diagnosis of parkinsonism with [18F]fluorodeoxyglucose and PET. *Mov. Disord.*, **13**(2), 268–74.

Antonini, A., Moresco, R. M., Gobbo, C. *et al.* (2001). The status of dopamine nerve terminals in Parkinson's disease and essential tremor: a PET study with the tracer [11-C]FE-CIT. *Neurol. Sci.*, **22**(1), 47–8.

Arahata, Y., Kato, T., Tadokoro, M. & Sobue, G. (1997). [18F-fluorodeoxyglucose positron emission tomography in Parkinson's disease]. *Nippon Rinsho*, **55**(1), 222–6.

Arahata, Y., Hirayama, M., Ieda, T. *et al.* (1999). Parieto-occipital glucose hypometabolism in Parkinson's disease with autonomic failure. *J. Neurol. Sci.*, **163**(2), 119–26.

Aylward, E. H., Codori, A. M., Rosenblatt, A. *et al.* (2000). Rate of caudate atrophy in presymptomatic and symptomatic stages of Huntington's disease. *Mov. Disord.*, **15**(3), 552–60.

Barthel, H., Sorger, D., Kuhn, H. J., Wagner, A., Kluge, R. & Hermann, W. (2001). Differential alteration of the nigrostriatal dopaminergic system in Wilson's disease investigated with [123I]ss-CIT and high-resolution SPET. *Eur. J. Nucl. Med.*, **28**(11), 1656–63.

Berding, G., Odin, P., Brooks, D. J. *et al.* (2001). Resting regional cerebral glucose metabolism in advanced Parkinson's disease studied in the off and on conditions with [(18)F]FDG-PET. *Mov. Disord.*, **16**(6), 1014–22.

Booij, J., Speelman, J. D., Horstink, M. W. & Wolters, E. C. (2001). The clinical benefit of imaging striatal dopamine transporters with [123I]FP-CIT SPET in differentiating patients with presynaptic parkinsonism from those with other forms of parkinsonism. *Eur. J. Nucl. Med.*, **28**(3), 266–72.

Brooks, D. J., Ibanez, V., Sawle, G. V. *et al.* (1990). Differing patterns of striatal 18F-dopa uptake in Parkinson's disease, multiple system atrophy, and progressive supranuclear palsy [see comments]. *Ann. Neurol.*, **28**(4), 547–55.

Carbon, M. & Eidelberg, D. (2002). Modulation of regional brain function by deep brain stimulation: studies with positron emission tomography. *Curr. Opin. Neurol.*, **15**(4), 451–5.

Dhawan, V. & Eidelberg, D. (2001). SPECT imaging in Parkinson's disease. *Adv. Neurol.*, **86**, 205–13.

Dhawan, V., Ishikawa, T., Patlak, C. *et al.* (1996). Combined FDOPA and 3OMFD PET studies in Parkinson's disease. *J. Nucl. Med.*, **37**(2), 209–16.

Dhawan, V., Ma, Y., Pillai, V., Spetsieres, P., Chaly, T. & Eidelberg, D. (2002). Comparative analysis of striatal FDOPA uptake in Parkinson's disease: ratio method versus graphical approach. *J. Nucl. Med.*, in press.

During, M. J., Kaplitt, M. G., Stern, M. B. & Eidelberg, D. (2001). Subthalamic GAD gene transfer in Parkinson disease patients who are candidates for deep brain stimulation. *Hum. Gene Ther.*, **12**(12), 1589–91.

Eidelberg, D., Moeller, J. R., Dhawan, V. *et al.* (1990). The metabolic anatomy of Parkinson's disease: complementary [18F]fluorodeoxyglucose and [18F]fluorodopa positron emission tomographic studies. *Mov. Disord.*, **5**(3), 203–13.

Eidelberg, D., Takikawa, S., Dhawan, V. *et al.* (1993). Striatal 18F-dopa uptake: absence of an aging effect. *J. Cereb. Blood Flow. Metab.*, **13**(5), 881–8.

Eidelberg, D., Moeller, J. R., Dhawan, V. *et al.* (1994). The metabolic topography of parkinsonism. *J. Cereb. Blood Flow. Metab.*, **14**(5), 783–801.

Eidelberg, D., Moeller, J. R., Ishikawa, T. *et al.* (1995a). Early differential diagnosis of Parkinson's disease with 18F-fluorodeoxyglucose and positron emission tomography. *Neurology*, **45**(11), 1995–2004.

Eidelberg, D., Moeller, J. R., Ishikawa, T. *et al.* (1995b). Assessment of disease severity in parkinsonism with fluorine-18-fluorodeoxyglucose and PET. *J. Nucl. Med.*, **36**(3), 378–83.

Eidelberg, D., Moeller, J. R., Ishikawa, T. *et al.* (1996). Regional metabolic correlates of surgical outcome following unilateral pallidotomy for Parkinson's disease. *Ann. Neurol.*, **39**(4), 450–9.

Eidelberg, D., Moeller, J. R., Kazumata, K. *et al.* (1997). Metabolic correlates of pallidal neuronal activity in Parkinson's disease. *Brain*, **120**(Pt 8), 1315–24.

Eidelberg, D., Edwards, C., Mentis, M., Dhawan, V. & Moeller, J. R. (2000). Movement disorders: Parkinson's disease. In *Brain Mapping: The Disorders*, ed. J. C., Mazziotta, A. W., Toga & R. S. J., Frackowiak, pp. 241–61. San Diego: Academic Press.

Feigin, A., Fukuda, M., Dhawan, V. *et al.* (2001a). Metabolic correlates of levodopa response in Parkinson's disease. *Neurology*, **57**, 2083–8.

Feigin, A., Fukuda, M., Zgaljardic, D. *et al.* (2001b). Metabolic brain networks in presymptomatic Huntington's disease. *Mov. Disord.*, **16**(5), 985–6.

Feigin, A., Leenders, K. L., Moeller, J. R. *et al.* (2001c). Metabolic network abnormalities in early Huntington's disease: an [(18)F]FDG PET study. *J. Nucl. Med.*, **42**(11), 1591–5.

Feigin, A., Antonini, A., Fukuda, M. *et al.* (2002). Tc-99m ethylene cysteinate dimer SPECT in the differential diagnosis of parkinsonism. *Mov. Disord.*, **17**(6), 1265–70.

Feigin, A., Ma, Y., Zgaljardic, D., Carbon, M., Dhawan, V. & Eidelberg, D. (2003). PET measures of longitudinal progression in presymptomatic Huntington's disease. *55th Annual Meeting of the American Academy of Neurology*, Honolulu, Hawaii: Lippincott, Williams, and Wilkins.

Frey, K., Koeppe, R., Kilbourn, M. *et al.* (1996). Presynaptic monoaminergic vesicles in Parkinson's disease and normal aging. *Ann. Neurol.*, **40**(6), 873–4.

Frey, K. A., Koeppe, R. A. & Kilbourn, M. R. (2001). Imaging the vesicular monoamine transporter. *Adv. Neurol.*, **86**, 237–47.

Fukuda, M., Mentis, M. J., Ma, Y. *et al.* (2001). Networks mediating the clinical effects of pallidal brain stimulation for Parkinson's disease: A PET study of resting-state glucose metabolism. *Brain*, **124**(8), 1601–9.

Gerschlager, W., Bencsits, G., Pirker, W. *et al.* (2002). [123I]beta-CIT SPECT distinguishes vascular parkinsonism from Parkinson's disease. *Mov. Disord.*, **17**(3), 518–23.

Gjedde, A., Reith, J., Dyve, S. *et al.* (1991). Dopa decarboxylase activity of the living human brain. *Proc. Natl Acad. Sci., USA*, **88**(7), 2721–5.

Guttman, M., Stewart, D., Hussey, D., Wilson, A., Houle, S. & Kish, S. (2001). Influence of L-dopa and pramipexole on striatal dopamine transporter in early PD. *Neurology*, **56**(11), 1559–64.

Hayden, M. R., Martin, W. R., Stoessl, A. J. *et al.* (1986). Positron emission tomography in the early diagnosis of Huntington's disease. *Neurology*, **36**(7), 888–94.

Hayden, M. R., Hewitt, J., Stoessl, A. J., Clark, C., Ammann, W. & Martin, W. R. (1987). The combined use of positron emission tomography and DNA polymorphisms for preclinical detection of Huntington's disease. *Neurology*, **37**(9), 1441–7.

Hierholzer, J., Cordes, M., Venz, S. *et al.* (1998). Loss of dopamine-D2 receptor binding sites in Parkinsonian plus syndromes. *J. Nucl. Med.*, **39**(6), 954–60.

Hilker, R., Klein, C., Ghaemi, M. *et al.* (2001). Positron emission tomographic analysis of the nigrostriatal dopaminergic system in familial parkinsonism associated with mutations in the parkin gene. *Ann. Neurol.*, **49**(3), 367–76.

Hilker, R., Klein, C., Hedrich, K. *et al.* (2002). The striatal dopaminergic deficit is dependent on the number of mutant alleles in a family with mutations in the parkin gene: evidence for enzymatic parkin function in humans. *Neurosci. Lett.*, **323**(1), 50–4.

Hwang, W. J., Yao, W. J., Wey, S. P., Shen, L. H. & Ting, G. (2002). Downregulation of striatal dopamine D2 receptors in advanced Parkinson's disease contributes to the development of motor fluctuation. *Eur. Neurol.*, **47**(2), 113–17.

Innis, R. B., Marek, K. L., Sheff, K. *et al.* (1999). Effect of treatment with L-dopa/carbidopa or L-selegiline on striatal dopamine transporter SPECT imaging with [123I]beta-CIT. *Mov. Disord.*, **14**(3), 436–42.

Ishikawa, T., Dhawan, V., Chaly, T. *et al.* (1996a). Clinical significance of striatal DOPA decarboxylase activity in Parkinson's disease. *J. Nucl. Med.*, **37**(2), 216–22.

Ishikawa, T., Dhawan, V., Kazumata, K. *et al.* (1996b). Comparative nigrostriatal dopaminergic imaging with iodine-123-beta CIT-FP/SPECT and fluorine-18-FDOPA/PET. *J. Nucl. Med.*, **37**(11), 1760–5.

Jeon, B. S., Jeong, J. M., Park, S. S. *et al.* (1998). Dopamine transporter density measured by [123I]beta-CIT single-photon emission computed tomography is normal in dopa-responsive dystonia. *Ann. Neurol.*, **43**(6), 792–800.

Kaasinen, V., Nurmi, E., Bruck, A. *et al.* (2001). Increased frontal [(18)F]fluorodopa uptake in early Parkinson's disease: sex differences in the prefrontal cortex. *Brain*, **124**(Pt 6), 1125–30.

Kaasinen, V., Ruottinen, H. M., Nagren, K., Lehikoinen, P., Oikonen, V. & Rinne, J. O. (2000). Upregulation of putaminal dopamine D2 receptors in early Parkinson's disease: a comparative PET study with [11C] raclopride and [11C]N-methylspiperone. *J. Nucl. Med.*, **41**(1), 65–70.

Kazumata, K., Dhawan, V., Chaly, T. *et al.* (1998). Dopamine transporter imaging with fluorine-18-FPCIT and PET. *J. Nucl. Med.*, **39**(9), 1521–30.

Kim, Y. J., Ichise, M., Ballinger, J. R. *et al.* (2002). Combination of dopamine transporter and D2 receptor SPECT in the diagnostic evaluation of PD, MSA, and PSP. *Mov. Disord.*, **17**(2), 303–12.

Kish, S. J., Zhong, X. H., Hornykiewicz, O. & Haycock, J. W. (1995). Striatal 3,4-dihydroxyphenylalanine decarboxylase in aging: disparity between postmortem and positron emission tomography studies? *Ann. Neurol.*, **38**(2), 260–4.

Kuhl, D. E., Phelps, M. E., Markham, C. H., Metter, E. J., Riege, W. H. & Winter, J. (1982). Cerebral metabolism and atrophy in Huntington's disease determined by 18FDG and computed tomographic scan. *Ann. Neurol.*, **12**(5), 425–34.

Kuwert, T., Lange, H. W., Langen, K. J., Herzog, H., Aulich, A. & Feinendegen, L. E. (1990). Cortical and subcortical glucose consumption measured by PET in patients with Huntington's disease. *Brain*, **113**(Pt 5), 1405–23.

Kuwert, T., Ganslandt, T., Jansen, P. *et al.* (1992). Influence of size of regions of interest on PET evaluation of caudate glucose consumption. *J. Comput. Assist. Tomogr.*, **16**(5), 789–94.

Laureys, S., Salmon, E., Garraux, G. *et al.* (1999). Fluorodopa uptake and glucose metabolism in early stages of corticobasal degeneration. *J. Neurol.*, **246**(12), 1151–8.

Lozza, C., Marie, R. M. & Baron, J. C. (2002). The metabolic substrates of bradykinesia and tremor in uncomplicated Parkinson's disease. *Neuroimage*, **17**(2), 688–99.

Lozza, C., Marie, R.-M., Mentis, M., Eidelberg, D. & Baron, J.-C. (2001). Clues for metabolic topography of executive dysfunction in Parkinson's disease. *Parkinsonism Rel. Disord.*, **7**, S30.

Ma, Y., Dhawan, V., Mentis, M., Chaly, T., Spetsieris, P. G. & Eidelberg, D. (2002). Parametric mapping of [18F]FPCIT binding in early stage Parkinson's disease: a PET study. *Synapse*, **45**(2), 125–33.

Ma, Y., Feigin, A., Dhawan, V. *et al.* (2002). Dyskinesia after fetal cell transplantation for parkinsonism: a PET study. *Ann. Neurol.*, **52**(5), 628–34.

Maraganore, D. M., O'Connor, M. K., Bower, J. H. *et al.* (1999). Detection of preclinical Parkinson disease in at-risk family members with use of [123I]beta-CIT and SPECT: an exploratory study. *Mayo Clin. Proc.*, **74**(7), 681–5.

Marek, K., Innis, R., van Dyck, C. *et al.* (2001). [123I]beta-CIT SPECT imaging assessment of the rate of Parkinson's disease progression. *Neurology*, **57**(11), 2089–94.

Mazziotta, J. C., Phelps, M. E., Pahl, J. J. *et al.* (1987). Reduced cerebral glucose metabolism in asymptomatic subjects at risk for Huntington's disease. *N. Engl. J. Med.*, **316**(7), 357–62.

Mentis, M. J., McIntosh, A. R., Feigin, A. *et al.* (2002). Relationships between the metabolic patterns that correlated with mnemonic, visuospatial, and mood symptoms in Parkinson's disease. *Am. J. Psychiatry*, **159**(5), in press.

Moeller, J. R. & Eidelberg, D. (1997). Divergent expression of regional metabolic topographies in Parkinson's disease and normal ageing. *Brain*, **120**(Pt 12), 2197–206.

Moeller, J. R., Ishikawa, T., Dhawan, V. *et al.* (1996). The metabolic topography of normal aging. *J. Cereb. Blood Flow. Metab.*, **16**(3), 385–98.

Morrish, P. K., Sawle, G. V. & Brooks, D. J. (1996). An [18F]dopa-PET and clinical study of the rate of progression in Parkinson's Disease. *Brain*, **119**, 585–91.

Nakamura, T., Ghilardi, M. F., Mentis, M. *et al.* (2001). Functional networks in motor sequence learning: abnormal topographies in Parkinson's disease. *Hum. Brain Mapp.*, **12**(1), 42–60.

Nurmi, E., Ruottinen, H. M., Bergman, J. *et al.* (2001). Rate of progression in Parkinson's disease: a 6-[18F]fluoro-L-dopa PET study. *Mov. Disord.*, **16**(4), 608–15.

Pate, B. D., Kawamata, T., Yamada, T. *et al.* (1993). Correlation of striatal fluorodopa uptake in the MPTP monkey with dopaminergic indices. *Ann. Neurol.*, **34**(3), 331–8.

Piccini, P., Brooks, D., Bjorklund, A. *et al.* (1999). Dopamine release from nigral transplants visualized in vivo in a Parkinson's patient. *Nat. Neurosci.*, **2**(12), 1137–40.

Pirker, W., Djamshidian, S., Asenbaum, S. *et al.* (2002). Progression of dopaminergic degeneration in Parkinson's disease and atypical parkinsonism: a longitudinal beta-CIT SPECT study. *Mov. Disord.*, **17**(1), 45–53.

Prunier, C., Tranquart, F., Cottier, J. P. *et al.* (2001). Quantitative analysis of striatal dopamine D2 receptors with 123 I-iodolisuride SPECT in degenerative extrapyramidal diseases. *Nucl. Med. Commun.*, **22**(11), 1207–14.

Rakshi, J. S., Uema, T., Ito, K. *et al.* (1999). Frontal, midbrain and striatal dopaminergic function in early and advanced Parkinson's disease A 3D [(18)F]dopa-PET study. *Brain*, **122** (Pt 9), 1637–50.

Ribeiro, M. J., Vidailhet, M. & Remy, P. (2002). 18F-dopa vs dopamine transporter ligands in positron emission computed tomographic scans for Parkinson disease. *Arch. Neurol.*, **59**(12), 1973–4.

Rosas, H. D., Goodman, J., Chen, Y. I. *et al.* (2001). Striatal volume loss in HD as measured by MRI and the influence of CAG repeat. *Neurology*, **57**(6), 1025–8.

Ruottinen, H. M., Partinen, M., Hublin, C. *et al.* (2000). An FDOPA PET study in patients with periodic limb movement disorder and restless legs syndrome. *Neurology*, **54**(2), 502–4.

Sawle, G. V., Colebatch, J. G., Shah, A., Brooks, D. J., Marsden, C. D. & Frackowiak, R. S. (1990). Striatal function in normal aging: implications for Parkinson's disease. *Ann. Neurol.*, **28**(6), 799–804.

Seibyl, J. P., Marek, K., Sheff, K. *et al.* (1997). Test/retest reproducibility of iodine-123-betaCIT SPECT brain measurement of dopamine transporters in Parkinson's patients. *J. Nucl. Med.*, **38**(9), 1453–9.

Snow, B., Tooyama, I., McGeer, E. *et al.* (1993). Human positron emission tomographic [18F]fluorodopa studies correlate with dopamine cell counts and levels. *Ann. Neurol.*, **34**(3), 324–30.

Su, P., Ma, Y., Fukuda, M. *et al.* (2001). Metabolic changes following subthalamotomy for advanced Parkinson's disease. *Ann. Neurol.*, in press.

Tissingh, G., Bergmans, P., Booij, J. *et al.* (1997). [123I]beta-CIT single-photon emission tomography in Parkinson's disease reveals a smaller decline in dopamine transporters with age than in controls. *Eur. J. Nucl. Med.*, **24**(9), 1171–4.

Trenkwalder, C., Walters, A. S., Hening, W. A. *et al.* (1999). Positron emission tomographic studies in restless legs syndrome. *Mov. Disord.*, **14**(1), 141–5.

Trošt, M., Feigin, A. S., Ma, Y., Dhawan, V. & Eidelberg D. (2002). Increasing activity of abnormal metabolic brain networks with the progression of Parkinson's disease. *Neurology*, **58**(7), A202.

Turjanski, N., Weeks, R., Dolan, R., Harding, A. E. & Brooks, D. J. (1995). Striatal D1 and D2 receptor binding in patients with Huntington's disease and other choreas. A PET study. *Brain*, **118**(Pt 3), 689–96.

van Dyck, C. H., Seibyl, J. P., Malison, R. T. *et al.* (1995). Age-related decline in striatal dopamine transporter binding with iodine-123-beta-CITSPECT [see comments]. *J. Nucl. Med.*, **36**(7), 1175–81.

Varrone, A., Marek, K. L., Jennings, D., Innis, R. B. & Seibyl, J. P. (2001). [(123)I]beta-CIT SPECT imaging demonstrates reduced density of striatal dopamine transporters in Parkinson's disease and multiple system atrophy. *Mov. Disord.*, **16**(6), 1023–32.

Volkow, N. D., Ding, Y. S., Fowler, J. S. *et al.* (1996). Dopamine transporters decrease with age. *J. Nucl. Med.*, **37**(4), 554–9.

Weeks, R. A., Piccini, P., Harding, A. E. & Brooks, D. J. (1996). Striatal D1 and D2 dopamine receptor loss in asymptomatic mutation carriers of Huntington's disease. *Ann. Neurol.*, **40**(1), 49–54.

Wichmann, T. & DeLong, M. R. (1996). Functional and pathophysiological models of the basal ganglia. *Curr. Opin. Neurobiol.*, **6**(6), 751–8.

Wilson, J. M., Levey, A. I., Rajput, A. *et al.* (1996). Differential changes in neurochemical markers of striatal dopamine nerve terminals in idiopathic Parkinson's disease. *Neurology*, **47**(3), 718–26.

Young, A. B., Penney, J. B., Starosta-Rubinstein, S. *et al.* (1986). PET scan investigations of Huntington's disease: cerebral metabolic correlates of neurological features and functional decline. *Ann. Neurol.*, **20**(3), 296–303.

Young, A. B., Penney, J. B., Starosta-Rubinstein, S. *et al.* (1987). Normal caudate glucose metabolism in persons at risk for Huntington's disease. *Arch. Neurol.*, **44**(3), 254–7.

21

Magnetic resonance spectroscopy of neurodegenerative illness

Bruce G. Jenkins[1], Ji-Kyung Choi[1] and M. Flint Beal[2]

[1]Department of Radiology, Athinoula A. Martinos Center for Biomedical Imaging, Massachusetts General Hospital and Harvard Medical School
[2]Department of Neurology, Weill Medical College, Cornell University, NY, USA

Introduction

Since its introduction for human study in the early 1980s, magnetic resonance (MR) has proven itself an extremely versatile technique for evaluation of many different parameters of anatomic, physiologic, and metabolic interest. The number of phenomena amenable to analysis using magnetic resonance (MR) techniques is increasing every year. This versatility arises from the many different sources of magnetic contrast that can be generated using either endogenous or exogenous contrast, from the versatility of the techniques for manipulation of the nuclear spins that generate the observed signals, and from the extremely safe nature of MR that lends itself well to longitudinal studies and large patient populations.

MR techniques can now evaluate tissue parameters relevant to TCA cycle metabolism, anaerobic glycolysis, ATP levels, blood–brain barrier permeability, macrophage infiltration, cytotoxic edema, spreading depression, cerebral blood flow and volume, and neurotransmitter function. The paramagnetic nature of certain oxidation states of iron leads to the ability to map out brain function using deoxyhemoglobin as an endogenous contrast agent, and also allows for mapping of local tissue iron concentrations. In addition to these metabolic parameters, the number of ways to generate anatomic contrast using MR is also expanding, and in addition to conventional anatomic scans, mapping of axonal fiber tracts can also be performed using the anisotropy of water diffusion. A selective, non-exhaustive, summary of the various parameters of relevance to neurodegeneration (ND) that can be measured using MR techniques is presented in Table 21.1. A schematic representing the "phylogenetic tree" of MR techniques for chemical, physiological and structural purposes is shown in Fig. 21.1.

A competent review of all these various techniques would require more than just a chapter. Therefore, in what follows we will describe the use of magnetic resonance spectroscopy (MRS) for examination of neurodegeneration and potential therapeutic strategies. MRS techniques have much to offer for the evaluation of brain physiology, chemistry and function of neurodegenerative disorders. These types of studies can generally be divided into three main areas: studies of etiology, studies of the natural history and progression of the disease, and study of therapy. Our goal is not to provide an exhaustive review of MRS techniques and what has been done in prior work. Rather, we will discuss how a few select questions of interest to the study of neurodegeneration can be approached using various MRS techniques. We will provide examples of how best to integrate the potential of each MRS technique to answer specific questions related to a given question in both animal and human studies.

While a surprising convergence of evidence indicates that many neurodegenerative illnesses have a common etiologic origin in aberrant protein folding and aggregation (Schulz & Dichgans, 1999; Kopito, 2000), understanding the progression and finding potential therapies is still quite difficult. This is not surprising, as many of the pathways leading to neuronal death are common and progressive. Thus, for instance, the initial insult in focal ischemia is clear – an interruption of blood flow leading to cessation of ATP production. However, the cascade of events that results from this process is extremely complicated, and the ultimate neuronal destruction is a result of multiple interactive pathways. This fact is exemplified by the large number of different therapeutic approaches that prove efficacious in experimental ischemia. Aside from the obvious "clot busting" therapies such as TPA, effective reduction of final infarct size can be demonstrated using glutamate antagonism (e.g. MK-801) to ameliorate excitotoxicity, inhibition of

Table 21.1. Parameters of relevance to neurodegeneration amenable to MR analysis

Parameter and/or Chemical	Relevance to ND	MR Techniques and/or Parameters Used	MR References
ATP	ATP defects noted in mitochondrial disorders	^{31}P MRS	(Radda, 1992; Barbiroli *et al.*, 1993, 1998)
Lactate	Marker for impaired energy metabolism and/or reduced blood flow	^{1}H MRS	(Matthews *et al.*, 1993; Dager *et al.*, 1995; De Stefano *et al.*, 1995a,b; Brownell *et al.*, 1998)
Glucose	Can be used in labeled form (^{13}C) to examine TCA cycle flux	^{13}C MRS; ^{1}H MRS	(Gyngell *et al.*, 1991; Mason *et al.*, 1995; Gruetter *et al.*, 1994; Ross *et al.*, 2003)
Glutamate	Marker for potential excitotoxicity; in labeled form (^{13}C) marker for TCA cycle metabolism	^{13}C MRS; ^{1}H MRS	(Mason *et al.*, 1995; Pioro *et al.*, 1999; Rothman *et al.*, 1995)
Glutamine	Marker for determination of neuronal/glial glutamate/glutamine cycling or ammonia toxicity	^{13}C MRS; ^{1}H MRS	(Yudkoff *et al.*, 1993; Ross *et al.*, 1996; Sibson *et al.*, 1997)
N-acetylaspartate	Marker for neuronal number, integrity and health	^{1}H MRS	(Bates *et al.*, 1996; Kalra *et al.*, 1999; Jenkins *et al.*, 2000)
myo-Inositol	Marker for glial cells and cerebral osmolarity	^{1}H MRS	(Thurston *et al.*, 1989; Brand *et al.*, 1993; Shonk *et al.*, 1995)
Phosphoesters	May be markers for neuronal membrane integrity	^{31}P MRS	(Pettegrew *et al.*, 1997)
Macromolecular/ lipid resonances	Potential markers for macrophage/ microglial activity	^{1}H MRS	(Petroff *et al.*, 1992; Hwang *et al.*, 1996)
Apparent diffusion coefficient (ADC)	Markers for cytotoxic edema, cell swelling, and fiber tract mapping	Pulsed field gradient spin echoes	(Basser & Pierpaoli, 1996; Dijkhuizen *et al.*, 1996; Makris *et al.*, 1997; Pierpaoli *et al.*, 2001)
BBB permeability	Impairment during ischemia, tumors and possibly AD	Decreased T_1 after injection of contrast agents	(Kermode *et al.*, 1990; Tofts & Kermode, 1991)
Iron content	Can be used to look for evidence of increased iron in PD or FA	Mapping of T_2^* and T_2 relaxivity changes	(Antonini *et al.*, 1993; Ordidge *et al.*, 1994; Ye *et al.*, 1996)
Blood oxygenation level dependent contrast (BOLD)	Marker for neuronal activity; can derive relative oygen consumption	Fast gradient echo, or asymmetric spin echo imaging	(Kwong *et al.*, 1992; Ogawa *et al.*, 1992; Davis *et al.*, 1998)
Cerebral blood flow and volume (CBF, CBV)	Markers for tissue perfusion, neuronal and neurotransmitter activity	FAIR or arterial spin labelling (T_1-based), contrast injections (T_2^*-based)	(Belliveau *et al.*, 1991; Detre *et al.*, 1992; Bartenstein *et al.*, 1997; Nguyen *et al.*, 2000)

References are non-exhaustive and weighted towards those of direct relevance to in vivo study of neurodegenerative disorders.

apoptosis using caspase inhibitors, trapping of free radicals using spin traps (e.g. α-SPBN) to block the negative consequences of excess free radical production, energy repletion, calcium channel blockers to inhibit intracellular calcium influx – and the list goes on (see the other chapters in this book as well as recent reviews in (Siesjo, 1992; Hossmann, 1994; Fisher, 1995; Kogure & Kogure, 1997; Endres *et al.*, 1998; Keller *et al.*, 1998). Each of these various approaches targets one component of an interactive mesh. Similar observations have been made with acute MPP$^+$ toxicity, where the initial insult is impairment of ATP production via

blockade of complex I in the electron transport chain, yet multiple therapeutic strategies are effective in ameliorating the lesions (Beal *et al.*, 1994; Jenkins *et al.*, 1996, 1997).

It is easy to see why then, that many deleterious factors observed in a given neurodegenerative illness may be the result, rather than the cause of given disease. Once the initiation of the neurodegenerative process occurs, other negative factors, associated with natural aging, for instance, may accelerate the neurodegeneration. Thus, one needs to frame questions about etiology to address both the primary insult itself, as well as secondary consequences of the

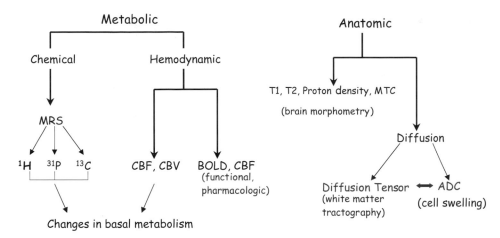

Fig. 21.1 Schematic for the "phylogenetic tree" of various MR techniques.

primary insult that may lead to further progressive degeneration. The secondary consequences can be considered part of the "natural history" of the disease. Such a parsing of primary, secondary and even tertiary effects with respect to energy metabolism has been proposed by Blass and colleagues previously (Blass *et al.*, 1988). Irrespective of questions related to etiology or natural history, the multiple factors involved in the "neurodegenerative cascade" provide many potentially efficacious therapeutic entry points for either preventing or slowing down the neurodegenerative process.

Thus, in this chapter we will cover the basics of in vivo MRS with an eye towards determining which parameters of relevance to the etiological and therapeutic questions can be addressed using in vivo MRS. In the interests of brevity, we will confine discussion to proton, carbon and phosphorus spectroscopy, with a focus on proton MRS as this is representative of the vast majority of in vivo studies.

Evaluation of neurochemistry

Magnetic Resonance Spectroscopy (MRS) is one of the few available techniques that can provide information on in vivo neurochemistry non-invasively. MRS is extremely versatile with respect to the different numbers of chemicals and brain processes that can be examined as can be seen in Tables 21.1 and 21.2. A number of different nuclei can be observed using MR, and those that are most commonly seen in brain disorders (in decreasing order of number of studies) are: ^{1}H, ^{31}P, ^{13}C, ^{19}F, ^{15}N, ^{23}Na, and ^{7}Li, with the first three nuclei accounting for approximately 99% of all studies. While only proton and phosphorous have been applied extensively to neurodegenerative conditions,

there are a number of potential studies of neurodegeneration that could be performed using both ^{13}C and ^{23}Na. In the former case one can assay TCA cycle dynamics and note the efficacy of a given neuroprotective compound in improving cellular energetics. In the latter case, it has been suggested that studies of ^{23}Na may be of use in studying stroke for examining changes in intracellular and extracellular sodium content (Hilal *et al.*, 1983; Kalyanapuram *et al.*, 1998; Thulborn *et al.*, 1999; Lin *et al.*, 2001).

Proton MRS is by far the most common application to the brain. The reason for this is that the gyromagnetic ratio of the proton is much larger than that of all other nuclei excluding tritium. Based upon three simple equations one readily predicts that the largest signal will arise from proton MRS. The three equations are:

(i) The Larmor equation, which describes the frequency at which a given nucleus resonates – $\omega_o = \gamma B_0$; where w_0 is the resonant frequency (in radians per second), γ is the gyromagnetic ratio (a fixed constant for each nucleus) and B_0 is the applied magnetic field;

(ii) The Planck–Einstein equation ($E = h\nu$), where E is the energy, h is Planck's constant and ν is the resonant frequency;

(iii) The Boltzmann distribution $N/N_0 = \exp(-\Delta E/kT)$ where N is the number of nuclei in the higher energy state, k is Boltzmann's constant and T is the temperature.

Since the MR signal is linearly proportional to N, as the energy increases the population of spins that can be excited is larger. These three equations also predict that in addition to the gyromagnetic ratio, that the MR signal will increase with increasing magnetic field strength. This latter fact is the major impetus for the constantly increasing magnetic

Table 21.2. Most commonly observed neurochemicals and their relevance to neurodegeneration

Compound (Chemical shifts and approximate brain concentration)	Structure	Relevance to Neurodegeneration and neuroprotection
N-acetylaspartate (NAA) 2.023 ppm (CH$_3$) 2.52 ppm (βCH) 2.70 ppm (β'CH) ~ 8–10 mM		Neuronal marker not present in glial cells. Synthesized in mitochondria, although role in the brain is not clear. Reflective of neuronal and mitochondrial health as well as neuronal loss.
Choline / phosphocholine (Cho) 3.23 ppm (CH$_3$)$_3$ ~ 1.5 mM		Can be composed of other trimethylamines, but is primarily glycerolphosphocholine. May represent lipid membrane breakdown or turnover products. Higher concentration in glial cells.
Creatine / phosphocreatine (Cr/PCr) 3.03 ppm (CH$_3$) 3.95 ppm (CH$_2$) ~7–10 mM		Peak represents sum of total creatine and remains constant in many pathologies. Hence, often used as denominator in ratio methods of quantification. Supplies phosphate for conversion of ADP to ATP in creatine kinase reaction.
γ-aminobutyrate (GABA) 1.91 ppm (βCH$_2$) 2.31 ppm (αCH$_2$) 3.02 ppm (gCH$_2$) ~ 3 mM		Can be modulated using vigabitrin. Does not seem to be changed in neurodegenerative conditions where examined.
Glutamate (Glu) 2.06 ppm (βCH) 2.10 ppm (β'CH) 2.36 ppm (γCH$_2$) 3.76 ppm (αCH) ~ 6–10 mM		Major excitatory neurotransmitter in brain. Potential excitotoxin. Separation of glutamate from glutamine is only possible at high fields (not at 1.5 T). Capable of being used in ^{13}C NMR to measure TCA cycle flux.
Glutamine (Gln) 2.14 ppm (βCH$_2$) 2.46 ppm (γCH$_2$) 3.78 ppm (αCH) ~ 3–5 mM		Source of glutamate for neurotransmission. Major endpoint for ammonia detoxification in the brain. Often elevated in hepatic encephalopathy. Capable of being used with ^{13}C labeling to measure neuronal-glial glutamate-glutamine cycling.
Myo-inositol (mI) 3.54 ppm ([1,3]CH) ~ 5 mM		Possible osmoregulator of brain glial volume Increases in mI may reflect glial proliferation.
Lactate 1.33 ppm (CH$_3$) ~ 0.5 mM		End product of anaerobic glycolysis. Barely detectable in normal brain but can be quite elevated in various mitochondrial encephalopathies.

field strengths pursued by the MR community, and is especially important in MRS where the signal to noise ratio is always at a premium.

Unfortunately, even though protons are the most sensitive nuclei, the inherent sensitivity of MR compared to, for instance, optical spectroscopy, is quite low (this is also why it is so safe – because the energies involved are so small). Thus, while it is no problem imaging the 80M in water protons in the brain, imaging the other neurochemicals of interest is another matter entirely. The end result of this is that one must use much lower spatial resolution (much larger voxels) to acquire MRS images compared to conventional MRI imaging of water. Often, only one voxel, of about 4–8 cc, is acquired from a

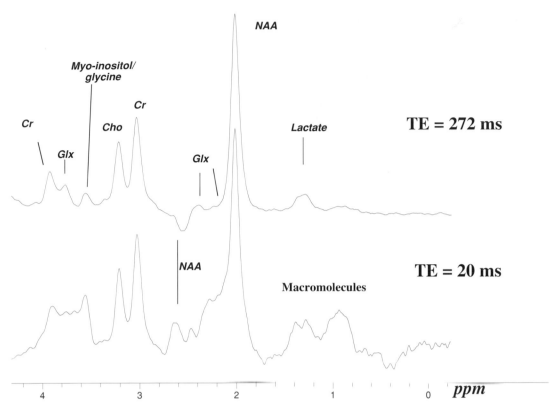

Fig. 21.2 Typical ^{1}H spectrum from cortex in Huntington's disease. The spectrum on top is an averaged spectrum from 38 patients. The spectra were acquired using a TR/TE of 2000/272 ms and an average voxel size of 5 cc. The only difference between the occipital cortex spectrum and that of a normal control is a slight, but significant, increase in the lactate peak at 1.33 ppm. On the bottom a spectrum is shown from an HD subject at an echo time of 20 ms. Note the spectrum on the bottom is from one subject showing the increased signal to noise available at a short echo time (20 ms). The major peaks are labeled.

brain region to avert the sensitivity problem. As shown in Table 21.2, there are a number of molecules of interest with concentrations between about 1–10 mM that can be observed using in vivo ^{1}H MRS. In order to orient the reader unfamiliar with MRS, typical brain spectra averaged from cortex are shown in Fig. 21.2 for patients with Huntington's disease at two different TE values. The most prominent peak in the spectrum is the methyl group from NAA at about 2 ppm. Also prominent are peaks at 3.0 and 3.2 ppm from the methyl groups of creatine and cholines. At the TE 20ms spectrum the myo-inositol/glycine peak is prominent and the peaks labeled "glx" (glutamate + glutamine) are also much larger. These effects are due to the fact that the observed signal will be proportional to exp(−TE/T2) and the T2 of glutamate/glutamine and myo-inositol are shorter than those of the methyl groups representing NAA, creatine and choline at 2, 3 and 3.2ppm, respectively. These spectra were acquired at 1.5 T. In addition to collection of data from a single voxel, one can collect data from multiple voxels simultaneously. The latter data sets are referred to as spectroscopic imaging or chemical shift imaging. An example of a spectroscopic image is shown in Fig. 21.3. In this case a patient had a lesion in the anterior cingulate that led to a huge decrease in NAA and an increase in macromolecular resonances. The macromolecular resonances have been associated histologically with microglial infiltration in stroke patients (Hwang *et al.*, 1996). Collection of data using spectroscopic imaging is far more time efficient than conventional single voxel techniques; however, it comes at some price with regards to accurate spatial localization due to the increased point spread function associated with a limited number of phase encoding steps.

At much higher fields, such as 7 T in humans and 9.4 T in animals, it is possible to quantitate even more chemicals (Pfeuffer *et al.*, 1999; Tkac *et al.*, 2001). As an example, we show the ultimate in neurochemical detection – in vitro MRS spectra of brain extracts at high field. Shown in Fig. 21.4 is a spectrum coming from a mouse at 600 MHz

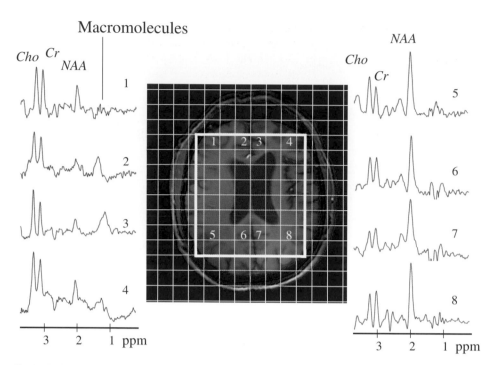

Fig. 21.3 Spectroscopic image from a patient after resolution of a lesion in the anterior cingulate. The water image is shown with a grid overlaid showing the spectroscopic voxels. The CSI data were collected with a TR/TE of 1500/135 ms. Spectra arising from the locations indicated are shown. Note that, in the frontal cortex there is a dramatic decrease in NAA and an increase in macromolecular intensities. The visibility of these resonances even at the long TE is indicative of macrophage/microglia infiltration (Hwang *et al.*, 1996).

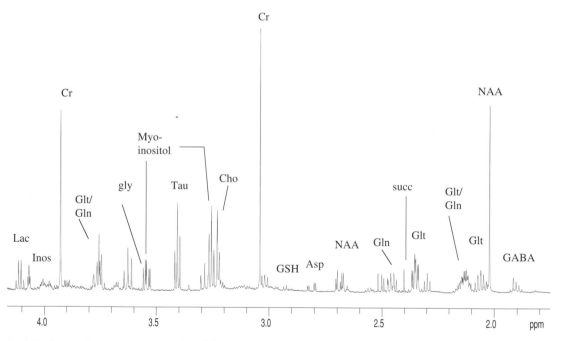

Fig. 21.4 Spectra from a brain extract of a wild-type mouse taken at 600 MHz (14 T). The high field provides incredible spectral dispersion and discrimination of many different neurochemicals. The TR in this spectrum is 10 s, so the peak areas are proportional to concentration directly after correction for the number of protons giving rise to a particular resonance.

(14 T). It is clear that many chemicals can be detected. A brief synopsis of the relevance of the major neurochemicals, and their utility as markers for neuroprotection, is given below.

NAA

There seems to be little doubt that NAA is a marker for neurons because it is found almost exclusively in neurons but not glial cells (Birken & Oldendorf, 1989; Simmons *et al.*, 1991; Urenjak *et al.*, 1992, 1993). The concentration of NAA is fairly spatially uniform within either gray or white matter; with the major distinction in NAA concentrations being that those neurons with extensive axonal projections, like the substantia nigra, have higher concentrations than those with shorter projections, like the striatum. The NAA concentration seems to be relatively similar among the major neurotransmitter neuronal subtypes including cholinergic, noradrenergic, GABAergic and glutamatergic neurons (Simmons *et al.*, 1991). The biochemical literature indicates that the NAA concentration is higher in gray matter than in white matter (by a factor of about 2). The MRS literature in this regard is rather controversial. Some studies seem to find the NAA higher in white matter, while others find it higher in gray matter. The resolution of the controversy may come from more detailed study of the relaxation times of NAA in gray and white matter than has hitherto been performed. Accurate relaxation times are the *sine qua non* for accurate metabolite concentrations, but their acquisition is time consuming and few studies have attempted adequate measurements. NAA seems to have a longer T_2 in white than in gray matter (Frahm *et al.*, 1989), thereby leading to overestimates of its concentration when using Cr as a denominator since Cr seems to have a similar T_2 in white versus gray matter.

Given the neuronal localization of NAA it is reasonable to expect NAA to be a marker for neuronal loss in neurodegenerative conditions – and this is exactly what one finds. The association is borne out by the data for Alzheimer's disease where a number of studies indicate diffuse neuronal loss in various regions in the cortex. In addition, comparisons of AD with other dementias indicated NAA loss in the patients with dementia as well (Shonk *et al.*, 1995). There is less inter-laboratory consistency about NAA loss in Parkinson's disease in the brain areas examined, though the substantia nigra has not been examined due to its small size. In PD a number of studies found no change in NAA levels in the putamen or lentiform nucleus (Holshouser *et al.*, 1995; Cruz *et al.*, 1997). However, these findings are not universal, for a number of other authors have found decreases

in NAA in either putamen or temporoparietal cortex (Ellis *et al.*, 1997; Choe *et al.*, 1998). What was most intriguing in the latter study is that the NAA reductions were largest on the side contralateral to the side most affected by the motor symptoms. Part of the problem in these studies is the possible progression of the disease process leading to dynamic changes in NAA levels. We have found in a long-term chronic MPTP Parkinson's primate model that both pre-synaptic dopamine transporters measured using PET and NAA levels in putamen continue to decrease over a time course of 2 years after cessation of MPTP treatment (Brownell *et al.*, 1998).

In the case of HD there is NAA loss in the striatum, as might be expected, but no significant loss in the cortex in the patient populations that were examined (Jenkins *et al.*, 1993, 1998). It might be expected that, in patients with late stage HD, there would be NAA loss in the cortex, as MR imaging and histopathology indicate considerable neuronal loss at this time. However, examination of these patients is complicated by their severe chorea and fragile health. *Postmortem* spectroscopy of tissue extracts in HD patients revealed about 50% NAA loss in the putamen (Dunlop *et al.*, 1992), and studies of HD transgenic mice showed extensive NAA loss in striatum (Jenkins *et al.*, 2000). Huntington's disease is caused by an expanded CAG repeat on a gene that codes for a 364 kD protein (huntingtin) of unknown function. A number of different transgenic mouse models have been created with varying numbers of CAG repeats. A spectrum from striatum comparing an HD mouse with 141 CAG repeats to a wild-type mouse is shown in Fig. 21.5. Also shown are spectra from a wild-type and HD mouse brain extract. There is extensive loss of NAA, and increases in taurine, choline and glutamine detectable in vivo. In the in vitro spectra the greatly increased spectral resolution and sensitivity demonstrate changes in other peaks such as increases in scyllo-inositol. In the case of the mitochondrial encephalopathies, NAA loss is consistently found in most patients. Thus in almost every neurodegenerative condition examined to date, there is extensive NAA loss in the region of the brains affected by the pathology. This is also true in conditions like infarcts after stroke where NAA decreases dramatically and irreversibly (Fenstermacher & Narayana, 1990; Higuchi *et al.*, 1996; Saunders, 2000).

Thus large decreases in NAA levels are almost surely a result of some neuronal loss and/or axonal damage in most pathologies. At the same time it should be kept in mind that, in certain conditions, NAA levels can drop and then return. This phenomenon has been demonstrated in the plaques found in multiple sclerosis and demyelinating lesions (Davie *et al.*, 1994; De Stefano *et al.*, 1995a, 1997).

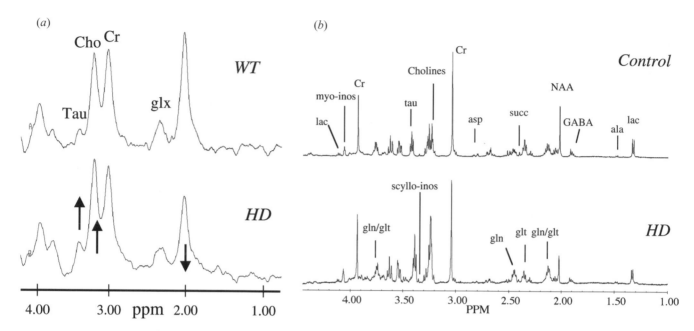

Fig. 21.5 (*a*) Typical ¹H spectrum from striata in a wild-type mouse and a transgenic HD mouse with 141 CAG repeats (TR/TE 2000/136 ms). Note the increases in taurine (tau) and choline and the decrease in NAA. (*b*) Comparison of ¹H spectra from striatal extracts of a wild-type and the same HD mouse model as in (*a*). The greatly increased spectral resolution and sensitivity lead to the ability to quantify many more resonances. The same pattern is detected as is found in vivo. Spectra were acquired at 500 MHz.

Furthermore, two recent comparisons of histopathological measurements of neuronal/glial content and NAA loss from hippocampal tissue resected for surgical treatment of temporal lobe epilepsy, showed a surprising lack of correlation between NAA loss and neuronal loss (Kuzniecky *et al.*, 2001; Petroff *et al.*, 2002). We performed a study of NAA levels in transgenic HD mice that showed that although there is extensive NAA loss in the striatum this is accompanied by a decrease in neuronal area, but not number (Ferrante *et al.*, 2000; Jenkins *et al.*, 2000). These findings lead to the important conclusion that NAA decreases can reflect a decline in neuronal health as well as number.

As a last word about NAA we will mention the postulated roles for this molecule. Since most studies of neurodegeneration have assumed it to be a neuronal marker, it could be of value to understand its role in the brain as this may shed light on the neurodegenerative process itself. NAA seems to play no role as a neurotransmitter as it is neither excitatory nor inhibitory to other neurons. Postulated roles include involvement in lipid synthesis in myelin, both precursor and breakdown product of *N*-acetylaspartylglutamate (NAAG), and as a storage form of aspartate (Birken & Oldendorf, 1989). While these roles for NAA are reasonable, they remain speculative for the most part. A recent study has indicated that NAA may play a role in osmoregulation (Taylor *et al.*, 1995). This study, using microdialysis, determined that hypoosmolarity caused an increase of NAA in the extracellular space. Because no other amino acids, except taurine, increased under these conditions this NAA increase was interpreted to be a specific response to hypoosmolarity. Taurine has already been shown to play a role in osmoregulation and it was reasoned that NAA may also serve this function to reduce osmotic stress and possibly prevent neuronal swelling. This hypothesis has been taken a step further with the proposal that NAA represents a "molecular water pump" to remove the metabolic water produced during both ordinary glucose oxidation as well as during pathological conditions (Baslow, 2002, 2003). Interestingly, the enzyme from which NAA is synthesized, L-*N*-acetylaspartyl transferase, seems to be localized in mitochondria. Thus, some of the postulated mitochondrial abnormalities in neurodegenerative disorders may also lead to changes in the concentration of NAA. Whatever the ultimate role of NAA in the brain, it seems fairly well established that, quantification problems notwithstanding, it will serve as a useful marker for neuronal loss in neurodegenerative illnesses.

Lactate

Lactate is the end product of anaerobic glycolysis. It is present in normal brain in barely detectable amounts by MRS (~ 0.5 mM). Therefore, when lactate is detected in measurable amounts, the result is significant. The question is – significant of what? Lactate increases can be stimulated by neuronal activation (Prichard *et al.*, 1991), and lactate can be used as a fuel by the brain (Schurr *et al.*, 1988). Lactate is postulated to play a role as a metabolic fuel by means of coupling glutamate reuptake in glial cells after neuronal stimulation to increased glycolysis in glial cells (Magistretti & Pellerin, 1997). The increase in lactate concentration caused by neuronal stimulation is, however, rather small – being only about a factor of two – which makes it still barely, albeit reliably, above the noise level. The amount of lactate detected in mitochondrial disorders, or in some HD patients, is quite a bit higher than this, in some cases being four to tenfold over baseline in normal controls. The amount of lactate detected by MRS represents the net balance between production and efflux and/or consumption. Therefore, it is difficult to decide whether these increases represent increased production rates or decreased rates of efflux; either through the blood brain barrier or by reconversion to pyruvate via lactate dehydrogenase. In this regard, it is usually more important to know the lactate/pyruvate ratio because this quantity truly represents the cellular redox state through its relationship to NADH and NAD$^+$ levels. Unfortunately, pyruvate concentrations are too low to be measured by in vivo MRS.

There are other sources of increased lactate in the brain that may not necessarily involve impaired oxidative phosphorylation. Increased macrophage activity in cerebral infarcts has been demonstrated to lead to elevated lactate levels as a result of the high glycolytic rates of the macrophages themselves (Petroff *et al.*, 1992). The lactate levels were highest, and NAA and Cr levels were lowest, in regions of high macrophage density. This type of process might be possible in late stage HD, but seems unlikely to occur in PD striatum or in other slowly progressing neurodegenerative conditions. Another possible source for elevated lactate levels is hyperventilation. It has recently been shown that hyperventilation can induce increases in lactate concentrations in normal subjects and even higher concentrations in subjects with panic disorders (Dager *et al.*, 1995). The mechanism by which this occurs is not yet clear; however, like neuronal stimulation, lactate concentrations only increase by about a factor of two. When the mechanism by which this increase occurs is found, it may prove to shed some light on the increases seen in the neurodegenerative disorders.

A final word about quantification of lactate is that increased lipids whose resonances are quite strong between 1 and 1.5 ppm may sometimes interfere with the lactate signal at 1.33 ppm – especially when the lactate concentrations are low. In addition, use of echo times of 136 ms can often lead to gross underestimates of lactate concentrations in STEAM sequences (Sotak & Alger, 1991). There can often be underestimates even in PRESS sequences with brain movement and at higher fields (B. G. Jenkins, unpublished observations). Thus, it is usually better to use TEs of 272 ms rather than 136 ms when in doubt. However, the inversion of the lactate doublet at 136 ms is convincing evidence that the peak there has a ~ 7 Hz coupling constant which can aid in identification of lactate as opposed to lipid or macromolecular components.

Glutamate and Aspartate

Glutamate and aspartate are amino acids that are excitatory neurotransmitters in the brain. The role of glutamate as an excitotoxin is well documented elsewhere in this book and it will not be recapitulated here. Aspartate could also presumably function in such a role, although its concentration in the brain is about five times lower than that of glutamate. Due to their large concentrations, which for glutamate range from ~ 5–10 mM at various locations within the brain, these neurotransmitters should be easy to detect using MRS. Detection, unfortunately, is not easy in vivo at the commonly used field strength of 1.5 T. The reasons for this have to do with the complicated spectral patterns induced by strong J-coupling at low fields and the severe overlap with other metabolites – especially glutamine, but including macromolecules as well. These reasons explain why one often sees glutamate and glutamine referred to in the MRS literature as Glx. Accurate quantification of glutamate and aspartate at these low field strengths is, in our opinion, nearly impossible. At 4 T, with an exceptionally good shim, it may be possible to separate glutamate from glutamine (Mason *et al.*, 1994). Almost nothing has been done with regards to quantification of aspartate, and this molecule will be a "very tough nut to crack" given its severe spectral overlap with the NAA methylene protons and its complicated coupling patterns.

Thus, elucidation of the role of glutamate and aspartate in neurodegenerative illness using MRS awaits higher field strengths. Because glutamate reuptake systems in the glial cells are so potent, it may be that elevations of neuronal glutamate will be difficult to detect, even in cases where there may actually be transient elevations. In a condition like amyotrophic lateral sclerosis (ALS) impaired glial uptake of glutamate is found via damage to the glutamate transporter EAAT2 (Rothstein *et al.*, 1995; Bristol & Rothstein, 1996). Thus, in ALS increases in glutamate might be postulated. This has been detected (as the sum of glutamate + glutamine) using MRS in both humans in medulla (Pioro *et al.*, 1999) and in transgenic mice with mutations in SOD1

(Andreassen *et al.*, 2001a). Certainly the presence of elevated glutamate, as a potential neurotoxin in early HD or PD would be amenable to testing using MRS techniques at high fields, presuming that increased iron concentrations found in the basal ganglia do not increase linewidths too much. We have detected elevations in glutamine in transgenic HD mice, possibly as a result of impaired glutamate/glutamine neuronal/glial cycling (Jenkins *et al.*, 2000); such a finding in humans remains to be seen. In addition, the elevations in ammonia seen in patients with hepatic encephalopathy lead to increased glutamine which is the end product of ammonia detoxification in the brain (for review, see Jenkins & Kraft (1999)).

Choline, creatine and myo-Inositol

For the sake of brevity we have lumped these chemicals together. As we have mentioned above, the peak labeled Cr at 3.03 ppm is composed of both Cr and PCr as well as smaller contributions from GABA and macromolecules. In conditions where there is impairment of energy metabolism, one expects hydrolysis of PCr to Cr. In this case the total resonance intensity would not change assuming that the relaxation times were the same for both molecules. Since most data indicate that the total PCr + Cr content is constant under a variety of conditions, it is reasonable to use this chemical as a denominator in ratio methods as long as it is realized that it may not really be constant.

Choline compounds are trimethylamines that may be chemically heterogeneous. What appears to be a singlet resonance at 1.5 T often appears more complicated at higher field strengths. The Cho observed in MRS may not be entirely water soluble because in vitro acid extracts of brain tissue often yield smaller intensities than in vivo measurements (Petroff *et al.*, 1995). Also, glial cells have a concentration of cholines that is 2–3 fold higher than that found in neurons (Urenjak *et al.*, 1993). Thus, the possibility of Cho serving as a marker for gliosis is reasonable; however this hypothesis will require histopathologic correlation. It is clear that many brain tumors derived from glial cells are highly enriched in choline as rapid membrane turnover leads to a high glycerolphosphocholine signal (Podo, 1999; Smith *et al.*, 2003).

Lastly, we discuss *myo*-inositol. We have examined our data from occipital cortex in 35 HD patients and found no significant change in this brain region compared to normal controls. The data in AD, however, seems to clearly indicate an increase in this compound in various cortical regions. By combining this increase with the decrease in NAA, Ross and colleagues were able to distinguish AD from other dementias (Shonk *et al.*, 1995). Numerous other studies have confirmed the increase in myo-inositol and decrease in NAA in AD (Klunk *et al.*, 1996; Pettegrew *et al.*, 1997). The possible significance of this increase is not clear at this time, though these authors have speculated that it may be involved in osmoregulation. A potential problem with measurement of *myo*-inositol is that glycine has its CH_2 resonance at 3.55 ppm. Although *myo*-inositol has an approximately two-three fold higher concentration than glycine, it may have a shorter T2. This should be kept in mind when analyzing purported changes in *myo*-inositol. Myo-inotsitol has a much higher concentration in glial cells than in neurons (Brand *et al.*, 1993), thus it may also serve as a good marker for gliosis. It is also has a well-established role in osmoregulation as proposed by Thurston (Thurston *et al.*, 1989) and verified in many subsequent studies (Isaacks *et al.*, 1999).

Quantification of proton spectroscopy

Almost all proton spectra are acquired using some variation on what is known as a 'spin-echo' experiment. The spin-echo sequence starts with nutation of the magnetization vector from the *z*-axis to the *x*,*y* plane by use of a 90° pulse. This is followed by a time usually called TE/2 where the magnetization vector undergoes dephasing due to T_2^* processes. If one then applies a 180° pulse, the direction of motion of the spins will be reversed (slower ω_{effs} appear to be faster and vice versa) and, if we wait another TE/2 interval, the magnetization will rephase and form what is aptly called an 'echo' (Hahn, 1950). One must then wait for the magnetization to reach close to thermal equilibrium (i.e. to realign along the *z*-axis) to repeat the process again – this time is generally called TR (TE being the time to echo and TR being the time of repetition). From these spin echo experiments one can collect either a spectroscopic image (MRSI or chemical shift image (CSI)) or just a single large voxel. The most common collection of data involves the use of what are known as the STEAM (stimulated echo acquisition mode (Granot, 1986; Frahm *et al.*, 1987) or PRESS (point resolved spectroscopy (Bottomley, 1987)) sequences. Both rely upon the use of three orthogonal slice selective pulses which make use of the fact that application of a linear magnetic field gradient causes a spreading of effective Larmor frequencies and a radiofrequency pulse applied at a narrow band of those frequencies will select a slice orthogonal to the gradient. By combining three of these pulses in a spin-echo sequence, selection of a volume is attained at the intersection of the three slices. The size can be adjusted at will. Additional gradient encoding periods (called phase encoding) between the 90° and 180° pulses can be specified to create a spectroscopic image with N_x, N_y and N_z steps. A diagram of the spin echo sequence, along with the STEAM and PRESS sequences, is shown below

Spin-echo   TR – {180° – TI} – 90° – TE/2 – 180° – TE/2 – Acquire

STEAM   TR – {180° – TI} – 90° – TE/2 – 90° – TM – 90° – TE/2 – Acquire

PRESS   TR – {180° – TI} – 90° – TE/4 – 180° – TE/2 – 180° – TE/4 – Acquire

The curly brackets indicate the option of including an inversion pulse before the sequence to start from the $-z$-axis instead of the $+z$-axis, followed by the inversion time TI. The differential equations which describe the return to equilibrium (T_1) and the dephasing (T_2^*) are called the Bloch equations. The solution to the simple case of the spin echo sequence described above is:

$$M(TR) = M_0*(1-\exp(-TR/T_1))*\exp(-TE/T_2^*)$$
$$M(TI) = M_0*(1-2*\exp(-TI/T_1))*\exp(-TE/T_2^*)$$

where M(T) is the magnetization at time T and M_0 is the equilibrium magnetization. The equations above indicates the solution to the case where one uses a preceding 180° pulse. Other pulse sequences will all have similar looking exponential solutions with slight differences depending upon the sequence of pulses in the acquisition scheme. An additional pulse, or set of pulses, must be added at the beginning of the sequence to perform water suppression or the small metabolite signals ($\sim$ 1–10 mM) will be buried under the large water peak ($\sim$ 80 M). This is usually performed by presaturating the water using a series of rf pulses followed by gradients to dephase the magnetization vector in the x,y plane.

Because the NMR signal is directly proportional to the number of nuclei absorbing the radiofrequency energy, the possibility exists for direct determination of molecular concentrations. However in order to do this, one must also know the T_1 and T_2 of each molecular species, and how the resonances of each species might overlap. This latter problem is especially important because most of the most highly concentrated neurochemicals have resonances between only 1–5 ppm, and some suffer from severe overlap. It turns out that the absolute concentration problem is quite difficult to solve in practice, though one can, in principle, come quite close. Thus, to avert these problems, one often sees brain spectra results reported as ratios of one compound to another.

Most often the denominator is chosen to be the creatine/phosphocreatine peak at 3.0 ppm due to its supposed insensitivity to the state of the tissue. It has also become common practice to report "absolute" concentrations using water as an internal standard due to its relative molar invariance. This practice is also fraught with some difficulty, especially in neurodegenerative diseases. As much brain tissue in older subjects and subjects with neurodegenerative diseases will be somewhat atrophied, the possibility of CSF contamination is high. Since CSF has T_1 and T_2 properties quite different from tissue, water and neurochemicals, the degree to which it contaminates your voxel must be known. Further, metabolite relaxation times can vary between white and gray matter (Frahm *et al.*, 1989; Hetherington *et al.*, 1996), which means one must know how much each of the large spectroscopic voxels is composed of white and gray matter. In addition, due to severe overlap of metabolites with tissue macromolecules the unique determination of T_1 and T_2 for each neurochemical is quite difficult. Going to higher magnetic field strength helps in this regard as there are now more Hz per ppm. This means that our spectral resolution will increase leading to better discrimination of slightly overlapping chemicals.

A terse, but general, discussion of the quantification problem is described below. To convert the observed resonance intensity at a given frequency (here chosen to be NAA at 2.0 ppm) into a concentration using water (at 4.7 ppm) as an internal standard we would arrive at an equation which looks something like the following (for a simple spin echo sequence:

$$[2.0\,ppm] = \frac{A(2.0\,ppm)}{A(4.7\,ppm)} * 80M$$

$$\frac{A(2.0\,ppm)}{A(4.7\,ppm)} = \frac{\sum_{i=1}^{n} M_0^i \left(1 - \exp\left(-TR/T_1^i\right)\right)\exp\left(-TR/T_2^i\right)}{\sum_{j=1}^{n} M_0^j \left(1 - \exp\left(-TR/T_1^j\right)\right)\exp\left(-TR/T_2^j\right)}$$

where A(ppm) is the area at a given frequency, M_0^i is the magnetization of the ith resonance at that frequency (necessary because so many neurochemical resonances overlap – like NAA and glutamate at 2.0 ppm), and likewise the T_0^i and T_2^i are the longitudinal and transverse relaxation times of the *i*th components, M_0^j is the water magnetization of the *j*th compartment, with its longitudinal and transverse relaxation times (necessary because a given voxel may contain white matter, gray matter and CSF in differing amounts and these all have different relaxation times) and we have assumed that the molar proton concentration of water in the brain is $\sim$80 M. It is apparent that this is a tricky problem, and this is notwithstanding the fact that a further complication relating to the splitting of resonances by "J-coupling" is ignored in the equation above.

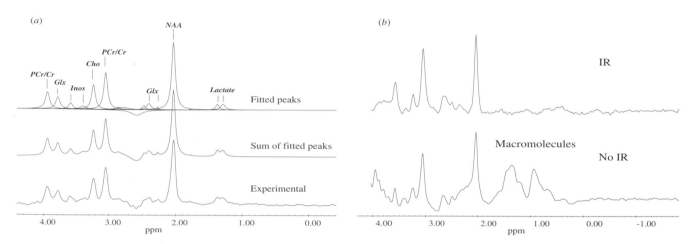

Fig. 21.6 (*a*) Spectra from an HD subject in occipital cortex showing fits to the spectra. On the top is the modeled spectrum on the bottom is the original data. (*b*) STEAM spectra from occipital cortex in a normal control at a TE of 17 ms. On the top is the spectrum with a preceding inversion pulse of 210 ms to null the lipids. Note the macromolecules disappear. On the bottom is a normal spectrum without the preceding inversion pulse.

Currently, it is fair to say that these problems are often glossed over in the literature. For instance, one common approach to quantification fits linear combinations of metabolite sub-spectra to the observed spectra (the LCModel approach (Provencher, 1993)). This is an eminently reasonable approach, however it suffers from the problem that the relaxation times for both metabolites and water go undetermined (indeed they have to for a reasonable total acquisition time) and the macromolecule contributions are undetermined except as baseline noise. We discuss this problem extensively elsewhere (Jenkins *et al.*, 1997). It has been shown that without incorporation of prior knowledge of the macromolecules it is impossible to obtain concentrations of metabolites consistent with the biochemical literature (Bartha *et al.*, 1999). Since the macromolecular components are largely undetermined biochemically, and it is not known how they may change in disease, it is very difficult to remove them using a priori information from "template" spectra of controls. It is apparent that this is a major problem, and most "absolute" quantifications reported in the literature should be taken with a grain of salt. That this is true can be seen from "absolute" concentration determinations of NAA in cortex by MRS ranging from 7–11 mM in the literature.

On the other hand, if one wishes merely to compare control populations to patient populations or patient populations longitudinally then as long as one uses consistent methods, useful and statistically significant data can be obtained. Most often this problem is dealt with by taking ratios of peaks rather than absolute concentrations. Usually the peak called creatine (Cr) at 3.0 ppm, is used as

the denominator due to its relative invariance in multiple pathologies compared to the other major peaks. When comparing the ratios it is important to note that, due to the complexity of the equations above, the ratios will very likely change at different TE values. Thus, the NAA/Cr ratio, for instance, is greater at 272 ms than at 136 ms. This means direct conversion of a decrease in NAA/Cr ratios to percent neuronal loss is dangerous.

To illustrate these concepts shown in Fig. 21.6 are fits of spectra acquired from a voxel in occipital cortex in a Huntington's disease patient at a long echo time where the macromolecular contamination is absent. The spectra fits well to combinations of individual resonance lines. Shown in Fig. 21.6(b) are spectra acquired from occipital cortex in a normal control before and after use of a preceding inversion pulse to suppress the macromolecular resonances (these have much shorter T_1 values than the metabolites). It is clear that significant macromolecular intensity lies under the methyl resonances of NAA and Cr at 2ppm, as well as under lactate and glutamate resonances.

^{31}P spectroscopy

Using ^{31}P spectroscopy, one can readily measure ATP, phosphocreatine (PCr), inorganic phosphate (Pi), and phosphomono- and di-esters. The difference in chemical shift between PCr and Pi allows one to measure tissue pH (Gadian & Radda, 1981). The ability to readily measure ATP levels makes this an attractive technique. Unfortunately, ATP levels are maintained at a near constancy under almost

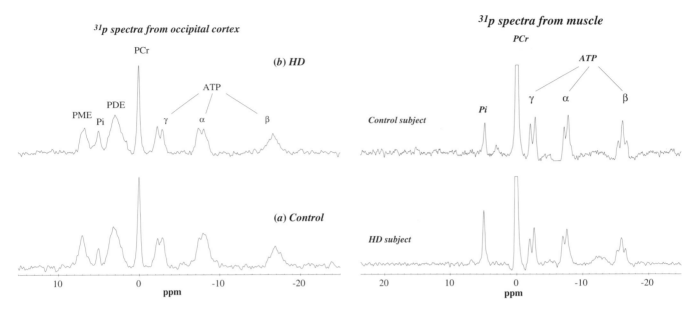

Fig. 21.7 *Left* [31]P spectra (1.5 T) taken from occipital cortex in an HD patient and a normal control. Peaks corresponding to ATP, phosphocreatine, inorganic phosphate, and phosphomonoesters and diesters are visible. No major differences between the HD and control subject are seen in this brain region implying that any energetic defects seen are less severe than those found in ischemic regions or in patients with mitochondrial disorders. *Right* [31]P spectra (1.5 T) taken from muscle in an HD and control subject. In this case a decrease in the PCr/Pi ratio is detected that is significant. No change in pH was noted (Koroshetz *et al.*, 1997).

all but the most extreme metabolic conditions. Some workers attempt to calculate ADP levels (since ADP concentrations are usually too low to observe directly) based upon ATP and PCr and Pi concentrations using the equilibrium constant for the creatine kinase reaction below:

$$PCr + ADP + {}^+H \rightleftharpoons Cr + ATP$$

The ATP thus formed can then be used as a fuel:

$$ATP \xrightarrow{\text{ATPase}} ADP + pi + energy$$

Unfortunately, it is not clear that the creatine kinase reaction is always at equilibrium. It is certain that ATP levels are not held constant during ischemia or in the direct injection of a neurotoxin; however, it is more than likely that the neurodegenerative disorders manifest metabolic defects less severe than this. Most ^{31}P studies to date have examined muscle in mitochondrial disorders. These studies have long shown defects in many measures of high energy phosphate metabolism that in some cases are refractory to treatment with CoQ or vitamin therapy (Chance *et al.*, 1986; Argov & Bank, 1991; Bendahan *et al.*, 1992; Radda, 1992). Although we have shown defects in phosphocreatine levels in resting muscle using ^{31}P in HD (Koroshetz *et al.*, 1997) and these have also been found to a small degree in PD (Penn *et al.*, 1995) it is possible that use of exercise protocols could elicit larger differences between controls and neurodegenerative disease patients (Argov & Bank, 1991; Bendahan *et al.*, 1992; Argov, 1998). Differences are seen in both resting PCr/Pi ratios and recovery of ATP in exercised muscle in HD (Lodi *et al.*, 2000).

In brain many studies have shown no decrease in ATP levels in AD or PD. We, and others (Hoang *et al.*, 1998), have found the same thing in HD brain as shown in Fig. 21.7, where no changes are observed in ATP or even PCr. Even in mitochondrial disorders, the primary observation is decreased PCr levels, not decreased ATP levels (Barbiroli *et al.*, 1993, 1997). However brain studies are complicated by the necessity of using large voxels due to the lower sensitivity of ^{31}P compared to [1]H. This means that there is quite a bit of partial volume averaging, which tends to decrease sensitivity for detection of focal changes. It would be of interest, for example, to examine the hippocampus in AD or the striatum in HD, however these studies will likely require higher fields such as 4 or 7 T in order to gain the increased sensitivity necessary for detection of focally specific changes. In any case even if small changes in ATP or PCr levels were to be detected, the low signal to noise ratios of ^{31}P compared to ^{1}H spectroscopy would render this technique to be less useful as a marker for possible therapeutic interventions. This is not true in the mitochondrial disorders where larger changes are noted.

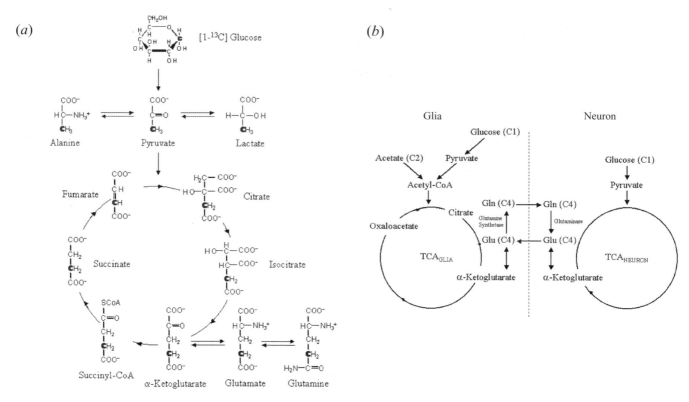

Fig. 21.8 (*a*) Schematic for the metabolism of glucose and its conversion to observable ^{13}C-labeled compounds. The Cs in bold represent the carbon as it is passed through the TCA cycle. Note that, on the first pass, the glutamate and glutamine are labeled at the C-4 position. If the TCA cycle is blocked by, for instance, 3-nitropropionic acid, one will see an increase in lactate and alanine, as well as a buildup of succinate. (*b*) Schematic of neuronal/glial metabolism and glutamate/glutamine cycle. Neurotransmitter release of glutamate is taken up by the astrocyte where it is converted to glutamine and shuttled back to the neuron where it is reconverted to glutamate. Also shown is the metabolism of acetate which is only taken up by glial cells, and hence can provide a means to discriminate neuronal from glial metabolism using ^{13}C MRS.

^{13}C NMR spectroscopy

Although carbon is less sensitive than even phosphorus (the relative sensitivities of proton : phosphorus : carbon is 100 : 6.7 : 0.018) it makes a useful marker for a number of interesting biological pathways. Because the natural abundance of the carbon-13 isotope (the NMR active isotope with spin 1/2) is only 1.1%, one can label molecules and see them as they are metabolized. In such cases the background signal will be quite low as carbon-12 is NMR invisible. Such studies can be performed using glucose as a label to watch as it passes through the TCA cycle. Usually the C1 position of glucose is labeled using ^{13}C, then the metabolism of the glucose molecule is followed as the glucose gets metabolized through the glycolytic pathway, and then through the TCA cycle. A schematic for this process is shown in Fig. 21.8. On the first pass through the TCA cycle the primary detectable molecule is ^{13}C-labeled glutamate

in the C4 position, followed rather quickly by glutamine at the C4 position. Subsequent passes through the TCA cycle produce labeling at the C3 and C2 positions of glutamate and glutamine. One can also detect the absolute amount of ^{13}C-labeled glucose in the brain at the same time. At later time points other metabolites start to appear, such as lactate, gaba and *N*-acetylaspartate (NAA).

In addition to labeling glucose, one can label acetate as well. This provides an interesting comparison with glucose labeling since acetate is only taken up by the glial cells and can be used to probe altered glial metabolism as shown in Fig. 21.8 (Badar-Goffer *et al.*, 1990; Hassel *et al.*, 1995; Bluml *et al.*, 2002; Lebon *et al.*, 2002).

Much work has gone into trying to model the kinetics of the reactions and determining, for instance, TCA cycle flux and glutamate-glutamine cycling from these numbers. Space precludes a full discussion here, however most researchers who study brain make the assumption that the

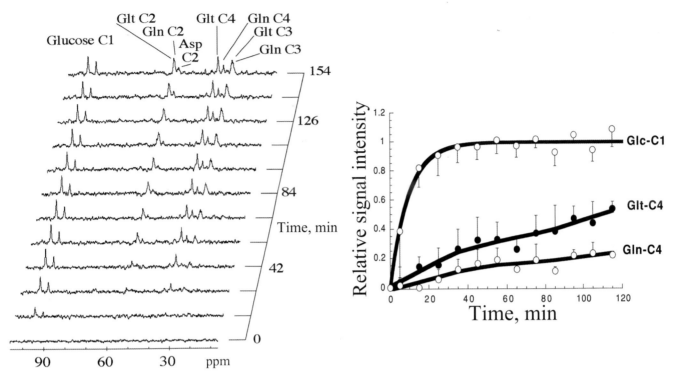

Fig. 21.9 Glucose metabolism using ^{13}C NMR. *Left*: Serial ^{13}C, [1]H-decoupled spectra acquired from a single rat from frontal cortex. Each spectrum is collected in 14 min and yields adequate SNR for temporal analysis of TCA cycle flux rates when combined with the metabolic modeling. *Right*: Average time courses for enrichment of glucose (C1), glut and gln (C4) carbons in seven halothane anesthetized rats.

reaction from oxo-glutarate to glutamate is much faster than the rate at which the substrate comes in (i.e. TCA cycle flux) and therefore the rate of C4 labeling is thus essentially the rate of TCA cycle flux. While this approach is somewhat controversial, its validity does not affect our qualitative understanding here. As an example of the type of information possible, we show data in Fig. 21.9 from a ^{13}C labeling experiment in a rat. The major metabolites observed, along with the corresponding time curves are shown. The rate at which the various TCA cycle intermediates gets labeled yields the desired information in the context of a metabolic model (Mason *et al.*, 1992; Gruetter *et al.*, 1994; Mason *et al.*, 1995; Sibson *et al.*, 1997; Van Zijl *et al.*, 1997)). Thus, administration of ^{13}C-labeled glucose to a patient with a suspected defect in glycolysis would yield a slower rate for labeling of glutamate compared to a control subject. At this point, such an observation would be indistinguishable from a defect in the TCA cycle. Preliminary data on such an experiment have been obtained for Alzheimer's disease, and the result was reduced glutamate labeling that correlated with measures of cognitive impairment obtained by NAA (Lin *et al.*, 2003). Large increases in lactate labeling, and decreased glutamate and NAA labeling were found ^{13}C spectra in two

patients with mitochondrial disorders (Bluml *et al.*, 2001). We have shown increased glutamate metabolism in mouse models of ALS and decreased glutamate and increased glutamine labeling in an HD mouse model (Choi *et al.*, 2003). These results are consistent with impaired neurons in HD and impaired glial function in ALS.

Although the biochemical specificity of carbon spectroscopy is tantalizing in its potential, it is unlikely to become anywhere nearly as well used as proton spectroscopy since the cost of ^{13}C-labeled glucose and the limited spatial resolution obtainable are likely to limit widespread application to humans. Nonetheless, it remains a very useful tool for investigation of etiological and symptomatic questions in neurodegenerative illness, especially when combined with proton MRS and other techniques such as PET.

Use of MRS in studies of therapeutics in humans

The use of MRS to study neuroprotection can only be defined as in its infancy for any number of reasons that are not worth digressing into here. Suffice it to say that, as the end point in any human therapeutic trial, MR spectroscopy can be considered, at this point, only as complementary to other end points including clinical metrics. On the other hand, there are numerous animal studies where MR spectroscopic data can be considered as a major criterion for evaluation of the animal's neurochemistry. Instead of cataloguing the various studies that have been performed, let us examine what major end points may prove useful in future studies.

Because NAA is typically the largest peak in the MR spectrum, it remains an attractive target for assessment of therapeutic interventions. There are two reasons for this, first in any trial, reproducibility from one time point to the next is quite important. Due to the low sensitivity of MRS as well as the relatively low concentrations of the neurochemicals such as NAA, it is imperative to maximize the intrasubject reliability. This is best attained using those resonances that have the highest signal to noise ratios. This is a useful, but hardly compelling, reason. Second, since NAA is a marker for the health of neurons, it can be imagined to be a therapeutic marker in any pathology that anticipates the loss of neurons such as Alzheimer's disease, Huntington's disease or amyotrophic lateral sclerosis. Since the neuronal loss in these pathologies proceeds fairly rapidly, NAA makes for a reasonable choice to follow the neuronal loss. Among the complications that make such a study difficult is the need for reproducibility of the voxels (whether they are acquired as single voxels or as multiple voxels from a spectroscopic image). Because gray and white matter have different amounts of NAA it is important to collect a high resolution 3-D MRI image to assess the amount of gray and white matter in each voxel as well as to properly register the voxels (Hetherington *et al.*, 1996).

A number of studies have used NAA as a therapeutic marker in humans. A study in epilepsy showed re-normalization of NAA in epileptic patients rendered seizure-free after surgery (this re-normalization was significant compared both to before surgery as well as compared to patients who were not rendered seizure free) (Serles *et al.*, 2001). NAA has also been used as a marker for recovery in treatment of ALS with riluzole (Kalra *et al.*, 1998, 1999). In this case a small increase in NAA levels (6%) was recorded in motor cortex in those patients treated with riluzole. The untreated group showed a decline in NAA of about 4%. Studies of other brain regions more affected, such as the medulla where NAA is decreased by 17% compared to controls (Pioro *et al.*, 1999), may prove to provide better sensitivity for such types of studies. Further, large increases in NAA/Cr ratios correlated with improved recovery from traumatic head injury (Signoretti *et al.*, 2002).

An intriguing example of the use of MRS has been proposed in following therapy in Parkinson's disease in both primate models (Jenkins *et al.*, 1994) and in human patients (Ross *et al.*, 1999) after grafting of dopaminergic fetal cells in the striatum. Since fetal cells possess very little NAA it is possible to measure changes in NAA levels longitudinally after grafting. Presumably such increases in NAA levels indicates the graft is surviving and generating axonal sprouting (Ross *et al.*, 1999). Evaluation of NAA levels may prove complementary in this regard to study of dopamine transporter levels and binding using both PET and pharmacologic MRI (phMRI).

Use of NAA could thus be a powerful adjunct to other techniques to assess neuroprotective strategies such as NMDA antagonists in stroke, anti-epileptic medications in epilepsy, and potential therapies in ALS, AD and HD. One could study any neurodegenerative condition where progression of symptoms is rapid enough to assess neuroprotection in a reasonable time window. One important issue that must be settled in such a study is that of the neuronal loss vs. neuronal health. In the former case one would expect to find the rate of NAA loss slower than in the untreated controls, in the latter case one may actually see an increase in NAA levels if the neurons have not actually died.

Other molecules can be studied in addition to NAA and are usually collected in the same spectrum anyway. One chemical studied extensively has been lactate. MRS may be an attractive probe to monitor (experimental) treatment in patients with mitochondrial disorders. These disorders are progressive degenerative disorders, which affect multiple organs. Among the most common of these disorders is mitochondrial myopathy, encephalopathy, lactic acidosis and stroke-like episodes (MELAS-syndrome). A hallmark of MELAS is elevated intracerebral lactate because of the dysfunctional oxidative metabolism. Therefore, monitoring lactate levels has potential as a therapeutic outcome measure. De Stefano *et al.* studied 11 patients with various mitochondrial disorders in a short term clinical treatment trial (De Stefano *et al.*, 1995b). The patients received sodium dichloroacetate in a placebo-controlled, double-blinded crossover study. Dichloroacetate can cause stimulation of pyruvate dehydrogenase activity and subsequent decreases in lactate. Seven of them showed a significant decrease of the Lac/Cr ratio after 1 week of treatment. However, their clinical disability remained unchanged, likely because a large fraction of the neuronal damage was not due to lactic acidosis (i.e. the lactate was a symptom not a cause of the encephalopathy). Pavlakis *et al.* studied one patient with MELAS over the course of several weeks of dichloroacetate therapy showing that the lactate levels decreased with time, and that NAA levels increased

(Pavlakis *et al.*, 1998). Unfortunately because of the variable clinical course of this disease the relapsing stroke-like episodes may resolve on their own and do not necessarily reflect responsiveness to treatment. Nonetheless, they did show that lactate levels were elevated even in tissue that showed no abnormalities in conventional MRI. In a similar disorder increased lactate has been observed in children with defects in pyruvate dehydrogenase complex (Harada *et al.*, 1996; Rubio-Gozalbo *et al.*, 1999). Rubio-Gozalbo *et al.*, 1999) determined that, in addition to increased lactate, there was increased alanine. Both these abnormalities correlated with changes in thiamine levels, lending support to the idea that MRS would be useful in following therapy. Harada *et al.* (1996) showed that the lactate levels renormalized in such patients upon treatment with dichloroacetate. One caveat to the dichloroacetate studies is that decreases in lactate may not be reflective of improved tissue metabolic status as it is the lactate/pyruvate ratio that truly reflects the cellular redox state, and lactate decreases induced via dichloroacetate are not always the result of stimulation of pyruvate dehydrogenase activity (Dimlich & Nielsen, 1992).

We also used treatment with coenzyme Q_{10} to lower lactate levels in HD in occipital cortex (Koroshetz *et al.*, 1997). In these subjects the small increase in lactate observed in occipital cortex (compared to controls) was lowered by about 28% in the HD subjects. As we discussed above, since the origins of the increased lactate in this population is not clear, the mechanism by which coenzyme Q_{10} is working remains to be elucidated.

Neuroprotection in animal models

The non-invasive nature of MR makes studies of neuroprotection quite attractive. The ability to follow an animal longitudinally, and as its own control, allows evaluation of neuroprotection with smaller numbers of animals than might be attempted from histological methods. These types of MRS experiments have been performed in many of the animal models discussed above including models of neurodegeneration generated using mitochondrial poisons (injected both systemically as well as intracerebrally) as well as transgenic mice. Examples of the neuroprotective strategies evaluated using magnetic resonance techniques have included:

(*a*) glutamate blockade by either antagonists such as MK-801 or by ablation of the cortical input of glutamate into the striatum via decortectomy (Storey *et al.*, 1992; Beal *et al.*, 1993; Henshaw *et al.*, 1994; Dijkhuizen *et al.*, 1996; Jenkins *et al.*, 1996; Lee *et al.*, 2000).

(*b*) blockade of free radical production using blockers of neuronal nitric oxide synthase or trapping of free radicals after they are formed with compounds such as n-tert-butyl-alpha-(2-sulfophenyl)-nitrone (S-PBN) (Schulz *et al.*, 1995a,b).

(*c*) Administration of neuronal growth factors such as basic fibroblast growth factor (bFGF) (Kirschner *et al.*, 1996).

(*d*) Energy repletion strategies whereby attempts are made to restore ATP levels with, for instance, mitochondrial electron transport chain substrates (e.g. coenzyme Q_{10} or ubiquinone) or creatine supplementation (Beal *et al.*, 1994; Jenkins *et al.*, 1996; Matthews *et al.*, 1998; Ferrante *et al.*, 2000; Andreassen *et al.*, 2000a,b).

Many of these same strategies have proved useful in models of focal ischemia.

Magnetic resonance spectroscopy can play a role in assessing the efficacy of such potential therapies by monitoring their effects on: neuronal health and number using NAA; on oxidative phosphorylation using lactate or ATP; and on lesion size as measured by water imaging. Shown in Fig. 21.10 are data showing a focal increase in lactate and T_2 signal after acute intrastriatal injection with 3-NP (an inhibitor of succinate dehydrogenase or complex II). The lactate and NAA are shown in the form of spectroscopic images. (We also show as well, spectra demonstrating the identification of succinate at 2.40 ppm using comparisons with phantom spectra.) One week later, there is no lactate detectable at the lesion site, however, there is a large decrease in NAA as well as a decrease in the size of altered T_2 signal. The NAA would thus prove to be a good marker to follow long term neuroprotection, as we discuss below. On the other hand, lactate proves to be a useful marker for following the acute neuroprotection. As an example of this we present data, in Fig. 21.11, culled from more than 4 years' worth of neuroprotective experiments in the animal models discussed above using azide (a blocker of complex IV in the electron transport chain), malonate, 3-NP (another blocker of complex II) and MPP$^+$ (a blocker of complex I in the electron transport chain). The protective agents that were used all have different mechanisms of action, and yet are all capable of producing neuroprotection to a varying degree. It is clear that MRS measurements of lactate correlate well with histological measures of neuroprotection in the majority of compounds studied. (One possible origin of this correlation is that the decrease in lactate measured in the striatum is actually due to the reduced size of the lesion while the actual concentration doesn't change (because the lactate measurements come from rather large voxels of greater than 2×2 mm)).

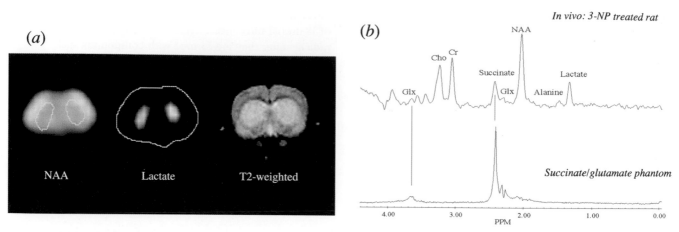

Fig. 21.10 MR images of focal energy impairment induced via systemic injections of 3-NP, an inhibitor of succinate dehydrogenase. (*a*) Spectroscopic images of decreased NAA, increased lactate and T_2-weighted signal intensity taken 3–4 hours after i.v. injection of 33 mg/kg. The CSI images of lactate and NAA were acquired with a spatial resolution of approximately 2 × 2 mm with a 6 mm slice thickness. (*b*) Spectra from the striatum showing increased lactate and succinate after 3-NP. For comparison a phantom with glutamate and succinate is shown illustrating the singlet assignment of the succinate resonance at 2.40 ppm. Ordinarily, this peak is barely observable.

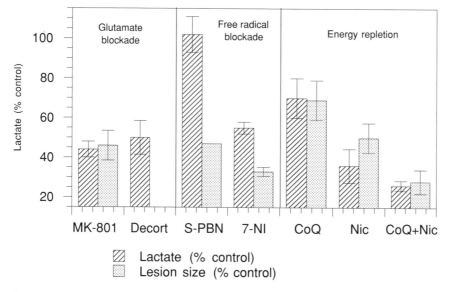

Fig. 21.11 Bar chart comparing measures of MRS lactate and lesion size determined histologically using either TTC or Nissl stain, as a function of neuroprotective strategies in the rat mitochondrial poison models of neurodegeneration. The MK-801 data are from intrastriatal MPP$^+$ injections, the decortectomies were performed in systemically treated 3-NP rats, and the other results come from intrastriatal malonate injections.

NAA has been shown to be a useful marker for neuroprotection against MPP$^+$ lesions using neuronal growth factors (Kirschner *et al.*, 1996). In this study, basic fibroblast growth factor (bFGF) was administered to neonatal rats (in whom the blood–brain barrier is not yet formed) and it was found that it could protect against neuronal loss as measured by NAA. A clear and marked protection was shown by measuring absolute NAA relative to water from proton density-weighted images (i.e. images in which the TR is long and the TE is short and in which CSF, edema and brain are nearly iso-intense) in the same animals. Using this method, it was shown that the NAA loss 2.5–3 months

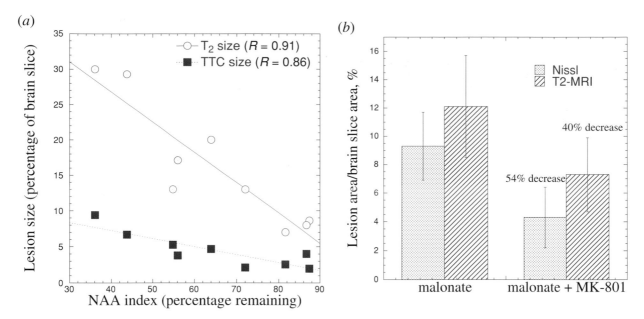

Fig. 21.12 Plots showing the relations between histology and T_2-weighted MRI measures of lesion sizes. (*a*) Plots of lesion areas/brain areas (percents) measured using either TTC or T_2-weighted MRI 2–3 months after lesioning with MPP$^+$. The lesion areas are correlated quite well with an NAA measurement of absolute NAA loss. The animals with smaller lesions and less NAA loss have been treated with bFGF. (*b*) Plots of the relations between lesion size measured using Nissl staining 24 hours after intrastriatal lesioning with malonate (either with or without MK-801 pre-treatment) or measured using T_2-weighted MRI 3–5 hours after lesioning. The T_2 measures lead to a larger lesion size, but the percentage reduction in lesion size between the two techniques is close.

after lesioning in the bFGF-treated animals was $85 \pm 3\%$ of the contralateral side compared to the untreated animals in which the loss in the lesioned side was $60 \pm 8\%$ (Kirschner *et al.*, 1996). These numbers also agreed with the histology and MRI measurements, and correlated with lactate measurements. These correlations are shown in Fig. 21.12(*a*). The lactate measurements also showed the protective effects of bFGF because the lactate concentration was lowered significantly. It is important to note that one can measure all the neurochemicals from one spectrum, and thus one can analyze neurodegeneration from a number of different perspectives with regards to neuronal loss and energy metabolism.

Numerous other animal studies have appeared using NAA as a marker for neuroprotective strategies. Our own studies have used NAA as a marker for neuroprotection in both neurotoxin models of neurodegenerative illness using blockade of mitochondrial complex II (succinate dehydrogenase) (Matthews *et al.*, 1998) or complex I (*N*-methyl-4-phenyl pyridinium (MPP$^+$)) (Kirschner *et al.*, 1996), as well as in transgenic mouse models of Huntington's disease (Ferrante *et al.*, 2000). In the latter study it was found that a dietary creatine supplementation (2% creatine in the food) leads to an increase in the life span of the R6/2 mice from about 15 weeks to about 17.5 weeks. Creatine

supplementation also led to a 30% increase in NAA in the striatum of these mice. These mice typically suffer loss of greater than 50% of the NAA in the striatum (Jenkins *et al.*, 2000). Typical spectra for HD and wild-type mice were shown in Fig. 21.5. MRS can simultaneously measure both the creatine increase in the brain, as well as the NAA and other neurochemicals by using, for instance, water as an internal reference standard. Thus, in this latter study we showed an increase in brain creatine levels of 21%. Most importantly, the increase in NAA levels correlated with the increase in creatine levels. The protection of NAA levels was also correlated with a protection of neuronal size (about 31%) by creatine supplementation. Since NAA has an exclusively neuronal localization, the decrease in neuronal size leads to a decrease in the total NAA signal detected. These results show that the time course of neuronal shrinkage is roughly parallel to that of the NAA loss in the absence of creatine treatment. Creatine supplementation delays the loss of both NAA and neuronal shrinkage to approximately the same degree. These are again reflective of the utility of NAA as a neuronal marker.

We also studied the ability of creatine to neuroprotect in a transgenic mouse model of ALS using a mutation in superoxide dismutase. In these mice lifespan was prolonged about 20% using 2% oral creatine supplementation

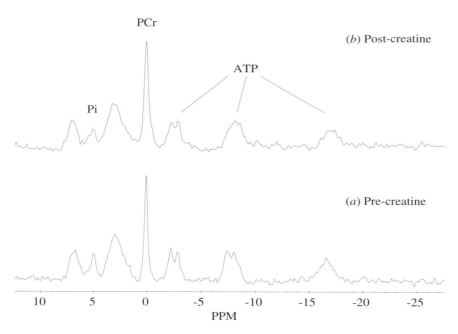

Fig. 21.13 ^{31}P spectra from occipital cortex in a Huntington's disease patient before and after treatment with oral creatine. Note that the spectra are quite similar with the exception of a decrease in the area of the peak labeled Pi. Spectra have been scaled to the PCr peak.

(Andreassen *et al.*, 2001). Further, the creatine lowered the elevated glutamate levels observed in these mice as measured by proton MRS. The peak labeled glx is smaller in the ALS mouse after creatine supplementation at about 80 days of age. Unfortunately, the effect wears off at 120 days in which the elevated glx reappears in spite of creatine supplementation (Andreassen *et al.*, 2001b).

Combined MRS and MRI of excitotoxicity

Use of MRI for examination of acute indirect excitotoxic insults using mitochondrial poisons was presented above. These studies are similar in nature to those used for the clinical aging of infarcts. In ischemia, as in the excitotoxic lesions, the first changes noted are decreases in the apparent diffusion coefficient (discussed below) that are consistent with redistribution of water from the extracellular to the intracellular space. At later time points (many hours to days) there is an increase in the T_2 relaxation time. The increased T_2 relaxation is believed to correlate with the cytotoxic edema, and more rapid rotational correlation times for the water. The lesion sizes determined using the T_2-weighted MRI can be used to measure the effects of neuroprotective strategies. We made extensive comparisons between measurements of lesion size using T_2-weighted

MRI and using TTC staining as well as Nissl staining postmortem. We found that the T_2-weighted MRI generally yielded slightly larger sizes (by about 30%, although the percentage changes induced by the various neuroprotective strategies was similar in the postmortem and in vivo techniques. While the MRI may include tissue that eventually recovers (i.e. penumbral tissue), it is also true that the histological techniques suffer from some degree of tissue shrinkage. Examples of these experiments are shown in Fig. 21.12. On the left in Fig. 21.12(*a*) are data showing correlations between T_2-weighted signal intensity, TTC staining lesion size and NAA decreases in a series of rats treated with MPP$^+$ and with or without bFGF (as discussed above). It is clear that there are good correlations between all three techniques. There is a larger increase in lesion area using T_2-weighted imaging than with TTC, however there is very good correlation between T_2 area and TTC area (R = 0.85). Shown in Fig. 21.12(*b*) are data showing the neuroprotective effects of MK-801 in acute excitotoxic lesions induced using malonate (Henshaw *et al.*, 1994; Jenkins *et al.*, 1996) compared using T_2-weighted MRI and Nissl staining. While again the T_2-weighted MRI lesion sizes are larger than the histologically measured lesion areas, the overall correlation between the two techniques, as far as percent decrease in lesion size is good.

Unfortunately, the acute nature of the neurodegenerative models above are not directly applicable to the T_2 contrast noted in the chronic neurodegenerative conditions. One possible exception to this is ALS. In this disease increased T_2 in the lateral cortical spinal tracts was measured in the cervical spine (Terao *et al.*, 1995). Other groups claimed there were no effects (Tanabe *et al.*, 1998). Our own studies indicate that the decreased volume of the cortical spinal tracts may lead to increased CSF signal in the region. Due to the exceptionally long T_2 of CSF this can be a potential confound.

^{31}P spectroscopy

To conclude, we will briefly discuss phosphorus spectroscopy. Most ^{31}P studies to date have examined muscle in mitochondrial disorders. These studies have long shown defects in many measures of high energy phosphate metabolism that in some cases are refractory to treatment with CoQ_{10} or vitamin therapy (Chance *et al.*, 1986; Argov & Bank, 1991; Bendahan *et al.*, 1992; Radda, 1992). The efficacy of coenzyme Q_{10} in improving abnormalities in high energy phosphates in patients with mitochondrial disorders has been claimed in both brain and muscle (Bendahan *et al.*, 1992; Barbiroli *et al.*, 1993, 1997, 1998); however other groups have claimed it is inefficacious (Matthews *et al.*, 1993). Due to the variable treatment times with coenzyme Q_{10}, variable clinical progression and courses in the various mitochondrial disorders, as well as the relative rarity of these diseases the question of efficacy remains open.

We have studied the ability of treatment with cyclocreatine and creatine to neuroprotect lesions induced by inhibitors of succinate dehydrogenase (electron transport chain complex II) using either systemic or intrastriatal injections (Matthews *et al.*, 1993). ^{31}P spectroscopy showed increases in both PCr and phosphocyclocreatine in the brain. In addition, treatment with cyclocreatine increased ATP levels in control animals in brain (creatine treatment did not). The MRS proved invaluable in assessing the amount of creatine that made it into the brain, and how much an increase in high energy phosphates there were. These data would be even easier to collect in humans due to their larger brains. Shown in Fig. 21.13 are ^{31}P spectra in an Huntington's disease patient before and after oral supplementation with 6 gms of creatine per day. Although the ^{31}P spectra are not dramatically different there does appear to be a decrease in the inorganic phosphate peak (Pi) consistent with an increase in PCr. The spectra are scaled to the PCr peak. The spectra are consistent with an increase in PCr. Such studies, however, need to be performed over long periods of time, since the normal variability of these chemicals in patient populations is not well characterized.

Acknowledgements

We would like to acknowledge the contributions of our many colleagues to the work presented here. In particular: Drs Diana Rosas, Alpaslan Dedeoglu, Ekkehardt Kuestermann, Iris Chen, Russell Matthews, Ole Andreassen, Jorg Schulz, and Bruce Rosen.

REFERENCES

Andreassen, O. A., Jenkins, B. G., Dedeoglu, A. *et al.* (2001a). Increases in cortical glutamate concentrations in transgenic amyotrophic lateral sclerosis mice are attenuated by creatine supplementation. *J. Neurochem.*, **77**, 383–90.

Andreassen, O. A., Dedeoglu, A., Ferrante, R. J. *et al.* (2001b). Creatine increase survival and delays motor symptoms in a transgenic animal model of Huntington's disease. *Neurobiol. Dis.*, **8**, 479–91.

Argov, Z. (1998). Functional evaluation techniques in mitochondrial disorders. *Eur. Neurol.*, **39**, 65–71.

Argov, Z. & Bank, W. J. (1991). Phosphorus magnetic resonance spectroscopy (31P MRS) in neuromuscular disorders. *Ann. Neurol.*, **30**, 90–7.

Badar-Goffer, R. S., Bachelard, H. S. & Morris P. G. (1990). Cerebral metabolism of acetate and glucose studied by 13C-n.m.r. spectroscopy. A technique for investigating metabolic compartmentation in the brain. *Biochem. J.*, **266**, 133–9.

Barbiroli, B., Montagna, P., Martinelli, P. *et al.* (1993). Defective brain energy metabolism shown by in vivo 31P MR spectroscopy in 28 patients with mitochondrial cytopathies. *J. Cereb. Blood Flow Metab.*, **13**, 469–74.

Barbiroli, B., Frassineti, C., Martinelli, P. *et al.* (1997). Coenzyme Q10 improves mitochondrial respiration in patients with mitochondrial cytopathies. An in vivo study on brain and skeletal muscle by phosphorous magnetic resonance spectroscopy. *Cell. Mol. Biol.*, **43**, 741–9.

Barbiroli, B., Iotti, S. & Lodi, R. (1998). Aspects of human bioenergetics as studied in vivo by magnetic resonance spectroscopy. *Biochimie*, **80**, 847–53.

Bartha, R., Drost, D. J. & Williamson, P. C. (1999). Factors affecting the quantification of short echo in-vivo 1H MR spectra: prior knowledge, peak elimination, and filtering. *NMR Biomed.*, **12**, 205–16.

Baslow, M. H. (2002). Evidence supporting a role for *N*-acetyl-L-aspartate as a molecular water pump in myelinated neurons in the central nervous system. An analytical review. *Neurochem. Int.*, **40**, 295–300.

(2003). Brain *N*-acetylaspartate as a molecular water pump and its role in the etiology of Canavan disease: a mechanistic explanation. *J. Mol. Neurosci.*, **21**, 185–90.

Beal, M. F., Brouillet, E., Jenkins, B. G. *et al.* (1993). Neurochemical and histologic characterization of striatal excitotoxic lesions produced by the mitochondrial toxin 3-nitropropionic acid. *J. Neurosci.*, **13**, 4181–92.

Beal, M. F., Henshaw, D. R., Jenkins, B. G., Rosen, B. R. & Schulz, J. B. (1994). Coenzyme Q10 and nicotinamide block striatal lesions produced by the mitochondrial toxin malonate. *Ann. Neurol.*, **36**, 882–8.

Bendahan, D., Desnuelle, C., Vanuxem, D. *et al.* (1992). ^{31}P NMR spectroscopy and ergometer exercise test as evidence for muscle oxidative performance improvement with coenzyme Q in mitochondrial myopathies. *Neurology*, **42**, 1203–8.

Birken, D. L. & Oldendorf, W. H. (1989). *N*-acetyl-L-aspartic acid: a literature review of a compound prominent in ^{1}H-NMR spectroscopic studies of brain. *Neurosci. Biobehav. Rev.*, **13**, 23–31.

Blass, J. P., Sheu, R. K. & Cedarbaum, J. M. (1988). Energy metabolism in disorders of the nervous system. *Rev. Neurol.*, **144**, 543–63.

Bluml, S., Moreno, A., Hwang, J. H. & Ross, B. D. (2001). 1-(13)C glucose magnetic resonance spectroscopy of pediatric and adult brain disorders. *NMR Biomed.*, **14**, 19–32.

Bluml, S., Moreno-Torres, A., Shic, F., Nguy, C. H. & Ross, B. D. (2002). Tricarboxylic acid cycle of glia in the in vivo human brain. *NMR Biomed.*, **15**, 1–5.

Bottomley, P. (1987). Spatial localization in NMR spectroscopy *in vivo*. *Ann. NY Acad. Sci.*, **508**, 333–8.

Brand, A., Richter-Landsberg, C. & Leibfritz, D. (1993). Multinuclear NMR studies on the energy metabolism of glial and neuronal cells. *Dev. Neurosci.*, **15**, 289–98.

Bristol, L. A. & Rothstein, J. D. (1996). Glutamate transporter gene expression in amyotrophic lateral sclerosis motor cortex. *Ann. Neurol.*, **39**, 676–9.

Brownell, A. L., Jenkins, B. G., Elmaleh, D. R., Deacon, T. W., Spealman, R. D. & Isacson, O. (1998). Combined PET/MRS brain studies show dynamic and long-term physiological changes in a primate model of Parkinson disease. *Nat. Med.*, **4**, 1308–12.

Chance, B., Leigh, J. S., Smith, D. S., Nioka, S. & Clark, B. J. (1986). Phosphorus magnetic resonance spectroscopy studies of the role of mitochondria in the disease process. *Ann. NY Acad. Sci.*, **488**, 140–53.

Choe, B. Y., Park, J. W., Lee, K. S. *et al.* (1998). Neuronal laterality in Parkinson's disease with unilateral symptom by in vivo 1H magnetic resonance spectroscopy. *Invest. Radiol.*, **33**, 450–5.

Choi J.-K., Kuestermann, E., Andreassen, O. A., Beal, M. F. & Jenkins, B. G. (2003). A tale of two mice: impaired glial-neuronal cycling in mouse models of Huntington's disease and amyotrophic lateral sclerosis. In *International Society of Magnetic Resonance in Medicine*, p. 437. Toronto, Canada.

Cruz, C. J., Aminoff, M. J., Meyerhoff, D. J., Graham, S. H. & Weiner, M. W. (1997). Proton MR spectroscopic imaging of the striatum in Parkinson's disease. *Magn. Reson. Imaging*, **15**, 619–24.

Dager, S. R., Strauss, W. L., Marro, K. I., Richards, T. L., Metzger, G. D. & Artru, A. A. (1995). Proton magnetic resonance spectroscopy investigation of hyperventilation in subjects with panic disorder and comparison subjects. *Am. J. Psychiatry*, **152**, 666–72.

Davie, C. A., Hawkins, C. P., Barker, G. J. *et al.* (1994). Serial proton magnetic resonance spectroscopy in acute multiple sclerosis lesions. *Brain*, **117**, 49–58.

De Stefano, N., Matthews, P. M. & Arnold, D. L. (1995a). Reversible decreases in *N*-acetylaspartate after acute brain injury. *Magn. Reson. Med.*, **34**, 721–7.

De Stefano, N., Matthews, P. M., Ford, B., Genge, A., Karpati, G. & Arnold, D. L. (1995b). Short-term dichloroacetate treatment improves indices of cerebral metabolism in patients with mitochondrial disorders. *Neurology*, **45**, 1193–8.

De Stefano, N., Matthews, P. M., Narayanan, S., Francis, G. S., Antel, J. P. & Arnold, D. L. (1997). Axonal dysfunction and disability in a relapse of multiple sclerosis: longitudinal study of a patient. *Neurology*, **49**, 1138–41.

Dijkhuizen, R. M., van Lookeren Campagne, M., Niendorf, T. *et al.* (1996). Status of the neonatal rat brain after NMDA-induced excitotoxic injury as measured by MRI, MRS and metabolic imaging. *NMR Biomed.*, **9**, 84–92.

Dimlich, R. V. & Nielsen, M. M. (1992). Facilitating postischemic reduction of cerebral lactate in rats. *Stroke*, **23**, 1145–52; discussion 1152–63.

Dunlop, D. S., McHale, D. M. & Lajtha, A. (1992). Decreased brain *N*-acetylaspartate in Huntington's disease. *Brain Res.*, **580**, 44–8.

Ellis, C. M., Lemmens, G., Williams, S. C. *et al.* (1997). Changes in putamen *N*-acetylaspartate and choline ratios in untreated and levodopa-treated Parkinson's disease: a proton magnetic resonance spectroscopy study. *Neurology*, **49**, 438–44.

Endres, M., Namura, S., Shimizu-Sasamata, M. *et al.* (1998). Attenuation of delayed neuronal death after mild focal ischemia in mice by inhibition of the caspase family. *J. Cereb. Blood Flow Metab.*, **18**, 238–47.

Fenstermacher, M. J. & Narayana, P. A. (1990). Serial proton magnetic resonance spectroscopy of ischemic brain injury in humans. *Invest. Radiol.*, **25**, 1034–9.

Ferrante, R. J., Andreassen, O. A., Jenkins, B. G. *et al.* (2000). Neuroprotective effects of creatine in a transgenic mouse model of Huntington's disease. *J. Neurosci.*, **20**, 4389–97.

Fisher, M. (1995). Potentially effective therapies for acute ischemic stroke. *Eur. Neurol.*, **35**, 3–7.

Frahm, J., Merboldt, K. D. & Hanicke, W. (1987). Localized proton spectroscopy using stimulated echoes. *J. Magn. Reson.*, **72**, 502–8.

Frahm, J., Bruhn, H., Gyngell, M. L., Merboldt, K. D., Hanicke, W. & Sauter, R. (1989). Localized proton NMR spectroscopy in different regions of the human brain in vivo. Relaxation times and concentrations of cerebral metabolites. *Magn. Reson. Med.*, **11**, 47–63.

Gadian, D. G. & Radda, G. K. (1981). NMR studies of tissue metabolism. *Annu. Rev. Biochem.*, **50**, 69–83.

Granot, J. (1986). Selected volume spectroscopy using stimulated echoes (VEST). Application to spatially localized spectroscopy and imaging. *J. Magn. Reson.*, **70**.

Gruetter, R., Novotny, E. J., Boulware, S. D. *et al.* (1994). Localized 13C NMR spectroscopy in the human brain of amino acid labeling from D-[1-13C]glucose. *J. Neurochem.*, **63**, 1377–85.

Hahn, E. (1950). Spin echoes. *Phys. Rev.*, **80**, 580–94.

Harada, M., Tanouchi, M., Arai, K., Nishitani, H., Miyoshi, H. & Hashimoto, T. (1996). Therapeutic efficacy of a case of pyruvate dehydrogenase complex deficiency monitored by localized proton magnetic resonance spectroscopy. *Magn. Reson. Imaging*, **14**, 129–33.

Hassel, B., Sonnewald, U. & Fonnum, F. (1995). Glial-neuronal interactions as studied by cerebral metabolism of [2–13C]acetate and [1-13C]glucose: an ex vivo 13C NMR spectroscopic study. *J. Neurochem.*, **64**, 2773–82.

Henshaw, R., Jenkins, B. G., Schulz, J. B. *et al.* (1994). Malonate produces striatal lesions by indirect NMDA receptor activation. *Brain Res.*, **647**, 161–6.

Hetherington, H. P., Pan, J. W., Mason, G. F. *et al.* (1996). Quantitative 1H spectroscopic imaging of human brain at 4.1 T using image segmentation. *Magn. Reson. Med.*, **36**, 21–9.

Higuchi, T., Fernandez, E. J., Maudsley, A. A., Shimizu, H., Weiner, M. W. & Weinstein, P. R. (1996). Mapping of lactate and N-acetyl-L-aspartate predicts infarction during acute focal ischemia: in vivo 1H magnetic resonance spectroscopy in rats. *Neurosurgery*, **38**, 121–9; discussion 129–30.

Hilal, S. K., Maudsley, A. A., Simon, H. E. *et al.* (1983). In vivo NMR imaging of tissue sodium in the intact cat before and after acute cerebral stroke. *AJNR Am. J. Neuroradiol.*, **4**, 245–9.

Hoang, T. Q., Bluml, S., Dubowitz, D. J. *et al.* (1998). Quantitative proton-decoupled 31P MRS and 1H MRS in the evaluation of Huntington's and Parkinson's diseases. *Neurology*, **50**, 1033–40.

Holshouser, B. A., Komu, M., Moller, H. E. *et al.* (1995). Localized proton NMR spectroscopy in the striatum of patients with idiopathic Parkinson's disease: a multicenter pilot study. *Magn. Reson. Med.*, **33**, 589–94.

Hossmann, K. A. (1994). Glutamate-mediated injury in focal cerebral ischemia: the excitotoxin hypothesis revised. *Brain Pathol.*, **4**, 23–36.

Hwang, J. H., Graham, G. D., Behar, K. L., Alger, J. R., Prichard, J. W. & Rothman, D. L. (1996). Short echo time proton magnetic resonance spectroscopic imaging of macromolecule and metabolite signal intensities in the human brain. *Magn. Reson. Med.*, **35**, 633–9.

Isaacks, R. E., Bender, A. S., Kim, C. Y., Shi, Y. F. & Norenberg, M. D. (1999). Effect of ammonia and methionine sulfoximine on myo-inositol transport in cultured astrocytes. *Neurochem. Res.*, **24**, 51–9.

Jenkins, B., Brouillet, E., Chen, Y. *et al.* (1996). Non-invasive neurochemical analysis of focal excitotoxic lesions in models of neurodegenerative illness using spectroscopic imaging. *J. Cereb. Blood Flow Metab.*, **16**, 450–61.

Jenkins B., Chen, Y. & Rosen, B. eds. (1997). *Investigating the Neurochemistry and Etiology of Neurodegenrative Disorders using Magnetic Resonance Spectroscopy.* New York, NY: Wiley-Liss.

Jenkins, B. G. & Kraft, E. (1999). Magnetic resonance spectroscopy in toxic encephalopathy and neurodegeneration. *Curr. Opin. Neurol.*, **12**, 753–60.

Jenkins, B. G., Koroshetz, W. J., Beal, M. F. & Rosen, B. R. (1993). Evidence for impairment of energy metabolism in vivo in Huntington's disease using localized 1H NMR spectroscopy. *Neurology*, **43**, 2689–95.

Jenkins, B. G., Burns, L., Pakzaban, P. *et al.* (1994). Spectroscopic studies of neurochemical changes in a primate model of neurodegeneration and neural transplantation. In: *Society of Magnetic Resonance*, p 1423. San Francisco.

Jenkins, B. G., Rosas, H. D., Chen, Y. C. *et al.* (1998). ^{1}H NMR spectroscopy studies of Huntington's disease: correlations with CAG repeat numbers. *Neurology*, **50**, 1357–65.

Jenkins, B. G., Klivenyi, P., Kustermann, E. *et al.* (2000). Nonlinear decrease over time in N-acetyl aspartate levels in the absence of neuronal loss and increases in glutamine and glucose in transgenic Huntington's disease mice. *J. Neurochem.*, **74**, 2108–19.

Kalra, S., Cashman, N. R., Genge, A. & Arnold, D. L. (1998). Recovery of N-acetylaspartate in corticomotor neurons of patients with ALS after riluzole therapy. *Neuroreport*, **9**, 1757–61.

Kalra, S., Arnold, D. L. & Cashman, N. R. (1999). Biological markers in the diagnosis and treatment of ALS. *J. Neurol. Sci.*, **165** Suppl. 1, S27–32.

Kalyanapuram, R., Seshan, V. & Bansal, N. (1998). Three-dimensional triple-quantum-filtered 23Na imaging of the dog head in vivo. *J. Magn. Reson. Imaging*, **8**, 1182–9.

Keller, J. N., Kindy, M. S., Holtsberg, F. W. *et al.* (1998). Mitochondrial manganese superoxide dismutase prevents neural apoptosis and reduces ischemic brain injury: suppression of peroxynitrite production, lipid peroxidation, and mitochondrial dysfunction. *J. Neurosci.*, **18**, 687–97.

Kirschner, P. B., Jenkins, B. G., Schulz, J. B. *et al.* (1996). NGF, BDNF and NT-5, but not NT-3 protect against MPP+ toxicity and oxidative stress in neonatal animals. *Brain Res.*, **713**, 178–85.

Klunk, W. E., Xu, C., Panchalingam, K., McClure, R. J. & Pettegrew, J. W. (1996). Quantitative ^{1}H and. ^{31}P MRS of PCA extracts of postmortem Alzheimer's disease brain. *Neurobiol. Aging*, **17**, 349–57.

Kogure, T. & Kogure, K. (1997). Molecular and biochemical events within the brain subjected to cerebral ischemia (targets for therapeutical intervention). *Clin. Neurosci.*, **4**, 179–83.

Kopito, R. R. (2000). Aggresomes, inclusion bodies and protein aggregation. *Trends Cell Biol.*, **10**, 524–30.

Koroshetz, W. J., Jenkins, B. G., Rosen, B. R. & Beal, M. F. (1997). Energy metabolism defects in Huntington's disease and effects of coenzyme Q10. *Ann. Neurol.*, **41**, 160–5.

Kuzniecky, R., Palmer, C., Hugg, J. *et al.* (2001). Magnetic resonance spectroscopic imaging in temporal lobe epilepsy: neuronal dysfunction or cell loss? *Arch. Neurol.*, **58**, 2048–53.

Lebon, V., Petersen, K. F., Cline, G. W. *et al.* (2002). Astroglial contribution to brain energy metabolism in humans revealed by ^{13}C nuclear magnetic resonance spectroscopy: elucidation of the dominant pathway for neurotransmitter glutamate repletion and measurement of astrocytic oxidative metabolism. *J. Neurosci.*, **22**, 1523–31.

Lee, W. T., Shen, Y. Z. & Chang, C. (2000). Neuroprotective effect of lamotrigine and MK-801 on rat brain lesions induced by 3-nitropropionic acid: evaluation by magnetic resonance imaging and in vivo proton magnetic resonance spectroscopy. *Neuroscience*, **95**, 89–95.

Lin, A. P., Shic, F., Enriquez, C. & Ross, B. D. (2003). Reduced glutamate neurotransmission in patients with Alzheimer's disease – an in vivo (13)C magnetic resonance spectroscopy study. *Magma*, **16**, 29–42.

Lin, S. P., Song, S. K., Miller, J. P., Ackerman, J. J. & Neil, J. J. (2001). Direct, longitudinal comparison of (1)H and (23)Na MRI after transient focal cerebral ischemia. *Stroke*, **32**, 925–32.

Lodi, R., Schapira, A. H., Manners, D. *et al.* (2000). Abnormal in vivo skeletal muscle energy metabolism in Huntington's disease and dentatorubropallidoluysian atrophy. *Ann. Neurol.*, **48**, 72–6.

Magistretti, P. J. & Pellerin, L. (1997). Metabolic coupling during activation. A cellular view. *Adv. Exp. Med. Biol.*, **413**, 161–6.

Mason, G. F., Behar, K. L., Rothman, D. L. & Shulman, R. G. (1992). NMR determination of intracerebral glucose concentration and transport kinetics in rat brain. *J. Cereb. Blood Flow Metab.*, **12**, 448–55.

Mason, G. F., Pan, J. W., Ponder, S. L., Twieg, D. B., Pohost, G. M. & Hetherington, H. P. (1994). Detection of brain glutamate and glutamine in spectroscopic images at 4.1 T. *Magn. Reson. Med.*, **32**, 142–5.

Mason, G. F., Gruetter, R., Rothman, D. L., Behar, K. L., Shulman, R. G. & Novotny, E. J. (1995). Simultaneous determination of the rates of the TCA cycle, glucose utilization, alpha-ketoglutarate/glutamate exchange, and glutamine synthesis in human brain by NMR. *J. Cereb. Blood Flow Metab.*, **15**, 12–25.

Matthews, P. M., Ford, B., Dandurand, R. J. *et al.* (1993). Coenzyme Q10 with multiple vitamins is generally ineffective in treatment of mitochondrial disease. *Neurology*, **43**, 884–90.

Matthews, R. T., Yang, L., Jenkins, B. G. *et al.* (1998). Neuroprotective effects of creatine and cyclocreatine in animal models of Huntington's disease. *J. Neurosci.*, **18**, 156–63.

Pavlakis, S. G., Kingsley, P. B., Kaplan, G. P., Stacpoole, P. W., O'Shea, M. & Lustbader, D. (1998). Magnetic resonance spectroscopy: use in monitoring MELAS treatment. *Arch. Neurol.*, **55**, 849–52.

Penn, A. M., Roberts, T., Hodder, J., Allen, P. S., Zhu, G. & Martin, W. R. (1995). Generalized mitochondrial dysfunction in Parkinson's disease detected by magnetic resonance spectroscopy of muscle. *Neurology*, **45**, 2097–9.

Petroff, O. A., Graham, G. D., Blamire, A. M. *et al.* (1992). Spectroscopic imaging of stroke in humans: histopathology correlates of spectral changes. *Neurology*, **42**, 1349–54.

Petroff, O. A., Pleban, L. A. & Spencer, D. D. (1995). Symbiosis between in vivo and in vitro NMR spectroscopy: the creatine, *N*-acetylaspartate, glutamate, and GABA content of the epileptic human brain. *Magn. Reson. Imaging*, **13**, 1197–211.

Petroff, O. A., Errante, L. D., Rothman, D. L., Kim, J. H. & Spencer, D. D. (2002). Neuronal and glial metabolite content of the epileptogenic human hippocampus. *Ann. Neurol.*, **52**, 635–42.

Pettegrew, J. W., Klunk, W. E., Panchalingam, K., McClure, R. J. & Stanley, J. A. (1997). Magnetic resonance spectroscopic changes in Alzheimer's disease. *Ann. NY Acad. Sci.*, **826**, 282–306.

Pfeuffer, J., Tkac, I., Provencher, S. W. & Gruetter, R. (1999). Toward an in vivo neurochemical profile: quantification of 18 metabolites in short-echo-time (1)H NMR spectra of the rat brain. *J. Magn. Reson.*, **141**, 104–20.

Pioro, E. P., Majors, A. W., Mitsumoto, H., Nelson, D. R. & Ng, T. C. (1999). 1H-MRS evidence of neurodegeneration and excess glutamate + glutamine in ALS medulla. *Neurology*, **53**, 71–9.

Podo F. (1999). Tumour phospholipid metabolism. *NMR Biomed.*, **12**, 413–39.

Prichard, J., Rothman, D., Novotny, E. *et al.* (1991). Lactate rise detected by 1H NMR in human visual cortex during physiologic stimulation. *Proc. Natl Acad. Sci., USA*, **88**, 5829–31.

Provencher, S. W. (1993). Estimation of metabolite concentrations from localized in vivo proton NMR spectra. *Magn. Reson. Med.*, **30**, 672–9.

Radda, G. K. (1992). Control, bioenergetics, and adaptation in health and disease: noninvasive biochemistry from nuclear magnetic resonance. *FASEB J.*, **6**, 3032–8.

Ross, B. D., Hoang, T. Q., Bluml, S. *et al.* (1999). In vivo magnetic resonance spectroscopy of human fetal neural transplants. *NMR Biomed.*, **12**, 221–36.

Rothstein, J. D., Van Kammen, M., Levey, A. I., Martin, L. J. & Kuncl, R. W. (1995). Selective loss of glial glutamate transporter GLT-1 in amyotrophic lateral sclerosis. *Ann. Neurol.*, **38**, 73–84.

Rubio-Gozalbo, M. E., Heerschap, A., Trijbels, J. M., Meirleir, L. D., Thijssen, H. O. & Smeitink, J. A. (1999). Proton MR spectroscopy in a child with pyruvate dehydrogenase complex deficiency. *Magn. Reson. Imaging*, **17**, 939–44.

Saunders, D. E. (2000). MR spectroscopy in stroke. *Br. Med. Bull.*, **56**, 334–45.

Schulz, J. B. & Dichgans, J. (1999). Molecular pathogenesis of movement disorders: are protein aggregates a common link in neuronal degeneration? *Curr. Opin. Neurol.*, **12**, 433–9.

Schulz, J. B., Matthews, R. T., Jenkins, B. G., Brar, P. & Beal, M. F. (1995a). Improved therapeutic window for treatment of histotoxic hypoxia with a free radical spin trap. *J. Cereb. Blood Flow Metab.*, **15**, 948–52.

Schulz, J. B., Henshaw, D. R., Siwek, D. *et al.* (1995b). Involvement of free radicals in excitotoxicity in vivo. *J. Neurochem.*, **64**, 2239–47.

Schurr, A., West, C. A. & Rigor, B. M. (1988). Lactate-supported synaptic function in the rat hippocampal slice preparation. *Science*, **240**, 1326–8.

Serles, W., Li, L. M., Antel, S. B. *et al.* (2001). Time course of postoperative recovery of *N*-acetyl-aspartate in temporal lobe epilepsy. *Epilepsia.*, **42**, 190–7.

Shonk, T. K., Moats, R. A., Gifford, P. *et al.* (1995). Probable Alzheimer disease: diagnosis with proton MR spectroscopy [see comments]. *Radiology*, **195**, 65–72.

Sibson, N. R., Dhankhar, A., Mason, G. F., Behar, K. L., Rothman, D. L. & Shulman, R. G. (1997). In vivo 13C NMR measurements of cerebral glutamine synthesis as evidence for glutamate-glutamine cycling. *Proc. Natl Acad. Sci., USA*, **94**, 2699–704.

Siesjo, B. K. (1992). Pathophysiology and treatment of focal cerebral ischemia. Part II: Mechanisms of damage and treatment. *J. Neurosurg.*, **77**, 337–54.

Signoretti, S., Marmarou, A., Fatouros, P. *et al.* (2002). Application of chemical shift imaging for measurement of NAA in head injured patients. *Acta. Neurochir. Suppl.*, **81**, 373–5.

Simmons, M., Frandoza, C. & Coyle, J. (1991). Immunocytochemical localization of *N*-acetyl-aspartate with monoclonal antibodies. *Neuroscience*, **45**, 37–45.

Smith, J. K., Castillo, M. & Kwock, L. (2003). MR spectroscopy of brain tumors. *Magn. Reson. Imaging Clin. N. Am.*, **11**, 415–29, v–vi.

Sotak, C. H. & Alger, J. R. (1991). A pitfall associated with lactate detection using stimulated-echo proton spectroscopy. *Magn. Reson. Med.*, **17**, 533–8.

Storey, E., Hyman, B., Jenkins, B. *et al.* (1992). MPP$^+$ produces excitotoxic lesions in rat striatum due to impairment of oxidative metabolism. *J. Neurochem.*, **58**, 1271–8.

Tanabe, J. L., Vermathen, M., Miller, R., Gelinas, D., Weiner, M. W. & Rooney, W. D. (1998). Reduced MTR in the corticospinal tract and normal T2 in amyotrophic lateral sclerosis. *Magn. Reson. Imaging*, **16**, 1163–9.

Taylor, D. L., Davies, S. E., Obrenovitch, T. P. *et al.* (1995). Investigation into the role of *N*-acetylaspartate in cerebral osmoregulation. *J. Neurochem.*, **65**, 275–81.

Terao, S., Sobue, G., Yasuda, T., Kachi, T., Takahashi, M. & Mitsuma, T. (1995). Magnetic resonance imaging of the corticospinal tracts in amyotrophic lateral sclerosis. *J. Neurol. Sci.*, **133**, 66–72.

Thulborn, K. R., Gindin, T. S., Davis, D. & Erb, P. (1999). Comprehensive MR imaging protocol for stroke management: tissue sodium concentration as a measure of tissue viability in non-human primate studies and in clinical studies. *Radiology*, **213**, 156–66.

Thurston, J. H., Sherman, W. R., Hauhart, R. E. & Kloepper, R. F. (1989). Myo-inositol: a newly identified nonnitrogenous osmoregulatory molecule in mammalian brain. *Pediatr. Res.*, **26**, 482–5.

Tkac, I., Andersen, P., Adriany, G., Merkle, H., Ugurbil, K. & Gruetter, R. (2001). In vivo 1H NMR spectroscopy of the human brain at 7 T. *Magn. Reson. Med.*, **46**, 451–6.

Urenjak, J., Williams, S. R., Gadian, D. G. & Noble, M. (1992). Specific expression of *N*-acetylaspartate in neurons, oligodendrocyte-type-2 astrocyte progenitors, and immature oligodendrocytes in vitro. *J. Neurochem.*, **59**, 55–61.

Urenjak, J., Williams, S. R., Gadian, D. G. & Noble, M. (1993). Proton nuclear magnetic resonance spectroscopy unambiguously identifies different neural cell types. *J. Neurosci.*, **13**, 981–9.

Van Zijl, P. C., Davis, D., Eleff, S. M., Moonen, C. T., Parker, R. J. & Strong, J. M. (1997). Determination of cerebral glucose transport and metabolic kinetics by dynamic MR spectroscopy. *Am. J. Physiol.*, **273**, E1216–27.

Part III

Therapeutic approaches in neurodegeneration

22

Gene therapy

Chamsy Sarkis and Jacques Mallet

Laboratoire de Génétique Moléculaire de la Neurotransmission et des Processus, Neurodégénératifs (LGN) – Centre National de la Recherche Scientifique UMR 7091, Hôpital Pitié-Salpétrière (Bâtiment CERVI), Paris, France

In the past 20 years, the development of molecular biology and genetic engineering has led to new horizons in therapy. Introducing therapeutic nucleic sequences into the organism for curing a disease is a very attractive approach for treating both inherited and acquired diseases for which classical drug therapy is not satisfactory. Although the idea is simple, many hurdles have to be overcome before clinical applications can be envisaged. The transfer vector and the therapeutic gene are the major determinants for successful therapy. An ideal vector would be easy to produce, and safe for the patient and the environment. Ideally, it must transduce only the target cells and do so efficiently. It should be possible to readminister the vector to the patients without triggering a deleterious immune reaction from the host, and the transgene has to be expressed at an appropriate level for the desired duration. The optimal characteristics of the gene depend on the disease. For a recessive monogenic disease, a wild-type allele of the mutated gene is generally required. For a dominant monogenic disease, sequences that inhibit the expression of the mutated allele, or that counter its physiological effect may be used. For many complex diseases, whether inherited or acquired, there are several potentially therapeutic genes. A therapeutic gene must be effective, but have minimal side effects. In particular, it should not lead to an immune response from the host organism, and this can be a major problem for recessive monogenic diseases, where the patient had never been in contact with the wild-type gene product.

In this chapter, we will address the development of the viral vectors most widely used for gene transfer into the nervous system. The principles of vector production will be described, with the advantages and limitations of the various vectors, with particular attention to gene transfer to the nervous system. We will also describe preclinical studies of gene transfer for treating two model diseases affecting the central nervous system (CNS): Parkinson's disease, a pro-gressive neurodegeneration of a restricted area in the brain; and mucopolysaccharidosis type VII (MPS VII), a global enzymatic deficiency affecting all cells in the CNS.

Delivery vectors for gene transfer into the nervous system

The particular constraints on gene transfer into the nervous system have hampered its development. The complexity of the nervous system itself has been a psychological barrier inhibiting research in this field. There has also been a shortage of vectors for efficient transduction of quiescent cells, particularly neural cells. The first vectors were derived from the murine leukaemia virus (MLV) and they were unable to transduce non-dividing cells such as neurones. Vectors were then developed from a naturally neurotropic virus, the herpes simplex virus (HSV), but the complexity of its genome initially prevented the development of a transfer vector. A breakthrough came in 1993 with the idea of using a vector derived from a virus, adenovirus, that did not generally infect neural cells naturally, and the proof of principle of transferring genetic material in the CNS in this way (Le Gal La Salle *et al.*, 1993). Since then, HSV and adenovirus-derived vectors have been improved repeatedly and many other vectors have been developed, including the widely used adeno-associated-virus (AAV) and lentivirus. Another factor that limited the development of gene therapy for the nervous system was the high complexity of neurological affections, such as neurodegenerative diseases and trauma. Recent advances in the understanding of the pathophysiological mechanisms underlying these diseases have led to the identification of several endogenous factors that could be of therapeutic value. They include neurotrophic factors, enzymes involved in the clearing of free radicals and enzymes involved in the regulation of cell death or apoptosis. Many of these factors have now been shown to protect neurones from decay or death and could be used as the basis for protective therapies.

There are various specific features that make gene therapy of CNS attractive. First, the CNS is isolated from the peripherial organs by physical barriers: a dense endothelial microvascular network known as the brain–blood barrier (BBB), the arachnoid epithelial membrane covering the surface of the brain, and the choroid plexus epithelium, which forms the blood–cerebrospinal fluid (CSF) barrier. These barriers block the entry of external factors including viruses and prevent the use of most vectors via the vascular route, unless special strategies are used involving penetrating or permeabilising them, or using retrograde transport of the vector. Nevertheless, this barrier confers a privileged immunological status on the CNS, helping prevent any immune reaction against either the vector or the therapeutic product of the transgene (Lowenstein, 2002). These barriers may also prevent side effects of the vector or the gene product in peripheral organs. A second advantage of the CNS for gene therapy is that many therapeutic products with potential clinical effects are diffusible and thus may be secreted from non-neuronal cells, such as astrocytes, and nevertheless act to prevent the pathological alteration of neuronal homeostasis and functions. The therapeutic molecules (or the vector) can also be captured by neurone terminals and transported to the neuronal soma by axonal retrograde transport. A third advantage is that the CNS is totally bathed in the cerebrospinal fluid (CSF) that can be used to deliver the vector or the gene product widely across the CNS. This can be done by intraventricular, intrathecal or intracisternal injection of the vector. Finally, the nervous system is structured and organized into many nuclei and layers that can be specifically targeted by locally, stereotactically, injecting the vector. Moreover, many neurological diseases affect a restricted area of the brain, such as the substantia nigra or the striatum, and such structures are relatively easy to target as compared to muscles and the intestine, for example. With all these characteristics, the nervous system is an organ particularly suited to experimental gene transfer.

Two approaches have been used to deliver genes to the nervous system. The first, called direct or in vivo gene delivery is the injection of the vector and thus the gene directly into the target organ. Although synthetic delivery systems may be appealing, the most efficient vectors currently available for this strategy are derived from viruses. The second approach is indirect or ex vivo gene delivery: the transplantation of genetically modified cells into the nervous system. These cells may be transplanted directly or may be encapsulated. The genetic

modification is performed using the same vectors as for in vivo delivery. In this chapter we will describe only the first delivery mode. Transplantation strategies are dealt with elsewhere.

Adenovirus derived vectors

Adenoviruses have a broad tropism, meaning that they can infect many species and cell types. They can infect both dividing and quiescent cells making them particularly useful for gene transfer to the nervous system. In 1993 we showed that adenovirus-derived vectors can transduce all cell types in the CNS after direct injection into the brain or the ventricles (Le Gal La Salle et al., 1993). More than 100 adenoviruses have now been described, and about 50 different human serotypes have been found. They all contain a linear double-stranded DNA genome (30 to 38 kb long) encapsidated in an icosahedral protein shell measuring 60 to 100 nm in diameter. They enter cells via endocytosis following interaction with two distinct receptors. First, the protein fiber of the capsid interacts with CAR (coxsakievirus and adenovirus receptor), a cellular receptor (Bergelson et al., 1997). Then, the base of the penton interacts with the cellular αv integrins (Wickham et al., 1993). Two hours later, the DNA is transported to the nucleus and the first expression round starts with the immediate early genes (E1 to E4). The immediate early gene E1A is the first transcription unit to be expressed and it trans-activates a cascade of expression of other viral and cellular transcription units. The E1B products react with E1A products and transform the infected cell. E2 codes for proteins involved in viral replication, E3 products contribute to the inflammatory response by preventing the infected cells from being recognized by the host immune system and E4 products participate in viral DNA replication and the activation of late structural genes.

The first adenovirus-derived vectors were produced by deletion of the E1 region to prevent viral replication. A transcomplementing cell line (HEK 293 cells) was obtained by transforming embryonic human kidney cells with the E1 region of the Ad5 (Graham et al., 1977). Recombinant adenovirus vectors are obtained by homologous recombination between a shuttle plasmid (containing the gene of interest) and the ΔE1 adenoviral genome in HEK 293 cells. A recombinant genome in which the E1 region is replaced by the transgene is thereby obtained and can be propagated in HEK 293 cells. Clonal lysis plaques are selected, purified, analyzed and amplified in HEK 293 cells. This method of production is tedious and time consuming. Improved production techniques, avoiding lysis plaque selection have been developed based on homologous recombination in yeast using YAC (Ketner *et al.*, 1994) or in *E. coli* (Chartier *et al.*, 1996; Crouzet *et al.*, 1997).

All these methods present a major inconvenience as they allow the production of replication competent adenovirus (RCA), due to the possible reinsertion of the E1 region of the HEK 293 cell into the vector genome during the amplification step. New transcomplementation cell lines have been produced by transformation with an E1 region that has no homology with the vector genome (Fallaux *et al.*, 1996, 1998). Nevertheless, all these first-generation ΔE1 vectors present several other limitations. First, their cloning capacity is limited to 7–8 kb as the total vector genome cannot exceed 105% of the wild type genome length. The E3 region was deleted to increase the cloning capacity, but this resulted in higher immune reaction from the host. Second, the direct injection of these vectors induces a local inflammation dependent on the dose because of a residual expression of viral genes, despite the E1 region being deleted. The expression of the viral genes induces cytotoxicity and specific cellular and humoral immune reactions, the consequence of which is the death of the transduced cells and therefore only short-term expression of the transgene.

Thus, second-generation adenovirus vectors were produced by introducing a thermosensitive mutation in the E2A gene. These vectors gave a smaller inflammatory reaction and greater transgene persistence, but the thermosensitive mutation was reversible and the improved efficacy did not seem to be consistently obtained (Fang *et al.*, 1996).

Third-generation adenovirus vectors were developed by deleting other regions of the viral genome: the E1 region, the E4 region and the E3 region. New transcomplementation cell lines derived from 293 and expressing a minimal E4 unit are used for their production. Although these vectors give reduced cytotoxicity and improved transgene stability, the persistence of transgene expression is not improved in all cases, production remains tedious and the generation of RCA is still possible.

The latest generation of adenovirus-derived vectors are called *helper-dependent* or *gutless* vectors. They are devoid of all viral coding sequences. They were first designed in 1995 (Mitani *et al.*, 1995), and several more or less complex systems of production have been developed since (Fisher *et al.*, 1996; Hardy *et al.*, 1997; Hillgenberg *et al.*, 2001; Kochanek *et al.*, 1996; Ng *et al.*, 2001). The process is based on the utilization of a helper virus providing in *trans* all the functions needed for production and amplification of defective recombinant vectors. The main difficulty is eliminating the helper virus from recombinant stocks. Currently, the best method consists in preventing encapsidation of helper genome by inducible recombination of the encapsidation signal (Ψ region) using Cre/Lox or FLP/FRT

systems. Although production is still laborious, the cytotoxicity of these vectors is much lower than that of earlier generation vectors. Inflammatory and immune responses in the host are lower, resulting in sustained high-level expression in many organs, including the brain (Thomas *et al.*, 2000; Zou *et al.*, 2000, 2001). Nevertheless, they retain a transient capsid-mediated inflammatory response (Thomas *et al.*, 2001). These latest vectors can be produced devoid of RCA and have an increased cloning capacity (up to 37 kb). The production process for this latest generation of adenoviral vectors will have to be scaled-up at low cost before clinical application can become routine.

The efficacy of adenovirus delivery to patients might be hampered because most people have been exposed to natural adenovirus infection. Classical vectors are derived from Ad2 and Ad5, for which most people have neutralizing antibodies. Several strategies have been proposed to overcome this problem. The simplest is to reduce the dose, as it has been shown that direct cellular toxicity increases linearly with vector dose (Thomas *et al.*, 2001). Another strategy consists of using adenoviral vectors derived from non-human serotypes or from rare serotypes in humans, or by using chimeric adenoviruses containing an ectopic fibre derived from rare serotype. Alternatively, the surface of vector particles could be coated with polymers such as PEG (Croyle *et al.*, 2002) or pHPMA (Fisher *et al.*, 2001). The use of different serotypes and the coating process also allow the repeated administration, an important factor for clinical applications.

Another important feature is the targeting of the vector to transduce specific cell types. Adenoviral vectors efficiently transduce most of the cells in the nervous system (Akli *et al.*, 1993; Bajocchi *et al.*, 1993; Davidson *et al.*, 1993; Le Gal La Salle *et al.*, 1993). Some serotypes are more efficient in certain cells and could thus be used to obtain relative specificity. For example, type D adenovirus (Ad17), and chimeric type C adenovirus (Ad2) containing a type D fiber, are more efficient for the infection of primary neurones (Chillon *et al.*, 1999). The re-routing of adenoviral vectors is also feasible by incorporating a ligand in the fiber (Krasnykh *et al.*, 2001; Magnusson *et al.*, 2001; Sosnowski *et al.*, 1999) or in a polymer used to coat the viral particles, thus combining both immune reaction prevention and specificity of interaction with a membrane receptor of the target cell (Fisher *et al.*, 2001). It is also possible to use a molecular adaptor (bi-allelic antibody) to create a specific interaction between the viral particle and the target cell (Goldman *et al.*, 1997; Wickham *et al.*, 1997). These techniques should permit very specific targeting of the vector, but they also make production more complex. Thus, it might be preferable to use the simpler approach of restricting the expression of the transgene instead of restricting the entry of the particle. Transcriptional targeting can be obtained by using cellular or chimeric promoters specifically active in a certain type or subtype of cells of the nervous system (Hashimoto *et al.*, 1996; Kugler *et al.*, 2001; Lee *et al.*, 2000; Millecamps *et al.*, 1999; Navarro *et al.*, 1999; Robert *et al.*, 1997).

Another specific feature of adenovirus-derived vectors for gene transfer into the nervous system is that they can be transported via the axonal transport system of neurones. Thus, inoculation of the muscle with a vector targets the innervating motor neurones and sensory neurones (Finiels *et al.*, 1995; Ghadge *et al.*, 1995). Similarly, intranasal inoculation targets olfactory neurones (Zhao *et al.*, 1996) and administration may be possible in the area of projection of neurones for which the cell bodies are difficult or hazardous to reach in humans. An example is the dopaminergic neurones in the substantia nigra which can be accessed by injecting the vectors into the striatum (Kuo *et al.*, 1995). The efficacy of retrograde uptake of the vector particles is dependent on the synaptic sprouting of the innervating terminals and it can be enhanced by using botulinum toxin (Millecamps *et al.*, 2001, 2002). Another alternative route of inoculation of adenovirus-derived vectors is injection into the CSF, which leads to the transduction of meninges cells and vascular cells (Christenson *et al.*, 1998), ependymal cells (Ghodsi *et al.*, 1998) and motor neurones (Mannes *et al.*, 1998). Systemic hyperosmolality can be induced by mannitol before inoculation of the vector into the CSF (Ghodsi *et al.*, 1999) to enhance the spreading of the virus in the parenchyma.

In summary, the latest generations of adenoviral vectors are thus particularly promising for long-term gene transfer into both the CNS and the PNS for treating chronic diseases.

Herpes simplex virus (HSV)-derived vectors

The herpes simplex virus 1 has features making it attractive as the basis for gene therapy vectors, especially for applications in the nervous system. It is large and has a broad host range, high infectivity, and ability to infect quiescent cells. Most of all, it has a natural tropism for the CNS and PNS neuronal cells and can be transported retrogradely through axons. Moreover, it has a latent phase of its life cycle in neurones, which might be exploited for long-term expression of transgenes in these cells. The genome of this enveloped virus is 160 kb and has been sequenced. Following wild-type HSV primary cutaneous or mucosal inoculation, the virus replicates. Its replication is controlled by regulated temporal expression of its genes. The cycle starts with the transcription of five immediate early genes (ICP0, ICP4, ICP22, ICP27 and ICP47), which initiate a cascade of transcription of the early and late genes. From the primary infection site, the virus may enter sensory neurones. The nucleocapsid and tegument are carried by retrograde axonal transport to the neuronal soma in the dorsal root ganglia or trigeminal ganglia where the viral genome enters the nucleus. At this point, lytic replication may occur. Alternatively, the virus can become latent and its genome persists as a stable episomal element, potentially for many years. During latency only the latency-associated transcripts (LATs) are expressed.

Two types of vectors can be obtained from this virus. First, recombinant HSV vectors deficient for replication can be constructed by the deletion of one or several immediate early genes and non-essential genes from wild-type HSV to prevent lytic viral replication. The production process is very similar to that of adenovirus-derived vectors. A transcomplementation cell line stably expressing the deleted immediate early genes is co-transfected with the deleted viral plasmid and a shuttle plasmid containing the transgene expression cassette flanked with viral sequences. An important advantage of these vectors is the cloning capacity, which is as high as 50 kb. When homologous recombination occurs, a recombinant defective HSV vector is obtained and packaged in empty virions. The next step consists of purification of vector stocks, as both deleted viral genome and recombinant vector are present. This requires selection of lysis plaques and further amplification on transcomplementation cells.

A major problem encountered with these vectors is their toxicity due to residual expression of viral genes. The toxicity can be greatly diminished by deletion of ICP0, ICP4, ICP22 and ICP47 (Samaniego *et al.*, 1998). Unfortunately, in the absence of ICP0, the vectors grow poorly and the transgene expression is low in most cells (Samaniego *et al.*, 1997). However, it seems that ICP0 retention is not deleterious in neurones, which simplifies the design and production of the vectors for many neurological gene therapy applications. Another important issue is the level and stability of the transgene expression in transduced cells. In many cases, expression is downregulated when ectopic promoters are used. As the latency potential of the HSV is potentially useful for sustained expression of the vector, latency promoters have been exploited to drive long-term expression of a transgene in neurones in vivo. Promoter elements of the LATs can be used at ectopic positions in the vector genome, combined with other strong viral immediate–early promoters or used in their original position by replacing a latency gene with the transgene. These approaches have been successfully used to obtain long-term expression of transgenes in the PNS motor and sensory neurones (Goins *et al.*, 1994, 1999; Lachmann & Efstathiou, 1997; Palmer *et al.*, 2000), and in CNS neurones (Lachmann & Efstathiou, 1999; Scarpini *et al.*, 2001; Smith *et al.*, 2000).

The second type of vectors that can be obtained from HSV are called amplicons and were first generated by the transfection of an amplicon plasmid (containing the transgene expression cassette, the origin of replication of HSV (Ori$_s$) and a Ψ encapsidation signal), and the co-infection with an HSV helper virus (Geller & Breakefield, 1988). The amplicon plasmid replicates in a *rolling circle* mode forming a concatemer of about 150 kb containing several copies of the transgene (Leib & Olivo, 1993). Thus, amplicons can have a genome length up to 150 kb. However, the production technique for these forms gives stocks that are rich in wild-type helper virus, and thus are not adequate for safe gene transfer because of their toxicity. In 1996, Fraefel *et al.* proposed a method for producing amplicon stocks devoid of helper virus. The genome of HSV-1 has been deleted of the encapsidation signal and subcloned in several cosmids. The co-transfection of the cosmids and the amplicon plasmid give rise to amplicon vector stocks uncontaminated with helper virus (Fraefel *et al.*, 1996). Several teams have subsequently improved this method by using a bacterial artificial chromosome instead of cosmids (Saeki *et al.*, 1998; Stavropoulos & Strathdee, 1998). Recently, Logvinoff *et al.* designed a new process to ensure production of high titre stocks of helper-free amplicon vectors with a Cre/LoxP system excising the Ψ encapsidation signal from a helper virus (Logvinoff & Epstein, 2001). However, all these methods are limited by the fact that amplicon vectors cannot be amplified directly in a transcomplementation cell line.

Like adenoviruses, HSV vectors may be limited for use in human clinical applications because of the existence of wild-type virus in most patients. The injection of a HSV vector might reactivate endogenous virus, potentially causing encephalitis. Nevertheless, no reactivation was observed in two murine models of latent infection of HSV after intracerebral injection of HSV vectors (Wang *et al.*, 1997), or after intratumoral administration of HSV vectors in nine patients treated for gliomas in a gene therapy trial (Rampling *et al.*, 2000). Although pre-existing antibodies do not seem to impair HSV vector efficacy in murine models (Brockman & Knipe, 2002; Delman *et al.*, 2000), repeated administration of the vector might be problematic. To overcome this problem, HSV vectors have been delivered through liposome formulation, but efficiency was lower than that of non-formulated vectors (Fu & Zhang, 2001).

HSV vectors are able to infect many kinds of different cells, particularly in the nervous system. Virus entry depends on the interactions of its numerous glycoproteins with cellular receptors which are still poorly characterised. Various strategies have been considered for modifying the tropism of the vectors. Engineered virions in which the viral gC glycoprotein is replaced by a gC-erythropoietin (EPO) fusion protein, and the viral gB partially deleted, have acquired specific binding properties to the EPO receptor (Laquerre *et al.*, 1998). An alternative strategy used consisted in pseudotyping the vectors with an ectopic glycoprotein (VSV-G) and deleting the gB or gD from the vector (Anderson *et al.*, 2000).

Applications in the nervous system for HSV-derived vectors are very similar to those for adenoviruses. Their ability to carry large DNA fragments and to be transported via the axonal retrograde pathway and their latency properties make them potentially valuable for chronic neurological diseases, particularly of the PNS. However, their toxicity must be reduced and their production facilitated for clinical applications.

Adeno-associated virus (AAV) derived vectors

The adeno-associated virus (AAV) is a dependovirus of the *Parvoviridae* family. It is one of the smallest and simplest of eucaryotic viruses. It is unique in the world of animal viruses in that it needs the co-infection with a helper virus (adenovirus or herpesvirus) for a productive cycle of infection (Atchison *et al.*, 1965; Buller *et al.*, 1981). This non-enveloped virus has an icosahedral structure of about 20 nm in diameter constituted only of proteins and DNA. Three proteins (VP1, VP2 and VP3) form a very stable capsid, resistant to pH inactivation, solvents and high temperatures (up to 50 °C). In the absence of helper virus, the AAV integrates specifically into a particular locus in humans (19q13.3-qter) (Kotin *et al.*, 1990). Its genome is a linear single-strand non-segmented DNA of 4.7 kb. Two terminal sequences (ITR) flank its two genes: *rep*, coding for the proteins controlling viral replication and integration into the host genome, and *cap* coding for the structural proteins. The wild-type AAV is not pathogenic for humans and is able to infect both dividing and quiescent cells making it particularly suitable for the development of transfer vectors for neurological applications.

The first method for producing AAV-derived vectors involved the co-transfection of a plasmid expressing *cap* and *rep* and a plasmid containing the transgene expression cassette flanked with the ITRs in cells infected with an adenovirus. After virus production, the adenovirus is heat-inactivated and the AAV vectors are purified on a CsCl gradient. This method gives only low-titre stocks and helper adenovirus contamination is frequent. Purification has been improved by using HPLC (Drittanti *et al.*, 2001) or column purification (Auricchio *et al.*, 2001) to avoid contamination with helper virus. Several teams expressed *rep* and *cap* stably in transcomplementation cell lines and/or subcloned the AAV vector genome in a shuttle vector (adenovirus or baculovirus) to bypass the unreliable transfection step (Liu *et al.*, 1999; Sollerbrant *et al.*, 2001). The best approach however for preventing contamination with helper virus and by obtaining high titers stocks is to isolate the necessary adenoviral genes on a plasmid and to co-transfect this plasmid with the AAV vector plasmid and the *cap/rep* plasmid (Matsushita *et al.*, 1998; Xiao *et al.*, 1998). This protocol has been further improved by reducing the number of plasmids to two (Collaco *et al.*, 1999). AAV vectors are reliably and efficiently produced and purified in an increasing number of laboratories, making it one of the most popular vectors for in vivo applications. Indeed, with high titre stocks devoid of helper adenovirus, AAV vectors are very effective for the transduction of many cell types including neural cells. They drive stable and strong expression of the transgene with a very low toxicity and immune/inflammatory reaction (Chamberlin *et al.*, 1998; McCown *et al.*, 1996; Okada *et al.*, 2002; Peel & Klein, 2000). Another advantage of AAV vectors is their great stability, which allows the lyophilisation of stocks, which is useful for clinical applications (Croyle *et al.*, 2001). Finally, the harmlessness of wild-type AAV in humans makes it particularly suited for human applications.

However, AAV vectors have several drawbacks. First, their cloning capacity is very limited (about 4.5 kb), such that the use of several genes or long transgenes (for example a long cDNA or a long segment of a cellular promoter) cannot be used in AAV vectors. Some have bypassed the problem by using mini-genes (Wang *et al.*, 2000), or reconstituting a protein from different subunits expressed from several vectors (Burton *et al.*, 1999). A more generally applicable approach is to exploit the in vivo concatemerization of AAV genomes before their integration (episomal AAV genomes persist in a variety of molecular forms including concatemers (Duan *et al.*, 1999; Nakai *et al.*, 1999)). By splitting an expression cassette between two vectors, a functional cassette can be reconstituted after concatemerization in the cell nucleus (Duan *et al.*, 2001; Nakai *et al.*, 2000; Yan *et al.*, 2000).

Another issue for AAV vectors is their integration property. Although wild-type AAVs integrate into a specific locus due to the rep proteins, the recombinant vector integrates more or less randomly and the integration ratio depends on the cell type and cell cycle stage (Alexander *et al.*, 1994; Podsakoff *et al.*, 1994; Ponnazhagan *et al.*, 1997; Rutledge & Russell, 1997; Wu *et al.*, 1998). Integration of the vector

genome into the host genome may cause an insertional mutagenesis that could be tumorogenic. Moreover, recombinant AAV genome integration preferentially occurs in active genes and is usually associated with chromosomal rearrangements including deletions and translocations (Miller *et al.*, 2002; Nakai *et al.*, 2003). To make AAV vectors safer, several teams are developing new vectors which specifically integrate into the human chromosome 19 locus, using various approaches including chimeric vectors (Kogure *et al.*, 2001; Palombo *et al.*, 1998; Recchia *et al.*, 1999; Rinaudo *et al.*, 2000; Rizzuto *et al.*, 1999; Satoh *et al.*, 2000; Tsunoda *et al.*, 2000; Ueno *et al.*, 2000).

Another hurdle is the pre-existing immunity in the population. The immune reaction to AAV2 is very variable between individuals. Although anti-AAV2 immunoglobulins are common, most are not neutralizing antibodies (Chirmule *et al.*, 1999). The repeated administration of AAV vectors may be problematic, but switching capsid serotypes (Halbert *et al.*, 2000) or using vectors derived from nonhuman parvoviruses may avoid the potential impediments (Gao *et al.*, 2002).

The tropism of AAV vectors can be targeted by modification of the capsid. Not all serotypes have the same efficacy for a given cell type. For example, vectors derived from AAV4 and AAV5 are more efficient than AAV2-derived vectors for the transduction of ependymal cells after intraventricular injection. When injected into the striatal parenchyma of rodents, AAV4 has a selective tropism for ependymal cells, whereas AAV2 seems to transduce mainly parenchymal neurones and AAV5 transduces both neurones and astrocytes (Davidson *et al.*, 2000). Some serotypes diffuse more than others into the brain parenchyma (Mastakov *et al.*, 2002). Nevertheless, as for adenoviruses, diffusion can be enhanced by mannitol injection (Mastakov *et al.*, 2001), heparin co-infusion (Mastakov *et al.*, 2002) or by the use of *convection enhanced delivery* (Bankiewicz *et al.*, 2000; Nguyen *et al.*, 2001). Targeting can also be achieved by modifying the capsid with a ligand (Girod *et al.*, 1999; Grifman *et al.*, 2001; Nicklin *et al.*, 2001) or with a bispecific antibody (Bartlett *et al.*, 1999). The use of tissue-specific regulatory sequences (cellular promoters or chimeric promoters) can also direct expression to a given cell type or subtype (Peel & Klein, 2000). Unlike adenovirus and HSV-derived vectors, AAV-derived vectors are not transported retrogradely through axons. However, they can be administered via the CSF route to efficiently transduce neural cells (Elliger *et al.*, 1999).

All these properties give AAV-derived vectors great potential for chronic neurological affections although they cannot be used easily for applications needing a large transgene. The increasing number of gene therapy clinical trials for various diseases reflects the potential of these vectors.

Retrovirus derived vectors

The retrovirus family is divided into seven genders of which two have been extensively used for gene transfer purposes: mammal type C retroviruses (such as the murine leukaemia virus, MLV) and lentiviruses (such as the human immunodeficiency virus, HIV). Retroviruses are enveloped particles of about 100nm in diameter presenting an internal conical core (capsid) protecting a genome of two molecules of RNA. The viral replication cycle involves the adsorption of the virions through specific receptor and fusion to the cell membrane, reverse transcription leading to the formation of a linear double stranded DNA (provirus) and integration of the provirus into the host genome. Two viral RNA molecules are packaged into an assembled capsid and the virion buds from the cell membrane which expresses the envelope protein at its surface. The RNA (+) genome of retroviruses is about 7–12 kb long, and is composed of two long terminal repeats (LTRs) flanking three coding genes and several *cis* acting elements involved in the genome replication, transportation and encapsidation. The *gag* gene codes for the matrix, the capsid and the nucleocapsid proteins. The *pol* gene codes for two enzymes necessary for the viral replication cycle: the retrotranscriptase and the integrase. The *env* gene codes for the glycoprotein present at the surface of the virions (envelope). A Ψ encapsidation signal ensures the specific packaging of the retroviral RNAs into the capsid. Some of the complex retroviruses such as lentiviruses contain additional accessory genes (for example, Vpr, Vif, Nef) important for viral infectivity and pathogenicity. They also contain regulatory proteins such as Tat and Rev, governing the expression of the viral gene at both transcriptional and post-transcriptional levels. The LTRs have many important functions involved in retrotranscription, integration and replication.

Retroviruses have potentially valuable properties for gene transfer. They are relatively easy to manipulate and they integrate stably into the host genome. The first retroviral vectors were derived from MLV, by a relatively simple method. A proviral genome is subcloned into a plasmid and the *gag*, *pol* and *env* genes are replaced by the transgene. Recombinant retroviral particles are obtained by co-transfection of this plasmid with a transcomplementing plasmid encoding all the structural proteins. To facilitate production, encapsidation cell lines have been generated by stable transformation of cells with *gag*, *pol* and *env* genes. To prevent the risk of creating replication competent retroviral vectors, the three genes can be introduced at different loci into the transcomplementation cell's genome (Bosselman *et al.*, 1987; Cosset *et al.*, 1995; Danos & Mulligan, 1988; Miller *et al.*, 1991).

MLV-derived vectors cannot be used for most neurological applications because they are unable to cross the nuclear membrane to integrate, preventing them from transducing non-dividing cells in which the nuclear membrane is complete. However, lentiviruses can transduce quiescent cells including neurones, and thus have potential for developing transfer vectors. The development of efficient lentiviral vectors has been delayed by production problems. The first HIV1-derived vectors were generated in exactly the same way as MLV vectors, but the titers were low (Page *et al.*, 1990; Poznansky *et al.*, 1991; Richardson *et al.*, 1995). Replacing the HIV *env* gene with a VSV-G envelope, i.e. by pseudotyping the vector, was a substantial step forward. The VSV envelope is resistant to ultracentrifugation, allowing concentration of the virions to high titers (Akkina *et al.*, 1996; Naldini *et al.*, 1996a,b). It is also able to attach to the majority of the mammal cells, broadening the tropism of the vectors. Such vectors have proved very efficient for transducing many tissues, but are particularly efficient for the CNS.

Because of the high risk inherent to wild-type lentiviruses, the bio-safety of lentivirus-derived vectors has been optimized. Many non-human lentiviral vectors have been engineered from the simian SIV (Nakajima *et al.*, 2000), feline FIV (Poeschla *et al.*, 1998), equine EIAV (Mitrophanous *et al.*, 1999), bovine BIV (Berkowitz *et al.*, 2001), or ovin Visna virus (Berkowitz *et al.*, 2001) for this reason. However, it is still unclear whether non-primate lentiviruses are safer than primate lentivirus-derived vectors. The main risk is possible interactions between the vector and endogenous retrovirus in the patient leading to rescue of a vector RNA by wild-type virions. A vector RNA molecule and a wild-type RNA molecule could be recruited into the same particle, enhancing the risk of recombination and the generation of novel viruses. It has been shown that FIV RNA could be rescued by HIV viruses (Browning *et al.*, 2001) and the risk might be greater if HIV-derived vectors are used to transduce wild-type-HIV-infected cells. However, thanks to knowledge of MLV vectors, the development of lentiviral vectors has been extremely fast, and researchers have focused particularly on safety issues. In the latest production systems for HIV vectors, using transient transfections, the *trans* functions are supplied by three or four separate plasmids to reduce the risk of formation of replication competent vectors. Moreover, four accessory genes have been deleted from the packaging plasmids with no effect on transduction efficacy (Zufferey *et al.*, 1997), and several packaging cell lines have been generated to facilitate production (Dull *et al.*, 1998; Kafri *et al.*, 1998, 1999; Xu *et al.*, 2001). Thus, with the latest generation of vectors, it is theoretically impossible to form wild-type lentivirus during the production process, because this would require at least three recombination events, and because some of the accessory genes, important for the pathogenocity of lentiviruses, are missing from the packaging plasmids. Nevertheless, it is also important to optimize the design of the vector genome, carrying the transgene between the LTRs, in terms of safety as well as efficiency. The basic vector genome comprises the LTRs flanking the packaging sequences, an intron, the RRE sequence (rev responsive element, important for the export of the RNA) and the expression cassette. Because LTRs contain enhancer and promoter functions that may possibly activate cellular genes or disturb the activity of the internal expression cassette, vectors with a deletion in the U3 regulatory region of the LTRs have been developed, and show improved expression in the brain (Iwakuma *et al.*, 1999; Miyoshi *et al.*, 1998; Zufferey *et al.*, 1998). Also, excisable lentivirus could be developed with a Cre/LoxP system (Salmon *et al.*, 2000). Using an inducible recombinase system, the deletion of the Ψ encapsidation signal could prevent the rescue of vector RNA molecules by endogenous retroviruses. Although such systems might be efficient in vitro, their use in vivo may be limited by the relatively poor efficiency of the Cre recombinase.

In contrast to MLV vectors, lentiviral vectors seem to maintain long-term expression of a transgene in many tissues, and particularly in the nervous system (Blomer *et al.*, 1997; Kafri *et al.*, 1997) including the retina (Lotery *et al.*, 2002; Miyoshi *et al.*, 1997; Takahashi *et al.*, 1999). This may be due to the absence of immune/inflammatory reactions to lentiviral vectors which also allows repeated injection of the vector into the same animal (Kafri *et al.*, 1997) (C. Sarkis, personal data). Expression can be further increased by optimizing the expression cassette by using different promoters, or the *woodchuck post-transcriptional regulatory element* (WPRE), which enhances the expression of transgene by RNA processing (Brun *et al.*, 2003; Ramezani *et al.*, 2000; Zufferey *et al.*, 1999). The transduction efficacy of lentivirus is limited in most tissues by the lack of nuclear transportation functions of the provirus. The incorporation into the vector genome of the flap cis element that was previously deleted, re-established the normal level of nuclear transport of provirus genome, and thus improved the transduction efficiency by a factor of 2 to 10, including in the brain in vivo (Follenzi *et al.*, 2000; Zennou *et al.*, 2000, 2001).

The tropism of VSV pseudotyped lentiviral vectors in the brain has been reported as being mainly neuronal (Blomer *et al.*, 1997). However, in our hands it seems that the tropism depends on the promoter used for the expression of the transgene (C. Sarkis, personal data). Also, discordant results have been published concerning the retina, suggesting that VSV-HIV preferentially infects the retina pigment epithelium or the photoreceptors after subretinal injection, depending on the promoter (Auricchio *et al.*, 2001; Miyoshi *et al.*, 1997). Several factors may influence the type of cells transduced, such as the dose of vector, the preparation protocol, and the injection procedure. Like other enveloped vectors, lentiviral vectors can be pseudotyped using various envelopes, of which the lyssavirus (rabies) glycoproteins are the most interesting for neural applications (Auricchio *et al.*, 2001; Desmaris *et al.*, 2001; Mitrophanous *et al.*, 1999; Mochizuki *et al.*, 1998; Reiser, 2000). The pseudotyping of an EIAV vector with the rabies glycoprotein seems to target the transduction to neuronal cells, and to allow the retrograde transport of the vectors, which does not occur with other vectors (Mazarakis *et al.*, 2001). VSV pseudotyped lentiviral vectors do not undergo axonal transport, and it is not clear if lyssavirus glycoprotein pseudotyping can confer axonal transportation properties to non-EIAV lentiviral vectors.

Lentiviral vectors are very suitable for the transduction of neuronal cells. The lack of toxicity and the stability of expression of the transgene make them, like AAV vectors, valuable tools for chronic neurological applications. Moreover, their cloning capacity is higher than that of AAV vectors (around 7 kb). However, continued efforts are required to reduce as far as possible all risks associated with these vectors. As for all randomly integrative vectors, the risk of insertional mutagenesis exists, and must be addressed. Engineered specific integrases constructed by fusing specific binding domains to the HIV integrase (Holmes-Son *et al.*, 2001; Holmes-Son & Chow, 2000, 2002) or ectopic integrase such as the ΦC31 integrase (Olivares *et al.*, 2002) could be used.

Examples of therapeutic strategies

Gene transfer methods can be envisaged for therapy in the nervous system for both chronic and acute affections. However, the complexity of the brain, the variable and often poorly understood pathological basis of the diseases, the availability of animal models, the difficulty of targeting neural genes, the limitations of vectors and many other difficulties have impeded successful application of these techniques.

As examples, we will describe the use of gene transfer strategies on two chronic affections of the central nervous system: Parkinson's disease; and mucopolysaccharidosis type VII (MPS-VII). For both diseases, both in vivo and ex vivo strategies have been explored. We will focus on the direct transfer strategy, because another chapter is dedicated to transplantation procedures.

Parkinson's disease

PD is a neurological disorder which involves the progressive loss of dopaminergic neurones from the SN (substantia nigra), a brain structure which innervates the striatum, leading to specific motor impairment (tremor, rigidity and akinesia) sometimes associated with cognitive impairment (Poewe & Wenning, 1996). Usually, clinical symptoms do not appear until about 70% of the dopaminergic neurones have been lost (McGeer *et al.*, 1977). Standard oral administration of L-dopa (a substance that crosses the blood–brain barrier and is transformed into the neurotransmitter dopamine) can significantly improve motor function during the first years of treatment. However, as the neurodegeneration progresses, higher doses of L-dopa are required leading to deleterious side effects such as dyskinesia. L-dopa or other related drugs can prevent the apparition of symptoms (tremor, rigidity), but these drugs do not treat the cause or progress of the disease. Electrical deep brain stimulation of the subthalamic nucleus reduces dyskinesia and the amount of drugs needed for PD treatment by 50% (Benabid *et al.*, 1998; Limousin *et al.*, 1998). However, this method has drawbacks: the stimulating apparatus requires battery charging and can be perturbed by magnetic waves. Thus, a gene therapy treatment that could be administered once and work for a long period of time would be a major leap forward.

Gene therapy studies for PD have been facilitated by the availability of animal models in rats and primates. Both restorative and protective strategies have been investigated. The restorative approach consists of focal and sustained delivery of L-dopa or dopamine into the striatum. This has been done by transfer of the genes encoding the L-dopa and/or dopamine synthetic enzymes. The tyrosine hydroxylase gene, coding the enzyme that transform tyrosine to L-dopa, has been introduced into the striatum of PD animal models (Horellou *et al.*, 1994), and the system optimized by regulating the level of enzyme synthesized (Corti *et al.*, 1999) and by combining different enzymes such as AADC (transforming L-dopa into dopamine) and GCH (synthesizing BH4, the cofactor of TH) using various vectors (adenovirus, AAV, HSV and lentivirus) to obtain physiological levels of dopamine (for review see (Costantini *et al.*, 2000) and (Hsich *et al.*, 2002)). Delivery by AAV vectors of the genes coding for the three enzymes resulted

in functional recovery (reduced rotational behavior) lasting at least 12 months and elevated striatal dopamine production in the rat PD model (Shen *et al.*, 2000). Alternatively, transfer of AADC coupled with L-dopa administration could counteract the loss of AADC activity during the progression of the disease which results in increasingly high L-dopa requirements and associated side effects (Bankiewicz *et al.*, 2000). These approaches address the reduction of motor symptoms after the onset of the disease. However, a preferred solution would be to prevent the death of the dopaminergic neurones before the disease onset or to protect the remaining neurones immediately after diagnosis. This requires protective strategies.

The protective strategy offers a better prospect for the long-term treatment of the disease. Many genes have been envisaged to protect against neuronal death, including those coding for neurotrophic factors, anti-apoptotic factors or anti-oxidative enzymes. The genetic transfer of GDNF, a neurotrophic factor, has been the most studied and results in many animal models of PD are encouraging. GDNF promotes the survival and neurite outgrowth of embryonic dopaminergic (DA) neurones in vitro (Lin *et al.*, 1993). Intracerebral administration of GDNF into the substantia nigra (SN) via adenoviral gene transfer completely prevents nigral cell death and atrophy in a rat model of Parkinson's disease (Sauer *et al.*, 1995). GDNF acts on several levels. It can prevent neuronal death of dopaminergic neurones if expressed directly in the neurones of the SN. It can also prevent axonal degeneration when expressed in the projection area of the degenerating neurones (striatum), and induces sprouting, compensating for the deficit of dopaminergic neurones. Work in animal models of PD suggests that the intrastriatal delivery of the GDNF is the best strategy. The proof of principle of this strategy was obtained by intrastriatal injection of an adenoviral vector encoding the GDNF into a rat model of PD. When Ad-GDNF was injected into the same site 6 days before the 6-OHDA lesion, production of GDNF was observed at both the DA nerve terminal and nigral cell bodies following retrograde transport of the virus. Three weeks after the lesion, there were twice as many TH-immunoreactive cell bodies in the SN of the Ad-GDNF treated animals than in control animals. Furthermore, amphetamine-induced behavioral asymmetry (a behavioral marker for DA depletion) was markedly reduced in the Ad-GDNF treated rats (Bilang-Bleuel *et al.*, 1997). Recently, Kordower *et al.* injected lentiviral vector expressing GDNF (lenti-GDNF) into the striatum and substantia nigra of nonlesioned aged rhesus monkeys and young adult rhesus monkeys treated 1 week prior with 1-methyl-4-phenyl-1,2,3,6-tetrahydropyridine (MPTP)

(Kordower *et al.*, 2000). Extensive GDNF expression with anterograde and retrograde transport was observed in all animals. In aged monkeys, lenti-GDNF augmented dopaminergic function. In MPTP-treated monkeys, lenti-GDNF reversed functional deficits and completely prevented nigrostriatal degeneration. Additionally, lenti-GDNF injections to intact rhesus monkeys resulted in long-term gene expression (8 months). In MPTP-treated monkeys, lenti-GDNF treatment reversed motor deficits in a hand-reach task.

As GDNF can be secreted and subsequently captured by the neuronal terminals of the dopaminergic neurones, it does not need to be expressed inside the neurones. Astrocytic expression was compared to neuronal expression in the striatum in a rat model of PD, by injection of Ad-GDNF under the control of either a glial (GFAP) or a neuronal promoter (NSE). The Ad-GFAP-GDNF was more effective than Ad-NSE-GDNF in inducing sprouting of the innervating dopaminergic terminations and behavioral recovery (A. Do Thi, personal data). Thus, the expression of the GDNF in striatal astrocytes is preferable to expression in neurones.

Both restorative and protective approaches might be viable therapeutic strategies for PD patients. The choice of the strategy will be governed by the onset of detection of the disease.

Mucopolysaccharidosis type VII (MPS-VII)

In mammals, recessive mutations in the autosomal β-glucuronidase gene and the consequent loss of protein activity induce a lysosomal distension due to the storage of undegraded products. This defect affects both systemic and central tissues, and is associated with growth and mental retardation, hepatosplenomegaly and skeletal deformity. MPS-VII has also been described in mice (Birkenmeier *et al.*, 1989), cats (Schultheiss *et al.*, 2000) and dogs (Haskins *et al.*, 1984), with common manifestations, thus providing various animal models for preclinical applications of gene transfer. Another interesting feature of the syndrome is that the β-glucuronidase is a secreted enzyme that can be captured by distant cells through the ubiquitous mannose-6-phosphate receptor (M6PR) (Kornfeld & Mellman, 1989). Moreover, partial activity of the enzyme (about 10%) is sufficient to reverse the lysosomal storage. This phenomenon has been used in various experimental works to provide the missing enzyme in animal models, including by gene transfer. However, there is a major hurdle to the success of pharmacological treatment: β-glucuronidase cannot cross the blood–brain barrier. Thus, two independent therapies could be used: one for peripheric tissues (by bone marrow transplantation, enzyme replacement, gene transfer), and another for the CNS.

The blood–brain barrier is completed in mammals after birth, during the first weeks of postnatal development in humans. This postnatal window of opportunity has been used for gene transfer into the CNS by intravenous injection of newborn MPS-VII mice with an AAV encoding the β-glucuronidase. Distribution of the vector at therapeutic levels was widespread throughout the body, including in the brain, and there was phenotypic improvement (Daly *et al.*, 1999, 2001). If these results can be repeated in large animals (dog), it could be clinically relevant for humans. A single injection would treat both peripheral and central tissues. However, success would require lifetime expression of the transgene, and very early detection of the disease (preferably before birth). Gene transfer could be performed in utero to bypass the blood–brain barrier. Recent findings have proven the relevance of the murine model for embryonic onset of MPS-VII, and gene transfer in utero could be tested in this model (Casal & Wolfe, 2000). Although in utero gene transfer is feasible with several viral and non-viral vectors (Gallot *et al.*, 2002; Lai *et al.*, 2002; MacKenzie *et al.*, 2002; Saito & Nakatsuji, 2001; Shen *et al.*, 2002; Waddington *et al.*, 2003), it still needs optimization for high-level transduction in the brain. In addition, this strategy raises ethical concerns (Would germ-line cells be transduced? Is it dangerous for the mother?).

Once the BBB is formed, gene transfer could be performed by direct injection of a vector to transduce the CNS cells. It should not be necessary to transduce every cell because of the recapture of secreted β-glucuronidase by surrounding cells, but the transduction should ideally be widely spread throughout the CNS. Intraparenchymal injections have been performed using a variety of vectors and led to lysosomal clearance in the brain and the elimination of related neurological deficits, but the effect was relatively local because both the virus and the enzyme cannot diffuse sufficiently in the parenchyma (Bosch *et al.*, 2000a,b; Brooks *et al.*, 2002; Ghodsi *et al.*, 1998). To improve diffusion of the enzyme, mannitol can be injected after viral infection, as it induces wider diffusion of the enzyme. Injection of a vector into the CSF might then be more efficient in terms of distribution of the transduced cells. Combining intraventricular injection of adenoviral vector and mannitol treatment led to wide distribution of the enzyme in the brain (Ghodsi *et al.*, 1999). Similarly, intrathecal injection of AAV led to a global distribution of the enzyme in the CNS (Elliger *et al.*, 1999). However, such approaches may not be relevant in larger animals because of the much greater size of the brain and spinal cord.

Another approach would be to give a vector the ability to cross the blood-brain barrier. There are several ways to do this, as summarized by Pardridge (Pardridge, 2002a,b). Plasmid DNA encapsulated inside a nanocontainer composed of PEGylated immunoliposome (PILs) targeted across both the blood–brain barrier and the neuronal cell membrane by receptor-specific monoclonal antibodies can be delivered intravenously and transduce the whole CNS (Shi *et al.*, 2001a,b; Zhang *et al.*, 2002, 2003). Although this approach does not allow long-term expression because the formulated DNA is not stable, it might be applicable to the formulation of PILs containing a stable vector such as AAV, lentivirus or transposons. This appraoch may allow rapid progress towards global and stable gene transfer into the CNS.

Conclusions

The development of a succesful gene therapy for any application is dependent on the many critical issues described above: choice of vector, choice of therapeutic gene, vector production process, immune reaction and safety concerns. Moreover, depending on the pathology, several other issues have to be addressed such as the duration of the expression, the targeting of the vector and the regulation of the transgene expression. The duration of the expression can be achieved by the use of stable viral vectors such as AAV or lentivirus-derived vectors and the optimization of the expression cassette by the inclusion of sequences that stabilize the expression such as MARs or SARs. In contrast, short-term expression might be wanted (for seizure or trauma for example) and can be achieved by the use of transient vectors derived from poliovirus or alphavirus or the use of synthetic vectors. Although we did not describe these vectors in the previous chapters, they are gaining importance in terms of development and potentiality of use. The duration of expression can be regulated by turning off or on the transgene expression using regulatable expression systems such as the tetracycline or the rapamycin systems. These systems also have the advantage of regulating the level of transgene expression by external factors to obtain physiological levels of the therapeutic product.

Great efforts from the scientific community involved in the field of gene therapy have led to the first successful human trial for the correction of the SCID (severe combined immunodeficiency) phenotype in two patients (Cavazzana-Calvo *et al.*, 2000). Since then, this result has been confirmed in four of five patients with the disease (Hacein-Bey-Abina *et al.*, 2003), but a severe adverse event tempered the initial excitement. Two patients developed symptoms similar to acute lymphoblastic leukemia, resulting from insertional mutagenesis of the retroviral vector used in this therapy. Thus, although the proof of the principle of successful gene therapy for humans was established, it is essential for the researchers and clinicians to work with caution.

Very few clinical trials concerning in vivo gene therapy have been initiated for neurological affections, except for gliomas. A database of gene therapy clinical trials can be accessed on the web site of the *Journal of Gene Medicine* (http://www.wiley.co.uk/genetherapy/clinical/). Ongoing phase I clinical trials for neurological affections concern the treatment of Canavan disease using adenovirus-mediated transfer of the aspartoacylase gene and PD involving subthalamic AAV-mediated GAD (glutamic acid decarboxylase 65–67) gene transfer to patients who are candidates for deep brain stimulation. Another trial involves the intrathecal administration of AAV carrying the EEAT2 gene for the treatment of the amyotrophic lateral sclerosis (ALS). For the treatment of age-related macular degeneration, intravitreal delivery of an adenoviral vector coding the PEDF gene is being tested for inducing neovascularisation.

Gene therapy must be considered as the ultimate solution for treating diseases for which "classical" treatment is either not available or unsatisfactory. Efforts are still needed to obtain feasability of gene therapy for many applications, and its scaling-up will require further developments.

REFERENCES

Akkina, R. K., Walton, R. M., Chen, M. L., Li, Q. X., Planelles, V. & Chen, I. S. (1996). High-efficiency gene transfer into CD34+ cells with a human immunodeficiency virus type 1-based retroviral vector pseudotyped with vesicular stomatitis virus envelope glycoprotein G. *J. Virol.*, **70**, 2581–5.

Akli, S., Caillaud, C., Vigne, E. *et al.* (1993). Transfer of a foreign gene into the brain using adenovirus vectors. *Nat. Genet.*, **3**, 224–8.

Alexander, I. E., Russell, D. W. & Miller, A. D. (1994). DNA-damaging agents greatly increase the transduction of nondividing cells by adeno-associated virus vectors. *J. Virol.*, **68**, 8282–7.

Anderson, D. B., Laquerre, S., Ghosh, K. *et al.* (2000). Pseudotyping of glycoprotein D-deficient herpes simplex virus type 1 with vesicular stomatitis virus glycoprotein G enables mutant virus attachment and entry. *J. Virol.*, **74**, 2481–7.

Atchison, R. W., Casto, B. C. & Hammon, W. (1965). Adenovirus-associated defective virus particles. *Science*, **149**, 754.

Auricchio, A., Hildinger, M., O'Connor, E., Gao, G. P. & Wilson, J. M. (2001). Isolation of highly infectious and pure adeno-associated virus type 2 vectors with a single-step gravity-flow column. *Hum. Gene Ther.*, **12**, 71–6.

Auricchio, A., Kobinger, G., Anand, V. *et al.* (2001). Exchange of surface proteins impacts on viral vector cellular specificity and transduction characteristics: the retina as a model. *Hum. Mol. Genet.*, **10**, 3075–81.

Bajocchi, G., Feldman, S. H., Crystal, R. G. & Mastrangeli, A. (1993). Direct in vivo gene transfer to ependymal cells in the central nervous system using recombinant adenovirus vectors. *Nat. Genet.*, **3**, 229–34.

Bankiewicz, K. S., Eberling, J. L., Kohutnicka, M. *et al.* (2000). Convection-enhanced delivery of AAV vector in parkinsonian monkeys; in vivo detection of gene expression and restoration of dopaminergic function using pro-drug approach. *Exp. Neurol.*, **164**, 2–14.

Bartlett, J. S., Kleinschmidt, J., Boucher, R. C. & Samulski, R. J. (1999). Targeted adeno-associated virus vector transduction of nonpermissive cells mediated by a bispecific F(ab'gamma)2 antibody. *Nat. Biotechnol.*, **17**, 181–6.

Benabid, A. L., Benazzouz, A., Hoffmann, D., Limousin, P., Krack, P. & Pollak, P. (1998). Long-term electrical inhibition of deep brain targets in movement disorders. *Mov. Disord.*, **13** Suppl 3, 119–25.

Bergelson, J. M., Cunningham, J. A., Droguett, G. *et al.* (1997). Isolation of a common receptor for Coxsackie B viruses and adenoviruses 2 and 5. *Science*, **275**, 1320–3.

Berkowitz, R., Ilves, H., Lin, W. Y. *et al.* (2001a). Construction and molecular analysis of gene transfer systems derived from bovine immunodeficiency virus. *J. Virol.*, **75**, 3371–82.

Berkowitz, R. D., Ilves, H., Plavec, I. & Veres, G. (2001b). Gene transfer systems derived from Visna virus: analysis of virus production and infectivity. *Virology*, **279**, 116–29.

Bilang-Bleuel, A., Revah, F., Colin, P. *et al.* (1997). Intrastriatal injection of an adenoviral vector expressing glial-cell-line-derived neurotrophic factor prevents dopaminergic neuron degeneration and behavioral impairment in a rat model of Parkinson disease. *Proc. Natl, Acad. Sci., USA*, **94**, 8818–23.

Birkenmeier, E. H., Davisson, M. T., Beamer, W. G. *et al.* (1989). Murine mucopolysaccharidosis type VII. Characterization of a mouse with beta-glucuronidase deficiency. *J. Clin. Invest.*, **83**, 1258–6.

Blomer, U., Naldini, L., Kafri, T., Trono, D., Verma, I. M. & Gage, F. H. (1997). Highly efficient and sustained gene transfer in adult neurons with a lentivirus vector. *J. Virol.*, **71**, 6641–9.

Bosch, A., Perret, E., Desmaris, N. & Heard, J. M. (2000a). Long-term and significant correction of brain lesions in adult mucopolysaccharidosis type VII mice using recombinant AAV vectors. *Mol. Ther.: J. Am. Soc. Gene Ther.*, **1**, 63–70.

Bosch, A., Perret, E., Desmaris, N., Trono, D. & Heard, J. M. (2000b). Reversal of pathology in the entire brain of mucopolysaccharidosis type VII mice after lentivirus-mediated gene transfer. *Hum. Gene Ther.*, **11**, 1139–50.

Bosselman, R. A., Hsu, R. Y., Bruszewski, J., Hu, S., Martin, F. & Nicolson, M. (1987). Replication-defective chimeric helper proviruses and factors affecting generation of competent virus: expression of Moloney murine leukemia virus structural genes via the metallothionein promoter. *Mol. Cell Biol.*, **7**, 1797–806.

Brockman, M. A. & Knipe, D. M. (2002). Herpes simplex virus vectors elicit durable immune responses in the presence of preexisting host immunity. *J. Virol.*, **76**, 3678–87.

Brooks, A. I., Stein, C. S., Hughes, S. M. *et al.* (2002). Functional correction of established central nervous system deficits in an animal model of lysosomal storage disease with feline immunodeficiency virus-based vectors. *Proc. Natl Acad. Sci., USA*, **99**, 6216–21.

Browning, M. T., Schmidt, R. D., Lew, K. A. & Rizvi, T. A. (2001). Primate and feline lentivirus vector RNA packaging and propagation by heterologous lentivirus virions. *J. Virol.*, **75**, 5129–40.

Brun, S., Faucon-Biguet, N. & Mallet, J. (2003). Optimization of transgene expression at the posttranscriptional level in neural cells: implications for gene therapy. *Mol. Ther.*, **7**, 782–9.

Buller, R. M., Janik, J. E., Sebring, E. D. & Rose, J. A. (1981). Herpes simplex virus types 1 and 2 completely help adenovirus-associated virus replication. *J. Virol.*, **40**, 241–7.

Burton, M., Nakai, H., Colosi, P., Cunningham, J., Mitchell, R. & Couto, L. (1999). Coexpression of factor VIII heavy and light chain adeno-associated viral vectors produces biologically active protein. *Proc. Natl Acad. Sci., USA*, **96**, 12725–30.

Casal, M. L. & Wolfe, J. H. (2000). Mucopolysaccharidosis type VII in the developing mouse fetus. *Pediatr Res.*, **47**, 750–6.

Cavazzana-Calvo, M., Hacein-Bey, S., de Saint Basile, G. *et al.* (2000). Gene therapy of human severe combined immunodeficiency (SCID)-X1 disease. *Science*, **288**, 669–72.

Chamberlin, N. L., Du, B., de Lacalle, S. & Saper, C. B. (1998). Recombinant adeno-associated virus vector: use for transgene expression and anterograde tract tracing in the CNS. *Brain Res.*, **793**, 169–75.

Chartier, C., Degryse, E., Gantzer, M., Dieterle, A., Pavirani, A. & Mehtali, M. (1996). Efficient generation of recombinant adenovirus vectors by homologous recombination in *Escherichia coli. J. Virol.*, **70**, 4805–10.

Chillon, M., Bosch, A., Zabner, J. *et al.* (1999). Group D adenoviruses infect primary central nervous system cells more efficiently than those from group C. *J. Virol.*, **73**, 2537–40.

Chirmule, N., Propert, K., Magosin, S., Qian, Y., Qian, R. & Wilson, J. (1999). Immune responses to adenovirus and adeno-associated virus in humans. *Gene Ther.*, **6**, 1574–83.

Christenson, S. D., Lake, K. D., Ooboshi, H. *et al.* (1998). Adenovirus-mediated gene transfer in vivo to cerebral blood vessels and perivascular tissue in mice. *Stroke*, **29**, 1411–15; discussion 1416.

Collaco, R. F., Cao, X. & Trempe, J. P. (1999). A helper virus-free packaging system for recombinant adeno-associated virus vectors. *Gene*, **238**, 397–405.

Corti, O., Sanchez-Capelo, A., Colin, P., Hanoun, N., Hamon, M. & Mallet, J. (1999). Long-term doxycycline-controlled expression of human tyrosine hydroxylase after direct adenovirus-mediated gene transfer to a rat model of Parkinson's disease. *Proc. Natl Acad. Sci., USA*, **96**, 12120–5.

Cosset, F. L., Takeuchi, Y., Battini, J. L., Weiss, R. A. & Collins, M. K. (1995). High-titers packaging cells producing recombinant retroviruses resistant to human serum. *J. Virol.*, **69**, 7430–6.

Costantini, L. C., Bakowska, J. C., Breakefield, X. O. & Isacson, O. (2000). Gene therapy in the CNS. *Gene Ther.*, **7**, 93–109.

Crouzet, J., Naudin, L., Orsini, C. *et al.* (1997). Recombinational construction in *Escherichia coli* of infectious adenoviral genomes. *Proc. Natl Acad. Sci., USA*, **94**, 1414–19.

Croyle, M. A., Cheng, X. & Wilson, J. M. (2001). Development of formulations that enhance physical stability of viral vectors for gene therapy. *Gene Ther.*, **8**, 1281–90.

Croyle, M. A., Chirmule, N., Zhang, Y. & Wilson, J. M. (2002). PEGylation of E1-deleted adenovirus vectors allows significant gene expression on readministration to liver. *Hum. Gene Ther.*, **13**, 1887–900.

Daly, T. M., Okuyama, T., Vogler, C., Haskins, M. E., Muzyczka, N. & Sands, M. S. (1999). Neonatal intramuscular injection with recombinant adeno-associated virus results in prolonged beta-glucuronidase expression in situ and correction of liver pathology in mucopolysaccharidosis type VII mice. *Hum. Gene Ther.*, **10**, 85–94.

Daly, T. M., Ohlemiller, K. K., Roberts, M. S., Vogler, C. A. & Sands, M. S. (2001). Prevention of systemic clinical disease in MPS VII mice following AAV-mediated neonatal gene transfer. *Gene Ther.*, **8**, 1291–8.

Danos, O. & Mulligan, R. C. (1988). Safe and efficient generation of recombinant retroviruses with amphotropic and ecotropic host ranges. *Proc. Natl Acad. Sci., USA*, **85**, 6460–4.

Davidson, B. L., Allen, E. D., Kozarsky, K. F., Wilson, J. M. & Roessler, B. J. (1993). A model system for in vivo gene transfer into the central nervous system using an adenoviral vector. *Nat. Genet.*, **3**, 219–23.

Davidson, B. L., Stein, C. S., Heth, J. A. *et al.* (2000). Recombinant adeno-associated virus type 2, 4 & 5 vectors: transduction of variant cell types and regions in the mammalian central nervous system. *Proc. Natl Acad. Sci., USA*, **97**, 3428–32.

Delman, K. A., Bennett, J. J., Zager, J. S. *et al.* (2000). Effects of pre-existing immunity on the response to herpes simplex-based oncolytic viral therapy. *Hum. Gene Ther.*, **11**, 2465–72.

Desmaris, N., Bosch, A., Salaun, C. *et al.* (2001). Production and neurotropism of lentivirus vectors pseudotyped with lyssavirus envelope glycoproteins. *Mol. Ther.*, **4**, 149–56.

Drittanti, L., Jenny, C., Poulard, K. *et al.* (2001). Optimised helper virus-free production of high-quality adeno-associated virus vectors. *J. Gene Med.*, **3**, 59–71.

Duan, D., Yan, Z., Yue, Y. & Engelhardt, J. F. (1999). Structural analysis of adeno-associated virus transduction circular intermediates. *Virology*, **261**, 8–14.

Duan, D., Yue, Y. & Engelhardt, J. F. (2001). Expanding AAV packaging capacity with trans-splicing or overlapping vectors: a quantitative comparison. *Mol. Ther.: J. Am. Soc. Gene Ther.*, **4**, 383–91.

Dull, T., Zufferey, R., Kelly, M. *et al.* (1998). A third-generation lentivirus vector with a conditional packaging system. *J. Virol.*, **72**, 8463–71.

Elliger, S., Elliger, C., Aguilar, C., Raju, N. & Watson, G. (1999). Elimination of lysosomal storage in brains of MPS VII mice treated by intrathecal administration of an adeno-associated virus vector. *Gene Ther.*, **6**, 1175–8.

Fallaux, F. J., Kranenburg, O., Cramer, S. J. *et al.* (1996). Characterization of 911: a new helper cell line for the titration and propagation of early region 1-deleted adenoviral vectors. *Hum. Gene Ther.*, **7**, 215–22.

Fallaux, F. J., Bout, A., van der Velde, I. *et al.* (1998). New helper cells and matched early region 1-deleted adenovirus vectors prevent generation of replication-competent adenoviruses. *Hum. Gene Ther.*, **9**, 1909–17.

Fang, B., Wang, H., Gordon, G. *et al.* (1996). Lack of persistence of E1- recombinant adenoviral vectors containing a temperature-sensitive E2A mutation in immunocompetent mice and hemophilia B dogs. *Gene Ther.*, **3**, 217–22.

Finiels, F., Gimenez y Ribotta, M., Barkats, M. *et al.* (1995). Specific and efficient gene transfer strategy offers new potentialities for the treatment of motor neurone diseases. *Neuroreport*, **7**, 373–8.

Fisher, K. D., Stallwood, Y., Green, N. K., Ulbrich, K., Mautner, V. & Seymour, L. W. (2001). Polymer-coated adenovirus permits efficient retargeting and evades neutralising antibodies. *Gene Ther.*, **8**, 341–8.

Fisher, K. J., Choi, H., Burda, J., Chen, S. J. & Wilson, J. M. (1996). Recombinant adenovirus deleted of all viral genes for gene therapy of cystic fibrosis. *Virology*, **217**, 11–22.

Follenzi, A., Ailles, L. E., Bakovic, S., Geuna, M. & Naldini, L. (2000). Gene transfer by lentiviral vectors is limited by nuclear translocation and rescued by HIV-1 pol sequences. *Nat. Genet.*, **25**, 217–22.

Fraefel, C., Song, S., Lim, F. *et al.* (1996). Helper virus-free transfer of herpes simplex virus type 1 plasmid vectors into neural cells. *J. Virol.*, **70**, 7190–7.

Fu, X. & Zhang, X. (2001). Delivery of herpes simplex virus vectors through liposome formulation. *Mol. Ther. J. Am. Soc. Gene Ther.*, **4**, 447–53.

Gallot, D., Seifer, I., Lemery, D. & Bignon, Y. J. (2002). Systemic diffusion including germ cells after plasmidic in utero gene transfer in the rat. *Fetal Diag. Ther.*, **17**, 157–62.

Gao, G. P., Alvira, M. R., Wang, L., Calcedo, R., Johnston, J. & Wilson, J. M. (2002). Novel adeno-associated viruses from rhesus monkeys as vectors for human gene therapy. *Proc. Natl Acad. Sci., USA*, **99**, 11854–9.

Geller, A. I. & Breakefield, X. O. (1988). A defective HSV-1 vector expresses Escherichia coli beta-galactosidase in cultured peripheral neurons. *Science*, **241**, 1667–9.

Ghadge, G. D., Roos, R. P., Kang, U. J. *et al.* (1995). CNS gene delivery by retrograde transport of recombinant replication-defective adenoviruses. *Gene Ther.*, **2**, 132–7.

Ghodsi, A., Stein, C., Derksen, T., Yang, G., Anderson, R. D. & Davidson, B. L. (1998). Extensive beta-glucuronidase activity in murine central nervous system after adenovirus-mediated gene transfer to brain. *Hum. Gene Ther.*, **9**, 2331–40.

Ghodsi, A., Stein, C., Derksen, T., Martins, I., Anderson, R. D. & Davidson, B. L. (1999). Systemic hyperosmolality improves beta-glucuronidase distribution and pathology in murine

MPS VII brain following intraventricular gene transfer. *Exp. Neurol.*, **160**, 109–16.

Girod, A., Ried, M., Wobus, C. *et al.* (1999). Genetic capsid modifications allow efficient re-targeting of adeno-associated virus type 2. *Nat. Med.*, **5**, 1052–6.

Goins, W. F., Sternberg, L. R., Croen, K. D. *et al.* (1994). A novel latency-active promoter is contained within the herpes simplex virus type 1 UL flanking repeats. *J. Virol.*, **68**, 2239–52.

Goins, W. F., Lee, K. A., Cavalcoli, J. D. *et al.* (1999). Herpes simplex virus type 1 vector-mediated expression of nerve growth factor protects dorsal root ganglion neurons from peroxide toxicity. *J. Virol.*, **73**, 519–32.

Goldman, C. K., Rogers, B. E., Douglas, J. T. *et al.* (1997). Targeted gene delivery to Kaposi's sarcoma cells via the fibroblast growth factor receptor. *Cancer Res.*, **57**, 1447–51.

Graham, F. L., Smiley, J., Russell, W. C. & Nairn, R. (1977). Characteristics of a human cell line transformed by DNA from human adenovirus type 5. *J. Gen. Virol.*, **36**, 59–74.

Grifman, M., Trepel, M., Speece, P. *et al.* (2001). Incorporation of tumor-targeting peptides into recombinant adeno-associated virus capsids. *Mol. Ther.*, **3**, 964–75.

Hacein-Bey-Abina, S., von Kalle, C., Schmidt, M. *et al.* (2003). A serious adverse event after successful gene therapy for X-linked severe combined immunodeficiency. *N. Engl. J. Med.*, **348**, 255–6.

Halbert, C. L., Rutledge, E. A., Allen, J. M., Russell, D. W. & Miller, A. D. (2000). Repeat transduction in the mouse lung by using adeno-associated virus vectors with different serotypes. *J. Virol.*, **74**, 1524–32.

Hardy, S., Kitamura, M., Harris-Stansil, T., Dai, Y. & Phipps, M. L. (1997). Construction of adenovirus vectors through Cre-lox recombination. *J. Virol.*, **71**, 1842–9.

Hashimoto, M., Aruga, J., Hosoya, Y., Kanegae, Y., Saito, I. & Mikoshiba, K. (1996). A neural cell-type-specific expression system using recombinant adenovirus vectors. *Hum. Gene Ther.*, **7**, 149–58.

Haskins, M. E., Desnick, R. J., DiFerrante, N., Jezyk, P. F. & Patterson, D. F. (1984). Beta-glucuronidase deficiency in a dog: a model of human mucopolysaccharidosis VII. *Pediatr. Res.*, **18**, 980–4.

Hillgenberg, M., Schnieders, F., Loser, P. & Strauss, M. (2001). System for efficient helper-dependent minimal adenovirus construction and rescue. *Hum. Gene Ther.*, **12**, 643–57.

Holmes-Son, M. L. & Chow, S. A. (2000). Integrase-lexA fusion proteins incorporated into human immunodeficiency virus type 1 that contains a catalytically inactive integrase gene are functional to mediate integration. *J. Virol.*, **74**, 11548–56.

Holmes-Son, M. L. & Chow, S. A. (2002). Correct integration mediated by integrase-LexA fusion proteins incorporated into HIV-1. *Mol. Ther.*, **5**, 360–70.

Holmes-Son, M. L., Appa, R. S. & Chow, S. A. (2001). Molecular genetics and target site specificity of retroviral integration. *Adv. Genet.*, **43**, 33–69.

Horellou, P., Vigne, E., Castel, M. N. *et al.* (1994). Direct intracerebral gene transfer of an adenoviral vector expressing tyrosine hydroxylase in a rat model of Parkinson's disease. *Neuroreport*, **6**, 49–53.

Hsich, G., Sena-Esteves, M. & Breakefield, X. O. (2002). Critical issues in gene therapy for neurologic disease. *Hum. Gene Ther.*, **13**, 579–604.

Iwakuma, T., Cui, Y. & Chang, L. J. (1999). Self-inactivating lentiviral vectors with U3 and U5 modifications. *Virology*, **261**, 120–32.

Kafri, T., Blomer, U., Peterson, D. A., Gage, F. H. & Verma, I. M. (1997). Sustained expression of genes delivered directly into liver and muscle by lentiviral vectors. *Nat. Genet.*, **17**, 314–17.

Kafri, T., van Praag, H., Ouyang, L., Gage, F. H. & Verma, I. M. (1999). A packaging cell line for lentivirus vectors. *J. Virol.*, **73**, 576–84.

Kaul, M., Yu, H., Ron, Y. & Dougherty, J. P. (1998). Regulated lentiviral packaging cell line devoid of most viral cis-acting sequences. *Virology*, **249**, 167–74.

Ketner, G., Spencer, F., Tugendreich, S., Connelly, C. & Hieter, P. (1994). Efficient manipulation of the human adenovirus genome as an infectious yeast artificial chromosome clone. *Proc. Natl Acad. Sci., USA*, **91**, 6186–90.

Kochanek, S., Clemens, P. R., Mitani, K., Chen, H. H., Chan, S. & Caskey, C. T. (1996). A new adenoviral vector: Replacement of all viral coding sequences with 28 kb of DNA independently expressing both full-length dystrophin and beta-galactosidase. *Proc. Natl Acad. Sci., USA*, **93**, 5731–6.

Kogure, K., Urabe, M., Mizukami, H. *et al.* (2001). Targeted integration of foreign DNA into a defined locus on chromosome 19 in K562 cells using AAV-derived components. *Int. J. Hematol.*, **73**, 469–75.

Kordower, J. H., Emborg, M. E., Bloch, J. *et al.* (2000). Neurodegeneration prevented by lentiviral vector delivery of GDNF in primate models of Parkinson's disease. *Science*, **290**, 721–4.

Kornfeld, S. & Mellman, I. (1989). The biogenesis of lysosomes. *Annu. Rev. Cell Biol.*, **5**, 483–525.

Kotin, R. M., Siniscalco, M., Samulski, R. J. *et al.* (1990). Site-specific integration by adeno-associated virus. *Proc. Natl Acad. Sci., USA*, **87**, 2211–5.

Krasnykh, V., Belousova, N., Korokhov, N., Mikheeva, G. & Curiel, D. T. (2001). Genetic targeting of an adenovirus vector via replacement of the fiber protein with the phage T4 fibritin. *J. Virol.*, **75**, 4176–83.

Kugler, S., Meyn, L., Holzmuller, H. *et al.* (2001). Neuron-specific expression of therapeutic proteins: evaluation of different cellular promoters in recombinant adenoviral vectors. *Mol. Cell Neurosci.*, **17**, 78–96.

Kuo, H., Ingram, D. K., Crystal, R. G. & Mastrangeli, A. (1995). Retrograde transfer of replication deficient recombinant adenovirus vector in the central nervous system for tracing studies. *Brain Res.*, **705**, 31–8.

Lachmann, R. H. & Efstathiou, S. (1997). Utilization of the herpes simplex virus type 1 latency-associated regulatory region to drive stable reporter gene expression in the nervous system. *J. Virol.*, **71**, 3197–207.

(1999). Use of herpes simplex virus type 1 for transgene expression within the nervous system. *Clin. Sci.*, **96**, 533–41.

Lai, L., Davison, B. B., Veazey, R. S., Fisher, K. J. & Baskin, G. B. (2002). A preliminary evaluation of recombinant adeno-associated virus biodistribution in rhesus monkeys after intrahepatic inoculation in utero. *Hum. Gene Ther.*, **13**, 2027–39.

Laquerre, S., Anderson, D. B., Stolz, D. B. & Glorioso, J. C. (1998). Recombinant herpes simplex virus type 1 engineered for targeted binding to erythropoietin receptor-bearing cells. *J. Virol.*, **72**, 9683–97.

Le Gal La Salle, G., Robert, J. J., Berrard, S. *et al.* (1993). An adenovirus vector for gene transfer into neurons and glia in the brain. *Science*, **259**, 988–90.

Lee, E. J., Thimmapaya, B. & Jameson, J. L. (2000). Stereotactic injection of adenoviral vectors that target gene expression to specific pituitary cell types: implications for gene therapy. *Neurosurgery*, **46**, 1461–8; discussion 1468–9.

Leib, D. A. & Olivo, P. D. (1993). Gene delivery to neurons: is herpes simplex virus the right tool for the job? *Bioessays*, **15**, 547–54.

Limousin, P., Krack, P., Pollak, P. *et al.* (1998). Electrical stimulation of the subthalamic nucleus in advanced Parkinson's disease. *N. Engl. J. Med.*, **339**, 1105–11.

Lin, L. F., Doherty, D. H., Lile, J. D., Bektesh, S. & Collins, F. (1993). GDNF: a glial cell line-derived neurotrophic factor for midbrain dopaminergic neurons. *Science*, **260**, 1130–2.

Liu, X. L., Clark, K. R. & Johnson, P. R. (1999). Production of recombinant adeno-associated virus vectors using a packaging cell line and a hybrid recombinant adenovirus. *Gene Ther.*, **6**, 293–9.

Logvinoff, C. & Epstein, A. L. (2001). A novel approach for herpes simplex virus type 1 amplicon vector production, using the Cre-loxP recombination system to remove helper virus. *Hum. Gene Ther.*, **12**, 161–7.

Lotery, A. J., Derksen, T. A., Russell, S. R. *et al.* (2002). Gene transfer to the nonhuman primate retina with recombinant feline immunodeficiency virus vectors. *Hum. Gene Ther.*, **13**, 689–96.

Lowenstein, P. R. (2002). Immunology of viral-vector-mediated gene transfer into the brain: an evolutionary and developmental perspective. *Trends Immunol.*, **23**, 23–30.

MacKenzie, T. C., Kobinger, G. P., Kootstra, N. A. *et al.* (2002). Efficient transduction of liver and muscle after in utero injection of lentiviral vectors with different pseudotypes. *Mol. Ther.*, **6**, 349–58.

Magnusson, M. K., Hong, S. S., Boulanger, P. & Lindholm, L. (2001). Genetic retargeting of adenovirus: novel strategy employing 'deknobbing' of the fiber. *J. Virol.*, **75**, 7280–9.

Mannes, A. J., Caudle, R. M., O'Connell, B. C. & Iadarola, M. J. (1998). Adenoviral gene transfer to spinal-cord neurons: intrathecal vs. intraparenchymal administration. *Brain Res.*, **793**, 1–6.

Mastakov, M. Y., Baer, K., Xu, R., Fitzsimons, H. & During, M. J. (2001). Combined injection of rAAV with mannitol enhances gene expression in the rat brain. *Mol. Ther.: J. Am. Soc. Gene Ther.*, **3**, 225–32.

Mastakov, M. Y., Baer, K., Kotin, R. M. & During, M. J. (2002). Recombinant adeno-associated virus serotypes 2- and 5-mediated gene transfer in the mammalian brain: quantitative analysis of heparin co-infusion. *Mol. Ther.*, **5**, 371–80.

Matsushita, T., Elliger, S., Elliger, C. *et al.* (1998). Adeno-associated virus vectors can be efficiently produced without helper virus. *Gene Ther.*, **5**, 938–45.

Mazarakis, N. D., Azzouz, M., Rohll, J. B. *et al.* (2001). Rabies virus glycoprotein pseudotyping of lentiviral vectors enables retrograde axonal transport and access to the nervous system after peripheral delivery. *Hum. Mol. Genet.*, **10**, 2109–21.

McCown, T. J., Xiao, X., Li, J., Breese, G. R. & Samulski, R. J. (1996). Differential and persistent expression patterns of CNS gene transfer by an adeno-associated virus (AAV) vector. *Brain Res.*, **713**, 99–107.

McGeer, P. L., McGeer, E. G. & Suzuki, J. S. (1977). Aging and extrapyramidal function. *Arch. Neurol.*, **34**, 33–5.

Millecamps, S., Kiefer, H., Navarro, V. *et al.* (1999). Neuron-restrictive silencer elements mediate neuron specificity of adenoviral gene expression. *Nat. Biotech.*, **17**, 865–9.

Millecamps, S., Nicolle, D., Ceballos-Picot, I., Mallet, J. & Barkats, M. (2001). Synaptic sprouting increases the uptake capacities of motoneurons in amyotrophic lateral sclerosis mice. *Proc. Natl Acad. Sci., USA*, **98**, 7582–7.

Millecamps, S., Mallet, J. & Barkats, M. (2002). Adenoviral retrograde gene transfer in motoneurons is greatly enhanced by prior intramuscular inoculation with botulinum toxin. *Hum. Gene Ther.*, **13**, 225–32.

Miller, A. D., Garcia, J. V., von Suhr, N., Lynch, C. M., Wilson, C. & Eiden, M. V. (1991). Construction and properties of retrovirus packaging cells based on gibbon ape leukemia virus. *J. Virol.*, **65**, 2220–4.

Miller, D. G., Rutledge, E. A. & Russell, D. W. (2002). Chromosomal effects of adeno-associated virus vector integration. *Nat. Genet.*, **30**, 147–8.

Mitani, K., Graham, F. L., Caskey, C. T. & Kochanek, S. (1995). Rescue, propagation and partial purification of a helper virus-dependent adenovirus vector. *Proc. Natl Acad. Sci., USA*, **92**, 3854–8.

Mitrophanous, K., Yoon, S., Rohll, J. *et al.* (1999). Stable gene transfer to the nervous system using a non-primate lentiviral vector. *Gene Ther.*, **6**, 1808–18.

Miyoshi, H., Takahashi, M., Gage, F. H. & Verma, I. M. (1997). Stable and efficient gene transfer into the retina using an HIV-based lentiviral vector. *Proc. Natl Acad. Sci., USA*, **94**, 10319–23.

Miyoshi, H., Blomer, U., Takahashi, M., Gage, F. H. & Verma, I. M. (1998). Development of a self-inactivating lentivirus vector. *J. Virol.*, **72**, 8150–7.

Mochizuki, H., Schwartz, J. P., Tanaka, K., Brady, R. O. & Reiser, J. (1998). High-titers human immunodeficiency virus type 1-based vector systems for gene delivery into nondividing cells. *J. Virol.*, **72**, 8873–83.

Nakai, H., Iwaki, Y., Kay, M. A. & Couto, L. B. (1999). Isolation of recombinant adeno-associated virus vector-cellular DNA junctions from mouse liver. *J. Virol.*, **73**, 5438–47.

Nakai, H., Storm, T. A. & Kay, M. A. (2000). Increasing the size of rAAV-mediated expression cassettes in vivo by intermolecular joining of two complementary vectors. *Nat. Biotechnol.*, **18**, 527–32.

Nakai, H., Montini, E., Fuess, S., Storm, T. A., Grompe, M. & Kay, M. A. (2003). AAV serotype 2 vectors preferentially integrate into active genes in mice. *Nat. Genet.*, **34**, 297–302.

Nakajima, T., Nakamaru, K., Ido, E., Terao, K., Hayami, M. & Hasegawa, M. (2000). Development of novel simian immunodeficiency virus vectors carrying a dual gene expression system. *Hum. Gene Ther.*, **11**, 1863–74.

Naldini, L., Blomer, U., Gage, F. H., Trono, D. & Verma, I. M. (1996a). Efficient transfer, integration and sustained long-term expression of the transgene in adult rat brains injected with a lentiviral vector. *Proc. Natl Acad. Sci., USA*, **93**, 11382–8.

Naldini, L., Blomer, U., Gallay, P. *et al.* (1996b). In vivo gene delivery and stable transduction of nondividing cells by a lentiviral vector [see comments]. *Science*, **272**, 263–7.

Navarro, V., Millecamps, S., Geoffroy, M. C. *et al.* (1999). Efficient gene transfer and long-term expression in neurons using a recombinant adenovirus with a neuron-specific promoter. *Gene Ther.*, **6**, 1884–92.

Ng, P., Beauchamp, C., Evelegh, C., Parks, R. & Graham, F. L. (2001). Development of a FLP/frt system for generating helper-dependent adenoviral vectors. *Mol. Ther.*, **3**, 809–15.

Nguyen, J. B., Sanchez-Pernaute, R., Cunningham, J. & Bankiewicz, K. S. (2001). Convection-enhanced delivery of AAV-2 combined with heparin increases TK gene transfer in the rat brain. *Neuroreport*, **12**, 1961–4.

Nicklin, S. A., Buening, H., Dishart, K. L. *et al.* (2001). Efficient and selective aav2-mediated gene transfer directed to human vascular endothelial cells. *Mol. Ther.*, **4**, 174–81.

Okada, T., Nomoto, T., Shimazaki, K. *et al.* (2002). Adeno-associated virus vectors for gene transfer to the brain. *Methods*, **28**, 237–47.

Olivares, E. C., Hollis, R. P., Chalberg, T. W., Meuse, L., Kay, M. A. & Calos, M. P. (2002). Site-specific genomic integration produces therapeutic Factor IX levels in mice. *Nat. Biotechnol.*, **20**, 1124–8.

Page, K. A., Landau, N. R. & Littman, D. R. (1990). Construction and use of a human immunodeficiency virus vector for analysis of virus infectivity. *J. Virol.*, **64**, 5270–6.

Palmer, J. A., Branston, R. H., Lilley, C. E. *et al.* (2000). Development and optimization of herpes simplex virus vectors for multiple long-term gene delivery to the peripheral nervous system. *J. Virol.*, **74**, 5604–18.

Palombo, F., Monciotti, A., Recchia, A., Cortese, R., Ciliberto, G. & La Monica, N. (1998). Site-specific integration in mammalian cells mediated by a new hybrid baculovirus-adeno-associated virus vector. *J. Virol.*, **72**, 5025–34.

Pardridge, W. M. (2002a). Drug and gene delivery to the brain: the vascular route. *Circulation*, **106**, e220–1; author reply e220–1.

(2002b). Drug and gene targeting to the brain with molecular Trojan horses. *Nat. Rev. Drug Discovery*, **1**, 131–9.

Peel, A. L. & Klein, R. L. (2000). Adeno-associated virus vectors: activity and applications in the CNS. *J. Neurosci. Methods.*, **98**, 95–104.

Podsakoff, G., Wong, K. K., Jr. & Chatterjee, S. (1994). Efficient gene transfer into nondividing cells by adeno-associated virus-based vectors. *J. Virol.*, **68**, 5656–66.

Poeschla, E. M., Wong-Staal, F. & Looney, D. J. (1998). Efficient transduction of nondividing human cells by feline immunodeficiency virus lentiviral vectors. *Nat. Med.*, **4**, 354–7.

Poewe, W. H. & Wenning, G. K. (1996). The natural history of Parkinson's disease. *Neurology*, **47**, S146–52.

Ponnazhagan, S., Erikson, D., Kearns, W. G. *et al.* (1997). Lack of site-specific integration of the recombinant adeno-associated virus 2 genomes in human cells. *Hum. Gene Ther.*, **8**, 275–84.

Poznansky, M., Lever, A., Bergeron, L., Haseltine, W. & Sodroski, J. (1991). Gene transfer into human lymphocytes by a defective human immunodeficiency virus type 1 vector. *J. Virol.*, **65**, 532–6.

Ramezani, A., Hawley, T. S. & Hawley, R. G. (2000). Lentiviral vectors for enhanced gene expression in human hematopoietic cells. *Mol. Ther.*, **2**, 458–69.

Rampling, R., Cruickshank, G., Papanastassiou, V. *et al.* (2000). Toxicity evaluation of replication-competent herpes simplex virus (ICP 34.5 null mutant 1716) in patients with recurrent malignant glioma. *Gene Ther.*, **7**, 859–66.

Recchia, A., Parks, R. J., Lamartina, S. *et al.* (1999). Site-specific integration mediated by a hybrid adenovirus/adeno-associated virus vector. *Proc. Natl Acad. Sci., USA*, **96**, 2615–20.

Reiser, J. (2000). Production and concentration of pseudotyped HIV-1-based gene transfer vectors. *Gene Ther.*, **7**, 910–13.

Richardson, J. H., Kaye, J. F., Child, L. A. & Lever, A. M. (1995). Helper virus-free transfer of human immunodeficiency virus type 1 vectors. *J. Gen. Virol.*, **76**, 691–6.

Rinaudo, D., Lamartina, S., Roscilli, G., Ciliberto, G. & Toniatti, C. (2000). Conditional site-specific integration into human chromosome 19 by using a ligand-dependent chimeric adeno-associated virus/Rep protein. *J. Virol.*, **74**, 281–94.

Rizzuto, G., Gorgoni, B., Cappelletti, M. *et al.* (1999). Development of animal models for adeno-associated virus site-specific integration. *J. Virol.*, **73**, 2517–26.

Robert, J. J., Geoffroy, M. C., Finiels, F. & Mallet, J. (1997). An adenoviral vector-based system to study neuronal gene expression: analysis of the rat tyrosine hydroxylase promoter in cultured neurons. *J. Neurochem.*, **68**, 2152–60.

Rutledge, E. A. & Russell, D. W. (1997). Adeno-associated virus vector integration junctions. *J. Virol.*, **71**, 8429–36.

Saeki, Y., Ichikawa, T., Saeki, A. *et al.* (1998). Herpes simplex virus type 1 DNA amplified as bacterial artificial chromosome in *Escherichia coli*: rescue of replication-competent virus progeny and packaging of amplicon vectors. *Hum. Gene Ther.*, **9**, 2787–94.

Saito, T. & Nakatsuji, N. (2001). Efficient gene transfer into the embryonic mouse brain using in vivo electroporation. *Dev. Biol.*, **240**, 237–46.

Salmon, P., Oberholzer, J., Occhiodoro, T., Morel, P., Lou, J. & Trono, D. (2000). Reversible immortalization of human primary cells by lentivector-mediated transfer of specific genes. *Mol. Ther.: J. Am. Soc. Gene Ther.*, **2**, 404–14.

Samaniego, L. A., Wu, N. & DeLuca, N. A. (1997). The herpes simplex virus immediate-early protein ICP0 affects transcription from the viral genome and infected-cell survival in the absence of ICP4 and ICP27. *J. Virol.*, **71**, 4614–25.

Samaniego, L. A., Neiderhiser, L. & DeLuca, N. A. (1998). Persistence and expression of the herpes simplex virus genome in the absence of immediate-early proteins. *J. Virol.*, **72**, 3307–20.

Satoh, W., Hirai, Y., Tamayose, K. & Shimada, T. (2000). Site-specific integration of an adeno-associated virus vector plasmid mediated by regulated expression of rep based on Cre-loxP recombination. *J. Virol.*, **74**, 10631–8.

Sauer, H., Rosenblad, C. & Bjorklund, A. (1995). Glial cell line-derived neurotrophic factor but not transforming growth factor beta 3 prevents delayed degeneration of nigral dopaminergic neurons following striatal 6-hydroxydopamine lesion. *Proc. Natl Acad. Sci., USA*, **92**, 8935–9.

Scarpini, C. G., May, J., Lachmann, R. H. *et al.* (2001). Latency associated promoter transgene expression in the central nervous system after stereotaxic delivery of replication-defective HSV-1-based vectors. *Gene Ther.*, **8**, 1057–71.

Schultheiss, P. C., Gardner, S. A., Owens, J. M., Wenger, D. A. & Thrall, M. A. (2000). Mucopolysaccharidosis VII in a cat. *Vet. Pathol.*, **37**, 502–5.

Shen, J. S., Meng, X. L., Ohashi, T. & Eto, Y. (2002). Adenovirus-mediated prenatal gene transfer to murine central nervous system. *Gene Ther.*, **9**, 819–23.

Shen, Y., Muramatsu, S. I., Ikeguchi, K. *et al.* (2000). Triple transduction with adeno-associated virus vectors expressing tyrosine hydroxylase, aromatic-L-amino-acid decarboxylase and GTP cyclohydrolase I for gene therapy of Parkinson's disease. *Hum. Gene Ther.*, **11**, 1509–19.

Shi, N., Boado, R. J. & Pardridge, W. M. (2001a). Receptor-mediated gene targeting to tissues in vivo following intravenous administration of pegylated immunoliposomes. *Pharmaceut. Res.*, **18**, 1091–5.

Shi, N., Zhang, Y., Zhu, C., Boado, R. J. & Pardridge, W. M. (2001b). Brain-specific expression of an exogenous gene after i.v. administration. *Proc. Natl Acad. Sci., USA*, **98**, 12754–9.

Smith, C., Lachmann, R. H. & Efstathiou, S. (2000). Expression from the herpes simplex virus type 1 latency-associated promoter in the murine central nervous system. *J. Gen. Virol.*, **81** (3), 649–62.

Sollerbrant, K., Elmen, J., Wahlestedt, C. *et al.* (2001). A novel method using baculovirus-mediated gene transfer for production of recombinant adeno-associated virus vectors. *J. Gen. Virol.*, **82**, 2051–60.

Sosnowski, B. A., Gu, D. L., D'Andrea, M., Doukas, J. & Pierce, G. F. (1999). FGF2-targeted adenoviral vectors for systemic and local disease. *Curr. Opin. Mol. Ther.*, **1**, 573–9.

Stavropoulos, T. A. & Strathdee, C. A. (1998). An enhanced packaging system for helper-dependent herpes simplex virus vectors. *J. Virol.*, **72**, 7137–43.

Takahashi, M., Miyoshi, H., Verma, I. M. & Gage, F. H. (1999). Rescue from photoreceptor degeneration in the rd mouse by human immunodeficiency virus vector-mediated gene transfer. *J. Virol.*, **73**, 7812–16.

Thomas, C. E., Birkett, D., Anozie, I., Castro, M. G. & Lowenstein, P. R. (2001). Acute direct adenoviral vector cytotoxicity and chronic, but not acute, inflammatory responses correlate with decreased vector-mediated transgene expression in the brain. *Mol. Ther.: J. Am. Soc. Gene Ther.*, **3**, 36–46.

Thomas, C. E., Schiedner, G., Kochanek, S., Castro, M. G. & Lowenstein, P. R. (2000). Peripheral infection with adenovirus causes unexpected long-term brain inflammation in animals injected intracranially with first-generation, but not with high-capacity, adenovirus vectors: toward realistic long-term neurological gene therapy for chronic diseases. *Proc. Natl Acad. Sci., USA*, **97**, 7482–7.

(2001). Preexisting antiadenoviral immunity is not a barrier to efficient and stable transduction of the brain, mediated by novel high-capacity adenovirus vectors. *Hum. Gene Ther.*, **12**, 839–46.

Tsunoda, H., Hayakawa, T., Sakuragawa, N. & Koyama, H. (2000). Site-specific integration of adeno-associated virus-based plasmid vectors in lipofected HeLa cells. *Virology*, **268**, 391–401.

Ueno, T., Matsumura, H., Tanaka, K. *et al.* (2000). Site-specific integration of a transgene mediated by a hybrid adenovirus/adeno-associated virus vector using the Cre/loxP-expression-switching system. *Biochem. Biophys. Res. Commun.*, **273**, 473–8.

Waddington, S. N., Mitrophanous, K. A., Ellard, F. M. *et al.* (2003). Long-term transgene expression by administration of a lentivirus-based vector to the fetal circulation of immunocompetent mice. *Gene Ther.*, **10**, 1234–40.

Wang, B., Li, J. & Xiao, X. (2000). Adeno-associated virus vector carrying human minidystrophin genes effectively ameliorates muscular dystrophy in mdx mouse model. *Proc. Natl Acad. Sci., USA*, **97**, 13714–19.

Wang, Q., Guo, J. & Jia, W. (1997). Intracerebral recombinant HSV-1 vector does not reactivate latent HSV-1. *Gene Ther.*, **4**, 1300–4.

Wickham, T. J., Haskard, D., Segal, D. & Kovesdi, I. (1997). Targeting endothelium for gene therapy via receptors up-regulated during angiogenesis and inflammation. *Cancer Immunol. Immunother.*, **45**, 149–51.

Wickham, T. J., Mathias, P., Cheresh, D. A. & Nemerow, G. R. (1993). Integrins alpha v beta 3 and alpha v beta 5 promote adenovirus internalization but not virus attachment. *Cell*, **73**, 309–19.

Wu, P., Phillips, M. I., Bui, J. & Terwilliger, E. F. (1998). Adeno-associated virus vector-mediated transgene integration into neurons and other nondividing cell targets. *J. Virol.*, **72**, 5919–26.

Xiao, X., Li, J. & Samulski, R. J. (1998). Production of high-titers recombinant adeno-associated virus vectors in the absence of helper adenovirus. *J. Virol.*, **72**, 2224–32.

Xu, K., Ma, H., McCown, T. J., Verma, I. M. & Kafri, T. (2001). Generation of a stable cell line producing high-titers self-inactivating lentiviral vectors. *Mol. Ther.*, **3**, 97–104.

Yan, Z., Zhang, Y., Duan, D. & Engelhardt, J. F. (2000). Trans-splicing vectors expand the utility of adeno-associated virus for gene therapy. *Proc. Natl Acad. Sci., USA*, **97**, 6716–21.

Zennou, V., Petit, C., Guetard, D., Nerhbass, U., Montagnier, L. & Charneau, P. (2000). HIV-1 genome nuclear import is mediated by a central DNA flap. *Cell*, **101**, 173–85.

Zennou, V., Serguera, C., Sarkis, C. *et al.* (2001). The HIV-1 DNA flap stimulates HIV vector-mediated cell transduction in the brain. *Nat. Biotechnol.*, **19**, 446–50.

Zhang, Y., Jeong Lee, H., Boado, R. J. & Pardridge, W. M. (2002). Receptor-mediated delivery of an antisense gene to human brain cancer cells. *J. Gene Med.*, **4**, 183–94.

Zhang, Y., Calon, F., Zhu, C., Boado, R. J. & Pardridge, W. M. (2003). Intravenous nonviral gene therapy causes normalization of striatal tyrosine hydroxylase and reversal of motor impairment in experimental parkinsonism. *Hum. Gene Ther.*, **14**, 1–12.

Zhao, H., Otaki, J. M. & Firestein, S. (1996). Adenovirus-mediated gene transfer in olfactory neurons in vivo. *J. Neurobiol.*, **30**, 521–30.

Zou, L., Yuan, X., Zhou, H., Lu, H. & Yang, K. (2001). Helper-dependent adenoviral vector-mediated gene transfer in aged rat brain. *Hum. Gene Ther.*, **12**, 181–91.

Zou, L., Zhou, H., Pastore, L. & Yang, K. (2000). Prolonged transgene expression mediated by a helper-dependent adenoviral vector (hdAd) in the central nervous system. *Mol. Ther.*, **2**, 105–13.

Zufferey, R., Nagy, D., Mandel, R. J., Naldini, L. & Trono, D. (1997). Multiply attenuated lentiviral vector achieves efficient gene delivery in vivo. *Nat. Biotechnol.*, **15**, 871–5.

Zufferey, R., Dull, T., Mandel, R. J. *et al.* (1998). Self-inactivating lentivirus vector for safe and efficient in vivo gene delivery. *J. Virol.*, **72**, 9873–80.

Zufferey, R., Donello, J. E., Trono, D. & Hope, T. J. (1999). Woodchuck hepatitis virus posttranscriptional regulatory element enhances expression of transgenes delivered by retroviral vectors. *J. Virol.*, **73**, 2886–92.

23

Stem cells and cell-based therapy in neurodegenerative disease

Eva Chmielnicki[1] and Steven A. Goldman[2]

[1]Department of Neurology and Neuroscience, Cornell University Medical College, USA
[2]Department of Neurology, University of Rochester Medical Center, NY, USA

Neurodegenerative diseases are characterized by the gradual loss of functional neuronal populations within the nervous system (Cummings *et al.*, 1998; Jenner & Olanow, 1998; Kowall *et al.*, 1987). While all other organs of the body typically replace lost cells by proliferation and differentiation of resident tissue-specified stem cell populations, the adult central nervous system does not appear capable of regenerating dying neurons to any clinically significant degree. Historically, this inability of the mammalian nervous system to regenerate had led to the conclusion that the adult CNS did not contain competent neuronal progenitor or stem cells. However, a number of studies over the past two decades have refuted this dogma, by identifying significant and heterogeneous populations of both neural stem and progenitor cells in the adult brain (Altman & Das, 1966; Bayer *et al.*, 1982; Goldman & Nottebohm, 1983; Goldman *et al.*, 1992; Kirschenbaum *et al.*, 1994; Lois & Alvarez-Buylla, 1993; Luskin, 1993; Reynolds & Weiss, 1992; Richards *et al.*, 1992). These discoveries have led to the suggestion that induced compensatory neurogenesis by endogenous progenitor cells should be experimentally and therapeutically feasible, regardless of whether compensatory neurogenesis proves to be a natural occurrence of any clinical significance (Gage, 2000; Goldman *et al.*, 2002; Goldman & Luskin, 1998; Weiss *et al.*, 1996b). A number of recent studies have supported this concept, in that neurogenesis from resident progenitors has now been induced in the rodent forebrain in response to exogenous factor administration (Aberg *et al.*, 2000; Benraiss *et al.*, 2001; Chmielnicki & Goldman, 2002; Kuhn *et al.*, 1997; Pencea *et al.*, 2001), injury (Arvidsson *et al.*, 2002; Magavi *et al.*, 2000), or both (Fallon *et al.*, 2000; Nakatomi *et al.*, 2002).

This chapter will discuss the potential utility of both resident and introduced neural progenitor cells in the treatment of neurodegenerative disease. After presenting a synopsis of our current understanding of neural progenitor cell phenotypes in mammals, and of the persistence and distribution of each in adults, we will focus on transplant-based strategies for neural repair. We will then consider current strategies for inducing neuronal replacement from endogenous stem cells, and disease settings within which induced neuronal replacement might be therapeutically efficacious.

Neural stem cells of the mammalian forebrain

Tissue-specified stem cells are multipotential cells capable of giving rise to the resident phenotypes of a given organ, which retain the capacity for long-term self-renewal. Neural stem cells, the resident multipotential progenitors of the central nervous system, have been isolated from various regions of the fetal and adult mammalian nervous system (Gritti *et al.*, 1996; Kilpatrick & Bartlett, 1993; Palmer *et al.*, 1997; Reynolds & Weiss, 1992; Temple & Davis, 1994; Weiss *et al.*, 1996a). Neural stem cells can give rise to neural progenitor cells, which possess a more limited capacity for self-renewal, and may have a more restricted differentiation potential (Kilpatrick & Bartlett, 1995). These neural progenitors may include multipotential progenitors incapable of sustained self-renewal (Nunes *et al.*, 2003b), or committed neuronal (Luskin, 1998; Roy *et al.*, 2000a,b; Wang *et al.*, 2000) or glial progenitors (Rao & Mayer-Proschel, 1997).

To determine the lineage potential of putative stem and progenitor cells, single cells can be infected with a genetic tag, typically by means of a genomically integrating retroviral or lentiviral infection, and their progeny monitored for the expression of markers characteristic of oligodendrocytes, astrocytes, or neurons. In vitro, self-renewal capacity may be then monitored by clonal analysis, in which primary neurospheres derived from a single stem/progenitor cell are then re-dissociated to determine whether sphere-generating cells can be formed again from clonogenic founders (Morshead *et al.*, 1998; Reynolds & Weiss, 1996). By such clonal lineage analysis, resident multipotential neural progenitor cells have now been identified and isolated from both the fetal (Keyoung *et al.*, 2001; Uchida *et al.*, 2000) and adult human forebrain (Arsenijevic *et al.*, 2001; Nunes *et al.*, 2003b). In each, a mixture of uncommitted stem cells and phenotypically restricted progenitors appears to reside within the wall, in the ventricular/subventricular zone of fetal development, or in its adult derivative, the subependymal zone.

Neuronal progenitor cells of the adult brain

Three major populations of neural progenitor cells persist into adulthood: the subgranular zone in the dentate gyrus of the hippocampus, the subventricular zone (SVZ) of the lateral ventricle (Alvarez-Buylla *et al.*, 2000; Alvarez-Buylla & Lois, 1995; Goldman & Luskin, 1998; Palmer *et al.*, 1997), and the nominally glial progenitor pool of the brain parenchyma. Although the latter have traditionally been considered glial progenitors, these cells have recently been shown to be neurogenic as well. This population thus at least includes a pool of multipotential progenitors, and as such may serve as an additional source of neuronal progenitor cells in the adult brain. Among these diverse reservoirs of potentially neurogenic progenitors, only two pools appear to generate neuronally committed progenitors and their neuronal daughters in vivo in the adult. First, the subependymal zone of the anterior surface of the lateral ventricle (SVZa; Luskin, 1993) generates neurons that migrate in closely associated chains via the rostral migratory stream to the olfactory bulb, where they differentiate into GABAergic interneurons (Goldman & Luskin, 1998). Second, the progenitor pool of the hippocampal dentate gyrus, localized to the subgranular zone (SGZ) of the hippocampus, is similarly neurogenic, with neurons arising from what appear to be phenotypically restricted neuronal progenitors (Roy *et al.*, 2000a,b; Seaberg & van der Kooy, 2002). In both the forebrain SVZa and the hippocampal SGZ, however, residual multipotential stem cells can be demonstrated in vitro (Seri *et al.*, 2002), and likely give rise to the neuronally restricted progenitor pools of these loci. Thus, while potentially neurogenic progenitor cells are distributed throughout the rostral two-thirds of the SVZ, the regions of actual neuronal recruitment are very few and are segregated from one another (Kirschenbaum & Goldman, 1995). The establishment of neurogenesis in vivo in these few discrete niches, despite the prevalence and widespread distribution of potentially neurogenic progenitor cells, suggests the establishment and maintenance of discrete

niches for neurogenesis (Lim *et al.*, 2000; Louissaint *et al.*, 2002; Palmer *et al.*, 2000), similar to those that have been described for hematopoesis in the bone marrow (Lim *et al.*, 2000).

Stem cell-based transplant strategies in the neurodegenerative diseases

Derivation and expansion of implantable human neural stem cells

Neurogenesis persists through mid-gestational ontogeny in humans. The fetal human brain thus represents a plentiful source of both neural stem cells and more lineage-restricted neuronal and glial progenitor cells (Keyoung *et al.*, 2001). As a result, the implantation of both gross tissue dissociates and specifically extracted neural progenitors has become an important strategy for the experimental therapy of a variety of CNS disease models (Bjorklund & Lindvall, 2000). In addition, propagated neural stem cells have been derived from both fetal and adult human brain tissue (Arsenijevic *et al.*, 2001; Caldwell *et al.*, 2001; Keyoung *et al.*, 2001; Nunes *et al.*, 2003b; Pincus *et al.*, 1996; Roy *et al.*, 2000b; Svendsen *et al.*, 1999; Vescovi *et al.*, 1999). Each constitute a potential source of transplantable cells, since the persistent propagation and expansion of these cells mitigates the ongoing need for new tissue acquisition. If cultured in the presence of appropriate growth factor mitogens, such as fibroblast growth factor-2 (FGF-2) or epidermal growth factor (EGF), neural stem cells can be induced to divide (Gritti *et al.*, 1996; Kilpatrick & Bartlett, 1995). Importantly, propagated neural stem cells may be biased strongly towards neuronal differentiation and survival, most notably by the neurotrophins NT3 (Collazo *et al.*, 1992; Ghosh & Greenberg, 1995) and brain-derived neurotrophic factor (BDNF) (Ahmed *et al.*, 1995; Goldman *et al.*, 1997; Kirschenbaum & Goldman, 1995; Shetty & Turner, 1998). As a result, propagated neural stem cells may represent a renewable source from which to derive implantable neural cell populations.

Huntington's disease as a prototypic target for neural stem cell-based therapy

Among the degenerative disease targets of greatest interest for transplantation-based therapy has been Huntington's disease. Pathologically, this uniformly fatal condition is characterized by a progressive motor deficit resulting from the degeneration of neostriatal medium spiny neurons, and by severe cognitive and behavioral deficits accompanied by both cortical and subcortical neuronal loss (Kowall *et al.*, 1987). The motor deficits of Huntington's disease have been considered a feasible target for transplantation-based repair, because the region of relevant neuronal degeneration is initially delimited, both geographically and phenotypically, to the medium spiny neurons of the caudateputamen (Mitchell *et al.*, 1999). Huntington's disease is characterized by the expansion of CAG repeats in the Huntington's disease gene, resulting in long polyglutamine stretches that are toxic to their host neurons (Gusella *et al.*, 1983). Implanted wild-type cells may escape this CAG repeat-associated toxicity, since it appears to be cell-autonomous (Bjorklund & Lindvall, 2000), although deleterious effects of Huntington's disease cortical neurons on their striatal targets – including implanted wild-type neurons – may result from deficient neurotrophic support from the Huntington's disease cortical efferents (Canals *et al.*, 2001). Notwithstanding the latter caveat, several groups have attempted stem and progenitor cell transplantation as a strategy for treating Huntington's disease.

Initial attempts at stem and progenitor cell transplantation were in excitotoxic models of Huntington's disease, in which neuronal destruction was induced by intrastriatal injections of ibotenic acid (IA) (Isacson *et al.*, 1984). IA-lesioned rats exhibit motor abnormalities similar to those seen in Huntington's disease, and as such, represent a model whereby the effect of transplantation therapy on the motor deficit can be tested. On that basis, neural stem and progenitor cells derived and cultured from the embryonic rat striatum were grafted into IA-lesioned rats. The neurons that developed from these grafts were found to receive appropriate dopaminergic afferent connections from the host substantia nigra, and to make appropriate efferent connections to the globus pallidus and substantia nigra pars reticulata (Campbell *et al.*, 1993; Pritzel *et al.*, 1986). In addition, a significant attenuation of motor abnormalities was seen in IA-lesioned animals that received these striatal progenitor implants (Isacson *et al.*, 1984).

On the basis of these initial studies in rats, fetal striatal progenitor cells were then implanted into IA-lesioned primates. The implanted recipients were reported to exhibit a significant decrease in the incidence of abnormal motor behaviors, including dyskinesia, chorea and dystonia (Hantraye *et al.*, 1992). When fetal human striatal progenitor cells were also noted to ameliorate symptoms in IA-lesioned rats (Pundt *et al.*, 1996), human clinical trials were then initiated to assess the potential utility of progenitor transplantation in the treatment of Huntington's disease. In the first such study reported, an open-label unblinded and uncontrolled trial, human fetal neuronal progenitor cells derived from the ganglionic eminence were implanted bilaterally into the striata of five Huntington's disease patients. Two years after the initial grafting, motor and cognitive improvement was seen in three of the five (Bachoud-Levi *et al.*, 2000). Striatal glucose metabolism in these three patients remained steady or increased, as assessed by ^{18}F-fluorodeoxyglucose PET. Moreover, PET and MRI showed small regions of elevated metabolic activity, which suggested the presence of "metabolically active neural grafts" (Bachoud-Levi *et al.*, 2000). The improvement of these three patients compared with the progressive decline of a matched cohort of non-grafted control Huntington's disease patients, as well as with the two grafted patients who did not show any clinical benefit (Bachoud-Levi *et al.*, 2000). However, the unblinded nature and small size of this initial trial demands cautious interpretation. Tellingly, in a subsequent study in which seven patients received bilateral human fetal progenitor implants, three subjects experienced subdural hemorrhages, and no amelioration of Huntington's disease symptoms was observed (Hauser *et al.*, 2002).

Many variables may account for the overall lack of efficacy thus far observed in transplanted Huntington's disease in these patients. First, the donor cell populations used thus far have been notably heterogeneous. Human striatal primordia contain progenitor cells for a variety of neuronal cell types, including medium spiny projection neurons as well as striatal interneurons. As such, it has been unclear how many medium spiny cells at what developmental stages, and with what neuronal and glial accompaniments, have been implanted in the transplant trials thus far conducted. Furthermore, the adult human striatum may lack developmentally restricted signals necessary for the appropriate differentiation and functional integration of the implanted fetal progenitor cells. As such, the progenitor cells may have to be primed first in vitro before implantation.

These are approachable issues, which would bear further evaluation before future trials of experimental transplantation. For instance, transplant homogeneity, or at least high-grade enrichment, may now be achieved through several means of phenotypic selection. Techniques such as promoter-based antibiotic selection (Li *et al.*, 1998), or fluorescence-activated cell sorting (Keyoung *et al.*, 2001; Roy *et al.*, 2000b; Wang *et al.*, 2000), are readily adapted to the preimplantation enrichment of defined progenitor pools, such as those for medium spiny cells. That being said, it is not yet clear if purified cell populations are actually optimal as transplant vehicles, or whether instead mixed populations intentionally spiked with glial and endothelial elements might prove superior graft populations. To date, surprisingly few studies have systematically assessed the role of such variables in determining neural transplant efficacy.

For now then, the ability of implanted progenitors to restore normal structure and function to a region of brain disease or injury remains to be demonstrated in humans. Thus, although stem and progenitor cell transplantation may yet prove a useful modality for the treatment of Huntington's disease and PD, the need for developing alternative strategies for striatal restoration, such as inducing neurogenesis from endogenous progenitors (see below), has become clear.

Progenitor cell-mediated restoration of striatal dopamine: Parkinson's as a disease target

Fetal cell and tissue grafts have also been studied extensively in Parkinson's disease (Bjorklund & Lindvall, 2000). Several distinct strategies of introducing fetal mesencephalic grafts to the diseased striatum have been attempted, and each has thus far yielded disappointing results, characterized in broad terms by both unimpressive efficacy and overt iatrogenic morbidity. This is particularly disappointing since Parkinson's disease is a better-understood and anatomically more discrete degeneration than Huntington's. Parkinson's is characterized by the progressive deterioration of dopaminergic neurons in the substantia nigra (Jenner & Olanow, 1998). As these midbrain dopaminergic neurons project to the striatum, there is a significant decrease in striatal dopamine levels over time. Therapeutic transplantation has thus far focused on implantation of fetal ventral midbrain progenitor cells heterotopically into the neostriatum (Lindvall, 1999; Olanow et al., 1996). These donor dopaminergic neurons are able to ameliorate Parkinsonian symptoms only when a sufficient number of them survive, avoid immune rejection and make appropriate postsynaptic connections with striatal neurons (Bjorklund & Lindvall, 2000). Despite promising studies in experimental models, fetal mesencephalic tissue and cell grafts to adult Parkinson's patients have yielded poor results thus far, characterized by limited efficacy and significant morbidity, the latter manifested as refractory, medication-independent dyskinesias (Hagell et al., 2002). To date, the cause of these morbid side effects of dopaminergic engraftment is unclear, as is the overall lack of therapeutic efficacy of fetal mesencephalic transplantation, which has yielded limited benefit despite FDG-PET and histological data suggesting significant striatal dopaminergic engraftment (Hauser et al., 1999; Kordower et al., 1995, 1998).

The potential causes of this disappointment are legion; they include donor cell heterogeneity, inhomogeneities in the tissue distributions of the successfully implanted cells, a lack of appropriate afferent control, of the engrafted nigral cells, and disturbed presynaptic receptive thresholds on the part of the implanted dopaminergic cells, among others. At the very least though, the heterotopic nature of these grafts, which are delivered to the striatum rather than to their native substantia nigra, suggests that the implanted cells may fail to acquire appropriate afferent control. This, in turn, suggests that strategies based upon implanting dopaminergic neurons into diseased striatal targets, whether tissue or stem-cell derived, may be doomed to failure. Rather, in order to achieve physiologically appropriate dopaminergic function by engrafted cells, donor cells may need to be implanted into recipient substantia nigra. As a result, long-distance nigrostriatal axogenesis and reformation of the nigrostriatal tract may well be needed to assure proper regulation of the implanted dopaminergic cells. That being said, no technology currently permits the long-distance extension of tracts within the adult brain, at least not over the many cm distances that separate the ventral mesencephalon and the caudate-putamen. Until this capability is achieved, one must be circumspect about the potential for tissue or stem cell-derived dopaminergic neurons for safely mediating functional restoration in human Parkinson's disease.

Embryonic stem cells as a replenishable source of dopaminergic neurons

The failure of fetal nigral grafts to ameliorate Parkinson's disease symptoms or progression has, if anything, spurred research into generating more homogeneous and accessible populations of human dopaminergic neurons. Weaknesses of tissue-derived progenitor grafts included not only the heterogeneity of the implants, which included not only non-dopaminergic as well as dopaminergic neurons, but also both glial and vascular cells, all in relative proportions that varied from one donor to the next. Most troubling perhaps was the relatively low proportion of dopaminergic neurons in the mixture, which may have varied significantly as a function of the gestational age and dissection accuracy of each sample. These factors conspired to limit the extent to which one donor sample could be compared to the next, and made comparisons between recipient patients – whose variability was already high by virtue of their unique disease histories – difficult.

To address this issue of the non-uniformity of donor cell populations, and their minor representation of dopaminergic derivatives, a number of groups explored the possibility of generating highly enriched populations of dopaminergic neurons from mesencephalic progenitors (Sawamoto et al., 2001; Studer et al., 1998). These studies demonstrated that tissue-derived mesencephalic progenitors were capable of giving rise to functional dopaminergic neurons, in sufficient numbers and uniformity so as to permit the functional recovery of rats rendered Parkinsonian by 6-hydroxydopamine (6-OHDA) injection (Sawamoto *et al.*, 2001; Studer *et al.*, 1998). Yet enriching engraftable quantities of primary dopaminergic progenitors from human fetal tissue has proven difficult, because of both the small numbers of mesencephalic neural stem cells that may be purified as such from first trimester human abortuses, and the impracticability of high-volume sampling of human abortuses for this purpose.

To address these concerns, a number of groups have begun to assess the feasibility of using human embryonic stem cells as a potential source of dopaminergic progenitor cells. This possibility was opened by an elegant series of developmental studies, in which FGF8 and sonic hedgehog (SHH) were implicated as tandem initiators of dopaminergic neurogenesis during early midbrain development (Ye *et al.*, 1998). On this basis, McKay and colleagues first attempted to generate dopaminergic neurons from embryonic stem cells, by recapitulating the environment of the developing midbrain in vitro (Lee *et al.*, 2000). To this end, they added FGF8, SHH and ascorbate to cultures of embryonic stem cells. By this means, cultures were generated in which over 30% of the total neuronal population expressed tyrosine hydroxylase, a marker of catecholaminergic neurons (Lee *et al.*, 2000). In subsequent studies, these authors achieved even greater degrees of dopaminergic enrichment in ES culture by also mimicking the oxygen tension and redox state of the developing midbrain (Studer *et al.*, 2000). When implanted into 6OHDA-lesioned rats, in which nigrostriatal dopaminergic afferents are largely lost, these ES cells restored functional normalcy to the dopamine-depleted animals (Kim *et al.*, 2002). This result suggested that the dopaminergic neuronal cohort within the engrafted ES cell pool were at least sufficient to ameliorate the effects of catecholaminergic deafferentation on the adult rodent striatum. However, whether and to what degree the induction of dopaminergic phenotype is needed prior to implantation remains controversial, since naïve ES cells injected into the lesioned striatum may also become dopaminergic, and in sufficient numbers as to ameliorate amphetamine-induced rotational behavior after 6-OHDA lesion (Bjorklund *et al.*, 2002).

The use of ES cell-derived and FGF8/SHH-induced dopaminergic neurons, although both elegant and operationally significant, remains limited by some of the same caveats discussed in regards to tissue-derived progenitor implantation. First, the ES-derived dopaminergic cell populations achieved are by no means purified, and at the very least may be contaminated with serotonergic and GABAergic neurons, as well as by glia. Second, the cells must still be injected into the recipient striatum, given their apparent inability to extend processes through normal adult brain parenchyma. Other considerations unique to the use of ES cells may also limit the utility of directed dopaminergic differentiation. Induction of ventral midbrain phenotypes by FGF8/SHH is associated not only with dopaminergic neurogenesis, but also with the generation of GABAergic and serotonergic neurons (Goridis & Rohrer, 2002). The co-introduction of these other transmitter phenotypes, without further dopaminergic selection, might yield as yet unpredictable interactions among the engrafted cells, both synaptic and presynaptic. These interactions might serve at the very least to minimize the efficacy of the engrafted dopaminergic neurons. In addition, undifferentiated ES cells that have escaped the differentiating steps of embryoid body formation and FGF8/SHH induction may produce teratomas upon implantation, with such high frequency that their complete abolition from donor cell grafts would appear a reasonable prerequisite to the use of ES-derived dopaminergic neurons. The advent of promoter-based selection strategies, based on both GFP-based sorting and antibiotic selection (Wang *et al.*, 1998), has made high-grade purification of prospectively identified target phenotypes possible. Nonetheless, whether either of these approaches is sufficient to achieve the complete abolition of undesired phenotypes – such as undifferentiated ES cells – remains to be seen.

Stem and progenitor cell-mediated treatment of Alzheimer's and the cholinergic depletions

In Alzheimer's disease, degeneration of neurons in the basal forebrain cholinergic system, as well as in the cortex and hippocampus, results in a progressive dementia characterized by memory loss and dysphasia, often accompanied by personality changes and spatial disorientation (Cummings *et al.*, 1998). Since cholinergic neurons in the basal forebrain innervate the cortex and hippocampus, acetylcholine levels in these regions fall in Alzheimer's patients, and are inversely correlated with their degree of dementia (Wilcock *et al.*, 1982). As a result, central acetylcholinesterase inhibition has become the principal treatment for human Alzheimer's disease; the efficacy of this approach is limited, however, emphasizing the need for additional therapeutic strategies.

In animals, heterotopic transplantation of fetal forebrain cholinergic neurons into the neocortex results in significant behavioral improvements in animals subjected to lesions of the basal forebrain cholinergic projection, a traditional model of Alzheimer's disease (Dunnett, 1990; Fine *et al.*, 1985; Welner *et al.*, 1988). Despite these early promising studies, little effort has been made since to attempt the structural reconstitution of the basal forebrain cholinergic projection, even though subsequent studies served only to emphasize the importance of the cholinergic innervation of the neocortex to memory consolidation and recall (Winkler *et al.*, 1995). However, any past experimental therapeutic strategy based upon cholinergic progenitor implantation would have been limited by the unavailability of appropriately enriched populations of human cholinergic neuronal progenitors. Yet recent studies have begun to define the developmental environment in which cholinergic neurons are generated, with the intent of being able to selectively generate them from both embryonic and neural stem cells (Blackshaw & Cepko, 2002; Wu *et al.*, 2002).

Indeed, spinal motor neurons, another ventral cholinergic neuronal population, can already be specifically induced from undifferentiated ES cells, under the tandem influences of retinoic acid and sonic hedgehog activation (Wichterle *et al.*, 2002). These neurons, of critical importance in any cell-based strategy for treating amyotrophic lateral sclerosis and the primary motor neuron diseases, may share ontogenetic determinants with their more rostrally-situated forebrain counterparts. One might expect that as we better understand the patterning factors regulating cholinergic neurogenesis in the telencephalon, then basal forebrain cholinergic neurons may prove as amenable to in vitro production as their spinal counterparts. In addition, our evolving understanding of transcripts specifically expressed by developing cholinergic progenitors – forebrain as well as spinal – should permit their promoter-based isolation, from fetal tissue as well as from ES cell culture. The acquisition of cholinergic progenitor cells by either of these means – induction, selection, or both – may open up entirely new avenues in the treatment of diseases of the cholinergic neuron. Diseases as distinct yet related as the cortical dementias and ALS may prove approachable via cell-based therapy, as position-defined human cholinergic neuronal progenitors become available in both purity and quantity.

Neurogenesis from endogenous progenitor cells in the adult brain

Compensatory neurogenesis as a predictor of inducible neuronal replacement

As a result of the regionally heterogeneous nature of stem and progenitor cells within both the forebrain subependyma and hippocampal subgranular zone (Seaberg & van der Kooy, 2002), compensatory neurogenesis in response to injury or disease may be limited by the regionally-specified inhibition of migration, differentiation, or survival of SVZ progenitor cells and their neuronal progeny. That being said, examples now abound of such compensatory neurogenesis from resident progenitor cells in higher vertebrates. In birds, lesion of the adult song nucleus HVC, a highly neurogenic region of the songbird brain (Goldman, 1998; Goldman & Nottebohm, 1983), leads to compensatory neurogenesis with regeneration of lost HVC projection neurons to its efferent target, nucleus RA (Scharff *et al.*, 2000). In mice, similar phototoxic lesion of cortical callosal projection neurons leads to the recruitment of new cortical neurons, though in small numbers (Magavi *et al.*, 2000). Similarly, striatal neurogenesis has been demonstrated in response to middle cerebral artery occlusion, even though neither experimental nor clinical stroke appear to be associated with clinically significant neuronal replacement (Arvidsson *et al.*, 2002; Nakatomi *et al.*, 2002). Indeed, none of these mammalian instances of attempted compensatory neurogenesis appears to be of sufficient quantitative magnitude to afford clinical benefit. Yet infusion of neurotrophic mitogens during the degenerative process may potentiate the replenishment of the dying neurons, sufficiently so to yield significant structural and behavioral recovery. Nakatomi *et al.* (2002) reported in this regard that concurrent administration of FGF2 and EGF permitted the recruitment of new hippocampal pyramidal neurons after ischemia, in numbers sufficient to mediate both structural and behavioral recovery. Fallon and colleagues similarly demonstrated that concurrent administration of TGFα, a membrane-linked congener of EGF, was associated with compensatory striatal neurogenesis in response to 6-OHDA-induced nigrostriatal deafferentation (Fallon *et al.*, 2000). In this study, animals infused with TGFα after 6-OHDA lesion exhibited not only the local proliferation of SVZ cells, but also the directed migration of SVZ progeny to the TGFα infusion site. These cells expressed neuronal βIII-tubulin, and some co-expressed the dopamine transporter protein and tyrosine hydroxylase, markers of dopaminergic cells. Most remarkably, the TGFα-treated 6-OHDA-lesioned animals exhibited functional improvement in apomorphine-induced rotational behavior, that was significantly improved relative to that exhibited by their untreated controls. Thus, growth factor application in this disease environment resulted in the expansion and local recruitment of new neurons from SVZ progenitor cells (Fallon *et al.*, 2000). Together, these studies suggest that neuronal degeneration may be associated with the release of signals competent to induce otherwise latent local progenitor cells to generate new neurons able to replace their dying kindreds. They also show that the environment in which a progenitor resides might be dramatically changed in injury or disease, and that this alone may substantially alter the response of resident progenitor cells to both endogenous and introduced neurotrophic growth factors.

To capitalize upon the neurogenic capability of endogenous progenitor cells, several strategies have been proposed. First, redirection of SVZ progenitor-derived neurons from the olfactory stream to the septum and striatum have been employed to achieve neuronal recruitment to otherwise non-neurogenic regions of the adult forebrain (Nait-Oumesmar *et al.*, 1999; Parent *et al.*, 2002). Second, since the local recruitment and survival of newly generated neurons may be limited by the availability of postmitotic neurotrophic factors, the provision of these agents might achieve heterotopic neuronal addition in response to injury or disease (Benraiss *et al.*, 2001; Pencea *et al.*, 2001). Third, since most SVZ progenitor cells appear to give rise to glial cells, an inhibition of glial differentiation provided in tandem with neuronal instructive signals might provide another means by which to potentiate neuronal recruitment (Chmielnicki & Goldman, 2002; Lim *et al.*, 2000; Shah *et al.*, 1996). Indeed, recent evidence suggests that targeted ventricular administration of growth factors known to induce neuronal differentiation and survival from SVZ progenitors, as well as the redirected migration of their neuronal progeny, may be viable strategies for inducing neuronal replacement in the adult mammalian brain (Benraiss *et al.*, 2001; Pencea *et al.*, 2001).

Forebrain progenitor cells can be induced to expand and generate neurons in vivo

Neuroepithelial stem cells have been found to proliferate in response to EGF, FGF, or TGFα in vitro (Anchan *et al.*, 1991; Gensburger *et al.*, 1987; Reynolds *et al.*, 1992). On the basis of these studies, several groups have assessed the effects of these growth factors on mobilizing progenitor cell populations in the adult rodent SVZ (Craig *et al.*, 1996; Kuhn *et al.*, 1997). Intraventricular infusions of both EGF and FGF have each been found to increase SVZ cell proliferation. However, whereas EGF infusion has been associated only with astrocytic expansion, FGF does appear to increase neuronal addition to the olfactory bulb, a normally neurogenic region (Craig *et al.*, 1996; Kuhn *et al.*, 1997). Nonetheless, FGF administration has failed to induce the recruitment of neurons to any other regions of the adult forebrain. Thus, neither EGF nor FGF, at least when used in isolation, have yet proven useful in

inducing heterotopic neuronal addition to the uninjured brain.

In contrast, the neurotrophin BDNF has been found by several groups to induce heterotopic neuronal addition to the normal adult brain. In broad terms, members of the neurotrophin family, which includes NGF, BDNF, NT3, and NT4/5, are capable of enhancing progenitor-derived neuronal differentiation and/or survival throughout development, and over the entire geographic extent of the nervous system (Hyman *et al.*, 1991; Lindsay *et al.*, 1985; Tuszynski, 2000). On this basis, the specific role of neurotrophin family members on SVZ progenitor-derived neurogenesis and recruitment was assessed in explants of the adult rat SVZ. In this model, BDNF, but not NGF or NT3, promoted both the maturation and survival of SVZ-derived neurons in a dose-dependent fashion, for as long as 2 months in vitro (Kirschenbaum & Goldman, 1995). Accordingly, full-length trkB, the high affinity BDNF receptor, was heavily expressed by the SVZ progenitor-derived neurons. Since virtually none of these neurons incorporated [^{3}H]thymidine in vitro, BDNF appeared to exert its effects on the postmitotic neuronal progeny of SVZ cells, rather than upon the dividing progenitors themselves (Kirschenbaum & Goldman, 1995).

As further studies corroborated the role of BDNF as a differentiation and/or survival factor for neurons newly generated from the adult subependyma (Ahmed *et al.*, 1995; Shetty & Turner, 1998), an important question in the field became whether BDNF administration might mediate neuronal commitment and recruitment from SVZ progenitors in vivo. To address this issue, Zigova *et al.* (1998) postulated that intraventricular administration of BDNF protein would be sufficient to induce neuronal recruitment in vivo. They first established that full-length trkB is expressed in the SVZ and rostral migratory stream, suggesting that SVZ progenitors and their progeny would be BDNF responsive in vivo as in vitro. Zigova *et al.* (1998) then showed that intraventricular infusion of BDNF resulted in a doubling in the rate of addition of BrdU$^+$/βIII-tubulin$^+$ neurons to the olfactory bulb. These data demonstrated that the infusion of BDNF, a prototypic neurotrophic growth factor, could be used to augment neuronal addition to neurogenic regions of the adult CNS.

Intraventricular viral expression vectors can target subependymal progenitor cells

BDNF's potentiation of adult neuronal recruitment suggested the potential utility of maintaining BDNF administration over prolonged periods of time in vivo. Yet chronic infusion of proteins necessitates transcranial implantation of intraventricular mini-pumps, whose useful life is delimited by the quantity of protein that may be stored therein, the stability of that protein at body temperatures, and the inefficient bioavailability of protein delivered to the ventricular lumen. In addition, chronic infusion via minipump is a more practicable experimental than clinical strategy for drug delivery, since chronic intraventricular protein administration to adult patients may be complicated by both infection and catheter occlusion, both of which typically limit the effective life of ventricular catheters. Parenchymal protein delivery is not a viable option for targeting subependymal progenitor cells with neurotrophins. Subependymal cells and subventricular glia express high amounts of truncated trkB, which limit the access of parenchymally-delivered BDNF access to the subventricular zone progenitor population (Biffo *et al.*, 1995; Yan *et al.*, 1994). Thus, too much brain tissue would be nonspecifically and unnecessarily accessed by the delivered drug, while the periventricular target region would be insufficiently accessed.

To devise a better means of protein delivery to the restricted region of the subependymal cell population, we chose to infect the ependymal wall with a replication-defective adenovirus engineered to overexpress the gene encoding BDNF (AdBDNF) (Bajocchi *et al.*, 1993; Yoon *et al.*, 1996). By this means, the ventricular wall was subrogated to serve as a secretory source of high levels of BDNF for the subependymal progenitor population – thereby utilizing the transduced ependymal layer as a drug delivery vehicle, yet without having to transduce the progenitors themselves. As a proof-of-principle, AdBDNF, containing hGFP as a reporter gene, was injected into the lateral ventricles of adult rats. *In situ* hybridization of sagittal brain sections three weeks after the adenoviral injections showed that BDNF mRNAs were restricted to the ventricular wall (Benraiss *et al.*, 2001). The selective targeting of viral transgene expression to the ventricular wall was thus accomplished by the spatial restriction of adenoviral infection, which was limited to the ependymal cells. ELISA then confirmed that while BDNF was undetectable in the CSF of control rats, the AdBDNF-injected animals averaged >2 ng BDNF/ml (Benraiss *et al.*, 2001), a level sufficient to elicit neurotrophic effects in vitro (Kirschenbaum & Goldman, 1995; Lindsay *et al.*, 1994). CSF BDNF levels remained elevated relative to controls for up to 2 months after injection, with a steady decline in the second month. Thus, a single intraventricular injection of an adenoviral vector proved able to target viral transgene expression to the ventricular wall, effectively recruiting the ventricular ependyma to serve as a source of a secreted protein intended to activate subependymal progenitor cells (Benraiss *et al.*, 2001).

This strategy may be extended to include serial infections by different viruses, encoding transgenes that sequentially influence SVZ progenitor division, differentiation, neurotransmitter phenotype, migration, and neurite extension. By so doing, we may hope to direct neuronal recruitment and fiber projection to pre-specified targets in the injured or diseased brain.

BDNF overexpression induces heterotopic neuronal recruitment to the adult neostriatum

On this basis, Benraiss *et al.* (2001) then asked if the periventricular overexpression of BDNF might be associated with neuronal recruitment to otherwise non-neurogenic regions of the adult brain, such as the striatum and cortex. They assessed whether adenovirally delivered BDNF stimulated the production of new neurons in nominally non-neurogenic brain regions, by tagging mitotic SVZ progenitor cells with bromodeoxyuridine (BrdU), a thymidine analogue, and then following these BrdU-tagged SVZ cells after either AdBDNF or control AdNull injection. In particular, all BrdU-tagged cortical, septal and striatal cells were individually assessed for their expression of neuron-specific markers. Whereas no BrdU$^+$/βIII-tubulin$^+$ cells were found in the septum or cortex of AdBDNF-injected animals, the neostriata of these animals harbored >140 newly generated neurons/mm3. This contrasted to the absence of any such neuronal addition to the striata of animals that had received PBS as a control (Benraiss *et al.*, 2001).

Thus, adenoviral overexpression of BDNF led to the induction of neuronal addition to the adult neostriatum. BDNF's effect in this regard appeared to derive from its signaling of neuronal differentiation and survival (Ahmed *et al.*, 1995; Kirschenbaum & Goldman, 1995), as well as its direct promotion of migration into the subjacent parenchyma (Behar *et al.*, 1997; Borghesani *et al.*, 2002). Of note, Luskin and colleagues similarly demonstrated that chronic intraventricular infusions of BDNF protein yielded striatal neurogenesis (Pencea *et al.*, 2001). Using much larger effective doses of BDNF than those used by Benraiss *et al.* (100 μg/ml CSF, in contrast to the 2 ng/ml achieved in the CSF of rats given AdBDNF), Pencea *et al.* noted other sites of heterotopic subcortical neurogenesis. These included the otherwise non-neurogenic septum and thalamus, as well as the hypothalamus. The latter observation, if otherwise confirmed, opens the possibility that broader subcortical neurogenesis may be achieved through the parenchymal delivery or overexpression of BDNF.

Induced neurogenesis may be a therapeutic strategy in animal models of Huntington's disease

The BDNF-induced addition of new neurons to the adult neostriatum may prove of specific therapeutic interest in regards to Huntington's disease. Huntington's disease is characterized by the gradual loss of striatal medium spiny neurons (Mitchell *et al.*, 1999). BDNF overexpression has already been found to decrease striatal neuronal loss in animal models of Huntington's disease (Martinez-Serrano and Bjorklund, 1996; Perez-Navarro *et al.*, 2000), an effect that has been attributed to the improved survival of BDNF-exposed striatal neurons. Yet since BDNF overexpression can also induce the addition of new neurons to the adult neostriatum, we postulated that it might be competent to induce the specific replacement of striatal neurons lost to Huntington's disease. We further postulated that new neurons arising from the endogenous progenitor pool of the striatal subependyma might contribute meaningfully to the BDNF-associated attenuation of neuronal loss that had previously been noted in experimental Huntington's disease, and which had been attributed to the trophic dependence of DARPP32$^+$ medium spiny cells upon BDNF (Nakao *et al.*, 1995; Ivkovic & Ehrlich, 1999; Ivkovic *et al.*, 1997).

A key assumption of these postulates is that a significant portion of newly generated striatal neurons must integrate as medium spiny neurons, the major striatal victim of Huntington's disease, which normally serve as the pallidal projection neuron of the caudate-putamen. Benraiss *et al.* (2001) first reported that most AdBDNF-induced striatal neurons in adult rats, as defined by their incorporation of BrdU and co-expression of neuronal antigens, indeed expressed the phenotypic markers characteristic of medium spiny neurons. Moreover, these investigators reported that the overwhelming majority of AdBDNF-induced neurons were recruited as MSNs. Perhaps this should not have been surprising: Although the neostriatum includes a complex array of phenotypes, the overwhelming majority of caudate-putamen neurons are GABAergic medium spiny projection neurons to the globus pallidus (Mitchell *et al.*, 1999). These cells are defined by their expression of calbindin, a calcium binding protein, and DARPP-32, a dopamine- and cAMP-regulated phosphoprotein (Ouimet *et al.*, 1998). Thus, BDNF appeared to play an important role not only in the recruitment of new neurons from striatal precursors, but in their specific recruitment as medium spiny cells. As such, most BrdU$^+$ cells in AdBDNF-treated brains co-expressed GAD, calbindin, and/or DARPP-32, prototypic markers of these cells

(Benraiss *et al.*, 2001). Together, these observations suggest that BDNF overexpression may be a viable means of triggering the addition of new medium spiny neurons to the adult neostriatum.

Thus far, the effect of BDNF overexpression in experimental Huntington's disease has only been assessed in a single transgenic line, that of the R6-2 mouse. R6-2 is a relatively dramatic model of Huntington's disease, in which the affected mice harbor a roughly 150-polyglutamine repeat in the huntingtin gene (Mangiarini *et al.*, 1996; Samdani *et al.*, 2002). Their disease course is truncated such that they become symptomatically ill by 6–8 weeks of age, and typically die by 12–14 weeks. When these mice were treated with AdBDNF, a substantial number of BrdU/βIII-tubulin$^+$-defined newly generated neurons were recruited to their neostriata. These newly-generated neurons expressed DARPP-32 as well as other markers of medium spiny neurons. In addition, they were found to backfill with FluoroGold introduced into the globus pallidus, indicating their establishment of appropriate efferent connections. These observations suggested to us that the functional replacement of striatal cells lost in Huntington's disease might be accomplished through such a strategy of induced medium spiny neurogenesis (Mitchell *et al.*, 1999). Although the critical studies testing this hypothesis are ongoing, preliminary studies strongly suggest that AdBDNF-induced striatal neuronal recruitment from endogenous progenitor cells may prove a viable experimental therapeutic strategy for Huntington's disease.

Synergistic strategies for inducing striatal neurogenesis from endogenous progenitor cells

Striatal neuronal addition may therefore be accomplished through the BDNF-mediated mobilization and neuronal differentiation of SVZ progenitor cells. Yet as a corollary strategy, the inhibition of glial differentiation by SVZ cells may also serve to enhance neuronal production from endogenous progenitor cells. Several agents have been shown to induce astroglial differentiation from VZ progenitor cells in vitro (Hughes *et al.*, 1988; Lillien *et al.*, 1988). The bone morphogenetic proteins (BMPs) in particular have been found to instruct late fetal VZ progenitors to the glial lineage (Mehler *et al.*, 2000). Since both the BMPs and their receptors are present in high concentrations in the adult forebrain subependyma, the abrogation of BMP signaling by these cells might effectively inhibit astroglial differentiation, allowing instead neuronal differentiation (Gross *et al.*, 1996). On this basis, we postulated that the glial differentiation of ventricular zone progenitor cells might be disrupted and the cells redirected to neuronal lineage, if the dividing progenitors and their daughters were exposed to a suitable neuronal differentiation agent during glial suppression.

To test this hypothesis, noggin protein was overexpressed, with the intention of actively suppressing glial differentiation. Noggin is one of a class of diffusible competitive antagonists that prevent BMPs from binding to their receptors (Zimmerman et al., 1996). It is synthesized tonically in neurogenic regions of the adult rat SVZ (Lim et al., 2000), and may provide a critical aspect of the periventricular niche for adult neurogenesis. We found that ventricular noggin overexpression indeed led to a substantial fall in gliogenesis within the adult subependyma, and was associated with a sharp and concomitant increase in olfactory neuronal recruitment from the SVZ. Moreover, this effect was accentuated by BDNF overexpression, such that the concurrent suppression of gliogenesis and promotion of neuronal differentiation by SVZ progenitor cells proved a powerful means of potentiating neuronal addition to both the neostriatum and olfactory bulb in vivo. Indeed, intraventricular noggin and BDNF co-overexpression resulted in a two- to threefold increase in the number of new neurons recruited in response to BDNF alone (Chmielnicki et al., 2001). As in response to BDNF alone, most of these noggin/BDNF-stimulated neurons were recruited as medium spiny neurons, and projected to the globus pallidus. In light of BDNF and noggin's collaborative effects on striatal SVZ progenitor cells, their co-overexpression would seem a reasonable strategy by which to induce and maximize neuronal addition to the diseased Huntington's neostriatum.

Additional strategies for mobilizing striatal progenitor cells

A variety of soluble differentiation agents may prove suitable candidates for inducing neuronal addition to the adult neostriatum. EGF- or FGF-mediated expansion of endogenous progenitor cells may potentiate neuronal replacement in the presence of permissive signals for neuronal differentiation (Kuhn et al., 1997). This may occur in the setting of injury, or in concert with factors such as BDNF, which can independently stimulate neuronal recruitment from endogenous progenitor cells (Benraiss et al., 2001). TGFα has also been shown to achieve a similar effect in the adult striatum, in which TGFα exposure in the setting of catecholaminergic cell injury appears sufficient to induce the heterotopic recruitment of new dopaminergic neurons to the striatum (Fallon et al., 2000).

Among agents not yet studied in the context of striatal regeneration, IGF1 may have particular promise as a co-agonist for neuronal recruitment. IGF1, classically designated as somatomedin C, has been found to be an important agent in neuronal recruitment in both adult birds (Jiang et al., 1997) and rodents (Arsenijevic & Weiss, 1998; Brooker et al., 2000; Jiang et al., 1998). IGF-1 mutant mice display neocortical hypoplasia despite a thickening of the VZ, while transgenic IGF1-overexpressors display neocortical hyperplasia (D'Ercole, 1993). In addition, IGF1 is expressed selectively by neurogenic radial cells of the adult avian forebrain, and its addition to explants of the neurogenic ventricular zone substantially increases in vitro neuronal recruitment (Jiang et al., 1998). As noted, IGF1 mobilizes endogenous dentate progenitors, and can thereby potentiate hippocampal neurogenesis (Aberg et al., 2000). Moreover, since IGF1 induces expression of trkB in SVZ progenitor cells (Arsenijevic & Weiss, 1998), mmIGF and BDNF might operate synergistically to induce neuronal production from resident progenitors of the adult striatum, as they appear to do in vitro (E. Chmielnicki, Harrison & S. A. Goldman, unpublished data). Together, these data across multiple species and models suggest that IGF1 overexpression might stimulate or enhance neuronal production from SVZ progenitor cells (Arsenijevic & Weiss, 1998; Liu et al., 1993). Accordingly, the co-expression of these two agents might be predicted to enhance the induction of striatal neurons from resident VZ progenitor cells. Since IGF1 and noggin-mediated enhancement of BDNF's induced-neuronal recruitment appear to utilize different mechanisms, the concurrent overexpression of all three of these agents may prove a viable means of achieving clinically useful numbers of neurons to the diseased adult neostriatum.

Beyond the VZ: induction of non-striatal progenitor cell pools

Induction of resident progenitors as a means of restoring dopaminergic input to the striatum

Just as in Huntington's disease, nigral neurons lost to Parkinson's disease might optimally be regenerated from a patient's own store of endogenous progenitors, rather than delivered as an allograft. But in regions discontiguous with a source of ventricular zone progenitors, it remains unclear whether an inductive approach to regeneration is biologically feasible. The mesencephalic ventricular zone continues to harbor neural stem cells (Weiss et al., 1996a,b), and these are especially biased towards dopaminergic neurogenesis (Sawamoto et al., 2001). When isolated and expanded in vitro, mesencephalic neural stem cells give rise to dopaminergic neurons in sufficient numbers and proportions that they may be used to restore dopaminergic innervation to the 6-OHDA-lesioned striatum. Nonetheless, no means of inducing the endogenous mesencephalic stem cell pool to *in situ* neurogenesis has yet been identified, so that no strategy of induced neuronal recruitment comparable to that established in the neostriatum has yet been defined.

As an alternative approach, a number of groups have begun to focus on inducing dopaminergic neurogenesis from resident progenitors within the parenchyma of the substantia nigra. As noted, parenchymal progenitor cells able to generate neurons persist throughout the adult brain (Kondo & Raff, 2000; Palmer *et al.*, 1997), in humans as well as in rodents (Nunes *et al.*, 2003a). These cells persist in the substantia nigra (Lie *et al.*, 2002) as well as the forebrain, and can readily be stimulated to generate neurons, despite their nominally glial phenotype in vivo. However, whether these cells may be induced to generate neurons in vivo remains unknown, and moreover, whether they may be stimulated specifically to generate dopaminergic neurons is even more problematic. While astrocytes derived from fetal ventral mesencephalon have been shown to potentiate the maturation of dopaminergic neurons (Johansson & Stromberg, 2002), specific factors that are necessary and sufficient for dopaminergic induction from parenchymal progenitors have not yet been elucidated. As noted previously, embryonic stem cells can be induced to differentiate as dopaminergic neurons upon treatment with SHH and FGF8, and these cells can ameliorate amphetamine-induced rotational behavior in an animal model of Parkinson's disease (Kim *et al.*, 2002). One might predict that the co-overexpression of FGF8 and SHH in the ventral midbrain might induce dopaminergic differentiation from neural progenitor cells in the substantia nigra. However, whether these parenchymal progenitors may respond to the same signals as their much less differentiated ES cells counterparts is unknown. Moreover, one can only presume that additional factors may prove necessary to guide the axons of any such newly generated nigral neurons to their neostriatal targets.

Progenitor stimulation as a restorative strategy for the hippocampal atrophies

The adult dentate gyrus exhibits persistent constitutive neurogenesis throughout life in animals and appears to do so as well in humans (Altman & Das, 1965; Eriksson *et al.*, 1998; Roy *et al.*, 2000b), although the natural history of hippocampal neurogenesis in adult humans remains largely unexplored. New neurons are added to the adult dentate from progenitors in the subgranular zone of the hippocampus, a layer which is developmentally contiguous with the most posterior reaches of the subependymal zone of the lateral ventricle (Gage *et al.*, 1998). The subgranular zone progenitors appear committed to neuronal phenotype, although they may derive from less committed multipotential progenitors (Seaberg & van der Kooy, 2002). The regulatory control of these cells remains unclear. Although they respond to both FGF2 and IGF1 with mitotic expansion, neither of these agents seems to exert robust effects in vivo, although their relative potency may increase in the setting of antecedent factor depletion or injury (Aberg *et al.*, 2000; Palmer *et al.*, 1995). Sonic hedgehog, a prototypic morphogen more often implicated in phenotypic induction and regionalization of the developing nervous system, also appears able to regulate both the proliferation and differentiation of adult neural progenitor cells (Rowitch *et al.*, 1999). SHH remains active in the adult forebrain, where it is transported from the septum to the hippocampus, in which it appears to regulate neurogenesis from endogenous subgranular progenitor cells (Lai *et al.*, 2003). Other than SHH though, little has been learned of protein growth factors necessary or sufficient for hippocampal neurogenesis in vivo.

Besides the peptide growth factors, hippocampal neurogenesis may be normally regulated – and therefore potentially modified – by a great number of pharmacological agents and processes. Negative regulators of hippocampal neurogenesis include stress, corticosteroids, and alcohol, all of which may be associated with deficits in memory acquisition and storage (Cameron & Gould, 1994; Gould *et al.*, 1992; Nixon & Crews, 2002; Pham *et al.*, 2003). Positive regulators include environmental enrichment, exercise, and serotonin agonists, all of which have been associated with mood elevation and improved cognitive performance in a variety of memory-dependent tasks (Brezun & Daszuta, 2000; Gould, 1999; Nilsson *et al.*, 1999; van Praag *et al.*, 1999). The malleability of hippocampal neurogenesis in adult animals, and the persistence of competent dentate neuronal progenitors in the adult human hippocampus, argue that therapeutic stimulation of endogenous progenitor cells in the adult human hippocampus should be feasible. Current investigation is proceeding on precisely those lines with regards to the potentiation of hippocampal neurogenesis by serotonin reuptake inhibitors (Malberg *et al.*, 2000). Such an approach may prove beneficial not only in the affective disorders, but also as adjunctive therapy in the degenerative dementias associated with hippocampal atrophy.

Conclusions

Neural stem and progenitor cells comprise a potential source of new neurons to replace those lost in neurodegenerative diseases. Both transplanted and endogenous progenitor cells can be induced to divide, differentiate as neurons, survive and make appropriate postsynaptic and presynaptic connections. Experimentally, both implanted and resident progenitor cells have proved able to replace neurons lost to either experimental injury or disease. Yet the marginal results of neural cell and tissue grafts in Parkinson's disease provide a cautionary tale, and serve to remind clinicians of the unpredictable nature of perturbing the circuitry of the adult brain. To be sure, contemporary advances in both embryonic and neural stem cell biology, as well as in targeted progenitor isolation, serve to assure us more uniform and well-characterized populations of donor cells for future engraftment studies. Nonetheless, the compromised and compensated neural circuits of the diseased brain may prove even more fragile and prone to iatrogenic disruption than their healthy counterparts. As such, the future may prove brighter for strategies intended to induce endogenous progenitor cells. The studies discussed in the latter half of this chapter suggest that targeted periventricular delivery of diffusible factors, rationally designed to capitalize upon the known responsiveness of resident progenitor cells, will prove a viable strategy for inducing neuronal production from endogenous progenitor cells in the adult mammalian brain.

Acknowledgements

Dr. Goldman is supported by the NIH, the Cure Huntington's disease Project of the Hereditary Disease Foundation, Project ALS, the Michael J. Fox Foundation, the National Multiple Sclerosis Society, the Christopher Reeve Paralysis Foundation, the New York State Spinal Cord Research Program, and Aventis Pharmaceuticals.

REFERENCES

Aberg, M., Aberg, D., Hedbacker, H., Oscarsson, J. & Eriksson, P. (2000). Peripheral infusion of IGF-1 selectively induces neurogenesis in the adult rat hippocampus. *J. Neurosci.*, **20**, 2896–903.

Ahmed, S., Reynolds, B. A. & Weiss, S. (1995). BDNF enhances the differentiation but not the survival of CNS stem cell-derived neuronal precursors. *J. Neurosci.*, **15**, 5765–78.

Altman, J. & Das, G. D. (1965). Autoradiographic and histological evidence of postnatal hippocampal neurogenesis in rats. *J. Comp. Neurol.*, **124**, 319–35.

Altman, J. & Das, G. D. (1966). Autoradiographic and histological studies of postnatal neurogenesis. I. A longitudinal investigation of the kinetics, migration and transformation of cells incorporating tritiated thymidine in neonate rats, with special reference to postnatal neurogenesis in some brain regions. *J. Comp. Neurol.*, **127**, 337–90.

Alvarez-Buylla, A., Herrera, D. G. & Wichterle, H. (2000). The subventricular zone: source of neuronal precursors for brain repair. *Prog. Brain Res.*, **127**, 1–11.

Alvarez-Buylla, A. & Lois, C. (1995). Neuronal stem cells in the brain of adult vertebrates. *Stem Cells*, **13**, 263–72.

Anchan, R. M., Reh, T. A., Angello, J., Balliet, A. & Walker, M. (1991). EGF and TGF-alpha stimulate retinal neuroepithelial cell proliferation in vitro. *Neuron*, **6**, 923–36.

Arsenijevic, Y., Villemure, J., Brunet, J. *et al.* (2001). Isolation of multipotent neural precursors residing in the cortex of the adult human brain. *Exp. Neurol.*, **170**, 48–62.

Arsenijevic, Y. & Weiss, S. (1998). Insulin-like growth factor-I is a differentiation factor for postmitotic CNS stem cell-derived neuronal precursors: distinct actions from those of brain-derived neurotrophic factor. *J. Neurosci.*, **18**, 2118–28.

Arvidsson, A., Collin, T., Kirik, D., Kokaia, Z. & Lindvall, O. (2002). Neuronal replacement from endogenous precursors in the adult brain after stroke. *Nat. Med.*, **8**, 963–70.

Bachoud-Levi, A. C., Remy, P., Nguyen, J. P. *et al.* (2000). Motor and cognitive improvements in patients with Huntington's disease after neural transplantation. *Lancet*, **356**, 1975–9.

Bajocchi, G., Feldman, S., Crystal, R. & Mastrangeli, A. (1993). Direct in vivo gene transfer to ependymal cells in the central nervous system using recombinant adenovirus vectors. *Nat. Genet.*, **3**, 229–34.

Bayer, S., Yackel, J. & Puri, P. (1982). Neurons in the rat dentate gyrus granular layer substantially increase during juvenile and adult life. *Science*, **216**, 890–2.

Behar, T., Dugich-Djordjevic, Li, Y. *et al.* (1997). Neurotrophins stimulate chemotaxis of embryonic cortical neurons. *Eur. J. Neurosci.*, **9**, 2561–70.

Benraiss, A., Chmielnicki, E., Lerner, K., Roh, D. & Goldman, S. A. (2001). Adenoviral brain-derived neurotrophic factor induces both neostriatal and olfactory neuronal recruitment from endogenous progenitor cells in the adult forebrain. *J. Neurosci.*, **21**, 6718–31.

Biffo, S., Offenhauser, N., Carter, B. D. & Barde, Y. A. (1995). Selective binding and internalisation by truncated receptors restrict the availability of BDNF during development. *Development*, **121**, 2461–70.

Bjorklund, A. & Lindvall, O. (2000). Cell replacement therapies for central nervous system disorders. *Nat. Neurosci.*, **3**, 537–44.

Bjorklund, L., Sanchez-Pernaute, R., Chung, S. *et al.* (2002). Embryonic stem cells develop into functional dopaminergic neurons after transplantation in a Parkinson rat model. *Proc. Natl Acad. Sci., USA*, **99**, 2344–9.

Blackshaw, S. & Cepko, C. (2002). Stem cells that know their place. *Nat. Neurosci.*, **5**, 1251–2.

Borghesani, P. R., Peyrin, J. M., Klein, R. *et al*. (2002). BDNF stimulates migration of cerebellar granule cells. *Development*, **129**, 1435–42.

Brezun, J. & Daszuta, A. (2000). Serotonin may stimulate granule cell proliferation in the adult hippocampus, as observed in rats grafted with foetal raphe neurons. *Eur. J. Neurosci.*, **12**, 391–6.

Brooker, G. J., Kalloniatis, M., Russo, V. C., Murphy, M., Werther, G. A. & Bartlett, P. F. (2000). Endogenous IGF-1 regulates the neuronal differentiation of adult stem cells. *J. Neurosci. Res.*, **59**, 332–41.

Caldwell, M. A., He, X., Wilkie, N. *et al*. (2001). Growth factors regulate the survival and fate of cells derived from human neurospheres. *Nat. Biotechnol.*, **19**, 475–9.

Cameron, H. & Gould, E. (1994). Adult neurogenesis is regulated by adrenal steroids in the dentate gyrus. *Neuroscience*, **61**, 203–9.

Campbell, K., Kalen, P., Wictorin, K., Lundberg, C., Mandel, R. J. & Bjorklund, A. (1993). Characterization of GABA release from intrastriatal striatal transplants: dependence on host-derived afferents. *Neuroscience*, **53**, 403–15.

Canals, J., Checa, N., Marco, S. *et al*. (2001). Expression of BDNF in cortical neurons is regulated by striatal target area. *J. Neurosci.* **21**, 117–24.

Chmielnicki, E., Benraiss, A., Rosenow, J. *et al*. (2001). Adenoviral infection of the adult rat ventricular zone to overexpress noggin and BDNF increases neuronal recruitment from endogenous progenitor cells. *Soc. Neurosci. Abstr.*, 361–4.

Chmielnicki, E. & Goldman, S. A. (2002). Induced neurogenesis by endogenous progenitor cells in the adult mammalian brain. *Prog. Brain Res.*, **138**, 451–64.

Collazo, D., Takahashi, H. & McKay, R. D. (1992). Cellular targets and trophic functions of neurotrophin-3 in the developing rat hippocampus. *Neuron*, **9**, 643–56.

Craig, C. G., Tropepe, V., Morshead, C. M., Reynolds, B. A., Weiss, S. & van der Kooy, D. (1996). In vivo growth factor expansion of endogenous subependymal neural precursor cell populations in the adult mouse brain. *J. Neurosci.*, **16**, 2649–58.

Cummings, J. L., Vinters, H. V., Cole, G. M. & Khachaturian, Z. S. (1998). Alzheimer's disease: etiologies, pathophysiology, cognitive reserve, and treatment opportunities. *Neurology*, **51**, S2–17; discussion S65–17.

D'Ercole, A. J. (1993). Expression of insulin-like growth factor-I in transgenic mice. *Ann. NY Acad. Sci.*, **692**, 149–60.

Dunnett, S. (1990). Neural transplantation in animal models of dementia. *Eur. J. Neurosci.*, **2**, 567–87.

Eriksson, P. S., Perfilieva, E., Bjork-Eriksson, T. *et al*. (1998). Neurogenesis in the adult human hippocampus. *Nat. Med.*, **4**, 1313–17.

Fallon, J., Reid, S., Kinyamu, R. *et al*. (2000). In vivo induction of massive proliferation, directed migration, and differentiation of neural cells in the adult mammalian brain. *Proc. Natl Acad. Sci., USA*, **97**, 14686–91.

Fine, A., Dunnett, S. B., Bjorklund, A. *et al*. (1985). Cholinergic ventral forebrain grafts into the neocortex improve passive avoidance memory in a rat model of Alzheimer disease. *Proc. Natl Acad. Sci., USA*, **82**, 5227–30.

Gage, F. (2000). Mammalian neural stem cells. *Science*, **287**, 1433–8.

Gage, F. H., Kempermann, G., Palmer, T. D., Peterson, D. A. & Ray, J. (1998). Multipotent progenitor cells in the adult dentate gyrus. *J. Neurobiol.*, **36**, 249–66.

Gensburger, C., Labourdette, G. & Sensenbrenner, M. (1987). Brain basic fibroblast growth factor stimulates the proliferation of rat neuronal precursor cells in vitro. *FEBS Lett.*, **217**, 1–5.

Ghosh, A. & Greenberg, M. (1995). Distinct roles for bFGF and NT3 in the regulation of neurogenesis. *Neuron*, **15**, 89–103.

Goldman, S. (1998). Adult neurogenesis: from canaries to the clinic. *J. Neurobiol.*, **36**, 267–86.

Goldman, S., Benraiss, A., Chmielnicki, E. *et al*. (2002). Isolation and induction of adult neural progenitor cells. *Clin. Neurosci. Res.*, **2**, 70–9.

Goldman, S. A., Kirschenbaum, B., Harrison-Restelli, C. & Thaler, H. T. (1997). Neuronal precursors of the adult rat subependymal zone persist into senescence, with no decline in spatial extent or response to BDNF. *J. Neurobiol.*, **32**, 554–66.

Goldman, S. A. & Luskin M. B. (1998). Strategies utilized by migrating neurons of the postnatal vertebrate forebrain. *Trends Neurosci.*, **21**, 107–14.

Goldman, S. A. & Nottebohm, F. (1983). Neuronal production, migration, and differentiation in a vocal control nucleus of the adult female canary brain. *Proc. Natl. Acad. Sci., USA*, **80**, 2390–4.

Goldman, S. A., Zaremba, A. & Niedzwiecki, D. (1992). In vitro neurogenesis by neuronal precursor cells derived from the adult songbird brain. *J. Neurosci.*, **12**, 2532–41.

Goridis, C. & Rohrer, H. (2002). Specification of catecholaminergic and serotonergic neurons. *Nat. Neurosci.*, **3**, 531–41.

Gould, E. (1999). Serotonin and hippocampal neurogenesis. *Neuropsychopharmacology*, **21**, 46S–51S.

Gould, E., Cameron, H., Daniels, D., Wooley, C. & McEwen, B. (1992). Adrenal hormones suppress cell division in the adult rat dentate gyrus. *J. Neurosci.*, **12**, 3642–50.

Gritti, A., Parati, E. A., Cova, L. *et al*. (1996). Multipotential stem cells from the adult mouse brain proliferate and self-renew in response to basic fibroblast growth factor. *J. Neurosci.*, **16**, 1091–100.

Gross, R. E., Mehler, M. F., Mabie, P. C., Zang, Z., Santschi, L. & Kessler, J. A. (1996). Bone morphogenetic proteins promote astroglial lineage commitment by mammalian subventricular zone progenitor cells. *Neuron*, **17**, 595–606.

Gusella, J., Wexler, N., Conneally, P. *et al*. (1983). A polymorphic DNA marker genetically linked to Huntington's disease. *Nature*, **306**, 234–8.

Hagell, P., Piccini, P., Bjorklund, A. *et al*. (2002). Dyskinesias following neural transplantation in Parkinson's disease. *Nat. Neurosci.*, **5**, 627–8.

Hantraye, P., Riche, D., Maziere, M. & Isacson, O. (1992). Intrastriatal transplantation of cross-species fetal striatal cells reduces abnormal movements in a primate model of Huntington disease. *Proc. Natl Acad. Sci., USA*, **89**, 4187–91.

Hauser, R., Freeman, T., Snow, B. *et al.* (1999). Long-term evaluation of bilateral fetal nigral transplantation in Parkinson disease. *Arch. Neurol.*, **56**, 179–87.

Hauser, R. A., Furtado, S., Cimino, C. R. *et al.* (2002). Bilateral human fetal striatal transplantation in Huntington's disease. *Neurology*, **58**, 687–95.

Hughes, S. M., Lillien, L. E., Raff, M. C., Rohrer, H. & Sendtner, M. (1988). Ciliary neurotrophic factor induces type-2 astrocyte differentiation in culture. *Nature*, **335**, 70–3.

Hyman, C., Hofer, M., Barde, Y. A. *et al.* (1991). BDNF is a neurotrophic factor for dopaminergic neurons of the substantia nigra. *Nature*, **350**, 230–2.

Isacson, O., Brundin, P., Kelly, P., Gage, F. & Bjorklund, A. (1984). Functional neuronal replacement by grafted striatal neurons in the ibotenic acid-lesioned rat striatum. *Nature*, **311**, 458–60.

Ivkovic, S. & Ehrlich, M. (1999). Expression of the striatal DARPP-32/ARPP-21 phenotype in GABAergic neurons requires neurotrophins in vivo and in vitro. *J. Neurosci.*, **19**, 5409–19.

Ivkovic, S., Polonskaia, O., Farinas, I. & Ehrlich, M. E. (1997). Brain-derived neurotrophic factor regulates maturation of the DARPP-32 phenotype in striatal medium spiny neurons: studies in vivo and in vitro. *Neuroscience*, **79**, 509–16.

Jenner, P. & Olanow, C. W. (1998). Understanding cell death in Parkinson's disease. *Ann. Neurol.*, **44**, S72–84.

Jiang, J., McMurtry, J., Niedzwiecki, D. & Goldman, S. A. (1998). Insulin-like growth factor-1 is a radial cell-associated neurotrophin that promotes neuronal recruitment from the adult songbird edpendyma/subependyma. *J. Neurobiol.*, **36**, 1–15.

Jiang, W., McMurtry, J. & Goldman, S. A. (1997). IGF-1 is a radial cell-associated neurotrophin in the adult songbird forebrain. *Soc. Neurosci. Abstr.*, **23**.

Johansson, S. & Stromberg, I. (2002). Guidance of dopaminergic neuritic growth by immature astrocytes in organotypic cultures of rat fetal ventral mesencephalon. *J. Comp. Neurol.*, **443**, 237–49.

Keyoung, H. M., Roy, N., Louissant, A. *et al.* (2001). Specific identification, selection and extraction of neural stem cells from the fetal human brain. *Nat. Biotechnol.* **19**, 843–50.

Kilpatrick, T. J. & Bartlett, P. F. (1993). Cloning and growth of multipotential neural precursors: requirements for proliferation and differentiation. *Neuron*, **10**, 255–65.

Kilpatrick, T. J. & Bartlett, P. F. (1995). Cloned multipotential precursors from the mouse cerebrum require FGF-2, whereas glial restricted precursors are stimulated with either FGF-2 or EGF. *J. Neurosci.*, **15**, 3653–61.

Kim, J., Auerbach, J., Rodriguez-Gomez, J. *et al.* (2002). Dopamine neurons derived from embryonic stem cells function in an animal model of Parkinson's disease. *Nature*, **418**, 50–6.

Kirschenbaum, B. & Goldman, S. A. (1995). Brain-derived neurotrophic factor promotes the survival of neurons arising from the adult rat forebrain subependymal zone. *Proc. Natl Acad. Sci.*, **92**, 210–14.

Kirschenbaum, B., Nedergaard, M., Preuss, A., Barami, K., Fraser, R. A. & Goldman, S. A. (1994). In vitro neuronal production and differentiation by precursor cells derived from the adult human forebrain. *Cereb. Cortex*, **4**, 576–89.

Kondo, T. & Raff, M. (2000). Oligodendrocyte precursor cells reprogrammed to become multipotential CNS stem cells. *Science*, **289**, 1754–7.

Kordower, J., Freeman, T., Chen, E. *et al.* (1998). Fetal nigral grafts survive and mediate clinical benefit in a patient with Parkinson's disease. *Mov. Disord.*, **13**, 383–93.

Kordower, J., Freeman, T., Snow, B. *et al.* (1995). Neuropathological evidence of graft survival and striatal reinnervation after the transplantation of fetal mesencephalic tissue in a patient with Parkinson's disease. *N. Engl. J. Med.*, **332**, 1118–24.

Kowall, N. W., Ferrante, R. & Martin, J. B. (1987). Patterns of cell loss in Huntington's disease. *Trends in Neurosci.*, **10**, 24–9.

Kuhn, H. G., Winkler, J., Kempermann, G., Thal, L. & Gage, F. (1997). Epidermal growth factor and fibroblast growth factor-2 have different effects on neural progenitors in the adult rat brain. *J. Neurosci.*, **17**, 5820–9.

Lai, K., Kaspar, B., Gage, F. & Schaffer, D. (2003). Sonic hedgehog regulates adult neural progenitor proliferation in vitro and in vivo. *Nat. Neurosci.*, **6**, 21–7.

Lee, S.-H., Lumelsky, N., Studer, L., Auerbach, J. & McKay, R. (2000). Efficient generation of midbrain and hindbrain neurons from mouse embryonic stem cells. *Nat. Biotechnol.*, **18**, 675–9.

Li, M., Pevny, L., Lovell-Badge, R. & Smith, A. (1998). Generation of purified neural precursors from embryonic stem cells by lineage selection. *Curr. Biol.*, **8**, 971–4.

Lie, D., Dziewczapolski, G., Willhoite, A., Kaspar, B., Shults, C. & Gage, F. (2002). The adult substantia nigra contains progenitor cells with neurogenic potential. *J. Neurosci.*, **22**, 6639–49.

Lillien, L. E., Sendtner, M., Rohrer, H., Hughes, S. M. & Raff, M. C. (1988). Type-2 astrocyte development in rat brain cultures is initiated by a CNTF-like protein produced by type-1 astrocytes. *Neuron*, **1**, 485–94.

Lim, D., Tramontin, A., Trevejo, J., Herrera, D., Garcia-Verdugo, J. & Alvarez-Buylla, A. (2000). Noggin antagonizes BMP signaling to create a niche for adult neurogenesis. *Neuron*, **28**, 713–26.

Lindsay, R. M., Thoenen, H. & Barde, Y. A. (1985). Placode and neural crest-derived sensory neurons are responsive at early developmental stages to brain-derived neurotrophic factor. *Dev. Biol.*, **112**, 319–28.

Lindsay, R. M., Wiegand, S. J., Altar, C. A. & DiStefano, P. S. (1994). Neurotrophic factors: from molecule to man. *Trends in Neurosci.*, **17**, 182–90.

Lindvall, O. (1999). Cerebral implantation in movement disorders: state of the art. *Mov. Disord.*, **14**, 201–5.

Liu, J. P., Baker, J., Perkins, A. S., Robertson, E. J. & Efstratiadis, A. (1993). Mice carrying null mutations of the genes encoding insulin-like growth factor I (Igf-1) and type 1 IGF receptor (Igf1r). *Cell*, **75**, 59–72.

Lois, C. & Alvarez-Buylla, A. (1993). Proliferating subventricular zone cells in the adult mammalian forebrain can differentiate into neurons and glia. *Proc. Natl Acad. Sci., USA*, **90**, 2074–7.

Louissaint, A., Rao, S., Leventhal, C. & Goldman, S. A. (2002). Coordinated interaction of angiogenesis and neurogenesis in the adult songbird brain. *Neuron*, **34**, 945–60.

Luskin, M. B. (1993). Restricted proliferation and migration of post-natally generated neurons derived from the forebrain subventricular zone. *Neuron*, **11**, 173–89.

Luskin, M. B. (1998). Neuroblasts of the postnatal mammalian forebrain: their phenotype and fate. *J. Neurobiol.*, **36**, 221–33.

Magavi, S., Leavitt, B. & Macklis, J. (2000). Induction of neurogenesis in the neocortex of adult mice. *Nature*, **405**, 951–5.

Malberg, J., Eisch, A., Nestler, E. & Duman, R. (2000). Chronic antidepressant treatment increases neurogenesis in adult rat hippocampus. *J. Neurosci.*, **20**, 9104–10.

Mangiarini, L., Sathasivam, K., Seller, M. *et al.* (1996). Exon 1 of the HD gene with an expanded CAG repeat is sufficient to cause a progressive neurological phenotype in transgenic mice. *Cell*, **87**, 493–506.

Martinez-Serrano, A. & Bjorklund, A. (1996). Protection of the neostriatum against excitotoxic damage by neurotrophin-producing, genetically modified neural stem cells. *J. Neurosci.*, **16**, 4604–16.

Mehler, M. F., Mabie, P. C., Zhu, G., Gokhan, S. & Kessler, J. A. (2000). Developmental changes in progenitor cell responsiveness to bone morphogenetic proteins differentially modulate progressive CNS lineage fate. *Dev. Neurosci.*, **22**, 74–85.

Mitchell, I. J., Cooper, A. J. & Griffiths, M. R. (1999). The selective vulnerability of striatopallidal neurons. *Prog. Neurobiol.*, **59**, 691–719.

Morshead, C. M., Craig, C. G. & van der Kooy, D. (1998). In vivo clonal analyses reveal the properties of endogenous neural stem cell proliferation in the adult mammalian forebrain. *Development*, **125**, 2251–61.

Nait-Oumesmar, B., Decker, L., Lachapelle, F., Avellana-Adalid, V., Bachelin, C. & Van Evercooren, A. B. (1999). Progenitor cells of the adult mouse subventricular zone proliferate, migrate and differentiate into oligodendrocytes after demyelination. *Eur. J. Neurosci.*, **11**, 4357–66.

Nakao, N., Brundin, P., Funa, K., Lindvall, O. & Odin, P. (1995). Trophic and protective actions of brain-derived neurotrophic factor on striatal DARPP-32-containing neurons in vitro. *Brain Res. Dev. Brain Res.*, **90**, 92–101.

Nakatomi, H., Kuriu, T., Okbe, S. *et al.* (2002). Regeneration of hippocampal pyramidal neurons after ischemic brain injury by recruitment of endogenous progenitors. *Cell*, **110**, 429–41.

Nilsson, M., Perfilieva, E., Johansson, U., Orwar, O. & Eriksson, P. (1999). Enriched environment increases neurogenesis in the adult rat dentate gyrus and improves spatial memory. *J. Neurobiol.*, **39**, 569–78.

Nixon, K. & Crews, F. (2002). Binge ethanol exposure decreases neurogenesis in adult rat hippocampus. *J. Neurochem.*, **83**, 1087–93.

Nunes, M., Roy, N. S., Keyoung, H. M. *et al.* (2003). Identification and isolation of multipotential neural progenitor cells from the subcortical white matter of the adult human brain. *Nat. Med.*, **9**, 439–47.

Olanow, C., Kordower, J. & Freeman, T. (1996). Fetal nigral transplantation as a therapy for Parkinson's disease. *Trends Neurosci.*, **19**, 102–9.

Ouimet, C. C., Langley-Gullion, K. C. & Greengard, P. (1998). Quantitative immunocytochemistry of DARPP-32-expressing neurons in the rat caudatoputamen. *Brain Res.*, **808**, 8–12.

Palmer, T., Willhoite, A. & Gage, F. (2000). Vascular niche for adult hippocampal neurogenesis. *J. Comp. Neurol.*, **425**, 479–94.

Palmer, T. D., Ray, J. & Gage, F. H. (1995). FGF-2-responsive neuronal progenitors reside in proliferative and quiescent regions of the adult rodent brain. *Mol. Cell Neurosci.*, **6**, 474–86.

Palmer, T. D., Takahashi, J. & Gage, F. H. (1997). The adult rat hippocampus contains primordial neural stem cells. *Mol. Cell Neurosci.*, **8**, 389–404.

Parent, J., Vexler, Z., Gong, C., Derugin, N. & Ferriero, D. (2002). Rat forebrain neurogenesis and striatal neuron replacement after focal stroke. *Ann. Neurol.*, **52**, 802–13.

Pencea, V., Bingaman, K. D., Wiegand, S. J. & Luskin, M. B. (2001). Infusion of brain-derived neurotrophic factor into the lateral ventricle of the adult rat leads to new neurons in the parenchyma of the striatum, septum, thalamus, and hypothalamus. *J. Neurosci.*, **21**, 6706–17.

Perez-Navarro, E., Canudas, A. M., Akerund, P., Alberch, J. & Arenas, E. (2000). Brain-derived neurotrophic factor, neurotrophin-3, and neurotrophin-4/5 prevent the death of striatal projection neurons in a rodent model of Huntington's disease. *J. Neurochem.*, **75**, 2190–9.

Pham, K., Nacher, J., Hof, P. & McEwen, B. (2003). Repeated restraint stress suppresses neurogenesis and induces biphasic PSA-NCAM expression in the adult rat dentate gyrus. *Eur. J. Neurosci.*, **17**, 879–86.

Pincus, D., Harrison, C., Goodman, R. *et al.* (1996). Sequential treatment with FGF2 and BDNF permits the production of new neurons by precursors derived from the adult human epileptic temporal lobe. *Ann. Neurol.*, **40**, 550.

Pritzel, M., Isacson, O., Brundin, P., Wiklund, L. & Bjorklund, A. (1986). Afferent and efferent connections of striatal grafts implanted into the ibotenic acid lesioned neostriatum in adult rats. *Exp. Brain Res.*, **65**, 112–26.

Pundt, L. L., Kondoh, T., Conrad, J. A. & Low, W. C. (1996). Transplantation of human fetal striatum into a rodent model of Huntington's disease ameliorates locomotor deficits. *Neurosci. Res.*, **24**, 415–20.

Rao, M. & Mayer-Proschel, M. (1997). Glial-restricted precursors are derived from multipotential neuroepithelial stem cells. *Dev. Biol.*, **188**, 48–63.

Reynolds, B. A. & Weiss, S. (1992). Generation of neurons and astrocytes from isolated cells of the adult mammalian central nervous system. *Science*, **255**, 1707–10.

(1996). Clonal and population analyses demonstrate that an EGF-responsive mammalian embryonic CNS precursor is a stem cell. *Dev. Biol.*, **175**, 1–13.

Reynolds, B. A., Tetzlaff, W. & Weiss, S. (1992). A multipotent EGF-responsive striatal embryonic progenitor cell produces neurons and astrocytes. *J. Neurosci.*, **12**, 4565–74.

Richards, L. J., Kilpatrick, T. J. & Bartlett, P. F. (1992). *De novo* generation of neuronal cells from the adult mouse brain. *Proc. Natl Acad. Sci., USA*, **89**, 8591–5.

Rowitch, D. H., B, S. J., Lee, S. M., Flax, J. D., Snyder, E. Y. & McMahon, A. P. (1999). Sonic hedgehog regulates proliferation and inhibits differentiation of CNS precursor cells. *J. Neurosci.*, **19**, 8954–65.

Roy, N. S., Benraiss, A., Wang, S. *et al.* (2000a). Promoter-targeted selection and isolation of neural progenitor cells from the adult human ventricular zone. *J. Neurosci. Res.*, **59**, 321–31.

Roy, N. S., Wang, S., Jiang, L. *et al.* (2000b). In vitro neurogenesis by progenitor cells isolated from the adult human hippocampus. *Nat. Med.*, **6**, 271–7.

Samdani, A., Chmielnicki, E., Benraiss, A. & Goldman, S. A. (2002). Adenoviral BDNF induces neostriatal neuronal recruitment from endogenous progenitor cells in transgenic R6/2 huntingtin mice. *Mol. Ther* (Abstr) **5**.

Sawamoto, K., Nakao, N., Kakishita, K. *et al.* (2001). Generation of dopaminergic neurons in the adult brain from mesencephalic precursor cells labeled with a nestin-GFP transgene. *J. Neurosci.*, **21**, 3895–903.

Scharff, C., Kirn, J., Grossman, M., Macklis, J. & Nottebohm, F. (2000). Targeted neuronal death affects neuronal replacement and vocal behavior in adult songbirds. *Neuron*, **25**, 481–92.

Seaberg, R. M. & van der Kooy, D. (2002). Adult rodent neurogenic regions: the ventricular subependyma contains neural stem cells, but the dentate gyrus contains restricted progenitors. *J. Neurosci.*, **22**, 1784–93.

Shah, N. M., Groves, A. K. & Anderson, D. J. (1996). Alternative neural crest cell fates are instructively promoted by TGFbeta superfamily members. *Cell*, **85**, 331–43.

Shetty, A. K. & Turner, D. A. (1998). In vitro survival and differentiation of neurons derived from epidermal growth factor-responsive postnatal hippocampal stem cells: inducing effects of brain-derived neurotrophic factor. *J. Neurobiol.*, **35**, 395–425.

Studer, L., Tabar, V. & McKay, R. (1998). Transplantation of expanded mesencephalic precursors leads to recovery in Parkinsonian rats. *Nat. Neurosci.*, **1**, 290–5.

Studer, L., Csete, M., Lee, S. *et al.* (2000). Enhanced proliferation, survival and dopaminergic differentiation of CNS precursors in lowered oxygen. *J. Neurosci.*, **20**, 7377–8.

Svendsen, C., Caldwell, M. & Ostenfeld, T. (1999). Human neural stem cells: isolation, expansion and transplantation. *Brain Pathol.*, **9**, 499–513.

Temple, S. & Davis, A. A. (1994). Isolated rat cortical progenitor cells are maintained in division in vitro by membrane-associated factors. *Development*, **120**, 999–1008.

Tuszynski, M. H. (2000). Intraparenchymal NGF infusions rescue degenerating cholinergic neurons. *Cell Transpl.*, **9**, 629–36.

Uchida, N., Buck, D. W., He, D. *et al.* (2000). Direct isolation of human central nervous system stem cells. *Proc. Natl Acad. Sci., USA*, **97**, 14720–5.

van Praag, H., Kempermann, G. & Gage, F. (1999). Running increases cell proliferation and neurogenesis in the adult mouse dentate gyrus. *Nat. Neurosci.*, **2**, 266–70.

Vescovi, A., Parati, E., Gritti, A. *et al.* (1999). Isolation and cloning of multipotential stem cells from the embryonic human CNS and establishment of transplantable human stem cells lines by epigenetic stimulation. *Exp. Neurol.*, **156**, 71–83.

Wang, S., Wu, H., Jiang, J., Delohery, T. M., Isdell, F. & Goldman, S. A. (1998). Isolation of neuronal precursors by sorting embryonic forebrain transfected with GFP regulated by the T alpha 1 tubulin promoter [published erratum appears in *Nat. Biotechnol.* 1998 May; 16(5):478]. *Nat. Biotechnol.*, **16**, 196–201.

Wang, S., Roy, N., Benraiss, A., Harrison-Restelli, C. & Goldman, S. (2000). Promoter-based isolation and purification of mitotic neuronal progenitor cells from the adult mammalian ventricular zone. *Dev. Neurosci. in press.*

Weiss, S., Dunne, C., Hewson, J. *et al.* (1996a). Multipotent CNS stem cells are present in the adult mammalian spinal cord and ventricular neuroaxis. *J. Neurosci.*, **16**, 7599–609.

Weiss, S., Reynolds, B. A., Vescovi, A. L., Morshead, C., Craig, C. G. & van der Kooy, D. (1996b). Is there a neural stem cell in the mammalian forebrain? Trends Neurosci., **19**, 387–93.

Welner, S., Dunnett, S., Salamone, J. *et al.* (1988). Transplantation of embryonic ventral forebrain grafts to the neocortex of rats with bilateral lesions of the nucleus basalis magnocellularis ameliorates a lesion-induced deficit in spatial memory. *Brain Res.*, **463**, 192–7.

Wichterle, H., Lieberam, I., Porter, J. & Jessell, T. (2002). Directed differentiation of embryonic stem cells into motor neurons. *Cell*, **110**, 385–97.

Wilcock, G., Esiri, M., Bowen, D. & Smith, C. (1982). Alzheimer's disease. Correlation of cortical choline acetyltransferase activity with the severity of dementia and histological abnormalities. *J. Neurol. Sci.*, **57**, 407–17.

Winkler, J., Suhr, S., Gage, F. *et al.* (1995). Essential role of neocortical acetylcholine in spatial memory. *Nature*, **375**, 484–7.

Wu, P., Tarasenko, Y., Gu, Y., Huang, L., Coggeshall, R. & Yu, Y. (2002). Region-specific generation of cholinergic neurons from fetal human neural stem cells grafted into adult rat. *Nat. Neurosci.*, **12**, 1271–8.

Yan, Q., Matheson, C., Sun, J., Radeke, M. J., Feinstein, S. C. & Miller, J. A. (1994). Distribution of intracerebral ventricularly administered neurotrophins in rat brain and its correlation with trk receptor expression. *Exp. Neurol.*, **127**, 23–36.

Ye, W., Shimamura, K., Rubenstein, J., Hynes, M. & Rosenthal, A. (1998). FGF and Shh signals control dopaminergic and serotinergic cell fate in the anterior neural plate. *Cell*, **93**, 755–66.

Yoon, S. O., Lois, C., Alvirez, M., Alvarez-Buylla, A., Falck-Pedersen, E. & Chao, M. V. (1996). Adenovirus-mediated gene delivery into neuronal precursors of the adult mouse brain. *Proc. Natl Acad. Sci., USA*, **93**, 11974–9.

Zimmerman, L., Jesus-Escobar, J. & Harlan, R. (1996). The Spemann organizer signal Noggin binds and inactivates bone morphogenetic protein 4. *Cell*, **86**, 599–606.

24

Necessary methodological and stem cell advances for restoration of the dopaminergic system in Parkinson's disease patients

Ole Isacson[1,2,4], Kwang-Soo Kim[1,3], Ivar Mendez[5], Craig van Horne[1,2],
Lars M. Bjorklund[1,2] and Rosario Sanchez-Pernaute[1,2]

[1]Udall Parkinson's Disease Research Center of Excellence
[2]Neuroregeneration Laboratories
[3]Molecular Neurobiology Laboratory, McLean Hospital/Harvard Medical School, Belmont, MA, USA
[4]Program in Neuroscience, Harvard Medical School, Boston, MA 02114, USA
[5]Division of Neurosurgery, Dalhousie University, Halifax, NS, Canada

Introduction

New therapeutic non-pharmacological methodology involves cell and synaptic renewal or replacement in the living brain to restore function of neuronal systems, including the dopaminergic (DA) system in Parkinson's disease. Understanding the cell biological principles for generating functional DA neurons in lieu of the diseased can provide many new avenues for better treatment of patients with PD. Recent laboratory work has focused on using stem cells as a starting point for exogenous or endogenous derivation of the optimal DA cells for repair (Fig. 24.1). Using fetal DA cell therapy in PD patients (Piccini *et al.*, 1999, 2000; Freed *et al.*, 2001; Isacson *et al.*, 2001; Mendez *et al.*, 2002a) and stem cell-derived DA neurons in animal models (Bjorklund *et al.*, 2002; Kim *et al.*, 2002), it has been demonstrated that functional motor deficits associated with PD can be reduced after application of this new technology. Evidence shows that the underlying disease process does not destroy the transplanted fetal DA cells, although the patient's original DA system degeneration progresses (Piccini *et al.*, 1999, 2000). The optimal DA cell regeneration system would reconstitute a normal network capable of restoring feedback-controlled release of DA in the nigro-striatal system (Bjorklund & Isacson, 2002). The success of cell therapy for neurological diseases is limited by access to preparation and development of highly specialized dopaminergic neurons found in the A9 and A10 region of the substantia nigra (SN) in the ventral mesencephalon,

as well as technical and surgical steps associated with transplantation.

New neurons can grow to replace adult brain damaged or degenerated neuronal pathways. In clinical trials (Table 24.1), despite technical shortcomings, human fetal dopamine (DA) specified phenotypic ventral mesencephalic (VM) neurons have shown functional capacity in Parkinson's disease patients (Piccini *et al.*, 1999, 2000; Lindvall & Hagell, 2000; Freed *et al.*, 2001; Mendez *et al.*, 2002a; Ramachandran *et al.*, 2002 (Fig. 24.2)). Recently, it has been suggested that unregulated production of DA from grafted fetal neurons is the cause of unwanted dyskinesias seen in a subset of transplanted PD patients (Freed *et al.*, 2001; Olanow, 2002a) (Table 24.1). This is quite possible in a scenario of a "primed" dyskinetic circuitry produced by prior L-dopa treatment in a patient. Nonetheless, preclinical and clinical transplantation work demonstrates that striatal DA terminal release from appropriately grafted fetal DA neurons is regulated by both cell intrinsic and extrinsic synaptic and autoreceptor mechanisms and therefore, at least theoretically, the risk for dyskinesias should be less than with drug treatments (Piccini *et al.*, 1999; Bjorklund & Isacson, 2002). In animal models, fetal DA grafted neurons can reduce L-dopa induced dyskinesias (Lee *et al.*, 2000a). In grafted DA neurons, pre-synaptic DA auto-receptors regulate excess DA release and in vivo infusion of the full DA agonist apomorphine can block spontaneous DA release (Zetterstrom & Ungerstedt, 1984; Strecker *et al.*, 1987; Bjorklund & Isacson, 2002).

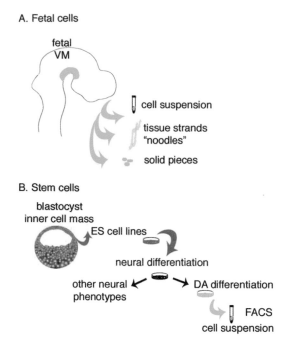

A. Fetal cells

fetal
VM

cell suspension

tissue strands
"noodles"

solid pieces

B. Stem cells

blastocyst
inner cell mass

ES cell lines

neural differentiation

other neural
phenotypes

DA differentiation

FACS
cell suspension

Fig. 24.1 Cell sources of dopamine neurons for neural transplantation into Parkinson's disease patients. (A) From the fetal brain dopamine neurons are obtained from the ventral midbrain (VM) at 6 to 9 weeks post-conceptional age. The VM is dissected and the tissue is prepared for transplantation following different methods, such as enzymatic and mechanical trituration to obtain a cell suspension, mincing into minute solid pieces or extruding through a glass pipette to form tissue strands. In any of these forms, the dopamine neurons are only a small fraction of the cells. Fetal VM can be maintained for some time (hours to days) in vitro (strands) or under special conditions such as hibernation media and be exposed to trophic factors and anti-apoptotic agents to promote survival. (B) From embryonic stem cell lines dopamine neurons (and other neural phenotypes with therapeutic potential) can be obtained in vitro through inductive protocols combining co-culture systems and sequential exposure to signaling and trophic factors that mimic the normal events during brain development. These cells can be characterized extensively in vitro and purified, using fluorescence activated cell sorting (FACS) or magnetic cell separation, before transplantation.

It is necessary to obtain structural reconstitution of terminal synaptic function and regulated dopamine release by new dopamine neurons

The scientific and clinical field of neural and cell repair has experienced the typical conceptual hurdles of major discoveries. The primary conceptual challenge is the idea that drugs (substance delivery) are a panacea for treatment of brain disorders. The initial success of L-dopa for PD and growth of pharmacology as a discipline in some ways may have retarded the development of molecular, cell biological and regenerative strategies. Simplistic reasoning suggesting that a "biological pump" of dopamine would be sufficient for functional recovery in PD led to several unsuccessful clinical trials, for example those involving autologous transplantation of catecholamine-containing adrenal medulla cells (Backlund *et al.*, 1985; Madrazo *et al.*, 1988). The absence of objective reductions of PD signs, the low adrenal medulla graft survival and the reported morbidity of patients strengthened, however, the scientific rationale for using dopamine producing and striatally adapted fetal neural mesencephalic donor cells (instead of adrenal medulla that produces minute non-synaptic DA even after NGF stimulation). Since the 1990s, some success has been achieved by using such a fetal DA prototype cell replacement treatment, but the quality of cell implantation technology and cell preparations using fetal DA cells have so far been variable (Fig. 24.1, Table 24.1), and highly experimental.

The development of brain cell transplantation with embryonic neurons and glia is innovative both from a technical and biological standpoint and thus will require much work to optimize. The scaling up of this method from rodents to primates and humans has proved very challenging, particularly in obtaining an acceptable, abundant and reliable donor cell source and preparation (Table 24.1). Early studies indicated some motor improvement in association with increased fluorodopa uptake (Widner *et al.*, 1992). Longitudinal and validated data from Lindvall and colleagues indicate stable DA cell survival and function in patients for almost a decade after surgery and substantially reduced need for pharmacological substitution by dopaminergic drugs (Piccini *et al.*, 1999, 2000). The transplantation of non-dissociated human VM tissue pieces has also provided benefits to many patients (Freed *et al.*, 1992; Freeman *et al.*, 1995). In a series of pilot transplantation studies carried out by Olanow and colleagues in the US, autopsy from two bilaterally transplanted (6.5–9 week human fetal VM) patients who died 18–19 months after surgery showed over 200 000 surviving DA neurons, which *partially* reinnervated the right putamen (about 50%) and the left putamen (only about 25%) (Kordower *et al.*, 1996). Electron microscopy revealed axo-dendritic and occasional axo-axonic synapses between graft and host was possible, and analysis of tyrosine hydroxylase (TH) mRNA revealed higher expression within the fetal neurons than within the residual host nigral cells (Kordower *et al.*, 1996). Autopsy of another patient in this surgical group showed over 130 000 surviving DA neurons, reinnervating almost 80% of the putamen (Kordower *et al.*, 1998).

Table 24.1. Transplantation clinical trials for Parkinson's disease

GROUP	REF	CASES	TYPE	DONOR AGE (weeks)	DONORS per SIDE	SITE	IS	CLINICAL BENEFIT (% in OFF)	PET F-DOPA UPTAKE	Dyskinesias	Autopsy TH cell number and reinervation
Lund/London	(Lindvall et al., 1989)	2 (open)	SUSP	7–9	4	C+P	yes	–	–(6mo)	14 cases reviewed by Hagell 2002 Off-phase dyskinesias were minimal to mild in 8; moderate in 5 and severe in 1 patient. Peak on–phase dyskinesias improved and time on without dyskinesias increased (although non significantly).	
	(Lindvall et al., 1990)	2 (open)	SUSP	6–7	4	P	yes	+	+		
	(Lindvall et al., 1992)	2 (open)	SUSP	6–7	4	P	yes	+/+++	+		
	(Widner et al., 1992)	2 (MPTP)	SUSP	6–8	4	P/C+P (Bi)	yes	+++	++ (200%)		
	(Wenning et al., 1997)	6*	SUSP	6–8	4	P/C+P	yes	+ (~30%) 4/6	++ (60%)		
	(Hagell et al., 1999)	5*	SUSP	6–8	4–8	P/C+P (Bi)	yes	+ 3/5	++ (85%) see also (Piccini et al., 1999) (dopamine release) and (Piccini et al., 2000) (motor activation)		
Creteil	(Brundin et al., 2000)	5 (open)	SUSP (lazaroids)	5–7	3–5	C+P (Bi)	yes	+ (~40%)	+ (~60%)		
	(Peschanski et al., 1994)	2 (open)	SUSP	6–8	2–3	P	yes	+	+	Worse in on	
	(Defer et al., 1996)	5* (open)	SUSP	6–8	2–3	P/C+P	yes	+	+ (~60%)	Worse in on (3/5)	
Brussels	(Levivier et al., 1997)	3 (open, safety study)	SUSP	6–8	3–4	P	yes	+	+/++		
Cuba	(Molina et al., 1994)	7 (open)	SUSP	10	1	C+P	yes	+	NA		
Denver	(Freed et al., 1990)	2 (open)	SOLID	5–6	1	C+P	yes	+/–	NA		
	(Freed et al., 1992)	7* (open)	SOLID	5–6	1	P (Bi)	4/7	+	+		

(cont.)

Table 24.1. (cont.)

GROUP	REF	CASES	TYPE	DONOR AGE (weeks)	DONORS per SIDE	SITE	IS	CLINICAL BENEFIT (% in OFF)	PET F-DOPA UPTAKE	Dyskinesias	Autopsy TH cell number and reinervation
	(Freed et al., 2001)	Double blind sham 19 +14 open	SOLID (up to 28 d in vitro)	7–8	2	P (Bi)	no	+ (~30%)	+ (~40%) (Nakamura et al., 2001) And (Ma et al., 2002) (dyskinesia related PET changes)	Severe off phase dysk 5/33	2 TH+ cells (2000–22 000 per track)
Tampa	(Freeman et al., 1995)	4 (open)	SOLID	6.5–9	6–8	P (Bi)	yes	+ (~30%)	+ (~40%)		2 TH+ cells 80 000 & 1 35 000 (5000–50 000 per track) 2–7 mm reinervation (Kordower et al., 1995; Kordower et al., 1996)
	(Hauser et al., 1999)	6* (open)	SOLID (hiber 2d)	6.5–9	3–4	P (Bi)	yes	+ (30%)	+ (55%)	Improved	
	(Olanow 2002b) (abstract)	Double blind sham (34)	SOLID	6.5–9	4/1	P (Bi)	yes	+ (?)	+ (?)	Dyskinesias?	
LA	(Kopyov et al., 1996)	22 (open)	SOLID	6–10	2–4	P (Bi)	yes	+ (18/22)	NA		
	(Kopyov et al., 1997)	13 (blind volume)	SOLID	6–9	2 vs 3–4	P (Bi)	yes	low 10%–high 50%	NA		
	(Jacques et al., 1999)	60* (retrospective)	SOLID	6–10	2–4	P (Bi)	yes	+	NA		
Halifax	(Mendez et al., 2000a)	8 (open)	SUSP (GDNF)	6–9	3–4	P (Bi)	no	+	+		1 graft volume 4–25 mm³/track (Mendez et al. unpublished data)
	(Mendez et al., 2002a)	3 (open)	SUSP (GDNF)	6–9	3–4	P+SN (Bi)	no	+ (~40%)	+ (~40% in putamen)		

Not included are trials from New Haven, US, using cryopreserved tissue (no TH cells in autopsy). (Redmond et al., 1990; Spencer et al., 1992) and Birmingham, UK, using tissue from embryos over 10 weeks old, as well as open procedures.

* Includes patients previously reported. Susp: cell suspension, solid tissue pieces or strands. IS = immunosuppression. C: Caudate nucleus; P: Putamen; SN: Substantia nigra reticulata; Bi: bilateral. Clinical benefit was rated in most studies as mild or moderate (+) corresponding roughly to 30% improvement in the UPDRS motor scores in OFF, – however, different studies based outcome on scores or % time in ON or in OFF and rating was performed on different medication regimes. In general, all studies reported a decrease in the amount of L-DOPA and dopaminomimetic drugs, although there is great variability in the amount of the reduction and the time after transplantation when it happened; only exceptionally patients have been off medication (3 in the Lund series although in one it was reintroduced 3.5 years after the transplant and the other 2 had MPTP-induced parkinsonism).

F-DOPA PET uptake was increased (+) in most studies (average 40–60%) but again PET studies were performed at variable time points. Although F-DOPA PET is considered a good indicator of dopamine cell survival in the graft, the sensitivity is debated because of lack of good clinical and pathological correlation (one of the patients in Freed's study who died had symmetric uptake in spite of a five-fold difference (6000/30 000) in the number of TH+ cells between sides, (Freed et al., 2001)).

Notably, both patients had shown major improvements in motor function and increases in fluorodopa uptake in the putamen on PET scanning (Table 24.1). Nevertheless, these and other detailed observations indicate that many specific regions of the human putamen may not be innervated by such non-specific VM grafts unless they contain the appropriate number and type of the A9 dopamine neuronal phenotype (Isacson, unpublished observations).

The most important factor in obtaining optimal functional effects (and minimal side effects) in PD by brain repair is in our opinion the presence of new synapses or DA transmission that adequately adapt to the local milieu and provide physiologically appropriate DA release in the host caudate-putamen and substantia nigra (Piccini *et al.*, 1999, 2000; Bjorklund & Isacson 2002). Fetal DA neurons have been shown to accomplish functional connections with the mature host striatal neurons. Synaptic contacts between transplanted fetal DA cells and host cells, as well as afferent contact by host neurons to transplanted cells, have been extensively documented (Mahalik *et al.*, 1985; Doucet *et al.*, 1989). Of both theoretical and practical relevance are analyses showing that pharmacological delivery into the striatum may not be as effective in ameliorating the motor symptom of PD, as regulated, synaptic release obtained with transplanted DA neurons (Bjorklund & Isacson, 2002). When DA is directly administered into the ventricle of PD patients, serious psychosis and motor abnormalities can develop (Venna *et al.*, 1984). The biological necessity for normal range DA release is illustrated by molecular differential display experiments that show abnormal upregulation of over ten genes within the striatum after abnormal DA exposure in vivo (Gerfen *et al.*, 1998). Complications associated with unregulated DA levels are obvious when observing effects of long-term L-dopa administration in patients as PD progresses, and the DA neuron and its synapses continue to degenerate, the non-physiological levels of DA within the striatum and abnormal down-stream activity in the basal ganglia seem to produce severe motor abnormalities such as dyskinesias. In neurophysiological recordings, it is clear that dopamine provides a modulatory role for the glutamate-mediated transmission, so that it appears to have a form of a gating function at that important striatal synapse (Freeman *et al.*, 1985; Strecker & Jacobs, 1985; Grace, 1991; Johnson *et al.*, 1992; Ljungberg *et al.*, 1992; Nutt *et al.*, 2000; Onn *et al.*, 2000). Physiologically appropriate DA functions can be achieved by normal DA synapses or, alternatively, cells which express the complete set of feedback elements required to regulate release and uptake of DA (Zetterstrom *et al.*, 1986; Strecker *et al.*, 1987; Isacson

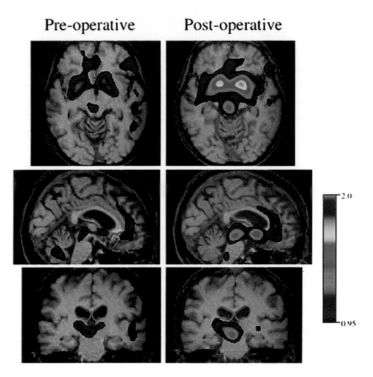

Pre-operative   **Post-operative**

Fig. 24.2 Preoperative and postoperative fluorodopa PET scans obtained in a patient with Parkinson's disease who received simultaneous intrastriatal and intranigral fetal VM grafts. These images consist of parametric maps of fluorodopa K_i transformed into stereotactic space and overlaid on the patient's MR image (also in stereotactic space). The parametric maps were smoothed using an 8 mm gaussian filter. The axial, coronal, and sagittal sections demonstrate an increase in K_i in the midbrain and putamen bilaterally, likely resulting from surviving grafted dopamine neurons (Mendez *et al.*, 2002, with permission).

& Deacon, 1997). The evidence for the importance of DA-mediated regulation of striatal neuronal and network interactions indicate that, unless there is a regulated and tonic release of DA that is approximately regulated at the synaptic cleft by afferents, glutamatergic synapses will be less effective in control of the striatal GABAergic output neurons (Nutt *et al.*, 2000; Onn *et al.*, 2000). Discontinuous stimulation of dopamine receptors such that may occur after degeneration and L-dopa treatment is probably a major cause of dyskinesia induction. Normally, there are small basal increases in firing by mesencephalic dopamine neurons in a number of situations, at least as has been tested in animal models (Strecker & Jacobs, 1985; Ljungberg *et al.*, 1992). Nonetheless, such frequency stimulation does not raise the extracellular concentration of dopamine because the synaptic network and terminals work to reduce fluctuations in DA concentration by reuptake mechanisms and possibly other autoreceptor mediated functions (Freeman *et al.*, 1985; Strecker & Jacobs 1985; Grace, 1991; Johnson *et al.*, 1992; Ljungberg *et al.*, 1992; Nutt *et al.*, 2000; Onn *et al.*, 2000). Fetal DA transplants have been shown to reduce the incidence of L-dopa induced dyskinesias in animal models (Lee *et al.*, 2000a). Several clinical studies have also shown normalized metabolic and brain functional activity throughout the basal ganglia after DA neural transplantation (Piccini *et al.*, 1999, 2000). In rodent studies, using cytochrome oxidase histochemistry as an indicator of neuronal metabolism in the 6-OHDA-lesioned rat; the lesion-induced increases in cytochrome oxidase activity of the entopeduncular nucleus and SN reticulata were finally eliminated by intrastriatal VM grafts, whereas the lesion-induced increases in globus pallidus and subthalamic nucleus were not changed by grafting (Nakao *et al.*, 1998). Similarly, in MPTP-treated monkey receiving VM transplants, DA cell implants increased the metabolic activity of the implanted striatum, particularly in the region of grafts containing greater numbers and innervation by DA neurons (Collier *et al.*, 1997).

Positron emission tomography (PET) and carbon-11-labeled 2B-carbomethoxy-3B-(4-fluorophenyl)tropane (11C-CFT) can also be used to visualize and quantify striatal presynaptic DA transporters in PD patients and PD degeneration models. In one such study of unilateral lesion of the SN DA system in rodents, the binding ratio was initially reduced to 15–35% of an intact side. After fetal DA neuronal transplantation, behavioral recovery occurred gradually and only after the 11C-CFT binding ratio had increased to 75–85% of the intact side, revealing a threshold for functional recovery in the lesioned nigrostriatal system after neural transplantation that fits our understanding of the normal DA system requirements (Brownell *et al.*, 1998). Importantly, autoregulation of DA release and metabolism by intrastriatal DA cell containing grafts has been shown by in vivo microdialysis in the striatum. Infusion of a non-selective DA agonist (apomorphine) almost abolishes endogenous DA release in the DA neuron-grafted striatum (Strecker *et al.*, 1987; Galpern, 1996), showing a normal auto-regulation of DA levels by the implanted cells. Further proof for the formation of functional DA terminals and synapses and appropriate DA release and regulation of transplanted fetal DA neurons have been studied in rodents after repeated L-dopa injections (Gaudin *et al.*, 1990; Lee *et al.*, 2000a). L-dopa-induced dyskinesias in non-human primates are also reduced after fetal DA cell transplantation (H. Widner, personal communication). These data indicate that DA levels within the transplanted striatum can be regulated in a functional manner by

correctly transplanted DA neurons if they appropriately innervate and form functional cellular communication with their normal target areas (Isacson & Deacon, 1997; Bjorklund & Isacson, 2002). Below, we describe some of these important variables in detail as they have been evaluated in animal model experiments and early observations in clinical applications.

Therefore, the current state of the art cell therapy for PD appears to require transfer of appropriate and selectively placed DA neurons in patients that are responsive to DA substitution therapy. Possibly, the emergence of stem cell generated DA neurons in concert with improved surgical and technical approaches may provide a more optimal intervention.

Technical developments of a new technology for regeneration of neural function and pathways in patients

The specific preparations of donor cells and associated procedures are very important in cell-based therapies and there are major differences in cell preparations for transplantation in Parkinson's disease in clinical trials to date (Fig. 24.1). The most successful method involves freshly dissected fetal tissue pieces (minute cubic millimeter pieces) that can be treated with proteolytic enzymes, then dissociated into a cell suspension (Brundin *et al.*, 1985; Piccini *et al.*, 1999; Lindvall & Hagell 2000; Piccini *et al.*, 2000; Mendez *et al.*, 2002a; Ramachandran *et al.*, 2002) (Fig. 24.1, Table 24.1). Other less effective procedures have included untreated tissue pieces, minced from the ventral mesencephalon of aborted fetuses (Henderson *et al.*, 1991; Freeman *et al.*, 1995; Kordower *et al.*, 1995; Olanow, 2002b). A third type, the so-called "noodle" technique (Freed *et al.*, 2001) includes a cell culture step. Such culture steps may alter the cells and select for cell types that are different than the populations obtained by fresh preparations, since storing or cell culture of DA neurons prior to transplantation may cause in vitro based selection favoring the A10 neurons that are less sensitive to oxidative stress than A9 (German *et al.*, 1992). These three different techniques produce different grafts. Only the cell suspension grafts grow to slender deposits that do not disrupt or displace the host target tissue (Brundin *et al.*, 1985; Piccini *et al.*, 1999, 2000; Mendez *et al.*, 2002a,b; Ramachandran *et al.*, 2002). In any event, all the current PD transplantation studies have employed rather crude cell preparations, since the starting point for all work are the pieces dissected from fetal tissue, which only contain about 10% newborn dopamine (DA) neurons; the rest are cells of types not generally relevant to PD degeneration (Brundin *et al.*, 1985). In addition, while there is selective degeneration of substantia nigra pars compacta (SNc; A9) neurons, with a relative sparing of ventral tegmental area (VTA; A10) neurons in PD (Iacopino & Christakos, 1990; Yamada *et al.*, 1990; Gibb, 1992; Ito *et al.*, 1992), both of these DA cell groups are currently transplanted as a mixture (Lindvall *et al.*, 1988; Kordower *et al.*, 1996; Hauser *et al.*, 1999; Freed *et al.*, 2001). Notably, these two subpopulations of DA neurons within the SN have very different functions and project to different brain areas (importantly also within the SN through dendritic release). The midline positioned DA neurons (known as area A10) (Dahlstrom & Fuxe, 1964) selectively send axons to limbic and cortical regions (Gerfen *et al.*, 1987) while the adjacent A9 DA neurons (the major dysfunction in PD) grow selectively to putamen motor areas (Damier *et al.*, 1999). Thus, the differences between A10 and A9 DA neurons (Costantini *et al.*, 1997; Haque *et al.*, 1997) are potentially very important for understanding how to make cell replacement strategies work in patients. In summary, while current work demonstrates a clear capacity of fetal dopamine cell transplants to repair PD brains (Piccini *et al.*, 1999; Mendez *et al.*, 2000a; Piccini *et al.*, 2000), there are technical limitations with available prototypes of this technique. Both animal model experiments and clinical trials are limited by today's mixed cell preparations of low DA neuronal yield, inappropriate surgical placements and potentially the loss of DA cell subpopulations of therapeutic interest during tissue incubation, cell culture and preparation steps. Practically and ethically it is not possible to use fetal tissue as a source for transplantation for PD in more than rare experimental situations. For example, to replace a sufficient number of DA neurons, one needs 6–8 fetal tissue pieces per patient, primarily due to low post-transplantational survival of the grafted fetal DA neurons. In addition, current surgical techniques are inconsistent with respect to placement, volume and type of cells grafted. It is, however, encouraging that recent research in stem cell biology may provide a solution to this problem of low cell access and yield (Bjorklund *et al.*, 2002; Kim *et al.*, 2002).

Subpopulations of midbrain dopaminergic neurons perform different functions and reach different targets: its potential relevance to repair of PD brains

An important question in neural transplantation is the capacity for specific neuronal cell types to selectively reinnervate denervated host target regions (Schultzberg *et al.*, 1984; Nilsson *et al.*, 1988; Isacson *et al.*, 1995; Isacson &

Deacon, 1996). Neurons developed from fetal or embryonic stem cell stages, when transplanted into host targets display a relative specificity in axonal outgrowth into regions typical of their mature phenotype (Schultzberg *et al.*, 1984; Nilsson *et al.*, 1988; Isacson *et al.*, 1995; Isacson & Deacon, 1996). Midbrain DA neurons can be clearly categorized into subpopulations based on differences in the expression of certain proteins such as the dopamine transporter, TH, calbindin and cholecystokinin (CCK) and target neuron selection (Schultzberg *et al.*, 1984; Blanchard *et al.*, 1994; Haber *et al.*, 1995). The biochemical markers used reflect specific projection areas reached by the different categories of DA SN neurons. In rodents, Schultzberg *et al.* (1984) demonstrated, by grafting embryonic VM tissue into the dorsal deafferented striatum, that subsets of SN DA neurons have specific final patterns of axonal terminal networks. CCK-negative/TH (A9) cells extend their axons into the motor striatum, while CCK-positive/TH neurons (A10) do not. Instead, A10 DA neurons project their axons in cortical areas and limbic striatal regions. Another interesting protein is the retinoic acid-generating enzyme, aldehyde dehydrogenase 2 (AHD2), which is expressed only in a subset of A9 DA neurons in the substantia nigra (McCaffery & Drager, 1994). The AHD2 DA neurons project to the dorsal and rostral regions of the striatum and have a reduced DA terminal density gradient ventrally. Transplanted DA neurons at first appear to extend fibers in a non-specific heliocentric fashion around the graft; however we have shown that the subset of transplanted DA fibers expressing AHD2 preferentially reinnervate the dorsolateral part of striatum (Haque *et al.*, 1997). Histological observations of post-mortem patient tissue (O. Isacson, unpublished data) also indicate that transplanted human DA neurons will only seek their normal targets; and actively avoid innervation of other caudate-putamen regions according to their specific neuronal phenotype. The AHD2 enzyme is very sensitive to oxidation, which may correlate with increased vulnerability of A9 neurons seen in PD (McCaffery & Drager, 1994). Since only 2–10% of neurons normally in the dissected VM are of a phenotype DA, hypothetically after transplantation they may compete for trophic support with the majority of the transplanted non-DA neurons. It is well known that midbrain DA neurons are positively influenced by growth factors such as bFGF (Mayer *et al.*, 1993) and GDNF (Granholm *et al.*, 1997; Meyer *et al.*, 1999). Such trophic dependency may vary between midbrain DA cell subpopulations, and it is likely that a limited supply of trophic molecules influences DA cell survival and growth. In addition, 20–80% of the SN cell population normally undergoes a period of programmed cell death between P2 and P14 (Janec & Burke, 1993).

Transplanted fetal VM derived DA neurons develop extensive axonal terminal networks, in the host striatum and nucleus accumbens in a normal, dense, homogeneous fashion (Bjorklund *et al.*, 1980; Dunnett *et al.*, 1984). In contrast, identical phenotypic DA neurons (from fetal or stem cell derivation) only extend a few axons into the host brain when transplanted into non-target areas such as cortex, thalamus and hypothalamus (Abrous *et al.*, 1988). Ultrastructural data show that grafted DA neurons are able to form appropriate and abundant synaptic connections with medium-sized spiny striatal neurons, which are the primary target of the mesencephalic DA afferents (Clarke *et al.*, 1988). The molecular mechanisms defining anatomical specificity of the DA projections have not been fully elucidated but they are likely to involve target-derived trophic signals and recognition of target-specific cell surface molecules by growth-cones (Isacson & Deacon, 1997).

Evidence that tissue type, surgical cell preparation or specific surviving dopaminergic neuronal phenotype influence the degree of functional recovery

We have demonstrated (Haque *et al.*, 1997) that a non-linear regression function exists between DA neuron survival and extent of functional motor recovery. For example, approximately 590 rat-derived DA cells in the graft were necessary to obtain a 50% reduction in motor asymmetry using solid piece VM transplants. A plateau in motor recovery was reached at about 1200 TH-positive neurons. Using pieces (non-dissociated grafts), the number of cells required for a 50% reduction in rotation is higher than comparable values in the literature for cell suspension grafts (Haque *et al.*, 1997). There may be several reasons for differences in efficacy between single cell suspension grafts and tissue pieces. Single cell suspension grafts become more vascularized than multiple-fragment transplants (Leigh *et al.*, 1994). Further, Nikkah *et al.* (1994) showed that smaller suspension grafts show relatively better axonal coverage of the striatum compared to larger grafts. Large grafts, whether transplanted as cell suspensions or as tissue pieces, may actually limit the direct access to host tissue cues causing grafted cells to have less interaction with the host and integrate more within the actual transplanted tissue. These data and reasons indicate that single fetal cells in smaller deposits or possibly endogenous progenitor cells integrate better into the host brain and elicit behavioral recovery more efficiently (Brundin *et al.*, 1985; Sotelo & Alvarado-Mallart, 1987; Hernit-Grant & Macklis, 1996). Co-grafting

of embryonic striatal tissue with fetal VM show that such grafts result in enhanced DA neuronal survival and function through trophic support (Costantini & Snyder-Keller, 1997). Thus, graft–host interaction and graft–graft interaction are both factors regulating fetal VM transplant development. We established that the percentage reduction in rotations at 10 weeks post-transplantation is mostly associated with the proportion of AHD2-positive A9 DA neurons in the grafts (Haque *et al.*, 1997). An inverse tendency was also apparent with the presence of A10 neurons. This observation suggests that the greater the proportion of A9 neurons in cell transfer or repair, the greater the degree of symptomatic recovery of motor signs or abnormalities.

The importance of proper development of appropriate molecular and phenotypic cell characteristics can be observed in the functional effects of transplanted xenogeneic DA neurons. In xenografting experiments in a rat model of parkinsonism, recovery from amphetamine induced motor asymmetry is tightly linked to the normal developmental rate of the species from where the grafted DA neurons are derived (Isacson & Deacon, 1997; Bjorklund *et al.*, 2002). Galpern *et al.* (1996) reported that between 80–120 TH-positive neurons were required to see the same effect using 120–140 rodent DA neurons, which is consistent with larger species-determined axonal growth areas in animals with larger brains.

Can we produce better therapies with fewer side-effects by accomplishing a more specific cellular and synaptic dopamine replacement?

Recently, it has been postulated that excess and unregulated production of DA from grafted fetal neurons could be responsible for some unwanted side effects seen in transplanted PD patients (Freed *et al.*, 2001). However, it has been convincingly demonstrated that striatal DA release normally is tightly regulated by both intrinsic and extrinsic mechanisms. Presynaptic dopamine autoreceptors regulate excess DA release and administration of the DA agonist apomorphine can inhibit spontaneous DA release up to 100% (Zetterstrom & Ungerstedt, 1984). It is believed that approximately 50% of this inhibition can be contributed to a direct effect on DA autoreceptors and 50% involves postsynaptic neurons engaged in short and long distance feedback circuits (Zetterstrom & Ungerstedt, 1984). Subsequently, it has been shown that grafted fetal DA neurons display similar autoinhibition mechanisms as demonstrated by a 40% reduction in spontaneous DA release when grafted animals are treated with apomorphine (Strecker *et al.*, 1987;

Bjorklund & Isacson, 2002). These basic studies are important as they provide evidence contrary to current theories that implanted DA neurons may release excess amounts of DA in an unregulated manner, thereby contributing to side effects such as dyskinesias (Freed *et al.*, 2001). Instead, such side effects may have several alternative explanations (Isacson *et al.*, 2001). DA released from nerve terminals into the synaptic cleft is normally rapidly taken up and transported back into the terminals by the dopamine transporter (DAT). This mechanism is important for appropriate temporal regulation of DA concentration in the synaptic cleft. When the DAT is blocked by agents such as cocaine, DA will remain in the synaptic cleft in higher concentrations and for longer time periods than normal thus allowing increased binding and activation of postsynaptic receptors. When fetal ventral midbrain is dissected prior to transplantation, most published protocols do not make any distinction between the DA neurons residing in the VTA (A10) and those in the SNc (A9) (Lindvall *et al.*, 1988; Kordower *et al.*, 1996; Hauser *et al.*, 1999; Freed *et al.*, 2001). These two midbrain subpopulations of DA neurons express different levels of the DAT (Blanchard *et al.*, 1994), project to different areas (Graybiel *et al.*, 1990) and show different response to growth factors (Johansson *et al.*, 1995; Meyer *et al.*, 1999). In addition Parkinson's disease patients show a relative sparing of DA neurons in the VTA compared to the SNc indicating that the VTA DA neurons are less vulnerable compared to their SNc counterparts (Iacopino & Christakos, 1990; Yamada *et al.*, 1990; Gibb, 1992; Ito *et al.*, 1992). One possible explanation for the reported dyskinesias in five out of 37 patients in the study by Freed *et al.* (2001) and 13 out of 23 patients in the study by Olanow (2002b) could be that unselective preparations of fetal tissue pieces containing fetal dopamine neurons prior to implantation may result in selective survival of the less vulnerable, but inappropriate VTA DA neurons (Isacson *et al.*, 2001). When such neurons are implanted into the putamen of PD patients, they may form inappropriate connections with, or avoid, the projection neurons of the putamen, since these are not their normal targets (Isacson & Deacon, 1997; Isacson *et al.*, 2001). In addition, differences in DAT expression between subpopulations of DA neurons (Blanchard *et al.*, 1994; Sanghera *et al.*, 1997; Ciliax *et al.*, 1999) may also result in abnormal dendritic DA release in the putamen (Falkenburger *et al.*, 2001) and uptake patterns that could cause suboptimal DA transmission. Another likely reason for uncontrolled motor response after transplantation is that location and size of tissue pieces implanted may in some cases create small lesions in the putamen with subsequent dysregulation of the GABAergic output neurons (as seen in Huntington's chorea). This theory is supported by the fact that small lesions in the striatum of primates (modeling Huntington's disease) make these animals severely dyskinetic in response to DA agonist treatment (Hantraye *et al.*, 1990, 1992; Burns *et al.*, 1995), that would also occur in a situation of diffuse release from inappropriate DA neurons placed as tissue pieces in the lateral putamen (Freed *et al.*, 2001; Olanow, 2002a). Supporting such a view is the relative absence of side effects from transplanted fetal DA cells to humans, when donor cells are prepared and placed as liquid cell suspension into PD putamen (Lindvall & Hagell, 2000; Mendez *et al.*, 2000a,b; Schumacher *et al.*, 2000; Ramachandran *et al.*, 2002). Such grafts typically reach less destructive size, but are better integrated in the host with more extensive axonal and synaptic outgrowth into appropriate target zones (I. Mendez, O. Isacson *et al.*, in preparation).

Finally, of significance, the importance of appropriate cellular and biochemical characteristics of transplanted DA cells has also been shown by behavioral experiments. In a rodent model of parkinsonism, recovery from movement asymmetry is correlated with the rate of cellular maturation of the donor species (Isacson & Deacon 1997; Bjorklund & Isacson, 2002). Embryonic stem (ES) cells generating DA neurons also abide by such biological principles (Bjorklund & Isacson, 2002; Bjorklund *et al.*, 2002). Multiple anatomical analyses have demonstrated that specific axon guidance and cell differentiation factors remain in the adult and degenerating brain, providing growth and axonal guidance cues for fetal or ES cells (Isacson *et al.*, 1995; Isacson & Deacon 1996; Haque *et al.*, 1997).

In summary, the pathology of PD reveals a relatively selective loss of DA neurons in the substantia nigra pars compacta (SNc; A9) with a relative sparing of ventral tegmental area (VTA; A10) neurons. Our preliminary studies and reasoning suggest that selective repair by A9 DA cells in the putamen is more likely to contribute to symptomatic relief and prevent motor side effects compared to implantation of the A10 DA cell group (Haque *et al.*, 1997; Isacson & Deacon, 1997). For example, transplanted A9 (AHD2+ and dopamine D2 receptor+) neurons selectively reinnervate the appropriate motor regions of the affected putamen and correlate better with improved behavioral function in rodent models (Haque *et al.*, 1997) than non-A9 SN DA neurons. Since the A9 DA neurons have a better capacity to downregulate dopamine release than A10 DA neurons by synaptic mechanisms, the A9 neurons are also *a priori* less likely to have unregulated DA release, that may cause too high or low and unstable DA levels provoking motor side effects, such as dyskinesia in patients as typically seen after long-term L-dopa or DA agonist treatment (Olanow & Obeso, 2000; Olanow & Tatton, 2000; Isacson *et al.*, 2001).

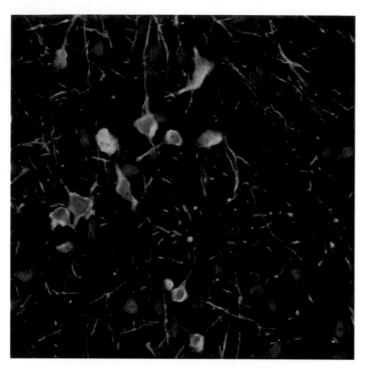

Fig. 24.3 Dopamine neurons derived in vivo from mouse embryonic stem (ES) cells. This confocal image shows numerous dopamine cells in the striatum of a 6-OHDA-lesioned rat, 11 weeks post-transplantation of undifferentiated ES cells (∼2000 cells). Dopamine neurons co-expressed the synthetic enzymes tyrosine hydroxylase (TH, green) and aromatic amino acid decarboxylase (AADC, blue) and the neuronal nuclei marker (NeuN, red). Animals with ES cells derived dopamine neurons in the grafts showed recovery of motor asymmetry (Bjorklund *et al.*, 2002).

Generation of a stem cell derived therapy for Parkinson's disease

Previous work has shown that DA neurons can be expanded in a cell culture dish from growth factor expanded embryonic day 12 (E12) VM precursor cells (Studer *et al.*, 1998) or ES cells (Kawasaki *et al.*, 2000; Lee *et al.*, 2000b), as well as from Nurr-1 transfected mouse progenitor clones cultured with midbrain type 1 astrocytes (Wagner *et al.*, 1999). Remarkably, by injecting the undifferentiated ES cell directly into living tissue (brain or kidney capsule) ES cells or embryoid body cells can spontaneously differentiate into neurons (Deacon *et al.*, 1998). We have recently demonstrated that naïve ES cells implanted in low numbers into a DA depleted striatum can develop and function as replicas of the DA neurons lost in PD (Fig. 24.3). These new cells restore amphetamine induced motor symmetry and cortical activation (Bjorklund *et al.*, 2002) lost both in

PD and PD animal models. Such findings suggest that ES cells are a reasonable cell source for PD transplantation and could overcome the problem associated with using fetal primary neuron (predifferentiated) or the fetal VM expanded precursor cells (Studer *et al.*, 1998), which both show low in vivo survival rates after transplantation (3–5% of the grafted DA neurons)(Brundin & Bjorklund, 1998; Studer *et al.*, 1998). In contrast, the direct ES cell transfer to brain has a high in vivo yield (up to four-fold) expansion and differentiation into DA neurons from a small number of implanted cells (1000 ES cells) (Bjorklund *et al.*, 2002) (Fig. 24.3). Vigorous basic research that defines the developmental sequences and repair mechanisms involved in fetal and stem cell derived DA neuron cell therapy will likely provide a future modality for the treatment of PD. Nonetheless, the growth potential of the cell source (ES) also needs to be tempered and controlled (Bjorklund *et al.*, 2002). The risk for growth of non-neural tissues from the endodermal and mesodermal germ-layers needs to be eliminated (Bjorklund *et al.*, 2002). This can be accomplished by blocking activation or influence of meso- and endodermal cell fate inducers (Bjorklund *et al.*, 2002).

How can stem cell biology research help Parkinson patients?

Most living systems undergo continuous growth. In humans, bone marrow stem cells are capable of dividing into most of the cells necessary for blood and immune systems. Even entire tissues or organs, such as the liver, can be regrown. Cells in the lining of the gut are shed and replaced on a daily basis, and in the skin, the basal cell layers of the dermis provide a continuous supply of growth. In adult mature mammalian cell systems, it is however typical that only organ-specific and specialized progenitor cells divide to maintain growth of organ systems in the body, while pathological processes can limit such replenishment. A fertilized cell is capable of cell divisions that grow logarithmically and in the early cluster of cells (in the range of 250 cells) each cell is capable of (or appears to be) forming any germ layer and part of the body plan (Hemmati-Brivanlou & Melton, 1997). This type of cell is therefore denoted stem cell, or in this case, embryonic stem cells. Recently, such divisible (yet non-malignant and non-carcinogenic) cells have gained increased attention. In a more limited scientific context, the concept and methodology of stem cell-derived dopamine cells intrigues both neurobiologists and clinically oriented scientists, insofar as it could both explain the biology of the developing dopamine cells and what controls its function, as well as generating a

Table 24.2. Candidate fate-determining factors that may play critical role in development and phenotypic specification of dopaminergic neurons

Factor	Embryonic day (mouse)	Comments	References
Wnt	8.0	Homozygous mutant mice lack the midbrain and adjacent cerebellar component of the metencephalon. Transgenic mice expressing En1 under the Wnt1 promoter rescues the phenotype of Wnt$^{-/-}$ mice, indicating that En1 gene may be downstream of Wnt.	(Danielian & McMahon, 1996) (McMahon *et al.*, 1992)
Engrailed−1 (En−1)	8.0	En 1$^{-/-}$ mice die shortly after birth and lack most of the colliculi and cerebellum and third and fourth cranial nerves. The absence of mid-hindbrain areas is evident as early as E9.5 and the phenotype resembles that of Wnt$^{-/-}$ mice.	(Wurst *et al.*, 1994)
Engrailed−2 (En−2)	8.5	En 2$^{-/-}$ mice viable but have an altered adult cerebellar foliation pattern. A recent analysis of En 1$^{-/-}$, En 2$^{-/-}$ double null mutant mouse showed that the midbrain DA neurons are generated and differentiate their dopaminergic phenotype but disappear soon thereafter. Thus, En1/En2 genes may be important for maintenance of DA phenotypes.	(Millen *et al.*, 1994) (Simon *et al.*, 2001)
Nurr1	10.5	Gene inactivation studies have established that Nurr1 is a critical fate-determining factor for DA neurons. In Nurr1$^{-/-}$ mice, precursors are developed but DA phenotype such as TH is not expressed. In a gain-of-function analysis in mouse embryonic stem cells, Nurr1 overexpression resulted in upregulation of all known DA marker genes such as TH, DDC, and DAT. Nurr1 appears to transactivate the 5′ promoter activity of the TH gene.	(Zetterstrom *et al.*, 1997) (Saucedo-Cardenas *et al.*, 1998) (Castillo *et al.*, 1998) (Chung *et al.*, 2002) (Kim *et al.*, 2003)
Lmx1b	7.5	Lmx1b is a LIM homeodomain transcription factor that is critical for dorsoventral patterning of the developing limbs and is involved in the nail patella syndrome. Re-evaluation of Lmx1b$^{-/-}$ null mice showed that TH$^+$ midbrain neurons form but soon disappear. Ptx3 gene is not induced indicating that Lmx1b is upstream of Ptx3. Thus, Lmx1b along with Pitx3 may constitute a molecular cascade independent of Nurr1 and TH.	(Smidt *et al.*, 2000)
Pitx3	11.5	Pitx3 and its rat homologue Ptx3 are selectively expressed in developing lens and in the midbrain. Pitx3 was mapped to the aphakia region on mouse chromosome 19 and the homozygous ak mouse was characterized by a small eye missing the lens. The human homologue PITX3 gene was mutated in two unrelated families with congenital cataracts and anterior segment mesenchymal dysgenesis. In regard to its potential role for DA development, loss-of-function or gain-of-function data are not yet available.	(Semina *et al.*, 1997; Semina *et al.*, 1998) (Smidt *et al.*, 1997)

procedure for obtaining such cells in abundance for clinical applications.

Starting at the genetic level, a number of genes related to the development or control of dopaminergic identity and specialization (e.g. sonic hedgehog protein, Pitx3 and Nurr-1) (Table 24.2) act in concert with other transcription factors to activate specific transmitter enzymes (for instance TH, DAT and dopa-decarboxylase) (Fig. 24.3) in dopaminergic neurons (Marsden, 1982; Montgomery *et al.*, 1996; Mandel *et al.*, 1998). An alternative or different route to cell repair is the possibility of manipulating inherent neurogenesis in the adult brain (Rakic, 2002). For example, in the adult brain exists neural precursor cells embedded in the subventricular zone (SVZ) that are capable of migration and differentiation into different neural cell types (Alvarez-Buylla & Garcia-Verdugo, 2002). These neural progenitor cells can be expanded and studied, possibly even as a neuronal repair tool (Flax *et al.*, 1998). The expansion of SVZ neuroprecursor cells is stimulated by delivery of basic fibroblast growth factor (bFGF), brain-derived neurotrophic factor (BDNF) (Benraiss *et al.*, 2000), noggin (Lim *et al.*, 2000), ciliary neurotrophic factor (CNTF) (Shimazaki *et al.*, 2001) or epidermal growth factor (EGF) (Craig *et al.*, 1996) to the CSF. Migration into the parenchyma can be stimulated by infusion of transforming growth factor-alpha (TGF-α) into a target region (Fallon *et al.*, 2000). Neuronal differentiation from precursors is enhanced by GDNF, BDNF (Zurn *et al.*, 2001) and natural BMP receptor antagonists (Lim *et al.*, 2000). Expression of a dopaminergic phenotype can be driven by transcription factors such as Pitx3 (Lebel *et al.*, 2001) and Nurr1 which drive genes of the full DA neuronal phenotype such as TH, DAT and components of trophic factor receptors (Saucedo-Cardenas *et al.*, 1998; Wallen *et al.*, 2001; Tornqvist *et al.*, 2002) (Table 24.2). Further, release of GDNF or BDNF by genetically modified cells in the caudate-putamen can increase survival of precursor cells and of dopaminergic neurons in the SN following lesions (Akerud *et al.*, 2001), and the programmed cell death process can also be temporarily suspended by anti-apoptotic factors, e.g. XIAP (Eberhardt *et al.*, 2002). Interestingly for novel therapies, genetically modified cells can also serve as biologic pumps to produce growth factors that sustain neurons on site in the striatum or projecting dopaminergic neurons from the SN (Schumacher *et al.*, 1991; Frim *et al.*, 1994; Akerud *et al.*, 2001).

In summary, stem cell biology is valuable in a discovery process of several new and potential treatments for Parkinson's disease. For example, research on ES cells may demonstrate the genetic transcription factors that control the specific genes participating in DA orchestrated neuronal function and cell development (Table 24.2). Genetic programs have dynamic components; for example, concerted actions of growth factors or neurotrophic factors that act as molecular switches required for initiating and maintaining the function of a DA neuron. The knowledge of how DA neurons can be formed would allow a reasonable process to be established for industrially producing a large number of such cells for transplantation or their regeneration inside the living brain. The stem cell biology related to brain development and repair can be approached by methods using either adult or embryonic stem cells potentially capable of generating new neurons, after selective engineering, expansion in cell culture systems or in the living brain. The investigation of embryonic stem cells also pro-

vides a system in which transcription factors responsible for directing the typical dopaminergic cell fate in the nigrostriatal systems can be determined. This allows a sophisticated understanding of the factors controlling the specialization and health of such cells. All of these investigations help clarify pathological, toxic or genetically induced cell dysfunction.

In conclusion, recent discoveries elucidating the cell biology of dopaminergic neurons allow both sequential and parallel strategies for protection of remaining cells and treating with new cells to restore function in Parkinson's patients (Check, 2002). The rapidly developing understanding of pathological mechanisms in Parkinson's disease and the life cycle of the dopamine neuron from stem cells, via progenitor cells, to adult and later aging dopamine neurons provides reasonable opportunities for new interventions to reverse the effects of this disease. Nonetheless, detailed knowledge is necessary about the appropriate neurons, correct brain locations for repair and responsive PD patients for these regeneration therapies to become successful.

Acknowledgements

This work is supported by the following US federal grant awards to O.I.: Udall Parkinson's Disease Research Center of Excellence (P50 NS39793), DAMD17-01-1-0762, RO1-NS-41263 and RO1-NS-30064. Support from the Kinetics Foundation, the Parkinson Foundation of the National Capital Area, the Anti-Aging Foundation, and the Orchard Foundation is also gratefully acknowledged.

REFERENCES

Abrous, N., Guy, J., Vigny, A., Calas, A., LeMoal, M. & Herman, J.-P. (1988). Development of intracerebral dopaminergic grafts: A combined immunohistochemical and autoradiographic study of its time course and environmental influences. *J. Comp. Neurol.*, **273**, 26–41.

Akerud, P., Canals, J. M., Snyder, E. Y. & Arenas, E. (2001). Neuroprotection through delivery of glial cell line-derived neurotrophic factor by neural stem cells in a mouse model of Parkinson's disease. *J. Neurosci.*, **21**, 8108–18.

Alvarez-Buylla, A. & Garcia-Verdugo, J. M. (2002). Neurogenesis in adult subventricular zone. *J. Neurosci.*, **22**, 629–34.

Backlund, E., Granberg, P. & Hamberger, B. (1985). Transplantation of adrenal medullary tissue to striatum in parkinsonism. *J. Neurosurg.*, **62**, 169–73.

Benraiss, A., Lerner, K., Chmielnicki, E. *et al.* (2000). Adenoviral transduction of the ventricular wall with a BDNF expression vector induces neuronal recruitment from endogenous progenitor cells in the adult forebrain. *Mol. Ther.*, **1**, S35–6.

Bjorklund, A., Schmidt, R. H. & Stenevi, U. (1980). Functional reinnervation of the neostriatum in the adult rat by use of intraparenchymal grafting of dissociated cell suspensions from the substantia nigra. *Cell Tissue Res.*, **212**, 39–45.

Bjorklund, L. M. & Isacson, O. (2002). Regulation of dopamine cell type and transmitter function in fetal and stem cell transplantation for Parkinson's disease. *Prog. Brain Res.*, **138**, 411–20.

Bjorklund, L. M., Sánchez-Pernaute, R., Chung, S. *et al.* (2002). Embryonic stem cells develop into functional dopaminergic neurons after transplantation in a Parkinson rat model. *Proc. Natl Acad. Sci., USA*, **99**, 2344–9.

Blanchard, V., Raisman-Vozari, R., Vyas, S. *et al.* (1994). Differential expression of tyrosine hydroxylase and membrane dopamine transporter genes in subpopulations of dopaminergic neurons of the rat mesencephalon. *Brain Res. Mol. Brain Res.*, **22**, 29–38.

Brownell, A. L., Livni, E., Galpern, W. & Isacson, O. (1998). In vivo *PET* imaging in rat of dopamine terminals reveals functional neural transplants. *Ann. Neurol.*, **43**, 387–90.

Brundin, P. & Bjorklund, A. (1998). Survival of expanded dopaminergic precursors is critical for clinical trials. *Nat. Neurosci.*, **1**, 537.

Brundin, P., Isacson, O. & Björklund, A. (1985). Monitoring of cell viability in suspensions of embryonic CNS tissue and its use as a criterion for intracerebral graft survival. *Brain Res.*, **331**, 251–9.

Brundin, P., Pogarell, O., Hagell, P. *et al.* (2000). Bilateral caudate and putamen grafts of embryonic mesencephalic tissue treated with lazaroids in Parkinson's disease. *Brain*, **123** (7), 1380–90.

Burns, L. H., Pakzaban, P., Deacon, T. W. *et al.* (1995). Selective putaminal excitotoxic lesions in non-human primates model the movement disorder of Huntington disease. *Neuroscience*, **64**, 1007–17.

Castillo, S. O., Baffi, J. S., Palkovits, M. *et al.* (1998). Dopamine biosynthesis is selectively abolished in substantia nigra/ventral tegmental area but not in hypothalamic neurons in mice with targeted disruption of the Nurr1 gene. *Mol. Cell Neurosci.*, **11**, 36–46.

Check, E. (2002). Parkinson's patients show positive response to implants. *Nature*, **416**, 666.

Chung, S., Sonntag, K. C., Andersson, T. *et al.* (2002). Genetic engineering of mouse embryonic stem cells by Nurr1 enhances differentiation and maturation into dopaminergic neurons. *Eur. J. Neurosci.*, **16**, 1829–38.

Ciliax, B. J., Drash, G. W., Staley, J. K. *et al.* (1999). Immunocytochemical localization of the dopamine transporter in human brain. *J. Comp. Neurol.*, **409**, 38–56.

Clarke, D. J., Brundin, P., Strecker, R. E., Nilsson, O. G., Bjorklund, A. & Lindvall, O. (1988). Human fetal dopamine neurons grafted in a rat model of Parkinson's disease: ultrastructural evidence for synapse formation using tyrosine hydroxylase immunocytochemistry. *Exp. Brain Res.*, **73**, 115–26.

Collier, T., Redmond, D. J., Roth, R., Elsworth, J., Taylor, J. & Sladek, J. J. (1997). Metabolic energy capacity of dopaminergic grafts and the implanted striatum in parkinsonian nonhuman primates as visualized with cytochrome oxidase histochemistry. *Cell Transpl.*, **6**, 135–40.

Costantini, L. C., Lin, L. & Isacson, O. (1997). Medial fetal ventral mesencephalon: a preferred source for dopamine neuron grafts. *Neuroreport*, **8**, 2253–7.

Costantini, L. C. & Snyder-Keller, A. (1997). Co-transplantation of fetal lateral ganglionic eminence and ventral mesencephalon can augment function and development of intrastriatal transplants. *Exp. Neurol.*, **145**, 214–27.

Craig, C. G., Tropepe, V., Morshead, C. M., Reynolds, B. A., Weiss, S. & van der Kooy, D. (1996). In vivo growth factor expansion of endogenous subependymal neural precursor cell population in the adult mouse brain. *J. Neurosci.*, **16**, 2649–58.

Dahlstrom, A. & Fuxe, K. (1964). Localization of monoamines in the lower brain stem. *Experientia*, **20**, 398–9.

Damier, P., Hirsch, E. C., Agid, Y. & Graybiel, A. M. (1999). The substantia nigra of the human brain. I. Nigrosomes and the nigral matrix, a compartmental organization based on calbindin D(28K) immunohistochemistry. *Brain*, **122**, 1421–36.

Danielian, P. S. & McMahon, A. P. (1996). Engrailed-1 as a target of the Wnt-1 signalling pathway in vertebrate midbrain development. *Nature*, **383**, 332–4.

Deacon, T., Dinsmore, J., Costantini, L., Ratliff, J. & Isacson, O. (1998). Blastula-stage stem cells differentiate into dopaminergic and serotonergic neurons after transplantation. *Exp. Neurol.*, **149**, 28–41.

Defer, G. L., Geny, C., Ricolfi, F. *et al.* (1996). Long-term outcome of unilaterally transplanted parkinsonian patients. I. Clinical approach. *Brain*, **119**, 41–50.

Doucet, G., Murata, Y., Brundin, P. *et al.* (1989). Host afferents into intrastriatal transplants of fetal ventral mesencephalon. *Exp Neurol.*, **106**, 1–19.

Dunnett, S. B., Bunch, S. T., Gage, F. H. & Bjorklund, A. (1984). Dopamine-rich transplants in rats with 6-OHDA lesions of the ventral tegmental area. 1. Effects on spontaneous and drug-induced locomotor activity. *Behav. Brain Res.*, **13**, 71–82.

Eberhardt, O., Coelin, R. V., Kugler, S. *et al.* (2002). Protection by synergistic effects of adenovirus-mediated X-linked chromosome-linked inhibitor of apoptosis and glial-derived neurotrophic factor gene transfer in the 1-methyl-4-pheyl-1,2,3,6-tetrahydropyridine model of Parkinson's disease. *J. Neurosci.*, **20**, 9126–34.

Falkenburger, B. H., Barstow, K. L. & Mintz, I. M. (2001). Dendrodendritic inhibition through reversal of dopamine transport. *Science*, **293**, 2465–70.

Fallon, J., Reid, S., Kinyamu, R. *et al.* (2000). In vivo induction of massive proliferation, directed migration, and differentiation of neural cells in the adult mammalian brain. *Proc. Natl Acad. Sci., USA*, **97**, 14686–91.

Flax, J. D., Aurora, S., Yang, C. *et al.* (1998). Engraftable human neural stem cells respond to developmental cues, replace neurons, and express foreign genes. *Nat. Biotechnol.*, **16**, 1033–9.

Freed, C. R., Breeze, R. E., Rosenberg, N. L. *et al.* (1990). Transplantation of human fetal dopamine cells for Parkinson's disease. Results at 1 year. *Arch. Neurol.*, **47**, 505–12.

Freed, C. R., Breeze, R. E., Rosenberg, N. L. *et al.* (1992). Survival of implanted fetal dopamine cells and neurologic improvement 12 to 46 months after transplantation for Parkinson's disease. *N. Engl. J. Med.*, **327**, 1549–55.

Freed, C. R., Greene, P. E., Breeze, R. E. *et al.* (2001). Transplantation of embryonic dopamine neurons for severe Parkinson's disease. *N. Engl. J. Med.*, **344**, 710–19.

Freeman, A. S., Meltzer L. T. & Bunney B. S. (1985). Firing properties of substantia nigra dopaminergic neurons in freely moving rats. *Life Sci.*, **36**, 1983–94.

Freeman, T. B., Olanow, C. W., Hauser, R. A. *et al.* (1995a). Bilateral fetal nigral transplantation into the postcommissural putamen in Parkinson's disease. *Ann. Neurol.*, **38**, 379–88.

Frim, D. M., Uhler T. A., Galpern W. R., Beal M. F., Breakefield X. O. & Isacson O. (1994). Biologically delivered BDNF increases dopaminergic neuronal survival in a rat model of Parkinson's disease. *Proc. Natl Acad. Sci., USA*, **91**, 5104–8.

Galpern, W. R., Burns, L. H., Deacon, T. W., Dinsmore, J. & Isacson, O. (1996). Xenotransplantation of porcine fetal ventral mesencephalon in a rat model of Parkinson's disease: functional recovery and graft morphology. *Exp. Neurol.*, **140**, 1–13.

Gaudin, D., Rioux, L. & Bedard, P. (1990). Fetal dopamine neuron transplants prevent behavioral supersensitivity induced by repeated administration of L-Dopa in the rat. *Brain Res.*, **506**, 166–8.

Gerfen, C., Keefe, K. & Steiner, H. (1998). Dopamine-mediated gene regulation in the striatum. *Adv. Pharmacol.*, **42**, 670–3.

Gerfen, C. R., Herkenham M. & Thibault J. (1987). The neostriatal mosaic: II. Patch- and matrix-directed mesostriatal dopaminergic and non-dopaminergic systems. *J. Neurosci.*, **7**, 3915–34.

German, D. C., Manaye K. F., Sonsalla P. K. & Brooks B. A. (1992). Midbrain dopaminergic cell loss in Parkinson's disease and MPTP-induced parkinsonism: sparing of calbindin-D28k-containing cells. *Ann. NY Acad. Sci.*, **648**, 42–62.

Gibb, W. R. (1992). Melanin, tyrosine hydroxylase, calbindin and substance P in the human midbrain and substantia nigra in relation to nigrostriatal projections and differential neuronal susceptibility in Parkinson's disease. *Brain Res.*, **581**, 283–91.

Grace, A. A. (1991). Phasic versus tonic dopamine release and the modulation of dopamine system responsivity: a hypothesis for the etiology of schizophrenia. *Neuroscience*, **41**, 1–24.

Granholm, A., Mott, J., Bowenkamp, K. *et al.* (1997). Glial cell line-derived neurotrophic factor improves survival of ventral mesencephalic grafts to the 6-hydroxydopamine lesioned striatum. *Exp. Brain Res.*, **116**, 29–38.

Graybiel, A. M., Hirsch, E. & Agid, Y. (1990). The nigrostriatal system in Parkinson's disease. In *Advances in Neurology*, ed. M. B. Streifler, A. D. Korczyn, E. Melamed & M. B. H. Youdim, pp. 17–29. New York: Raven Press.

Haber, S. N., Ryoo, H., Cox, C. & Lu, W. (1995). Subsets of midbrain dopaminergic neurons in monkeys are distinguished by different levels of mRNA for the dopamine transporter: comparison with the mRNA for the D2 receptor, tyrosine hydroxylase and calbindin immunoreactivity. *J. Comp. Neurol.*, **362**, 400–10.

Hagell, P., Schrag, A., Piccini, P. *et al.* (1999). Sequential bilateral transplantation in Parkinson's disease: effects of the second graft. *Brain*, **122** (6), 1121–32.

Hagell, P., Piccini, P., Bjorklund, A. *et al.* (2002). Dyskinesias following neural transplantation in Parkinson's disease. *Nat. Neurosc.*, **5**, 627–8.

Hantraye, P., Riche, D., Maziere, M. & Isacson, O. (1990). A primate model of Huntington's disease: behavioral and anatomical studies of unilateral excitotoxic lesions of the caudate-putamen in the baboon. *Exp. Neurol.*, **108**, 91–104.

(1992). Intrastriatal transplantation of cross-species fetal striatal cells reduces abnormal movements in a primate model of Huntington disease. *Proc. Natl Acad. Sci., USA*, **89**, 4187–91.

Haque, N. S., LeBlanc, C. J. & Isacson, O. (1997). Differential dissection of the rat E16 ventral mesencephalon and survival and reinnervation of the 6-OHDA-lesioned striatum by a subset of aldehyde dehydrogenase-positive TH neurons. *Cell Transpl.*, **6**, 239–48.

Hauser, R. A., Freeman, T. B., Snow, B. J. *et al.* (1999). Long-term evaluation of bilateral fetal nigral transplantation in Parkinson disease. *Arch. Neurol.*, **56**, 179–87.

Hemmati-Brivanlou, A. & Melton, D. (1997). Vertebrate embryonic cells will become nerve cells unless told otherwise. *Cell*, **88**, 13–17.

Henderson, B. T., Clough, C. G., Hughes, R. C., Hitchcock, E. R. & Kenny, B. G. (1991). Implantation of human fetal ventral mesencephalon to the right caudate nucleus in advanced Parkinson's disease. *Arch. Neurol.*, **48**, 822–7.

Hernit-Grant, C. S. & Macklis, J. D. (1996). Embryonic neurons transplanted to regions of targeted photolytic cell death in adult mouse somatosensory cortex re-form specific callosal projections. *Exp. Neurol.*, **139**, 131–42.

Iacopino, A. M. & Christakos, S. (1990). Specific reduction of calcium-binding protein (28-kilodalton calbindin-D) gene expression in aging and neurodegenerative diseases. *Proc. Natl Acad. Sci., USA*, **87**, 4078–82.

Isacson, O. & Deacon, T. W. (1996). Specific axon guidance factors persist in the mature rat brain: evidence from fetal neuronal xenografts. *Neuroscience*, **75**, 827–37.

Isacson, O. & Deacon, T. W. (1997). Neural transplantation studies reveal the brain's capacity for continuous reconstruction. *Trends in Neurosci.*, **20**, 477–82.

Isacson, O., Deacon, T. W., Pakzaban, P., Galpern, W. R., Dinsmore, J. & Burns, L. H. (1995). Transplanted xenogeneic neural cells in neurodegenerative disease models exhibit remarkable axonal target specificity and distinct growth patterns of glial and axonal fibres. *Nat. Med.*, **1**, 1189–94.

Isacson, O., Bjorklund, L. & Pernaute, R. S. (2001). Parkinson's disease: interpretations of transplantation study are erroneous. *Nat. Neurosci.*, **4**, 553.

Ito, H., Goto, S., Sakamoto, S. & Hirano, A. (1992). Calbindin-D28k in the basal ganglia of patients with parkinsonism. *Ann. Neurol.*, **32**, 543–50.

Jacques, D. B., Kopyov, O. V., Eagle, K. S., Carter, T. & Lieberman, A. (1999). Outcomes and complications of fetal tissue transplantation in Parkinson's disease. *Stereotact. Funct. Neurosurg.*, **72**, 219–24.

Janec, E. & Burke, R. E. (1993). Naturally occuring cell death during postnatal development of the substantia nigra pars compacta of rat. *Mol. Cell Neurosci.*, **4**, 30–5.

Johansson, M., Friedemann, M., Hoffer, B. & Stromberg, I. (1995). Effects of glial cell line-derived neurotrophic factor on developing and mature ventral mesencephalic grafts in oculo. *Exp. Neurol.*, **134**, 25–34.

Johnson, S. W., Seutin, V. & North, R. A. (1992). Burst firing in dopamine neurons induced by *N*-methyl-D-aspartate: role of electrogenic sodium pump. *Science*, **258**, 665–7.

Kawasaki, H., Mizuseki, K., Nishikawa, S. *et al.* (2000). Induction of midbrain dopaminergic neurons from ES cells by stromal cell-derived inducing activity. *Neuron*, **28**, 31–40.

Kim, J. H., Auerbach, J. M., Rodriguez-Gomez, J. A. *et al.* (2002). Dopamine neurons derived from embryonic stem cells function in an animal model of Parkinson's disease. *Nature*, **418**, 50–6.

Kim, K. S., Kim, C. H., Hwang, D. Y. *et al.* (2003). The orphan nuclear receptor Nurr1 directly transactivates the promotor of the tyrosine hydroxylase gene, but not the dopamine b-hydroxylase gene, in a cell-specific manner. *J. Neurochem.*, **85**, 622–34.

Kopyov, O. V., Jacques, D., Lieberman, A., Duma, C. M. & Rogers, R. L. (1996). Clinical study of fetal mesencephalic intracerebral transplants for the treatment of Parkinson's disease. *Cell Transpl.*, **5**, 327–37.

Kopyov, O. V., Jacques, D. S., Lieberman, A., Duma, C. M. & Rogers, R. L. (1997). Outcome following intrastriatal fetal mesencephalic grafts for Parkinson's patients is directly related to the volume of grafted tissue. *Exp. Neurol.*, **146**, 536–45.

Kordower, J., Freeman, T., Chen, E. *et al.* (1998). Fetal nigral grafts survive and mediate clinical benefit in a patient with Parkinson's disease. *Mov. Disord.*, **13**, 383–93.

Kordower, J. H., Freeman, T. B., Snow, B. J. *et al.* (1995). Neuropathological evidence of graft survival and striatal reinnervation after the transplantation of fetal mesencephalic tissue in a patient with Parkinson's disease. *N. Engl. J. Med.*, **332**, 1118–24.

Kordower, J. H., Rosenstein, J. M., Collier, T. J. *et al.* (1996). Functional fetal nigral grafts in a patient with Parkinson's disease: chemoanatomic, ultrastructural, and metabolic studies. *J. Comp. Neurol.*, **370**, 203–30.

Lebel, M., Gauthier, Y., Moreau, A. & Drouin, J. (2001). Pitz3 activates mouse tyrosine hydroxylase promoter via a high-affinity binding site. *J. Neurochem.*, **77**, 558–67.

Lee, C. S., Cenci, M. A., Schulzer, M. & Bjorklund, A. (2000a). Embryonic ventral mesencephalic grafts improve levodopa-induced dyskinesia in a rat model of Parkinson's disease. *Brain*, **123**, 1365–79.

Lee, S. H., Lumelsky, N., Studer, L., Auerbach, J. M. & McKay, R. D. (2000b). Efficient generation of midbrain and hindbrain neurons from mouse embryonic stem cells. *Nat. Biotechnol.*, **18**, 675–9.

Leigh, K., Elisevich, K. & Rogers, K. A. (1994). Vascularisation and microvascular permeability in solid versus cell-suspension embryonic neural grafts. *J. Neurosurg.*, **81**, 272–83.

Levivier, M., Dethy, S., Rodesch, F. *et al.* (1997). Intracerebral transplantation of fetal ventral mesencephalon for patients with advanced Parkinson's disease. Methodology and 6-month to 1-year follow-up in 3 patients. *Stereotact. Funct. Neurosurg.*, **69**, 99–111.

Lim, D. A., Tramontin, A. D., Trevejo, J. M. & Alverez-Buylla, A. (2000). Noggin antagonizes BMP signaling to create a niche for adult neurogenesis. *Neuron*, **28**, 713–26.

Lindvall, O., Brundin, P., Widner, H. *et al.* (1990). Grafts of fetal dopamine neurons survive and improve motor function in Parkinson's disease. *Science*, **247**, 574–7.

Lindvall, O. & Hagell P. (2000). Clinical observations after neural transplantation in Parkinson's disease. *Prog. Brain Res.*, **127**, 299–320.

Lindvall, O., Rehncrona, S., Gustavi, B. *et al.* (1988). Fetal dopamine-rich mesencephalic grafts in Parkinson's disease. *Lancet*, **ii**, 1483–4.

Lindvall, O., Rehncrona, S., Brundin, P. *et al.* (1989). Human fetal dopamine neurons grafted into the striatum in two patients with severe Parkinson's disease. A detailed account of methodology and a 6-month follow-up. *Arch. Neurol.*, **46**, 615–31.

Lindvall, O., Widner, H., Rehncrona, S. *et al.* (1992). Transplantation of fetal dopamine neurons in Parkinson's disease: one-year clinical and neurophysiological observations in two patients with putaminal implants. *Ann. Neurol.*, **31**, 155–65.

Ljungberg, T., Apicella, P. & Schultz W. (1992). Responses of monkey dopamine neurons during learning of behavioral reactions. *J. Neurophysiol.*, **67**, 145–63.

Ma, Y., Feigin, A., Dhawan, V. *et al.* (2002). Dyskinesia after fetal cell transplantation for parkinsonism: a PET study. *Ann. Neurol.*, **52**, 628–34.

Madrazo, I., Leon, V. & Torres, C. (1988). Transplantation of fetal substantia nigra and adrenal medulla to the caudate putamen in two patients with Parkinson's disease. *N. Engl. J. Med.*, **318**, 51.

Mahalik, T., Finger, T., Stromberg, I. & Olson, L. (1985). Substantia nigra transplants into denervated striatum of the rat: ultrastructure of graft and host interconnections. *J. Comp. Neurol.*, **240**, 60–70.

Mandel, R., Rendahl, K., Spratt, S., Snyder, R., Cohen, L. & Leff, S. (1998). Characterization of intrastriatal recombinant adeno-associated virus-mediated gene transfer of human tyrosine hydroxylase and human GTP-cyclohydrolase I in a rat model of Parkinson's disease. *J. Neurosci.*, **18**, 4271–84.

Marsden, C. D. (1982). Basal ganglia disease. *Lancet*, **ii** (8308), 1141–7.

Mayer, E., Fawcett, J. W. & Dunnett, S. B. (1993). Basic fibroblast growth factor promotes the survival of embryonic ventral mesencephalic dopaminergic neurons. II. Effects on nigral transplants in vivo. *Neuroscience*, **56**, 389–98.

McCaffery, P. & Drager U. C. (1994). High levels of a retinoic acid-generating dehydrogenase in the meso-telencephalic dopamine system. *Proc. Natl Acad. Sci., USA*, **91**, 7772–6.

McMahon, A. P., Joyner A. L., Bradley A. & McMahon J. A. (1992). The midbrain-hindbrain phenotype of Wnt-1-/Wnt-1- mice results from stepwise deletion of engrailed-expressing cells by 9.5 days postcoitum. *Cell*, **69**, 581–95.

Mendez, I., Dagher A. & Hong M. (2000a). Simultaneous intra-putaminal and intranigral fetal dopaminergic grafts in Parkinson's disease: first clinical trials. *Exp. Neurol.*, **164**, 464.

Mendez, I., Hong, M., Smith, S., Dagher, A. & Desrosiers, J. (2000b). Neural transplantation cannula and microinjector system: experimental and clinical experience. Technical note. *J. Neurosurg.*, **92**, 493–9.

Mendez, I., Dagher, A., Hong, M. *et al.* (2002a). Simultaneous intrastriatal and intranigral fetal dopaminergic grafts in patients with Parkinson disease: a pilot study. Report of three cases. *J. Neurosurg.*, **96**, 589–96.

Meyer, M., Zimmer, J., Seiler, R. W. & Widmer, H. R. (1999). GDNF increases the density of cells containing calbindin but not of cells containing calretinin in cultured rat and human fetal nigral tissue. *Cell Transpl.*, **8**, 25–36.

Millen, K. J., Wurst, W., Herrup, K. & Joyner, A. L. (1994). Abnormal embryonic cerebellar development and patterning of postnatal foliation in two mouse Engrailed-2 mutants. *Development*, **120**, 695–706.

Molina, H., Quinones-Molina, R., Munoz, J. *et al.* (1994). Neurotransplantation in Parkinson's disease: from open microsurgery to bilateral stereotactic approach: first clinical trial using microelectrode recording technique. *Stereotact. Funct. Neurosurg.*, **62**, 204–8.

Montgomery, R., Warner, M., Lum, B. & Spear, P. (1996). Herpes simplex virus-1 entry into cells mediated by a novel member of the TNF/NGF receptor family. *Cell*, **87**, 427–36.

Nakamura, T., Dhawan, V., Chaly, T. *et al.* (2001). Blinded positron emission tomography study of dopamine cell implantation for Parkinson's disease. *Ann. Neurol.*, **50**, 181–7.

Nakao, N., Ogura, M., Nakai, K. & Itakura, T. (1998). Intrastriatal mesencephalic grafts affect neuronal activity in basal ganglia nuclei and their target structures in a rat model of Parkinson's disease. *J. Neurosci.*, **18**, 1806–17.

Nikkah, G., Cunningham, M. G., Jodicke, A., Knappe, U. & Bjorklund, A. (1994). Improved graft survival and striatal reinnervation by microtransplantation of fetal nigral cell suspensions in the rat Parkinson model. *Brain Res.*, **633**, 133–43.

Nilsson, O. G., Clarke, D. J., Brundin, P. & Bjorklund, A. (1988). Comparison of growth and reinnervation properties of cholinergic neurons from different brain regions grafted to the hippocampus. *J. Comp. Neurol.*, **268**, 204–22.

Nutt, J. G., Obeso, J. A. & Stocchi, F. (2000). Continuous dopamine-receptor stimulation in advanced Parkinson's disease. *Trends Neurosci.*, **23**, S109–15.

Olanow, C. W. (2002a). Surgical therapy for Parkinson's disease. *Eur. J. Neurol.*, **9 Suppl 3**, 31–9.

Olanow, C. W. (2002b). Transplantation for Parkinson's disease: pros, cons, and where do we go from here? *Mov. Disord.*, **17**, S15.

Olanow, C. W. & Obeso J. A. (2000). Preventing levodopa-induced dyskinesias. *Ann. Neurol.*, **47**, 167–78.

Olanow, C. W. & Tatton W. G. (2000). Etiology and pathogenesis of Parkinson's disease. *Annu. Rev. Neurosci.*, **22**, 123–44.

Onn, S.-P., West, A. R. & Grace, A. A. (2000). Dopamine-mediated regulation of striatal neuronal and network interactions. *Trends Neurosci.*, **23**, S45–56.

Peschanski, M., Defer, G., N'Guyen, J. P. *et al.* (1994). Bilateral motor improvement and alteration of L-dopa effect in two patients with Parkinson's disease following intrastriatal transplantation of foetal ventral mesencephalon. *Brain*, **117** (3), 487–99.

Piccini, P., Brooks, D. J., Bjorklund, A. *et al.* (1999). Dopamine release from nigral transplants visualized in vivo in a Parkinson's patient. *Nat. Neurosci.*, **2**, 1137–40.

Piccini, P., Lindvall, O., Bjorklund, A. *et al.* (2000). Delayed recovery of movement-related cortical function in Parkinson's disease after striatal dopaminergic grafts. *Ann. Neurol.*, **48**, 689–95.

Rakic, P. (2002). Adult neurogenesis in mammals: an identity crisis. *J. Neurosci.*, **22**, 614–18.

Ramachandran, A. C., Bartlett, L. E. & Mendez I. M. (2002). A multiple target neural transplantation strategy for Parkinson's disease. *Rev. Neurosci.*, **13**, 243–56.

Redmond, D. E., Jr., Leranth, C., Spencer, D. D. *et al.* (1990). Fetal neural graft survival. *Lancet*, **336**, 820–2.

Sanghera, M. K., Manaye, K., McMahon, A., Sonsalla, P. K. & German, D. C. (1997). Dopamine transporter mRNA levels are high in midbrain neurons vulnerable to MPTP. *Neuroreport*, **8**, 3327–31.

Saucedo-Cardenas, O., Quintana-Hau, J. D., Le W. D. *et al.* (1998). Nurr1 is essential for the induction of the dopaminergic phenotype and the survival of ventral mesencephalic late dopaminergic precursor neurons. *Proc. Natl Acad. Sci., USA*, **95**, 4013–18.

Schultzberg, M., Dunnett, S. B., Bjorklund, A. *et al.* (1984). Dopamine and cholecystokinin immunoreactive neurones in mesencephalic grafts reinnervating the neostriatum: evidence for selective growth regulation. *Neuroscience*, **12**, 17–32.

Schumacher, J. M., Short, M. P., Hyman, B. T., Breakefield, X. O. & Isacson, O. (1991). Intracerebral implantation of nerve growth factor-producing fibroblasts protects striatum against neurotoxic levels of excitatory amino acids. *Neuroscience*, **45**, 561–70.

Schumacher, J., Ellias, S., Palmer, E. *et al.* (2000). Transplantation of embryonic porcine mesencephalic tissue in patients with Parkinson's disease. *Neurology*, **54**, 1042–50.

Semina, E. V., Ferrell, R. E., Mintz-Hittner, H. A. *et al.* (1998). A novel homeobox gene PITX3 is mutated in families with autosomal-dominant cataracts and ASMD. *Nat. Genet.*, **19**, 167–70.

Semina, E. V., Reiter, R. S. & Murray, J. C. (1997). Isolation of a new homeobox gene belonging to the Pitx/Rieg family: expression during lens development and mapping to the aphakia region on mouse chromosome 19. *Hum. Mol. Genet.*, **6**, 2109–16.

Shimazaki, T., Shingo T. & Weiss S. (2001). The ciliary neurotrophic factor/leukemia inhibitory factor/gc130 receptor complex operates in the maintenance of mammalian forebrain neural stem cells. *J. Neurosci.*, **21**, 7642–53.

Simon, H. H., Saueressig, H., Wurst, W., Goulding, M. D. & O'Leary, D. D. (2001). Fate of midbrain dopaminergic neurons controlled by the engrailed genes. *J. Neurosci.*, **21**, 3126–34.

Smidt, M. P., van Schaick, H. S., Lanctot, C. *et al.* (1997). A homeodomain gene Ptx3 has highly restricted brain expression in mesencephalic dopaminergic neurons. *Proc. Natl Acad. Sci., USA*, **94**, 13305–10.

Smidt, M. P., Asbreuk, C. H., Cox, J. J., Chen, H., Johnson, R. L. & Burbach, J. P. (2000). A second independent pathway for development of mesencephalic dopaminergic neurons requires Lmx1b. *Nat. Neurosci.*, **3**, 337–41.

Sotelo, C. & Alvarado-Mallart, R. M. (1987). Embryonic and adult neurons interact to allow Purkinje cell replacement in mutant cerebellum. *Nature*, **327**, 421–3.

Spencer, D. D., Robbins, R. J., Naftolin, F. *et al.* (1992). Unilateral transplantation of human fetal mesencephalic tissue into the caudate nucleus of patients with Parkinson's disease. *N. Engl. J. Med.*, **327**, 1541–8.

Strecker, R. E. & Jacobs, B. L. (1985). Substantia nigra dopaminergic unit activity in behaving cats: effects of arousal on spontaneous discharge and sensory evoked activity. *Brain Res.*, **361**, 339–50.

Strecker, R. E., Sharp, T., Brundin, P., Zetterstrom, T., Ungerstedt, U. & Bjorklund A. (1987). Autoregulation of dopamine release and metabolism by intrastriatal nigral grafts as revealed by intracerebral dialysis. *Neuroscience*, **22**, 169–78.

Studer, L., Tabar, V. & McKay, R. D. (1998). Transplantation of expanded mesencephalic precursors leads to recovery in parkinsonian rats. *Nat. Neurosci.*, **1**, 290–5.

Tornqvist, N., Hermanson, E., Perlmann, T. & Stromberg, I. (2002). Generation of tyrosine hydroxylase-immunoreactive neurons in ventral mesencephalic tissue of Nurr1 deficient mice. *Brain Res. Dev. Brain Res.*, **133**, 37–47.

Venna, N., Sabin, T., Ordia, J. & Mark, V. (1984). Treatment of severe Parkinson's disease by intraventricular injection of dopamine. *Appl. Neurophysiol.*, **47**, 62–4.

Wagner, J., Akerud, P., Castro, D. S. *et al.* (1999). Induction of a midbrain dopaminergic phenotype in Nurr1-overexpressing neural stem cells by type 1 astrocytes. *Nat. Biotechnol.*, **17**, 653–9.

Wallen, A. A., Castro, D. S., Zetterstrom, R. H. *et al.* (2001). Orphan nuclear receptor Nurr1 is essential for Ret expression in midbrain dopamine neurons and in the brain stem. *Mol. Cell. Neurosci.*, **18**, 649–63.

Wenning, G. K., Odin, P., Morrish, P. *et al.* (1997). Short- and long-term survival and function of unilateral intrastriatal dopaminergic grafts in Parkinson's disease. *Ann. Neurol.*, **42**, 95–107.

Widner, H., Tetrud, J., Rehncrona, S. *et al.* (1992). Bilateral fetal mesencephalic grafting in two patients with parkinsonism induced by 1-methyl-4-phenyl-1,2,3,6-tetrahydropyridine. *N. Engl. J. Med.*, **327**, 1556–63.

Wurst, W., Auerbach, A. B. & Joyner, A. L. (1994). Multiple developmental defects in Engrailed-1 mutant mice: an early mid-hindbrain deletion and patterning defects in forelimbs and sternum. *Development*, **120**, 2065–75.

Yamada, T., McGeer, P. L., Baimbridge, K. G. & McGeer, E. G. (1990). Relative sparing in Parkinson's disease of substantia nigra dopamine neurons containing calbindin-D28K. *Brain Res.*, **526**, 303–7.

Zetterstrom, R. H., Solomin, L., Jansson, L., Hoffer, B. J., Olson, L. & Perlmann T. (1997). Dopamine neuron agenesis in Nurr1-deficient mice. *Science*, **276**, 248–50.

Zetterstrom, T., Brundin, P., Gage, F. H. *et al.* (1986). In vivo measurement of spontaneous release and metabolism of dopamine from intrastriatal nigral grafts using intracerebral dialysis. *Brain Res.*, **362**, 344–9.

Zetterstrom, T. & Ungerstedt, U. (1984). Effects of apomorphine on the in vivo release of dopamine and its metabolites, studied by brain dialysis. *Eur. J. Pharmacol.*, **97**, 29–36.

Zurn, A. D., Widmer, H. R. & Aebischer, P. (2001). Sustained delivery of GDNF: towards a treatment for Parkinson's disease. *Brain Res.*, **36**, 222–9.

Part IV

Normal aging

25

Clinical aspects of normal aging

Marilyn S. Albert

Department of Neurology, Johns Hopkins University School of Medicine, Baltimore, MD, USA

Overview

It is now widely understood that the number of persons living into old age increased dramatically during the last century. In 1900, the average life expectancy at birth was 47 years. By 1950, this had increased to 68 years. In the year 2000, the average life expectancy for males was estimated at slightly over 74 years, and for females it was almost 80 years of age. There is thus increasing interest in understanding the normal changes that occur with age. Along with this has come an interest in developing ways to maintain function at its maximum. This chapter will describe epidemiological aspects of aging, cognitive and motor changes that are associated with aging, the underlying neurobiologic alterations that are thought to be responsible for age-related changes in cognitive and motor function, and the implications of these alterations for the clinical evaluation of an older person.

Epidemiologic aspects of aging

The numbers of persons living to an old age has risen dramatically, and this is expected to continue until at least 2050, as noted above. During the first half of the twentieth century, the increase in life expectancy was largely the result of decreased mortality early in life. The continued expansion of life expectancy during the last half of the twentieth century was largely the result of increased survival during middle and old age. At the same time, virtually all developed countries experienced decreases in the birth rate. Therefore, older persons became an ever-increasing portion of the population, as shown in Table 25.1, which provides data for the US population in particular. In 1900, slightly over 4% of the population was 65 and older. This percentage had doubled by 1950, when 8% of the population was 65 or above, and in the year 2000 almost 13% was in this age range (Guralnik & Ferrucci, 2003). The projections for the year 2050, when the baby boomer generation will be 65 and over, are equally dramatic. Estimates indicate that one in five Americans will be 65 and older by 2050.

The portion of the population represented by those 85 and over, the so-called "oldest old," shows a similarly striking pattern. In 1900, those 85 years of age and older represented 0.1% of the population. In 1950, this percentage continued to be low, at 0.6%. In 2000, almost $4\frac{1}{2}$% of the population was 85 and older. By 2050, this number is expected to grow exponentially, and is estimated to be almost 20% of the population (Guralnik & Ferrucci, 2003).

The number of individuals aged 100 and older is projected to follow similar trends in the next 50 years. In the USA, the number has doubled every decade since 1980. In 2050, it is estimated that there will be 1 million centenarians in the USA (Guralnik & Ferrucci, 2003).

This increased aging of the population is seen most clearly in developed countries, and is most striking in Europe. Twenty-four of the 25 oldest countries are in eastern or western Europe, with Japan being the 25th. Italy has the oldest population, with over 18% aged 65 and older. The percentage of older persons in underdeveloped countries (such as Asia, Latin America, and North Africa) although low at the present time, is expected to double by the year 2030.

The speed with which countries have aged varies widely. One can see this by examining the time it has taken (or will take) for 14% of the population to be 65 and older. Some countries, such as Sweden and the United Kingdom, reached this level in the mid 1970s, taking approximately 85 years to double in size (from 7% to 14%). Japan took 26 years to do so. The USA is expected to reach this

Table 25.1. Actual and projected growth of the US population, 1900–2050 (millions)

Year	Total population (all ages)	65 years and older		85 years and older	
		Number	Percent of total population	Number	Percent of 65 years and older population
1900	76.1	3.1	4.1	0.1	3.2
1950	152.3	12.3	8.2	0.6	4.9
2000	276.1	34.9	12.6	4.4	12.6
2050	403.7	82.0	20.3	19.4	23.7

Source: Population Division. US Census Bureau, Washington, DC. Reprinted with permission from Guralnik & Ferucci, *Demography and Epidemiology*, 2003.

level by 2013, taking 69 years. The developing countries are expected to have a pattern much like Japan's, and are expected to reach the 14% level by 2030 (Guralnik & Ferrucci, 2003).

Females have a greater life expectancy than males at all ages. At birth this differential is estimated to be about 5 1/2 years. Whites have a greater life expectancy than blacks until age 75. However, once individuals have lived to age 75, life expectancy is similar for whites and blacks. It is assumed that the differential in life expectancy between whites and blacks relates to the higher prevalence of illnesses among blacks, such as heart disease and diabetes, as well as access to health care and the use of healthcare prevention strategies. Information concerning Hispanics is less clear, since Hispanic status has been ascertained in varying ways in recent years.

When one has lived to age 75, life expectancy remains substantial. The average 75-year-old will live another 10–12 years. The average 85-year-old will live another 5–6 years (Guralnik & Ferrucci, 2003).

Changes in cognitive function with age

A number of aspects of cognitive function show alterations with advancing age. The focus of this section will be on age-related changes in memory and executive function because these have been the focus of intense investigation in recent years. Moreover, these two areas of cognition are the two that have been studied across species. This makes it possible to determine the degree to which age-related changes in cognition found in one species are corroborated in another. When such parallels are found, it strengthens the likelihood that the cognitive change is related to age, and not to early signs of a neurodegenerative disorder, such as Alzheimer's disease. Since there is an increas-

ing focus on identifying patients as early as possible in the course of AD (for example, see Chapter 27), distinctions between age-related and disease-related changes in cognition are of great practical, as well as theoretical, interest. Other aspects of age-related changes in cognition, such as alterations in language, visuospatial processing, and general intelligence are reviewed elsewhere (Albert & Moss, 1999).

Memory

Workers in the field of memory have concluded that memory is not a unitary phenomenon, and most models of memory function hypothesize that memory consists of a series of specific yet interactive stores (e.g. Waugh & Norman, 1965; Tulving, 1972). They include, at a minimum: sensory memory, primary memory, and secondary memory. In addition, a distinction has been made between information that is consciously learned (called explicit or declarative memory) and information that is acquired over time, unrelated to specific conscious effort of episodes (called implicit or procedural memory) (Reber & Squire, 1994).

Memory in humans

There are minimal changes with age in sensory and primary memory, but substantial age-related changes occur in secondary memory (for a review, see Craik, 1977 and Poon, 1985). The age at which changes in secondary memory occur depends upon the methods that are used to test the memory store. Difficult explicit memory tasks (e.g. delayed recall) demonstrate statistically significant differences by subjects in their 50s, in comparison to younger individuals (Albert *et al.*, 1987).

A close examination of memory performance in the older individuals shows, however, that they are not more rapidly forgetting what they learned, but rather they are taking longer to learn the new information. For example, if one compares the difference between immediate and delayed recall over the lifespan, there are no statistically significant age differences (Petersen *et al.*, 1992). Thus, if one allows older subjects to learn material well (i.e. to the point where few errors are made), they do not forget what they have learned more rapidly than the young. However, if older subjects are not given the ability to learn material to the same level of proficiency as younger individuals, after a delay, less information will be retained by the average older person.

However, there is considerable variability among older subjects on tasks of this sort. There are many healthy older subjects who have test scores that overlap those of subjects many years younger than themselves (e.g. about one-third of healthy 70-year-old humans have delayed recall scores that overlap those of 30-year-olds, equated for education).

Memory in non-human primates

Similar findings have emerged from studies in monkeys. Since free recall cannot be easily tested in monkeys, considerable effort has gone into developing a memory task that uses recognition, but determines the quantity of information aging monkeys can retain across varying delay intervals. The delayed non-matching to sample task (DNMS) is the most widely used method for assessing recognition memory in the nonhuman primate. This task relies upon a two-alternative forced choice paradigm in which the monkey is required to discriminate which of two objects was recently presented. By using the delayed non-matching to sample task, many studies have shown that aged monkeys are impaired at learning the non-matching principle but are, at best, only mildly impaired across the delay conditions of the test (Moss *et al.*, 1988; Arnsten & Goldman-Rakic, 1990; Bachevalier *et al.*, 1991; Presty *et al.*, 1987; Rapp & Amaral, 1989). Thus, like humans, the old monkeys take longer to learn something new but do not appear to forget this information more rapidly over lengthening delays than younger monkeys.

Moreover, on a very difficult memory task, such as the delayed recognition span test (DRST) (Moss, 1983), age-related changes are seen among middle-aged monkeys. This test requires a monkey to identify a novel stimulus from an increasingly large array of previously presented stimuli. The goal is to keep track of as many stimuli as possible without making a mistake. Middle-aged monkeys (16–23 years) are impaired on the spatial version of the DRST but not on the color version (Moss *et al.*, 1988). Aged

monkeys (25–27 years) are impaired relative to young adults (5–7 years) under both conditions of the task. This suggests that the performance of monkeys on the spatial version of the DRST may be functionally equivalent to the performance of humans on difficult delayed recall tasks. Longitudinal assessment of young and aged monkeys (after an interval of 4 years) confirm the findings of the cross-sectional data (Moss, 1993). Young animals show either slight improvements or slight declines on the DRST, while aged monkeys show either slight declines or severe declines over time.

A more recently developed task, the visual paired-comparison test (VPC), was developed to study memory without requiring the subject to make a conscious response. Subjects are first shown a picture of a stimulus item (e.g. an object); after a delay, they are shown the same image paired with a novel image. By measuring the length of time the subject looks at a stimulus (by recording their eye movements) one can show that normal subjects spend more time looking at a novel stimulus than a familiar one (McKee & Squire, 1993). Young monkeys spend longer looking at a novel stimulus than aged monkeys (Eriksson & Barnes, 2003).

Like aging humans, there is also considerable variability in the performance of aging monkeys. Among the oldest animals there are subjects who perform within the range of younger animals, even though the mean performance of the group declines significantly. For example, on DNMS, the number of trials to criterion ranges from 50 to 220 and the number of errors range from 29–60. Among the older monkeys, the trials to criterion range from 200–516 and the number of errors range from 50 to 115.

Memory in rodents

Since rats can be trained on tasks that are almost identical tasks to those given to monkeys, parallels between the two species are clear. When young, middle-aged and elderly rats are tested on the delayed non-matching to position task, older rats show age-related deficits with increasing delay intervals (Dunnett *et al.*, 1988). Aged rats show less exploration than young rats in a task that is similar to the Visual Paired Comparison task (Cavoy & Delacour, 1993). Aged rodents are also impaired, relative to young and middle-aged rats, on the Morris water maze (Gallagher *et al.*, 1993), in which animals are required to find a platform that is submerged under water, after having first learned its location when it was visible (Morris, 1981). These deficits are highly stable over time, when a specific combination of learning trials and probe trials are used. Moreover, as with humans, there is considerable variability in performance among older animals. A substantial subgroup shows age-related declines in performance, but some aged animals perform on a par with young animals (Gallagher & Rapp, 1997).

Executive function

The complex set of abilities sometimes referred to as "executive functions" include abilities such as: abstraction, maintenance of set, shifting of set, and cognitive flexibiity. The term "executive function" derives from the fact that these abilities play a major role in problem solving, planning and adaptation to one's environment.

Executive function in humans

Tests evaluating concept formation and set shifting uniformly show significant changes with age, primarily when subjects are in their late 60s or 70s. For example, the similarities subtest of the Wechsler Adult Intelligence Scale (WAIS), which asks subjects to identify how two objects (e.g. a table and a chair) are similar to each other, is the subtest on the Verbal scale of the WAIS that shows the greatest decline with age (Heaton et al., 1986). Education appears to be a modifier of this decline, in that subjects with lower amounts of education demonstrate declines at younger ages; however, all subjects in the oldest group (mean age 68 years), regardless of educational level, show significant declines in performance.

Series completion tests also show substantial age declines. These tests generally require the subject to examine a series of letters or numbers and determine the rule that governed the sequencing of the items in the series. Cross-sectional and longitudinal data demonstrate age-related declines on tasks of this sort (e.g. Lachman & Jelalian, 1984; Schaie, 1983).

Proverb interpretation tests, which require the subject to provide the general meaning of a proverb (e.g. "barking dogs seldom bite"), also demonstrate age-related declines (Albert et al., 1990). This is true whether or not subjects are asked to provide the meaning of the proverb themselves or are given alternate choices among which to choose. Similarly, set shifting tasks, such as the Visual–Verbal test (in which subjects are asked to look at a series of cards and indicate how three of the four objects on each card are alike in one way, and then how three of the objects are alike in another way), also show substantial age-related declines. These changes appear to be related to the fact that older subjects have difficulty switching from one abstract answer to another (i.e. they tend to get the first item in the set correct but the second one wrong). Slowness in establishing mental set (i.e. getting the first item in the set wrong but the

second one right) and failure to establish set (i.e. getting both items in the set wrong) did not increase differentially with age (Albert et al., 1990).

Executive function in monkeys

Changes in executive function in monkeys have been examined primarily by using reversal learning paradigms (Bartus et al., 1979; Rapp, 1990), or a form of delayed response (Bachevalier, 1993). Reversal learning involves responding to a change in reinforcement contingencies by first "unlearning" or breaking the initial stimulus-reinforcement bond, and then acquiring, or "shifting" to a new one. In this way, reversal learning can be considered a measure of executive function. Data have accumulated to suggest that aged monkeys have difficulty in reversing established stimulus-reward contingencies, particularly when based on spatial location. Thus, compared to young adult monkeys, aged monkeys, as a group, are impaired on spatial, but not on object reversal learning (Lai et al., 1995). Moreover, aged monkeys tend to make more perseverative responses than young adults on both spatial and object reversal learning.

Recently, a task called the Conceptual Set Shifting Task (CSST) was developed for non-human primates, as an equivalent of the Wisconsin Card Sorting task in humans (Moore et al., 2003). In the monkey version, a pattern of responding is developed on the basis of rewards for responses to a specific visual pattern, the animal maintains this response pattern for a while, and then the reward contingency changes. One can therefore examine the number of errors prior to attainment of the initial "abstraction rule", as well as the number of perseverative responses after the rule changes. Aged monkeys are impaired, in comparison to young, on both the concept formation and set shifting aspects of the task (Moore et al., 2003).

Imaging studies of age-related changes in cognition

Recent advances in brain imaging have begun to provide insights into the changes in brain structure and function that underly age-related changes in cognition. These include studies using magnetic resonance imaging (MRI) scans, as well as positron emission tomography (PET) and functional MRI (fMRI).

Structural imaging – MRI

MRI studies of healthy adults across the age range have shown that, regardless of the sequence type, overall brain volume shows a decrease with age, while the amount of

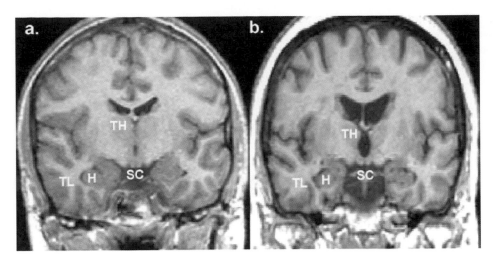

Fig. 25.1 An example of a structural MRI (*a*) in a healthy young and (*b*) healthy older individual. H-hippocampus, TH-thalamus, SC-suprasellar cistern.

CSF increases, even if individuals are healthy (Christiansen *et al.*, 1994; Coffey *et al.*, 1992; Harris *et al.*, 1994; Jernigan *et al.*, 1990, 1991; Lim *et al.*, 1992; Murphy *et al.*, 1992; Matsumae *et al.*, 1996; Pfefferbaum *et al.*, 1994; Tanna *et al.*, 1991) (see Fig. 25.1).

The volume of brain tissue decreases with advancing age. Several structural MRI studies have shown that the prefrontal cortex undergoes disproportionate shrinkage as people get older (Raz *et al.*, 1998; Resnick *et al.*, 2003). The largest declines in volume are seen in the lateral prefrontal cortex (Tisserand *et al.*, 2002). Studies using diffusion tensor imaging have also shown selectively greater declines in white matter tracts in the prefrontal cortex (Head *et al.*, 2004). These findings are consistent with the theory that normal aging is associated with declines in frontal-striatal systems (see Hedden & Gabrieli, 2004). The underlying neurobiological alterations responsible for this brain atrophy is, however, unlikely to be neuronal loss, as discussed below.

Functional imaging – PET and fMRI

One of the most important innovations for the study of brain–behavior relationships has been the development of functional imaging, initially using PET and more recently fMRI. In PET scanning, a radioactive isotope is either injected or inhaled by the subject, and the scanning machine evaluates the differential decay of radioactivity in order to assess regional changes in blood flow in the brain. The blood flow is considered a surrogate for neuronal activity. Likewise, fMRI uses the magnetic qualities of water molecules to evaluate the differential distribution of oxygenated blood in the brain, and the ratio of oxygenated to deoxygenated blood is thought to be an indirect measure of neuronal activity. Since fMRI does not involve exposure to radioactivity, and measurements are closer to real time, many investigators who previously employed PET are turning to fMRI.

To obtain information about how the brain performs cognitive tasks, these imaging techniques are combined with cognitive paradigms, which produce a range of brain activations. Through careful design of such paradigms, it becomes possible to obtain information about the brain regions that are involved in a specific cognitive activity. Perceptual and emotional experience can also be interrogated in a similar manner. When such functional imaging procedures are combined with structural imaging, one can obtain data with highly accurate anatomical detail. The newest of these approaches, fMRI, provides such information in close to real time (i.e. the latency between stimulus onset and fMRI response is typically 2 seconds).

The most important general concept to emerge from such studies is that multiple brain regions are essential for encoding or retrieving new information. Moreover, some of the brain regions that appear to be integral to "memory networks" have not been easy to evaluate by other imaging modalities. The most important in this regard is the frontal lobes, which are activated during both encoding and retrieval in normal young individuals (Kapur *et al.*, 1994, 1996; Demb *et al.*, 1995; Fletcher *et al.*, 1995; Wagner *et al.*, 1998a; Madden *et al.*, 1999; Buckner *et al.*, 1999).

The hippocampus, known to be essential for normal memory based primarily on lesion studies (Squire *et al.*, 1988), was initially more difficult to activate than many other brain regions, for reasons that are not entirely clear.

Nevertheless, many recent PET and fMRI studies have shown that significant activations of the hippocampus may be demonstrated when an individual is attempting to learn or retrieve new information. (Schacter & Wagner, 1999; Gabrieli *et al.*, 1997; Brewer *et al.*, 1998; Martin *et al.*, 1997; Stern *et al.*, 1996; Wagner *et al.*, 1998a), as is the prefrontal cortex (e.g. Haxby *et al.*, 1996; Wagner *et al.*, 1998b).

The most consistent finding to emerge from PET and fMRI studies of aging is that there are alterations in the activation of the frontal lobes during encoding and/or retrieval of new information (e.g. Cabeza *et al.*, 1997, 2000; Hazlett *et al.*, 1998; Grady *et al.*, 1999; Stebbins *et al.*, 2002; Logan *et al.*, 2002). Some have found increased activity, while others have found decreases. The increases in prefrontal activity are often observed in areas contralateral to those activated in the young. This has been interpreted as evidence of age-related reductions in hemispheric asymmetry (Cabeza, 2002).

An age-related reduction in hippocampal activation has also been demonstrated during episodic memory tasks, but the differences are much less striking than what is seen in the frontal lobes. Reductions have been seen primarily in the left parahippocampal gyrus (Daselaar *et al.*, 2003; Morcom *et al.*, 2003).

Taken together, these findings indicate that normal memory function requires integrated activation of a network of brain regions that involves the hippocampus and the prefrontal cortex. It has been hypothesized for some time that alterations in frontal systems play a major role in cognitive changes with age (Albert & Kaplan, 1980), and the recent imaging findings cited above, support this hypothesis. It has been hypothesized that the functional impact of these changes is that elderly subjects, in comparison to young, use differing strategies to perform memory tasks (e.g. Cabeza, 2002; Rosen *et al.*, 2002). This is consistent with numerous previous reports showing that elderly individuals are less likely to spontaneously use mnemonic strategies than the young, when trying to learn new information (for reviews see Craik, 1977; Arenberg & Robertson-Tchabo, 1977). An alternative possibility is that the same strategy is being applied in different ways by the two age groups. (For a more detailed discussion of hypotheses regarding age-related alterations in frontal systems and their impact on cognition see Hedden & Gabrieli, 2004 and Tisserand & Jolles, 2003.)

It should also be noted that some investigators have reported differences between the young and the elderly in hemodynamic response (D'Esposito *et al.*, 1999, 2003). While the nature of these changes is still controversial, ranging from the possibility of decreased hemodynamic response (and therefore signal change) in the elderly, to increased noise with no absolute reduction in the magnitude of signal change, it is possible that these differences are, at least in part, responsible for some of the fMRI differences between healthy young and older individuals.

Changes in motor function with age

As people get older, they also have increasing difficulty with mobility, including the ability to perform common tasks, such as walking, rising from a chair, or regaining balance when it has been disturbed. Although there are age-related changes in muscle reaction time, proprioception, range of motion and muscle strength and power, it is the latter that appears to be most strongly related to declines in mobility.

Several factors related to muscle strength decline with age, even in healthy and physically active older adults (Schultz, 1992). Many of these declines are related to the ability to recover one's balance after some perturbation, and thus are likely related to falls. There is a decline in muscle strength of approximately 30% by age 65 (with women having less strength than men at all ages, even when normalized for body size). For example, hip flexor muscles, that are critical for recovery of balance, decline with age. There is also a decline in fast motor units with age, which are important for hip flexion. Joint torque (or the strength developed about a joint) is also necessary for the restoration of balance after instability. Healthy older adults are slower to develop joint torque than young adults, and older women are slower than older men. Declines also occur in the ability of muscles to produce power. For example, well-trained runners over 70 years of age are 30% slower than younger runners with equivalent training. Healthy rodents, likewise, show a decline in muscle output with advancing age. Impairments in muscle strength also affect the ability to rise from a chair. Taken together, these findings suggest that it is important to assess and train muscle power in order to maintain muscle function that is critical for a variety of daily activities (Ashton-Miller & Alexander, 2003).

Despite the fact that there are systematic increases in reaction time as people get older, it has been argued that these are not sufficient to interfere with rapid responses in time-critical situations. For example, healthy older adults require about 400 ms to fully contract a muscle and 200–400 ms to take a quick step. However, myoelectric reaction times (or the time from the stimulus cue to the first measurable change in electrical activity in a muscle) are about 10–20 ms longer in healthy older adults than in young adults. Likewise, movement-to-target reaction times increase about 2 ms per decade from the 20s to the 90s. Thus, these differences are not considered critical for mobility function (Ashton-Miller & Alexander, 2003).

A number of studies have shown that body joint range of motion decreases with advancing age. For example, there is a 20% decline in hip rotation between the ages of 45 and 70, and a 10% decline in wrist and shoulder range of motion. These types of decreases appear related to limitations in activities of daily living. The ability to bend down correlates with hip flexion range of motion and ability to do activities involving the hands and arms correlates with range of motion of these upper extremities.

Studies of proprioception (one's awareness of body position and orientation) have shown slight decreases in joint position sense in the knee and declines in vibration sense. As these studies are few in number, it remains unclear if these declines have functional consequences.

Among adults free of overt disease, there are also changes in gait (Odenheimer et al., 1994). After approximately aged 60, self-selected gait speed (i.e. comfortable gait) declines by 1–2% per year. Most of the decline in speed is attributable to a decline in stride length. Muscle strength may be a factor in this decline in gait speed as well, since walking speed is related in a non-linear fashion to leg muscle strength (Buchner et al., 1996). Reductions in gait speed do not appear to be related to falls, but increases in stride time variability are associated with a five times greater risk of falls.

Finally, there are changes in postural control with advancing age that have a functional impact in daily life. Postural tasks that are demanding (e.g. standing on one leg with eyes open) show declines by aged 50 (Bohannon et al., 1984). Postural tasks that are relatively undemanding (e.g. standing on two feet with eyes open) show minimal changes until aged 70, and decrease thereafter.

Thus, the primary age-related changes that have substantial impact on function are alterations in gait and postural control. The reasons for these changes are not entirely clear, but it has been hypothesized that age-related decreases in dopamine play an important role (Odenheimer et al., 1994). These declines in dopamine also appear to play a role in cognitive changes with age, as described below.

Underlying neural mechanisms that contribute to age-related changes in cognitive and physical function

Neuronal number

Given the cognitive and motor changes discussed above, it is striking that the wealth of recent morphological data in humans (Haug, 1984; Leuba & Garey, 1989; Terry et al., 1987), indicate that, with advancing age, neuronal loss in the cortex is either not significant or not as extensive as reports prior to 1984 had suggested (Brody, 1955, 1970; Colon, 1972; Shefer, 1973; Henderson et al., 1980; Anderson et al., 1983). While large neurons appear to shrink, few are lost (Terry et al., 1987).

There are, in addition, comparable data in monkeys. Minimal neuronal cortical loss with age in monkeys has now been demonstrated in the striate cortex (Vincent et al., 1989), motor cortex (Tigges et al., 1992), frontal cortex (Peters et al., 1994: O'Donnell et al., 1999), and the entorhinal cortex (Amaral, 1993). These general conclusions have been reached not only on the basis of a comparison of counts of neurons in young (5 to 6 years) and old (over 25 years of age) monkeys, but also on the basis of an examination of the cortical tissue by electron microscopy (Peters et al., 1994). Beyond an accumulation of lipofuscin granules in the cell body of some neurons and some cellular debris in neuroglial cells, there is very little evidence of changes with age in the neurons of these cortical regions (Peters et al., 1991). Morphological studies in rodents have reported comparable findings (Rapp et al., 2000).

The weight of the evidence from postmortem studies also supports the conclusion that the hippocampus shows minimal structural change with advancing age. The postmortem data in humans and monkeys indicate that neuronal loss is surprisingly low in most subfields of the hippocampus. For example, the subiculum shows a significant age-related loss in humans, with a similar trend in monkeys, however, the CA1, CA2 and CA3 subfields of the hippocampus show no evidence of age-related neuronal loss (Amaral, 1993; Rosene, 1993; West et al., 1994; Gomez-Isla et al., 1996). Equivalent data have been reported in rodents, where it has been shown that even in the subset of animals with declines on a memory task, there was no decrease in the number of neurons in the various hippocampal subfields (Rapp & Gallagher, 1996; Rapp et al., 1999). (See Morrison & Hof, 1997 for a more detailed discussion of these issues.)

Neuronal loss and neurotransmitter changes

There is substantial neuronal loss in selected subcortical regions that is likely responsible for decreases in the production of neurotransmitters important for cognitive function, such as in the basal forebrain and the locus coeruleus (e.g. Chan-Palay & Asan, 1989; Rosene, 1993). For example, in humans and monkeys there is approximately a 50% neuronal loss with age in the basal forebrain and 35–40% loss in the locus coeruleus and dorsal raphe (Kemper, 1993). This compares with an approximate loss of 5% in the CA1 subfield of the hippocampus. The neuronal loss in these subcortical nuclei may be very important for memory function, as these brain regions influence the production of several neurotransmitters important for memory (such as acetylcholine, dopamine and serotonin). Though subcortical, these nuclei have extensive connections with the cortex, and thus are responsible for the level of many neurotransmitters within the cortex. For example, treatment of rhesus monkeys with a D2 receptor agonist improves performance on a delayed memory task in aged monkeys (Arnsten *et al.*, 1995). As mentioned above, age-related declines in dopamine may also play a role in the alterations in motor function seen with advancing age.

Synaptic integrity

Even though there does not appear to be enough neuronal loss to account for age-related cognitive change, there are changes in other aspects of neuronal function, specifically the number and/or function of synapses. Most of the studies that have explored this question with respect to aging pertain to learning and memory in rodents. It has been demonstrated that there are synaptic changes in the CA3 region of the hippocampus when one compares older rodents who are memory impaired with younger rodents (Smith *et al.*, 2000). Specifically, older rodents with spatial learning deficits display significant reductions in synaptophysin immunoreactivity in the CA3 region of the hippocampus, but not in other subfields. This region receives its input from layer II of the entorhinal cortex. Thus, it has been hypothesized that there are circuit-specific changes involving the entorhinal input to CA3 that influence the computational function of the hippocampus and are thereby related to age-related memory change (Smith *et al.*, 2000). There are, in addition, alterations in long-term potentiation and long-term depression in aged rodents with learning deficits (Barnes, 2003; Norris *et al.*, 1996), and alterations in at least one receptor type (i.e. NMDA receptors) (Gazzaley *et al.*, 1996; Barnes *et al.*, 1997). These results suggest that the variability seen in memory changes with advancing age among healthy individuals is related to variations in synaptic integrity and activity-dependent synaptic plasticity in specific brain circuits related to learning and memory. (See Rosensweig & Barnes, 2003 for a detailed discussion of this issue.)

Neuronal proliferation in the adult brain

One of the most strongly held dogmas of neurobiology was the concept that once nerve cells were formed they could only die. There was no such thing as endogenous neuronal replacement. There is increasing evidence that concept is incorrect. The work of Altman over 30 years ago suggested that, in the rodent, neurogenesis could continue in selected regions of the brain into adulthood, particularly the dentate region of the hippocampus, the olfactory and cerebellum (Altman & Das, 1965). In recent years, this issue has been revisited in rodents and there is ample evidence, based on the DNA marker, bromodeoxyuridine, that neurogenesis occurs in the hippocampus and olfactory system. Similar findings have also been demonstrated in monkeys (Kornack & Rakic, 1999; Gould *et al.*, 1999), and even in the human (Eriksson *et al.*, 1998).

In the dentate gyrus of the macaque monkey, labeled cells are thought to proliferate in the border zone between the hilus and granular cell layer, and then to migrate and differentiate in the granule cell layer. The proliferation of new neurons decreases with age. In the rodent there appears to be a gradual increase in total numbers of neurons; in primates, such an accumulation is less certain. It has been suggested (Kornack & Rakic, 1999) that the number of neurons in the hippocampus is constant, but with a fixed replacement rate – neurogenesis balanced by the rate of apoptosis and cell removal.

The source of these new neurons may be pluripotential stem cells. In the rodent it has been shown that physical activity stimulates this neurogenesis from stem cells (Kemperman *et al.*, 2000). Since pluripotential stem cells have been identified in areas other than the hippocampus, where neurogenesis has not been demonstrated to occur normally, investigators are exploring ways to cause these cells to produce new neurons. This is an active area of research in neurodegeneration.

White matter changes

In addition, age-related alterations in the white matter have recently been described in some detail (Peters *et al.*, 1994; Peters, 1996; Nielson & Peters, 2000). At first glance, the data suggesting loss of white matter in the brain but only loss of synapses (with minimal loss of neurons cortex) can be difficult to understand. Conventional knowledge suggests that white matter consists of the axons of neurons and that if there is a loss of axons, there should be cell death and a substantial loss of grey matter. However, the white matter of the brain is also composed of a number of glial elements, particularly oligodendrocytes. Evidence from the non-human primate suggests that the oligodendrocytes, that are responsible for forming the myelin sheath surrounding the axons, may be less efficient with age. For example, when the oligodendrocytes of young and old monkeys were compared (Peters, 1996) it was found that the myelin sheaths in the old monkeys were abnormal and appeared to be degenerating. However, when the number of axons in old and young monkeys was compared by the same investigators (Nielsen & Peters, 2000) relatively few degenerating axons were found in the old monkeys. Taken together, these findings suggest changes in myelin, rather than axonal loss, are at least in part responsible for age-related changes in white matter observed with advancing age. As mentioned above, imaging studies in humans suggests that these alterations may be greater in some regions, such as the frontal lobes, than in others. Thus, having a selective impact on cognition.

Implications for clinical evaluation of older persons

As the foregoing review demonstrates, there are significant cognitive and motor changes as people get older. The fact that comparable changes are found among healthy non-human primates and rodents emphasizes the likelihood that they are not the result of a neurodegenerative disorder such as Alzheimer's disease.

Perhaps surprisingly, these changes in function are not associated with frank neuronal loss, but rather with changes in synaptic function and plasticity that have an impact on the integrated function within neuronal networks. These alterations have a clear impact on the learning and retention of new information. It is likely that alterations in executive function are the result of similar age-associated changes.

The practical implication of these findings is that very mild declines in memory and executive function should be considered within the normal range. Very high functioning older persons are often aware of such changes, despite the fact that they do not have an impact on instrumental activities in daily life. This complicates the ability to detect declines that are a harbinger of disease, suggesting that it might be very beneficial to include a simple memory test as part of a routine annual evaluation to improve the ability to detect disease-related declines, if they occur.

The increased prevalence of medical diseases among older individuals adds to the difficulty of conducting a clinical evaluation. The average 75-year-old suffers from at least three chronic diseases. The distinguishing feature of the evaluation of an older person is, therefore, the presence of multiple chronic conditions, each of which must be evaluated and weighed for importance. This is because these diseases often interact, so that clinical manifestations are less straightforward. Some symptoms, such as a cognitive disorder, may result from more than one disease. When multiple diseases coexist, it is often difficult to assess the severity of one particular disease, and to determine how that disease effects overall functional status. Likewise, the treatment of one disease may make another worse.

There are several additional factors that complicate the clinical evaluation of an older person. First is the under-reporting of symptoms. This may occur because older persons, as well as their physicians, conclude that a symptom which may be treatable is an age-related change for which no treatment is warranted. Cognitive impairment and/or depressive symptoms may also reduce the ability of the individual to accurately report symptoms that are present. Moreover, diseases often present differently in the elderly than in the young. For example, pneumonia or a urinary tract infection may present as confusion. Finally, advancing age brings with it general predisposing factors, such as a gait disorder, which predisposes the individual to an acute disorder (such as fall, which can precipitate a subdural hematoma, causing confusion). It has, therefore, been suggested that evaluation of an older person should focus less on the "chief complaint" and instead on a general review of systems (Tinetti, 2003).

REFERENCES

Albert, M. & Kaplan, E. (1980). Organic implications of neuropsychological deficits in the elderly. In *New Directions in Memory and Aging: Proceedings of the George Talland Memorial Conference*, ed. L. Poon, J. L. Fozard, L. Cermak, D. Ehrenberg & L. W. Thompson, pp. 403–3. New Jersey: L. Erlbaum Assoc.

Albert, M. & Moss, B. (1999). Early features of Alzheimer's disease. In *Cerebral Cortex*, ed. A. Peters & J. Morrison, pp. 461–71. Vol 14, New York: Plenum.

Albert, M., Heller, H. & Milberg, W. (1987). Changes in naming ability with age. *Psychol. Aging*, **41**, 141–57.

Albert, M., Wolfe, J. & Lafleche, G. (1990). Differences in abstraction ability with age. *Psychol. Aging*, **5**, 94–100.

Altman, J. & Das, G. D. (1965). Autoradiographic and histologic evidence of postnatal hippocampal neurogenesis. *J. Comp. Neurol.*, **124**, 319–36.

Amaral, D. (1993). Morphological analyses of the brains of behaviorally characterized aged nonhuman primates. *Neurobiol Aging*, **14**, 671–2.

Anderson, J. M., Hubbard, B. M., Coghill, G. R. & Slidders, W. (1983). The effect of advanced old age on the neurone content of the cerebral cortex. Observations with an automatic image analyser point counting method. *J. Neurol. Sci.*, **58**, 233–44.

Arenberg, D. & Robertson-Tchabo, E. (1977). Learning and aging. In *Handbook of the Psychology of Aging*, ed. J. Birren & K. Schaie, pp. 421–49. New York: Van Nostrand Reinhold.

Arnsten, A. & Goldman-Rakic, P. (1990). Analysis of alpha-2 adrenergic agonist effects on the delayed non-matching-to-sample performance of aged rhesus monkeys. *Neurobiol. Aging*, **11**, 583–90.

Arnsten, A., Cai, J., Steere, J. & Goldman-Rakic, P. (1995). Dopamine D2 receptor mechanisms in the cognitive performance of young adult and aged monkeys. *Psychopharmacology*, **116**, 143–51.

Ashton-Miller, J. & Alexander, N. (2003). Biomechanics of mobility in older adults. In *Principles of Geriatric Medicine and Gerontology*, ed. W. Hazzard, J. Blass, J. Halter, J. Ouslander & M. Tinetti, pp. 905–18. New York: McGraw-Hill.

Bachevalier, J. (1993). Behavioral changes in aged rhesus monkeys. *Neurobiol. Aging*, **14**, 619–21.

Bachevalier, J., Landis, L., Walker, M. *et al.* (1991). Aged monkeys exhibit behavioral deficits indicative of widespread cerebral dysfunction. *Neurobiol. Aging*, **12**, 99–111.

Barnes, C. A., Suster, M. S., Shen, J. & McNaughton, B. L. (1997). Multistability of cognitive maps in the hippocampus of old rats. *Nature*, **388**, 272–5.

Barnes, C. (2003). Long-term potentiation and the ageing brain. *Phil. Trans. Roy. Soc. Lond.*, **358**, 765–72.

Bartus, R., Dean, R. & Fleming, D. (1979). Aging in the rhesus monkey: effects on visual discrimination learning and reversal learning. *J. Gerontol.*, **34**, 209–19.

Bohannon, R. W., Larkin, P. A., Cook, A. M., Gear, J. & Singer, J. (1984). Decrease in timed balance test scores with aging. *Phys. Ther.*, **64**, 1067–70.

Brewer, J., Zhao, Z., Desmond, J., Glover, G. & Gabrieli, J. (1998). Making memories: brain activity that predicts how well visual experience will be remembered. *Science*, **281**, 1185–7.

Brody, H. (1955). Organization of cerebral cortex III. A study of aging in the human cerebral cortex. *J. Comp. Neurol.*, **102**, 511–56.

   (1970). Structural changes in the aging nervous system. *Interdiscipl. Top. Gerontol.*, **7**, 9–21.

Buchner, D., Larson, E., Wagner, Koepsell T., de Lateur (1996). Evidence for a non-linear relationship between leg strength and gait speed. *Age Ageing*, **25**, 386–91.

Buckner, R., Kelley, W. & Petersen, W. (1999). Frontal cortex contributes to human memory formation. *Nat. Neurosci.*, **2**, 1–4.

Cabeza, R. (2002). Hemispheric asymmetry reduction in older adults: the HAROLD model. *Psychol. Aging*, **17**, 85–100.

Cabeza, R., Grady, C., Nyberg, L. *et al.* (1997). Age-related differences in neural activity during memory encoding and retrieval: A positron emission tomography study. *J. Neurosci.*, **17**, 391–400.

Cabeza, R., Anderson, N., Houle, S., Mangels, J. & Nyberg, L. (2000). Age-related differences in neural activity during item and temporal-order memory retrieval: a positron emission tomography study. *J. Cogn. Neurosci.*, **12**, 197–206.

Cavoy, A. & Delacour, J. (1993). Spatial but not object recognition is impaired by aging in rats. *Physiol. Behav.*, **53**, 527–30.

Chan-Palay, V. & Asan, E. (1989). Quantitation of catecholamine neurons in the locus ceruleus in human brains of normal young and older adults in depression. *J. Comp. Neurol.*, **287**, 357–72.

Christiansen, P., Larsson, H. B., Thomsen, C., Wieslander, S. B. & Henriksen, O. (1994). Age dependent white matter lesions and brain volume changes in healthy volunteers. *Acta Radiol.*, **35**, 117–22.

Coffey, C. E., Wilkinson, W. E., Parashos, I. A. *et al.* (1992). Quantitative cerebral anatomy of the aging human brain: a cross-sectional study using magnetic resonance imaging. *Neurology*, **42**, 527–36.

Colon, E. (1972). The elderly brain. A quantitative analysis of the cerebral cortex in two cases. *Psychiatr. Neurol Neurochir.*, **75**, 261–70.

Craik, F. (1977). Age differences in human memory. In *Handbook of the Psychology of Aging*, ed. J. Birren & K. Schaie, pp. 384–420. New York: Van Nostrand Reinhold.

Daselaar, S. M., Veltman, D. J., Rombouts, S. A., Raaijmakers, J. G. & Jonker, C. (2003). Neuroanatomical correlates of episodic encoding and retrieval in young and elderly subjects. *Brain*, **126**, 43–56.

Demb, J., Desmond, J., Wagner, A., Waidya, C., Glover, G. & Gabrieli, J. (1995). Semantic encoding and retrieval in the left inferior prefrontal cortex: a functional MRI study of task difficulty and process specificity. *J. Neurosci.*, **15**, 5870–8.

D'Esposito, M., Zarahn, E., Aguirre, G. & Rypma, B. (1999). The effect of normal aging on the coupling of neural activity to the BOLD hemodynamic response. *Neuroimage*, **10**, 6–14.

D'Esposito, M., Deouell, L. & Gazzaley, A. (2003). The impact of alterations of neurovascular coupling on BOLD fMRI signal: implications for studies of aging and disease. *Nat. Rev. Neurosci.*, **4**, 863–72.

Dunnett, S., Evenden, J. & Iversen, S. (1988). Delay-dependent short-term memory deficits in aged rats. *Psychopharmacology*, **96**, 174–80.

Eriksson, C. A. & Barnes., C. A. (2003). The neurobiology of memory changes in normal aging. *Exper. Gerontol.*, **38**, 61–9.

Eriksson, P. S., Perfilieva, E., Bjork-Eriksson, T. *et al.* (1998). *Nat. Med.*, **4**, 1313–17.

Fletcher, P., Frith, C., Grasby, P., Shallice, T., Frackowiack, R. & Dolan, R. (1995). Brain systems for encoding and retrieval of auditory-verbal memory: an in vivo study in humans. *Brain*, **118**, 401–16.

Gabrieli, J., Brewer, J., Desmond, J. & Glover, G. (1997). Separate neural bases of two fundamental memory processes in the human medial temporal lobe. *Science*, **276**, 264–6.

Gallagher, M. & Rapp, P. (1997). The use of animal models to study the effects of aging on cognition. *Annu. Rev. Psychol.*, **48**, 339–70.

Gallagher, M., Burwell, R. & Burchinal, M. (1993). Severity of spatial learning impairment in aging: development of a learning index for performance in the Morris water maze. *Behav. Neurosci.*, **107**, 618–26.

Gazzaley, A., Siegel, R., Kordowe, J., Mufson, E. & Morrison, J. (1996). Circuit-specific alterations of *N*-methyl-D-aspartate receptor subunit 1 in the dentate gyrus of aged monkeys. *Proc. Natl Acad. Sci., USA*, **93**, 3121–5.

Gomez-Isla, T., Price, J. L., McKeel, D. W., Morris, J. C., Growdon, J. H. & Hyman, B. T. (1996). Profound loss of layer II entorhinal cortex neurons occurs in very mild Alzheimer's disease. *J. Neurosci.*, **16**, 4491–500.

Gould, E., Reeves, A., Fallah, M., Tanapat, P., Gross, C. & Fuchs, E. (1999). Hippocampal neurgenesis in old world primates *Proc. Natl Acad. Sci., USA*, **27**, 5263–7.

Grady, C., McIntosh, A., Rajah, N., Beig, S. & Craik, F. (1999). The effects of age on the neural correlates of episodic encoding. *Cereb. Cortex*, **9**, 805–14.

Guralnik, J. & Ferrucci, L. (2003). *Demography and Epidemiology*, ed. W. Hazzard, J. Blass, J. Halter, J. Ouslander & M. Tinetti, pp. 53–76. New York: McGraw-Hill.

Harris, G. J., Schlaepfer, T. E., Peng, L. W., Lee, S., Federman, E. B. & Pearlson, G. (1994). Magnetic resonance imaging evaluation of the effects of ageing on grey–white ratio in the human brain. *Neuropath. Appl. Neurobiol.*, **20**, 290–3.

Haug, H. (1984). Macroscopic and microscopic morphometry of the human brain and cortex. A survey in the light of new results. *Brain Pathol.*, **1**, 123–49.

Haxby, J., Ungerleider, L., Horwitz, B., Maisog, J., Rapaport, S. & Grady, C. (1996). Face encoding and recognition in human brain. *Proc. Natl Acad. Sci., USA*, **93**, 922–7.

Hazlett, E., Buchsbaumm, M., Mohs, R. *et al.* (1998). Age-related shift in brain region activity during successful memory performance. *Neurobiol. Aging*, **19**, 437–45.

Head, D., Buckner, R. L., Shimony, J. S. *et al.* (2004). Differential vulnerability of anterior white matter in nondemented aging with minimal acceleration in dementia of the Alzheimer type: evidence from diffusion tenor imaging. *Cereb. Cortex*, **14**, 410–23.

Heaton, R., Grant, I. & Matthes, C. (1986). Differences in neuropsychological function test performance associated wtih age, education, and sex. In *Neuropsychological Assessment of Neuropsychiatric Disorders*, ed. I. Grant & K. Adams, pp. 100–20. New York: Oxford.

Hedden, T. & Gabrieli, J. (2004). Insights into the ageing mind: A view from cognitive neuroscience. *Nat. Rev. Neurosci.*, **5**, 87–95.

Henderson, G., Tomlinson, B. & Gibson, P. (1980). Cell counts in human cerebral cortex in normal aduls throughout life, using an image analyzing computer. *J. Neurol. Sci.*, **46**, 113–36.

Jernigan, T. L., Press, G. A. & Hesselink, J. R. (1990). Methods for measuring brain morphologic features on magnetic resonance images. *Arch. Neurol.*, **47**, 27–32.

Jernigan, T. L., Archibald, S., Berhow, M., Sowell, E., Foster, D. & Hesselink, J. (1991). Cerebral structure on MRI. I. Localization of age-related changes. *Biol. Psychiatr.*, **29**, 55–67.

Kapur, S., Craik, F., Tulving, E., Wilson, A., Houle, S. & Brown, G. (1994). Neuroanatomical correlates of encoding in episodic memory: levels of processing effects. *Proc. Natl Acad. Sci., USA*, **91**, 2008–11.

Kapur, S., Tulving, E., Cabeza, R., McIntosh, A., Houle, S. & Craik, F. (1996). The neural correlates of intentional learning of verbal materials: a PET study in humans. *Cogn. Brain Res.*, **4**, 243–9.

Kemper, T. (1993). The relationship of cerebral cortical changes to nuclei in the brainstem. *Neurobiol. Aging*, **14**, 659–60.

Kemperman, G., vanPraag, H. & Gage, F. (2000). Activity-dependent regulation of neuronal plasticity and self repair. *Prog. Brain Res.*, **127**, 35–48.

Kornack, D. & Rakic, P. (1999). Continuation of neurogenesis in the hippocampus of the adult macaque monkey. *Proc. Natl Acad. Sci., USA*, **96**, 5768–73.

Lachman, M. & Jelalian, E. (1984). Self-efficacy and attributions for intellectual performance in young and elderly adults. *J. Gerontol.*, **39**, 577–82.

Lai, Z., Moss, M., Killiany, R. & Rosene, D. (1995). Executive system dysfunction in the aged monkeys: spatial and object reversal learning. *Neurobiol. Aging*, **16**, 947–54.

Leuba, G. & Garey, L. (1989). Comparison of neuronal and glial numerical density in primary and secondary visual cortex. *Exp. Brain Res.*, **77**, 31–8.

Lim, K. O., Zipursky, R. B., Watts, M. C. & Pfefferbaum, A. (1992). Decreased gray matter in normal aging: an in vivo magnetic resonance study. *J. Gerontol.*, **47**, B26–30.

Logan, J. M., Sanders, A. L., Snyder, A. Z., Morris, J. C. & Buckner, R. L. (2002). Under-recruitment and nonselective recruitment: dissociable neural mechanisms associated with aging. *Neuron*, **33**, 827–40.

Madden, D. J., Turkington, T. G., Provenzale, J. M. *et al.* (1999). Adult age differences in the functional neuroanatomy of verbal recognition memory. *Hum. Brain Map.*, **7**, 115–35.

Martin, J., Wiggs, C. & Weisberg, J. (1997). Modulation of human medial temporal lobe activity by form, meaning and experience. *Hippocampus*, **7**, 587–93.

Matsumae, M., Kikinis, R., Morocz, I. A. *et al.* (1996). Age-related changes in intracranial compartment volumes in normal adults assessed by magnetic resonance imaging. *J. Neurosurg.*, **84**, 982–91.

McKee, R. & Squire, L. (1993). On the development of declarative memory. *J. Exp. Psychol. Learn. Mem. Cogn.*, **19**, 397–404.

Morcom, A., Good, C., Frackowiak, R. & Rugg, M. (2003). Age effects on the neural correlates of successful memory encoding. *Brain*, **126**, 213–29.

Moore, T., Killiany, R., Herndon, J., Rosene, D. & Moss, M. (2003). Impairment in abstraction and set shifting in aged Rhesus monkeys. *Neurobiol. Aging*, **24**, 125–34.

Morris, R. G. M. (1981). Spatial localization does not require the presence of local cues. *Learn Motiv.*, **12**, 239–61.

Morrison, J. H. & Hof, R. P. (1997). Life and death of neurons in the aging brain. *Science*, **278**, 412–19.

Moss, M. (1983). Assessment of memory in amnesic and dementia patients: Adaptation of behavioral tests used with non-human primates. *INS Bull.*, **5**, 15.

Moss, M. (1993). The longitudinal assessment of recognition memory in aged rhesus monkeys. *Neurobiol. Aging*, **14**, 635–6.

Moss, M., Rosene, D. & Peters, A. (1988). Effects of aging on visual recognition memory in the rhesus monkey. *Neurobiol. Aging*, **9**, 495–502.

Murphy, D. G., DeCarli, C., Schapiro, M. B., Rapoport, S. I. & Horwitz, B. (1992). Age-related differences in volume of subcortical nuclei, brain matter, and cerebrospinal fluid in healthy men as measured with magnetic resonance imaging. *Arch. Neurol.*, **49**, 839–45.

Nielsen, K. & Peters, A. (2000). The effects on the frequency of nerve fibers in rhesus monkey striate cortex. *Neurobiol. Aging*, **21**, 621–8.

Norris, C., Korol, D. & Foster, T. (1996). Increased susceptibility to induction of long-term depression and long-term potentiation reversal during aging. *J. Neurosci.*, **16**, 5382–92.

Odenheimer, G., Funkenstein, H., Beckett, L. *et al.* (1994). Comparison of neurologic changes in successfully aging persons vs the total aging population. *Arch. Neurol.*, **51**, 573–80.

O'Donnell, K. A., Rapp, P. R. & Hof, P. R. (1999). Preservation of prefrontal cortical volume in behaviorally characterized aged macaque monkeys. *Exp. Neurol.*, **160**, 300–10.

Peters, A. (1996). Age-related changes in oligodendrocytes in monkey cerebral cortex. *J. Comp. Neurol.*, **371**, 153–63.

Peters, A., Josephson, K. & Vicent, S. (1991). Effects of aging on the neuroglial cells and pericytes within area 17 of the rhesus monkey (*Macaca mulatta*). *Anat. Rec.*, **229**, 384–98.

Peters, A., Leahu, D., Moss, M. & McNally, K. (1994). The effects of aging on Area 46 of the frontal cortex of the rhesus monkey. *Cereb. Cortex*, **6**, 621–35.

Petersen, R., Smith, G., Kokmen, E., Ivnik, R. & Tangalos, E. (1992). Memory function in normal aging. *Neurology*, **42**, 396–401.

Pfefferbaum, A., Mathalon, D. H., Sullivan, E. V., Rawles, J. M., Zipursky, R. B. & Lim, K. O. (1994). A quantitative magnetic resonance imaging study of changes in brain morphology from infancy to late adulthood. *Arch. Neurol.*, **51**, 874–87.

Poon, L. (1985). Differences in human memory with aging. In *Handbook of the Psychology of Aging*, ed. J. E. Birren & K. W. Schaie, pp. 427–62. New York: Van Nostrand Reinhold.

Presty, S., Bachevalier, J., Walker, L. *et al.* (1987). Age differences in recognition memory of the Rhesus monkey (macaca mulatta). *Neurobiol. Aging*, **8**, 435–40.

Rapp, P. (1990). Visual discrimination and reversal learning in the aged monkey (*Macaca mulatta*). *Behav. Neurosci.*, **104**, 876–88.

Rapp, P. & Amaral, D. (1989). Evidence for task-dependent memory dysfunction in the aged monkey. *J. Neurosci.*, **9**, 3568–76.

Rapp, P. R. & Gallagher, M. (1996). Preserved neuron number in the hippocampus of aged rats with spatial learning deficits. *Proc. Natl Acad. Sci., USA*, **93**, 9926–30.

Rapp, P., Stack, E. & Gallagher, M. (1999). Morphometric studies of the aged hippocampus: I. Volumetric analysis in behaviorally characterized rats. *J. Comp. Neurol.*, **403**, 459–70.

Rapp, P., Deroche, P. & Burwell, R. (2000). Preserved neuron number in the entorhinal, perirhinal, and postrhinal cortices of behaviorally characterized rats. *Abstr. Soc. Neurosci.*, **26**, 470.

Raz, N., Gunning-Dixon, F. M., Head, D., Dupuis, J. H. & Acker, J. D. (1998). Neuroanatomical correlates of cognitive aging: evidence from structural magnetic resonance imaging. *Neuropsychology*, **12**, 95–114.

Reber, P. & Squire, L. (1994). Parallel brain systems for learning with and without awareness. *Learn. Mem.*, **4**, 217–19.

Resnick, S. M., Pharm, D. L., Kraut, M. A., Zonderman, A. B. & Davatzikos, C. (2003). Longitudinal magnetic resonance imaging studies of older adults: a shrinking brain. *J. Neurosci.*, **23**, 3295–301.

Rosen, A. C., Prull, M. W., O'Hara, R. *et al.* (2002). Variable effects of aging on frontal lobe contributions to memory. *NeuroReport*, **13**, 2425–8.

Rosene, D. (1993). Comparing age-related changes in the basal forebrain and hippocampus of the rhesus monkey. *Neurobiol. Aging*, **14**, 669–70.

Rosenzweig, E. S. & Barnes, C. A. (2003). Impact of aging on hippocampal function: plasticity, network dynamics, and cognition. *Prog. Neurobiol.*, **69**, 143–79.

Schacter, D. & Wagner, A. (1999). Medial temporal lobe activations in fMRI and PET studies of episodic encoding and retrieval. *Hippocampus*, **9**, 7–24.

Schaie, K. (1983). The Seattle longitudinal study: a 21 year exploration of psychometric intelligence in adulthood. In *Longitudinal Studies of Adult Psychological Development*, ed. K. W. Schaie, pp. 64–135. New York: Guilford.

Schultz, A. B. (1992). Mobility impairment in the elderly: challenges for biomechanics research. *J. Biomech.*, **25**, 519–28.

Shefer, V. (1973). Absolute number of neurons and thickness of the cerebral cortex during aging, senile and vascular dementia, and Pick's and Alzheimer's diseases. *Neurosci. Behav. Physiol.*, **6**, 319–24.

Smith, T., Adams, M., Gallagher, M., Morrison, J. & Rapp, P. (2000). Circuit-specific alterations in hippocampal synaptophysin immunoreactivity predict spatial learning impairment in aged rats. *J. Neurosci.*, **20**, 6587–93.

Squire, L., Zola-Morgan, S. & Chen, K. (1988). Human amnesia and animal models of amnesia: performance of amnesic patients on tests designed for the monkey. *Behav. Neurosci.*, **11**, 210–21.

Stebbins, G. T., Carrillo, M. C., Dorfman, J. *et al.* (2002). Aging effects on memory encoding in the frontal lobes. *Psychol. Aging*, **17**, 44–55.

Stern, C., Corkin, S., Gonzalez, R. *et al.* (1996). The hippocampus participates in novel picture encoding: evidence from functional magnetic resonance imaging. *Proc. Natl Acad. Sci., USA*, **93**, 8660–5.

Tanna, N. K., Kohn, M. I., Horwich, D. N. *et al.* (1991). Analysis of brain and cerebrospinal fluid volumes with MR imaging: Impact on PET data correction for atrophy. Part II. Aging and Alzheimer's dementia. *Radiology*, **178**, 123–30.

Terry, R., Deteresa, R. & Hansen, L. (1987). Neocortical cell counts in normal human adult aging. *Ann. Neurol.*, **21**, 530–9.

Tigges, J., Herndon, J. & Peters, A. (1992). Neuronal population of area 4 during life span of rhesus monkeys. *Neurobiol. Aging*, **11**, 201–8.

Tinetti, M. (2003). Clinical evaluation of older persons. In *Principles of Geriatric Medicine and Gerontology*, ed. W. Hazzard, J. Blass, J. Halter, J. Ouslander & M. Tinetti, pp. 1028–32. New York: McGraw-Hill.

Tisserand, D. J. & Jolles, J. (2003). On the involvement of prefrontal networks in cognitive ageing. *Cortex*, **39**, 1107–28.

Tisserand, D. J., Pruessner, J. C., Sanz Argita, E. J. *et al.* (2002). Regional frontal cortical volumes decrease differentially in aging: an MRI study to compare volumetric approaches and voxel-based morphometry. *NeuroImage*, **17**, 657–69.

Tulving, E. (1972). Episodic and semantic memory. In: *Organization of Memory*, ed. E. Tulving & W. Donaldson, pp. 381–403. New York: Academic Press.

Vincent, S., Peters, A. & Tigges, J. (1989). Effects of aging on neurons within area 17 of rhesus monkey cerebral cortex. *Anat Rec.*, **223**, 329–41.

Wagner, A., Poldrack, R., Eldridge, L., Desmond, J., Glover, G. & Gabrieli, J. (1998a). Material-specific lateralization of prefrontal activation during episodic encoding and retrieval. *NeuroReport*, **9**, 3711–17.

Wagner, A., Schacter, D., Rotte, M. *et al.* (1998b). Building memories: remembering and forgetting verbal experiences as predicted by brain activity. *Science*, **281**, 1188–91.

Waugh, N. & Norman, D. (1965). Primary memory. *Psychol. Rev.*, **72**, 89–104.

West, M., Coleman, P., Flood, D. & Troncoso, J. (1994). Differences in the pattern of hippocampal neuronal loss in normal ageing and Alzheimer's disease. *Lancet*, **344**, 769–72.

26

Neuropathology of normal aging in cerebral cortex

John H. Morrison[1,2], Patrick R. Hof[1,2,3], and Peter R. Rapp[1,2]

[1]Department of Neuroscience [2]Department of Geriatrics and Adult Development [3]Department of Ophthalmology, Mount Sinai School of Medicine, NY, USA

Introduction

In order to understand the neuropathology of normal aging, it is instructive to review the major elements of circuit degeneration associated with Alzheimer's disease. AD is characterized by senile plaque (SP) and neurofibrillary tangle (NFT) formation and extensive, yet selective, neuron death in the hippocampus and neocortex that leads to dramatic decline in cognitive abilities and memory. A more modest disruption of memory, referred to as mild cognitive impairment (MCI) or age-associated memory impairment (AAMI), occurs often in the context of normal aging, in humans, monkeys and rodents. However, unlike AD, significant neuron death does not appear to be the cause of AAMI. In AD, the neurons providing the connection between the entorhinal cortex and the dentate gyrus (e.g. the perforant path) are devastated, as are the neurons providing corticocortical circuits that interconnect association regions. Whereas the death of these same neurons appears to be minimal in normal aging, these same circuits and the corresponding circuits in animal models are vulnerable to sublethal age-related alterations in morphology, neurochemical phenotype and synaptic integrity that might impair function. Biochemical alterations of the synapse, such as shifts in distribution or abundance of NMDA receptors, may also contribute to memory impairment. The same brain regions are also responsive to circulating estrogen levels, and thus, critical interactions between reproductive senescence and brain aging may affect excitatory synaptic transmission in the hippocampus. Importantly, some of the effects of estrogen on these neurons imply that certain synaptic alterations that accompany aging may be reversible. Thus, the aging spine and synapse may be the key to age-related memory decline, whereas the loss of select cortical circuits is the more prominent substrate for functional decline in AD.

Selective vulnerability in Alzheimer's disease

Overview

Both structurally and functionally, AD is predominantly a disease of the cerebral cortex. However, only certain populations of neurons and circuits are affected, whereas other neuron types are spared. Generally, interneurons are spared whereas pyramidal neurons are vulnerable, yet the vulnerability is confined to key subsets of pyramidal cells. Clues as to which circuits are vulnerable are provided by the distribution of pathologic changes in AD and the correlation with specific elements of cortical circuitry. The vulnerable neurons also have a unique neurochemical phenotype, particularly with respect to cytoskeletal proteins such as neurofilament and tau. Through linking human neuropathology with animal data in experimental preparations, correlations have emerged between distribution of cellular pathologic changes, neurochemical characteristics related to vulnerability, and cortical circuits at risk (for review, see Morrison & Hof, 2002).

Hippocampal pathology in AD

The entorhinal cortex, subiculum, and CA1 within hippocampus represent particularly vulnerable regions that consistently display very high NFT densities and resultant neuron death in AD. The most consistent observation in AD cases is the presence of large numbers of NFT in layers II and V of the entorhinal cortex (Hyman et al., 1984; Morrison & Hof, 1997). The distribution of SP in the hippocampal formation is variable, but often parallels the termination of vulnerable projections, such as a high density of SP in the molecular layer of the dentate gyrus, and the terminal zone of the projection from entorhinal cortex (Hyman et al., 1990). Thus, the perforant pathway that projects from layers II and III of the entorhinal cortex is severely compromised in AD, as reflected by NFT in the neurons of origin of this pathway and SP in the termination zone in the dentate gyrus (Hyman *et al.*, 1984). Extensive amyloid accumulation in the perforant path terminal zone has also been described in a transgenic mouse model of AD (Reilly *et al.*, 2003).

In the absence of AD, there does not appear to be significant neuron loss in entorhinal cortex (West, 1993; Gómez-Isla *et al.*, 1996; Hof *et al.*, 2003), nor is there loss of neurons in the entorhinal cortex in aged monkeys (Gazzaley *et al.*, 1997). However, a lack of quantifiable neuron loss does not necessarily mean that no degenerative changes are occurring in a given brain region and it does not negate nondegenerative changes that lead to compromised function. For example, while the neurons in layer II of entorhinal cortex are clearly devastated early in AD, their status in cognitively normal aged individuals and those with MCI has been more difficult to pinpoint. Neuron counts in neurologically normal individuals suggest that there is no neuron loss in entorhinal cortex (Gómez-Isla *et al.*, 1996); however, analyses of NFT, the classic reflection of a degenerating neuron in AD, suggest that virtually all humans over the age of 50 have some NFT in layer II of entorhinal cortex (Bouras *et al.*, 1994), making it difficult to distinguish qualitatively between age-related degenerative events in the entorhinal cortex that represent early progressive AD and those that are more stable. This distinction is critically important for patients with MCI where it is unclear whether their condition represents early AD or a more stable level of AAMI. The key to understanding the presence of NFT in this region lies in the "transitional neurons", i.e., neurons that are still intact and included in an analysis of total neuron counts, yet have transitional intraneuronal pathology (Hof *et al.*, 2003). When neurons in layer II of entorhinal cortex are counted in three categories – ghost tangles, transitional neurons containing an intracellular NFT, and healthy neurons – the data are far more revealing with respect to early pathologic events in layer II of entorhinal cortex. Such transitional neurons may represent only 10% of the total in layer II of patients with MCI, but the majority of neurons in AD. However, the degree to which such "transitional" neurons are functional or able to be rescued is unclear, yet important to determine as interventions are introduced. Even a more precise delineation of the events surrounding degeneration will not provide a full understanding of the vulnerability of this circuit, because as described below, this circuit displays age-related changes short of degeneration that would also impact its function. In addition, as described below, the fully developed dementia of AD is unlikely to result from even mass destruction

of this circuit, if it occurs in the absence of neocortical involvement.

Neocortical pathology in AD

Lesion types and cortical distribution

The distribution and density of NFT and SP have been analyzed in great detail and constitute the basis of the neuropathologic diagnosis of AD (Arnold *et al.*, 1991; Mirra *et al.*, 1993). NFT are characterized by the accumulation of abnormal components of the neuronal cytoskeleton that form paired helical filaments, whereas SP are composed of dystrophic neurites and glial elements with or without a central amyloid core (Hof *et al.*, 1999). Both lesions are predominant in the cerebral cortex, where NFT are located in the perikarya of large pyramidal neurons, and SP are distributed throughout the cortical regions, but are particularly numerous in association areas (Rogers & Morrison, 1985; Arnold *et al.*, 1991; Hof *et al.*, 1999).

These visible reflections of pathology are particularly important in the degree to which each of them reflects neuron or synapse loss that amounts to the circuit disruption underlying dementia. Considerable neuronal loss occurs in the association regions of the neocortex in AD, leaving primary sensory and motor areas relatively spared (Morrison & Hof, 1997). Many studies of NFT and SP distribution have demonstrated strong correlations between the regional and laminar distribution of SP and NFT, and the presumed neurons of origin of certain long corticocortical and hippocampal projections (Pearson *et al.*, 1985; Rogers & Morrison, 1985; Hyman *et al.*, 1986; Lewis *et al.*, 1987; Hof *et al.*, 1990; Hof & Morrison, 1990). Overall, the distribution and severity of neuron loss follows closely that of NFT in the neocortex (Gómez-Isla *et al.*, 1996, 1997; Morrison & Hof, 1997). The regional and laminar distribution of SP suggests that they may be related to NFT formation. It has been proposed that SP reflect the degeneration of the terminations of projections from neurons that contain NFT (Pearson *et al.*, 1985; Lewis *et al.*, 1987; Vickers *et al.*, 2000), and that the slightly higher incidence of SP in the supragranular layers and in layer IV in the association cortex reflects the involvement of feedforward corticocortical projections (Lewis *et al.*, 1987). It is likely that degeneration of presumed corticocortical circuits within the neocortex is required for the clinical expression of dementia in AD (Morrison & Hof, 1997), since elderly individuals can maintain a high level of cognitive performance though with accompanied memory deficits, while sustaining significant compromise of hippocampal circuits. Thus, they may rely more on neocortical than on hippocampal circuits for memories essential for daily activities (Albert, 1996).

Neurofilament protein is a marker of neuronal vulnerability in Alzheimer's disease

Certain pyramidal neurons in the neocortex of both human and monkeys have been shown to be enriched in nonphosphorylated epitopes of neurofilament protein (Campbell & Morrison, 1989; Hof *et al.*, 1990; Hof & Morrison, 1990, 1995). This pattern in the primate neocortex is restricted to the perikarya and dendrites of a subpopulation of large pyramidal neurons and is more concentrated in the cell body and dendrites of the largest of these neurons (Campbell & Morrison, 1989). Neurofilaments as well as other cytoskeletal proteins have been implicated in NFT formation (Morrison *et al.*, 1987; Trojanowski *et al.*, 1993; Morrison & Hof, 1997; Hof *et al.*, 1999), and pyramidal cells with a high content of non-phosphorylated neurofilament protein emerge as a neuron type highly susceptible to NFT formation (Bussière *et al.*, 2003).

The distribution of neurofilament protein-enriched neurons corresponds to the distribution of corticocortically projecting cells as demonstrated by transport studies in the macaque monkey cortex (Hof *et al.*, 1995, 1996, 1997; Nimchinsky *et al.*, 1996). Of direct relevance to AD, we have shown that, in the macaque monkey, many long association corticocortical projections originate from neurofilament protein-enriched neurons, and that in circuits interconnecting key prefrontal and temporal regions, 90–100% of the neurons of origin of the projection are neurofilament-enriched (Hof *et al.*, 1995). These circuits are known to be involved in networks subserving many aspects of cognition (Goldman-Rakic, 1988).

In AD, neurofilament protein-enriched neurons in certain neocortical and hippocampal areas are dramatically affected and die through NFT formation (Morrison *et al.*, 1987; Hof *et al.*, 1990; Hof & Morrison, 1990; Vickers *et al.*, 1992, 1994; Morrison & Hof, 1997; Vickers, 1997; Vickers *et al.*, 2000). The laminar distribution of neurofilament protein-enriched neurons in visual association, prefrontal, and anterior cingulate cortices in human is very similar to the distribution of NFT. Furthermore, the layers that have high NFT density in an AD brain no longer contain a high density of neurofilament protein-immunoreactive neurons (Hof *et al.*, 1990, 1999; Hof & Morrison, 1990). If the monkey data are considered within the context of the distribution of neurofilament protein-enriched neurons and NFT in human, it is likely that the human homologues of the neurofilament protein-enriched corticocortically projecting neurons in the macaque monkey are those that are highly vulnerable in human AD.

To test this correlation more directly in human aging and AD, we targeted layer III of area 9 as a focus for quantitative analysis in which total neuron counts were obtained, as well as NPNFP-immunoreactive neurons with no trace of tau accumulation and NPNFP-immunoreactive neurons with tau accumulation. All profile counts were correlated with clinical assessment as reflected in the Clinical Dementia Rating Scale (CDR). A CDR rating of 0.5 amounts to MCI, CDR 1 reflects probable AD, CDR 2 is mild AD, CDR 3 is moderate AD, and CDR 5 is severe AD (Hof *et al.*, 2003). The most recent data obtained indicate that, in area 9, neurofilament protein-enriched pyramidal cells are unaffected in CDR 0.5 cases, yet undergo notable tau accumulation in CDR 2 cases, and virtually all neurofilament-enriched neurons are in the process of degenerating by CDR 3 (Fig. 26.1) (Bussière *et al.*, 2003). However, the remaining non-neurofilament labelled neurons remain relatively unaffected even with well-established AD. This result suggests that tangle formation affects a well-defined subset of neurons, and CDR 2, which corresponds to mild AD, represents the clinical transition stage at which this subset of highly vulnerable neurons is profoundly affected (Hof *et al.*, 2003) in the prefrontal cortex.

Summary: AD and cortical circuitry

The relevance and impact of pathologic changes in AD have to be understood within the context of organized systems that underlie neocortical function. For instance, integrated processing in a given sensory modality such as vision involves the simultaneous activity of numerous separable visual areas that have extensive highly ordered interconnections that establish a distributed system subserving the proper integration of visual information. Similarly, cognition and language, which are not modality-specific functions, presumably depend strongly on the complex communication among neocortical regions provided by the corticocortical circuits which degenerate in AD, leading to a global neocortical disconnection syndrome that presents clinically as dementia (Morrison & Hof, 1997). Other degenerative processes occur in AD, and they may also contribute to the clinical characteristics of the disease, but the generalized loss of long corticocortical projections emerges functionally as the most devastating component of AD, and the pathologic outcome most directly related to dementia.

This interpretation of the pathological features of AD suggests that the debilitating dementia results from changes restricted to the association neocortex, whereas extensive hippocampal alterations can exist in absence of neocortical involvement and with only minor disruptions in activities of daily living of the individual, whose memory deficits could be revealed by formal testing, but are not compatible with the diagnosis of dementing illness. As the elements of the biochemical and anatomical phenotype that are linked to differential cellular vulnerability in AD are increasingly recognized, hopefully it will be possible to develop therapeutic interventions to protect or rescue the neurons that are at high risk in AD. The protection of these neurons appears to be an attractive strategy for the management of AD, that may have the advantage of being more achievable than the development of a cure.

Age-associated memory impairment: functional decline without neuron loss

While NFT and SP are also present in the brains of humans without clinical AD, their presence is not associated with measurable neuron loss. While layer II of entorhinal cortex shows some pathology in virtually all humans over 55 years old (Bouras *et al.*, 1993, 1994), it is not sufficient to register as decreased neuron number in neurologically normal elderly subjects. In addition, CA1 and other hippocampal fields as well as neocortex do not display significant neuron loss in normal aging. If neuron loss cannot account for memory loss with aging in this population, then what is the neurobiological complement of such functional decline? Insight on this issue has been gained from animal studies of aging, where AAMI can be analyzed without the potential confound of early AD. Studies from both non-human primates and rodents have illuminated both neocortical and hippocampal changes associated with aging. These studies (reviewed below) suggest that age-related changes in key excitatory synaptic connections in the absence of frank circuit degeneration may be the primary neurobiological correlate of AAMI.

The aging synapse: non-human primate studies

Morphologic analyses of corticocortical circuits

As described above, a distinct subpopulation of neurons forming long corticocortical projections in the association neocortex is highly vulnerable to the degenerative process in AD (Lewis *et al.*, 1987; Morrison & Hof, 1997). However, the degree to which age-related molecular and morphologic alterations of these same circuits might lead to functional decline has not been investigated until recently. Whereas, no neuronal loss in neocortex is observed in the course of normal aging in non-human primates (Peters *et al.*, 1998b), significant cognitive

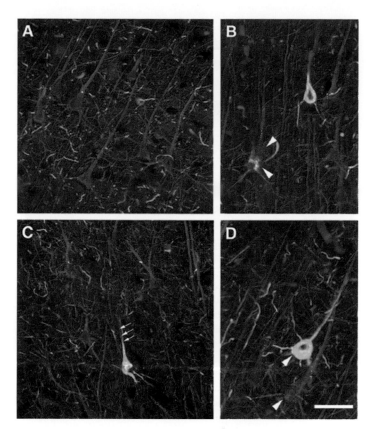

Fig. 26.1 Typical immunohistochemical patterns observed with an antibody to non-phosphorylated neurofilament protein (SMI-32, red fluorescence) and phosphorylated tau (antibody 988, green fluorescence). (A) Large SMI-32-immunoreactive neurons are seen in layer IIIc of a CDR 0.5 case with many neuropil threads but no NFT. Panels (**B–D**) display neurons with different degrees of NFT formation. Two intracellular NFT are seen in a CDR 2 case (layer IIIc; B). The tangled neuron in panel C shows faint immunoreactivity in its apical dendrite (arrows; CDR 2, layer Va). Panel D shows a large endstage NFT next to intact SMI-32-immunoreactive neurons (CDR 2, layer IIIc). Scale bar (on D) = 30 μm. (Adapted from Bussière *et al.*, 2003.)

changes can be observed in animals older than 19 years of age (Gallagher & Rapp, 1997). Are the same corticocortical circuits that degenerate in human AD vulnerable to sublethal alterations in normal aging? Electron microscopic investigations have demonstrated consistent changes in oligodendrocyte and axonal myelin sheath morphology in aged non-human primates (Peters *et al.*, 1996, 1998a, 2000), pointing to the possible involvement of certain cortical projection systems in aging. Several studies indicate that the cognitive processes mediated by the prefrontal cortex are impaired during the normal aging processes (Bartus *et al.*, 1978; Bachevalier *et al.*, 1991; Peters *et al.*, 1996; Rapp &

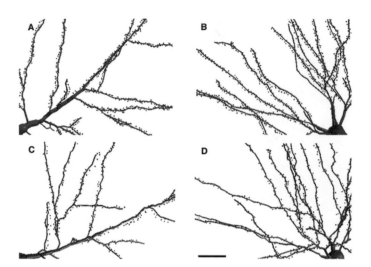

Fig. 26.2 Examples of apical and basal dendritic segments with spines plotted onto them from young and aged animals showing age-related differences in spine density. These neurons provide corticocortical connections between temporal and prefrontal association cortices. The dendritic segments shown are rendered at the same scaling factor. (A) and (B) are from the apical and basal dendritic trees, respectively, of a neuron from a young animal. (C) and (D) are from the apical and basal dendritic trees, respectively, of a neuron from an old animal. There are visible decreases in spine numbers on the apical and basal dendrites in the aged animals. Quantitative analyses of this material showed a 30–40% loss of spines in these neurons with aging. Scale bar (on D) = 20 μm. Adapted from Duan *et al.*, 2003.

Gallagher, 1997; O'Donnell *et al.*, 1999). In particular, aged macaque monkeys show consistently lower performance in delayed response (DR) tasks, which are sensitive to prefrontal cortical damage, when compared to young animals (Rapp & Gallagher, 1997). These and other data indicate that age-related cognitive deficits in nonhuman primates may be a consequence of abnormalities in cortical circuits that clearly do not include loss of neurons but rather involve subcellular compartments. In order to identify potential sublethal circuit-specific alterations, we quantified age-related morphological changes at the single cell level in identified populations of corticocortically-projecting neurons in monkeys (Page *et al.*, 2002; Duan *et al.*, 2003).

Neurons furnishing long corticocortical projections from parietal and temporal regions to area 46 in prefrontal cortex were targeted for these studies. These neurons were targeted through retrograde transport of fluorescent dyes following injections in area 46, followed by intracellular filling and 3-dimensional reconstruction of the retrogradely filled neurons (Fig. 26.2). This approach results in detailed quantitative data on the dendritic arbor and spine density

of the same corticocortically projecting neurons that we hypothesize to be vulnerable to AD in human cortex. Based on the three-dimensional reconstructions of these neurons, indices of dendritic arbor such as total dendritic length and number of dendritic segments were similar across ages, demonstrating that general dendritic morphology and extent in the neurons was not vulnerable to aging. However, aged animals showed a consistent reduction in dendritic spine numbers and densities along the dendritic branches (Fig. 26.2). Total spine number on these corticocortically-projecting neurons decreased by approximately 35% in the basal and apical dendrites of aged animals compared to young ones. The spine densities per μm of dendritic length decreased by about 25% overall and this decrease occurred throughout the entire dendritic arborization on apical dendrites and was more pronounced on distal dendrites in the basal dendrites (Page *et al.*, 2002; Duan *et al.*, 2003).

The observed change in spine numbers may lead to a potential deficit in the excitatory drive on the neurons that receive these inputs, leading to cognitive deficits such as those described in aged monkeys in the absence of neuron loss. These neurons also show decreases in glutamate receptors with aging (Hof *et al.*, 2002), which is a further reflection of alterations in excitatory inputs to these neurons with aging, and is excitatory related to the spine loss.

Circuit-specific shifts in NMDA receptors in hippocampus of aged monkeys

Spatial memory is vulnerable to aging (Gallagher & Rapp, 1997), and is also disrupted by pharmacological blockade of NMDA receptor function (Kentros *et al.*, 1998) or hippocampal knockout of NR1 (Tsien *et al.*, 1996). NMDA-receptor mediated functions such as maintenance and induction of long-term potentiation and maintaining stability of spatial information coding by "place cells" are compromised in aging (Barnes *et al.*, 1997). Given the selective vulnerability displayed by both neocortical and hippocampal circuits in aging and AD, high resolution analyses of receptors can be particularly informative, since the changes are very likely to be cell, circuit, and synapse specific and therefore difficult to resolve at the regional level.

Age-related shifts in NR1, the obligatory subunit of the NMDA receptors, in the molecular layer of the dentate gyrus have been reported in monkeys (Gazzaley *et al.*, 1996a). The projection from entorhinal cortex to the dentate gyrus is strictly confined to the outer molecular layer (OML), i.e. to the distal dendrites of granule cells, whereas other excitatory inputs terminate in a non-overlapping fashion in the inner molecular layer (IML), on the proximal dendrites (Witter & Amaral, 1991). This quantitative

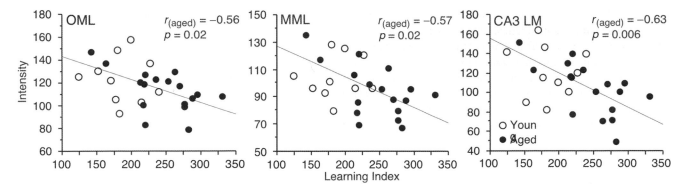

Fig. 26.3 Scatter plots relating individual spatial learning index scores to levels of hippocampal synaptophysin–immunoreactivity (SYN-IR) in young and aged rats. Lower learning index scores, indicative of better learning, correlated with higher SYN-IR intensity values selectively in the dentate gyrus MML, OML, and CA3-LM, all termination zones for the perforant path. The statisitical correlations refer to the relationship between individual performance and SYN-IR for the aged subjects alone. (Taken from Smith *et al.*, 2000.)

analysis demonstrated that aged monkeys, compared to young adult monkeys, exhibit a decrease in the fluorescence intensity for NR1 in the OML of the dentate gyrus as compared to the IML. Given the tight laminar organization of these circuits, this suggests that the decreased NR1 levels primarily affect the input from the entorhinal cortex, pointing to the entorhinal cortex input to the hippocampus as a key element in age-related changes. Parallel qualitative and quantitative studies with antibodies to AMPA and kainate subunits demonstrated that the intradendritic alteration in NR1 occurs without a similar alteration of non-NMDA receptor subunits. Further analyses, using markers for presynaptic terminals and dendritic markers demonstrated that the circuit is not grossly interrupted in these aged monkeys. These findings suggest that the intradendritic distribution of a neurotransmitter receptor can be modified in an age-related and circuit-specific manner.

Age-related changes in rat hippocampus

While neuroanatomic datasets and behavioral datasets can be compared across experiments, it is most powerful when the neuroanatomic and cellular analyses are done in the same animals that have been behaviorally characterized. This approach is also useful for behavioral screening of aged animals, so that the behaviorally impaired aged animals can be considered as a distinct group from those that are not behaviorally impaired (Gallagher & Rapp, 1997; Peters *et al.*, 1998a). This interdisciplinary approach has been applied with great success to the rat hippocampus and aging, and has led to the conclusion that, just as in AD in humans and aging in monkeys, the projection from entorhinal cortex to

dentate gyrus (i.e. the perforant path) is highly vulnerable to aging and directly linked to age-related memory defects.

Recently, a comprehensive analysis of several synaptic indices was performed in the hippocampus of behaviorally characterized young and aged rats (Smith *et al.*, 2000; Adams *et al.*, 2001). Young and aged rats were tested on a hippocampal-dependent version of the Morris water maze that reveals substantial variability in spatial learning ability among aged rats (Gallagher & Rapp, 1997). A quantitative confocal method was used to quantify changes in immunofluorescence staining for the presynaptic vesicle glycoprotein, synaptophysin, which is an established marker for presynaptic terminals and is required for synaptic release. Individual differences in spatial learning capacity correlated with levels of synaptophysin staining in three of the regions examined; the OML and MML of the dentate gyrus, and the CA3 stratum lacunosum-moleculare (Fig. 26.3). These changes in relative synaptophysin immunofluorescence intensity occur in the absence of any evidence of structural degeneration of the innervated dendrites, and thus would affect synaptic transmission perhaps through compromised glutamate release rather than degeneration of pre- or postsynaptic elements. Most importantly, all three of the regions displaying decreased levels of synaptophysin expression receive a major projection from layer II of entorhinal cortex, offering further evidence that this circuit is exquisitely sensitive to aging. These findings suggest that circuit-specific alterations in glutamate release in the rat hippocampus may contribute to the effects of aging on learning and memory, in the absence of frank degeneration.

In these same animals, the AMPA receptor subunit, GluR2, and the NMDA receptor subunit NR1 were investigated as well, to determine whether or not postsynaptic shifts in receptors such as those observed in monkey (Gazzaley *et al.*, 1996b) might also be occurring in the context of aging that would further impact the functional status of the entorhinal inputs to dentate gyrus and CA3 (Adams *et al.*, 2001). There was no statistically significant decrease in NR1 directly associated with age-related memory impairment in rat hippocampus, although there was a direct correlation between NR fluorescence intensity and behavioral performance across all animals. While these studies require extensive ultrastructural analysis to confirm the synaptic nature of the receptor changes, it appears that both pre- and postsynaptic proteins (including GluRs) in specific circuits can be correlated with performance under many conditions, including decrements in performance associated with aging.

Interactions between neural and endocrine senescence

One of the most difficult challenges for research on brain aging over the next several decades will be to determine the critical points of interaction and influence between neural senescence and the aging of other systems. For example, it is particularly critical that we understand the interaction of reproductive senescence with the aging of the nervous system. At the turn of the century, the life expectancy of American women was roughly equivalent to the average age of onset of menopause. Currently, there is a 30-year discrepancy between these two demographic indices, with a life expectancy of approximately 80 years and the average onset of menopause remaining in the early 50s, making the issue of endocrine senescence particularly relevant to human aging.

The role of estrogen in controlling the reproductive axis at the level of the hypothalamus has been studied for many years and characterized in great detail (Fink, 1986). However, estrogens also impact synaptic communication in brain regions involved in cognitive processing, such as the hippocampus (Woolley, 1998), and these effects may be of particular importance in the context of aging when both circulating estrogen levels change and hippocampal-dependent functions decline (Sherwin, 2000). However, until recently, our understanding of estrogen effects on synaptic plasticity in the hippocampus was based primarily on data from young animals. For example, dendritic spine density in CA1 pyramidal cells is sensitive to naturally occurring estrogen fluctuations in young animals (Woolley *et al.*, 1990), as well as experimentally induced estrogen depletion and replacement (Gould *et al.*, 1990; Woolley & McEwen, 1992, 1993).

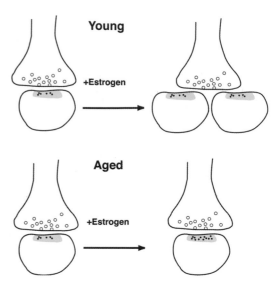

Fig. 26.4 A schematic of estrogen-induced plasticity in young and aged animals. Estrogen treatment increases NR1 expression per synapse in aged hippocampus, whereas it increases spine number but not synaptic NR1 in young female rat hippocampus. Small black dots represent immunogold particles labelling NR1 associated with the postsynaptic density, and open circles are synaptic vesicles. The grey zone indicates the postsynaptic density. (Adapted from Adams et al., 2001.)

These effects of estrogen on hippocampal circuitry are NMDA receptor-dependent (McEwen, 2002), and estrogen replacement directly increases levels NMDA receptor levels in CA1 dendrites and soma (Gazzaley *et al.*, 1996a). Using quantitative postembedding immunogold electron microscopy, a recent study investigated estrogen's effects on axospinous synapse density and the synaptic distribution of the NMDA receptor subunit, NR1, within the context of aging (Adams *et al.*, 2001). As shown before (Woolley & McEwen, 1992) estrogen induced an increase in axospinous synapse density in young animals. However, it did not alter the synaptic representation of NR1 in young animals, in that the amount of NR1 molecules per synapse was equivalent across groups. Estrogen replacement in aged female rats failed to increase axospinous synapse density, however, estrogen upregulated synaptic NR1 expression compared to aged animals not receiving estrogen (Adams *et al.*, 2001). Therefore, the young and aged hippocampus react differently to estrogen replacement, with the aged animals unable to mount a plasticity response generating additional synapses, yet responsive to estrogen with respect to additional NMDA receptor content per synapse (Fig. 26.4) (Adams *et al.*, 2001). Thus, while estrogen affects the aged CA1 synapse in a manner that might enhance hippocampal function, it does so in the context of a synaptic

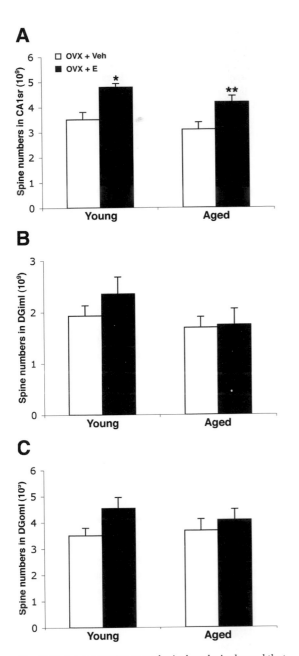

Fig. 26.5 A quantitative stereological analysis showed that estrogen significantly increased the total spine number of CA1sr (A) by 37% ($p < 0.005$) in young ovariectomized female rhesus monkeys and 35% in aged ovariectomized female monkeys ($p < 0.05$). No significant estrogen-induced changes in spine number were observed in the inner molecular layer of dentate gyrus (Dgiml) (B) and or the outer molecular layer of dentate gyrus (Dgoml), though a similar trend was observed in the young animals (C). Values represent means ± SEM. Asterisk indicates a statistically significant difference between young OVX + Veh and young OVX + E, $p < 0.005$, two asterisks indicate statistically significant difference between aged OVX + Veh and aged OVX + E, $p < 0.05$. (Taken from Hao *et al.*, 2003.)

density compromised by age. What change in CA1 spines occurs with aging that makes the aged rat CA1 spine less responsive to estrogen? It was recently demonstrated that the key estrogen receptor, ERα is present in CA1 spines and synapses (Milner *et al.*, 2001; Adams *et al.*, 2002), and presumably has local effects on synaptic transmission in this case, rather than its more traditional role in gene regulation in the nucleus (McEwen, 2002). We recently demonstrated that the number of spines in CA1 that contain ERα decreases dramatically with age (Adams *et al.*, 2002), and this decrease may be the cause of the decreased sensitivity to estrogen with respect to formation of new spines that we reported in the aged rats.

Importantly, our early results in non-human primates show a similar increase in spines in CA1 in response to estrogen, however aged monkeys were just as responsive as young monkeys (Hao *et al.*, 2003, Fig. 26.5). In addition, prefrontal cortex in monkeys also displays an estrogen-induced increase in spine number (Tang *et al.*, 2003). A recent behavioral analysis in estrogen-induced demonstrated a significant enhancement of cognitive function in aged rhesus monkeys (Rapp *et al.*, 2003). Aged female rhesus monkeys were ovariectomized, and then treated with either vehicle or 100 μg of estradiol cypionate every 21 days during an extended course of behavioral testing. The estrogen treated group showed enhanced performance on both a hippocampal-dependent task, delayed non-matching to sample, and on DR, the prefrontal task demonstrated to be sensitive to age. In fact, estrogen treatment restored performance to that of young animals (Fig. 26.6). These data are not only important as a demonstration of estrogen's impact on cognition in a non-human primate model, but also suggest that age-related decline in cognitive performance, is potentially reversible through pharmaceutical intervention.

Conclusions and future directions

The transition from fairly circumscribed memory impairment sometimes referred to as mild cognitive impairment to the dramatic loss of cognitive abilities that accompanies AD likely requires progressive development of neocortical pathology. The key vulnerable neocortical cell class has been characterized morphologically, neurochemically, and with respect to its connections. The demise of this cell class begins early in the transition to dementia; thus, interventions for AD should be aimed at protecting this cell class. Age-related memory impairment likely involves alternative mechanisms that do not involve frank neuron death, but rather involve alterations of spines and synapses. A

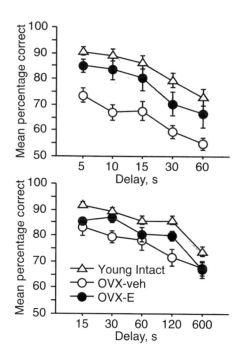

Fig. 26.6 Neuropsychological performance of aged OVX-veh and
OVX-E monkeys relative to young intact subjects. *Top*: delay
component of delayed response (DR). *Bottom*: delayed
non-matching to sample (DNMS). Note that the estrogen treated
group performed at a level nearly equivalent to young animals in
the DR task. In the DNMS task, estrogen treated animals
displayed enhanced performance at two delay intervals, 30 and
120 seconds. Error bars = SEM. (Modified from Rapp *et al.*,
2003.)

number of potential molecular and synaptic targets for
such age-related decline have been identified, and the key
circuits in which such changes occur have been delineated. An important interface exists between reproductive
and neural senescence, with estrogen levels influencing
many of the same circuits implicated in age-related memory impairment. Some of the synaptic alterations at this
interface have been identified.

Future studies will require interdisciplinary approaches
that reveal cellular and synaptic alterations that can be
quantitatively linked to endocrine status and/or behavioral
performance.

Acknowledgements

Collective thanks to members of the Morrison Hof and Rapp
laboratories. Supported by NIH grants AG02219, AG05138,
AG06647 AG16765, AG10606, and AG09973.

REFERENCES

Adams, M. M., Smith, T. D., Moga, D., *et al.* (2001). Hippocampal dependent learning ability correlates with *N*-methyl-D-
aspartate (NMDA) receptor levels in CA3 neurons of young
and aged rats. *J. Comp. Neurol.*, **432**, 230–43.

Adams, M. M., Fink, S. E., Shah, R. A. *et al.* (2002). Estrogen and
aging affect the subcellular distribution of estrogen receptor-
alpha in the hippocampus of female rats. *J. Neurosci.*, **22**, 3608–
14.

Albert, M. S. (1996). Cognitive and neurobiologic markers of early
Alzheimer disease. *Proc. Natl Acad. Sci., USA*, **93**, 13547–
51.

Arnold, S. E., Hyman, B. T., Flory, J., Damasio, A. R. & Van Hoesen,
G. W. (1991). The topographical and neuroanatomical distribution of neurofibrillary tangles and neuritic plaques in the cerebral cortex of patients with Alzheimer's disease. *Cereb. Cortex*,
1, 103–16.

Bachevalier, J., Landis, L. S., Walker, L. C. *et al.* (1991). Aged monkeys
exhibit behavioral deficits indicative of widespread cerebral
dysfunction. *Neurobiol. Aging*, **12**, 99–111.

Barnes, C. A., Suster, M. S., Shen, J. & McNaughton, B. L. (1997).
Multistability of cognitive maps in the hippocampus of old
rats. *Nature*, **388**, 272–5.

Bartus, R. T., Fleming, D. & Johnson, H. R. (1978). Aging in the rhesus
monkey: debilitating effects on short-term memory. *J. Gerontol.*, **33**, 858–71.

Bouras, C., Hof, P. R. & Morrison, J. H. (1993). Neurofibrillary tangle
densities in the hippocampal formation in a non-demented
population define subgroups of patients with differential early
pathologic changes. *Neurosci. Lett.*, **153**, 131–5.

Bouras, C., Hof, P. R., Giannakopoulos, P., Michel, J. P. & Morrison,
J. H. (1994). Regional distribution of neurofibrillary tangles and
senile plaques in the cerebral cortex of elderly patients: a quantitative evaluation of a one-year autopsy population from a
geriatric hospital. *Cereb. Cortex*, **4**, 138–50.

Bussière, T., Giannakopoulos, P., Bouras, C., Perl, D. P., Morrison,
J. H. & Hof, P. R. (2003). Progressive degeneration of non-
phosphorylated neurofilament protein-enriched pyramidal
neurons predicts cognitive impairment in Alzheimer's disease: Stereologic analysis of prefrontal cortex area 9. *J. Comp.
Neurol.*, **463**, 281–302.

Campbell, M. J. & Morrison, J. H. (1989). Monoclonal antibody
to neurofilament protein (SMI-32) labels a subpopulation of
pyramidal neurons in the human and monkey neocortex.
J. Comp. Neurol., **282**, 191–205.

Duan, H., Wearne, S. L., Rocher, A. B., Macedo, A., Morrison, J. H.
& Hof, P. R. (2003). Age-related dendritic and spine changes
in corticocortically projecting neurons in macaque monkeys.
Cereb. Cortex, **13**, 950–61.

Fink, G. (1986). The endocrine control of ovulation. *Sci. Prog.*, **70**,
403–23.

Gallagher, M. & Rapp, P. R. (1997). The use of animal models to
study the effects of aging on cognition. *Annu. Rev. Psychol.*, **48**,
339–70.

Gazzaley, A. H., Weiland, N. G., McEwen, B. S. & Morrison, J. H. (1996a). Differential regulation of NMDAR1 mRNA and protein by estradiol in the rat hippocampus. *J. Neurosci.*, **16**, 6830–8.

Gazzaley, A. H., Siegel, S. J., Kordower, J. H., Mufson, E. J. & Morrison, J. H. (1996b). Circuit-specific alterations of *N*-methyl-D-aspartate receptor subunit 1 in the dentate gyrus of aged monkeys. *Proc. Natl. Acad. Sci., USA*, **93**, 3121–5.

Gazzaley, A. H., Thakker, M. M., Hof, P. R. & Morrison, J. H. (1997). Preserved number of entorhinal cortex layer II neurons in aged macaque monkeys. *Neurobiol. Aging*, **18**, 549–53.

Goldman-Rakic, P. S. (1988) Topography of cognition: parallel distributed networks in primate association cortex. *Annu. Rev. Neurosci.*, **11**, 137–56.

Gómez-Isla, T., Price, J. L., McKeel, D. W., Jr., Morris, J. C., Growdon, J. H. & Hyman, B. T. (1996). Profound loss of layer II entorhinal cortex neurons occurs in very mild Alzheimer's disease. *J. Neurosci.*, **16**, 4491–500.

Gómez-Isla, T., Hollister, R., West, H. *et al.* (1997). Neuronal loss correlates with but exceeds neurofibrillary tangles in Alzheimer's disease. *Ann. Neurol.*, **41**, 17–24.

Gould, E., Woolley, C. S., Frankfurt, M. & McEwen, B. S. (1990). Gonadal steroids regulate dendritic spine density in hippocampal pyramidal cells in adulthood. *J. Neurosci.*, **10**, 1286–91.

Hao, J., Janssen, W. G. M., Tang, Y. *et al.* (2003). Estrogen increases the number of spinophilin-immunoreactive spines in the hippocampus of young and aged female rhesus monkeys. *J. Comp. Neurol.*, **465**, 540–50.

Hof, P. R. & Morrison, J. H. (1990). Quantitative analysis of a vulnerable subset of pyramidal neurons in Alzheimer's disease: II. Primary and secondary visual cortex. *J. Comp. Neurol.*, **301**, 55–64.

(1995). Neurofilament protein defines regional patterns of cortical organization in the macaque monkey visual system: a quantitative immunohistochemical analysis. *J. Comp. Neurol.*, **352**, 161–86.

Hof, P. R., Cox, K. & Morrison, J. H. (1990). Quantitative analysis of a vulnerable subset of pyramidal neurons in Alzheimer's disease: I. Superior frontal and inferior temporal cortex. *J. Comp. Neurol.*, **301**, 44–54.

Hof, P. R., Nimchinsky, E. A. & Morrison, J. H. (1995). Neurochemical phenotype of corticocortical connections in the macaque monkey: quantitative analysis of a subset of neurofilament protein-immunoreactive projection neurons in frontal, parietal, temporal, and cingulate cortices. *J. Comp. Neurol.*, **362**, 109–33.

Hof, P. R., Ungerleider, L. G., Webster, M. J. *et al.* (1996). Neurofilament protein is differentially distributed in subpopulations of corticocortical projection neurons in the macaque monkey visual pathways. *J. Comp. Neurol.*, **376**, 112–27.

Hof, P. R., Ungerleider, L. G., Adams, M. M. *et al.* (1997). Callosally projecting neurons in the macaque monkey V1/V2 border are enriched in nonphosphorylated neurofilament protein. *Vis. Neurosci.*, **14**, 981–7.

Hof, P. R., Bouras, C. & Morrison, J. H. (1999). Cortical neuropathology in aging and dementing disorders: neuronal typology, connectivity, and selective vulnerability. In *Cerebral Cortex*, Vol. 14, *Neurodegenerative and Age-Related Changes in Cerebral Cortex*, ed. A. Peters & J. H. Morrison, pp. 175–312. New York: Kluwer Academic-Plenum.

Hof, P. R., Duan, H., Page, T. L. *et al.* (2002). Age-related changes in GluR2 and NMDAR1 glutamate receptor subunit protein immunoreactivity in corticocortically projecting neurons in macaque and patas monkeys. *Brain Res.*, **928**, 175–86.

Hof, P. R., Bussière, T., Gold, G. *et al.* (2003). Stereologic evidence for persistence of viable neurons in layer II of the entorhinal cortex and the CA1 field in Alzheimer disease. *J. Neuropathol. Exp. Neurol.*, **62**, 55–67.

Hyman, B. T., Van Horsen, G. W., Damasio, A. R. & Barnes, C. L. (1984). Alzheimer's disease: cell-specific pathology isolates the hippocampal formation. *Science*, **225**, 1168–70.

Hyman, B. T., Van Hoesen, G. W., Kromer, L. J. & Damasio, A. R. (1986). Perforant pathway changes and the memory impairment of Alzheimer's disease. *Ann. Neurol.*, **20**, 472–81.

Hyman, B. T., Van Hoesen, G. W. & Damasio, A. R. (1990). Memory-related neural systems in Alzheimer's disease: an anatomic study. *Neurology*, **40**, 1721–30.

Kentros, C., Hargreaves, E., Hawkins, R.D., Kandel, E. R., Shapiro, M. & Muller, R. V. (1998). Abolition of long-term stability of new hippocampal place cell maps by NMDA receptor blockade. *Science*, **280**, 2121–6.

Lewis, D. A., Campbell, M. J., Terry, R. D. & Morrison, J. H. (1987). Laminar and regional distributions of neurofibrillary tangles and neuritic plaques in Alzheimer's disease: a quantitative study of visual and auditory cortices. *J. Neurosci.*, **7**, 1799–808.

McEwen, B. (2002). Estrogen actions throughout the brain. *Rec. Prog. Horm. Res.*, **57**, 357–84.

Milner, T. A., McEwen, B. S., Hayashi, S., Li, C. J., Reagan, L. P. & Alves, S. E. (2001). Ultrastructural evidence that hippocampal alpha estrogen receptors are located at extranuclear sites. *J. Comp. Neurol.*, **429**, 355–71.

Mirra, S. S., Hart, M. N. & Terry, R. D. (1993). Making the diagnosis of Alzheimer's disease. A primer for practicing pathologists. *Arch. Pathol. Lab. Med.*, **117**, 132–44.

Morrison, J. H., & Hof, P. R. (1997). Life and death of neurons in the aging brain. *Science*, **278**, 412–19.

(2002). Selective vulnerability of corticocortical and hippocampal circuits in aging and Alzheimer's disease. *Prog. Brain Res.*, **136**, 467–86.

Morrison, J. H., Lewis, D. A., Campbell, M. J., Huntley, G. W., Benson, D. L. & Bouras, C. (1987). A monoclonal antibody to non-phosphorylated neurofilament protein marks the vulnerable cortical neurons in Alzheimer's disease. *Brain Res.*, **416**, 331–6.

Nimchinsky, E. A., Hof, P. R., Young, W. G. & Morrison, J. H. (1996). Neurochemical, morphologic, and laminar characterization of cortical projection neurons in the cingulate motor areas of the macaque monkey. *J. Comp. Neurol.*, **374**, 136–60.

O'Donnell, K. A., Rapp, P. R. & Hof, P. R. (1999). Preservation of prefrontal cortical volume in behaviorally characterized aged macaque monkeys. *Exp. Neurol.*, **160**, 300–10.

Page, T. L., Einstein, M., Duan, H., *et al.* (2002). Morphological alterations in neurons forming corticocortical projections in the neocortex of aged Patas monkeys. *Neurosci. Lett.*, **317**, 37–41.

Pearson, R. C., Esiri, M. M., Hiorns, R. W., Wilcock, G. K. & Powell, T. P. (1985). Anatomical correlates of the distribution of the pathological changes in the neocortex in Alzheimer disease. *Proc. Natl Acad. Sci., USA*, **82**, 4531–4.

Peters, A., Rosene, D. L., Moss, M. B. *et al.* (1996). Neurobiological bases of age-related cognitive decline in the rhesus monkey. *J. Neuropathol. Exp. Neurol.*, **55**, 861–74.

Peters, A., Sethares, C. & Moss, M. B. (1998a). The effects of aging on layer 1 in area 46 of prefrontal cortex in the rhesus monkey. *Cereb. Cortex*, **8**, 671–84.

Peters, A., Morrison, J. H., Rosene, D. L. & Hyman, B. T. (1998b). Feature article: are neurons lost from the primate cerebral cortex during normal aging? *Cereb. Cortex*, **8**, 295–300.

Peters, A., Moss, M. B. & Sethares, C. (2000). Effects of aging on myelinated nerve fibers in monkey primary visual cortex. *J. Comp. Neurol.*, **419**, 364–76.

Rapp, P. R. & Gallagher, M. (1997). Toward a cognitive neuroscience of normal aging. In *Advances in Cell Aging and Gerontology*, Vol. 2 (ed. P. S. Timiras & E. E. Bittar, pp. 1–21, Mattson Geddes.

Rapp, P. R., Morrison, J. H. & Roberts, J. A. (2003). Cyclic estrogen replacement improves cognitive function in aged ovariectomized rhesus monkeys. *J. Neurosci.*, **23**, 5708–14.

Reilly, J. F., Games, D., Rydel, R. E. *et al.* (2003). Amyloid deposition in the hippocampus and entorhinal cortex: quantitative analysis of a transgenic mouse model. *Proc. Natl Acad. Sci. USA*, **100**, 4837–42.

Rogers, J. & Morrison, J. H. (1985). Quantitative morphology and regional and laminar distributions of senile plaques in Alzheimer's disease. *J. Neurosci.*, **5**, 2801–8.

Sherwin, B. B. (2000). Oestrogen and cognitive function throughout the female lifespan. *Novartis Found Symp.*, **230**, 188–96; discussion 196–201.

Smith, T. D., Adams, M. M., Gallagher, M., Morrison, J. H. & Rapp, P. R. (2000). Circuit-specific alterations in hippocampal synaptophysin immunoreactivity predict spatial learning impairment in aged rats. *J. Neurosci.*, **20**, 6587–93.

Tang, Y., Janssen, W. G. M., Hao, J. *et al.* (2003). Estrogen replacement increases spinophilin-immunoreactive spine number in the prefrontal cortex of female rhesus monkeys. *Cereb. Cortex*, **14**, 215–23.

Trojanowski, J. Q., Schmidt, M. L., Shin, R. W., Bramblett, G. T., Rao, D. & Lee, V. M. (1993). Altered tau and neurofilament proteins in neuro-degenerative diseases: diagnostic implications for Alzheimer's disease and Lewy body dementias. *Brain Pathol.*, **3**, 45–54.

Tsien, J. Z., Huerta, P. T. & Tonegawa, S. (1996). The essential role of hippocampal CA1 NMDA receptor-dependent synaptic plasticity in spatial memory. *Cell*, **87**, 1327–38.

Vickers, J. C. (1997). A cellular mechanism for the neuronal changes underlying Alzheimer's disease. *Neuroscience*, **78**, 629–39.

Vickers, J. C., Delacourte, A. & Morrison, J. H. (1992). Progressive transformation of the cytoskeleton associated with normal aging and Alzheimer's disease. *Brain Res.*, **594**, 273–8.

Vickers, J. C., Riederer, B. M., Marugg, R. A. *et al.* (1994), Alterations in neurofilament protein immunoreactivity in human hippocampal neurons related to normal aging and Alzheimer's disease. *Neuroscience*, **62**, 1–13.

Vickers, J. C., Dickson, T. C., Adlard, P. A., Saunders, H. L., King, C. E. & McCormack, G. (2000). The cause of neuronal degeneration in Alzheimer's disease. *Prog. Neurobiol.*, **60**, 139–65.

West, M. J. (1993). Regionally specific loss of neurons in the aging human hippocampus. *Neurobiol. Aging*, **14**, 287–93.

Witter, M. P. & Amaral, D. G. (1991). Entorhinal cortex of the monkey: V. Projections to the dentate gyrus, hippocampus, and subicular complex. *J. Comp. Neurol.*, **307**, 437–59.

Woolley, C. S. (1998). Estrogen-mediated structural and functional synaptic plasticity in the female rat hippocampus. Horm. Behav., **34**, 140–8.

Woolley, C. S. & McEwen, B. S. (1992). Estradiol mediates fluctuation in hippocampal synapse density during the estrous cycle in the adult rat. *J. Neurosci.*, **12**, 2549–54.

(1993). Roles of estradiol and progesterone in regulation of hippocampal dendritic spine density during the estrous cycle in the rat. *J. Comp. Neurol.*, **336**, 293–306.

Woolley, C. S., Gould, E., Frankfurt, M. & McEwen, B. S. (1990). Naturally occurring fluctuation in dendritic spine density on adult hippocampal pyramidal neurons. *J. Neurosci.*, **10**, 4035–9.

Part V

Alzheimer's disease

27

Mild cognitive impairment

Keith A. Josephs[1], David F. Tang-Wai[2]
and Ronald C. Petersen[3]

[1,3]Department of Neurology, Mayo Clinic, Rochester, MN, USA
[2]Division of Neurology, University Health Network, Toronto Western Hospital, ON, Canada

Overview

As research in aging and dementia moves toward an earlier identification of individuals with a cognitive impairment, the concept of mild cognitive impairment (MCI) has received considerable attention. Mild cognitive impairment refers to an intermediate stage between the cognitive changes that are felt to be part of normal aging and those that represent the very earliest features of a dementia such as Alzheimer's disease. This stage of intermediate impairment is believed to be important, since several studies have indicated that these subjects are likely to progress to AD at an accelerated rate over the general population (Petersen *et al.*, 1999). The initial literature on the concept of MCI pertained to individuals with memory impairment beyond what would be expected for normal aging (Petersen, 1995). These subjects may have a mild impairment in other cognitive domains but performance is felt to be within the range of normal. Similarly, they may have slight difficulties with activities of daily living, but these are generally felt not to be significant. More recently, the construct of MCI has been broadened to include other presentations of persons with transitional cognitive impairment and these will be discussed below. Implicit in the discussion of MCI is an understanding of the concept of normal cognitive function. While we are learning a great deal about aging and cognitive function, this still remains an area of uncertainty.

Normal aging and evolution to MCI

Normal cognitive function has been the subject of a great deal of research and development in the last few decades (Rowe & Kahn, 1987). Yet, the concept of normal aging and what constitutes abnormal aging have remained controversial. "Successful aging" can describe individuals without any functional impairment or significant medical comorbidities but probably does not represent the majority of elderly (Kaye *et al.*, 1994). "Typical aging" therefore can describe individuals who have comorbid medical illnesses and are functioning normally in society (Petersen *et al.*, 1990). However, performance in this group tends to decline with age, and is associated with both neuroradiologic and neuropathologic changes.

While a great deal of research has been conducted characterizing cognitive changes with aging, there is no agreement on the nature or degree of impairment or the pathophysiologic substrate for that clinical picture. Consequently, the lack of precise knowledge of cognitive changes in normal aging makes the characterization of very early changes of MCI challenging. Normal cognitive aging can be defined based on neuropsychological tests with published normative data on a variety of neuropsychological tests for individuals up to age 100 (Ivnik *et al.*, 1992). However, criticisms of these data exist including arguments that normative data are contaminated by the inclusion of persons with incipient cognitive impairment (Sliwinski *et al.*, 1996). Consequently, some investigators argue for the elimination of those people from the norms, as they incorporate more of an impairment than would be the case had these subjects not been included.

Several descriptive terms were used over the past 40 years to address memory and cognitive impairment that develops with aging. An early term that was used to draw attention to memory changes in aging was "benign senescent forgetfulness" (Kral, 1962), describing a condition whereby persons can experience a decline in memory function with aging that did not progress to a dementia. This was followed by the term, "age-associated memory impairment" (AAMI) by a National Institute of Mental Health work group (Crook *et al.*, 1986). One difficulty of this concept was an

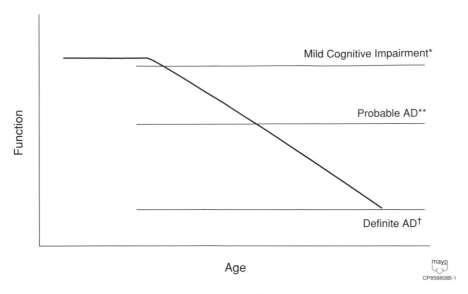

Fig. 27.1 Hypothetical continuum from normal aging through mild cognitive impairment to dementia.

overinclusion of most of the population as having a memory impairment when these individuals were compared to younger adults. Revision of AAMI led to "age-associated cognitive decline" (AACD), which included impairment of cognitive domains other than memory. Finally, the Canadian Study of Health and Aging developed the concept of "cognitive impairment – no dementia" (Graham *et al.*, 1997) to capture intermediate stages of impairment.

Longitudinal studies of aging and dementia in various communities have identified individuals who developed memory impairment but did not satisfy the criteria for AD (Petersen & Morris, 2003). Over time, however, many of these individuals progress to probable AD. MCI is a clinical diagnosis describing the transitional state between normal aging and mild dementia. In this transitional stage, there are objective signs of mild memory impairment with preservation of other cognitive functions. These patients, who during neurological evaluation, were found to have objective mild episodic memory impairment, that is neither severe enough nor affecting lifestyle to warrant a diagnosis of dementia. More recently, however, the concept of MCI has become more heterogeneous in terms of etiology and clinical presentation (see below).

The actual transition between normal aging and MCI is also not well understood and remains in an area of debate. It is important, however, not to consider MCI as being a rigid separation between normal aging and mild dementia but rather a continuum or a transitional zone between normal and abnormal function in those subjects who are destined to develop dementia. This hypothetical functional decline from normal aging to dementia is depicted in Fig. 27.1. The

current challenge is to identify patients at the earliest point on this slope and try to prevent or alter progression.

Clinical description

The Mayo Clinic and others have been involved with studies on aging and dementia for at least the past decade (Ivnik *et al.*, 1992, Smith *et al.*, 1992). From these studies and vast clinical experience, others and we have devised clinical criteria for the diagnosis of amnestic MCI. The criteria used for diagnosis of MCI include the following:

- memory complaint, preferably corroborated by an informant
- memory dysfunction for age and education
- essentially normal general cognitive function
- largely intact activities of daily living
- not demented.

Other researchers have used rating scales to characterize subjects with intermediate impairment. The two most common alternative approaches involve the use of: the Clinical Dementia Rating scale (CDR) (Morris, 1993) and the Global Deterioration Scale (GDS) (Reisberg *et al.*, 1982). The CDR is a scale that classifies patients along a continuum from normal (CDR 0), to questionable dementia (CDR 0.5), mild dementia (CDR 1), moderate dementia (CDR 2) and severe dementia (CDR 3). The GDS is another scale similar to the CDR that classifies patients from normal (GDS 1), normal with subjective memory impairment

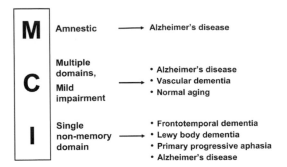

Fig. 27.2 Heterogeneity of mild cognitive impairment.

(GDS 2), mild dementia (GDS 3), up to very severe dementia (GDS 7). Some researchers have contended that MCI as defined above is equivalent to CDR 0.5 and GDS 3. On a sample of 76 consecutively evaluated patients with MCI, Mayo investigators showed that MCI patients with a CDR of 0.5 and AD patients with a CDR of 0.5 differed significantly on all measures of general cognitive functioning. From that study and others, some have concluded that all patients with MCI are CDR 0.5; however, not all patients classified as CDR 0.5 will be MCI, as some will be demented. Similarly, it was shown that MCI patients could either be categorized as GDS 2 or GDS 3 (Petersen *et al.*, 1999).

Heterogeneity of MCI

In its original description MCI implied mild dysfunction affecting only episodic memory. However, there has been concern about patients who present with either mild impairment in multiple cognitive domains or impairment in one non-amnestic cognitive domain. This has led to the conceptualization of three clinical subcategories or three variants of MCI (Fig. 27.2): amnestic MCI, multiple domain MCI and non-amnestic single domain MCI.

Amnestic MCI refers to patients with MCI, with cognitive impairment limited primarily to episodic memory. This form of MCI is the one most referenced in the literature and when it occurs on a degenerative basis most probably progresses to early AD. Multiple domain MCI, as the term implies, defines a group of patients with mild impairment in multiple domains without sufficient overall deficit to warrant a diagnosis of dementia. Patients with multiple domain MCI may have mild behavioral changes, executive dysfunction, dysphasia, apperceptive agnosia or visuospatial deficits. Causes of the multiple domain MCI include AD or vascular dementia. Single non-amnestic domain MCI is defined by mild isolated cognitive impairment of behavior, executive function, language, visuospatial or visuo-perceptual processing, but not episodic memory. When non-amnestic domain MCI occurs on a degenerative basis, it may represent a precursor of dementia with Lewy bodies, or a frontotemporal lobar degeneration (frontotemporal dementia, primary progressive aphasia, semantic dementia or progressive non-fluent dysphasia).

Therefore, one can approach the diagnosis of MCI from a clinical perspective much the same as one would make the diagnosis of dementia. That is, if the subject meets the criteria for one of the subtypes of MCI, then a search for a likely etiology is pursued. Ultimately, a suspected cause for the clinical impairment is determined and this likely represents a precursor of one of the dementias.

Approach to the diagnosis of MCI

The concept of MCI is important as it currently defines a group of patients at the earliest stage in the development of AD. This group of patients most likely will be the focus of pharmaceutical therapeutic measures and therefore it is important that we develop highly sensitive and specific measures to correctly identify them. An accurate medical and neurological history, and clinical examination, needs to be completed. Ancillary testing is necessary and will complement clinical and physical examination. Ancillary testing also helps to eliminate other conditions that could mimic presentation of MCI, and aids in better identification of the subset of MCI patients that may be the ones at risk for future development of dementia.

History and examination

The history should focus on determining if there is any evidence for mild episodic memory impairment (Petersen, 2003b). From studies on familial AD, we know that verbal episodic memory is affected first (Newman *et al.*, 1994). Therefore, during history taking and cognitive examination, there should be emphases on determining the patient's ability for detailed recall. Episodic memory should be accessed by discussing specific recent events over the past weeks to months. Education and familiarity with subject matter is very important. It is important to remember that, when evaluating patients with MCI, only subtle abnormalities may be found. The fact that a patient looks to his or her spouse when asked a specific question should be considered a red flag. Patients must be thoroughly evaluated and questions should cover a broad range of topics that the patient should be familiar with.

The neurological examination should include at least mental status testing that can evaluate learning, recall, attention, language, problem solving, executive functioning and visuospatial function. Some of the screening measures recommended include the Mini-Mental State Examination (MMSE) (Folstein *et al.*, 1975) and the Short Test of Mental Status (STMS)(Kokmen *et al.*, 1991). Although both measures are effective, the STMS may provide additional sensitivity to determine and to predict those individuals with MCI because there are four words to recall with longer delayed recall (Tang-Wai *et al.*, 2003). Attention to behavior, dysexecutive symptoms, language difficulties, alien limb-like complaints, hallucinations, Parkinsonism and visuospatial complaints are also important. A complete neurological examination must be undertaken as some dementing illnesses may present with signs of motor and sensory deficits. It is particularly important to look for fasciculations, parkinsonism, signs of cerebral infarction, asymmetry, eye movement abnormalities, frontal release phenomena (including a snout and palmomental) and dysarthrias, dyspraxias and visual disorientation.

Laboratory tests

In addition to a thorough history and physical examination, we recommend the following routine screening studies (in uncomplicated cases) in all patients who are being evaluated for a possible diagnosis of MCI: chemistry panel, complete blood count, erythrocyte sedimentation rate (ESR), thyroid function studies, liver function tests, folic acid, vitamin B12 levels and syphilis serology. Additional testing may be necessary depending upon the clinical presentation of the individual patient and whether abnormalities are found on initial screening.

Neuropsychometric test

Neuropsychometric testing complements and extends the bedside mental status testing and provides an additional level of security in the diagnosis of MCI. Studies have demonstrated that patients with mild AD perform poorly on test of memory, delayed recall, language and executive functioning compared to controls. (Knopman & Ryberg, 1989; Storandt & Hill, 1989; Welsh *et al.*, 1991, 1992; Petersen *et al.*, 1994; Masur *et al.*, 1994). In amnestic MCI, clinicians should be interested in both learning and delayed recall as patients demonstrate slightly depressed learning curve and deficit in delayed recall. These measures may also be able to predict which normal subjects are at risk to progress to MCI or from MCI to AD (Petersen *et al.*, 2003). Because only mild cognitive deficits may be present, it is important that thorough neuropsychometric tests be performed in all patients.

The neuropsychological testing does not make the diagnosis of MCI. It is the clinician who must combine the features of the history, bedside mental status examination, the neurological and general medications examination, results of laboratory, neuropsychological, and imaging tests to arrive at a diagnosis.

Neuroimaging

Neuroimaging is another tool that can aid with the diagnosis of MCI (Jack, 2003). Computer tomography (CT) or magnetic resonance imaging (MRI) is useful in excluding structural causes of cognitive decline including brain tumors, subdural hematoma, ischemic and hemorrhagic infarcts and can also give us an idea of the density of silent vascular damage that may be present in both cortical and subcortical areas. They help us to localize anatomical damage that may be critical to the presenting complaint. Small thalamic damage, which may not be apparent on neurological examination, may be seen on MR imaging. Similarly, we are able to get a better understanding of changes that may be occurring in mesiotemporal lobe structures. Enlargement of focal peri-hippocampal spaces would be consistent with hippocampal atrophy and could explain subtle complaints of episodic memory impairment while findings, for example, of perisylvian atrophy or parietal atrophy would be in keeping with non-fluent aphasia and apraxia, respectively. Even though no imaging finding is specific for a diagnosis of MCI, a recent longitudinal study has shown that MRI hippocampal volumes in MCI are predictive of conversion to AD even when multivariate prediction equation has controlled for age, estrogen use, neuropsychological testing, apolipoprotein E status, history of ischemic heart disease, and hypertension (Jack *et al.*, 1999) and correlates with pathological evidence of atrophy and neuronal drop out (Bobinski *et al.*, 1998). Others and we have also demonstrated that measurements of the entorhinal cortex may be a better measure of early cognitive impairment (Bobinski *et al.*, 1999; Killiany *et al.*, 2000, Xu *et al.*, 2000). Functional neuroimaging is also an additional useful tool and aids with the detection of subtle abnormalities in patients with MCI (Johnson & Albert, 2000, 2003; Holman *et al.*, 1992; Johnson *et al.*, 1998). More recently, magnetic resonance spectroscopy (Kantarci *et al.*, 2000) and fMRI (Machulda *et al.*, 2003) have been assessed as a possible tool in evaluating MCI, but unfortunately studies have been limited.

Biomarkers

To date, there is no definitive test that allows us to predict which patients with a diagnosis of MCI will go on to develop

AD even though there are some suggestive findings on neuropsychometric testing and neuroimaging. Two biomarkers that have been used in studies in AD are tau and Aβ42 in the cerebrospinal fluid (CSF). Both biomarkers have been assessed in patients with MCI and may improve positive predictive value (Graff-Radford *et al.*, 2003). CSF tau levels have been found not to be increased in patients with AD (Galasko *et al.*, 1997). However, recent longitudinal studies have demonstrated that tau level is increased in patients with MCI who later convert to AD but is not increased in the patients with MCI that do not convert (Sunderland *et al.*, 1990). Longitudinal analysis of plasma Aβ42 in patients progressing from normal through MCI to AD revealed that plasma Aβ42 declines in the year before MCI develops and continues to decline throughout the MCI stage (Graff-Radford *et al.*, 2003). These findings may later prove to be important prognosticators. As in amnestic MCI, one could speculate about similar findings with other biomarkers in non-amnestic and multiple domain MCI that may prove to be useful in the subclassification of MCI as well as in predicting which patients will later dement.

Neuropathology

Neuropathological substrate of MCI is uncertain. Patients with a diagnosis of MCI do not die unless from accidents or incidents unrelated to their disease. By the time they die, most have converted to having a dementia. One study from the Mayo Clinic on 15 subjects who died while their clinical classification was MCI reported that many subjects did not have the neuropathological features of AD at the time of death but were found to have heterogeneous pathologies including argyrophilic grain disease, hippocampal sclerosis and vascular disease (Petersen, 2002). Data from the Religious Orders Study indicated that approximately 60% of subjects with multi-domain MCI had AD changes at autopsy (DeKosky *et al.*, 2002).

Genetics and predictors of progression

The genetic features of amnestic MCI are also similar to those of clinically probable AD. In particular, there appears to be a higher representation of Apo E ε 4 carriers in MCI and in some studies, the presence of an E4 allele may predict progression (Petersen *et al.*, 1994; Grundman *et al.*, 2004). However, these data are only mildly positive and it is currently not recommended to use Apo E for either a diagnostic tool for MCI or as an indicator of progression. Additional research is progressing on this topic.

Clinical trials

Currently, there are no treatments available for arresting or reversing the progression that occur in patients with MCI. However, therapeutic clinical trials will continue to focus on this group of patients, as we know that by 6 years approximately 80% will have converted to AD. Current clinical trials in MCI are focusing on treatments that have demonstrated possible efficacy in slowing progression in patients with AD.

One class of drugs currently being tested is the cholinesterase inhibitors. Studies on cholinesterase inhibitors in patients with AD have shown some benefit in slowing progression (Rogers *et al.*, 1998). The cholinesterase inhibitors that are currently available for use with AD include tacrine, donepezil, rivastigmine and galantamine, and are currently being evaluated for efficacy in patients with MCI. Estrogens are another class of drugs that have shown to be associated with slowing progression of cognitive dysfunction in patients with AD (Yaffe *et al.*, 1998, Waring *et al.*, 1999). Another class of drugs includes the anti-inflammatory agents and clinical trials on the effect of cyclooxygenase-2 (COX-2) inhibitory are underway (Petersen, 2003a). One current study is the Alzheimer's disease Cooperative Study MCI trail, a placebo control trial, involving 68 centres; comparing therapeutic benefit of vitamin E vs donepezil vs placebo (Grundman *et al.*, 2004).

Finally, in the current era of amyloid and tau genetics, it is worth considering medications that can either prevent the formation of tau and amyloidal aggregates or destroy the abnormal soluble protein polymers. An example is the recent vaccine trial that unfortunately was discontinued prematurely after many patients treated with the vaccine developed an encephalitis (Orgogozo *et al.*, 2003). Studies on these agents as well as other anti-amyloid agents are currently being developed and tested.

AAN practice parameters

In early 2001 the Quality Standards Subcommittee of the American Academy of Neurology (AAN) met to develop scientifically sound measures in evaluating patients with dementia. A work group was created to focus on two main questions that were felt very important for the enhancement of the field of dementia. First, they wanted to determine if the presence of MCI predict the development of dementia and second, whether screening at-risk subjects with a specific instrument in a specific setting led to the diagnosis of dementia. This group, after completing an evidence-based medicine literature search, put forth the following guidelines (Petersen *et al.*, 2001). They felt that patients with MCI should be recognized and monitored for functional decline due to their increased risk for subsequent development of dementia. This risk was determined to be between 6% and 25% per year, much higher than the risk to conversion of the general population that ranges from 0.2% to 3.9% depending on the age group being studied. They also felt that general cognitive screening instruments should be considered for the detection of dementia in MCI. Some of the screening measures recommended included the Mini-Mental State Examination (Folstein *et al.*, 1975), the Short Test of Mental Status (Kokmen *et al.*, 1991), 7-Minute Screening Test (Solomon *et al.*, 1998) and the Memory Impairment Screen (Buschke *et al.*, 1999). They found that neuropsychological batteries should be considered in identifying patients with dementia, especially when the subpopulation in which one practises has an increased risk of cognitive impairment.

Future directions

The concept of MCI is an important one for all neurodegenerative disorders. It allows us to conceptualize a transitional zone, not only in dementing diseases, but also in disorders of motor dysfunction, for example, idiopathic Parkinson's disease where early theraputic intervention my halt further development of end-stage disease. The concept of MCI is evolving. We are in the process of identifying normal patients who are at risk for the later development of MCI and dementia. Our ability to predict which group of the population is at risk for developing MCI will allow early detection and intervention.

Further development in better imaging techniques, neuropsychological batteries and biomarkers are currently under way and will further refine and improve our diagnostic sensitivities and specificities.

REFERENCES

Bobinski, M., de Leon, M. J., Tarnawski, M. *et al.* (1998). Neuronal and volume loss in CA1 of the hippocampal formation uniquely predicts duration and severity of Alzheimer's disease. *Brain Res.*, **805**, 267–9.

Bobinski, M., de Leon, M. J., Convit, A. *et al.* (1999). MRI of entorhinal cortex in mild Alzheimer's disease. *Lancet*, **353**, 38–40.

Buschke, H., Kuslansky, G., Katz, M. *et al.* (1999). Screening for dementia with the memory impairment screen. *Neurology*, **52**, 231–8.

Crook, T., Bartus, R. T., Ferris, S. H., Whitehouse, P., Cohen, G. D. & Gershon, S. (1986). For the National Institute of Mental Health Work Group. Age-associated memory impairment: proposed diagnostic criteria and measures of clinical change. *Dev. Neuropsychol.*, **2**, 261–7.

De Kosky, S. T., Ikonomovi, M. D., Styren, S. D. *et al.* (2002). Upregulation of choline acetyltransferase activity in hippocampus and frontal cortex of elderly subjects with mild cognitive impairment. *Ann. Neurol.*, **51**, 145–55.

Folstein, M. F., Folstein, S. E. & MCHugh, P. R. (1975). 'Mini-Mental State'. A practical method for grading the cognitive state of patients for the clinician. *J. Psychiatr. Res.*, **12**, 189–98.

Galasko, D., Clark, C., Chang, L. *et al.* (1997). Assessment of CSF levels of tau protein in mildly demented patients with Alzheimer's disease. *Neurology*, **48**, 632–5.

Graff-Radford, N., Lucas, J., Younkin, L. & Younkin, S. (2003). Longitudinal analysis of plasma Aß42 in patients progressing from normal through MCI to AD. *Neurology*, **60**(S1), A245.

Graham, J. E., Rockwood, K., Beattie, B. L. *et al.* (1997). Prevalence and severity of cognitive impairment with and without dementia in an elderly population. *Lancet*, **349**, 1793–6.

Grundman, M., Petersen, R. C., Ferris, S. H. *et al.* (2004). Alzheimer's Disease Cooperative Study. *Arch. Neurol.*, **61**, 59–66.

Holman, B. L., Johnson, K. A., Gerada, B., Carvalho, P. A. & Satlin, A. (1992). The scintigraphic appearance of Alzheimer's disease: a prospective study using technetium-99m-HMPAO SPECT. *J. Nuc. Med.*, **33**, 181–5.

Ivnik, R. J., Malec, J. F., Smith, G. E. *et al.* (1992). Mayo's older American normative studies: WAIS-R, WMS-R and AVLT norms for ages 56 through 97. *Clin. Neuropsychol.*, **6**(suppl), 1–104.

Jack, C. R. Jr. (2003). Magnetic resonance imaging. In *Mild Cognitive Impairment: Aging to Alzheimer's Disease.* ed. R. C. Petersen, pp. 105–32. New York: Oxford University Press, Inc.

Jack, C. R. Jr., Petersen, R. C., Xu, Y. C. *et al.* (1999). Prediction of AD with MRI-based hippocampal volume in mild cognitive impairment. *Neurology*, **52**, 1397–403.

Johnson, K. A. & Albert, M. S. (2000). Perfusion abnormalities in prodromal AD. *Neurobiol. Aging*, **21**, 289–92.

(2003). Functional Imaging. In *Mild Cognitive Impairment: Aging to Alzheimer's Disease*, ed. R. C. Petersen, pp. 133–48. New York: Oxford University Press, Inc.

Johnson, K. A., Jones, K. J., Becker, J. A., Satlin, A., Holman, B. L. & Albert, M. S. (1998). Preclinical prediction of Alzheimer's disease using SPECT. *Neurology*, **50**, 1563–71.

Kantarci, K., Jack, C. R. Jr., Xu, Y. C. *et al.* (2000). Regional metabolic patterns in mild cognitive impairment and Alzheimer's disease: a 1H MRS study. *Neurology*, **55**, 210–17.

Kaye, J. A., Oken, B. S., Howieson, D. B., Howieson, J., Holm, L. A. & Dennison, K. (1994). Neurologic evaluation of the optimally healthy oldest old. *Arch. Neurol.*, **51**, 1205–11.

Killiany, R. J., Gomez-Isla, T., Moss, M. *et al.* (2000). Use of structural magnetic resonance imaging to predict who will get Alzheimer's disease. *Ann. Neurol.*, **47**, 430–9.

Knopman, D. S. & Ryberg, S. (1989). A verbal memory test with high predictive accuracy for dementia of the Alzheimer type. *Arch. Neurol.*, **46**, 141–5.

Kokmen, E., Smith, G. E., Petersen, R. C., Tangalos, E. & Ivnik, R. J. (1991). The short test of mental status: Correlations with standardized psychometric testing. *Arch. Neurol.*, **48**, 725–8.

Kral, V. A. (1962). Senescent forgetfulness: benign and malignant. *Can. Med. Assoc. J.*, **86**, 257–60.

Machulda, M. M., Ward, H. A., Borowski, B. *et al.* (2003). Comparison of memory fMRI response among normal, MCI, and Alzheimer's patients. *Neurology*, **61**, 500–6.

Masur, D. M., Sliwinski, M., Lipton, R. B., Blau, A. D. & Crystal, H. A. (1994). Neuropsychological prediction of dementia and the absence of dementia in healthy elderly persons. *Neurology*, **44**, 1427–32.

Morris, J. C. (1993). The Clinical Dementia Rating (CDR): current version and scoring rules. *Neurology*, **43**, 2412–14.

Newman, S. K., Warrington, E. K., Kennedy, A. M. & Rossor, M. N. (1994). The earliest cognitive change in a person with familial Alzheimer's disease: presymptomatic neuropsychological features in a pedigree with familial Alzheimer's disease confirmed at necropsy. *J. Neurol. Neurosurg. Psychiatry*, **57**, 967–72.

Orgogozo, J. M., Gilman, S., Dartigues, J. F. *et al.* (2003). Subacute meningoencephalitis in a subset of patients with AD after Abeta42 immunization. *Neurology*, **61**, 46–54.

Petersen, R. C. (1995). Normal aging, mild cognitive impairment, and early Alzheimer's disease. *Neurologist*, **1**, 326–44.

(2002). Mild cognitive impairment. *Neurobiol. Aging*, **23**, S145.

(2003a). Mild cognitive impairment clinical trials. *Nat. Rev. Drug Discov.*, **2**, 646–53.

(2003b). Clinical evaluation. In *Mild Cognitive Impairment: Aging to Alzheimer's Disease*, ed. R. C. Petersen, pp. 229–42. New York: Oxford University Press, Inc.

Petersen, R. C. & Morris, J. C. (2003). Clinical features. In Petersen, R. C., ed. *Mild Cognitive Impairment: Aging to Alzheimer's Disease*, ed. R. C. Petersen, pp. 15–40. New York: Oxford University Press, Inc.

Petersen, R. C., Kokmen, E., Tangalos, E., Ivnik, R. J. & Kurland, L. T. (1990). Mayo Clinic Alzheimer's Disease, Patient Registry. *Aging*, **2**, 408–15.

Petersen, R. C., Smith, G. E., Ivnik, R. J., Kokmen, E. & Tangalos, E. G. (1994). Memory function in very early Alzheimer's disease. *Neurology*, **44**, 867–72.

Petersen, R. C., Smith, G. E., Waring, S. C., Ivnik, R. J., Tangalos, E. G. & Kokmen, E. (1999). Mild cognitive impairment: clinical characterization and outcome. *Arch. Neurol.*, **56**, 303–8.

Petersen, R. C., Stevens, J. C., Ganguli, M., Tangalos, E. G., Cummings, J. L. & DeKosky, S. T. (2001). Practice parameter: early detection of dementia: mild cognitive impairment (an evidence-based review). Report of the Quality Standards Subcommittee of the American Academy of Neurology. *Neurology*, **56**, 1133–42.

Petersen, R. C., Tang-Wai, D. F., Boeve, B. F. *et al.* (2003). Predictors of mild cognitive impairment. *Neurology*, **60**, A244.

Reisberg, B., Ferris, S., deLeon, M. J. & Crook, T. (1982). The Global Deterioration Scale for assessment of primary degenerative dementia. *Am. J. Psychiatry*, **139**, 1136–9.

Rogers, S. L., Farlow, M. D., Doody, R. S., Mohs, R. & Friedhoff, L. T. (1998). A 24-week, double-blind placebo-controlled trial of donepezil in patients with Alzheimer's disease. Donezepil Study Group. *Neurology*, **50**, 136–45.

Rowe, J. W. & Kahn, R. L. (1987). Human aging: usual and successful. *Science*, **237**, 143–9.

Sliwinski, M., Lipton, R. B., Buschke, H. & Stewart, W. (1996). The effect of pre-clinical dementia on estimates of normal cognitive function in aging. *J. Gerontol. Psychol. Sci.*, 51B, 217–25.

Smith, G. E., Ivnik, R. J., Malec, J. F., Petersen, R. C., Tangalos, E. G. & Kurland, L. T. (1992). Mayo's older Americans normative studies (MOANS): factors structure of a core battery. *Psychol. Assessm.: J. Cons. Clin. Psychology*, **4**, 382–90.

Solomon, P. R., Hirschoff, A., Kelly, B. *et al.* (1998). A 7 minute neurocognitive screening battery highly sensitive to Alzheimer's disease. *Arch. Neurol.*, **55**, 349–55.

Storandt, M. & Hill, R. D. (1989). Very mild senile dementia of the Alzheimer type. II. Psychometric test performance. *Arch. Neurol.*, **46**, 383–6.

Sunderland, T., Wolozin, G. & Galasko, D. (1990). Longitudinal stability of CSF tau levels in Alzheimer patients. *Biol. Psychiatry*, **46**, 750–5.

Tang-Wai, D. F., Knopman, D. S., Geda, Y. E., *et al.* (2003). A comparison of the short test of mental status and the mini-mental status examination in determining mild cognitive impairment. *Arch. Neurol.*, **60**, 1777–81.

Waring, S. C., Rocca, W. A., Petersen, R. C., O'Brien, P. C., Tangalos, E. G. & Kokmen, E. (1999). Postmenopausal estrogen replacement therapy and risk of AD: a population-based study. *Neurology*, **52**, 965–70.

Welsh, K., Butters, N., Hughes, J., Mohs, R. & Heyman, A. (1991). Detection of abnormal memory decline in mild cases of Alzheimer's disease using CERAD neuropsychological measures. *Arch. Neurol.*, **48**, 278–81.

Welsh, K., Butters, N., Hughes, J., Mohs, R. & Heyman, A. (1992). Detection and staging of dementia in Alzheimer's disease. Use of the neuropsychological measures developed for the Consortium to Establish a Registry for Alzheimer's Disease. *Arch. Neurol.*, **49**, 448–52.

Xu, Y. C., Jack, C. R., Jr., Petersen, R. C. *et al.* (2000). Usefulness of MRI measures of entorhinal cortex vs. hippocampus in AD. *Neurology*, **54**, 1760–7.

Yaffe, K., Sawaya, G., Liebergurg, I. & Grady, D. (1998). Estrogen therapy in postmenopausal women: effects on cognitive function and dementia. *J. Am. Med. Assoc.*, **279**, 688–95.

28

Alzheimer's disease – overview

David F. Tang-Wai,[1] Keith A. Josephs,[2]
and Ronald C. Petersen[2]

[1]Division of Neurology, University Health Network, Toronto Western Hospital, Canada, ON
[2]Department of Neurology, Mayo Clinic, Rochester MN, USA

Dementia

Dementia, itself, neither implies a specific disease nor implies a specific underlying pathology. It refers to a change in cognitive function that is severe enough to compromise an individual's daily function. The *Diagnostic and Statistical Manual of Mental Disorders*, fourth edition (DSM-IV) defines dementia as an acquired impairment of cognitive function that includes a decline in memory beyond what would be expected for age and at least one other cognitive function, such as attention, visuospatial skills or language, or a decline in executive functioning such as planning, organization, sequencing, or abstracting. The decline cannot only affect emotional abilities, but must also interfere with work or social activities. The deficits should not be accompanied by an impairment of arousal (delirium) or be accounted for by another psychiatric condition, such as depression or schizophrenia. Dementia can further be defined by a *possible*, *probable*, or *definite* etiologic diagnosis. A degenerative dementia implies disease progression over time.

While the DSM-IV criteria are generally useful, one problem with the criteria is that memory impairment is an essential feature. While this is common in most dementias, other dementias may present with impairment in a non-memory cognitive domain. If the initial presentation is a change in personality or behavior, rather than memory, a frontotemporal dementia may be the diagnosis. In subjects with parkinsonism, hallucinations and fluctuations in behavior, dementia with Lewy bodies may be more likely than AD. Vascular dementia can involve abrupt changes in function for large vessel or embolic disease or can present insidiously if subcortical ischemia is responsible for the changes in function. A prominent anomia with other features of language impairment can signal a primary progressive aphasia. A dementia evolving rapidly over weeks to months with psychiatric symptoms and motor function abnormalities suggests a prion disorder such as Creutzfeldt–Jakob disease.

First description/historical overview

The current understanding of AD evolved in three stages (Munoz & Feldman, 2002): (i) the initial description of AD, (ii) the association between the degree of pathology and disease severity, and (iii) the genetic and biochemical advances.

In 1907, Dr Alois Alzheimer published a report concerning "an usual illness of the cerebral cortex" (Stelzmann *et al.*, 1995). He described the case of a 51-year-old woman, Auguste D, who initially developed a delusional disorder but then developed a "rapid loss of memory." Postmortem examination of her brain revealed an atrophic brain without evidence for focal degeneration. Microscopically, he described neuronal cell loss and "only a tangle of fibrils [that] indicates the place where the neuron was previously located." In addition, "distributed all over the cortex . . . are minute military foci which are caused by the deposition of a special substance in the cortex" (Förstl & Levy, 1991; Stelzmann *et al.*, 1995; Klünemann *et al.*, 2002).

In the 1960s, Blessed and colleagues (Blessed *et al.*, 1968) reported the association between the number of senile plaque counts in sections of the cerebral cortex and decline in measures of intellectual functioning among the elderly. He also recognized that AD was the most common cause of dementia.

Recently, genetic advances further impacted on the current knowledge of AD. Mutations of the β-amyloid precursor protein on chromosome 21 and the *presenilin* genes 1 and 2 were associated with familial autosomal dominant AD (Sherrington *et al.*, 1995; Alzheimer's Disease

Collaborative Group, 1995; St George-Hyslop et al., 1996; Hardy & Gwinn-Hardy, 1998). The inheritance of the E4 allele of apolipoprotein E (ApoE) is considered as a risk factor for the late-onset inheritance and/or pathogenesis of AD (Corder et al., 1993). Furthermore, there may be other genetic contributors to AD such as chromosome 10 (Ertekin-Taner et al., 2000).

Epidemiology

AD is an age-related phenomenon and is the most common cause of dementia in the elderly, accounting for more than half of all cases (Small et al., 1997). It is estimated that there will be 360 000 incident cases of AD each year and is expected to rise over the subsequent 50 years to 1.14 million in 2047 (Brookmeyer et al., 1998). There is a greater prevalence of AD in women than in men (1.2–1.5: 1) reflecting the greater longevity of women (Evans et al., 1989; Kokmen et al., 1989; Bachman et al., 1992; Canadian Study of Health and Aging Working Group, 1994a; Hendrie et al., 1995; White et al., 1996; Hofman et al., 1997; Gao et al., 1998). Both the incidence and prevalence of AD increases dramatically with age and exponentially increases after the age of 65 (Kokmen et al., 1996; von Strauss et al., 1999; Kukull & Ganguli, 2000). It is estimated that the prevalence of dementia over the age of 65 years is 4% and 20% over the age of 85 years. It is rare below the age of 40 but can be seen and in such circumstances, consideration to a mutation in *presenilin-1* is entertained. It is uncertain as to whether the actual incidence of AD continues to rise into the 90s, but the incidence of dementia increases rapidly in that age range.

The combination of the facts that AD is an age-related disease and increasing numbers of individuals are living longer, has made this disease a common and important public-health problem. Some estimate that the present day cost of AD is $100 billion per year. (Small et al., 1997).

Risk factors for Alzheimer's disease

Increasing age is the most important risk factor of AD. Following age, the presence of the apolipoprotein E $\varepsilon 4$ (ApoE $\varepsilon 4$) allele is another major risk factor. There are 3 forms of ApoE alleles, $\varepsilon 2$, $\varepsilon 3$ and $\varepsilon 4$, but only the $\varepsilon 4$ allele increases the risk of both familial late-onset (Corder et al., 1993) and sporadic cases (Saunders et al., 1993) of AD, while $\varepsilon 2$ allele decreases risk (Corder et al., 1994). A similar pattern of age-related risk for decline associated with the $\varepsilon 4$ allele and the apparent protective effect of the $\varepsilon 2$ allele is observed in

African-Americans (Graff-Radford et al., 2002). The lifetime risk of AD in an individual without a family history is 9% without an Apo E $\varepsilon 4$; however, the lifetime risk increases to 29% if an individual is carrying at least 1 $\varepsilon 4$ allele (Seshadri et al., 1995).

Other putative risk factors of AD are implicated and include cardiovascular disease, traumatic brain injury, depression, lower educational achievement and/or occupational status, parental age at time of birth, smoking, first-degree relative with Down syndrome, low levels of folate and vitamin B12, and elevated plasma and total homocysteine levels (Mortimer, 1995; Clarke et al., 1998; Evans et al., 1997; Hofman et al., 1997; Fratiglioni et al., 1993; Guo et al., 2000; Launer et al., 1999; Seshadri et al., 2002; Green et al., 2003).

Putative protective factors include higher educational status, regular use of anti-inflammatory agents, use of cholesterol lowering agents (statins), estrogen replacement therapy in postmenopausal women, antihypertensive therapy, and diet of fish (Wolozin et al., 2000; in't Veld et al., 2001; Cummings & Cole, 2002; Qiu et al., 2003).

Currently, controversy exists with estrogen and progestin and subsequent development of AD. Prior long-term hormone replacement therapy use was associated with reduced risk of AD (Zandi et al., 2002). Recently, however, the Women's Health Initiative Memory Study revealed that estrogen and progestin therapy increased the risk of probable dementia in postmenopausal women aged 65 years or older and did not prevent mild cognitive impairment (MCI) (Shumaker et al., 2003). Included in the causes of probable dementia were vascular dementia, mixed-type dementia, normal pressure hydrocephalus, frontal lobe type, alcohol related, other/unknown, and AD. It is uncertain if estrogen and progestin have an effect on AD alone. This controversy will probably continue as additional studies will likely be published that examine the effects of estrogen or estrogen and progestin on AD and other dementias.

Clinical features

The clinical evolution of AD can be divided into three categories: (i) progressive memory impairment, (ii) progressive cortical dysfunction (aphasia, apraxia, visuospatial dysfunction) and (iii) neuropsychiatric disturbances. The typical clinical scenario of AD is the insidious onset and gradual progression of an amnestic memory disturbance with difficulties of learning and recall. In the initial stages of the disease, the memory impairment is for newly acquired information with relative sparing for remote events. The patient is typically unaware of memory or cognitive compromise (anosagnosia). Memory impairment alone, however, is not sufficient to make the diagnosis of dementia. NINCDS-ARDA criteria require that two or more other spheres of cognition be compromised, such as aphasia, apraxia and agnosia (McKhann *et al.*, 1984). The diagnosis of dementia is made on the basis of the fulfilment of clinical criteria, and as such constitutes a positive diagnosis rather than one of exclusion (Small *et al.*, 1997). The clinical–pathological correlation is actually quite high, in the 80–90% range (Galasko *et al.*, 1994; Gearing *et al.*, 1995).

As the disease evolves, patients will typically develop a progressive language disturbance beginning with anomia ("word finding difficulties") and progressing to a fluent aphasia. The patient may be unable to multitask or perform complex mental tracking tasks as other cognitive domains become impaired. This may be reported as diminished concentration, difficulty with mental arithmetic or tendency to become confused. Patients become less able to carry out the more demanding tasks of daily living, such as managing finances and driving, as disturbance of abstract reasoning, executive dysfunction (such as planning, insight and judgment), and disturbance of visuospatial skills (manifested by geographic or environmental disorientation and difficulty copying figures) evolve.

All cognitive deficits worsen over time. The patient will become progressively more dependent on the caregiver for feeding and hygiene. Plateaus can occur where cognitive impairment may not change for a period of 1 to 2 years, but resumption of progression does occur.

Neuropsychiatric symptoms are common in patients with AD (Chung & Cummings, 2000). There are four major groups of neuropsychiatric symptoms in AD: (i) mood disturbance, (ii) delusions and hallucinations, (iii) personality change, and (iv) disorders of behavior.

Personality change may be the first clinical change seen in AD and can be seen in at least 75% of patients. Most prominent is the apathy that appears early in the course with symptoms of diminished interests and concerns and may be associated with depression.

As the disease progresses, agitation and aggression may appear. Behavioral disturbance can be observed in 30–85% of patients and positively correlates with severity of dementia. Among all the neuropsychiatric symptoms, this may be the most difficult to manage. Patients may be both physically and verbally abusive, may wander, and may be incontinent of urine.

As dementia progresses, delusions, hallucinations and other psychotic behaviors may develop. Simple delusions of theft and suspicion are common, as are visual, auditory hallucinations. Misidentification of persons can also occur (for example, claiming one's spouse is an imposter) and incorrect identification of place is also reported.

Mood disorders can occur at any point throughout the illness, especially depression. Rates of depression can range from 25–30% with probable and possible AD to as high as 50% (Zubenko *et al.*, 2003). It is speculated that depression may be related to both structural and biochemical degenerative changes in the brain with neuronal loss in adrenergic, cholinergic and serotonergic systems (Tekin & Cummings 2001).

Motor abnormalities are absent in AD until the last few years of the disease. The presence of focal abnormalities, gait abnormalities, or seizures early in the clinical course makes AD unlikely.

Patients with AD usually survive 7 to 10 years (range 2–20 years) after the onset of symptoms. Average annual rate of reported decline on the MMSE is 4 to 5 points. Patients typically die from medical complications (bronchitis or pneumonia).

Clinical diagnosis

Clinical criteria of Alzheimer's disease

Diagnosis of AD can be made using criteria from either the National Institute of Neurologic, Communicative Disorders and Stroke/Alzheimer's Disease and Related Disorders Association (NINCDS-ADRDA) work group (Table 28.1) (McKhann *et al.*, 1984) or *Diagnostic and Statistical Manual*, Fourth Revision (DSM-IV). Assessment and diagnosis of AD require identifying the core clinical features and excluding other common causes of dementia. The American Academy of Neurology guidelines report that the DSM-IIIR and the NINCDS-ARDA criteria for the diagnosis of AD have sufficient reliability and validity and should be used (Knopman *et al.*, 2001).

History, bedside mental status examination, neurological examination

An essential element in establishing the diagnosis of dementia is obtaining the history from not only the patient themselves but also from someone who knows the patient quite well. Information to obtain in the history include a change and a decline in the level of a patient's ability to execute decisions, to plan (e.g. meals/recipes), to manage finances (e.g. payment of bills, balancing chequebook, payment of taxes), and to drive (e.g. getting lost while driving, new accidents or traffic tickets). Also pertinent is a history

Table 28.1. National Institute of Neurological and Communicative Disorders and Stroke and the Alzheimer's and Related Diseases Association (NINCDS-ARDA) Criteria

---

Clinical diagnosis of **probable** Alzheimer's disease
- Dementia established by clinical examination and mental status testing and confirmed by neuropsychological testing
- Deficits in at least two cognitive domains
- Progressive cognitive decline, including memory
- Normal level of consciousness
- Onset between ages 40 and 90 (most common after 65) years
- No other possible medical or neurological explanation

Probable Alzheimer's disease diagnosis supported by
- Progressive aphasia, apraxia, and agnosia
- Impaired activities of daily living
- Family history of similar disorder
- Brain atrophy on CT/MRI, especially if progressive
- Normal CSF, EEG

Other clinical features consistent with probable Alzheimer's disease
- Plateau in course
- Associated symptoms: depression, insomnia, incontinence, illusions, hallucinations, catastrophic verbal, emotional, or physical outbursts; sexual disorders; weight loss; during more advanced stages increased muscle tone, myoclonus, and abnormal gait
- Seizures in advance disease
- CT normal for age

Features that make Alzheimer's disease uncertain or unlikely
- Acute onset
- Focal sensorimotor signs
- Seizures or gait disorder early in course

Clinical diagnosis of **possible** Alzheimer's disease
- Dementia with atypical onset or course in the absence of another medical/neuropsychiatric explanation
- Dementia with another disease not felt otherwise to be the cause of dementia
- For research purposes, a progressive focal cognitive deficit

Definite Alzheimer's disease
- Meets clinical criteria for **probable** Alzheimer's disease
- Tissue confirmation (autopsy or brain biopsy)

Research classification of Alzheimer's disease should specifiy
- Familial?
- Early onset (before age 65))?
- Down's syndrome (trisomy 21)?
- Co-existent with other neurodegenerative disease?

McKhann, G. *et al.* (1984).

---

of the patient repeating himself. Although there are several instruments which can be used to obtain this information, one can inquire about the patient's ability and new onset difficulties to carry out typical activities of daily living.

In addition to the history, a cognitive assessment with an instrument designed for assessing mental function can be quite useful. Instruments designed for this purpose include the Mini-Mental State Examination (MMSE) (Folstein *et al.*, 1975), the modified Mini-Mental State (3MS) (Teng & Chui, 1987), the Blessed Orientation Memory Concentration Test (Katzman *et al.*, 1983) and the Short Test of Mental Status (Kokmen *et al.*, 1991). The structured interview provided by the Clinical Dementia Rating scale (CDR) (Morris, 1993) is helpful to further characterize the demented patient's ability in various domains of cognitive and functional performance. While these can be useful, none is superior to the others.

Individuals being evaluated for dementia should also have a general neurologic examination. Typically in early AD, this exam is largely normal with the exception of the mental status evaluation. However, in the course of the examination, other features suggesting other contributing factors to the dementia can be elucidated. For example, the findings of parkinsonism can suggest a Lewy body component or the presence of asymmetric reflexes or a visual field cut or other lateralizing signs can suggest a vascular component. Similarly, if there are other neurologic features such as a peripheral neuropathy, these may suggest toxic or metabolic problems. Assessment of sensory function is important since sensory deprivation can affect the mental status and neurologic examination. Finally, the neurologic examination should be complemented by a general medical examination looking for other systemic contributions to the cognitive impairment.

Laboratory evaluation

The utility of a variety of laboratory tests in evaluating a patient with dementia was assessed by the American Academy of Neurology practice parameter paper. Both vitamin B12 levels and thyroid functions should be assessed in cases of dementia since these are common co-morbidities that appear in the elderly. They can influence cognitive function and, while the treatment of these disorders may not completely reverse the dementia, their recognition and assessment are important. Screening for syphilis in patients with dementia is not justified unless there is a clinical suspicion for neurosyphilis. It is uncertain if routine screening for homocysteine is warranted at this time (Knopman *et al.*, 2001).

Table 28.2. Laboratory evaluation of patients with dementia

Routine	Optional
Chemistry group	Sedimentation rate
Complete blood count	Chest x-ray
Vitamin B$_{12}$ level*	Electrocardiogram
Thyroid function studies*	Urinalysis
Syphilis serology	Drug levels
CT/MRI*	HIV testing
	Lyme serology
	24hr -urine for heavy metal
	Electroencephalogram
	Cerebrospinal fluid
	PET/SPECT

* Suggested by the American Academy of Neurology.

It has been common practice, however, to assess a variety of tests to determine if there are other contributing factors. Table 28.2 lists suggested tests for a dementia evaluation. However, it should be emphasized once again that a few of these have been demonstrated to have an impact on improving the dementia; nevertheless, since other medical conditions can present with alterations in cognitive function, consideration to these tests can be given in the appropriate clinical setting.

Spinal fluid examination

There is little evidence to recommend the routine use of a lumbar puncture in the routine evaluation of elderly patients for dementia (Becker *et al.*, 1985). However, in the absence of contraindications, there may be certain clinical circumstances where spinal fluid examination is recommended. The clinician may suspect an alternative contributing process in dementias characterized by a sub-acute change in mental status, chronic encephalopathy, unusual clinical presentation, young onset (<65 years), the presence of fever and/or nuchal rigidity, systemic cancer, immunocompromised host or collagen vascular diseases. If spinal fluid examination is performed, in addition to routine tests such as total protein, glucose, cell count, cytology, and syphilis serology, consider cultures for bacteria, fungus and mycobacteria and immunological indices such as IgG index, IgG synthesis rate and oligoclonal bands. Positivity of any of the immunological indices would indicate inflammation and not AD. Opening pressure should also be recorded especially in patients with suspected communicating hydrocephalus.

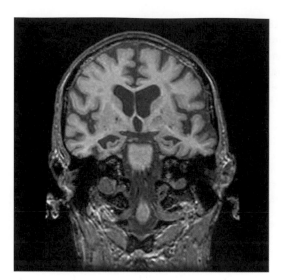

Fig. 28.1 Coronal T$_1$-weighted MRI image of the brain demonstrating hippocampal atrophy in a patient with clinically probable AD.

Other testing

Additional testing may be necessary in evaluating a patient with dementia and include EEG, overnight oximetry, psychiatric evaluation, small bowel biopsy, and paraneoplastic serologies. EEG abnormalities can be seen in toxic, metabolic, inflammatory, infectious and neoplastic encephalopathies. Overnight oximetry is a useful screening test for obstructive sleep apnea where patients may present with hypersomnolence, inattentiveness and mild memory impairment. Depression is common among individuals with coexistent cognitive impairment and should be screened (Knopman *et al.*, 2001). Psychiatric evaluation should be considered if depression is suspected or if psychotic symptoms complicate the clinical picture. If CNS Whipple's disease is suspected, small bowel biopsy should be considered.

Neuroimaging

Structural neuroimaging with either a non-contrast computer tomography (CT) or magnetic resonance imaging (MRI) scan is recommended in the routine evaluation of patients with dementia and can be useful in excluding reversible and treatable causes of dementias (Knopman *et al.*, 2001). Findings of subdural hematomas, neoplasms, infarct prior traumatic encephalomalacia, relevant focal atrophy and meningeal enhancement would lend a diagnosis other than AD. Bilateral atrophy of medial temporal lobe structures, such as the hippocampus, has been found in patients with AD (Fig. 28.1) (Jack *et al.*, 1997; Fox *et al.*, 2001). However, this atrophy may be non-specific and may be seen in other conditions but is certainly consistent with AD and is a fairly sensitive marker of the pathologic AD stage and consequent cognitive status (Fox *et al.*, 1999; Jack *et al.*, 2002). Recent data on longitudinal volumetric measurements of the hippocampal formation have also indicated that the rate of progression of atrophy of persons with AD exceeds that of normal controls (Jack *et al.*, 1999) and may precede the clinical symptoms of cognitive decline (Fox *et al.*, 1996). Investigations assessing the utility of volumetric measurements of the entorhinal cortex have been controversial (Killiany *et al.*, 2000; Xu *et al.*, 2000). Some investigators feel that the entorhinal cortex is superior in assessing early changes in the AD process, while others have found that the hippocampus and entorhinal cortex are equally efficacious (Xu *et al.*, 2000). Nevertheless, a structural imaging test of the brain should be done early in the assessment of persons with suspected AD.

Functional imaging with either single photon emission computed tomography (SPECT) or positron emission tomography (PET) typically reveal bilateral temporoparietal and posterior cingulate hypoperfusion and hypometabolism in AD. Several of SPECT studies have been suggestive of functional imaging's value in augmenting the clinician's acumen in the diagnosis of AD and may also correlate with Braak pathological stage (Van Gool *et al.*, 1995; Clauss *et al.*, 1994; Johnson *et al.*, 1990, 1993; Bartenstein *et al.*, 1997; Jagust *et al.*, 2001; Bradley *et al.*, 2002). Yet, based on Class II studies, the sensitivity of SPECT was lower than that of the clinical diagnosis (Knopman *et al.*, 2001). PET scanning has shown promise in its ability to differentiate among dementias and there is some evidence to indicate that FDG-PET may be useful in assessing the people who are at risk for developing AD but the longitudinal outcome of these persons is not yet known. One additional functional imaging modality to consider in the future is the use of functional MRI to discriminate normal subjects from those with either the prodromal stages of AD or MCI (Machulda *et al.*, 2003).

Functional imaging tests may also be particularly useful in the differential diagnosis of dementia. In particular, the ability of SPECT and PET to differentiate frontotemporal dementia from AD can be useful with the frontotemporal dementia subjects showing predominant hypoperfusion and hypometabolism in the frontal lobes with relative sparing of posterior structures.

While functional imaging tests are intriguing and show great potential, at present, the American Academy of Neurology practice parameter paper indicated that neither SPECT nor PET were recommended for routine use in the initial or differential diagnosis of dementias (Knopman *et al.*, 2001).

Neuropsychological testing

Neuropsychological testing can be particularly useful in evaluating cognitive function in a suspected dementia and can also be useful in providing a baseline for a subject who might be re-evaluated at some point in the future. Neuropsychological testing can help determine if the subject is experiencing cognitive changes of normal aging, MCI, or the earliest signs of AD. The particular profile of cognitive function can also be useful in differential diagnosis. While not diagnostic, the various clinical profiles can be useful to the clinician in helping to distinguish among various dementias.

Neuropsychological findings of AD mirror what one sees clinically. In the typical early stages, there is difficulty remembering or rapidly forgetting word lists, stories, designs after a delay, and possibly naming (which may be clinically elicited with word-finding difficulties). As the disease progresses from mesial temporal lobe to surrounding association areas, cognitive impairment becomes more widespread with decline in other areas of higher cortical function (Kramer & Miller, 2000). Visuospatial skills deteriorate and they may have impairment with copying designs. Reasoning becomes more concrete with impairment of novel-problem solving or abstract thinking. Problems with executive functioning becomes evident as patients lose inhibition abilities and the capacity to coordinate simultaneously storage and processing of information. Impairment of remote memory emerges with relative preservation of oldest memories. In severe stages, patients become apraxic, agnostic and aphasic (Kramer & Miller, 2000).

Pathogenesis/mechanisms of disease

Pathogenesis of AD can be subdivided into several interacting mechanisms: (i) aging influences, (ii) environmental influences (including inflammation, toxic exposures, infection, homocysteine), (iii) genetic influences (amyloid precursor protein, apolipoprotein E, presenilins), (iv) cerebral infarcts, (v) microscopic structural changes. There is no single mechanism that causes AD but rather it is the relative contributions of each component known this far that influences an individual to develop the symptoms of AD.

The major pathological findings in AD are generalized cerebral atrophy (Fig. 28.2) and widespread cortical

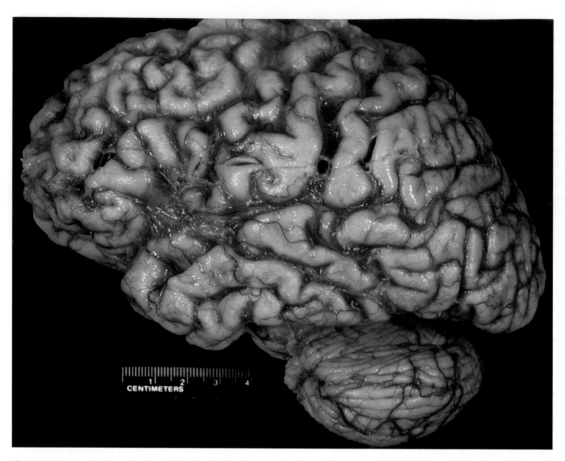

Fig. 28.2 Generalized cerebral cortical atrophy in Alzheimer's disease (Courtesy of D. W. Dickson M. D., Mayo Clinic, Jacksonville FL.)

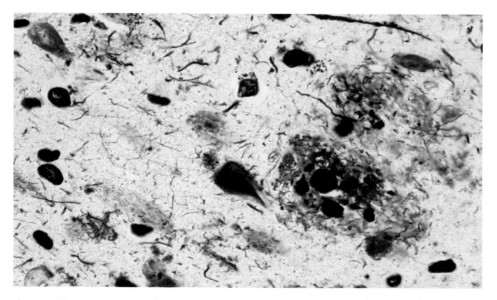

Fig. 28.3 Photomicrograph demonstrating a neuritic plaque composed of amyloid core surrounded by dystrophic neurites and dense flame-shaped neurofibillary tangles in the entorhinal cortex in Alzheimer's disease. Bielschowsky silver stain; 200X. (Courtesy D. W. Dickson M. D., Mayo Clinic, Jacksonville FL.)

neuritic amyloid plaques and neurofibrillary tangles (Fig. 28.3). Other neuropathological findings include neuropil threads, granuovacuolar degeneration, lipochrome accumulation, and Hirano bodies.

A major theory in the pathogenesis of AD is all or in part due to abnormal processing or deposition of amyloid (Selkoe, 2000). Aβ40 and Aβ42 are derived from differential proteolytic cleavage of the amyloid precursor protein (βAPP), a transmembrane protein with an extracellular amino terminal and intracellular carboxyl terminus. After initial cleavage of βAPP by β-secretase at amino acid 671, γ-secretase can cleave at either amino acid 711 or 713 resulting in the formation of Aβ42 and Aβ40, respectively. Although both species are detected in plasma and CSF, it is the Aβ40 which is found more often with a small component being Aβ42. However, it is the lesser common species, Aβ42, that is important in the pathogenesis of AD in that in vitro fibrils composed of Aβ42 form more rapidly than those composed on Aβ40, and Aβ42 may be deposited earlier in the genesis of an insoluble senile plaque. This deposition presumably initiates a cascade of events which result in inflammatory responses and cell destruction. While this may not be the only pathologic process, it is believed to be an important component of the degenerative cascade.

The other primary pathologic feature of AD involves the abnormal processing of tau and neurofibrillary tangle formation. Tau is an axonal phosphoprotein important for the binding and stabilization of microtubules (Spillantini & Goedert, 1998; Lee et al., 2001). Alternative splicing of the tau mRNA, from the *tau* gene on chromosome 17q21.2, produces six isoforms in the central nervous system with either 3 tandem repeat sequences (3-repeat or 3R-tau) or with 4 tandem-repeat sequences (4-repeat or 4R-tau) (van Slegtenhorst et al., 2000). The tandem repeat sequences represent key microtubule-binding sites. It is through both alternative splicing and degree of phosphorylation of tau that regulates its binding to microtubules. Neurodegeneration and pathology occur when one or both of these mechanisms are disrupted, either through mutations or other mechanisms, resulting in abnormal tau aggregation. In AD, neurofibrillary tangles are composed of paired helical filaments which, in turn, have been found to be mainly composed of hyperphosphorylated tau (Lee *et al.*, 2001). In other disorders, the normal 1:1 ratio of 3R- and 4R-tau in the human adult brain is disrupted, producing other neurodegenerative disorders, such as corticobasal degeneration, progressive supranuclear palsy and argyrophilic grain disease where the predominant form of is 4R tau (Dickson, 1999).

Biomarkers

An AD biomarker would provide clinicians increased accuracy of diagnosis of the disorder, identify those individuals at risk in the hopes of employing early therapy, and to determine if treatment is effective. A working group on biological markers for AD described the features of an ideal biomarker (The Ronald and Nancy Reagan Research Institute of the Alzheimer's Association and National Institute on Aging Working of Group, 1998):

- to be able to detect a fundamental feature of Alzheimer's neuropathology
- to be validated in neuropathologically confirmed cases
- to be able to detect AD early in its course and distinguish it from other dementias
- to be reliable
- to be non-invasive
- to be simple to perform
- to be inexpensive.

Several biomarkers have been investigated thus far and include CSF tau, plasma and CSF Aβ levels, platelet APP isoforms, and neuronal thread protein.

CSF Aβ and tau

Several studies have shown that CSF levels of Aβ42 are reduced in AD relative to normal control subjects (Andreasen *et al.*, 1999a; Galasko *et al.*, 1998; Hulstaert *et al.*, 1999; Shoji *et al.*, 1998), but it is unclear whether these levels are useful in the very early diagnosis. Similarly, CSF tau levels have been shown to be elevated in AD relative to controls (Arai *et al.*, 1997; Galasko *et al.*, 1997; Kurz *et al.*, 1998; Andreasen *et al.*, 1999b). The simultaneous measurement of CSF Aβ42 and tau may be a useful diagnostic marker, and studies have indicated sensitivities and specificities of 85 and 87%, respectively. However, it is not known if these biomarkers augment the diagnostic accuracy of the clinician.

Amyloid precursor protein isoforms in platelets

The βAPP can also be found in peripheral tissues, including platelets. Three major APP isoforms are present in membranes of resting platelets (Bush *et al.*, 1990) and patients with AD show specific alteration of levels of these platelet APP isoforms. Measurement of the ratio of the isoforms have been shown (i) to differentiate AD from normal controls and non-AD dementias (Di Luca *et al.*, 1998), (ii) to correlate with decline in cognition in AD and thus may be a biological index of the severity of cognitive loss in AD (Baskin *et al.*, 2000) and (iii) to change with administration of cholinesterase inhibitors, such as donepezil, suggesting it may be a marker for pharmacological activity (Padovani *et al.*, 2001; Borroni *et al.*, 2001). While a promising biomarker, it also has some drawbacks. Patients on medication that affects platelet function, such anticholinergic, antiplatelet agents, serotoninergic medications, anticoagulants and steroids, need to be off the medication for at least 2 weeks. Drawing the blood for harvesting platelets is complicated. Nonetheless, this test is certainly worthy of further study.

Neuronal thread protein (NTP)

The neural thread proteins are a family of proteins that is normally expressed in the brain and, especially, brains of AD patients (de la Monte & Wands 1992). Increased levels of NTP were found in advanced AD cases and correlated with progression of dementia (de la Monte *et al.*, 1992, 1997). NTP can be measured in both spinal fluid and urine and is higher in AD patients than controls (de la Monte *et al.*, 1992; Ghanbari *et al.*, 1998). Furthermore, NTP may distinguish individuals without dementia from those with AD and non-AD pathology (Kahle *et al.*, 2000).

AAN guidelines on biomarkers

Although promising, the American Academy of Neurology states that no biomarkers have emerged as being appropriate for routine use in the clinical evaluation of patients with suspected AD. While several of the approaches mentioned above including quantitative neuroimaging, genotyping and biomarkers are being actively investigated, at this point, none has achieved sufficient stature that it replaces or significantly augments the ability of the clinician to use the standard DSM IV or NINCDS/ADRDA criteria to diagnose AD (Knopman *et al.*, 2001).

Clinical variants of Alzheimer's disease

The typical presentation of AD is impairment of anterograde episodic memory. However, AD can present as a focal degenerative disease (Caselli 1995). In addition to the focal amnestic form, three other focal patterns of presentation have been described: (i) progressive aphasia, (ii) progressive visual dysfunction, and (iii) progressive biaparietal/apraxic motor dysfunction. Variants of AD can be clinically similar and have overlap among other neurodegenerative diseases, such as corticobasal degeneration and frontotemporal dementia. Yet despite the varied presentations, the pathology can reveal findings of typical AD (Galton *et al.*, 2000). It is the distribution of the AD pathology that dictates the clinical syndrome and not the disease itself (Galton *et al.*, 2000; Tang-Wai *et al.*, 2003a,b). Understanding the progression of typical AD from the initial amnestic syndrome to latter involvement of visual, language, executive impairment, praxis, it is not surprising that the disease can present with one of those impairments and yet can still be AD. AD should be clinically considered in any focal cortical syndrome.

Progressive aphasia

Although pathologies of progressive aphasia syndromes either reveals dementia lacking distinctive histology or Pick's disease, there are postmortem cases of AD. AD presenting as a focal language disturbance can be either a fluent or non-fluent syndrome. Non-fluent forms can mimic the clinical presentation of primary progressive aphasia (PPA) and can fulfil the diagnostic criteria of PPA (Mesulam, 1982, 2001). Over time, there is a general cognitive decline with progressive memory and visuospatial impairment. Fluent forms can mimic the clinical presentation of semantic dementia, however, they would not have met diagnostic criteria as there is typically evidence for additional impairments in episodic and working memory and deficits in visuospatial functioning (Hodges *et al.*, 1992; Garrard & Hodges, 2000). As the disease progresses, the patient becomes mute and memory becomes impaired. Neuroimaging typically reveals left temporal or more general asymmetric left hemisphere atrophy. Functional imaging mirrors the structural findings with temporal hypoperfusion. Pathologically, there is widespread involvement of plaques and tangles in the temporal lobe (Galton *et al.*, 2000).

Progressive visual disturbance

Posterior cortical atrophy (PCA) or the "visual variant" of AD is a clinical syndrome of visual agnosia, some or all of the components of Balint's syndrome, transcortical sensory aphasia, and Gerstmann's syndrome (Benson *et al.*, 1988). There have been other terms used to describe this syndrome, including the "visual variant of AD" (Levine *et al.*, 1993) and asymmetric cortical degeneration syndrome of the visuoperceptual subtype (Caselli, 1995). The syndrome is dictated by the prominent dysfunction of biparietal and occipital cortices. By the time PCA has run its course, many patients develop dementia more typical of

Alzheimer's disease. Neither ApoE allele nor *Tau* halplotype frequencies differ between PCA and AD (Tang-Wai *et al.*, 2003c). Although pathologically heterogeneous, several postmortem studies on PCA have shown AD pathology. The greatest involvement of plaques and tangles have been found in the primary and visual association cortices in the occipital lobes with lesser involvement in the parietal lobes (Hof *et al.*, 1997). Other documented neuropathologic findings of PCA include non-specific degenerative changes, with gliosis, neuronal loss, and vacuolation of superficial cortical layers, Creutzfeldt–Jakob disease (CJD) (Victoroff *et al.*, 1994), and corticobasal degeneration (Tang-Wai *et al.*, 2003b).

Progressive apraxic syndrome

Ross Mackenzie *et al.* (1996) published a case of a man with progressive difficulties performing manual tasks and an inability to write. Memory was initially preserved; however, over time he progressed from the initial biparietal syndrome to a more global dementia. MRI revealed left parietal and temporal atrophy while SPECT revealed biparietal hypoperfusion. Neuropathology revealed changes of AD affecting predominantly the superior parietal lobes. Predominant left focal anterior parietal dysfunction can lead to symptoms of ideomotor apraxia. Although apraxia is commonly seen in advanced stages of AD, it can be a presenting feature of the disease and can cause confusion with corticobasal degeneration (Boeve *et al.*, 1999). Unlike AD, corticobasal degeneration commonly presents with asymmetric parkinsonism, ideomotor apraxia and alien limb phenomenon with less severe memory deficits. Although the presence of a significant memory disturbance may differentiate AD from CBD or other neurodegenerative cases, this is not always the case.

Treatments of Alzheimer's disease

The strategies of pharmacological treatment of AD are (i) disease prevention, (ii) symptomatic treatment, and (iii) disease modification. Currently, only two types of treatment of AD are in use: disease modifying, with the use of antioxidants, and symptomatic treatment with anticholinesterase inhibitors (AChEI) (Table 28.3). Although other potential medications, such as cholesterol lowering agents, memantine and non-steroidal anti-inflammatory drugs, have shown an association to slow or delay the onset of AD, randomized blinded drugs trials are currently under way to evaluate their efficacy. Estrogen replacement therapy has not been shown to slow disease progression or improve cognitive function in women (Henderson *et al.*, 2000; Mulnard *et al.*, 2000).

Symptomatic treatment: *acetylcholinesterase inhibitors*

Acetylcholine is involved in many aspects of cognition, including memory and attention. The use of anticholinergic medications, however, can produce learning and recall deficit that is similar to the cognitive changes seen in AD (Petersen, 1977). Patients with AD have a cholinergic deficit due to reduction of choline acetyltransferase, the synthetic enzyme for acetylcholine (Bowen *et al.*, 1976; Davies & Maloney, 1976) and deposition of plaques and tangles causing damage and loss of cholinergic neurons in the basal forebrain (Whitehouse *et al.*, 1981, 1982). Based on these findings, there has been a longstanding effort to try to augment cholinergic functioning in the brains of patients with AD. By administering an AChEI, the acetylcholine increases and memory improves. Currently, the only approved Food and Drug Administration (FDA) medication for the treatment of clinically probable AD are AChEIs, tacrine, donepezil, rivastigmine, and galantamine. All of the AChEI have similar clinical profiles and have been shown in careful, double-blind, placebo-controlled studies to significantly improve memory in AD patients.

Tacrine (Cognex) was the first approved compound for the symptomatic treatment of AD. Although helpful, it was cumbersome to use with four times a day dosing and liver toxicity, necessitating regular monitoring of liver functions. Tacrine is rarely used for the treatment of AD currently as newer drugs without these limiting features have been introduced.

Donepezil (Aricept) was the next AChEI approved by the FDA in the mid-1990s. Its single daily dose and no laboratory monitoring requirement provide advantages over tacrine. The typical starting dose is 5 mg per day and if well tolerated in 4 to 6 weeks, the dose is increased to 10 mg per day. There have been several studies on the efficacy of donepezil and most show a modest improvement in cognitive function as measured by scales such as the Alzheimer's Disease Assessment Scale–Cognitive Subscale (ADAS–Cog) and the Clinician's Interview-Based Impression of Change (CIBIC Plus) (Rogers *et al.*, 1998; Doody *et al.*, 2001). The drug has been approved for mild to moderate AD and the length of the response has been documented up to 52 weeks. However, studies have indicated that, when donepezil is discontinued, performance of the subject returns to the same as in the untreated state. Furthermore, when used for 1 year, patients on donepezil revealed continued progression of the disease but it was

Table 28.3. Pharmacological treatment of Alzheimer's disease

Drug	Mechanism	Initial dose	Target dose	Titration interval	Side effects
Tacrine (Cognex)	AChEI	10 mg QID	40 mg QID	4 wks	Liver function test evaluations, diarrhea, anorexia, nausea, vomiting, myalgia
Donepezil (Aricept)	AChEI	5 mg QD	10 mg QD	4–6 wks	Nausea, vomiting, diarrhea, muscle cramps, anorexia, vivid dreaming
Rivastigmine (Exelon)	AChEI	1.5 mg BID	6 mg BID	2–4 wks	Nausea, vomiting, diarrhea, weight loss, dizziness
Galantamine (Reminyl)	AChEI	4 mg BID	12 mg BID	4–6 wks	Nausea, vomiting, diarrhea, anorexia, dizziness
Vitamin E	Antioxidant	1000 IU QD	1000 IU BID	2–4 wks	Liver function, hemorrhage
Memantine*	NMDA receptor antagonist	5 mg QD	10 mg BID or 20 mg QD	2–4 wks	Agitation, urinary incontinence, urinary tract infection, nausea, diarrhea, insomnia, tachycardia

* Not FDA approved.

associated with a reduction in the risk of functional decline compared to placebo (Mohs *et al.*, 2001). These indicate that donepezil has a symptomatic effect on the disease but does not affect the underlying pathophysiologic process.

The other AChEIs, rivastigmine (Exelon) and galatamine (Reminyl) have been approved by the FDA as well (Rosler *et al.*, 1999; Tariot *et al.*, 2000). While galantamine is a reversible inhibitor of acetyl cholinesterase, rivastigmine is pseudo-irreversible as it dissociates from the enzyme slowly. Unique biochemical features to either AchEI are that rivastgimine is also an inhibitor of butyrylcholinesterase and galantamine has some nicotinic receptor activity. These features are proposed to provide additional benefits of one AChEI over another. Both rivastigmine and galantamine are dosed twice daily and have similar dosing schemes. The dosing of rivastigmine begins with 1.5 mg twice a day and increases in increments of 1.5 mg per dose to a maximum of 6 mg twice daily. The starting dose of galantamine is 4 mg twice daily and increases in increments of 4 mg per dose twice a day to a maximum of 12 mg twice daily if tolerated. Dose escalation of either medication should be done on a 4-week basis to minimize side effects. Both of these medications afford greater dosing flexibility but may be somewhat more difficult for the patients because of the twice daily dosing schedule. Although they may provide greater cholinesterase inhibition at the highest dose, they are also prone to have an increased frequency of side effects. The effect size of either rivastigmine or galatamine on the ADAS–Cog and the CIBIC Plus is approximately the same as donepezil (Doody *et al.*, 2001).

All AChEI have a similar side effect profile including increase in bowel frequency, nausea and vomiting. Theoretically, all AChEI can influence cardiac rhythm but this is not commonly encountered unless a person has an underlying disturbance in cardiac conduction. An electrocardiogram prior to initiating an AChEI may be recommended. Cholinesterase inhibitors may also have an effect on respiratory conditions, such as chronic obstructive pulmonary disease or asthma, or gastrointestinal diseases, such as gastic ulcer. Occasionally, patients experience vivid dreaming and cholinesterase inhibitors can theoretically interfere with the administration of anesthesia during surgery. The absorption of AChEI is not influenced by food intake.

There have been few studies in which these drugs have been compared to each other so there is little to recommend one over the other. While the effects are modest, they do appear to enhance the cognitive function in subjects with AD and are recommended for the treatment for patients with mild to moderate AD (Doody *et al.*, 2001).

Disease modifying

Selegiline and alpha-tocopherol (vitamin E)

In a two-year double-blind study, 341 moderately severe AD patients (average MMSE of 12) participated in a placebo-controlled study comparing placebo with 2000 IU of alpha-tocopherol, 10 mg of selegiline and both medications (Sano *et al.*, 1997). In each of the three treatment groups compared to the placebo group, there was a significant delay in reaching the primary endpoints of death, institutionalization, loss of basic activities of daily living, or severe dementia, defined as progression from CDR-2 to CDR-3. However, the results for selegiline were less convincing and with its potential toxicities and drug interactions, large dose of vitamin E was recommend in AD patients. Long-term side effects of large doses of vitamin E are still unknown but it is generally well tolerated. However, in a recent study, small doses (50 mg) of vitamin E in almost 30 000 Finnish men, decreased heart attacks, strokes and prostate cancer but increased cerebral hemorrhage (The Alpha-Tocopherol Beta Carofene Cancer Prevention Study Group 1994). Vitamin E thus has anticoagulant properties and interacts with warfarin. The American Academy of Neurology has indicated that vitamin E, 1000 IU p.o. b.i.d. can be considered in an attempt to slow the progression of AD (Doody et al., 2001). The risk to benefit ratio for selegiline was felt to be less favorable.

Memantine

The glutamatergic hypothesis of dementia forms the rationale in the use of memantine, a non-competitive N-methyl-D-aspartate (NMDA) antagonist, in the treatment of AD (Müller et al., 1995). The basis for the glutamatergic hypothesis of dementia is based on the following facts (i) glutamate is the main fast excitatory neurotransmitter in regions associated with cognition and memory (the cerebral cortex and hippocampus); (ii) cortical and subcortical structures that contain glutamatergic receptors are structurally damaged during the course of AD; (iii) glutamate acts as an excitotoxin causing neuronal death when excessive levels are chronically released; (iv) the neurochemical changes and some of the clinical symptoms seen can be induced experimentally with potent glutamate agonists; and (v) clinical signs of dementia correlate with deficits of glutaminergic association fibers (Winblad & Poritis, 1999). Memantine blocks NMDA receptor channels in the resting state and can leave the channel upon physiological activation during memory formation but does not leave under pathological activation (Winblad & Poritis, 1999). Memantine treatment of 10 mg per day has been shown in a few double-blind, placebo-controlled trials to maintain or improve functional level in patients with severe dementia (Winblad & Poritis, 1999; Reisberg et al., 2003). Side effects of memantine were comparable to placebo. The most frequent side effects included vertigo, restlessness, hyperexcitation and fatigue.

Secretases and immunotherapy

Since the role of beta amyloid (Aβ) is considered to be paramount in the development of AD, several research strategies have been undertaken to alter the biochemistry of Aβ in the brain through interference of either the forma-tion or the deposition of Aβ. Beta amyloid is processed by several proteases to various non-amylogenic (α-secretase) and amylogenic pathways (β-secretase and γ-secretase) (Selkoe, 2000). Consequently, strategies have been developed in an attempt to inhibit the activities of both β-secretase and γ-secretase (Hussain et al., 1999; Sinha et al., 1999; Vassar et al., 1999; Yan et al., 1999) and thus inhibit the formation of Aβ. The β-secretase enzyme termed BACE is one target and γ-secretase is another. Clinical trials are being designed to assess the viability of these approaches, but currently no data are available.

Another therapeutic approach involves immunization therapy. When transgenic mice over-expressing a human mutant form of APP and demonstrating many of the pathologic features of AD were actively immunized against Aβ at birth, they demonstrated significantly reduced Aβ plaque formation later in life (Schenk et al., 1999). In addition, mice immunized in mid-life showed a reduction in further progression of the disease with a suggestion of regression of the underlying pathology.

Recently, a double-blind Phase II clinical trial was initiated testing the active immunization therapy approach in humans with mild to moderate AD. Despite the initial Phase I human safety trials revealing minimal side effects (Schenk, 2002), the trial was discontinued early due to development of postvaccination subacute meningoencephalitis in 18 of the 298 patients who received the active vaccine 3 to 6 months after their last injection (Senior, 2002; Orgogozo et al., 2003). The development and severity of the aseptic meningoencephalitis did not correlate with levels of antibody titres. Postmortem examination of a brain from one patient who received the active vaccine in the Phase I trial revealed widespread T-lymphocyte meningoencephalitis but, when compared to unimmunized cases of AD, there were extensive areas of neocortex with very few Aβ plaques (Nicoll et al., 2003). In areas of the cortex devoid of Aβ plaques, there were densities of tangles, neuropil threads and cerebral amyloid angiopathy similar to unimmunized AD, but lacking plaque-associated dystrophic neurites and astrocyte clusters; and in some regions, Aβ-immunoreactivity was associated with microglia (Nicoll et al., 2003). Although this postmortem case may have had an unusual pattern of AD pathology, the authors also report that these findings were similar to the murine models of Aβ immunotherapy and suggest an immune response was generated and elicited clearance of Aβ plaques in this patient (Nicoll et al., 2003).

Passive immunization can be another approach, as passively immunized mice also revealed reversal of memory deficits but not brain Aβ burden (Dodart et al., 2002) but with increased cerebral hemorrhages (Pfiefer et al.,

2002). Immunotherapy may remain a potential therapeutic option; however, there are concerns related to this approach and the potential side effects from the chronic immunization against Aβ in humans.

Conclusions

AD is a common disorder of aging and can be reliably diagnosed clinically. Since Alois Alzheimer's initial description of the disease, research on diagnosis, etiology and treatments is advancing. Although the clinical description will unlikely change, our understanding of this disorder will likely expand and change as various theories and observations continue to evolve.

REFERENCES

Alzheimer's Disease Collaborative Group (1995). The structure of the presenilin 1 (S1282) gene and identification of six novel mutations in early onset AD families. *Nat. Genet.*, **11**, 219–22.

American Psychiatric Association (1994). *Diagnostic and Statistical Manual of Mental Disorders*, 4th ed. Washington, DC: American Psychiatric Association.

Andreasen, N., Hesse, C., Davidsson, P. *et al.* (1999a). Cerebrospinal fluid beta-amyloid(1–42) in Alzheimer disease: differences between early- and late-onset Alzheimer disease and stability during the course of disease. *Arch. Neurol.*, **56**, 673–80.

Andeasen, N., Minthon, L., Clarberg, A. *et al.* (1999b). Sensitivity, specificity, and stability of CSF-tau in AD in a community-based patient sample. *Neurology*, **53**, 1488–94.

Arai, H., Higuchi, S. & Saskai, H. (1997). Apolipoprotein E genotyping and cerebrospinal fluid tau protein: implications for the clinical diagnosis of Alzheimer's disease. *Gerontology*, **43** (**suppl 1**), 2–10.

Bachman, D. L. , Wolf, P. A. , Linn, R. *et al.* (1992). Prevalence of dementia and probable senile dementia of the Alzheimer type in the Framingham Study. *Neurology*, **42**, 115–19.

Bartenstein, P., Minoshima, S., Hirsch, C. *et al.* (1997). Quantitative assessment of cerebral blood flow in patients with Alzheimer's disease by SPECT. *J. Nucl. Med.*, **38**, 1095–101.

Baskin, F., Rosenberg, R. N., Iyler, L., Hynan, L. & Cullum, C. M. (2000). Platelet APP isoform ratios correlate with declining cognition in AD. *Neurology*, **54** (10), 1907–9.

Becker, P. M., Feussner, J. R., Mulrow, C. D., Williams, B. C. & Vokaty, K. A. (1985). The role of lumbar puncture in the evaluation of dementia: the Durham Veterans Administration/Duke University Study. *J. Am. Geriat. Soc.*, **33**, 392–6.

Benson, D. F., Davis, R. J. & Snyder, B. D. (1988). Posterior cortical atrophy. *Arch. Neurol.*, **45** (7), 789–93.

Blessed, G., Tomlinson, B. E. & Roth, M. (1968). The association between quantitative measures of dementia and of senile changes in the cerebral gray matter of elderly subjects. *Br. J. Psychiat.*, **114**, 797–811.

Boeve, B. F., Maraganore, D. M., Parisi, J. E. *et al.* (1999). Pathologic heterogeneity in clinically diagnosed corticobasal degeneration. *Neurology*, **53**, 795–800.

Borroni, B., Colciaghi, F., Pastorino, L. *et al.* (2001). Amyloid precursor protein in platelets of patients with Alzheimer's disease: effect of acetylcholinerase inhibitor treatment. *Arch. Neurol.*, **58**, 442–6.

Bowen, D. M., Smith, C. B., White, P. & Davison, A. N. (1976). Neurotransmitter-related enzymes and indices of hypoxia in senile dementia and other abiotrophies. *Brain*, **99**, 459–96.

Bradley, K. M., O'Sullivan, V. T., Soper, N. D. W. *et al.* (2002). Cerebral perfusion SPEC T correlated with Braak pathological stage in Alzheimer's disease. *Brain*, 2002; **125**, 1772–81.

Brookmeyer, R., Gray, S. & Kawas, C. (1998). Projections of Alzheimer's disease in the United States and the public health impact of delaying disease onset. *Am. J. Public Hlth*, **88**, 1337–42.

Bush, A. I., Martins, R. N., Rumble, B. *et al.* (1990). The amyloid precursor protein of Alzheimer's disease is released by human platelets. *J. Biol. Chem.*, **265** (26), 15977–83.

Canadian Study of Health and Aging (1994). Study methods and prevalence of dementia. *Can. Med. Assoc. J.*, **150**, 899–913.

Caselli, R. J. (1995). Focal and asymmetric cortical degeneration syndromes. *The Neurologist*, **1** (1), 1–19.

Chung, J. A. & Cummings J. L. (2000). Neurobehavioral and neuropsychiatric symptoms in Alzheimer's disease: characteristics and treatment. *Neurologic Clinics*, **18** (4), 829–46.

Clarke, R., Smith, A. D., Jobst, K. A., Refsum, H., Sutton, L. & Ueland, P. M. (1998). Folate, vitamin B12, and total homocyteine levels in confirmed Alzheimer's disease. *Arch. Neurol.*, **55**, 1449–55.

Clauss, J. J., van Harskamp, F., Breteler, M. M. *et al.* (1994). The diagnostic value of SPECT with Tc 99m HMPAO in Alzheimer's disease: a population-based study. *Neurology*, **44**, 454–61.

Corder, E. H., Saunders, A. M., Strittmatter, W. J. *et al.* (1993). Gene dose of apolipoprotein E type 4 allele and the risk of Alzheimer's disease in late onset-families. *Science*, **261**, 921–3.

Corder, E. H., Saunders, A. M., Risch, N. J. *et al.* (1994). Protective effect of apolipoprotein E allele 2 for late onset Alzheimer's disease. *Nat. Genet.*, **7**, 180–4.

Cummings, J. L. & Cole, G. (2002). Alzheimer's disease. *J. Am. Med. Assoc.*, **287** (18), 2335–8.

Davies, P. & Maloney, A. J. (1976). Selective loss of central cholinergic neurons in Alzheimer's disease. *Lancet*, **4**, 1403.

de la Monte, S. M. & Wands, J. (1992). Neuronal thread protein overexpression in brains with Alzheimer's disease lesions. *J. Neurol. Sci.*, **113**, 153–64.

de la Monte, S. M., Volicer, L., Hauser, S. L. & Wands, J. R. (1992). Increased levels of neuronal thread protein in cerebrospinal fluid of patients with Alzheimer's disease. *Ann. Neurol.*, **32**, 733–42.

de la Monte, S. M., Ghanbari, K., Frey, W. H. *et al.* (1997). Characterization of the AD7C-NTP DNA cDNA expression in Alzheimer's disease and measurement of a 41-kD protein in the cerebrospinal fluid. *J. Clin. Invest.*, **100** (12), 3093–104.

Dickson, D. W. (1999). Neuropathologic differentiation of progressive supranuclear palsy and corticobasal degeneration. *J. Neurol.*, **246** (S2), 6–15.

Di Luca, M., Pastorino, L., Bianchetti, A. *et al.* (1998). Differential levels of platelet amyloid β precursor protein isoforms. *Arch. Neurol.*, **55**, 1195–200.

Dodart, J. C., Bales, K. R., Gannon, K. S. *et al.* (2002). Immunization reverses memory deficits without reducing brain Aβ burden in Alzheimer's disease model. *Nat. Neurosci.*, **5** (5), 452–7.

Doody, R. S., Stevens, J. C., Beck, C. *et al.* Practice parameter: management of dementia (an evidence-based review), Report of the Quality Standards Subcommittee of the American Academy of Neurology. *Neurology*, **56**, 1154–66.

Ertekin-Taner, N., Graff-Radford, N., Younkin, L. H. *et al.* (2000). Linkage of plasma Abeta42 to a quantitative locus on chromosome 10 in late-onset Alzheimer's disease pedigrees. *Science*, **290** (5500), 2303–4.

Evans, D. A., Funkenstein, H. H., Albert M. S. *et al.* (1989). Prevalence of Alzheimer's disease in a community population of older persons: higher than previously reported. *J. Am. Med. Assoc.*, **262**, 2551–6.

Evans, D. A., Hebert, L. E., Beckett, L. A. *et al.* Education and other measures of socioeconomic status and risk of incipient Alzheimer's disease in a defined population of older persons. *Arch. Neurol.*, **54**, 1399–1405.

Folstein, M. F., Folstein, S. E. & McHugh, P. R. (1975). 'Mini-Mental State'. A practical method for grading the cognitive state of patients for the clinician. *J. Psychiatr. Res.*, **12**, 189–98.

Förstl, H. & Levy, R. (1991). On certain peculiar diseases of old age. *Hist. Psychiatry*, **2** (5, 1), 71–101.

Fox, N. C., Warrington, E. K., Freeborough, P. A. *et al.* (1996). Presymptomatic hippocampal atrophy in Alzheimer's disease: a longitudinal study. *Brain*, **119** (6), 2001–7.

Fox, N. C., Scahill, F. I., Crum, W. R. & Rossor, M. N. (1999). Correlation between rates of brain atrophy and cognitive decline in AD. *Neurology*, **52** (8), 1687–9.

Fox, N. C., Crum, W. R., Scahill, R. I., Stevens, J. M., Janssen, J. C. & Rossor, M. N. (2001). Imaging of onset and progression of Alzheimer's disease with voxel-compression mapping of serial magnetic resonance images. *Lancet*, **358** (9277), 201–5.

Fratiglioni, L., Albom, A., Viitanen, M. & Winblad, B. (1993). Risk factors for late-onset Alzheimer's disease. *Ann. Neurol.*, **33**, 258–66.

Galasko, D., Hansen, L. A., Katzman, R. *et al.* (1994). Clinical–neuropathological correlations in Alzheimer's disease and related dementias. *Arch. Neurol.*, **51** (9), 888–95.

Galasko, D., Clark, C., Chang. L. *et al.* (1997). Assessment of CSF levels of tau protein in mildly demented patients with Alzheimer's disease. *Neurology*, **48**, 632–5.

Galasko, D., Chang, L., Motter, R. *et al.* (1998). High cerebrospinal fluid tau and low amyloid beta42 levels in the clinical diagnosis of Alzheimer disease and relation to apolipoprotein E genotype. *Arch. Neurol.*, **55**, 937–45.

Galton, C. J., Patterson, K., Xuereb, J. H. & Hodges, J. R. (2000). Atypical and typical presentations of Alzheimer's disease: a clinical, neuropsychological, neuroimaging and pathological study of 13 cases. *Brain*, **123**, 484–98.

Gao, S., Hendrie, H. C., Hall, K. S. & Hui, S. (1998). The relationships between age, sex, and the incidence of dementia and Alzheimer's disease. *Arch. Gen. Pyschiatry*, **55**, 809–15.

Garrard, P. & Hodges, J. R. (2000). Semantic dementia: clinical, radiological and pathological perspectives. *J. Neurol.*, **247**, 409–22.

Gearing, M., Mirra, S. S., Hedreen, J. C., Sumi, S. M., Hansen, L. A. & Heyman, A. (1995). The Consortium to Establish a Registry for Alzheimer's disease (CERAD). Part X. Neuropathology confirmation of the clinical diagnosis of Alzheimer's disease. *Neurology*, **45**, 461–6.

Ghanbari, H., Ghanbari, K., Beheshti, I., Munzar, M., Vasauskas, A. & Averback, P. (1998). Biochemical assay for AD7C-NTP in urine as an Alzheimer's disease marker. *J. Clin. Lab. Anal.*, **12**, 285–8.

Graff-Radford, N. R., Green, R. C., Go, R. C. *et al.* (2002). Association between apolipoprotein E genotype and Alzheimer's disease in African American subjects. *Arch. Neurol.*, **59** (4), 594–600.

Green, R. C., Cupples, L. A., Kurz, A. *et al.* (2003). Depression as a risk factor for Alzheimer's disease: the MIRAGE study. *Arch. Neurol.*, **60**, 753–9.

Guo, Z., Cupples, L. A., Kurz, A. *et al.* (2000). Head injury and the risk of AD in the MIRAGE study. Neurology, **54**, 1316–23.

Hardy, J. & Gwinn-Hardy, K. (1998). Genetic classification of primary neurodegenerative disease. *Science*, **282**, 1075–9.

Henderson, V. W., Paganini-Hill, A., Miller, B. L. *et al.* (2000). Estrogen for Alzheimer's disease in women: randomized, double-blind, placebo-controlled trial. *Neurology*, **54** (2), 295–301.

Hendrie, H. C., Osuntokun, B. O., Hall, K. S. *et al.* (1995). Prevalence of Alzheimer's disease and dementia in two communities: Nigerian Africans and African Americans. *Am. J. Psychiatry*, **152**, 1485–92.

Hodges, J. R., Patterson, K., Oxbury, S. & Funnell, E. (1992). Semantic dementia. *Brain*, **115**, 1783–806.

Hof, P. R., Vogt, B. A., Bouras, C. & Morrison, J. H. (1997). Atypical form of Alzheimer's disease with prominent posterior cortical atrophy: a review of lesion distribution and circuit disconnection in cortical visual pathways. *Vision Res.*, **37** (24), 3609–25.

Hofman, A., Ott, A., Breteler, M. M. *et al.* (1997). Atherosclerosis, apolipoprotein E and the prevalence of dementia and Alzheimer's disease in the Rotterdam Study. *Lancet*, **349**, 151–4.

Hulstaert, F., Blennow, K., Ivanoiu, A. *et al.* (1999). Improved discrimination of AD patients using beta-amyloid(1–42) and tau levels in CSF. *Neurology*, **52**, 1555–62.

Hussain, I., Powell, D., Howlett, D. R. *et al.* (1999). Identification of a novel aspartic protease (Asp 2) as beta-secretase. *Mol. Cell Neurosci.*, **14**, 419–27.

in't Veld, B. A., Ruitenberg, A., Hofman, A. *et al.* (2001). Nonsteroidal anti-inflammatory drugs and the risk of Alzheimer's disease. *N. Engl. J. Med.*, **325** (21), 1515–21.

Jack, C. R. Jr, Petersen, R. C., Xu, Y. C. *et al.* (1997). Medial temporal atrophy on MRI in normal aging and very mild Alzheimer's disease. *Neurology*, **49**, 786–94.

Jack, C. R. Jr, Petersen, R. C., Xu, Y. C. *et al.* (1999). Prediction of AD with MRI-based hippocampal volume in mild cognitive impairment. *Neurology*, **52**, 1397–403.

Jack, C. R., Dickson, D. W., Parisi, J. E. *et al.* (2002). Antemortem MRI findings correlate with hippocampal neuropathology in typical aging and dementia. *Neurology*, **58**, 750–7.

Jagust, W., Thisted, R., Devous, Sr. M. D. *et al.* (2001). SPECT perfusion imaging in the diagnosis of Alzheimer's disease: a clinical-pathologic study. *Neurology*, **56**, 950–6.

Johnson, K. A., Holman, B. L., Rosen, T. J., Nagel, J. S., English, R. J. & Growdon, J. H. (1990). Iofetamine I 123 single photon emission computed tomography is accurate in the diagnosis of Alzheimer's disease. *Arch. Intern. Med.*, **150**, 752–6.

Johnson, K. A., Kijewski, M., Becker, J., Garada, B., Satlin, A. & Holman, B. L. (1993). Quantitative brain SPECT in Alzheimer's disease and normal aging. *J. Nucl. Med.*, **34**, 2044–8.

Kahle, P. J., Jakowec, M., Teipel, S. J. *et al.* (2000). Combined assessment of tau and neuronal thread protein in Alzheimer's disease CSF. *Neurology*, **54**, 1498–504.

Katzman, R., Brown, T., Fuld, P., Peck, A., Schechter, R. & Schimmel, H. (1983). Validation of a short orientation-memory-concentration test of cognitive impairment. *Am. J. Psychiatr.*, **140**, 734–9.

Killiany, R. J., Gomez-Isla, T., Moss, M. *et al.* (2000). Use of structural magnetic resonance imaging to predict who will get Alzheimer's disease. *Ann. Neurol.*, **47**, 430–9.

Klünemann, H. H., Fronhöfer, W., Wurster, H., Fischer, W., Ibach, B. & Klein, H. E. (2002). Alzheimer's second patient: Johann F and his family. *Ann. Neurol.*, **52**, 520–3.

Knopman, D. S., DeKosky, S. T., Cummings, J. L. *et al.* (2001). Practice parameter: diagnosis of dementia (an evidence-based review). Report of the quality standards subcommittee of the American Academy of Neurology. *Neurology*, **56**, 1143–53.

Kokmen, E., Beard, C. M., Offord, K. & Kurland, L. T. (1989). Prevalence of medically diagnosed dementia in a defined United States population: Rochester, Minnesota, January 1, 1975. *Neurology*, **39**, 773–6.

Kokmen, E., Smith, G. E., Petersen, R. C., Tangalos, E. & Ivnik, R. J. (1991). The short test of mental status: correlations with standardized psychometric testing. *Arch. Neurol.*, **48**, 725–8.

Kokmen, E. K., Beard, C. M., O'Brien, P. C. & Kurland, L. T. (1996). Epidemiology of dementia in Rochester, Minnesota. *Mayo Clin. Proc.*, **71**, 275–82.

Kramer, J. H. & Miller, B. L. (2000). Alzheimer's disease and its focal variants. *Sem. Neurol.*, **20** (4), 447–54.

Kukull, W. A. & Ganguli, M. (2000). Epidemiology of dementia: concepts and overview. In *Neurologic Clinics* ed. S. DeKosky, Vol. 18, pp. 923–49. Philadelphia: W. B. Saunders.

Kurz, A., Riemenschneider, M., Buch, K. *et al.* (1998). Tau protein in cerebrospinal fluid is significantly increased at the earliest clinical stage of Alzheimer disease. *Alzheimer Dis. Assoc. Disord.*, **12**, 372–7.

Launer, L. J., Andersen, K., Dewey, M. E. *et al.* (1999). Rates and risk factors for dementia and Alzheimer's disease: results from EURODEM pooled analyses. EURODEM Incidence Research Group and Work Groups. European Studies of Dementia. *Neurology*, **52**, 78–84.

Lee, V. Y. M., Goedert, M. & Trojanowski, J. Q. (2001). Neurodegenerative tauopathies. *Ann. Rev. Neurosci.*, **24**, 1121–59.

Levine, D. N., Lee, J. M. & Fisher, C. M. (1993). The visual variant of Alzheimer's disease: a clinicopathologic case study. *Neurology*, **43** (2), 305–13.

Machulda, M. M., Ward, H. A., Borowski, B. *et al.* (2003). Comparison of memory fMRI response among normal, MCI and Alzheimer's patients. *Neurology*, **61**, 500–6.

McKhann, G., Drachman, D., Folstein, M., Katzman, R., Price, D. & Stadlan, E. M. (1984). Clinical Diagnosis of Alzheimer's Disease: Report of the NINCDS-ADRDA work group under the auspices of Department of Health and Human Services Task Force on Alzheimer's Disease. *Neurology*, **34**, 939–44.

Mesulam, M. M. (1982). Slowly progressive aphasia without generalized dementia. *Ann. Neurol.*, **11**, 592–8.

(2001). Primary progressive aphasia. *Ann. Neurol.*, **49**, 425–32.

Mohs, R. C., Doody, R. S., Morris, J. C. *et al.* (2001). A 1-year, placebo-controlled preservation of function survival study of donepezil in AD patients. *Neurology*, **57**, 481–8.

Morris, J. C. (1993). The Clinical Dementia Rating (CDR): Current version and scoring rules. *Neurology*, **43**, 2412–14.

Mortimer, J. A. (1995). The epidemiology of Alzheimer's Disease: Beyond risk factors. In *Research Advances in Alzheimer's Disease and Associated Disorders*, ed. I. Iqbal, J. Mortimer, B. Winblad & H. Wisniewski. Chichester, UK: John Wiley.

Müller, W. E., Mutschler, E. & Riederer, P. (1995). Noncompetitive NMDA receptor antagonists with fast open-channel blocking kinetics and strong voltage-dependency as potential therapeutic agents for Alzheimer's dementia. *Pharmacopsychiatry*, **28**, 113–24.

Mulnard, R. A., Cotman, C. W., Kawas, C. *et al.* (2000). Estrogen replacement therapy for treatment of mild to moderate Alzheimer disease: a randomized controlled trial. Alzheimer's Disease Cooperative Study. *J. Am. Med. Assoc.*, **283** (8), 1007–15.

Munoz, D. & Feldman, H. (2002). Causes of Alzheimer's disease. *Can. Med. Assoc. J.*, **162** (1), 65–72.

Nicoll, J. A., Wilkinson, D., Holmes, C., Steart, P., Markham, H. & Weller, R. O. (2003). Neuropathology of human Alzheimer's disease following immunization with amyloid beta peptide: a case report. *Nat. Med.*, **9**, 448–52.

Orgogozo, J. M., Gilman, S., Dartigues, J. F. *et al.* (2003). Subacute meningoencephalitis in a subset of patients with AD after Aβ42 immunization. *Neurology*, **61**, 46–54.

Padovani, A., Borroni, B., Colciaghi, F. *et al.* (2001). Platelet amyloid precursor protein forms in AD: a peripheral diagnostic and pharmacological target. *Mech. Aging Devel.*, **122**, 1997–2004.

Petersen, R. C. (1977). Scopolamine induced learning failures in man. *Psychopharmacology*, **52**, 283–9.

Pfiefer, M., Boncristiano, S., Bondolfi, L. *et al.* (2002). Cerebral hemorrhage after passive anti-Ab immunotherapy. *Science*, **298**, 1379.

Qiu, C., Winblad, B., Fastbom, J. & Fratiglioni, L. (2003). Combined effects of *APOE* genotype, blood pressure, and antihypertensive drug use on incident AD. *Neurology*, **61**, 655–60.

Reisberg, B., Doody, R., Stöffler, A., Schmitt, F., Ferris, S. & Möbius, H. J. (2003). Memantine in moderate-to-severe Alzheimer's disease. *N. Engl. J. Med.*, **348**, 1333–41.

Rogers, S., Farlow, M., Doody, R., Mohs, R. & Friedhoff, L. D. (1998). A 24-week, double-blind, placebo-controlled trial of donepezil in patients with Alzheimer's disease. Neurology, **50**, 136–45.

Rosler, M., Anand, R., Cicin-Sain, A. *et al.* (1999). Efficacy and safety of rivastigmine in patients with Alzheimer's disease: international randomised controlled trial. *B. Med. J.*, **318**, 633–8.

Ross Mackenzie, S. J., Graham, N., Stuart-Green, L. *et al.* (1996). Progressive biparietal atrophy: an atypical presentation of Alzheimer's disease. *J. Neurol. Neurosurg. Psychiatry*, **61** (4), 388–95.

Sano, M., Ernesto, C., Thomasm, R. *et al.* (1997). A controlled trial of selegiline, alpha-tocopherol, or both as treatment for Alzheimer's disease. The Alzheimer's Disease Cooperative Study. *N. Engl. J. Med.*, **336**, 1216–22.

Saunders, A. M., Strittmatter, W. J., Schmechel, D. *et al.* (1993). Association of apolipoprotein E allele 4 with late onset familial and sporadic Alzheimer's disease. *Neurology*, **43**, 1467–72.

Schenk, D., Barbour, R., Dunn, W. *et al.* (1999). Immunization with amyloid-beta attenuates Alzheimer-disease-like pathology in the PDAPP mouse. *Nature*, **400**, 173–7.

Schenk, D. (2002). Opinion. Amyloid-beta immunotherapy for Alzheimer's disease: the end of the beginning. *Nat. Rev. Neurosci.*, **3**, 824–8.

Selkoe, D. J. (2000). The genetics and molecular pathology of alzheimer's disease: roles of amyloid and the presenilins. In *Neurologic Clinics*, ed. S. DeKosky, pp. 903–21. Vol. 18. Philadelphia: W. B. Saunders.

Senior, K. (2002). Dosing in phase II trial of Alzheimer's vaccine suspended. *Lancet Neurol.* **1**, 3.

Seshadri, S., Drachman, D. A. & Lippa, C. F. (1995). Apolipoprotein E ε4 allele and the lifetime risk of Alzheimer's disease. *Arch. Neurol.*, **52**, 1074–9.

Seshadri, S., Beiser, A., Selhub, J. *et al.* (2002). Plasma homocysteine as a risk factor for dementia and Alzheimer's disease. *N. Engl. J. Med.*, **346** (7), 476–83.

Sherrington, R., Rogaev, E. I., Liang, Y. *et al.* (1995). Cloning of a gene bearing mis-sense mutations in early-onset familial Alzheimer's disease. *Nature*, **375**, 754–60.

Shoji, M., Matsubara, E., Kanai, M. *et al.* (1998). Combination assay of CSF tau, A beta 1–40 and A beta 1–42(43) as a biochemical marker of Alzheimer's disease. *J. Neurol. Sci.*, **158**, 134–40.

Shumaker, S. A., Legault, C., Rapp, S. R. *et al.* (2003). Estrogen plus progestin and the incidence of dementia and mild cognitive impairment in postmenopausal women: the Women's Health Initiative Memory Study: a randomized controlled trial. *J. Am. Med. Assoc.*, **289**, 2651–62.

Sinha, S., Anderson, J. P., Barbour, R. *et al.* (1999). Purification and cloning of amyloid precursor protein beta-secretase from human brain. *Nature*, **402**, 537–40.

Small, G., Rabins, P., Barry, P. *et al.* (1997). Diagnosis and treatment of Alzheimer's disease and related disorders. Consensus Statement of the American Association for Geriatric Psychiatry, the Alzheimer's Association, and the American Geriatrics Society. *J. Am. Med. Assoc.*, **278**, 1363–71.

Spillantini, M. G. & Goedert, M. (1998). Tau protein pathology in neurodegenerative diseases. *Trends Neurosci.*, **21**, 428–33.

St. George-Hyslop, P. H., Levesque, G., Levesque, L., Rommens, J., Westaway, D. & Fraser, P. E. (1996). Two homologous genes causing early-onset familial Alzheimer's disease. *Cold Spring Harbor Symp. Quant. Biol.*, **61**, 559–64.

Stelzmann, R. A., Schnitzlein, H. N. & Murtagh, F. R. (1995). An English translation of Alzheimer's 1907 paper 'Über eine eigenartige Erkankung der Hirnrinde'. *Clin. Anat.*, **8** (6), 429–31.

Tang-Wai, D. F., Josephs, K. A., Boeve, B. F., Dickson, D. K., Parisi, J. E. & Petersen, R. C. (2003a). Coexistent Lewy body disease in a case of 'visual variant Alzheimer's disease'. *J. Neurol. Neurosurg. Psychiatry*, **74**, 389.

(2003b). Pathologically confirmed corticobasal degneration presenting with visuospatial dysfunction. *Neurology*, **61** (8), 1134–5.

Tang-Wai, D. F., Graff-Radford, N. R., Boeve, B. F. *et al.* (2003c). Clinical and neuropathological characteristics of posterior cortical atrophy. *Neurology*, **60**, A264–5.

Tariot, P. N., Solomon, P. R., Morris, J. C., Kershaw, P., Lilienfeld, S. & Ding, C. (2000). A 5-month, randomized, placebo-controlled trial of galantamine in AD. The Galantamine USA-10 Study Group. *Neurology*, **54**, 2269–76.

Tekin, S. & Cummings, J. L. (2001). Depression in dementia. *The Neurologist*, **7**, 252–9.

Teng, E. L. & Chui, H. C. (1987). The Modified Mini-Mental State (3MS) examination. *J. Clin. Psychiatry*, **48**, 314–18.

The Alpha-Tocopherol, Beta Carotene Cancer Prevention Study Group (1994). The effect of vitamin E and beta carotene on the incidence of lung cancer and other cancers in male smokers. *N. Engl. J. Med.*, **330** (15), 1029–35.

The Ronald and Nancy Reagan Research Institute of the Alzheimer's Association and the National Institute on Aging Working Group (1998). Consensus report of the Working Group on: molecular and biochemical markers of Alzheimer's disease. *Neurobiol. Aging*, **19** (2), 109–16.

Van Gool, W. A., Walstra, G. J., Teunisse, S., Van der Zant, F. M., Weinstein, H. C. & Van Royen, E. A. (1995). Diagnosing Alzheimer's disease in elderly, mildly demented patients: the impact of routine single photon emission computed tomography. *J. Neurol.*, **242**, 401–5.

van Slegtenhorst, M., Lewis, J. & Hutton, M. (2000). The molecular genetics of the tauopathies. *Exp. Geront.*, **35**, 461–71.

Vassar, R., Bennett, B. D., Babu-Khan, S. *et al.* (1999). Beta-secretase cleavage of Alzheimer's amyloid precursor protein by the transmembrane aspartic protease BACE. *Science*, **286**, 735–41.

Victoroff, J., Ross, G. W., Benson, D. F., Verity, M. A. & Vinters, H. V. (1994). Posterior cortical atrophy, Neuropathologic correlations. *Arch. Neurol.*, **51** (3), 269–74.

von Strauss, E., Viitanen, M., De Ronchi, D., Winblad, B. & Fratiglioni, L. (1999). Aging and the occurrence of dementia: findings from a population-based cohort with a large sample of nonagenarians. *Arch. Neurol.*, **56**, 587–92.

White, L., Petrovitch, H., Ross, G. W. *et al.* (1996). Prevalence of dementia in older Japanese-American men in Hawaii: The Honolulu-Asia Aging Study. *J. Am. Med. Assoc.*, **276**, 955–60.

Whitehouse, P. J., Price, D. L., Clark, A. W., Coyle, J. T. & DeLong, M. R. (1981). Alzheimer disease: evidence for selective loss of cholinergic neurons in the nucleus basalis. *Ann. Neurol.*, **10**, 122–6.

Whitehouse, P. J., Price, D. L., Struble, R. G., Clark, A. W., Coyle, J. T. & Delon, M. R. (1982). Alzheimer's disease and senile dementia: loss of neurons in the basal forebrain. *Science*, **215**, 1237–9.

Winblad, B. & Poritis, N. (1999). Memantine in severe dementia: results of the 9M-BEST study (benefit and efficacy in severely demented patients during treatment with memantine). *Int. J. Geriat. Psychiatry*, **14**, 135–46.

Wolozin, B., Kellman, W., Ruosseau, P., Celesia, G. G. & Siegel, G. (2000). Decreased prevalence of Alzheimer's disease associated with 3-hydroxy-3-methylglutaryl coenzyme A reductase inhibitors. *Arch. Neurol.*, **57**, 1439–43.

Xu, Y., Jack, C. R. Jr, O'Brien, P. C. *et al.* (2000). Usefulness of MRI measures of entorhinal cortex versus hippocampus in AD. *Neurology*, **54**, 1760–7.

Yan, R., Bienkowski, M. J., Shuck, M. E. *et al.* (1999). Membrane-anchored aspartyl protease with Alzheimer's disease beta-secretase activity. *Nature*, **402**, 533–7.

Zandi, P. P., Carlson, M. C., Plassman, B. L. *et al.* (2002). Hormone replacement therapy and the incidence of Alzheimer's disease in older women: the Cache County study. *J. Am. Med. Assoc.*, **288**, 2123–9.

Zubenko, G. S., Zubenko, W. N., McPherson, S. *et al.* (2003). A collaborative study of the emergence and clinical features of the major depressive syndrome of Alzheimer's disease. *Am. J. Psychiatry*, **160** (5), 857–66.

29

The neuropathology of Alzheimer's disease in the year 2005

Colin L. Masters[1] and Konrad Beyreuther[2]

[1]Department of Pathology, The University of Melbourne and the Mental Health Research Institute of Victoria, Parkville, Australia
[2]Centre for Molecular Biology, the University of Heidelberg, Heidelberg, Germany

Introduction

The current molecular era of the neuropathology of Alzheimer's disease began in the early 1970s with the first attempts to characterize the biochemical basis of the amyloid deposits (now designated Aβ), which remain the pathognomic feature of this illness (Nikaido *et al.*, 1971). Subsequent dramatic progress in amino acid sequencing (Glenner & Wong, 1984; Masters *et al.*, 1985), gene cloning (Kang *et al.*, 1987), and elucidation of the biogenesis of the Aβ amyloid protein (for recent reviews see Beyreuther *et al.*, 2001; Cummings & Cole, 2002; Hardy & Selkoe, 2002; Ines Dominguez & DeStrooper, 2002; McLean *et al.*, 2001; Sisodia & St George-Hyslop, 2002) have led to a coherent picture of the pathogenesis of AD. However, this explosion of knowledge on AD still has not been fully translated back into the clinic, the pathology laboratory, or the mortuary, where diagnostic criteria remain subjective and ambiguous. As the natural history of AD becomes better understood at the molecular level, it would be highly desirable to develop standardized protocols for diagnosis based around the principal biochemical pathway: the biogenesis and accumulation of Aβ amyloid in susceptible areas of the brain (Fig. 29.1). This chapter outlines the traditional methods of neuropathologic diagnosis, together with some approaches to the contemporary molecular diagnosis of AD both during life and after death (Fig. 29.2), which should have general applicability to the other major diseases caused by the toxic gains-of-function of α-synuclein (Parkinson's disease; diffuse Lewy body disease; multiple system atrophy), prion protein (Creutzfeldt–Jakob and related diseases); Cu–Zu superoxide dismutase (amyotrophic lateral sclerosis); polyglutamine expansions (Huntington's disease and mechanistically related illnesses) and the tau microtubule associated protein (frontotemporal degenerations; Pick's disease; cortico-basal degeneration; progressive supranuclear palsy).

The Aβ theory of Alzheimer's disease and the problem of selective vulnerability

One of the dominant themes of classical neuropathology has been that of selective vulnerability, incorporating the Vogts' concept of "pathoclisis", in which the spectrum of regional-to-cellular graduation of vulnerability requires explanation. As the severity and duration of AD increases, the areas of brain involved appear to spread from temporal to frontal/parietal, then move posteriorly towards the occipital regions. In the more aggressive cases (particularly those with an early age of onset, often on a background of a pathogenic mutation in the APP/PS1,2 genes), then other subcortical structures (striatum, thalamus, cerebellum) become involved. This pattern of topographic vulnerability has eluded a rational explanation. The only clue that has emerged involves the glutamatergic system and the distribution of free vesicular zinc required for its operation (Hashemzadeh-Gargari & Guilarte, 1999; Weiss & Sensi, 2000). There is at least a superficial correspondence between the tissue content of free zinc ions and the regional vulnerability in AD. Our studies over the last eight years (Bush *et al.*, 1993, 1994; Cherny *et al.*, 1999, 2001; Jobling *et al.*, 2001; Opazo *et al.*, 2002) have indicated that Zn^{2+} and other metal ions have the capacity to induce aggregation of Aβ. These properties have recently been confirmed using biological models in which Aβ-overexpressing mice, when crossed into a background deficient in a synaptic veside zinc transporter (ZnT3), have decreased amounts of Aβ plaques (Lee JY *et al.*, 2002). The metal-induced aggregation of Aβ is therefore suggested to be the initial event which leads to the toxic-gain-of-function of Aβ. The immobilized

Aβ theory of Alzheimer's disease

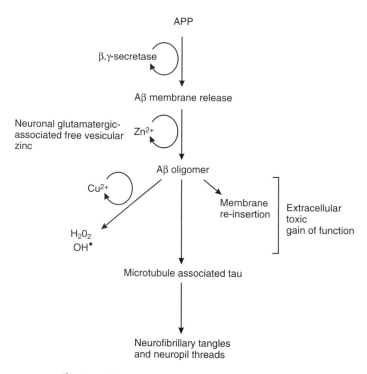

Fig. 29.1 The pathway downstream of APP (amyloid precursor protein), which leads to the neurodegeneration characteristic of Alzheimer's disease. Aβ is generated and released from the membrane through the actions of β- and γ-secretases; in a zinc-rich microenvironment, Aβ may oligomerize and either re-insert into a membrane or radicalize to form toxic reactive oxygen species. Further downstream, tau polymerizes to form tangles and threads.

Aβ can then react with redox-active ions such as Cu^{2+} or Fe^{3+}, generating H_2O_2 or OH^- or potentially interact with lipid membranes (Curtain *et al.*, 2001). In both cases the neuron is subjected to damaging stresses which, over time, result in dysfunction. How neurons develop neurofibrillary tangles and neuropil threads (containing polymerized tau) remains unclear, but we would suggest that this process lies downstream of the Aβ-induced toxic insult. Again, partial confirmation of this pathway has emerged from cell and animal models (Rapoport *et al.*, 2002).

The basic neuropathology of Alzheimer's disease

The neuropathologic diagnosis of Alzheimer's disease still revolves around the morphologic assessment of Aβ amyloid accumulation within the brain, either as "senile" plaques or as perivascular amyloid angiopathy. Quantitative biochemical assays of Aβ accumulation may eventually replace the standard morphologic approach, but this is unlikely to occur in the near future. In vivo neuroimaging techniques for Aβ amyloid, rather than biochemical assays, may well supersede the traditional neuropathologic assessment within the next decade.

Macroscopic changes

There are no macroscopic changes that are specific for AD. The brain may appear quite normal, or may show extreme atrophy in most cortical areas with concomitant dilation of the ventricular system. The degree of atrophy does seem to correlate partially with the "aggressiveness" of the disease process, being more pronounced in the younger, often familial, cases with rapid deterioration and prolonged vegetative state. Loss of white matter may also be apparent in such cases. Variation in regional areas of atrophy may also be related in some cases to the type of clinical presentation (frontal, temporal, left or right hemispheric predominance).

In cases where small vessel β-amyloid angiopathy is a feature, evidence of focal, old or fresh cortical and subpial hemorrhages may be seen. Concomitant large vessel atherosclerotic disease occurs at a rate expected in the general population, and does not appear to be particularly associated with AD.

Classical histological changes – Aβ amyloid plaques

The cardinal, pathognomic, feature of AD is the accumulation of Aβ amyloid, which with today's technology, is best evaluated by using sensitive immunocytochemical methods. There is still no agreement on what constitutes a "normal" or "threshold" level of Aβ deposition beyond which a diagnosis of AD can be entertained. Working backwards, however, the complete absence of Aβ deposits in the presence of other major histologic changes (neurofibrillary tangles, gliosis, neuronal loss) should mandate that a diagnosis of AD cannot be made.

The Aβ-amyloid plaque is the most easily identifiable structure using light microscopy. Attempts to classify these plaques as "senile," "neuritic," "amorphous," "diffuse," "cotton-wool," "primitive/early," "classical/mature," "burned-out/compact" remind us of the proverbial blind person describing an elephant. Immunocytochemistry has identified Aβ-amyloid at the nidus of all these structures, which have been partially re-created in the transgenic mouse models of AD. A seminal recent observation has been that some aspects of the "amorphous/ diffuse/

Contemporary neuropathology of Alzheimer's disease

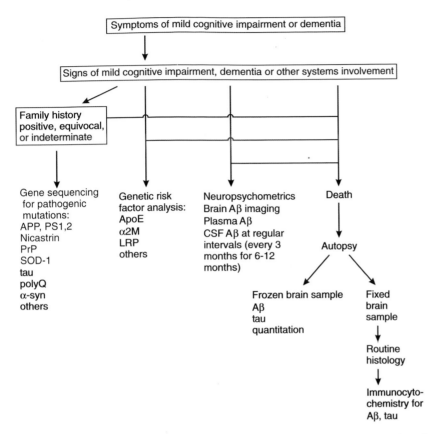

Fig. 29.2 A scheme of the clinical neuropathological work-up in the current time, with application of quantitative and qualitative molecular techniques to assign a diagnosis.

cotton-wool" morphology may actually represent intracellular Aβ aggregates. This would be consistent with the lack of any appreciable surrounding glial or microglial change. If confirmed, the presence of aggregated Aβ intraneuronally may provide the missing-link for an explanation of how the tau protein aggregates into the neurofibrillary tangle. At the very least, the tau-positive neuritic changes surrounding the extracellular Aβ deposits confirm the current theory that tau aggregation is down-stream of Aβ deposition/accumulation. It is sobering to recall that most of these morphological changes associated with Aβ plaques have been described for many years (for example, neuritic changes by Cajal, Drusige Entartung by Scholtz), and yet the molecular bases underlying them remain elusive.

Use of sensitive and specific immunocytochemical techniques for visualization of Aβ amyloid deposition has also disclosed the vast, unanticipated, extent of Aβ deposition in the subpial extracellular spaces, together with the perpendicular streaking patterns seen in the molecular layers of the cerebellum, and the laminar patterns within the central cortex, consistent with current ideas on the bulk flow of Aβ in the extracellular and perivascular spaces of the brain. These morphologic changes also support the idea that neuronally generated Aβ can be transported across the blood-brain-barrier into the general circulation.

Tau-related neurofibrillary tangles (NFT)

Often thought of as an hallmark of AD, these NFT structures (which also include neuritic changes in the neuropil and the Drusige Entartung around the Aβ amyloid plaques) are now seen as rather non-specific changes provoked by the upstream toxic effects of Aβ amyloid. They occur in other unrelated conditions (for example, the tauopathies including progressive supranuclear palsy). The intracellular tangles and neurites contain filamentous aggregates of the tau microtubule-associated protein, which also have the tinctorial properties of an amyloid substance. By electron microscopy, a very characteristic paired helical (twisted) filament substructure is seen, together with straight filaments. The structural basis for the differences between a twisted and straight filament remains unanswered, as both appear to be composed solely of the tau protein.

Granulovacuolar degeneration (GVD) and Hirano bodies

The GVD of Simchowicz and Hirano bodies are often seen in hippocampal neurons in AD, changes which still remain enigmatic in nature, and of little diagnostic value.

Neuronal and synaptic loss

As part of the Aβ-induced neurodegenerative process, synaptic dysfunction occurs at an early stage. The morphologic correlate of this may lie in the loss of markers of synapses (e.g. synaptophysin). As the disease progresses, neuronal death occurs, but is often difficult to quantitate, being apparent only in the more severe cases with extensive gliosis.

Astrocytic and microglial changes

The Aβ-induced damage to neurons provokes secondary glial and microglial reactive changes, easily observed with appropriate immunocytochemical markers, but rarely necessary for diagnosis. It is also possible that the soluble and insoluble forms of Aβ directly activate glial and microglial responses, as seen by the vigorous glial changes which often surround the "neuritic" plaque. More recent evidence of the reactive nature of microglia has come from the studies of immunization of experimental animals and humans with Aβ itself, as a method of promoting its clearance from the brain (Nicoll et al., 2003; Orgogozo et al., 2003).

The morphometric approach to the neuropathology of AD

The mainstay of current neuropathologic evaluation is still the microscopic demonstration of Aβ and tau accumulation. Utilization of specific immunocytochemical labels has permitted the unequivocal identification and semi-quantitation of these lesions (Gold et al., 2001; Kraszpulski et al., 2001; Parvathy et al., 2001). With the widespread availability of specific Aβ and tau antibodies, most cases coming to biopsy or autopsy can be categorized on these histologic criteria. Similarly, for the other major classes of neurodegeneration, the immunocytochemical demonstration of aggregates of α-synuclein, PrP, SOD-1, polyglutamine and tau should permit an efficient method for diagnosis and classification.

There is still a need, however, for more accurate and quantitative estimates of the degrees of cerebral involvement with Aβ. The spectrum of Aβ accumulation varies widely, ranging from subtle intracellular immunoreactivity of uncertain significance through to massive clouds of Aβ in the neuropil (amorphous or cotton wool plaques, Davies et al., 1988; Smith et al., 2001) or to perivascular congophilic deposits (Revesz et al., 2002). At the morphometric level, image analysis and stereologic techniques may have some useful properties (Bussière et al., 2002; Fishman et al., 2001), but practically the methods are too time consuming and require a large input of effort in cross-validation from one laboratory to the next.

The clinical biochemistry of Aβ in AD

Since Aβ lies in the centre of the pathway, it seems irrefutable that biochemical measurements of Aβ loads in the brain should provide the best estimate of disease activity. The physical forms of Aβ being assayed (soluble vs insoluble (McLean et al., 1999); monomer, dimer, oligomer (Walsh et al., 2002); oxidized or reduced (Kanski et al., 2002); metallated vs non-metallated (Cherny et al., 2000; Curtain et al., 2001); lipid-associated or -free (Oshima et al., 2001); and length of peptide, $A\beta_{x-40/42}$) and the tissue sources of Aβ (brain grey matter; CSF; plasma, etc.) need to be defined and validated in the clinical context.

While we and others have demonstrated the feasibility of measuring brain levels of Aβ (McLean et al., 1999), such measurements have yet to be trialled in a practical way. We would propose, in the first instance, a simple ELISA-based measure of total Aβ species ($A\beta_{\xi-40/42}$) in the soluble and insoluble fractions of grey matter homogenate. Our preliminary studies do not suggest that the area of cortex sampled is critical, but for the sake of consistency, a limited number of easily accessible and identifiable cortical sites could be selected (inferior temporal; superior frontal; parietal).

For obvious reasons, much attention has been given to assaying Aβ levels in CSF (Andreasen et al., 2001a, b; Maruyama et al., 2001; Mehta et al., 2001; Okamura et al., 2001; Riemenschneider et al., 2002a; Rösler et al., 2001; Shoji & Kanai 2001; Shoji et al., 2001; Sjögren et al., 2001) with a consensus emerging that while elevated levels may exist in the early phases of AD (especially an increased ratio of $A\beta_{42}$ to $A\beta_{40}$, Jensen *et al.*, 1999), and as the disease progresses, CSF levels of $A\beta$ decease and tau levels increase. The value of CSF $A\beta$ levels in discriminating AD from other causes of dementia is beginning to emerge (Kapaki *et al.*, 2001; Riemenschneider *et al.*, 2002b; Sjögren *et al.*, 2002; Tschampa *et al.*, 2001). Much larger data sets need to be reported, and comparisons made between in vivo levels and diagnostic outcomes obtained post mortem.

Better than CSF, plasma $A\beta$ could yet prove to be an accurate surrogate marker for cerebral $A\beta$. While early studies were disappointing, with large inter-subject variability (Mehta *et al.*, 2001), more recent results suggest that plasma $A\beta_{40/42}$ is in a dynamic equilibrium with cerebral $A\beta$ turnover (DeMattos *et al.*, 2001, 2002 a, b), and that the inter-subject variability of plasma $A\beta$ levels is under genetic control (Ertekin-Taner *et al.*, 2001; Schupf *et al.*, 2001). Understanding this genetic variability may lead to processes that determine cerebral $A\beta$ turnover and clearance mechanisms. Our own preliminary observations suggest that plasma $A\beta$ will prove to be a valuable guide to therapeutic intervention (Ritchie *et al.*, 2003), and others are also beginning to evaluate this aspect (Tokuda *et al.*, 2001). The early indications are that serial estimations of plasma $A\beta$ over a period (possibly 3 to 12 months) will provide a guide to cerebral $A\beta$ turnover, both for steady-state levels and for a guide to $A\beta$-targeted therapeutic interventions.

Besides $A\beta$ levels, estimates of markers upstream or downstream of $A\beta$ could prove to be complimentary. Upstream, γ-secretase and β-secretase (BACE1) can now be measured using both functional assays and immunoassays. Since β-secretase activity appears to be increased in sporadic AD (Holsinger *et al.*, 2002), this would be an obvious candidate for an upstream assay, particularly in CSF or plasma if this enzyme were released from the cerebral compartment. There is, as yet, no evidence for an increased function in the γ-secretase complex (presenilin 1,2; nicastrin; APH-2; PEN2) in any form of AD, so this would appear to be an unlikely object of assay development.

The place of genetic diagnostics in the neuropathology of AD

A full family history is now essential for a complete evaluation of anyone with adult-onset dementia, but it is disappointing to see how poorly this is documented in most neuropathologic reports on individual subjects. In most (if not all) pedigrees in which a clear history of autosomal dominant inheritance is obtained, a pathogenic mutation in one of the genes for APP, PS1,2 will be found. Screening of other relevant genes (Prnp, tau, SOD, Htt, α-syn) should be considered when an AD-causative mutation is not evident in an autosomal dominant pedigree.

While genetic risk factors such as ApoE allotype have a clear impact on the age of expression of AD, the full spectrum of risk factors (such as polymorphisms in the genes encoding IDE, α2Macroglobulin and LRP) have yet to be elucidated, and their practical contributions to diagnosis have yet to be demonstrated, both during life and at postmortem. It could be envisaged that a full evaluation of these risk factors in any given individual will eventually have a major role to play in neuropathologic diagnosis.

Neuroimaging of Aβ

Persistent attempts to develop labelled-ligands for $A\beta$ which can cross the blood-brain-barrier are beginning to yield encouraging results (Helmuth, 2002). Beginning with compounds which share properties with Congo Red or thioflavin-T (Klunk *et al.*, 2001; Lee C. W. *et al.*, 2001; Mathis *et al.*, 2002; Schmidt *et al.*, 2001; Zhuang *et al.*, 2001a,b), which have long been known to have an increased affinity for all types of amyloid, other $A\beta$ ligands have emerged (Bading *et al.*, 2002; Kung *et al.*, 2001; Lee H. J. *et al.*, 2002; Shoghi-Jadid *et al.*, 2002). The physical properties of $A\beta$ have suggested many possible leads, including $A\beta$ (or subfragments thereof) itself. As a proof-of-concept, the imaging of $A\beta$ (Helmuth, 2002) will now open a major avenue of diagnostic evaluation, with immense therapeutic-monitoring implications.

REFERENCES

Andreasen, N., Minthon, L., Davidsson, P. *et al.* (2001a). Evaluation of CSF-tau and CSF-Aβ42 as diagnostic markers for Alzheimer disease in clinical practice. *Arch. Neurol.*, **58**, 373–9.

Andreasen, N., Gottfries, J., Vanmechelen, E. *et al.* (2001b). Evaluation of CSF biomarkers for axonal and neuronal degeneration, gliosis, and β-amyloid metabolism in Alzheimer's disease. *J. Neurol. Neurosurg. Psychiatry*, **71**, 557–8.

Bading, J. R., Yamada, S., Mackic, J. B. *et al.* (2002). Brain clearance of Alzheimer's amyloid-β40 in the squirrel monkey: A SPECT study in a primate model of cerebral amyloid angiopathy. *J. Drug Targeting*, **10**, 359–68.

Beyreuther, K., Christen, Y. & Masters, C. L. (eds.) (2001). *Neurodegenerative Disorders: Loss of Function Through Gain of Function*. Berlin: Springe, 189pp.

Bush, A. I., Multhaup, G., Moir, R. D. *et al.* (1993). A novel zinc (II) binding site modulates the function of the βA4 amyloid protein precursor of Alzheimer's disease. *J. Biol. Chem.*, **268**, 16109–12.

Bush, A. I., Pettingell, W. H., Multhaup, G. *et al.* (1994). Rapid induction of Alzheimer Aβ amyloid formation by zinc. *Science*, **265**, 1464–7.

Bussière, T., Friend, P. D., Sadeghi, N. *et al.* (2002). Stereologic assessment of the total cortical volume occupied by amyloid deposits and its relationship with cognitive status in aging and Alzheimer's disease. *Neuroscience*, **112**, 75–91.

Cherny, R. A., Legg, J. T., McLean, C. A. *et al.* (1999). Aqueous dissolution of Alzheimer's disease Aβ amyloid deposits by biometal depletion. *J. Biol. Chem.*, **274**, 23223–8.

Cherny, R. A, Barnham, K., Lynch, T. *et al.* (2000). Chelation and intercalation: complementary properties in a compound for the treatment of Alzheimer's disease. *J. Struct. Biol.*, **130**, 209–16.

Cummings, J. L. & Cole, G. (2002). Alzheimer disease. *J. Am. Med. Assoc.*, **287**, 2335–8.

Curtain, C. C., Ali, F., Volitakis, I. *et al.* (2001). Alzheimer's disease amyloid-β binds copper and zinc to generate an allosterically ordered membrane-penetrating structure containing superoxide dismutase-like subunits. *J. Biol. Chem.*, **276**, 20466–73.

Davies, L., Wolska, B., Hilbich, C. *et al.* (1988). A4 amyloid protein deposition and the diagnosis of Alzheimer's disease: prevalence in aged brains determined by immunocytochemistry compared with conventional neuropathlogic techniques. *Neurology*, **38**, 1688–93.

DeMattos, R. B., Bales, K. R., Cummins, D. J., Dodart, J. C., Paul, S. M. & Holtzman, D. M. (2001). Peripheral anti-Aβ antibody alters CNS and plasma Aβ clearance and decreases brain Aβ burden in a mouse model of Alzheimer's disease. *Proc. Natl Acad. Sci., USA*, **98**, 8850–5.

DeMattos, R. B., Bales, K R., Parsadanian, M. and Holtzman DM (2002a). Plaque-associated disruption of CSF and plasma amyloid-β (Aβ) equilibrium in a mouse model of Alzheimer's disease. *J. Neurochem.*, **81**, 229–36.

DeMattos, R. B., Bales, K. R., Cummins, D. J., Paul, S. M. & Holtzman, D. M. (2002b). Brain to plasma amyloid-beta efflux: a measure of brain amyloid burden in a mouse model of Alzheimer's disease. *Science*, **295**, 2264–7.

Ertekin-Taner, N., Graff-Radford, N., Younkin, L. H. *et al.* (2001). Heritability of plasma amyloid β in typical late-onset Alzheimer's disease pedigrees. *Genet. Epidemiol.*, **21**, 19–30.

Fishman, C. E., Cummins, D. J., Bales, K. R. *et al.* (2001). Statistical aspects of quantitative image analysis of β-amyloid in the APP^{V717F} transgenic mouse model of Alzheimer's disease. *J. Neurosci. Methods*, **108**, 145–52.

Glenner, G. G. & Wong, C. W. (1984). Alzheimer's disease: initial report of the purification and characterization of a novel cerebrovascular amyloid protein. *Biochem. Biophys. Res. Commun.*, **120**, 885–90.

Gold, G., Kövari, E., Corte, G. *et al.* (2001). Clinical validity of Aβ-protein deposition staging in brain aging and Alzheimer disease. *J. Neuropathol. Exp. Neurol.*, **60**, 946–52.

Hardy, J. & Selkoe, D. J. (2002). The amyloid hypothesis of Alzheimer's disease: progress and problems on the road to therapeutics. *Science*, **297**, 353–6.

Hashemzadeh-Gargari, H. & Guilarte, T. R. (1999). Divalent cations modulate *N*-methyl-D-aspartate receptor function at the glycine site. *J. Pharmacol. Exp. Ther.*, **290**, 1356–62.

Holsinger, R. M. D. , McLean, C. A., Beyreuther, K., Masters, C. L. & Evin, G. (2002). Increased expression of the amyloid precursor β-secretase in Alzheimer's disease. *Ann. Neurol.*, **51**, 783–6.

Helmuth, L. (2002). Long-awaited techniques spots Alzheimer's toxin. *Science*, **297**, 752–3.

Ines Dominguez, D. & DeStrooper, B. (2002). Novel therapeutic strategies provide the real test for the amyloid hypothesis of Alzheimer's disease. *Trends Pharm. Sci.*, **23**, 324–30.

Jensen, M., Schröder, J., Blomberg, M. *et al.* (1999). Cerebrospinal fluid Aβ42 is increased early in sporadic Alzheimer's disease and declines with disease progression. *Ann. Neurol.*, **45**, 504–11.

Jobling, M. F., Huang, X., Stewart, L. R. *et al.* (2001). Copper and zinc binding modulates the aggregation and neurotoxic properties of the prion peptide PrP106–126. *Biochemistry*, **40**, 8073–84.

Kang, J., Lemaire, H., Unterbeck, A. *et al.* (1987). The precursor of Alzheimer's disease amyloid A4 protein resembles a cell-surface receptor. *Nature*, **325**, 733–6.

Kanski, J., Varadarajan, S., Aksenova, M. & Butterfield, D. A. (2002). Role of glycine-33 and methionine-35 in Alzheimer's amyloid β-peptide 1–42 associated oxidative stress and neurotoxicity. *Biochim. Biophys. Acta*, **1586**, 190–8.

Kapaki, E., Kilidireas, K., Paraskevas, G. P., Michalopoulou, M. & Patsouris, E. (2001). Highly increased CSF tau protein and decreased β-amyloid (1–42) in sporadic CJD: a discrimination from Alzheimer's disease? *J. Neurol. Neurosurg. Psychiatry*, **71**, 401–3.

Klunk, W. E., Wang, Y., Huang, G. F., Debnath, M. L., Holt, D. P. & Mathis, C. A. (2001). Uncharged thioflavin-T derivatives bind to amyloid-beta protein with high affinity and readily enter the brain. *Life Sci.*, **69**, 1471–84.

Kraszpulski, M., Soininen, H., Helisalmi, S. & Alafuzoff, I. (2001). The load and distribution of [beta]-amyloid in brain tissue of patients with Alzheimer's disease. *Acta Neurol. Scand.*, **103**, 88–92.

Kung, H. F., Lee, C. W., Zhuang, Z. P., Kung, M. P., Hou, C. & Plossl, K. (2001). Novel stilbenes as probes for amyloid plaques. *J. Am. Chem. Soc.*, **123**, 12740–1.

Lee, C. W., Zhuang, Z. P., Kung, M. P. *et al.* (2001). Isomerization of (*Z,Z*) to (*E,E*)1-bromo-2,5-bis-(3-hydroxycarbonyl-4-hydroxy)styrylbenzene in strong base: probes for amyloid plaques in the brain. *J. Med. Chem.*, **44**, 2270–5.

Lee, H. J., Zhang, Y., Zhu, C., Duff, K. & Pardridge, W. M. (2002). Imaging brain amyloid of Alzheimer disease *in vivo* in transgenic mice with an Aβ peptide radiopharmaceutical. *J. Cereb. Blood Flow Metab.*, **22**, 223–31.

Lee, J. Y., Cole, T. B., Palmiter, R. D., Suh, S. W. & Koh, J. Y. (2002). Contribution by synaptic zinc to the gender-disparate plaque formation in human Swedish mutant APP transgenic mice. *Proc. Natl Acad. Sci., USA*, **99**, 7705–10.

McLean, C. A., Cherny, R. A., Fraser, F. W. *et al.* (1999). Soluble pool of Aβ amyloid as a determinant of severity of neurodegeneration in Alzheimer's disease. *Ann. Neurol.*, **46**, 860–6.

McLean, C. A., Beyreuther, K. & Masters, C. L. (2001). Amyloid Aβ?levels in Alzheimer's disease – a diagnostic tool and the key to understanding the natural history of Aβ? *J. Alzheimer's Dis.*, **3**, 305–12.

Maruyama, M., Arai, H., Sugita, M. *et al.* (2001). Cerebrospinal fluid amyloid β(1–42) levels in the mild cognitive impairment stage of Alzheimer's disease. *Exp. Neurol.*, **172**, 433–6.

Masters, C. L., Simms, G., Weinman, N. A., McDonald, B. L., Multhaup, G. & Beyreuther, K. (1985). Amyloid plaque core protein in Alzheimer disease and Down syndrome. *Proc. Natl Acad. Sci., USA*, **82**, 4245–9.

Mathis, C. A., Bacskai, B. J., Kajdasz, S. T. *et al.* (2002). A lipophilic thioflavin-T derivative for positron emission tomography (PET) imaging of amyloid in brain. *Bioorg. Med. Chem. Lett.*, **12**, 295–8.

Mehta, P. D., Pirttila, T., Patrick, B. A., Barshatzky, M. & Mehta, S. P. (2001). Amyloid β protein 1–40 and 1–42 levels in matched cerebrospinal fluid and plasma from patients with Alzheimer disease. *Neurosci. Lett.*, **304**, 102–6.

Nicoll, J. A. R., Wilkinson, D., Holmes, C., Steart, P., Markham, H. & Weller, R. O. (2003). Neuropathology of human Alzheimer disease after immunization with amyloid-β peptide: a case report. *Nat. Med.*, **9**, 448–52.

Nikaido, T., Austin, J., Rinehart, R. *et al.* (1971). Studies in aging of the brain I. Isolation and preliminary characterization of Alzheimer plaques and cores. *Arch. Neurol.*, **25**, 198–211.

Okamura, N., Arai, H., Maruyama, M. *et al.* (2001). Serum cholesterol and cerebrospinal fluid amyloid β protein in Alzheimer's disease. *J. Am. Geriat. Soc.*, **49**, 1738–9.

Opazo, C., Huang, X., Cherny, R. A. *et al.* (2002). Metalloenzyme-like activity of Alzheimer's disease β-amyloid: Cu-dependent catalytic conversion of dopamine, cholesterol and biological reducing agents to neurotoxic H_2O_2. *J. Biol. Chem.*, **277**, 40302–8.

Orgogozo, J.-M., Gilman, S., Dartigues, J.-F. *et al.* (2003). Subacute meningoencephalitis in a subset of patients with AD after Aβ42 immunization. *Neurology*, **61**, 46–54.

Oshima, N., Morishima-Kawashima, M., Yamaguchi, H. *et al.* (2001). Accumulation of amyloid β-protein in the low-density membrane domain accurately reflects the extent of β-amyloid deposition in the brain. *Am. J. Pathol.*, **158**, 2209–18.

Parvathy, S., Davies, P., Haroutunian, V. *et al.* (2001). Correlation between Aβx-40-, Aβx-42-, and Aβx-43- containing amyloid plaques and cognitive decline. *Arch. Neurol.*, **58**, 2025–32.

Rapoport, M., Dawson, H. N., Binder, L. I., Vitek, M. P. & Ferreira, A. (2002). Tau is essential to β-amyloid-induced neurotoxicity. *Proc. Natl Acad. Sci., USA*, **99**, 6364–9.

Revesz, T., Holton, J. L., Lashley, T. *et al.* (2002). Frangione B. Sporadic and familial cerebral amyloid angiopathies. *Brain. Pathol.*, **12**, 343–57.

Riemenschneider, M., Schmolke, M., Lautenschlager, N. *et al.* (2002a). Association of CSF apolipoprotein E, Aβ42 and cognition in Alzheimer's disease. *Neurobiol. Aging*, **23**, 205–11.

Riemenschneider, M., Wagenpfeil, S., Diehl, J. *et al.* (2002b). Tau and Aβ42 protein in CSF of patients with frontotemporal degeneration. *Neurology*, **58**, 1622–8.

Ritchie, C. W., Bush, A. I., Mackinnon, A. *et al.* (2003). Metal–protein attenuation with iodochlorhydroxyquin (clioquinol) targeting Aβ amyloid deposition and toxicity in Alzheimer's disease: a pilot Phase 2 clinical trial. *Arch. Neurol.*, **60**, 1685–91.

Rösler, N., Wichart, I. & Jellinger, K. A. (2001). CSF Aβ40 and Aβ42: Natural course and clinical usefulness. *J. Alzheimer's Dis.*, **3**, 599–600.

Schmidt, M. L., Schuck, T., Sheridan, S. *et al.* (2001). The fluorescent Congo red derivative, (*trans, trans*)-1-bromo-2,5-bis-(3-hydroxycarbonyl-4-hydroxy) styrylbenzene (BSB), labels diverse β-pleated sheet structures in postmortem human neurodegenerative disease brains. *Am. J. Pathol.*, **159**, 937–43.

Schupf, N., Patel, B., Silverman, W. *et al.* (2001). Elevated plasma amyloid β-peptide 1–42 and onset of dementia in adults with Down syndrome. *Neurosci. Lett.*, **301**, 199–203.

Shoghi-Jadid, K., Small, G. W., Agdeppa, E. D. *et al.* (2002). Localization of neurofibrillary tangles and beta-amyloid plaques in the brains of living patients with Alzheimer disease. *Am. J. Geriatr. Psychiatry*, **10**, 24–35.

Shoji, M. & Kanai, M. (2001). Cerebrospinal fluid Aβ40 and Aβ42: natural course and clinical usefulness. *J. Alzheimer's Dis.*, **3**, 313–21.

Shoji, M., Kanai, M., Matsubara, E. *et al.* (2001). The levels of cerebrospinal fluid Aβ40 and Aβ42(43) are regulated age-dependently. *Neurobiol. Aging*, **22**, 209–15.

Sisodia, S. S. & St George-Hyslop, P. H. (2002). γ-Secretase, Notch, Abeta and Alzheimer's disease: where do the presenilins fit in? *Nat. Rev. Neurosci.* **3**, 281–90.

Sjögren, M., Vanderstichele, H., Ågren, H. *et al.* (2001). Tau and Aβ42 in cerebrospinal fluid from healthy adults 21–93 years of age: establishment of reference values. *Clin. Chem.*, **47**, 1776–81.

Sjögren, M., Davidsson, P., Wallin, A. *et al.* (2002). Decreased CSF-β-amyloid 42 in Alzheimer's disease and amyotrophic lateral sclerosis may reflect mismetabolism of β-amyloid induced by disparate mechanisms. *Dement. Geriatr. Cogn. Disord.*, **13**, 112–18.

Smith, M. J., Kwok, J. B. J., McLean, C. A. *et al.* (2001). Variable phenotype of Alzheimer's disease with spastic paraparesis. *Ann. Neurol.*, **49**, 125–9.

Tokuda, T., Tamaoka, A., Matsuno, S. *et al.* (2001). Plasma levels of amyloid β proteins did not differ between subjects taking statins and those not taking statins. *Ann. Neurol.*, **49**, 546–7.

Tschampa, H. J., Schulz-Schaeffer, W., Wiltfang, J. *et al.* (2001). Decreased CSF amyloid β42 and normal tau levels in dementia with Lewy bodies. *Neurology*, **56**, 576.

Walsh, D. M., Klyubin, I., Fadeeva, J. V. *et al.* (2002). Naturally secreted oligomers of amyloid β protein potently inhibit hippocampal long-term potentiation in vivo. *Nature*, **416**, 535–9.

Weiss, J. H. & Sensi, S. L. (2000). Ca^{2+}-Zn^{2+} permeable AMPA or kainite receptors: possible key factors in selective neurodegeneration. *Trends Neurosci.*, **23**, 365–71.

Zhuang, Z. P., Kung, M. P., Hou, C. *et al.* (2001a). Radioiodinated styrylbenzenes and thioflavins as probes for amyloid aggregates. *J. Med. Chem.*, **44**, 1905–14.

Zhuang, Z. P., Kung, M. P., Hou, C. *et al.* (2001b). IBOX(2-(4-dimethylaminophenyl)-6-iodobenzoxazole): a ligand for imaging amyloid plaques in the brain. *Nucl. Med. Biol.*, **28**, 887–94.

30

Genetics of Alzheimer's disease

Lars Bertram and Rudolph E. Tanzi

Genetics and Aging Research Unit, Department of Neurology, Massachusetts General Hospital, Charlestown, MA, USA

Introduction

Alzheimer's disease, the most common form of age-related dementia, is characterized by progressive and insidious neurodegeneration of the central nervous system eventually leading to a gradual decline of cognitive function and dementia. The key neuropathological features of AD are abundant amounts of neurofibrillary tangles and β-amyloid (Aβ) deposited in the form of senile plaques. Although the knowledge of disease pathophysiology still remains fragmentary, it is now widely accepted that, similar to other common diseases like diabetes, coronary artery disease, or breast cancer, genes play an essential role in predisposing to onset and/or in modifying the progress of the disease.

Genetically, AD is a complex and heterogeneous disorder: it is complex because there is no single mode of inheritance that accounts for its heritability. Moreover, disease inheritance shows an age-related dichotomy in which rare but highly penetrant mutations transmitted in an autosomal dominant manner are almost exclusively responsible for the early-onset familial forms of AD (EOFAD), while common polymorphisms with low penetrance appear to have their greatest effect on the more frequent late-onset form of the disease (LOAD; Tanzi, 1999). It is heterogeneous because genetic variants in multiple genes on several chromosomes throughout the genome are involved together with non-genetic factors. All of the known factors contribute to the increased accumulation of Aβ (more specifically: $A\beta_{42}$) owing to an imbalance in production vs degradation/clearance in the cell (Fig. 30.1, 30.2). Several additional characteristics aggravate the identification and consistent replication of AD genes or other complex disease genes across studies and populations (Bertram & Tanzi, 2001a; see also Chapter 17: "Strategies for molecular genetics in neurodegenerative disease"). These difficulties are evidenced by the fact that of almost 100 potential AD genes analyzed in the literature to date, only four have been proven to either play a direct role in AD pathogenesis (*APP*, *PSEN1*, *PSEN2*) or to significantly increase disease susceptibility in almost every study population worldwide (*APOE*; Table 30.1; for review see Bertram & Tanzi, 2001b).

Despite the complexities of AD genetics, tremendous progress has been made over the past two decades. The knowledge gained from genetic studies of AD was and remains the essential prerequisite for our current understanding of the etiological and pathophysiological mechanisms leading to neurodegeneration in AD as well as for the development of novel approaches for disease treatment and prevention. In this chapter we present a brief history of the genetics of Alzheimer's and discuss its current status and future outlook, focusing on recent findings suggesting the existence of several novel AD genes.

Early-onset Alzheimer's disease

Only a fraction of all AD cases can be explained by familial early-onset AD (EOFAD; Tanzi, 1999). Unlike the situation for the much more common late-onset form of AD, genetic studies of EOFAD are considerably facilitated by the availability of large multigenerational pedigrees allowing genetic linkage analysis and subsequent positional cloning to be carried out successfully. In 1987, initial results showed EOFAD linkage to the long arm of chromosome 21 encompassing a region that harbored the gene encoding the amyloid precursor protein (APP; gene: *APP*), a compelling candidate gene for AD (Tanzi *et al.*, 1987). The same chromosomal area also overlapped with the obligate region for Down's syndrome (DS), a disease where affected individuals almost invariably develop AD after a certain age. In

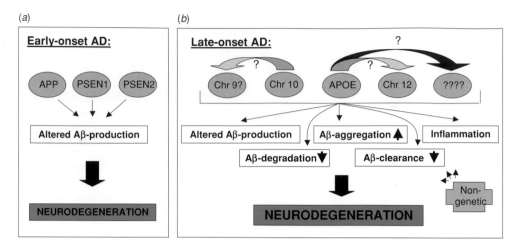

Fig. 30.1 Scheme of contribution and interaction pattern of known and putative AD genes. (*a*) Mutations in the early-onset AD genes *APP*, *PSEN1*, *PSEN2* all lead to an increase in Aβ-production without any known interaction with other factors.
(*b*) Simplified scheme of the interaction pattern of known and proposed late-onset AD genes. It is likely, these risk-factor genes each affect one or more of the known pathogenic mechanisms leading to neurodegeneration in AD. Their effects are further influenced by gene-gene interactions and the contribution of non-genetic risk-factors. Note that none of the interaction patterns outlined here for didactic purposes has actually been established. (Reproduced from Bertram & Tanzi, 2003, with permission.)

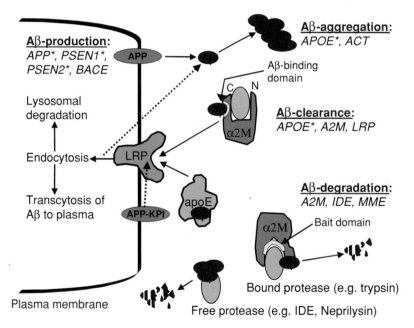

Fig. 30.2 Possible pathogenetic routes of Aβ production, clearance, and degradation. Early-onset AD genes *APP*, *PSEN1*, and *PSEN2* along with *BACE* (β-secretase) are involved in the production of Aβ. The late-onset AD gene *APOE* and the putative AD gene, α-1-antichymotrypsin (*ACT*) have been proposed to play roles in the aggregation and fibrillogenesis of Aβ. *APOE* and putative AD genes, *LRP* and *A2M* may play roles in the clearance of Aβ as follows. Once α2M-Aβ or apoE-Aβ complexes are internalized by LRP they may be targeted for endosomal recycling, lysosomal degradation, or undergo trancytosis across the blood–brain barrier to the plasma. Membrane APP containing an alternatively spliced Kunitz protease inhibitor (KPI) domain may also undergo internalization by LRP and generate Aβ (dotted-arrows) via the endocytic pathway (*Note:* APP has also been shown to undergo LRP-independent endocytosis). Extracellular degradation of Aβ can occur via binding of the peptide to α2M followed by degradation by an active protease (e.g. trypsin) bound to the bait region of α2M. Alternatively, Aβ may be degraded by "free" proteases such as the insulin degrading enzyme (*IDE*) or neprilysin (*MME*). Asterisk (*) denotes established AD genes. (Reproduced from Tanzi & Bertram, 2001, with permission.)

Table 30.1. Overview of the established Alzheimer's genes and their functional relevance

Gene (Protein)	Chromosomal location	Mode of inheritance	Number of pathogenic mutations (affected families)[a]	Mean familial onset age[a,b] (range)	Relevance to AD pathogenesis
APP (β-amyloid precursor protein)	21q21.3	autosomal-dominant	15(39)	51.5 years (35–60)	increase in Aβ ($A\beta_{42}/A\beta_{40}$-ratio); mutations close to γ-secretase site
PSEN1 (presenilin 1)	14q24.3	autosomal-dominant	128(258)	44.1 years (24–60)	increase in Aβ ($A\beta_{42}/A\beta_{40}$-ratio); essential for γ-secretase activity
PSEN2 (presenilin 2)	1q31–42	autosomal-dominant	9(15)	57.1 years (46–71)	increase in Aβ ($A\beta_{42}/A\beta_{40}$-ratio); essential for γ-secretase activity (?)
APOE (apolipoprotein E, ε4-allele)	19q13.32	complex (risk increase)	n.a.	onset-age modifier	increase in Aβ aggregation; via lipid/cholesterol transport (?)

[a] Source: "AD Mutation Database" (as of 04/01/2003).

[b] Not all familial onset ages were available for these genes.

1991, the first *APP* missense mutation in patients with EOFAD was described (Goate *et al.*, 1991), shortly after a report on a different variant in the same exon leading to Dutch-type hereditary cerebral hemorrhage with amyloidosis (for review see Hardy, 1997; Tanzi, 1999). Since then, 15 additional AD mutations have been reported in *APP* which, in total, account for approximately one-tenth of all early-onset AD families with known mutations (Table 30.1). Most of the *APP*-variants occur near the putative γ-secretase site between residues 714 and 717 ('AD Mutation Database'), suggesting that especially the γ-cleavage event of APP and/or its (dys-)regulation are critical for the development of AD.

A second AD linkage region, on chromosome 14q24, was reported almost simultaneously by four independent laboratories only 1 year after the discovery of the first *APP* mutation (Mullan *et al.*, 1992; Schellenberg *et al.*, 1992; St George-Hyslop *et al.*, 1992; Van Broeckhoven *et al.*, 1992). However, it took 3 more years to clone the responsible gene (*PSEN1*) and identify the first disease-causing mutations (Sherrington *et al.*, 1995). It is now known that *PSEN1* encodes a highly conserved polytopic membrane protein, presenilin 1 (PS1, for review, see Haass & De Strooper, 1999), which is required for γ-secretase activity necessary to liberate Aβ from APP (see below). Even a decade after the discovery of *PSEN1*, there are new AD-causing mutations reported in this gene almost every month, currently counting a total of nearly 130 (Table 30.1; "AD mutation database"). But despite the observation that, by far, most AD mutations are located in *PSEN1*, it soon became obvious that this gene together with *APP* does not account for all cases of EOFAD. A database search initiated in 1995 revealed a second member of the PS family of proteins that displayed very high homology to *PSEN1* at the genomic as well as at the

protein level (Levy-Lahad *et al.*, 1995; Rogaev *et al.*, 1995), and consequently, this gene was named "*PSEN2*" (protein: PS2). *PSEN2* maps to the long arm of chromosome 1 and mutations in this gene account for the smallest fraction of all EOFAD cases. On average, they also display a later age of onset and slower disease progression than *APP* or *PSEN1* mutations (Table 30.1).

Despite these seminal advances in understanding the genetics and pathophysiology of EOFAD, several lines of evidence suggest that additional genetic factors remain to be identified for this form of the disease: (i) numerous early-onset families do not show mutations in any of the three EOFAD genes despite extensive sequencing efforts of open reading frames and adjacent intronic regions; (ii) beyond APP and PS1 there are several additional key proteins involved in the γ- and β-secretase cleavage events and other aspects leading to the aggregation and deposition of Aβ (e.g. nicastrin, aph-1, pen-2, BACE; see below), as well as the hyperphosphorylation of tau and the development of neurofibrillary tangles; (iii) a recent full genome screen has identified at least four early-onset AD linkage regions in addition to chromosome 14q24 (Blacker *et al.*, 2003), some of which coincide with the pathophysiological factors mentioned above. Of these, two deserve particular attention. First, the gene encoding nicastrin (*NCSTN*) located on the long arm of chromosome 1. Nicastrin is a type 1 transmembrane glycoprotein and an essential component of the γ-secretase complex that cleaves APP and notch (Yu *et al.*, 2000). Although analyses aimed at identifying functionally important sequence variants in early- as well as late-onset AD patients were largely unsuccessful to date (e.g. Dermaut *et al.*, 2002; Orlacchio *et al.*, 2002), a four-locus haplotype that appears to be associated with EOFAD was identified (Dermaut *et al.*,

2002). Interestingly, no association with the same haplotype was observed in LOAD patients in the same study, despite previous positive linkage (Blacker *et al.*, 2003) and association (Hiltunen *et al.*, 2001) results with LOAD in the region. The second gene, encoding "β-secretase" or BACE (β-site APP-cleavage enzyme; gene: *BACE*), is an aspartic protease located within cell membranes and is highly expressed in brain (for review, see Vassar, 2001). Although a recent genome screen reports linkage only ~20 million base-pairs (Mb) upstream of *BACE* on chromosome 11q25 (Blacker *et al.*, 2003), none of the six independent association studies have found evidence for a genetic involvement of variants in this gene and AD (consult *AlzGene* database http://www.alzgene.org/). None withstanding, further research is needed to clarify whether or not possibly rare variants in these two genes may play a significant role in individual AD families, preferably those linked to the respective chromosomal regions, and confer risk similar to the other three established EOFAD genes.

Late-onset Alzheimer's disease

As outlined above and also in Fig. 30.1, late-onset Alzheimer's (LOAD) is characterized by a considerably more multifaceted and interwoven pattern of genetic and non-genetic factors that is only poorly understood. Adding to these complexities are methodological difficulties inherent to common diseases in general and late-onset diseases like AD in particular. Family data, for instance, is more often than not incomplete (e.g. owing to relatives who died before the family-specific age of risk and/or the lack of genotypic information for parents). Another complication is the unknown number of "phenocopies", i.e. subjects with a non-genetic form of the disease or subjects suffering from other forms of age-related cognitive decline. These and other characteristics largely reduce the power to detect new loci in reasonably sized samples and make the identification and, equally important, independent replication of genetic factors of only moderate or small effect very difficult if not impossible. This is evidenced by the fact that even 10 years after the first reports suggesting genetic association between AD and the common ε4-variant in the gene encoding apolipoprotein E (apoE; gene: *APOE*), no other genetic risk factor has been found to consistently confer susceptibility to AD, despite intensive efforts in many laboratories worldwide (Bertram & Tanzi, 2001b). And although none of the almost 100 genes that have been tested for association with AD have yielded consistent results, yet a recent study (Daw *et al.*, 2000), modeling AD as a quantitative trait locus, suggests that further gene hunting in LOAD is worthwhile: the authors found evidence for the existence of four to seven additional AD susceptibility loci (or onset age modifiers) besides *APOE*. This is in agreement with recent full genome screens in AD, in which regions on at least nine chromosomes emerge that show evidence for genetic linkage or association with *P*-values ≤0.01 in at least two studies (Table 30.2). In the remainder of this chapter we will discuss the relevance of *APOE* and then focus on two additional, novel AD candidate gene regions on chromosomes 10 and 12. An up-to-date overview on the status of all published case-control AD association studies can be found at the Alzheimer's Research Forum Genetic database, http://www.alzgene.org.

The APOE locus on chromosome 19

The first and, to date only, proof of principle for applying the "positional candidate gene strategy" (i.e. testing biologically plausible candidate genes in promising linkage regions, see also chapter 17) to identify novel AD loci was provided by the identification of genetic association between *APOE* and AD. The positional evidence arrived almost simultaneously with the identification of the first APP mutations, when Pericak-Vance and colleagues reported suggestive linkage of a locus on chromosome 19q to predominantly late-onset AD (Pericak-Vance *et al.*, 1991). Two years later, after Aβ was found to bind apoE (Strittmatter *et al.*, 1993a) which was the first evidence for a functional involvement of apoE in AD, a common polymorphism in its gene, which maps near the linkage region, was tested and shown to be associated with increased risk for AD (Saunders *et al.*, 1993; Strittmatter *et al.*, 1993). In contrast to all other reports of genetic association in AD, this result has been overwhelmingly replicated in a large number of studies across many ethnic groups worldwide (for a meta-analysis see: Farrer *et al.*, 1997). Three major alleles occur at the *APOE* locus, ε2, ε3 and ε4, which translate into combinations of two amino acid changes at residues 112 and 158 of the apoE-protein (ε2: Cys/Cys; ε3: Cys/Arg; ε4: Arg/Arg, respectively), and it is the phylogenetically oldest variant, ε4, that is over-represented in cases of AD. The least frequent allele, ε2, has been associated with a decreased risk for AD, although these findings were replicated in fewer studies than the more predominant ε4 effect (Farrer *et al.*, 1997).

Although the association between ε4 and AD is robust, it is not specific. In contrast to the genetic variants in EOFAD, the presence of ε4 is neither necessary nor sufficient to actually cause the disease. Rather, it appears to

Table 30.2. Overview of concordant linkage/association regions observed in full genome screens published to date

Chromosome	Linkage-Studies					Association-studies	
	Pericak-Vance (1997)	Pericak-Vance (2000)	Kehoe/Myers[a] (1999/2002)	Li et al. (2002)	Blacker et al. (2003)	Zubenko (1998)	Hiltunen et al. (2001)
1p36	–	–	TLS = 1.7	–	–	–	$P = 0.006$
4q35	–	TLS = 2.3	–	–	MLS = 1.8	–	-
5p13–15	–	TLS = 2.2	TLS = 2.8	–	MLS = 1.4	–	$P = 0.001$
6p21	*TLS > 1.0*	–	MLS = 2.0*	–	TLS = 1.9	–	$P = 0.003$
q15	TLS > 1.5	–	TLS = 1.9	–		–	–
9p21	–	MLS = 4.3	TLS = 1.8	–	MLS = 1.3	–	–
q22	–	–	MLS = 2.4*	–	MLS = 2.9	–	–
10q21–22	–	–	TLS = 4.1	–	MLS = 1.8	–	–
q24–25	–	–	–	MLS = 2.4	TLS = 1.9		
12p11	MLS = 3.7	–	MLS = 1.4	–		–	–
19q13	–	TLS = 3.6	MLS = 1.8*	MLS = 3.3	MLS = 7.7	$P < 0.0001$	–
Xp21	–	–	MLS = 1.5*	–	TLS = 1.6		
q21–26	–	–	MLS = 1.9*	–		$P = 0.0002$	–

Only results reflecting a *P*-value ≤ 0.01 (i.e. TLS or MLS ≥ 1.4) in at least two studies were considered. TLS = two-point lod score, MLS = multi-point lod score. Shading indicates chromosomes with significant findings using published criteria (Lander & Kruglyak, 1995). Note that samples in Pericak-Vance (2000), Myers (2002), Li *et al.* (2002) and Blacker *et al.* (2003) partly overlap.

[a] Stage-I linkage results from this group (Kehoe *et al.*, 1999) were used whenever they exceeded the results of the Stage II findings. (Current on 04/01/2003. For a more up-to-date overview, please consult the *AlzGene* database, http://www.alzgene.org.)

be a genetic risk-modifier (or susceptibility factor), that predominantly acts through decreasing the age of onset in a dose-dependent manner, in the sense that homozygous carriers on average show a younger onset age than carriers of just a single copy (Blacker *et al.*, 1997; Meyer *et al.*, 1998). Expressed in terms of overall disease risk, this effect translates into an increased relative risk (as measured by the odds ratio [OR]) of roughly threefold for heterozygous, and almost 15-fold for homozygous carriers as compared to the ε3/3 genotype in Caucasians (Farrer *et al.*, 1997). Similar trends can be seen across different ethnic groups, ranging from ORs of around twofold in Hispanic to more than 33-fold in Japanese ε4/4 individuals. However, due to the non-specific nature of the ε4-effect, there is widespread consensus within research as well as clinical communities to not use *APOE* genotyping as a sole diagnostic or prognostic test for AD, but only for scientific purposes (Burke *et al.*, 2001).

Despite the established genetic role of *APOE* in AD, only little is known about its potential pathophysiological effects and mechanisms. The most straightforward hypothesis assumes that the different variants directly influence Aβ-accumulation (Strittmatter *et al.*, 1993), and several lines of evidence support this notion, e.g. an increase of the number of Aβ-plaques in the brain of ε4-allele carriers

vs. non-carriers, and marked differences in the deposition of Aβ-plaques depending on the presence or absence of human *APOE* in transgenic mice over expressing *APP* (for a recent review on *Apoe* function, see Poirier, 2000). Further, there is evidence for a decrease in onset age depending on *APOE*-ε4 in EOFAD caused by *PSEN1* mutations (Nacmias *et al.*, 1995). No consensus has yet been reached regarding the predominant mechanism(s) underlying these effects, although systemic dysfunction in lipid transport, and more specifically cholesterol homeostasis are likely pathways, especially since high plasma cholesterol levels are associated with increased β-amyloid in the brain (Poirier, 2000). Thus, it is possible that *APOE*-ε4 confers risk for AD via mechanisms that are shared with its effects on cardiovascular disease, e.g. by increasing a carrier's risk for hypercholesterolemia.

Chromosome 12

Of the novel putative AD loci to be discussed in the remainder of this chapter, the locus on chromosome 12 was described first, when in 1997 and 1998 three independent laboratories reported evidence for linkage with AD near the p-telomere and the centromeric region of this chromosome (Pericak-Vance *et al.*, 1997; Rogaeva *et al.*, 1998; Wu *et al.*, 1998). Subsequent analyses revealed strong association with biologically highly plausible and related candidate genes in both regions, which are separated by ~50 Mb. The first gene, located on the proximal end of chromosome 12 (at approx. 10 Mb), encodes alpha2-macroglobulin (α2M; gene: *A2M*) a pan-protease inhibitor that has been found to potentially modify Aβ-catabolism in several ways, including the prevention of Aβ-fibril formation and fibril associated neurotoxicity, protease mediated degradation of Aβ, and LRP (see below) mediated endocytosis and subsequent lysosome degradation of Aβ (Fig. 30.2; for a recent review of α2M function, see Saunders *et al.*, 2003). Almost simultaneously, two papers were published shortly after the initial linkage findings reporting strong and significant association with separate polymorphisms in *A2M*. The first one used family-based methodologies and found an overrepresentation of a 5-bp deletion just upstream of exon 18, near the "bait" region of α2M, i.e. near the potentially functional region of the protein in mostly small LOAD families (Blacker *et al.*, 1998). The second study employed a case-control design, and reported association with an amino acid substitution at residue 1000 (Val→Ile), near the thiolester active site of α2M. In a small series of cases, this study also showed a small but significant increase in Aβ-burden in carriers of the risk allele, i.e. Val (Liao *et al.*, 1998).

The combination of promising and independent linkage and association findings has initiated a huge set of follow-up investigations, only exceeded in number by the studies on *APOE*. However, more often than not, subsequent attempts to corroborate the original findings in independent laboratories have failed. A recent meta-analysis even concluded that "*A2M* is not genetically associated with LOAD in white patients or mixed populations as found in the United States" (Koster *et al.*, 2000). This conclusion stands in contrast to at least ten independent reports beyond the two initial papers demonstrating significant association between polymorphisms in *A2M* and AD in US Caucasians and other ethnic groups, using both case-control and family-based designs (see *AlzGene* for an up-to-date overview). Eventually, more detailed and sufficiently-sized analyses will be necessary to indicate the extent to which variations in *A2M*, or possibly a gene nearby, confer risk for AD. The growing number of confirmatory reports, even amidst multiple refutations, make it unlikely that the initial findings are due to type I error alone. Further analyses in a greatly enlarged sample of NIMH families, including those for which the initial association was described, have revealed novel exonic and intronic polymorphisms in *A2M* that appear to be equally or stronger associated with disease than the 5-bp deletion upstream of exon 18 (Saunders *et al.*, 2003). In addition, haplotype analyses including all or only subsets of these polymorphisms, revealed even more pronounced association signals than the individual polymorphisms alone. Along these lines, recent case-control as well as family-based studies using SNP-haplotypes in or around *APOE* revealed strongly positive findings for polymorphisms that, individually, were either not or only weakly associated with AD (Martin *et al.*, 2000; Fallin *et al.*, 2001). It is noteworthy that the only haplotype-based case-control study on *A2M* in the AD literature to date supports an association of this locus and AD (Verpillat *et al.*, 2000).

The second gene reported to be associated with AD on chromosome 12 encodes the low-density lipoprotein receptor-related protein (LRP; gene: *LRP*), and resides approximately 50 Mb downstream of *A2M* in the more centromeric region of the chromosome (Kang *et al.*, 1997). LRP exerts its potentially pathophysiological effects by participating in two opposing mechanisms: first, by mediating the internalization of APP which can subsequently lead to an increase in Aβ-production, second, it has been shown that LRP also mediates the internalization of extra cellular Aβ bound to α2M and apoE, followed by lysosomal degradation, endosomal recycling or transcytosis via the blood-brain barrier (Fig. 30.2; for recent review, see Ulery & Strickland, 2000). Initial reports showing significant association between polymorphisms in this gene and AD (Kang *et al.*, 1997), remained largely unconfirmed in follow-up analyses (see *AlzGene* for an up-to-date overview). It was, once again, the analysis of multi-locus haplotypes that recently led to significant positive findings in the same sample (Scott *et al.*, 2000) that had previously yielded only negative results analyzing polymorphisms individually (Scott *et al.*, 1998). Mapping only ~7 Mb proximal of *LRP1* is the gene encoding the transcriptional factor LBP-1c/CP2/LSF (*TFCP2*), which has been found to be significantly decreased in AD patients in three independent case-control series (Lambert *et al.*, 2000; Taylor *et al.*, 2001; Luedecking-Zimmer *et al.*, 2003). Suggested roles for this protein in AD neuropathogenesis are the regulation of transcription/expression of other AD-related proteins, APP binding and internalization (via Fe65) or the regulation of inflammatory processes.

Although the findings on chromosome 12 require further investigation and clarification in larger samples, it is unlikely that the positive associations reported for the genes associated with AD to date (*A2M*, *LRP*, and *TFCP2*) reflect linkage disequilibrium between the two loci, i.e. *A2M* on the one and *LRP1* and/or *TFCP2* on the other end, given the large chromosomal distance in between the implicated regions (i.e. ~50 Mb). More likely, these results suggest the existence of two separate AD genes on chromosome 12, one near *A2M*, or *A2M* itself, and one near *LRP1*. Along these lines, only *TFCPZ* (L.B. and R.E.T., unpublished observations), but not *LRP1* (Bertram *et al.*, 2000a) appear to be associated in the same family sample (NIMH AD Genetics Initiative Study Sample) which continues to show strong association with *A2M* (see above).

Chromosome 10

There is emerging evidence that the long arm of chromosome 10 also harbors one or more AD loci. The situation is reminiscent of that encountered on chromosome 12; three independent laboratories initially reported significant linkage of AD to two general and possibly distinct regions on chromosome 10. The study by Myers and colleagues (Myers *et al.*, 2000) followed up on their own prior suggestive linkage results around ~65 Mb on 10q21–22 by genotyping additional markers and increasing the size of the study population. Interestingly and importantly, the linkage peak in this enlarged sample was found to be stronger than the linkage signal around *APOE* on chromosome 19 in the same dataset. A second study (Ertekin-Taner *et al.*, 2000) showed that upon using plasma Aβ_{42} levels as quantitative phenotype in five large and multi-generational pedigrees, there is strong evidence for linkage in a very similar region on chromosome 10. In this study the same phenotype yielded no linkage within or near the *APOE* region on chromosome 19, nor in three other previously reported linkage regions on chromosomes 1, 5 and 9. Our group (Bertram *et al.*, 2000b) performed a hypothesis-driven linkage analysis on six genetic markers in a region some 30–40 Mb distal, in between 93 and 106 Mb on chromosome 10q23–24. Markers in this region were chosen because they map close to the gene encoding insulin-degrading enzyme (*IDE*; protein: IDE), for which several studies have suggested a principal role in the degradation and clearance of Aβ in brain (for a recent review, see Selkoe, 2001). Two of the six markers showed significant linkage to AD by parametric and non-parametric analyses independent of the mode of inheritance, and one marker also showed evidence for association in the full and unstratified sample, a finding that was recently replicated in an independent case-control study (Ait-Ghezala *et al.*, 2002). The linkage findings, in combination with the positive association results, could be an indication of linkage disequilibrium with a disease modifying variant located nearby. Specifically, three genes (*IDE, KNSL1, HHEX*) are known in the immediate vicinity of

these markers and could be responsible for the observed effects.

Almost 2 years after the initial linkage reports, a second linkage study lent support to the more distal putative AD locus; as a matter of fact, the peak region of this most recent paper (Li *et al.*, 2002) coincides almost precisely with the distal bounds of the region implied by our study (Bertram *et al.*, 2000b), i.e. between 102 and 115 Mb. This study is also interesting because instead of using a conventional binary phenotype definition, the authors chose to analyze age at onset as quantitative trait. The linkage signal on chromosome 10 was not only the strongest observed in their full genome screen (excluding linkage at the *APOE* locus), but also emerged as an onset age modifying locus for Parkinson's disease, which was evaluated simultaneously. In fact, the linkage signal was strongest when both disease populations were combined into one analysis. At this time, it cannot be excluded that methodological or sampling/stratification differences across studies are responsible for the discrepant localization of the two linkage peaks which, in fact, could all be caused by the same gene. Another possible explanation is the presence of two loci, of which one primarily influences disease risk while the other acts more like a modifier of onset age (Li *et al.*, 2002). In any event, even though the actual disease gene(s) and its function remain(s) elusive, the fact that several independent laboratories have reported similar findings using different methodologies considerably increase the likelihood of at least one major late-onset AD locus on chromosome 10q.

Literally hundreds of genes have been mapped or predicted in the chromosomal stretch between 60 and 115 Mb, several of which are functionally plausible candidate genes for AD and are currently under investigation. Two of these candidates encode enzymes involved in the degradation of Aβ: *IDE* and *PLAU* (urokinase-type plasminogen activator [uPA]). According to some investigators, IDE displays the strongest Aβ degrading activity in vitro (Selkoe, 2001). It is a 110 kDa thiol zinc-metalloendopeptidase located in the cytosol, peroxisomes and the cell surface and degrades several small proteins all of which share the characteristic to form β-pleated sheet-rich amyloid fibrils, including Aβ and insulin (Kurochkin, 2001). In addition to Aβ, IDE has also been reported to degrade the APP intracellular domain (AICD), a fragment liberated after the γ-secretase cleavage of APP that has been suggested to play an important role in the regulation of transcriptional activity in the cell nucleus (Edbauer *et al.*, 2002). Besides the well characterized in vitro data, there is also growing evidence that IDE plays a role in the degradation of Aβ in vivo. First, naturally occurring missense mutations in *IDE* in a diabetic rat-model (GK rat) lead to a decrease in Aβ degrading activity in cultured fibroblasts and brain membranes (Farris *et al.*, 2002). Secondly and more importantly, *IDE* knockout mice not only show a significant decrease in Aβ-degradation in vivo, but also a significant increase in brain Aβ and AICD levels as compared to wild-type animals (Farris *et al.*, 2003). Finally, thus far, two groups have reported evidence for genetic association of haplotypes in *IDE* with AD in human study populations as well, although no single disease-modifying variants or mutations have been identified to date (Bertram *et al.*, 2002; Feuk *et al.*, 2002). These positive reports stand opposed by two fairly small negative case-control studies which did not see any evidence of association (Abraham *et al.*, 2001; Boussaha *et al.*, 2002, see *AlzGene* for an up-to-date overview).

Similar arguments have been put forward for *PLAU*, although in particular the evidence of in vivo relevance on Aβ-catabolism is less well established. *PLAU* encodes uPA which is a serine protease that converts plasminogen to plasmin, which in return is able to degrade both monomeric and oligomeric forms of Aβ, although the efficiency to carry out the latter is only about 1% as compared to monomeric Aβ. Both proteins are highly expressed in the brain, and uPA activity to generate plasmin is actually triggered by Aβ aggregates (for review, see Selkoe, 2001). Thus far, there exist only meeting reports both suggesting and refuting genetic association of this candidate gene with AD in human populations. Eventually, only sufficiently sized and appropriately designed studies will reveal whether or not *IDE* or *PLAU* (or both) are functionally, epidemiologically, and clinically relevant genetic risk factors for AD.

Findings on other chromosomes

In addition to the putative AD loci mentioned above, there have been several reports suggesting the existence of additional AD genes on various other chromosomes. Only a fraction of these can be considered positional candidate genes, i.e. not only has a biological relevance in AD pathogenesis been suggested, but they also map in or near previously reported linkage regions (Table 30.1). Examples of these are the tumor necrosis factor-α (*TNFA*) on chromosome 6q15 (Collins *et al.*, 2000), ubiquilin-1 (gene: *UBQLN1*) on 9q21 (Bertram *et al.*, 2003), or as mentioned earlier, nicastrin (*NCSTN*) on 1q23 (Dermaut *et al.*, 2002). The majority of the published AD association analyses targeted candidate genes solely on biological grounds, i.e. usually by testing functionally plausible candidates that do not map near any of the proposed linkage peaks. Examples of suggested associations are with the genes encoding cathepsin D (located on chromosome 11p15, proposed to display

γ-secretase like activities), α-synuclein (chromosome 4q22, involved in the binding and aggregation of Aβ), members of the interleukin-1 cluster genes (chromosome 2, involved in inflammatory processes) and the angiotensin-converting enzyme (chromosome 17, possibly also involved in inflammation and the regulation of the brain's renin–angiotensin system). In fact, by the end of 2001, over 60 candidate genes on 21 chromosomes had been tested for genetic association with AD, most of these involving fairly small case-control studies. With the exception of *APOE*, none of these risk factors has yet been shown to play a more than minor role in contributing to population-wide AD risk, and it is likely that most of the initial results will in fact prove to be false-positive findings (i.e. type I errors). More systematic and rigorous criteria for the design and publication of future genetic studies are needed to keep the research community focused on confirming and elucidating the most promising of the putative candidate genes, because it is these genes that will eventually broaden our understanding of the pathophysiology of AD neurodegeneration and allow the development of potential treatment strategies.

Conclusions

Despite the great progress in the field of AD genetics that has led to the discovery and confirmation of three autosomal-dominant early-onset genes and a late-onset risk factor, at least four additional major AD loci are predicted to exist. The hunt for these putative AD genes is aggravated by several factors that generally complicate the identification of complex disease genes: locus and/or allelic heterogeneity; only minor to modest effect size of any given variant; unknown, and difficult to model, interaction patterns; population differences and stratification; insufficient sample sizes/sampling strategies; the possibility of false positive results and, last but not least, linkage disequilibrium among polymorphisms other than those initially associated with the disease. The emergence of more powerful and efficient genotyping and analytic tools will ultimately enable us to disentangle the genetics of this and other complex diseases to the point where reliable and responsible genetic risk profiling will be possible. At that time, systematic assessment of individual genetic risk will dovetail with new and powerful means for therapeutically delaying or even preventing the onset of this devastating disease. This will enable a strategy of "early prediction, early prevention" forming the cornerstone of the genomic medical approach.

REFERENCES

Abraham, R., Myers, A., Wavrant-DeVrieze, F. *et al.* (2001). Substantial linkage disequilibrium across the insulin-degrading enzyme locus but no association with late-onset Alzheimer's disease. *Hum. Genet.*, **109**(6), 646–52.

AD Mutation Database (2003). *http://molgen-www.uia.ac.be/ADMutations/*

Ait-Ghezala, G., Abdullah, L., Crescentini, R. *et al.* (2002). Confirmation of association between D10S583 and Alzheimer's disease in a case-control sample. *Neurosci. Lett.*, **325**, 87–90.

AlzGene, AD genetic association database: http://www.alzgene.org.

Bertram, L. & Tanzi, R. E. (2001a). Dancing in the dark? The status of late-onset Alzheimer's disease genetics. *J. Mol. Neurosci.*, **17**(2), 127–36.

(2001b). Of replications and refutations: the status of Alzheimer's disease genetic research. *Curr. Neurol. Neurosci. Rep.*, **1**(5), 442–50.

Bertram, L., Blacker, D., Crystal, A. *et al.* (2000a). Candidate genes showing no evidence for association or linkage with Alzheimer's disease using family-based methodologies. *Exp. Gerontol.*, **35**(9–10), 1353–61.

Bertram, L., Blacker, D., Mullin, K. *et al.* (2000b). Evidence for genetic linkage of Alzheimer's disease to chromosome 10q. *Science*, **290**(5500), 2302–3.

Bertram, L., Mullin, K., Parkinson, M. *et al.* (2003). Search for novel Alzheimer's genes using family based methodologies. *Society for Neuroscience, Online*: http://www.sfn.org.

Bertram, L. & Tanzi, R. (2003). Genetics of Alzheimer's disease. In *Neurodegeneration: The Molecular Pathology of Dementia and Movement Disorders*, ed. D. Dickson. Basel: ISN Neuropath Press.

Blacker, D., Haines, J. L., Rodes, L. *et al.* (1997). ApoE-4 and age at onset of Alzheimer's disease: the NIMH genetics initiative. *Neurology*, **48**(1), 139–47.

Blacker, D., Wilcox, M. A., Laird, N. M. *et al.* (1998). Alpha-2 macroglobulin is genetically associated with Alzheimer disease. *Nat. Genet.*, **19**(4), 357–60.

Blacker, D., Bertram, L., Saunders, A. J. *et al.* (2003). Results of a high-resolution genome screen of 437 Alzheimer's Disease families. *Hum. Mol. Genet.*, **12**(1), 23–32.

Boussaha, M., Hannequin, D., Verpillat, P. *et al.* (2002). Polymorphisms of insulin degrading enzyme gene are not associated with Alzheimer's disease. *Neurosci. Lett.*, **329**(1), 121–3.

Burke, W., Pinsky, L. E. & Press, N. A. (2001). Categorizing genetic tests to identify their ethical, legal, and social implications. *Am. J. Med. Genet.*, **106**(3), 233–40.

Collins, J. S., Perry, R. T., Watson, B., Jr. *et al.* (2000). Association of a haplotype for tumor necrosis factor in siblings with late-onset Alzheimer disease: the NIMH Alzheimer Disease Genetics Initiative. *Am. J. Med. Genet.*, **96**(6), 823–30.

Daw, E. W., Payami, H., Nemens, E. J. *et al.* (2000). The number of trait loci in late-onset Alzheimer disease. *Am. J. Hum. Genet.*, **66**(1), 196–204.

Dermaut, B., Theuns, J., Sleegers, K. *et al.* (2002). The gene encoding nicastrin, a major gamma-secretase component, modifies risk for familial early-onset Alzheimer disease in a Dutch population-based sample. *Am. J. Hum. Genet.*, **70**(6), 1568–74.

Edbauer, D., Willem, M., Lammich, S. *et al.* (2002). Insulin-degrading enzyme rapidly removes the beta-amyloid precursor protein intracellular domain (AICD). *J. Biol. Chem.*, **277**(16), 13389–93.

Ertekin-Taner, N., Graff-Radford, N., Younkin, L. H. *et al.* (2000). Linkage of plasma Abeta42 to a quantitative locus on chromosome 10 in late-onset Alzheimer's disease pedigrees. *Science*, **290**(5500), 2303–4.

Fallin, D., Cohen, A., Essioux, L. *et al.* (2001). Genetic analysis of case/control data using estimated haplotype frequencies: application to APOE locus variation and Alzheimer's disease. *Genome Res.*, **11**(1), 143–51.

Farrer, L. A., Cupples, L. A., Haines, J. L. *et al.* (1997). Effects of age, sex, and ethnicity on the association between apolipoprotein E genotype and Alzheimer disease. A meta-analysis. APOE and Alzheimer Disease Meta Analysis Consortium. *J. Am. Med. Assoc.*, **278**(16), 1349–56.

Farris, R., Mansourian, S., Leissring, M. *et al.* (2002). Missense mutations in insulin-degrading enzyme associated with a diabetic phenotype in rats decrease A-beta degradation in brain. *Society for Neuroscience Meeting, Orlando, FL*, Abstract No 19.8.

Farris, W., Mansourian, S., Chang, Y. *et al.* (2003). Insulin-degrading enzyme regulates the levels of insulin, amyloid {beta}-protein, and the {beta}-amyloid precursor protein intracellular domain in vivo. *Proc. Natl Acad. Sci., USA* (**Early Edition**: www.pnas.org/cgi/dio/10.1073/pnas.0230450100)

Feuk, L., Prince, J., Graziano, C. *et al.* (2002). Multiple genes may be involved in explaining the linkage peak on chromosome 10: evidence from SNP-based association studies. *Neurobiol. Aging*, **23**, S424.

Goate, A., Chartier-Harlin, M. C., Mullan, M. *et al.* (1991). Segregation of a missense mutation in the amyloid precursor protein gene with familial Alzheimer's disease. *Nature*, **349**(6311), 704–6.

Haass, C. & De Strooper, B. (1999). The presenilins in Alzheimer's disease – proteolysis holds the key. *Science*, **286**(5441), 916–19.

Hardy, J. (1997). Amyloid, the presenilins and Alzheimer's disease. *Trends Neurosci.*, **20**(4), 154–9.

Hiltunen, M., Mannermaa, A., Thompson, D. *et al.* (2001). Genome-wide linkage disequilibrium mapping of late-onset Alzheimer's disease in Finland. *Neurology*, **57**(9), 1663–8.

Kang, D. E., Saitoh, T., Chen, X. *et al.* (1997). Genetic association of the low-density lipoprotein receptor-related protein gene (LRP), an apolipoprotein E receptor, with late-onset Alzheimer's disease. *Neurology*, **49**(1), 56–61.

Kehoe, P., Wavrant-De Vrieze, F., Crook, R. *et al.* (1999). A full genome scan for late onset Alzheimer's disease. *Hum. Mol. Genet.*, **8**(2), 237–45.

Koster, M. N., Dermaut, B., Cruts, M. *et al.* (2000). The alpha2-macroglobulin gene in AD: a population-based study and meta-analysis. *Neurology*, **55**(5), 678–84.

Kurochkin, I. V. (2001). Insulin-degrading enzyme: embarking on amyloid destruction. *Trends Biochem. Sci.*, **26**(7), 421–5.

Lambert, J. C., Goumidi, L., Vrieze, F. W. *et al.* (2000). The transcriptional factor LBP-1c/CP2/LSF gene on chromosome 12 is a genetic determinant of Alzheimer's disease. *Hum. Mol. Genet.*, **9**(15), 2275–80.

Lander, E. & Kruglyak, L. (1995). Genetic dissection of complex traits: guidelines for interpreting and reporting linkage results. *Nat. Genet.*, **11**(3), 241–7.

Levy-Lahad, E., Wasco, W. Poorkaj, P. *et al.* (1995). Candidate gene for the chromosome 1 familial Alzheimer's disease locus. *Science*, **269**(5226), 973–7.

Li, Y. J., Scott, W. K., Hedges, D. J. *et al.* (2002). Age at onset in two common neurodegenerative diseases is genetically controlled. *Am. J. Hum. Genet.*, **70**(4), 985–93.

Liao, A., Nitsch, R. M., Greenberg, S. M. *et al.* (1998). Genetic association of an alpha2-macroglobulin (Val1000Ile) polymorphism and Alzheimer's disease. *Hum. Mol. Genet.*, **7**(12), 1953–6.

Luedecking-Zimmer, E., DeKosky, S. T., Nebes, R. *et al.* (2003). Association of the 3' UTR transcription factor LBP-1c/CP2/LSF polymorphism with late-onset Alzheimer's disease. *Am. J. Med. Genet.*, **117B**(1), 114–17.

Martin, E. R., Lai, E. H., Gilbert, J. R. *et al.* (2000). SNPing away at complex diseases: analysis of single-nucleotide polymorphisms around APOE in Alzheimer disease. *Am. J. Hum. Genet.*, **67**(2), 383–94.

Meyer, M. R., Tschanz, J. T., Norton, M. C. *et al.* (1998). APOE genotype predicts when – not whether – one is predisposed to develop Alzheimer disease. *Nat. Genet.*, **19**(4), 321–2.

Mullan, M., Houlden, H., Windelspecht, M. *et al.* (1992). A locus for familial early-onset Alzheimer's disease on the long arm of chromosome 14, proximal to the alpha 1-antichymotrypsin gene. *Nat. Genet.*, **2**(4), 340–2.

Myers, A., Holmans, P., Marshall, H. *et al.* (2000). Susceptibility locus for Alzheimer's disease on chromosome 10. *Science*, **290**(5500), 2304–5.

Nacmias, B., Latorraca, S., Piersanti, P. *et al.* (1995). ApoE genotype and familial Alzheimer's disease: a possible influence on age of onset in APP717 Val–>Ile mutated families. *Neurosci. Lett.*, **183**(1–2), 1–3.

Orlacchio, A., Kawarai, T., Polidoro, M. *et al.* (2002). Association analysis between Alzheimer's disease and the Nicastrin gene polymorphisms. *Neurosci. Lett.*, **333**(2), 115–18.

Pericak-Vance, M. A., Bass, M. P., Yamaoka, L. H. *et al.* (1997). Complete genomic screen in late-onset familial Alzheimer disease. Evidence for a new locus on chromosome 12. *J. Am. Med. Assoc.*, **278**(15), 1237–41.

Pericak-Vance, M. A., Bebout, J. L., Gaskell, P. C. *et al.* (1991). Linkage studies in familial Alzheimer disease: evidence for chromosome 19 linkage. *Am. J. Hum. Genet.*, **48**(6), 1034–50.

Poirier, J. (2000). Apolipoprotein E and Alzheimer's disease. A role in amyloid catabolism. *Ann. NY Acad. Sci.*, **924**, 81–90.

Rogaev, E. I., Sherrington, R., Rogaeva, E. A. *et al.* (1995). Familial Alzheimer's disease in kindreds with missense mutations in a gene on chromosome 1 related to the Alzheimer's disease type 3 gene. *Nature*, **376**(6543), 775–8.

Rogaeva, E., Premkumar, S., Song, Y. *et al.* (1998). Evidence for an Alzheimer disease susceptibility locus on chromosome 12 and for further locus heterogeneity. *J. Am. Med. Assoc.*, **280**(7), 614–8.

Saunders, A. J., Bertram, L., Mullin, K. *et al.* (2003). Genetic association of Alzheimer's disease with multiple polymorphisms in alpha-2-macroglobulin. *Hum. Mol. Genet.*, **12**, 2765–76.

Saunders, A. M., Strittmatter, W. J., Schmechel, D. *et al.* (1993). Association of apolipoprotein E allele epsilon 4 with late-onset familial and sporadic Alzheimer's disease. *Neurology*, **43**(8), 1467–72.

Schellenberg, G. D., Bird, T. D. Wijsman, E. M. *et al.* (1992). Genetic linkage evidence for a familial Alzheimer's disease locus on chromosome 14. *Science*, **258**(5082), 668–71.

Scott, W. K., Grubber, J., Coneally, P. M. *et al.* (2000). Fine-mapping of the chromosome 12 Alzheimer disease locus using family-based association tests of microsatellite markers. *Neurobiol. Aging*, **21** (abstract), S129.

Scott, W. K., Yamaoka, L. H., Bass, M. P. *et al.* (1998). No genetic association between the LRP receptor and sporadic or late- onset familial Alzheimer disease. *Neurogenetics*, **1**(3), 179–83.

Selkoe, D. J. (2001). Clearing the brain's amyloid cobwebs. *Neuron*, **32**(2), 177–80.

Sherrington, R., Rogaev, E. I., Liang, Y. *et al.* (1995). Cloning of a gene bearing missense mutations in early-onset familial Alzheimer's disease. *Nature*, **375**(6534), 754–60.

St George-Hyslop, P., Haines, J., Rogaev, E. *et al.* (1992). Genetic evidence for a novel familial Alzheimer's disease locus on chromosome 14. *Nat. Genet.*, **2**(4), 330–4.

Strittmatter, W. J., Saunders, A. M., Schmechel, D. *et al.* (1993). Apolipoprotein E: high-avidity binding to beta-amyloid and increased frequency of type 4 allele in late-onset familial Alzheimer disease. *Proc. Natl Acad. Sci.*, *USA*, **90**(5), 1977–81.

Tanzi, R. E. (1999). A genetic dichotomy model for the inheritance of Alzheimer's disease and common age-related disorders. *J. Clin. Invest.*, **104**(9), 1175–9.

Tanzi, R. E. & Bertram, L. (2001). New frontiers in Alzheimer's disease genetics. *Neuron*, **32**(2), 181–4.

Tanzi, R. E., Gusella, J. F., Watkins, P. C. *et al.* (1987). Amyloid beta protein gene: cDNA, mRNA distribution, and genetic linkage near the Alzheimer locus. *Science*, **235**(4791), 880–4.

Taylor, A. E., Yip, A., Brayne, C. *et al.* (2001). Genetic association of an LBP-1c/CP2/LSF gene polymorphism with late onset Alzheimer's disease. *J. Med. Genet.*, **38**(4), 232–3.

Ulery, P. G. & Strickland, D. K. (2000). LRP in Alzheimer's disease: friend or foe? *J. Clin. Invest.*, **106**(9), 1077–9.

Van Broeckhoven, C., Backhovens, H., Cruts, M. *et al.* (1992). Mapping of a gene predisposing to early-onset Alzheimer's disease to chromosome 14q24.3. *Nat. Genet.*, **2**(4), 335–9.

Vassar, R. (2001). The beta-secretase, BACE: a prime drug target for Alzheimer's disease. *J. Mol. Neurosci.*, **17**(2), 157–70.

Verpillat, P., Bouley, S., Hannequin, D. *et al.* (2000). Alpha2-macroglobulin gene and Alzheimer's disease: confirmation of association by haplotypes analyses. *Ann. Neurol.*, **48**(3), 400–2.

Wu, W. S., Holmans, P., Wavrant-DeVrieze, F. *et al.* (1998). Genetic studies on chromosome 12 in late-onset Alzheimer disease. *J. Am. Med. Assoc.*, **280**(7), 619–22.

Yu, G., Nishimura, M., Arawaka, S. *et al.* (2000). Nicastrin modulates presenilin-mediated notch/glp-1 signal transduction and betaAPP processing. *Nature*, **407**(6800), 48–54.

The role of ß-amyloid in Alzheimer's disease

Roger M. Nitsch

Division of Psychiatry Research, University of Zurich, Switzerland

Introduction

ß-Amyloid is a central element of the histopathology of Alzheimer's disease. It damages neurons and it causes the formation of neurofibrillary tangles. It is genetically linked to mutations that cause familial Alzheimer's disease, and it is associated with polymorphisms that increase the risk for developing Alzheimer's disease. ß-Amyloid can be imaged by positron emission tomography in living people, and it is a major therapeutic target for the development of disease-modifying therapies (Selkoe, 2004).

ß-amyloid plaques are major histophathological hallmarks of Alzheimer's disease

The neuropathological diagnosis of Alzheimer's disease is based upon the presence in brain of ß-amyloid plaques and neurofibrillary tangles (Duyckaerts & Dickson, 2003). ß-Amyloid deposits occur within the neuropil in several forms depending upon the degree of aggregation and fibrillization of the amyloid ß-peptides $A\beta_{40}$ and $A\beta_{42}$, their principal proteinaceous components. The two most abundant, albeit different, forms of amyloid plaques are neuritic ß-amyloid plaques and diffuse plaques. Neuritic, or "senile," ß-amyloid plaques occur rarely in healthy subjects, they are an early histopathological sign of Alzheimer's disease (Tiraboschi *et al.*, 2004). Neuritic ß-amyloid plaques are composed of higher-order ß-amyloid fibrils that can be detected by Thioflavin S or Congo red, as well as by silver-based stains and by immunohistochemistry. Amyloid fibrils within the cores of neuritic ß-amyloid plaques visualized by electron microscopy have diameters of up to 10 nm, and often occur in radiating, star-like assemblies. Neuritic ß-amyloid plaques are closely associated with dystrophic neurites, with defective cell membranes and with cystoskeletal abnormalities pointing to the possibility that their components have neurotoxic activities. Neuritic ß-amyloid plaques are surrounded by reactive, GFAP-positive astrocytes. Frequently, these form a cellular outer layer separating the plaques from the surrounding tissue. In this form, reactive astrocytes may function as part of a physiological defence mechanism that protects healthy tissue from ß-amyloid-related pathology. In addition, activated microglia, the brain-resident macrophages, are frequently found within the plaques, and in close association with amyloid fibrils. Sometimes, microglia are filled with ß-amyloid fibrils. This association has led to the idea that microglia could possess a capacity of phagocytosing ß-amyloid fibrils, and thus may have a role in the natural turnover of brain ß-amyloid. In addition to Aß peptides, there are many other non-amyloid components associated with ß-amyloid plaques. This is due to the hydrophobic, sticky, nature of ß-amyloid that gives rise to hydrophobic interaction with multiple other proteins, proteogycans, lipoproteins, cholesterol and lipids. The non-amyloid proteins include proinflammatory cytokines that are most likely microglia-derived, pointing to two parallel roles of ß-amyloid-associated microglia: phagocytosis and proinflammatory signalling. The possible beneficial or toxic consequences of this dual microglia function are still controversial.

Additional forms of ß-amyloid deposits include cotton-wool plaques, these are large spherical structures composed of $A\beta_{42}$ with dense cores that are stained by H&E stains. Like neuritic plaques, cotton wool plaques are often accompanied by neuritic dystrophy, and they are infiltrated by microglia. In contrast, diffuse plaques, also referred to as "preamyloid," are deposits of soluble and oligomeric forms of Aß peptides with low degrees of fibrillization. In the histophathological routine, diffuse plaques are detected only by immunohistochemistry; they are negative for ß-amyloid-staining dyes including Thioflavin S or Congo red. Diffuse plaques often have irregular contours; some forms are fleecy and lake-like, they are usually not accompanied by dystrophic neurites or other obvious signs of neuronal pathology, and they can also occur in healthy aged subjects without Alzheimer's disease (Delaère *et al.*, 1991, 1993).

In four out of five patients with Alzheimer's disease, ß-amyloid fibrils are also deposited around cerebral blood vessels at the external face of perivascular smooth muscle cells. Perivascular ß-amyloid fibrils lead to cerebral amyloid angiopathy, replace perivascular smooth muscle cells, causing vessel wall fragility, with occasional leakage and microhemorrhages. Moreover perivascular ß-amyloid deposits may hinder periavascular interstitial fluid drainage into the cervical lymph system (Nicoll *et al.*, 2004).

Neurofibrillary tangles

A histophathological diagnosis of Alzheimer's disease is made in a case of progressive dementia when ß-amyloid plaques co-occur with neurofibrillary tangles. These are intracellular accumulations of paired helical filaments composed of the microtubule-binding protein tau. Under physiological conditions, tau plays a role in stabilizing axonal microtubules that are essential for axonal transport. Paired helical filament formation is associated with detachment of tau from their axonal microtubule binding sites, re-localization to the cell bodies and dendrites, abnormal phosphorylation and fibril formation. Neurons with neurofibrillary tangles degenerate and die, leaving within the neuropil a residual "ghost tangle," sometimes with flame-shaped contours reminding of the pyramidal cell body in which it was initially formed. Dendritic tau filaments often occur as "neuropil threads." Both neurofibrillary tangles and neuropil threads are readily stained with silver-based protocols, as well as with antibodies against phosphorylated tau. NFT occur in many neurodegenerative diseases, in a group of diseases that is referred to as "taupathies" (Giasson *et al.*, 2003). These include frontotemporal dementia, Pick's disease and boxer's dementia. This broad spectrum of diseases suggests that tau pathology along with the formation of NFT is a fairly general reaction of neurons to damage, and that many different toxic events can end up in the formation of neurofibrillary tangle. The co-occurrence of neurofibrillary tangles and ß-amyloid plaques in Alzheimer's disease suggests the possibility that ß-amyloid-related toxicity could be the toxic event that triggers the formation of neurofibrillary tangles.

ß-amyloid-related toxicity causes the formation of neurofibrillary tangles

The formation of ß-amyloid plaques occurs early in the pathophysiological cascade leading to Alzheimer's disease. ß-Amyloid plaque formation precedes the onset of clinical signs by a long pre-clinical time period of several decades, and ß-amyloid plaque burden reaches a maximum by the time the initial clinical signs begin to show (Ingelsson *et al.*, 2004). Overwhelming experimental evidence suggests that accumulation of ß-amyloid is paralleled by neurotoxicity that causes many – if not all – of the multiple abnormalities observed in Alzheimer's disease. These include neurodegeneration, inflammation, oxidative stress, cytoskeletal abnormalities, synaptic dysfunction, deficits in neurotransmission, homeostasis of ions and metabolism (Greeve *et al.*, 2004; Dudal *et al.*, 2004; Lewis *et al.*, 2001; Götz *et al.*, 2001; Stern *et al.*, 2004; Chapman *et al.*, 1999; Walsh *et al.*, 2002; Mattson and Chan, 2003; Mattson, 2004). In the brains of transgenic mice both endogenously expressed Aß as well as microinjected synthetic ß-amyloid fibrils can cause the formation of neurofibrillary tangles (Götz *et al.*, 2001; Lewis *et al.*, 2001). Other models using triple transgenic mice or tissue culture support this mechanism (Ferrari *et al.*, 2003; Oddo *et al.*, 2003, 2004). In human brains with Alzheimer's disease, a pathomechanistic link between ß-amyloid and neurofibrillary tangles is underscored by clinico-pathological correlations suggesting that ß-amyloid-induced cognitive decline is mediated by the formation of neurofibrillary tangles (Bennett *et al.*, 2004). Microinjections of ß-amyloid into brains of transgenic mice have demonstrated a special separation of ß-amyloid and neurofibrillary tangles formed in the cell bodies of neurons projecting with their axons to the microinjection sites of ß-amyloid. This observation suggested that ß-amyloid-related neurotoxicity is causing retrograde axonal degeneration, and formation of neurofibrillary tangles within the bodies of the neurons projecting to ß-amyloid. Neuropathological evidence in human patients demonstrating neurofibrillary tangles in subcortical projection neurons that project to cortical areas with high ß-amyloid burden supports this view of anatomical separation (Duyckaerts & Dickson, 2003). The molecular mechanisms of ß-amyloid-related toxicity are not well understood. They may involve the generation of reactive oxygen species as well as increased cytoplasmic Ca^{2+} concentrations within neurons caused either by increased influx or increased release from the ER or by mitochondrial dysfunction (Mattson, 2004).

Genetic evidence links ß-amyloid formation to familial Alzheimer's disease

Familial forms of Alzheimer's disease are caused by mutations in the APP, presenilin 1 and 2 genes (Tanzi & Bertram, 2001). These mutations cause the formation of more, or C-terminally extended, Aß peptides that lead to accelerated aggregation and ß-amyloid formation. The triplication of the APP gene in Down's syndrome invariably results in a histopathology of Alzheimer's disease in adults, with both ß-amyloid and neurofibrillary tangles. Moreover, several susceptibility genes including ApoE, leading to an increased risk for Alzheimer's disease, are also associated with accelerated ß-amyloid formation. Thus, the available genetic evidence points to the possibility that increased generation of ß-amyloid caused by genetic variations increases the risk for Alzheimer's disease. It is noteworthy that mutations that cause increased ß-amyloid are also associated with the formation of neurofibrillary tangles, whereas mutations in the tau gene cause "tangle-only" frontotemporal dementia, without ß-amyloid plaques. Thus, while neurofibrillary tangles are clearly related to neurodegeneration in the tauopathies, they hardly induce ß-amyloid plaque formation.

Aß peptides are generated by ß-and γ-secretases that function in APP signalling

The generation of Aß from its precursor, the ß-amyloid precursor protein (APP) was extensively reviewed (Marjaux *et al.*, 2004; Koo & Kopan, 2004; Aguzzi & Haass, 2003; Selkoe & Kopan, 2003). Briefly, Aß is generated by proteolytic processing of APP by a sequential cleavage event mediated by ß-secretase, or ß-APP cleaving enzyme (BACE) and γ-secretase, a transmembrane multiprotein complex composed of presenilin, nicastrin, Aph-1, and Pen-2. Amyloidogenic APP processing initiated by BACE-mediated cleavage at the ectodomain, resulting in ectodomain shedding and in the generation of a membrane-bound carboxyl-terminal fragment that is a substrate for γ-secretase processing within the membrane via a proteolytic mechanism referred to as regulated intramembraneous proteolysis. Regulated intramembraneous processing by γ-secretase is non-selective as it cleaves many substrates including the E- and N-cadherins, notch1–4, delta, jagged, CD44, EbrB4

and many others. γ-secretase cleavage of the membrane-bound APP carboxyl-terminal fragment results in the secretion of Aß, that can potentially aggregate and form ß-amyloid fibrils. as well as in the liberation of the APP intracellular domain (AICD) into the cytoplasm where it binds to the adaptor proteins Fe65, Jip 1b or X11α – MINT1 that result either in cytoplamic retention or translocation into the nucleus where the shuttle complex associates with Tip60 to function in transcriptional regulation (Von Rotz *et al.*, 2004). The AICD complex increases the transcription of the APP gene, thereby regulating the concentrations of its own precursor (Von Rotz *et al.*, 2004). Other functions of the APP include a potential neurotrophic, growth-promoting activity of its ectodomain. The ectodomain includes, at its N-terminal end, a heparin-binding domain with possible roles in interacting with components of the extracellular matrix and with cell-surface molecules. It is also possible that this domain functions in cell surface-associated full-length APP in forming *trans*-homodimers with a role in cell–cell interactions (Rossjohn *et al.*, 1999).

Aggregation of soluble Aß into insoluble ß-amyloid fibrils

The formation of ß-amyloid fibrils found in ß-amyloid plaques from the soluble monomeric Aß peptides $Aß_{40}$ and $Aß_{42}$ involves oligomerization and nucleation leading to larger-order aggregates with conformational changes that are associated with increasing insolubility and ultimately, the precipitation of ß-amyloid fibrils that can grow further by the addition of soluble Aß peptides or oligomers.

The temporal sequence of aggregation into oligomers, proto-fibrils and fibrils is paralleled by increasing signs of neurodegeneration in human brains. Early, diffuse Aß deposits are often present in brains of cognitively healthy aged subjects, and they are not associated with neuropathology, but their further aggregation into insoluble fibrils is accompanied by neuritic dystrophy, neurodegeneration and functional loss (Knopman *et al.*, 2003). Thus, the neurotoxicity of the various forms of Aß aggregates is related to their degree of fibrillization. This does not exclude the possibility that soluble oligomers of Aß can also be causing neuronal dysfunction as suggested by their suppressing activities on long-term potentiation in experimental animals (Walsh *et al.*, 2002). The principle of confirmation-dependent insolubility paralleled by neurotoxicity may be a more general principle of neurodegenerative diseases underlying many other disorders as exemplified by α-synuclein deposits in Lewy bodies in

Parkinson's disease, Huntingtin inclusions in Huntington's disease, PrP^{Sc} plaques in BSE, scapie and CJD, as well as neurofibrillary tangles in taupathies including fronto-temporal dementia.

Imaging of ß-amyloid in living people

ß-amyloid can be imaged by PET in living people (Klunk *et al.*, 2004). This possibility puts researchers in the fortunate position of testing whether treatments designed to reduce brain ß-amyloid work as expected. When correlated with clinical efficacy, PET imaging of ß-amyloid will become an important primary outcome variable for future clinical trials designed to reduce brain ß-amyloid. Moreover, preclinical detection of ß-amyloid by PET in preclinical AD may ultimately identify an aged population with brain ß-amyloidosis who is at high risk for developing clinical signs of AD. If safe, ß-amyloid-lowering treatments could be a future option for prevention in these subjects at risk.

ß-Amyloid is a therapeutic target for the treatment and prevention of AD

The reduction of ß-amyloid is a major goal for the current development of novel strategies for the treatment and prevention of Alzheimer's disease. The principal idea common to these therapeutic approaches is based upon the hypothesis that lowering in brain the amount of ß-amyloid will lead to reduced ß-amyloid-related toxicity, and ultimately, to the disruption of the cascade leading to neuronal damage, neurofibrillary tangles, and neurodegeneration. In the absence of ß-amyloid-related toxicity, regeneration may occur to repair some of the tissue damage previously caused by ß-amyloid. A large variety of diverse possibilities to reach this goal is being currently pursued. It ranges from inhibitors of BACE and γ-secretase inhibitors, to stimulators of α-secretase by neurotransmitter receptor agonists (Nitsch *et al.*, 1992, 2000), acceleration of Aß degradation by Aß-cleaving enzymes including neprilysin and insulin-degrading enzyme, inhibition of Aß-aggregation with Aß-binding compounds or metal ion chelators, and removal of ß-amyloid by antibodies against ß-amyloid, to name just a few. Initial early phase studies of ß-amyloid-lowering treatments with either the metal ion chelator clioquinol or the glycosaminoglycan mimetic Alzhemed, or ß-amyloid immunotherapy consistently show signs of clinical efficacy (Aisen *et al.*, 2004; Ritchie *et al.*, 2003; Hock *et al.*, 2003; Gilman *et al.*, 2004). Larger studies are now performed to

confirm these initial positive findings. Moreover, the developments of BACE- and γ-secretase inhibitors are reaching clinical study phases.

Despite the fact that the toxic mechanisms linking ß-amyloid to neurodegeneration are incompletely understood, several therapeutic approaches were designed to block such suspected toxic consequences of ß-amyloid as oxidation and inflammation. Vitamin E alone, or together with vitamin C, tested in human trials had some, albeit small, degree of clinical efficacy (Sano *et al.*, 1997; Zandi *et al.*, 2004). In contrast, cinical trials of anti-inflammatory agents including either steroidal or non-steroidal anti-inflammatory agents were consistently negative (van Gool *et al.*, 2003). These results clearly emphasize the need for better understanding of the molecular mechanisms of ß-amyloid-related toxicity, as well as the need for identifying therapeutic targets within this cascade.

Immunization against ß-amyloid

Immunotherapy protocols are currently developed both in experimental animals and in initial clinical trials. Either active immunization with ß-amyloid-related epitopes or passive antibody transfer consistently reduce brain ß-amyloid load, followed by reductions in tau phosphorylation, protection of neurons and by improvements in ß-amyloid-related behavioral deficits. (Schenk *et al.*, 1999; Bard *et al.*, 2000; Morgan *et al.*, 2000; Mohajeri *et al.*, 2002, Lombardo et al., 2003; Wilcock *et al.*, 2004; Oddo *et al.*, 2004; Lemere *et al.*, 2004). Moreover, initial data from the first clinical immunotherapy trial suggest clinical efficacy in human patients with Alzheimer's disease. In this trial, ß-amyloid fibrils generated by aggregation of synthetic Aß$_{42}$ peptides were used as an immunogen to stimulate a humeral immune response and the generation of antibodies against ß-amyloid. Episodes of meningoencephalitis in some of the participants unfortunately caused the trial to be interrupted, but careful analyses of the immunized patients showed clinical efficacy in patients with Alzheimer's disease (Hock *et al.*, 2003; Gilman *et al.*, 2004). In particular, the presence of antibodies against ß-amyloid was associated with clinical stabilization and with slowed rates of cognitive decline over more than 2 years. Remarkably, a fraction of the IgG antibodies against ß-amyloid were present in CSF, suggesting that they are able to cross the blood-brain barrier (Hock *et al.*, 2003). The mechanisms for blood-brain barrier passage of plasma-derived IgG are incompletely understood, they may include increased blood-brain barrier permeability, possibly related to disease- or vaccination-induced inflammatory responses, passive diffusion, and active shuttling, possibly via F$_{cN}$-mediated transcytosis. These initial clinical data are supported by neuropathological analyses in four brains obtained at autopsy. Consistently, these studies showed reduced ß-amyloid pathology in extended brain areas, accompanied by reduced astrogliosis and maintained tangle pathology (Nicoll *et al.*, 2003; Ferrer *et al.*, 2004). Together with the stabilization of the clinical signs, these data could be indicative of initial proof of principle that links removal of ß-amyloid with clinical efficacy. Importantly, removal of ß-amyloid was also observed in the absence of prior episodes of meningoencephalitis strongly suggesting that meningoencephalitis is not required for ß-amyloid removal. Therefore, the previously raised speculation that clinical inflammation is required to clear ß-amyloid is not supported by the existing clinical and neuropathological data. There are three mechanisms currently discussed to explain the therapeutic response to immunotherapy, and all involve removal, or reduction, of brain ß-amyloid: microglia-mediated removal of amyloid, removal by peripheral amyloid sink, and antibody-mediated disaggregation of amyloid. These mechanisms may play in concert, but microglia-mediated uptake is almost certainly involved as indicated by the presence of microglia filled with ß-amyloid in brain areas that have been cleared of ß-amyloid following immunotherapy (Nicoll *et al.*, 2003).

Possibly related, exciting new features of antibodies against ß-amyloid are their effects on brain volume in patients with Alzheimer's disease. Results from two studies independently demonstrated that hippocampal volumes decrease more rapidly in the presence of antibodies against ß-amyloid during the initial year following vaccination, as compared to patients without antibodies against ß-amyloid (Fox *et al.*, 2004; Hock *et al.*, submitted). At first glance, these results may be counterintuitive. But they also raise the possibility of reflecting clearance of ß-amyloid plaques accompanied by a concurrent loss in astrocyte activation. Brain ß-amyloid burden in brain cortex can exceed 5% of the cortical volume, and reactive astrocytes in AD are hypertrophic with volumes that exceed many-fold their volumes in dormant states, therefore clearance of ß-amyloid and reduction in astrocyte hypertrophy may sufficiently explain initial volume losses. An additional factor that may underlie initial volume losses following immunotherapy was recently observed in transgenic mice where antibodies against Aß straightened out neurites that had been previously curvy and distorted due to an Alzheimer's disease-causing mutation (Lombardo *et al.*, 2003). Thus, initial brain volume losses in patients with Alzheimer's disease after vaccination may prove to be the first objective signs of relief: It should be followed, however, after a first clearance phase of ß-amyloid, by a second phase of stabilization, or even slight increases in brain volume, as signs of recovery and regeneration. In the first long-term follow-up analyses of hippocampal volumes in patients with antibodies against ß-amyloid, this pattern of initial volume loss followed by compensatory increases was actually observed. Combined with MRI volumetry, amyloid PET imaging will allow to address this possibility further during the upcoming clinical immunotherapy trials.

Other treatments of Alzheimer's disease

Novel disease-modifying approaches for the treatment and the prevention of Alzheimer's disease has replaced the attitude of therapeutic nihilism that clouded the field for a long time. Neurotransmitter-based therapies with Acetylcholine esterase inhibitors and NMDA receptor antagonists are now in current use; anti-inflammatory and anti-oxidative approaches as well as compounds that inhibit Aß aggregation, passive transfer of antibodies against ß-amyloid as well as active immunization against ß-amyloid are being tested in the clinic; ß- and γ-secretase inhibitors designed to reduce generation of Aß peptides are under development and will reach the clinic soon. Together, and possibly combined, these efforts are likely to generate better treatments for Alzheimer's disease in the near future.

Acknowledgements

I thank my many colleagues who participated in generating a wealth of knowledge on the role of ß-amyloid in Alzheimer's disease, and Dr. Christoph Hock for continued collaboration. This work was supported by grants from the NCCR on Neural Plasticity and Repair, EU-APOPIS and the Stammbach foundation.

REFERENCES

Aguzzi, A. & Haass, C. (2003). Games played by rogue proteins in prion disorders and Alzheimer's disease. *Science*, **302**, 814–18.

Aisen, P. S., Mehran, M., Poole, R. *et al.* (2004). Clinical data on Alzhemed™ after 12 months of treatment in patients with mild to moderate Alzheimer's disease. *Neurobiol. Aging*, **25S2**, 20 (abstract)

Bard, F., Cannon, C., Barbour, R. *et al.* (2000). Peripherally administered antibodies against amyloid beta-peptide enter the central nervous system and reduce pathology in a mouse model of Alzheimer disease. *Nat. Med.* **6**, 916–19.

Bennett, D. A., Schneider, J. A., Wilson, R. S., Bienias, J. L. & Arnold, S. E. (2004). Neurofibrillary tangles mediate the association of amyloid load with clinical Alzheimer disease and level of cognitive function. *Arch. Neurol.*, **61**, 378–84.

Chapman, P. F., White, G. L., Jones, M. W. *et al.* (1999). Impaired synaptic plasticity and learning in aged amyloid precursor protein transgenic mice. *Nat. Neurosci.*, **2**, 271–6.

Delaere, P., Duyckaerts, C., He, Y., Piette, F. & Hauw, J. J. (1991). Subtypes and differential laminar distributions of beta A4 deposits in Alzheimer's disease: relationship with the intellectual status of 26 cases. *Acta Neuropathol.*, **81**, 328–35.

Delaere, P., He, Y., Fayet, G., Duyckaerts, C. & Hauw, J. J. (1993). Beta A4 deposits are constant in the brain of the oldest old: an immunocytochemical study of 20 French centenarians. *Neurobiol. Aging*, **14**, 191–4.

Dudal, S., Krzywkowski, P., Paquette, J. *et al.* (2004). P, Gervais F. Inflammation occurs early during the Abeta deposition process in TgCRND8 mice. *Neurobiol. Aging*, **25**, 861–71.

Duyckaerts, C. & Dickson, D. W. (2003). Neuropathology in Alzheimer's disease. In *Neurodegeneration. The Molecular Pathology of Dementia and Movement Disorders*, ed. Dickson Basel: ISN Neuropath Press. pp. 47–65.

Ferrari, A., Hoerndli, F., Baechi, T., Nitsch, R. M. & Götz, J. (2003). Beta-amyloid induces PHF-like tau filaments in tissue culture. *J. Biol. Chem.*, **278**, 40162–8.

Ferrer, I., Boada Rovira, M., Sanchez Guerra, M. L., Rey, M. J. & Costa-Jussa, F. (2004). Neuropathology and pathogenesis of encephalitis following amyloid-beta immunization in Alzheimer's disease. *Brain Pathol.*, **14**, 11–20.

Fox, N. C., Black, R. S., Gilman, S. *et al.* (2004). Effects of a-beta immunotherapy (AN1792) on MRI measures of brain, ventricle and hippocampal volumes in Alzheimer's disease. *NeuroBiol. Aging*, **25S2**, 84.

Giasson, B. I., Lee, V. M. & Trojanowski, J. Q. (2003). Interactions of amyloidogenic proteins. *Neuromolec. Med.*, 49–58.

Gilman, S., Koller, M., Black, R. S. *et al.* (2004). Neuropsychological, CSF, and neuropathological effects of a-beta immunotherapy (AN1792) of Alzheimer's disease in an interrupted trial. *Neurobiol. Aging*, **25S2**, 84 (abstract).

Götz, J., Chen, F., Van Dorpe, J. & Nitsch, R. M. (2001). Abeta42 fibrils induce the formation of neurofibrillary tangles in P301L tau transgenic mice. *Science*, **293**, 1491–5.

Greeve, I., Kretzschmar, D., Beyn, A. *et al.* (2004). Age-dependent neurodegeneration and Alzheimer-amyloid plaque formation in transgenic *Drosophila*. *J. Neurosci.*, **24**, 3899–906.

Hock, C., Konietzko, U., Papassotiropoulos, A. *et al.* (2002). Generation of antibodies specific for beta-amyloid by vaccination of patients with Alzheimer disease. *Nat. Med.*, **8**, 1270–5.

Hock, C., Konietzko, U., Streffer, J. R. *et al.* (2003). Antibodies against beta-amyloid slow cognitive decline in Alzheimer's disease. *Neuron*, **38**, 547–54.

Ingelsson, M., Fukumoto, H., Newell, K. L. *et al.* (2004). Early A-beta accumulation and progressive synaptic loss, gliosis, and tangle formation in AD brain. *Neurology*, **62**, 925–31.

Klunk, W. E., Engler, H., Nordberg, A. *et al.* (2004). Imaging brain amyloid in Alzheimer's disease with Pittsburgh Compound-B. *Ann. Neurol.*, **55**, 306–19.

Knopman, D. S., Parisi, J. E., Salviati, A. *et al.* (2003). Neuropathology of cognitively normal elderly. *J. Neuropathol. Exp. Neurol.*, **62**, 1087–95.

Koo, E. H. & Kopan, R. (2004). Potential role of presenilin-regulated signaling pathways in sporadic neurodegeneration. *Nat. Med.*, 10 Suppl:S26–33.

Lemere, C. A., Beierschmitt, A., Iglesias, M. *et al.* (2004). Alzheimer's disease abeta vaccine reduces central nervous system abeta levels in a non-human primate, the Caribbean vervet. *Am. J. Pathol.*, **165**, 283–97.

Lewis, J., Dickson, D. W., Lin, W. L. *et al.* (2001). Enhanced neurofibrillary degeneration in transgenic mice expressing mutant tau and APP. *Science*, **293**, 1487–91.

Lombardo, J. A., Stern, E. A., McLellan, M. E. *et al.* (2003). Amyloid-beta antibody treatment leads to rapid normalization of plaque-induced neuritic alterations. *J. Neurosci.*, **23**, 10879–83.

Marjaux, E., Hartmann, D. & De Strooper, B. (2004). Presenilins in memory, Alzheimer's disease, and therapy. *Neuron*, **42**(2), 189–92.

Mattson, M. P. (2004). Pathways towards and away from Alzheimer's disease. *Nature*, **430**, 631–9.

Mattson, M. P. & Chan, S. L. (2003). Neuronal and glial calcium signaling in Alzheimer's disease. *Cell Calcium*, **34**, 385–97.

Mohajeri, H. M., Saini, K., Schultz, J. G., Wollmer, M. A., Hock, C. & Nitsch, R. M. (2002). Passive immunization against β-amyloid peptide protects CNS neurons from increased vulnerability associated with an Alzheimer's disease-causing mutation *J. Biol. Chem.*, **277**, 33012–17.

Morgan, D., Diamond, D. M., Gottschall, P. E. *et al.* (2000). A beta peptide vaccination prevents memory loss in an animal model of Alzheimer's disease. *Nature*, **408**, 982–5.

Nicoll, J. A., Wilkinson, D., Holmes, C., Steart, P., Markham, H. & Weller, R. O. (2003). Neuropathology of human Alzheimer disease after immunization with amyloid-beta peptide: a case report. *Nat. Med.*, **9**, 448–52.

Nicoll, J. A., Yamada, M., Frackowiak, J., Mazur-Kolecka, B. & Weller, R. O. (2004). Cerebral amyloid angiopathy plays a direct role in the pathogenesis of Alzheimer's disease. Pro-CAA position statement. *Neurobiol. Aging*, **25**, 589–97

Nitsch, R. M., Slack, B. E., Wurtman, R. J. & Growdon, J. H. (1992). Release of Alzheimer amyloid precursor derivatives stimulated by activation of muscarinic acetylcholine receptors. *Science*, **258**, 304–7.

Nitsch, R. M., Deng, M., Tennis, M., Schoenfeld, D. & Growdon, J. H. (2000). The selective muscarinic M1 agonist AF102B decreases levels of total Abeta in cerebrospinal fluid of patients with Alzheimer's disease. *Ann. Neurol.*, **48**, 913–18.

Oddo, S., Caccamo, A., Shepherd, J. D. *et al.* (2003). Triple-transgenic model of Alzheimer's disease with plaques and tangles: intracellular Abeta and synaptic dysfunction. *Neuron*, **39**, 409–21.

Oddo, S., Billings, L., Kesslak, J. P., Cribbs, D. H. & LaFerla, F. M. (2004). Abeta immunotherapy leads to clearance of early, but not late, hyperphosphorylated tau aggregates via the proteasome. *Neuron*, **43**, 321–32.

Ritchie, C. W., Bush, A. I., Mackinnon, A. *et al.* (2003). Metal–protein attenuation with iodochlorhydroxyquin (clioquinol) targeting Abeta amyloid deposition and toxicity in Alzheimer disease: a pilot phase 2 clinical trial. *Arch. Neurol.*, **60**, 1685–91.

Rossjohn, J., Cappai, R., Feil, S. C. *et al.* (1999). Crystal structure of the N-terminal, growth factor-like domain of Alzheimer amyloid precursor protein. *Nat. Struct. Biol.*, **6**(4), 327–31.

Sano, M., Ernesto, C., Thomas, R. G. *et al.* (1997). A controlled trial of selegiline, alpha-tocopherol, or both as treatment for Alzheimer's disease. The Alzheimer's Disease Cooperative Study. *N. Engl. J. Med.*, **336**, 1216–22.

Schenk, D., Barbour, R., Dunn, W. *et al.* (1999). Immunization with amyloid-beta attenuates Alzheimer-disease-like pathology in the PDAPP mouse. *Nature*, **400**, 173–7.

Selkoe, D. J. (2004). Alzheimer disease: mechanistic understanding predicts novel therapies. *Ann. Intern. Med.*, **140**, 627–38.

Selkoe, D. & Kopan, R. (2003). Notch and Presenilin: regulated intramembrane proteolysis links development and degeneration. *Annu. Rev. Neurosci.*, **26**, 565–97.

Stern, E. A., Bacskai, B. J., Hickey, G. A., Attenello, F. J., Lombardo, J. A. & Hyman, B. T. (2004). Cortical synaptic integration in vivo is disrupted by amyloid-beta plaques. *J. Neurosci.*, **24**, 4535–40.

Tanzi, R. E. & Bertram, L. (2001). New frontiers in Alzheimer's disease genetics. *Neuron*, **32**, 181–4.

Tiraboschi, P., Hansen, L. A., Thal, L. J & Corey-Bloom, J. (2004). The importance of neuritic plaques and tangles to the development and evolution of AD. *Neurology*, **62**, 1984–9.

van Gool, W. A., Aisen, P. S. & Eikelenboom, P. (2003). Anti-inflammatory therapy in Alzheimer's disease: is hope still alive? *J. Neurol.*, **250**, 788–92.

Von Rotz, R. C., Kohli, B. M., Bosset, J. *et al.* (2004). The APP intracellular domain forms nuclear multiprotein complexes and regulates the transcription of its own precursor. *J. Cell Sci.*, **117**, 4435–48.

Walsh, D. M., Klyubin, I., Fadeeva, J. V. *et al.* (2002). Naturally secreted oligomers of amyloid beta protein potently inhibit hippocampal long-term potentiation in vivo. *Nature*, **416**, 535–9.

Wilcock, D. M., Rojiani, A., Rosenthal, A. *et al.* (2004). Passive amyloid immunotherapy clears amyloid and transiently activates microglia in a transgenic mouse model of amyloid deposition. *J. Neurosci.*, **24**, 6144–51.

Zandi, P. P., Anthony, J. C., Khachaturian, A. S. *et al.* (2004). Cache County Study Group. Reduced risk of Alzheimer disease in users of antioxidant vitamin supplements: the Cache County Study. *Arch. Neurol.*, **61**, 82–8.

32

Treatment of Alzheimer's disease

Mary Sano

Alzheimer's Disease Research Center, Department of Psychiatry, Mount Sinai School of Medicine, New York NY and Bronx VA Medical Center, Bronx, NY, USA

Overview

Over the past decade medications have been approved for the treatment of Alzheimer's disease (AD). The first of these worked via cholinergic stimulation, and targeted the symptoms of attention and memory. More recently Memantine, an NMDA receptor antagonist, has been added to the list of approved medications for AD. These treatments provide symptomatic benefits. Initiative for new therapeutics target the characteristic neuropathological features of AD or other biological mechanisms that may reflect the etiology of the disease in the hope of identifying preventative or curative agents.

Research into treatment of AD tends to focus on interventions at the earliest stage of the disease and the concept of mild cognitive impairment (MCI), a prodrome to dementia, has become the target of many interventions. This approach has the added challenge of determining diagnostic specificity of an entity, which does not yet constitute a diagnosis. At the same time, interest in treating the more impaired patient has grown with the approval of the first drug with an indication for moderate to severe AD and with new studies examining cholinesterase inhibitors in more advanced patients.

Awareness that AD may coexist with other CNS diseases or be difficult to distinguish from dementia of other etiologies may have contributed to the interest in treatments for individuals with other conditions including vascular and mixed dementia.

The neurobiology of AD, models of disease mechanisms, and epidemiological data, have been the backbone of many hypotheses for etiology and the basis for both planned and completed trials of AD treatment and prevention. The greatest hope lies in exploring these mechanisms to find better treatments and possibly preventative strategies.

Introduction

Alzheimer's disease is a devastating illness characterized by loss of memory and other cognitive functions, leading to functional disability and significant dependence. While there are a growing number of approved treatments, there is no cure and little is known about prevention. The prevalence of AD increases with age with estimates of 2.8 to 9.4 million over the next 50 years (Brookmeyer et al., 1998). AD is associated with an increase in the need for healthcare services (Torian et al., 1992) and is the third most costly disease in the United States behind heart disease and cancer (Kirchstein, 2002). While nearly 60% of all care to AD patients is delivered by informal caregivers, the projected costs may underestimate the true cost of the disease. As the population ages, finding treatment and prevention for Alzheimer's disease becomes a compelling public health mandate.

The first treatment for AD received regulatory approval over a decade ago. Some improvements have been made in this first class of agents and a drug from another class has also been approved. The progress has been aided by regulatory definition of efficacy and safety. For an indication of symptomatic benefit in the treatment of AD, the Food and Drug Administration (FDA) requires evidence of cognitive and 'clinical global' benefit. European approval requires benefit in two of three domains; the third is functional benefit usually assessed with a measure of activities of daily living. As awareness of the breadth of symptomatology and social and economic impact has grown, clinical trials for AD have come to include measures of behavioral disturbance, quality of life, and cost effectiveness.

Several studies have examined the breadth of efficacy of approved agents and trials have been reported in advanced stages of Alzheimer's, vascular, and mixed dementia. One limitation of the studies examining non-AD dementia is that outcome measures are typically those used in mild to moderate AD, which may not be the most appropriate for capturing benefit to other diseases.

Interest in the prevention of AD has grown and the identification of mildly symptomatic individuals typically labelled with the condition mild cognitive impairment (MCI) has provided a model for trials of secondary prevention of AD. While few results of these trials are currently available, early methodological reports describe these individuals and have estimated the likelihood of their progression. There are few studies that examine treatments of mild cognitive impairment and clinical practice is often directed by anecdotes, impressions, and untested hypotheses. The absence of adequate data makes it difficult to assess efficacy and safety. By and large, the agents under study have been agents that have been used to treat AD or which theoretically could treat AD.

Treatment with agents approved for Alzheimer's disease

Cholinergic stimulation

Tacrine

The first approved treatments for AD were cholinesterase inhibitors which enhance cholinergic transmission by inhibiting the breakdown of acetylcholine in the synaptic cleft. At this writing there are four agents approved in the US. Tacrine, the first approved agent in this class, required multiple daily dosing (QID), slow titration of dose into the effective range (i.e. 16 weeks), had limited tolerability of about 65% at the highest dose, and required monitoring of liver enzymes (Knapp *et al.*, 1994).

Donepezil

The second agent, Donepezil (Rogers *et al.*, 1998), has several advantages including once daily dosing, with no required medical monitoring for toxicity. Donepezil is a pseudo-irreversible acetyl cholinesterase inhibitor. It is well absorbed with oral bioavailability of 100% and the pharmacokinetics are linear in the 1 to 10 mg dose ranges. The elimination half life is approximately 70 h; with multiple doses it accumulates in plasma four- to sevenfold, reaching a steady state in 15 days. Efficacy has been demonstrated at 5 and 10 mg. Dosing recommendations indicate initiation with 5 mg/day and escalating dosage only after 4 to 6 weeks at the lower dose. Adverse events include diarrhea, nausea, vomiting, insomnia, muscle cramps,

and anorexia with more study withdrawals from those on 10 mg than 5 mg. However, side effect rates were reduced at the 10 mg dose when the interval between 5 and 10 mg was increased from 1 to 6 weeks. Postmarketing information has identified sleep disturbance as a possible phenomenon, perhaps because recommended dosing instructions suggest evening administration (Geldmacher, 1997). A review examining 16 double-blind clinical trials of Donepezil in patients with mild, moderate, or severe AD summarized data involving 4365 participants in studies ranging from 12 to 52 weeks duration (Birks & Harvey, 2003). Outcome data from each trial covered at minimum, cognitive function, and global clinical state. This review found systematic support for cognitive benefit with evidence of statistically significant improvement for both 5 and 10 mg/day of Donepezil. Clinical global measures also showed systematic benefit and some studies reported benefit in activities of daily living and behaviour.

Rivastigmine

The next agent to appear on the market was Rivastigmine, which reports both acetyl and butyrl cholinesterase inhibition, but there is little information on the relationship of each mechanism to the clinical impact of the drug. Rivastigmine is a reversible, acetylcholinesterase inhibitor. It is well absorbed and at a 3 mg dose the oral bioavailability is 40%. It has a half-life of 1.5 hours and recommended doses are from 6 to 12 mg/day, administered twice daily. Dose titration begins at 1.5 mg b.i.d. with a minimum of 2-week intervals between dose increases and longer intervals may reduce tolerability problems. If medication is discontinued at any point for more than a few days, it is recommended that the treatment be re-initiated at the lowest dose and titrated as described above.

A review of eight trials, involving 3450 participants, with a treatment interval of 26 weeks found high-dose Rivastigmine (6 to 12 mg daily) provided benefit in cognition, clinical global measures, and activities of daily living. At lower doses (4 mg daily or lower) differences were in the same direction but were statistically significant only for cognitive function. High dose Rivastigmine was associated with nausea, vomiting, diarrhea, anorexia, headache, syncope, abdominal pain, and dizziness. There is some evidence that adverse events might be less common with dosing regimens that use smaller doses more frequently (Birks *et al.*, 2004).

Galantamine

The newest of the cholinesterase inhibitors to receive approval in the United States for use for AD is Galantamine. The drug was originally isolated from several plants, including daffodil bulbs, but is now synthesized. Galantamine is a specific, reversible, competitive acetyl-cholinesterase inhibitor. It is also an allosteric modulator at nicotinic cholinergic receptor sites potentiating cholinergic nicotinic neurotransmission. It is well absorbed with high oral bioavailability (90%). It has a half-life of about 7 hours and recommended doses are 16 to 24 mg/day administered twice daily. A review of seven trials of various lengths from 12 weeks to 6 months yielded similar results to those seen with other cholinesterase inhibitors. In general, daily doses of 16 to 32 mg demonstrated efficacy over placebo in cognitive and functional abilities. Doses of 8 mg/day consistently failed to show statistically significant benefit. Adverse effects appear similar to those of other cholinesterase inhibitors, in that it tends to produce gastrointestinal symptoms acutely and with dosage increases. In clinical trials, dosage increases were associated with greater discontinuation in the Galantamine treated groups compared to the placebo groups. However, in the one trial with a slow rate of titration (4 weeks vs. 2 weeks) the discontinuation rate was not significantly greater than placebo for the 16 mg/day dose (Olin & Schneider, 2004).

Quality of life and economic benefit of cholinesterase inhibitors

There is no agreed upon method for assessing quality of life (QOL) in clinical trials of AD. Few AD specific measures of QOL exist, and those that have been published focus on domains that may not be modified by pharmacologic interventions (Logsdon et al., 2002). These scales observe mood, social interaction, or behavior to make an estimate of QOL. However, since measures of behavioral symptoms and functional measures such as those assessing activities of daily living are commonly included in clinical trials, QOL is often assessed by examining these outcome measures. In a systematic review of randomized clinical trials of cholinesterase inhibitors in AD, published between 1966 and 2001, the authors identified 29 reports that assessed functional impairment ($N = 18$) and behavioral symptoms ($N = 16$) (Trinh et al., 2003). For behavioral outcomes, ten trials included the ADAS-noncog and six included the NPI. Compared with placebo, patients randomized to cholinesterase inhibitors improved 1.72 points on the NPI (95% CI, 0.87–2.57 points), and 0.03 points on the ADAS-cog (95% CI, 0.00–0.05 points). For functional outcomes, 14 trials used ADL and 13 trials used instrumental ADL (IADL) scales. Compared with placebo, patients randomized to cholinesterase inhibitors improved 0.1 SDs on ADL scales (95% CI, 0.00–0.19 SDs), and 0.09 SDs on IADL scales (95% CI, 0.01 to 0.17 SDs). There was no difference in efficacy among various cholinesterase inhibitors, although there is very little power to observe such effects. There are several limitations to this review including the incorporation of trials of agents that failed in the development process, the absence of trials with Rivastigmine, and the consideration of relatively few measures of behavior and function. Despite this, it appears that cholinesterase inhibitors may affect these domains that are so relevant to QOL.

Much of the economic assessment of benefit of cholinesterase inhibitors is predicated on models which examine delay to nursing home placement. Longitudinal data from open label follow-up of clinical trials have been used to support a benefit for delaying nursing home placement for Tacrine and Donepezil (Knopman et al., 1996; Geldmacher et al., 2003). This type of data is seriously confounded by the large number of cases that discontinue from the treatment group leaving the remaining cases to inflate the apparent affect. Reduction of caregiver time has been associated with treatment with a cholinesterase inhibitor (Sano et al., 2003), though this effect is more observable as disease severity increases. Other studies have reported longitudinal effect on delaying cognitive decline and have used these cognitive benefits to model time savings by caregivers (Marin et al., 2003) and delay to need for full-time care (Caro et al., 2002). A single double-blind trial of long-term outcomes has been published and, while this indicates small but persistent cognitive and functional benefit for up to 2 years, no effect was observed in outcomes such as delaying stage of disease, need for nursing home placement or caregiver outcomes (AD 2000 Collaborative Group, 2004). While this study may have been underpowered to observe benefit in important clinical outcomes, it does cast doubt on many of the models of disease progression and economic impact.

Considerations for cholinesterase inhibitor use in AD

In general, clinical improvement with the cholinesterase inhibitors is robust though the effect size is modest. The side effect profile is relatively benign with gastrointestinal disturbances the most likely problem. These drugs are currently approved for the treatment of individuals in the mild to moderate stages of the disease. Given that these treatments have proven efficacy, it is reasonable to initiate a trial of cholinesterase inhibitors in patients with AD. There are no guidelines for selecting among the available agents. Since all medications have only been tested in situations where a caregiver administers the drug and monitors side effects, practical issues, such as the availability of someone to administer medication multiple times a day, may be a limiting factor for choosing an agent. At this writing, only a single agent, Donepezil, is administered once a day.

In general, it appears that slower titration may minimize cholinergic side effects. Most patients demonstrate stabilization or mild improvement and, in most studies, these benefits are not seen until 3 to 6 months of exposure. Therefore, it is important to attempt a reasonable length of treatment exposure before making a decision about continuing on a given agent. In addition, objective, placebo-controlled data from exposure of up to 1 year indicates that benefits continue though they may be smaller (Winblad *et al.*, 2001). Several agents may need to be tried since tolerance of side effects of each agent may differ among patients. Generally, the experience of the family members as well as patients will play a key role in weighing benefits of any treatment. While data supports benefits in areas that should have an important impact on quality of life and indications of an economic value, no such result has yet been observed and greater exposure may be needed to provide convincing evidence of benefit.

Glutamate and the NMDA receptor

Memantine

Memantine, a newly approved agent for the treatment of moderate to severe AD, has a novel mechanism of action. It is a low to moderate affinity uncompetitive (open-channel) NMDA receptor antagonist which selectively binds to the cation channels. Glutamate excitotoxicity may be mediated through the post synaptic NMDA receptor. Memantine is an uncompetitive NMDA-receptor antagonist and presumably this antagonism blocks glutamate damage. The half-life is 60 to 80 hours with the peak concentration reached in 3–7 hours. The recommended starting dose is 5 mg once a day with an increment of 5 mg/day at weekly intervals until the maximum dose of 20 mg/day is achieved. With the first dose escalation it is recommended that BID dosing be observed.

Three trials, including 973 patients with moderate to severe AD, lasting 12 to 28 weeks have been published. In one, Memantine alone demonstrated benefits in cognition over placebo (Reisberg *et al.*, 2003). Additionally, in a randomized trial of Memantine plus Donepezil compared to Donepezil alone, the combination demonstrated benefits in cognition, a clinical global measure, and behavior (Tariot *et al.*, 2004). While a third study did not have a cognitive measure (Winblad & Poritis, 1999), all three studies assessed clinical global benefits and 2 of 3 demonstrated a statistically significant benefit of Memantine over placebo (or Donepezil plus placebo) in ITT analysis and all three demonstrated efficacy in completers analyses. In clinical trials Memantine was well tolerated. An increase in confusion (7.9 vs 2%) was reported in one study (Tariot *et al.*, 2004) but no consistent pattern of side effects has emerged. Clinical exposure to this agent is minimal compared to cholinesterase inhibitors and it may be too early to know the complete side effect profile.

The effect of Memantine in mild to moderate AD is not yet clear. Early reports of the use of Memantine in mild to moderate AD in combination with a cholinesterase inhibitor failed to demonstrate efficacy, though the details of the study are not available at this writing. A study examining the effect of Memantine in this patient population in the absence of other treatments yields small but significant effect on cognition and on clinical global measures (Peskind *et al.*, 2004). Additional studies are needed to provide support for the use of this agent in patients at these stages of the disease.

Treatment of vascular and mixed dementia with agents approved for AD

The ability to distinguish between different types of dementia is complicated by the lack of biomarkers. Thus much of the diagnosis is based on clinical evaluation and while the research diagnostic criteria required in clinical trials may provide some added assurance, it is unclear if such criteria can be practical in a typical clinical setting. One of the most difficult distinctions to make clinically is between AD and vascular disease, primarily because the two entities frequently coexist and it is not obvious to what degree each contributes to the dementia symptomatology. Given this dilemma of clinical practice, it is important to know to what degree the agents approved in the treatment of AD may have efficacy in other conditions To this end, several studies have examined agents in patients with AD and some degree of vascular disease as well as in individuals described as having probable or possible vascular disease. Perhaps the largest data base exists for Donepezil, with published clinical trials including over 1200 individuals with possible or probable vascular dementia or cognitive decline (Birks *et al.*, 2003). Donepezil, at doses of 5 or 10 mg a day, was compared with placebo for 24 weeks. In general, significant effects on cognition, measured with the ADAS-cog, have been observed in ITT analyses at nearly every time point. Clinical global improvement in the ITT analysis was observed in one study (Wilkinson *et al.*, 2003) but not in others, although significance was observed at 5 mg but not at 10 mg in an observed case analysis. In a trial of patients with AD plus vascular disease and vascular dementia alone Galantamine was shown to be superior to placebo on cognitive outcomes but not on clinical global outcomes. Subgroup analysis suggested that the effect was more pronounced in the AD plus vascular disease group than in the VAD group (Erkinjuntti, 2002).

Taken together, these studies suggest a beneficial effect of approved AD treatments in patients with vascular dementia. However, these effects are small and there is a need for instruments better suited for assessing vascular dementia.

Other pharmacologic approaches to treating AD

Anti-oxidants

The role for oxidative stress as a pathological mechanism in aging and dementia is supported by several lines of evidence. Biological studies demonstrate that the accumulation of free radicals is associated with damage to lipids, cell membranes, and proteins including DNA and RNA. These oxidative byproducts induce the production of the Amyloid Precursor Protein (APP), the protein precursor to the amyloid plaque, the hallmark of AD pathology. The accumulation of Aβ fragments may reduce compensatory anti-oxidant ability resulting in further increases in Aβ deposition, synapse loss, DNA damage, neuronal dysfunction, and cell death. Free radical scavengers sequester free radicals rendering them impotent, minimizing oxidative reactions, and minimizing cellular damage. (For a review of these potential mechanisms see Butterfield, 2002.)

Compelling support for the link between oxidative stress and Aβ comes from a recent study which crossed mice with a knockout of one allele of a critical anti-oxidant enzyme (manganese superoxide dismutase: MnSOD) with a mouse that overexpressed a doubly mutated human β-amyloid precursor protein (i.e. Tg19959). Previous work established the MnSOD to cause elevated oxidative stress and the mice of the resulting cross demonstrated increases in both amyloid plaque burden and amyloid levels (Li *et al.*, 2004).

Evidence for a benefit of anti-oxidant agents comes from observational studies. Most recently, two prospective studies examined the association of dietary anti-oxidants and incident AD and provided evidence of reduced risk of Alzheimer's disease (Morris *et al.*, 2002; Engelhart *et al.*, 2002). Daily intake of antioxidants including vitamin E, vitamin C, beta carotene, and flavenoids was assessed with food frequency questionnaires. In one study of over 800 subjects followed for a mean of nearly 4 years the group in the highest quintile of vitamin E intake had a relative risk of AD of 0.36 (95% CI: 0.11–1.17) compared to the group in the lowest quintile (Morris *et al.*, 2002). Other anti-oxidants had no effect. In another study

of more than 5000 individuals followed for a mean of 6 years, a reduced risk of AD was reported with vitamin E and with vitamin C intake (RR = 0.82; 95% CI: 0.66–1.00). Both reports failed to demonstrate a benefit to the use of anti-oxidant supplements, though they increased the intake levels by 50% or more (Sano, 2002). Data from the multi-ethnic cohort of Washington Heights, in New York City, examined both dietary intake and supplemental use of antioxidant vitamins. Elderly subjects (N = 980) were followed for a mean of 4 years and nutrient data was gathered with a standardized food-frequency questionnaire which also gathered data on supplement intake. This report found no evidence of risk reduction nor a trend toward reduction with vitamin E, C, or carotenoids in any combination. Recently, a study from the well-described cohort from Cache County of Utah, examined the effect of supplement intake on both prevalent and incident dementia. This report described a reduction in both prevalence and incidence with the combination of vitamins C and E, but not with either alone (Zandi *et al.*, 2004). A trend toward lower incidence of AD was associated with vitamin E in combination with a multi-vitamin possibly containing C, but not with a multivitamin alone.

Typically, we move from observational studies to clinical trials to test hypotheses about potential treatments. A range of agents has been tried in clinical trials for the treatment of AD. As described below, early trials provided promising evidence of benefit with anti-oxidant therapies, but longer and larger trials have been disappointing.

Vitamin E

As evidence for a benefit to AD, vitamin E was found to delay clinical milestones in moderately impaired patients with AD though no benefit was observed on standardized cognitive tests (Sano *et al.*, 1997). In the same study, Selegiline, a selective inhibitor of monoamine oxidase-B, was also effective but the combination of drugs had no additional benefit. Physicians commonly recommend vitamin E as treatment for AD. While no data is available for the combination, it is often given along with cholinesterase inhibitors, probably based on its perceived safety.

Two trials have reported the outcome of cognitive add-ons to other studies. One is the anti-oxidant arm of the Heart Protection Study (Heart Protection Study Collaborative Group 2002). This large trial of over 20 000 enrollees, aged 40 to 80 years, selected subjects who were at risk for cardiovascular disease. The study used a 2 × 2 factorial design in which one agent was Simvastatin and the other was an anti-oxidant combination of vitamin E (600 mg), vitamin C (250 mg), and beta carotene (20 mg). While no initial cognitive assessment was conducted, at the final visit the modified Telephone Interview for Cognitive Status (TICS-m) questionnaire was administered. Using an established cut-off score to identify cognitive impairment (22 of 39) no significant difference was found between the treatment groups in the percentages of the cognitively impaired (23.4% vitamin group vs. 24.4% vitamin placebo group). There was also no difference in the mean TICS-m score and similar numbers of participants in each treatment group were reported to have developed dementia (0.3%) or other psychiatric disorder (0.6%). This rate of incident cases appears quite low, given the age range of the subject population, suggesting that this methodology may have been inadequately sensitive to cognitive change. Interestingly, these supplemental doses are far above the range in which dietary anti-oxidants were reported to have an effect.

The DATATOP study was a trial of over 800 subjects, newly diagnosed with Parkinson's disease, who were treated with Selegiline or vitamin E (2000 International Units (IU)) in a 2×2 factorial design. Cognitive assessments consisted of a battery of tests, including memory tests. No significant difference was noted among the groups (Kieburtz *et al.*, 1994). Whether these results from this specialized population can be generalized is difficult to know since the study population was relatively young and all had early/mild Parkinson's disease. Nevertheless, in this cognitively fragile cohort, high dose vitamin E was unable to modify cognition.

An ongoing study known as PREADVISE is an 'add-on' study, which will examine the preventative effect of various anti-oxidants on prostate cancer. The parent study recruits men, age of 60 or greater who are randomly assigned to receive 200 micrograms of selenium and 400 IU of vitamin E per day and monitors for prostate cancer. Participants randomized to assess anti-oxidant effects on prostate cancer may enroll in this cognitive 'add-on' study which will assess cognition and dementia with a brief screen followed by a more comprehensive work-up. The relatively young age of the cohort may make it difficult to observe a cognitive change and follow-up may be confounded by results or new findings with bearing on prostate treatment. Nevertheless, this represents an opportunity to observe cognition in this unique cohort.

Gingko biloba

Gingko biloba is a plant extract containing flavenoids which act as free radical scavengers that may protect cells from excessive lipid peroxidation and neuronal membrane breakdown (Scholtyssek *et al.*, 1997). Clinical trials of this drug in cognitively impaired populations have yielded mixed results with reports of benefit in some but not all outcomes (van Dongen *et al.*, 2000). Benefits on

cognitive measures in patients with AD have been demonstrated with Gingko biloba (Le Bars *et al.*,1997). These trials suggest that anti-oxidants, which appear to be well tolerated, may have a role in the treatment of AD, though sufficient evidence is not yet available (Oken *et al.*, 1998). However, a recent randomized, double-blind, placebo-controlled trial evaluated elderly individuals with memory impairment, living in a residential setting and compared two doses of Ginkgo biloba (160 mg/day and 240 mg/day) to placebo and found no significant effect on cognition, function, or mood (van Dongen *et al.*, 2000). A systematic review of published trials identified 33 studies using double-blind placebo-controlled designs in a range of cognitively impaired populations, most of which had a dementia resembling AD. The studies used treatment exposure intervals from 3 to 52 weeks, with a modal exposure of 12 weeks. Few studies used rigorous Intent to Treat analysis and thus conclusions were based on a completers analysis. In general, doses less than 200 mg per day were associated with benefits in cognition, mood and improved activities of daily living. Longer exposures and higher doses did not systematically increase these benefits. There was no significant difference between Ginkgo biloba and placebo in adverse events and no data on quality of life, depression, or dependency (Birks *et al.*, 2002).

Laboratory studies indicate that Gingko biloba may maintain neuronal function in the hippocampus with evidence of neurotrophic effects in mossy fibers and maintenance of age-related adrenergic and serotonergic receptor loss (Barkats *et al.*, 1995). A primary prevention trial sponsored by the National Center for Complementary and Alternative Medicine and the National Institute on Aging is ongoing. The trial (Ginkgo for the Evaluation of Memory study; GEMS) is recruiting those over 75 years of age into a double-blind placebo-controlled study of Gingko biloba (240 mg/day) for 3 years or more. The primary outcome measure is dementia with a specified analysis for the diagnosis of Alzheimer's disease and secondary outcome measures include a cognitive battery and other domains typically used in clinical trials for AD.

In general, while anti-oxidant treatments appear safe, results from supplement trials in the area of cognition have been disappointing. There appears to be many methodological challenges to previously reported trials, so hopefully future studies will focus on definitive trial designs.

Anti-inflammatory agents

Several lines of evidence support the notion that locally mediated, non-immune, chronic, inflammatory processes may play a role in AD pathology. A wide range of inflammation-related proteins appear in proximity to Aβ plaque including α1-antichymotripsin, ICAM-1, α2-macroglobuline and they are presumed to be locally produced, as they do not pass the blood–brain barrier. In addition, mRNA for complement factors and complement proteins are found in neurons but not in glial cells, supporting the notion that they are in response to the neural injury. Data from animal studies using human APP transgenic mice suggests that (i) inflammation related proteins are associated with higher amyloid load (Nilsson *et al.*, 2001) and (ii) inhibition of complement factors lowers amyloid burden (Bales *et al.*, 1997). Human postmortem tissue analysis has identified correlations with microglial cells and plaque deposits in the cerebral cortex of AD brains but not with Aβ or tau markers of disease progression (Arends *et al.*, 2000). One interpretation of these data is that the inflammatory process is an early response to disease (Eikelenboom & van Gool, 2004).

Epidemiologic data supporting the connection between inflammatory mechanisms and AD is based on the finding of reduced dementia in cohorts using nonsteroidal anti-inflammatory drugs (NSAIDs) (in t' Veld *et al.*, 2001; Zandi *et al.*, 2002; Etminan *et al.*, 2003). One study, which examined pharmacy records of a cohort of over 2000 elders, demonstrated a reduction in dementia among those with 2 or more years of exposure to NSAIDS (in t' Veld *et al.*, 2001). Similar results were reported by Zandi *et al.* (2002) in the Cache County cohort. The strength of the association in both studies was best observed when the analysis only included NSAID exposure 1 to 2 years prior to the onset of disease, leading to the impression that NSAID protection can only be observed in the intact brain and is not likely to be apparent as a treatment effect. A recent meta-analysis of six cohort studies totalling over 13 000 individuals projects that the effect size for dementia protection is approximately 30% reduction in incidence with significant results in those with use greater than 24 months (Etminan *et al.*, 2003).

It is possible that the epidemiological effect observed with the NSAIDs is not due to the anti-inflammatory properties. In a recent paper, Weggen *et al.* (2001) reported that, in cell cultures Ibuprofen and Indomethacen, but neither Naproxen nor the COX 2 inhibitors, reduced the amyloidagenic Aβ 42 formation in a variety of cell culture models (Weggen *et al.*, 2001). These authors postulate that this effect may come from subtle mediation of secretase activity. Unfortunately, the epidemiologic data is not available to make distinctions between the NSAIDs.

Clinical trials to date have been disappointing, although many have been designed as treatment studies in patients with AD rather than as prevention trials. Glucocorticoids, which are known to be effective anti-inflamatory agents in the CNS, acting on several of the hypothesized inflammatory processes, have not been proven to be beneficial in treating AD in clinical trials. In a multicenter, randomized clinical trial of Prednisone no benefit was seen and significant side effect was observed (Aisen *et al.*, 2000). Non-steroidal agents have been studied in several trials. An early, single site trial demonstrated borderline benefit in the presence of significant side effect with Indomethacin (Rogers *et al.*, 1993). A more recent study examined the NSAID Diclofenac in combination with Misoprostol and also found no benefit and reported nearly a 50% withdrawal rate (Scharf *et al.*, 1999). A recent multi-center trial of Naproxen was also unable to demonstrate benefit in patients with AD (Aisen *et al.*, 2003a,b). Selective COX 2 inhibitors, effective anti-inflammatory agents with minimal gastrointestinal disturbances, have reasonable CNS penetrability. However, well-designed, year-long, multicentre trials of these agents have not demonstrated efficacy in the treatment of AD (Aisen *et al.*, 2003; Reines *et al.*, 2004).

Taken together, the present state of knowledge provides no data to support the use of anti-inflammatory agents for the treatment of AD, and the known side effect profile suggests that the risks may be considerable, particularly in an elderly population. Interest in these agents for the prevention of AD has led to several secondary and primary prevention trials. The selective COX II inhibitor, Rofecoxib, was used in a trial of prevention of AD among individuals with Mild Cognitive Impairment (MCI) and results indicated no benefit either in reduced conversion or in performance on cognitive testing (Visser *et al.*, 2003).

It has been suggested that, despite failure in treatment and secondary prevention, there is hope that primary prevention may be the challenge for demonstrating efficacy with anti-inflammatory agents. A primary prevention trial known as Alzheimer Disease Anti-inflammatory Prevention Trial (ADAPT), is a multicentre trial based on observational data (Martin *et al.*, 2002). The primary outcomes are to reduce incident dementia and cognitive decline. The study will enrol 2625 individuals aged 70 and older with a family history of AD in a first-degree relative. This study will examine two anti-inflammatory agents, the conventional NSAID, Naproxen sodium (220 mg bid) and the selective COX 2 inhibitor Celecoxib (200 mg bid) and to achieve 80% power to detect a 30% reduction in AD incidence, will follow subjects over 7 years.

Lowering homocysteine

Homocysteine, an amino acid involved in methionine and cysteine metabolism, plays a role in methylation reactions.

The role of homocysteine as a cardiac disease and stroke risk factor has been well established. Several studies have demonstrated that hyperhomocysteinemia is associated with Alzheimer's disease (AD) in the absence of folate or B_{12} deficiency. When age-based norms for plasma homocysteine are divided into tertiles, the risk of AD in subjects in the highest tertile of homocysteine levels is more than four times higher than those in the lowest (McCaddon et al., 1998; Seshadri et al., 2002). Other evidence for a role for homocysteine in AD comes from data indicating that elevated plasma homocysteine occurs in neuropathologically confirmed cases of AD, in the absence of any vascular neuropathology (Clarke, 1998). Also, among AD cases, higher levels of homocysteine are associated with more rapid radiological disease progression.

Folate, as well as vitamins B_{12} and B_6 are cofactors in metabolic reactions involving homocysteine and are very effective in lowering homocysteine levels. In addition, folate improves nitric oxide availability in the brain. It also plays a number of other roles, such as acting as a coenzyme in the synthesis of serotonin and catecholamine neurotransmitters and also of S-adenosylmethionine, and these have been reported to have antidepressant properties. Thus, the use of folate may have benefit through several mechanisms. It is therefore reasonable to postulate that lowering homocysteine with these vitamins would provide cognitive benefit or protection from cognitive decline. It has been demonstrated that supplementation with folate, vitamin B_{12} and vitamin B_6 can lower homocysteine in patients with AD even in those with already normal levels, although the ability to affect cognition has not yet been demonstrated.

Several clinical trials have assessed folate effects on cognition in a range of populations. Four randomized trials were identified in a recent review; one enrolled healthy women only and three others recruited people with mild to moderate cognitive impairment or dementia. While folic acid plus vitamin B_{12} was effective in reducing serum homocysteine concentrations, a meta-analysis of these studies found no benefit from folic acid with or without vitamin B_{12} in comparison with placebo on any measures of cognition or mood for healthy, cognitively impaired, or demented people. Folic acid was well tolerated and no adverse effects were reported. Several limitations of these studies include brief exposure periods, lack of standardized diagnosis, and lack of surety about appropriate outcome measures.

Effective lowering of homocysteine levels can be achieved with folate, vitamins B_{12} and B_6, even when levels are in the relatively normal range and in the presence of fortified grain (Aisen et al., 2003). On this basis and given its relative safety it is reasonable to hypothesize vitamin supplementation may lower the risks of cognitive decline and dementia in the elderly. Since ongoing trials of high doses of supplementation continue to prove to be safe in aging populations, intervention with these supplements are worthy of study as a treatment strategy for primary prevention of cognitive loss and dementia in aging.

Lowering lipids

There is compelling evidence from laboratory research in animal model and cell culture systems, observational epidemiological studies, and small clinical trials that lowering cholesterol may reduce the pathology of Alzheimer's disease (AD). In support of the link between cholesterol and AD there are in vitro studies demonstrating that cholesterol levels modulate the enzymatic processing of the amyloid precursor protein (APP) and consequently, $A\beta$ production. Dietary manipulation to increase cholesterol in rabbits, rats, and transgenic mice demonstrate that high cholesterol yields increased secretion of amyloidagenic $A\beta 1$–40 and 1–42, as well as increasing size and number of amyloid plaques. Lipid lowering agents can reduce these findings both in cell cultures and in animals. It is not clear that cholesterol lowering can help patients with AD, and retrospective studies have not supported that connection. However, well-controlled clinical trials could answer this question directly.

Recent epidemiological data have suggested that use of some lipid lowering drugs was associated with a reduced risk of Alzheimer's disease. Observational studies using existing clinical practice registries have reported an inverse association between statin use and risk of AD. Wolozin et al. (2000) reported cross-sectional examination of computerized medical records from three hospitals and demonstrated that the prevalence of diagnosed AD in patients taking Lovastatin or Pravastatin was 60–73% lower than the entire patient population during the period from 1996–1998. Jick and colleagues (2000) examined the General Practice Research Database in the United Kingdom and reported reduced risk of AD with statin use. In this study, the 284 cases were patients who developed a first-time diagnosis of dementia or Alzheimer's disease between 1992 and 1998. Rockwood and colleagues reported a reduced risk of AD among those using statins and other lipid lowering agents (OR = 0.26; 95% CI 0.08–0.88) (Rockwood et al., 2002). These authors noted no effect of statins among those over 80, though very few in that age group were taking statins.

Despite these epidemiological findings, two recent large scaled trials conducted 'add-on' studies to assess cognition.

The Heart Protection Study (HPS) also examined the effect of Simvastatin, a cholesterol lowering agent, on the large cohort with the Telephone Interview for Cognition (TIC) as described above (Heart Protection Study Collaborative Group, 2002). There was no difference in the percentages of participants classified as cognitively impaired, (23.7% simvastatin allocated vs. 24.2% placebo allocated) or having incident dementia during follow-up (0.3% vs. 0.3%). In a trial of Pravastatin in over 5000 individuals age 70 to 82, cognitive testing administered before and after found no effect on measures of learning, memory, attention, speed of processing, mental status, or activities of daily living (Shepherd *et al.*, 2002). While these studies use large sample sizes, the observation study may be too brief to observe the transition from normal cognition to dementia, resulting in insufficient power to observe an effect in this intact population.

The relative safety of these drugs has led to their use in trials to slow disease progression in AD. A single site study of Atorvastatin in patients with mild to moderate AD was recently presented suggesting a beneficial effect in cognitive and clinical global outcome measures (Sparks *et al.*, 2004). At this writing there are two ongoing multicentre trials of statins that will examine the rate of change on cognition and clinical global benefit over an 18-month period with patients with mild to moderate disease. The advantage to trials conducted with patients with AD is that the rate of progression in cognition and other clinical measures is relatively well established and rapid enough to permit sufficient power to observe an effect, if it exists.

Theoretical approaches based on attacking amyloid

The amyloid plaque in neurons remains the hallmark pathology of AD and the formation of the plaque is nearly universally considered the primary underlying mechanism and etiology of the disease. As such, interventions that could reduce amyloid plaque burden either by altering amyloid metabolism or by maximizing clearance are widely proposed though not so widely realized. Metabolism of amyloid precursor protein (APP) may determine the likelihood of the plaque formation. Cleavage of APP by the enzyme, α-secretase, leads to the formation of non-amyloidagenic, soluble APP (sAPP). Aβ, the building block of amyloid plaque is the result of APP cleavage by β-secretase. It also appears that the enzyme, γ-secretase, has a cleavage site within the intramembranous domain and it results in the formation of a small but potent peptide A-β 42, which is highly likely to aggregate. From this scenario, at least in theory, modulation of these enzymes might result

in differential rate of amyloid plaque formation. Unfortunately, these enzymes have many components and many substrates making it difficult to select a manipulation that will yield efficacy and avoid mechanism-related toxicity. To this end, selective enzyme inhibitors have been proposed, but to date none have advanced to clinical trials for efficacy.

Protein phosphorylation apparently regulates APP cleavage, by stimulating the α-secretase pathway leading to the relatively non-toxic sAPP. Stimulation of protein kinase-C through steroid hormones such as 17-b-estradiol or DHEA have been shown to stimulate this pathway and similar signal transduction systems have been proposed as treatment intervention, despite the fact that clinical trials examining these approaches have not yielded benefits (Gandy *et al.*, 2003).

Vaccination strategies have focused on vaccination with A-β. It is clear that A-β antibodies can be generated and can achieve clearance of plaque with some behavioral benefit in animal models and there is implication of clearance in pathology reports from human trials. While clinical benefit in humans has not yet been confirmed, anecdotal reports suggest an association between anti-amyloid response and slowed cognitive decline. These strategies have been associated with significant side effect probably resulting from pathologic immune response.

Conclusions: the challenge of managing a neurodegenerative disease

A growing awareness of the impact of cognitive impairment has led to our ability and willingness to diagnose and offer treatment to individuals with Alzheimer's disease. However, disease detection remains inadequate and it is estimated that only a third to a half of prevalent cases are identified. The initiation of clinical attention is often via a concerned family member or friend and seldom by any routine screening. This illustrates the lack of prominence given to this disease in the overall context of medical evaluation and management of the elderly. Elevating the importance of diagnosing this disease may encourage a willingness to acknowledge cognitive deficits at early stages of dementia and increase public motivation for prevention.

Understanding the pathology and how to manipulate it in a clinically relevant way remains elusive. However, the efforts of basic scientists to elucidate disease mechanisms is an essential requirement for progress in developing interventions. One emerging theme is that results of clinical trials in AD do not match results of risk reduction reported in observational studies. This dichotomy occurs with anti-inflammatories, anti-oxidants, and statins. While mechanisms have been proposed to explain observational findings of well known agents in AD, direct use of these agents in AD patients have provided disappointing results. This has led to the idea that once the disease is present, manipulation of the pathology cannot provide a benefit and an inevitable cascade of deterioration is in place. This reasoning does not adequately value the clinical observation that patients with AD may live for years, some leading relatively independent lives. Clinical progression is well characterized and theories of pathology and mechanisms of intervention must model a continuum of disease from presymptomatic through early and middle disease stages. Biological models, which address the full spectrum of disease, may provide drugs for common targets both in treatment and prevention.

Acknowledgement

The author is supported in this work in part by Federal Grants RO1AG 15922 and UO1 AG 10483 and P50 AG005138.

REFERENCES

AD2000 Collaborative Group (2004). Long-term donepezil treatment in 565 patients with Alzheimer's disease (AD2000): randomized double-blind trial. *Lancet*, **363**, 2105–15.

Aisen, P. S., Davis, K. L., Berg, J. D. *et al.* (2000). A randomized controlled trial of prednisone in Alzheimer's disease. *Neurology*, **54**, 588–92.

Aisen, P. S., Egelko, S., Andrews, H. *et al.* (2003a). A pilot study of vitamins to lower plasma homocysteine levels in Alzheimer disease. *Am. J. Geriatr. Psychiatry*, **11**(2), 246–9.

Aisen, P. S., Schafer, K. A., Grundman, M . *et al.* (2003b). Alzheimer's disease cooperative study. Effects of rofecoxib or naproxen vs placebo on Alzheimer disease progression: a randomized controlled trial. *J. Am. Med. Assoc.*, **289**(21), 2819–26.

Arends, Y. M., Duyckaerts, C., Rozemuller, J. M., Eikelenboom, P. & Hauw, J. (2000). Microglia, amyloid and dementia in Alzheimer's disease. A correlative study. *Neurobiol. Aging*, **21**, 39–47.

Bales, K. R., Verina, T., Dodel, R. C. *et al.* (1997). Lack of apolipoprotein E dramatically reduces amyloid b-peptide deposition. *Nat. Genet*, **17**, 263–4.

Barkats, M., Venault, P., Christen, Y. & Cohen-Salmon, C. (1995). Effect of long-term treatment with EGb 761 on age-dependent structural changes in the hippocampi of three inbred mouse strains. *Life Sci.*, **56**, 213–22.

Birks, J., Grimley, E. V. & Van Dongen, M. (2002). Ginkgo biloba for cognitive impairment and dementia. *Cochrane Database Syst. Rev.*, (4), CD003120.

Birks, J., Grimley Evans, J., Iakovidou, V. & Tsolaki, M. (2003). Rivastigmine for Alzheimer's disease. [systematic review] Cochrane Dementia and Cognitive Improvement Group. *Cochrane Database of Systematic Reviews*, **2**.

Birks, J. S. & Harvey, R. (2003). Donepezil for dementia due to Alzheimer's disease. *Cochrane Database of Systematic Reviews*, (3), CD001190.

Brookmeyer, R., Gray, S. & Kawas, C. (1998). Projections of Alzheimer's disease in the United States and the public health impact of delaying disease onset. *Am. J. Public Hlth.*, **88**, 1337–42.

Butterfield, D. A. (2002). Amyloid beta-peptide (1–42)-induced oxidative stress and neurotoxicity: implications for neurodegeneration in Alzheimer's disease brain. A review. *Free Radic Res.*, **36**, 1307–13.

Caro, J. J., Salas, M., Ward, A., Getsios, D. & Mehnert, A. & AHEAD Study Group (2002). Assessment of Health Economics in Alzheimer's Disease Economic analysis of galantamine, a cholinesterase inhibitor, in the treatment of patients with mild to moderate Alzheimer's disease in the Netherlands. *Dement. Geriatr. Cogn. Disord.*, **14**(2), 84–9.

Clarke, R., Smith, A. D., Jobst, K. A. *et al.* (1998). Vitamin B_{12}, and serum total homocysteine levels in confirmed Alzheimer disease. *Arch. Neurol.*, **55**, 1449–55.

Eikelenboom, P. & van Gool, W. A. (2004). Neuroinflammatory perspectives on the two faces of Alzheimer's disease. *J. Neural. Transm.*, **111**, 281–94.

Engelhart, M. J., Geerlings, M. I., Ruitenberg, A. *et al.* (2002). Dietary intake of antioxidants and risk of Alzheimer disease. *J. Am. Med. Assoc.*, **287**(24), 3223–9.

Erkinjuntti, T., Kurz, A., Gauthier, S., Bullock, R., Lilienfeld, S. & Damaraju, C. V. (2002). Efficacy of galantamine in probable vascular dementia and Alzheimer's disease combined with cerebrovascular disease: a randomised trial. *Lancet*, **359**, 1283–90.

Etminan, M., Gill, S. & Samii, A. (2003). Effect of non-steroidal anti-inflammatory drugs on risk of Alzheimer's disease: systematic review and meta-analysis of observational studies. *Br. Med. J.*, **327**, 128.

Gandy, S., Martins, R. N. & Buxbaum, J. (2003). Molecular and cellular basis for anti-amyloid therapy in Alzheimer disease. *Alzheimer. Dis. Assoc. Disord.*, **17**, 259–66.

Geldmacher, D. (1997). Donepezil (Aricept) therapy for Alzheimer's disease. *Compr. Ther.*, **23**(7), 492–3.

Geldmacher, D. S., Provenzano, G., McRae, T., Mastey, V. & Ieni, D. E. G. Jr. (2003). Donepezil is associated with delayed nursing home placement in patients with Alzheimer's disease. *J. Am. Geriatr. Soc.*, **51**, 937–44.

Heart Protection Study Collaborative Group (2002). MRC/BHF Heart Protection Study of antioxidant vitamin supplementation in 20 536 high-risk individuals: a randomised placebo-controlled trial. *Lancet*, **360**, 23–33.

in t' Veld, B. A., Ruitenberg, A., Hofman, *et al.* (2001). Nonsteroidal antiinflammatory drugs and the risk of Alzheimer's disease. *N. Engl. J. Med.*, **345**, 1515–21.

Jick, H., Zornberg, G. L., Jick, S. S., Seshadri, S. & Drachman, D. A. (2000). Statins and the risk of dementia. *Lancet*, **356**, 1627–31.

Kieburtzk, K., McDermott, M., Como, P. *et al.* (1994). The effect of deprenyl and tocopherol on cognitive performance in early untreated Parkinson's disease. Parkinson Study Group. *Neurology*, **44**, 1756–9.

Kirschstein, R. (2002). Disease-specific estimates of direct and indirect costs of illness and NIH support. *National Institutes of Health*, 6–11. http://www1.od.nih.gov/osp/ospp/ecostudies/COIreportweb.

Knapp, M. J., Knopman, D. S., Solomon, P. R., Pendlebury, W. W., Davis, C. S., Gracon, S. I. (1994). A 30-week randomized controlled trial of high-dose tacrine in patients with Alzheimer's disease. The Tacrine Study Group. *J. Am. Med. Assoc.*, **271**(13), 985–91.

Knopman, D., Schneider, L., Davis, K. *et al.* (1996). Long-term tacrine (Cognex) treatment: effects on nursing home placement and mortality, Tacrine Study Group. *Neurology*, **47**(1), 166–77.

Le Bars, P. L., Katz, M. M., Berman, N., Itil, T. M., Freedman, A. M. & Schatzberg, A. F. (1997). A placebo-controlled, double-blind, randomized trial of an extract of Ginkgo biloba for dementia. North American EGb Study Group. *J. Am. Med. Assoc.*, **278**, 1327–32.

Li, F., Calingasan, N., Yo, F. *et al.* (2004). Increased plaque burden in brains of APP mutant MnSOD heterozygous knockout mice. *J. Neurochem.*, **89**, 1308–12.

Logsdon, R. G., Gibbons, L. E., McCurry, S. M. & Teri, L. (2002). Assessing quality of life in older adults with cognitive impairment. *Psychosom. Med.*, **64**(3), 510–19.

Marin, D., Amaya, K., Casciano, R. *et al.* (2003). Impact of rivastigmine on costs and on time spent in caregiving for families of patients with Alzheimer's disease. *Int. Psychogeriatr.*, **15**(4), 385–98.

Martin, B. K., Meinert, C. L. & Breitner, J. C. S. (2002). Double placebo design in a prevention trial for Alzheimer's disease. *Controlled Clin. Trials*, **23**, 93–9.

McCaddon, A., Davies, G., Hudson, P., Tandy, S. & Cattell, H. (1998). Total serum homocysteine in senile dementia of Alzheimer type. *Int. J. Geriatr. Psychiatry*, **13**, 235–9.

Morris, M. C., Evans, D. A., Bienias, J. L. *et al.* (2002). Dietary intake of antioxidant nutrients and the risk of incident Alzheimer disease in a biracial community study. *Am. Med. Assoc.*, **287**, 3230–7.

Nilsson, I. N., Bales, K. R., DiCarlo, G. *et al.* (2001). Alpha-1-antichymotrypsin promotes beta-sheet amyloid plaque deposition in a transgenic mouse model of Alzheimer's disease. *J. Neurosci.*, **21**(5), 1444–51.

Oken, B. S., Storzbach, D. M. & Kaye, J. A. (1998). The efficacy of Ginkgo biloba on cognitive function in Alzheimer disease. *Arch. Neurol.*, **55**, 1409–15.

Olin, J. & Schneider, L. (2004). Galantamine for dementia due to Alzheimer's disease. [systematic review] Cochrane Dementia and Cognitive Improvement Group Cochrane Database of Systematic Reviews, **2**.

Peskind, E. R., Potkin, S. G., Pomara, N., McDonald, D., Xie, Y. & Gergel, I. (2004). Memantine monotherapy is elective and safe for the treatment of mild to moderate AD. *Am. J. Geriatr. Psychiatry*.

Reines, S. A., Block, G. A., Morris, J. C. *et al.* (2004). Rofecoxib Protocol 091 Study Group. No effect on Alzheimer's disease in a 1-year, randomized, blinded, controlled study. *Neurology*, **62**(1), 66–71.

Reisberg, B., Doody, R., Stoffler, A., Schmitt, F., Ferris, S. & Mobius, H. J. Memantine Study Group (2003). Memantine in moderate-to-severe Alzheimer's disease. *N. Engl. J. Med.* **348**(14), 1333–41.

Rockwood, K., Kirkland, S., Hogan, D. B. *et al.* (2002). Use of lipid-lowering agents, indication bias, and the risk of dementia in community-dwelling elderly people. *Arch. Neurol.*, **59**, 223–7.

Rogers, J., Kirby, L. C., Hempelman, S. R. *et al.* (1993). Clinical trial of indomethacin in Alzheimer's disease. *Neurology*, **43**, 1609–11.

Rogers, S. L., Farlow, M. R., Doody, R. S., Mohs, R. & Friedhoff, L. T. Donepezil Study Group (1998). A 24-week, double-blind, placebo-controlled trial of donepezil in patients with Alzheimer's disease. *Neurology*, **50**(1), 136–45.

Sano, M. (2002). Prevention of Alzheimer's disease: the problem of the drugs and the designs. *Curr. Neurol. Neurosci. Rep.*, **2**, 392–9.

Sano, M., Ernesto, C., Thomas, R. G. *et al.* The Alzheimer's Disease Cooperative Study. (1997). A controlled trial of selegiline, alpha-tocopherol, or both as treatment for Alzheimer's disease. *N. Engl. J. Med.*, **24**(336), 1216–22.

Sano, M., Wilcock, G., van Baelen, B. & Kavanagh, S. (2003). The effects of galantamine treatment on caregiver time in Alzheimer's disease. *Int. J. Geriatr. Psychiatry*, **18**, 1–9.

Scharf, S., Mander, A., Ugoni, A., Vajda, F. & Christophidis, N. (1999). A double-blind, placebo-controlled trial of diclofenac/misoprostol in Alzheimer's disease. *Neurology*, **53**, 197–201.

Scholtyssek, H., Damerau, W., Wessel, R. & Schimke, I. (1997). Antioxidative activity of ginkgolides against superoxide in an aprotic environment. *Chem.-Biol. Interactions*, **106**, 83–90.

Seshadri, S., Beiser, A., Selhub, J. *et al.* (2002). Plasma homocysteine as a risk factor for dementia and Alzheimer's disease. *N. Engl. J. Med.*, **14**(346), 476–83.

Shepherd, J., Blauw, G. J., Murphy, M. B. *et al.* PROSPER study group (2002). PROspective Study of Pravastatin in the Elderly at Risk. Pravastatin in elderly individuals at risk of vascular disease (PROSPER): a randomised controlled trial. *Lancet*, **360**, 1623–30.

Tariot, P. N., Farlow, M. R., Grossberg, G. T., Graham, S. M., McDonald, S., Gergel, I.; Memantine Study Group (2004). Memantine treatment in patients with moderate to severe Alzheimer disease already receiving donepezil: a randomized controlled trial. *J. Am. Med. Assoc.*, **291**(3), 317–24.

Torian, I., Davidson, E., Fulop, G., Sell, I. & Fillit, H. (1992). The effect of dementia on acute care in a geriatric medical unit. *Int. Psychogeriatr.*, **4**(2), 231–9.

van Dongen, M. C., van Rossum, E., Kessels, A. G., Sielhorst, H. J. & Knipschild, P. G. (2000). The efficacy of ginkgo for elderly people with dementia and age-associated memory impairment: new results of a randomized clinical trial. *J. Am. Geriatr. Soc.*, **48**, 1183–94.

Visser, H., Thal, L., Ferris, S. *et al.* (2003). A randomized double-blind placebo controlled trial of Rofecoxib in patients with MCI. ACNP Annual Meeting 12-10-03. San Juan, Puerto Rico.

Weggen, S., Eriksen, J. L., Das, P. *et al.* (2001). A subset of NSAIDs lower amyloidogenic Abeta42 independently of cyclooxygenase activity. *Nature*, **414**, 212–16.

Wilkinson, D., Doody, R., Helme, R. *et al.* (2003). Donepezil in vascular dementia: a randomized, placebo-controlled study. *Neurology*, **61**(4), 479–86.

Winblad, B., & Poritis, N. (1999). Memantine in severe dementia: results of the 9M-Best Study (benefit and efficacy in severely demented patients during treatment with memantine). *Int. J. Geriatr. Psychiatry*, **14**(12), 135–46.

Winblad, B., Engedal, K., Soininen, H. *et al.* (2001). A 1-year, randomized, placebo-controlled study of donepezil in patients with mild to moderate AD. *Neurology*, **57**, 489–95.

Wolozin, B., Kellman, W., Ruosseau, P., Celesia, G. G. & Siegel, G. (2000). Decreased prevalence of Alzheimer disease associated with 3-hydroxy-3-methyglutaryl coenzyme A reductase inhibitors. *Arch. Neurol.*, **57**, 1439–43.

Zandi, P. P., Anthony, J. C., Hayden, K. M., Mehta, K., Mayer, L. & Breitner, J. C; Cache County Study Investigators (2002). Reduced incidence of AD with NSAID but not H2 receptor antagonists: the Cache County Study. *Neurology*, **59**, 880–6.

Zandi, P. P., Anthony, J. C., Khachaturian, A. S. *et al.* Cache County Study Group (2004). Reduced risk of Alzheimer disease in users of antioxidant vitamin supplements. *Arch. Neurol.*, **61**, 82–8.

Part VI

Other dementias

33

Dementia with Lewy bodies

Norman Relkin

Weill Cornell Medical College, New York, NY, USA

Introduction

"Lewy bodies" are proteinaceous intraneuronal inclusions that were first described by F. H. Lewy in 1912 in neurons of the basal forebrain and thalamus of patients with Parkinson's disease (PD) (Lewy, 1913). More than eight decades after Dr. Lewy's original report, international consensus criteria (see Table 33.1) were created that formally acknowledged the existence of a syndrome of dementia with parkinsonism associated with LBs in other brain areas such as the limbic system and neocortex (McKeith et al., 1996). This condition, known as Dementia with Lewy bodies (DLB), is now recognized to be the second most common cause of neurodegenerative dementia in older adults. Lewy body neuropathology is found in the brains of 15% to 28% of dementia patients that undergo autopsy (Jellinger, 2003; Rahkonen et al., 2003), and DLB accounts for nearly half as many cases of dementia as Alzheimer's disease (Barker et al., 2002). Despite its considerable prevalence and morbidity, DLB is a relatively unknown entity to a large segment of the general public as well as many physicians.

In its most recognizable form, DLB presents as a hypokinetic movement disorder associated with progressive cognitive decline. Other core features include delirium-like fluctuations of attention/arousal, autonomic and sleep disturbances as well as idiosyncratic delusions and hallucinations. While the clinical features of DLB can resemble those of Alzheimer's and Parkinson's disease, possible demographic distinctions have been reported among these disorders. In one autopsy series, DLB was found to be over-represented in men relative to women (Rahkonen et al., 2003), the reverse of the gender ratio generally observed for Alzheimer's disease. However, this finding has not been generally replicated in subsequent clinical studies. DLB has a predilection to take onset in the seventh and eighth decades of life, similar to Alzheimer's disease but later than is typical for idiopathic Parkinson's disease (McKeith, 2000). A recent study found comparable life expectancies in Alzheimer's disease and DLB, as well as similar age of onset and duration of illness until death (Weiner et al., 2003). Across studies there has been sufficient overlap between Alzheimer's, Parkinson's and DLB to suggest they might be part of a single disease continuum rather than discrete diseases, although there is no clear consensus on that issue.

It is very important from a clinical standpoint to distinguish DLB from diseases such as Alzheimer's and Parkinson's disease because of differences in the course of DLB and its response to treatment. From the onset, DLB patients often exhibit hallucinosis and behavior disturbances that are unexpected at a comparably early stage of Alzheimer's or Parkinson's disease. These psychiatric disturbances can be especially difficult to treat because DLB patients exhibit idiosyncratic reactions to medications that can be prescribed with relative impunity in other conditions. For example, up to a half of patients with DLB show a pathologic sensitivity to the types of antipsychotic medications that are typically used to treat hallucinations and delusions (Ballard et al., 1998). Although the risk is greatest for conventional high-potency neuroleptics, even newer antipsychotics may cause adverse events such as coma after a single dose of clozapine reported in a DLB patient (Sadek & Rockwood, 2003). Anti-parkinsonian medications, particularly dopamine agonists, may worsen confusion in DLB patients and tend to be less effective in treating rigidity and postural instability than in patients with Parkinson's disease (Kaufer, 2002). These and other treatment distinctions underscore the importance of recognizing DLB in the clinical setting and managing it appropriately.

Table 33.1. Lewy body consensus criteria

1. Progressive cognitive decline of sufficient magnitude to interfere with normal social function.
   - Memory loss may not be persistent or prominent in earliest stages but generally becomes evident with disease progression.
   - Deficits on tests of attention, frontal executive and visuospatial abilities may be especially prominent.

2. Two core features necessary for a diagnosis of probable DLB, one for possible DLB:
   (a) fluctuating cognition with pronounced variations in attention and alertness.
   (b) recurrent visual hallucinations which are typically well formed and detailed.
   (c) spontaneous motor features of parkinsonism.

3. Features supportive of diagnosis:
   (a) repeated falls
   (b) syncope
   (c) transient loss of consciousness
   (d) neuroleptic sensitivity
   (e) systematized delusions
   (f) hallucinations in other modalities.

4. A diagnosis of DLB is less likely if:
   (a) stroke disease is evident as focal neurological signs or on brain imaging.
   (b) evidence on physical examination and investigation of any physical illness or other brain disorder is sufficient to account for the clinical picture.

From McKeith *et al.* (1996).

While DLB can present difficult treatment challenges, it can also be gratifyingly amenable to certain interventions. Acetylcholinergic deficiency is reportedly more profound in DLB than in Alzheimer's disease, and alterations in both the muscarinic and nicotinic cholinergic system have been reported (Ballard *et al.*, 2002). Treatment with acetylcholinesterase inhibitors such as tacrine, rivastigmine and donepezil have been reported to reduce the behavioral and cognitive symptoms associated with DLB without a marked proclivity to worsen extrapyramidal symptoms or cause other severe side effects (Wild *et al.*, 2003). Unfortunately, the use of cholinesterase inhibitors to treat DLB has not been formally approved by major regulatory bodies at this time. Treatment of DLB with this class of medications is often delayed or neglected. For these and other reasons, it is important to increase recognition of DLB as well as the awareness of availability of effective pharmacologic interventions.

Pathogenesis and heritability

Despite ongoing studies of its molecular pathogenesis, relatively little is known about the primary causes of DLB. The constituents of Lewy bodies include several cytoskeletal elements and components of proteosomal degradation pathways such as alpha-synuclein, ubiquitin and intermediate neurofilament proteins. This may imply that DLB, like several other central neurodegenerative disorders, is associated with disturbances in protein folding and aggregation. However, more research is needed to identify the precise mechanisms involved.

Genetic studies often provide clues to the pathogenic mechanisms underlying human disorders. Because DLB was not commonly diagnosed before the 1980s, data on familial inheritance patterns and genetic linkage is more limited than for disorders such as Parkinson's and Alzheimer's disease. There is emerging evidence of heritable factors in DLB based on linkage studies carried out in a limited number of reported familial cohorts (Trembath *et al.*, 2003). To date, only one autosomal dominant genetic mutation (the E46K mutation of the α-synuclein gene) has been identified as a specific cause of DLB (Zarranz *et al.*, 2004). This was discovered in a Spanish family in which multiple affected individuals developed parkinsonism, dementia, and visual hallucinations. At postmortem, the brains of those affected showed lack of Alzheimer pathology and numerous Lewy bodies which were immunoreactive to α-synuclein and ubiquitin in cortical and subcortical areas. The mutation that was found in all affected family members results in substitution of lysine for glutamate in the α-synuclein protein. The alpha-synuclein protein is a central component of the Lewy bodies, and other mutations in the alpha-synuclein gene have been previously reported to cause early onset forms of parkinsonism associated with dementia. Transgenic animal models using alpha-synuclein mutations have been created in mice and flies that manifest several of the features of human DLB neuropathology (for review, see Sommer *et al.*, 2000).

The APOE-ε4 allele is modestly over-represented among patients with DLB, although the strength of the association is less than with Alzheimer's disease. Autopsy studies have suggested a correlation between Alzheimer's disease pathology in DLB patients and possession of the APOE-ε4 allele, but have failed to demonstrate a dose-dependent effect on either senile plaque burden or neurofibrillary tangle density (Singleton *et al.*, 2002). Other genetic polymorphisms have been studied in relation to DLB, but as yet none has been strongly associated with risk of this disorder.

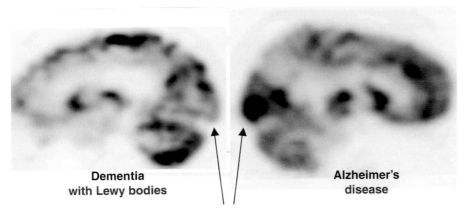

**Dementia
with Lewy bodies**

**Alzheimer's
disease**

Fig. 33.1 [18]Fluorodeoxyglucose PET scans in patients with dementia with Lewy bodies and Alzeimer's disease respectively. Sagittal images of cerebral glucose metabolism in severity matched patients imaged with eyes open using identical scanner. Arrows denote area of hypometabolism in occipital cortex of DLB patient and occipital sparing in Alzheimer's disease case. Hypoperfusion and hypometabolism in the occipital lobe has been found in more than half of DLB patients, and can assist in differential diagnosis of DLB from Alzheimer's disease.

Neuropathology

The acceptance of DLB as a clinical disease entity over the last two decades is in part a consequence of improvements in the techniques used to identify its associated neuropathology. Brainstem LBs were readily detected by the conventional histochemical stains of the kind available to Dr. Lewy in the 1910s (see Fig. 33.1). However, cortical LBs have different staining properties that make them harder to detect by these methods. Immunohistochemical methods for identifying ubiquitin and other minor LB components became available in the 1980s. These immunostains helped to better identify the burden of Lewy bodies in individual cases and revealed other elements of DLB pathology such as "Lewy neurites," dystrophic neuronal elements that classically stain positive for ubiquitin and occur prominently in the CA2/CA3 region of the hippocampus. In addition to a central core of α-synuclein, LBs contain ubiquitin, neurofilament protein, tubulin, microtubule associated protein (MAP) and amyloid precursor protein.

Use of ubiquitin stains and characterization of the distribution of Lewy bodies and associated pathology are part of the recommended procedures for the neuropathological diagnosis of DLB. Consensus criteria have drawn distinctions between cases in which Lewy bodies are found predominately in the brainstem vs. limbic structures vs. the neocortex. A recent study in Japan (Marui *et al.*, 2002) suggests that Lewy body neuropathology may progress in a spatially and cytopathologically specific pattern. Postmortem examination of the brains of 27 patients indicated that the earliest occurrence of Lewy neurites was in the amygdala, followed by limbic cortex and subsequently the neocortex. Within the neocortex, there was evidence of a sequential involvement of cortical layers V–VI, then layer III followed by layer II. Intraneuronal alterations were seen first in the axonal terminal, followed by the cell body and ultimately dendrites. Further studies are needed to establish the reproducibility of these findings and their relevance to the symptomatic progression of DLB.

Clinical characterization

DLB is diagnosed directly based on findings derived from the clinical history and neurologic examination. Consensus clinical criteria are listed in Table 33.1, and include primary as well as supportive symptoms. The features that are most typical of DLB include a parkinsonian extrapyramidal movement disturbance, visuospatial and executive functional cognitive impairments that wax and wane over time, and neuropsychiatric symptoms such as visual hallucinations with fixed delusions. The order of emergence of these symptoms is variable, but by convention cognitive disturbances and parkinsonism are usually expected to appear within a year of one another in DLB. In contrast, the very similar form of dementia associated with idiopathic Parkinson's disease can emerge several years after the onset of the movement disorder. Extrapyramidal abnormalities in Alzheimer's disease are expected predominantly in late stages of the disease.

The extrapyramidal disturbance in DLB is typically described as parkinsonism without tremor. The complete absence of resting tremor in DLB is not uniformly observed, but in most cases tremor is not a prominent feature. Other extrapyramidal symptoms may include increased tone, retropulsion or other postural instability, shortened steps, bradykinesia and masked facies. The reported frequency of parkinsonian symptoms at onset of DLB ranges from 10–100%, which varies with the referral base of the clinical population studied (e.g. greatest in Neurologic clinics, least in General Practice) (McKeith et al., 2003). Parkinsonian symptoms may be symmetric or asymmetric in DLB, and may wax and wane in much the same manner as cognitive and behavioral disturbances. Myoclonus is infrequently observed in DLB patients, and in rare cases supranuclear gaze palsies have been observed. DLB symptoms sometimes respond positively to levo-dopa therapy, but the therapeutic window is generally narrow. Confusion and other cognitive changes can be exacerbated by dopaminergic treatments, particularly with dose escalation (Kaufer, 2002).

Patients with DLB show a variety of cognitive symptoms that overlap with those observed in Alzheimer's disease and the dementia of Parkinson's disease, as well as some features that are relatively distinctive. Performance on verbal memory tests and tests of orientation are often better in DLB than at comparable stages of Alzheimer's disease, but may be worse than in patients with Parkinson's disease at otherwise comparable stages of disease. DLB patients often do less well than Alzheimer's disease patients on performance-based tests and visual recognition tasks, while Parkinson's disease patients may show even greater weaknesses on such tests. Frontal executive functions are generally impaired in all of these disorders, but tend to fluctuate more in patients with DLB. Fluctuation in attention can be detected by repeated administration of timed tests in a clinical setting, and reportedly show a greater degree of variation in DLB and Parkinson's disease than Alzheimer's disease (Ballard et al., 2002a,b).

With progression of disease, dementia in DLB can progress through mild to moderate and severe stages characterized by progressively greater cognitive deficits as well as increasing functional dependency. Eventually, patients tend to lose all independent function in the disease's final stages. Rate of decline has been reported to be slightly greater in DLB than Alzheimer's disease, averaging 4–5 minimental state exam (MMSE) points per year in comparison to the expected 3 points per year decline on the MMSE in Alzheimer's disease (Helmes et al., 2003). Formal testing by a neuropsychologist familiar with disorders such as DLB can be helpful in characterizing the cognitive status of patients with presumed DLB, which can be difficult in the context of fluctuation arousal and co-morbid psychiatric symptoms.

Fluctuations in attention and arousal occur on multiple time scales in patients with DLB. This includes millisecond to millisecond variations in the EEG and long latency evoked response measurements to changes in state spanning weeks to months in some cases. While specific tests can be brought to bear to document these fluctuations, their physiologic and neurochemical basis remains uncertain. It has been observed that treatment with cholinesterase inhibitors may dampen the oscillations in some patients with DLB, suggesting a role for the cholinergic system in their etiology (Ballard et al., 2002a,b). Disease-related fluctuations can be mistaken for willful dissemblance on the part of patients, and may confound assessment of progression of disease and response to treatment over time. Patients and caregivers should be alerted to the tendency of DLB symptoms to fluctuate and encouraged not to assume disease progression has been accelerated when symptoms wax as part of this cycle.

The neuropsychiatric manifestations of DLB are among the most fascinating aspects of the illness and can provide extremely useful clues to the diagnosis. A majority of patients with DLB experience some psychiatric disturbance, and at least half develop characteristic visual hallucinations during the course of their illness. These hallucinations are most commonly fully formed and animate, often involving deceased relatives, complete strangers or animals. In most cases the hallucinations are not perceived as threatening by the patient, but there are clear exceptions. It is unusual although not unprecedented for these visual hallucinations to have auditory components, and some DLB patients express their frustration that their hallucinations do not respond to their overtures to conversation. The hallucinations are occasionally triggered by comparably shaped or patterned objects in the immediate environment, and may move away or disappear when approached. The so-called "extracampine" hallucination is another common occurrence, in which affected individuals have the sense that someone else is in the room with them, or perhaps briefly glimpsed out of the corner of their eye (Chan & Rossor, 2002). A common feature of DLB is the elaboration of systematized delusions that often center around the hallucinations. Patients may acknowledge that the hallucinated relative is deceased, but nevertheless treat them as though they are alive. The combined occurrence of visual hallucinosis and circumscribed delusions in the context of dementia and/or an extrapyramidal disorder should trigger consideration of DLB. Depression, apathy, anxiety, insomnia, paranoia and paramnestic phenomena also occur in DLB with some frequency and require sensitive management particularly owing to the pharmacological sensitivities DLB patients often manifest.

A number of other findings have been associated with DLB but are variable in their occurrence. When present these features are considered supportive of the diagnosis, but are not required according to consensus criteria. This includes Rapid Eye Movement Sleep Behavior Disorder (REMSBD), orthostatic hypotension and other autonomic dysfunction, unexplained falls or syncopy, and neuroleptic sensitivity.

Onset of REMSBD may precede symptoms of DLB by several years, and is more likely to be associated with DLB than any other form of dementia (Boeve *et al.*, 2001; Turner, 2002). This disorder is characterized by a failure of the normal mechanisms of sleep paralysis resulting in vocalizations, gesticulations and other behaviors associated with patients acting out their dreams while asleep. One proposed mechanism is loss of neurons in monoaminergic brainstem nuclei such as the locus ceruleus and substantia nigra causing decreased inhibition of the cholinergic pedunculopontine nucleus which is a mediator of the atonia of sleep (Turner *et al.*, 2000). Treatment with the cholinesterase inhibitor donepezil has been reported to decrease symptoms of REMSBD in some cases (Ringman & Simmons, 2000).

Orthostatic hypotension may be a contributing factor in syncope and falls among DLB patients, and can be treated with pressure stockings, increased salt intake and if necessary, mineralocorticoids. Increased neuroleptic sensitivity is frequently observed but is not something that should be tested for provocatively, since relatively dire consequences have been reported in some DLB patients after receiving even a single dose of antipsychotics. Some of the symptoms of DLB have been found to correlate with the burden of LB in relatively circumscribed neuranatomic regions (McKeith *et al.*, 2003). Cortical LB in DLB tend to be found in the greatest density in the anterior cingulated gyrus, the transentorhinal region of the medial temporal lobe and portions of the frontal lobes. Overall dementia severity has been found to correlate with LB burden in frontal and temporal cortices. Visual hallucinations have been found to correlate with LB density in the amygdala, parahippocampal gyrus and inferior temporal cortex. Degenerative changes in the cholinergic peduncolopontine nucleus may be associated with postural instability and with REM Sleep Behavior Disorder.

Advanced stages of DLB are associated with relatively global cognitive and functional impairments. Death, as in other central neurodegenerative disorders, is usually not the direct consequence of progressive brain failure but rather the co-morbid medical conditions to which it predisposes the patient, such as aspiration pneumonia and sepsis.

Laboratory evaluations and brain imaging

While blood tests are a part of the routine evaluation of DLB, they are primarily used for identifying co-morbid conditions rather than direct diagnosis. Despite the reported association between APOE-ε4 and DLB, genetic testing is not part of the routine diagnosis of DLB. APOE genotyping could conceivably provide information relevant to differential diagnosis of Parkinson's disease and DLB. Lumbar puncture and analysis of cerebrospinal fluid (CSF) is not currently recommended for routine evaluation since as yet there are no CSF markers that have been unequivocally linked to DLB.

Both structural and functional brain imaging can provide information supportive of a DLB diagnosis. For example, SPECT studies of clinically diagnosed DLB patients have identified resting occipital hypoperfusion in some patients, in addition to a pattern of temporoparietal and prefrontal hypoperfusion typically seen in Alzheimer's disease (Lobotesis *et al.*, 2001) (see Fig. 33.1). Occipital hypoperfusion on HMPAO SPECT scans was also found in 57% of DLB patients with visual hallucinations (Pasquier *et al.*, 2002). Although occipital hypoperfusion and hypometabolism does not occur ubiquitously in patients with DLB, it is useful when present for distinguishing suspected DLB from Alzheimer's, since occipital metabolism is generally preserved in Alzheimer's. Use of dopaminergic ligands for functional brain imaging in this context is under study and may further assist in the differentiation of DLB and Alzheimer's (Marshall & Grosset, 2003).

Cerebral atrophy is a feature of both Alzheimer's and DLB. Annualized rates of atrophy are comparable in the two conditions. Voxel-based morphometry, an image quantification technique that is less prone to operator bias than manual volumetric measurements, has been used to demonstrate regional differences in the pattern of cerebral atrophy in Alzheimer's disease and DLB (Marshall & Grosset, 2003). Hippocampal atrophy in DLB is reported to be greater than that of age-matched normal controls but less than that of Alzheimer's disease patients with a comparable duration of disease. As many as 40% of DLB patients have no discernable hippocampal atrophy relative to age-matched controls. VBM also shows greater preservation of the medial temporal lobe, amygdala and thalamus in DLB relative to Alzheimer's. This "sparing" of the hippocampus may explain the relative preservation of verbal

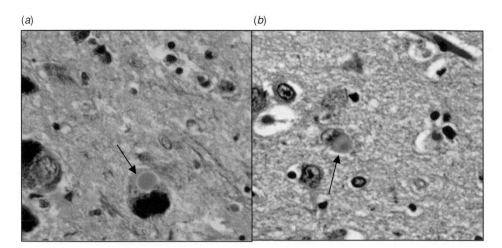

Fig. 33.2 (*a*) Hematoxylin and eosin staining of a Lewy body (arrow) within a pigmented neuron of the substantia nigra in Parkinson's disease. (*b*) Hematoxylin and eosin staining of a cortical Lewy body (arrow) in dementia with Lewy bodies.

memory observed early in the course of DLB compared to Alzheimer's at the same stage of illness.

Management

Optimal management of DLB is facilitated by early and accurate diagnosis. While patients at any stage of the disease may still be responsive to treatment, early diagnosis can help to reduce the likelihood of adverse occurrences such as inappropriate neuroleptic exposure, wandering and other risky behaviors, as well as caregiver burnout. Patients with DLB may already have been treated by other physicians under the mistaken belief that they were suffering from another disorder such Alzheimer's, Parkinson's or a primary psychiatric disturbance. It is therefore good practice to review the medications already prescribed to confirm their appropriateness, and when indicated, judiciously reduce or withdraw those medications known to adversely affect cognition in DLB patients. A brief drug holiday (e.g. 3–7 days) may be a useful means of assessing the degree to which individual medications are contributing positively or negatively to the patient's clinical status, but must be carefully considered based on whether those medications are medical necessities. For maintenance therapy, high potency neuroleptics such as haloperidol should generally be discontinued if possible, substituting other medications as needed to address the patient's behavioral state. Dopaminergic therapies such as levodopa, dopamine agonists and COM-T inhibitors can in some cases exacerbate DSLB symptoms and should be reduced in dose or temporarily withdrawn if problematic behaviors are present. If withdrawal of these medications fails to yield behavioral improvement, low doses of novel neuroleptics such as quetiapine that have a relatively low propensity for EPS can be prescribed on a temporary or as need basis. However, other medications such as cholinesterase inhibitors (see below) should be considered for long-term treatment.

Only one large-scale double-blind, placebo-controlled treatment trial with DLB patients was completed prior to 2004, and in this study rivastigmine was found to significantly improve behavior but not cognition (McKeith *et al.*, 2000) Based on the results of a limited number of open label prospective treatment trials completed to date, cholinesterase inhibitors such as donepezil, galanthamine and tacrine administered at the same doses as are used to treat Alzheimer's disease may improve cognition and behavior in DLB patients. Delusions tend to be more refractory to treatment but in some cases improve considerably over time. Improvements in MMSE scores can be dramatic as can restoration of functional and behavioral status. In studies completed to date, speed of movement increased and only minimal evidence of worsening of parkinsonism has been observed after cholinesterase treatment, largely confined to exaggeration of existing tremors. The symptomatic improvement observed in some DLB patients after treatment with cholinesterase inhibitors has been documented to persist for up to one year (Grace *et al.*, 2001). Although longer-term benefits can be expected in analogy to Alzheimer's disease, this has yet to be demonstrated in controlled clinical trials. As of 2004, the NMDA receptor antagonist Memantine, which has been approved in the United States and Europe for treatment of advanced

Alzheimer's, has yet to be tested as a treatment for DLB in a large-scale randomized prospective study. Based on the available data, cholinesterase inhibitors should be considered the current treatment of choice for symptoms of DLB and should be initiated as soon as possible after diagnosis.

In addition to cholinesterase therapy, treatment must be individualized to the needs of the particular patient. A profoundly depressed DLB patient may not improve from cholinesterase inhibitors alone, but may benefit from the combined use of these agents with a conventional antidepressant such as an SSRI that has relatively little cholinergic side effects. While benzodiazepines are generally not recommended in the context of dementia, there are advocates of the use of low doses of clonazepam to treat symptoms of REM Sleep Behavior Disorder that are refractory to cholinesterase inhibitors or melatonin (McKeith et al., 2003). There is only limited experience in using mood stabilizing anticonvulsants such as depakote and topiramate in the treatment of DLB, and while they may worsen cognitive impairments and EPS in some cases, they may have a role in reducing aggressive and other socially inacceptable behaviors. Other symptoms such as apathy, insomnia and agitation may be targeted for treatment, keeping in mind that DLB patients may exhibit altered dose responses to conventional medications and should be treated with the lowest effective dose whenever possible.

Conclusions

Although acceptance of DLB as a clinical entity has increased in the past two decades, there are many issues that remain unresolved. One major question is whether cortical LBs actually cause dementia. There is not a one-to-one relationship between DLB symptoms during life and LB neuropathology at autopsy. Postmortem studies have documented extensive numbers of cortical LBs in the brains of some individuals who survived to advanced ages without developing dementia. Likewise, patients meeting clinical criteria for probable DLB are sometimes found to have exclusively Alzheimer's or Parkinson's neuropathology at autopsy in the absence of cortical LBs. Only limited reports have documented exclusively neocortical LBD pathology in association with dementia in the absence of Alzheimer's pathology (Uchikado et al., 2002). The pathophysiological relevance of LBs is incompletely understood, and some lines of evidence even suggest that LBs may be the byproduct of mechanisms that protect neurons against toxic injury rather than an actual cause of neurodegeneration (McNaught et al., 2002).

Another ambiguity about DLB is its relationship to other neurodegenerative disorders. Although LB pathology can occur in isolation, it is more commonly found in combination with Alzheimer-related brain changes. One recent review of cases from a Florida brain bank found concomitant Alzheimer pathology in 66% of DLB cases at autopsy (Jellinger, 2003). Some authors have even advocated use of the term "Lewy body Variant of Alzheimer's" as an expression of the frequency with which Alzheimer's neuropathology accompanies that of DLB. Hardy has argued that Alzheimer's, DLB and Parkinson's disease should be considered disease processes on a continuum rather than separate diagnostic entities (Rahkonen et al., 2003). While this viewpoint is consistent with evidence from a variety of molecular, genetic and neuropathological studies, it is difficult to operationalize in clinical practice.

Until molecular diagnostic techniques permit more objective diagnoses in individual cases, the accurate clinical diagnosis of DLB will continue to require clinical acumen. By following the formal clinical diagnostic guidelines, accuracy in the range of 75–80% relative to autopsy can be expected. While this may seem a less than satisfying percentage, it represents a sizeable number of cases in which management and outcome can be improved as a result of a previously unrecognized disorder being properly identified. In light of its prevalence, the difficulties inherent in management of untreated cases, the adverse effects of neuroleptics observed in this population, and the responsiveness to treatment with cholinergic agents, DLB is unquestionably an important disease entity meriting increasing efforts towards diagnosis, treatment and future study.

REFERENCES

Ballard, C., O'Brien, J. et al. (1998). A prospective study of dementia with Lewy bodies. *Age Ageing*, **27**(5), 631–6.

Ballard, C., Aarsland, D. et al. (2002a). Fluctuations in attention: Parkinson's disease dementia vs DLB with parkinsonism. *Neurology*, **59**(11), 1714–20.

Ballard, C., Court, J. et al. (2002b). Disturbances of consciousness in dementia with Lewy bodies associated with alteration in nicotinic receptor binding in the temporal cortex. *Conscious Cogn.*, **11**(3), 461–74.

Barker, W. W., Luis, C. A., Kashuba, A. et al. (2002). Relative frequencies of Alzheimer disease, Lewy body, vascular and frontotemporal dementia, and hippocampal sclerosis in the State of Florida Brain Bank. *Alzheimer Dis. Assoc. Disord.*, **16**(4), 203–12.

Boeve, B. F., Silber, M. H., Ferman, T. J. et al. (2001). Association of REM sleep behavior disorder and neurodegenerative disease may reflect an underlying synucleinopathy. *Mov. Disord.*, **16**(4), 622–30.

Burton, E. J., Karas, G. & Paling, S. M. (2002). Patterns of cerebral atrophy in dementia with Lewy bodies using voxel-based morphometry. *Neuroimage*, **17**(2), 618–30.

Chan, D. & Rossor, M. (2002). -but who is that on the other side of you? Extracampine hallucinations revisited. *Lancet*, **360**(9350), 2064–6.

Grace, J., Daniel, S. & Stevens, T. (2001). Long-term use of rivastigmine in patients with dementia with Lewy bodies: an open-label trial. *Int. Psychogeriatr.*, **13**(2), 199–205.

Helmes, E., Bowler, J. *et al.* (2003). Rates of cognitive decline in Alzheimer's disease and dementia with Lewy bodies. *Dement. Geriatr. Cogn. Disord.*, **15**(2), 67–71.

Jellinger, K. A. (2003). Age-associated prevalence and risk factors of Lewy body pathology in a general population. *Acta Neuropathol. (Berl.)*, **106**(4), 374–82.

Kaufer, D. (2002). Pharmacologic therapy of dementia with Lewy bodies. *J. Geriatr. Psychiatry Neurol.*, **15**(4), 224–32.

Lewy, F. H. (1913). Zur pathologischen anatomie der paralysis agitans. Dtsch. Z. Nervenheilkd., **50**, 50–5.

Lobotesis, K., Fenwick, J. D., Phipps, A. *et al.* (2001). Occipital hypoperfusion on SPECT in dementia with Lewy bodies but not Alzheimer's disease. *Neurology*, **56**(5), 643–9.

Marshall, V. & Grosset, D. (2003). Role of dopamine transporter imaging in routine clinical practice. *Mov. Disord.*, **18**(12), 1415–23.

Marui, W., Iseki, E., Nakai, T. *et al.* (2002). Progression and staging of Lewy pathology in brains from patients with dementia with Lewy bodies. *J. Neurol. Sci.*, **195**(2), 153–9.

McKeith, I. G. (2000). Clinical Lewy body syndromes. *Ann. NY Acad. Sci.*, **920**, 1–8.

McKeith, I. G., Galasko, D., Kosaka, K. *et al.* (1996). Consensus guidelines for the clinical and pathologic diagnosis of dementia with Lewy bodies (DLB): report of the consortium on DLB international workshop. *Neurology*, **47**(5), 1113–24.

McKeith, I., Del Ser, T. & Spano, P. (2000). Efficacy of rivastigmine in dementia with Lewy bodies: a randomised, double-blind, placebo-controlled international study. *Lancet*, **356**(9247), 2031–6.

McKeith, I. G., Burns, D. J., Ballard, C. G. *et al.* (2003). Dementia with Lewy bodies. *Sem. Clin. Neuropsychiatry*, **8**(1), 46–57.

McNaught, K. S., Shashidharan, P., Perl, D. P. *et al.* (2002). Aggresome-related biogenesis of Lewy bodies. *Eur. J. Neurosci.*, **16**(11), 2136–48.

Pasquier, J., Michel, B. *et al.* (2002). Value of (99m)Tc-ECD SPET for the diagnosis of dementia with Lewy bodies. *Eur. J. Nucl. Med. Mol. Imaging*, **29**(10), 1342–8.

Rahkonen, T., Eloniemi-Sulkava, U., Rissanen, S. *et al.* (2003). Dementia with Lewy bodies according to the consensus criteria in a general population aged 75 years or older. *J. Neurol. Neurosurg. Psychiatry*, **74**, 720–4.

Ringman, J. M. & Simmons, J. H. (2000). Treatment of REM sleep behavior disorder with donepezil: a report of three cases. *Neurology*, **55**(6), 870–1.

Sadek, J. & Rockwood, K. (2003). Coma with accidental single dose of an atypical neuroleptic in a patient with Lewy Body dementia. *Am. J. Geriatr. Psych.*, **11**(1), 112–13.

Singleton, A., Wharton, A. *et al.* (2002). Clinical and neuropathological correlates of apolipoprotein E genotype in dementia with Lewy bodies. *Dement. Geriatr. Cogn. Disord.*, **14**(4), 167–75.

Sommer, B., Barbieri, S., Hofele, K. *et al.* (2000). Mouse models of alpha-synucleinopathy and Lewy pathology. *Exp. Gerontol.*, **35**(9–10) 1389–403.

Trembath, Y., Rosenberg, C. *et al.* (2003). Lewy body pathology is a frequent co-pathology in familial Alzheimer's disease. *Acta Neuropathol. (Berl.)*, **105**(5), 484–8.

Turner, R. (2002). Idiopathic rapid eye movement sleep behavior disorder is a harbinger of dementia with Lewy bodies. *J. Geriatr. Psychiatry Neurol.*, **15**(4), 195–9.

Turner, R., D'Amato, C., Chervin, R. *et al.* (2000). The pathology of REM sleep behavior disorder with comorbid Lewy body dementia. *Neurology*, **55**(11), 1730–2.

Uchikado, H., Iseki, E. & Tsuchiya, K. (2002). Dementia with Lewy bodies showing advanced Lewy pathology but minimal Alzheimer pathology – Lewy pathology causes neuronal loss inducing progressive dementia. *Clin. Neuropathol.*, **21**(6), 269–77.

Weiner, M. F., Hynan, L. S., Parikh, B. *et al.* (2003). Can Alzheimer's disease and Dementias with Lewy bodies be distinguished clinically? *J. Geriatr. Psych. Neurol.*, **16**(4), 245–50.

Wild, R., Pettit, T. *et al.* (2003). Cholinesterase inhibitors for dementia with Lewy bodies. *Cochrane Database Syst. Rev.*

Zarranz, J. J., Alegre, J., Gomez-Esteban, J. C., *et al.* (2004). The new mutation, E46K, of alpha-synuclein causes Parkinson and Lewy body dementia. *Ann. Neurol.*, **55**(2), 164–73.

34

Frontotemporal lobar degeneration

Adam L. Boxer,[1] John Q. Trojanowski,[2] Virginia M.-Y. Lee[2] and Bruce L. Miller[1]

[1]Memory and Aging Center, Department of Neurology, University of California at San Francisco, CA, USA
[2]Center for Neurodegenerative Disease Research, University of Pennsylvania School of Medicine, Philadelphia, PA, USA

Introduction

Frontotemporal lobar degeneration, formerly called Pick's disease, is a progressive dementia that is associated with focal atrophy of the frontal and/or temporal lobes. For over 100 years, the key clinical and pathological feature of this disease has been recognized to be focal, often asymmetric cortical involvement. Histopathologically, frontotemporal lobar degeneration (FTLD) is distinct from Alzheimer's disease but heterogeneous, even among similar clinical syndromes. Recently, with the advent of specialized immunohistochemical stains and insights gained from molecular genetics, it has been recognized that FTLD is closely related to, and sometimes overlaps with three other neurodegenerative diseases: corticobasal ganglionic degeneration (CBD), progressive supranuclear palsy (PSP), and motor neuron disease (MND). The central role of the microtubule-associated protein, tau, in the pathogenesis of FTLD, has led to classification as a "tauopathy."

First description and history of FTLD

The first case of what is now called frontotemporal lobar degeneration (FTLD) was described by Arnold Pick in 1892 (Pick, 1892). His subsequent description of six similar patients emphasized a language impairment, which he termed "amnestic aphasia," and a focal pattern of brain atrophy involving the temporal and/or frontal lobes. A lack of senile plaques and tangles in the brains of similar patients was noted by Alzheimer in 1911. He and Altman provided the first histopathological description of argyrophilic inclusions (later termed Pick bodies) and swollen achromatic cells (later termed Pick cells) (Altman, 1923). Onari and Spatz, two of Pick's students, later introduced the term Pick's disease to describe cases of

circumscribed atrophy lacking plaques and tangles (Onari & Spatz, 1926). The later insistence by some researchers that a diagnosis of Pick's disease requires the presence of Pick bodies on histopathology led to an underestimation of the prevalence of cases of FTLD and most likely hindered research into this disorder.

In 1974, Constantinidis et al. (1974) documented three types of histopathology in cases clinically defined as having Pick's disease. The first group of patients had classic Pick bodies and Pick cells. The second group of patients had pathology similar to what is now called corticobasal ganglionic degeneration (CBD). The last group was more heterogeneous, and would include what is now termed dementia lacking distinctive histopathology. The recognition that it was difficult to distinguish histological subtypes of Pick's disease eventually led to a focus on clinical symptoms associated with circumscribed lobar atrophy.

In the late 1980s, Arne Brun and Lars Gustafson, working in Lund, Sweden, and David Neary and Julie Snowden working in Manchester, England began studying non-Alzheimer's degenerative dementias. Both groups described clinical, neuroimaging and histopathological features of dementia patients with progressive frontal lobar degeneration (Snowden et al., 1996a). Although the patients studied by both groups clinically resembled those originally described by Pick, most lacked classic Pick bodies. Instead, Brun noted the presence of prominent astrocytic gliosis and spongiosis of layers I–III in the frontal cortex in typical cases, without the plaques and tangles found in AD (Brun, 1987). He suggested the name *frontal dementia of the non-Alzheimer type* for these patients, while Neary coined the term *dementia of the frontal type* (Miller et al., 1998a). In 1994, the Lund and Manchester groups published consensus research criteria for what they termed frontotemporal dementia (FTD) (Lund & Manchester Groups, 1994).

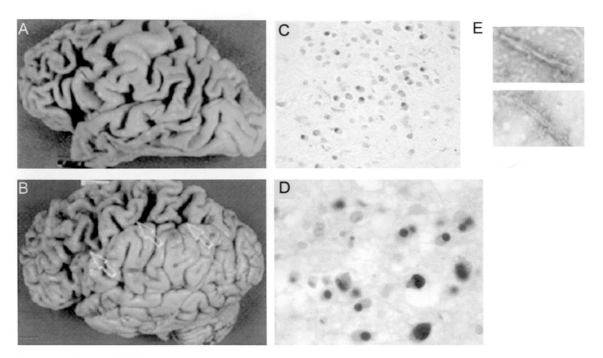

Fig. 34.1 Pathology of FTLD.

A. Gross pathological specimen from patient with Pick's disease. Note frontal and temporal lobar atrophy, with less significant atrophy of inferior parietal lobule and sparing of pre- and post-central gyri.

B. Gross pathological specimen from a patient with corticobasal ganglionic degeneration demonstrating circumscribed atrophy of the parasagittal superior frontal gyrus and superior parietal lobule, including the pre- and post-central gyri (arrows).

C. Tissue section from the hippocampus of a patient with Pick's disease demonstrating Pick bodies stained with an anti-ubiquitin monoclonal antibody.

D. Tissue section from layer IV frontal cortex of a patient with Pick's disease demonstrating Pick bodies stained with an anti-tau antibody (Mab PHF1).

E. Electron micrograph of isolated tau filaments stained with uranyl acetate from a Pick's disease brain.

(A & B from (Trojanowski and Dickson, 2001), C–E from (Zhukareva *et al.*, 2002) with permission)

Also during the 1980s, Mesulam described a group of patients who developed a progressive aphasia with few other cognitive symptoms, which he termed primary progressive aphasia (Mesulam, 1982). He noted that there were two subtypes of patients, one with a primary non-fluent aphasia associated with atrophy of the left frontal lobe, and a second type with a primary fluent aphasia associated with degeneration of the left anterior temporal lobe. This latter group was similar to the original patients described by Pick. The majority of patients in both groups lacked Alzheimer's pathology, and instead showed neuropathological features similar to the frontal disease described by Brun. During the same period of time, Snowden and colleagues described the linguistic deficits of patients with left anterior temporal lobe degeneration (Snowden *et al.*, 1992). These patients also lacked Alzheimer's disease pathology and instead resembled FTD. Because the language disorder was primarily due to a loss of semantic information in these patients, the disorder was later termed semantic dementia (Hodges *et al.*, 1992).

Taking into account the clinical and pathological similarities between frontotemporal dementia, semantic dementia and primary progressive aphasia, the Lund-Manchester criteria were further refined by Neary *et al.* in 1998 to provide descriptions of these three common clinical presentations of FTD, which was renamed frontotemporal lobar degeneration (FTLD) (Neary *et al.*, 1998). Recent evidence of pathological and genetic overlap between FTLD and corticobasal ganglionic degeneration (CBD) suggested to Kertesz and colleagues that these clinical syndromes may be one pathological entity (Kertesz *et al.*, 2000). The most recent clinicopathological criteria for FTLD reflect this association, as well as the overlap between FTLD and Progressive Supranuclear Palsy (PSP), and FTLD and motor neuron disease (MND) (McKhann *et al.*, 2001).

Gross morphological pattern of vulnerability

Focal brain atrophy is apparent both macroscopically and microscopically in FTLD brains. Severe brain atrophy may result in postmortem brain weights as low as 750 grams (Dickson, 2001). Quantitative volumetric assessments of brain atrophy have demonstrated tissue loss in the frontal lobes, the anterior, medial and inferior temporal lobes, including the amygdala and hippocampus, the insula, and variably in subcortical structures such as the caudate, putamen, thalamus and substantia nigra (Mann *et al.*, 1993). Of these regions, the frontal and anterior temporal lobes usually show the largest volume losses. Based on patterns of brain atrophy measured at autopsy in patients with fvFTD, four stages of disease severity have been proposed: (i) mild atrophy of the orbital and superior medial frontal cortices and hippocampus, (ii) progression of mild atrophy to the anterior frontal and temporal cortices and basal ganglia, (iii) progression of mild atrophy to other cortical regions and (iv) severe, cortical atrophy (Broe *et al.*, 2003).

In classic Pick's disease, gross pathology demonstrates predominantly frontal and/or temporal atrophy (Figure 34.1(*a*)). Primary motor and sensory cortex are invariably spared in Pick's disease. Pathological changes similar to that seen in corticobasal ganglionic degeneration (CBD) may be found in most FTLD clinical syndromes, however CBD pathology is most commonly associated with patients who present with language impairment (Kertesz *et al.*, 2000). Gross pathology usually demonstrates superior frontal and parietal atrophy in these patients (Fig. 34.1(*b*)).

Biochemical findings (microscopic pattern of vulnerability)

Pick's disease

A minority of patients who are clinically diagnosed with FTLD will be found to have classic Pick's disease pathology. Microscopically, areas of cortex most severely affected in Pick's disease show a severe loss of large pyramidal neurons with diffuse spongiosis and gliosis. Pick cells, ballooned neurons that stain weakly with silver stains, are found in the deeper cortical layers. These ballooned neurons are filled with granulofilamentous material that is best demonstrated with antibodies to phosphorylated neurofilament, low molecular weight stress protein, αβ-crystallin and ubiquitin hydrolase. Focal tau and/or ubiquitin hydrolase immunoreactivity is sometimes present in ballooned neurons (Dickson, 2001).

In Pick's disease, superficial cortical layers in affected areas contain small neurons with round inclusions that are intensely argyrophilic on silver stains called Pick bodies (Fig. 34.1(*c*), (*d*)). Brain regions rich in Pick bodies show extensive loss of large neurons as well as evidence of synapse loss as demonstrated by loss of synaptophysin immunoreactivity (Masliah *et al.*, 1990). Pick bodies are most commonly found in limbic, paralimbic and ventral temporal lobe cortex. Smaller numbers of Pick bodies are found in the anterior frontal and dorsal temporal lobes, and are rarely found elsewhere. Like the neurofibrillary tangles found in Alzheimer's disease (AD), the hippocampus and amygdala have the largest numbers of Pick bodies. Unlike the neurofibrillary tangles in Alzheimer's disease, which spare the dentate gyrus, Pick bodies are frequently found there. Also in contrast to AD, the nucleus basalis of Meynert is relatively spared in Pick's disease. Consistent with this observation, cholinergic markers are relatively preserved in Pick's disease (Wood *et al.*, 1983). In contrast, dopaminergic neurons in the substantia nigra are frequently affected in Pick's disease.

Pick bodies stain with antibodies to the paired helical filaments (PHF) that make up the neurofibrillary tangles observed in AD and progressive supranuclear palsy (PSP), although ultrastructurally the arrangement of tau filaments is different. Pick bodies are composed of randomly arranged filaments of tau, as opposed to PHF (Fig. 34.1(*e*)) (Pollock *et al.*, 1986). The most sensitive stain for Pick bodies is the anti-tau antibody (Dickson, 2001). Western blot analysis of hyperphosphorylated tau protein in Pick's brains demonstrates a different pattern of abnormal variants than in AD. In Pick's disease, there are two abnormal bands that migrate at 55 and 66 kDa, whereas in AD there are three bands: 55, 66, and 69 kDa. Recent analysis of Pick's brains, using phosphorylation-state specific antisera to tau, has demonstrated large amounts of insoluble tau protein in subcortical white matter, consistent with the predominantly axonal localization of tau in normal neurons (Zhukareva *et al.*, 2002).

Corticobasal ganglionic degeneration (CBD; see also Chapter 45)

CBD brains have ballooned neurons similar to classic Pick's brains, however there are no Pick bodies. Atrophy and ballooned neurons are found throughout the neocortex, and are most abundant in the superior frontal and parietal lobes, unlike Pick's disease, which tends to spare these regions. Unlike Pick's disease, ballooned cells may be found in primary motor or sensory cortex. There is prominent neuronal loss and gliosis in areas most affected by CBD pathology. In many cases, there is significant involvement of basal ganglia structures. Astrocytic plaques that stain with anti-tau antibodies are a hallmark of CBD (Dickson *et al.*, 2002).

Dementia lacking distinctive histopathology (DLDH)

DLDH is a common pathological finding in patients with the clinical symptoms of sporadic FTLD (Knopman *et al.*, 1990; Bird & Schellenberg, 2001). There is a variable pattern of brain involvement in DLDH. These patients have significant neuronal loss and gliosis, without Pick bodies, ballooned neurons, neurofibrillary tangles or other inclusion bodies. There may be spongiform changes in the superficial cortical layers. In contrast to classic Pick's disease, in which there are abnormal accumulations of tau protein, there is a dramatic reduction of tau protein expression in DLDH brains. This most likely represents a post-transcriptional effect on tau gene expression, since mRNA for tau is present in these brains (Zhukareva *et al.*, 2001).

Frontotemporal dementia with motor neuron disease (FTD-MND)

Frontal lobe degeneration may occur in patients with motor neuron disease (MND; amyotrophic lateral sclerosis). In addition, two series of FTLD patients, one with semantic dementia (Rossor *et al.*, 2000), the other with frontotemporal dementia (Forno *et al.*, 2002), both lacking clinical features of MND, were found to have this pattern of neuropathology. Three families with autosomal dominantly inherited frontotemporal dementia, lacking mutations in tau, have also been described with FTD-MND pathology (Rosso *et al.*, 2001). Like DLDH, there are no Pick bodies or ballooned neurons, however immunohistochemical stains reveal ubiquitin-positive, tau-negative neuronal inclusions in affected areas of cerebral cortex, as well as in anterior horn cells (Jackson *et al.*, 1996).

Molecular biology

The role of tau protein in FTLD pathogenesis

Advances in the molecular biology of the tau protein have led to a better understanding of the molecular pathogenesis and histopathology of FTLD (Hutton, 2001). Tau is a neuronal protein that binds to microtubules, and is thought to be involved in assembly, and maintaining the stability of these cytoskeletal structural elements. In the normal adult human brain, tau is a soluble protein that is expressed as six major protein isoforms that are generated by alternative splicing of the tau gene. The alternative splicing of exon 10 controls the number of microtubule binding domains. If exon 10 is included in the mRNA (exon10+), there will be 4 microtubule binding domains in the translated protein (4R tau). If exon 10 is excluded in the mRNA (exon 10−), there will be 3 microtubule binding domains (3R tau). In the normal adult human brain, there is an approximately 1:1 ratio of 3R tau to 4R tau.

The tau gene is found on chromosome 17q21. Mutations in the tau gene lead to FTD and Parkinsonism linked to chromosome 17 (FTDP-17, see chapter 35 for a more detailed discussion). Most patients with tau gene mutations develop an autosomal dominantly inherited syndrome with features of FTLD. Analysis of tau mutations found in FTDP-17 has provided insight into the pathogenesis of FTLD. Tau gene mutations that produce this clinical syndrome are clustered around exon 10, and alter the microtubule binding affinity of the translated protein (missense mutations in exon 10) or the ratio of 3R to 4R tau (splice site mutations flanking exon 10) that is expressed (Hong *et al.*, 1998). Changes in tau isoform expression are thought to eventually result in the formation of insoluble protein aggregates, which in turn lead to neuronal dysfunction and death. Histopathologically, tau mutations (FTDP-17) may result in the formation of different forms of insoluble protein aggregates, including Pick bodies, ballooned neurons and neurofibrillary tangles.

Biochemical analysis of tau protein extracted from Pick's brains has suggested that Pick bodies consist of deposits of predominantly 3R tau. Ballooned neurons found in Pick's and CBD are thought to contain predominantly 4R tau, as are tau deposits identified in the brains of patients with progressive supranuclear palsy (PSP). Neurofibrillary tangles in AD contain an equal mixture of 3R and 4R tau. Other disorders, such as post-encephalitic parkinsonism (Bussiere *et al.*, 1999), neurofibrillary tangle dementia (Reed *et al.*, 1997), Lytico-bodig disease (Hof *et al.*, 1994), and Niemann Pick C disease (Love *et al.*, 1995) also produce insoluble protein aggregates containing equal ratios of 3R and 4R tau. FTLD and other primary neurodegenerative disorders with prominent tau pathology have been grouped together as "tauopathies," to distinguish them from other protein aggregate diseases such as Parkinson's and Lewy body disease, which display protein aggregates composed of alpha synuclein (Hardy & Gwinn-Hardy, 1998).

A recent consensus statement on clinical and pathological diagnosis of FTLD emphasized the composition of insoluble tau deposits found in brains at autopsy (McKhann *et al.*, 2001). For example, it was suggested that if the insoluble tau aggregates contained predominantly 3R tau, the most likely diagnosis would be Pick's disease or FTDP-17. However, a study of tau isoform expression in sporadic Pick's disease, using exon 10-specific tau antibodies has demonstrated cases with predominantly 3R tau, 4R tau or an equal ratio of both (Zhukareva *et al.*, 2002). This study calls into question the utility of classifying FTLD pathology by tau isoform expression ratio. Further studies will be necessary to fully understand the relationship between tau isoform expression and clinical disease.

Pathogenesis/mechanisms of disease (animal models)

The molecular pathogenesis of both sporadic FTLD and FTDP-17 is poorly understood. The discovery of pathogenic mutations in tau as a cause of FTLD has led to attempts to develop transgenic mouse models of the disease. Lines of transgenic mice have been constructed that overexpress a single tau protein isoform (3R or 4R), a mutant tau protein or protein kinases thought to be upstream in the development of hyperphosphorylated tau. So far, no transgenic model has been completely successful in recapitulating the FTLD phenotype and associated pathology observed in humans (Hutton *et al.*, 2001).

Transgenic mice that overexpress wild-type 4R tau at up to ten times the level of endogenous mouse tau develop motor disturbances in tasks involving balancing on a rod or hanging from a grid. Histopathologically, these mice display dilated axons containing neurofilament and tubulin and dystrophic neurites that stain with an antibody to hyperphosphorylated tau (Probst *et al.*, 2000). Transgenic mice that overexpress 3R tau also develop motor symptoms, however they do not show clear neuropathological abnormalities until late in life. These mice develop neurofibrillary tangles similar to those observed in AD (Ishihara *et al.*, 1999). A transgenic mouse line that overexpresses an exon 10 mutant tau (P301L) which causes FTDP-17 in humans, develops motor and behavioral deficits, with early hind limb dysfunction, followed by dystonic posturing, docility, reduced weight and decreased vocalization. These mice show profound neuronal loss in the spinal cord and tau-positive neurofibrillary tangles throughout the brain (Lewis *et al.*, 2000). Glial tau deposits and motor deficits, similar to those seen in CBD and PSP, have been observed in a transgenic mouse line that overexpresses human tau in both neurons and glia (Higuchi *et al.*, 2002).

A number of transgenic mouse lines have been developed that express protein kinases upstream of tau, and thus might serve as model systems for the molecular pathogenetic mechanisms that underlie sporadic tauopathies. One line expresses glycogen synthase kinase-3β (GSK-3β), under the control of an inducible promoter system targeted to CA1 hippocampal neurons. When GSK-3β expression is induced, the mice produce hyperphosphorylated tau and evidence of increased neuronal apoptosis, however no FTLD phenotype (Lucas *et al.*, 2001). A second transgenic line that expresses p25, a positive regulator of cyclin-dependent kinase 5 (cdk5), under the control of the platelet derived growth factor promoter, has increased cdk5 kinase activity and develops motor symptoms at 3 months of age. These p25 mice show widespread axonal degeneration, with focal accumulation of tau in multiple brain and spinal cord regions. However, ultrastructurally, the tau deposits do not resemble those found in AD or FTLD (Ahlijanian *et al.*, 2000).

Molecular genetic experiments performed in fruit flies (*Drosophila melanogaster*) transgenic for tau and protein kinases may prove to be a powerful system to dissect the molecular pathogenesis of FTLD. Recently, one such line that expresses wild type human tau has been shown to develop neurofibrillary tangles and progressive neurodegeneration by a mechanism involving the Wnt signaling pathway (Jackson *et al.*, 2002). A second transgenic *Drosophila* line expressing human tau, shows adult onset of progressive neurodegeneration leading to early death. These flies have accumulations of insoluble tau protein in anatomically appropriate regions (Wittmann *et al.*, 2001).

Clinical picture

Core clinical characteristics of FTLD

FTLD clinical syndromes

The 1998 consensus criteria for FTLD list three clinical syndromes: frontotemporal dementia (FTD; sometimes referred to as frontal variant FTD), semantic dementia (SD; sometimes referred to as temporal variant FTD) and progressive nonfluent aphasia (PNFA). One study has suggested that FTD and SD each account for approximately 40% of FTLD cases, and PNFA makes up the remaining 20% (Hodges & Miller, 2001). Patients with tau gene mutations are classified as having frontotemporal dementia with Parkinsonism linked to chromosome 17 (FTDP-17), although clinically they are often indistinguishable from patients with sporadic FTLD. Motor neuron disease (amyotrophic lateral sclerosis (ALS)), most commonly with prominent bulbar symptoms, is associated with FTD in approximately 10% of patients (Miller *et al.*, 1995a). In a series of 36 patients with FTLD, five met clinical criteria for FTLD, and an additional 11 patients had at least one clinical sign of ALS (Lomen-Hoerth *et al.*, 2002). Likewise, almost one third of a series of 100 ALS patients were found to meet clinical criteria for FTLD (Lomen-Hoerth *et al.*, 2003). Patients who meet clinical criteria for FTLD, especially those with prominent language impairment, and who develop movement disorder symptoms within 2–7 years after diagnosis are often found to have CBD at autopsy (Kertesz *et al.*, 2000).

Clinical presentation and differentiation from AD
Frontotemporal lobar degeneration is caused by progressive dysfunction of the frontal and/or anterior temporal lobes. The most severely involved areas are different in each patient, and may be initially unilateral or bilateral, with different degrees of frontal and/or temporal involvement. For this reason initial symptoms may be heterogeneous. Careful neurological examination of patients with FTLD often reveals mild ocular motor abnormalities (such as breakdown of smooth pursuit or mild ocular apraxia), subtle reflex asymmetry, primitive reflexes (grasp or snout), or mild Parkinsonism (slow finger tapping, slight rigidity or decreased arm swing). At the bedside, tasks such as the Luria (fist-hand-palm) and the Frontal Assessment Battery (Dubois *et al.*, 2000) often reveal abnormalities in these patients.

Historically, many cases of pathologically verified FTLD were diagnosed with AD during life (Mendez *et al.*, 1993). Two recent studies of pathologically verified cases of FTLD have identified clinical and neuropsychological features which differentiate FTLD from AD. The presence of a social conduct disorder, hyperorality or akinesia, and the absence of amnesia or a perceptual disorder correctly classified 93% of patients with FTLD in one series of 30 autopsy-proven cases of FTLD cases and 30 cases of AD (Rosen *et al.*, 2002b). Patients with autopsy-proven FTLD performed worse on letter and category fluency tests, but better on the Mattis Dementia Rating Scale memory subscale, block design test and clock drawing test than patients with AD (Rascovsky *et al.*, 2002).

Clinical variants

Frontotemporal dementia (frontal lobe variant FTLD; fvFTD)

The insidious onset of behavioral abnormalities and personality changes are initially the most prominent features of fvFTD. Patients with evidence of right brain involvement on neuroimaging studies tend to have the most severe behavioral symptoms (Mychack *et al.*, 2001). Orbitobasal (ventromedial) frontal lobe dysfunction leads to disinhibition, poor impulse control, antisocial behavior and stereotyped behaviors. Disinhibition or distractability may manifest as restlessness, pressured speech, impulsivity, irritability, aggressiveness, violent outbursts, or excessive sentimentality (Rosen *et al.*, 2000). Hypersexuality and sexual disinhibition are commonly seen in fvFTD. Other socially inappropriate behaviors include theft, assault, inappropriate or offensive speech, public urination or masturbation (Miller *et al.*, 1995a). Criminal behavior is common in fvFTD. Stereotyped or perseverative behaviors may include impulse buying, hoarding or compulsions. Other stereotyped behaviors include counting, repetitive cleaning, pacing, organizing objects into groups or rows or the use of a "catch phrase." Features of obsessive-compulsive disorder are very common in fvFTD, and some patients may initially be given this psychiatric diagnosis (Ames *et al.*, 1994). Compulsions were the presenting symptoms in 30–60% of patients in three clinical series of fvFTD patients (Perry & Miller, 2001). Delusions are common in fvFTD, and tend to be jealous, somatic, religious or bizarre, but are rarely persecutory. Euphoric symptoms, such as elevated mood, inappropriate jocularity and exaggerated self-esteem were found in 30% of fvFTD patients in one clinical series (Levy *et al.*, 1996).

Poor insight, loss of personal awareness, loss of social awareness and blunting of affect are common behavioral changes in fvFTD. Patients may deny the existence of deficits and often show a lack of concern about their illness (Rosen *et al.*, 2000). Increased submissiveness, a lack of empathy, self-centeredness, emotional coldness and decreased concern about family and friends is also common (Rankin *et al.*, 2003). Apathy is frequently seen in patients with fvFTD who have involvement of the anterior cingulate and medial frontal lobes. This may be mistaken for depression in some patients. Unlike in AD, depression is uncommon in fvFTD. Apathy and emotional withdrawal are often punctuated with outbursts of disinhibited behavior (Swartz *et al.*, 1997a). Patients with right frontal involvement may undergo dramatic changes in beliefs, attitudes and/or religious sentiment leading to the emergence of a new personality as the disease progresses (Miller *et al.*, 2001). With more advanced disease, many patients develop language dysfunction, with features of progressive nonfluent aphasia (see below) if disease involves left frontal/insular cortex, and/or akinetic mutism with progressive medial frontal/cingulate cortex involvement.

Dietary changes, especially cravings for sweets, are common in FTLD (Miller *et al.*, 1995b). Decreased satiety and food cravings often lead to a weight gain in many patients. As the disease progresses, features of the Kluver-Bucy syndrome, such as hyperorality and oral exploratory behaviors may arise. Reduced sexual drive is a common finding in FTLD, and impotence may be an early feature of disease in men (Miller *et al.*, 1995b).

Semantic dementia (temporal lobe variant FTD; SD)

Semantic dementia is a syndrome of progressive loss of semantic knowledge, or knowledge about people, objects, facts and words (Snowden *et al.*, 1996b). The syndrome was first described in patients with progressive anomia who were recognized to have lost not only the ability to name objects, but also fundamental information about each item, leading to difficulties with category-specific comprehension and object recognition (Warrington, 1975). Many of the patients with the fluent subtype of primary progressive aphasia, described by Mesulam (Mesulam, 2001), would now be classified as having SD (Grossman, 2002).

Most patients diagnosed with SD have prominent involvement of left temporal lobe structures. The most common presenting complaint in SD involves language, and is often described as a loss of memory for words or a loss of word meaning. While SD patients are aware of their expressive deficits, they are often unaware of their comprehension difficulties (Hodges, 2001). Speech is fluent but there are frequent semantic paraphrasias, and use of substitute phrases such as "thing" or "stuff." Repetition, prosody, syntax and verb generation are preserved. Associative agnosia may lead to difficulty with object recognition. This may manifest as misuse of or an inability to recognize household items such as a can-opener or pliers. An emergence of artistic talent has been observed in some patients with SD who have significant language impairment (Miller *et al.*, 1998b).

Patients with more significant right brain involvement may present with prosopagnosia (Evans *et al.*, 1995). Unlike the prosopagnosia caused by right occipito-temporal strokes, which is limited to the visual domain, the prosopagnosia of SD extends to other sensory modalities such as the association of names with voices (Hodges, 2001). Behavioral changes similar to those seen in fvFTD often arise as the disease progresses. Patients with right-sided disease tend to have more severe behavioral abnormalities than patients with left-sided disease (Edwards-Lee *et al.*, 1997).

In contrast to patients with AD, recent memory tends to be preserved early in the course of SD. Instead, there is more difficulty with distant memory, such as autobiographical events. Thus in SD there is a reversal of the temporal gradient of memory impairment that is observed in AD (Hodges and Graham, 2001).

Progressive non-fluent aphasia (PNFA)

Unlike other FTD syndromes, PNFA has been associated with either FTLD pathology or AD pathology in approximately 50% of cases (Weintraub *et al.*, 1990). PNFA may be the presenting complaint in patients with ALS (Rakowicz & Hodges, 1998; Caselli *et al.*, 1993). PNFA is also a frequent presenting symptom of CBD.

Patients typically present with complaints involving changes in fluency, pronunciation or word finding difficulty. Anomia in PNFA is more significant for verbs than for nouns, and has been associated with motor neuron disease pathology involving Brodman's areas 44 and 45 (Bak *et al.*, 2001). Unlike FTD and SD, PNFA patients do not display typical behavioral abnormalities until late in the course of the disease (Neary *et al.*, 1998). Insight and personal awareness are often normal. Depression and social withdrawal are common features of PNFA.

Time course of the disease

The mean age of onset for FTD has been estimated to be 52.8 to 56 years old (Miller *et al.*, 1998a). Mean duration of illness is approximately 8 years, with considerable variability depending on underlying pathology (Snowden *et al.*, 1996a). A study of presymptomatic family members of patients with FTDP-17, who carry the tau mutation, has demonstrated frontal-executive dysfunction on neuropsychological tests decades before the onset of FTLD symptoms (Geschwind *et al.*, 2001). This suggests that there may be a neurodevelopmental component in some cases of FTLD, and raises the question whether there is a premorbid phenotype.

Epidemiology

FTLD is a common cause of presenile dementia, or dementia that occurs in patients less than 65 years of age. FTLD is thought to account for up to 20% of all cases of dementia, irrespective of age (Grossman, 2001). The prevalence of FTLD in patients aged 45 to 64 from a population of approximately 300 000 individuals in Cambridgeshire, England has been estimated to be 15 (95% CI: 8.4 to 27) per 100 000 (Ratnavalli *et al.*, 2002). This was identical to the prevalence of early-onset AD in the same population. Overall, the proportion of AD cases to FTD cases was 1.6 : 1 in this study. A different study, using the older Lund–Manchester clinical criteria for FTD, found a similar prevalence of 9.3 (95% CI: 5.5 to 14.7) per 100 000 in a group of patients who were 65 or younger (Harvey, 1998). In most case series there is no gender predominance.

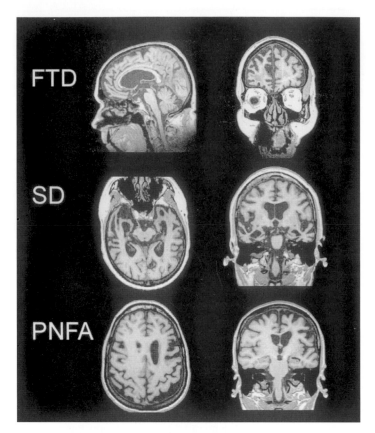

Fig. 34.2 MRI findings in FTLD. FTD: Parasagittal and coronal images from T_1-weighted MRI scan of a patient with frontotemporal dementia. Note asymmetric right frontal atrophy on coronal image, and lack of significant atrophy posterior to frontal lobe on saggital image. SD: Axial and coronal images from a patient with semantic dementia. Note that atrophy is most severe anteriorly and involves both medial and lateral temporal lobe structures. PNFA: Axial and coronal images from a patient with progressive nonfluent aphasia. Note asymmetric left frontal atrophy with minimal temporal lobe involvement.

Investigations

Imaging

Frontotemporal dementia (fvFTD)

Functional neuroimaging of blood flow abnormalities using Tc_{99}-hexamethylyl-propyleneamine (HMPAO)-SPECT shows bilateral frontal hypoperfusion early in the course of fvFTD, and reliably differentiates patients with FTD from patients with AD (Miller *et al.*, 1991; Miller & Gearhart, 1999; Miller *et al.*, 1997). Fluorodeoxy glucose (FDG)-PET demonstrates frontal hypometabolism in patients with FTD (Hoffman *et al.*, 2000). Unbiased analysis of T_1-weighted MRI scans from patients with fvFTD has identified regions of significant cortical atrophy in the ventromedial frontal cortex, the posterior orbital frontal regions bilaterally, the insula bilaterally, the left anterior cingulate cortex, the right dorsolateral frontal cortex and the left premotor cortex as compared with controls and patients with SD (Rosen *et al.*, 2002a) (see also Fig. 34.2).

Longitudinal measurements of MRI scans of patients with fvFTD show faster rates of frontal atrophy (4.1–4.5% per year), and similar rates of parieto-occipital atrophy (2.2–2.4% per year) as compared to patients with AD (2.4–2.8% per year, globally) (Chan *et al.*, 2001a). Parkinsonism in FTD has been associated with reduced uptake of the dopamine transporter ligand [11C]CFT in the caudate and putamen on PET imaging (Rinne *et al.*, 2002).

Semantic dementia (SD)

SD patients often have severe, bilateral, but asymmetric atrophy of anterior temporal lobe ("knife edge atrophy") as well as medial temporal lobe structures (Fig. 34.2). These findings may be preceded by hypoperfusion on HMPAO-SPECT (Edwards-Lee *et al.*, 1997; Garrard & Hodges, 2000). Anterior temporal lobe atrophy is easily appreciated on MRI scans, and visual inspection may be sufficient to accurately differentiate SD from AD patients (Galton *et al.*, 2001a). More detailed volumetric measurements of temporal lobe structures have demonstrated that hippocampal atrophy is often more severe in SD than in AD patients, but is usually more asymmetric, and accompanied by more severe atrophy of the amygdala, temporal pole, fusiform and inferolateral temporal gyri (Chan *et al.*, 2001b; Galton *et al.*, 2001b). Unbiased measurements of T_1-weighted MRI scans suggest that atrophy in SD is much more significant in temporal than extra-temporal brain regions (Rosen *et al.*, 2002a; Mummery *et al.*, 2000). FDG-PET studies during semantic memory tasks in SD patients show brain activation changes outside the areas of brain atrophy, suggesting that neuronal networks involving the temporal lobes are disrupted in SD (Mummery *et al.*, 1999).

Progressive non-fluent aphasia (PNFA)

Atrophy of the left frontal, insular, anterior parietal and superior temporal cortices is found in PNFA (Mesulam, 2001). Structural neuroimaging demonstrates left perisylvian atrophy in PNFA (Hodges & Patterson, 1996; Rosen *et al.*, 2002c) (Fig. 34.2).

Neuropsychology

Frontotemporal dementia (fvFTD)

Impairment on tests of executive function and working memory is the most common deficit in fvFTD. Memory and visuospatial function are relatively spared in fvFTD, and screening tests such as the Mini-Mental State Examination often remain normal even after patients require nursing home care (Gregory et al., 1999). This is in striking contrast to AD, where there is early impairment of memory and visuospatial function (Perry & Hodges, 2000). Patients may have difficulty with set shifting, concept formation, abstraction and reasoning, inhibition of over-learned responses, response generation, organization, planning, self-monitoring and using feedback to guide behavior (Rosen et al., 2000). Tasks such as the Wisconsin Card Sorting Test, Trailmaking Test, Stroop Category Test, verbal and design fluency, and proverb interpretation are sensitive to frontal executive dysfunction in patients with fvFTD (Hodges, 2001).

Semantic dementia (SD)

Due to their language difficulties, patients with SD may score poorly on bedside screening measures such as the Mini Mental State Exam. However, more detailed testing reveals a loss of semantic knowledge, with relatively preserved episodic memory for recent events (Graham et al., 2000). Patients are most impaired on tests such as category fluency (i.e. the number of animals or musical instruments generated in one minute), picture naming (Boston Naming Test), and generation of verbal definitions of words and pictures. Hodges and colleagues have shown that errors on these tasks initially reflect a loss of subordinate knowledge, or detailed items within categories, followed by a loss of more superordinate knowledge (the categories, themselves). For example, a patient may initially misidentify an orange as an apple; however with time, both are identified only as fruit, and eventually, only as food (Hodges et al., 1995). Non-verbal semantic knowledge may be assessed with tests such as the Pyramids and Palm Trees Test, in which the subject is asked to judge which of two pictures is related to a third picture. For example, a pyramid is shown, and the subject is asked whether a picture of a pine tree or a palm tree best goes with the pyramid (Bozeat et al., 2000).

Language testing in SD reveals preserved phonology and syntax. However, surface dyslexia is commonly found in SD patients, and presents as difficulty in reading or spelling irregular words that sound different than they are spelled ("pint" read as hint or lint). SD patients also have diffi-culty with generating past tenses from low frequency verbs, which has implications for the role of semantic knowledge in basic linguistic functions (Patterson et al., 2001).

Progressive non-fluent aphasia (PNFA)

Episodic memory, semantic memory and visuospatial function are preserved in PNFA. Executive function and working memory are often impaired. Language difficulties include aggramatism, phonemic paraphrasias and anomia. Aggramatism is defined as the presence of grammatical errors in speech, such as the omission or incorrect usage of articles ("cow jumped over moon"), prepositions ("dog walk bridge"), or verbs ("cat eated mouse"). Phonemic paraphrasias are errors involving use of the incorrect phoneme ("head" instead of "bed") or transposition of a phoneme ("efelant" for "elephant") (Hodges, 2001). Other language problems may include stuttering, impaired repetition, apraxia of speech, alexia and agraphia.

Genetics

Approximately 29% to 38% of patients with FTLD have a positive family history of dementia, and it has been estimated that first-degree relatives of patients with FTD are at a 3.5 times higher risk of developing dementia than the general population (Stevens et al., 1998). A more recent study suggests that 38% to 45% of patients with FTLD have a strong hereditary component, with an autosomal dominant inheritance pattern in 80% of cases (Chow et al., 1999). Chromosome 17 tau gene mutations are thought to be present in 10% to 50% of FTLD patients with a positive family history of dementia (Morris et al., 2001). To date, most cases of familial FTLD with tau pathology identified at autopsy have been found to have a tau mutation. In contrast, analysis of two series of sporadic FTLD patients suggests that only 5.9 to 13.6% of all FTLD patients will be found to have a tau mutation (Rosso & Van Swieten, 2002). At this time, routine clinical testing for tau mutations is not available.

In addition to tau mutations, mutations in other genes are likely to be involved in the development of FTLD. A different locus on chromosome 17q21–22 may lead to familial FTLD in one Dutch family (Rosso et al., 2001). Familial FTLD associated with motor neuron disease has been linked to chromosome 9q21–22 (Hosler et al., 2000). Hereditary FTLD associated with inclusion body myopathy and Paget's disease has been linked to a different locus on chromosome 9 (9p13.3–p12) (Kovach et al., 2001). A locus in the pericentromeric region of chromosome 3 has also been identified in a Danish FTLD family (Rosso & Van Swieten, 2002).

Treatment

Currently there are no treatments that alter the progression of FTLD. Instead, medications and behavioral interventions are targeted to specific neuropsychiatric symptoms. Although theoretically, acetylcholinesterase inhibitors developed for use in AD, such as donepezil, might be expected to improve attention and working memory in FTLD, most patients experience no benefit from these agents. This finding may be related to the relative sparing of cholinergic neurons in the nucleus basalis of Meynert in FTLD as compared to AD. Additionally, clinical experience suggests that many patients will become more agitated when placed on acetylcholinesterase inhibitors. Finally, acetylcholinesterase inhibitors may cause increased production of oral secretions, which is undesirable in patients with dysphagia due to MND or PSP symptoms. For these reasons, acetylcholinesterase inhibitors are not indicated in most cases of FTLD. A minority of PNFA patients, who are believed to have underlying AD pathology, may benefit from treatment with an acetylcholinesterase inhibitor.

Practical and theoretical evidence suggests that deficits in serotonergic neurotransmission may be responsibie for some of the behavioral abnormalities observed in FTLD (Perry & Miller, 2001). Compulsions and carbohydrate craving improved in a group of FTLD patients who were treated with a selective serotonin reuptake inhibitor (SSRI) and assessed for a change in behavior 3 months later (Swartz *et al.*, 1997b). SSRIs are well tolerated in patients with FTLD, and are currently the best available medications for behavioral control. Patients with aggressive or delusional behavior that does not respond to treatment with an SSRI may benefit from use of low doses of an atypical antipsychotic such as olanzepine, quetiapine or risperidone. Valproic acid and carbamazepine may also be useful in treating refractory agitation or aggressiveness in FTLD. Typical antipsychotics such as haloperidol should be avoided since FTLD patients are more likely to experience Parkinsonian side effects. The cognitive side effects of benzodiazepines outweigh their usefulness in FTLD. Although there are no studies of exercise in FTLD, clinical experience suggests that a regular cardiovascular exercise program may help to maintain motor function in these patients.

Behavioral symptoms, lack of empathy, poor insight and communication difficulties create a unique constellation of stressors for the caregivers of FTLD patients that is different from the stressors experienced by AD caregivers. Caregiver distress is associated with earlier nursing home placement of dementia patients (Litvan, 2001), and thus an important role of the physician is to support the caregiver as well as the patient. Caregivers should be educated about FTLD and given anticipatory guidance as to what problems will likely arise with time. Efforts to increase detection of caregiver depression, and to treat psychiatric morbidity in caregivers with support groups, psychiatric referrals and respite care may delay patient institutionalization and improve the quality of life for both patients and caregivers (Talerico & Evans, 2001). Environmental, behavioral and psychosocial strategies have been developed to aid in management of FTLD both at home and if institutionalization becomes necessary (Talerico & Evans, 2001).

Acknowledgements

ALB is a fellow of The John Douglas French Foundation. Supp. by NIA P01 AG19724-01A1 to BLM.

REFERENCES

Ahlijanian, M. K., Barrezueta, N. X., Williams, R. D. *et al.* (2000). Hyperphosphorylated tau and neurofilament and cytoskeletal disruptions in mice overexpressing human p25, an activator of cdk5. *Proc. Natl Acad. Sci., USA*, **97**, 2910–15.

Altman, E. (1923). Uber die eigenartige Krankheitsfalle des spateren Alters. *Zeitschrift fur die Gesamte Neurologie und Psychiatrie*, **4**, 356–85.

Alzheimer, A. (1911). Uber eigenartige Krankheitsfalle des spateren Alters. *Zeitschrift fur die Gesamte Neurologie und Psychiatrie*, **4**, 7–44.

Ames, D., Cummings, J. L., Wirshing, W. C., Quinn, B. & Mahler, M. (1994). Repetitive and compulsive behavior in frontal lobe degenerations. *J. Neuropsychiatry Clin. Neurosci.*, **6**, 100–13.

Bak, T. H., O'Donovan, D. G., Xuereb, J. H., Boniface, S. & Hodges, J. R. (2001). Selective impairment of verb processing associated with pathological changes in Brodmann areas 44 and 45 in the motor neurone disease- dementia-aphasia syndrome. *Brain*, **124**, 103–20.

Bird, T. D. & Schellenberg, G. D. (2001). The case of the missing tau, or, why didn't the mRNA bark? *Ann. Neurol.*, **49**, 144–5.

Bozeat, S., Gregory, C. A., Ralph, M. A. & Hodges, J. R. (2000). Which neuropsychiatric and behavioural features distinguish frontal and temporal variants of frontotemporal dementia from Alzheimer's disease? *J. Neurol. Neurosurg. Psychiatry*, **69**, 178–86.

Broe, M., Hodges, J. R., Schofield, E., Shepherd, C. E., Kril, J. J. & Halliday, G. M. (2003). Staging disease severity in pathologically confirmed cases of frontotemporal dementia. *Neurology*, **60**, 1005–11.

Brun, A. (1987). Frontal lobe degeneration of non-Alzheimer type. I. Neuropathology. *Arch. Gerontol. Geriatr.*, **6**, 193–208.

Bussiere, T., Hof, P. R., Mailliot, C. *et al.* (1999). Phosphorylated serine 422 on tau proteins is a pathological epitope found in several diseases with neurofibrillary degeneration. *Acta Neuropathol. (Berl.)*, **97**, 221–30.

Caselli, R. J., Windebank, A. J., Petersen, R. C. *et al.* (1993). Rapidly progressive aphasic dementia and motor neuron disease. *Ann. Neurol.*, **33**, 200–7.

Chan, D., Fox, N. C., Jenkins, R., Scahill, R. I., Crum, W. R. & Rossor, M. N. (2001a). Rates of global and regional cerebral atrophy in AD and frontotemporal dementia. *Neurology*, **57**, 1756–63.

Chan, D., Fox, N. C., Scahill, R. I. *et al.* (2001b). Patterns of temporal lobe atrophy in semantic dementia and Alzheimer's disease. *Ann. Neurol.*, **49**, 433–42.

Chow, T. W., Miller, B. L., Hayashi, V. N. & Geschwind, D. H. (1999). Inheritance of frontotemporal dementia. *Arch. Neurol.*, **56**, 817–22.

Constantinidis, J., Fichard, J. & Tissot, R. (1974). Pick's disease. Histological and clincial correlations. *Eur. Neurol.*, **11**, 208–17.

Dickson, D. W. (2001). Neuropathology of Pick's disease. *Neurology*, **56**(Suppl 4), S16–20.

Dickson, D. W., Bergeron, C., Chin, S. S. *et al.* (2002). Office of Rare Diseases neuropathologic criteria for corticobasal degeneration. *J. Neuropathol. Exp. Neurol.*, **61**, 935–46.

Dubois, B., Slachevsky, A., Litvan, I. & Pillon, B. (2000). The FAB: a Frontal Assessment Battery at bedside. *Neurology*, **55**, 1621–6.

Edwards-Lee, T., Miller, B. L., Benson, D. F. *et al.* (1997). The temporal variant of frontotemporal dementia. *Brain*, **120**, 1027–40.

Evans, J. J., Heggs, A. J., Antoun, N. & Hodges, J. R. (1995). Progressive prosopagnosia associated with selective right temporal lobe atrophy. A new syndrome? *Brain*, **118**, 1–13.

Forno, L. S., Langston, J. W., Herrick, M. K., Wilson, J. D. & Murayama, S. (2002). Ubiquitin-positive neuronal and tau 2-positive glial inclusions in frontotemporal dementia of motor neuron type. *Acta Neuropathol. (Berl.)*, **103**, 599–606.

Galton, C. J., Gomez-Anson, B., Antoun, N. *et al.* (2001a). Temporal lobe rating scale: application to Alzheimer's disease and frontotemporal dementia. *J. Neurol. Neurosurg. Psychiatry*, **70**, 165–73.

Galton, C. J., Patterson, K., Graham, K. *et al.* (2001b). Differing patterns of temporal atrophy in Alzheimer's disease and semantic dementia. *Neurology*, **57**, 216–25.

Garrard, P. & Hodges, J. R. (2000). Semantic dementia: clinical, radiological and pathological perspectives. *J. Neurol.*, **247**, 409–22.

Geschwind, D. H., Robidoux, J., Alarcon, M. *et al.* (2001). Dementia and neurodevelopmental predisposition: cognitive dysfunction in presymptomatic subjects precedes dementia by decades in frontotemporal dementia. *Ann. Neurol.*, **50**, 741–6.

Graham, K. S., Simons, J. S., Pratt, K. H., Patterson, K. & Hodges, J. R. (2000). Insights from semantic dementia on the relationship between episodic and semantic memory. *Neuropsychologia*, **38**, 313–24.

Gregory, C. A., Serra-Mestres, J. & Hodges, J. R. (1999). Early diagnosis of the frontal variant of frontotemporal dementia: how sensitive are standard neuroimaging and neuropsychologic tests? *Neuropsychiatry Neuropsychol. Behav. Neurol.*, **12**, 128–35.

Grossman, M. (2001). A multidisciplinary approach to Pick's disease and frontotemporal dementia. *Neurology*, **56**, S1–2.

Grossman, M. (2002). Progressive aphasic syndromes: clinical and theoretical advances. *Curr. Opin. Neurol.*, **15**, 409–13.

Hardy, J. & Gwinn-Hardy, K. (1998). Genetic classification of primary neurodegenerative disease. *Science*, **282**, 1075–9.

Harvey, R. J. (1998). Young onset dementia: epidemiology, clinical symptoms, family burden, support and outcome. Dementia Research Group, Imperial College School of Medicine, London.

Higuchi, M., Ishihara, T., Zhang, B. *et al.* (2002). Transgenic mouse model of tauopathies with glial pathology and nervous system degeneration. *Neuron*, **35**, 433–46.

Hodges, J. R. (2001). Frontotemporal dementia (Pick's disease): clinical features and assessment. *Neurology*, **56**, S6–10.

Hodges, J. R. & Graham, K. S. (2001). Episodic memory: insights from semantic dementia. *Phil. Trans. R. Soc. Lond. B. Biol. Sci.*, **356**, 1423–34.

Hodges, J. R. & Miller, B. (2001). The classification, genetics and neuropathology of frontotemporal dementia. Introduction to the special topic papers: Part I. *Neurocase*, **7**, 31–5.

Hodges, J. R. & Patterson, K. (1996). Nonfluent progressive aphasia and semantic dementia: a comparative neuropsychological study. *J. Int. Neuropsychol. Soc.*, **2**, 511–24.

Hodges, J. R., Patterson, K., Oxbury, S. & Funnell, E. (1992). Semantic dementia. Progressive fluent aphasia with temporal lobe atrophy. *Brain*, **115**, 1783–806.

Hodges, J. R., Graham, N. & Patterson, K. (1995). Charting the progression in semantic dementia: implications for the organisation of semantic memory. *Memory*, **3**, 463–95.

Hof, P. R., Nimchinsky, E. A., Buee-Scherrer, V. *et al.* (1994). Amyotrophic lateral sclerosis/parkinsonism–dementia complex of Guam: quantitative neuropathology, immunohistochemical analysis of neuronal vulnerability, and comparison with related neurodegenerative disorders. *Acta Neuropathol.*, **88**, 397–404.

Hoffman, J. M., Welsh-Bohmer, K. A., Hanson, M. *et al.* (2000). FDG PET imaging in patients with pathologically verified dementia. *J. Nucl. Med.*, **41**, 1920–8.

Hong, M., Zhukareva, V., Vogelsberg-Ragaglia, V. *et al.* (1998). Mutation-specific functional impairments in distinct tau isoforms of hereditary FTDP-17. *Science*, **282**, 1914–17.

Hosler, B. A., Siddique, T., Sapp, P. C. *et al.* (2000). Linkage of familial amyotrophic lateral sclerosis with frontotemporal dementia to chromosome 9q21–q22. *J. Am. Med. Assoc.*, **284**, 1664–9.

Hutton, M. (2001). Missense and splice site mutations in tau associated with FTDP-17: multiple pathogenic mechanisms. *Neurology*, **56**, S21–5.

Hutton, M., Lewis, J., Dickson, D., Yen, S. H. & McGowan, E. (2001). Analysis of tauopathies with transgenic mice. *Trends Mol. Med.*, **7**, 467–70.

Ishihara, T., Hong, M., Zhang, B. *et al.* (1999). Age-dependent emergence and progression of a tauopathy in transgenic mice overexpressing the shortest human tau isoform. *Neuron*, **24**, 751–62.

Jackson, G. R., Wiedau-Pazos, M., Sang, T. K. *et al.* (2002). Human wild-type tau interacts with wingless pathway components and produces neurofibrillary pathology in Drosophila. *Neuron*, **34**, 509–19.

Jackson, M., Lennox, G. & Lowe, J. (1996). Motor neurone disease-inclusion dementia. *Neurodegeneration*, **5**, 339–50.

Kertesz, A., Martinez-Lage, P., Davidson, W. & Munoz, D. G. (2000). The corticobasal degeneration syndrome overlaps progressive aphasia and frontotemporal dementia. *Neurology*, **55**, 1368–75.

Knopman, D. S., Mastri, A. R., Frey, W. H., 2nd, Sung, J. H. & Rustan, T. (1990). Dementia lacking distinctive histologic features: a common non-Alzheimer degenerative dementia. *Neurology*, **40**, 251–6.

Kovach, M. J., Waggoner, B., Leal, S. M. *et al.* (2001). Clinical delineation and localization to chromosome 9p13.3–p12 of a unique dominant disorder in four families: hereditary inclusion body myopathy, Paget disease of bone, and frontotemporal dementia. *Mol. Genet. Metab.*, **74**, 458–75.

Levy, M. L., Miller, B. L., Cummings, J. L., Fairbanks, L. A. & Craig, A. (1996). Alzheimer disease and frontotemporal dementias. Behavioral distinctions. *Arch. Neurol.*, **53**, 687–90.

Lewis, J., McGowan, E., Rockwood, J. *et al.* (2000). Neurofibrillary tangles, amyotrophy and progressive motor disturbance in mice expressing mutant (P301L) tau protein. *Nat. Genet.*, **25**, 402–5.

Litvan, I. (2001). Therapy and management of frontal lobe dementia patients. *Neurology*, **56**, S41–5.

Lomen-Hoerth, C., Anderson, T. & Miller, B. (2002) The overlap of amyotrophic lateral sclerosis and frontotemporal dementia. *Neurology*, **59**, 1077–9.

Lomen-Hoerth, C., Murphy, J., Langmore, S., Kramer, J. H., Olney, R. K. & Miller, B. (2003). Are amyotrophic lateral sclerosis patients cognitively normal? *Neurology*, **60**, 1094–7.

Love, S., Bridges, L. R. & Case, C. P. (1995). Neurofibrillary tangles in Niemann–Pick disease type C. *Brain*, **118**, 119–29.

Lucas, J. J., Hernandez, F., Gomez-Ramos, P., Moran, M. A., Hen, R. & Avila, J. (2001). Decreased nuclear beta-catenin, tau hyperphosphorylation and neurodegeneration in GSK-3beta conditional transgenic mice. *EMBO J.*, **20**, 27–39.

Lund and Manchester Groups (1994). Clinical and neuropathological criteria for frontotemporal dementia. *J. Neurol. Neurosurg. Psychiatry*, **57**, 416–18.

Mann, D. M., South, P. W., Snowden, J. S. *et al.* (1993). Dementia of frontal lobe type: neuropathology and immunohistochemistry, *J. Neurol. Neurosurg. Psychiatry*, **56**(6), 605–14.

Masliah, E., Terry, R. D., Alford, M. & DeTeresa, R. (1990). Quantitative immunohistochemistry of synaptophysin in human neocortex: an alternative method to estimate density of presynaptic terminals in paraffin sections. *J. Histochem. Cytochem.*, **38**, 837–44.

McKhann, G. M., Albert, M. S., Grossman, M., Miller, B., Dickson, D. & Trojanowski, J. (2001). Clinical and pathological diagnosis of frontotemporal dementia. *Arch. Neurol.*, **58**, 1803–9.

Mendez, M. F., Selwood, A., Mastri, A. R. & Frey, W. H., 2nd (1993). Pick's disease versus Alzheimer's disease: a comparison of clinical characteristics. *Neurology*, **43**, 289–92.

Mesulam, M. M. (1982). Slowly progressive aphasia without generalized dementia. *Ann. Neurol.*, **11**, 592–8.

Mesulam, M. M. (2001). Primary progressive aphasia. *Ann. Neurol.*, **49**, 425–32.

Miller, B., Cummings, J., Boone, K. *et al.* (1995a). Clinical and neurobehavioral characteristics of fronto-temporal dementia and Alzheimer disease. *Neurology*, **45**, A318.

Miller, B. L., Boone, K., Mishkin, F., Swartz, J. R., Koras, N. & Kushii, J. (1998a). Clinical and neuropsychological features of frontotemporal dementia. In *Pick's Disease and Pick Complex*, ed., A. Kertesz & D. Munoz. New York: Wiley-Liss. pp. 23–33.

Miller, B. L., Cummings, J., Mishkin, F. *et al.* (1998b). Emergence of artistic talent in frontotemporal dementia. *Neurology*, **51**, 978–82.

Miller, B. L., Cummings, J. L., Villanueva-Meyer, J. *et al.* (1991). Frontal lobe degeneration: clinical, neuropsychological, and SPECT characteristics. *Neurology*, **41**, 1374–82.

Miller, B. L., Darby, A. L., Swartz, J. R., Yener, G. G. & Mena, I. (1995b). Dietary changes, compulsions and sexual behavior in frontotemporal degeneration. *Dementia*, **6**, 195–9.

Miller, B. L. & Gearhart, R. (1999). Neuroimaging in the diagnosis of frontotemporal dementia. *Dement. Geriatr. Cogn. Disord.*, **10**, 71–4.

Miller, B. L., Ikonte, C., Ponton, M. (1997). A study of the Lund-Manchester research criteria for frontotemporal dementia: clinical and single-photon emission CT correlations. *Neurology*, **48**, 937–42.

Miller, B. L., Seeley, W. W., Mychack, P., Rosen, H. J., Mena, I. & Boone, K. (2001). Neuroanatomy of the self: evidence from patients with frontotemporal dementia. *Neurology*, **57**, 817–21.

Morris, H. R., Khan, M. N., Janssen, J. C. *et al.* (2001). The genetic and pathological classification of familial frontotemporal dementia. *Arch Neurol*, **58**, 1813–16.

Mummery, C. J., Patterson, K., Price, C. J., Ashburner, J., Frackowiak, R. S. & Hodges, J. R. (2000). A voxel-based morphometry study of semantic dementia: relationship between temporal lobe atrophy and semantic memory. *Ann. Neurol.*, **47**, 36–45.

Mummery, C. J., Patterson, K., Wise, R. J. S., Vandenbergh, R., Price, C. J. & Hodges, J. R. (1999). Disrupted temporal lobe connections in semantic dementia. *Brain*, **122**, 61–73.

Mychack, P., Kramer, J. H., Boone, K. B. & Miller, B. L. (2001). The influence of right frontotemporal dysfunction on social behavior in frontotemporal dementia. *Neurology*, **56**, S11–15.

Neary, D., Snowden, J. S., Gustafson, L. *et al.* (1998). Frontotemporal lobar degeneration: a consensus on clinical diagnostic criteria. *Neurology*, **51**, 1546–54.

Onari, K. & Spatz, H. (1926). Anatomische Beitrage zur Lehre von der Pickschen umschriebene-Grosshirnriden-Atrophie ('Picksche

Krankheit'). *Zeitschrift fur die Gesamte Neurologie und Psychiatrie*, **101**, 470–511.

Patterson, K., Lambon Ralph, M. A., Hodges, J. R. & McClelland, J. L. (2001). Deficits in irregular past-tense verb morphology associated with degraded semantic knowledge. *Neuropsychologia*, **39**, 709–24.

Perry, R. J. & Hodges, J. R. (2000). Differentiating frontal and temporal variant frontotemporal dementia from Alzheimer's disease. *Neurology*, **54**, 2277–84.

Perry, R. J. & Miller, B. L. (2001). Behavior and treatment in frontotemporal dementia. *Neurology*, **56**, S46–51.

Pick, A. (1892). Uber die Beziehungen der senilen Hirnantropie zur aphasie. *Prager Medizinishe Wochenschrift*, **17**, 165–7.

Pollock, N. J., Mirra, S. S., Binder, L. I., Hansen, L. A. & Wood, J. G. (1986). Filamentous aggregates in Pick's disease, progressive supranuclear palsy, and Alzheimer's disease share antigenic determinants with microtubule-associated protein, tau. *Lancet*, **2**, 1211.

Probst, A., Gotz, J., Wiederhold, K. H. *et al.* (2000). Axonopathy and amyotrophy in mice transgenic for human four-repeat tau protein. *Acta Neuropathol. (Berl.)*, **99**, 469–81.

Rakowicz, W. P. & Hodges, J. R. (1998). Dementia and aphasia in motor neuron disease: an underrecognised association? *J. Neurol. Neurosurg. Psychiatry*, **65**, 881–9.

Rankin, K. P., Kramer, J. H., Mychack, P. & Miller, B. L. (2003). Double dissociation of social functioning in frontotemporal dementia. *Neurology*, **60**, 266–71.

Rascovsky, K., Salmon, D. P., Ho, G. J. *et al.* (2002). Cognitive profiles differ in autopsy-confirmed frontotemporal dementia and AD. *Neurology*, **58**, 1801–8.

Ratnavalli, E., Brayne, C., Dawson, K. & Hodges, J. R. (2002). The prevalence of frontotemporal dementia. *Neurology*, **58**, 1615–21.

Reed, L. A., Grabowski, T. J., Schmidt, M. L. *et al.* (1997). Autosomal dominant dementia with widespread neurofibrillary tangles. *Ann. Neurol.*, **42**, 564–72.

Rinne, J. O., Laine, M., Kaasinen, V., Norvasuo-Heila, M. K., Nagren, K. & Helenius, H. (2002). Striatal dopamine transporter and extrapyramidal symptoms in frontotemporal dementia. *Neurology*, **58**, 1489–93.

Rosen, H. J., Gorno-Tempini, M. L., Goldman, W. P. (2002a). Patterns of brain atrophy in frontotemporal dementia and semantic dementia. *Neurology*, **58**, 198–208.

Rosen, H. J., Hartikainen, K. M., Jagust, W. *et al.* (2002b). Utility of clinical criteria in differentiating frontotemporal lobar degeneration (FTLD) from AD. *Neurology*, **58**, 1608–15.

Rosen, H. J., Kramer, J. H., Gorno-Tempini, M. L., Schuff, N., Weiner, M. & Miller, B. L. (2002c). Patterns of cerebral atrophy in primary progressive aphasia. *Am. J. Geriatr. Psychiatry*, **10**, 89–97.

Rosen, H. J., Lengenfelder, J. & Miller, B. (2000). Frontotemporal dementia. *Neurol. Clin.*, **18**, 979–92.

Rosso, S. M., Kamphorst, W., de Graaf, B. (2001). Familial frontotemporal dementia with ubiquitin-positive inclusions is linked to chromosome 17q21–22. *Brain*, **124**, 1948–57.

Rosso, S. M. & Van Swieten, J. C. (2002). New developments in frontotemporal dementia and parkinsonism linked to chromosome 17. *Curr. Opin. Neurol.*, **15**, 423–8.

Rossor, M. N., Revesz, T., Lantos, P. L. & Warrington, E. K. (2000). Semantic dementia with ubiquitin-positive tau-negative inclusion bodies. *Brain*, **123**, 267–76.

Snowden, J. S., Neary, D., Mann, D. M., Goulding, P. J. & Testa, H. J. (1992). Progressive language disorder due to lobar atrophy. *Ann. Neurol.*, **31**, 174–83.

Snowden, J. S., Neary, D. & Mann, D. M. A. (1996a). Fronto-temporal dementia. In *Fronto-Temporal Lobar Degeneration*, ed. J. S. Snowden, D. Neary & D. M. A. Mann, New York: Churchill Livingstone. pp. 1–41.

Snowden, J. S., Neary, D. & Mann, D. M. A. (1996b). Semantic dementia. In *Fronto-Temporal Lobar Degeneration*, ed. J. S. Snowden, D. Neary, & D. M. A. Mann, New York: Churchill Livingstone. pp. 91–114.

Stevens, M., van Duijn, C. M., Kamphorst, W. *et al.* (1998). Familial aggregation in frontotemporal dementia. *Neurology*, **50**, 1541–5.

Swartz, J. R., Miller, B. L., Lesser, I. M., Booth, R., Darby, A., Wohl, M. & Benson, D. F. (1997a). Behavioral phenomenology in Alzheimer's disease, frontotemporal dementia, and late-life depression: a retrospective analysis. *J. Geriatr. Psychiatry Neurol.*, **10**, 67–74.

Swartz, J. R., Miller, B. L., Lesser, I. M. & Darby, A. L. (1997b). Frontotemporal dementia: treatment response to serotonin selective reuptake inhibitors. *J. Clin. Psychiatry*, **58**, 212–16.

Talerico, K. A. & Evans, L. K. (2001). Responding to safety issues in frontotemporal dementias. *Neurology*, **56**, S52–5.

Trojanowski, J. Q. & Dickson, D. (2001). Update on the neuropathological diagnosis of frontotemporal dementias. *J. Neuropathol. Exp. Neurol.*, **60**, 1123–6.

Warrrington, E. (1975). Selective impairment of semantic memory. *Q. J. Exp. Psychol.*, **27**, 635–7.

Weintraub, S., Rubin, N. P. & Mesulam, M. M. (1990). Primary progressive aphasia. Longitudinal course, neuropsychological profile, and language features. *Arch. Neurol.*, **47**, 1329–35.

Wittmann, C. W., Wszolek, M. F., Shulman, J. M. *et al.* (2001). Tauopathy in *Drosophila:* neurodegeneration without neurofibrillary tangles. *Science*, **293**, 711–14.

Wood, P. L., Etienne, P., Lal, S. *et al.* (1983). A post-mortem comparison of the cortical cholinergic system in Alzheimer's disease and Pick's disease. *J. Neurol. Sci.*, **62**, 211–17.

Zhukareva, V., Mann, D., Pickering-Brown, S. *et al.* (2002). Sporadic Pick's disease: a tauopathy characterized by a spectrum of pathological tau isoforms in gray and white matter. *Ann. Neurol.*, **51**, 730–9.

Zhukareva, V., Vogelsberg-Ragaglia, V., Van Deerlin, V. M. *et al.* (2001). Loss of brain tau defines novel sporadic and familial tauopathies with frontotemporal dementia. *Ann. Neurol.*, **49**, 165–75.

35

Frontotemporal dementia with parkinsonism linked to chromosome 17

Mark S. Forman, Virginia M.-Y. Lee, and John Q. Trojanowski

Center for Neurodegenerative Disease Research, Department of Pathology and Laboratory Medicine
University of Pennsylvania, PA, USA

Introduction

A variety of sporadic and familial neurodegenerative disorders, characterized clinically by dementia and/or motor dysfunction, demonstrate intracellular accumulations of filamentous material composed of the microtubule-associated protein (MAP) tau (See chapters 29, 'Neuropathology of Alzheimer's disease', 34, 'Pick's and other frontotemporal dementias', 44, 'Progressive supranuclear palsy', and 45, 'Corticobasal degeneration'). The term 'tauopathies' was coined to refer to this seemingly heterogeneous group of neurodegenerative disorders with filamentous tau deposits as their predominant histopathological feature. The progressive accumulation of filamentous tau inclusions in the absence of other disease-specific neuropathological abnormalities provided circumstantial evidence implicating tau dysfunction in disease onset and/or progression. However, the discovery of pathogenic *tau* mutations in a heterogeneous group of disorders termed frontotemporal dementia with parkinsonism linked to chromosome 17 (FTDP-17) provided unequivocal confirmation of the central role of tau abnormalities in the etiology of neurodegenerative disorders (Foster *et al.*, 1997; Poorkaj *et al.*, 1998; Hutton *et al.*, 1998; Spillantini *et al.*, 1998c). This seminal finding has opened novel areas of investigation into the pathophysiologic mechanisms of tau dysfunction and the relationship of tau abnormalities to brain degeneration.

Familial frontotemporal dementia

In 1892, Arnold Pick described a woman with lobar brain atrophy, who presented clinically with presenile dementia and aphasia (Pick, 1892). Thus, this was the first description of what is now classified clinically as frontotemporal dementia (FTD) (McKhann *et al.*, 2001). The clinical syndromes of FTD are associated with several neuropathological abnormalities including disorders with tau pathology such as Pick's disease (PiD), corticobasal degeneration (CBD), progressive supranuclear palsy (PSP), neurofibrillary tangle dementia, argyrophilic grain disease, and FTDP-17, as well as several without tau aggregates including frontotemporal lobar degeneration (FTLD, also known as dementia lacking distinctive histopathology) and FTLD with motor neuron disease-type inclusions (FTLD-MND) (see chapter 34, Pick's and other frontotemporal dementias) (Lund and Manchester Groups, 1994; McKhann *et al.*, 2001). In addition, Alzheimer's disease (AD) and other neurodegenerative diseases such as dementia with Lewy bodies may manifest an FTD-like clinical picture. However, specific sets of pathological findings do not correlate with the particular clinical manifestations.

In 1939, Sanders provided the first description of familial FTD in a Dutch kindred with behavioral and language abnormalities including disinhibition, aggression, and an obsessive personality (Sanders *et al.*, 1939; Schenk, 1959). However, localization of a genetic abnormality in FTD was not identified until 1994 when Wilhelmsen *et al.* demonstrated linkage to chromosome 17q21–22 in a large family with an autosomal dominant disorder named 'disinhibition–dementia–parkinsonism–amyotrophy complex' (Wilhelmsen *et al.*, 1994). Subsequently, a number of related neurodegenerative disorders were linked to a similar locus on chromosome 17 and a consensus conference convened in Ann Arbor, Michigan, coined the term FTDP-17 (Wijker *et al.*, 1996; Foster *et al.*, 1997; Bird *et al.*, 1997; Heutink *et al.*, 1997; Murrell *et al.*, 1997; Baker *et al.*, 1997; Lendon *et al.*, 1998). Since the *tau* gene also mapped to chromosome 17q21–22, it was an obvious candidate gene for the disease locus. In 1998, several groups identified pathogenic mutations in the *tau* gene that

Table 35.1. Tau mutations identified in FTDP-17

Mutation	Location	Exon 10 splicing	MT binding	Tau aggregation	Reference
R5H	Exon 1	No change	Reduced	Increased	Hayashi *et al.* (2002)
R5L	Exon 1	No change	Reduced	ND	Poorkaj *et al.* (2002)
K257T	E9, R1	No change	Reduced	Increased (3Rtau)	Pickering-Brown *et al.* (2000) Rizzini *et al.* (2000)
I260V	E9, R1	ND	ND	ND	Reed *et al.* (2001)
G272V	E9, R1	No change	Reduced	Variable[#]	Hutton *et al.* (1998)
E9+33	I9	ND	NA	NA	Rizzu *et al.* (1999)
N279K	E10, IR1–2	Increased[*]	Variable	Variable	Clark *et al.* (1998)
Δ280K	E10, IR1–2	Decreased[+]	Reduced	Increased	Rizzu *et al.* (1999)
L284L	E10, IR1–2	Increased	NA	NA	D'Souza *et al.* (1999)
N296N	E10, R2	Increased	NA	NA	Spillantini *et al.* (2000)
N296H	E10, R2	Increased	Decreased	No Change	Iseki *et al.* (2001)
ΔN296±	E10, R2	No change	Decreased	Increased	Pastor *et al.* (2001)
P301L	E10, R2	No change	Reduced	Increased	Hutton *et al.* (1998)
P301S	E10, R2	No change	Reduced	Increased	Bugiani *et al.* (1999) Sperfeld *et al.* (1999)
S305N	E10, IR2–3	Increased	No effect	ND	Hasegawa *et al.* (1999) Iijima *et al.* (1999)
S305S	E10, IR2–3	Increased	NA	NA	Stanford *et al.* (2000)
E10+3	I10	Increased	NA	NA	Spillantini *et al.* (1998a)
E10+11	I10	Increased	NA	NA	Miyamoto *et al.* (2001)
E10+12	I10	Increased	NA	NA	Yasuda *et al.* (2000a)
E10+13	I10	Increased	NA	NA	Hutton *et al.* (1998)
E10+14	I10	Increased	NA	NA	Hutton *et al.* (1998)
E10+16	I10	Increased	NA	NA	Hutton *et al.* (1998)
S320F	E11	No change	Reduced	ND	Rosso *et al.* (2002)
V337M	E12, IR3–4	No change	Reduced	Increased	Poorkaj *et al.* (1998)
G342V	E12, IR3–4	Increased	ND	ND	Lippa *et al.* (2000)
K369I	E12, IR3–4	ND	Reduced	Reduced	Neumann *et al.* (2001)
G389R	E13	No change	Reduced	ND	Murrell *et al.* (1999)
R406W	E13	No change	Reduced	Increased	Hutton *et al.* (1998)

E = exon; I = intron; R = MT binding repeat; IR = inter-repeat regions; ND = not determined; NA = not applicable.
Effects on tau fibril formation in vitro.
±Homozygous mutation.
*Increased indicates enhanced exon 10 utilization.
+Decreased indicates reduced exon 10 utilization.
#Variable indicates conflicting data in literature.

segregated with affected individuals and not in control subjects (Table 35.1, Fig. 35.1) (Poorkaj *et al.*, 1998; Hutton *et al.*, 1998; Spillantini *et al.*, 1998c).

However, it is evident that *tau* mutations are not present in all kindreds with familial FTD. While there is a positive family history of a similar dementing illness in ~38–50% of patients with FTD (Knopman *et al.*, 1990; Stevens *et al.*, 1998; Chow *et al.*, 1999), the incidence of *tau* mutations in different studies is quite variable (Houlden *et al.*, 1999; Rizzu *et al.*, 1999; Fabre *et al.*, 2001; Poorkaj *et al.*, 2001; Morris *et al.*, 2001). For instance, in two studies of community-based practices, mutations were not identified in *tau* despite a positive family history in ~38% of patients (Houlden *et al.*, 1999; Fabre *et al.*, 2001). In contrast, in

studies of referral populations with FTD, the proportion of kindreds with *tau* mutations ranged from 3.6% to 17.8%, and if there was a positive family history of a similar dementing illness, the incidence increased to as much as 50% (range 9.4% to 50%) (Houlden *et al.*, 1999; Rizzu *et al.*, 1999; Poorkaj *et al.*, 2001; Morris *et al.*, 2001). Moreover, if tau pathology was present at autopsy, the incidence of *tau* mutations increased further, from 33% to 100% (Poorkaj *et al.*, 2001; Morris *et al.*, 2001).

While mutations in additional genes that lead to FTD have not been identified, linkage analysis implicated several other genetic loci in specific kindreds. Chromosome 3 was linked to a large Dutch kindred with FTD and autosomal dominant inheritance (Brown, 1998; Ashworth *et al.*,

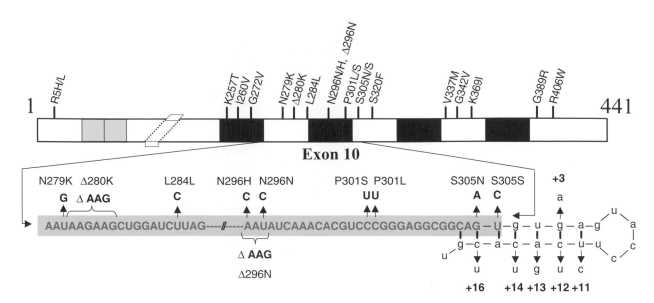

Fig. 35.1 Schematic representation of mutations in the tau gene identified in FTDP-17. The structure of the largest tau isoform is shown with known coding region mutations indicated above. The gray boxes near the amino terminus represent the alternatively spliced inserts encoded for by exons 2 and 3, while the black boxes represent each of the four MT binding repeats (not drawn to scale). The second MT binding repeat is encoded by exon 10. Part of the mRNA sequence encoding exon 10 and the intron following exon 10 is enlarged to visualize the 5′ splice site as well as the mutations in both exon 10 and within the 5′ splice site. Nucleotides that are part of intron 10 are shown in lower case. Nucleotides that are colored blue represent the approximate positions of the ESEs while those colored in red represent the ESS (see text).

1999). This pedigree shows anticipation suggestive of a trinucleotide repeat disorder. Hosler and colleagues demonstrated linkage to chromosome 9q21–q22 in a kindred with both ALS and FTD, but not ALS or FTD alone (Hosler *et al.*, 2000). A second genetic loci was identified on chromosome 9p13.3–p12 in 4 unrelated United States families (Kovach *et al.*, 2001). These kindreds also show autosomal dominant inheritance with a unique constellation of clinical findings including FTD, inclusion body myopathy, and Paget's disease of bone. Finally, two large kindreds with FTD showed linkage to chromosome 17q21–22, a locus which is similar to FTDP-17, but mutations in *tau* were not identified (Lendon *et al.*, 1998; Rosso *et al.*, 2001). These kindreds showed distinct pathology, one classified as FTLD-MND and the other as FTLD (Rosso *et al.*, 2001; Zhukareva *et al.*, 2001). Moreover, one of these kindreds that presented clinically with what has been termed 'hereditary dysphasic disinhibition dementia' showed reduced levels of tau protein, a biochemical feature of a FTLD (Zhukareva *et al.*, 2001). Currently, efforts are focused on identifying the genes implicated in these kindreds as well as identifying additional genetic factors involved in the pathogenesis of familial FTD. One candidate gene is the serine threonine protein kinase, myotonic dystrophy protein kinase (MDPK) (Kiuchi *et al.*, 1991; Sergeant *et al.*, 2001). In patients with myotonic

dystrophy type I, there is an unstable CTG repeat expansion in the 3-untranslated region of this protein kinase. Furthermore, there are abundant neurofibrillary tangles (NFTs) in the brains of many affected individuals, thus suggesting a relationship between the expanded trinucleotide repeats of MDPK and tau pathology.

Frontotemporal dementia with parkinsonism linked to chromosome 17

The initial identification of mutations in *tau* led to a flurry of research activity that attempted to identify additional FTDP-17 mutations. At least 28 distinct pathogenic mutations have been identified in *tau* in a large number of families with FTDP-17 (Table 35.1, Fig. 35.1). Sixteen missense mutations in coding regions of *tau* are known, including missense mutations in exon 1 (R5H (Hayashi *et al.*, 2002) and R5L (Poorkaj *et al.*, 2002)), exon 9 (K257T (Pickering-Brown *et al.*, 2000; Rizzini *et al.*, 2000), I260V (Reed *et al.*, 2001), and G272V (Hutton *et al.*, 1998; Spillantini *et al.*, 1998b)), exon 10 (N279K (Clark *et al.*, 1998; Yasuda *et al.*, 1999; Delisle *et al.*, 1999; Arima *et al.*, 2000), N296H (Iseki *et al.*, 2001), P301L (Dumanchin *et al.*, 1998; Hutton *et al.*, 1998; Clark *et al.*, 1998; Mirra *et al.*, 1999; Houlden

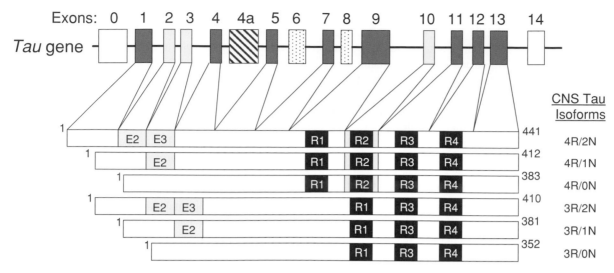

Fig. 35.2 Schematic representation of the human tau gene and six human CNS tau isoforms generated by alternative splicing. The human tau gene contains 16 exons, including exon 0 that is part of the promoter. Exons 1, 4, 5, 7, 9, and 11 to 13 (blue boxes) are constitutively expressed. Alternative splicing of exons 2 (E2), 3 (E3) and 10 (yellow boxes) produces the six tau isoforms observed in the CNS. Exons 6 and 8 (stippled boxes) are not transcribed in the human CNS. Exon 4a (striped box), which is also not transcribed in the human CNS, is expressed in the PNS leading to the larger tau isoforms, termed 'big tau'. The black bars depict the 18 amino acid MT binding repeats and are designated R1 to R4. The relative sizes of the exons and introns are not drawn to scale.

et al., 1999; Bird *et al.*, 1999; Kodama *et al.*, 2000; Tanaka *et al.*, 2000), P301S (Bugiani *et al.*, 1999; Sperfeld *et al.*, 1999; Yasuda *et al.*, 2000b), and S305N (Iijima *et al.*, 1999)), exon 11 (S320F (Rosso *et al.*, 2002)), exon 12 (V337M (Poorkaj *et al.*, 1998), E342V (Lippa *et al.*, 2000), and K369I (Neumann *et al.*, 2001)), and exon 13 (G389R (Murrell *et al.*, 1999; Pickering-Brown *et al.*, 2000) and R406W (Hutton *et al.*, 1998; Van Swieten *et al.*, 1999; Saito *et al.*, 2002)). Three silent mutations in exon 10 (L284L (D'Souza *et al.*, 1999), N296N (Spillantini *et al.*, 2000), and S305S (Stanford *et al.*, 2000)) as well as two single amino acid deletions (ΔK280 (Rizzu *et al.*, 1999) and ΔN296 (Pastor *et al.*, 2001)) have also been identified; however, the ΔN296 does not show autosomal dominant inheritance. In addition, seven different nucleotide substitutions were identified in the introns following exons 9 (+33 (Rizzu *et al.*, 1999)) and 10 (+3 (Spillantini *et al.*, 1998c; Tolnay *et al.*, 2000), +11 (Miyamoto *et al.*, 2001), +12 (Yasuda *et al.*, 2000a), +13 (Hutton *et al.*, 1998), +14 (Hutton *et al.*, 1998; Clark *et al.*, 1998), and +16 (Hutton *et al.*, 1998; Morris *et al.*, 1999; Hulette *et al.*, 1999; Goedert *et al.*, 1999b)) that presumably play a role in the regulation of the alternative splicing of exon 10, which will be discussed below.

Biology of the tau protein

Tau proteins are low-molecular-weight MAPs that are abundant in the central nervous system (CNS) where they are expressed predominantly in axons (Cleveland *et al.*, 1977; Binder *et al.*, 1985), and at low levels in astrocytes and oligodendrocytes (Shin *et al.*, 1991; LoPresti *et al.*, 1995). They are also expressed in axons of peripheral nervous system neurons (Couchie *et al.*, 1992). Human tau proteins are encoded by a single copy gene on chromosome 17q21 composed of 16 exons with the CNS isoforms generated by the alternative mRNA splicing of 11 of these exons (Fig. 35.2) (Neve *et al.*, 1986; Goedert *et al.*, 1988; Andreadis *et al.*, 1992). In adult human brain, alternative splicing of exons 2, 3, and 10 generates 6 tau isoforms ranging from 352 to 441 amino acids in length which differ by the presence of either 3 (3Rtau) or 4 (4Rtau) carboxy-terminal tandem MT binding motifs of 31 or 32 amino acids each that are encoded by exons 9 to 12 (Goedert *et al.*, 1989a,b). Additionally, alternative splicing of exons 2 and 3 leads to the absence (0N) or presence of inserted sequences of 29 (1N) or 58 (2N) amino acids in the amino-terminal third of the molecule. In the adult human brain, the ratio of 3Rtau to 4Rtau isoforms is approximately 1:1, while the 0N, 1N, and 2N tau isoforms comprise about 37%, 54%, and 9%, respectively, of total tau (Goedert & Jakes, 1990; Hong *et al.*, 1998).

Since its discovery over 25 years ago, a number of functions of tau have been characterized (for review see Buée *et al.*, 2000; Lee *et al.*, 2001). Most notably, tau binds to and stabilizes microtubules (MTs) and promotes MT polymerization (Weingarten *et al.*, 1975; Cleveland *et al.*, 1977). The

MT binding domains of tau are localized to the carboxy-terminal half of the molecule within the 4 MT binding motifs (Figs. 35.1 and 35.2). These motifs are composed of highly conserved 18-amino acid binding elements separated by less conserved 13 or 14 amino acid flexible inter-repeat sequences (Himmler *et al.*, 1989; Lee *et al.*, 1989; Butner & Kirschner, 1991). The binding of tau to MTs is a complex process that is mediated by a flexible array of weak binding sites that are distributed throughout the MT binding domain delineated by these repeats and their inter-repeat sequences (Lee *et al.*, 1989; Butner & Kirschner, 1991).

The function of tau as a MT binding protein is regulated by phosphorylation (Drechsel *et al.*, 1992; Yoshida & Ihara, 1993; Bramblett *et al.*, 1993; Biernat *et al.*, 1993). There are 79 potential serine (Ser) and threonine (Thr) phosphate acceptor residues in the longest tau isoform, and phosphorylation at approximately 30 of these sites has been reported in normal tau proteins (for review see Billingsley & Kincaid, 1997; Buée *et al.*, 2000; Hong *et al.*, 2000). Furthermore, at least 12 Ser/Thr protein kinases and 4 Ser/Thr protein phosphatases have been implicated in regulating the phosphorylation state and thus the function of tau. The phosphorylation sites are clustered in regions flanking the MT binding repeats, and increasing tau phosphorylation at multiple sites negatively regulates MT binding (Drechsel *et al.*, 1992; Yoshida & Ihara, 1993; Bramblett *et al.*, 1993; Biernat *et al.*, 1993). However, in both sporadic and familial tauopathies including AD and FTDP-17, tau is hyperphosphorylated, and it is this 'abnormal' tau that is the principal component of the filamentous aggregates in neurons and glia that are the pathological hallmarks of these disorders (Hasegawa *et al.*, 1996; Hoffmann *et al.*, 1997; Zheng-Fischhofer *et al.*, 1998).

Clinical features of FTDP-17

The term FTDP-17 was coined in 1997 to describe the common features found in the affected members of kindreds that demonstrated linkage to chromosome 17 (Foster *et al.*, 1997). The individuals in these FTDP-17 kindreds all exhibited autosomal dominant inheritance with age-dependent penetrance typically in the third to sixth decade of life. Duration of disease is approximately 10 years but with wide variability ranging from as little as 3 years to as long as 30 years. The disease commonly presents insidiously with behavioral, language, and/or motor abnormalities. However, in one study, cognitive deficits particularly involving executive function were observed in presymptomatic subjects decades before the onset of dementia in FTDP-17 patients (Geschwind *et al.*, 2001). The behavioral

abnormalities are typical of FTD, including alterations in personality, impaired social or occupation functioning, hyperorality, hyperphagia, and psychosis associated with disturbed executive function on neuropsychologic examination (Lund & Manchester Groups, 1994; McKhann *et al.*, 2001). In most patients, visuospatial function, orientation, and memory are preserved until late in the course of disease, features that are distinct from that of AD. Language disorders are typical of either an expressive or semantic aphasia, while motor abnormalities consist principally of L-dopa-unresponsive parkinsonism including bradykinesia, rigidity, and postural instability.

With reports of additional kindreds, it became apparent that the clinical presentation is highly variable, reflecting the specific pattern of neuronal loss in affected individuals (Table 35.2) (for review see Foster *et al.*, 1997; Spillantini *et al.*, 1998a; Reed *et al.*, 2001). The clinical phenotype of patients with different mutations, as well as occasionally with the same mutation, is quite variable ranging from FTD to CBD to PSP to AD to a multisystem degeneration. However, some *tau* mutations cause a relatively similar phenotype. For instance, the N279K missense mutation typically causes a phenotype reminiscent of PSP with superimposed dementia (Reed *et al.*, 1998; Yasuda *et al.*, 1999; Delisle *et al.*, 1999). Similarly, the +16 mutation in the intron following exon 10 described in at least ten kindreds causes a very characteristic FTD with disinhibition and affective disturbances presenting in the fourth to sixth decade of life (Baker *et al.*, 1997; Morris *et al.*, 1999; Hulette *et al.*, 1999; Goedert *et al.*, 1999b; Janssen *et al.*, 2002). In contrast, there are numerous clinical and pathologic descriptions of families with P301L mutations that demonstrate a highly variable clinical phenotype including PSP, CBD, and PiD (Spillantini *et al.*, 1998b; Mirra *et al.*, 1999; Nasreddine *et al.*, 1999; Bird *et al.*, 1999). Similarly, while several kindreds with the R406W mutation present with relatively late-onset, slowly progressive memory deficits similar to AD, other kindreds present with early-onset, rapidly progressive FTD (Reed *et al.*, 1997; Van Swieten *et al.*, 1999; Saito *et al.*, 2002). Even more perplexing is a FTDP-17 family with the P301S mutation in which one individual presented clinically with FTD while his son presented clinically with CBD (Bugiani *et al.*, 1999). The ΔN296 mutation is unique in that it gives rise to atypical progressive supranuclear palsy in individuals homozygous for the mutation, but in heterozygous individuals this mutation is incompletely penetrant and associated with a phenotype similar to idiopathic Parkinson's disease (Pastor *et al.*, 2001). These reports, albeit anecdotal, suggest tremendous overlap between the various tau-related disorders, and the clinical distinctions between them may be due to other genetic

Table 35.2. Tau pathology in FTDP-17

Mutation	Regional distribution	Neurons	Glia	Biochemistry[*]	Ultrastructure
R5H	FT, MT, SN	Pretangles (+/−)	Oligodendrocytes Astrocytes (+/−)	4Rtau	Straight tubules, 15–20 nm
R5L	BG, Th, STN, BS, CB	Globose tangles	Astrocytes (tufted) Oligodendrocytes	4Rtau	Straight filaments
K257T	FT, MT	Pick bodies Pretangles	Negative	3Rtau > 4Rtau	Twisted ribbons
I260V	NA	NA	NA	NA	NA
G272V	FT, MT, Ca, Th, SN	Pretangles Pick-body like	Oligodendrocytes (+/−)	NA	NA
E9+33	NA	NA	NA	NA	NA
N279K	FT, MT, BG, Th, STN, BS, CB	Pretangles Balloon neurons	Oligodendrocytes Astrocytes	4Rtau	Twisted ribbons Paired tubules
Δ280K	NA	NA	NA	NA	NA
L284L	FT, MT, BG, SN	Pretangles NFTs	Glia	NA	NA
N296N	FT, Hip, GP, BS	Pretangles Balloon neurons Corticobasal bodies	Oligodendrocytes	NA	NA
N296H	FT, MT, Ca, Th, SN	Pretangles Balloon neurons (+/−)	Astrocytes Oligodendrocytes	4Rtau	Straight tubules, 15 nm
ΔN296	NA	NA	NA	NA	NA
P301L	FT, MT, BG, SN	Pretangles Balloon neurons	Astrocytes Oligodendrocytes	4Rtau	Twisted ribbons Straight filaments
P301S	FT, Ca, SN	Pretangles	Astrocytes Oligodendrocytes	NA	Straight filaments, 10 nm
S305N	FT, MT	Pretangles NFTs, ring-shaped	Oligodendrocytes	NA	Straight tubules, 15 nm
S305S	PR, MT, GP, STN, SN	Pretangles Balloon neurons	Astrocytes, tufted Oligodendrocytes	NA	Twisted filaments, 15 nm Straight filaments, 15 nm
E10+3	FT, SN, CB	Pretangles NFTs	Oligodendrocytes Astrocytes (+/−)	4Rtau	Straight filaments Twisted filaments
E10+11	FT, BG, Th, BS, CB	Pretangles NFTs	Astrocytes (tufted) Oligodendrocytes	NA	NA
E10+12	FT, BG, Th, BS, CB	Pretangles	Glia	4Rtau	Twisted ribbons, 5–23 nm
E10+13	FT, BG, SN	Pretangles NFTs (+/−)	Oligodendrocytes	4Rtau > 3Rtau	Twisted filaments
E10+14	FT, MT, BG, SN	Pretangles NFTs Balloon neurons	Oligodendrocytes	4Rtau	NA
E10+16	FT, BG, SN	Pretangles NFTs (+/−) Pick bodies (+/−) Balloon neurons (+/−)	Astrocytes Oligodendrocytes	4Rtau	Twisted ribbons
S320F	Temp, Hip	Pick bodies Pretangles	Oligodendrocytes (+/−)	3Rtau = 4Rtau	Straight filaments (major) Twisted filaments (minor)
V337M	FT, MT, SN	NFTs Pretangles	ND	3Rtau = 4Rtau	PHF-like Straight filaments
G342V	FT	NFTs Pretangles Pick bodies (+/−) Balloon neurons (+/−)	Astrocytes	4Rtau > 3Rtau (4R0N)	PHF-like
K369I	FT, MT, Ca,	Pick bodies Balloon neurons	Astrocytes (tufted) (+/−) Oligodendrocytes (+/−)	3Rtau = 4Rtau	Twisted ribbons
G389R	FT, MT, Ca, SN	Pretangles Pick bodies NFTs	ND	3Rtau = 4Rtau	Twisted filaments Straight filaments
R406W	FT, MT	NFTs Pretangles	Oligodendrocytes (+/−)	3Rtau = 4Rtau	PHF-like Twisted ribbons Straight filaments

BG = basal ganglia; BS = brainstem; Ca = caudate; CB = cerebellum; FT = frontotemporal lobe; GP = globus pallidus; Hip = hippocampus; MT = medial temporal lobe (hippocampus, entorhinal cortex and amygdala); NFTs = neurofibrillary tangles; PHF = paired helical filaments; PR = peri-Rolandic cortex; SN = substantia nigra; STN = subthalamic nucleus; NA = not available; ND = not detected; Temp = temporal lobe; Th = thalamus; +/− = scattered tau positive inclusions. *Refers to the predominant tau isoforms detected in the analysis of insoluble (filamentous) tau extracts.

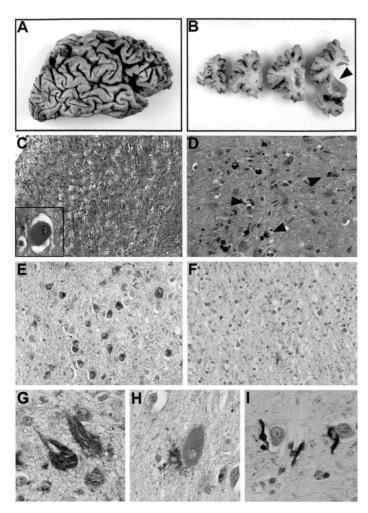

Fig. 35.3 Neuropathology of FTDP-17. **A-B**. FTDP-17 brain with intron 10, +16 mutation showing prominent frontal and temporal lobe atrophy with relative sparing of parietal and occipital lobes. Coronal sections (**B**) show marked hydrocephalus of the lateral ventricles and moderate atrophy of the head of the caudate nucleus (arrowhead). (**C**) Severe neuron loss with spongiosis of upper cortical lamina and prominent gliosis in frontal cortex of patient with P301L mutation (H&E). The surface of the brain is in the upper left corner while the subcortical white matter is in the lower right corner. Inset shows a ballooned neuron identified in the deep cortical layers. (**D**) Marked depletion of pigmented neurons in the substantia nigra of patient with N279K mutation. There is prominent gliosis with extravasation of neuromelanin and uptake into macrophages (arrowheads) (H&E). (**E**) Frontal cortex with numerous tau positive inclusions (pretangles) in patient with P301L mutation (IHC with anti-tau antibody). (**F**) Thread pathology in subcortical white matter of the frontal lobe in a patient with the P301L mutation (IHC with anti-tau antibody). (**G**) NFTs in the hippocampus of patient with R406W mutation (IHC with anti-tau antibody). (**H**) Granular astrocytic inclusion (left) and ballooned neuron (right) in the frontal cortex

and/or epigenetic factors that modify the effects of the *tau* mutations.

Neuropathology of FTDP-17

Similar to the clinical phenotypes, the neuropathology of FTDP-17 is quite variable (Table 35.2) (Reed *et al.*, 2001; Pickering-Brown *et al.*, 2002). The most characteristic gross neuropathologic feature is severe frontotemporal atrophy involving both cortex and the underlying white matter with relative sparing of the parietal and occipital lobes (Fig. 35.3) (Foster *et al.*, 1997). The pathology in the medial temporal lobe including the hippocampus, amygdala, and entorhinal cortex is highly variable ranging from minimal involvement to marked atrophy. The basal ganglia often exhibit severe degeneration, while involvement of the thalamus and subthalamus is typically not prominent. The substantia nigra is characteristically depigmented, while atrophy of the remainder of the brainstem and cerebellum is variable, typically mirroring the clinical phenotype of the patient (Fig. 35.3). Microscopically, there is marked neuron loss in effected brain regions similar to that observed for sporadic tauopathies (Fig. 35.3). In affected cortices, the neuron loss is associated with rarefaction and spongiosis of the superficial cortex with gliosis of both the gray and underlying white matter. Similarly, there is atrophy and neuron loss in the basal ganglia and substantia nigra (Fig. 35.3). Neuron loss in other brain regions is highly variable, paralleling both the clinical phenotype and pattern of gross atrophy. For instance, kindreds with the R406W mutation show profound neuron loss with severe gliosis in the medial temporal lobe including the amygdala, hippocampus, and entorhinal cortex with relative sparing of the basal ganglia and brainstem (Table 35.2) (Reed *et al.*, 1997; Van Swieten *et al.*, 1999; Rosso *et al.*, 2000; Saito *et al.*, 2002). In contrast, the N279K mutation causes neuron loss in subcortical and brainstem nuclei with variable pathology in the medial temporal lobe structures (Table 35.2) (Kawai *et al.*, 1993; Reed *et al.*, 1998; Delisle *et al.*, 1999; Arima *et al.*, 2000).

Despite the regional heterogeneity of the pathology of FTDP-17 kindreds, there is extensive neuronal or glial and neuronal fibrillary pathology composed of hyperphosphorylated tau protein in all cases, in the absence of β-amyloid (Aβ) deposits or other disease-specific brain

---

Fig. 35.3 (*cont.*) of a patient with intron 10, +16 mutation (IHC with anti-tau antibody). The astrocytic inclusion resembles the tufted astrocyte typical of PSP. (**I**) Coiled bodies and threads in the globus pallidus of patient with N279K mutation (IHC with anti-tau antibody).

lesions (Fig. 35.3) (for review see Spillantini *et al.*, 1998a; Reed *et al.*, 2001). These pathological inclusions are only variably identified with amyloid binding dyes such as Congo red and ThioflavinS as well as silver stains including Bodian, Bielschowsky and Gallyas. However, the inclusions are most consistently identified by immunohistochemistry (IHC) for tau protein, particularly with antibodies specific for phosphorylation-dependent epitopes that are characteristic of the insoluble inclusions.

The filamentous aggregates exhibit remarkable heterogeneity in both neurons and glia. The neuronal tau pathology frequently demonstrates a granular staining pattern, often referred to as 'pretangles' (Fig. 35.3) (Spillantini *et al.*, 1998a; Reed *et al.*, 2001). Classic NFTs, similar to that observed in AD, are abundant in several of the FTDP-17 mutations (Fig. 35.3) (Sumi *et al.*, 1992; Spillantini *et al.*, 1996; Foster *et al.*, 1997; Bird *et al.*, 1997; Reed *et al.*, 1997; Van Swieten *et al.*, 1999; Saito *et al.*, 2002). In addition, Pick bodies similar to those observed in PiD are a neuropathological feature associated with several mutations including K257V (Pickering-Brown *et al.*, 2000; Rizzini *et al.*, 2000), G272V (Spillantini *et al.*, 1998b), S320F (Rosso *et al.*, 2002), K369I (Neumann *et al.*, 2001), and G389R (Murrell *et al.*, 1999; Pickering-Brown *et al.*, 2000). Ballooned neurons and corticobasal bodies similar to those originally described in CBD are also detected with many of the mutations (Foster *et al.*, 1997; Spillantini *et al.*, 2000; Reed *et al.*, 2001). The tau pathology in astrocytes typically demonstrates a granular staining pattern (Fig. 35.3). However, occasional glial inclusions are observed that are reminiscent of the astrocytic plaques and tufted astrocytes described in CBD and PSP, respectively (Foster *et al.*, 1997; Spillantini *et al.*, 1998a; Komori, 1999; Reed *et al.*, 2001). With many *tau* mutations, there is abundant tau pathology in oligodendrocytes, similar to the coiled bodies observed in many sporadic tauopathies (Fig. 35.3) (Foster *et al.*, 1997; Spillantini *et al.*, 1998a; Komori, 1999; Reed *et al.*, 2001). Finally, tau-positive threads are abundant in either the gray matter or both the white and gray matter within the processes of both neurons and glia (Fig. 35.3) (Komori, 1999).

Ultrastructural analysis of the tau filaments in FTDP-17 also demonstrates marked heterogeneity in the tau pathology (Table 35.2). In two mutations, R406W and V337M, paired helical filaments (PHFs) with a diameter of 8 to 20 nm and a periodicity of 80 nm as well as straight filaments (SFs) nearly identical to those present in AD are observed (Sumi *et al.*, 1992; Spillantini *et al.*, 1996; Reed *et al.*, 1997). However, in the majority of mutations, the filaments demonstrate a range of morphologies including wide and narrow twisted ribbons, twisted filaments, paired tubules, and

SFs that range in width from 8 to 25 nm typically with longer periodicities than that observed in the PHFs of AD (Spillantini *et al.*, 1998a; Yen *et al.*, 1999b; Reed *et al.*, 2001).

Perhaps the most unique feature of the pathology of FTDP-17 is that the pattern and nature of the tau inclusions fail to fit neatly into any of the known categories of sporadic tauopathies. However, the FTDP-17 mutations can be loosely categorized based on the tau immunostaining and biochemical profile (Table 35.2 and Fig. 35.4). In one group, the tau aggregates are primarily within neurons. By IHC, the tau pathology is localized predominantly in gray matter, although biochemically there is aggregation of all 6 tau isoforms (or predominantly 3Rtau with the K257T mutation) within both gray and white matter (Table 35.2, Figs. 35.4 and 35.5). In contrast, the second group shows extensive tau pathology within both glia and neurons in gray and white matter that is composed of 4Rtau only (Table 35.2, Figs. 35.4 and 35.5).

Effects of FTDP-17 mutations

FTDP-17 mutations lead to tau dysfunction and presumably disease by several distinct mechanisms (Table 35.1). Intronic and some exonic mutations affect the alternative splicing of exon 10 and consequently alter the relative proportions of 3Rtau and 4Rtau. The other exonic mutations impair the ability of tau to bind MTs and to promote MT assembly. Some of the mutations also promote the assembly of tau into filaments. Moreover, additional mechanisms may play a role in the case of some coding region mutations (reviewed in Lee *et al.*, 2001). The intronic mutations clustered around the 5′ splice site of exon 10, as well as several mutations within or near exon 10 (N279K, L284L, N296N, N296H, S305N, S305S, and G342V), increase the ratio of 4Rtau to 3Rtau by altering the splicing of this exon (Hutton *et al.*, 1998; Yasuda *et al.*, 1999; Delisle *et al.*, 1999; Varani *et al.*, 1999; Grover *et al.*, 1999; D'Souza *et al.*, 1999; Hasegawa *et al.*, 1999; Stanford *et al.*, 2000; D'Souza & Schellenberg, 2000; Gao *et al.*, 2000; Spillantini *et al.*, 2000; Yasuda *et al.*, 2000a; Miyamoto *et al.*, 2001; Grover *et al.*, 2002). As a result of these mutations there is a relative increase in mRNA containing exon 10, reflecting increased utilization of the 5′ splice site of exon 10 as demonstrated in exon trapping experiments. Biochemical analysis of insoluble tau extracted from autopsied FTDP-17 brain tissue of patients with these mutations reveals predominantly 4Rtau isoforms (Figs. 35.4 and 35.5) (Clark *et al.*, 1998; Reed *et al.*, 1998; Hong *et al.*, 1998; Spillantini *et al.*, 1998c; Hulette *et al.*, 1999; Goedert *et al.*, 1999b; Arima *et al.*, 2000; Yasuda *et al.*, 2000a; Iseki *et al.*, 2001). Furthermore, 4Rtau

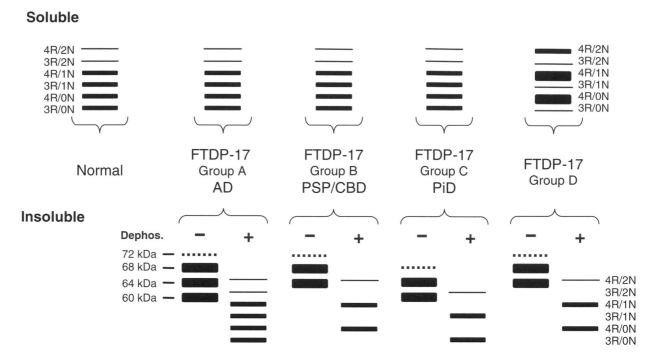

Fig. 35.4 Schematic representation of Western blot banding patterns of soluble and insoluble tau from different tauopathies. The cartoon depicts the typical banding pattern of soluble tau (top panels) and insoluble/filamentous tau (bottom panels) from the brains of patients with FTDP-17 as well as sporadic tauopathies following resolution with SDS-PAGE and immunoblotting with anti-tau antibodies. The FTDP-17 mutations show several different Western blot banding patterns of soluble and insoluble tau protein that are depicted as groups A to D. The soluble fraction from the brains of unaffected (normal) individuals, sporadic tauopathies, and FTDP-17 with mutations that do not effect tau splicing (Groups A, B, and C) show expression of all 6 tau isoforms. Non-dephosphorylated insoluble tau from the brains of patients with group A variants of FTDP-17 (S320F, V337M, K369I, G389R, and R406W) resolve as 3 major proteins of 68-, 64- and 60-kDa; and a minor band of 72 kDa similar to that observed in AD. When dephosphorylated, they resolve into 6 proteins that correspond to all 6 tau isoforms similar to the soluble fraction. In group B variants of FTDP-17 (R5H, P301L, and G342V) 2 prominent 68- and 64-kDa protein bands are detected (the 72 kDa minor band is variably detected) that align with 4Rtau following dephosphorylation similar to that observed in PSP and CBD indicating the selective aggregation of 4Rtau. In the group C variant of FTDP-17 (K257T) and PiD the 64 and 60 kDa insoluble tau protein isoforms predominate and align with 3Rtau isoforms following dephosphorylation indicating selective aggregation of 3Rtau. In contrast, in group D variants of FTDP-17 mutations that effect mRNA splicing (N279K, L284L, N296N, N296H, S305S, S305N, and intron 10 mutations), there is expression of predominantly 4Rtau throughout the entire brain which is reflected in the insoluble tau aggregates. Note that normal brains do not contain insoluble species of tau.

protein levels are increased in both affected and unaffected regions of FTDP-17 brains (Hong *et al.*, 1998; Spillantini *et al.*, 1998c; Goedert *et al.*, 1999b; Yasuda *et al.*, 2000a).

The regulation of splicing of exon 10 of *tau* is complex, and may involve multiple *cis*-acting regulatory elements that either enhance or inhibit the utilization of the 5′ splice site, many of which are affected by mutations identified in *tau* (Varani *et al.*, 1999; D'Souza *et al.*, 1999; Hasegawa *et al.*, 1999; D'Souza & Schellenberg, 2000; Jiang *et al.*, 2000; Gao *et al.*, 2000; Grover *et al.*, 2002). Splicing regulatory elements within exon 10 include an exon-splicing enhancer (ESE) and an exon-splicing silencer (ESS) (Fig. 35.1) (D'Souza *et al.*, 1999; D'Souza & Schellenberg, 2000; Gao *et al.*, 2000). The ESE consists of three domains, a potential SC35 binding

element, a purine rich sequence, and an AC-rich sequence (D'Souza & Schellenberg, 2000). Immediately downstream of the ESE within exon 10 is the purine-rich ESS followed by a second ESE. The flanking exons of *tau* also affect exon 10 splicing (Gao *et al.*, 2000). Exons 9 and 11 exert opposite effects; exon 9 promotes splicing of exon 10, while exon 11 suppresses it. Lastly, intronic sequences immediately downstream of exon 10 inhibit its splicing (Varani *et al.*, 1999; D'Souza *et al.*, 1999; Hasegawa *et al.*, 1999; D'Souza & Schellenberg, 2000; Jiang *et al.*, 2000; Gao *et al.*, 2000; Grover *et al.*, 2002). The inhibition may be secondary to the formation of a stem–loop structure that sequesters the 5′ splice site from the splicing machinery including the U1- and U6-snRNP (Fig. 35.1) (Varani *et al.*, 1999; Grover *et al.*, 1999;

A. Soluble Tau

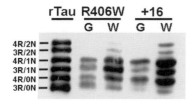

B. Insoluble Tau, R406W

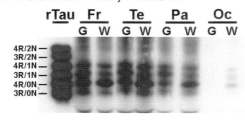

C. Insoluble Tau, Intron +16

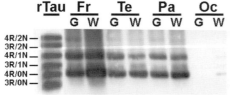

Fig. 35.5 Western blots of soluble and insoluble tau from FTDP-17 brains. Soluble (**A**) and insoluble (**B,C**) tau fractions extracted from gray (G) and white (W) matter of patients with FTDP-17 were dephosphorylated with *E. coli* alkaline phosphatase, resolved by SDS-PAGE and immunoblotted with phosphorylation-independent tau antibodies. (**A**) Soluble fractions from the frontal cortex of patients with the R406W show all 6 tau isoforms. In contrast, in patients with the intron 10, +16 mutation, there is selective overexpression of 4Rtau isoforms. (**B,C**) The insoluble tau protein from the indicated cortices are composed of either equimolar amounts of both 4Rtau and 3Rtau (R406W) or predominantly 4Rtau only (intron 10, +16). With both mutations the tau pathology is most abundant in the frontal and temporal lobes with relative sparing of the occipital lobe. In addition, there is abundant insoluble tau in the white matter of the brain with the R406W mutation that is not detected by IHC. Recombinant tau isoforms (rTau) are as indicated. Fr = frontal lobe; Te = temporal lobe; Pa = parietal lobe; Oc = occipital lobe.

Jiang *et al.*, 2000). The relative proportions of 3Rtau and 4Rtau from other species correlates with the predicted stability of this stem–loop structure (Grover *et al.*, 1999). However, another study concluded that the inhibitory effect of the intronic sequence is due to a linear sequence array that is independent of the stem–loop structure (D'Souza & Schellenberg, 2000).

FTDP-17 mutations in *tau* may alter exon 10 splicing by affecting several of the regulatory elements described above. For example, the intronic mutations as well as the exonic mutations at codon 305 (S305N and S305S) may destabilize the inhibitory stem–loop structure (Fig. 35.1) (Hutton *et al.*, 1998; Grover *et al.*, 1999; D'Souza *et al.*, 1999). The S305N and the +3 intronic mutations may also enhance exon 10 splicing by increasing the strength of the 5′ splice site (GUgugagu to AUgugagu) (Senapathy *et al.*, 1990). However, the finding that the S305S mutation weakens the 5′ splice site (GUgugagu to GCgugagu) and also leads to predominantly 4Rtau argues against this effect of the mutation (Stanford *et al.*, 2000). The N279K mutation may improve the function of the ESE by lengthening the purine-rich sequence within this regulatory element (UAAGAA to GAAGAA), and thus enhance exon 10 splicing (D'Souza & Schellenberg, 2000). Moreover, the thymidine nucleotide present in the wild-type (WT) sequence may function as an inhibitor of splicing (Tanaka *et al.*, 1994). This hypothesis is supported by the observation that the ΔK280 mutation, which deletes the three adjacent purine residues (AAG), reduces exon 10 splicing. The silent L284L mutation that enhances exon 10 splicing may do so by disrupting a potential exon splicing inhibitor (UUAG to UCAG) (Si *et al.*, 1998; D'Souza *et al.*, 1999). However, since mutation of this consensus sequence does not increase exon 10 splicing, a second possibility is that the mutation lengthens the AC-rich element within the ESE (Si *et al.*, 1998; D'Souza & Schellenberg, 2000). Thus, the L284L mutation may affect either an enhancing or inhibitory splicing element. Lastly, the effect of the N296N and N296H mutations on splicing of exon 10 is due to disruption of the ESS or conversely the creation of a novel splice enhancer sequence (D'Souza & Schellenberg, 2000; Grover *et al.*, 2002).

The mechanisms by which these changes in the ratio of 3Rtau to 4Rtau (3R/4Rtau) lead to neuronal and glial dysfunction and cell death remain unclear. However, 3Rtau and 4Rtau may bind to distinct sites on MTs (Goode & Feinstein, 1994), and it is possible that a specific ratio of tau isoforms is necessary for normal MT function (Goode *et al.*, 1997). Thus, the altered ratio of 3R/4Rtau may directly affect MT function. In addition, overproduction of 4Rtau isoforms may lead to an excess of free tau in the cytoplasm that is prone to aggregate and polymerize into filaments over time.

Another subset of the *tau* mutations has no effect on *tau* splicing but instead alters the ability of tau to interact with MTs. Specifically, missense mutations K257T, G272V, ΔK280, ΔN296, P301L, P301S, V337M, G389R, and R406W reduce the binding of tau to MTs and decrease its ability to promote MT stability and assembly in vitro (Hong *et al.*, 1998; Hasegawa *et al.*, 1998; Bugiani *et al.*, 1999; Rizzu *et al.*, 1999; Pickering-Brown *et al.*, 2000; Rizzini *et al.*, 2000; Barghorn *et al.*, 2000; Grover *et al.*, 2002). In contrast to other mutations that affect the splicing of *tau*, these mutations do not alter the expression pattern of 3Rtau and 4Rtau (Hong *et al.*, 1998). However, the P301L mutation causes a moderate (25%) decrease in soluble 4Rtau due to the selective aggregation of mutant 4Rtau isoforms (Hong *et al.*, 1998; Rizzu *et al.*, 2000; Miyasaka *et al.*, 2001). Biochemical analysis of insoluble tau extracted from brain tissue of patients with these mutations reveals a variety of patterns. Several mutations including S320F, V337M, K369I, G389R, and R406W are characterized by the aggregation of equal amounts of both 3Rtau and 4Rtau (Figs. 35.4 and 35.5) (Spillantini *et al.*, 1996; Hong *et al.*, 1998; Murrell *et al.*, 1999; Neumann *et al.*, 2001; Rosso *et al.*, 2002). A second group (R5H, R5L, P301L, and G342V) leads to the selective aggregation of 4Rtau isoforms similar to that observed in PSP and CBD (Fig. 35.4) (Clark *et al.*, 1998; Spillantini *et al.*, 1998b; Bugiani *et al.*, 1999; Mirra *et al.*, 1999; Nasreddine *et al.*, 1999; Lippa *et al.*, 2000; Hayashi *et al.*, 2002). In contrast, the K257T mutation causes the selective aggregation of 3Rtau similar to PiD (Fig. 35.4) (Rizzini *et al.*, 2000). This is intriguing because the neuropathology of both kindreds identified with the K257T mutation is characterized by the widespread deposition of Pick bodies comparable to those observed in PiD (Pickering-Brown *et al.*, 2000; Rizzini *et al.*, 2000).

The effects of these FTDP-17 mutations on MT binding, assembly, and stability are not observed with the tau missense mutations that directly affect exon 10 splicing (Hong *et al.*, 1998; D'Souza *et al.*, 1999; Hasegawa *et al.*, 1999). The effects of these FTDP-17 mutations on MT function are observed when mutant *tau* is expressed in a variety of cell lines including SHSY5Y neuroblastoma cells (Dayanandan *et al.*, 1999), Chinese hamster ovary (CHO) cells (Matsumura *et al.*, 1999; Dayanandan *et al.*, 1999; Vogelsberg-Ragaglia *et al.*, 2000), monkey kidney (COS) cells (Arawaka *et al.*, 1999; Sahara *et al.*, 2000), human embryonic kidney (HEK293) cells (Sahara *et al.*, 2000; Nagiec *et al.*, 2001), and SF9 insect cells (Frappier *et al.*, 1999). Expression of a variety of *tau* missense mutations including G272V, P301L, V337M, and R406W in these cells caused reduced MT binding, MT instability, disorganized MT morphology, and defects in MT assembly to varying degrees. However, in two studies, many mutations had either no or only a modest effect on MT binding and/or function both in in vitro assays and in transfected cell lines (DeTure *et al.*, 2000; Sahara *et al.*, 2000). The discrepancies between these and other studies are most likely due to either differences in the levels of tau expression, the specific cells in which the FTDP-17

mutations were expressed, and/or the binding of tau to MTs. Nevertheless, even if the FTDP-17 mutations cause only a modest reduction in MT binding affinity, this effect could lead to large cumulative effects on neurons over the human life span. Furthermore, increased cytosolic concentrations of unbound mutant tau may facilitate aggregation of these abnormal proteins into filamentous inclusions. In support of this hypothesis, Yen and colleagues demonstrated that several mutations lead to decreased susceptibility to calpain I digestion, an enzyme involved in the normal degradation of tau, which might lead to an increase in the concentration of cytosolic tau (Yen *et al.*, 1999a). The loss of function of tau could also cause a variety of toxic effects within affected cells. For example, the reduced capacity of these mutants to stabilize MTs might affect axonal transport in neurons. Alternatively, impairments in tau functions could lead to increased apoptotic vulnerability as suggested in a recent study in which 2 of the FTDP-17 mutations (N279K and V337M) showed increased cell death upon serum withdrawal in transfected neuroblastoma cell lines (Furukawa *et al.*, 2000).

A subset of missense *tau* mutations may cause FTDP-17, at least in part, by promoting tau aggregation (Table 35.1). Several studies demonstrated that numerous mutations, including K257T, G272V, ΔK280, ΔN296, P301L, P301S, V337M, and R406W, promote heparin- or arachidonic acid-induced tau filament formation in vitro relative to WT tau (Arrasate *et al.*, 1999; Nacharaju *et al.*, 1999; Goedert *et al.*, 1999a; Rizzini *et al.*, 2000; Barghorn *et al.*, 2000; Gamblin *et al.*, 2000; Grover *et al.*, 2002). The ΔK280 and P301L promote in vitro filament formation more readily than other missense mutations and WT tau (von Bergen *et al.*, 2001). This effect is most likely due to the enhancement of β-structure around 2 hexapeptide motifs that are strong promoters of tau fibrillization (von Bergen *et al.*, 2000). Additionally, the P301L mutation causes the selective deposition of mutant tau in the pathologic intracellular inclusions with corresponding depletion in the soluble fraction (Rizzu *et al.*, 2000; Miyasaka *et al.*, 2001). The aggregation of mutant tau in intact cells has also been demonstrated. Thus, CHO cells expressing tau with the ΔK280 mutation, but not other mutations (V337M, P301L and R406W), formed insoluble aggregates (Vogelsberg-Ragaglia *et al.*, 2000).

It is unclear whether the filaments composed of mutant tau proteins are similar to those composed of WT tau. Goedert *et al.* reported that, while a subset of the *tau* mutations stimulated filament formation, they were structurally identical to WT tau filaments as assessed by circular dichroism (Goedert *et al.*, 1999a). However, Jicha *et al.* reported altered physical and structural properties of filaments composed of mutant tau as assessed by both circular dichroism and reverse phase high performance liquid chromatography (Jicha et al., 1999).

The missense *tau* mutations may also effect tau function, and thus contribute to the pathogenesis of FTDP-17, by altering the phosphorylation of tau. Numerous mutations decreased the binding affinity of tau for protein phosphatase 2A, a major phosphatase implicated in the regulation of the MT-binding activity of tau (Goedert et al., 2000). Goedert and colleagues suggest that this leads to both tau hyperphosphorylation and dissociation of tau from MTs therefore altering the normal balance between free and MT-bound tau. However, expression of several mutations, particularly R406W, both in vitro and in transfected cell lines led to reduced levels of tau phosphorylation relative to WT tau, suggesting that increased tau phosphorylation is not required for pathogenesis of disease (Matsumura et al., 1999; Dayanandan et al., 1999; Sahara et al., 2000; Perez et al., 2000; Vogelsberg-Ragaglia et al., 2000; Connell et al., 2001).

The biochemical and structural characteristics of the tau aggregates in FTDP-17 are somewhat predictable based on our understanding of the functions of tau proteins and *tau* splicing. However, the basis for the clinical phenotypes and topographical distributions of pathology of individuals with the various FTDP-17 mutations remains enigmatic. This finding suggests that the phenotypic differences may be due to other genetic and/or epigenetic factors that modify the effects of the primary mutation. The specific modifiers that mediate the 'selective vulnerability' of specific regions and/or cells associated with either a specific mutation or even of a specific individual remain unknown, but these are fields of active investigation and the generation of animal models of tau-mediated neurodegeneration may facilitate this research.

Animal models of FTDP-17

Experimental and transgenic (TG) models of tauopathies will serve as informative systems for elucidating the role of abnormalities in tau in the onset and progression of disease as well as providing useful models for the development of novel therapies. Several models of tau pathology were produced by overexpressing human tau proteins in mice (for review see Götz, 2001). However, these mice were either asymptomatic or developed pathology that was localized to the spinal cord and/or lacked many of the key features of tau-based disorders. In contrast, the introduction of the P301L mutation led to the development of TG mice that develop age- and gene dose-dependent accumulation of tau tangles in the brain and spinal cord with

associated nerve cell loss and gliosis as well as behavioral abnormalities (Lewis et al., 2000; Götz et al., 2001a). Similar to human disease, the tau aggregates were composed of only mutant human tau further implicating the P301L change in promoting the selective aggregation of mutant tau. Gene expression profiling of brain tissue from these mice showed altered expression of genes contributing to the inhibition of apoptosis, inflammation, and intracellular transport (Ho et al., 2001). The co-expression or injection of Aβ in mice expressing P301L mutant tau led to enhanced neurofibrillary degeneration with preferential involvement of the limbic system similar to that observed in AD (Lewis et al., 2001; Götz et al., 2001b). This observation suggests that there may be a mechanistic interaction between the Aβ and tau pathologies that influence their distribution and abundance. Subsequently, TG mice were developed with different FTDP-17 mutations that also lead to neurodegeneration in either neurons (V337M) (Tanemura et al., 2001; Tanemura et al., 2002) or oligodendrocytes (G272V) (Götz et al., 2001c).

Other systems were also developed to model various aspects of human tauopathies. Overexpression of tau in lamprey reticulospinal neurons led to the formation of PHF-like tau inclusions with degeneration of a subset of neurons (Hall et al., 1997, 2000). In addition, overexpression of either WT or FTDP-17 mutant tau (R406W and V337M) in *Drosophila melanogaster* demonstrated key features of tauopathies including adult-onset progressive neurodegeneration with accumulation of abnormal tau (Wittmann et al., 2001). However, the neurodegeneration occurred in the absence of NFT formation. More recent studies demonstrated NFT-like pathology when tau was co-expressed with *shaggy* that is homologous to glycogen synthase 3-kinase implicated in tau phosphorylation (Jackson et al., 2002). Nonetheless, all of these models show various features of tau-related disorders that will hopefully facilitate an understanding of the molecular mechanisms underlying tau neurotoxicity.

Conclusions

The accumulation of filamentous tau inclusions is a common feature of a wide variety of sporadic and familial neurodegenerative disorders that present clinically with FTD. These tauopathies are distinguished by the distinct topographic and cell type-specific distribution of inclusions. The biochemical and ultrastructural characteristics of the tau pathology also reveal a significant phenotypic overlap. The discovery of multiple mutations in *tau* that lead to the abnormal aggregation of tau and cause FTDP-17 demonstrates that tau dysfunction is sufficient to produce neurodegenerative disease. The mutations lead to specific alterations in the expression, function, and biochemistry of the tau protein. Furthermore, in light of the similarities between FTDP-17 and other tauopathies, it is likely that elucidation of this perplexing enigma will provide important clues into mechanisms underlying the interaction between genetic and environmental factors in neurodegenerative disease. The identification of additional gene mutations or polymorphisms at distinct genetic loci in families with FTD that either cause or are risk factors for disease will provide additional insights into disease pathogenesis as well as in the development of novel strategies for treatment and prevention.

Acknowledgements

M. S. Forman is supported by a grant from the National Institute of Aging. V. M.-Y. Lee is the John H. Ware Third Professor of Alzheimer's Disease Research at the University of Pennsylvania. We would like to thank Dr. Victoria Zhukareva who generously provided Western blots of FTDP-17 patients. We would also like to thank the many patients studied and their families for making the research reviewed here possible.

REFERENCES

Andreadis, A., Brown, W. M. & Kosik, K. S. (1992). Structure and novel exons of the human tau gene. *Biochemistry*, **31**, 10626–33.

Arawaka, S., Usami, M., Sahara, N., Schellenberg, G. D., Lee, G. & Mori, H. (1999). The tau mutation (val337met) disrupts cytoskeletal networks of microtubules. *Neuroreport*, **10**, 993–7.

Arima, K., Kowalska, A., Hasegawa, M. *et al.* (2000). Two brothers with frontotemporal dementia and parkinsonism with an N279K mutation of the tau gene. *Neurology*, **54**, 1787–95.

Arrasate, M., Perez, M., Armas-Portela, R. & Avila, J. (1999). Polymerization of tau peptides into fibrillar structures. The effect of FTDP-17 mutations. *FEBS Lett.*, **446**, 199–202.

Ashworth, A., Lloyd, S., Brown, J. *et al.* (1999). Molecular genetic characterization of frontotemporal dementia on chromosome 3. *Dement. Geriatr. Cogn. Disord.*, **10** (Suppl 1), 93–101.

Baker, M., Kwok, J. B., Kucera, S. *et al.* (1997). Localization of frontotemporal dementia with parkinsonism in an Australian kindred to chromosome 17q21–22. *Ann. Neurol.*, **42**, 794–8.

Barghorn, S., Zheng-Fischhofer, Q., Ackmann, M. *et al.* (2000). Structure, microtubule interactions, and paired helical filament aggregation by tau mutants of frontotemporal dementias. *Biochemistry*, **39**, 11714–21.

Biernat, J., Gustke, N., Drewes, G., Mandelkow, E. M. & Mandelkow, E. (1993). Phosphorylation of Ser262 strongly reduces binding of tau to microtubules: distinction between PHF-like immunoreactivity and microtubule binding. *Neuron*, **11**, 153–63.

Billingsley, M. L. & Kincaid, R. L. (1997). Regulated phosphorylation and dephosphorylation of tau protein: effects on microtubule interaction, intracellular trafficking and neurodegeneration. *Biochem. J*, **323**, 577–91.

Binder, L. I., Frankfurter, A. & Rebhun, L. I. (1985). The distribution of tau in the mammalian central nervous system. *J. Cell. Biol.*, **101**, 1371–8.

Bird, T. D., Wijsman, E. M., Nochlin, D. *et al.* (1997). Chromosome 17 and hereditary dementia: linkage studies in three non-Alzheimer families and kindreds with late-onset FAD. *Neurology*, **48**, 949–54.

Bird, T. D., Nochlin, D., Poorkaj, P. *et al.* (1999). A clinical pathological comparison of three families with frontotemporal dementia and identical mutations in the tau gene (P301L). *Brain*, **122**, 741–756.

Bramblett, G. T., Goedert, M., Jakes, R., Merrick, S. E., Trojanowski, J. Q. & Lee, V. M.-Y. (1993). Abnormal tau phosphorylation at Ser396 in Alzheimer's disease recapitulates development and contributes to reduced microtubule binding. *Neuron*, **10**, 1089–99.

Brown, J. (1998). Chromosome 3-linked frontotemporal dementia. *Cell Mol. Life Sci.*, **54**, 925–7.

Buée, L., Bussière, T., Buée-Scherrer, V., Delacourte, A. & Hof, P. R. (2000). Tau protein isoforms, phosphorylation and role in neurodegenerative disorders. *Brain Res. Rev.*, **33**, 1–36.

Bugiani, O., Murrell, J. R., Giaccone, G. *et al.* (1999). Frontotemporal dementia and corticobasal degeneration in a family with a P301S mutation in tau. *J. Neuropathol. Exp. Neurol.*, **58**, 667–77.

Butner, K. A. & Kirschner, M. W. (1991). Tau protein binds to microtubules through a flexible array of distributed weak sites. *J. Cell Biol.*, **115**, 717–30.

Chow, T. W., Miller, B. L., Hayashi, V. N. & Geschwind, D. H. (1999). Inheritance of frontotemporal dementia. *Arch. Neurol.*, **56**, 817–22.

Clark, L. N., Poorkaj, P., Wszolek, Z. *et al.* (1998). Pathogenic implications of mutations in the tau gene in pallido-ponto-nigral degeneration and related neurodegenerative disorders linked to chromosome 17. *Proc. Natl Acad. Sci., USA*, **95**, 13103–7.

Cleveland, D. W., Hwo, S. Y. & Kirschner, M. W. (1977). Purification of tau, a microtubule-associated protein that induces assembly of microtubules from purified tubulin. *J. Mol. Biol.*, **116**, 207–25.

Connell, J. W., Gibb, G. M., Betts, J. C. *et al.* (2001). Effects of FTDP-17 mutations on the *in vitro* phosphorylation of tau by glycogen synthase kinase 3beta identified by mass spectrometry demonstrate certain mutations exert long-range conformational changes. *FEBS Lett.*, **493**, 40–4.

Couchie, D., Mavilia, C., Georgieff, I. S., Liem, R. K., Shelanski, M. L. & Nunez, J. (1992). Primary structure of high molecular weight tau present in the peripheral nervous system. *Proc. Natl Acad. Sci., USA*, **89**, 4378–81.

D'Souza, I. & Schellenberg, D. (2000). Determinants of 4 repeat tau expression: Coordination between enhancing and inhibitory splicing sequences for exon 10 inclusion. *J. Biol. Chem.*, **275**, 17700–9.

D'Souza, I., Poorkaj, P., Hong, M. *et al.* (1999). Missense and silent tau gene mutations cause frontotemporal dementia with parkinsonism-chromosome 17 type, by affecting multiple alternative RNA splicing regulatory elements. *Proc. Natl Acad. Sci., USA*, **96**, 5598–603.

Dayanandan, R., van Slegtenhorst, M., Mack, T. G. *et al.* (1999). Mutations in tau reduce its microtubule binding properties in intact cells and affect its phosphorylation. *FEBS Lett.*, **446**, 228–32.

Delisle, M. B., Murrell, J. R., Richardson, R. *et al.* (1999). A mutation at codon 279 (N279K) in exon 10 of the Tau gene causes a tauopathy with dementia and supranuclear palsy. *Acta Neuropathol.(Berl)*, **98**, 62–77.

DeTure, M., Ko, L. W., Yen, S. *et al.* (2000). Missense tau mutations identified in FTDP-17 have a small effect on tau- microtubule interactions. *Brain Res.*, **853**, 5–14.

Drechsel, D. N., Hyman, A. A., Cobb, M. H. & Kirschner, M. W. (1992). Modulation of the dynamic instability of tubulin assembly by the microtubule-associated protein tau. *Mol. Biol. Cell*, **3**, 1141–54.

Dumanchin, C., Camuzat, A., Campion, D. *et al.* (1998). Segregation of a missense mutation in the microtubule-associated protein tau gene with familial frontotemporal dementia and parkinsonism. *Hum. Mol. Genet.*, **7**, 1825–9.

Fabre, S. F., Forsell, C., Viitanen, M. *et al.* (2001). Clinic-based cases with frontotemporal dementia show increased cerebrospinal fluid tau and high apolipoprotein E epsilon4 frequency, but no tau gene mutations. *Exp. Neurol.*, **168**, 413–18.

Foster, N. L., Wilhelmsen, K., Sima, A. A., Jones, M. Z., D'Amato, C. J. & Gilman, S. (1997). Frontotemporal dementia and parkinsonism linked to chromosome 17: a consensus conference. *Ann. Neurol.*, **41**, 706–15.

Frappier, T., Liang, N. S., Brown, K. *et al.* (1999). Abnormal microtubule packing in processes of SF9 cells expressing the FTDP-17 V337M tau mutation. *FEBS Lett.*, **455**, 262–6.

Furukawa, K., D'Souza, I., Crudder, C. H. *et al.* (2000). Pro-apoptotic effects of tau mutations in chromosome 17 frontotemporal dementia and parkinsonism. *Neuroreport*, **11**, 57–60.

Gamblin, T. C., King, M. E., Dawson, H. *et al.* (2000). *In vitro* polymerization of tau protein monitored by laser light scattering: method and application to the study of FTDP-17 mutants. *Biochemistry*, **39**, 6136–44.

Gao, Q. S., Memmott, J., Lafyatis, R., Stamm, S., Screaton, G. & Andreadis, A. (2000). Complex regulation of tau exon 10, whose missplicing causes frontotemporal dementia. *J. Neurochem.*, **74**, 490–500.

Geschwind, D. H., Robidoux, J., Alarcon, M. *et al.* (2001). Dementia and neurodevelopmental predisposition: cognitive dysfunction in presymptomatic subjects precedes dementia by decades in frontotemporal dementia. *Ann. Neurol.*, **50**, 741–6.

Goedert, M. & Jakes, R. (1990). Expression of separate isoforms of human tau protein: correlation with the tau pattern in brain and effects on tubulin polymerization. *EMBO J*, **9**, 4225–30.

Goedert, M., Wischik, C. M., Crowther, R. A., Walker, J. E., and Klug, A. (1988). Cloning and sequencing of the cDNA encoding a core protein of the paired helical filament of Alzheimer disease: identification as the microtubule-associated protein tau. *Proc. Natl Acad. Sci., USA*, **85**, 4051–5.

Goedert, M., Spillantini, M. G., Jakes, R., Rutherford, D. & Crowther, R. A. (1989a). Multiple isoforms of human microtubule-associated protein tau: sequences and localization in neurofibrillary tangles of Alzheimer's disease. *Neuron*, **3**, 519–26.

Goedert, M., Spillantini, M. G., Potier, M. C., Ulrich, J. & Crowther, R. A. (1989b). Cloning and sequencing of the cDNA encoding an isoform of microtubule-associated protein tau containing four tandem repeats: differential expression of tau protein mRNAs in human brain. *EMBO J.*, **8**, 393–9.

Goedert, M., Jakes, R. & Crowther, R. A. (1999a). Effects of frontotemporal dementia FTDP-17 mutations on heparin-induced assembly of tau filaments. *FEBS Lett.*, **450**, 306–11.

Goedert, M., Spillantini, M. G., Crowther, R. A. *et al.* (1999b). Tau gene mutation in familial progressive subcortical gliosis. *Nat. Med.*, **5**, 454–7.

Goedert, M., Satumtira, S., Jakes, R. *et al.* (2000). Reduced binding of protein phosphatase 2A to tau protein with frontotemporal dementia and parkinsonism linked to chromosome 17 mutations. *J. Neurochem.*, **75**, 2155–62.

Goode, B. L. & Feinstein, S. C. (1994). Identification of a novel microtubule binding and assembly domain in the developmentally regulated inter-repeat region of tau. *J. Cell Biol.*, **124**, 769–82.

Goode, B. L., Denis, P. E., Panda, D. *et al.* (1997). Functional interactions between the proline-rich and repeat regions of tau enhance microtubule binding and assembly. *Mol. Biol. Cell*, **8**, 353–65.

Götz, J. (2001). Tau and transgenic animal models. *Brain Res. Rev.*, **35**, 266–86.

Götz, J., Chen, F., Barmettler, R. & Nitsch, R. M. (2001a). Tau filament formation in transgenic mice expressing P301L tau. *J. Biol. Chem.*, **276**, 529–34.

Götz, J., Chen, F., Van Dorpe, J. & Nitsch, R. M. (2001b). Formation of neurofibrillary tangles in P301L tau transgenic mice induced by Abeta 42 fibrils. *Science*, **293**, 1491–5.

Götz, J., Tolnay, M., Barmettler, R., Chen, F., Probst, A. & Nitsch, R. M. (2001c). Oligodendroglial tau filament formation in transgenic mice expressing G272V tau. *Eur. J. Neurosci.*, **13**, 2131–40.

Grover, A., Houlden, H., Baker, M. *et al.* (1999). 5' splice site mutations in tau associated with the inherited dementia FTDP-17 affect a stem–loop structure that regulates alternative splicing of exon 10. *J. Biol. Chem.*, **274**, 15134–43.

Grover, A., DeTure, M., Yen, S. H. & Hutton, M. (2002). Effects on splicing and protein function of three mutations in codon N296 of tau *in vitro*. *Neurosci. Lett.*, **323**, 33–6.

Hall, G. F., Yao, J. & Lee, G. (1997). Human tau becomes phosphorylated and forms filamentous deposits when overexpressed in lamprey central neurons *in situ. Proc. Natl Acad. Sci., USA*, **94**, 4733–8.

Hall, G. F., Chu, B., Lee, G. & Yao, J. (2000). Human tau filaments induce microtubule and synapse loss in an *in vivo* model of neurofibrillary degenerative disease. *J. Cell Sci.*, **113** (8), 1373–87.

Hasegawa, M., Jakes, R., Crowther, R. A., Lee, V. M.-Y., Ihara, Y. & Goedert, M. (1996). Characterization of mAb AP422, a novel phosphorylation-dependent monoclonal antibody against tau protein. *FEBS Lett.*, **384**, 25–30.

Hasegawa, M., Smith, M. J. & Goedert, M. (1998). Tau proteins with FTDP-17 mutations have a reduced ability to promote microtubule assembly. *FEBS Lett.*, **437**, 207–10.

Hasegawa, M., Smith, M. J., Iijima, M., Tabira, T. & Goedert, M. (1999). FTDP-17 mutations N279K and S305N in tau produce increased splicing of exon 10. *FEBS Lett.*, **443**, 93–6.

Hayashi, S., Toyoshima, Y., Hasegawa, M. *et al.* (2002). Late-onset frontotemporal dementia with a novel exon 1 (Arg5His) tau gene mutation. *Ann. Neurol.*, **51**, 525–30.

Heutink, P., Stevens, M., Rizzu, P. *et al.* (1997). Hereditary frontotemporal dementia is linked to chromosome 17q21–q22: a genetic and clinicopathological study of three Dutch families. *Ann. Neurol.*, **41**, 150–9.

Himmler, A., Drechsel, D., Kirschner, M. W. & Martin, D. W., Jr. (1989). Tau consists of a set of proteins with repeated C-terminal microtubule-binding domains and variable N-terminal domains. *Mol. Cell Biol.*, **9**, 1381–8.

Ho, L., Xiang, Z., Mukherjee, P. *et al.* (2001). Gene expression profiling of the tau mutant (P301L) transgenic mouse brain. *Neurosci. Lett.*, **310**, 1–4.

Hoffmann, R., Lee, V. M.-Y., Leight, S., Varga, I. & Otvos, L., Jr. (1997). Unique Alzheimer's disease paired helical filament specific epitopes involve double phosphorylation at specific sites. *Biochemistry*, **36**, 8114–24.

Hong, M., Zhukareva, V., Vogelsberg-Ragaglia, V. *et al.* (1998). Mutation-specific functional impairments in distinct tau isoforms of hereditary FTDP-17. *Science*, **282**, 1914–17.

Hong, M., Trojanowski, J. Q. & Lee, V. M.-Y., (2000). Tau-based neurofibrillary lesions. In: *Neurodegenerative Dementias*, ed. C. M.Clark & J. Q.Trojanowski, pp. 161–75. New York: McGrawHill.

Hosler, B. A., Siddique, T., Sapp, P. C. *et al.* (2000). Linkage of familial amyotrophic lateral sclerosis with frontotemporal dementia to chromosome 9q21–q22. *J. Am. Med. Assoc.*, **284**, 1664–9.

Houlden, H., Baker, M., Adamson, J. *et al.* (1999). Frequency of tau mutations in three series of non-Alzheimer's degenerative dementia. *Ann. Neurol.*, **46**, 243–8.

Hulette, C. M., Pericak-Vance, M. A., Roses, A. D. *et al.* (1999). Neuropathological features of frontotemporal dementia and parkinsonism linked to chromosome 17q21–22 (FTDP-17): Duke Family 1684. *J. Neuropathol. Exp. Neurol.*, **58**, 859–66.

Hutton, M., Lendon, C. L., Rizzu, P. *et al.* (1998). Association of missense and 5′-splice-site mutations in tau with the inherited dementia FTDP-17. *Nature*, **393**, 702–5.

Iijima, M., Tabira, T., Poorkaj, P. *et al.* (1999). A distinct familial presenile dementia with a novel missense mutation in the tau gene. *Neuroreport*, **10**, 497–501.

Iseki, E., Matsumura, T., Marui, W. *et al.* (2001). Familial frontotemporal dementia and parkinsonism with a novel N296H mutation in exon 10 of the tau gene and a widespread tau accumulation in glial cells. *Acta Neuropathol.*, **102**, 285–92.

Jackson, J. R., Wiedau-Pazos, M., Sang, T.-K. *et al.* (2002). Human wild-type tau interacts with *wingless* pathway components and produces neurofibrillary pathology in *Drosophila. Neuron*, **34**, 509–19.

Janssen, J. C., Warrington, E. K., Morris, H. R. *et al.* (2002). Clinical features of frontotemporal dementia due to the intronic tau 10(+16) mutation. *Neurology*, **58**, 1161–8.

Jiang, Z., Cote, J., Kwon, J. M., Goate, A. M. & Wu, J. Y. (2000). Aberrant splicing of tau pre-mRNA caused by intronic mutations associated with the inherited dementia frontotemporal dementia with parkinsonism linked to chromosome 17. *Mol.Cell Biol.*, **20**, 4036–48.

Jicha, G. A., Rockwood, J. M., Berenfeld, B., Hutton, M. & Davies, P. (1999). Altered conformation of recombinant frontotemporal dementia-17 mutant tau proteins. *Neurosci. Lett.*, **260**, 153–6.

Kawai, J., Sasahara, M., Hazama, F. *et al.* (1993). Pallidonigroluysian degeneration with iron deposition: a study of three autopsy cases. *Acta Neuropathol. (Berl.)*, **86**, 609–16.

Kiuchi, A., Otsuka, N., Namba, Y., Nakano, I. & Tomonaga, M. (1991). Presenile appearance of abundant Alzheimer's neurofibrillary tangles without senile plaques in the brain in myotonic dystrophy. *Acta Neuropathol. (Berl.)*, **82**, 1–5.

Knopman, D. S., Mastri, A. R., Frey, W. H., Sung, J. H. & Rustan, T. (1990). Dementia lacking distinctive histologic features: a common non-Alzheimer degenerative dementia. *Neurology*, **40**, 251–6.

Kodama, K., Okada, S., Iseki, E. *et al.* (2000). Familial frontotemporal dementia with a P301L tau mutation in Japan. *J. Neurol. Sci.*, **176**, 57–64.

Komori, T. (1999). Tau-positive glial inclusions in progressive supranuclear palsy, corticobasal degeneration and Pick's disease. *Brain Pathol.*, **9**, 663–79.

Kovach, M. J., Waggoner, B., Leal, S. M. *et al.* (2001). Clinical delineation and localization to chromosome 9p13.3–p12 of a unique dominant disorder in four families: hereditary inclusion body myopathy, Paget's disease of bone, and frontotemporal dementia. *Mol. Genet. Metab.*, **74**, 458–75.

Lee, G., Neve, R. L. & Kosik, K. S. (1989). The microtubule binding domain of tau protein. *Neuron*, **2**, 1615–24.

Lee, V. M.-Y., Goedert, M. & Trojanowski, J. Q. (2001). Neurodegenerative tauopathies. *Ann. Rev. Neurosci.*, **24**, 1121–59.

Lendon, C. L., Lynch, T., Norton, J. *et al.* (1998). Hereditary dysphasic disinhibition dementia: a frontotemporal dementia linked to 17q21–22. *Neurology*, **50**, 1546–55.

Lewis, J., McGowan, E., Rockwood, J. *et al.* (2000). Neurofibrillary tangles, amyotrophy and progressive motor disturbance in mice expressing mutant (P301L) tau protein. *Nat. Genet.*, **25**, 402–5.

Lewis, J., Dickson, D. W., Lin, W. L. *et al.* (2001). Enhanced neurofibrillary degeneration in transgenic mice expressing mutant tau and APP. *Science*, **293**, 1487–91.

Lippa, C. F., Zhukareva, V., Kawarai, T. *et al.* (2000). Frontotemporal dementia with novel tau pathology and a Glu342Val tau mutation. *Ann. Neurol.*, **48**, 850–8.

LoPresti, P., Szuchet, S., Papasozomenos, S. C., Zinkowski, R. P. & Binder, L. I. (1995). Functional implications for the microtubule-associated protein tau: localization in oligodendrocytes. *Proc. Natl Acad. Sci., USA*, **92**, 10369–73.

Lund and Manchester Groups (1994). Clinical and neuropathological criteria for frontotemporal dementia. *J. Neurol. Neurosurg. Psychiatry*, **57**, 416–18.

Matsumura, N., Yamazaki, T. & Ihara, Y. (1999). Stable expression in Chinese hamster ovary cells of mutated tau genes causing frontotemporal dementia and parkinsonism linked to chromosome 17 (FTDP-17). *Am. J. Pathol.*, **154**, 1649–56.

McKhann, G. M., Albert, M. S., Grossman, M., Miller, B., Dickson, D. & Trojanowski, J. Q. (2001). Clinical and pathological diagnosis of frontotemporal dementia: report of the Work Group on Frontotemporal Dementia and Pick's Disease. *Arch. Neurol.*, **58**, 1803–9.

Mirra, S. S., Murrell, J. R., Gearing, M. *et al.* (1999). Tau pathology in a family with dementia and a P301L mutation in tau. *J. Neuropathol. Exp. Neurol.*, **58**, 335–45.

Miyamoto, K., Kowalska, A., Hasegawa, M. *et al.* (2001). Familial frontotemporal dementia and parkinsonism with a novel mutation at an intron 10+11-splice site in the tau gene. *Ann. Neurol.*, **50**, 117–20.

Miyasaka, T., Morishima-Kawashima, M., Ravid, R., Kamphorst, W., Nagashima, K. & Ihara, Y. (2001). Selective deposition of mutant tau in the FTDP-17 brain affected by the P301L mutation. *J. Neuropathol. Exp. Neurol.*, **60**, 872–84.

Morris, H. R., Perez-Tur, J., Janssen, J. C. *et al.* (1999). Mutation in the tau exon 10 splice site region in familial frontotemporal dementia. *Ann. Neurol.*, **45**, 270–1.

Morris, H. R., Khan, M. N., Janssen, J. C. *et al.* (2001). The genetic and pathological classification of familial frontotemporal dementia. *Arch. Neurol.*, **58**, 1813–16.

Murrell, J. R., Koller, D., Foroud, T. *et al.* (1997). Familial multiple-system tauopathy with presenile dementia is localized to chromosome 17. *Am. J. Hum. Genet.*, **61**, 1131–8.

Murrell, J. R., Spillantini, M. G., Zolo, P. *et al.* (1999). Tau gene mutation G389R causes a tauopathy with abundant pick body-like inclusions and axonal deposits. *J. Neuropathol. Exp. Neurol.*, **58**, 1207–26.

Nacharaju, P., Lewis, J., Easson, C., Yen, S., Hackett, J., Hutton, M. & Yen, S. H. (1999). Accelerated filament formation from tau protein with specific FTDP-17 missense mutations. *FEBS Lett.*, **447**, 195–9.

Nagiec, E. W., Sampson, K. E. & Abraham, I. (2001). Mutated tau binds less avidly to microtubules than wildtype tau in living cells. *J. Neurosci. Res.*, **63**, 268–75.

Nasreddine, Z. S., Loginov, M., Clark, L. N. *et al.* (1999). From genotype to phenotype: a clinical pathological, and biochemical investigation of frontotemporal dementia and parkinsonism (FTDP-17) caused by the P301L tau mutation. *Ann. Neurol.*, **45**, 704–15.

Neumann, M., Schulz-Schaeffer, W., Crowther, R. A. *et al.* (2001). Pick's disease associated with the novel Tau gene mutation K369I. *Ann. Neurol.*, **50**, 503–13.

Neve, R. L., Harris, P., Kosik, K. S., Kurnit, D. M. & Donlon, T. A. (1986). Identification of cDNA clones for the human microtubule-associated protein tau and chromosomal localization of the genes for tau and microtubule-associated protein 2. *Brain Res.*, **387**, 271–80.

Pastor, P., Pastor, E., Carnero, C. *et al.* (2001). Familial atypical progressive supranuclear palsy associated with homozygosity for the delN296 mutation in the tau gene. *Ann. Neurol.*, **49**, 263–7.

Perez, M., Lim, F., Arrasate, M. & Avila, J. (2000). The FTDP-17-linked mutation R406W abolishes the interaction of phosphorylated tau with microtubules. *J. Neurochem.*, **74**, 2583–9.

Pick, A. (1892). Über die Bejiehungen der senilen Hirnatrophie zur Aphasie. *Prager. Med. Wochenschr.*, **17**, 165–7.

Pickering-Brown, S., Baker, M., Yen, S. H., *et al.* (2000). Pick's disease is associated with mutations in the tau gene. *Ann. Neurol.*, **48**, 859–67.

Pickering-Brown, S. M., Richardson, A. M., Snowden, J. S. *et al.* (2002). Inherited frontotemporal dementia in nine British families associated with intronic mutations in the tau gene. *Brain*, **125**, 732–51.

Poorkaj, P., Bird, T. D., Wijsman, E. *et al.* (1998). Tau is a candidate gene for chromosome 17 frontotemporal dementia. *Ann. Neurol.*, **43**, 815–25.

Poorkaj, P., Grossman, M., Steinbart, E. *et al.* (2001). Frequency of tau gene mutations in familial and sporadic cases of non-Alzheimer dementia. *Arch. Neurol.*, **58**, 383–7.

Poorkaj, P., Muma, N. A., Zhukareva, V. *et al.* (2002). An R5L tau mutation in a subject with a progressive supranuclear palsy phenotype. *Ann. Neurol.*, **52**, 511–16.

Reed, L. A., Grabowski, T. J., Schmidt, M. L. *et al.* (1997). Autosomal dominant dementia with widespread neurofibrillary tangles. *Ann. Neurol.*, **42**, 564–72.

Reed, L. A., Schmidt, M. L., Wszolek, Z. K. *et al.* (1998). The neuropathology of a chromosome 17-linked autosomal dominant parkinsonism and dementia ('pallido-ponto-nigral degeneration'). *J. Neuropathol. Exp. Neurol.*, **57**, 588–601.

Reed, L. A., Wszolek, Z. K. & Hutton, M. (2001). Phenotypic correlations in FTDP-17. *Neurobiol. Aging*, **22**, 89–107.

Rizzini, C., Goedert, M., Hodges, J. R. *et al.* (2000). Tau gene mutation K257T causes a tauopathy similar to Pick's disease. *J. Neuropathol. Exp. Neurol.*, **59**, 990–1001.

Rizzu, P., Van Swieten, J. C., Joosse, M. *et al.* (1999). High prevalence of mutations in the microtubule-associated protein tau in a population study of frontotemporal dementia in the Netherlands. *Am. J. Hum. Genet.*, **64**, 414–21.

Rizzu, P., Joosse, M., Ravid, R. *et al.* (2000). Mutation-dependent aggregation of tau protein and its selective depletion from the soluble fraction in brain of P301L FTDP-17 patients. *Hum. Mol. Genet.*, **9**, 3075–82.

Rosso, S. M., Kamphorst, W., de Graaf, B. *et al.* (2001). Familial frontotemporal dementia with ubiquitin-positive inclusions is linked to chromosome 17q21–22. *Brain*, **124**, 1948–57.

Rosso, S. M., Kamphorst, W., Ravid, R. & Van Swieten, J. C. (2000). Coexistent tau and amyloid pathology in hereditary frontotemporal dementia with tau mutations. *Ann. NY. Acad. Sci.*, **920**, 115–19.

Rosso, S. M., van Herpen, E., Deelen, W. *et al.* (2002). A novel tau mutation, S320F, causes a tauopathy with inclusions similar to those in Pick's disease. *Ann. Neurol.*, **51**, 373–6.

Sahara, N., Tomiyama, T. & Mori, H. (2000). Missense point mutations of tau to segregate with FTDP-17 exhibit site-specific effects on microtubule structure in COS cells: a novel action of R406W mutation. *J. Neurosci. Res.*, **60**, 380–7.

Saito, Y., Geyer, A., Sasaki, R. *et al.* (2002). Early-onset, rapidly progressive familial tauopathy with R406W mutation. *Neurology*, **58**, 811–13.

Sanders, J., Schenk, V. & van Veen, P. (1939). A family with Pick's disease. *Veerhandelingen de Koninklijke Nederlandse Akadamie van Wetenschappen.*

Schenk, V. (1959). Re-examination of a family with Pick's disease. *Ann. Hum. Genet.*, **23**, 325–33.

Senapathy, P., Shapiro, M. B. & Harris, N. L. (1990). Splice junctions, branch point sites, and exons: sequence statistics, identification, and applications to genome project. *Methods Enzymol.*, **183**, 252–78.

Sergeant, N., Sablonniere, B., Schraen-Maschke, S. *et al.* (2001). Dysregulation of human brain microtubule-associated tau mRNA maturation in myotonic dystrophy type 1. *Hum. Mol. Genet.*, **10**, 2143–55.

Shin, R. W., Iwaki, T., Kitamoto, T. & Tateishi, J. (1991). Hydrated autoclave pretreatment enhances tau immunoreactivity in formalin-fixed normal and Alzheimer's disease brain tissues. *Lab. Invest.*, **64**, 693–702.

Si, Z. H., Rauch, D. & Stoltzfus, C. M. (1998). The exon splicing silencer in human immunodeficiency virus type 1 Tat exon 3 is bipartite and acts early in spliceosome assembly. *Mol. Cell Biol.*, **18**, 5404–13.

Sperfeld, A. D., Collatz, M. B., Baier, H. *et al.* (1999). FTDP-17: an early-onset phenotype with parkinsonism and epileptic seizures caused by a novel mutation. *Ann. Neurol.*, **46**, 708–15.

Spillantini, M. G., Crowther, R. A. & Goedert, M. (1996). Comparison of the neurofibrillary pathology in Alzheimer's disease and familial presenile dementia with tangles. *Acta Neuropathol. (Berl.)*, **92**, 42–8.

Spillantini, M. G., Bird, T. D. & Ghetti, B. (1998a). Frontotemporal dementia and Parkinsonism linked to chromosome 17: a new group of tauopathies. *Brain Pathol.*, **8**, 387–402.

Spillantini, M. G., Crowther, R. A., Kamphorst, W., Heutink, P. & Van Swieten, J. C. (1998b). Tau pathology in two Dutch families with mutations in the microtubule-binding region of tau. *Am. J. Pathol.*, **153**, 1359–63.

Spillantini, M. G., Murrell, J. R., Goedert, M., Farlow, M. R., Klug, A. & Ghetti, B. (1998c). Mutation in the tau gene in familial multiple system tauopathy with presenile dementia. *Proc. Natl Acad. Sci., USA*, **95**, 7737–41.

Spillantini, M. G., Yoshida, H., Rizzini, C. *et al.* (2000). A novel tau mutation (N296N) in familial dementia with swollen achromatic neurons and corticobasal inclusion bodies. *Ann. Neurol.*, **48**, 939–43.

Stanford, P. M., Halliday, G. M., Brooks, W. S. *et al.* (2000). Progressive supranuclear palsy pathology caused by a novel silent mutation in exon 10 of the tau gene: expansion of the disease phenotype caused by tau gene mutations. *Brain*, **123**, 880–93.

Stevens, M., van Duijn, C. M., Kamphorst, W. *et al.* (1998). Familial aggregation in frontotemporal dementia. *Neurology*, **50**, 1541–5.

Sumi, S. M., Bird, T. D., Nochlin, D. & Raskind, M. A. (1992). Familial presenile dementia with psychosis associated with cortical neurofibrillary tangles and degeneration of the amygdala. *Neurology*, **42**, 120–7.

Tanaka, K., Watakabe, A. & Shimura, Y. (1994). Polypurine sequences within a downstream exon function as a splicing enhancer. *Mol. Cell Biol.*, **14**, 1347–54.

Tanaka, R., Kobayashi, T., Motoi, Y., Anno, M., Mizuno, Y. & Mori, H. (2000). A case of frontotemporal dementia with tau P301L mutation in the Far East. *J. Neurol.*, **247**, 705–7.

Tanemura, K., Akagi, T., Murayama, M. *et al.* (2001). Formation of filamentous tau aggregations in transgenic mice expressing V337M human tau. *Neurobiol. Dis.*, **8**, 1036–45.

Tanemura, K., Murayama, M., Akagi, T. *et al.* (2002). Neurodegeneration with tau accumulation in a transgenic mouse expressing V337M human tau. *J. Neurosci.*, **22**, 133–41.

Tolnay, M., Grazia, S. M., Rizzini, C., Eccles, D., Lowe, J. & Ellison, D. (2000). A new case of frontotemporal dementia and parkinsonism resulting from an intron 10 +3-splice site mutation in the tau gene: clinical and pathological features. *Neuropathol. Appl. Neurobiol.*, **26**, 368–78.

Van Swieten, J. C., Stevens, M., Rosso, S. M. *et al.* (1999). Phenotypic variation in hereditary frontotemporal dementia with tau mutations. *Ann. Neurol.*, **46**, 617–26.

Varani, L., Hasegawa, M., Spillantini, M. G. *et al.* (1999). Structure of tau exon 10 splicing regulatory element RNA and destabilization by mutations of frontotemporal dementia and parkinsonism linked to chromosome 17. *Proc. Natl Acad. Sci., USA*, **96**, 8229–34.

Vogelsberg-Ragaglia, V., Bruce, J., Richter-Landsberg, C. *et al.* (2000). Distinct FTDP-17 missense mutations in tau produce tau aggregates and other pathological phenotypes in transfected CHO cells. *Mol. Biol. Cell*, **11**, 4093–104.

von Bergen, M., Friedhoff, P., Biernat, J., Heberle, J., Mandelkow, E. M. & Mandelkow, E. (2000). Assembly of tau protein into Alzheimer paired helical filaments depends on a local sequence motif ((306)VQIVYK(311)) forming beta structure. *Proc. Natl Acad. Sci., USA*, **97**, 5129–34.

von Bergen, M., Barghorn, S., Li, L. *et al.* (2001). Mutations of tau protein in frontotemporal dementia promote aggregation of paired helical filaments by enhancing local beta-structure. *J. Biol. Chem.*, **276**, 48165–74.

Weingarten, M. D., Lockwood, A. H., Hwo, S. Y. & Kirschner, M. W. (1975). A protein factor essential for microtubule assembly. *Proc. Natl Acad. Sci., USA*, **72**, 1858–62.

Wijker, M., Wszolek, Z. K., Wolters, E. C. *et al.* (1996). Localization of the gene for rapidly progressive autosomal dominant parkinsonism and dementia with pallido-ponto-nigral degeneration to chromosome 17q21. *Hum. Mol. Genet.*, **5**, 151–4.

Wilhelmsen, K. C., Lynch, T., Pavlou, E., Higgins, M. & Nygaard, T. G. (1994). Localization of disinhibition-dementia-parkinsonism-amyotrophy complex to 17q21–22. *Am. J. Hum. Genet.*, **55**, 1159–65.

Wittmann, C. W., Wszolek, M. F., Shulman, J. M. *et al.* (2001). Tauopathy in Drosophila: neurodegeneration without neurofibrillary tangles. *Science*, **293**, 711–14.

Yasuda, M., Kawamata, T., Komure, O. *et al.* (1999). A mutation in the microtubule-associated protein tau in pallido-nigro-luysian degeneration. *Neurology*, **53**, 864–8.

Yasuda, M., Takamatsu, J., D'Souza, I. *et al.* (2000a). A novel mutation at position +12 in the intron following exon 10 of the tau gene in familial frontotemporal dementia (FTD-Kumamoto). *Ann. Neurol.*, **47**, 422–9.

Yasuda, M., Yokoyama, K., Nakayasu, T. *et al.* (2000b). A Japanese patient with frontotemporal dementia and parkinsonism by a tau P301S mutation. *Neurology*, **55**, 1224–7.

Yen, S., Easson, C., Nacharaju, P., Hutton, M. & Yen, S. H. (1999a). FTDP-17 tau mutations decrease the susceptibility of tau to calpain I digestion. *FEBS Lett.*, **461**, 91–5.

Yen, S. H., Hutton, M., DeTure, M., Ko, L. W. & Nacharaju, P. (1999b). Fibrillogenesis of tau: insights from tau missense mutations in FTDP-17. *Brain Pathol.*, **9**, 695–705.

Yoshida, H. & Ihara, Y. (1993). Tau in paired helical filaments is functionally distinct from fetal tau: assembly incompetence of paired helical filament-tau. *J. Neurochem.*, **61**, 1183–6.

Zheng-Fischhofer, Q., Biernat, J., Mandelkow, E. M., Illenberger, S., Godemann, R. & Mandelkow, E. (1998). Sequential phosphorylation of Tau by glycogen synthase kinase-3beta and protein kinase A at Thr212 and Ser214 generates the Alzheimer-specific epitope of antibody AT100 and requires a paired-helical-filament-like conformation. *Eur. J. Biochem.*, **252**, 542–52.

Zhukareva, V., Vogelsberg-Ragaglia, V., Van Deerlin, V. M. *et al.* (2001). Loss of brain tau defines novel sporadic and familial tauopathies with frontotemporal dementia. *Ann. Neurol.*, **49**, 165–75.

36

PRION DISEASES

I The clinical approach to human prion diseases

Hayrettin Tumani and Albert C. Ludolph

Department of Neurology, University of Ulm, Germany

Introduction

Prion diseases represent a disease complex that is clinically rare. However, they are epidemiologically important severe diseases, and very likely to be important for our basic understanding of neurodegeneration in principle. This is reflected in this introductory clinical overview, which presents the clinical diagnostic and differential diagnostic approach to the patient; then a review follows which focuses on the current status of the field of basic sciences of prion diseases.

The history of prion diseases started in the year 1920 when Hans Gerhard Creutzfeldt described a mysterious focal disease of the central nervous system of a 22-year-old female patient, which clinically was characterized by progressive psychomotor disturbances and cortical symptoms (Creutzfeldt, 1920). In his autopsy he observed a pronounced gliosis which accompanied non-inflammatory focal lesions of the cortex. One year later, Alfons Jakob saw three similar cases which he also considered a new entity – he described a spastic pseudosclerosis and encephalomyelitis with disseminated focal degeneration (Jakob, 1921). Based on the similarity of the reported cases, Walter Spielmeyer suggested the name Creutzfeldt–Jakob disease (CJD). In 1936, the Gerstmann–Sträussler–Schenker (GSS) syndrome was first described and in 1957 fatal familial insomnia (FFI) (Gerstmann & Sträussler 1936; Lugaresi *et al.*, 1986). In the 1960s, interest in the epidemiology of prion diseases increased when Gajdusek and Gibbs showed that Kuru – a disease first observed by the German Walter Zigas and Carleton Gajdusek among the Fore in Papua New Guinea and thought to be associated with cannibalism – could be transmitted to non-human primates and had similarities with the spongiform encephalopathy of sheep-scrapie (Zigas & Gajdusek, 1957; Hadlow,

1959; Gajdusek & Gibbs, 1966). However, studies in the United Kingdom showed no evidence that sporadic CJD is in any way related to scrapie (Harries-Jones *et al.*, 1988).

Nevertheless, knowledge of the transmissibility of spongiform encephalopathies stimulated research into iatrogenic CJD, which comprises more than 180 cases following medical manipulations ranging from surgical procedures such as epilepsy surgery and cornea transplants to the administration of human growth factor. The prion diseases once again came into the center of public interest when in the late 1990s evidence accumulated that the bovine spongiform encephalopathy (BSE) in the United Kingdom was causally related to a new variant of CJD (vCJD) which predominantly affected young adults (Will *et al.*, 2000). In the year 2004, it seems that the threat of a large vCJD epidemic – which was predicted by many – is getting smaller (Andrews *et al.*, 2003; Collins *et al.*, 2004).

Epidemiology

The epidemiological assessment of cases of CJD is most reliable in countries that have set up a surveillance unit. Subsequent prospective studies conducted by surveillance units allowed a reliable assessment of incidence, prevalence, mortality, clinical symptoms and ultimately risk factors. Since CJD patients die within a few months, the annual statistics for incidence, prevalence and mortality are very similar. In general, the worldwide incidence is estimated as 1/million/year; however, experience shows that, in countries with a high autopsy rate or with a surveillance unit, incidence rates may reach 1.3 or 1.4 patients/1 million inhabitants/year. Based on prospective epidemiological

Table 36.1. Types of Creutzfeldt–Jakob Disease (CJD)

CJD type	Prevalence	Age (years)	Disease duration (months)
Sporadic (sCJD)	90%	60	4–5
Genetic (gCJD)	10%	50	21
Iatrogenic (iCJD)	$n = 180$	4–60	10
Variant (vCJD)	$n = 153^*$	30	14

* reported by December 2003 worldwide.

studies, there has been a clear increase of annual incidence rates of CJD from less than 0.4 before 1990 to more than 1.0 after 1995 in many European countries (Poser *et al.*, 1999; Mollenhauer *et al.*, 2002). The increased incidence is primarily a consequence of improved diagnostic criteria as well as of increased awareness of CJD since the onset of BSE.

Overall, the incidence is not sex specific. Both males and females are affected equally, with a slight female excess reported in some studies. CJD is predominantly a disease of late middle age with highest mortality rates in the age groups between 60 and 70 years. Cases below 50 and above 80 years are very rare.

Four CJD phenotypes are known (Table 36.1):

- **Sporadic CJD** is the most common (85–90%) human prion disease with unknown cause.
- **Genetic CJD** is the second most common type (15–10%) comprising familial CJD, Gerstmann Sträussler–Schenker syndrome (GSS), fatal familial insomnia (FFI) which is always related to an underlying prion protein gene (*PRNP*) mutation. Meanwhile, more than 20 *PRNP* mutations are known with an autosomal dominant pattern of inheritance.
- **Iatrogenic CJD** cases are much more rare and are induced by accidental transmission of CJD during surgical or medical treatment (human dura mater implants, corneal grafting, contaminated neurosurgical instruments, human cadaveric growth hormone and human pituitary gonadotropine). The – few – iatrogenic cases cannot be clinically distinguished from the genetic and sporadic forms.
- **Variant CJD** ("human BSE") is a relatively new disease known since 1996 and showing a striking geographical distribution. From 153 registered cases worldwide, only 14 patients were outside UK (France, Ireland, Italy, Canada, USA) (http://www.doh.gov.uk/cjd/stats/feb04).

Transmissibility and neuropathology

All human prion diseases are progressive and fatal neurodegenerative disorders with transmissibility to a range of laboratory animal hosts and with broadly similar neuropathological features consisting of neuronal degeneration, reactive astrogliosis and extensive vacuoles subsuming in spongiform changes (Kretzschmar *et al.*, 1996). The most specific immunohistochemical feature is the PrP^{Sc} deposition. Intracerebral inoculation of minor concentration of PrP^{Sc} containing tissue material will induce a spongiform encephalopathy in various animal hosts. A horizontal transmissibility has been postulated only in cases of Kuru.

Transmissibility has been successfully achieved after inoculation of the following tissues from CJD patients: brain, eye, spinal cord, lung, CSF and lymphoreticular organs. Other organs proved to be non-infectious: peripheral nerves, whole blood and blood components, bone marrow, muscle, sputum, urine and milk (Kretzschmar *et al.*, 1996).

Despite the uniformity in certain aspects, the human prion diseases are associated with diverse clinicopathological phenotypes, mainly dependent upon two factors: (i) the specific confirmation of the Scrapie protein PrP^{Sc} and (ii) the genotype at codon 129 of the prion protein gene. In sCJD two isotypes of PrP^{Sc} are known, with differing electrophoretic patterns.

At codon 129 there is a polymorphism coding for valine (V) or methionine (M). In the normal population the distribution is 40% MM, 10% VV, and 50%MV. All variant CJD cases so far, and 80% of sCJD victims, were homozygous for MM. This indicates that MM homozygotes are at higher risk for CJD, while MV heterozygotes seem relatively protected.

The combination of the PrP^{Sc} isoform pattern and the codon 129 polymorphisms results in six different molecular phenotypes (Fig. 36.1), which correlate with clinical, neuropathological and diagnostic (EEG and CSF) findings, and which allow a new classification of the clinico-pathological diversity on the molecular basis (Parchi *et al.*, 1999).

Clinical diagnostic features

Sporadic CJD

Early symptomatology (Table 36.2., Brown *et al.*, 1994)
Early symptoms of sCJD are quite non-specific comprising various prodromi, including depressive alterations

Table 36.2. Clinical features in sCJD ($n = 232$ Pat.) (Brown *et al.*, 1994)

Features	early (%)	late (%)
Cognitive impairment	69	100
• Memory deficits	48	100
• Behavioral alteration	29	57
• Decline in cortical functions	16	73
Cerebellar disturbance	33	86
Visual defects (cortical blindness)	17	42
Dizziness	13	19
Headaches	11	18
Vegetative symptoms	3	7
Extrapyramidal signs	2	73
Myoclonus	5	90
Typical periodic EEG	0	60

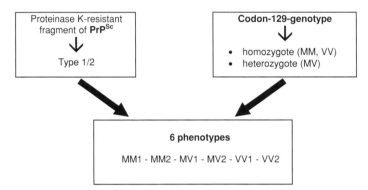

Fig. 36.1 Molecular classification of sCJD resulting from the combination of polymorphism at codon 129 of the prion protein gene and the electrophoretic pattern of PrP^{Sc}.

of personality, sleep and appetite disturbance, loss of body weight, anxiety and social regression. None of these symptoms is specific for CJD. In the majority of the patients, the presenting neurological symptoms consist of psychopathological alterations, including memory deficits and behavioral alterations subsumed in a rapidly progressive global encephalopathy. About one-third of the patients present with pure neurological symptoms – mostly cerebellar gait ataxia. The remaining patients present with mixed features consisting of cognitive decline and focal neurological deficits.

Patients may first see a neurologist when they complain of visual disturbances – mostly cortical blindness, gait ataxia or psychotic episodes. Psychotic disturbances consist of optic hallucinations with scenic pictures occurring primarily at night. After a mean time of 4 months, patients are admitted to a neurological department where CJD is

first considered. The combination of rapidly progressive cognitive impairment and myoclonus leads in most cases to the suspect diagnosis of CJD.

Clinical variants

There are two – but relatively rare – particularly known CJD variants (Heidenheim and Brownell–Oppenheimer). The Heidenheim variant is associated with neuropathological changes most predominantly occurring in the occipital cortex resulting in primarily visual symptoms (cortical blindness, optic hallucinations, agnosia). The Brownell–Oppenheimer variant presents with a pure cerebellar syndrome related to extensive neuropathological involvement of the cerebellum.

Late symptomatology, course of the disease

The subsequent clinical course is represented by a rapidly progressing disease surprising the clinician and dismaying the relatives. The evolving clinical picture always includes dementia, myoclonus, and ataxia. Depending on the CNS region involved, additional symptoms may occur such as primitive reflexes, paratonic rigidity, cortical blindness, oculomotor disturbances, and other pyramidal and extrapyramidal (e.g. parkinsonism, chorea, dystonia) signs. In the terminal state, patients often show an akinetic mutism (lack of spontaneous movement or verbal utterance, lack of voluntary reaction to external stimuli) accompanied by stimulus-sensitive myoclonus and less often vegetative disturbances and epileptic events. Eventually, CJD patients suffer from respiratory infections and thrombembolic complications, which mostly are the immediate cause of death. The mean disease duration is around 7 months. In less than 15% of cases patients show a relatively long duration of more than 12 months. Disease duration of more than 2 years is extremely rare (<5%).

Major pyramidal weakness, lower motor features, sensory disturbance and epileptic seizures are uncommon clinical features with a frequency of less than 20%.

Diagnostic procedures

While none of the above-mentioned single clinical features is specific for CJD, a typical pattern of symptoms has been identified to be helpful in the clinical diagnosis of CJD. Based on these clinical patterns and on typical EEG findings, diagnostic criteria were developed first by Masters *et al.*, 1979. These criteria were later extended by addition of the CSF parameter 14-3-3 (WHO, 1998; Zerr *et al.*, 2000b).

According to these criteria the diagnosis of CJD can be categorized as in Table 36.3:

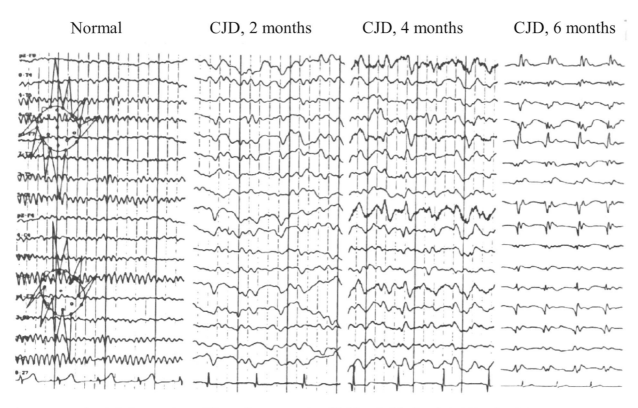

Fig. 36.2 Typical EEG-findings in sCJD at different disease stages (modified from Steinhoff *et al.*, *Arch Neurol*, 1996).

Table 36.3. Diagnostic criteria for sporadic CJD according to (Masters *et al.*, 1979; WHO, *Weekly Epidemiol Rec.* 1998; 47:361–365)

I	Neuropathological confirmation including immunohistochemical detection of PrP^{Sc}
II	Rapidly progressing dementia (duration < than 2 years)
III	• Myoclonus • Visual and cerebellar features • Pyramidal and extrapyramidal signs • Akinetic mutism
IV	Typical periodic EEG
V	Positive proteins 14-3-3 in CSF
Definite:	I
Probable:	II and 2 of III and IV or V
Possible:	II and 2 of III (EEG and CSF normal)

- **definite** (neuropathologically confirmed);
- **probable** (dementia with a course less than 2 years, two of four defined neurological symptoms and presence of typical EEG pattern and/or 14-3-3 proteins in CSF);
- **possible** (typical clinical features and absence of typical EEG and CSF findings).

Probable and possible CJD are clinical diagnoses based on the exclusion of alternative diseases and the presence of supportive findings in EEG or CSF. A probable classification according to these criteria is quite reliable with a certainty of 95%. However, since there is no pathognomonic clinical test, confirmation by autopsy or biopsy is still necessary to achieve diagnostic certainty.

EEG (Fig. 36.2)
The EEG shows characteristic discharges (periodic bi- and triphasic sharp wave complexes (PSWC)), originally described in the 1950s, at some stage of the disease (Levy *et al.*, 1986). A standardized evaluation showed that typical EEG findings in patients with CJD are found with a sensitivity of 67% and specificity of 86% if the following criteria were present (Steinhoff *et al.*, 1996):

Stereotypic sharp-wave complexes occurring at least 5 times with an interval of 500–2000 ms and duration of 100–600 ms. These data can be improved by standardized repeat recordings. In early stages of the illness these characteristic EEG findings may be absent so that repeat EEG recordings may be necessary. The characteristic EEG changes occur after a median of 12 weeks from disease onset, and they do not correlate with clinical severity of CJD. Their absence does not exclude the diagnosis of CJD, however, a persistently normal EEG despite clinical progression is incompatible with CJD. On the other hand, the characteristic EEG discharges may also be seen in conditions other than CJD, such as viral encephalitis, hepatic encephalopathy, epileptic seizures, Alzheimer disease, etc. (Zerr *et al.*, 2000a).

Magnetic resonance imaging (MRI)

MRI findings contribute to the diagnosis and differential diagnosis of CJD. Progressive global cerebral atrophy is a consistent finding, which is often accompanied by symmetric hyperintensities in the putamen and the caudate nuclei (up to 67%). These alterations are best demonstrated by using T_2-, proton-density, FLAIR and diffusion-weighted sequences. A major advantage of the diffusion-weighted sequence is its short investigation time allowing brain images in agitated patients with less artefacts. The MRI signal alterations correlate significantly with brain regions neuropathologically characterized by extensive astrocytosis and vacuoles. A significant decrease of brain volume related to cortical atrophy is seen after a disease course of 4 months. In early disease stages (<3 months) MRI may often reveal normal brain imaging despite rapidly progressing and devastating illness (Finkenstedt *et al.*, 1996; Gertz *et al.*, 1988; Röther *et al.*, 1992; Tartaro *et al.*, 1993; Urbach *et al.*, 1998; Samman *et al.*, 1999; Schröter *et al.*, 2000).

Cerebrospinal fluid (CSF) analysis

The routine CSF parameters reveal mostly normal results. Signs of inflammation such as oligoclonal IgG bands or lymphocytic pleocytosis occur in about 7% and are not a typical feature of CJD. However, a disturbed blood–CSF barrier function or elevated total protein level is more common (up to 25%) (Jacobi *et al.*, 2000). Elevated CSF concentration of specific brain derived proteins such as 14-3-3 (Harrington *et al.*, 1986; Hsich *et al.*, 1996; Zerr *et al.*, 1996 and 1998), neuron-specific enolase (Zerr *et al.*, 1995), tau-protein (Otto *et al.*, 1997) and S100b (Otto *et al.*, 1998) represent valuable supportive investigation and thereby contribute significantly to the diagnosis and differential diagnosis of CJD. The increase of their CSF concentrations is related to the rapid neuronal destruction and reactive astrogliosis inherent to the neuropathological disease process. Increased CSF levels of these markers may also be found in conditions other than CJD such as viral encephalitis, intracerebral bleeding, subarachnoid hemorrhage and several other neurodegenerative diseases. Although these surrogate markers are not causally related to the pathogenetic process, in the appropiate clinical context they show a remarkably high diagnostic sensitivity and speci-

Table 36.4. Diagnostic value of various paraclinical tests

Test	Sensitivity (%)	Specificity (%)
MRI ($n = 208$) (symmetrical SI in basal ganglia)	67	93
EEG ($n = 805$)(PSWC)	65	86
Cerebrospinal fluid markers		
• 14-3-3 proteins ($n = 1532$)(Western blot)	94	93
• Tau-Protein ($n = 290$)(>1400 pg/ml)	93	91
• NSE ($n = 1276$) (>35 ng/ml)	81	92
• S100b ($n = 135$)(>4.2 ng/ml)	84	91
• PrP^{Sc} ($n = 34$)	20	100

ficity (>90%) even in early disease stages of CJD (Table 36.4) (Zerr *et al.*, 2000a).

The diagnostic certainty of suspect CJD cases can be improved significantly if the CSF 14-3-3 is included as a diagnostic test. According to the extended diagnostic criteria (WHO, 1998; Zerr *et al.*, 2000b) a probable CJD can be established based on typical clinical features and a positive CSF 14-3-3 despite absence of typical EEG changes. A test to detect the abnormal prion protein (PrP^{Sc}) would be a valuable specific diagnostic tool, which could allow confirmation of CJD without neuropathological analysis of brain tissue. There are new and ultrasensitive methods (fluorescence correlated spectroscopy, capillary electrophoresis, plasminogen precipitation, prion protein amplification) in experimental or developmental stages aiming to detect very low concentrations of PrP^{Sc} in bodily fluids including CSF and urine (Bieschke *et al.*, 2000; Schmerr *et al.*, 1999; Maissen *et al.*, 2001; Saborio *et al.*, 2001; Shaked *et al.*, 2001). So far, their sensitivity is still too low (20%) to reach sufficient clinical significance (Zerr *et al.*, 2002).

Detection of PrP^{Sc} in extracerebral compartment has been possible in tonsils of patients with vCJD but not in those with sCJD (Brown *et al.*, 2001).

Genetic CJD (gCJD)

About 15–10% of the CJD patients have a positive family history. The autosomal-dominant pattern of inheritance dictates that 50% of the children of the victim will suffer from the disease. More than 20 mutations of the prion protein gene are responsible for the phenotype. The Gerstmann–Sträussler–Scheinker (GSS) syndrome and fatal familial insomnia are also hereditary forms of prion diseases. An HD-like disease in a single pedigree was mapped to chromosome 20p12 (Moore *et al.*, 2001), the site of the prion protein PrP gene, and found to segregate with a 192 nucleotide insertion in the PrP gene, encoding eight octapeptide repeats. This disease was called HD-like 1 (HDL1). In the future, it is likely that these diseases will be reclassified according to their genotype. The transmissibility of genetic CJD to non-human primates was first reported in 1973.

The clinical presentation depends on the underlying mutation and other factors such as the polymorphism in codon 129. Genetic CJD tends to occur in clusters. Most known geographical concentrations involving the E200K mutation are (i) a community of Libyan Jews in Israel with annual incidence of 50 per million and (ii) two foci in Slovakia with annual incidences ranging between 4 and 17 per million.

The spectrum of symptoms of gCJD is mostly similar to that of sCJD. However, a sensory–motor polyneuropathy is an additional clinical feature. Since apparently sCJD cases occasionally turn out to have an underlying mutation, prion protein gene sequencing is the only method to exclude genetic cause of CJD.

GSS

GSS was first described around 1930 in a large Austrian family with several affected generations (Gerstmann, 1928; Gerstmann & Sträussler, 1936). However, its classification as prion disease was achieved much later (Masters *et al.*, 1981). Originally, GSS was clinically described as predominantly progressive cerebellar ataxia. Meanwhile it has been associated with a more diverse clinical spectrum including dementia, spastic paraparesis and extrapyramidal symptoms. Neuropathological findings include, in addition to spongiform changes that occur most extensively in patients with the mutation P102L, large multicentric amyloid plaques containing PrP^{Sc}. Furthermore, neurofibrillary tangles (mainly in those with the mutations Y145*, F198S, and Q217R) and amyloid angiopathy (mutation Y145*) have been described to be part of the neuropathologic phenotype. The considerable phenotypic heterogeneity varying from typical CJD to classic GSS even within a pedigree can be partly explained by the genetic heterogeneity comprising several prion protein gene mutations. The more typical GSS cases may have their disease onset in the early middle age, and their mean illness duration is around 5–6 years. Diagnostic tools such as MRI brain imaging and EEG are not helpful in the diagnosis of GSS revealing normal or non-specific findings.

Fatal familial insomnia (FFI)

FFI was first described in 1986 afflicting five members of a large Italian family. The initial pathological classification was "selective thalamic degeneration" (Lugaresi *et al.*, 1986). A few years later it was reported to be a genetically determined prion disease with a mutation at codon 178 (Medori *et al.*, 1992). Soon after it was confirmed to be transmissible (Tateishi *et al.*, 1995). Since then, a number of additional pedigrees manifesting with FFI have been described; nevertheless this remains a very rare disorder.

According to the name of the disease, the main clinical feature of FFI is a profound disruption of the sleep–wake cycle. Additional symptoms are dysautonomia (most prominent sympathetic overactivity), diverse endocrine disturbances and cognitive impairment (mnestic difficulties).

The autonomic dysfunction occurs early in the disease course and may be the presenting symptom. The sleep disturbance may initially be minor, but progresses over weeks to months accompanied with vivid dreams and somnolence. Prompt arousal with light stimuli is characteristic. A variety of hallucinations occur in addition to the parasomnias contributing to the bizarre nocturnal behaviors. A range of motor abnormalities (cerebellar and pyramidal dysfunction, spontaneous and reflex myoclonus) evolve in variable combinations.

Eventually, patients become confused and disoriented, progressing to stupor and coma. The routine EEG in the early stages is usually normal, while in progressed stages it becomes non-specifically altered with slower frequencies and generalised less responsive alpha activity. PSWC are not typically associated with FFI. Routine laboratory parameters including CSF analysis are typically normal. Circadian oscillations of various hormones including growth hormone, prolactin, gonadotrophins and thyrotrophin-releasing hormone are disturbed. Polysomnographic recordings reveal reduced total sleep time and absence of REM periods. Pharmacologic agents such as benzodiazepines and barbiturates seem unable to induce sleep-like EEG activity.

vCJD

Epidemiology

The current public interest in CJD is explained by the accumulating evidence on the causal relationship between BSE and vCJD. The most remarkable epidemiological feature of vCJD is its geographical distribution. By December 2003, 153 cases had been confirmed worldwide, from which 139 were registered in UK with a decreasing north–south

Table 36.5. Differences between sCJD and vCJD

	vCJD	sCJD
Early symptoms	Sensory disturbance, psychiatric symptoms	Dementia, focal neurological signs
Disease duration (months)	14	7
Age at death (years)	30	67
EEG (PSWC)	0%	67%
MRI (symmetrical SI)	"Pulvinar sign"	Nucl. Caudatus, Putamen
14-3-3 (positive)	45%	94%
Neuropathology (amyloid plaques)	Prominent and diffuse	Sparse (10%)
Extracerebral distribution of PrP^{Sc}	Tonsil, appendix, spleen, lymph node	Negative
PrP^{Sc}-Pattern in Western blot	Type 4 (as in BSE)	Type 1 and 2

gradient (http://www.doh.gov.uk/cjd/stats/feb04). In contrast to sCJD, vCJD patients are younger with an age range of 14–53 years, and the median age of onset is 28 years. Females and males are affected equally (Will *et al.*, 2000).

Early symptomatology (dysesthesias, psychiatric symptomatology) (Table 36.5.)

In contrast to sCJD presenting with rapidly progressive cognitive impairment, vCJD presents with relatively slowly progressive clinical features comprising sensory and psychiatric symptoms. The most common symptoms are psychiatric/behavioral disturbances (depressive states requiring antidepressant treatment, anxiety, agitation, delusions and hallucinations), and unpleasant sensory features including pain, mostly worse at night. Neurological abnormalities are not usually evident at disease onset. Affected individuals are mostly referred to a psychiatrist by their family doctors. While nerve conduction is usually normal, somato-sensory evoked potentials may show minor abnormalities suggesting central affection of the sensory pathways and thalamic origin of the pain.

Course of the disease – late stages

Subsequent symptoms include neurological features which develop more than 6 months after onset of first symptoms. Most commonly, gait ataxia is a prominent feature, followed by involuntary movements (myoclonus,

chorea, dystonia), dementia and upgaze paresis. The terminal state of vCJD with predominant dementia, multiple neurological deficits and akinetic mutism resembles that seen in sCJD. The median disease duration in vCJD is twice as long as in sCJD with a median of 14 months (range 6–38 months).

Relation to BSE

There is now increasing evidence from experimental studies that BSE and vCJD have a causal link. It seems most likely that vCJD is due to infection of humans with the BSE agent via contaminated food. The greatest incidence of BSE in UK is a relevant epidemiological clue, indicating that the agent passed from cattle to man. However, an absolute proof that the zoonotic link was via food has not been provided to date. The most reasonable hypothesis is that the agent was transmitted via mechanically recovered meat containing spinal cord material from infected cattle (Brown *et al.*, 2001).

Diagnostic procedures (MRI, tonsil biopsy, neuropathology)

The cerebral MRI scan appears to be very useful in vCJD with bilateral signal intensities in the dorsal thalamus ("pulvinar sign") in the majority of cases (Zeidler *et al.*, 2000). Unlike the diagnostic criteria for sCJD, the diagnostic criteria for vCJD include MRI features.

Cerebral biopsy shows, in addition to the spongiform changes, extensive PrP^{Sc} deposition with the so-called "florid-plaque" diffusely occurring throughout the cerebrum and cerebellum. Based on the extracerebral distribution of PrP^{Sc} mainly in lymphoreticular organs, tonsillar biopsy has been proposed potentially useful in the ante mortem diagnosis of vCJD (Ghani *et al.*, 2000; Brown *et al.*, 2001).

CSF, EEG

CSF and EEG measures are less helpful in the diagnosis of vCJD as compared to sCJD. CSF 14-3-3 is less sensitive being positive in only half of the affected individuals. EEG recordings do not show the typical PSWC typical of sCJD.

Kuru

Kuru is the only human prion disease with a naturally occurring horizontal transmission from man-to-man. It was first identified in the mid-1950s in Papua New Guinea and was recognized to be endemic among the Fore tribe resident in the Eastern Highlands of New Guinea (Zigas & Gajdusek, 1957; Hadlow, 1959).

The majority of the Kuru victims were adult females and children of either sex. Eventually, epidemiological and scientific data suggested that Kuru had been transmitted by cannibalistic rituals observed in funeral ceremonies. It is hypothesized that a cannibalistic passage of a sporadic CJD case most likely occurred, although the ultimate cause remains unclear (Gajdusek *et al.*, 1966).

Epidemiological data from pregnant women delivering healthy infants remaining asymptomatic do not provide evidence for vertical transmission. At the end of the 1960s, after ritual cannibalism was not practiced any longer, Kuru disappeared almost completely.

The clinical picture was characterized by the insidious onset of a predominant progressive cerebellar dysfunction. Symptoms of pyramidal or extrapyramidal functions were not prominent, and cognitive functions remained relatively spared or were impaired in terminal disease stages. Within a few months, affected patients were not able to sit unsupported and became bedridden, totally dependent for feeding and personal care. Patients died from complications such as bronchopneumonia, infected pressure sores or undernutrition. The total disease duration was reported to be around 6–9 months ranging from 4–24 months, a little longer than sCJD.

There are no typical changes of routine biochemical laboratory parameters or of CSF analysis as for other prion diseases. For unequivocal confirmation of Kuru, a neuropathological examination is required. Neuropathological findings are dominated by mainly cerebellar spongiform changes containing so called "Kuru-plaques," which are found in Kuru cases more frequently than in CJD types. This may be explained by the relatively higher frequency of valin at codon 129 of the prion protein gene. Kuru plaques are detectable by HE and PAS staining as homogenous and eosinophilic PrP-depositions. They are mainly found in the granular cell layer of the cerebellum. In sCJD cases Kuru plaques occur exclusively in certain molecular phenotypes: MV-heterozygotes and PrP^{Sc}-type 2 (Kretzschmar, 1996).

Differential diagnosis (Table 36.6)

The differential diagnosis of sCJD is of clinical importance. Depending on the disease stage and on the initially prominent symptom a number of different differential diagnoses with psychiatric and neurological origin have to be considered.

Table 36.6. Spectrum of important differential diagnoses in cases of suspect sCJD

Degenerative brain disorders	**Alzheimer dementia**
	Parkinson syndromes with dementia
	Frontotemporal dementia
	Chorea Huntington
	Multisystem atrophy
	Cerebellar atrophy
Inflammatory encephalopathies	**Encephalitis (viral, autoimmune)**
	AIDS-encephalopathy
	multiple sclerosis
	progressive mutifocal leukencephalopathy
Metabolic encephalopathies	Hepatopathic, uremic, Korsakow syndrome, Wernicke-encephalopathy
Toxic encephalopathy	Intoxication with metals and drugs
Paraneoplastic encephalopathies	Limbic encephalomyelitis paraneoplastic cerebellar atrophy

The rapidly progressive Alzheimer disease, Lewy body dementia and frontotemporal dementia represent the most frequent differential diagnosis in clinically advanced cases. In patients with predominant cerebellar dysfunction or extrapyramidal symptoms other neurodegenerative disorders such as multiple system atrophy, PSP or CBD have to be considered (Lopez *et al.*, 1999; Verghese *et al.*, 1999; Zerr *et al.*, 2000b and 2002). In younger patients with suspect CJD chronic encephalitis or Hashimoto encephalopathy as a potentially treatable cause may be important differential diagnoses (Seipelt *et al.*, 1999).

Therapeutic aspects

Symptomatic treatment

Current therapy is confined to symptomatic treatment. Myoclonus may respond to benzodiazepines. Agitation and psychotic features can be treated wth neuroleptic drugs, whereby drug-induced rigidity may appear and cause difficulties in interpretation of disease-related rigidity.

Disease-specific treatment, anti-prion approach

There are a number of promising anti-prion agents that are effective in animal models and are shown in cell culture experiments to influence aggregation of PrP^{Sc}. In cell culture even "clearance" of PrP^{Sc} has been shown to be possible. However none of these substances has shown convincing therapeutic results in clinical trials in CJD victims.

A partial list of potential anti-prion compounds includes:

acridine and phenothiazine derivatives (Korth *et al.*, 2001),

amphotericin B (Pocchiari *et al.*, 1987),

anti-Prion antibodies (Peretz *et al.*, 2001; Enari *et al.*, 2001),

branched polyamines (Supattapone *et al.*, 2001),

Congo red (Caughey & Race, 1992)

quinacrin (Collins *et al.*, 2002).

synthetic beta-sheet breaker peptides (Soto *et al.*, 2000).

REFERENCES

Andrews, N. J., Farrington, C. P., Ward, H. J. T., *et al.* (2003). Deaths from variant Creutzfeldt–Jakob disease in the UK. *Lancet*, **361**, 751–2.

Bieschke, J., Giese, A., Schulz-Schaeffer, W. *et al.* (2000). Ultrasensitive detection of pathological prion protein aggregates by dual – color scanning for intensely fluorescent targets. *Proc. Natl Acad. Sci., USA*, **97**, 5468–73.

Brown, P., Gibbs, C. J., Rodgers-Johnson, P. *et al.* (1994). Human spongiform encephalopathy: the National Institutes of Health series of 300 cases of experimentally transmitted disease. *Ann. Neurol.*, **35**, 513–29.

Brown, P., Will, R. G., Bradley, R., Asher, D. M. & Detwiler, L. (2001). Bovine spongiform encephalopathy and variant Creutzfeldt–Jakob disease: background, evolution, and current concerns. *Emerg. Infect. Dis.* **7**, 6–16.

Caughey, B. & Race, R. E. (1992). Potent inhibition of scrapie-associated PrP accumulation by congo red. *J. Neurochem.*, **59**, 768–71.

Collins, P. S., Lawson, V. A. & Masters, P. C. (2004). Transmissible spongiform encephalopathies. *Lancet*, **363**, 51–61.

Collins, S. J., Lewis, V., Brazier, M. *et al.* (2002). Quinacrine does not prolong survival in a murine Creutzfeldt–Jakob disease model. *Ann. Neurol.*, **52**, 503–6.

Creutzfeld, H. G. (1920). Über eine eigenartige herdförmige Erkrankung des Zentralnervensystems. *Z. Neurol. Psychiatr.*, **57**, 1–18.

Enari, M., Flechsig, E. & Weissmann, C. (2001). Scrapie prion protein accumulation by scrapie-infected neuroblastoma cells abro-gated by exposure to a prion protein antibody. *Proc. Natl Acad. Sci., USA*, **98**, 9295–9.

Finkenstedt, M., Szurdra, A., Zerr, I. *et al.* (1996). MR imaging of Creutzfeldt–Jakob disease. *Radiology*, **199**, 793–8.

Gajdusek, D. C., Gibbs, C. J. & Alpers, M. (1966). Experimental transmission of a kuru-like syndrome to chimpanzees. *Nature*, **209**, 794–6.

Gerstmann, J. (1928). Über ein noch nicht beschriebenes Reflexphänomen beieiner Erkrankung des zerebellären Systems. *Wien Med. Wochenschr.*, **78**, 906–8.

Gerstmann, J. & Sträussler, E. (1936). Über eine eigenartige hereditär-familiäre Erkrankung des Zentralnervensystems. Zugleich ein Beitrag zur Frage des vorzeitigen lokalen Alterns. *Z. Neurol.*, **154**, 736–62.

Gertz, H. J., Henkes, H. & Cervos, N. J. (1988). Creutzfeldt–Jakob disease: correlation of MRI and neuropathologic findings. *Neurology*, **38**, 1481–2.

Ghani, A. C., Donnelly, C. A., Ferguson, N. M. *et al.* (2000). Assessment of the prevalence of vCJD through testing tonsils and appendices for abnormal prion protein. *Proc. R. Soc. Lond. B. Biol. Sci.*, **267**, 23–9.

Hadlow, W. J. (1959). Scrapie and Kuru. *Lancet*, **2**, 289–90.

Harries-Jones, R., Knight, R., Will, R. G. *et al.* (1988). Creutzfeldt–Jakob disease in England and Wales, 1980–1984: a case-control study of potential risk factors. *J. Neurol. Neurosurg. Psychiatry*, **51**, 1113–19.

Harrington, M. G., Merril, C. R., Asher, D. M. *et al.* (1986). Abnormal proteins in the cerebrospinal fluid of patients with Creutzfeldt–Jakob disease. *N. Engl. J. Med.*, **315**, 279–83.

Hsich, G., Kenney, K., Gibbs, C. J. *et al.* (1996). The 14-3-3 brain protein in cerebrospinal fluid as a marker for transmissible spongiform encephalopathies. *N. Engl. J. Med.*, **335**, 924–30.

Jakob, A. (1921). Über eine eigenartige Erkrankung des Zentralnervensystems mit bemerkenswertem anatomischen Befund (Spastische Pseudosklerose – Encephalopathie mit disseminierten Degenerationsherden). *Z. Ges. Neurol. Psychiat.*, **64**, 147–228.

Jacobi, C., Zerr, I., Arlt, S. *et al.* (2000). Cerebrospinal fluid pattern in patients with definite Creutzfeldt–Jakob disease. *J. Neurol.*, **247**, III/14.

Korth, C., May, B. C., Cohen, F. E. *et al.* (2001). Acridine and phenothiazine derivatives as pharmacotherapeutics for prion disease. *Proc. Natl Acad. Sci., USA*, **98**, 9836–41.

Kretzschmar, H. A., Ironside, J. W., DeArmond, S. J. *et al.* (1996). Diagnostic criteria for sporadic Creutzfeldt–Jakob disease. *Arch. Neurol.*, **53**, 913–20.

Levy, S. R., Chiappa, K. H., Burke, C. J. *et al.* (1986). Early evolution and incidence of electroencephalographic abnormalities in Creutzfeldt–Jakob disease. *J. Clin. Neurophysiol.*, **3**, 1–21.

Lopez, O. L., Litvan, I., Catt, K. E. *et al.* (1999). Accuracy of four clinical diagnostic criteria for the diagnosis of neurodegenerative dementias. *Neurology*, **53**, 1292–9.

Lugaresi, E., Medori, R., Montagna, P. *et al.* (1986). Fatal familial insomnia and dysautonomia with selective degeneration of thalamic nuclei. *N. Engl. J. Med.*, **315**, 997–1003.

Maissen, M., Roeckl, C., Glatzel, M. *et al.* (2001). Plasminogen binds to disease-associated prion protein of multiple species. *Lancet*, **357**, 2026–8.

Masters, C. L., Harris, J. O., Gajdusek, D. C., Gibbs, C. J., Bernoulli, C. & Asher, D. M. (1979). Creutzfeldt–Jakob disease: patterns of worldwide occurrence and the significance of familial and sporadic clustering. *Ann. Neurol.*, **5**, 177–88.

Masters, C. L., Gajdusek, D. C. & Gibbs, C. J. (1981). Creutzfeldt–Jakob disease virus isolations from the Gerstmann–Sträussler syndrome with an analysis of the forms of amyloid plaque deposition in the virus-induced spongiform change. *Brain*, **104**, 559–88.

Medori, R., Tritschler, H. J., LeBlanc, A. *et al.* (1992). Fatal familial insomnia, a prion disease with a mutation at codon 178 of the prion protein gene. *N. Engl. J. Med.*, **326**, 444–9.

Mollenhauer, B., Zerr, I., Ruge, D. *et al.* (2002). Epidemiologie und klinische Symptomatik der Creutzfeldt–Jakob–Krankheit. [Epidemiology and clinical symptomatology of Creutzfeldt–Jakob disease]. *Dtsch. Med. Wochenschr.*, **127**, 312–17.

Moore, R. C., Xiang, F., Monaghan, J. *et al.* (2001). Huntington disease phenocopy is a familial prion disease. *Am. J. Hum. Gen.*, **69**, 1385–8.

Otto, M., Wiltfang, J., Tumani, H. *et al.* (1997). Elevated levels of tau-protein in cerebrospinal fluid of patients with Creutzfeldt–Jakob disease. *Neurosci. Lett.*, **225**, 210–12.

Otto, M., Wiltfang, J., Schütz, E. *et al.* (1998). Diagnosis of Creutzfeldt–Jakob disease by measurement of S100 protein in serum: prospective case-control study. *Br. Med. J.* **316**, 577–82.

Parchi, P., Giese, A., Capellari, S. *et al.* (1999). Classification of sporadic Creutzfeldt–Jakob disease based on molecular and phenotypic analysis of 300 subjects. *Ann. Neurol.*, **46**, 224–33.

Peretz, D., Williamson, R. A., Kaneko, K. *et al.* (2001). Antibodies inhibit prion propagation and clear cell cultures of prion infectivity. *Nature*, **412**, 739–43.

Pocchiari, M., Schmittinger, S. & Masullo, C. (1987). Amphotericin B delays the incubation period of scrapie in intracerebrally inoculated hamsters. *J. Gen. Virol.*, **68**, 219–23.

Poser, S., Mollenhauer, B., Krauß, A. *et al.* (1999). How to improve the clinical diagnosis of Creutzfeldt–Jakob disease. *Brain*, **122**, 2345–51.

Röther, J., Schwartz, A., Harle, M. *et al.* (1992). Magnetic resonance imaging follow-up in Creutzfeldt–Jakob disease. *J. Neurol.*, **239**, 404–6.

Saborio, G. P., Permanne, B. & Soto, C. (2001). Sensitive detection of pathological prion protein by cyclic amplification of protein misfolding. *Nature*, **411**, 810–13.

Samman, I., Schulz-Schaeffer, W. J., Wohrle, J. C. *et al.* (1999). Clinical range and MRI in Creutzfeldt–Jakob disease with heterozygosity at codon 129 and prion protein type 2. *J. Neurol. Neurosurg. Psychiatry*, **67**, 678–81.

Schmerr, M. J., Jenny, A. L., Bulgin, M. S. *et al.* (1999). Use of capillary electrophoresis and fluorescent labeled peptides to detect abnormal prion protein in the blood of animals that are infected with a transmissible spongiform encephalopathy. *J. Chromatogr. A.*, **853**, 207–14.

Schröter, A., Zerr, I., Henkel, K. *et al.* (2000). Magnetic resonance imaging (MRI) in the clinical diagnosis of Creutzfeldt–Jakob disease. *Arch. Neurol.*, **57**, 1751–7.

Seipelt, M., Zerr, I., Nau, R. *et al.* (1999). Hashimoto encephalitis as a differential diagnosis of Creutzfeldt–Jakob disease. *J. Neurol. Neurosurg. Psychiatry*, **66**, 172–6.

Shaked, G. M., Shaked, Y. & Kariv-Inbal, Z. (2001). A protease-resistant prion protein isoform is present in urine of animals and humans affected with prion diseases. *J. Biol. Chem.*, **276**, 31479–82.

Soto, C., Kascsak, R. J., Saborio, G. P. *et al.* (2000). Reversion of prion protein conformational changes by synthetic beta-sheet breaker peptides. *Lancet*, **355**, 192–7.

Steinhoff, B. J., Räcker, S., Herrendorf, G. *et al.* (1996). Accuracy and reliability of periodic sharp wave complexes in Creutzfeldt–Jakob disease. *Arch. Neurol.*, **53**, 162–6.

Supattapone, S., Wille, H., Uyechi, L. *et al.* (2001). Branched polyamines cure prion-infected neuroblastoma cells. *J. Virol.*, **75**, 3453–61.

Tartaro, A., Fulgente, T., Delli-Pizzi, C. *et al.* (1993). MRI alterations as an early finding in Creutzfeld–Jakob disease. *Eur. J. Radiol.*, **17**, 155–8.

Tateishi, J., Brown, P., Kitamoto, T. *et al.* (1995). First experimental transmission of fatal familial insomnia. *Nature*, **376**, 434–5.

Urbach, H., Klisch, J. & Wolf, H. K. (1998). MRI in sporadic Creutzfeldt–Jakob disease: correlation with clinical and neuropathological data. *Neuroradiology*, **40**, 65–70.

Verghese, J., Crystal, H. A. & Dickson, D. W. (1999). Validity of clinical criteria for the diagnosis of dementia with Lewy bodies. *Neurology*, **53**, 1974–82.

WHO (1998). Human transmissible spongiform encephalopathies. *Weekly Epidemiol. Rec.*, **47**, 361–5.

Will, R. G., Zeidler, M., Stewart, G. E. *et al.* (2000). Diagnosis of new variant Creutzfeldt–Jakob disease. *Ann. Neurol.*, **47**, 575–82.

Zeidler, M., Sellar, R. J., Collie, D. A. *et al.* (2000). The pulvinar sign on magnetic resonance imaging in variant Creutzfeldt–Jakob disease. *Lancet*, **355**, 1412–18.

Zerr, I., Bodemer, M., Räcker, S. *et al.* (1995). Cerebrospinal fluid concentration of neuron-specific enolase in diagnosis of Creutzfeldt–Jakob disease. *Lancet*, **345**, 1609–10.

Zerr, I., Bodemer, M., Otto, M. *et al.* (1996). Diagnosis of Creutzfeldt–Jakob disease by two-dimensional gel electophoresis of cerebrospinal fluid. *Lancet*, **348**, 846–9.

Zerr, I., Bodemer, M., Gefeller, O. *et al.* (1998). Detection of 14-3-3 protein in cerebrospinal fluid supports the diagnosis of Creutzfeldt–Jakob disease. *Ann. Neurol.*, **43**, 32–40.

Zerr, I., Pocchiari, M., Collins, S. *et al.* (2000a). Analysis of EEG and CSF 14-3-3 proteins as aids to the diagnosis of Creutzfeldt–Jakob disease. *Neurology*, **55**, 811–15.

Zerr, I., Schulz-Schaeffer, W. J., Giese, A. *et al.* (2000b). Current clinical diagnosis in CJD; identification of uncommon variants. *Ann. Neurol.*, **48**, 323–9.

Zerr, I., Mollenhauer, B., Werner, C. *et al.* (2002). Früh- und Differenzialdiagnose der Creutzfeldt–Jakob Krankheit1 [Early and differential diagnosis of Creutzfeldt–Jakob disease]. *Dtsch. Med. Wochenschr.*, **127**, 323–7.

Zigas, W. & Gajdusek, D. C. (1957). Kuru: clinical study of a new syndrome resembling paralysis agitans in natives of the Eastern Highlands of Australian New Guinea. *Med. J. Austr.*, **2**, 745–54.

II The pathogenesis and mechanisms of prion diseases

Adriano Aguzzi

Institute of Neuropathology, University of Zürich, Switzerland

Introduction

For more than two decades it has been contended that prion infection does not elicit immune responses: transmissible spongiform encephalopathies do not go along with conspicuous inflammatory infiltrates, and antibodies to the prion protein are typically undetectable. Why is it, then, that prions accumulate in lymphoid organs, and that various states of immune deficiency prevent peripheral prion infection? This review revisits the current evidence of the involvement of the immune system in prion diseases, while attempting to trace the elaborate mechanisms by which peripherally administered prions invade the brain and ultimately provoke damage. The investigation of these questions leads to unexpected detours, including the neurophysiology of lymphoid organs, and even the function of a prion protein homologue in male fertility.

Prion biology: some basic facts

Prion diseases are inevitably fatal neurodegenerative conditions that affect humans and a wide variety of animals (Aguzzi et al., 2001c). Although prion diseases may present with certain morphological and pathophysiological parallels to other progressive encephalopathies, such as Alzheimer's and Parkinson's disease (Aguzzi & Raeber, 1998), they are unique in that they are transmissible. Homogenization of brain tissue from affected individuals and intracerebral inoculation into another individual of the same species will typically reproduce the disease. This important fact was recognized more than half a century ago in the case of scrapie (Cuille & Chelle, 1939), a prototypic prion disease that affects sheep and goats.

In the 1960s and 1970s, the work of Gajdusek on Kuru and Creutzfeldt–Jakob disease (Gajdusek et al., 1966; Gibbs et al., 1968), partly inspired by a suggestion of Hadlow (Hadlow, 1959) on the similarity of scrapie and Kuru, established that these diseases are also transmissible to primates, to mice, and in some unfortunate iatrogenic instances, also to other humans (Brown P. et al., 2000). Therefore, prion diseases are also called transmissible spongiform encephalopathies (TSEs), a term that emphasizes their infectious character.

While only less than 1% of all reported cases of Creutzfeldt-Jakob disease (CJD) can be traced to a defined infectious source, the identification of bovine spongiform encephalopathy (BSE) (Wells et al., 1987) and its subsequent epizootic spread has highlighted prion-contaminated meat-and-bone meal as a tremendously efficient vector for bovine prion diseases (Weissmann & Aguzzi, 1997), which does not completely lose its infectious potential even after extensive autoclaving (Taylor, 2000). BSE is most likely transmissible to humans, too, and strong circumstantial evidence (Aguzzi, 1996; Aguzzi & Weissmann, 1996b; Collinge et al., 1996; Bruce et al., 1997; Hill et al., 1997a) suggests that BSE is the cause of variant Creutzfeldt–Jakob disease (vCJD) which has claimed more than 130 lives in the United Kingdom (Will R. G. et al., 1996; http://www.doh.gov.uk/cjd/stats/aug02.htm, 2002) and, to a much smaller extent, in some other countries (Chazot et al., 1996). When transmitted to primates, BSE produces a pathology strikingly similar to that of vCJD (Aguzzi & Weissmann, 1996b; Lasmezas et al., 1996b). While there is no direct indication yet that variant Creutzfeldt–Jakob disease has been transmitted from one human to another, this is certainly a very worrying scenario (Aguzzi, 2000). Not only surgical instruments may represent potential vectors of transmission, but possibly also transfusions. Significantly, sheep infected with BSE can efficiently transmit the agent to other sheep via blood transfusion (Houston et al., 2000; Hunter et al., 2002).

Several aspects of CJD epidemiology continue to be enigmatic. For example, CJD incidence in Switzerland has risen two-fold in 2001, and appears to be increasing even further in the year 2002 (Glatzel *et al.*, 2002). A screen for recognized or hypothetical risk factors for CJD has, to date, not exposed any causal factors. Several scenarios may account for the increase in incidence, including improved reporting, iatrogenic transmission, and transmission of a prion zoonosis.

Prion diseases typically exhibit a very long latency period between the time of infection and the clinical manifestation: this is the reason why these diseases were originally thought to be caused by "slow viruses". From the viewpoint of interventional approaches, this peculiarity may be exploitable, since it opens a possible window of intervention after infection has occurred, but before brain damage is being initiated. Prions spend much of this latency time executing neuroinvasion, which is the process of reaching the central nervous system after entering the body from peripheral sites (Aguzzi, 1997a; Nicotera, 2001). During this process, little or no damage occurs to brain, and one might hope that its interruption may prevent neurodegeneration.

Stanley Prusiner's protein-only hypothesis

The most widely accepted hypothesis on the nature of the infectious agent causing TSEs (which was termed prion by Stanley B. Prusiner) (Prusiner, 1982) predicates that it consists essentially of PrP^{Sc}, an abnormally folded, protease-resistant, beta-sheet rich isoform of a normal cellular protein termed PrP^{C}. According to this fascinating theory, the prion does not contain any informational nucleic acids, and its infectivity propagates simply by recruitment and "auto-catalytic" conformational conversion of cellular prion protein into disease-associated PrP^{Sc} (Aguzzi & Weissmann, 1997).

A large body of experimental and epidemiological evidence is compatible with the protein-only hypothesis, and very stringently designed experiments have failed to disprove it. It would go well beyond the scope of this article to review all efforts that have been undertaken to this effect. Perhaps most impressively, knockout mice carrying a homozygous deletion of the *Prnp* gene that encodes PrP^{C}, fail to develop disease upon inoculation with infectious brain homogenate (Büeler *et al.*, 1993), nor does their brain carry prion infectivity (Sailer *et al.*, 1994). Reintroduction of *Prnp* by transgenesis – even in a shortened, redacted form – restores infectibility and prion replication in *Prnp*$^{\%}$ mice (Fischer *et al.*, 1996; Shmerling *et al.*, 1998; Supattapone *et al.*, 1999; Flechsig *et al.*, 2000). In addition, all familial

cases of human TSEs are characterized by *Prnp* mutations (Aguzzi & Weissmann, 1996a; Prusiner *et al.*, 1998).

Informational nucleic acids of >50 nucleotides in length do not participate in prion infectivity (Kellings *et al.*, 1993; Riesner *et al.*, 1993), but shorter non-coding oligonucleotides have not been formally excluded – a fact that may have some relevance in view of the surprising discoveries related to RNA-mediated gene silencing. *Prnp* exhibits a long reading frame on its non-coding strand (Moser *et al.*, 1993) which is conserved among mammals (Aguzzi, 1997b; Rother *et al.*, 1997), suggesting that it may be transcribed – maybe only in specific pathological situations. One might wonder, therefore, whether this peculiar property of *Prnp* might result in the production of double-stranded transcripts with silencing properties. However, *bona fide* antisense transcription of the *Prnp* locus has never been demonstrated in vivo, nor in cultured cells.

Some major open questions in prion biology

In recent years, prion research has progressed at a faster pace than many of us would have thought possible. As a consequence, many enigmas surrounding prion diseases have now been solved. However, the areas that are still obscure do not relate only to the details: some of these concern the core of the prion concept (Chesebro, 1998). In my opinion, there are four large groups of questions regarding the basic science of prion replication and of development of transmissible spongiform encephalopathies diseases that deserve to be addressed with a vigorous research effort.

- Which are the molecular mechanisms of prion replication? How does the disease-associated prion protein, PrP^{Sc}, achieve the conversion of its cellular sibling, PrP^{C}, into a likeness of itself? Which other proteins assist this process? Can we inhibit this process? If so, how?
- What is the essence of prion strains, which are operationally defined as variants of the infectious agent capable of retaining stable phenotypic traits upon serial passage in syngeneic hosts? The existence of strains is very well known in virology, but it was not predicted to exist in the case of an agent that propagates epigenetically.
- How do prions reach the brain after having entered the body? Which molecules and which cell types are involved in this process of neuroinvasion? Which inhibitory strategies are likely to succeed?
- The mechanisms of neurodegeneration in spongiform encephalopathies is not understood. Which are the pathogenetic cascades that are activated upon accumulation of disease-associated prion protein, and ultimately lead to brain damage?

• What is the physiological function of the highly conserved, normal prion protein, PrP^C? The *Prnp* gene encoding PrP^C was identified in 1985 (Oesch *et al.*, 1985; Basler *et al.*, 1986), *Prnp* knockout mice were described in 1992 (Büeler *et al.*, 1992), and some PrP^C-interacting proteins have been identified (Oesch *et al.*, 1990; Rieger *et al.*, 1997; Yehiely *et al.*, 2002; Zanata *et al.*, 2002). Yet the function of PrP^C remains unknown.

The present review article will discuss some of the progress recently achieved in some of the areas delineated above, with special reference to the topics that have directly interested my laboratory.

Brain damage in prion diseases

An interesting question regards the molecular mechanism underlying neuropathological changes, in particular cell death, resulting from prion disease. Depletion of PrP^C is an unlikely cause, in view of the finding that abrogation of PrP does not cause scrapie-like neuropathological changes (Büeler *et al.*, 1992), even when elicited postnatally (Mallucci *et al.*, 2002). More likely, toxicity of PrP^{Sc} or some PrP^C-dependent process is responsible.

To address the question of neurotoxicity, brain tissue of *Prnp$^%$* mice was exposed to a continuous source of PrP^{Sc}. To this purpose, telencephalic tissue from transgenic mice overexpressing PrP (Fischer *et al.*, 1996) was transplanted into the forebrain of *Prnp$^%$* mice and the "pseudochimeric" brains were inoculated with scrapie prions. All grafted and scrapie-inoculated mice remained free of scrapie symptoms for at least 70 weeks; this exceeded at least sevenfold the survival time of scrapie-infected donor mice (Brandner *et al.*, 1996a). Therefore, the presence of a continuous source of PrP^{Sc} and of scrapie prions does not exert any clinically detectable adverse effects on a mouse devoid of PrP^C. On the other hand, the grafts developed characteristic histopathological features of scrapie after inoculation. The course of the disease in the graft was very similar to that observed in the brain of scrapie-inoculated wild-type mice (Brandner *et al.*, 1998). Importantly, grafts had extensive contact with the recipient brain, and prions could navigate between the two compartments, as shown by the fact that inoculation of wild-type animals engrafted with PrP-expressing neuroectodermal tissue resulted in scrapie pathology in both graft and host tissue. Nonetheless, histopathological changes never extended into host tissue, even at the latest stages (>450 days), although PrP^{Sc} was detected in both grafts and recipient brain, and immunohistochemistry revealed PrP deposits in the hippocampus, and occasionally in the parietal cortex, of all

animals (Brandner *et al.*, 1996a). Thus, prions moved from the grafts to some regions of the PrP-deficient host brain without causing pathological changes or clinical disease. The distribution of PrP^{Sc} in the white matter tracts of the host brain suggests diffusion within the extra-cellular space (Jeffrey *et al.*, 1994) rather than axonal transport.

These findings suggest that the expression of PrP^C by an infected cell, rather than the extracellular deposition of PrP^{Sc}, is the critical prerequisite for the development of scrapie pathology. Perhaps PrP^{Sc} is inherently non-toxic and PrP^{Sc} plaques found in spongiform encephalopathies are an epiphenomenon rather than a cause of neuronal damage. This hypothesis appears to be supported by the recent data (Ma and Lindquist, 2002; Ma *et al.*, 2002) indicating that exaggerated retrograde transport of the prion protein from the endoplasmatic reticulum into the cytosol, or functionally equivalent inhibition of proteasome function, might induce a self-propagating, extremely cytotoxic cellular form, which may ultimately be responsible for neuronal damage. These results are very exciting, and it will be important to validate them by investigating whether the aggregated self-propagating material can also be transmitted between individual animals in a classic transmission experiment.

One may therefore propose that availability of PrP^C for some intracellular process elicited by the infectious agent, perhaps the formation of a toxic form of PrP (PrP* (Weissmann, 1991)) other than PrP^{Sc} is responsible for spongiosis, gliosis, and neuronal death. This would be in agreement with the fact that in several instances, and especially in fatal familial insomnia, spongiform pathology is detectable although very little PrP^{Sc} is present (Aguzzi & Weissmann, 1997).

Peripheral entry sites of prions

The fastest and most efficient method for inducing spongiform encephalopathy in the laboratory is intracerebral inoculation of brain homogenate. Inoculation of 1 000 000 infectious units (defined as the amount of infectivity that will induce TSE with 50% likelihood in a given host) will yield disease in approximately half a year; a remarkably strict inverse relationship can be observed between the logarithm of the inoculated dose and the incubation time (Prusiner *et al.*, 1982) (Fig. 36.3).

However, the above situation does not correspond to what typically happens in the field. There, acquisition of prion infectivity through any of several peripheral routes is the rule. However, prion diseases can also be initiated by feeding (Wells *et al.*, 1987; Kimberlin & Wilesmith, 1994;

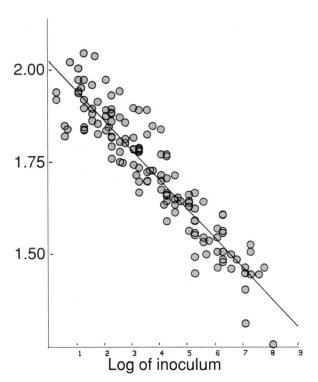

Fig. 36.3 Prion bioassay by the incubation time method. This Figure is reproduced from an important study by Prusiner and colleagues that demonstrates an inverse logarithmic relationship between size of infectious inoculum and latency period of scrapie in experimental animals (Prusiner *et al.*, 1982). The relationship is so precise that incubation time can actually be used to back-calculate the prion titer of a test article, e.g. for inactivation studies. Measurement of prion titers by the incubation time method has become a standard procedure which can be used for both wild-type and transgenic animals.

Anderson *et al.*, 1996), by intravenous and intraperitoneal injection (Kimberlin & Walker, 1978) as well as from the eye by conjunctival instillation (Scott *et al.*, 1993), corneal grafts (Duffy *et al.*, 1974) and intraocular injection (Fraser, 1982).

The pathway of orally administered prions

Upon oral challenge, an early rise in prion infectivity can be observed in the distal ileum of infected organisms: this applies to several species but was most extensively investigated in the sheep (Wells *et al.*, 1994; Vankeulen *et al.*, 1996). There, Peyer's patches acquire strong immunopositivity for the prion protein. Immunohistochemical stains with antibodies to the prion protein typically reveal a robust signal in primary B-cell follicles and germinal centers, which roughly colocalizes with the complement receptor, CD35,

in a wide variety of secondary lymphoid organs including appendix and tonsils (Hill *et al.*, 1997b). Although conventional light microscopy does not allow differentiating between PrP^C and PrP^{Sc}, Western blot analysis has not left any doubt about the fact that Peyer's patches do accumulate the disease-associated form of the prion protein.

The latter is true also in the mouse model of scrapie, which is being used as a convenient experimental paradigm by many laboratories including ours. Administration of mouse-adapted scrapie prions (Rocky Mountain Laboratory or RML strain, originally derived from the Chandler sheep scrapie isolate) induces a surge in intestinal prion infectivity as early as a few days after inoculation (Marco Prinz, Gerhard Huber and AA, unpublished results).

All of the above evidence conjures the suggestion that Peyer's patches may represent a portal of entry for orally administered prions on their journey from the luminal aspect of the gastroenteric tube to the central nervous system. However, the question as to whether the same applies for BSE-affected cattle has been answered less unambiguously.

In a monumental study of BSE pathogenesis in cattle carried out at the UK Veterinary Laboratory Agency, cows of various ages were fed with 100 g, 10 g, 1 g, or 100 mg of brain homogenate derived from BSE-sick cows (Bradley, 2000). A large variety of tissues was taken at various points in time, homogenized, and transmitted intracerebrally to indicator organisms in order to assess their prion content. This study was designed to be performed over a time frame of more than a decade and is still underway at the time of writing: it has uncovered a transient surge in infectivity in the distal ileum of cows at approximately 6 months postinfection. Infectivity then subsides, but it appears to return to the terminal ileum at the end stages of disease, maybe by means of some sort of retrograde transport (Wells *et al.*, 1998). Although this was not formally confirmed, it appears likely that Peyer's patches are the sites of prion accumulation in the gastrointestinal tract of cattle challenged orally with prions.

Oral prion susceptibility correlates with number but not structure of Peyer's patches

Reduced mucosal lymphocyte trafficking does not impair, as expected, the susceptibility to orally initiated prion disease. In contrast, mice deficient in both tumor necrosis factor and lymphotoxin-α ($TNF\alpha^{-/-} \times LT\alpha^{-/-}$) or in lymphocytes ($RAG-1^{-/-}$, μMT), in which numbers of Peyer's patches are reduced in number, are highly resistant to oral challenge, and their intestines were virtually devoid of prion infectivity at all times after challenge. Therefore, lymphoreticular requirements for enteric and for intraperitoneal uptake of prions differ from each other and that susceptibility to prion infection following oral challenge correlates with the number of Peyer's patches, but is independent of the number of intestinal mucosa-associated lymphocytes (Prinz *et al.*, 2003).

Diagnosis of prion disease: identification of the infectious agent

As explained in the glossary, the term "prion" is used here in an operational meaning: it is not meant to be necessarily identical with PrP^{Sc}, but it simply denotes the infectious agent, whatever this agent exactly consists of (Aguzzi & Weissmann, 1997). If one takes this viewpoint, PrP^{Sc} defined originally as the protease-resistant moiety associated with prion disease would be a mere surrogate marker for the prion. Even if this position may seem all too negativistic in view of the wealth of compelling evidence in favor of the protein-only hypothesis, it is still advisable to maintain that we do not understand any of the molecular details of prion replication. In other words, we still need to be open to the possibility that infectivity might be brought about by a conformer of PrP^{C} that is not identical with what was originally defined as PrP^{Sc} (see Glossary). This position appears to gain increasing acceptance, as documented by the recent description of "protease sensitive PrP^{Sc}" by the group of Stanley Prusiner (Safar *et al.*, 1998, 2000).

Because protease resistance and infectivity of PrP^{Sc} may not necessarily be congruent, it is desirable to expand the range of reagents that will interact specifically with disease-associated prion protein, but not (or to a lesser degree) with its counterpart, PrP^{C}. One IgM monoclonal antibody termed 15B3 has been described a few years ago to fulfill the above conditions (Korth *et al.*, 1997), but this antibody has not become generally available, and no follow-up studies have been published. Disappointingly, expression of the complementarity-determining regions of 15B3 in the context of a phage, as well as expression of its heavy chain variable region in transgenic mice, failed to reproduce the specificity of PrP^{Sc} binding (Heppner *et al.*, 2001b).

We have described the puzzling phenomenon that a prevalent constituent of blood serum, plasminogen, captures efficiently PrP^{Sc} but not PrP^{C} when immobilized onto the surface of magnetic beads (Fischer *et al.*, 2000; Maissen *et al.*, 2001). The significance of this phenomenon in vivo has yet to be addressed, and it has been claimed on the basis of experiments that binding occurs only in the presence of specific detergents (Shaked *et al.*, 2002). While the latter study was performed only in vitro, and related only to the binding of a mixture of serum proteins rather than puri-

fied plasminogen, this does not detract from the usefulness of the binding phenomenon for diagnostic purposes: plasminogen binds to PrP^{Sc} from a variety of species and genotypes (Maissen *et al.*, 2001), and the captured PrP^{Sc} retains the glycotype profile characteristic of the prion strain from which it was isolated (M. Maissen and AA, unpublished data).

Transepithelial enteric passage of prions: a role for M cells?

We have set out to investigate some of the preconditions of transepithelial passage of prions. Membranous epithelial cells (M cells) are key sites of antigen sampling for the mucosal-associated lymphoid system (MALT) and have been recognized as major ports of entry for enteric pathogens in the gut via transepithelial transport (Neutra *et al.*, 1996). Interestingly, maturation of M cells is dependent on signals transmitted by intraepithelial B cells. The group of Jean-Pierre Kraehenbuhl (Lausanne) has developed efficient in vitro systems, in which epithelial cells can be instructed to undergo differentiation to cells that resemble M cells by morphological and functional–physiological criteria. Therefore, we investigated whether M cells are a plausible site of prion entry in a co-culture model (Kerneis *et al.*, 1997) in which colon carcinoma cells are seeded with B-lymphoblastoid cells, inducing differentiation of M cells. After 24h, scrapie infectivity was determined within the basolateral compartment by bioassay with *tg*a20 mice, which overexpress a *Prnp* transgene and develop scrapie rapidly after infection (Fischer *et al.*, 1996). Even at low prion doses (3 logLD$_{50}$), we found infectivity in at least one M cell-containing co-culture. In contrast, there was hardly any prion transport in Caco-2 cultures without M cells (Heppner *et al.*, 2001a).

These findings indicate that M cell differentiation is necessary and sufficient for active transepithelial prion transport in vitro. M cell-dependent uptake of foreign antigens or particles is known to be followed by rapid transcytosis directly to the intraepithelial pocket, where key players of the immune system, e.g. macrophages, dendritic cells and lymphocytes (Neutra *et al.*, 1996), are located. Therefore, prions may exploit M cell-dependent transcytosis to gain access to the immune system.

While these findings suggest that M cells are a plausible candidate for the mucosal portal of prion infection, it still remains to be established whether the pathway delineated above does indeed represent the first portal of entry of orally administered prions into the body. This will necessitate in vivo experimentation, for example by ablation of M-cells

Table 36.7. Susceptibility of various strains of immunodeficient mice to intracerebrally or intraperitoneally administered prions (Klein *et al.*, 1997)

Defect	Genotype	Intracerebral route		Intraperitoneal route	
		Scrapie	Time to terminal disease	Scrapie	Time to terminal disease
T	CD-4$^{\%\,\$}$	7/7	159±11	8/8	191±1
T	CD-8$^{\%\,\$}$	6/6	157± 15	6/6	202±5
T	ß$_2$-μ$^{\%\,\$}$	8/8	162±11	7/7	211±6
T	Perforin$^{-/-\,\$}$	3/4*	171±2	4/4	204±3
T and B	SCID$^{\$}$	7/8*	160±11	6/8**	226±15
T and B	RAG 2$^{\%\,\$}$	7/7	167±2	0/7	healthy (>504)
T and B	RAG 1$^{\%\,\$}$	3/3	175±2	0/5	healthy (>258)
T and B	AGR$^{\%\,@}$	6/6	184±10	0/7	healthy (>425)
B	IgM$^{\%\,\$}$	8/8	181±6	0/8	healthy (>510)
IgG	t11umt $	5/5	170±3	4/4	223±2
FDC	TNFR1$^{\%\,£}$	7/7	165±3	9/9	216±4
Controls	129Sv	4/4	167±9	4/4	193±3
	C57BL/6	4/4	166±2	4/4	206±2

One perforin-deficient and one SCID mouse suffered from intercurrent death 135 and 141 days after inoculation, respectively.

$: genetic background was C57BL/6; £: genetic background was 129sv; @: genetic background was C57BL/6 x 129sv; ** two SCID mice remained healthy and were sacrificed 303 and 323 days after inoculation

through suicide transgenetic strategies, or by M-cell specific expression of *Prnp* transgenes.

Lymphocytes and prion pathogenesis

Innate or acquired deficiency of lymphocytes impairs peripheral prion pathogenesis, whereas no aspects of pathogenesis are affected by the presence or absence of lymphocytes upon direct transmission of prions to the central nervous system (Kitamoto *et al.*, 1991; Lasmezas *et al.*, 1996a). Klein and colleagues were then able to pinpoint the lymphocyte requirement to B-cells (Klein *et al.*, 1997; Aguzzi, 1997a): at first blush this was very surprising, since there had been no suggestions that any aspect of humoral immunity would be involved in prion diseases. In the same study, it was shown that T-cells deficiency brought about by ablation of the T-cell receptor α (TCRα) chain did not affect prion pathogenesis (Table 36.7). We measured the latency of scrapie (days from inoculation to terminal disease) upon delivery of a standard prion inoculum. All mice developed spongiform encephalopathy after *i.c.* inoculation. In contrast, all mice that carried a defect in B-cell differentiation stayed healthy after *i.p.* inoculation of RML scrapie prions. Intriguingly, in this any in several subsequent study, TNF

receptor I deficient mice developed disease with the same kinetics as wild-type mice, although there are no morphologically detectable follicular dendritic cells in the spleens of TNFRI$^{-/-}$ mice.

TCRα deficient mice, however, still contain TCRγδ T-lymphocytes. Although the latter represent a subpopulation of T-cells, the experiments described did not allow to exclude a role for TCRγδ T-lymphocytes. Therefore, we challenged also TCR TCRβ/δ deficient mice with prions. Incubation times after intracerebral and intraperitoneal inoculation of limiting or saturating doses of prions, however, elicited disease in these mice with the same kinetics as in wild-type mice (M. Klein and AA, unpublished data). Also, accumulation of PrP^{Sc} and development of histopathological changes in the brain were indistinguishable in these two strains of mice. We therefore conclude that the complete absence of T-cells has no measurable impact on prion diseases. Therefore, it is unlikely that the T-cell infiltrates which have been reported to occur in the central nervous system during the course of prion infections (Betmouni *et al.*, 1996; Betmouni & Perry, 1999; Perry *et al.*, 2002) represent more than an epiphenomenon.

In 1996–7, when the results of the studies described above were being collected, we had no precise idea of what the mechanistic role of B-cells might be in prion pathogenesis.

It had become rather clear, on the other hand, that lymphocytes alone could not account for the entirety of prion pathogenesis, and an additional sessile compartment had to be involved: adoptive transfer of *Prnp*⁺/⁺ bone marrow to *Prnp*ᵒ recipient mice did not suffice to restore infectibility of *Prnp*-expressing brain grafts, indicating that neuroinvasion was still defective (Blättler *et al.*, 1997).

It then emerged that peripheral prion pathogenesis required the physical presence of B-cells, yet intraperitoneal infection occurred efficiently even in B-cell deficient hosts that had been transferred with B-cell from *Prnp* knockout mice (Klein *et al.*, 1998). Therefore, presence of B-cells – but not expression of the cellular prion protein by these cells – is indispensable for pathogenesis upon intraperitoneal infection in the mouse scrapie model (Aguzzi *et al.*, 2001a).

The above results have been reproduced and confirmed several times over the years by many laboratories in various experimental paradigms: the requirement for B-cells in particular appears to be very stringent in most instances investigated. However, it has emerged that not all strains of prions induce identical patterns of peripheral pathogenesis, even when propagated in the same, isogenic strain of host organism.

Straining the lymphocytes

Another interesting discrepancy that remains to be addressed concerns the actual nature of the cells that replicate and accumulate prions in lymphoid organs. Four series of rigorously controlled experiments over five years (Aguzzi *et al.*, 2000; Kaeser *et al.*, 2001; Klein *et al.*, 2001; Prinz *et al.*, 2002) unambiguously reproduced the original observation by Thomas Blättler and colleagues that transfer of wild-type bone marrow cells (or fetal liver cells) to *Prnp* deficient mice restored accumulation and replication of prions in spleen (Blättler *et al.*, 1997). By contrast, Karen Brown and colleagues reported a diametrically opposite outcome of similar experiments when mice were inoculated with prions of the ME7 strain (Brown *et al.*, 1999). Maybe this discrepancy may identify yet another significant difference in the cellular tropism of different prion strains.

Bone marrow transplantation may (1) transfer an ill-defined population with the capability to replenish splenic stroma and to replicate prions, or – less probably – (2) donor-derived PrP^C expressing hematopoietic cells may confer prion replication capability to recipient stroma by virtue of "GPI painting", i.e. the post-translational cell-to-cell transfer of glycophosphoinositol linked extracellular membrane proteins (Kooyman *et al.*, 1998). Some evidence might be accrued for either possibility: stromal splenic

follicular dendritic cells have been described by some authors to derive possibly from hematopoietic precursors, particularly when donors and recipients were young (Szakal *et al.*, 1995; Kapasi *et al.*, 1998). Conversely, instances have been described in which transfer of GPI-linked proteins occurs in vivo with suprisingly high efficiency (Kooyman *et al.*, 1995). Most recently, GPI painting has been described specifically for the cellular prion protein (Liu *et al.*, 2002).

The paradox described above may uncover an analogous phenomenon in peripheral prion pathogenesis. The latter question may be important, *since the molecular and cellular basis of peripheral tropism of prion strains is* likely to be *directly* linked *to* the potential danger of *BSE in sheep* (Glatzel and Aguzzi, 2001; Bruce *et al.*, 2002; Kao *et al.*, 2002), as well the potential presence of *v*CJD prions in human blood (Aguzzi, 2000).

Prion hideouts in lymphoid organs

Prion infectivity rises in a matter of days in the spleen of intraperitoneally infected mice. Although B-lymphocytes are crucial for neuroinvasion, the bulk of infectivity is not contained in lymphocytes. Instead, most splenic prion infectivity resides in a "stromal" fraction. Lymphocytes may be important for trafficking prions within lymphoid organs, but follicular dendritic cells are the prime candidate prion reservoir. Recently, elegant immuno electron microscopic studies have evidenced that prion immunoreactivity is situated in the immediate neighborhood of iccosomes (Jeffrey *et al.*, 2000).

A definitive assessment of the contribution of FDCs to prion pathogenesis continues to be problematic since the histogenesis and the molecular characteristics of these cells are ill-defined. FDCs express S-100 proteins, as well as the complement receptors 2 (CD35) and 4 (identical to the marker FDC-M2). All of these markers, however, are also expressed by additional cell types, even within lymphoid organs (Bofill *et al.*, 2000). The FDC-M1 marker recognized by hybridoma clone 4C11 appears somewhat more specific.

Gene deletion experiments in mice have shown that signaling by both TNF and lymphotoxins is required for FDC development (Fu *et al.*, 1997; Koni *et al.*, 1997; Endres *et al.*, 1999). Membrane-bound lymphotoxin-α/β (LT-α/β) heterotrimers signal through the LT-β receptor (LT-βR) (Ware *et al.*, 1995) thereby activating a signaling pathway required for the development and maintenance of secondary lymphoid organs (Mackay *et al.*, 1997; Matsumoto *et al.*, 1997). Membrane LT-α/β heterotrimers are mainly expressed by activated lymphocytes (Browning *et al.*, 1993, 1995).

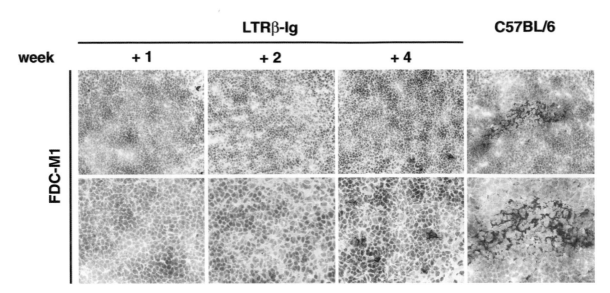

Fig. 36.4 Depletion of follicular dendritic cells by pharmacological inhibition of lymphotoxin signalling. Time course of FDC depletion in spleen of LTβR-Ig treated mice. Frozen sections of treated (left) and control mice (right) immunostained with follicular dendritic cell specific antibody FDC-M1 at different times points after injection of LTβR-Ig (original magnifications: upper row 8x25; lower row 8x63). Germinal centers FDCs networks were depleted already one week after treatment as described (Mackay and Browning, 1998; Montrasio et al., 2000). Some FDC-M1 positive cells, which may represent residual FDCs or tingible body macrophages, were still detectable in the spleens of treated mice.

Maintenance of pre-existing FDCs in a differentiated state requires continuous interaction with B lymphocytes expressing surface LT-α/β (Gonzalez et al., 1998). Inhibition of the LT-α/β pathway in mice by treatment with LTβR-immunoglobulin fusion protein (LTβR-Ig) (Crowe et al., 1994) leads to the disappearance of mature, functional FDCs (defined as cells that express markers such as FDC-M1, FDC-M2 or CD35) within one day, both in spleen and in lymph nodes (Mackay et al., 1997; Mackay & Browning, 1998). Prolonged administration of the LTβR-Ig protein leads to disruption of B cell follicles.

All of the above prompted us to study the effect of selective ablation of functional FDCs on the pathogenesis of scrapie in mice. FDC-depletion was maintained by weekly administration of the LTβR-Ig fusion protein for 8 weeks. Histological examination of spleen sections revealed that FDC networks had disappeared one week after treatment(Fig. 36.4), as expected.

In mice, following peripheral inoculation, infectivity in the spleen rises within days and reaches a plateau after a few weeks (Bruce, 1985; Rubenstein et al., 1991; Büeler et al., 1993). Even after intracerebral inoculation, spleens of C57BL/6 animals contain infectivity already 4 days post-infection (p.i.), (Büeler et al., 1993). However, Western blot analysis (Fig. 36.5) revealed that 8 weeks after inoculation spleens of control mice showed strong bands of protease-resistant PrP, whereas mice injected weekly with LTβR-Ig, starting either one week before or one week after inoculation, showed no detectable signal (<1/50th of the controls).

Prion infectivity in three spleens for each time point was assayed by intracerebral inoculation into indicator mice (Fischer et al., 1996). In spleens of mice treated with LTβR-Ig 1 week before intraperitoneal inoculation no infectivity could be detected after 3 or 8 weeks (<1.0 log ID50 units/ml 10% homogenate). Traces of infectivity, possibly representing residual inoculum, were present in the 1-week samples. In mice treated with LTβR-Ig 1 week after inoculation the titers were about 2.2 and 4.1 logID50 units/ml 10% homogenate at 3 weeks and at borderline detectability at 8 weeks after infection, suggesting that some prion accumulation took place in the first weeks after inoculation but was reversed under treatment with LTβR-Ig by 8 weeks. Spleens of scrapie-inoculated control mice treated with unspecific pooled human immunoglobulins (huIgG) 1 week after inoculation had 4.5 and 5.5 logID$_{50}$ units/ml 10% homogenate 8 weeks after intraperitoneal inoculation.

To assess whether prolonged depletion of mature FDCs would perturb the progression of the disease, C57BL/6 mice were subjected to weekly administration of the fusion protein up to eight weeks post inoculation and observed for more than 340 days. Mice receiving LTβR-Ig starting one

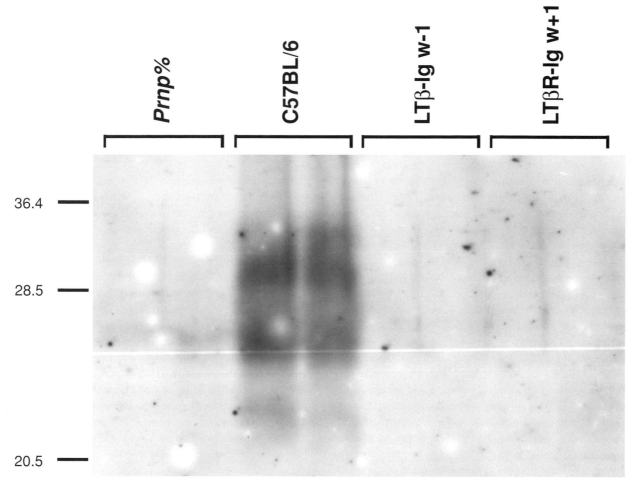

Fig. 36.5 Inhibition of lymphotoxin signalling blocks prion replication in lymphoid organs. Accumulation of PrP^Sc in spleens of LTβR-Ig treated mice eight weeks after inoculation. Immunoblot analysis of spleen extracts (200 μg total protein) from LTβR-Ig-treated and control mice sacrificed 8 weeks after inoculation. All spleen samples were treated with proteinase K. Mice analyzed (left to right): *Prnp^%*; untreated, LTβR-Ig treated C57BL/6 mice either 1 week before (LTβR-Ig w-1) or after (LTβR-Ig w+1) prion inoculation. Spleens of two mice for each group were analyzed. Immunoreactive PrP was detected using a rabbit antiserum against mouse-derived PrP (1B3) (Farquhar *et al.*, 1994) and enhanced chemiluminescence. The position of the molecular weight standards (in kDa) is indicated on the left side of the fluorogram. The three diagnostic bands of PrP^Sc are only recognized in untreated mice. LTβR-Ig treatment led to complete disappearance of the signal (reduction >50 fold).

week after inoculation developed the disease with about 25 days delay as compared to control mice. Whenever FDC depletion was initiated 1 week before inoculation, the effect on incubation time was even more pronounced. Immunofluorescence analysis of spleen sections of terminally sick animals revealed that the FDC networks were reconstituted after interruption of LTβR-Ig administration at 8 weeks and that PrP^C and/or PrP^Sc co-localized with FDCs. Immunoblot analysis showed that PrP^Sc accumulation was restored upon reappearance of FDCs in the spleens of terminal sick LTβR-Ig treated mice.

Therefore, FDCs are essential for the deposition of PrP^Sc and generation of infectivity in the spleen and suggest that they participate in the process of neuroinvasion. PrP knock-out mice expressing PrP transgenes only in B cells do not sustain prion replication in the spleen or elsewhere, suggesting that prions associated with splenic B cells (Raeber *et al.*, 1999a) may be acquired from FDCs. Finally, these results suggest that strategies aimed at depleting FDCs might be envisaged for post-exposure prophylaxis (Aguzzi & Collinge, 1997) of prion infections initiated at extracerebral sites.

Additional experimentation appears to indicate that PrP^C-expressing hematopoietic cells are required in addition to FDCs for efficient lymphoreticular prion propagation (Blättler *et al.*, 1997; Kaeser *et al.*, 2001). This apparent discrepancy called for additional studies of the molecular requirements for prion replication competence in lymphoid stroma. We therefore set out to study peripheral prion pathogenesis in mice lacking TNFα, LTα/β, or their receptors.

After intracerebral inoculation, all treated mice developed clinical symptoms of scrapie with incubation times, attack rates, and histopathological characteristics similar to those of wild-type mice, indicating that TNF/LT signaling is not relevant to cerebral prion pathogenesis. Upon intraperitoneal prion challenge, mice defective in LT signaling (LTα$^{-/-}$, LTβ$^{-/-}$, LTβR$^{-/-}$, or LTαTNFα$^{-/-}$) proved virtually non-infectible with ≤5 logLD$_{50}$ scrapie infectivity, and establishment of subclinical disease (Frigg *et al.*, 1999) was prevented. In contrast, TNFR1$^{-/-}$ mice were almost fully susceptible to all inoculum sizes, and TNFα$^{-/-}$ mice showed dose-dependent susceptibility. TNFR2$^{-/-}$ mice had intact FDCs and germinal centers, and were fully susceptible to scrapie. Unexpectedly, all examined lymph nodes of TNFR1$^{-/-}$ and TNFα$^{-/-}$ mice had consistently high infectivity titers. Even inguinal lymph nodes, which are distant from the injection site and do not drain the peritoneum, contained infectivity titers equal to all other lymph nodes. Therefore, TNF deficiency prevents lymphoreticular prion accumulation in spleen but not in lymph nodes.

Why is susceptibility to peripheral prion challenge preserved in the absence of TNFR1 or TNFα, whereas deletion of LT signalling components confers high resistance to peripheral prion infection? After all, each of these defects (except TNFR2$^{-/-}$) abolishes FDCs. For one thing, prion pathogenesis in the lymphoreticular system appears to be compartmentalized, with lymph nodes (rather than spleen) being important reservoirs of prion infectivity during disease. Second, prion replication appears to take place in lymph nodes even in the absence of mature FDCs.

In *Prnp*$^{\%}$ mice grafted with TNFR1$^{-/-}$ hematopoietic cells, high infectivity loads were detectable in lymph nodes but not spleens, indicating that TNFR1 deficient, PrP^C expressing hematopoietic cells may support prion propagation within lymph nodes. The PrP signal colocalized with a subset of macrophages in TNFR1$^{-/-}$ lymph nodes. Since marginal zone macrophages are in close contact to FDCs and also interact with marginal zone B cells, this cell type is certainly a candidate supporter in prion uptake and replication. On the other hand, it has been reported that in short-time infection experiments depletion of macrophages appears to enhance the amount of recoverable infectivity, implying that macrophages may degrade prions rather than transport them (Beringue *et al.*, 2000). The finding that a cell type other than mature FDCs is involved in prion replication and accumulation within lymph nodes may be relevant to the development of post-exposure prophylaxis strategies.

Neuroinvasion proper: the role of sympathetic nerves

In the last several years, a model has emerged that predicts prion neuroinvasion to consist of two distinct phases (Aguzzi *et al.*, 2001c). The details of the first phase are discussed above: widespread colonization of lymphoreticular organs is achieved by mechanisms that depend on B-lymphocytes (Klein *et al.*, 1997, 1998), follicular dendritic cells (Montrasio *et al.*, 2000), and complement factors (Klein *et al.*, 2001). The second phase has long been suspected to involve peripheral nerves, and possibly the autonomic nervous system, and may depend on expression of PrP^C by these nerves (Glatzel & Aguzzi, 2000). We have been attempting to test the requirement for expression of PrP^C in peripheral nerves for several years, and have developed a gene transfer protocol to spinal ganglia aimed at resolving this question (Glatzel *et al.*, 2000); however, we were never able to recover infectivity in spinal cords of *Prnp*$^{\%}$ mice whose spinal nerves had been transduced by Prnp-expressing adenoviruses (M. Glatzel and A. Aguzzi, unpublished results). Also, fast axonal transport does not appear to be involved in prion neuroinvasion, since mice that are severely impaired in this transport mechanism experience prion pathogenesis with kinetics similar to that of wild-type mice (Künzi *et al.*, 2002).

There is substantial evidence suggesting that prion transfer from the lymphoid system to the CNS occurs along peripheral nerves in a PrP^C dependent fashion (Blättler *et al.*, 1997; Glatzel & Aguzzi, 2000; Race *et al.*, 2000). Studies focusing on the temporal and spatial dynamics of neuroinvasion have suggested that the autonomic nervous system might be responsible for transport from lymphoid organs to the CNS (Clarke & Kimberlin, 1984; Cole & Kimberlin, 1985; Beekes *et al.*, 1998; McBride & Beekes, 1999).

The innervation pattern of lymphoid organs is mainly sympathetic (Felten & Felten, 1988). Markus Glatzel and colleagues have shown that denervation by injection of the drug 6-hydroxydopamine (6-OHDA), as well as "immunosympathectomy" by injection of antibodies against nerve growth factor (NFG) leads to a rather dramatic decrease in the density of sympathetic innervation of lymphoid organs, and significantly delayed the development

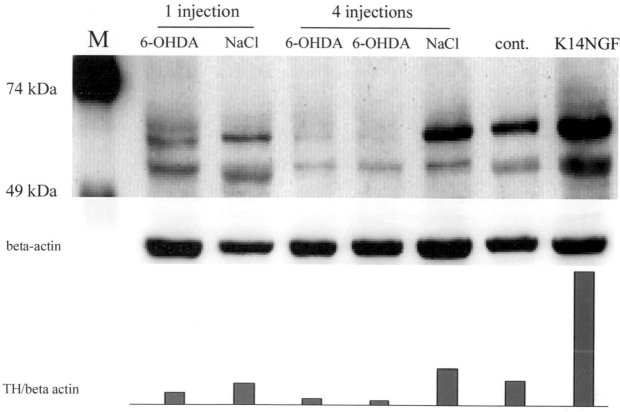

Fig. 36.6 The sympathetic innervation of the spleen can be ablated by 6-hydroxydopamine. The density of sympathetic innervation correlates with the concentration of tyrosine hydroxylase, which was measured by Western blot analysis in spleens of adult 6-OHDA treated mice, K14NGF transgenic mice and controls. The two main tyrosine hydroxylase bands are visible at ca. 55 kDa. While, there is a certain increase in sympathetic innervation with age, it is obvious that 6-OHDA treatment depletes, and the K14NGF transgene increases sympathetic innervation. Lower panel: quantification of tyrosine hydroxylase content by chemiluminescence scanning. The bars represent the ratio between signal intensity of the tyrosine hydroxylase band and that of the corresponding beta-actin bands (arbitrary units).

of scrapie (Glatzel *et al.*, 2001). Sympathectomy appears to delay the transport of prions from lymphatic organs to the thoracic spinal cord, which is the entry site of sympathetic nerves to the CNS. Transgenic mice overexpressing NGF under control of the K14 promoter, whose spleens are hyperinnervated, developed scrapie significantly earlier than non-transgenic mice. No alteration in lymphocyte subpopulations was detected in spleens at any time point investigated. In particular, we did not detect any significant differences in the content of FDCs of treated and untreated mice, which negates the possibility that the observed protection may be due to modulation of FDC microanatomy.

While the sympathetic nervous system may represent a major component of the second phase of prion neuroinvasion, many details remain to be elucidated. It is not known whether prions can be transferred directly from FDCs to sympathetic endings, or whether additional cell types are involved. The latter possibility is particularly enticing, since FDCs have not been shown to entertain physical contact with sympathetic nervous system terminals.

Moreover, it is unclear how prions are actually transported within peripheral nerves. Axonal and non-axonal transport mechanisms may be involved, and non-neuronal cells (such as Schwann cells) may play a role. Within the framework of the protein-only hypothesis, one may hypothesize a "domino" mechanism, by which incoming PrP^{Sc} converts resident PrP^{C} on the axolemmal surface, thereby propagating spatially the infection. While speculative, this model is attractive since it may accommodate the finding that the velocity of neural prion spread is extremely slow (Kimberlin *et al.*, 1983) and may not follow the canonical mechanisms of fast axonal transport. Indeed, recent studies may favor a non-axonal transport mechanism that results in periaxonal deposition of PrP^{Sc} (Hainfellner & Budka, 1999; Glatzel & Aguzzi, 2000).

The fact that denervated mice eventually developed scrapie may be due to an alternative, low-efficiency route of entry that may become uncovered by the absence of sympathetic fibers. Entry through the vagal nerve has been proposed in studies of the dynamics of vacuolation following oral and intraperitoneal challenge with prions (Baldauf et al., 1997; Beekes et al., 1998).

The surprising finding that infectious titers in hyperinnervated spleens are at least two logs higher and show enhanced PrP^{Sc} accumulations compared to control mice suggests that sympathetic nerves, besides being involved in the transport of prions, may also accumulate and replicate prions in lymphatic organs (Clarke & Kimberlin, 1984). Obviously this finding has implications related to the permanence and possibly eradication of prions in subclinically infected hosts (Fig. 36.6).

Spread of prions within the central nervous system

Ocular administration of prions has proved particularly useful to study neural spread of the agent, since the retina is a part of the central nervous system and intraocular injection does not produce direct physical trauma to the brain, which may disrupt the blood-brain barrier and impair other aspects of brain physiology. The assumption that spread of prions occurs axonally rests mainly on the demonstration of diachronic spongiform changes along the retinal pathway following intraocular infection (Fraser, 1982).

To investigate whether spread of prions within the CNS is dependent on PrP^C expression in the visual pathway, PrP-producing neural grafts were used as sensitive indicators of the presence of prion infectivity in the brain of an otherwise PrP-less host. Following inoculation with prions into the eye of grafted Prnp$^\%$ mice, none of the grafts showed signs of scrapie. Therefore, it was concluded that infectivity administered to the eye of PrP-deficient hosts cannot induce scrapie in a PrP-expressing brain graft (Brandner et al., 1996b).

Engraftment of Prnp$^\%$ mice with PrP^C-producing tissue might lead to an immune response to PrP which, in turn, was shown to be in principle capable of neutralizing infectivity (Heppner et al., 2001b). In order to definitively rule out the possibility that prion transport was disabled by a neutralizing immune response, Prnp$^\%$ mice were rendered tolerant by expressing PrP^C under the control of the lck promoter. These mice overexpress PrP on T-lymphocytes, but are resistant to scrapie and do not replicate prions in brain, spleen and thymus after intraperitoneal inocula-

tion with scrapie prions (Raeber et al., 1999b). Engraftment of these mice with PrP-overexpressing neuroectoderm did not lead to the development of antibodies to PrP after intracerebral or intraocular inoculation, presumably due to clonal deletion of PrP-immunoreactive T-lymphocytes. As before, intraocular inoculation with prions did not provoke scrapie in the graft, supporting the conclusion that lack of PrP^C, rather than immune response to PrP, prevented prion spread (Brandner et al., 1996b). Therefore, PrP^C appears to be necessary for the spread of prions along the retinal projections and within the intact CNS.

These results indicate that intracerebral spread of prions is based on a PrP^C-paved chain of cells, perhaps because they are capable of supporting prion replication. When such a chain is interrupted by interposed cells that lack PrP^C, as in the case described here, no propagation of prions to the target tissue can occur. Perhaps prions require PrP^C for propagation across synapses: PrP^C is present in the synaptic region (Fournier et al., 1995) and certain synaptic properties are altered in Prnp$^\%$ mice (Collinge et al., 1994; Whittington et al., 1995). Perhaps transport of prions within (or on the surface of) neuronal processes is PrP^C-dependent. Within the framework of the protein-only hypothesis (Griffith, 1967; Prusiner, 1989), these findings may be accommodated by a "domino-stone" model in which spreading of scrapie prions in the CNS occurs per continuitatem through conversion of PrP^C by adjacent PrP^{Sc} (Aguzzi, 1997a).

Innate immunity and antiprion defense

Macrophages and toll-like receptors

Cells of the monocyte/macrophage lineage typically represent the first line of defense against an extremely broad variety of pathogens. In the case of prions, it might be conceivable that macrophages protect against prions. However, it would be equally conceivable that macrophages, by virtue of their phagocytic properties and of their intrinsic mobility, may function as Trojan horses that transport prion infectivity between sites of replication within the body. This interesting question has not yet been fully resolved.

In a short-term prion infection paradigm, Beringue and colleagues administered dichloromethylene disphosphonate encapsulated into liposomes to mice: this eliminates for a short period of time all spleen macrophages. Accumulation of newly synthesized PrP^{Sc} was accelerated, suggesting that macrophages participate in the clearance of prions, rather than being involved in PrP^{Sc} synthesis.

On the basis of the results presented above, Beringue and colleagues have suggested that activation or targeting of macrophages may represent a therapeutic pathway to explore in TSE infection. This suggestion was taken up by Sethi and Kretzschmar, who recently reported that activation of Toll like receptors (TLRs), which function as general stimulators of innate immunity by driving expression of various sets of the immune regulatory molecules, can effect postexposure prophylaxis in an experimental model of intraperitoneal scrapie infection (Sethi *et al.*, 2002). In this experimental paradigms, administration of prions intraperitoneally elicited disease after approximately 180 days, whereas the administration of CpG oligodeoxynucleotides 7 hours after prion inoculation and daily for 20 days led to disease-free intervals of "more than 330 days" – although it appears that all inoculated mice died of scrapie shortly thereafter (communicated by H. Kretzschmar at the TSE conference in Edinburgh, September 2002).

This finding is very surprising, since most available evidence indicates that general activation of the immune system would typically sensitize mice to prions, rather than protect them. The mechanism by which activation of toll-like receptor can result in post-exposure prophylaxis are wholly unclear at present, particularly in view of the fact that mice lacking Myd88 (Adachi *et al.*, 1998), which is an essential mediator of TLR signaling, develop prion disease with exactly the same sensitivity and kinetics as wild-type mice [Prinz *et al.*, 2003].

The role of the complement system

Another prominent component at the crossroad between innate and adaptive immunity is represented by the complement system. Opsonization by complement system components also appears to be relevant to prion pathogenesis: mice genetically engineered to lack complement factors (Klein *et al.*, 2001), or mice depleted of the C3 complement component by administration of cobra venom (Mabbott *et al.*, 2001), exhibit a remarkable resistance to peripheral prion inoculation. This phenomenon may, once again, be related to the pathophysiology of FDCs, which typically function as antigen traps. Trapping mechanisms essentially consist of capture of immune complexes by Fcγ receptors, and binding of opsonized antigens (linked covalently to C3d and C4b complement adducts) to the CD21/CD35 complement receptors.

Capture mediated by Fcγ receptors does not appear to be very important in prion disease: for one thing, knock-out mice lacking Fcγ receptors (Takai *et al.*, 1994, 1996; Hazenbos *et al.*, 1996; Park *et al.*, 1998) are just as susceptible to intraperitoneally administered scrapie as wild-type

mice. Further, introduction into μMT mice of a generic immunoglobulin μ chain fully restored prion neuroinvasion irrespective of whether this heavy chain allowed for secretion of immunoglobulins, or only for production of membrane-bound immunoglobulins. We therefore conclude that circulating immunoglobulins are certainly not crucial to prion replication in lymphoid organs and to neuroinvasion.

A second mechanism exploited by FDCs for antigen trapping involves covalent linking of proteolytic fragments of the complement components C3 and C4 (Szakal & Hanna, 1968; Carroll, 1998). The CD21/CD35 complement receptors on FDCs bind C3b, iC3b, C3d, and C4b through short consensus repeats in their extracellular domain. Ablation of C3, or of its receptor CD21/CD35, as well as C1q (alone or combined with BF/C2$^{-/-}$), delayed neuroinvasion significantly after *intraperitoneal* inoculation when a limiting dose of prions was administered. These effects suggest that opsonization of the infectious agent may enhance its accessibility to germinal centers by facilitating docking to FDCs.

Very large prion inocula ($\geq 10^6$ infectious units) appear to override the requirement for a functional complement receptor in prion pathogenesis. This is similar to systemic viral infections and coreceptor-dependent retention within the follicular compartment, whose necessity can be overridden by very high affinity antigens (Fischer *et al.*, 1998) or adjuvants (Wu *et al.*, 2000). Additional retention mechanisms for prions may therefore exist in FDCs, which are not complement-dependent, or depend on hitherto unidentified complement receptors.

Adaptive immunity and pre-exposure prophylaxis against prions

For many conventional viral agents, vaccination is the most effective method of infection control. But is it at all possible to induce protective immunity in vivo against prions? Prions are extremely sturdy and their resistance against sterilization is proverbial. Pre-incubation with anti-PrP antisera was reported to reduce the prion titer of infectious hamster brain homogenates by up to 2 log units (Gabizon *et al.*, 1988) and an anti-PrP antibody was found to inhibit formation of PrP^{Sc} in a cell-free system (Horiuchi & Caughey, 1999). Also, antibodies (Klein *et al.*, 2001) and F(ab) fragments raised against certain domains of PrP (Peretz *et al.*, 2001) can suppress prion replication in cultured cells. However, it is difficult to induce humoral immune responses against PrP^C and PrP^{Sc}. This is most likely due to tolerance of the mammalian immune system to PrP^C, which is an endogenous protein expressed rather ubiquitously. Ablation of the

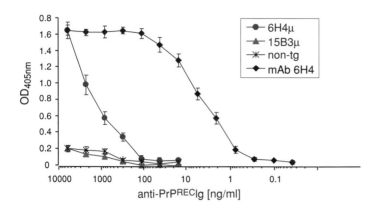

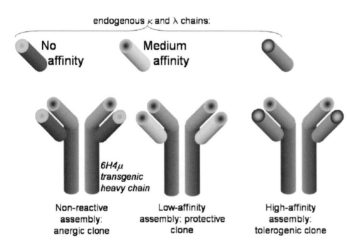

Fig. 36.7 Affinity and avidity of antibodies against the prion protein. While the heavy chain is kept constant in the transgene, it may pair with a large repertoire of endogenous light chains. Some of the pairs will yield very high affinity antibodies, others will have low affinity, but the majority may have no affinity at all for the prion protein. It is possible that some degree of clonal deletion occurs, and that combinations with the highest affinity are eliminated.

Prnp gene (Büeler *et al.*, 1992), which encodes PrP^C, renders mice highly susceptible to immunization with prions (Brandner *et al.*, 1996b), and many of the best available monoclonal antibodies to the prion protein have been generated in *Prnp*^% mice (Prusiner *et al.*, 1993). However, *Prnp*^% mice are unsuitable for testing vaccination regimens since they do not support prion pathogenesis (Büeler *et al.*, 1993).

We have therefore asked whether genes encoding high-affinity anti-PrP antibodies (originally generated in *Prnp*^% mice) may be utilized to reprogram B cell responses of prion-susceptible mice that express PrP^C. Indeed, introduction of the epitope-interacting region the heavy chain of 6H4, a high-affinity anti-PrP monoclonal antibody

(Korth *et al.*, 1997) into the germ line of mice sufficed to produce high-titer anti-PrP^C immunity. The 6H4μ heavy chain transgene induced similar anti-PrP^C titers in *Prnp*^%, *Prnp*^{o/+} and *Prnp*^{+/+} mice, indicating that deletion of autoreactive B-cells does not prevent anti-PrP immunity. The buildup of anti-PrP^C titers, however, was more sluggish in the presence of endogenous PrP^C, suggesting that some clonal deletion is actually occurring.

How can these observations be interpreted? The total anti-PrP^C titer results from pairing of one transgenic μ heavy chain with a large repertoire of endogenous κ and λ chains: some pairings may lead to reactive moieties, while others may be anergic (Fig. 36.7). Maybe the B cell clones with the highest affinity to PrP^C are being eliminated by the immune tolerization machinery, and only clones with medium affinity are retained. This would explain the delay in titer buildup in the presence of PrP^C, and would be in agreement with our affinity measurements – which indicate that the total molar avidity of 6H4m serum is approximately 100-fold lower that that of the original 6H4 antibody from which the transgene was derived. But most intriguingly, expression of the 6H4μ heavy chain sufficed to block peripheral prion pathogenesis upon intraperitoneal inoculation of the prion agent (Heppner *et al.*, 2001a).

PrP^C is a normal protein expressed by most tissues of the body. Therefore an anti-PrP immune response may conceivably induce an autoimmune disease, and defeat any realistic prospect for prion vaccination. We did not observe any blatant autoimmune disease as a consequence of anti-prion immunization – unless PrP^C was artificially transgenically expressed at non-physiological, extremely high levels.

The strategy outlined above delivers proof-of-principle that a protective humoral response against prions can be mounted by the mammalian immune system, and suggests that B cells are not intrinsically tolerant to PrP^C. If the latter is generally true, lack of immunity to prions may be due to T-helper tolerance. The latter problem is not trivial, but may perhaps be overcome by presenting PrP^C to the immune system along with highly active adjuvants. These findings, therefore, encourage a reassessment of the possible value of active and passive immunization (Westaway and Carlson, 2002), and perhaps of reprogramming B cell repertoires by μ chain transfer, in prophylaxis or in therapy of prion diseases.

Prion immunization and its reduction to practice

Approximately one year later, a first example of a reduction to practice of the approach proposed by Heppner was demonstrated by the laboratory of Thomas Wisnieswki

(Sigurdsson *et al.*, 2002). The authors have explored whether immunization with recombinant prion protein might be protective against prion diseases. Two paradigms where chosen: prophylactic immunization, and rescue after infection (post-exposure prophylaxis).

The first remarkable surprise of the study was that it was indeed possible to induce antibody responses in wild-type mice – although the actual titers were not determined. Immunization was simply achieved by injecting 50 µg of recombinant prion protein emulsified in Freund's adjuvant. This procedure had been utilized extensively in the Zurich laboratory (F. L. Heppner, M. Polymenidou, E. Pellicioli, M. Bachmann, & A. Aguzzi, unpublished observations), but had never produced any reasonable titers in wild-type mice.

Upon inoculation with a high dose or with a lower dose of prion inoculum, vaccinated mice exhibited a modest delay in development of prion disease. Although the success of the study, from the viewpoint of survival of the mice, might be regarded as limited, the study is in my view very promising in that it shows that vaccination approaches can be translated into models that are closer to the real-life situation than immunoglobulin-transgenic mice. The possibility of producing protective immunity against prions has captured the imagination of a considerable number of scientists, and additional reports are appearing of original ways to break tolerance and induce an immune response in animals that express the normal prion protein, including mixing of the immunogenic moiety with bacterial chaperons, among others (Koller *et al.*, 2002).

The prion doppelganger

Despite considerable efforts, the physiological function of PrP^C is still unclear. PrP^C was reported to have weak superoxide dismutase activity *in vitro* (a report that awaits independent confirmation) and evidence for a physiological relevance is scant (Brown *et al.*, 2001). PrP^C can bind copper (Brown *et al.*, 1997; Wadsworth *et al.*, 1999), but reports of increased copper content of neurons lacking PrP^C have been questioned by contradictory findings (Waggoner *et al.*, 2000). Similarly, a proposed role for PrP^C in synaptic function has been questioned by other investigators (Collinge *et al.*, 1994; Lledo *et al.*, 1996) and a possible regulation of circadian rhythm by PrP^C has remained more-or-less anecdotal (Tobler *et al.*, 1996). It is fair to say that if it was not for its role in prion diseases, the significance of PrP^C would be obscure and it might be viewed as just another one among many poorly understood GPI-linked proteins.

After the advent of large scale sequencing efforts and genome projects, it was realized that there is an open reading frame (ORF) directly adjacent of *Prnp* that encodes a protein sharing significant homology with PrP^C (Moore *et al.*, 1999). The novel gene, *Prnd*, is located 16 kb downstream *Prnp* in the mouse genome, and encodes a protein of 179 residues, which was termed Dpl ('downstream of the *Prnp* locus' or 'doppel', German for 'double') (Moore *et al.*, 1999; Weissmann & Aguzzi, 1999; Behrens & Aguzzi, 2002). The *Prnd* gene is evolutionarily conserved from humans to sheep and cattle, and shows roughly 25% identity with the carboxy-proximal two thirds of PrP^C. Structural studies indicate that Dpl contains three alpha helices like PrP^C and two disulphide bridges between the second and third helix (Lu *et al.*, 2000; Silverman *et al.*, 2000; Mo *et al.*, 2001).

Dpl mRNA is expressed at high levels in testis, less in other peripheral organs and, notably, at very low levels in brain of adult wild-type mice. However, significant *Prnd* mRNA transcripts were detected during embryogenesis and in the brains of newborn mice, arguing for a possible function of Dpl in brain development (Li *et al.*, 2000).

To better understand the function of Dpl, we have inactivated the *Prnd* gene in embryonic stem (ES) cells (Behrens *et al.*, 2001). Similarly to mice lacking PrP^C, mice devoid of Dpl survive to adulthood and do not show obvious phenotypical alterations, suggesting that Dpl is dispensable for embryogenesis and postnatal development (Behrens *et al.*, 2002). The similarities between PrP^C and Dpl in primary amino acid sequence, structure and subcellular localization suggest related biological functions. Therefore a possible role of PrP^C and Dpl during development may be masked by functional redundancy. To address this question it will be necessary to generate mice lacking *Prnp* as well as *Prnd* and to study whether the lack of both PrP^C and Dpl will result in an exacerbation of the mutant phenotypes. These double-mutant mice may finally reveal the true physiological function of PrP^C and Dpl, and pave the way for the long-awaited understanding of these proteins.

The Dpl protein resembles an N-terminally truncated PrP^C protein lacking the octamer repeats. But the latter version of PrP^C is actually capable of supporting PrP^{Sc} propagation (Flechsig *et al.*, 2000), suggesting that the Dpl protein may in principle be susceptible to conversion into "Dpl^{Sc}". However, presently there is no evidence whether upon scrapie inoculation Dpl can be converted into a misfolded beta-strand-rich, protease-resistant conformation.

Embryonic stem (ES) cells carrying a homozygous null mutation of the *Prnd* locus, and a normal *Prnp* locus, were found to be capable of giving rise to all neural cell lineages when transplanted into host brains. After inoculation with scrapie prions, Dpl-deficient neural grafts showed spongiosis, gliosis and unimpaired accumulation of PrP^{Sc} and infectivity similar to wild-type neuroectodermal grafts (Behrens *et al.*, 2001). Therefore in neural grafts *Prnd* deficiency does not prevent prion pathogenesis. It is important to note, however, that this experimental approach does not rule out a role for Dpl in peripheral prion pathogenesis and in PrP^{Sc} transport to the brain. The latter possibility is worth studying, because *Prnd* is expressed in the spleen, a major peripheral reservoir of PrP^{Sc} and prion infectivity (Li *et al.*, 2000).

Four polymorphisms in human *PRND* were detected, but no strong association was found between any of these polymorphisms and human prion diseases (Mead *et al.*, 2000; Peoc'h *et al.*, 2000). These findings further argue against an important function of Dpl in neurons during prion disease, at least in genetically determined forms of these diseases.

Phenotypes of Prnp deficient mice: a paradox resolved

Although this was not realized for quite some time, a Dpl-associated phenotype had been accidentally produced in knock-out mice lacking PrP^C. Several mouse lines with targeted disruptions of *Prnp* were independently generated. All mutant mouse lines lacked significant portions of the *Prnp* ORF and did not produce PrP^C protein, but showed two strikingly different phenotypes. Zrch *Prnp$^{%}$* and Edbg *Prnp$^{-/-}$* (termed after the city of origin) showed only minor defects (Büeler *et al.*, 1992; Collinge & Palmer, 1994; Manson *et al.*, 1994; Tobler *et al.*, 1996) whereas Ngsk *Prnp$^{-/-}$*, Zürich II and Rcm0 mice develop cerebellar Purkinje cell degeneration causing ataxia with advancing age (Sakaguchi *et al.*, 1996; Moore *et al.*, 1999; Rossi *et al.*, 2001). This conundrum was solved when David Westaway and colleagues realized that in the brain of ataxic, but not of healthy *Prnp*-mutant mice, *Prnd* mRNA was upregulated (Moore *et al.*, 1999; Li *et al.*, 2000). An intergenic splicing event places the Dpl locus under the control of the *Prnp* promoter, probably due to the deletion of the *Prnp* intron 2 sequence including its splicing acceptor (Moore *et al.*, 1999). This intergenic splicing event could be detected at very low levels also in wild-type mice, but was greatly enhanced by the absence of the intron 2 splice acceptor (Moore *et al.*, 1999). Whereas the *Prnp* promoter is strongly expressed in neuronal cells, the *Prnd* promoter is not (Moore *et al.*, 1999; Li *et al.*, 2000; Rossi *et al.*, 2001) and therefore *Prnd* expression from the *Prnp* promoter results in overproduction of Dpl in the brain (Moore *et al.*, 1999; Li *et al.*, 2000; Rossi *et al.*, 2001). Further experiments have demonstrated an inverse correlation between the mRNA levels of *Prnd* and the onset of ataxia. Disease progression was accelerated by increasing *Prnd* levels, supporting the notion that ectopic Dpl expression, but not functional loss of PrP^C, may be responsible for neuronal degeneration in ataxic *Prnp*-deficient mice (Rossi *et al.*, 2001).

Consequences of Doppel deficiency: a detour to reproductive pathology

We then inactivated the *Prnd* gene. However, we have not been able to generate any progeny from intercrosses of *Prnd$^{-/-}$* mice. Female *Prnd$^{-/-}$* mice, when crossed to *Prnd$^{-/-}$* or *Prnd$^{+/-}$* mice, yielded litter sizes similar to those of wild-type. In contrast, male *Prnd$^{-/-}$* mice were infertile. Their sexual activity was similar to that of controls, as shown by a normal number of copulation plugs. However, the number of spermatozoa in the cauda epididymis of *Prnd$^{-/-}$* males was reduced, and motility of mutant sperm was decreased. Therefore, sterility of Dpl-mutant males is not due to behavioral abnormalities, but may be due to a spermatogenesis defect. Indeed, *Prnd$^{-/-}$* sperm heads were severely malformed and lacked a discernible well-developed acrosome (Fig. 36.8). As the acrosome is essential for sperm–egg interaction, this defect could explain the sterility of *Prnd* deficient males.

In vitro fertilization (IVF) experiments confirmed that spermatozoa isolated from *Prnd$^{-/-}$* males were unable to fertilize wild-type oocytes. Spermatozoa of *Prnd$^{-/-}$* males never penetrated the zona pellucida. However, if the zona pellucida was partially dissected and IVF was performed with sperm suspension from *Prnd$^{-/-}$* males, fertility was partially rescued. These data indicate that *Prnd$^{-/-}$* spermatozoa are capable of oocyte fertilization, albeit at a lower frequency than controls, but that they cannot overcome the barrier imposed by the zona pellucida (Fig. 36.9).

A significant amount of PrP^C is expressed in mature spermatozoa. The PrP protein found in testes was truncated in its C terminus in the vicinity of residue 200 (Shaked *et al.*, 1999). A protective role for PrP against copper toxicity has been proposed: sperm cells originating from *Prnp* ablated mice were more susceptible to high copper concentrations than wild-type sperm. However, male *Prnp$^{%}$* knock-out mice are not sterile and produce normal litter sizes. PrP expressed in testes is clearly not capable of compensating for the absence of Dpl, suggesting non-redundant functions for the two proteins. However, Dpl may mask a minor function of PrP^C in testes development or spermiogenesis: therefore it will be very interesting to explore whether males lacking both PrP^C and Dpl might display a more severe defect than *Prnd$^{-/-}$* single mutant mice.

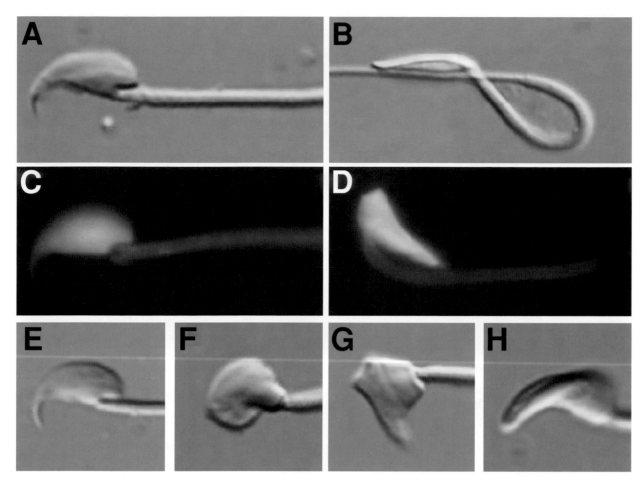

Fig. 36.8 Morphology of sperms in mice lacking the Doppel gene. Spermatozoa from Dpl-deficient mice are often heavily malformed. (A, B) Photographs of bright field images of spermatozoa isolated from wild-type (A) and *Prnd*⁻/⁻ mice (B). (C, D) Spermatozoa isolated from *Prnd*⁺/⁺ (C) and *Prnd*⁻/⁻ mice (D) were stained with mitotracker to detect mitochondria (in green) and with the DNA stain Hoechst (in blue). (E–H) Photographs of bright field images of sperm heads from *Prnd*⁺/⁺ (E) and *Prnd*⁻/⁻ mice (F–H).

At present the molecular mechanism of Dpl-regulated acrosome development is unclear. Dpl may be present on the acrosomic vesicles through its GPI-anchor, and possibly participate in acrosome morphogenesis. Alternatively, Dpl may regulate acrosome function in a more indirect way. We have also observed that sperm isolated from *Prnd*⁻/⁻ mice is greatly impaired in sperm–egg interaction and that *Prnd*⁻/⁻ spermatozoa fail to trigger the acrosomal reaction. Oligosaccharides have been implicated in sperm binding and signaling for the acrosome reaction, but the composition and structure of the essential carbohydrate moieties remain controversial (Wassarman *et al.*, 2001). Dpl is a highly glycosylated protein located at the outside of the plasma membrane (Moore *et al.*, 1999; Silverman *et al.*, 2000). It is possible that Dpl present on the sperm plasma membrane is directly involved in sperm-egg interaction.

In this context, it is interesting to mention that the laboratory of David Melton in Edinburgh has reported a slightly different phenotype of Dpl deficient mice (communicated by Derek Paisley and David Melton at the international TSE conference in Edinburgh, September 2002). In contrast to the mice generated in Zurich, Doppel deficient homozygous males in Edinburgh appear to be able to fertilize eggs. In a series of in vitro fertilizations, the Melton laboratory has reported that progression to the early cleavage divisions occurred, but was soon thereafter followed by death of the embryos at the preimplantation stage. Instead, there were no obvious malformations of sperms. Whether this discrepancy is related to a divergent genetic background

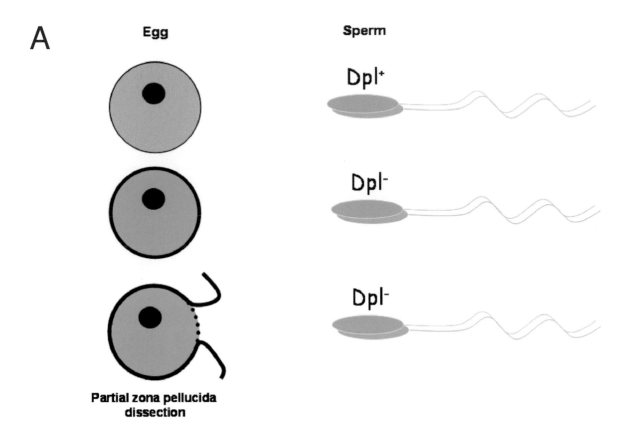

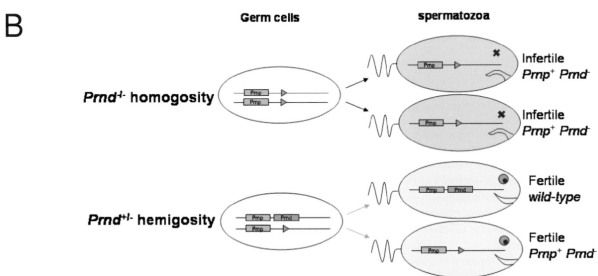

Fig. 36.9 A possible model for the function of Dpl in fertilization. (A) Male sterility in mice that lack the Doppel protein appears to come about because Doppel deficient sperms are incapable of fertilizing eggs. The process that appears to be disturbed relates to the acrosomal reaction and to the penetration of the zona pellucida. In fact, mechanical dissection of the zona pellucida restores, at least in part, fertility. (B) Interestingly, haploid spermatozoa lacking the Doppel gene (*Prnd⁻*) are perfectly fertile when generated in the context of a heterozygous *Prnd⁺/⁻* mouse. Instead, *Prnd⁻* sperms are infertile when generated in a *Prnd⁻/⁻* mouse. This may be because sperms spend much of the maturation time in the form of syncytia, with maturing cells connected to each other by cytoplasmic bridges. This may allow sufficient amounts of Doppel protein to be transferred from *Prnd⁺* to *Prnd⁻* spermatids, and rescue fertility in *trans*.

of the mice utilized, whether it points to slightly different targeting strategies, or finally whether it might uncover yet another surprising phenomenon in the genetics of prion-related genes, is – at the time of writing – wholly unclear.

With regard to the keen interest in the development of new methods of contraception (in particular those targeting the male) the phenotype of $Prnd^{-/-}$ mutant mice suggests that inhibition of Dpl function may provide a novel target for contraceptive intervention.

Perspectives in prion therapy

On the long run, one would hope that this accrued knowledge will be put into useful practice. To that effect, it is encouraging to note that a sizeable number of the steps in prion transport which have been discussed above appears to be rate-limiting. Because of that, these steps lend themselves as a target for interventions, which may be therapeutic or prophylactic (Aguzzi et al., 2001b).

A number of substances appear capable of influencing the outcome of a contact of mammalian organisms with prions: a non-exhaustive list includes compounds as diverse as Congo red (Caughey & Race, 1992), amphotericin B (Pocchiari et al., 1987), anthracyclin derivatives (Tagliavini et al., 1997), sulfated polyanions (Caughey & Raymond, 1993), pentosan polysulphate (Farquhar et al., 1999), soluble lymphotoxin-ß receptors (Montrasio et al., 2000), porphyrins (Priola et al., 2000), branched polyamines (Supattapone et al., 2001), and beta-sheet breaker peptides (Soto et al., 2000). However, it is sobering that none of the substances have yet made it to any validated clinical use: quinacrine appears to represent the most recent unfulfilled promise (Collins et al., 2002). On the other hand, the tremendous interest in this field has attracted researchers from various neighboring disciplines, including immunology, genetics, and pharmacology, and therefore it is to hope that rational and efficient methods for managing prion infections will be developed in the future.

A prion glossary

Prion: agent of transmissible spongiform encephalopathy (TSE), with unconventional properties. The term does not have structural implications other than that a protein is an essential component.

'Protein-only' hypothesis: Maintains that the prion is devoid of informational nucleic acid, and that the essential pathogenic component is protein (or glycoprotein). Genetic evidence indicates that the protein is an abnormal form of PrP (perhaps identical with PrP^{Sc}). The association with other 'non-informational' molecules (such as lipids, glycosamino glycans, or maybe even short nucleic acids) is not excluded.

PrP^C: the naturally occurring form of the mature *Prnp* gene product. Its presence in a given cell type is necessary, but not sufficient, for replication of the prion.

PrP^{Sc}: an 'abnormal' form of the mature *Prnp* gene product found in tissue of TSE sufferers, defined as being partly resistant to digestion by proteinase K under standardized conditions. It is believed to differ from PrP^C only (or mainly) conformationally, and is often considered to be the transmissible agent or prion.

These definitions (Aguzzi & Weissmann, 1997) describe our terminology which is, however, not agreed on by convention and is not necessarily used by others.

Acknowledgments

The work of my laboratory is supported by the Canton of Zurich, the Faculty of Medicine at the University of Zurich, the Swiss Federal Offices of Education and Science, of Health, and of Animal Health, the Swiss National Foundation, the National Center for Competence in Research on neural plasticity and repair, the Migros foundation, the Coop foundation, the UK Department for Environment, Food and Rural Affairs, and the Stammbach foundation.

REFERENCES

Adachi, O., Kawai, T., Takeda, K. et al. (1998). Targeted disruption of the MyD88 gene results in loss of IL-1- and IL-18-mediated function. *Immunity*, **9**, 143–50.

Aguzzi, A. (1996). Between cows and monkeys. *Nature*, **381**, 734.

(1997a). Neuro-immune connection in spread of prions in the body? *Lancet*, **349**, 742–3.

(1997b). Prions and antiprions. B. C., **378**, 1393–5.

(2000). Prion diseases, blood and the immune system: concerns and reality. *Haematologica*, **85**, 3–10.

Aguzzi, A. & Collinge, J. (1997). Post-exposure prophylaxis after accidental prion inoculation. *Lancet*, **350**, 1519–20.

Aguzzi, A. & Heppner, F. L. (2000). Pathogenesis of prion diseases: a progress report. *Cell Death Differentiation*, **7**, 889–902.

Aguzzi, A. & Raeber, A. J. (1998). Transgenic models of neurodegeneration. Neurodegeneration: of (transgenic) mice and men. *Brain Pathol.*, **8**, 695–7.

Aguzzi, A. & Weissmann, C. (1996a). Sleepless in Bologna: transmission of fatal familial insomnia. *Trends Microbiol.*, **4**, 129–31.

(1996b). Spongiform encephalopathies: a suspicious signature. *Nature*, **383**, 666–7.

(1997). Prion research: the next frontiers. *Nature*, **389**, 795–8.

Aguzzi, A., Klein, M. A., Montrasio, F. *et al.* (2000). Prions: pathogenesis and reverse genetics. *Ann. N. Y. Acad. Sci.*, **920**, 140–57.

Aguzzi, A., Brandner, S., Fischer, M. B. *et al.* (2001a). Spongiform encephalopathies: insights from transgenic models. *Adv. Virus Res.*, **56**, 313–52.

Aguzzi, A., Glatzel, M., Montrasio, F., Prinz, M. & Heppner, F. L. (2001b). Interventional strategies against prion diseases. *Nat. Rev. Neurosci.*, **2**, 745–9.

Aguzzi, A., Montrasio, F. & Kaeser, P. S. (2001c). Prions: health scare and biological challenge. *Nat. Rev. Mol. Cell. Biol.* **2**, 118–26.

Anderson, R. M., Donnelly, C. A., Ferguson, N. M. *et al.* (1996). Transmission dynamics and epidemiology of BSE in British cattle. *Nature*, **382**, 779–88.

Aucouturier, P., Geissmann, F., Damotte, D. *et al.* (2001). Infected splenic dendritic cells are sufficient for prion transmission to the CNS in mouse scrapie. *J. Clin. Invest.*, **108**, 703–8.

Baldauf, E., Beekes, M. & Diringer, H. (1997). Evidence for an alternative direct route of access for the scrapie agent to the brain bypassing the spinal cord. *J. Gen. Virol.*, **78**, 1187–97.

Basler, K., Oesch, B., Scott, M. *et al.* (1986). Scrapie and cellular PrP isoforms are encoded by the same chromosomal gene. *Cell*, **46**, 417–28.

Beekes, M., McBride, P. A. & Baldauf, E. (1998). Cerebral targeting indicates vagal spread of infection in hamsters fed with scrapie. *J. Gen. Virol.*, **79** (3), 601–7.

Behrens, A. & Aguzzi, A. (2002). Small is not beautiful: antagonizing functions for the prion protein PrP(C) and its homologue Dpl. *Trends Neurosci.*, **25**, 150–4.

Behrens, A., Brandner, S., Genoud, N. & Aguzzi, A. (2001). Normal neurogenesis and scrapie pathogenesis in neural grafts lacking the prion protein homologue Doppel. *EMBO Rep.*, **2**, 347–52.

Behrens, A., Genoud, N., Naumann, H. *et al.* (2002). Absence of the prion protein homologue Doppel causes male sterility. *EMBO J.*, **21**, 3652–8.

Beringue, V., Demoy, M., Lasmezas, C. I. *et al.* (2000). Role of spleen macrophages in the clearance of scrapie agent early in pathogenesis. *J. Pathol.*, **190**, 495–502.

Betmouni, S. & Perry, V. H. (1999). The acute inflammatory response in CNS following injection of prion brain homogenate or normal brain homogenate [In Process Citation]. *Neuropathol. Appl. Neurobiol.*, **25**, 20–8.

Betmouni, S., Perry, V. H. & Gordon, J. L. (1996). Evidence for an early inflammatory response in the central nervous system of mice with scrapie. *Neuroscience*, **74**, 1–5.

Blättler, T., Brandner, S., Raeber, A. J. *et al.* (1997). PrP-expressing tissue required for transfer of scrapie infectivity from spleen to brain. *Nature*, **389**, 69–73.

Bofill, M., Akbar, A. N. & Amlot, P. L. (2000). Follicular dendritic cells share a membrane-bound protein with fibroblasts. *J. Pathol.*, **191**, 217–26.

Bradley, R. (2000). Veterinary research at the Central Veterinary Laboratory, Weybridge, with special reference to scrapie and bovine spongiform encephalopathy. *Rev. Sci. Tech.*, **19**, 819–30.

Brandner, S., Isenmann, S., Kuhne, G. & Aguzzi, A. (1998). Identification of the end stage of scrapie using infected neural grafts. *Brain Pathol.*, **8**, 19–27.

Brandner, S., Isenmann, S., Raeber, A. *et al.* (1996a). Normal host prion protein necessary for scrapie-induced neurotoxicity. *Nature*, **379**, 339–43.

Brandner, S., Raeber, A., Sailer, A. *et al.* (1996b). Normal host prion protein (PrPC) is required for scrapie spread within the central nervous system. *Proc. Natl. Acad. Sci. USA*, **93**, 13148–51.

Brown, D. R., Qin, K., Herms, J. W. *et al.* (1997). The cellular prion protein binds copper in vivo. *Nature*, **390**, 684–7.

Brown, K. L., Stewart, K., Ritchie, D. L. *et al.* (1999). Scrapie replication in lymphoid tissues depends on prion protein-expressing follicular dendritic cells. *Nat. Med.*, **5**, 1308–12.

Brown, P, P. M., Brandel, J. P., Sato, T. *et al.* (2000). Iatrogenic Creutzfeldt–Jakob disease at the millennium. *Neurology*, **55**, 1075–81.

Brown, D. R., Clive, C. & Haswell, S. J. (2001). Antioxidant activity related to copper binding of native prion protein. *J. Neurochem.*, **76**, 69–76.

Browning, J. L., Ngam-ek, A., Lawton, P. *et al.* (1993). Lymphotoxin beta, a novel member of the TNF family that forms a heteromeric complex with lymphotoxin on the cell surface. *Cell*, **72**, 847–56.

Browning, J. L., Dougas, I., Ngam-ek, A. *et al.* (1995). Characterization of surface lymphotoxin forms. Use of specific monoclonal antibodies and soluble receptors. *J. Immunol.*, **154**, 33–46.

Bruce, M. E. (1985). Agent replication dynamics in a long incubation period model of mouse scrapie. *J. Gen. Virol.*, **66**, 2517–22.

Bruce, M. E., Will, R. G., Ironside, J. W. *et al.* (1997). Transmissions to mice indicate that 'new variant' CJD is caused by the BSE agent [see comments]. *Nature*, **389**, 498–501.

Bruce, M. E., Boyle, A., Cousens, S. *et al.* (2002). Strain characterization of natural sheep scrapie and comparison with BSE. *J. Gen. Virol.*, **83**, 695–704.

Büeler, H. R., Fischer, M., Lang, Y. *et al.* (1992). Normal development and behaviour of mice lacking the neuronal cell-surface PrP protein. *Nature*, **356**, 577–82.

Büeler, H. R., Aguzzi, A., Sailer, A. *et al.* (1993). Mice devoid of PrP are resistant to scrapie. *Cell*, **73**, 1339–47.

Carp, R. I. (1982). Transmission of scrapie by oral route: effect of gingival scarification [letter]. *Lancet*, **1**, 170–1.

Carroll, M. C. (1998). CD21/CD35 in B cell activation. *Semin. Immunol.*, **10**, 279–86.

Cashman, N. R., Loertscher, R., Nalbantoglu, J. *et al.* (1990). Cellular isoform of the scrapie agent protein participates in lymphocyte activation. *Cell*, **61**, 185–92.

Caughey, B. & Race, R. E. (1992). Potent inhibition of scrapie-associated PrP accumulation by congo red. *J. Neurochem.*, **59**, 768–71.

Caughey, B. & Raymond, G. J. (1993). Sulfated polyanion inhibition of scrapie-associated PrP accumulation in cultured cells. *J. Virol.*, **67**, 643–50.

Chazot, G., Broussolle, E., Lapras, C., Blättler, T., Aguzzi, A. & Kopp, N. (1996). New variant of Creutzfeldt–Jakob disease in a 26-year-old French man [letter]. *Lancet*, **347**, 1181.

Chesebro, B. (1998). BSE and prions: uncertainties about the agent. *Science*, **279**, 42–3.

Clarke, M. C. & Kimberlin, R. H. (1984). Pathogenesis of mouse scrapie: distribution of agent in the pulp and stroma of infected spleens. *Vet. Microbiol.*, **9**, 215–25.

Cole, S. & Kimberlin, R. H. (1985). Pathogenesis of mouse scrapie: dynamics of vacuolation in brain and spinal cord after intraperitoneal infection. *Neuropathol. Appl. Neurobiol.*, **11**, 213–27.

Collinge, J. & Palmer, M. S. (1994). Human prion diseases. *Baillieres Clin. Neurol.*, **3**, 241–7.

Collinge, J., Sidle, K. C., Meads, J., Ironside, J. & Hill, A. F. (1996). Molecular analysis of prion strain variation and the aetiology of 'new variant' CJD. *Nature*, **383**, 685–90.

Collinge, J., Whittington, M. A., Sidle, K. C. *et al.* (1994). Prion protein is necessary for normal synaptic function. *Nature*, **370**, 295–7.

Collins, S. J., Lewis, V., Brazier, M., Hill, A. F., Fletcher, A. & Masters, C. L. (2002). Quinacrine does not prolong survival in a murine Creutzfeldt-Jakob disease model. *Ann. Neurol.*, **52**, 503–6.

Crowe, P. D., VanArsdale, T. L., Walter, B. N. *et al.* (1994). A lymphotoxin-beta-specific receptor. *Science*, **264**, 707–10.

Cuille, J. & Chelle, P. L. (1939). Experimental transmission of trembling to the goat. *C R Seances Acad. Sci.*, **208**, 1058–60.

Duffy, P., Wolf, J., Collins, G., DeVoe, A. G., Streeten, B. & Cowen, D. (1974). Possible person-to-person transmission of Creutzfeldt–Jakob disease. *N. Engl. J. Med.*, **290**, 692–3.

Endres, R., Alimzhanov, M. B., Plitz, T. *et al.* (1999). Mature follicular dendritic cell networks depend on expression of lymphotoxin beta receptor by radioresistant stromal cells and of lymphotoxin beta and tumor necrosis factor by B cells. *J. Exp. Med.*, **189**, 159–68.

Farquhar, C., Dickinson, A. & Bruce, M. (1999). Prophylactic potential of pentosan polysulphate in transmissible spongiform encephalopathies [letter]. *Lancet*, **353**, 117.

Farquhar, C. F., Dornan, J., Somerville, R. A., Tunstall, A. M. & Hope, J. (1994). Effect of Sinc genotype, agent isolate and route of infection on the accumulation of protease-resistant PrP in non-central nervous system tissues during the development of murine scrapie. *J. Gen. Virol.*, **75**, 495–504.

Felten, D. L. & Felten, S. Y. (1988). Sympathetic noradrenergic innervation of immune organs. *Brain Behav. Immun.*, **2**, 293–300.

Fischer, M., Rülicke, T., Raeber, A. *et al.* (1996). Prion protein (PrP) with amino-proximal deletions restoring susceptibility of PrP knockout mice to scrapie. *EMBO J.*, **15**, 1255–64.

Fischer, M. B., Goerg, S., Shen, L. *et al.* (1998). Dependence of germinal center B cells on expression of CD21/CD35 for survival. *Science*, **280**, 582–5.

Fischer, M. B., Roeckl, C., Parizek, P., Schwarz, H. P. & Aguzzi, A. (2000). Binding of disease-associated prion protein to plasminogen. *Nature*, **408**, 479–83.

Flechsig, E., Shmerling, D., Hegyi, I. *et al.* (2000). Prion protein devoid of the octapeptide repeat region restores susceptibility to scrapie in PrP knockout mice. *Neuron*, **27**, 399–408.

Fournier, J. G., Escaig Haye, F., Billette de Villemeur, T. & Robain, O. (1995). Ultrastructural localization of cellular prion protein (PrPc) in synaptic boutons of normal hamster hippocampus. *C. R. Acad. Sci. III*, **318**, 339–44.

Fraser, H. (1982). Neuronal spread of scrapie agent and targeting of lesions within the retino-tectal pathway. *Nature*, **295**, 149–50.

Frigg, R., Klein, M. A., Hegyi, I., Zinkernagel, R. M. & Aguzzi, A. (1999). Scrapie pathogenesis in subclinically infected B-cell-deficient mice. *J. Virol.*, **73**, 9584–8.

Fu, Y. X., Huang, G., Matsumoto, M., Molina, H. & Chaplin, D. D. (1997). Independent signals regulate development of primary and secondary follicle structure in spleen and mesenteric lymph node. *Proc. Natl. Acad. Sci. USA*, **94**, 5739–43.

Gabizon, R., McKinley, M. P., Groth, D. & Prusiner, S. B. (1988). Immunoaffinity purification and neutralization of scrapie prion infectivity. *Proc. Natl Acad. Sci. USA*, **85**, 6617–21.

Gajdusek, D. C., Gibbs, C. J. & Alpers, M. (1966). Experimental transmission of a Kuru-like syndrome to chimpanzees. *Nature*, **209**, 794–6.

Gibbs, C. J., Jr., Gajdusek, D. C., Asher, D. M. *et al.* (1968). Creutzfeldt–Jakob disease (spongiform encephalopathy): transmission to the chimpanzee. *Science*, **161**, 388–9.

Glatzel, M. & Aguzzi, A. (2000). PrP(C) expression in the peripheral nervous system is a determinant of prion neuroinvasion. *J. Gen. Virol.*, **81**, 2813–21.

(2001). The shifting biology of prions. *Brain Res. Brain Res. Rev.*, **36**, 241–8.

Glatzel, M., Flechsig, E., Navarro, B. *et al.* (2000). Adenoviral and adeno-associated viral transfer of genes to the peripheral nervous system. *Proc. Natl Acad. Sci. USA*, **97**, 442–7.

Glatzel, M., Heppner, F. L., Albers, K. M. & Aguzzi, A. (2001). Sympathetic innervation of lymphoreticular organs is rate limiting for prion neuroinvasion. *Neuron*, **31**, 25–34.

Glatzel, M., Rogivue, C., Ghani, A., Streffer, J., Amsler, L. & Aguzzi, A. (2002). Incidence of Creutzfeldt–Jakob disease in Switzerland. *Lancet*, **360**, 139–41.

Gonzalez, M., Mackay, F., Browning, J. L., Kosco-Vilbois, M. H. & Noelle, R. J. (1998). The sequential role of lymphotoxin and B cells in the development of splenic follicles. *J. Exp. Med.*, **187**, 997–1007.

Griffith, J. S. (1967). Self-replication and scrapie. *Nature*, **215**, 1043–4.

Hadlow, W. J. (1959). Scrapie and kuru. *Lancet*, **2**, 289–90.

Hainfellner, J. A. & Budka, H. (1999). Disease associated prion protein may deposit in the peripheral nervous system in human transmissible spongiform encephalopathies. *Acta Neuropathol.* (Berl.), **98**, 458–60.

Hazenbos, W. L., Gessner, J. E., Hofhuis, F. M. *et al.* (1996). Impaired IgG-dependent anaphylaxis and Arthus reaction in Fc gamma RIII (CD16) deficient mice. *Immunity*, **5**, 181–8.

Heppner, F. L., Christ, A. D., Klein, M. A. *et al.* (2001a). Transepithelial prion transport by M cells. *Nat. Med.*, **7**, 976–7.

Heppner, F. L., Musahl, C., Arrighi, I. *et al.* (2001b). Prevention of Scrapie Pathogenesis by transgenic expression of anti-prion protein antibodies. *Science*, **294**, 178–82.

Hill, A. F., Desbruslais, M., Joiner, S. *et al.* (1997a). The same prion strain causes vCJD and BSE [letter] [see comments]. *Nature*, **389**, 448–50.

Hill, A. F., Zeidler, M., Ironside, J. & Collinge, J. (1997b). Diagnosis of new variant Creutzfeldt–Jakob disease by tonsil biopsy. *Lancet*, **349**, 99.

Horiuchi, M. & Caughey, B. (1999). Specific binding of normal prion protein to the scrapie form via a localized domain initiates its conversion to the protease-resistant state [In Process Citation]. *EMBO J.*, **18**, 3193–203.

Houston, F., Foster, J. D., Chong, A., Hunter, N. & Bostock, C. J. (2000). Transmission of BSE by blood transfusion in sheep. *Lancet*, **356**, 999–1000.

http://www.doh.gov.uk/cjd/stats/aug02.htm. (2002). Monthly Creutzfeldt–Jakob disease statistics. In Department of Health.

Huang, F. P., Farquhar, C. F., Mabbott, N. A., Bruce, M. E. & MacPherson, G. G. (2002). Migrating intestinal dendritic cells transport PrP(Sc) from the gut. *J. Gen. Virol.*, **83**, 267–71.

Hunter, N., Foster, J., Chong, A. *et al.* (2002). Transmission of prion diseases by blood transfusion. *J. Gen. Virol.*, **83**, 2897–905.

Jeffrey, M., Goodsir, C. M., Bruce, M., McBride, P. A., Scott, J. R. & Halliday, W. G. (1994). Correlative light and electron microscopy studies of PrP localisation in 87V scrapie. *Brain Res.*, **656**, 329–43.

Jeffrey, M., McGovern, G., Goodsir, C. M., K, L. B. & Bruce, M. E. (2000). Sites of prion protein accumulation in scrapie-infected mouse spleen revealed by immuno-electron microscopy [In Process Citation]. *J. Pathol.*, **191**, 323–32.

Kaeser, P. S., Klein, M. A., Schwarz, P. & Aguzzi, A. (2001). Efficient lymphoreticular prion propagation requires prp(c) in stromal and hematopoietic cells. *J. Virol.*, **75**, 7097–106.

Kao, R. R., Gravenor, M. B., Baylis, M. *et al.* (2002). The potential size and duration of an epidemic of bovine spongiform encephalopathy in British sheep. *Science*, **295**, 332–5.

Kapasi, Z. F., Qin, D., Kerr, W. G. *et al.* (1998). Follicular dendritic cell (FDC) precursors in primary lymphoid tissues. *J. Immunol.*, **160**, 1078–84.

Kellings, K., Meyer, N., Mirenda, C., Prusiner, S. B. & Riesner, D. (1993). Analysis of nucleic acids in purified scrapie prion preparations. *Arch. Virol.* Suppl **7**, 215–25.

Kerneis, S., Bogdanova, A., Kraehenbuhl, J. P. & Pringault, E. (1997). Conversion by Peyer's patch lymphocytes of human enterocytes into M cells that transport bacteria. *Science*, **277**, 949–52.

Kimberlin, R. H., Hall, S. M. and Walker, C. A. (1983). Pathogenesis of mouse scrapie. Evidence for direct neural spread of infection to the CNS after injection of sciatic nerve. *J. Neurol. Sci.*, **61**, 315–25.

Kimberlin, R. H. & Walker, C. A. (1978). Pathogenesis of mouse scrapie: effect of route of inoculation on infectivity titres and dose-response curves. *J. Comp. Pathol.*, **88**, 39–47.

Kimberlin, R. H. & Wilesmith, J. W. (1994). Bovine spongiform encephalopathy. Epidemiology, low dose exposure and risks. *Ann. NY Acad. Sci.*, USA, **724**, 210–20.

Kitamoto, T., Muramoto, T., Mohri, S., Dohura, K. & Tateishi, J. (1991). Abnormal isoform of prion protein accumulates in follicular dendritic cells in mice with Creutzfeldt–Jakob disease. *J. Virol.*, **65**, 6292–5.

Kitamura, D., Roes, J., Kuhn, R. & Rajewsky, K. (1991). A B cell-deficient mouse by targeted disruption of the membrane exon of the immunoglobulin mu chain gene. *Nature*, **350**, 423–6.

Klein, M. A., Frigg, R., Flechsig, E. *et al.* (1997). A crucial role for B cells in neuroinvasive scrapie. *Nature*, **390**, 687–90.

Klein, M. A., Frigg, R., Raeber, A. J. *et al.* (1998). PrP expression in B lymphocytes is not required for prion neuroinvasion. *Nat. Med.*, **4**, 1429–33.

Klein, M. A., Kaeser, P. S., Schwarz, P. *et al.* (2001). Complement facilitates early prion pathogenesis. *Nat. Med.*, **7**, 488–92.

Koller, M. F., Grau, T. & Christen, P. (2002). Induction of antibodies against murine full-length prion protein in wild-type mice. *J. Neuroimmunol.*, **132**, 113–16.

Koni, P. A., Sacca, R., Lawton, P., Browning, J. L., Ruddle, N. H. & Flavell, R. A. (1997). Distinct roles in lymphoid organogenesis for lymphotoxins alpha and beta revealed in lymphotoxin beta-deficient mice. *Immunity*, **6**, 491–500.

Kooyman, D. L., Byrne, G. W., McClellan, S. *et al.* (1995). In vivo transfer of GPI-linked complement restriction factors from erythrocytes to the endothelium. *Science*, **269**, 89–92.

Kooyman, D. L., Byrne, G. W. & Logan, J. S. (1998). Glycosyl phosphatidylinositol anchor. *Exp. Nephrol.*, **6**, 148–51.

Korth, C., Stierli, B., Streit, P. *et al.* (1997). Prion (PrPSc)-specific epitope defined by a monoclonal antibody. *Nature*, **390**, 74–7.

Künzi, V., Glatzel, M., Nakano, M. Y., Greber, U. F., Van Leuven, F. & Aguzzi, A. (2002). Unhampered prion neuroinvasion despite impaired fast axonal transport in transgenic mice overexpressing four-repeat tau. *J. Neurosci.*, in Press.

Lasmezas, C. I., Cesbron, J. Y., Deslys, J. P. *et al.* (1996a). Immune system-dependent and -independent replication of the scrapie agent. *J. Virol.*, **70**, 1292–5.

Lasmezas, C. I., Deslys, J. P., Demaimay, R. *et al.* (1996b). BSE transmission to macaques. *Nature*, **381**, 743–4.

Li, A., Sakaguchi, S., Shigematsu, K. *et al.* (2000). Physiological expression of the gene for PrP-like protein, PrPLP/Dpl, by brain endothelial cells and its ectopic expression in neurons of PrP- deficient mice ataxic due to purkinje cell degeneration [In Process Citation]. *Am. J. Pathol.*, **157**, 1447–52.

Liu, T., Li, R., Pan, T. *et al.* (2002). Intercellular transfer of the cellular prion protein. *J. Biol. Chem.*

Lledo, P. M., Tremblay, P., Dearmond, S. J., Prusiner, S. B. & Nicoll, R. A. (1996). Mice deficient for prion protein exhibit normal neuronal excitability and synaptic transmission in the hippocampus. *Proc. Natl Acad. Sci., USA*, **93**, 2403–7.

Lu, K., Wang, W., Xie, Z. *et al.* (2000). Expression and structural characterization of the recombinant human doppel protein(,) [In Process Citation]. *Biochemistry*, **39**, 13575–83.

Ma, J. & Lindquist, S. (2002). Conversion of PrP to a self-perpetuating PrPSc-like conformation in the cytosol. *Science.*

Ma, J., Wollmann, R. & Lindquist, S. (2002). Neurotoxicity and neurodegeneration when PrP accumulates in the cytosol. *Science.*

Mabbott, N. A., Bruce, M. E., Botto, M., Walport, M. J. & Pepys, M. B. (2001). Temporary depletion of complement component C3 or genetic deficiency of C1q significantly delays onset of scrapie. *Nat. Med.*, **7**, 485–7.

Mackay, F. & Browning, J. L. (1998). Turning off follicular dendritic cells. *Nature*, **395**, 26–7.

Mackay, F., Majeau, G. R., Lawton, P., Hochman, P. S. & Browning, J. L. (1997). Lymphotoxin but not tumor necrosis factor functions to maintain splenic architecture and humoral responsiveness in adult mice. *Eur. J. Immunol.*, **27**, 2033–42.

Maissen, M., Roeckl, C., Glatzel, M., Goldmann, W. & Aguzzi, A. (2001). Plasminogen binds to disease-associated prion protein of multiple species. *Lancet*, **357**, 2026–8.

Mallucci, G. R., Ratte, S., Asante, E. A. *et al.* (2002). Post-natal knock-out of prion protein alters hippocampal CA1 properties, but does not result in neurodegeneration. *EMBO J.*, **21**, 202–10.

Manson, J. C., Clarke, A. R., Hooper, M. L., Aitchison, L., McConnell, I. & Hope, J. (1994). 129/Ola mice carrying a null mutation in PrP that abolishes mRNA production are developmentally normal. *Mol. Neurobiol.*, **8**, 121–7.

Matsumoto, M., Fu, Y. X., Molina, H. *et al.* (1997). Distinct roles of lymphotoxin alpha and the type I tumor necrosis factor (TNF) receptor in the establishment of follicular dendritic cells from non-bone marrow-derived cells. *J. Exp. Med.*, **186**, 1997–2004.

McBride, P. A. & Beekes, M. (1999). Pathological PrP is abundant in sympathetic and sensory ganglia of hamsters fed with scrapie. *Neurosci. Lett.*, **265**, 135–8.

Mead, S., Beck, J., Dickinson, A., Fisher, E. M. & Collinge, J. (2000). Examination of the human prion protein-like gene doppel for genetic susceptibility to sporadic and variant Creutzfeldt–Jakob disease. *Neurosci. Lett.*, **290**, 117–20.

Mo, H., Moore, R. C., Cohen, F. E. *et al.* (2001). Two different neurodegenerative diseases caused by proteins with similar structures. *Proc. Natl Acad. Sci. USA*, **98**, 2352–7.

Montrasio, F., Frigg, R., Glatzel, M. *et al.* (2000). Impaired prion replication in spleens of mice lacking functional follicular dendritic cells. *Science*, **288**, 1257–9.

Moore, R. C., Lee, I. Y., Silverman, G. L. *et al.* (1999). Ataxia in prion protein (PrP)-deficient mice is associated with upregulation of the novel PrP-like protein doppel [In Process Citation]. *J. Mol. Biol.*, **292**, 797–817.

Moser, M., Oesch, B. & Bueler, H. (1993). An anti-prion protein? *Nature*, **362**, 213–14.

Neutra, M. R., Frey, A. & Kraehenbuhl, J. P. (1996). Epithelial M cells: gateways for mucosal infection and immunization. *Cell*, **86**, 345–8.

Nicotera, P. (2001). A route for prion neuroinvasion. *Neuron*, **31**, 345–8.

Oesch, B., Teplow, D. B., Stahl, N., Serban, D., Hood, L. E. & Prusiner, S. B. (1990). Identification of cellular proteins binding to the scrapie prion protein. *Biochemistry*, **29**, 5848–55.

Oesch, B., Westaway, D., Walchli, M. *et al.* (1985). A cellular gene encodes scrapie PrP 27–30 protein. *Cell*, **40**, 735–46.

Park, S. Y., Ueda, S., Ohno, H. *et al.* (1998). Resistance of Fc receptor-deficient mice to fatal glomerulonephritis. *J. Clin. Invest.*, **102**, 1229–38.

Peoc'h, K., Guerin, C., Brandel, J. P., Launay, J. M. & Laplanche, J. L. (2000). First report of polymorphisms in the prion-like protein gene (PRND): implications for human prion diseases. *Neurosci. Lett.*, **286**, 144–8.

Peretz, D., Williamson, R. A., Kaneko, K. *et al.* (2001). Antibodies inhibit prion propagation and clear cell cultures of prion infectivity. *Nature*, **412**, 739–43.

Perry, V. H., Cunningham, C. & Boche, D. (2002). Atypical inflammation in the central nervous system in prion disease. *Curr. Opin. Neurol.*, **15**, 349–54.

Pocchiari, M., Schmittinger, S. & Masullo, C. (1987). Amphotericin B delays the incubation period of scrapie in intracerebrally inoculated hamsters. *J. Gen. Virol.*, **68**, 219–23.

Prinz, M., Huber, G., Macpherson, A. J. S. *et al.* (2003). Oral prion infection requires normal numbers of Peyer's patches but not of enteric lymphocytes. submitted.

Prinz, M., Montrasio, F., Klein, M. A. *et al.* (2002). Lymph nodal prion replication and neuroinvasion in mice devoid of follicular dendritic cells. *Proc. Natl Acad. Sci. USA*, **99**, 919–24.

Priola, S. A., Raines, A. & Caughey, W. S. (2000). Porphyrin and phthalocyanine antiscrapie compounds [see comments]. *Science*, **287**, 1503–6.

Prusiner, S. B. (1982). Novel proteinaceous infectious particles cause scrapie. *Science*, **216**, 136–44.

(1989). Scrapie prions. *Annu. Rev. Microbiol.*, **43**, 345–74.

Prusiner, S. B., Cochran, S. P., Groth, D. F., Downey, D. E., Bowman, K. A. & Martinez, H. M. (1982). Measurement of the scrapie agent using an incubation time interval assay. *Ann. Neurol.*, **11**, 353–8.

Prusiner, S. B., Groth, D., Serban, A. *et al.* (1993). Ablation of the prion protein (PrP) gene in mice prevents scrapie and facilitates production of anti-PrP antibodies. *Proc. Natl Acad. Sci. USA*, **90**, 10608–12.

Prusiner, S. B., Scott, M. R., DeArmond, S. J. and Cohen, F. E. (1998). Prion protein biology. *Cell*, **93**, 337–48.

Race, R., Oldstone, M. & Chesebro, B. (2000). Entry versus blockade of brain infection following oral or intraperitoneal scrapie administration: role of prion protein expression in peripheral nerves and spleen. *J. Virol.*, **74**, 828–33.

Race, R. E., Priola, S. A., Bessen, R. A. *et al.* (1995). Neuron-specific expression of a hamster prion protein minigene in transgenic mice induces susceptibility to hamster scrapie agent. *Neuron*, **15**, 1183–91.

Raeber, A. J., Klein, M. A., Frigg, R., Flechsig, E., Aguzzi, A. & Weissmann, C. (1999a). PrP-dependent association of prions with splenic but not circulating lymphocytes of scrapie-infected mice. *EMBO J.*, **18**, 2702–6.

Raeber, A. J., Sailer, A., Hegyi, I. *et al.* (1999b). Ectopic expression of prion protein (PrP) in T lymphocytes or hepatocytes of PrP knockout mice is insufficient to sustain prion replication. *Proc. Natl Acad. Sci. USA*, **96**, 3987–92.

Rieger, R., Edenhofer, F., Lasmezas, C. I. & Weiss, S. (1997). The human 37-kDa laminin receptor precursor interacts with the prion protein in eukaryotic cells [see comments]. *Nat. Med.*, **3**, 1383–8.

Riesner, D., Kellings, K., Wiese, U., Wulfert, M., Mirenda, C. & Prusiner, S. B. (1993). Prions and nucleic acids: search for "residual" nucleic acids and screening for mutations in the PrP-gene. *Dev. Biol. Stand.*, **80**, 173–81.

Rossi, D., Cozzio, A., Flechsig, E., Klein, M. A., Aguzzi, A. & Weissmann, C. (2001). Onset of ataxia and Purkinje cell loss in PrP null mice inversely correlated with Dpl level in brain. *EMBO J.*, **20**, 1–9.

Rother, K. I., Clay, O. K., Bourquin, J. P., Silke, J. & Schaffner, W. (1997). Long non-stop reading frames on the antisense strand of heat shock protein 70 genes and prion protein (PrP) genes are conserved between species [see comments]. *Biol. Chem.*, **378**, 1521–30.

Rubenstein, R., Merz, P. A., Kascsak, R. J. *et al.* (1991). Scrapie-infected spleens: analysis of infectivity, scrapie-associated fibrils, and protease-resistant proteins. *J. Infect. Dis.*, **164**, 29–35.

Safar, J., Wille, H., Itri, V. *et al.* (1998). Eight prion strains have PrP(Sc) molecules with different conformations [see comments]. *Nat. Med.*, **4**, 1157–65.

Safar, J., Cohen, F. E. & Prusiner, S. B. (2000). Quantitative traits of prion strains are enciphered in the conformation of the prion protein. *Arch. Virol. Suppl.*, **16**, 227–35.

Sailer, A., Büeler, H., Fischer, M., Aguzzi, A. & Weissmann, C. (1994). No propagation of prions in mice devoid of PrP. *Cell*, **77**, 967–8.

Sakaguchi, S., Katamine, S., Nishida, N. *et al.* (1996). Loss of cerebellar Purkinje cells in aged mice homozygous for a disrupted prp gene. *Nature*, **380**, 528–31.

Scott, J. R., Foster, J. D. & Fraser, H. (1993). Conjunctival instillation of scrapie in mice can produce disease. *Vet. Microbiol.*, **34**, 305–9.

Sethi, S., Lipford, G., Wagner, H. & Kretzschmar, H. (2002). Postexposure prophylaxis against prion disease with a stimulator of innate immunity. *Lancet*, **360**, 229–30.

Shaked, Y., Rosenmann, H., Talmor, G. & Gabizon, R. (1999). A C-terminal-truncated PrP isoform is present in mature sperm. *J. Biol. Chem.*, **274**, 32153–8.

Shaked, Y., Engelstein, R. & Gabizon, R. (2002). The binding of prion proteins to serum components is affected by detergent extraction conditions. *J. Neurochem.*, **82**, 1–5.

Shlomchik, M. J., Radebold, K., Duclos, N. & Manuelidis, L. (2001). Neuroinvasion by a Creutzfeldt–Jakob disease agent in the absence of B cells and follicular dendritic cells. *Proc. Natl Acad. Sci. USA*, **98**, 9289–94.

Shmerling, D., Hegyi, I., Fischer, M. *et al.* (1998). Expression of amino-terminally truncated PrP in the mouse leading to ataxia and specific cerebellar lesions. *Cell*, **93**, 203–14.

Sigurdsson, E. M., Brown, D. R., Daniels, M. *et al.* (2002). Immunization delays the onset of prion disease in mice. *Am. J. Pathol.*, **161**, 13–17.

Silverman, G. L., Qin, K., Moore, R. C. *et al.* (2000). Doppel is an *N*-glycosylated, glycosylphosphatidylinositol-anchored protein. Expression in testis and ectopic production in the brains of Prnp(0/0) mice predisposed to Purkinje cell loss. *J. Biol. Chem.*, **275**, 26834–41.

Soto, C., Kascsak, R. J., Saborio, G. P. *et al.* (2000). Reversion of prion protein conformational changes by synthetic beta-sheet breaker peptides. *Lancet*, **355**, 192–7.

Supattapone, S., Bosque, P., Muramoto, T. *et al.* (1999). Prion protein of 106 residues creates an artifical transmission barrier for prion replication in transgenic mice. *Cell*, **96**, 869–78.

Supattapone, S., Wille, H., Uyechi, L. *et al.* (2001). Branched polyamines cure prion-infected neuroblastoma cells. *J. Virol.*, **75**, 3453–61.

Szakal, A. K. & Hanna, M. G., Jr. (1968). The ultrastructure of antigen localization and viruslike particles in mouse spleen germinal centers. *Exp. Mol. Pathol.*, **8**, 75–89.

Szakal, A. K., Kapasi, Z. F., Haley, S. T. & Tew, J. G. (1995). Multiple lines of evidence favoring a bone marrow derivation of follicular dendritic cells (FDCs). *Adv. Exp. Med. Biol.*, **378**, 267–72.

Tagliavini, F., McArthur, R. A., Canciani, B. *et al.* (1997). Effectiveness of anthracycline against experimental prion disease in Syrian hamsters. *Science*, **276**, 1119–22.

Takai, T., Li, M., Sylvestre, D., Clynes, R. & Ravetch, J. V. (1994). FcR gamma chain deletion results in pleiotrophic effector cell defects. *Cell*, **76**, 519–29.

Takai, T., Ono, M., Hikida, M., Ohmori, H. & Ravetch, J. V. (1996). Augmented humoral and anaphylactic responses in Fc gamma RII-deficient mice. *Nature*, **379**, 346–9.

Taylor, D. M. (2000). Inactivation of transmissible degenerative encephalopathy agents: a review [see comments]. *Vet. J.*, **159**, 10–7.

Taylor, D. M., McConnell, I. & Fraser, H. (1996). Scrapie infection can be established readily through skin scarification in immunocompetent but not immunodeficient mice. *J. Gen. Virol.*, **77**, 1595–9.

Tobler, I., Gaus, S. E., Deboer, T. *et al.* (1996). Altered circadian activity rhythms and sleep in mice devoid of prion protein. *Nature*, **380**, 639–42.

Vankeulen, L. J. M., Schreuder, B. E. C., Meloen, R. H., M. E. W. & Langeveld, J. P. M. (1996). Immunohistochemical detection of prion protein in lymphoid tissues of sheep with natural scrapie. *J. Clin. Microbiol.*, **34**, 1228–31.

Wadsworth, J. D., Hill, A. F., Joiner, S., Jackson, G. S., Clarke, A. R. & Collinge, J. (1999). Strain-specific prion–protein conformation determined by metal ions [see comments]. *Nat. Cell. Biol.*, **1**, 55–9.

Waggoner, D. J., Drisaldi, B., Bartnikas, T. B. *et al.* (2000). Brain copper content and cuproenzyme activity do not vary with prion protein expression level. *J. Biol. Chem.*, **275**, 7455–8.

Wagner, N., Lohler, J., Kunkel, E. J. *et al.* (1996). Critical role for beta7 integrins in formation of the gut-associated lymphoid tissue. *Nature*, **382**, 366–70.

Ware, C. F., VanArsdale, T. L., Crowe, P. D. & Browning, J. L. (1995). The ligands and receptors of the lymphotoxin system. *Curr. Top. Microbiol. Immunol.*, **198**, 175–218.

Wassarman, P. M., Jovine, L. & Litscher, E. S. (2001). A profile of fertilization in mammals. *Nat. Cell. Biol.*, **3**, E59–64.

Weissmann, C. (1991). Spongiform encephalopathies. The prion's progress. *Nature*, **349**, 569–71.

Weissmann, C. & Aguzzi, A. (1997). Bovine spongiform encephalopathy and early onset variant Creutzfeldt–Jakob disease. *Curr. Opin. Neurobiol.*, 7, 695–700.

Weissmann, C. & Aguzzi, A. (1999). Perspectives: neurobiology. PrP's double causes trouble. *Science*, **286**, 914–15.

Wells, G. A., Scott, A. C., Johnson, C. T. *et al.* (1987). A novel progressive spongiform encephalopathy in cattle. *Vet. Rec.*, **121**, 419–20.

Wells, G. A., Dawson, M., Hawkins, S. A. *et al.* (1994). Infectivity in the ileum of cattle challenged orally with bovine spongiform encephalopathy. *Vet. Rec.*, **135**, 40–1.

Wells, G. A., Hawkins, S. A., Green, R. B. *et al.* (1998). Preliminary observations on the pathogenesis of experimental bovine spongiform encephalopathy (BSE): an update. *Vet. Rec.*, **142**, 103–6.

Westaway, D. & Carlson, G. A. (2002). Mammalian prion proteins: enigma, variation and vaccination. *Trends Biochem. Sci.*, **27**, 301–7.

Whittington, M. A., Sidle, K. C., Gowland, I. *et al.* (1995). Rescue of neurophysiological phenotype seen in PrP null mice by transgene encoding human prion protein. *Nat. Genet*, **9**, 197–201.

Will R. G., Ironside J. W., Zeidler M. *et al.* (1996). A new variant of Creutzfeldt–Jakob disease in the UK. *Lancet*, **347**, 921–5.

Wu, X., Jiang, N., Fang, Y. F. *et al.* (2000). Impaired affinity maturation in Cr2−/− mice is rescued by adjuvants without improvement in germinal center development. *J. Immunol.*, **165**, 3119–27.

Yehiely, F., Bamborough, P., Costa, M. D. *et al.* (2002). Identification of candidate proteins binding to prion protein. *Neurobiol. Dis.*, **10**, 67–8.

Zanata, S. M., Lopes, M. H., Mercadante, A. F. *et al.* (2002). Stress-inducible protein 1 is a cell surface ligand for cellular prion that triggers neuroprotection. *EMBO J.*, **21**, 3307–16.

Part VII

Parkinson's and related movement disorders

37

Approach to the patient presenting with parkinsonism

Katie Kompoliti and Christopher G. Goetz

Section of Movement Disorders, Department of Neurological Sciences, Rush University Medical Center, Chicago, IL, USA

General symptomatology of patients with parkinsonism

In the nearly 200 years since James Parkinson's original essay on 'shaking palsy' (Parkinson, 1817), clinicians have learned that he described a syndrome rather than a specific disease and that Parkinson's has many imitators. As a syndrome, parkinsonism is characterized by tremor, bradykinesia, rigidity and postural reflex compromise. Parkinson's disease is one of many parkinsonian syndromes and is defined by the same clinical signs in association with a distinct type and pattern of cellular degeneration. Parkinsonism can occur as an isolated clinical syndrome, classified as primary when it is due to hereditary or idiopathic causes or secondary when it has another identifiable underlying etiology. When parkinsonism occurs in association with other neurological signs, it is classified as one of the well-defined parkinsonism-plus syndromes or as parkinsonism associated with defined hereditodegenerative disorders (Table 37.1). Parkinson's disease is the archetype of primary parkinsonism. A thorough history and comprehensive examination can usually differentiate Parkinson's disease from other parkinsonian syndromes. Nevertheless, clinicopathological studies have shown that 20% of patients thought clinically to have Parkinson's disease turn out to have pathological cellular changes suggestive of other diagnoses, and 5–10% of parkinsonian subjects with an atypical clinical picture for Parkinson's disease have the typical cellular changes of Parkinson's disease at autopsy (Hughes *et al.*, 2001).

Unilateral tremor is the most common initial symptom resulting in medical consultation for Parkinson's disease. Tremor is not the usual presenting sign in parkinsonism of other etiologies, and instead, gait impairment and slowness of movement are more typical early features. When the patient with parkinsonism first presents for evaluation, more careful interview will often reveal that other symptoms of parkinsonism have been present for months and sometimes years. These components of the history include difficulty performing finger movements that require dexterity, uncomfortable sensations of tightness, stiffness, and aches, difficulty getting up, especially from deep chairs or couches, difficulty turning in bed, alteration in handwriting (micrographia), dragging of the involved leg(s), and a 'frozen shoulder' on the side of an affected limb that has led to prior orthopedic consultation, lack of spontaneous smile (masked face), absence of blinking (reptilian stare), 'bent over' (simian) posture, or simply the acknowledgement that there is an overall slowing and early fatigue when performing the activities of daily life (Weiner & Lang, 1989).

The earliest manifestation of gait involvement in parkinsonism is usually a subjective sense of imbalance resulting in stumbling, near-falls and falls. In Parkinson's disease, objective gait impairment is not a typical early disease manifestation. When present at the onset of the illness, the clinician should immediately consider diseases other than Parkinson's disease. Over time, however, Parkinson's disease patients start walking with a stooped posture and develop short-stepped, shuffling, uncertain steps, especially when pivoting. Gait initiation becomes particularly cumbersome, but once walking, the patient attains a forward momentum in a festinating manner. Freezing occurs often in late Parkinson's disease and can be especially pronounced at initiation of gait, turning, approaching a narrow or crowded space, and reaching an intended target.

When parkinsonian symptomatology is overshadowed by other complaints, alternative diagnoses involving multiple neuronal systems should be considered. These problems can be recurrent infections, speech and swallowing difficulties, vision problems, orthostatic dizziness, urinary urgency/frequency or incontinence, severe constipation, early impotence, cognitive impairment, depression,

Table 37.1. Parkinsonism

Primary parkinsonism
Dopa-responsive dystonia
Idiopathic Parkinson's disease
Juvenile parkinsonism
Secondary parkinsonism
Drugs
    Antipsychotics, anti-emetics, tetrabenazine, reserpine,
    alpha-methyl-dopa, calcium channel blockers, lithium
Hemiparkinsonism–hemiatrophy syndrome
Hydrocephalus
Infectious
    Encephalitis lethargica, acquired immune deficiency
    syndrome (AIDS), fungal, syphilis, subacute sclerosing
    panencephalitis (SSPE), subacute spongiform encephalopathy
Metabolic
    Symptomatic basal ganglia calcification / parathyroid
    abnormalities
    Acquired hepatolenticular degeneration
Neoplastic
Psychogenic parkinsonism
Toxins
    1-methyl-4-phenyl-4-propionoxypiperidine (MPTP), Carbon
    monoxide (CO), manganese (Mn), cyanide, carbon disulfide,
    mercury (Hg), methanol, ethanol
Traumatic
    'Punch drunk' syndrome
Vascular
Parkinsonism-plus syndromes
Corticobasal degeneration
Dementia syndromes
    Alzheimer's disease, Dementia with Lewy bodies
    Frontotemporal dementia–parkinsonism linked to
    chromosome 17
Multiple system atrophy
    Olivopontocerebellar degeneration
    Shy-Dragger syndrome
    Striatonigral degeneration
Parkinsonism–dementia–amyotrophic lateral sclerosis complex
    of Guam
Progressive pallidal, pallidonigral, and pallidoluysionigral
    degenerations
Progressive supranuclear palsy
Hereditodegenerative disorders
    Ceroid lipofuscinosis
    Familial basal ganglia calcification (Fahr's disease)
    GM_1 gangliosidosis
    Gaucher's disease
    Hallervorden Spatz disease
    Huntington's disease
    Mitochondrial encephalopathies
    Neuroacanthocytosis
    Spinocerebellar ataxia
    Wilson's disease
    X-linked dystonia–parkinsonism (Lubag)
    Premutation carriers of fragile X

hallucinations or psychotic symptomatology and marked sleep disturbance. At times, the initial presentation of the patient with parkinsonism will suggest a specific diagnosis involving multiple neural pathways, but at other times, the full picture will remain obscure for some time. Even if patients are seen when their disease is already advanced, it may be difficult to arrive at the correct diagnosis, especially when the historical data regarding the sequence and time frame of events are lacking. The most instrumental tool available to the clinician in order to make the diagnosis of a parkinsonian patient is direct longitudinal observation over a period of years.

Clinical signs constituting the syndrome of parkinsonism

The four cardinal features of parkinsonism are tremor, bradykinesia, rigidity and postural reflex compromise. Tremor is the first motor manifestation in 75% of patients with Parkinson's disease, usually beginning in the distal limb unilaterally, in most cases an arm (Parkinson, 1817). The tremor of Parkinson's disease is termed rest tremor, because it is present when the involved body part is completely relaxed, and usually abates when the affected limb performs a motor task. Patients with Parkinson's disease commonly also have a postural or kinetic component to their tremor, and the presence of combined tremor types is consistent with the diagnosis, especially in more advanced stages of the disease. In contrast, tremor is not a prominent feature of other parkinsonian syndromes with the exception of drug-induced parkinsonism, and the parkinsonism associated with Wilson's disease.

Akinesia/bradykinesia refers to the difficulty patients with parkinsonism have in initiating and executing a motor plan. Early signs of bradykinesia may be confined to distal muscles (micrographia, difficulty buttoning a shirt, or executing movements with fine motor manipulations that require dexterity). Facial and vocal manifestations of bradykinesia begin early in the course of parkinsonism and masked facies, decreased blink rates and a hypophonic voice may be apparent to the clinician even before the formal examination begins. Sequential or rapid alternating movements are impaired with decreased amplitude and frequency (Weiner & Lang, 1989).

Rigidity is the increase in muscle tone that affects all muscle groups, axial and appendicular, flexors and extensors. In early Parkinson's disease, rigidity is more appendicular than axial. The opposite is true in several other parkinsonian syndromes, the classic being progressive supranuclear palsy, where axial rigidity occurs far out of proportion to involvement of appendicular muscles. The rigidity in parkinsonism can be either smooth (lead pipe) or ratchety (cogwheel). Cogwheeling is felt by some to reflect in part the superimposed rest tremor. Rigidity can be reinforced by voluntary movements of the contralateral limb (Paulson & Sten, 1997).

Postural instability underlies much of the gait disorder or parkinsonism. It is the last cardinal feature of idiopathic Parkinson's disease to appear, but carries the most morbidity. In advanced disease, it is among the least responsive signs to pharmacological manipulation (Agid *et al.*, 1989). The examiner can elicit this finding by standing behind the patient and pulling backwards from the shoulders. In a normal response, patients will remain steady or take two steps backwards to catch themselves. With impaired postural reflexes, patients will take several steps or will fall if not caught by the examiner. Whereas bradykinesia and postural reflex impairment account for most aspects of the gait disorder of Parkinson's disease, when additional neurological signs are present and impede standing or ambulation, other syndromes should be considered more likely. In cases of multiple system atrophy of the olivopontocerebellar variant, additional midline ataxia with wide based gait and inability to stand with the feet together occurs. In corticobasal degeneration, a dystonic limb and dyspraxia can impair gait (Quinn, 1989). In progressive supranuclear palsy, poor downward control of eye movements causes added walking impairment.

Other signs to evaluate

The presence of early axial dystonia before initiation of levodopa treatment questions the diagnosis of idiopathic Parkinson's disease. Disproportionate anterocollis is suggestive of multiple system atrophy, while a retrocollic neck is suggestive of progressive supranuclear palsy (Colosimo *et al.*, 1995). Appendicular dystonia not associated with antiparkinsonian medication regimens can be seen in drug-induced parkinsonism, corticobasal degeneration and hereditodegenerative disorders (Table 37.1).

Cerebellar signs can herald the involvement of multiple neuronal systems typical of metabolic and toxic illnesses or be a clue to the specific diagnosis of multiple system atrophy. In the latter, cerebellar involvement presents as gait ataxia with less frequent appendicular dysmetria (Shulman & Weiner, 1997). Dysarthria is present in most patients, but the speech is not necessarily scanning. Ocular findings, such as nystagmus, jerky pursuit, ocular dysmetria, and fixation instability are common in patients with multiple system atrophy. Elderly men who carry the premutation

for fragile x have been reported to develop a mixed syndrome of parkinsonism, ataxia, dystonia and mild cognitive impairment. Pyramidal signs, including exaggerated deep tendon reflexes, extensor plantar responses, pseudobulbar palsy, and spasticity can be seen in multiple system atrophy, progressive supranuclear palsy, and vascular parkinsonism. The presence of prominent extrapyramidal rigidity and bradykinesia can often mask both the pyramidal and cerebellar findings.

Supranuclear ophthalmoplegia, initially affecting saccadic eye movements in the downward direction, is the hallmark of progressive supranuclear palsy (Golbe, 1997). In a study of 14 patients with Parkinson's disease, 14 patients with striatonigral degeneration, 10 patients with corticobasal degeneration, and 10 patients with progressive supranuclear palsy, vertical saccade paralysis was observed in 9 out of 10 patients with progressive supranuclear palsy but none in the other groups (Vidailhet *et al.*, 1994). In the corticobasal degeneration group, saccade latency was significantly decreased and correlated to an 'apraxia' score, whereas in the progressive supranuclear palsy group, saccade amplitude was significantly decreased. The percentage of errors in the anti-saccade task, an index of prefrontal dysfunction, was markedly increased only in the progressive supranuclear palsy group (Vidailhet *et al.*, 1994).

Autonomic dysfunction in a patient with signs and symptoms of parkinsonism does not immediately imply the diagnosis of multiple system atrophy, since it may also occur in Parkinson's disease. In a retrospective review of autonomic dysfunction in pathologically confirmed cases of multiple system atrophy and Parkinson's disease, autonomic failure occurred in 84% of the multiple system atrophy cases and 26% of the Parkinson's disease cases (Wenning *et al.*, 2000). Autonomic dysfunction in multiple system atrophy involved more autonomic functions and was more severe than that seen in Parkinson's disease, particularly with regard to inspiratory stridor (Magalhaes *et al.*, 1995). Although autonomic disturbance alone does not distinguish between multiple system atrophy and Parkinson's disease, the presence of severe autonomic dysfunction, preceding parkinsonism, and the specific occurrence of inspiratory stridor are more suggestive of multiple system atrophy (Magalhaes *et al.*, 1995). Signs of autonomic failure include orthostatic hypotension, urinary disturbance, constipation, male impotence, and dysphagia.

Mental status remains relatively intact in early idiopathic Parkinson's disease, although executive memory impairment can be detected with appropriate tests. Dementia occurs late in the course of idiopathic Parkinson's disease in approximately 20 to 30% of patients (Mayeux *et al.*, 1981, 1990). Parkinsonian features in a patient associated with early-onset dementia should raise the possibility of dementia with Lewy bodies or, less commonly, atypical parkinsonian syndromes, including multiple system atrophy, progressive supranuclear palsy and corticobasal degeneration. Although prominent dementia or behavioral changes are uncommon early in multiple system atrophy and progressive supranuclear palsy, corticobasal degeneration and Alzheimer's disease with extrapyramidal features can often present as dementia or aphasia (Bergeron *et al.*, 1998).

Differential diagnosis of parkinsonism

During life, the diagnosis of the different parkinsonian syndromes relies on the clinician's expertise, but the ultimate diagnosis is made by neuropathological evaluation. For research purposes, arriving at the right diagnosis is important in order to be able to study neuroprotective treatments and conduct epidemiological studies. For patient care purposes, because the prognosis is different for the various disorders, an accurate diagnosis permits the physician to relay the most pertinent information to the patient and the family. Furthermore, treatment outcomes are different in the various parkinsonian syndromes and with an accurate diagnosis, the neurologist can tailor the management to address the specific disease entity and its clinical elements. Unfortunately, misdiagnosis is especially high during the early stages, even among movement disorder specialists, so continual vigilance and rethinking of diagnoses are essential in all parkinsonian patients (Hughes *et al.*, 1992; Rajput *et al.*, 1991; Litvan *et al.*,1996, 1998; Hughes *et al.*, 1992).

Rajput *et al.* (1991) reported autopsy results in 59 patients with parkinsonism, followed longitudinally by a single neurologist, who based his original diagnosis on the presence of two out of three cardinal features (tremor, bradykinesia, rigidity). He excluded cases with evidence of any other identifiable cause of parkinsonism or other central nervous system lesions. Patients with postural instability as an original sign were also excluded, as the sign is not generally present in early Parkinson's disease. From this cohort, the clinical diagnosis of Parkinson's disease was retained over the study period in 41/59 but only 31 (75%) showed histopathological signs of Parkinson's disease at autopsy.

Another clinicopathological study found that only 69–75% of patients with autopsy-confirmed diagnosis of Parkinson's disease had at least two of the three cardinal features listed above, while 20–25% of patients who showed

two of these cardinal features had a pathological diagnosis other than Parkinson's disease. Furthermore, 13–19% of patients with all three cardinal features had another pathological diagnosis (Gelb *et al.*, 1990).

Based on multiple studies, the best predictive diagnostic variables for idiopathic Parkinson's disease compared to other diagnoses in studies with clinico-pathological correlation appear to be: asymmetrical parkinsonism, rest tremor, and levodopa response (moderate to excellent response or levodopa-induced dyskinesias) (Hughes *et al.*, 2001; Litvan *et al.*, 1998). Other significant predictors are the absence of atypical features, such as: extensor plantar response, early dementia, early marked autonomic disturbance, supranuclear gaze palsy, and bulbar palsy (Hughes *et al.*, 2001).

The epidemiology of the differential forms of parkinsonism

Signs of parkinsonism are frequently found on neurologic examination of older people. A stratified random sample of 467 residents of East Boston, Massachusetts, 65 years or older, was given structured neurological examinations in order to estimate the prevalence of parkinsonism in a community population (Bennett *et al.*, 1996). Parkinsonism was defined as at least two of the four cardinal features (bradykinesia, rigidity, tremor, and gait disturbance). The overall prevalence estimates of parkinsonism were 14.9% for people 65 to 74 years of age, 29.5% for those 75 to 84, and 52.4% for those 85 and older. Adjusted for age and sex, the overall risk of death among people with parkinsonism was 2.0 times that among people without it. Gait disturbance was the sign associated with this increased risk of death.

Although there is abundant literature on the epidemiology of idiopathic Parkinson's disease (Tanner & Goldman, 1996), the frequency of specific forms of atypical parkinsonism has rarely been estimated (Golbe, 1994; Bower *et al.*, 1997; Rajput *et al.*, 1984; Schrag *et al.*, 1999; Vanacore *et al.*, 2001a,b). In a postmortem cohort of 620 cases, with parkinsonian syndromes, parkinsonism-plus syndromes accounted for 10.2% and secondary parkinsonism for 10.8% (Jellinger, 1996). More specifically, progressive supranuclear palsy accounted for 2.7% of this series, multiple system atrophy 2.4%, Alzheimer's disease 3.5%, other degenerative syndromes (dementia with Lewy bodies, corticobasal degeneration, Pick's disease, and parkinsonism-dementia complex of Guam) 1.5%, vascular parkinsonism 3.2%, post-encephalitic 2.6%, toxic and drug-induced 1%, post-traumatic 0.6%, and symptomatic parkinsonism from tumor, hydrocephalus and prion disease 0.8%. This series was collected from 1957–1993 and this time frame accounts for the higher than usual prevalence of post-encephalitic cases (Jellinger, 1996). This series is of interest in regards to the referenced population, but carries the limitation of referral bias.

Studies of the prevalence of progressive supranuclear palsy have estimated the age-adjusted prevalence rate between 1.4–6.4 per 100 000 (Schrag, 1999; Golbe, 1996). Since the diagnosis of progressive supranuclear palsy is frequently made several years after onset of symptoms, this figure probably underestimates the prevalence of progressive supranuclear palsy. The incidence of progressive supranuclear palsy has been measured directly in two populations: Perth, Australia (population 1 million) over 2 years and Rochester, Minnesota (population 50 000) over 13 years, giving crude incidences of 3.0–4.0 per million per year, approximately 5% of that of idiopathic Parkinson's disease (Rajput et al., 1984; Mastaglia et al., 1973).

Multiple system atrophy accounts for 8–22% of brains in parkinsonian brain banks (Colosimo et al., 1995; Rajput et al., 1991). The prevalence rate has been estimated to be 4–5 cases per 100 000 persons (Schrag et al., 1999; Vanacore et al., 2001a) and the incidence rate 0.6 cases per 100 000 persons per year (Vanacore et al., 2001a). Data on other parkinsonism-plus syndromes, like corticobasal degeneration are largely based on biased samples derived from small autopsy series with cases originating from specialty clinics rather than from more widely dispersed or population-based sources.

Drug-induced parkinsonism is one of the most frequent causes of symptomatic parkinsonism (Bower et al., 1999). The most commonly associated offending agents are neuroleptics. The reported prevalence of drug-induced parkinsonism in patients receiving neuroleptics is 10–15% (Moleman et al., 1986). Infectious causes of parkinsonism are extremely rare with the obvious exception of post-encephalitic parkinsonism associated with encephalitis lethargica. It is remarkable that the encephalitis lethargica epidemic, reaching dimensions that justify the description of a pandemic, has all but completely disappeared. Other causes of secondary parkinsonism, such as vascular and trauma-related, have been a subject of debate, preventing any clarification of their prevalence and incidence. Finally, although the list is long (see Table 37.1), parkinsonism associated with hereditometabolic diseases is extremely rare with the exception of Wilson's disease. Estimates of the prevalence of Wilson's disease vary widely, but the most frequently quoted figure is 30 cases per million (Saito, 1981).

Anatomy, physiology and biochemistry as they apply to the clinical signs of parkinsonism

Advances in molecular genetics and pathology are leading to a new classification for degenerative diseases that damage the basal ganglia. Many forms of parkinsonism can now be viewed as being caused predominantly by the genetic or sporadic occurrence of conditions associated with either alpha-synuclein or tau protein deposition. For some parkinsonian syndromes, autosomal-dominant mutations have been identified with links to the genes encoding for these proteins (Polymeropoulos et al., 1997; Hutton et al., 1998). For the sporadic disorders, abnormal deposition of these proteins correlates with cell loss. Therefore, in both hereditary and sporadic diseases, abnormal protein–protein interaction and/or lesions that result from the aggregation of pathological protein fibrils could play a mechanistic role in the dysfunction and death of neurons or glial cells in neurodegenerative diseases (Trojanowski & Lee, 2000). In a large number of seemingly diverse neurodegenerative disorders, abnormal interactions among normal brain proteins alter their conformation and promote their assembly into filaments that progressively accumulate as intracellular or extracellular fibrous deposits in the central nervous system. Whether inclusion body formation is an adaptive response or is directly related to degeneration of neuronal and glial cells is a topic of current research.

Tau is a microtubule associated protein that plays an important role in neuronal axonal transport. Abundant tau-positive inclusions are found in several diseases presenting with parkinsonism. These include: progressive supranuclear palsy, corticobasal degeneration, postencephalitic parkinsonism, Alzheimer's disease, dementia pugilistica, Down syndrome, frontotemporal dementia-parkinsonism linked to chromosome 17, Pick's disease, subacute sclerosing panencephalitis, amyotrophic lateral sclerosis–parkinsonism–dementia complex of Guam, and Niemann–Pick disease type C. (Dickson, 1999; Feany & Dickson, 1996; Morris et al., 1999; Lee et al., 2000). Its specific role in the development of clinical signs of parkinsonism is under active investigation.

The synucleins are a family of soluble proteins that often occur in the brain of subjects with parkinsonian signs, but their specific function is not well understood. Beginning with the isolation of the fragment of alpha-synuclein known as the non-Abeta component of amyloid plaques from Alzheimer's disease brains, alpha-synuclein has been increasingly implicated in the pathogenesis of neurodegenerative diseases, which are now classified as synucleopathies (Duda et al., 2000). Shortly thereafter, alpha-synuclein was shown to be a major component of Lewy bodies and Lewy neurites in sporadic idiopathic Parkinson's disease (Dickson, 1999; Duda *et al.*, 2000; Galvin *et al.*, 2001). Diseases associated with abnormal alpha-synuclein depositions include: idiopathic Parkinson's disease, dementia with Lewy bodies, Alzheimer's disease, Down syndrome, multiple system atrophy, neurodegeneration with brain iron accumulation, type 1 (Hallervorden-Spatz, neuroaxonal dystrophy), Pick's disease, and traumatic brain injury (Galvin *et al.*, 2001). For several parkinsonism-plus syndromes, neuropathological criteria have been established, and clinical signs that best predict the neuropathological findings have been tested.

Neuropathological criteria for progressive supranuclear palsy have been outlined by a task force organized by the National Institute of Neurological Disorders and Stroke (NINDS). Typical, atypical and combined progressive supranuclear palsy has been distinguished. Typical progressive supranuclear palsy is marked by variable neuronal loss and gliosis with widespread neurofibrillary tangles and neuropil threads in the basal ganglia, brainstem, including oculomotor complex, inferior olives, and dentate nucleus. Involvement of the cerebral cortex mainly involves prefrontal/precentral regions with sparing of the association areas predominantly affected in Alzheimer's disease. In atypical progressive supranuclear palsy either the severity or the distribution of the lesions, or both, deviates from the typical pattern. In combined progressive supranuclear palsy, the typical pathology of progressive supranuclear palsy is accompanied by findings from other neurodegenerative diseases (Hauw *et al.*, 1994). The neurofibrillary tangles seen in progressive supranuclear palsy contain straight filaments composed of abnormally phosphorylated tau proteins (tau 64, 69) and ubiquitin, with few paired helical filaments, distinguishing them from neurofibrillary tangles in Alzheimer's disease, postencephalitic parkinsonism, and amyotrophic lateral sclerosis–parkinsonism–dementia complex of Guam, which are composed of paired helical filaments with few straight filaments (Jellinger, 1996).

Based on these pathological changes, clinical signs that best correlate with a final, accurate postmortem diagnosis of PSP have been studied. Two clinical categories, possible PSP and probable PSP, have differing sensitivity and specificity profiles (Litvan *et al.*, 1996). In the case of probable PSP, defined as a progressive disorder with onset at age 40 or greater and the presence of vertical gaze paresis, prominent postural instability, and falls in the first year of disease, these criteria accurately differentiate PSP from other parkinsonian syndromes. The sensitivity of this set of clinical criteria is only 50%, but the specificity and positive predictive value are both 100%.

In multiple system atrophy there is gross atrophy and gliosis in substantia nigra and striatum, accompanied by deposition of granular lipofusin-iron pigment. Additional findings may include olivopontocerebellar and other brainstem nuclei degeneration, as is the case in olivopontocerebellar atrophy, or intermediolateral neuron loss combined with damage to the peripheral autonomous nervous system, as is the case in Shy–Drager syndrome (Jellinger, 1998). The characteristic inclusions of multiple system atrophy are cytoplasmic oligodendroglial inclusions, consisting of 25 nm tubules, reacting with antibodies to tau, ubiquitin, tubulin, α–β-crystallin, and rare ubiquitin-positive neuronal inclusions (Jellinger, 1998).

Clinical criteria to establish a high correlation with neuropathological changes typical of multiple system atrophy have also been studied (Quinn, 1989; Wenning *et al.*, 2000; Litvan *et al.*, 1997; Gilman *et al.*, 1999). Using a list of 17 clinical signs or symptoms, Wenning demonstrated that when at least 11 items were positive, the sensitivity of this criterion was 90% with a specificity of 93% (Wenning *et al.*, 2000). This study shows that, when a large series of clinical signs are assembled and analysed, accurate diagnosis during life is possible for this condition.

In corticobasal degeneration there is gross circumscribed/lobar frontal or parietal atrophy. Histologically, there is severe neuronal loss and astrogliosis in the frontal/parietal cortex, substantia nigra and basal ganglia. The cortex shows severe neuronal loss, astrogliosis, spongiosis and ballooned or achromatic tau and ubiquitin-positive neurons, neurofibrillary tangles and neuropil threads. Substantia nigra and basal ganglia reveal severe degeneration, and basophilic skein-like tau-positive, ubiquitin-negative inclusions composed of 15 nm straight filaments are distributed in the substantia nigra, subthalamic nucleus, striatum and pallidum (Wakabayashi *et al.*, 1994).

The clinical characteristics and the pathological lesions of vascular parkinsonism are still debatable (Yamanouchi & Nagura, 1997). While cerebrovascular lesions occur in 6–10% of idiopathic Parkinson's disease patients, vascular parkinsonism has a distinct clinical presentation characterized by predominantly lower body parkinsonism, early gait impairment and lack of response to levodopa (Jankovic, 1989). In autopsy series of patients with parkinsonism, vascular brain lesions are seen in 1–3.2% (Jellinger, 1996). These include multilacunar state, Binswanger's subcortical vascular lesions, and/or strategically placed infarcts in the basal ganglia or substantia nigra with little or no degeneration in the substantia nigra.

In parkinsonism due to carbon monoxide, carbon disulfide and cyanide lesions are found in globus pallidus, substantia nigra and other areas. In manganese-induced parkinsonism, there is neuronal loss and gliosis in the pallidum and striatum with little nigral damage with or without Lewy bodies. Parkinsonism associated with chronic lead intoxication if associated to lesions in the substantia nigra. The neuropathology of MPTP-induced parkinsonism shows neuronal loss and gliosis in the substantia nigra pars compacta without typical Lewy bodies and selective damage to the dopamine-containing neurons of A9 area with variable involvement of the other regions (Snow *et al.*, 2000). The neuropathology of neuroleptic-induced parkinsonism is poorly understood (Jellinger, 1998). Pugilistic encephalopathy or boxer's dementia shows diffuse cortical atrophy, severe cell loss in the substantia nigra, locus ceruleus and striatum with widespread neurofibrillary tangles and β-amyloid, similar to the ones seen in Alzheimer's disease, throughout the central nervous system (Jellinger, 1996).

Clinical approach to the investigation of parkinsonism

The diagnosis of the patient presenting with parkinsonism begins with a careful history and physical examination. One should view the first encounter with the patient as a snapshot of an evolving disease, revealing an isolated point in time. Knowledge on disease progression and response to treatment complement the picture and enhance more accurate conclusions. Laboratory and radiological surrogate investigations may help establish the diagnosis, especially when atypical features are seen in either the history or physical examination.

In a young patient presenting with parkinsonism, considerations include hereditodegenerative diseases as outlined in Table 37.1. Laboratory tests, investigating metabolic or genetic abnormalities can help diagnose most of the disease entities listed depending on the context of the patient's presentation and the age group. One important consideration when dealing with a patient with young onset parkinsonism is to rule out Wilson's disease, since it requires specific treatment. Serum ceruloplasmin, 24-hour urine collection for copper determination, and slit-lamp examination for Kayser–Fleischer ring detection can help reach the diagnosis most of the time. Additional tests include determination of the rate of incorporation of radiocopper into ceruloplasmin, neuroimaging studies, neurophysiological studies, free serum copper, and cerebrospinal fluid copper levels. If all of the above are inconclusive, determination of hepatic copper content via liver biopsy is the single most sensitive and accurate test for Wilson's disease.

The role of structural imaging in the understanding and diagnosis of the patient with a hypokinetic movement disorder is a limited one. Computed tomography/magnetic resonance imaging (CT/MRI) findings rarely help establish the diagnosis in neurodegenerative diseases. An inconsistent finding in Parkinson's disease is increased signal on T_2-weighted images in the substantia nigra (Duguid *et al.*, 1986; Rutledge *et al.*, 1987). In striatonigral degeneration, significant hypointensity is observed in the putamen in T_2-weighted images, consistent with magnetic susceptibility effects of iron or other paramagnetic substances (Gorell *et al.*, 1995; Pastakia *et al.*, 1986). In the early stages of the olivopontocerebellar variant of multiple system atrophy, there is atrophy of the pons in the midline sagittal section in T_1-weighted images, seen as flattening of the inferior part, with loss of its normal bulging over the medulla oblongata. With advancing disease, proton density and T_2-weighted images show mild to moderate increases in signal intensity in the transverse pontine fibres, middle cerebellar peduncles, and cerebellar cortex. If the above findings are mild or poorly appreciable in transverse sections, coronal sections allow for easy comparison with the normal signal intensity of the supratentorial structures (Savoiardo *et al.*, 1990, 1993). Obvious midbrain atrophy is present in approximately half of the clinically diagnosed cases with progressive supranuclear palsy. This finding is better visualized in sagittal than in transverse sections. Also, a concaved floor of the third ventricle observed in axial sections, reflects atrophy of the diencephalon (Savoiardo *et al.*, 1994). The MRI findings of patients with corticobasal degeneration are consistent with cerebral atrophy, most marked in the superior frontal and parietal regions, and asymmetrical, with more marked degeneration on the side contralateral to the prominent clinical symptoms (Savoiardo *et al.*, 2000).

Two main abnormalities are expected on MRI scans of patients with Wilson's disease. The first is high signal intensity on proton density and T_2-weighted images in the putamen, lateral thalami, red nuclei and periaqueductal area, and pons. These abnormalities are caused by neuronal loss, gliosis and vacuolization. The second type of MRI changes consist of a decrease or loss of signal intensity on T_2-weighted images in the putamen, pallidum, and, more rarely, head of the caudate, likely caused by deposition of copper (van Wassenaer-van Hall *et al.*, 1996). Finally, MRI can be very helpful in establishing the diagnosis in parkinsonian syndromes associated with cerebrovascular disease, hydrocephalus, neoplasms, trauma, symptomatic basal ganglia calcifications/parathyroid abnormalities or

Fahr's disease, hemiparkinsonism–hemiatrophy syndrome and certain infections.

Functional imaging techniques provide a new means of detecting and characterizing regional changes in brain metabolism and receptor binding. Although these neuroimaging tools offer future hope to explain the clinical symptomatology of parkinsonism in different diseases, they remain research strategies and offer only suggestive data for the individual patient. Among the several different approaches to functional imaging, positron emission tomography (PET) allows for quantitative examination of regional cerebral blood flow, glucose and oxygen metabolism, dopamine metabolism (the presynaptic and postsynaptic components of the dopaminergic system), and brain pharmacology. Single photon emission computed tomography (SPECT) is less sensitive but more widely available and can give estimates of regional blood flow, the function of the presynaptic dopaminergic system through measurements of the dopamine transporter, and receptor binding. Magnetic resonance spectroscopy (MRS) has a lower resolution than both of the above-mentioned techniques and provides measures of metabolite levels (*N*-acetyl-aspartate, lactate, phospholipids, adenosine triphosphate). Finally, functional MRI can be used to measure changes in brain activation (Brooks, 1997). Future refinements in functional imaging techniques may be valuable in the diagnosis of the patient presenting with parkinsonism and define the pathophysiology underlying the specific syndromes. Because the four primary features of parkinsonism are clinically distinct and may not present or progress in unison, these tools may help to track the specific lesions associated with individual parkinsonian signs. Furthermore, they may provide a means of detecting subclinical disease, measuring disease progression and investigating treatments designed to alter disease progression.

REFERENCES

Agid, Y., Cervera, P., Hirsch, E. *et al.* (1989). Biochemistry of Parkinson's disease 28 years later: a critical review. *Mov. Disord.*, **4**, S126–44.

Bennett, D. A., Beckett, L. A., Murray, A. M. *et al.* (1996). Prevalence of parkinsonian signs and associated mortality in a community population of older people. *N. Engl. J. Med.*, **334**, 71–6.

Bergeron, C., Davis, A. & Lang, A. E. (1998). Corticobasal ganglionic degeneration and progressive supranuclear palsy presenting with cognitive decline. *Brain Pathol.*, **8**, 355–65.

Bower, J. H., Maraganore, D. M., McDonnell, S. K. & Rocca, W. A. (1997). Incidence of progressive supranuclear palsy and multiple system atrophy in Olmsted County, Minnesota, 1976 to 1990. *Neurology*, **49**, 1284–8.

Bower, J. H., Maraganore, D. M., McDonnell, S. K. & Rocca, W. A. (1999). Incidence and distribution of parkinsonism in Olmsted County, Minnesota, 1976–1990. *Neurology*, **52**, 1214–20.

Brooks, D. J. (1997). Neuroimaging of movement disorders. In *Movement Disorders, Neurologic Principles and Practice*, ed. R. L. Watts & W. C. Koller, pp. 31–48. New York, NY: McGraw-Hill.

Colosimo, C., Albanese, A., Hughes, A. J., de Bruin, V. M. & Lees, A. J. (1995). Some specific clinical features differentiate multiple system atrophy (striatonigral variety) from Parkinson's disease. *Arch. Neurol.*, **52**, 294–8.

Dickson, D. W. (1999). Tau and synuclein and their role in neuropathology. *Brain Pathol.*, **9**, 657–61.

Duda, J. E., Lee, V. M. & Trojanowski, J. Q. (2000). Neuropathology of synuclein aggregates. *J. Neurosci. Res.*, **61**, 121–7.

Duguid, J. R., De La Paz, R. & DeGroot, J. (1986). Magnetic resonance imaging of the midbrain in Parkinson's disease. *Ann. Neurol.*, **20**, 744–7.

Feany, M. B. & Dickson, D. W. (1996). Neurodegenerative disorders with extensive tau pathology: a comparative study and review. *Ann. Neurol.*, **40**, 139–48.

Galvin, J. E., Lee, V. M. & Trojanowski, J. Q. (2001), Synucleinopathies: clinical and pathological implications. *Arch. Neurol.*, **58**, 186–90.

Gelb, D. J., Oliver, E. & Gilman, S. Research diagnostic criteria for Parkinson's disease. In *Parkinson's Disease: Anatomy, Pathology, and Therapy*, ed. M. Streifler, A. Korczyn, E. Melamed & M. Youdim. New York: Raven Press.

Gilman, S., Low, P. A. & Quinn, N. P. (1999). Consensus statement on the diagnosis of multiple system atrophy. *J. Neurol. Sci.*, **163**, 94–8.

Golbe, L. I. (1994). The epidemiology of PSP. *J. Neural. Transm.* Suppl **42**, 263–73.

Golbe, L. I. (1996). The epidemiology of progressive supranuclear palsy. *Adv. Neurol.*, **69**, 25–31.

Golbe, L. I. (1997). Progressive supranuclear palsy. In *Movement Disorders: Neurologic Principles and Practice*, ed. R. L. Watts & W. C. Koller, pp. 279–95. New York, NY: McGraw-Hill.

Gorell, J. M., Ordidge, R. J., Brown, G. G., Deniau, J. C., Buderer, N. M. & Helpern, J. A. (1995). Increased iron-related MRI contrast in the substantia nigra in Parkinson's disease. *Neurology*, **45**, 1138–43.

Hauw, J. J., Daniel, S. E., Dickson, D. *et al.* (1994). Preliminary NINDS neuropathologic criteria for Steele–Richardson–Olszewski syndrome (progressive supranuclear palsy). *Neurology*, **44**, 2015–19.

Hughes, A. J., Daniel, S. E., Kilford, L. & Lees, A. J. (1992). Accuracy of clinical diagnosis of idiopathic Parkinson's disease: a clinico-pathological study of 100 cases. *J. Neurol. Neurosurg. Psychiatry*, **55**, 181–4.

Hughes, A. J., Ben-Shlomo, Y., Daniel, S. E. & Lees, A. J. (2001). What features improve the accuracy of clinical diagnosis in Parkinson's disease: a clinicopathologic study 1992. *Neurology*, **57**, S34–8.

Hutton, M., Lendon, C. L., Rizzu, P. *et al.* (1998). Association of missense and 5'-splice-site mutations in tau with the inherited dementia FTDP-17. *Nature*, **393**, 702–5.

Jankovic, J. (1989). Parkinsonism-plus syndromes. *Mov. Disord.*, **4** Suppl 1, S95–119.

Jellinger, K. A. (1998). Neuropathology of movement disorders. *Neurosurg. Clin. N. Am.*, **9**, 237–62.

Jellinger, K. A. (1996). The neuropathologic diagnosis of secondary parkinsonian syndromes. In *Parkinson's Disease*, ed. L. Battistin, G. Scarlato, T. Caraceni & S. Ruggieri, pp. 293–303. Philadelphia, PA: Lippincott-Raven.

Lee, V. M., Goedert, M. & Trojanowski, J. Q. (2001). Neurodegenerative tauopathies. *Annu. Rev. Neurosci.*, **24**, 1121–59.

Litvan, I., Agid, Y., Jankovic, J. *et al.* (1996). Accuracy of clinical criteria for the diagnosis of progressive supranuclear palsy (Steele–Richardson–Olszewski syndrome). *Neurology*, **46**, 922–30.

Litvan, I., Goetz, C. G. & Jankovic, J. (1997). What is the accuracy of the clinical diagnosis of multiple system atrophy. *Arch. Neurol.*, **54**, 937–44.

Litvan, I., MacIntyre, A., Goetz, C. G. *et al.* (1998). Accuracy of the clinical diagnoses of Lewy body disease, Parkinson disease, and dementia with Lewy bodies: a clinicopathologic study. *Arch. Neurol.*, **55**, 969–78.

Mayeux, R., Stern, Y., Rosen, J. & Leventhal, J. (1981). Depression, intellectual impairment, and Parkinson disease. *Neurology*, **31**, 645–50.

Mayeux, R., Chen, J., Mirabello, E. *et al.* (1990). An estimate of the incidence of dementia in idiopathic Parkinson's disease. *Neurology*, **40**, 1513–17.

Magalhaes, M., Wenning, G. K., Daniel, S. E. & Quinn, N. P. (1995). Autonomic dysfunction in pathologically confirmed multiple system atrophy and idiopathic Parkinson's disease – a retrospective comparison. *Acta Neurol. Scand.*, **91**, 98–102.

Mastaglia, F. L., Grainger, K., Kee, F., Sadka, M. & Lefroy, R. (1973). Progressive supranuclear palsy (the Steele–Richardson–Olszewski syndrome): clinical and electrophysiological observations in eleven cases. *Proc. Aust. Assoc. Neurol.*, **10**, 35–44.

Moleman, P., Janzen, G., von Bargen, B. A., Kappers, E. J., Pepplinkhuizen, L. & Schmitz, P. I. (1986). Relationship between age and incidence of parkinsonism in psychiatric patients treated with haloperidol. *Am. J. Psychiatry*, **143**, 232–4.

Morris, H. R., Lees, A. J. & Wood, N.W. (1999). Neurofibrillary tangle parkinsonian disorders – tau pathology and tau genetics. *Mov. Disord.*, **14**, 731–6.

Parkinson, J. (1817). *An Essay on the Shaking Palsy*. London, Whittingham and Rowland for Sherwood, Neely and Jones.

Pastakia, B., Polinsky, R., Di Chiro, G., Simmons, J. T., Brown, R. & Wener, L. (1986). Multiple system atrophy (Shy–Drager syndrome): MR imaging. *Radiology*, **159**, 499–502.

Paulson, H. L. & Stern, M. B. (1997). Clinical manifestations of Parkinson's disease. In *Movement Disorders: Neurologic Principles and Practice*, ed. R. L. Watts & W. C. Koller, pp. 183–99. New York, NY: McGraw-Hill.

Pfeiffer, R. F. (1997). Wilson's disease. In *Movement Disorders, Neurologic Principles and Practice*, ed. R. L. Watts & W. C. Koller, pp. 623–37. New York, NY: McGraw-Hill.

Polymeropoulos, M. H., Lavedan, C., Leroy, E. *et al.* (1997). Mutation in the alpha-synuclein gene identified in families with Parkinson's disease [see comments]. *Science*, **276**, 2045–7.

Quinn, N. (1989). Multiple system atrophy – the nature of the beast. *J. Neurol. Neurosurg. Psychiatry*, Suppl, 78–89.

Rajput, A. H., Offord, K. P., Beard, C. M. & Kurland, L. T. (1989). Epidemiology of parkinsonism: incidence, classification, and mortality. *Ann. Neurol.*, **16**, 278–82.

Rajput, A. H., Rozdilsky, B. & Rajput, A. (1991). Accuracy of clinical diagnosis in parkinsonism – a prospective study. *Can. J. Neurol. Sci.*, **18**, 275–8.

Rutledge, J. N., Hilal, S. K., Silver, A. J., Defendini, R. & Fahn, S. (1987). Study of movement disorders and brain iron by MR. *Am. J. Roentgenol.*, **149**, 365–79.

Saito, T. (1981). An assessment of efficiency in potential screening for Wilson's disease. *J. Epidemiol. Commun. Hlth.*, **35**, 274–80.

Savoiardo, M., Strada, L., Girotti, F. *et al.* (1990). Olivopontocerebellar atrophy: MR diagnosis and relationship to multisystem atrophy. *Radiology*, **174**, 693–6.

Savoiardo, M., Halliday, W. C., Nardocci, N. *et al.* (1993). Hallervorden–Spatz disease: MR and pathologic findings. *Am. J. Neuroradiol.*, **14**, 155–62.

Savoiardo, M., Girotti, F., Strada, L. & Ciceri, E. (1994). Magnetic resonance imaging in progressive supranuclear palsy and other parkinsonian disorders. *J. Neural. Transm. Suppl*, **42**, 93–110.

Savoiardo, M., Grisoli, M. & Girotti, F. (2000). Magnetic resonance imaging in CBD, related atypical parkinsonian disorders, and dementias. *Adv. Neurol.* **82**, 197–208.

Schrag, A., Ben-Shlomo, Y. & Quinn, N. P. (1999). Prevalence of progressive supranuclear palsy and multiple system atrophy: a cross-sectional study. *Lancet*, **354**, 1771–5.

Shulman, L. M. & Weiner, W. J. (1997). Multiple-system atrophy. In *Movement Disorders, Neurologic Principles and Practice*, ed. R. L. Watts & W. C. Koller, pp. 297–306. New York, NY: McGraw-Hill.

Snow, B. J., Vingerhoets, F. J., Langston, J. W., Tetrud, J. W., Sossi, V. & Calne, D. B. (2000). Pattern of dopaminergic loss in the striatum of humans with MPTP induced parkinsonism. *J. Neurol. Neurosurg. Psychiatry*, **68**, 313–16.

Tanner, C. M. & Goldman, S. M. (1996). Epidemiology of Parkinson's disease. *Neurol. Clin.*, **14**, 317–35.

Trojanowski, J. Q. & Lee, V. M. (2000). 'Fatal attractions' of proteins. A comprehensive hypothetical mechanism underlying Alzheimer's disease and other neurodegenerative disorders. *Ann. NY Acad. Sci.*, **924**, 62–7.

Vanacore, N., Bonifati, V., Fabbrini, G. *et al.* (2001a). Epidemiology of multiple system atrophy. ESGAP Consortium. European Study Group on Atypical Parkinsonisms. *Neurol. Sci.*, **22**, 97–9.

Vanacore, N., Bonifati, V., Colosimo, C. *et al.* (2001b). Epidemiology of progressive supranuclear palsy. ESGAP Consortium. European Study Group on Atypical Parkinsonisms. *Neurol. Sci.*, **22**, 101–3.

van Wassenaer-van Hall, H. N., van den Heuvel, A. G., Algra, A., Hoogenraad, T. U. & Mali, W. P. (1996). Wilson disease: findings at MR imaging and CT of the brain with clinical correlation. *Radiology*, **198**, 531–6.

Vidailhet, M., Rivaud, S., Gouider-Khouja, N. *et al.* (1994). Eye movements in parkinsonian syndromes. *Ann. Neurol.*, **35**, 420–6.

Wakabayashi, K., Oyanagi, K., Makifuchi, T. *et al.* (1994). Corticobasal degeneration: etiopathological significance of the cytoskeletal alterations. *Acta Neuropathol. (Berl.)*, **87**, 545–53.

Weiner, W. J. & Lang, A. E. (1989). *Movement Disorders: A Comprehensive Survey*. New York, NY: Futura Publishing Company.

Wenning, G. K., Ben-Shlomo, Y., Hughes, A., Daniel, S. E., Lees, A. & Quinn, N. P. (2000). What clinical features are most useful to distinguish definite multiple system atrophy from Parkinson's disease? *J. Neurol. Neurosurg. Psychiatry*, **68**, 434–40.

Yamanouchi, H. & Nagura, H. (1997). Neurological signs and frontal white matter lesions in vascular parkinsonism. A clinicopathologic study. *Stroke*, **28**, 965–9.

38

Parkinson's disease

Christopher G. Goetz and Katie Kompoliti

Department of Neurological Sciences Rush University Medical Center, Chicago, IL, USA

Historical background

James Parkinson, a London physician, first described Parkinson's disease in 1817, using the term *paralysis agitans* (Parkinson, 1817; Roberts, 1997). The distinctive features of tremor, rigidity, and gait difficulties were appreciated in this early monograph (Goetz *et al.*, 2001). Over 50 years later, in his teaching at the Salpêtrière Hospital, the world renown French neurologist, Jean-Martin Charcot, was more thorough in describing the varied features of the illness and distinguished the hallmark of bradykinesia (Charcot, 1879). He recognized the arthritic changes, dysautonomia, and pain that can accompany the disease. Brissaud (1895) drew attention to midbrain lesions, but Greenfield and Bosanquet (1953) performed the most complete delineation of the selective cell loss, depigmentation and degeneration of the substantia nigra. In the 1960s, the biochemical and pharmacologic discoveries that dopamine was depleted in Parkinson's disease and that levodopa, as the precursor to this neurotransmitter, could improve Parkinson's disease signs were described in landmark studies (Barbeau, 1962; Birkmayer & Hornikewicz, 1962; Cotzias *et al.*, 1967). Besides pharmacological therapy, surgical interventions likewise have a long-standing history in Parkinson's disease treatment (Speelman & Bosch, 1998). Although public awareness of Parkinson's disease has been heightened by recognition of the disease in certain actors, political leaders, and public figures, probably the most notorious historical figure afflicted with parkinsonism was Adolph Hitler (Gerstenbrand & Karamat, 1999; Horowski *et al.*, 2000).

Morphological patterns of vulnerability (pathology)

Pathological findings of Parkinson's disease are discreetly dispersed in highly specific regions of the central nervous system (see Chapter 39). The primary focus of disease involvement is the *pars compacta* portion of the substantia nigra in the midbrain where marked depigmentation and neuronal loss occur (Jankovic & Stacy, 1999). These cells project predominantly to the putamen. In addition to degeneration, intracytoplasmic eosinophilic inclusion bodies, termed Lewy bodies, are a hallmark of Parkinson's disease and occur in the substantia nigra as well as other pigmented nuclei like the locus ceruleus and the dorsal motor nucleus of the vagus nerve (Andersen, 2000). Lewy bodies are composed of neurofilament tubulin components, alpha-synuclein, ubiquitin and Torsin A, a protein product of the DYT1 gene (Lucking & Brice, 2000). Pale bodies are also characteristic of Parkinson's disease, are composed of neurofilament interspersed with vacuolar granuels, and distribute themselves in the substantia nigra as well as the basal ganglia, cortex, brainstem and spinal cord (Shashidharan *et al.*, 2000). Because of the relatively discreet areas of neuronal loss, research efforts have been directed towards specific biochemical features of nigrostriatal cells in an effort to understand their selective vulnerability.

Biochemical patterns of vulnerability (neurochemistry)

Because the degenerating cells of the substantia nigra produce the neurochemical, dopamine, Parkinson's disease has become the prototypic disorder of a single neurochemical deficiency affecting a single primary anatomical system (see Chapter 39). Anatomical and physiological studies of parkinsonian animals and patients with Parkinson's disease confirm the important balance between two dopaminergic systems, termed the direct and indirect (Obeso *et al.*, 2000; Smith & Kieval, 2000; Beal, 2001). The protypic construct posits that in Parkinson's disease, activity in the direct pathway, linked to the D1 receptors, is diminished and activity in the indirect pathway, linked to D2 receptors, is enhanced (Graybiel, 2000). These effects cause aberrant outflow from the globus pallidus, subthalamic nucleus, and thalamus to decrease thalamo-cortical activation. Several other nuclei and transmitter receptor systems play indirectly into this basic system. Some inconsistencies in this archetypic schema exist and have prompted continual studies and resultant modifications (Blandini *et al.*, 2000; Rodriquez *et al.*, 2000).

A number of intertwining biochemical clues have suggested that Parkinson's disease involves free radical toxicity from oxidative reactions (Olanow, 1990). MPTP, a designer drug self-injected by drug addicts, causes a clinical syndrome closely resembling Parkinson's disease and represents the single best example of an environmental compound that can induce parkinsonism without marked accompanying signs of diffuse or multifocal neurotoxicity (Langston *et al.*, 1983). With the discoveries that MPTP is a protoxin, that MPP+ is the actual toxin, and that the conversion of MPTP to MPP+ involves the enzyme monoamine oxidase B, oxidative biochemistry gained increasing attention (Heikkila *et al.*, 1984). Based on the observation that animals treated with both MPTP and a monoamine oxidase B inhibitor did not develop parkinsonian toxic signs, a potential protective effect of monoamine oxidase B inhibition was suggested for Parkinson's disease.

Free radicals react almost instantaneously with membrane lipids and cause lipid peroxidation, membrane injury, and cell death (Grunblatt *et al.*, 2000). Dopamine is metabolized by oxidation reactions capable of generating free radical byproducts. Whereas the substantia nigra of Parkinson's disease patients contains high levels of iron, a facilitator of oxidation, and decreased levels of glutathione, a protector against free radical formation, these two features may explain in part the selective degeneration of nigral cells in Parkinson's disease (Youdim *et al.*, 1993). The specific interaction of dopamine and metal ions has been posited to activate an ordered cascade of events leading to cell death (Jimenez del Rio & Velez-Pardo, 2000). Mitochondrial respiratory failure and oxidative stress appear to be two important contributors to neuronal death in the substantia nigra of patients with Parkinson's disease. Complex I deficiency, reported by many investigators, appears to be one of the basic abnormalities related to this respiratory failure. It is not established whether Complex I deficiency is primary and inherited or secondary to environmental influences, and the deficiency may develop from a combination of the two. Second, it is still not established whether the identified Complex I deficiency is isolated,

diffuse, but more pronounced in the nigrostriatal system or equally distributed in all systemic cells. It is known that high dopamine content is in itself a high oxidative stress environment, suggesting at least one mechanism whereby the nigrostriatal system may be particularly vulnerable to degeneration by these mechanisms (Mizuno *et al.*, 1998b). These observations suggest that oxidative stress is a pivotal part of the biological basis of Parkinson's disease and that antioxidant therapies may slow down nigral degeneration in Parkinson's disease.

Other neurotransmitters besides dopamine, including norepinephrine and serotonin, are affected in Parkinson's disease, but unlike animal models of parkinsonism, human Parkinson's disease is not associated with changes in striatal expression of Substance P and methionine enkephalin (Levy *et al.*, 1995). New attention has particularly focused on the adenosine A2A receptor (Richardson, 2001), glutamate (Chase & Oh, 2000; Greenamyre *et al.*, 2001), neurotrophic factors (Howells *et al.*, 2000; Siegel & Chauhan, 2000), and more detailed analyses of the multiple subtypes of dopamine receptors (Oak *et al.*, 2000; Sealfon & Olanow, 2000). The pedunculopontine nucleus, predominantly under cholinergic control, is a current focus of physiologic studies of the initiation of programmed movements and sleep function (Pahapill & Lozano, 2000).

Concepts regarding etiology

In the past, neuroscientists implicitly held to the concept that Parkinson's disease was a single and specific morbid entity with a particular, though not yet identified, etiology. This pillar has been questioned (Duvoisin, 1989), with suggestions that nigral cells can be killed from multidimensional factors that include genetic, endogenous biochemical derangements, and exogenous toxins (see Chapters 1 and 2). The role of genetics in Parkinson's disease has been argued for decades, and the follow-up study from the World War II Veteran Twins Registry demonstrated an overall similarity in concordance for monozygotic and dizygotic twins. The study concluded that genetic influences were not important to the etiology of typical Parkinson's disease with onset after age 50, but among the few pairs of early-onset Parkinson's disease, these genetic influences appeared to be stronger (Tanner *et al.*, 1999). Nonetheless, in the past several years, well-described pedigrees with Mendelian dominant inheritance have been reported, but this pattern is clearly exceptional (Barbeau & Pourcher, 1982; Golbe *et al.*, 1990). Several pedigrees of familial parkinsonism have been linked to a mutation of alpha-synuclein (Polymeropoulos *et al.*, 1997; Krüger *et al.*,

2001; Spira *et al.*, 2001). Alpha-synuclein catalyses the formation of hydrogen peroxide, a product known to damage neuronal membranes (Saha *et al.*, 2000; Turnbull *et al.*, 2001) and accumulation is associated with neuronal death in laboratory models of Parkinson's disease. These observations led to the logical search for this same defect among Parkinson's disease patients. Several other groups have failed to find this defect in subjects with nonfamilial and other familial forms of Parkinson's disease (Chan *et al.*, 1998; Wang *et al.*, 1998; Khan *et al.*, 2001). These studies have suggested that synuclein may be a key factor to a variety of neurodegenerative disorders, collectively termed synucleinopathies (Galvin *et al.*, 2001). Recessively inherited juvenile parkinsonism appears to be linked to the gene termed PARKIN (Leroy *et al.*, 1998; Mizuno *et al.*, 1998a; Tassin *et al.*, 1998). Exonic deletion mutations of the same gene have also been reported in some series of patients with typical sporadic Parkinson's disease (Wang *et al.*, 1999; Klein *et al.*, 2000; Kobayashi *et al.*, 2000), although other investigators have not found these associations.

The new appreciation of mitochondrial genetics, whereby inheritance of DNA is strictly maternal, may provide clues to the role of genetically determined alterations in the mitochondrial respiratory chain and detoxication pathways (Mizuno *et al.*, 1988; DiMauro, 1993; de la Fuente-Fernandez, 2000). In this context, among five families in which Parkinson's disease occurred in a parent and multiple offspring, the proband parent was always a woman. Furthermore, the age of Parkinson's disease onset in the offspring was younger than in the mother whereas this 'anticipation' pattern is not seen with paternal inheritance (Wooten *et al.*, 1997). The manganese superoxide dismutase gene (Grasbon-Frodl *et al.*, 1999), the E_2 subunit of the alpha-ketoglutarate complex (Kobayashi *et al.*, 1998), alpha-1-antichymotrypsin gene polymorphisms (Munoz *et al.*, 1999), monamine oxidase B intron 13 allele polymorphisms (Checkoway *et al.*, 1998), the alpha-2 macroglobulin gene (Kruger *et al.*, 2000), and the catechol-*o*-methyltransferase gene (Mizuto *et al.*, 2000) are among the current areas of active research interest. A number of observations suggest a link between mitochondrial genetic and environmental etiologic hypotheses in Parkinson's disease. First, Complex I activity of the respiratory chain is reduced in the brains of Parkinson's disease patients; second, MPP+ acts directly on Complex I to inhibit activity and produce synaptosomal adenosine triphosphate depletion (Nicklas *et al.*, 1985). Involvement of the mitochondria in Parkinson's disease could relate to putative mutations in mitochondrial DNA (DiMauro, 1993). Despite this interest in mitochondrial genetics, however, data do not support a maternal mode of inheritance for most patients with Parkinson's disease. The polymorphic cytochrome P450 gene has been examined in numerous studies but also does not show a consistent pattern of defect (Bordet *et al.*, 1996; Diederich *et al.*, 1996). These studies underscore the likely complex genetic heterogeneity of Parkinson's disease, and each identified mutation may point towards an eventual common pathogenetic mechanism.

A major area of budding research is the identification of early diagnostic markers that might detect Parkinson's disease patients at a time when they are asymptomatic. The reports of diminished Complex I in platelets of Parkinson's disease patients are an example of these attempts, and numerous approaches with various biochemical products are being investigated (Parker *et al.*, 1989). The hypothesis that genetic susceptibility to Parkinson's disease was linked to chromosome 22q13 and the cytochrome P450 monooxygenase gene CYP2D6 has been argued for several years (Christensen *et al.*, 1998). Whereas most studies show no association between polymorphisms of CYP2D6 (Tsuneoka *et al.*, 1998), linkage disequilibrium with dinucleotide repeat markers mapping near CYP2D6 on ch22q13 may still be important (Wilhelmsen *et al.*, 1997; Kobayashi *et al.*, 1998). CYP2D6 polymorphisms have been associated with aging, a factor that may confound analyses of Parkinson's disease (Payami *et al.*, 2001). A meta-analysis of numerous prior publications suggested that polymorphisms of *N*-acetyltransferase-2, monoamine oxidase B, glutathione transferase and the mitochondrial gene tRNAGlu should be the primary focus of future linkage studies (Tan *et al.*, 2000). In one study of 137 Parkinson's disease patients, those with epsilon-4 apolipoprotein allele had a significantly earlier onset of parkinsonism than patients with epsilon3/epsilon 3 or epsilon2/epsilon 2. Such findings suggest apolipoprotein E genotypes may modulate age of onset of Parkinson's disease (Zareparsi *et al.*, 1998). In contrast to Alzheimer disease, Apolipoprotein E_4 does not appear to be associated with dementia in Parkinson's disease (Inzelberg *et al.*, 1998). A new focus of study has been delineation of the pro-apototic protein, Bax. This protein accumulates in substantia nigra cells after MPTP treatment and in Parkinson's disease (Tatton, 2000; Hartmann *et al.*, 2001). Furthermore, in animals treated with the dopamine cell toxin MPTP, ablation of Bax prevents dopaminergic degeneration (Vila *et al.*, 2001). These combined observations suggest that Bax ablation strategies may be a future therapeutic aim in Parkinson's disease (Ploix & Spier, 2001). Special attention has been placed on homovanillic acid levels in the cerebrospinal fluid, since this chemical is the breakdown product of central dopamine. Although the absolute levels of homovanillic acid do not correlate with disease severity, the ratio of homovanillic acid/xanthine is significantly different between patients with mild Parkinson's disease compared with controls (Litvan *et al.*, 1998).

Cardinal motor features

Parkinsonism is a clinical diagnosis based on the signs of resting tremor, bradykinesia or slowness of movement, rigidity, and loss of postural reflexes. Several diseases can be associated with these signs and are termed parkinsonian syndromes as a group; Parkinson's disease is the prototype, and in this condition, parkinsonian signs occur in isolation without other marked evidence of major neuropathologic change (Litvan *et al.*, 1998).

Of all the parkinsonian signs, tremor is the most distinctive. Tremor is a to-and-fro rhythmic involuntary movement, and the typical parkinsonian tremor occurs prominently at rest when the body part is completely relaxed. During activity or the maintenance of a posture, tremor may be modestly present, but these activities do not induce marked shaking. Resting tremor is primarily seen in the jaw, and extremities and when it affects the hands, the term 'pill-rolling' has been historically honored. Whereas the prototypic tremor occurs at rest, the tremor that can occur during activity may contribute to physiologic changes underlying bradykinesia (Carboncini *et al.*, 2001). Bradykinesia means slowness of movement in the absence of weakness and patients with Parkinson's disease initiate and carry out movements at a slow speed and with intermittent interruptions in the smooth rhythm of normal tasks. Buttoning buttons, writing, and performing fine motor tasks are affected as well as large body movements like rising from a soft chair or car seat. The third cardinal feature of Parkinson's disease is rigidity, or increased muscle tone that affects both agonist and antagonist muscles simultaneously. As the examiner moves the patient's arm, wrist or leg through the given joint's full range, the extremity moves with passive resistance and a give-and-take or ratchet-like movement, termed cogwheel rigidity. The final cardinal feature of parkinsonism is compromised postural reflexes with balance difficulties. The patient may experience this sign with a sense of unsteadiness, stumbling or falls. The examiner tests this feature by standing behind the patient and pulling briskly on the shoulders in order to displace the patient's frame of gravity. Whereas the normal response is one or two steps backwards, the parkinsonian subject takes several steps backwards and may even fall.

Whereas these cardinal signs are seen in Parkinson's disease as well as other parkinsonian syndromes distinct from Parkinson's disease, signs that additionally help the clinician to distinguish Parkinson's disease clinically are asymmetry of parkinsonian signs, marked rest tremor, a clinically significant response to the dopaminergic medications, usually levodopa (see Chapter 42), and little or no balance problems in the first months and years of the disease (Lang & Lozano, 1998). The pattern of asymmetry persists throughout the disease, even as late as 15 years after onset (Lee *et al.*, 1995). These features are guidelines and although not foolproof, until an accurate biological marker of Parkinson's disease is discovered, clinical features are the best criteria for diagnosing the neurologic disorder during life (Weiner & Lang, 1989). Among Parkinson's disease specialists who diagnosed early Parkinson's disease in a large cohort of untreated patients, 8.1% were later found to have another diagnosis after 7.6 years of follow-up (Jankovic, 2000).

Especially in the early months of Parkinson's disease, parkinsonian signs may be particularly subtle and patients may only complain of slowness, stiffness, and trouble with handwriting, usually noting that their script has become small, cramped and tremulous (micrographia). Physicians are often tempted to diagnose arthritis, depression, or normal aging unless rest tremor is evident. Particular attention to the history of tremor, even if not visible in the office, to slowness of fine motor control, and to a hunched and slightly flexed posture may permit the clinician to diagnose Parkinson's disease in its very early phases.

Moderate and advanced Parkinson's disease patients develop increasing gait difficulty, bradykinesia and tremor, plus a number of motor and non-motor complications that relate to both the progressive disease and its treatment (see section 'Time course of the disease'). In the very late stages of the illness, sometimes tremor decreases. Although most aspects of Parkinson's disease are managed in an outpatient ambulatory setting, physicians can see Parkinson's disease patients in the emergency room because of falls, freezing, malignant neuroleptic-like syndromes due to decreasing or stopping medications, psychosis, and panic episodes (Factor & Molho, 2000). Falls can be associated with fractures, and resultant imposed immobility and pain medication utilization that can collectively compromise patient autonomy and independence (Gray & Hildebrand, 2000).

Other clinical features

Among the behavioral and cognitive troubles experienced by Parkinson's disease patients, depression occurs in approximately one third of patients, especially in

Parkinson's disease patients who have akinesia and rigidity as their predominant symptoms (Hoogendijk et al., 1998; Starkstein et al., 1998). Dementia occurs in approximately one-third of patients and hallucinations and psychotic behavior in approximately one fourth of chronically treated patients (Gotham et al., 1986). Hallucinations in Parkinson's disease usually involve vivid images of people often familiar to the patient (Goetz, 1999; Fenelon et al., 2000; Holroyd et al., 2001). Several studies have linked hallucinations to co-existent REM-related sleep disorders (Pappert et al., 1999; Arnulf et al., 2000b). The biological basis of hallucinations has been studied with molecular biology techniques and, among Parkinson's disease patients with hallucinations, dopamine receptor gene polymorphisms do not differ from patients without hallucinations (Makoff et al., 2000). Parkinson's disease patients with hallucinations do not have the dopamine receptor polymorphisms seen in hallucinating patients with Alzheimer's disease (Goetz et al., 2001).

Dementia is more likely to develop in patients whose parkinsonism did not include tremor in the early phases of clinical disease (Roos et al., 1996). A recent study showed that non-demented patients with Parkinson's disease had impaired ability to incrementally learn associations, which is a prerequisite for habit learning. This impairment is reversed by administration of levodopa, suggesting that association learning involves dopaminergic neostriatal pathways (Knowlton et al., 1996). Tests that involve maintenance of attention, executive function, and working memory are particularly affected in Parkinson's disease (Dujardin et al., 2001).

The retina is rich in dopamine, and contrast sensitivity and color discrimination are impaired in Parkinson's disease patients (Buttner et al., 2000). Parkinson's disease subjects experience both physical and mental fatigue (Lou et al., 2001). Quality of life measures demonstrate the marked impact of Parkinson's disease on the patient's life; and depression, stress, and insomnia or other sleep disorders account for many of these compromises (Tandberg et al., 1998; Karlsen et al., 1999; Schrag et al., 2000b). Daytime sleepiness, due to Parkinson's disease itself, or secondary to poor nocturnal sleep or drug effects, can be particularly problematic and may affect driving safety (Frucht et al., 2000; Lachenmayer, 2000; Olanow et al., 2000; Razmy & Shapiro, 2000). Olfactory disturbances in odor identification, recognition, and detection thresholds occur in Parkinson's disease and resemble patterns seen in Alzheimer disease patients (Mesholam et al., 1998; Liberini et al., 2000; Tissingh et al., 2001). Several studies have suggested that even before motor signs of parkinsonism develop, distinc-

tive personality traits, including introversion and low risk-taking, may be more frequent among Parkinson's disease subjects compared to other family members or the general population (Menza, 2000).

The autonomic nervous system is also affected by Parkinson's disease, and orthostatic hypotension, abnormal cardiac reflexes and aberrant perspiration responses are frequently encountered (Goetz et al., 1986). Urological problems including urgency and nocturia, as well as sexual dysfunction, both impotence and hypersexual behaviour, can significantly impact on overall function and require pharmacological interventions (Araki et al., 2000; Jacobs et al., 2000). Dysautonomia is an inherent part of Parkinson's disease, but is also induced by dopaminergic and anticholinergic medications used to treat the motor elements of the disease.

Subtypes of Parkinson's disease

In a large US–Canadian database on 800 early Parkinson's disease subjects, three clinical subgroups were apparent early in the disease: those with tremor-predominance, those with bradykinesia, postural instability and gait difficulty, and the largest group with no specific predominance of symptoms. Postural instability and gait difficulty patients were motorically more functionally impaired early in their disease, and those who experienced balance problems within 1-year of symptom onset recalled experiencing gait and balance problems from the onset of their disease (Jankovic et al., 1990). Whereas very early gait impairment can occur in Parkinson's disease, other parkinsonian syndromes, such as progressive supranuclear palsy, should be considered in subjects with this clinical presentation (Litvan et al., 1996).

Clinical subgroups often used for comparisons include tremor-predominant versus akinetic/rigid-predominant variants, and young-onset (usually onset between age 21 and 40 years) vs. later onset Parkinson's disease. As a group, tremor-predominant patients progress in motor impairment slower than the akinetic/rigid patients, and young-onset patients have more preserved cognitive function and fewer falls than subjects with elderly disease onset (Schrag et al., 1998; Colcher & Simuni, 1999). On the other hand, subjects with younger onset Parkinson's disease appear to be especially prone to dyskinesias or involuntary movements, although whether this problem relates to their early and prolonged use of medications or relates specifically to their Parkinson's disease has not been specifically determined.

Time course of the disease

Parkinson's disease is known to be a slowly progressive disorder (Poewe & Wenning, 1998; Muller *et al.*, 2000). The classic study by Hoehn and Yahr (1967) documented that disease duration is closely associated with progressive disability. Marttila and Rinne examined a large cohort of Parkinson's disease subjects and concluded that patients remain at mild stages (unilateral or bilateral, but with retained postural reflex responses) for approximately 5 years. One index of progression is the need for levodopa, the primary symptomatic treatment for Parkinson's disease. Among 100 consecutive patients with Parkinson's disease who were not receiving levodopa at their first university centre evaluation, the mean duration of symptoms until levodopa was needed was 48 months, but half the cohort met this milestone by 3 years. The primary reason for starting therapy was progression of balance and gait impairment (Goetz *et al.*, 1987). Other elements of disease progression that lead to the introduction of dopaminergic therapy include job insecurity, enhanced bradykinesia, and disabling tremor. Certain subgroups may have a more indolent course than others, and studies have suggested that young age of onset and tremor-predominant disease are less rapidly progressive (Wooten & Jankovic, 1992).

In addition to progressive tremor, slowness, and balance difficulties, the major problems that patients experience after 5 years of treatment for Parkinson's disease are motor fluctuations, dyskinesias and behavioural or cognitive changes. The mechanisms behind these complications relate both to the underlying Parkinson's disease and to the effects of medications. There are several forms of motor fluctuations. Most commonly, a predictable decline in motor performance occurs near the end of each medication dose. Patients change gradually from 'on' meaning a good medication response into an 'off' period motorically declining 30 minutes to 1 hour before the next medication dose is due. Often patients experience involuntary movements, termed dyskinesias, as a peak-dose complication, and sometimes similar movements occur at the end of the dose. Rarely, sudden and severe cataclysms of motor fluctuation occur, with ambulatory patients becoming immobilized over seconds (de Jong *et al.*, 1987). Because these fluctuations occur throughout the day, accurate detection requires cooperation by the patient who must be trained to complete diaries of functions (Hauser *et al.*, 2000). These journals generally divide the 24-hour day into 30-minute segments to detect good medication response ('on'), poor medication response ('off'), disabling dyskinesias and sleep. Some, but not all, dyskinesias and fluctuations correlate with alterations in plasma levodopa levels (Kurth *et al.*, 1993), although the pharmacologic mechanisms underlying relief of parkinsonism and the production of dyskinesia appear to be different (Schuh & Bennett, 1993). Patients with motor fluctuations show presynaptic and postsynaptic central changes that occur in the dopaminergic striatal system (Colosimo & DeMichele, 1999). Studies have suggested that alterations of basal ganglion physiology in association with dyskinesia include overt changes in average firing rates of neurons and modulations of cell-to-cell communication within subregions of the basal ganglion circuitry (Brotchie, 2000; Hirsch, 2000). Additionally, the NMDA–glutamate system and striatal opioid transmission is involved in the pathophysiology of dyskinesia in Parkinson's disease (Greenamyre & O'Brien, 1991; Piccini *et al.*, 1997).

Whereas the cumulative medical literature derived largely from university-based populations suggests that dyskinesia and motor fluctuation are common among chronically treated patients with Parkinson's disease, one community-based study found that 78% of Parkinson's disease subjects did not have fluctuations (Larsen *et al.*, 2000; Ahlskog & Muenter, 2001).

Progressive compromise in quality of life occurs with prolonged Parkinson's disease (Schrag *et al.*, 2000). Over a 4-year period, 111 patients were examined with standardized measures and significantly declined in quality of life indices that reflected physical disability, but also emotional function, pain and social interaction (Karlsen *et al.*, 2000). Because the risk for dementia is approximately sixfold in Parkinson's disease compared with the general population, this factor impacts on caregiver stress and patient consent to medical treatment because of competency issues (Aarsland *et al.*, 2001; Dymek *et al.*, 2001). Progressive disease places patients at particular risk for hip fractures (Sato *et al.*, 2001) and nursing home placement especially when hallucinations are prominent (Goetz & Stebbins, 1992; Aarsland *et al.*, 2000).

After the discovery of specific therapy for Parkinson's disease (see Chapter 42), mortality figures changed. Prior to the availability of levodopa, observed-to-expected death ratio was 2.9, but with drug treatment, later reports argued that life expectancy in Parkinson's disease was normal (Joseph *et al.*, 1978). More recent studies, however, suggest that mortality may still be increased in Parkinson's disease relative to the general population (Uitti *et al.*, 1993; Clarke, 1995). Added dementia is the highest risk factor for shortened life (Louis *et al.*, 1996). In a community-based study, Parkinson's disease patients died more frequently from pneumonia and less frequently from cardiac disease than control subjects (Beyer *et al.*, 2001). Concerns that selegeline exposure could enhance cardiac-related mortality in Parkinson's disease subjects has been refuted (Donnan *et al.*, 2000).

Numerous strategies have been suggested to attempt an interruption in the natural progression of Parkinson's disease (see Chapter 42). Treatment with monoamine oxidase inhibitors, selegiline, delayed the need to start levodopa by approximately 9 months, although the biochemical mechanism of this effect has been debated (Parkinson Study Group, 1993). Because clinical signs of Parkinson's disease do not develop until dopamine levels reach only 20% of the normal level at birth, a long preclinical period likely exists, suggesting that such strategies could be useful.

Epidemiology

Besides essential tremor, Parkinson's disease is the most common movement disorder and affects approximately 500 000 people in the United States (Kessler, 1978). It is most frequently seen after the age of 50, and approximately 1% of this age group has the disorder. There is a modest (1.5:1) male predominance (Kessler, 1978; Knopio *et al.*, 1999). The gender prevalence differences are not explained, although in animal models of parkinsonism, testosterone does not potentiate damage to the nigrostriatal system and estrogen has inconsistent effects (Gao & Dluzen, 2001). Among women with Parkinson's disease and motor fluctuations, estrogen and progesterone shifts that coincide with the normal menstrual cycles bear no relationship to clinical motor impairments (Kompoliti *et al.*, 2000a). Several studies have suggested that Caucasians are affected more often than African-Americans, but this question is unsettled (Schoenberg *et al.*, 1988). Joint analysis of five European communities identified no substantial difference in prevalence of Parkinson's disease across European countries. The overall prevalence was 1.6 per 100 population, and a substantial proportion of patients with clear-cut clinical Parkinson's disease had never sought medical attention or been previously diagnosed (de Rijk *et al.*, 1997).

Numerous population studies have documented that Parkinson's disease is more common in highly industrialized countries than in agricultural societies, and more frequent in Europe and North America than in the Far East (Tanner *et al.*, 1989; Rajput, 1993). Several studies suggest that exposure to chronic well water drinking and living near or working with industrial chemicals and pesticide or herbicide products increase the risk for early-onset Parkinson's disease (Tanner *et al.*, 1989; Rajput, 1993). Using an urban United States multiethnic community, logistic regression models demonstrated that rural living, area farming, and well water drinking were associated with Parkinson's disease only in African-Americans, whereas in Hispanic areas, farming was protective, and drinking unfiltered water was a risk factor (Marder *et al.*, 1998a). In Denmark, a consistent pattern of high Parkinson's disease morbidity was found among occupational groups employed in agriculture and horticulture (Tuchsen & Jensen, 2000). The concept that well water might accumulate chemical products more readily than free-flowing water has indirectly supported an environmental hypothesis of Parkinson's disease. Of interest, MPTP, a selective dopaminergic cell toxin associated with parkinsonism, was industrially developed as a potential herbicide, but was never produced commercially. The herbicide, rotenone, with potent inhibitory activity on Complex I mitochondrial activity, is of particular current research interest (Adam, 2000; Greenamyre *et al.*, 2001; Jenner, 2001).

Epidemiological studies have confirmed that smoking is less frequent among subjects with Parkinson's disease (Benedetti *et al.*, 2000; Elbaz *et al.*, 2000). Coffee consumption was likewise less frequent among Parkinson's disease subjects (Benedetti *et al.*, 2000), whereas tea drinking has been reported to be more frequent (Preux *et al.*, 2000). Based on the observations that genetic polymorphisms of dopamine D2 receptors influence dopamine response and are associated with cigarette smoking, genetic and environmental factors have been suggested to interact in the pathogenesis of Parkinson's disease (Costa-Mallen *et al.*, 2000). Exposure to hydrocarbons has also been linked to Parkinson's disease (Pezzoli *et al.*, 2000) and the issue of chronic manganese exposure as a risk factor has been debated (Racette *et al.*, 2000).

Because epidemiology research usually involves the screening of large numbers of subjects, efforts have focused on the development of special assessment tools that maximize diagnostic sensitivity and specificity (Chan *et al.*, 2000; Reider & Hubble, 2000). These tests range from questionnaires to brief examinations or involve videotaping protocols that can be performed in the field and then evaluated by experts (Camicioli *et al.*, 2001).

Neuroimaging

PET is among the most important tools for studying the biological basis of changes in dopamine neurochemistry in sporadic Parkinson's disease and familial parkinsonism associated with the PARKIN gene (Eldelberg *et al.*, 1995; Hilker *et al.*, 2001). The development of radioligands for dopamine transporters and receptors permits the study of both presynaptic and postsynaptic mechanisms in Parkinson's disease (Volkow *et al.*, 1998). For Parkinson's disease, PET studies of the effect of levodopa (L-[11C]-dopa) reflux show marked differences between patients with early versus late Parkinson's disease. In mildly affected patients, decreased putaminal influx occurs, whereas in advanced disease, a significant upregulation develops (Torstenson *et al.*, 1997). In subjects with motor fluctuations, putaminal [18F]Dopa uptake is reduced compared to non-fluctuators (Brooks, 2000a). As such, loss of striatal dopamine storage capacity in association with pulsatile exposure to exogenous levodopa may result in fluctuating and often aberrant synaptic dopamine levels, deranged basal ganglionic function, and both peak-dose dyskinesias and end-of-dose wearing off. Further studies using dopamine receptor ligands demonstrate that extrastriatal D2 receptor binding and D3 receptor binding markedly decrease in the dorsolateral prefrontal cortex, anterior cingulate cortex, and medial thalamus among patients with advanced Parkinson's disease (Kaasinen *et al.*, 2000). Additional PET studies of patients undergoing mental tasks that stress frontostriatal circuitry demonstrate marked deficits in Parkinson's disease patients and suggest that the dopamine depletion of Parkinson's disease disrupts basal gangliar outflow to the cortex through this pathway (Owen *et al.*, 1998).

Because an individual's severity of impairment in tremor, bradykinesia, rigidity, gait and balance are not equal, investigators have searched for the clinical signs that best correlate with the dopamine nigrostriatal lesion. In a combined clinical and PET analysis, bradykinesia was better correlated with changes in fluorodopa PET reduction than tremor, rigidity or postural disturbance. As an index of bradykinesia, performance in the Purdue Pegboard Test was the best indicator of fluorodopa PET changes (Vingerhoets *et al.*, 1997). Studies with dopamine transporter probes demonstrate reduced activity in the caudate nucleus and orbitofrontal cortex in association with walking in Parkinson's disease subjects (Ouchi *et al.*, 2001).

With SPECT scans, [123I]beta-CIT has been used as a ligand to measure presynaptic dopaminergic activity. In untreated Parkinson's disease patients, dopamine and serotonin transporter activity are decreased compared to healthy controls (Haapaniemi *et al.*, 2001). Decrements of approximately 10% each year occur in Parkinson's disease. Furthermore, dopamine transporter deficits correlate with motor impairment and disease duration. Similar dopamine transporter changes and correlation with clinical severity and disease duration occur in treated Parkinson's disease subjects as well (Benamer *et al.*, 2000). Scans differentiate patients with Parkinson's disease from those with essential tremor and with clinically diagnosed progressive supranuclear palsy (Asenbaum *et al.*, 1998; Messa *et al.*, 1998).

Future perspectives

In light of the significant advances that have developed in the past 5 years, it is reasonable to hypothesize that the primary chemical cascade of biochemical reactions leading to nigrostriatal death in Parkinson's disease will be discovered shortly. Once this series of reactions is delineated, 'designer drugs' aimed at interrupting this sequence at one or many steps can be envisioned. The extent to which these lessons will be extrapolated to other neurodegenerative disorders will depend on whether the biochemical cascade that leads to cell death is a general neuronal one or highly specific to the cellular function of nigrostriatal cells. It is likely that some chemical reactions are shared by all neurons, but the relatively selective nigrostriatal dopaminergic cell loss of Parkinson's disease suggests that chemical reactions specific to these cells are important determinants of the pathogenesis of this unique neurodegenerative disease.

REFERENCES

Aarsland, D., Larsen, J. P., Tandberg, E. & Laake, K. (2000). Predictors of nursing home placement in Parkinson's disease: a population-based, prospective study. *J. Am. Geriatr. Soc.*, **48**, 938–42.

Aarsland, D., Anderson, K., Larsen, J. P., Lolk, A., Nielsen, H. & Kragh-Sorenson, P. (2001). Risk of dementia in Parkinson's disease: a community-based, prospective study. *Neurology*, **56**, 736–6.

Adam, D. (2000). Pesticide use linked to Parkinson's disease. *Nature*, **408**, 125.

Ahlskog, J. E. & Muenter, M. D. (2001). Frequency of levodopa-related dyskinesias and motor fluctuations as estimated from the cumulative literature. *Mov. Disord.*, **16**, 448–58.

Andersen, J. K. (2000). What causes the build-up of ubiquitin-containing inclusions in Parkinson's disease? *Mech Ageing Dev.*, **118**, 15–22.

Araki, I., Kitahara, M., Oida, T. & Kuno, S. (2000). Voiding dysfunction and Parkinson's disease: urodynamic abnormalities and urinary symptoms. *J. Urol.*, **164**, 1640–3.

Arnulf, I., Bonnet, A. M., Damier, P. *et al.* (2000b). Hallucinations, REM sleep, and Parkinson's disease: a medical hypothesis. *Neurology*, **55**, 281–8.

Asenbaum, S., Pirker, W., Angelberger, P., Bencsits, G., Pruckmayer, M. & Brucke, T. (1998). [123I]beta-CIT and SPECT in essential tremor and Parkinson's disease. *J. Neural Transm.*, **105**, 1213–28.

Barbeau, A. (1962). The pathogenesis of Parkinson's disease: a new hypothesis. *Can. Med. Assoc. J.*, **87**, 802–7.

Barbeau, A. & Pourcher, E. (1982). New data on the genetics of Parkinson's disease. *Can. J. Neurol. Sci.*, **9**, 53–60.

Beal, M. F. (2001). Experimental models of Parkinson's disease. *Nat. Rev. Neurosci.*, **2**, 325–34.

Benamer, H. T., Patterson, J., Wyper, D. J., Hadley, D. M., Macphee, G. J. & Grosset, D. G. (2000). Correlation of Parkinson's disease severity and duration with 123I-FP-CIT SPECT striatal uptake. *Mov. Disord.*, **15**, 692–8.

Benedetti, M. D., Bower, J. H., Maraganore, D. M. *et al.* (2000). Smoking, alcohol, and coffee consumption preceding Parkinson's disease: a case-control study. *Neurology*, **55**, 1350–8.

Beyer, M. K., Herlofson, K., Arsland, D. & Larsen, J. P. (2001). Causes of death in a community-based study of Parkinson's disease. *Acta Neurol. Scand.*, **103**, 7–11.

Birkmayer, W. & Hornikewicz, O. (1961). Der L-dioxyphenylalanin (=L-Dopa) effekt bei der Parkinson-Akinesie. *Wien. Klin. Wochenschr.*, **73**, 787–8.

Blandini, F., Nappi, G., Tassorelli, C., F. & Martignoni, E. (2000). Functional changes of the basal ganglia circuitry in Parkinson's disease. *Prog. Neurobiol.*, **62**, 63–88.

Bordet, R., Broly, F. & Destée, A. (1996). Debrisoquine hydroxylation genotype in familial forms of idiopathic Parkinson's disease. *Adv. Neurol.*, **65**, 97–100.

Brissaud, E. (1895). *Leçons sur les Maladies Nerveuses*. Paris: Masson.

Brooks, D. J. (2000a). PET studies and motor complications in Parkinson's disease. *Trends Neurosci.*, **23** (Suppl 10), S101–8.

Brotchie, J. M. (2000). The neural mechanisms underlying levodopa-induced dyskinesia in Parkinson's disease. *Ann. Neurol.*, **47**, S105–12.

Buttner, T., Muller, T. & Kuhn, W. (2000). Effects of apomorphine on visual functions in Parkinson's disease. *J. Neural. Transm.*, **107**, 87–94.

Camicioli, R., Grossmann, S. J., Spencer, P. S., Hudnell, K. & Anger, W. K. (2001). Discriminating mild parkinsonism: methods for epidemiological research. *Mov. Disord.*, **16**, 33–40.

Carboncini, M. C., Manzoni, D., Strambi, S. *et al.* (2001). The relation between EMG activity and kinematic parameters strongly supports a role of the action tremor in parkinsonian bradykinesia. *Mov. Disord.*, **16**, 47–57.

Chan, P., Tanner, C. M., Jiang, X. & Langston, J. W. (1998). Failure to find the alpha-synuclein gene missense mutation (G209A) in 100 patients with younger onset Parkinson's disease. *Neurology*, **50**, 513–14.

Chan, D. K., Hung, W. T., Wong, A., Hu, E. & Beran, R. G. (2000). Validating a screening questionnaire for parkinsonism in Australia. *J. Neurol. Neurosurg. Psychiatry*, **69**, 117–20.

Charcot, J. M. (1879). Lecture V. on paralysis agitans. In *Lectures on Diseases of the Nervous system*, ed. J. M. Charcot (translator G. Sigerson). Philadelphia: HC Lea.

Chase, T. N. & Oh, J. D. (2000). Striatal dopamine- and glutamate-mediated dysregulation in experimental parkinsonism. *Trends Neurosci.*, **23**(Suppl 10), S86–91.

Checkoway, H., Franklin, G. M. & Costa-Mallen, P. (1998). A genetic polymorphism of MAO-B modifies the association of cigarette smoking and Parkinson's disease. *Neurology*, **50**, 1458–61.

Christensen, P. M., Gotzsche, P. C. & Brosen, K. (1998). The sparteine/debrisoquine (CYP2D6) oxidation polymorphism and the risk of Parkinson's disease: a meta-analysis. *Pharmacogenetics*, **8**, 473–9.

Clarke, C. E. (1995). Does levodopa therapy delay death in Parkinson's disease? A review of the evidence. *Mov. Disord.*, **10**(3), 250–6.

Colcher, A. & Simuni, T. (1999). Clinical manifestations of Parkinson's disease. *Med. Clin. North Am.*, **83**, 327–47.

Colosimo, C. & DeMichele, M. (1999). Motor fluctuations in Parkinson's disease: pathophysiology and treatment. *Eur. J. Neurol.*, **6**, 1–21.

Cotzias, G. C., Van Woert, M. H. & Schiffer, L. M. (1967). Aromatic amino acids and modification of parkinsonism. *N. Engl. J. Med.*, **276**, 374–9.

Costa-Mallen, P., Costa, L. G., Smith-Weller, T., Franklin, G. M., Swanson, P. D. & Checkoway, H. (2000). Genetic polymorphism of dopamine D2 receptors in Parkinson's disease and interactions with cigarette smoking and MAO-B intron 13 polymorphism. *J. Neurol. Neurosurg. Psychiatry*, **69**, 535–7.

de Jong, G. J., Meerwaldt, J. D. & Schmitz, P. I. M. (1987). Factors that influence the occurrence of response variations in Parkinson's disease. *Ann. Neurol.*, **22**, 4–7.

de la Fuente-Fernandez, R. (2000). Maternal effect on Parkinson's disease. *Ann. Neurol.*, **48**, 782–7.

de Rijk, M. C., Tzourio, C., Breteler, M. M. *et al.* (1997). Prevalence of parkinsonism and Parkinson's disease in Europe: the EUROPARKINSON Collaborative Study. European Community Concerted Action on the Epidemiology of Parkinson's Disease. *J. Neurol. Neurosurg. Psychiatry*, **62**, 10–15.

Diederich, N. J., Hilder, C., Goetz, C. G., Keipes, M., Hentges, F. & Metz, H. (1996). Genetic variability of the CYP2D6 gene is not a risk factor for sporadic Parkinson's disease. *Ann. Neurol.*, **40**, 233–4.

DiMauro, S. (1993). Mitochondrial involvement in Parkinson's disease. *Neurology*, **43**, 2170–2.

Donnan, P. T., Steinke, D. T., Stubbings, C., Davey, P. G. & MacDonald, T. M. (2000). Selegiline and mortality in subjects with Parkinson's disease: a longitudinal community study. *Neurology*, **55**, 1785–9.

Dujardin, K., Defebvre, L., Grunberg, C., Becquet, E. & Destee, A. (2001). Memory and executive function in sporadic and familial Parkinson's disease. *Brain*, **124**, 89–98.

Duvoisin, R. C. (1989). Is there a Parkinson's disease? In *Disorders of Movement*, ed. N. P. Quinn & P. G. Jenner, London: Academic Press.

Dymek, M. P., Atchison, P., Harrell, L. & Marson, D. C. (2001). Competency to consent to medical treatment in cognitively impaired patients with Parkinson's disease. *Neurology*, **56**, 17–24.

Eidelberg, D., Moeller, J. R., Ishikawa, T. *et al.* (1995). Early differential diagnosis of Parkinson's disease with ^{18}F-fluorodeoxyglucose and positron emission tomography. *Neurology*, **45**, 1195–2004.

Elbaz, A., Manubens-Bertran, J. M., Baldereschi, M. *et al.* (2000). Parkinson's disease, smoking, and family history. Europarkinson Study Group. *J. Neurol.*, **247**, 793–8.

Factor, S. A. & Molho, E. S. (2000). Emergency department presentations of patients with Parkinson's disease. *Am. J. Emerg. Med.*, **18**(2), 209–15.

Fenelon, G., Mahieux, F., Huon, R. & Ziegler, M. (2000). Hallucinations in Parkinson's disease. Prevalence, phenomenology and risk factors. *Brain*, **123**, 733–45.

Fleming, L., Mann, J. B., Bean, J., Briggle, T. & Sanchez-Ramos, J. R. (1994). Parkinson's disease and brain levels of organochlorine pesticides. *Ann. Neurol.*, **36**(Suppl 1), 100–3.

Frucht, S. J., Greene, P. E. & Fahn, S. (2000). Sleep disorders in Parkinson's disease: a wake-up call. *Mov. Disord.*, **15**, 601–3.

Galvin, J. E., Lee, V. M. & Trojanowski, J. Q. (2001). Synucleinopathies: clinical and pathological implications. *Arch. Neurol.*, **58**, 186–90.

Gao, X. & Dluzen, D. E. (2001). The effect of testosterone upon methamphetamine neurotoxicity of the nigrostriatal dopaminergic system. *Brain Res.*, **892**, 63–9.

Gerstenbrand, F. & Karamat, E. (1999). Adolf Hitler's Parkinson's disease and an attempt to analyze his personality structure. *Eur. J. Neurol.*, **6**, 121–7.

Goetz, C. G. (1999). Hallucinations in Parkinson's disease: the clinical syndrome. In *Advances in Neurology: Parkinson's Disease*, ed. G. M. Stern, vol. **80**, pp. 419–23. Philadelphia: Lippincott, Williams & Wilkins.

Goetz, C. G. & Stebbins, G. T. (1992). Risk factors for nursing home placement in Parkinson's disease. *Ann. Neurol.*, **32**, 250.

Goetz, C. G., Lutge, W. & Tanner, C. M. (1986). Autonomic dysfunction in Parkinson's disease. *Neurology*, **36**, 73–5.

Goetz, C. G., Tanner, C. M. & Shannon, K. M. (1987). Progression of Parkinson's disease without levodopa. *Neurology*, **37**, 695–8.

Goetz, C. G., Burke, P. F., Leurgans, S. *et al.* (2001). Genetic variation analysis in Parkinson's disease patients with and without hallucinations: case control study. *Arch. Neurol.*, **58**, 209–13.

Goetz, C. G., Chmura, T. A. & Lanska, D. J. (2001). The history of Parkinson's disease: Part 2 of the MDS-sponsored history of movement disorders exhibit, Barcelona, June 2000. *Mov. Dis.*, **16**(1), 156–61.

Golbe, L. I., Di Iorio, G., Bonavita, V., Miller, D. C. & Duvoisin, R. C. (1990). A large kindred with autosomal dominant Parkinson's disease. *Ann. Neurol.*, **27**, 276–82.

Gotham, A. M., Brown, R. G. & Marsden, C. D. (1986). Depression in Parkinson's disease: a quantitative and qualitative analysis. *J. Neurol. Neurosurg. Psychiatry*, **49**, 381–9.

Grasbon-Frodl, E. M., Kosel, S., Riess, O. & Muller, U. (1999). Analysis of mitochondrial targeting sequence and coding region polymorphisms of the manganese superoxide dismutase gene in German Parkinson's disease patients. *Biochem. Biophys. Res. Commun.*, **255**, 749–52.

Gray, P. & Hildebrand, K. (2000). Fall risk factors in Parkinson's disease. *J. Neurosci. Nurs.*, **32**, 222–8.

Graybiel, A. M. (2000). The basal ganglia. *Curr. Biol.*, **10**, R509–11.

Greenamyre, J. T. & O'Brien, C. F. (1991). NMDA antagonists in the treatment of Parkinson's disease. *Arch. Neurol.*, **48**, 977–81.

Greenfield, J. G. & Bosanquet, F. D. (1953). The brain-stem lesions in parkinsonism. *J. Neurol. Neurosurg. Psychiatry*, **16**, 213–26.

Greenamyre, J. T., Betarbet, R., Sherer, T. & Panov, A. (2001). Response: Parkinson's disease, pesticides and mitochondrial dysfunction. *Trends Neurosci.*, **24**, 247.

Grunblatt, E., Mandel, S. & Youdim, M. B. (2000). Neuroprotective strategies in Parkinson's disease using the models of 6-hydroxydopamine and MPTP. *Ann. NY Acad. Sci.*, **899**, 262–73.

Haapaniemi, T. H., Ahonen, A., Torniainen, P., Sotaniemi, K. A. & Myllyla, V. V. (2001). [123I]beta-CIT SPECT demonstrates decreased brain dopamine and serotonin transporter levels in untreated parkinsonian patients. *Mov. Disord.*, **16**, 124–30.

Hartmann, A., Michel, P. P., Troadec, J. D. *et al.* (2001). Is Bax a mitochondrial mediator in apoptotic death of dopaminergic neurons in Parkinson's disease? *J. Neurochem.*, m76, 1785–93.

Hauser, R. A., Friedlander, J., Zesiewicz, T. A. *et al.* (2000). A home diary to assess functional status in patients with Parkinson's disease with motor fluctuations and dyskinesia. *Clin. Neuropharmacol.*, **23**, 75–81.

Heikkila, R. E., Manzino, L., Cabbat, F. S. & Duvoisin, R. C. (1984). Protection against the dopaminergic neurotoxicity of MPTP by monoamine oxidase inhibitors. *Nature*, **311**, 467–9.

Hilker, R., Klein, C., Ghaemi, M. *et al.* (2001). Positron emission tomographic analysis of the nigrostriatal dopaminergic system in familial parkinsonism associated with mutations in the parkin gene. *Ann. Neurol.*, **49**, 367–76.

Hirsch, E. C. (2000). Nigrostriatal system plasticity in Parkinson's disease: effect of dopaminergic denervation and treatment. *Ann. Neurol.*, **47**, S115–20.

Hoehn, M. M. & Yahr, M. D. (1967). Parkinsonism: onset, progression and mortality. *Neurology*, **17**, 427–42.

Holroyd, S., Currie, L. & Wooten, G. F. (2001). Prospective study of hallucinations and delusions in Parkinson's disease. *J. Neurol. Neurosurg. Psychiatry*, **70**, 734–8.

Hoogendijk, W. J., Sommer, I. E., Tissingh, G. & Deeg, D. J. (1998). Depression in Parkinson's disease. The impact of symptom overlap on prevalence. *Psychosomatics*, **39**, 416–21.

Horowski, R., Horowski, L., Calne, S. M. & Calne, D. B. (2000). From Wilhelm von Humboldt to Hitler – are prominent people more prone to have Parkinson's disease? *Parkinsonism Relat. Disord.*, **6**, 205–14.

Howells, D. W., Porritt, M. J., Wong, J. Y. *et al.* (2000). Reduced BDNF mRNA expression in the Parkinson's disease substantia nigra. *Exp. Neurol.*, **166**, 127–35.

Inzelberg, R., Chapman, J., Treves, T. A. *et al.* (1998). Apolipoprotein E4 in Parkinson's disease and dementia: new data and meta-analysis of published studies. *Alzheimer Dis. Assoc. Disord.*, **12**, 45–8.

Jacobs, H., Vieregge, A. & Vieregge, P. (2000). Sexuality in young patients with Parkinson's disease: a population based comparison with healthy controls. *J. Neurol. Neurosurg. Psychiatry*, **69**, 550–2.

Jankovic, J. (2000). Parkinson's disease therapy: tailoring choices for early and late disease, young and old patients. *Clin. Neuropharmacol.*, **23**, 252–61.

Jankovic, J. & Stacy, M. (1999). Movement disorders. In *Textbook of Clinical Neurology*, pp. 655–79. Philadelphia: W. B. Saunders.

Jankovic, J., McDermott, M., Parkinson Study Group (1990). Variable expression of Parkinson's disease: a base-line analysis of the DATATOP cohort. *Neurology*, **40**, 1529–34.

Jenner, P. (2001). Parkinson's disease, pesticides and mitochondrial dysfunction. *Trends Neurosci.*, **24**, 245–6.

Jimenez del Rio, M. & Velez-Pardo, C. (2000). Molecular mechanism of monoamine toxicity in Parkinson's disease: hypothetical cell death model. *Med. Hypotheses*, **54**, 269–74.

Joseph, C., Chassan, J. B. & Koch, M. L. (1978). Levodopa in Parkinson's disease: a long-term appraisal of mortality. *Ann. Neurol.*, **3**, 116–18.

Kaasinen, V., Någren, K., Hietala, J. *et al.* (2000). Extrastriatal dopamine D2 and D3 receptors in early and advanced Parkinson's disease. *Neurology*, **54**, 1482–7.

Karlsen, K. H., Larsen, J. P., Tandberg, E. & Maeland, J. G. (1999). Influence of clinical and demographic variables on quality of life in patients with Parkinson's disease. *J. Neurol. Neurosurg. Psychiatry*, **66**, 431–5.

Karlsen, K. H., Tandberg, E., Aarsland, D. & Larsen, J. P. (2000). Health related quality of life in Parkinson's disease: a prospective longitudinal study. *J. Neurol. Neurosurg. Psychiatry*, **69**, 584–9.

Kessler, I. (1978). Parkinson's disease in epidemiologic perspective. *Adv. Neurol.*, **19**, 355–84.

Khan, N., Graham, E., Dixon, P. *et al.* (2001). Parkinson's disease is not associated with the combined alpha-synuclein/apolipoprotein E susceptibility genotype. *Ann. Neurol.*, **49**, 665–8.

Klein, C., Schumacher, K., Jacobs, H. *et al.* (2000). Association studies of Parkinson's disease and parkin polymorphisms. *Ann. Neurol.*, **48**, 126–7.

Knowlton, B. J., Mangels, J. A. & Squire L. R. (1996). A neostriatal habit learning system in humans. *Science*, **273**, 1399–402.

Kobayashi, T., Matsumine, H., Matuda, S. & Mizuno, Y. (1998). Association between the gene encoding the E2 subunit of the alpha-ketoglutarate dehydrogenase complex and Parkinson's disease. *Ann. Neurol.*, **43**, 120–3.

Kobayashi, T., Wang, M., Hattori, N., Matsumine, H., Kondo, T. & Mizuno, Y. (2000). Exonic deletion mutations of the Parkin gene among sporadic patients with Parkinson's disease. *Parkinsonism Relat. Disord.*, **6**, 129–31.

Kompoliti, K., Comella, C. L., Jaglin, J. A., Leurgans, S., Raman, R. & Goetz, C. G. (2000a). Menstrual-related changes in motoric function in women with Parkinson's disease. *Neurology*, **55**, 1572–5.

Kruger, R., Menezes-Saecker, A. M., Schols, L. *et al.* (2000). Genetic analysis of the alpha2-macroglobulin gene in early- and late-onset Parkinson's disease. *Neuroreport*, **11**, 2439–42.

Krüger, R., Kuhn, W., Leenders, K. L. *et al.* (2001). Familial parkinsonism with synuclein pathology. *Neurology*, **56**, 1355–62.

Kuopio, A. M., Marttila, R. J., Helenius, H. & Rinne, U. K. (1999). Changing epidemiology of Parkinson's disease in southwestern Finland. *Neurology*, **52**, 302–8.

Kurth, M. C., Tetrud, J. W., Irwin, I., Lyness, W. H. & Langston, J. W. (1993). Oral levodopa/carbidopa solution versus tablets in Parkinson's patients with severe fluctuations: a pilot study. *Neurology*, **43**, 1036–9.

Lachenmayer, L. (2000). Parkinson's disease and the ability to drive. *J. Neurol.*, **247** (Suppl 4), IV/28–30.

Lang, A. E. & Lozano, A. M. (1998). Parkinson's disease. First of two parts. *N. Engl. J. Med.*, **339**, 1044–53.

Langston, J. W., Ballard P., Tetrud, J. W. & Irwin, I. (1983). Chronic parkinsonism in humans due to a product of meperidine-analog synthesis. *Science*, **219**, 979–80.

Larsen, J. P., Karlsen K. & Tandberg, E. (2000). Clinical problems in non-fluctuating patients with Parkinson's disease: a community-based study. *Mov. Disord.*, **15**, 826–9.

Lee, C. S., Schulzer, M., Mak, E., Hammerstad, J. P., Calne, S. & Calne, D. B. (1995). Patterns of asymmetry do not change over the course of idiopathic parkinsonism: implications for pathogenesis. *Neurology*, **45**, 435–9.

Leroy E., Anastasopoulos, D., Konitsiotis, S., Lavedan, C. & Polymeropoulos, M. H. (1998). Deletions in the Parkin gene and genetic heterogeneity in a Greek family with early onset Parkinson's disease. *Hum. Genet.*, **103**, 424–7.

Levy, R., Vila, M., Herrero, M. T., Faucheux, B., Agid, Y. & Hirsch, E. C. (1995). Striatal expression of substance P and methionine-enkephalin in genes in patients with Parkinson's disease. *Neurosci. Lett.*, **199**, 220–4.

Liberini, P., Parola, S., Spano, P. F. & Antonini, L. (2000). Olfaction in Parkinson's disease: methods of assessment and clinical relevance. *J. Neurol.*, **247**, 88–96.

Litvan, I., Agid, Y., Jankovic, J. *et al.* (1996). Accuracy of clinical criteria for the diagnosis of progressive supranuclear palsy (Steele–Richardson–Olszewski syndrome). *Neurology*, **46**, 922–30.

Litvan, I., MacIntyre, A., Goetz, C. G. *et al.* (1998). Accuracy of the clinical diagnoses of Lewy body disease, Parkinson disease, and dementia with Lewy bodes: a clinicopathologic study. *Arch. Neurol.*, **55**, 969–78.

LeWitt, P. A., Galloway, M. P., Matson, W. & Milbury, P. (1992). Markers of dopamine metabolism in Parkinson's disease: the Parkinson Study Group. *Neurology*, **42**, 2111–17.

Lou, J. S., Kearns, G., Oken, B., Sexton, G. & Nutt, J. (2001). Exacerbated physical fatigue and mental fatigue in Parkinson's disease. *Mov. Disord.*, **16**, 190–6.

Louis, E. D., Marder, K., Coté, L. & Mayeux, R. (1996). Age at death is significantly younger in patients with Parkinson's disease who have dementia. *Neurology*, **46**(Suppl), A377.

Lucking, C. B. & Brice, A. (2000). Alpha-synuclein and Parkinson's disease. *Cell Mol. Life Sci.*, **57**, 1894–908.

Makoff, A. K., Graham, J. M., Arranz, M. J. *et al.* (2000). Association study of dopamine receptor gene polymorphisms with drug-induced hallucinations in patients with idiopathic Parkinson's disease. *Pharmacogenetics*, **10**, 43–8.

Marder, K., Logroscino, G., Alfaro, B. *et al.* (1998a). Environmental risk factors for Parkinson's disease in an urban multiethnic community. *Neurology*, **50**, 279–81.

Menza, M. (2000). The personality associated with Parkinson's disease. *Curr. Psychiatry Rep.*, **2**, 421–6.

Mesholam, R. I., Moberg, P. J., Mahr, R. N. & Doty, R. L. (1998). Olfaction in neurodegenerative disease: a meta-analysis of olfactory functioning in Alzheimer's and Parkinson's diseases. *Arch. Neurol.*, **55**, 84–90.

Messa, C., Volonte, M. A., Fazio, F. *et al.* (1998). Differential distribution of striatal [123I]beta-CIT in Parkinson's disease and progressive supranuclear palsy, evaluated with single-photon emission tomography. *Eur. J. Nucl. Med.*, **25**, 1270–6.

Mizuno, Y. K., Sone, N. & Suzuki, K. (1988). Inhibition of mitochondrial respiration by MPTP in mouse brain in vivo. *Neurosci. Lett.*, **91**, 349–53.

Mizuno, Y., Hattori, N. & Matsumine, H. (1998a) Neurochemical and neurogenetic correlates of Parkinson's disease. *J. Neurochem.*, **71**, 893–902.

Mizuno, Y., Yoshino, H., Ikebe, S. *et al.* (1998b). Mitochondrial dysfunction in Parkinson's disease. *Ann. Neurol.*, **44**, S99–109.

Mizuta, I., Mizuta, E., Yamasaki, S., Kuno, S., Yasuda, M. & Tanaka, C. (2000). Meta-analysis of polymorphism of the catechol-O-methyltransferase gene in relation to the etiology of Parkinson's disease in Japan. *Mov. Disord.*, **15**, 1013–14.

Muller, J., Wenning, G. K., Jellinger, K., McKee, A., Poewe, W. & Litvan, I. (2000). Progression of Hoehn and Yahr stages in parkinsonian disorders: a clinicopathologic study. *Neurology*, q**55**, 888–91.

Munoz, E., Obach, V., Oliva, R. *et al.* (1999). Alpha1-antichymotrypsin gene polymorphism and susceptibility to Parkinson's disease. *Neurology*, **52**, 297–301.

Nicklas, W. J., Vyas, I. & Heikkila, R. E. (1985). Inhibition of NADH-linked oxidation in brain mitochondria by MPTP. *Life Sci.*, **36**, 2503–8.

Oak, J. N., Oldenhof, J. & Van Tol, H. H. (2000). The dopamine D(4) receptor: one decade of research. *Eur. J. Pharmacol.*, **405**, 303–27.

Obeso, J. A., Rodriguez-Oroz, M. C., Rodriguez, M. *et al.* (2000). Pathophysiology of the basal ganglia in Parkinson's disease. *Trends Neurosci.*, **23**(Suppl 10), S8–19.

Olanow, C. W. (1990). Oxidative reactions in Parkinson's disease. *Neurology*, **40**(Suppl 3), 32–7.

Olanow, C. W., Schapira, A. H. & Roth, T. (2000). Waking up to sleep episodes in Parkinson's disease. *Mov. Disord.*, **15**, 212–15.

Ouchi, Y., Kanno, T., Okada, H. *et al.* (2001). Changes in dopamine availability in the nigrostriatal and mesocortical dopaminergic systems by gait in Parkinson's disease. *Brain*, **124**, 784–92.

Owen, A. M., Doyon, J., Dagher, A., Sadikot, A. & Evans, A. C. (1998). Abnormal basal ganglia outflow in Parkinson's disease identified with PET. Implications for higher cortical functions. *Brain*, **121**, 949–65.

Pahapill, P. A. & Lozano, A. M. (2000). The pedunculopontine nucleus and Parkinson's disease. *Brain*, **123**, 1767–83.

Pappert, E. J., Goetz, C. G., Niederman, F. G., Raman, R. & Leurgans, S. (1999). Hallucinations, sleep fragmentation, and altered dream phenomena in Parkinson's disease. *Mov. Disord.*, **14**, 117–21.

Parkinson, J. (1817). An essay on the shaking palsy. *Med. Classics*, **10**(2), 964–97.

Parker, W. D. Jr, Boyson, S. J. & Parks, J. K. (1989). Abnormalities of the electron transport chain in idiopathic Parkinson's disease. *Ann. Neurol.*, **26**, 719–23.

Parkinson Study Group (1993). Effects of tocopherol and deprenyl on the progress disability in early Parkinson's disease. *N. Engl. J. Med.*, **328**, 17.

Payami, H., Lee, N., Zareparsi, S. *et al.* (2001). Parkinson's disease, CYP2D6 polymorphism, and age. *Neurology*, **56**, 1363–70.

Pezzoli, G., Canesi, M., Antonini, A. *et al.* (2000). Hydrocarbon exposure and Parkinson's disease. *Neurology*, **55**, 667–73.

Piccini, P., Weeks, R. A. & Brooks, D. J. (1997). Alterations in opioid receptor binding in Parkinson's disease patients with levodopa-induced dyskinesias. *Ann. Neurol.*, **42**, 720–6.

Ploix, C. & Spier, A. D. (2001). Fighting Bax: towards a Parkinson's disease therapy. *Trends Neurosci.*, **24**, 255.

Poewe, W. H. & Wenning, G. K. (1998). The natural history of Parkinson's disease. *Ann. Neurol.*, **44**, S1–9.

Polymeropoulos, M. H., Lavedan, C., Leroy, E. *et al.* (1997). Mutation in the alpha-synuclein gene identified in families with Parkinson's disease. *Science*, **276**, 2045–7.

Preux, P. M., Condet, A., Anglade, C. *et al.* (2000). Parkinson's disease and environmental factors. Matched case-control study in the Limousin region, France. *Neuroepidemiology*, **19**, 333–7.

Racette, B. A., McGee-Minnich, L., Moerlein, S. M., Mink, J. W., Videen, T. O. & Permutter, J. S. (2000). Welding-related parkinsonism: clinical features, treatment, and pathophysiology. *Neurology*, **56**, 8–13.

Rajput, A. H. (1993). Environmental causation of Parkinson's disease. *Arch. Neurol.*, **50**, 651–2.

Razmy, A. & Shapiro, C. M. (2000). Interactions of sleep and Parkinson's disease. *Semin. Clin. Neuropsychiatry*, **5**(1), 20–32.

Reider, C. R. & Hubble, J. P. (2000). Test-retest reliability of an epidemiolgical instrument for Parkinson's disease. *J. Clin. Epidemiol.*, **53**, 863–5.

Richardson, P. J. (2001). The adenosine A2A receptor of the basal ganglia. *J. Physiol.*, **523**, 284.

Roberts, S. (1997). *James Parkinson 1755–1824; From Apothecary to General Practitioner.* London: Roy. Soc. Med. Press.

Rodriquez, M., Abdala, P. & Obeso, J. A. (2000). Excitatory responses in the 'direct' striatonigral pathway: effect of nigrostriatal lesion. *Mov. Disord.*, **15**, 795–803.

Roos, R. A. C., Jongen, J. C. F. & van der Velde, E. A. (1996). Clinical course of patients with Parkinson's disease. *Mov. Disord.*, **11**, 236–42.

Sato, Y., Kaji, M., Tsuru, T. & Oizumi, K. (2001). Risk factors for hip fracture among elderly patients with Parkinson's disease. *J. Neurol. Sci.*, **182**, 89–93.

Saha, A. R., Ninkina, N. N., Hanger, D. P., Anderton, B. H., Davies, A. M. & Buchman, V. L. (2000). Induction of neuronal death by alpha-synuclein. *Eur. J. Neurosci.*, **12**, 3073–7.

Schoenberg, B. S., Osentokun, B. O., Adeuja, A. O. G. *et al.* (1988). Comparison of the prevalence of Parkinson's disease in black populations in rural United States and in rural Nigeria: door to door community studies. *Neurology*, **38**, 645–6.

Schrag, A., Ben-Shlomo, Y., Brown, R., Marsden, C. D. & Quinn, N. (1998). Young-onset Parkinson's disease revisited – clinical features, natural history, and mortality. *Mov. Disord.*, **13**, 885–94.

Schrag, A., Jahanshahi, M. & Quinn, N. (2000). How does Parkinson's disease affect quality of life? A comparison with quality of life in the general population. *Mov. Disord.*, **15**, 1112–18.

Schuh, L. A. & Bennett, J. P. (1993). Suppression of dyskinesias in advanced Parkinson's disease. *Neurology*, **43**, 1545–50.

Sealfon, S. C. & Olanow, C. W. (2000). Dopamine receptors: from structure to behavior. *Trends Neurosci.*, **23**(Suppl 10), S34–40.

Shashidharan, P., Good, P. F., Hsu, A., Perl, D. P., Brin, M. F. & Olanow, C. W. (2000). TorsinA accumulation in Lewy bodies in sporadic Parkinson's disease. *Brain Res.*, **877**, 379–81.

Siegel, G. J. & Chauhan, N. B. (2000). Neurotrophic factors in Alzheimer's and Parkinson's disease brain. *Brain Res. Rev.*, **33**, 199–227.

Smith, Y. & Kieval, J. Z. (2000). Anatomy of the dopamine system in the basal ganglia. *Trends Neurosci.*, **23**(Suppl 10), S28–33.

Speelman, J. D. & Bosch, D. A. (1998). Resurgence of functional neurosurgery for Parkinson's disease: a historical perspective. *Mov. Disord.*, **13**, 582–8.

Spira, P. J., Sharpe, D. M., Halliday G., Cavanagh, J. & Nicholson, G. A. (2001). Clinical and pathological features of a parkinsonian syndrome in a family with an Ala53Thr alpha-synuclein mutation. *Ann. Neurol.*, **49**, 313–19.

Starkstein, S. E., Petracca, G., Chemerinski, E. *et al.* (1998). Depression in classic versus akinetic-rigid Parkinson's disease. *Mov. Disord.*, **13**, 29–33.

Tan, E. K., Khajavi, M., Thornby, J. I., Nagamitsu, S., Jankovic, J. & Ashizawa, T. (2000). Variability and validity of polymorphism association studies in Parkinson's disease. *Neurology*, **55**, 533–8.

Tandberg, E., Larsen, J. P. & Karlsen, K. (1998). A community-based study of sleep disorders in patients with Parkinson's disease. *Mov. Disord.*, **13**, 895–9.

Tanner, C. M. & Aston, D. A. (2000). Epidemiology of Parkinson's disease and akinetic syndromes. *Curr. Opin. Neurol.*, **13**, 427–30.

Tanner, C. M., Chen, B., Wang, W. *et al.* (1989). Environmental factors and Parkinson's disease: a case-control study in China. *Neurology*, **39**, 660–3.

Tanner, C. M., Ottman, R., Goldman, S. M. *et al.* (1999). Parkinson's disease in twins: an etiologic study. *J. Am. Med. Assoc.*, **281**, 341–6.

Tassin, J., Durr, A., deBroucker, T. *et al.* (1998). Chromosome 6-linked autosomal recessive early-onset Parkinsonism: linkage in European and Algerian families, extension of the clinical spectrum, and evidence of a small homozygous deletion in one family. The French Parkinson's Disease Genetics Study Group, and the European Consortium on Genetic Susceptibility in Parkinson's Disease. *Am. J. Hum. Genet.*, **63**, 88–94.

Tatton, N. A. (2000). Increased caspase 3 and Bax immunoreactivity accompany nuclear GAPDH translocation and neuronal apoptosis in Parkinson's disease. *Exp. Neurol.*, **166**, 29–43.

Tissingh, G., Berendse, H. W., Bergmans, P. *et al.* (2001). Loss of olfaction in de novo and treated Parkinson's disease: possible implications for early diagnosis. *Mov. Disord.*, **16**, 41–6.

Torstenson, R., Hartvig, P., Langstrom, B., Westerberg, G. & Tedroff, J. (1997). Differential effects of levodopa on dopaminergic function in early and advanced Parkinson's disease. *Ann. Neurol.*, **41**, 334–40.

Tsuneoka, Y., Matsuo, Y., Ichikawa, Y. & Watanabe, Y. (1998). Genetic analysis of the CYP2D6 gene in patients with Parkinson's disease. *Metabolism*, **47**, 94–6.

Tuchsen, F. & Jensen, A. A. (2000). Agricultural work and the risk of Parkinson's disease in Denmark, 1981–1993. *Scand. J. Work Environ. Hlth*, **26**, 359–62.

Turnbull, S., Tabner, B. J., El-Agnaf, O. M., Moore, S., Davies, Y. & Allsop, D. (2001). Alpha-synuclein implicated in Parkinson's disease catalyses the formation of hydrogen peroxide in vitro. *Free Radic. Biol. Med.*, **30**, 1163–70.

Uitti, R. J., Ahlskog, J. E., Maraganore, D. M. *et al.* (1993). Levodopa therapy and survival in idiopathic Parkinson's disease: Olmstead County project. *Neurology*, **43**, 1918–26.

Vila, M., Jackson-Lewis, V. V., Vukosavic, S. *et al.* (2001). Bax ablation prevents dopaminergic neurodegeneration in the 1-methyl-4-phenyl-1,2,3,6-tetrahydropyridine mouse model of Parkinson's disease. *Proc. Natl Acad. Sci., USA*, **98**, 2837–42.

Vingerhoets, F. J., Schulzer M., Calne, D. B. & Snow, B. J. (1997). Which clinical sign of Parkinson's disease best reflects the nigrostriatal lesion? *Ann. Neurol.*, **41**, 58–64.

Volkow, N. D., Wang, G. J., Fowler, J. S. *et al.* (1998). Parallel loss of presynaptic and postsynaptic dopamine markers in normal aging. *Ann. Neurol.*, **44**, 143–7.

Wang, W. W., Khajavi, M., Patel, B. J., Beach J. & Jankovic, J. (1998). The G209A mutation in the alpha-synuclein gene is not detected in familial cases of Parkinson's disease in non-Greek and/or Italian populations. *Arch. Neurol.*, **55**, 1521–3.

Wang, M., Hattori, N., Matsumine, H. *et al.* (1999). Polymorphism in the parkin gene in sporadic Parkinson's disease. *Ann. Neurol.*, **45**, 655–8.

Weiner, W. J. & Lang, A. E. (1989). *Movement Disorders*. New York: Futura Publ.

Wilhelmsen, K., Mirel, D., Marder, K. *et al.* (1997). Is there a genetic susceptibility locus for Parkinson's disease on chromosome 22q13? *Ann. Neurol.*, **41**, 813–17.

Wooten, M. P. & Jankovic, J. (1992). Movement disorders. In *Prognosis of Neurological Disorders*, ed. R. W. Evans, D. S. Baskin & F. M. Yatsu. New York: Oxford Univ. Press.

Wooten, G. F., Currie, L. J., Bennett, J. P., Harrison, M. B., Trugman, J. M. & Parker, W. D. Jr. (1997). Maternal inheritance in Parkinson's disease. *Ann. Neurol.*, **41**, 265–8.

Youdim, M. B. H., Ben-Shachar, D. & Riederer, P. (1993). The possible role of iron in the etiopathology of Parkinson's disease. *Mov. Disord.*, **8**(Suppl 1), 1–12.

Zareparsi, S., Kay, J., Camicioli, R. *et al.* (1998). Analysis of the alpha-synuclein G209A mutation in familial Parkinson's disease. *Lancet*, **351**, 37–8.

39

Neuropathology of Parkinson's disease

Dennis W. Dickson

Departments of Neuroscience and Pathology (Neuropathology), Mayo Clinic Jacksonville, FL, USA

Introduction

The clinical features of Parkinson's disease (PD) are bradykinesia, rigidity, tremor and postural instability, but increasingly recognized are non-motor manifestations, such as anosmia, autonomic dysfunction, sleep disorders, psychiatric symptoms (e.g. depression) and cognitive impairment. The typical clinical features of PD reflect well-known pathology in the dopaminergic nigrostriatal system, while extra-nigral pathology accounts for many of the non-motor features of PD. As will be subsequently discussed, the most characteristic pathologic feature of PD is neurodegeneration with Lewy body (LB) formation, but it must be acknowledged that occasionally other pathologic processes cause clinical features typical of PD. In particular, some cases of multiple system atrophy (MSA) or even progressive supranuclear palsy (PSP) may be clinically mistaken for PD (Bower et al., 2002). More problematic are cases of PD with juvenile onset or those associated with an autosomal recessive pattern of inheritance, such as cases with Parkin and DJ-1 mutations (see below), in which LBs may not be present. Other early onset familial cases present with atypical clinical features such as early dementia and psychosis, which are not characteristic of typical PD (Gwinn-Hardy et al. 2000). Another diagnostic challenge is the relationship of cognitive dysfunction in PD to concurrent Alzheimer's disease and dementia with Lewy bodies (DLB) (McKeith et al. 1996).

As in all neurologic syndromes, the clinical presentation reflects the neuroanatomy of the disease process more than the nature of the underlying pathology. The typical and defining clinical features of PD stem from the fact that the pathology responsible for the typical clinical syndrome is due to selective involvement of the nigrostriatal dopaminergic neurons (Jellinger, 1999), but these neurons are vulnerable to degeneration in other disorders (Fig. 39.1).

Moreover, postmortem neuropathologic studies clearly show that neurodegeneration in clinically typical PD is more extensive than merely the substantia nigra dopaminergic neurons. The early and late clinical manifestations of PD may bear little resemblance to the typical clinical picture of PD. For example, the olfactory bulb and brainstem reticular neurons are affected in almost all cases early in the disease, while neocortical involvement is almost universal later in the disease (Braak et al., 2003). Involvement of these structures may account for anosmia or autonomic features early and dementia later in the disease course, respectively.

Pathology of PD

The brain is usually grossly unremarkable until the brainstem is sectioned, and then loss of neuromelanin pigmentation in the substantia nigra and locus ceruleus becomes apparent (Fig. 39.2). Increase in rust color pigment is not uncommon in the substantia nigra and sometimes in the globus pallidus. Many cases, especially older patients, have varying degrees of frontal atrophy with mild dilation of the frontal horns of the lateral ventricle. None of these gross features is specific. Loss of pigment in the substantia nigra can be detected in many Parkinsonian disorders (Fig. 39.1). On the other hand, the relative involvement of the substantia nigra and locus ceruleus is sometimes helpful in the differential diagnosis. Many cases of Alzheimer's disease have pigment loss in the locus ceruleus, with normal pigmentation in the substantia nigra. In contrast, other Parkinsonian disorders have pigment loss in the substantia nigra with relatively normal pigmentation of the locus ceruleus (Table 39.1).

The histologic correlate of pigment loss in the substantia nigra and locus ceruleus is neuronal loss and gliosis with hyaline cytoplasmic inclusions (Fig. 39.3) first described

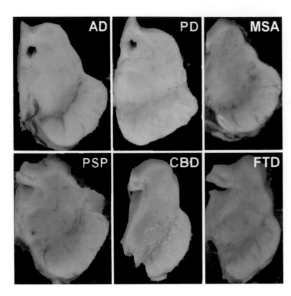

Fig. 39.1 Gross appearance of the midbrain is several disorders associated with Parkinsonism. Note normal pigment in substantia nigra in AD, but variable loss of nigral pigment in PD, MSA, PSP, CBD and FTD.

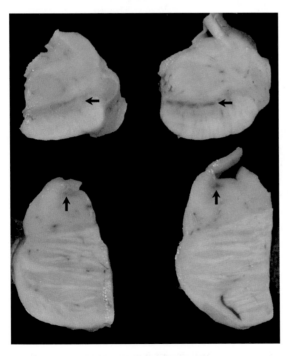

Fig. 39.2 Gross appearance of the midbrain (top pair) and pons (bottom pair) in typical PD (left) compared to age-matched control (right). Pigment loss is noted in both the locus ceruleus (vertical arrows) and the substantia nigra (horizontal arrows) in PD compared to normal.

Table 39.1. Differential diagnosis of Parkinsonism with respect to neuronal loss in the locus ceruleus and the substantia nigra

	Locus ceruleus	Substantia nigra
AD	↓↓	–
PD	↓↓	↓↓
PSP	↓	↓↓↓
CBD	↓	↓↓↓
MSA	–	↓↓
FTD	–	↓

(Severity of neuronal loss is indicated by '↓'. No significant neuronal loss is indicated by '–'.)

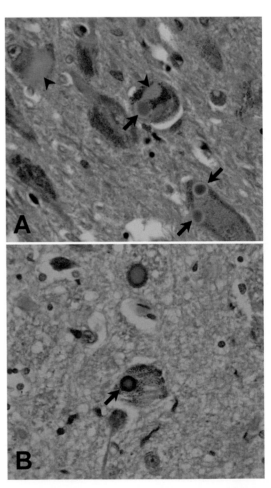

Fig. 39.3 Hyaline cytoplasmic inclusions, LBs (arrows), in substantia nigra with H&E (A) and synuclein immunostaining (B). Note also pale bodies considered to be precursors to LBs (arrow heads).

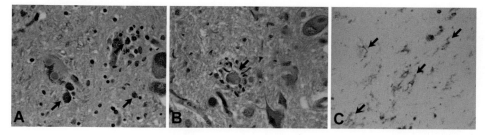

Fig. 39.4 Neuronal loss in substantia nigra. (A) extraneuronal neuromelanin in macrophages (arrows). (B) neuronophagia of a neuron with a LB (arrow). (C) microgliosis (reactive microglia – arrows) in the substantia nigra with HLA-DR immunostaining.

by Lewy in the early part of the twentieth century (Gibb & Poewe 1986). In typical PD, as in most other disorders associated with Parkinsonism, the neuronal loss in the substantia nigra is usually most marked in the ventrolateral tier of neurons (A9 dopaminergic neurons), which projects to the striatum, especially the putamen (Gibb & Lees, 1991). The more medial group of neurons (A10 dopaminergic neurons), which project to mesolimbic structures, is affected to a variable degree. Loss of neurons in the dorsal tier of the pars compacta may be more common in aging (Fearnley & Lees, 1991).

Neuronal loss in the substantia nigra is accompanied by astrocytosis and microglial activation (McGreer *et al.* 1998) (Fig. 39.4). The latter can be demonstrated with immunohistochemistry for class II major histocompatibility antigen, HLA-DR. The presence of HLA-DR in microglia indicates a state of functional activation typical of neuroinflammation, which may play a role in the progressive neuronal loss in the substantia nigra, although neuroinflammation is not currently considered to be a primary cause of degeneration (McGeer *et al.*, 2001). Neuromelanin pigment is often found in the cytoplasm of macrophages, which is a direct marker of loss of pigmented dopaminergic neurons, and occasionally neurons can be detected undergoing neuronophagia, or phagocytosis, by macrophages (Fig. 39.4). In most cases there is increased iron in the substantia nigra, which can be detected as a brown granular pigment and confirmed with special staining methods, such as Prussian blue stain. Iron pigment is almost always accompanied by swollen granular/foamy axonal spheroids (Fig. 39.5). The latter features are not specific to PD, but are also present in other parkinsonian disorders, most notably neuroaxonal dystrophies such as neurodegeneration with brain iron, formerly known as Hallervorden-Spatz disease (Jellinger & Duda, 2003).

The striatum is usually grossly normal in PD and with routine histologic methods there is usually no significant pathology. In contrast, immunohistochemical methods for synuclein often show lesions in the striatum in PD

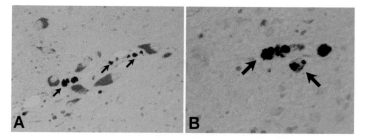

Fig. 39.5 Iron pigment in the substantia nigra. (A) Iron pigment (arrows) in the neuropil amongst pigmented neurons. (B) Perivascular iron pigment within macrophages (arrows). (Prussian blue stain)

(Duda *et al.*, 2002). This applies not only to PD with Lewy bodies, but to virtually all of the other disorders associated with clinical Parkinsonism, including PSP, MSA, corticobasal degeneration (CBD) and frontotemporal degeneration (Fig. 39.6). Striatal synuclein lesions increase with disease duration in PD and are especially dense in cases with dementia and diffuse Lewy bodies (Tsuboi *et al.*, 2003).

Lewy bodies (LBs) and Lewy neurites (LNs)

As noted above, concentric hyaline cytoplasmic inclusions or LBs are the most characteristic neuronal alteration in PD and are considered by some to be a *sine qua non* for the pathologic diagnosis of Parkinsonism (Hughes *et al.*, 2001). The latter is now a topic of current debate since some of the genetically determined causes of early onset Parkinsonism, such as PARK2 and PARK 7 (Table 39.2), which are autosomal recessive disorders with mutations in *Parkin* and *DJ-1*, respectively, are not always associated with LBs (Hardy *et al.*, 2003).

While most LBs are single and spherical, some neurons have multiple or pleomorphic LBs (Fig. 39.7). In some regions of the brain, such as the dorsal motor nucleus of the vagus and the basal nucleus of Meynert, similar inclusions are more often detected within neuronal processes.

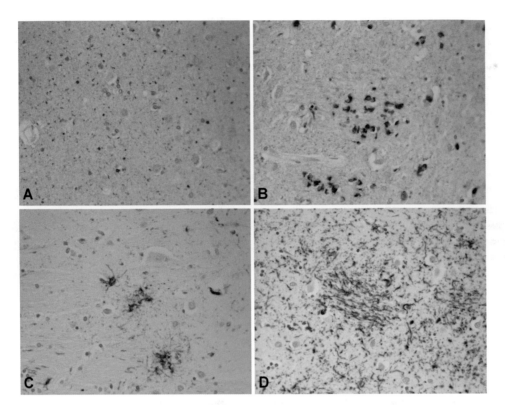

Fig. 39.6 Striatal pathology in parkinsonian disorders. (A) neuritic pathology revealed with synuclein immunohistochemistry in LBD. (B) Glial cytoplasmic inclusions in white matter bundles in multiple system atrophy revealed with synuclein immunohistochemistry. (C) Tufted astrocyte and threads in progressive supranuclear palsy revealed with tau immunohistochemistry. (D) Numerous threads in corticobasal degeneration revealed with tau immunohistochemistry.

The latter are sometimes referred to as 'intra-neuritic' LBs (Fig 39.8). Intra-neuritic-LBs can be detected in routine histopathologic preparations and should be distinguished from Lewy neurites (LNs), which are not visible in routine histopathology. Lewy neurites were first described in the hippocampus (Dickson *et al.*, 1991), but are also found in other regions of the brain, including the amygdala, cingulate gyrus and temporal cortex (Fig. 39.8). The density of LNs correlates with cognitive impairment (Churchyard & Lees, 1997).

Ultrastructural studies of LBs demonstrate non-membrane-bound, granulofilamentous structures within the cytoplasm of neurons. The central region of the LB usually contains amorphous dense material that lacks discernible detail, while the periphery has radially arranged 10 nm diameter filaments (Galloway *et al.*, 1992). At the electron microscopic level, LNs also have 10 nm filaments, but they lack a dense core and the filaments are more haphazardly arranged (Dickson *et al.*, 1991). LBs are also detected in cortical neurons and the latter, so-called

'cortical LBs' (cLBs) may be difficult to detect with routine histologic preparations (Fig. 39.9). They tend to be found in small non-pyramidal neurons in lower cortical layers, but can also be detected in pyramidal neurons. Occasionally, cLBs have a hyaline appearance similar to brainstem LBs (Masliah *et al.*, 1990). Ultrastructural studies of cortical LBs demonstrate poorly organized granulofilamentous structures, rather than the radial arrangement of filaments in classical LBs.

Composition of LBs

Immunohistochemical methods have indicated that, in addition to synuclein, LBs have other components (Pollanen *et al.*, 1993) (Table 39.3). Antibodies to neurofilament were first to be shown to label LBs (Goldman *et al.*, 1983), but most neurofilament antibodies label only a subset of LBs (Galvin *et al.*, 1997). Ubiquitin is present in most classical and cortical LBs (Kuzuhara *et al.*, 1988), but the

Table 39.2. Genetics and pathologic features of familial PD

Name	Locus and gene	Inheritance and clinical notes	Pathology	Comment
PARK1	4q21 α-synuclein	AD; early onset PD	LBD; diffuse cortical type	2 mutations (A53T, A30P); presynaptic protein
PARK2	6q25.2–27 Parkin	AR; juvenile onset PD; atypical features (dystonia & sleep benefit)	Nonspecific nigral loss; rare cases with LBs	Many mutations (substitutions, deletions, insertions); loss of function; ubiquitin E3 ligase
PARK3	2p13 unknown	AD; variable age of onset	LBD; typical brainstem type	
PARK4	4q21 α-synuclein	AD; early onset PD; dementia & dysautonomia	LBD; diffuse cortical type	Erroneous initial linkage to 4p15; SNCA multiplication & over-expression of α-synuclein
PARK5	4p14 ubiquitin C-terminal hydrolase	AD; late-onset PD	Unknown	Disputed as true linkage versus gene variant
PARK6	1p35–36 unknown	AR; early onset PD	Unknown	Compare PARK7 & PARK9 for linkage
PARK7	1p36DJ-1	AR; early onset PD	Unknown; heterozygous cases have LBs	DJ-1 function is unknown
PARK8	12p11.2–13.1 unknown	AD; late-onset PD	Variable pathology; some may have LBD, but nonspecific nigral degeneration may be more common	
PARK9	1p36 unknown	AR; early onset; parkinsonism with pyramidal syndrome	Unknown	Atypical parkinsonism phenotype; imaging studies
PARK10	1p32 unknown	Late-onset PD	Unknown	Population-based analysis (Icelandic)
PARK11	2q36–q37 unknown	AD; late-onset PD	Unknown	Sib-pair analysis

AR = autosomal recessive; AD = autosomal dominant; LBD = Lewy body disease.

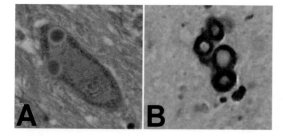

Fig. 39.7 Multiple LBs (A) and an atypical cluster of LBs (B) in brainstem neurons.

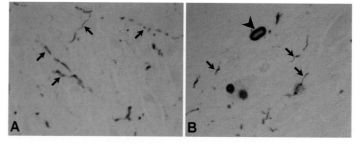

Fig. 39.8 Neuritic pathology in LBD. (A) LNs (arrows) in CA2 region of hippocampus. (B) LBs within cell processes (intra-neuritic LBs – arrowhead) in basal nucleus of Meynert. Note presence of LNs (arrows), as well.

most specific method of detecting LBs and LNs is synuclein immunocytochemistry (Irizarry *et al.*, 1998). Other molecules shown to be present in a variable number of LBs include components of the ubiquitin-proteolytic pathway, certain kinases and stress or chaperone proteins (for review, see Pollanen *et al.*, 1993).

Only a few biochemical studies on LBs have been reported, due to the paucity of LBs in a given volume of brain tissue and their solubility properties. Specifically, LBs are structurally unstable and disrupted upon attempted

biochemical purification (Iwatsubo *et al.*, 1996). Initial biochemical studies suggested that a major protein constituent of LBs was a 68 kDa protein that had cross reactivity with neurofilament protein (Pollanen *et al.*, 1992). The latter study raised the possibility that the microtubule associated protein tau, which is the major structural component of neurofibrillary tangles, was also a component of the LB, but subsequent studies indicated that the major structural

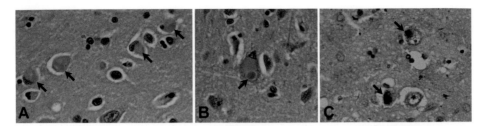

Fig. 39.9 Cortical LBs. (A) Round to pleomorphic inclusions within small non-pyramidal neurons (arrows). (B) Brainstem type LB (arrow) within a swollen pyramidal neuron. (C) Synuclein immunostain reveals cortical LBs (arrows).

Table 39.3. Components of Lewy bodies in addition to α-synuclein

Structural proteins

Synaptic proteins: α-synuclein, synaptophysin, chromogranin A
    Cytoskeletal elements: neurofilament, tau protein, MAP1,
    MAP2, tubulin, tropomyosin

Ubiquitin-proteasomal components

Ubiquitin, ubiquitin C-terminal hydrolase, multi-catalytic
    proteinase, Parkin (E3 ubiquitin ligase)

Stress-related proteins/chaperones

Chaperones: torsinA, αB-crystallin, heat shock proteins (HSP70),
    14-3-3
Stress-related: p38, glutathione S-transferase, heme oxygenase,
    superoxide dismutase-1

Neuroinflammatory

Immunoglobulins, complement, α2-macroglobulin

Kinases

Cdk-5, calcium-calmodulin kinase, extracellular receptor kinase
    (ERK)

Miscellaneous

gelsolin-related amyloid protein, βAPP, calbindin, tyrosine
    hydroxylase, retinoblastoma protein, ubiquitin,
    sphingomyelin, Bcl-2

component of LBs is α-synuclein (Baba *et al.*, 1998), rather than neurofilament or tau. In support of their importance to LBs in vitro studies have demonstrated that α-synuclein forms filaments similar to those seen in LBs (Conway *et al.*, 1998). On the other hand, recent immunohistochemical studies have shown tau in some LBs (Ishizawa *et al.*, 2003) and recent biochemical studies indicate that tau can promote α-synuclein fibrillogenesis and vice versa (Giasson *et al.*, 2003).

Biochemical changes in synuclein in PD

Changes in solubility of synuclein in PD and related disorders such as MSA and DLBD have been noted (Dickson *et al.*, 1999; Tu *et al.*, 1998). In brain tissue homogenates, synuclein is normally a soluble protein, with an electrophoretic profile consistent with a molecular weight of about 19 kDa. In LBD and MSA it becomes increasingly insoluble and is found in detergent extracts, whereas little or no synuclein from normal brains is detected in similar extracts. Moreover, in the detergent extracts synuclein has a higher molecular weight suggestive of post-translational modification, covalent cross-linking or an abnormal conformation leading to stable aggregates. Biochemical studies have demonstrated a number of post-translational modifications in synuclein, including phosphorylation, nitration and oxidative cross-linking (for review, see Dickson, 2001). It remains unclear if these modifications are directly linked to neurodegeneration or are merely epiphenomena.

What is the earliest pathology in PD?

PD is a progressive neurodegeneration, and at the cellular level synuclein modifications that eventually lead to fibrillar aggregates are reflective of this process. The use of immunostaining, with antigen retrieval methods such as protease treatment, reveals the earliest changes in neuronal cell processes and later LB in neuronal cell bodies (Neumann *et al.*, 2002; Braak *et al.*, 2003). While it has long been known that the neurons most vulnerable to LBs are monoaminergic neurons of the substantia nigra, locus ceruleus and dorsal motor nucleus of the vagus, as well as cholinergic neurons in the basal forebrain, immunohistochemistry with synuclein antibodies shows lesions in other areas not previously suspected, and at the earliest stage LNs are detected in the absence of LBs (Braak *et al.*, 2003).

While LBs are rarely detected in the basal ganglia or thalamus, synuclein immunohistochemistry often reveals neuritic changes in these areas (Duda *et al.*, 2002). LBs are common in the hypothalamus, especially the posterior and lateral hypothalamus, and in the brainstem reticular formation. The oculomotor nuclear complex is also vulnerable to LBs. In the pons, the dorsal raphe and subpeduncular

Table 39.4. Proposed staging of Lewy body PD

Stage	Anatomical distribution of LBs and LNs
1	Medullary tegmentum and the dorsal motor nucleus of the vagus; olfactory bulb
2	Locus ceruleus, caudal raphe and reticular nucleus of medullary and pontine tegmentum
3	Substantia nigra
4	Medial temporal (limbic) cortices, including the amygdala and CA2 region of the hippocampus
5	Multimodal association cortices, especially frontal and temporal lobes
6	Unimodal association cortices and occasionally primary cortices

nuclei are often affected, but neurons of the pontine base are not. LBs have not been described in the cerebellar cortex. In the spinal cord, the neurons of the intermediolateral cell column are most vulnerable. LBs can be found in the autonomic ganglia, including submucosal ganglia of the lower esophagus.

While LBs are increasingly recognized in the cortex, not all cortical regions are equally vulnerable. The frontal and temporal multimodal association and limbic cortices are most vulnerable. The amygdala is the most vulnerable of limbic structures. LBs are very uncommon in primary cortices, but neuritic pathology can be found in even the primary visual cortex. The cortical areas with the most cortical LBs are the insular cortex and the parahippocampal and cingulate gyri.

The selective vulnerability of various brain regions to LBs and LNs has been the focus of several recent studies. Of particular note is the attempt to develop a staging system for PD by Braak and co-workers (Braak *et al.*, 2003). In this staging system substantia nigra pathology occurs at a mid-stage of PD, whereas involvement of medulla and pontine tegmentum occur earlier (Table 39.4). The anterior olfactory nucleus is also affected early in the course. In the endstage PD, LBs involve cortical areas, and at this stage many patients with PD are expected to have significant cognitive problems. The pathology at this stage is similar to that found in diffuse LBD, an increasingly recognized late-life dementing disorder (Kosaka, 1990). Several studies suggest that the most common cause of later-developing dementia in patients who initially had typical PD is in fact diffuse LBD (Mattila *et al.*, 1998; Hurtig *et al.*, 2000; Apaydin *et al.*, 2002).

Despite the heuristic value of the Braak staging system for PD, it requires validation. A large cross-sectional study by Parkkinen and co-workers (Parkkinen *et al.*, 2003) of 904 brains studied with synuclein immunohistochemistry

largely concurred with the Braak staging scheme; however, in a small number of cases LBs were found in the substantia nigra without involvement of the medulla. These cases would seem to be exceptions. Another recent report by Jellinger of a large autopsy series also confirmed the general findings of the proposed staging, but also noted that there were some exceptions. Most notably were cases that had involvement of nigra and pons without medullary involvement. Medial temporal lobe pathology was also associated with variable involvement of lower parts of the neuraxis (Jellinger, 2003).

Another area in which the staging scheme breaks down is the presence of LBs in advanced Alzheimer's disease (AD). It is increasingly recognized that many cases of AD have LBs (Hamilton, 2000) and that the most common location for LBs in advanced AD is the amygdala (Lippa *et al.*, 1998). In a cross sectional study of 345 consecutive cases of AD in the Mayo Clinic Jacksonville neuropathology files, LBs were found in 94 cases in multiple brainstem, diencephalic and forebrain regions, but in the remaining 251 AD cases no brainstem LBs were detected. The amygdala was screened with synuclein immunohistochemistry in this group and 38 (15%) had Lewy bodies (DeLucia *et al.*, 2002). On re-examination the brainstem had only isolated and sparse LNs in eight cases, but the other cases did not have brainstem LBs. Thus, LBs in advanced AD begin *de novo* in the amygdala without progressing through the several brainstem stages that have been described for PD.

Other pathology in PD

Application of modern neuropathologic techniques has revealed additional pathology in PD that was not previously known. In particular, immunohistochemical stains for synuclein have shown that there is sometimes glial, as well as neuronal, pathology in PD (Wakabayashi *et al.*, 2000, Gwinn-Hardy *et al.*, 2000). Synuclein immunoreactive glial inclusions are the defining histopathologic lesions in MSA (Lantos, 1998). Occasionally, neuronal inclusions are detected in MSA (Kato & Nakamura, 1990; Dickson, 1999), and they have a number of features in common with cortical type Lewy bodies, including irregular shape, indistinct appearance of routine stains, cytoplasmic location and immunoreactivity with synuclein. While glial inclusions are not widely recognized in PD, they have been reported in previous studies using sensitive silver impregnation methods and more recently immunocytochemistry for synuclein (Wakabayashi *et al.*, 2000). They are within oligodendroglia, since they are negative for GFAP and positive with markers of pathologic oligodendrocytes, such as complement factor 4d (Gwinn-Hardy *et al.*, 2000).

Clinicopathologic correlations in PD

As discussed previously, the extrapyramidal motor signs of PD are best attributed to pathology in the nigrostriatal system. It has been estimated that pars compacta neuronal loss must exceed 50%, as estimated by loss of dopamine in the basal ganglia in PET scans, to be clinically apparent (Jellinger & Mizuno, 2003). This implies that considerable amount of pathology can be found in the substantia nigra and yet be subclinical. If the staging scheme proposed by Braak and coworkers is correct, then this stage of disease should also have been preceded by pathology in lower brainstem regions and by non-motor manifestations. In other words, PD patients should have had a history of non-motor signs and symptoms. The list of non-motor manifestations in PD is long and the correlation is imprecise and deserving of more detailed and ideally prospective clinicopathologic studies.

Anosmia is an early clinical feature of PD, although it is not specific and also detected in AD (Hawkes et al., 1997). Neurodegeneration with LB formation is common in the anterior olfactory nucleus in the olfactory bulb, but also in the medial temporal lobe olfactory cortical areas, as well as the amygdala. These are areas that might have pathology before the substantia nigra.

Autonomic dysfunction is common in PD and can manifest as constipation, urinary frequency, impotence or orthostatic hypotension (Goetz et al., 1986). Imaging studies of the heart show early involvement in PD (Taki et al., 2000). The autonomic nervous system is diffusely affected, with neuronal loss and LBs in autonomic ganglia, spinal cord preganglionic nuclei, the medullary tegmentum and the hypothalamus.

Depression is common in PD and may antedate extrapyramidal motor problems (Koller, 1992), although this hypothesis has been difficult to test. The pathoanatomic basis for depression is unknown in general, but involvement of brainstem monoaminergic nuclei, in particular noradrenergic neurons in the locus ceruleus and serotonergic neurons in the raphe nuclei, have been implicated. These nuclei are also involved in sleep cycles. PD patients often experience insomnia, parasomnias, daytime somnolence and REM sleep behavior disorder (RBD) and it is intriguing to hypothesize that involvement of these nuclei may also be involved in sleep disorders. In addition, sleep is regulated by the hypothalamus and several neurotransmitters such as adenosine, dopamine, GABA, histamine and hypocretin, have been implicated (Salin-Pascual et al., 2001). The relationship of pathology in these neuronal systems to sleep disorders in PD remains to be determined.

PD patients often have visuospatial dysfunction. The role of hypoperfusion in the primary visual cortex has not been systematically studied, but functional imaging studies show such deficits in DLB more often than in PD (Abe et al., 2003).

Psychiatric manifestations, in particular visual hallucinations, which are not related to anti-PD drugs such as L-DOPA, are common in PD, especially in older patients or those with cognitive impairments. The pathologic correlate of visual hallucinations is unknown, but studies suggest that pathology in the temporal lobe and amygdala may be responsible (Harding et al., 2002). There is also a correlation between sleep disorders and hallucinations and it has been hypothesized that visual hallucinations may be dream-like intrusions into wakefulness (dream intrusions) (Pappert et al., 1999).

Dementia is common in PD and its relationship to dementia with LBs is an ongoing debate. In the London Parkinson brain bank series, pathological findings considered to account for dementia in PD included subcortical pathology (39%), coexistent AD (29%) and DLBD (26%) (Hughes et al., 1993). The basal forebrain cholinergic system is the subcortical region most often implicated in dementia, and neurons in this region are damaged in both AD and LBD. Neuronal loss in the basal nucleus is consistently found in PD, especially PD with dementia (Whitehouse et al., 1993). As previously mentioned, the basal nucleus is also vulnerable to LBs. Not surprisingly, cholinergic deficits are found in LBD (Dickson et al., 1987). Cholinergic deficits may contribute to dementia in PD in those cases that do not have concurrent AD or cortical LBs.

While recent studies have shown that virtually all PD brains have a few cortical LBs, they are usually not widespread and not numerous in nondemented PD cases. When found in PD, cortical LBs are usually detected in the limbic cortices (e.g., cingulate gyrus) and not detected in association cortices of the frontal, temporal and parietal lobes (Harding & Halliday, 2001). In contrast, several studies have shown that cortical LBs can be numerous and widespread in PD with dementia. Furthermore, the density of cortical LBs has been shown to correlate with severity of dementia in some studies (Lennox et al., 1989). Cases with widespread cortical Lewy bodies are referred to as diffuse Lewy body disease (DLBD). Kosaka and coworkers were the first to use the term DLBD, and he subsequently subdivided DLBD into pure and common forms (Kosaka et al., 1984; Kosaka, 1990). The latter is associated with coexistent Alzheimer type pathology. Some investigators use of the term DLBD for cases in which cortical LBs are found in the absence of any Alzheimer type pathology, referring to cases with LBs and Alzheimer type pathology as Lewy body variant of AD (Hansen *et al.*, 1990). Brains with cortical LBs confined to the limbic lobe are classified as 'transitional LBD', while cases with LBs confined to brainstem and diencephalon are referred to as 'brainstem LBD' (Kosaka *et al.*, 1984). Non-demented PD subjects have brainstem or occasionally transitional LBD, while PD with dementia have DLBD or transitional LBD.

Acknowledgements

Supported by NIH grants: AG16574, AG17216, AG14449, AG03949 and NS40256; Mayo Foundation; State of Florida Alzheimer Disease Initiative; Society for Progressive Supranuclear Palsy; and Metropolitan Life Foundation.

REFERENCES

Abe, Y., Kachi, T., Kato, T. *et al.* (2003). Occipital hypoperfusion in Parkinson's disease without dementia: correlation to impaired cortical visual processing. *J. Neurol. Neurosurg., Psychiatry*, **74**, 419–22.

Apaydin, H., Ahlskog, J. E., Parisi, J. E., Boeve, B. F. & Dickson, D. W. (2002). Parkinson's disease neuropathology: later-developing dementia and loss of the levodopa response. *Arch. Neurol.*, **59**, 102–12.

Baba, M., Nakajo, S., Tu, P. H. *et al.* (1998). Aggregation of alpha-synuclein in Lewy bodies of sporadic Parkinson's disease and dementia with Lewy bodies. *Am. J. Pathol.*, **152**, 879–84.

Bower, J. H., Dickson, D. W., Taylor, L., Maraganore, D. M. & Rocca, W. A. (2002). Clinical correlates of the pathology underlying parkinsonism: A population perspective. *Mov. Disord.*, **17**, 910–16.

Braak, H., Del Tredici, K., Rüb, U., de Vos, R. A. I., Jansen Steur, E. N. H. & Braak, E. (2003). Staging of brain pathology related to sporadic Parkinson's disease. *Neurobiol. Aging*, **24**, 197–211.

Churchyard, A. & Lees, A. (1997). The relationship between dementia and direct involvement of the hippocampus and amygdala in Parkinson's disease. *Neurology*, **49**, 1570–6.

Conway, K. A., Harper, J. D. & Lansbury, P. T. (1998). Accelerated in vitro fibril formation by a mutant alpha-synuclein linked to early-onset Parkinson disease. *Nat. Med.*, **4**, 1318–20.

DeLucia, M. W., Cookson, N. & Dickson, D. W. (2002). Synuclein-immunoreactive Lewy bodies are detected in the amygdala in less than 20% of Alzheimer's disease (AD) cases. *J. Neuropathol. Exp. Neurol.*, **61**, 454.

Dickson, D. W., Davies, P., Mayeux, R. *et al.* (1987). Diffuse Lewy body disease: neuropathological and biochemical studies of six patients. *Acta Neuropathol.*, **75**, 8–15.

Dickson, D. W. (1999). Tau and synuclein and their role in neuropathology. *Brain Pathol.*, **9**, 657–61.

(2001). α-Synuclein and the Lewy body disorders. *Curr. Opin. Neurol.*, **14**, 423–32.

Dickson, D. W., Ruan, D., Crystal, H., Kress, Y. & Yen S.-H. (1991). Hippocampal degeneration differentiates diffuse Lewy body disease (DLBD) from Alzheimer's disease: light and electron microscopic immunocytochemistry of CA2–3 neurites specific to DLBD. *Neurology*, **41**, 1402–9.

Dickson, D. W., Liu, W.-K., Hardy, J. *et al.* (1999). Widespread alterations of alpha-synuclein in multiple system atrophy. *Am. J. Pathol.*, **155**, 1241–51.

Duda, J. E., Giasson, B. I., Mabon, M. E., Lee, V. M. & Trojanowski, J. Q. (2002). Novel antibodies to synuclein show abundant striatal pathology in Lewy body diseases. *Ann. Neurol.*, **52**, 205–10.

Fearnley, J. M. & Lees, A. J. (1991). Ageing and Parkinson's disease: substantia nigra regional selectivity. *Brain*, **114**, 2283–301.

Galloway, P. G., Mulvihill, P. & Perry, G. (1992). Filaments of Lewy bodies contain insoluble cytoskeletal elements. *Am. J. Pathol.*, **140**, 809–15.

Galvin, J. E., Lee, V. M., Baba, M. *et al.* (1997). Monoclonal antibodies to purified cortical Lewy bodies recognize the mid-size neurofilament subunit. *Ann. Neurol.*, **42**, 595–603.

Giasson, B. I., Forman, M. S., Higuchi, M., *et al.* (2003). Initiation and synergistic fibrillization of tau and alpha-synuclein. *Science*, **300**, 636–40.

Gibb, W. R. & Lees, A. J. (1991). Anatomy, pigmentation, ventral and dorsal subpopulations of the substantia nigra, and differential cell death in Parkinson's disease. *J. Neurol. Neurosurg. Psychiatry*, **54**, 388–96.

Gibb, W. R. & Poewe, W. H. (1986). The centenary of Friederich H. Lewy 1885–1950. *Neuropathol. Appl. Neurobiol.*, **12**, 217–22.

Goetz, C. G., Luthe, W. & Tanner, C. M. (1986). Autonomic dysfunction in Parkinson's disease. *Neurology*, **36**, 73–5.

Goldman, J. E., Yen, S.-H., Chiu, F.-C. & Peress, N. S. (1983). Lewy bodies of Parkinson's disease contain neurofilament antigens. *Science*, **221**, 1082–4.

Gwinn-Hardy, K., Mehta, N. D., Farrer, M. *et al.* (2000). Distinctive neuropathology revealed by α-synuclein antibodies in hereditary Parkinsonism and dementia linked to chromosome 4p. *Acta Neuropathol.*, **99**, 663–72.

Hamilton, R. L. (2000). Lewy bodies in Alzheimer's disease: a neuropathological review of 145 cases using alpha-synuclein immunohistochemistry. *Brain Pathol.*, **10**, 378–84.

Hansen, L., Salmon, D., Galasko, D. *et al.* (1990). Lewy body variant of Alzheimer's disease: a clinical and pathological entity. *Neurology*, **40**, 1–8.

Harding, A. J. & Halliday, G. M. (2001). Cortical Lewy body pathology in the diagnosis of dementia. *Acta Neuropathol.*, **102**, 355–63.

Harding, A. J., Broe, G. A. & Halliday, G. M. (2002). Visual hallucinations in Lewy body disease relate to Lewy bodies in the temporal lobe. *Brain*, **125**, 391–403.

Hardy, J., Cookson, M. R. & Singleton, A. (2003). Genes and parkinsonism. *Lancet Neurol.*, **2**, 221–8.

Hawkes, C. H., Shepard, B. C. & Daniel, S. E. (1997). Olfactory dysfunction in Parkinson's disease. *J. Neurol. Neurosurg., Psychiatry*, **62**, 436–46.

Hughes, A. J., Daniel, S. E., Blankson, S. & Lees, A. J. (1993). A clinicopathologic study of 100 cases of Parkinson's disease. *Arch. Neurol.*, **50**, 140–8.

Hughes, A. J., Daniel, S. E. & Lees, A. J. (2001). Improved accuracy of clinical diagnosis of Lewy body Parkinson's disease. *Neurology*, **57**, 1497–9.

Hurtig, H. I., Trojanowski, J. Q., Galvin, J. *et al.* (2000). Alpha-synuclein cortical Lewy bodies correlate with dementia in Parkinson's disease. *Neurology*, **54**, 1916–21.

Irizarry, M. C., Growdon, W., Gomez-Isla, T. *et al.* (1998). Nigral and cortical Lewy bodies and dystrophic nigral neurites in Parkinson's disease and cortical Lewy body disease contain α-synuclein immunoreactivity. *J. Neuropathol. Exp. Neurol.*, **57**, 334–337.

Ishizawa, T., Mattila, P., Davies, P., Wang, D. & Dickson, D. W. (2003). Colocalization of tau and alpha-synuclein epitopes in Lewy bodies. *J. Neuropathol. Exp. Neurol.*, **62**, 389–97.

Iwatsubo, T., Yamaguchi, H., Fujimuro, M. *et al.* (1996). Purification and characterization of Lewy bodies from the brains of patients with diffuse Lewy body disease. *Am. J. Pathol.*, **148**, 1517–29.

Jellinger, K. A. (1999). Post mortem studies in Parkinson's disease – is it possible to detect brain areas for specific symptoms? *J. Neural. Transm. Suppl.*, **56**, 1–29.

(2003). α-Synuclein pathology in Parkinson's and Alzheimer's disease brain: incidence and topographic distribution – a pilot study. *Acta Neuropathol.*, **106**, 191–201.

Jellinger, K. A. & Duda, J. (2003). Neurodegeneration with brain iron accumulation, type 1 (Hallervorden-Spatz disease). In *Neurodegeneration: The Molecular Pathology of Dementia and Movement Disorders*, ed. D. W. Dickson, pp. 394–9. Basel: ISN Neuropath Press.

Jellinger, K. A. & Mizuno, Y. (2003). Parkinson's disease. In *Neurodegeneration: the molecular pathology of dementia and movement disorders*, ed. D. W. Dickson, pp. 159–187. Basel: ISN Neuropath Press.

Kato, S. & Nakamura, H. (1990). Cytoplasmic argyrophilic inclusions in neurons of pontine nuclei in patients with olivopontocerebellar atrophy: immunohistochemical and ultrastructural studies. *Acta Neuropathol*, **79**, 584–94.

Koller, W. C. (1992). When does Parkinson's disease begin? *Neurology* **42**(4 Suppl 4), 27–31.

Kosaka, K. (1990). Diffuse Lewy body disease in Japan. *J. Neurol.* **237**, 197–204.

Kosaka, K., Yoshimura, M., Ikeda, K. & Budka, H. (1984). Diffuse type of Lewy body disease: progressive dementia with abundant cortical Lewy bodies and senile changes of varying degree – a new disease? *Clin. Neuropathol.*, **3**, 185–92.

Kuzuhara, S., Mori, H., Izumiyama, N., Yoshimura, M. & Ihara, Y. (1988). Lewy bodies are ubiquitinated: a light and electron microscopic immunocytochemical study. *Acta Neuropathol.*, **75**, 345–53.

Lantos, P. L. (1998). The definition of multiple system atrophy: a review of recent developments. *J. Neuropathol. Exp. Neurol.*, **57**, 1099–111.

Lennox, G., Lowe, J. S., Landon, M., Byrne, E. J., Mayer, R. J. & Godwin-Austen, R. B. (1989). Diffuse Lewy body disease: correlative neuropathology using anti-ubiquitin immunocytochemistry. *J. Neurol. Neurosurg., Psychiatry*, **52**, 1236–47.

Lippa, C. F., Fujiwara, H., Mann, D. M. A. *et al.* (1998). Lewy bodies contain altered α-synuclein in brains of many familial Alzheimer's disease patients with mutations in presenilin and amyloid precursor protein genes. *Am. J. Pathol.*, **153**, 1365–70.

Masliah, E., Galasko, D., Wiley, C. A. & Hansen, L. A. (1990). Lobar atrophy with dense-core (brain stem type) Lewy bodies in a patient with dementia. *Acta Neuropathol.*, **80**, 453–8.

Mattila, P. M., Roytta, M., Torikka, H., Dickson, D. W. & Rinne, J. O. (1998). Cortical Lewy bodies and Alzheimer-type changes in patients with Parkinson's disease. *Acta Neuropathol.*, **95**, 576–82.

McGreer, P. L., Itagaki, S., Boyes, B. E. & McGeer, E. G. (1998). Reactive microglia are positive for HLA-DR in the substantia nigra of Parkinson's and Alzheimer's disease brains. *Neurology*, **38**, 1285–91.

McGreer, P.L., Yasojima, K. & McGeer, E. G. (2001). Inflammation in Parkinson's disease. *Adv. Neurol.*, **86**, 83–9.

McKeith, I. G., Galasko, D., Kosaka, K. *et al.* (1996). Clinical and pathological diagnosis of dementia with Lewy bodies (DLB): Report of the Consortium on Dementia with Lewy Bodies International Workshop. *Neurology*, **47**, 1113–24.

Neumann, M., Kahle, P. J., Giasson, B. I. *et al.* (2002). Misfolded proteinase K-resistant hyperphosphorylated alpha-synuclein in aged transgenic mice with locomotor deterioration and in human alpha-synucleinopathies. *J. Clin. Invest.*, **110**, 1429–39.

Pappert, E. J., Goetz, C. G., Niederman, F. G., Raman, R. & Leurgans, S. (1999). Hallucinations, sleep fragmentation, and altered dream phenomena in Parkinson's disease. *Mov. Disord.*, **14**, 117–21.

Parkkinen, L., Soininen, H. & Alafuzoff, I. (2003). Regional distribution of alpha-synuclein pathology in unimpaired aging and Alzheimer disease. *J. Neuropathol. Exp. Neurol.*, **62**, 363–7.

Pollanen, M. S., Bergeron, C. & Weyer, L. (1992). Detergent-insoluble Lewy body fibrils share epitopes with neurofilament and tau. *J. Neurochem.*, **58**, 1953–6.

Pollanen, M. S., Dickson, D. W. & Bergeron, C. (1993). Pathology and biology of the Lewy body. *J. Neuropathol. Exp. Neurol.*, **52**, 183–91.

Salin-Pascual, R., Gerashchenko, D., Greco, M., Blanco-Centurion, C. & Shiromani, P. J. (2001). Hypothalamic regulation of sleep. *Neuropsychopharmacology*, **25**(5 Suppl), S21–27.

Taki, J., Nakajima, K., Hwang, E. H. *et al.* (2000). Peripheral sympathetic dysfunction in patients with Parkinson's disease without autonomic failure is heart selective and disease specific. *Eur. J. Nucl. Med.*, **27**, 566–73.

Tsuboi, Y., Iwatsubo, T. & Dickson, D. W. (2003). Striatal α-synuclein burden correlates with disease duration in Parkinson's disease (PD), but not in dementia with Lewy bodies (DLB). *Brain Pathol.*, **13**, S32.

Tu, P. H., Galvin, J. E., Baba, M. *et al.* (1998). Glial cytoplasmic inclusions in white matter oligodendrocytes of multiple system atrophy brains contain insoluble alpha-synuclein. *Ann. Neurol.*, **44**, 415–22.

Wakabayashi, K., Hayashi, S., Yoshimoto, M., Kudo, H. & Takahashi, H. (2000). NACP/alpha-synuclein-positive filamentous inclusions in astrocytes and oligodendrocytes of Parkinson's disease brains. *Acta Neuropathol.*, **99**, 14–20.

Whitehouse, P. J., Hedreen, J. C., White, C. L., III & Price, D. L. (1993). Basal forebrain neurons in dementia of Parkinson disease. *Ann. Neurol.*, **13**, 243–8.

40

Genetics of parkinsonism

Thomas Gasser

Department of Neurodegenerative Disorders, Hertie-Institute for Clinical Brain Research Center of Neurology,
University of Tübingen, Germany, thomas.gasser@med.uni-tuebingen.de

Overview

Over the last few years, several genes for monogenically inherited forms of Parkinson's disease have been mapped and/or cloned. In a small number of families with autosomal dominant inheritance and typical Lewy body pathology, mutations have been identified in the gene for α-synuclein. Aggregation of this protein in Lewy bodies may be a crucial step in the molecular pathogenesis of familial and sporadic PD. On the other hand, mutations in the *parkin* gene cause autosomal recessive parkinsonism of early onset. In this form of PD, nigral degeneration is not accompanied by Lewy body formation. *Parkin* mutations appear to be a common cause of PD in patients with very early onset. Parkin has been implicated in the cellular protein degradation pathways, as it has been shown that it functions as a ubiquitin ligase. This potential importance of this pathway is also highlighted by the finding of a mutation in the gene for ubiquitin C-terminal hydrolase L1 in another small family with PD. The most recently identified PD-genes are DJ-1 and PINK1, again in families with autosomal-recessive inheritance and early onset. Other loci have been mapped to chromosome 2p and 12p, respectively, in a small number of families with dominantly inherited PD, but those genes have not yet been identified. These findings prove that there are several genetically distinct forms of PD that can be caused by mutations in single genes.

On the other hand, there is at present no strong evidence that any of these genes have a direct role in the etiology of the common sporadic form of PD. Epidemiologic, case control, and twin studies, although supporting a genetic contribution to the development of PD, all suggest a clear familial clustering only in a minority of cases. It is therefore widely believed that a combination of interacting genetic and environmental causes may be responsible in the majority of PD cases.

Introduction and historical background

Parkinson's disease is traditionally defined as a clinico-pathologic entity, characterized clinically by a core syndrome of akinesia, rigidity, tremor and postural instability, and pathologically by a more or less selective degeneration of dopaminergic neurons of the substantia nigra, leading to a deficiency of dopamine in the striatal projection areas of these neurons. Characteristic eosinophilic inclusions, the Lewy bodies, are found in surviving dopaminergic neurons but also, although less abundantly, in other parts of the brain in most cases, and have been considered to be essential for the pathologic diagnosis of PD (Gibb & Lees, 1989).

Although early descriptions of the disease mentioned a familial aggregation in at least a subgroup of patients (Gowers, 1888), hereditary factors have until relatively recently been considered to play a minor, if any, role in the etiology of the disorder (Duvoisin, 1986).

The change of opinion that occurred mostly during the 1990s was based primarily on three different lines of evidence.

(i) Case-control studies consistently showed that a positive family history is a major risk-factor towards the development of the disease (Bonifati *et al.*, 1995; Vieregge & Heberlein, 1995; Lazzarini *et al.*, 1994), with relative risks ranging from about 2.3 in a population-based sample (Marder *et al.*, 1996) to as high as 14 in a sample drawn from specialty clinics (De Michele *et al.*, 1995).

Table 40.1. Genetically defined forms of Parkinson's disease and parkinsonism

Locus/gene	Inheritance	Onset	Pathology	Map position	Gene	Reference
PARK1	dominant	40s	nigral degeneration with Lewy bodies	4q21	α-synuclein	(Polymeropoulos *et al.*, 1997)
PARK2	recessive	20s	nigral degeneration without Lewy bodies	6q25	Parkin	(Kitada *et al.*, 1998)
PARK3	dominant	60s	nigral degeneration with Lewy bodies, Plaques and tangles in some	2p13	?	(Gasser *et al.*, 1998)
PARK4	dominant	30s	nigral degeneration with Lewy bodies, vacuoles in neurons of the hippocampus	4q21	α-synuclein	(Singleton *et al.*, 2003)
PARK5	dominant	~ 50	No pathology	4p14	Ubiquitin C-terminal hydrolase L1	(Leroy *et al.*, 1998)
PARK6	recessive	~ 40	No pathology	1p35–37	PINK1	(Valente *et al.*, 2004)
PARK7	recessive	~ 40	No pathology	1p38	DJ-1	(Bonifati *et al.*, 2002)
PARK8	dominant	~ 50	Degeneration of dopaminergic neurons without specific inclusions	12cen	?	(Funayama *et al.*, 2002)
PARK10	dominant	50–60	unknown	1p32	?	(Hicks *et al.*, 2002)

(ii) New twin studies using ^{18}F-fluorodopa PET to identify individuals with subclinical disturbances of their nigrostriatal dopaminergic system demonstrated significantly higher concordance rate in monozygous as compared to dizygous twins (Burn *et al.*, 1992), contrary to previous studies (Ward *et al.*, 1983).

(iii) Finally, several families were described in whom Parkinson's disease (or at least a disorder closely resembling PD) segregated as an apparently dominant (Golbe *et al.*, 1990; Wszolek *et al.*, 1993) or recessive (Takahashi *et al.*, 1994) trait with high penetrance.

It was the growing awareness of those families, combined with a rapid progress in molecular genetic techniques of gene identification, that led to one of the major breakthroughs in recent years in PD research: the mapping and cloning of an increasing number of genes that cause monogenically inherited forms parkinsonism with different associated pathologies and a variable, but overlapping, spectrum of clinical signs and symptoms (Gasser, 2003). In only a few years, these discoveries not only led to a reclassification of parkinsonian syndromes based on the underlying genetic defect, but also to an astonishing expansion of our knowledge of the molecular events that led to neurodegeneration in these disorders.

It has to be kept in mind, however, that all of the mutations and loci identified so far appear to be responsible in only a relatively small number of families, and their relationship to the vast majority of sporadic patients with PD and other parkinsonian syndromes is still unknown. Nevertheless, there is considerable promise that the elucidation of the molecular pathways leading to monogenically inherited forms of parkinsonism will also allow important insight into the common sporadic disorders, and eventually allow the development of novel protective and therapeutic strategies.

Monogenic forms of Parkinson's disease

A relatively small minority of patients with a more or less typical clinical picture of Parkinson's disease have a positive family history compatible with a Mendelian (autosomal-dominant or autosomal-recessive) inheritance. As a rule, age at onset in most of these cases is earlier as compared to sporadic PD. In many of these families, clinical signs and symptoms are found, in addition to parkinsonism, which would be considered unusual, or in some cases even incompatible, with a diagnosis of classic idiopathic PD (Muenter *et al.*, 1998; Perry *et al.*, 1990). In other cases the disease seems to be indistinguishable clinically, and sometimes also pathologically, from typical PD (Wszolek *et al.*, 1993, 1995). It should therefore be kept in mind that monogenic forms of parkinsonism may serve as valuable models for studying the molecular pathways involved in dopaminergic degeneration, but are not necessarily identical to the sporadic disease.

Autosomal dominant parkinsonism

Several genetic loci have been identified by linkage studies to cosegregate with parkinsonism in families with dominant inheritance.

PARK1: Parkinson's disease caused by mutations in the gene for α-synuclein (PARK1)

Mutations in the gene for α-synuclein on the long arm of chromosome 4 cause a disorder that resembles idiopathic PD in many ways, both clinically and pathologically (Polymeropoulos *et al.*, 1997). Patients have L-dopa-responsive parkinsonism, and neuropathological studies show the characteristic pattern of neuronal degeneration with α-synuclein-positive Lewy bodies in the substantia nigra. In the early descriptions it appeared that only the relatively early age at onset (with a mean 44 years in the large 'Contursi'-kindred) distinguished this disease from sporadic PD (Golbe *et al.*, 1996). Recently, it became clear, however, that patients with the most common mutation in the α-synuclein gene (the Ala53Thr mutation) can also exhibit clinical features, such as prominent dementia, hypoventilation and autonomic disturbances, which clearly exceed what is usually found in typical PD (Spira *et al.*, 2001). There are also differences in the pathologic picture (Duda *et al.*, 2002).

Despite these differences, the fact that the most conspicuous feature of the pathology in sporadic PD is the intracellular accumulation and aggregation of α-synuclein in a ß-sheet configuration (Spillantini *et al.*, 1997) points to the central role of this protein in the disease process of PD in general. α-Synuclein is a relatively small protein that is abundantly expressed in many parts of the brain and localized mostly to presynaptic nerve terminals. Many aspects of the normal function of α-synuclein are still unknown. The protein may functionally be involved in brain plasticity and has been shown to bind to brain vesicles (Jensen *et al.*, 1998) and other cell membranes (McLean *et al.*, 2000). However, knockout mice for α-synuclein show only very subtle alterations in dopamine release under certain experimental conditions, but no other phenotype (Abeliovich *et al.*, 2000).

The currently favoured hypothesis states that the amino acid changes in the α-synuclein protein associated with PD may favor the ß-pleated sheet conformation, which in turn may lead to an increased tendency to form aggregates. This has been demonstrated in vitro (Biere *et al.*, 2000; Conway *et al.*, 2000; Conway *et al.*, 1998). However, the precise relationship between the formation of aggregates and cell death is unknown. It is possible that a failure of proteasomal degradation of α-synuclein and other proteins may lead to an accumulation of toxic compounds, ultimately leading to cell death (McNaught *et al.*, 2001). Formation of α-synuclein-containing aggregates would then be only a secondary effect (McNaught & Jenner, 2001).

However, other mechanisms of pathogenesis may also be important. Known α-synuclein mutations appear to alter the vesicle-binding properties of the protein (Jensen *et al.*, 1998), and the functional homology of α-synuclein to the 14-3-3 protein, a ubiquitously expressed chaperone, may indicate a more profound role for this protein in cellular metabolism and suggests still other possible pathogenic mechanisms.

Mutations in the α-synuclein gene clearly appear to be a very rare cause of the disease. Only three point mutations have been recognized (Polymeropoulos *et al.*, 1997; Krüger *et al.*, 1998; Zarranz *et al.*, 2004). The mutation that was found in the original Contursi family (Ala53Thr) has also been identified in several Greek kindreds (Polymeropoulos *et al.*, 1997; Markopoulou *et al.*, 1995; Papadimitriou *et al.*, 1999). Haplotype analyses support the hypothesis that this is due to a founder effect (Papadimitriou *et al.*, 1999).

Recently, the role of α-synuclein aggregation in PD was further substantiated by the finding of a triplication of a 2 Mb genomic region containing the α-synuclein gene in a large autosomal-dominant family with PD (Singleton *et al.*, 2003). This genomic aberration leads to an overexpression of the intact α-synuclein gene, indicating the susceptibility of neurons to an overload with this amyloidogenic protein. Interestingly, several affected members of this kindred, as well as later reported individuals with an A53T (Spira *et al.*, 2001) and B46K point mutation (Zarranz *et al.*, 2004) had prominent dementia and pathologic findings consistent with Lewy body dementia, supporting the close relationship of this disease entity with PD.

Cellular and animal models

To study the effect of α-SYN mutations in vivo, transgenic mice overexpressing this gene, both the normal and the mutated human sequence, under different promotors have been generated.

Some of the first transgenic mouse lines generated showed somatodendritic accumulation of α-synuclein, but no fibrillar inclusions resembling Lewy bodies (Kahle *et al.*, 2000a; Matsuoka *et al.*, 2001; Masliah *et al.*, 2000).

Other transgenic lines, however, recapitulated human Lewy pathology more faithfully (Giasson *et al.*, 2002; Lee *et al.*, 2002; Neumann *et al.*, 2002). These mice showed age-dependent formation of amyloid-like αSYN fibrils within neuronal perikarya (Lewy bodies) and dystrophic neurites, and developed a progressive locomotor phenotype characterized by dystonia, rigidity, paralysis, and ultimately death. However, neurodegeneration affected predominantly the brainstem and spinal cord, while dopaminergic neurons were spared. This observation may indicate that mice have developed mechanisms protecting their dopaminergic neurons from α-SYN toxicity. The identification of putative defence mechanisms that protect DA neurons throughout the relatively short life span of mice may also be effective in humans. Such cellular defence mechanisms might lose activity in the elderly, ultimately leading to PD in affected patients.

A lot of interest has been generated by an animal model expressing mutant and wt-human α-SYN in the fruitfly *Drosophila* (Feany & Bender, 2000). Not only do these flies show degeneration of dopaminergic neurons and filamentous inclusions resembling LBs, but also a progressive motor phenotype that can be partially corrected by pharmacologic dopaminergic stimulation (Pendleton *et al.*, 2002). The relative ease of developing a *Drosophila* model of α-synucleinopathy might be due to the fact that invertebrate genomes do not code for any synucleins. Thus, flies may not have evolved cellular defence mechanisms to suppress αSYN fibrilization. The *Drosophila* phenotype could be rescued by gene transfer of the molecular chaperone Hsp70 (Auluck *et al.*, 2002), pointing to the cellular protein folding machinery as a therapeutic target.

PARK3: Parkinson's disease linked to chromosome 2

Another autosomal-dominant locus has been described (PARK3), located on chromosome 2p13, in a subset of families with typical PD and Lewy body pathology (Gasser *et al.*, 1998). Clinical features resembling those of sporadic Parkinson's disease (Wszolek *et al.*, 1993) include a similar mean age of onset (59 years in these families). Follow-up examination of these families over the years showed that, in addition to parkinsonism, several members of chromosome 2-linked families showed signs of dementia, and neuropathology revealed, in addition to neuronal loss in the substantia nigra and typical brainstem Lewy bodies, the presence of neurofibrillary tangles and Alzheimer plaques (Wszolek *et al.*, 2002). Therefore, the underlying mutation may be associated with a range of phenotypes, that includes varying degrees of dementia and Alzheimer's disease pathology, as is also known for a subset of patients with idiopathic Parkinson's disease.

The disease gene has not yet been identified (West *et al.*, 2001; Zink *et al.*, 2001). However, two independent recent reports implicate the PARK3-locus as a disease modifying locus influencing age at onset in sib pair cohorts with PD (DeStefano *et al.*, 2002; Pankratz *et al.*, 2003).

PARK4: Parkinsonism-dementia caused by α-synuclein triplication

In a family with parkinsonism with autosomal-dominant inheritance, originally described in detail by Muenter *et al.* (1998) evidence for linkage was found on the short arm of chromosome 4 (Farrer *et al.*, 1999). Affecteds in this family have L-dopa-responsive parkinsonism, but age at onset is considerably younger (mean 33.6 years), and several atypical features are present, such as early weight loss, dysautonomia and dementia. Neuropathologic changes include, in addition to nigral degeneration and Lewy body formation, conspicuous vacuoles in the hippocampus and several other brain areas. Reinvestigation of this family showed that the original mapping to the short arm of chromosome 4 was due to a typing error. The disease locus was then located to the α-synuclein region, and a triplication in the α-synuclein gene was identified as causative in this family (Singleton *et al.*, 2003).

PARK5: Parkinsonism associated with a mutation in the gene for ubiquitin hydrolase L1

A missense mutation in the gene for ubiquitin carboxy-terminal hydrolase L1 gene (UCH-L1) has been identified in two affecteds of a single family of German ancestry (Leroy *et al.*, 1998). This mutation reduces the enzymatic activity in vitro, which could be consistent with a causative role of this alteration, as an important role of the proteasomal ubiquitination – protein degradation pathway is suggested by the study of parkin-related parkinsonism (see below). To date, however, no other potentially pathogenic mutations of this gene have been identified (Harhangi *et al.*, 1999a; Lincoln *et al.*, 1999). Another rare variant has been found in a family with PD, which did not segregate with the disease (Farrer *et al.*, 2000).

The observation of a polymorphism in the UCHL1-gene (S18Y) and its possible protective role in patients with sporadic PD (Maraganore *et al.*, 1999; Wintermeyer *et al.*, 2000) has been controversial (Mellick & Silburn, 2000). A recent meta-analysis, however, has again strengthened the link between this gene and PD (Maraganore *et al.*, 2004). A naturally occurring mouse mutant (the GAD-mouse), which shows a phenotype of neuronal degeneration (although predominantly of the peripheral nervous system), has been found to be due to a deletion in the mouse homologue of the UCHL-1 gene (Saigoh *et al.*, 1999).

PARK8, PARK10

In a large Japanese family with dominant inheritance, the locus has been recently mapped to chromosome 12 (PARK8) (Funayama *et al.*, 2002). Affecteds in this family show typical PD with onset in the late forties and a relatively benign course. Autopsy in four affecteds revealed unspecific neuronal degeneration in the substantia nigra, but no LB-formation. Other dominant families are linked to this locus (Zimprich *et al.*, 2004), but no gene has yet been identified.

The Icelandic population is considered by many to be a genetic isolate, which may lend itself particularly to the study of genetically complex diseases. A clinico-genetic study has provided evidence for a significant familial aggregation of PD which may be caused, at least in part, by the segregation of a dominant gene with reduced penetrance (which may or may not be specific to this population) (Sveinbjornsdottir *et al.*, 2000). Linkage studies allowed the mapping of this locus to chromosome 1p32 (PARK10, (Hicks *et al.*, 2002)). Very recently the gene has been identified as a lencine-rich repeat kinase (LRRKZ) (Zimprich *et al.*, 2004).

Autosomal-recessive forms of parkinsonism

One of the surprising developments of recent years was the recognition of the relatively high proportion of patients with early-onset parkinsonism being caused by recessive mutations in a number of genes. So far, three of them, parkin (PARK2), PARK6 (PINK1) and DJ-1 (PARK7) have been cloned.

PARK2: autosomal recessive juvenile parkinsonism (AR-JP) caused by mutations in the gene for parkin

Juvenile cases of parkinsonism with recessive inheritance (families with affected siblings, but usually no transmission from one generation to the next), were first recognized in Japan (Ishikawa & Tsuji, 1996). Clinically, these patients suffer from L-dopa-responsive parkinsonism and some show diurnal fluctuations with symptoms becoming worse later in the day. Dystonia at onset of the disease is quite common. In contrast to patients with dopa-responsive dystonia, which is caused by mutations in the gene for GTP-cyclohydrolase (Ichinose *et al.*, 1994), one of the genes involved in dopamine biosynthesis, patients with recessive parkinsonism develop early and severe levodopa-

induced motor-fluctuations and dyskinesias (Ishikawa & Tsuji, 1996).

The genetic locus for AR-JP has been mapped to chromosome 6 (Matsumine *et al.*, 1997), and mutations have been identified in a large gene in that region that was called *parkin* (Kitada *et al.*, 1998).

Parkin mutations turned out to be a common cause of parkinsonism with early onset, particularly in those with evidence for recessive inheritance. Nearly 50% of families from a population of sibling pairs collected by the European Consortium on Genetic Susceptibility in PD showed parkin mutations (Lücking *et al.*, 2000). The clinical picture is frequently indistinguishable from that of the sporadic disease, with the exception of an earlier mean age-at-onset. While parkin mutations seem to be responsible for the majority of sporadic cases with onset before age 20, and are still rather common (25%) when onset is between 20 and 30, prevalence in older patients is almost certainly well below 5% (Lücking *et al.*, 2000).

The European study population allowed the characterization of the clinical spectrum of parkin-associated parkinsonism. Mean age at onset in a European population was 32 years, progression of the disease was slow but L-dopa associated fluctuations and dyskinesias occurred frequently. Dystonia (usually in a lower extremity) at disease-onset was found in about 40% of patients and brisk reflexes of the lower limbs were present in 44% (Lücking *et al.*, 2000). There was no discernable difference in the clinical phenotype between patients with missense mutations, truncating point mutations or deletions, suggesting that a complete loss of parkin function is associated with all of these mutations and with the full phenotype of early-onset parkinsonism.

The question of whether heterozygous mutations in the parkin gene can cause parkinsonism, or are able to confer an increased susceptibility for typical late-onset PD, is still unsettled. There is evidence from imaging studies (Hilker *et al.*, 2001) that heterozygotes may have mildly reduced uptake of Fluorodopa in the basal ganglia. Furthermore, occasional families with heterozygous mutation carriers manifesting symptoms of PD have been described (Klein *et al.*, 2000a; Farrer *et al.*, 2001). In these cases, however, it is difficult to prove the causal relationship between genotype and phenotype. The obvious study to answer this question, the systematic examination of (heterozygous) parents of patients with parkin mutations, has not been performed.

There is still relatively little information available on the neuropathology of molecularly confirmed cases of AR-JP. Severe and selective degeneration of dopaminergic neurons and gliosis in the substantia nigra, but usually no Lewy bodies have been described (Takahashi *et al.*, 1994).

The fact that Lewy bodies do not appear to be necessary for the selective degeneration of nigral neurons raises the question whether this neuropathologic feature should be regarded as an essential component of the disease process. The recent observation of typical ubiquitin-positive LBs in a patient with a parkin mutation (Farrer *et al.*, 2001) is difficult to reconcile with present concepts of the molecular pathogenesis of the disorder (see below).

As mutations in parkin cause parkinsonism, in all likelihood, by a loss-of-function mechanism, the study of the normal function of parkin, should provide insight into the molecular pathogenesis of the disorder. Several groups have now shown that parkin, a protein that has been found in the cytosole, but also associated with membranes, functions in the cellular ubiquitination/protein degradation pathway as a ubiquitin ligase (Shimura *et al.*, 2000; Zhang *et al.*, 2000). It is therefore conceivable that the loss of parkin function may lead to the accumulation of a non-ubiquitinated substrate which is deleterious to the dopaminergic cell, but due to its non-ubiquitinated nature, does not accumulate in typical Lewy bodies (Kahle *et al.*, 2000b). Several proteins have been shown to interact with parkin and could possibly be its crucial partner with regard to neurodegeneration; an O glycosylated form of alpha-synuclein (Shimura *et al.*, 2001), a protein associated with synaptic vesicles, CDCrel-1 (Zhang *et al.*, 2000), and a transmembrane protein, called the pael-receptor (Imai *et al.*, 2001) and synphillin (Chung *et al.*, 2001). The possible interaction with α-synuclein and synphillin is intriguing, as it may provide the link between parkin-associated juvenile parkinsonism and typical late-onset PD (Shimura *et al.*, 2001; Chung *et al.*, 2001). However, as both parkin and α-synuclein are widely expressed in the brain, this does not explain the striking selectivity of the degenerative process for dopaminergic neurons. However, regional selectivity may well be caused by other factors, for example, the high burden of oxidative stress in dopaminergic neurons, or by the lack of some, as yet undefined, compensatory mechanisms.

Recessive early-onset parkinsonism linked to chromosome 1 (PARK6 and PARK7)

Two other recessive loci have been linked in families with early-onset L-dopa-responsive parkinsonism, both to chromosome 1: one (PARK6) in a large Sicilian family with four definitely affected members (the Marsala kindred). The phenotype was characterized by early-onset (range 32–48 years) parkinsonism, with slow progression and sustained response to levodopa (Valente *et al.*, 2001), which is similar to parkin-associated parkinsonism. Preliminary analyses suggest that this gene may also be reponsible in more than a limited number of patients and families.

A second novel recessive locus, PARK7 has been mapped by van Duijn and coworkers (van Duijn *et al.*, 2001), also in a consanguinous Italian family. Again, the clinical picture is that of early-onset, L-dopa-responsive parkinsonism.

The gene responsible for PARK7-linked parkinsonism was the first of the two to be identified (Bonifati *et al.*, 2002). It was called DJ-1 and had originally been discovered as an oncogene. The reason why loss-of-function mutations in DJ-1 cause dopaminergic neurons to degenerate is unclear. The protein may play a role in the cellular response to oxidative stress, which may render dopaminergic neurons particularly vulnerable.

Very recently, a gene for a third form of autosomal-dominantly inherited early-onset parkinsonism has been identified (Valente *et al.*, 2004). Interestingly, it encodes a protein, which is likely to be located in the mitochondria, and possibly functions as a protein kinase. It is known as PINK1 (PTEN-induced kinase 1). The phenotype of patients carrying mutations in this gene resembles that of the other early-onset recessive forms of parkinsonism, in that the progression is slow, L-dopa response is often excellent, and dementia is not usually a part of the phenotype (in contrast to the dominant, α-synuclein-linked forms of parkinsonism.

Non-monogenic forms of familial PD

Monogenic forms of PD are rare and probably account for less than 5% of all of PD, with young-onset cases being clearly over-represented in this group. A larger proportion of cases, probably 10 to 15%, have affected family members, but a clear Mendelian pattern of inheritance cannot be demonstrated.

Segregation analyses have produced conflicting results suggesting autosomal dominant, autosomal-recessive (Maher *et al.*, 2002; Moilanen *et al.*, 2001) or non-Mendelian (Zareparsi *et al.*, 1998) inheritance of disease susceptibility or age at onset. It is therefore widely believed that typical PD is a 'genetically complex' disorder with several common susceptibility genes, each conferring only a relatively slight increase of risk, possibly interacting with each other and/or with non-genetic risk factors. Depending on age-at-onset or other clinical characteristics, the relative contribution of these genetic risk factors may vary between different populations.

Several linkage studies have been conducted in large cohorts of small families with PD (mostly nuclear families and/or affected sib pairs) with interesting, but still

Table 40.2. Association studies in Parkinson's disease. Only a few studies are cited as representative examples

Candidate gene	Locus	Positive (or negative) association	No association
Dopaminergic transmission			
Dopamine-D2-receptor	11q22–23	(Plante Bordeneuve et al., 1997)	(Nanko et al., 1994)
Dopamine-D3-receptor	3q13.3		(Nanko et al., 1994)
Dopamine-D4-receptor	11p15.5		(Nanko et al., 1994)
Dopamine transporter	5p15.3	(Le Couteur et al., 1997)	(Plante Bordeneuve et al., 1997) (Leighton et al., 1997)
Tyrosine hydroxylase	11p15.5		(Plante Bordeneuve et al., 1997)
Catechol-O-methyltransferase	22q12.1	(Yoritaka et al., 1997)	(Xie et al., 1997)
Monoamine oxidase A	X		(Hotamisligil et al., 1994)
Monoamine oxidase B	Xp11.3	(Costa et al., 1997; Kurth et al., 1993)	(Ho et al., 1995)
Heme oxygenase-1	22q12		(Kimpara et al., 1997)
Xenobiotic metabolism			
Debrisoquine-4-hydroxylase	22q13	(Wilhelmsen & Wszolek, 1995) (Armstrong et al., 1992; Smith et al., 1992)	(Diederich et al., 1996) (Gasser et al., 1996)
Cytochrome P4501A1	5q22–24		(Takakubo et al., 1996)
Paraoxonase 1	7q21.3	(Akhmedova et al., 2001)	(Wang & Liu, 2000; Taylor et al., 2000)
N-Acetyltransferase 2	8p23.1	(Agundez et al., 1998; Bandmann et al., 1998)	(Harhangi et al., 1999b)
Protein aggregation			
Apolipoprotein E	19q13.2	(Kruger et al., 1999)	(Whitehead et al., 1996)
α-synuclein	4q21.3–22	(Kruger et al., 1999)	(Parsian et al., 1998)
UCH-L1	4p15	(Maraganore et al., 2004)	(Mellick & Silburn, 2000)

inconclusive, results. Five different total genome screens in populations of 150 to 250 families have been performed (Scott et al., 2001; DeStefano et al., 2001; Pankratz et al., 2002; Li et al., 2002), and European Consortium on Genetic Susceptibility in PD (Martinez et al., 2004). None of these genome screens could unequivocally map a novel locus. This may be due to a still insufficient statistical power of the studies in the face of the high degree of genetic heterogeneity that has to be assumed. In all of these studies, several regions were identified with some evidence for increased allele sharing, but failing to reach statistical significance. Except for a locus on chromosome 5, 9q, and on the X-chromosome, none of these loci showed any overlap between different studies.

One of those loci, however, on the long arm of chromosome 2, has been followed up in an expanded group of small families with an inheritance pattern, compatible (but not proving) autosomal-dominant inheritance. In this population, a lod score of > 5 has been calculated, assuming autosomal-dominant inheritance. Fine mapping of a linked region in a population of small families can be much more difficult than in large multicase pedigrees, as no individual recombination events can be used for narrowing the region.

Another approach to identify genes contributing to the etiology of familial PD is the investigation of candidate genes. One recent example is the gene for the nuclear receptor Nurr1. Nurr1 is a member of the nuclear receptor superfamily of transcription factors that is expressed predominantly in the central nervous system, including developing and mature dopaminergic neurons. Recent studies have demonstrated that Nurr1 is essential for the induction of phenotypic markers of ventral mid-brain dopaminergic neurons (Saucedo-Cardenas et al., 1998). This gene, also called NR4A2 has been sequenced in individuals affected with Parkinson's disease and in controls. Two sequence variants have been identified (−291Tdel and -245T−>G), located in the first exon of NR4A2 to affect one allele in 10 of 107 individuals with familial Parkinson's disease but not in any individuals with sporadic Parkinson's disease ($n = 94$) or in unaffected controls ($n = 221$). These variants resulted in a marked decrease in NR4A2 mRNA levels and also affected transcription of the gene encoding tyrosine hydroxylase. This observation supports the assumption (but does not prove) that the observed sequence variants are in fact functionally relevant (Le et al., 2003).

However, other studies have failed to find any potentially pathogenic sequence variants in the Nurr1-gene, so the relevance of the original finding remains to be determined (Nichols *et al.*, 2004; Zimprich *et al.*, 2003).

Genetic contribution to sporadic PD

Although molecular genetic analysis has produced significant progress in families with parkinsonian phenotypes with mendelian inheritance, it must be remembered that Parkinson's disease, in the great majority of cases, is a sporadic disorder. The type and the extent of a genetic contribution to non-mendelian PD is still controversial. A population based case-control study indicates that the relative risk for first-degree family members of PD patients is increased only in the order of 2 to 3 (Marder *et al.*, 1996).

Most attempts to identify the susceptibility genes in sporadic PD have followed a candidate gene approach. Based on pathological, pathobiochemical and epidemiologic findings, hypotheses on the etiology of Parkinson's disease can be generated and genetic polymorphisms within, or closely linked to, genes that are thought to be involved in these pathways have been examined (Table 40.2). Unfortunately, no consistent findings have emerged so far.

Studied genes include those identified in monogenic forms of PD, including α-synuclein and parkin (Kruger *et al.*, 1999; Maraganore *et al.*, 1999; Scott *et al.*, 1999; Satoh & Kuroda, 1999; Klein *et al.*, 2000b; Wang *et al.*, 1999; Parsian *et al.*, 1998), genes encoding enzymes involved in the detoxification of xenobiotic compounds, such as debrisoquine hydroxylase, *N*-acetyltransferase (Bandmann *et al.*, 1998) and paraoxonase (Akhmedova *et al.*, 2001), as well as genes involved in dopamine metabolism and neurotransmission. Despite a large number of initial positive results, findings have not been confirmed beyond doubt in any of these cases (Table 40.2), indicating that studies with improved methodology (e.g. transmission disequilibrium testing (Spielman & Ewens, 1998)), and the examination of haplotypes instead of single polymorphisms (Seltman *et al.*, 2001) are necessary.

Conclusions

The genetic findings in rare inherited forms of PD have contributed to our understanding of the clinical, neuropathologic and genetic heterogeneity of PD. The variability of clinical features, such as age at onset, occurrence of demen-

tia or other associated features that has been found within single families, suggests that a single genetic cause (the pathogenic mutation in a given family) can lead to a spectrum of clinical manifestations. On the other hand, individuals with different genetic defects and different neuropathology (e.g. some of those with mutations in the PARK1 and PARK2 genes) may be clinically indistinguishable from each other and fulfil all presently accepted criteria of idiopathic Parkinson's disease. It is therefore apparent that a new genetic classification of PD that is only partially congruent with the classic clinical–pathologic classification is about to emerge.

At present, there is convincing evidence that genetic factors play an important role in the etiology of at least a subset of patients with PD. Only a small percentage of cases with dominant or recessive inheritance can probably be explained by mutations in the genes that have been identified so far (the genes for α-synuclein, ubiquitin carboxy-terminal hydrolase L1, and parkin) or by mutations in the as yet unidentified genes on chromosome 1p, 2p and 4p, and 12. However, the study of wild-type and mutated gene products will provide important insight into the molecular pathogenesis of nigral degeneration and Lewy body formation. However, it appears that intense efforts are still needed to unravel the full spectrum of etiologic factors leading to the common sporadic form of this neurodegenerative disorder.

REFERENCES

Abeliovich, A., Schmitz, Y., Farinas, I. *et al.* (2000). Mice lacking alpha-synuclein display functional deficits in the nigrostriatal dopamine system. *Neuron*, **25**, 239–52.

Agundez, J. A., Jimenez-Jimenez, F. J., Luengo, A. *et al.* (1998). Slow allotypic variants of the NAT2 gene and susceptibility to early-onset Parkinson's disease. *Neurology*, **51**, 1587–92.

Akhmedova, S. N., Yakimovsky, A. K. & Schwartz, E. I. (2001). Paraoxonase 1 Met – Leu 54 polymorphism is associated with Parkinson's disease. *J. Neurol. Sci.* **184**, 179–82.

Armstrong, M., Daly, A. K., Cholerton, S., Bateman, D. N. & Idle, J. R. (1992). Mutant debrisoquine hydroxylation genes in Parkinson's disease. *Lancet*, **339**, 1017–18.

Auluck, P. K., Chan, H. Y., Trojanowski, J. Q., Lee, V. M. & Bonini, N. M. (2002). Chaperone suppression of alpha-synuclein toxicity in a Drosophila model for Parkinson's disease. *Science*, **295**, 865–8.

Bandmann, O., Vaughan, J. R., Holmans, P., Marsden, C. D. & Wood, N. (1998). Association of slow acetylator genotype for *N*-acetyltransferase 2 with familial Parkinson's disease. *Lancet*, **350**, 1136–9.

Biere, A. L., Wood, S. J., Wypych, J. *et al.* (2000). Parkinson's disease-associated alpha-synuclein is more fibrillogenic than beta- and gamma-synuclein and cannot cross-seed its homologs. *J. Biol. Chem.*, **275**, 34574–9.

Bonifati, V., Fabrizio, E., Vanacore, N., De Mari, M. & Meco, G. (1995). Familial Parkinson's disease: a clinical genetic analysis. *Can. J. Neurol. Sci.*, **22**, 272–9.

Bonifati, V., Rizzu, P., Van Baren, M. J. *et al.* (2002). Mutations in the DJ-1 gene associated with autosomal recessive early-onset parkinsonism. *Science*, **299**, 256–9.

Burn, D. J., Mark, M. H., Playford, E. D. (1992). Parkinson's disease in twins studied with 18F-dopa and positron emission tomography. *Neurology*, **42**, 1894–900.

Chung, K. K., Zhang, Y., Lim, K. L. *et al.* (2001). Parkin ubiquitinates the alpha-synuclein-interacting protein, synphilin-1: implications for Lewy-body formation in Parkinson disease. *Nat. Med.*, **7**, 1144–50.

Conway, K. A., Harper, J. D. & Lansbury, P. T. (1998). Accelerated in vitro fibril formation by a mutant alpha- synuclein linked to early-onset Parkinson disease. *Nat. Med.* **4**, 1318–20.

Conway, K. A., Lee, S. J., Rochet, J. C., Ding, T. T., Williamson, R. E. & Lansbury, P. T. J. (2000). Acceleration of oligomerization, not fibrillization, is a shared property of both alpha-synuclein mutations linked to early-onset Parkinson's disease: implications for pathogenesis and therapy. *Proc. Natl Acad. Sci., USA*, **97** (2), 571–6.

Costa, P., Checkoway, H., Levy, D. *et al.* (1997). Association of a polymorphism in intron 13 of the monoamine oxidase B gene with Parkinson disease. *Am. J. Med. Genet.*, **74**, 154–6.

De Michele, G., Filla, A., Marconi, R. *et al.* (1995). A genetic study of Parkinson's disease. *J. Neural. Transm. Suppl* **45**, 21–5.

DeStefano, A. L., Golbe, L. I., Mark, M. H. *et al.* (2001). Genome-wide scan for Parkinson's disease: the Gene PD Study. *Neurology*, **57**, 1124–6.

DeStefano, A. L., Lew, M. F., Golbe, L. I. *et al.* (2002). PARK3 Influences on age at onset in Parkinson disease: a genome scan in the genePD study. *Am. J. Hum. Genet.*, **70**, 1089–95.

Diederich, N., Hilger, C., Goetz, C. G. *et al.* (1996). Genetic variability of the CYP2D6 gene is not a risk factor for sporadic Parkinson's disease. *Ann. Neurol.*, **40**, 463–5.

Duda, J. E., Giasson, B. I., Mabon, M. E. *et al.* (2002). Concurrence of alpha-synuclein and tau brain pathology in the Contursi kindred. *Acta Neuropathol. (Berl.)*, **104**, 7–11.

Duvoisin, R. C. (1986). Etiology of Parkinson's disease: current concepts. *Clin. Neuropharmacol.*, **9** Suppl 1, S3–21.

Farrer, M., Chan, P., Chen, R. *et al.* (2001). Lewy bodies and parkinsonism in families with parkin mutations. *Ann. Neurol.*, **50**, 293–300.

Farrer, M., Gwinn-Hardy, K., Muenter, M. (1999). A chromosome 4p haplotype segregating with Parkinson's disease and postural tremor. *Hum. Mol. Genet.*, **8**, 81–5.

Farrer, M., Destee, T., Becquet, E. *et al.* (2000). Linkage exclusion in French families with probable Parkinson's disease. *Mov. Disord.*, **15**, 1075–83.

Feany, M. B. & Bender, W. W. (2000). A Drosophila model of Parkinson's disease. *Nature*, **404**, 394–8.

Funayama, M., Hasegawa, K., Kowa, H., Saito, M., Tsuji, S. & Obata, F. (2002). A new locus for Parkinson's disease (PARK8) maps to chromosome 12p11.2-q13.1. *Ann. Neurol.*, **51**, 296–301.

Gasser, T. (2003). Overview of the genetics of parkinsonism. *Adv. Neurol.* **91**, 143–52.

Gasser, T., Müller-Myhsok, B., Supala, A. *et al.* (1996). The CYP2D6B-allele is not over-represented in a population of German patients with idiopathic Parkinson's disease. *J. Neurol. Neurosurg. Psychiatry*, **61**, 518–20.

Gasser, T., Müller-Myhsok, B., Wszolek, Z. K. *et al.* (1998). A susceptibility locus for Parkinson's disease maps to chromosome 2p13. *Nat. Genet.*, **18**, 262–5.

Giasson, B. I., Duda, J. E., Quinn, S. M., Zhang, B., Trojanowski, J. Q. & Lee, V. M. (2002). Neuronal alpha-synucleinopathy with severe movement disorder in mice expressing A53T human alpha-synuclein. *Neuron*, **34**, 521–33.

Gibb, W. R. & Lees, A. J. (1989). The significance of the Lewy body in the diagnosis of idiopathic Parkinson's disease. *Neuropathol. Appl. Neurobiol.* **15**, 27–44.

Golbe, L. I., Di Iorio, G., Bonavita, V., Miller, D. C. & Duvoisin, R. C. (1990). A large kindred with autosomal dominant Parkinson's disease. *Ann. Neurol.*, **27**, 276–82.

Golbe, L. I., Di Iorio, G., Sanges, G. *et al.* (1996). Clinical genetic analysis of Parkinson's disease in the Contursi kindred. *Ann. Neurol.*, **40**, 767–75.

Gowers, W. R. (1888). *Diseases of the Nervous System*. pp. 996. Philadelphia: P. Blakiston, Son & Co.

Harhangi, B. S., Farrer, M. J., Lincoln, S. *et al.* (1999a). The Ile93Met mutation in the ubiquitin carboxy-terminal-hydrolase-L1 gene is not observed in European cases with familial Parkinson's disease. *Neurosci. Lett.*, **270**, 1–4.

Harhangi, B. S., Oostra, B. A., Heutink, P., van Duijn, C. M., Hofman, A. & Breteler, M. M. (1999b). *N*-acetyltransferase-2 polymorphism in Parkinson's disease: the Rotterdam study. *J. Neurol. Neurosurg. Psychiatry*, **67**, 518–20.

Hicks, A. A., Petursson, H., Jonsson, T. *et al.* (2002). A susceptibility gene for late-onset idiopathic Parkinson's disease. *Ann. Neurol.*, **52**, 549–55.

Hilker, R., Klein, C., Ghaemi, M. *et al.* (2001). Positron emission tomographic analysis of the nigrostriatal dopaminergic system in familial parkinsonism associated with mutations in the parkin gene. *Ann. Neurol.*, **49**, 367–76.

Ho, S. L., Kapadi, A. L., Ramsden, D. B. & Williams, A. C. (1995). An allelic association study of monoamine oxidase B in Parkinson's disease. *Ann. Neurol.*, **37**, 403–5.

Hotamisligil, G. S., Girmen, A. S., Fink, J. S., *et al.* (1994). Hereditary variations in monoamine oxidase as a risk factor for Parkinson's disease. *Mov. Disord.*, **9**, 305–10.

Ichinose, H., Ohye, T., Takahashi, E. *et al.* (1994). Hereditary progressive dystonia with marked diurnal fluctuation caused by mutations in the GTP cyclohydrolase I gene. *Nat. Genet.*, **8**, 236–42.

Imai, Y., Soda, M., Inoue, H., Hattori, N., Mizuno, Y. & Takahashi, R. (2001). An unfolded putative transmembrane polypeptide, which can lead to endoplasmic reticulum stress, is a substrate of Parkin. *Cell*, **105**, 891–902.

Ishikawa, A. & Tsuji, S. (1996). Clinical analysis of 17 patients in 12 Japanese families with autosomal-recessive type juvenile parkinsonism. *Neurology*, **47**, 160–6.

Jensen, P. H., Nielsen, M. S., Jakes, R., Dotti, C. G. & Goedert, M. (1998). Binding of alpha-synuclein to brain vesicles is abolished by familial Parkinson's disease mutation. *J. Biol. Chem.*, **273**, 26292–4.

Kahle, P. J., Neumann, M., Ozmen, L. *et al.* (2000a). Subcellular localization of wild-type and Parkinson's disease-associated mutant alpha-synuclein in human and transgenic mouse brain. *J. Neurosci.*, **20**, 6365–73.

Kahle, P. J., Leimer, U. & Haass, C. (2000b). Does failure of parkin-mediated ubiquitination cause juvenile parkinsonism? *Trends Biochem. Sci.*, **25**, 524–7.

Kimpara, T., Takeda, A., Watanabe, K. *et al.* (1997). Microsatellite polymorphism in the human heme oxygenase-1 gene promoter and its application in association studies with Alzheimer and Parkinson disease. *Hum. Genet.*, **100**, 145–7.

Kitada, T., Asakawa, S., Hattori, N. *et al.* (1998). Mutations in the parkin gene cause autosomal recessive juvenile parkinsonism. *Nature*, **392**, 605–8.

Klein, C., Pramstaller, P. P., Kis, B. *et al.* (2000a). Parkin deletions in a family with adult-onset, tremor-dominant parkinsonism: expanding the phenotype. *Ann. Neurol.*, **48**, 65–71.

Klein, C., Schumacher, K., Jacobs, H. *et al.* (2000b). Association studies of Parkinson's disease and parkin polymorphisms. *Ann. Neurol.*, **48**, 126–7.

Krüger, R., Vieira-Saecker, A. M., Kuhn, W. *et al.* (1999). Increased susceptibility to sporadic Parkinson's disease by a certain combined alpha-synuclein/apolipoprotein E genotype. *Ann. Neurol.*, **45**, 611–17.

Krüger, R., Kuhn, W., Müller, T. *et al.* (1998). Ala39Pro mutation in the gene encoding a-synuclein in Parkinson's disease. *Nat. Genet.* **18**, 106–8.

Kurth, J. H., Kurth, M. C., Poduslo, S. E. & Schwankhaus, J. D. (1993). Association of a monoamine oxidase B allele with Parkinson's disease. *Ann. Neurol.*, **33**, 368–72.

Lazzarini, A. M., Myers, R. H., Zimmerman, T. R., Jr. *et al.* (1994). A clinical genetic study of Parkinson's disease: evidence for dominant transmission. *Neurology*, **44**, 499–506.

Le Couteur, D. G., Leighton, P. W., McCann, S. J. & Pond, S. M. (1997). Association of a polymorphism in the dopamine-transporter gene with Parkinson's disease. *Mov. Disord.*, **12**, 760–3.

Le, W. D., Xu, P., Jankovic, J. *et al.* (2003). Mutations in NR4A2 associated with familial Parkinson disease. *Nat. Genet.*, **33**, 85–9.

Lee, M. K., Stirling, W., Xu, Y. *et al.* (2002). Human alpha-synuclein-harboring familial Parkinson's disease-linked Ala-53-Thr mutation causes neurodegenerative disease with alpha-synuclein aggregation in transgenic mice. *Proc. Natl Acad. Sci., USA*, **99**, 8968–73.

Leighton, P. W., Le Couteur, D. G., Pang, C. C. *et al.* (1997). The dopamine transporter gene and Parkinson's disease in a Chinese population. *Neurology*, **49**, 1577–9.

Leroy, E., Boyer, R., Auburger, G. *et al.* (1998). The ubiquitin pathway in Parkinson's disease (letter). *Nature*, **395**, 451–2.

Li, Y. J., Scott, W. K., Hedges, D. J. *et al.* (2002). Age at onset in two common neurodegenerative diseases is genetically controlled. *Am. J. Hum. Genet.*, **70**, 985–93.

Lincoln, S., Vaughan, J., Wood, N. *et al.* (1999). Low frequency of pathogenic mutations in the ubiquitin carboxy-terminal hydrolase gene in familial Parkinson's disease (In Process Citation). *Neuroreport*, **10**, 427–9.

Lücking, C. B., Dürr, A., Bonifati, V. *et al.* (2000). Association between early-onset Parkinson's disease and mutations in the parkin gene. *N. Engl. J. Med.*, **342**, 1560–7.

Maher, N. E., Currie, L. J., Lazzarini, A. M. *et al.* (2002). Segregation analysis of Parkinson disease revealing evidence for a major causative gene. *Am. J. Med. Genet.*, **109**, 191–7.

Maraganore, D. M., Farrer, M. J., Hardy, J. A., Lincoln, S. J., McDonnell, S. K., Rocca, W. A. (1999). Case-control study of the ubiquitin carboxy-terminal hydrolase L1 gene in Parkinson's disease. *Neurology*, **53**, 1858–60.

Maraganore, D. M., Lesnick, T. G., Elbaz, A. *et al.* (2004). UCHL1 is a Parkinson's disease susceptibility gene. *Ann. Neurol.*, **55**, 512–21.

Marder, K., Tang, M. X., Mejia, H., Alfaro, B., Cote, L., Louis, E., Groves, J., Mayeux, R. (1996). Risk of Parkinson's disease among first-degree relatives: a community-based study. *Neurology*, **47**, 155–160.

Martinez, M. M., Brice, A., Vaughan, J. R. *et al.* (2004). Genome-wide Scan linkage analysis for Parkinson's disease. The European Genetic Study of PD. *J. Med. Genet.*, **41**, 900–7.

Markopoulou, K., Wszolek, Z. K. & Pfeiffer, R. F. (1995). A Greek-American kindred with autosomal dominant, levodopa-responsive parkinsonism and anticipation. *Ann. Neurol.*, **38**, 373–8.

Masliah, E., Rockenstein, E., Veinbergs, I. *et al.* (2000). Dopaminergic loss and inclusion body formation in alpha-synuclein mice: implications for neurodegenerative disorders. *Science*, **287**, 1265–9.

Matsumine, H., Saito, M., Shimoda-Matsubayashi, S. *et al.* (1997). Localization of a gene for an autosomal recessive form of juvenile Parkinsonism to chromosome 6q25.2–27. *Am. J. Hum. Genet.*, **60**, 588–96.

Matsuoka, Y., Vila, M., Lincoln, S. *et al.* (2001). Lack of nigral pathology in transgenic mice expressing human alpha-synuclein driven by the tyrosine hydroxylase promoter. *Neurobiol. Dis.*, **8**, 535–9.

McLean, P. J., Kawamata, H., Ribich, S. L., Hyman, B. T. (2000). Membrane association and protein conformation of alpha-synuclein in intact neurons. Effect of parkinson's disease-linked mutations. *J. Biol. Chem.*, **275**, 8812–16.

McNaught, K. S. & Jenner, P. (2001). Proteasomal function is impaired in substantia nigra in Parkinson's disease. *Neurosci. Lett.*, **19** (297) 191–4.

McNaught, K. S., Olanow, C. W., Halliwell, B., Isacson, O. & Jenner, P. (2001). Failure of the ubiquitin-proteasome system in Parkinson's disease. *Nat. Rev. Neurosci.*, **2**, 589–94.

Mellick, G. D. & Silburn, P. A. (2000). The ubiquitin carboxy-terminal hydrolase-L1 gene S18Y polymorphism does not confer protection against idiopathic Parkinson's disease. *Neurosci. Lett.*, **293**, 127–30.

Moilanen, J. S., Autere, J. M., Myllyla, V. V. & Majamaa, K. (2001). Complex segregation analysis of Parkinson's disease in the Finnish population. *Hum. Genet.*, **108**, 184–9.

Muenter, M. D., Forno, L. S., Hornykiewicz, O. *et al.* (1998). Hereditary form of parkinsonism – dementia. *Ann. Neurol.*, **43**, 768–81.

Nanko, S., Ueki, A., Hattori, M. *et al.* (1994). No allelic association between Parkinson's disease and dopamine D2, D3, and D4 receptor gene polymorphisms. *Am. J. Med. Genet.*, **54**, 361–4.

Neumann, M., Kahle, P. J., Giasson, B. I. *et al.* (2002). Misfolded proteinase K-resistant hyperphosphorylated alpha-synuclein in aged transgenic mice with locomotor deterioration and in human alpha-synucleinopathies. *J. Clin. Invest.*, **110**, 1429–39.

Nichols, W. C., Uniacke, S. K., Pankratz, N. *et al.* (2004). Evaluation of the role of Nurr1 in a large sample of familial Parkinson's disease. *Mov. Disord.*, **19**, 649–55.

Pankratz, N., Nichols, W. C., Uniacke, S. K. *et al.* (2002). Genome screen to identify susceptibility genes for Parkinson disease in a sample without parkin mutations. *Am. J. Hum. Genet.*, **71**, 124–35.

Pankratz, N., Nichols, W. C., Uniacke, S. K. *et al.* (2003). PARK3 and PARK7 Linked to Age of Onset of Parkinson Disease. *Neurology*, **60**, Abstract P02.076.

Papadimitriou, A., Veletza, V., Hadjigeorgiou, G. M., Patrikiou, A., Hirano, M. & Anastasopoulos, I. (1999). Mutated alpha-synuclein gene in two Greek kindreds with familial PD: incomplete penetrance? *Neurology*, **52**, 651–4.

Parsian, A., Racette, B., Zhang, Z. H. *et al.* (1998). Mutation, sequence analysis, and association studies of alpha-synuclein in Parkinson's disease. *Neurology*, **51**, 1757–9.

Pendleton, R. G., Parvez, F., Sayed, M. & Hillman, R. (2002). Effects of pharmacological agents upon a transgenic model of Parkinson's disease in *Drosophila melanogaster*. *J. Pharmacol. Exp. Ther.*, **300**, 91–6.

Perry, T. L., Wright, J. M., Berry, K., Hansen, S. & Perry, T. L., Jr. (1990). Dominantly inherited apathy, central hypoventilation, and Parkinson's syndrome: clinical, biochemical, and neuropathologic studies of 2 new cases. *Neurology*, **40**, 1882–7.

Plante Bordeneuve, V., Taussig, D., Thomas, F. *et al.* (1997). Evaluation of four candidate genes encoding proteins of the dopamine pathway in familial and sporadic Parkinson's disease: evidence for association of a DRD2 allele. *Neurology*, **48**, 1589–93.

Polymeropoulos, M. H., Lavedan, C., Leroy, E. *et al.* (1997). Mutation in the α-synuclein gene identified in families with Parkinson's disease. *Science*, **276**, 2045–7.

Saigoh, K., Wang, Y. L., Suh, J. G. *et al.* (1999). Intragenic deletion in the gene encoding ubiquitin carboxy-terminal hydrolase in gad mice. *Nat. Genet.*, **23**, 47–51.

Satoh, J. & Kuroda, Y. (1999). Association of codon 167 Ser/Asn heterozygosity in the parkin gene with sporadic Parkinson's disease. *Neuroreport*, **10**, 2735–9.

Saucedo-Cardenas, O., Quintana-Hau, J. D., Le, W. D. *et al.* (1998). Nurr1 is essential for the induction of the dopaminergic phenotype and the survival of ventral mesencephalic late dopaminergic precursor neurons. *Proc. Natl Acad. Sci., USA*, **95**, 4013–18.

Scott, W. K., Yamaoka, L. H., Stajich, J. M. *et al.* (1999). The alpha-synuclein gene is not a major risk factor in familial Parkinson disease. *Neurogenetics*, **2**, 191–2.

Scott, W. K., Nance, M. A., Watts, R. L. *et al.* (2001). Complete genomic screen in Parkinson disease: evidence for multiple genes. *J. Am. Med. Assoc.*, **286**, 2239–44.

Seltman, H., Roeder, K. & Devlin, B. (2001). Transmission/disequilibrium test meets measured haplotype analysis: family-based association analysis guided by evolution of haplotypes. *Am. J. Hum. Genet.*, **68**, 1250–63.

Shimura, H., Hattori, N., Kubo, S. *et al.* (2000). Familial parkinson disease gene product, parkin, is a ubiquitin-protein ligase. *Nat. Genet.*, **25**, 302–5.

Shimura, H., Schlossmacher, M. G., Hattori, N. *et al.* (2001). Ubiquitination of a new form of alpha-synuclein by parkin from human brain: implications for Parkinson's disease. *Science*, **293**, 263–9.

Singleton, A. B., Farrer, M., Johnson, I. *et al.* alpha-synuclein locus triplication causes Parkinson's disease. *Science*, (2003), **302**, 841.

Smith, C. A., Gough, A. C., Leigh, P. N. *et al.* (1992). Debrisoquine hydroxylase gene polymorphism and susceptibility to Parkinson's disease. *Lancet*, **339**, 1375–7.

Spielman, R. S. & Ewens, W. J. (1998). A sibship test for linkage in the presence of association: the sib transmission/disequilibrium test. *Am. J. Hum. Genet.*, **62**, 450–8.

Spillantini, M. G., Schmidt, M. L., Lee, V. M., Trojanowski, J. Q., Jakes, R. & Goedert, M. (1997). Alpha-synuclein in Lewy bodies. *Nature*, **388**, 839–40.

Spira, P. J., Sharpe, D. M., Halliday, G., Cavanagh, J. & Nicholson, G. A. (2001). Clinical and pathological features of a Parkinsonian syndrome in a family with an Ala53Thr alpha-synuclein mutation. *Ann. Neurol.*, **49**, 313–19.

Sveinbjornsdottir, S., Hicks, A. A., Jonsson, T. *et al.* (2000). Familial aggregation of Parkinson's disease in Iceland. *N. Engl. J. Med.*, **343**, 1765–70.

Takahashi, H., Ohama, E., Suzuki, S. *et al.* (1994). Familial juvenile parkinsonism: clinical and pathologic study in a family. *Neurology*, **44**, 437–41.

Takakubo, F., Yamamoto, M., Ogawa, N., Yamashita, Y., Mizuno, Y. & Kondo, I. (1996) Genetic association between cytochrome P450IA1 gene and susceptibility to Parkinson's disease. *J. Neural Transm. Gen. Sect.*, **103**, 843–9.

Taylor, M. C., Le Couteur, D. G., Mellick, G. D. & Board, P. G. (2000). Paraoxonase polymorphisms, pesticide exposure and

Parkinson's disease in a Caucasian population. *J. Neural Transm.*, **107**, 979–83.

Valente, E. M., Bentivoglio, A. R., Dixon, P. H. *et al.* (2001). Localization of a novel locus for autosomal recessive early-onset parkinsonism, park6, on human chromosome 1p35–p36. *Am. J. Hum. Genet.*, **68**, 895–900.

Valente, E. M., Abou-Sleiman, P. M., Caputo, V. *et al.* (2004). Hereditary early-onset Parkinson's disease caused by mutations in PINK1. *Science*, **304**, 1158–60.

van Duijn, C. M., Dekker, M. C., Bonifati, V. (2001). Park7, a novel locus for autosomal recessive early-onset parkinsonism, on chromosome 1p36. *Am. J. Hum. Genet.*, **69**, 629–34.

Vieregge, P. & Heberlein, I. (1995). Increased risk of Parkinson's disease in relatives of patients. *Ann. Neurol.*, **37**, 685.

Wang, J. & Liu, Z. (2000). No association between paraoxonase 1 (PON1) gene polymorphisms and susceptibility to Parkinson's disease in a Chinese population. *Mov. Disord.*, **15**, 1265–7.

Wang, M., Hattori, N., Matsumine, H. *et al.* (1999). Polymorphism in the parkin gene in sporadic Parkinson's disease. *Ann. Neurol.*, **45**, 655–8.

Ward, C. D., Duvoisin, R. C., Ince, S. E., Nutt, J. D., Eldridge, R. & Calne, D. B. (1983). Parkinson's disease in 65 pairs of twins and in a set of quadruplets. *Neurology*, **33**, 815–24.

West, A. B., Zimprich, A., Lockhart, P. J. *et al.* (2001). Refinement of the PARK3 locus on chromosome 2p13 and the analysis of 14 candidate genes. *Eur. J. Hum. Genet.*, **9**, 659–66.

Whitehead, A. S., Bertrandy, S., Finnan, F., Butler, A., Smith, G. D. & Ben-Shlomo, Y. (1996). Frequency of the apolipoprotein E epsilon 4 allele in a case-control study of early onset Parkinson's disease. *J. Neurol. Neurosurg. Psychiatry*, **61**, 347–51.

Wilhelmsen, K. C. & Wszolek, Z. K. (1995). Is there a genetic susceptibility to idiopathic parkinsonism? *Parkinsonism Rel. Disord.*, **1**, 73–84.

Wintermeyer, P., Kruger, R., Kuhn, W. *et al.* (2000). Mutation analysis and association studies of the UCHL1 gene in German Parkinson's disease patients. *Neuroreport*, **11**, 2079–82.

Wszolek, Z. K., Cordes, M., Calne, D. B., Munter, M. D., Cordes, I. & Pfeifer, R. F. (1993). Hereditary Parkinson disease: report of 3 families with dominant autosomal inheritance. *Nervenarzt*, **64**, 331–5.

Wszolek, Z. K., Pfeiffer, B. & Fulgham, J. R. (1995). Western Nebraska family (family D) with autosomal dominant parkinsonism. *Neurology*, **45**, 502–5.

Wszolek, Z. K., Gwinn-Hardy, K. & Wszolek, E. K. (2002). Family C (German-American) with late onset parkinsonism: longitudinal observations including autopsy. *Acta Neuropathol. (Berl.)*, **103**, 344–50.

Xie, T., Ho, S. L., Li, L. S. & Ma, O. C. (1997). G/A1947 polymorphism in catechol-O-methyltransferase (COMT) gene in Parkinson's disease. *Mov. Disord.*, **12**, 426–7.

Yoritaka, A., Hattori, N., Yoshino, H. & Mizuno, Y. (1997). Catechol-O-methyltransferase genotype and susceptibility to Parkinson's disease in Japan (in process citation). *J. Neural Transm.*, **104**, 1313–17.

Zareparsi, S., Taylor, T. D., Harris, E. L. & Payami, H. (1998). Segregation analysis of Parkinson disease. *Am. J. Med. Genet.*, **80**, 410–17.

Zarranz, J. J., Alegre, J., Gomez-Esteban, J. C. *et al.* (2004). The new mutation, E46K, of alpha-synuclein causes Parkinson and Lewy body dementia. *Ann. Neurol.*, **55**, 164–73.

Zhang, Y., Gao, J., Chung, K. K., Huang, H., Dawson, V. L. & Dawson, T. M. (2000). Parkin functions as an E2-dependent ubiquitin-protein ligase and promotes the degradation of the synaptic vesicle-associated protein, CDCrel-1. *Proc. Natl Acad. Sci., USA*, **97**, 13354–9.

Zimprich, A., Asmus, E., Leitner, P. *et al.* (2003). Point mutations in exon 1 of the NR4A2 gene are not a major cause of familial Parkinson's disease. *Neurogenetics*, **4**, 219–20.

Zimprich, A., Biskup, S., Leitner, P. *et al.* (2004). Mutations in LRRK2 cause autosomal–dominant parkinsonism with pleomorphic pathology. *Neuron*, **44**, 601–607.

Zimprich, A., Muller-Myhsok, B., Farrer, M. *et al.* (2004). The PARK8 locus in autosomal-dominant parkinsonism: confirmation of linkage and further delineation of the disease-containing interval. *Am. J. Hum. Genet.*, **74**, 11–19.

Zink, M., Grimm, L., Wszolek, Z. K. & Gasser, T. (2001). Autosomal-dominant Parkinson's disease linked to 2p13 is not caused by mutations in transforming growth factor alpha (TGF alpha). *J. Neural Transm.*, **108**, 1029–34.

41

Pathophysiology: biochemistry of Parkinson's disease

Daniela Berg[1,2], Olaf Riess[2] and Peter Riederer[3]

[1]Hertie Institute for Clinical Brain Research, Tübingen, Germany
[2]Institute for Medical Genetics, Tübingen, Germany
[3]Clinic and Policlinic of Psychiatry and Psychotherapy, University of Wurzburg, Germany

Although the primary pathology and key defects of neurotransmission leading to the clinical picture of Parkinson's disease (PD) are known, initiation and nature of the neurodegenerative process are still obscure. However, it is becoming increasingly evident that the underlying pathophysiology is complex and in most cases probably multifactorial, differing among the individuals affected.

Only a very small percentage of Parkinsonian cases are caused by monogenic alterations (see Chapter 40). However, since the first description of a family in which 79 of 194 members suffered from PD (Mjörnes, 1949), it has become evident that the risk of developing the clinical picture of PD is three to four times higher in individuals with relatives with PD compared to those with a negative family history. Functional neuroimaging proved to be especially valuable for the detection of affected siblings: for monozygotic twins a concordance of 75% for PD or at least a subclinical dopaminergic deficit was detected by PET-studies, the rate for dizygotic was 22% (Piccini et al., 1999). These and other findings provide strong evidence of a genetic contribution to idiopathic PD (Gasser et al., 1998, 2001). However, only about 25% of PD patients report a relative affected by the same disease. Therefore, other factors are necessary to explain the selectivity and susceptibility of the disease on the basis of a genetic predisposition. Biochemical and histological investigations of the past decades have illuminated some of these factors.

Oxidative stress

Oxidative stress (OS) occurs when reactive oxygen species, such as the superoxide radical ($O_2^{\bullet -}$), nitric oxide (NO) and especially the hydroxyl radical ($^{\bullet}OH$) due to an excessive production overwhelm the protective defense mechanisms of a cell resulting in functional disruption and ultimately in cell death. OS is regarded as key event in the neurodegenerative process of PD. Because of their high reactivity, free radicals cannot be measured directly. However, there are a number of indices for OS in the substantia nigra (SN) of PD patients:

- increased levels of products of lipid peroxidation and decreased levels of polyunsaturated fatty acid levels, a peroxidation substrate (Dexter et al., 1989; Yoritakta et al., 1996),
- increased levels of 8-hydroxy-2' dexyguanosine, indicating DNA base damage (Sanchez-Ramos et al., 1994; Alam et al., 1997),
- detection of 3-nitrotyrosine, the marker of OS induced by peroxynitrite, in Lewy bodies (Giasson et al., 2000)
- decrease in the level of reduced glutathione in SN of PD (Sofic et al., 1992) and low activity of phospholipid-catabolizing enzymes in normal SN compared with other regions of the human brain, indicating a reduced repair capacity of oxidative damage (Ross et al., 1998)
- upregulation of antioxidant enzymes like Mn-dependent superoxide dismutase and nonselenium glutathione peroxidase (Martilla et al., 1988; Yoshida et al., 1994; Power et al., 2002)
- OS-dependent protein aggregation in the form of advanced glycation end products, already detectable within Lewy bodies at a time when no clinical sign of PD is obvious (Münch et al., 2000).

Moreover, peripheral markers for oxidative stress like altered superoxide dismutase (SOD) activity, reductions in glutamate uptake and increased levels of malondialdehyde as well as thiobarbituric acid reactive substances have been detected in erythrocytes, serum and plasma of PD patients (Bostantjopoulou et al., 1997; Nagatsu et al., 1999; Ferrarese et al., 2001; Serra et al., 2001). These findings, as well as the demonstration of primary and oxidative DNA damage

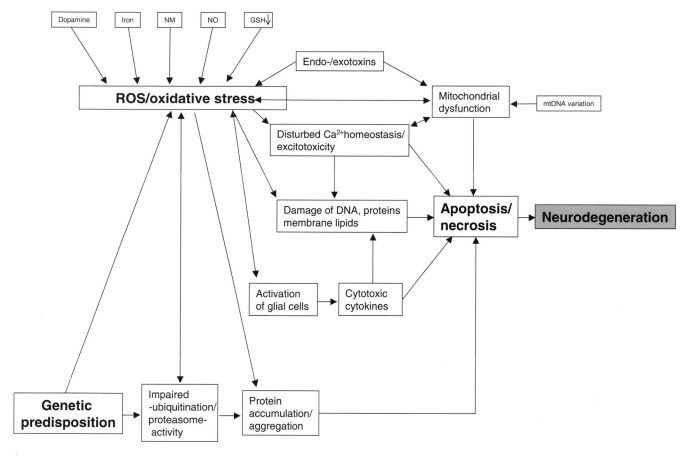

Fig. 41.1 Factors supposed to contribute to neurodegeneration in PD and their interaction. NM = neuromelanin, NO = nitric oxide, GSH = glutathione, ROS = reactive oxygen species.

in lymphocytes of untreated Parkinson patients (Migliore *et al.*, 2002), indicate a possible systemic affection related to the oxidative stress in the brain.

A number of factors have been shown to contribute to OS within the SN (Fig. 41.1).

Factors contributing to the generation of oxidative stress

Dopamine

Metabolism of dopamine, the main neurotransmitter of the neurons degenerating in PD, produces reactive oxygen species and might therefore account, at least in part, for the selective vulnerability of the SN pars compacta (SNc). After synthesis, dopamine is directly taken up into synaptic vesicles. Here dopamine is protected from catabolization, as there are no metabolizing enzymes (monoamine oxidase, MAO) and the pH is too low for autooxidation. In the cytoplasm, however, dopamine is either autooxidized or metabolized enzymatically (Lotharius & Brundin, 2002). Autooxida-

tion of dopamine leads to the production of dopaquinone and $O_2^{\bullet-}$. $O_2^{\bullet-}$ is either metabolized into H_2O_2 or it reacts with nitric oxide, generating the strongly reactive peroxynitrite ($ONOO^{\bullet-}$). Enzymatic metabolism of dopamine forms H_2O_2, which is converted into $^{\bullet}OH$ via the iron mediated Fenton reaction (Götz *et al.*, 1994; Antunes *et al.*, 2002; Maruyama & Naoi, 2002). Autooxidation may be increased in the early stages of the disease, when dopamine turnover increases to compensate for the dying dopaminergic neurons (Scherman *et al.*, 1989). Production of these reactive oxygen species has a detrimental effect on cellular macromolecules, damaging lipids, proteins and DNA (see above). Moreover, dopamine and various of its metabolites can inhibit complex I of the electron-transport chain (see below; Ben-Shachar *et al.*, 1995).

An additional toxic effect of the antiparkinsonian drug L-dopa has been the matter of discussion for many years. In vitro experiments seem to indicate an increase of OS and neurodegeneration after L-dopa administration (Spencer *et al.*, 1994; Walinshaw & Waters, 1995). In animal experiments, however, no increased toxicity was seen after L-dopa application (Perry *et al.*, 1984). Also, the ELLDOPA clinical trial has not substantiated an L-dopa induced toxicity (Fahn, 1999).

As in PD only selective dopaminergic neuron populations degenerate and other factors contributing to OS need also to be taken into account.

Iron

Iron content of the basal ganglia and SN is already under physiologic conditions higher than in most other regions of the brain (Hallgren & Sourander 1958). This is important, as iron is required as a co-factor for the synthesis of dopamine by the enzyme tyrosine hydroxylase. In PD, however, iron content of the SNc is about 35% higher, with an elevation of the Fe(III)/Fe(II)-ratio from 2:1 to almost 1:2 (Riederer *et al.*, 1988, 1989; Sofic *et al.*, 1988; Dexter *et al.*, 1993; Gerlach *et al.*, 1994). Increased levels of iron and Fe(II) enhance the conversion of H_2O_2 to $^\bullet OH$ via the Fenton reaction and favor a greater turnover in the Haber–Weiss cycle, which leads to an amplification of OS (Riederer & Youdim, 1993). Besides the contribution to the formation of highly reactive oxygen species iron has been shown to interact with α-synuclein (Hashimoto *et al.*, 1998, 1999; Paik *et al.*, 1999; Münch *et al.*, 2000; Osterova-Golts *et al.*, 2000; Golts *et al.*, 2002), one of the major components of Lewy bodies (see below). By catalyzing oxidative reactions, iron enhances the conversion of unfolded or α-helical conformation of α-synuclein to β-pleated sheet conformation, the primary form in Lewy bodies (Hashimoto *et al.*, 1998, 1999). Additionally, iron seems to play a pivotal role in the activation of NF-kappa B, a redox-sensitive transcription factor, which transactivates various genes of cytotoxic cytokines taking part in inflammatory responses (Youdim *et al.*, 1999). It is not entirely clear yet at what time in the pathophysiological cascade of PD iron accumulation occurs and whether it is a primary cause of neurodegeneration or rather reflects a secondary phenomenon. Iron accumulation induced by toxin-mediated neurodegeneration in animal models suggests it to be a secondary phenomenon (Mochizuki *et al.*, 1994; He *et al.*, 1996). However, high iron diet, fed to weanling mice, has been shown to lead to marked reduction of SN glutathione levels, a finding known to occur very early in PD (Lan and Jiang, 1997). Data from recent transcranial ultrasound studies also imply iron accumulation to occur very early in the disease process constituting rather a primary cause of the disease. In patients with PD a typical enhancement of SN echogenicity is visible on transcranial ultrasound, which has been shown to be caused by increased iron levels (Becker *et al.*, 1995; Berg *et al.*, 1999a, 2002). This marker occurs very early in life in a subgroup of the population and is associated with impaired nigrostriatal function detected by 18F-dopa PET in some young healthy individuals (Berg *et al.*, 1999b, 2002). The ultrasound marker, indicating increased iron levels, might therefore serve as a marker for vulnerability early in life. This early occurrence of increased iron levels indicates possible alterations in brain iron metabolism. Alterations have been found in proteins involved in the uptake, storage and release of iron (for review see Berg *et al.*, 2001). These alterations might be due to mutations and polymorphisms in genes encoding for iron metabolizing proteins (Berg *et al.*, 2002; Borie *et al.*, 2002).

Neuromelanin

The role of this very strong iron chelator in the pathogenesis of PD has been the matter of debate for many years (Youdim *et al.*, 1994). Neuromelanin (NM), consisting primarily of an aliphatic chain structure with a smaller aromatic backbone, is generally regarded to be the result of the spontaneous autoxidation of dopamine and noradrenaline (Zecca *et al.*, 1992; Double *et al.*, 2000). This, however, has been questioned due to the fact that (i) not all dopaminergic neurons of the SN contain neuromelanin and (ii) long-term L-Dopa treatment does not seem to enhance neuromelanin concentration in surviving neurons. As in PD, primarily NM-containing neurons degenerate (Hirsch *et al.*, 1988), leading to the typical depigmentation of the SN, a cytotoxic effect of NM contributing to OS has been proposed. Neuromelanin is an excellent chelator of metal ions, especially iron (Ben-Shachar *et al.*, 1991), therefore a neuroprotective role of neuromelanin is discussed (Zecca *et al.*, 1993; Gerlach *et al.*, 1994). Iron bound to NM accounts for 10–20% of the total iron in the SN in normal subjects aged 70–90 years (Shima *et al.*, 1997; Zecca *et al.*, 2001). In PD, however, the absolute concentration of NM within the SN is dramatically decreased (Zecca *et al.*, 2002). Moreover, iron levels of NM are higher than in controls (Good *et al.*, 1992; Jellinger *et al.*, 1992). The amount of iron determines the role of NM: in the situation of normal iron levels this redox active metal is sequestered. In the presence of excess iron, however, NM promotes the formation of reactive oxygen species and fosters the release of iron into the cytoplasm (Zareba *et al.*, 1995; Zecca *et al.*, 1996; Double *et al.*, 1999; Lopiano *et al.*, 2000). Additionally, NM can bind a variety of potentially toxic substances like MPP+, the neurotoxic metabolite of MPTP or pesticides suggesting a contribution to neurotoxin-mediated neurodegeneration (D'Amato *et al.*, 1986; Gerlach *et al.*, 1994).

Nitric oxide

Nitric oxide (NO) is produced in the reaction of arginine with molecular oxygen to generate citrulline and NO (Bredt, 1999). Besides its function in immune modulation, it plays an important role as neurotransmitter in the central and peripheral nervous system (Grisham et al., 1999). On one hand, NO acts as an antioxidant, scavenging free radicals (Rubanyi et al., 1991). On the other hand, NO may contribute to a selective neurotoxicity during brain development, rendering brain differentiation possible (Bredt, 1991). In PD enhanced production of NO by activated glial cells has been observed (Hunot et al., 1999). As a free radical, NO contributes to OS by reacting with proteins thereby altering their function and lipids, inducing lipid peroxidation (Beckmann, 1996; Iravani et al., 2002). Additionally, highly reactive intermediates like peroxynitrite are formed in the presence of superoxide, inducing DNA damage and lipid peroxidation (Beckmann et al., 1990; Liu et al., 2002). NO also mediates iron release from ferritin (Reif & Simmons, 1990), which again may contribute to OS. Direct interaction of NO and the respiratory chain can induce additional cell damage (Cleeter et al., 1994; Antunes et al., 2002). In these and other studies it has become obvious that NO is necessary but not sufficient to induce neurodegeneration. Only in concert with oxygen free radicals, other proinflammatory or cytotoxic substances, is induction of neurodegeneration achieved (Liu et al., 2002).

Factors diminishing oxidative stress

Protective defense mechanisms of cells against oxidative damage include enzymatic reactions by superoxide dismutase (SOD), glutathione peroxidase or catalase as well as non-enzymatic reactions by the antioxidants vitamin C and E, glutathione (GSH), cysteine or coenzyme Q (Gerlach et al., 2001). In situations of increased oxidative stress like in PD an increased activity of these systems would be expected to counteract toxicity of free radicals. However, no difference in the levels of antioxidative vitamins was found between PD patients and controls (Riederer et al., 1989). For catalase and glutathione peroxidase, almost equal or only slightly reduced levels and activities were found (Ambani et al., 1975; Kish et al., 1985; Martilla et al., 1988; Sian et al., 1994). However, increase of the antioxidant non-selenium glutathione peroxidase in astrocytes in PD brains (Power et al., 2002) and a specific and unique increase of SOD in the SNc were detected (Martilla et al., 1988; Yoshida et al., 1994). H_2O_2 generated in the detoxification process of free radicals by SOD is normally further converted by the enzymes catalase and glutathione peroxidase. The lack of increase of these enzymes in PD prevents this process leading to a deleterious increase of H_2O_2 (Foley & Riederer, 1999). Moreover, a reduction of total and reduced GSH is detectable in the SNc in PD (Riederer et al., 1989; Sofic et al., 1992) in the very early pathogenetic process rendering neurons more vulnerable to endo- or exotoxins (Jenner & Olanow, 1998). GSH depletion has been shown to cause a cascade of deleterious events like promoting the formation of defective proteins and thereby impairing the normal ubiquitin-proteasome pathway of protein degradation (Bharat et al., 2002). Additionally, release of arachidonic acid by GSH depletion may cause cellular damage through its metabolism by lipooxygenase (Kramer et al., 2002; Mytilineou et al., 2002). GSH depletion may also have an inhibitory affect of mitochondrial complex I activity (Bharat et al., 2002).

Mitochondrial dysfunction

A decline of about 30% in the activity of complex I, the first of five complexes of the mitochondrial respiratory chain, has been found in SNc of PD patients (Dexter et al., 1989; Mizuno et al., 1989; Reichmann & Riederer, 1989; Janetzky et al., 1994). Immunohistochemical studies revealed that dopaminergic neurons with high contents of NM were associated with low levels of complex I activity (Hattori et al., 1991). Because of the reduced activity less NAD is formed from NADH resulting in an impairment of proton pumping and electron transport, which in turn leads to an increase of reactive oxygen species, proteasome inhibition and cell death (Reichmann et al., 1993; Betarbet et al., 2000; Reichmann & Janetzky, 2000; Liu et al., 2002). Decline of complex I activity is also followed by reduced ATP production resulting in decreased energy for the cell and DNA damage. The cause of complex I impairment in PD is not clear yet. On the one hand, a secondary phenomenon resulting from radical formation, which may itself contribute to further radical formation, is discussed (Gu et al., 1998). On the other hand, changes in the mitochondrial genome have been found in the brain of PD patients with an increase of number and variety of mtDNA deletions/rearrangements compared to patients with other movement disorders, Alzheimer's disease and age-matched controls (Gu et al., 2002). Moreover, a variety of amino acid variations have been detected in cytochrome b of the mitochondrial genome in PD patients compared to only few variations in centenarians (Tanaka, 2002). This might indicate that deviations from standard amino sequence could be associated with increased production of reactive oxygen species. Besides an additional impairment of complex IV activity (Itoh *et al.*, 1997) no alterations in the functions of the other complexes of the respiratory chain have been detected, yet.

A specific role in determining survival and death in apoptosis induced by endogenous neurotoxins could be attributed to mitochondria (Naoi *et al.*, 2000, 2002). Additionally, exotoxins like the insecticide rotenone, a specific inhibitor of complex I, may produce features of PD, indicating that environmental exposure might lead to or superimpose with mitochondrial dysfunction resulting in neurodegeneration (Sherer *et al.*, 2002a,b).

Calcium homeostasis and excitotoxicity

Impaired calcium homeostasis with high levels of intracellular calcium may lead to uncontrolled stimulation of various calcium dependent enzymes and stimulation of mitochondrial generation of reactive oxygen species resulting in metabolic dysfunction and ultimately cell death (Gerlach *et al.*, 1996; Starkov *et al.*, 2002). The above mentioned loss of integrity of the cellular membrane due to destruction by free radicals and an increase of calcium influx due to disruption of the respiratory chain are sources of increased intracellular calcium levels. Another important cause is "excitotoxicity." Excitotoxicity means excitatory and toxic properties of a substance at the same time. Glutamate, the main excitatory transmitter in human central nervous system acts on NMDA, AMPA/kainate and metabotrophic receptors (Plaitakis & Shashidharan, 2000). These receptors are not only activated by glutamate, but also by specific endo- and exotoxins (Spencer *et al.*, 1987; Shaw & Bains, 2002). Lasting excitation may lead to cell death via an increase of intracellular calcium levels. Impairment of calcium homeostasis and excitotoxicity have been detected in a number of neurodegenerative diseases including Alzheimer's disease, Huntington and ALS (Landfield *et al.*, 1991; Beal *et al.*, 1993). The role of excitotoxicity in the pathogenesis of PD is not clear yet. However, neurons positive for the calcium binding protein calbindin appear less susceptible to the neurodegenerative changes occuring in PD (Yamada *et al.*, 1990; Hirsch *et al.*, 1992). The reported significant loss of calbindin in the SN of PD brains (Chan-Paley *et al.*, 1991) might therefore indirectly argue for the contribution of excess calcium to neurodegeneration in PD. High levels of expression of the neuron-specific glutamate carrier EAAT3 and high levels of the ATP-generating glutamate dehydrogenase in dopaminergic neurons of the SN demonstrate the need of high rates of energy. They may indicate a special vulnerability of these cells to excitotoxicity and impairment of glutamate metabolism (Plaitakis & Shashidharan, 2000). Studies on calcium binding to α-synuclein suggest that calcium ions may on the one hand participate in normal α-synuclein functioning, while on the other hand exercising pathological effects known to be involved in Lewy body formation (Nielsen *et al.*, 2001).

Exotoxins

First evidence of a contribution of exotoxins to the pathogenesis of PD came from the discovery of the toxicity of MPTP, an impurity formed during the preparation of meperidine, which provokes severe, progressive parkinsonism (David *et al.*, 1979; Langston *et al.*, 1983). Other substances known to cause or promote PD are CO, manganese, cyanide and methanol (Glass, 1983; Zayed *et al.*, 1990). Exposure to these substances might be at home, as seen in the case of drinking water from wells, polluted with heavy metals (Rajput *et al.*, 1986; Barbeau *et al.*, 1987). However, not all investigations corroborate these findings (Rajput *et al.*, 1987). At work, pesticides and herbicides are discussed to be the main substances of exposition (Sanchez-Ramos *et al.*, 1987; Secchi *et al.* 1992; Sherer *et al.*, 2002b). Chronic treatment with the insecticide rotenone has been shown to cause delayed oxidative damage and induce the formation of α-synuclein aggregates (Sherer *et al.*, 2002a). The latter, however, has not been confirmed in more recent studies (E. C. Hirsch, personal communication). Other toxins like chloralhydrate reacting with endogen amines (Bringmann *et al.*, 1998) and dieldrin (Kitazawa *et al.*, 2001) are still being investigated. As not all individuals exposed to the same environmental toxins develop PD, a genetically determined susceptibility is probable (see above; Jenner, 2001).

Infections have also been argued to contribute to the pathogenesis of PD in specific cases. Indices for a possible link between PD and infections are

- acute, mostly transient Parkinson syndromes in the course of virus infections (Walters, 1960; Isgreen *et al.*, 1976; Solbrig, 1993)
- detection of the influenza-A-antigen in postmortem brains of patients with postencephalitic parkinsonism (Gamboa *et al.*, 1974)
- increase of PD in certain generations after pandemics (Poskanzer & Schwab, 1963)

However, the clinical and histopathological pictures of infection-associated parkinsonism differ from idiopathic PD (Duvoisin *et al.*, 1963), rendering a contribution of infections to idiopathic PD unlikely (see also Riederer & Foley, 2002).

Glial cells and inflammation

Lower frequencies of infections and cancer in PD patients suggest a stimulation of the immune system in PD (Czlonkowska *et al.*, 2002). In the brain there are two types of glial cells involved in immunologic processes: microglia and astrocytes. Owing to their ability to secrete diffusible factors, these cells are capable of exerting either a protecting or a deleterious influence on dopaminergic neurons in PD. In the SN of PD patients glial cell distribution is lowest in areas where dopaminergic neurons degenerate and highest in those regions where they are preserved (Damier *et al.*, 1996). From this observation a protective effect of glial cells is assumed that is attributed to their production of glutathione peroxidase and pyruvate, protecting cells from highly toxic free radicals (Damier *et al.*, 1993; Desagher *et al.*, 1997), and neurotrophic factors exerting a neuroprotective influence. GDNF (glial cell line-derived neurotrophic factor) and BDNF (brain-derived neurotrophic factor) produced by glial cells have proven neuroprotective against different neurotoxic substances in vitro and in vivo (Beck *et al.*, 1993; Lin *et al.*, 1993; Gash *et al.*, 1996). Additionally, astrocytes maintain ionic homeostasis and buffer neurotransmission signals (Liu *et al.*, 2002). On the other hand, activated glial cells may exert a detrimental influence on dopaminergic neurons (Hirsch, 2000). Activated by brain damage, glial cells, especially microglia, produce various proinflammatory and neurotoxic substances. In PD brains the density of glial cells expressing tumor necrosis factor α, interferon γ and interleukin 1β is increased (Boka *et al.*, 1994; Mogi *et al.*, 1994; Hunot *et al.*, 1999). These findings as well as elevated concentrations of interleukin 2, interleukin 4 and interleukin 6 in the ventricular cerebrospinal fluid of PD patients (Blum-Degen *et al.*, 1995; Mogi *et al.*, 1996), indicate a contribution of these proinflammatory cytokines to neurodegeneration in PD. The detrimental effect of cytokines on neurons is achieved by the release of glutamate (McNaught *et al.*, 2000; Koutsilieri *et al.*, 2002) leading to an elevation of OS (Gao *et al.*, 2002) and excitotoxicity, by increased production of NO (Minghetti & Levi, 1998; Hunot *et al.*, 1999; Liu *et al.*, 2002) or by the activation of pro-apoptotic mechanisms.

Apoptosis

Apoptosis refers to "programmed cell death," a form of death in which intrinsic genetic programs of a cell act to attain its destruction (Jacobson *et al.*, 1997). Apoptosis of specific cells is not accompanied by negative effects, like inflammation, on other cells. The physiological function of apoptosis is elimination of cells either to enable differentiation during development or to get rid of noxious cells. Besides this physiological function, however, programmed cell death seems to play a role in different kinds of disorders either by insufficient (e.g. in cancer) or by enhanced apoptosis (e.g. in neurodegeneration) (Thompson, 1995). In PD the role of apoptosis remains controversial. In some studies typical evidence of apoptosis like fragmented nuclei and activation of caspase 3 has been detected (Mochizuki *et al.*, 1996; Anglade *et al.*, 1997; Tatton *et al.*, 1998; Tatton, 2000; Hartmann *et al.*, 2000). Other studies of end-stage PD patients, however, failed to demonstrate convincing evidence (Wüllner *et al.*, 1999; Jellinger, 2000). In vitro studies and animal models of PD, like the MPTP- or the NM(R)Sal-model, seem to favor the hypothesis of apoptosis mediated neurodegeneration in PD (for review see Burke & Kholodilov, 1998; Turmel *et al.*, 2001; Maruyama & Naoi, 2002; Nagatsu, 2002). The most corroborating evidence underlining that apoptosis might play an important role in PD comes from the investigation of chaperones. Chaperones are molecules with a multitude of different activities like mediation of proper protein folding, translocation of proteins across cellular membranes, signal transduction and mediation of transcriptional responses to stress (Muchowski, 2002). Immunohistochemical studies detected the 14–3–3 protein, a chaperone with seven known mammalian isoforms and 40% homology to α-synuclein (Osterova *et al.*, 1999), in Lewy bodies of PD brains (Kawamato *et al.*, 2002; Ubl *et al.*, 2002). Normally, the pro-apoptotic protein BAD prevents the anti-apoptotic function of other proteins in the mitochondria. This process can be prevented by binding of 14–3–3 proteins to BAD in the cytoplasm of cells (Muslin & Xing, 2000), relieving anti-apoptotic proteins for their function (Tzivion *et al.*, 2001). Association of 14–3–3 with α-synuclein in a complex however, reduces this anti-apoptotic activity by increasing free BAD or other pro-apoptotic binding partners (Welch & Yuan, 2002; Xu *et al.*, 2002). Indeed, Xu *et al.* could demonstrate a selective increase of the 14–3–3 / α-synuclein complex in the substantia nigra of PD patients, rendering the cell more susceptible to apoptosis (Xu *et al.*, 2002). Furthermore, application of the neurotoxin rotenone has been shown to induce selective oxidative damage in striatum (Sherer *et al.*, 2001) with chronic low dose application leading to low-level complex I inhibition resulting in delayed activation of the apoptotic pathway (Sherer *et al.*, 2002a).

Lewy bodies and protein aggregation

Lewy bodies are typical but not specific for PD. Lewy bodies or Lewy body-like inclusion bodies can also be found in other neurodegenerative diseases like multiple system atrophy, progressive supranuclear palsy, Alzheimer's disease, and other diseases affecting the brain like prion diseases, Down syndrome or subacute progressive panencephalitis (Lowe *et al.*, 1997; Goedert *et al.*, 1998; Trojanowski & Lee, 2001). More than 25 different protein components of Lewy bodies are known. One main group of components consists of neurofilaments, α-synuclein, β-amyloid, actin-like protein and many others, another group of proteins is expressed as a cellular response to the abnormal protein aggregation like ubiquitin, proteasome subunits and chaperones (Pollanen *et al.*, 1993; Galvin *et al.*, 1999). Dysbalance of protein accumulation/aggregation, on one hand, and impairment of protein degradation on the other seem to be responsible for the formation of Lewy bodies. Normally, proteins are ubiquitinated and degraded by proteasomes. This process becomes even more important under conditions of oxidative stress, when proteins are oxidized. However, under severe oxidative stress, particularly when GSH levels are reduced (Jahngen-Hodge *et al.*, 1997), the function of proteasomes may be insufficient. This might either be due to direct oxidative damage of the proteasomes, or to oxidative damage of the proteins, making them unrecognizable for the proteasomes or to an exceeding of the degrading capacity (Grune *et al.*, 1995; Jenner & Olanow, 1998). The result is an accumulation of oxidized proteins, which again can generate free radicals contributing to cell toxicity. Oxidative modified proteins are more prone to aggregation (Souza *et al.*, 2000). By further crosslinking, which may occur in the process of lipid peroxidation (Friquet & Szweda, 1997), oxidized proteins become insoluble with the result of protein deposition and ultimately cell death. Protein aggregation has also been shown to be induced by iron (Golts *et al.*, 2002) and by advanced glycation endproducts (AGEs) (Münch *et al.*, 2000). AGE formation is increased under conditions of increased iron levels and oxidative stress. Moreover, they contribute to OS by activating glial cells to produce superoxide and nitric oxide (Münch *et al.*, 1998). Besides OS, alteration of protein structure due to genetic variations may be another cause of protein aggregation. Genetic variations (see also Chapter 40) might either affect proteins that are usually degraded by the proteasomes, like α-synuclein, or those playing a role in the ubiquitin/proteasome degradation pathway like ubiquitin or parkin (Krüger *et al.*, 2002).

In PD, brain areas with the highest levels of α-synuclein are those associated with Lewy bodies. This is also a reason why it has been speculated that Lewy bodies result from altered handling of oxidized proteins and may at least initially represent a protective mechanism of the cell from the toxicity of protein accumulation (Jenner & Olanow, 1998). Also, the sequestration of toxic iron by Lewy bodies indicates a protective role of these inclusions (Castellani *et al.*, 2000). New lines of evidence indicate that by increased expression even α-synuclein itself might protect cells from oxidative stress by inactivation of a stress-signaling pathway (Hashimoto *et al.*, 2002). Some investigations, however, indicate that Lewy bodies might contribute to the pathological cascade. In analogy to a model with transgenic mice (Tu *et al.*, 1997), it has been hypothesized that proteins usually transported by axons are accumulated in Lewy bodies leading to a lack of function of neurons and ultimately to degeneration (Trojanowski *et al.*, 2001). Moreover, it has been shown that α-synuclein overexpression may contribute to the formation of free radicals, thereby exaggerating the vulnerability of neurons to dopamine-induced cell death (Turnbull *et al.*, 2001; Junn & Mouradian, 2002). In the case of α-synuclein mutations, impaired neurotransmitter storage could be the source of cytoplasmic accumulation of dopamine (Lotharius & Brundin, 2002) which again promotes OS. However, it needs to be noted that the majority of degenerating neurons do not contain Lewy bodies. Therefore, these inclusions do not seem to be necessary for neurodegeneration (Tompkins & Hill, 1997).

One might argue that mutations in the α-synuclein gene are very rare and therefore of limited relevance to PD. However, the recent identification of a triplication of the normal α-synuclein gene causing PD (Singleton *et al.*, 2003) and the association of α-synuclein promoter polymorphisms causing a higher expression of α-synuclein mRNA in sporadic PD (Holzmann *et al.*, 2003; Chiba-Falek & Nussbaum, 2001; Krüger *et al.*, 1999; Farrer *et al.*, 2001) points to a more casual role of α-synuclein in the pathogenesis of PD. Notably, overexpression of wildtype α-synuclein is neurotoxic to human dopaminergic neurons but neuroprotective to non-dopaminergic neurons (Xu *et al.*, 2002). Dopamine-dependent neurotoxicity is mediated by a protein complex which also contains 14–3–3 protein which in turn binds tyrosine hydroxylase (Ichimura *et al.*, 1987). Like α-synuclein, 14–3–3 proteins are aggregated in Lewy bodies (Ubl *et al.*, 2002; Berg *et al.*, 2003a). The implication of 14–3–3 proteins in PD clearly needs further investigation as 14–3–3 proteins might not only answer some questions on the selectivity of neurodegeneration in PD but also to neuronal apoptotic cell death (Berg *et al.*, 2003b). Alpha-synuclein itself is also upregulated by environmental factors such as herbicides (Manning-Bo *et al.*, 2001), which have been associated with an increased risk for PD (LeCouteur *et al.*, 2002). How these effects take place at the cellular level remains to be determined but it could be caused by an alteration of the ubiquitin-proteasome pathway therefore indirectly leading to a reduced clearance of α-synuclein finally leading to increased oxidative stress of dopaminergic neurons.

Taken together, different pathways seem to contribute to the pathogenesis of PD. Mounting evidence suggests that the marked heterogeneity in the clinical phenotype of PD patients might be caused by varying and sometimes multiple genetic factors rendering an individual susceptible to various endo- and environmental toxins. Then a pathological cascade is induced that includes oxidative stress, mitochondrial dysfunction, excitotoxicity, glial factors, protein aggregation and finally death of neurons (Fig. 41.1).

REFERENCES

Alam, Z. I., Jenner, A., Daniel, S. E. *et al.* (1997). Oxidative DNA damage in the parkinsonian brain: a selective increase in 8-hydroxyguanine in substantia nigra? *J. Neurochem.*, **69**, 1196–203.

Ambani, L. M., Van Woert, M. H. & Murphy, S. (1975). Brain peroxidase and catalase in Parkinson's disease. *Arch. Neurol.*, **32**, 114–18.

Anglade, P., Vyas, S., Hirsch, E. C. *et al.* (1997). Apoptosis and autophagy in nigral neurons of patients with Parkinson's disease. *Histol. Histopathol.*, **12**, 25–31.

Antunes, F., Han, D., Rettori, D. & Cadenas, E. (2002). Mitochondrial damage by nitric oxide potentiated by dopamine in PC12 cells. *Biochim. Biophys. Acta*, **1556**, 233–8.

Barbeau, A., Roy, M., Cloutier, T., Plasse, L. & Paris, S. (1987). Environmental and genetic factors in the etiology of Parkinson's disease. *Adv. Neurol.*, **45**, 299–306.

Beal, M. F., Hyman, B. T. & Koroshetz, W. (1993). Do defects in mitochondrial energy metabolism underlie the pathology of neurodegenerative diseases. *Trends Neurosci.*, **16**, 125–31.

Beck, K. D., Knusel, B. & Hefti, F. (1993). The nature of the trophic action of brain-derived neurotrophic factor, des(T-3)-insulin-like growth factor, and basic fibroblast growth factor on mesencephalic dopaminergic neurons developing in culture. *Neuroscience*, **52**, 855–66.

Becker, G., Seufert, J., Bogdahn, U., Reichmann, H. & Reiners, K. (1995). Degeneration of substantia nigra in chronic Parkinson's disease visualized by transcranial color-coded real-time sonography. *Neurology*, **45**, 182–4.

Beckmann, J. S. (1996). Oxidative damage and tyrosine nitration from peroxynitrite. *Chem. Res. Toxicol.*, **9**, 836–44.

Beckmann, J. S., Beckmann, T. W., Chen, J., Marshall, P. A. & Freeman, P. A. (1990). Apparent hydroxyl radical production by peroxynitrite: implications for endothilial injury from nitric oxide and superoxide. *Proc. Natl Acad. Sci., USA*, **87**, 1620–4.

Ben-Shachar, D., Riederer, P. & Youdim, M. B. (1991). Iron–melanin interaction and lipid peroxidation: implications for Parkinson's disease. *J. Neurochem.*, **57**, 1609–14.

Ben-Shachar, D., Zuk, R. & Glinka, Y. (1995). Dopamine neurotoxicity: inhibition of mitochondrial respiration. *J. Neurochem.*, **64**, 718–23.

Berg, D., Becker, G., Zeiler, B. *et al.* (1999a). Vulnerability of the nigrostriatal system as detected by transcranial ultrasound. *Neurology*, **53**, 1026–31.

Berg, D., Grote, C., Rausch, W.-D. *et al.* (1999b). Iron accumulation of the substantia nigra in rats visualized by ultrasound. *Ultrasound Med. Biol.*, **25**, 901–4.

Berg, D., Gerlach, M., Youdim, M. B. H. *et al.* (2001). Brain iron pathways and their relevance to Parkinson's disease. *J. Neurochem.*, **79**, 225–36.

Berg, D., Roggendorf, W., Schröder, U. *et al.* (2002). Echogenicity of the substantia nigra – association with increased iron content and marker for susceptibility to nigrostriatal injury. *Arch. Neurol.*, **35**, 999–1005.

Berg, D., Riess, O. & Bornemann, A. (2003a). Specification of 14–3–3 proteins in Lewy bodies. *Ann. Neurol.*, **54**, 135.

Berg, D., Holzmann, C. & Riess, O. (2003b). 14–3–3 proteins in the nervous system. *Nat. Rev. Neurosci.*, **4**, 1–11.

Betarbet, R., Sherer, T. B., MacKenzie, G., Garcia-Osuna, M., Panov, A. V. & Greenamyre, J. Z. (2000). Chronic systemic pesticide exposure reproduces features of Parkinson's disease. *Nat. Neurosci.*, **3**, 1301–6.

Bharat, S., Hsu, M., Kaur, D., Rajagopalan, S. & Andersen, J. K. (2002). Glutathione, iron and Parkinson's disease. *Biochem. Pharmacol.*, **64**, 1037–48.

Blum-Degen, D., Müller, T., Kuhn, W. *et al.* (1995). Interleukin-1-beta and interleukin 6 are elevated in the cerebrospinal fluid of Alzheimer's and *de novo* Parkinson's disease patients. *Neurosci. Lett.*, **202**, 17–20.

Boka, G., Anglade, P., Wallach, D., Javoy-Agid, F., Agdi, Y. & Hirsch, E. C. (1994). Immunocytochemical analysis of tumor necrosis factor and its receptors in Parkinson's disease. *Neurosci. Lett.*, **172**, 151–4.

Borie, C., Gasparini, F., Verpillat, P. *et al.* (2002). Association study between iron-related genes polymorphisms and Parkinson's disease. *J. Neurol.*, **249**, 801–4.

Bostantjopoulou, S., Kyriazis, G., Katsarou, Z., Kiosseoglou, G., Kazis, A. & Mentenopouplos, G. (1997). Superoxide dismutase activity in early and advanced Parkinson's disease. *Funct. Neurol.*, **12**, 63–8.

Bredt, D. S. (1999). Endogenous nitric oxide synthesis: biological functions and pathophysiology. *Free Radic. Res.*, **31**, 577–96.

Bringmann, G., Feineis, D., Grote, C. *et al.* (1998). Highly halogenated tetrahydro-β-carbolines as a new class of dopaminergic neurotoxins. In *Pharmacology of Endogenous Neurotoxins. A Handbook*, ed. A. Moser, pp. 151–69. Boston: Birkhäuser.

Burke, R. E. & Kholodilov, N. G. (1998). Programmed cell death: does it play a role in Parkinson's disease? *Ann. Neurol.*, **44**, S126–33.

Castellani, R. J., Siedlak, S. L., Perry, S. & Smith, M. A. (2000). Sequestration of iron by Lewy bodies in Parkinson's disease. *Acta Neuropathol.*, **100**, 111–14.

Chan-Palay, V., Zetsche, T. & Hochli, M. (1991). Parvalbumin neurons in the hippocampus in senile dementia of the Alzheimer type, Parkinson's disease and multi-infarct dementia. *Dementia*, **2**, 297–313.

Chiba-Falek, O. & Nussbaum, R. L. (2001). Effect of allelic variation at the NACP-Rep1 repeat upstream of the α-synuclein gene (SNCA) on transcription in a cell culture luciferase reporter system. *Hum. Mol. Genet.*, **10**, 3101–9.

Cleeter, M. W. J., Cooper, J. M., Darley Usmar, V. M., Moncada, S. & Schapira, A. H. V. (1994). Reversible inhibition of cytochrome c oxidase, the terminal enyzme of the mitochondrial respiratory chain, by nitric oxide: implications for neurodegenerative disorders. *Acta Biochem. Biophys.*, **288**, 481–7.

Czlonkowska, A., Kurkowska-Jastrzebska, I., Czlonkowski, A., Peter, D. & Stefano, G. B. (2002). Immune processes in the pathogenesis of Parkinson's disease – a potential role for microglia and nitric oxide. *Med. Sci. Monit.*, **8**, 165–77.

D'Amato, R. J., Lipman, Z. P. & Snyder, S. H. (1986). Selectivity of the Parkinson neurotoxin MPTP: toxic metabolite MPP+ binds to neuromelanin. *Science*, **231**, 987–9.

Damier, P., Hirsch, E. C., Zhang, P., Agid, Y. & Javoy-Agid, F. (1993). Glutathione peroxidase, glial cells and Parkinson's disease. *Neuroscience*, **52**, 1–6.

Damier, P., Kastner, A., Agid, Y. & Hirsch, E. C. (1996). Does monoamine oxidase type B play a role in dopaminergic nerve cell death in Parkinson's disease? *Neurology*, **46**, 1262–9.

David, G. C., Williams, A. C., Markey, S. P. *et al.* (1979). Chronic Parkinsonism secondary to intravenous injection of meperidine analogues. *Psychiat. Res.*, **1**, 249 – (PF Sz).

Desagher, S., Glowinski, J. & Premont, J. (1997). Pyruvate protects neurons against hydrogen peroxide-induced toxicity. *J. Neurosci.*, **17**, 9060–7.

Dexter, D. T., Cater, C. J., Wells, F. R. *et al.* (1989). Basal lipid peroxidation in substantia nigra is increased in Parkinson's disease. *J. Neurochem.*, **52**, 381–9.

Dexter, D. T., Sian, J., Jenner, P. & Marsden, C. D. (1993). Implications of alterations in trace element levels in brain in Parkinson's disease and other neurological disorders affecting the basal ganglia. *Adv. Neurol.*, **60**, 273–81.

Double, K. L., Riederer, P. & Gerlach, M. (1999). Significance of neuromelanin for neurodegeneration in Parkinson's disease. *Drug News Perspect.*, **12**, 333–40.

Double, K. L., Gerlach, M., Youdim, M. B. H. & Riederer, P. (2000). Impaired iron homeostasis in Parkinson's disease. *J. Neural Transm.*, **60**, 37–58.

Duvoisin, R. C., Zahr, M. D., Schweitzer, M. D. *et al.* (1963). Parkinsonism before and since the epidemic of encephalitis lethargica. *Arch. Neurol.*, **9**, 232–6.

Fahn, S. (1999). Parkinson disease, the effect of levodopa, and the ELLDOPA trial. Earlier vs later L-dopa. *Arch.Neurol.*, **56**, 529–35.

Farrer, M., Maraganore, D. M., Lockhart, P. *et al.* (2001). α-synuclein gene haplotypes are associated with Parkinson's disease. *Hum. Mol. Genet.*, **10**, 1847–51.

Ferrarese, C., Tremolizzo, L., Rigoldi, M., Sala, G. & Begni, B. (2001). Decreased platelet glutamate uptake and genetic risk factors in patients with Parkinson's disease. *Neurol. Sci.*, **22**, 65–6.

Foley, P. & Riederer, P. (1999). Pathogenesis and preclinical course of Parkinson's disease. *J. Neural. Transm.*, **56**, S31–74.

Friquet, B. & Szweda, L. I. (1997). Inhibition of the multicatalytic proteinase (proteasome) by the 4-hydroxy-2-nonenal cross linked protein. *FEBS Lett.*, **405**, 21–5.

Galvin, J. F., Lee, V. M. Y., Schmidt, L. *et al.* (1999). Pathology of the Lewy body. In *Advances in Neurology*, Vol 80, *Parkinson's Disease*, ed. G. Stern, pp. 313–24. Philadelphia: Lippincott Williams & Wilkins.

Gamboa, E. T., Wolf, A., Yahr, M. D. *et al.* (1974). Influenza virus antigen in postencephalic parkinsonism brain. *Arch. Neurol.*, **31**, 228–32.

Gao, H. M., Jiang, J., Wilson, B., Zhang, W., Hong, J. S. & Liu, B. (2002). Microglia activation-mediated delayed and progressive degeneration of rat nigral dopaminergic neurons: relevance to Parkinson's disease. *J. Neurochem.*, **81**, 1285–97.

Gash, D. M., Zhang, Z., Ovadia, A. *et al.* (1996). Functional recovery in parkinsonian monkeys treated with GDNF. *Nature*, **380**, 252–5.

Gasser, T. (1998). Genetics of Parkinson's disease. *Ann. Neurol.*, **44**, S53–7.

Gasser, T. (2001). Molecular genetics of Parkinson's disease. In *Advances in Neurology*, Vol 86, *Parkinson's Disease*, ed. D. Calne & S. Calne, pp. 23–32. Philadelphia: Lippincott Williams & Wilkins.

Gerlach, M., Ben-Shachar, D., Riederer, P. *et al.* (1994). Altered brain metabolism of iron as a cause of neurodegenerative diseases. *J. Neurochem.*, **63**, 793–807.

Gerlach, M., Riederer, P. & Youdim, M. B. H. (1996). Molecular mechanisms for neurodegeneration: synergism between reactive oxygen species, calcium and excitotoxic amino acids. In *Advances in Neurology*, Vol 69, *Parkinson's Disease.*, ed. L. Battistin, G. Scarlato, T. Caraceni & S. Ruggieri, pp. 177–94. Philadelphia: Lippincott-Raven.

Gerlach, M., Reichmann, H. & Riederer, P. (2001). *Die Parkinsonkrankheit, Grundlagen, Klinik, Therapie*. Wien, New York: Springer.

Giasson, B. I., Duda, J. E., Murray, I. V. *et al.* (2000). Oxidative damage linked to neurodegeneration by selective alpha-synuclein nitration in synucleinopathy lesions. *Science*, **3**, 985–9.

Glass, J. (1983). Untersuchung zur Bedeutung chemischer Noxen in der Ätiologie des Parkinson Syndroms. In *Pathophysiologie, Klinik und Therapie des Parkinsonismus*, pp. 103–7. Basel: Roches.

Goedert, M., Spillantini, M. G. & Davies, S. W. (1998). Filamentous nerve cell inclusions in neurodegenerative diseases. *Curr. Opin. Neurobiol.*, **8**, 619–32.

Golts, N., Snyder, H., Frasier, M., Theisler, C., Choi, P. & Wolozin, B. (2002). Magnesium inhibits spontaneous and iron-induced aggregation of alpha-synuclein. *J. Biol. Chem.*, **277**, 16116–23.

Good, P., Olanow, C. & Perl, D. (1992). Neuromelanin-containing neurons of the substantia nigra accumulate iron and aluminium in Parkinson's disease: a LAMMA study. *Brain*, **593**, 343–6.

Götz, M. E., Künig, G., Riederer, P. & Youdim, M. B. H. (1994). Oxidative stress. Free radical production in neural degeneration. *Pharmac. Ther.*, **63**, 37–122.

Grisham, M. B., Jourd'Heul, D. & Wink, D. A. (1999). Nitric oxide I. Physiological chemistry of nitric oxide and its metabolites: implications in inflammation. *Am. J. Physiol.*, **276**, 315–21.

Grune, T., Reinheckel, T., Joshi, M. & Davies, K. J. A. (1995). Proteolysis in cultured liver epithelial cells during oxidative stress. Role of multicatalytic proteinase complex proteasome. *J. Biol. Chem.*, **270**, 2344–51.

Gu, M., Cooper, J. M., Taanman, J. W. & Schapira, A. H. V. (1998). Mitochondrial DNA transmission of the mitochondrial defect in Parkinson's disease. *Ann. Neurol.*, **44**, 177–86.

Gu, G., Reyes, P. E., Golden, G. T. *et al.* (2002). Mitochondrial DNA deletions/rearrangements in Parkinson disease and related neurodegenerative disorders. *J. Neuropathol. Exp. Neurol.*, **61**, 634–9.

Hallgren, B. & Sourander, P. (1958). The effect of age on non-haem iron in the human brain. *J. Neurochem.*, **3**, 41–51.

Hartmann, A., Hunot, S., Michel, P. P., Muriel, M. P. & Vyas, S. (2002). Caspase-3 activation: a vulnerability factor and final effector in apoptotic death of dopaminergic neurons in Parkinson's disease. *Proc. Natl Acad. Sci., USA*, **97**, 2875–80.

Hashimoto, M., Hsu, L. J., Sisk, A. *et al.* (1998). Human recombinant NACP/alpha-synuclein is aggregated and fibrillated in vitro: relevance for Lewy body disease. *Brain. Res.*, **799**, 301–6.

Hashimoto, M., Hsu, L. J., Xia, Y. *et al.* (1999). Oxidative stress induces amyloid-like aggregate formation of NACP/α-synuclein *in vitro*. *NeuroReport*, **10**, 717–21.

Hashimoto, M., Hsu, L. J., Rockenstein, E., Takenouchi, T., Mallory, M. & Masliah, E. (2002). Alpha-synuclein protects against oxidative stress via inactivation of the c-Jun N-terminal kinase stress-signaling pathway in neuronal cells. *J. Biol. Chem.*, **277**, 11465–72.

Hattori, N., Tanaka, M., Ozawa, T. & Mizuno, Y. (1991). Immunohistochemical studies on complexes I, II, III and IV of mitochondria in Parkinson's disease. *Ann. Neurol.*, **30**, 563–71.

He, Y., Thong, P. S., Lee, T. *et al.* (1996). Increased iron in the substantia nigra of 6-OHDA induced parkinsonian rats: a nuclear microscopy study. *Brain. Res.*, **735**, 149–53.

Hirsch, E. C. (2000). Glial cells and Parkinson's disease. *J. Neurol.*, **247** (II) 58–62.

Hirsch, E. C., Graybiel, A. M. & Agid, Y. A. (1988). Melanid dopaminergic neurons are differentially susceptible to degeneration in Parkinson's disease. *Nature*, **334**, 345–8.

Hirsch, E. C., Mouatt, A., Thomasser, M., Javoy-Agid, F., Agid, Y. & Graybiel, A. M. (1992). Expression of calbindin D$_{28K}$-like immunoreactivity in catecholaminergic cell groups in the human midbrain. Normal distribution and distribution in Parkinson's disease. *Neurodegeneration*, **1**, 83–93.

Holzmann, C., Krüger, R., Saecker, A. M. *et al.* (2003). Polymorphisms of the α-synuclein promoter: expression analyses and association studies in Parkinson's disease. *J. Neural. Transm.*, **110**, 67–76.

Hunot, S., Dugas, N., Faucheux, B. *et al.* (1999). Fc epsilon-RII/CD23 is expressed in Parkinson's disease and induces, in vitro, production of nitric oxide and tumor necrosis factor-alpha in glial cells. *J. Neurosci.*, **19**, 3440–7.

Ichimura, T., Isobe, T., Okuyama, T., Yamauchi, T. & Fujisawa, H. (1987). Brain 14–3–3 protein is an activator protein that activates tryptophan 5-monooxygenase and tyrosine-3-monooxygenase in the presence of Ca^{2+}-, calmodulin-dependent protein kinase II. *FEBS Lett.*, **219**, 79–82.

Iravani, M. M., Kashefi, K., Mander, P., Rose, S. & Jenner, P. (2002). Involvement of inducible nitric oxide synthase in inflammation-induced dopaminergic neurodegeneration. *Neuroscience*, **110**, 49–58.

Isgreen, W. P., Chutorian, A. M. & Fahn, S. (1976). Sequential parkinsonism and chorea following 'mild' influenza. *Trans. Am. Neurol. Assoc.*, **101**, 56–9.

Itoh, K., Weis, S., Mehraein, P. & Muller-Hocker, J. (1997). Defects of cytochrome c oxidase in the substantia nigra of Parkinson's disease: an immunohistochemical and morphometric study. *Mov. Disord.*, **12**, 9–16.

Jacobson, M. D., Weil, M. & Raff, M. C. (1997). Programmed cell death in animal development. *Cell*, **88**, 347–54.

Janetzky, B., Hauck, S., Youdim, M. B. *et al.* (1994). Unaltered aconitase activity, but decreased complex I activity in substantia nigra pars compacta of patients with Parkinson's disease. *Neurosci. Lett.*, **169**, 126–8.

Jangen-Hodge, J., Obin, M. S., Gong, X. *et al.* (1997). Regulation of ubiquitin-conjugating enzymes by glutathione following oxidative stress. *J. Biol. Chem.*, **272**, 28218–26.

Jellinger, K. A. (2000). Cell death mechanisms in Parkinson's disease. *J. Neural Transm.*, **107**, 1–29.

Jellinger, K., Kienzel, E., Rumpelmair, G. *et al.* (1992). Iron–melanin complex in substantia nigra of Parkinsonian brains: an X-ray microanalysis. *J. Neurochem.*, **59**, 1168–71.

Jenner, P. (2001). Parkinson's disease, pesticides and mitochondrial dysfunction. *Trends Neurosci.*, **24**, 245–6.

Jenner, P. & Olanow, C. W. (1998). Understanding cell death in Parkinson's disease. *Ann. Neurol.*, **44**, S72–84.

Junn, E. & Mouradian, M. M. (2002). Human alpha-synuclein over-expression increases intracellular reactive oxygen species and susceptibility to dopamine. *Neurosci. Lett.*, **320**, 146–50.

Kawamato, Y., Akiguchi, S., Nakamura, Y., Honjyo, H., Shibasaki, H. & Budka, H. (2002). 14-3-3 proteins in Lewy bodies in Parkinson disease and diffuse Lewy body disease brain. *J. Neuropathol. Exp. Neurol.*, **61**, 245–53.

Kish, S. J., Morito, C. H. & Hornykiewics (1985). Glutathione peroxidase activity in Parkinson's disease brain. *Neurosci. Lett.*, **58**, 343–6.

Kitazawa, M., Anantharam, V. & Kanthasamy, A. G. (2001). Dieldrin-induced oxidative stress and neurochemical changes contribute to apoptotic cell death in dopaminergic cells. *Free Radic. Biol. Med.*, **31**, 1473–85.

Koutsilieri, E., Scheller, C., Tribl, F. & Riederer, P. (2002). Degeneration of neuronal cells due to oxidative stress – microglial contribution. *Parkinsonism Relat. Disord.*, **8**, 401–6.

Kramer, B. C., Yabut, J. A., Cheong, J. *et al.* (2002). Lipopolysaccharide prevents cell death caused by glutathione depletion: possible mechanism of protection. *Neuroscience*, **114**, 361–72.

Krüger, R., Vieira-Saecker, A. M. M., Kuhn, W. *et al.* (1999). *Ann Neurol.*, **45**, 611–17.

Krüger, R., Eberhardt, O., Riess, O. & Schulz, J. B. (2002). Parkinson's disease: one biochemical pathway to fit all genes? *Trends Mol. Med.*, **8**, 236–40.

Lan, J. & Jiang, D. H. (1997). Excessive iron accumulation in the brain: a possible potential risk of neurodegeneration in Parkinson's disease. *J. Neural. Transm.*, **104**, 649–60.

Landfield, P. W., Applegate, M. D., Schwitzer-Osborne, S. E. & Naylor, C. E. (1991). Phosphate/calcium alterations in the first stages of Alzheimer's disease: implications for etiology and pathogenesis. *J. Neurol. Sci.*, **106**, 221–9.

Langston, J. W., Ballard, P., Tetrud, J. W. & Irwin, I. (1983). Chronic parkinsonism in humans due to a product of meperidine-analog synthesis. *Science*, **219**, 989–90.

LeCouteur, D. G., Muller, M., Yang, M. C., Mellick, G. D. & McLean, A. J. (2002). Age–environment and gene–environment interactions in the pathogenesis of Parkinson's disease. *Rev. Environm. Hlth.*, **17**, 51–64.

Lin, L. F., Doherty, D. H., Lile, J. D., Bektesh, S. & Collins, F. (1993). GDNF: a glial cell line-derived neurotrophic factor for midbrain dopaminergic neurons. *Science*, **260**, 1130–2.

Liu, B., Gao, H., Wang, J., Jeohn, G., Cooper, C. & Hong, J. (2002). Role of nitric oxide in inflammation-mediated neurodegeneration. *Ann. NY Acad. Sci.* **962**, 318–31.

Liu, Y., Fiskum, G. & Schubert, D. (2002). Generation of reactive oxygen species by the mitochondrial electron transport chain. *J. Neurochem.*, **80**, 780–7.

Lopiano, L., Chiesa, M., Digilio, G. *et al.* (2000). Q-band EPR investigations of neuromelanin in control and Parkinson's disease patients. *Biochim. Biophys.*, **17**, 306–12.

Lotharius, J. & Brundin, P. (2002). Impaired dopamine storage resulting from alpha-synuclein mutations may contribute to the pathogenesis of Parkinson's disease. *Hum. Mol. Genet.*, **11**, 2395–405.

Lowe, J., Lennox, G. & Leigh, P. N. (1997). Disorders of movement and system degenerations. In *Greenfield's Neuropathology*, 6th edn. ed. D. Graham & P. L. Lantos, pp. 280–366. London: Edward Arnold.

Martilla, R. J., Lorentz, H. & Rinne, U. K. (1988). Oxygen toxicity protecting enzymes in Parkinson's disease: increase of superoxide-dismutase-like activity in the substantia nigra and basal nucleus. *J. Neurol. Sci.*, **86**, 321–31.

Maruyama, W. & Naoi, M. (2002). Cell death in Parkinson's disease. *J. Neurol.*, **249** (11), 6–10.

McNaught, K. S. P. & Jenner, P. (2000). Extracellular accumulation of nitric oxide, hydrogen peroxide and glutamate in astrocytic cultures following glutathione depletion, complex I inhibition and/or lipopolysaccharide-induced activation. *Biochem. Pharmacol.*, **60**, 979–88.

Migliore, L., Petrozzi, L., Lucetti, C. *et al.* (2002). Oxidative damage and cytogenetic analysis in leukocytes of Parkinson's disease patients. *Neurology*, **58**, 1809–15.

Minghetti, L. & Levi, G. (1998). Microglia as effector cells in brain damage and repair: focus on prostanoids and nitric oxide. *Prog. Neurobiol.*, **54**, 99–125.

Mizuno, Y., Ohta, S., Tanaka, M. *et al.* (1989). Deficiencies in complex I subunits of the respiratory chain in Parkinson's disease. *Biochem. Biophys. Res. Commun.*, **163**, 1450–5.

Mjörnes, H. (1949). Paralysis agitans: a clinical and genetic study. *Acta Psychiatr. Neurol.*, **54**, 1–95.

Mochizuki, H., Imai, H., Endo, K. *et al.* (1994). Iron accumulation in the substantia nigra of 1-methyl-4-phenyl-1,2,3,6-tetrahydropyridine (MPTP)-induced hemiparkinsonian monkeys. *Neurosci. Lett.*, **168**, 251–3.

Mochizuki, H., Goto, K., Mori, H. *et al.* (1996). Histochemical detection of apoptosis in Parkinson's disease. *J. Neurol. Sci.*, **137**, 120–3.

Mogi, M., Harada, M., Kondo, T. *et al.* (1994). Interleukin-1 beta, interleukin-6, epidermal growth factor and transforming growth factor-alpha are elevated in the brain from parkinsonian patients. *Neurosci. Lett.*, **180**, 147–50.

Mogi, M., Harada, M., Narabayashi, H., Inagaki, H., Minami, M. & Nagatsu, T. (1996). Interleukin (IL)-1 beta, IL-2, IL-4, IL-6 and transforming growth factor-alpha levels are elevated in ventricular cerebrospinal fluid in juvenile parkinsonism and Parkinson's disease. *Neurosci. Lett.*, **211**, 13–16.

Muchowski, P. J. (2002). Protein misfolding, amyloid formation, and neurodegeneration: a critical role for molecular chaperones? *Neuron*, **35**, 9–12.

Münch, G., Lüth, H. J., Wong, A. *et al.* (2000). Crosslinking of α-synuclein by advanced glycation endproducts – an early pathophysiological step in Lewy body formation. *J. Clin. Neuroanatomy*, **20**, 253–7.

Münch, G., Gerlach, M., Sian, J., Wong, A. & Riederer, P. (1998). Advanced glycation end products in neurodegeneration: more than early markers of oxidative stress? *Ann. Neurol.*, **44** (Suppl 1), S85–8.

Muslin, A. J. & Xing, H. (2000). 14–3–3 proteins: regulation of subcellular localization by molecular interference. *Cell. Signalling*, **12**, 703–9.

Mytilineou, C., Kramer, B. C. & Yabut, J. A. (2002). Glutathione depletion and oxidative stress. *Parkinsonism Relat Disord.*, **8**, 385–7.

Nagatsu, T. (2002). Parkinson's disease: changes in apoptosis-related factors suggesting possible gene therapy. *J. Neural Transm.*, **109**, 731–45.

Nagatsu, T., Mogi, M., Ichinose, H., Togari, A. & Riederer, P. (1999). Cytokines in Parkinson's disease. *NeuroSci. News*, **2**, 88–90.

Naoi, M., Maruyama, W., Akao, Y., Zhang, J. & Parvez, H. (2000). Apoptosis induced by an endogenous neurotoxin, N-methyl(R)salsolinol, in dopamine neurons. *Toxicology*, **153**, 123–41.

Naoi, M., Maruyama, W., Akao, Y. & Yi, H. (2002). Mitochondria determine the survival and death in apoptosis by an endogenous neurotoxin, N-methyl(R)salsolinol, and neuroprotection by propargylamines. *J. Neural Transm.*, **109**, 607–21.

Nielsen, M. S., Vorum, H., Lindersson, E. & Jensen, P. H. (2001). Ca^{2+} binding to alpha-synuclein regulates ligand binding and oligomerization. *J. Biol. Chem.*, **276**, 22680–4.

Osterova-Golts, N., Petrucelli, L., Hardz, J., Lee, J. M., Farer, M. & Wolozin, B. (2000). The A53T α-Synuclein mutation increases iron-dependent aggregation and toxicity. *J. Neurosci.*, **20**, 6048–54.

Osterova, N., Petrucelli, L., Farrer, M. *et al.* (1999). α-synuclein shares physical and functional homology with 14–3–3 proteins. *J. Neurosci.*, **19**, 5782–91.

Paik, S., Shin, H., Lee, J., Chang, C. & Kim, J. (1999). Copper(II)-induced self oligomerization of α-synuclein. *Biochem. J.*, **340**, 821–8.

Parent, A. & Cicchetti, F. (1998). The current model of basal ganglia organisation under scrutiny. *Mov. Disord.*, **13**, 199–202.

Perry, T. L., Young, V. W., Ito, M., *et al.* (1984). Nigrostriatal dopaminergic neurons remain undamaged in rats given high doses of L-Dopa and carbidopa chronically. *J. Neurochem.*, **43**, 990–3.

Piccini, P., Burn, D. J., Ceravolo, R., Maraganore, D. & Brooks, D. J. (1999). The role of inheritance in sporadic Parkinson's disease: evidence from a longitudinal study of dopaminergic function in twins. *Ann. Neurol.*, **45**, 577–82.

Plaitakis, A. & Shashidharan, P. (2000). Glutamate transport and metabolism in dopaminergic neurons of substantia nigra: implications for the pathogenesis of Parkinson's disease. *J. Neurol.*, **247**, S25–35.

Pollanen, M. S., Dickson, D. W. & Bergeron, C. (1993). Pathology and biology of the Lewy Body. *J. Neuropathol. Exp. Neurol.*, **52**, 183–91.

Poskanzer, D. C. & Schwab, R. S. (1963). Cohort analysis of Parkinson's syndrome: evidence for a single etiology related to subclinical infection about 1920. *J. Chron. Dis.*, **16**, 961–73.

Power, J. H., Shannon, J. M., Blumbergs, P. C. & Gai, W. P. (2002). Nonselenium glutathione peroxidase in human brain: elevated levels in Parkinson's disease and dementia with Lewy bodies. *Am. J. Pathol.*, **161**, 885–94.

Rajput, A. H., Uitti, R. J., Stern, W. & Laverty, W. (1986). Early onset Parkinson's disease and childhood environment. *Adv. Neurol.*, **45**, 295–7.

Rajput, A. H., Ryan, J., Uitti, W. *et al.* (1987). Geography, drinking water chemistry, pesticides and herbicides and the etiology of Parkinson's disease. *Can. J. Neurol. Sci.*, **14**, 414–18.

Reichmann, H. & Janetzky, B. (2000). Mitochondrial dysfunction – a pathogenetic factor in Parkinson's disease. *J. Neurol.*, **247**, S63–7.

Reichmann, H. & Riederer, P. (1989). Biochemical analyses of respiratory chain enzymes in different brain regions of patients with Parkinson's disease. BMFT Symposium 'Morbus Parkinson und andere Basalganglienerkrankungen', Bad Kissingen (Abstract S 44).

Reichmann, H., Lestienne, P., Jellinger, K. & Riederer, P. (1993). Parkinson's disease and the electron transport chain in post mortem brain. In *Advances in Neurology*, Vol 60, *Parkinson's Disease: From Basic Research to Treatment*, ed. H. Narabayashi, T. Nagatsu, N. Yanagisawa & Y. Mizuno, pp. 297–9. New York: Raven.

Reif, D. W. & Simmons, R. D. (1990). Nitric oxide mediates iron release from ferritin. *Arch. Biochem. Biophys.*, **283**, 537–41.

Riederer, P. & Foley, P. (2002). Mini-review: multiple developmental forms of parkinsonism. The basis for further research as to the pathogenesis of parkinsonism. *J. Neural Transm.*, **109**, 1469–75.

Riederer, P. & Youdim, M. B. H. (eds.) (1993). *Iron in Central Nervous System Disorders*. Vienna: Springer.

Riederer, P., Rausch, W. D., Schmidt, B. *et al.* (1988). Biochemical fundamentals of Parkinson's disease. *Mt. Sinai J. Med.*, **55**, 21–8.

Riederer, P., Sofic, E., Rausch, W. D. *et al.* (1989). Transition metals, ferritin, glutathione and ascorbic acid in Parkinsonian brains. *J. Neurochem.*, **52**, 515–20.

Ross, B. M., Moszczynska, A., Ehrlich, J. & Kish, S. J. (1998). Low activity of key phospholipid catabolic and anabolic enzymes in human substantia nigra: possible implications for Parkinson's disease. *Neuroscience*, **83**, 791–8.

Rubanyi, G. M., Ho, E. H., Cantor, E. H., Lumma, W. C. & Botelho, L. H. (1991). Cytoprotective function of nitric oxide: inactivation of superoxide radicals produced by human leukocytes. *Biochem. Biophys. Res. Commun.*, **181**, 1392–7.

Sanchez-Ramos, J. R., Hefti, F. & Weiner, W. J. (1987). Paraquat and Parkinson's disease. *Neurology*, **37**, 728.

Sanchez-Ramos, J. R., Övervik, E. & Ames, B. N. (1994). A marker of oxyradical-mediated DNA damage (8-hydroxy-2'-deoxyguanosine) is increased in nigro-striatum of Parkinson's disease brain. *Neurodegeneration*, **3**, 197–204.

Scherman, D., Desnos, C., Darchen, F., Javoy-Agid, F. & Agid, Y. (1989). Striatal dopamine deficiency in Parkinson's disease: role of aging. *Ann. Neurol.*, **26**, 551–7.

Secchi, G. P., Angetti, V., Piredda, M. *et al.* (1992). Acute and persistent parkinsonism after use of diquat. *Neurology*, **42**, 261–3.

Serra, J. A., Dominguez, R. O., de Lustig, E. S. *et al.* (2001). Parkinson's disease is associated with oxidative stress: comparison of peripheral antioxidant profiles in living Parkinson's, Alzheimer's and vascular dementia patients. *J. Neural Transm.*, **108**, 1135–48.

Shaw, C. A. & Bains, J. S. (2002). Synergistic versus antagonistic actions of glutamate and glutathione: the role of excitotoxicity and oxidative stress in neuronal disease. *Cell Mol. Biol.*, **48**, 127–36.

Sherer, T. B., Betarbet, R. & Greenamyre, J. T. (2001). The rotenone model of Parkinson's disease in vivo: selective striatal oxidative damage and caspase-3 activation in nigrostriatal neurons. *Soc. Neurosci. Abstr.*, **27**, 653–2.

(2002a). Environment, mitochondria, and Parkinson's disease. *Neuroscientist*, **8**, 192–7.

Sherer, T. B., Betarbet, R., Stout, A. K., Lund, S. & Baptista, M. (2002b). An *in vitro* model of Parkinson's disease: linking mitochondrial impairment to altered α-synuclein metabolism and oxidative damage. *J. Neurosci.*, **22**, 7006–15.

Shima, T., Sarna, T., Swartz, H., Stroppolo, A., Gerbasi, R. & Zecca, L. (1997). Binding of iron to neuromelanin of human substantia nigra and synthetic neuromelanin: an electron paramagnetic resonance spectroscopy study. *Free Radic. Biol. Med.*, **23**, 110–19.

Sian, J., Dexter, D. T., Lees, A. J., Daniel, S., Jenner, P. & Marsden, C. D. (1994). Glutathione-related enzymes in brain in Parkinson's disease. *Ann. Neurol.*, **36**, 356–61.

Singleton, A., Farrer, M., Johnson, J. *et al.* (2003). Triplication of the normal α-synuclein gene is a cause of hereditary Parkinson's disease. *Science*, **302**, 841.

Sofic, E., Riederer, P., Heinsen, H. *et al.* (1988). Increased iron (III) and total iron content in post mortem substantia nigra of parkinsonian brain. *J. Neural. Transm.*, **74**, 199–205.

Sofic, E., Lange, K. W., Jellinger, K. & Riederer, P. (1992). Reduced and oxidized glutathione in the substantia nigra of patients with Parkinson's disease. *Neurosci. Lett.*, **142**, 128–130.

Solbrig, M. V. (1993). Acute parkinsonism in suspected herpes simplex encephalitis. *Mov. Disord.*, **8**, 233–4.

Souza, J. M., Giasson, B. I., Chen, Q., Lee, V. M. & Ischiropoulos, H. (2000). Dityrosine cross-linking promotes formation of stable α-synuclein polymers. Implication of nitrative and oxidative stress in the pathogenesis of neurodegenerative synucleinopathies. *J. Biol. Chem.*, **275**, 18344–9.

Spencer, J. P. E., Jenner, A., Aruoma, O. I. *et al.* (1994). Intense oxidative DNA damage promoted by L-Dopa and its metabolites: implications for neurodegenerative disease(S?). *FEBS Lett.*, **353**, 246–50.

Spencer, P. S., Nunn, P. B., Hugon, J. *et al.* (1987). Guam amyotrophic lateral sclerosis-parkinsonism-dementia linked to a plant excitant neurotoxin. *Science*, **237**, 517–22.

Starkov, A. A., Polster, B. M. & Fiskum, G. (2002). Regulation of hydrogen peroxide production by brain mitochondria by calcium and Bax. *J. Neurochem.*, **83**, 220–8.

Tanaka, M. (2002). Mitochondrial genotypes and cytochrome b variants associated with longevity or Parkinson's disease. *J. Neurol.*, **249** (III), 1–8.

Tatton, N. A. (2000). Increased caspase 3 and Bax immunoreactivity accompany nuclear GAPDH translocation and neuronal apoptosis in Parkinson's disease. *Exp. Neurol.*, **166**, 29–43.

Tatton, N. A., Mallean-Fraser, A., Tatton, W. G. *et al.* (1998). A fluorescent double labeling method to detect and confirm apoptotic nuclei in Parkinson's disease. *Ann. Neurol.*, **44**, S142–8.

Thompson, C. B. (1995). Apoptosis in the pathogenesis of disease. *Science*, **267**, 1456–62.

Tompkins, M. M. & Hill, W. D. (1997). Contribution of somal Lewy bodies to neuronal death. *Brain Res.*, **775**, 24–9.

Trojanowski, J. Q. & Lee, V. M.-Y. (2001). Parkinson's disease and related neurodegenerative synucleinopathies linked to progressive accumulation of synuclein aggregates in brain. *Parkinsonism Rel. Disord.*, **7**, 247–51.

Tu, P. H., Robinson, K. A., de Snoo, F. *et al.* (1997). Selective degeneration of Purkinje cells with Lewy body-like inclusions in aged NFHLACZ transgenic mice. *J. Neurosci.*, **17**, 1064–74.

Turmel, H., Hartmann, A., Parain, K. (2001). Caspase-3 activation in 1-methyl-4-phenyl-1,2,3,6-tetrahydropyridine (MPTP)-treated mice. *Mov. Disord.*, **16**, 185–9.

Turnbull, S., Tabner, B. J., El-Agnaf, O. M. A., Moore, S., Davies, Y. & Allsop, D. (2001). α-synuclein implicated in Parkinson's disease catalyses the formation of hydrogen peroxide in vitro. *Free Radic. Biol. Med.*, **30**, 1163–70.

Tzivion, G., Shen, Y. H. & Zhu, J. (2001). 14–3–3 proteins; bringing new definitions to scaffolding. *Oncogene*, **20**, 6331–8.

Ubl, A., Berg, D., Holzmann, C. *et al.* (2002). 14–3–3 protein is a component of Lewy bodies in Parkinson's disease – mutation analysis and association studies of 14–3–3 eta. *Mol. Brain. Res.*, **108**, 33–9.

Walinshaw, G. & Waters, C. M. (1995). Induction of apoptosis in catecholaminergic PC12 cells by L-Dopa: implications for the treatment of Parkinson's disease. *J. Clin. Invest.*, **95**, 2458–64.

Walters, J. H. (1960). Postencephalitic Parkinson syndrome after meningoencephalitis due to Coxsacki virus group B, type 2. *N. Engl. J. Med.*, **263**, 744–7.

Welch, K. & Yuan, J. (2002). Releasing the nerve cell killers. *Nat. Med.* **8**, 564–5.

Wüllner, U., Kornhuber, J. & Weller, M. (1999). Cell death and apoptosis regulating proteins in Parkinson's disease – a cautionary note. *Acta Neuropathol.*, **97**, 408–12.

Xu, J., Kao, S. Y., Lee, F. J. S., Song, W., Jin, L. W. & Yankner, B. A. (2002). Dopamine-dependent neurotoxicity of α-synuclein: a mechanism for selective neurodegeneration in Parkinson disease. *Nat. Med.*, **8**, 600–6.

Yamada, T., McGeer, P. L., Baimbridge, K. G. & McGeer, E. G. (1990). Relative sparing in Parkinson's disease of substantia nigra neurons containing calbindin D28K. *Brain Res.*, **526**, 303–7.

Yoshida, E., Mokuno, K., Aoki, S. I. *et al.* (1994). Cerebrospinal fluid levels of superoxide dismutase. *Neurol. Sci.*, **124**, 25–31.

Youdim, M. B., Ben-Shachar, D. & Riederer, P. (1994). The enigma of neuromelanin in Parkinson's disease substantia nigra. *J. Neural Transm.*, **43**, S113–22.

Youdim, M. B., Grunblatt, E. & Mandel, S. (1999). The pivotal role of iron in NF-kappa B activation and nigrostriatal dopaminergic neurodegeneration. Prospects for neuroprotection in Parkinson's disease with iron chelators. *Ann. NY Acad. Sci.*, **890**, 7–25.

Zareba, M., Bober, A., Korytowski, W., Zecca, L. & Sarna, T. (1995). The effect of a synthetic neuromelanin on yield of free hydroxyl radicals generated in model systems. *Biochim. Biophys. Acta.*, **1271**, 343–8.

Zayed, J., Ducic, S., Campanella, G. *et al.* (1990). Facteurs environnementeaux dans la maladie de Parkinson. *Can. J. Neurol. Sci.*, **17**, 286–91.

Zecca, L. & Swartz, H. M. (1993). Total and paramagnetic metals in human substantia nigra and its neuromelanin. *J. Neural Transm.*, **5**, 203–13.

Zecca, L., Mecacci, O., Seraglia, R. & Parati, E. (1992). The chemical characterization of melanin contained in substantia nigra of human brain. *Biochim. Biophys. Acta*, **1138**, 6–10.

Zecca, L., Shima, T., Stroppolo, A. *et al.* (1996). Interaction of neuromelanin and iron in the substantia nigra and other areas of human brain. *Neuroscience*, **73**, 407–15.

Zecca, L., Gallorini, M., Schünemann, V. *et al.* (2001). Iron, neuromelanin and ferritin in substantia nigra of normal subjects at different ages. Consequences for iron storage and neurodegenerative processes. *J. Neurochem.*, **76**, 1766–73.

Zecca, L. Fariello, R., Riederer, P., Sulzer, D., Gatti, A. & Tampellini, D. (2002). The absolute concentration of nigral dopamine, assayed by a new sensitive method, increases throughout the life and is dramatically decreased in Parkinson's disease. *FEBS Lett.*, **510**, 216–20.

42

Current and potential treatments of Parkinson's disease

Clifford W. Shults

Department of Neurosciences, University of California, La Jolla, San Diego, CA, USA and VA San Diego Healthcare System, Dan Diego, CA, USA

Parkinson's disease (PD) is a progressive, degenerative neurological disorder characterized by rest tremor, bradykinesia, cogwheel rigidity and postural instability (Lang & Lozano, 1998). In the later stages of the illness approximately 30–40% of patients will develop cognitive compromise. The cardinal pathological features of PD are loss of neurons on the substantia nigra pars compacta (SNpc) and the presence of eosinophilic, intracytoplasmic inclusions, and Lewy bodies (Braak & Braak, 2000). The neurons of the SNpc project primarily to the caudate and putamen, which are referred to collectively as the striatum, and utilize the neurotransmitter dopamine. Dopamine is severely reduced in the SNpc and striatum in parkinsonian brains (Hornykiewicz, 2002). Although the loss of neurons is most conspicuous in the SNpc, neuronal loss and Lewy bodies are found in a number of brain regions, e.g. locus ceruleus, entorhinal region and amygdala (Braak & Braak, 2000). The neuronal loss and the presence of Lewy bodies in regions other than the SNpc suggest that although treatments that target only the nigrostriatal dopaminergic system may substantially benefit patients, they are unlikely to completely resolve the deficits of PD.

The following review presents a strategic framework through which to consider targets for therapies of PD. In some of the areas we are just beginning to have treatments, e.g. slowing the progression of the disease, and in others we have well-established therapies, e.g. augmentation of the function of the remaining dopaminergic system.

Slowing or stopping the progression of PD

No currently available treatments have been proven unequivocally to slow the degeneration of the nigrostriatal dopaminergic system and the functional decline of PD patients. However, recent research in PD has elucidated a number of processes that appear to contribute to the degenerative process, and researchers have begun to identify interventions in these processes. These pathogenic mechanisms include mitochondrial dysfunction, oxidative stress, impaired protein degradation, abnormal protein aggregation, inflammation and apoptosis.

Mitochondrial dysfunction

A role for mitochondrial dysfunction was first suggested by the discovery that methyl-4-phenyl-1,2,3,6-tetrahydropyridine (MPTP), which injures the nigral dopaminergic system and causes a parkinsonian syndrome in human and non-human primates (Langston *et al.*, 1983), acts by inhibition of complex I of the mitochondrial electron transport chain (see review by Przedborski & Jackson-Lewis, 1998). Complex I activity was subsequently found to be reduced in the substantia nigra in Parkinsonian brains and in platelets from PD patients with early, untreated disease (Schapira *et al.*, 1990; Haas *et al.*, 1995). Shults *et al.* (1997) reported that mitochondria from patients with early untreated PD had significantly reduced levels of coenzyme Q_{10}, which is the electron acceptor for complexes I and II of the mitochondrial electron transport chain and a potent antioxidant. Recently, Shults *et al.* (2002) reported on a phase II trial of three dosages of coenzyme Q_{10} (300, 600 and 1200 mg/d) vs. placebo in patients with early, untreated PD; all groups also received vitamin E at a dosage of 1200 IU/d. The study demonstrated a trend toward slowing the functional decline, as measured by the Unified Parkinson Disease Rating Scale (UPDRS); in patients treated with coenzyme Q_{10} and in the group receiving the highest doses of coenzyme Q_{10} (1200 mg/d) the difference from the placebo group was nominally significant ($P = 0.04$). These results need to be confirmed and extended in a larger trial before the recommendation can be made for widespread use of coenzyme Q_{10} in PD. Preclinical studies have indicated that other therapies directed at mitochondrial dysfunction, e.g. creatinine, might be neuroprotective in PD (Tarnopolsky & Beal, 2001).

Oxidative stress

Increased oxidative stress can lead to cellular dysfunction and death through oxidative damage to proteins, lipids and DNA (Halliwell, 2001; Beal, 2002). Studies from autopsy samples have revealed evidence of a number of markers of oxidative stress and damage in PD brains, including elevated malondialdehyde (an intermediate in lipid peroxidation) (Dexter *et al.*, 1989), decreased reduced glutathione in PD but not multiple system atrophy or progressive supranuclear palsy (Sian *et al.*, 1994), and increased 8-hydroxy-2′deoxyguanosine (a marker of DNA damage) (Sanchez-Ramos *et al.*, 1994). Alam *et al.* (1997) reported an increase in protein carbonyls in PD brains but not brains with incidental Lewy bodies and considered that the increase was a late phenomenon and perhaps due to levodopa treatment. Reaction of superoxide with nitric oxide (NO) forms peroxynitrite, which can nitrate tyrosines. Giasson *et al.* (2000) reported the presence of nitrated alpha-synuclein in Lewy bodies.

Brains in which incidental Lewy bodies are found are thought to represent a presymptomatic phase of PD. A study of indices of oxidative stress and mitochondrial function in brains with incidental Lewy bodies revealed reduced levels of glutathione in the nigra but not other brain regions (Sian *et al.*, 1994). No difference between the incidental Lewy body and control brains were found in levels of dopamine in the striatum or levels of iron, copper, manganese, zinc or ferritin in the substantia nigra. The activity of complex I of the mitochondrial electron transport chain was reduced to a level intermediate between those in control and Parkinsonian brains, but the difference did not reach statistical significance. There was no reduction in other components in the electron transport chain. These data suggest that oxidative stress plays an early role in the pathogenesis of PD.

Despite considerable data that oxidative stress plays a role in the pathogenesis of PD, relatively few trials of antioxidants in PD have been undertaken. The DATATOP study demonstrated a benefit of deprenyl, which reduces oxidative stress through inhibition of monoamine oxidase B, but not of alpha-tocopherol (vitamin E) (Parkinson Study Group, 1993). However, benefit from deprenyl was noted at 1 month, which suggested that the benefit was due to a "symptomatic" effect due to inhibition of the metabolism of dopamine. The study of coenzyme Q_{10} combined with vitamin E (Shults *et al.*, 2002; please see above) supports the concept that antioxidant therapy may affect the progression of PD. New antioxidant agents have been shown to be promising in PD (Matthews *et al.*, 1999; Drukarch & Muiswinkel, 2000). Further clinical trials of antioxidants in PD appear warranted.

Impaired protein degradation

The stimuli for study of abnormal protein degradation in PD were the discoveries by Mizuno and his colleagues that mutations in the Parkin gene were linked to an autosomal recessive form of PD and that Parkin acts as an E3 ligase in the ubiquitin/proteasome pathway (Kitada *et al.*, 1998; Shimura *et al.*, 2000; Mizuno *et al.*, 2001). These discoveries have led to extensive studies of protein degradation in PD (Chung *et al.*, 2001; Giasson & Lee, 2001; McNaught *et al.*, 2001). However, not all investigators have found impaired protein degradation in PD brains (Furukawa *et al.*, 2002). Pathogenic mechanisms, other than mutations in the Parkin gene, which lead to impaired protein degradation, remain to be defined and possible therapies to overcome impaired degradation remain to be developed.

Protein aggregation

The presence of abnormal, intracytoplasmic aggregates, the Lewy body, as a cardinal pathological feature of PD has been known for almost a century (Galvin *et al.*, 1999). However, Lewy bodies are not limited to PD and can be found in a number of other disorders, including Alzheimer's disease, amyotrophic lateral sclerosis, and Hallervoren–Spatz disease. Lewy bodies are composed of a number of proteins but a prominent component is alpha-synuclein. Shortly after the discovery that a rare, familial form of PD was associated with a mutation in the gene for alpha-synuclein (Polymeropoulos *et al.*, 1997), a number of groups reported that a major component of Lewy bodies is alpha-synuclein (Spillantini *et al.*, 1997; Takeda *et al.*, 1998; Wakabayashi *et al.*, 1997). This observation led to intensive study of the role of alpha-synuclein, and development of treatments to interfere with this aggregation is an active area of research.

Inflammation

The substantia nigra in PD brains contains activated microglia (McGeer & McGeer, 1997), which can produce a number of potentially injurious compounds such as cytokines and nitric oxide (Hirsch *et al.*, 1998). Nitric oxide can combine with superoxide to form peroxynitrite, a reactive oxygen species capable of nitration of proteins. Although there is little evidence that inflammation is a primary causative factor in PD, it is plausible that it may contribute to the ongoing injury to the nigral dopaminergic neurons injured by a primary insult. Also, it is conceivable that in some cases of PD there is an initial, limited insult to the nigral dopaminergic system that results in sustained inflammation in the substantia nigra, which persists past the initial insult. Langston *et al.* (1999) reported on three intravenous drug users, who had acutely become parkinsonian after exposure to MPTP. The three subjects died between 3 and 16 years after the presumed only exposure to MPTP but were found to have ongoing cell loss and microglia in the substantia nigra.

Preclinical studies have indicated that it may be possible to reduce inflammation associated with injury to the nigrostriatal dopaminergic system with minocycline (Du *et al.*, 2001; Wu *et al.*, 2002) or inhibitors of cyclooxygenases (COX) (Teismann & Ferger, 2001). Ascherio and colleagues (personal communication) studied the incidence of PD in two large cohorts (44 057 men in the Health Professionals Follow-Up Study and 98 845 women in the Nurses' Health Survey) and found that participants who reported regular use of nonsteroidal anti-inflammatory drugs (NSAIDS) at the beginning of the study had lower risk of PD than non-users (pooled relative risk 0.55, $P = 0.04$).

Apoptosis

The mechanisms that lead to death of the nigral, dopaminergic neurons are not fully understood. Evidence has accumulated to suggest that apoptosis is involved in this process, but this remains somewhat controversial (Kingsbury *et al.*, 1998; Anderson, 2001). Apoptosis is a part of the normal function of multicellular organisms (nearly one million cells commit "suicide" each second in the adult human body (Reed, 2002)) and plays a role in normal functions such as elimination of cells during development, removal of cells infected by viruses, and homeostasis in tissues in which production of new cells is balanced by elimination of older cells. Apoptosis is defined morphologically, and the characteristics of apoptosis include chromatin condensation, nuclear fragmentation, condensation of cell contents and formation of small membrane-bound vesicles, which are phagocytosed by nearby cells without accompanying inflammation (Zimmermann *et al.*, 2001; Nijhawan *et al.*, 2000).

Apoptosis can be triggered by external and internal pathways, which act through activation of cysteine aspartyl-specific proteases (caspases). The external pathways are activated through ligation of death receptors, such as tumor necrosis factor receptor-1, and the internal pathway works through mitochondria and release of proapoptotic factors, such as cytochrome c. The Bcl-2 family members serve as pro-apoptotic or anti-apoptotic factors. Development of anti-apoptotic drugs is an active area of research (Reed, 2002). Development of anti-apoptotic therapies for PD will need to be mindful of the possibility of neoplasia, and treatments will optimally be selectively directed toward cells that degenerate in PD. Although the degenerative process affects extranigral neurons (Braak & Braak, 2000), one would anticipate that the first target for anti-apoptotic therapies in PD would be directed toward the nigral, dopaminergic neurons.

Augmentation of the function of the remaining nigrostriatal dopaminergic system

Levodopa

The introduction of levodopa revolutionized treatment of PD (Hornykiewicz, 2002). The work of Cotzias and colleagues (1969) demonstrated the benefit of levodopa alone or in combination with peripheral dopa decarboxylase inhibitor, which did not cross the blood brain barrier. There are few studies in which the efficacy of levodopa has been compared in randomized, double-blinded studies to placebo. The benefit of levodopa has been best evaluated recently in comparison to other agents, most commonly dopaminergic agonists. In a randomized, controlled study Rascol *et al.* (2000) treated patients with early PD with either levodopa/benserazide or ropinirole. In subjects who completed the study, the subjects treated with levodopa/benserazide had a greater reduction in the activity of daily living score and motor score on the Unified Parkinson Disease Rating Scale (UPDRS) than did the ropinirole group. In a similar prospective, double-blinded study in which the dosage of carbidopa/levodopa or pramipexole was titrated to a dosage that the patient and treating neurologist considered to provide satisfactory benefit, at the end of 23.5 months levodopa reduced the score on the UPDRS by 30% from the baseline score versus a 14% reduction in subjects who received pramipexole (Parkinson Study Group, 2000).

Unfortunately, patients treated with levodopa will often develop motor fluctuations (wearing off and sudden on-off) and dyskinesia within five years of beginning treatment. The Parkinson's Disease Research Group in the United Kingdom found that approximately one third of patients begun on levodopa developed motor oscillations within 3 years (1993). Hely *et al.* (1994) reported that levodopa treated patients had an average incidence of newly arising dyskinesia of 7.4% for each 6 months of treatment with levodopa. Rascol *et al.* (2000) found that, after 5 years of treatment with levodopa, 34% of the patients had developed wearing off and 45% had developed dyskinesia. In the comparison of levodopa and pramipexole, the Parkinson Study Group (2000) reported that after 2 years of treatment 38% had developed wearing off and 31% had developed dyskinesia.

Standard formulations of levodopa have a short half-life of less than two hours. Controlled release formulations of levodopa were developed to reduce the number of doses needed and to overcome the problem of wearing off. A number of studies have documented that the controlled release formulations of levodopa do allow fewer doses to be taken. The increase of "on" time with controlled release levodopa is relatively modest (Hutton *et al.*, 1989; Wolters & Tesselaar, 1996). Two studies were carried out to determine whether initial treatment with controlled release formulations of levodopa could reduce the development of motor fluctuations, e.g. wearing off or on-off (Dupont *et al.*, 1996; Koller *et al.*, 1999). Neither study demonstrated any reduction in the incidence of fluctuations, and there is no reason to use controlled release levodopa for the initial treatment of PD.

Dopaminergic agonists

The first dopaminergic agonists used were ergoline compounds, such as bromocriptine and pergolide, and the ergots, in addition to being agonists for the D2 dopamine receptor, typically have mild 5-HT2 antagonistic effects and mild adrenergic effects. More recently, nonergot dopaminergic agonists have been developed, such as pramipexole and ropinirole.

Dopaminergic agonists were introduced into the treatment of PD in the 1970s (Calne *et al.*, 1974) as a means to reduce the dosage of levodopa, and investigators found that addition of a dopaminergic agonist could reduce the dosage of levodopa needed and that dopaminergic agonists could provide satisfactory amelioration of symptoms.

A number of studies have evaluated the ability of dopaminergic agonists to be used as monotherapy in the initial treatment of PD. Riopelle (1987) reported that bromocriptine caused an improvement in clinical signs and disability, as did levodopa during the first 5.5 months after beginning therapy. Barone *et al.* (1999) found that initial treatment with pergolide was clearly superior to placebo as measured by the percentage of patients who had at least a 30% improvement on the UPDRS and other indices such as the UPDRS and the Schwab and England

Disability scale. Kieburtz and his colleagues in the Parkinson Study Group (1997a) compared the efficacy of four doses of pramipexole (1.5, 3.0, 4.5 and 6.0 mg/d) vs. placebo in patients with early PD and found that the benefit was equivalent across the four doses of pramipexole, and they showed approximately a 20% greater improvement in measurements of motor function than placebo. Adler *et al.* (1998) and Brooks *et al.* (1998) reported that compared to placebo ropinirole caused approximately a 20% improvement in the motor portion of the UPDRS.

A number of open label studies that compared initial treatment with bromocriptine suggested that early use of an agonist might reduce the incidence of dyskinesia and motor fluctuations, which often occur with levodopa treatment (Parkinson's Disease Research Group in the UK, 1993; Hely *et al.*, 1994; Montastruc *et al.*, 1994). This possibility led to prospective, randomized, double blind studies that compared the long-term outcome in patients with early PD who were initially treated with ropinirole (Rascol *et al.*, 2000) or pramipexole (Parkinson Study Group, 2000) compared to those treated with levodopa. In both studies open label levodopa could be added after the initial period of titration, if the response to the assigned treatment was no longer satisfactory. Interestingly, in both studies levodopa was significantly more effective in reducing the score on the UPDRS than the agonist (see above). Rascol *et al.* (2000) found that, after 5 years, 20% of the subjects initially assigned to ropinirole had developed dyskinesia while 45% of the subjects assigned to levodopa had developed dyskinesia. Wearing off was less frequent in the group initially treated with ropinirole, but the difference did not reach statistical significance. Similarly, the Parkinson Study Group (2000) found that 10% of patients initially randomized to pramipexole developed dyskinesia while 31% of patients initially assigned to carbidopa/levodopa developed dyskinesia. A number of conclusions can be drawn from the studies of Rascol *et al.* (2000) and the Parkinson Study Group (2000). First, treatment with a dopaminergic agonist or levodopa ameliorated the symptoms of PD to a level that the patient and enrolling investigator considered satisfactory. Second, both dopaminergic agonists and levodopa were typically well tolerated but side effects (nausea, hallucinations) were not uncommon and side effects were more common with the agonists than with levodopa. Third, in both studies levodopa reduced the score on the UPDRS more than the agonist did. Fourth, initial use of a dopaminergic agonist resulted in a lower incidence of dyskinesia. The fourth conclusion has raised some controversy because the groups were not comparable for effect of therapy (levodopa treated patients improved more), and the question has been raised whether agonist treated patients would have had a lower incidence of dyskinesia if they had improvement commensurate to that of the levodopa-treated patients.

Dopaminergic agonists are often added to levodopa to treat PD, and a number of studies have demonstrated improvement. Guttman *et al.* (1997) added bromocriptine, pramipexole or placebo to patients treated with levodopa who fluctuated. They found that both bromocriptine and pramipexole significantly improved scores on the UPDRS part II (ADL) and part III (motor score) when compared to placebo. There was a nonsignificant trend for pramipexole to cause greater improvement than bromocriptine on the UPDRS, and pramipexole, but not bromocriptine, caused a significant reduction in the time spent in the off state. Olanow *et al.* (1994) conducted a randomized, parallel group comparison of pergolide and placebo in levodopa treated patients who had dyskinesia and end of dose deterioration and found that pergolide caused significant reduction in the daily dose of levodopa and a significantly greater improvement on ratings of parkinsonian findings and activities of daily living. Lieberman *et al.* (1997) and Wermuth *et al.* (1998) both reported that addition of pramipexole in patients with motor fluctuations significantly reduced the "off" time.

Similar to levodopa, dopaminergic agonists can cause nausea, vomiting, hypotension, confusion, dyskinesia and hallucinations. The agonists also appear to cause edema more commonly than levodopa. The ergot agonists can cause fibrosis. Clinicians have recently increasingly recognized that sleep disturbances are more frequent in PD patients (Kumar *et al.*, 2002) and that higher dosages of levodopa and particularly dopaminergic agonists, e.g. pramipexole and ropinirole, can cause somnolence and sudden sleepiness or sleep attacks (Etminan *et al.*, 2001; Tan *et al.*, 2002).

Catecholamine-o-methyl transferase (COMT) inhibitors

In the periphery dopa is metabolized by aromatic amino acid decarboxylase, which is inhibited by carbidopa and benserazide, and COMT. In the brain levodopa is also metabolized by monoamine oxidase B. Two COMT inhibitors are currently marketed, entacapone and tolcapone. At therapeutic doses entacapone works exclusively in the periphery, but at high doses tolcapone may also inhibit COMT in the brain. A number of studies have indicated that addition of tolcapone to patients on levodopa with fluctuations can decrease the percentage of off time by 2 to 3 hours (Rajput *et al.*, 1997; Adler *et al.*, 1998). Unfortunately, approximately 3–4% of patients on tolcapone developed an increase in liver function tests, and three deaths

from liver failure occurred in patients in the postmarketing period. This liver toxicity led to a ban of tolcapone in the European Union and to substantial controls over its use in the United States. The Parkinson Study Group (1997b) compared entacapone, at a dose of 200 mg with each dose of carbidopa/levodopa, and placebo in patients with wearing off and found that addition of entacapone caused a 5% increase in the on time (approximately one hour). The Nomecomt Study (Rinne *et al.*, 1998) reported a similar benefit. In both studies the dose of levodopa was reduced by approximately 12% with addition of entacapone. Common side effects of entacapone were an increase in dyskinesia and discoloration of the urine.

Monoamine oxidase B (MAO-B) inhibitors

A number of studies have evaluated the usefulness of MAO-B inhibitors both as monotherapy and as adjunctive therapy. Selegiline, which is also referred to as deprenyl, irreversibly inhibits MAO-B and thereby reduces the production of hydrogen peroxide by MAO-B. Because of its ability to reduce the formation of reactive oxygen species, selegiline was considered as a potential neuroprotective agent for dopaminergic neurons and a drug that might slow the progression of PD. Recently studies have indicated that deprenyl-like agents may have neuroprotective effects independent of MAO-B (Reed, 2002). The Parkinson Study Group (1993) carried out the DATATOP study, in which patients with early PD, who did not require treatment with levodopa, were randomly assigned to placebo, selegiline (5 mg twice each day), tocopherol (vitamin E; 1000 IU twice each day) or selegiline and tocopherol. The patients were followed until the point that they had reached disability sufficient to require treatment with levodopa. Selegiline delayed the time until levodopa was required by approximately nine months. However, improvement in the scores on the motor portion of the UPDRS 1 month after beginning selegiline (washin) and worsening after withdrawal of selegiline (washout) suggested that the effect was likely not due to a neuroprotective effect but more likely due to a symptomatic effect caused by reduction in the metabolism of dopamine in the brain. Olanow *et al.* (1995) used a different trial design and a 2-month washout period, but even this longer washout period might not have been sufficient. Pålhagen *et al.* (1998) conducted a study similar to the DATATOP study and found that again selegiline had a significant "washin" effect and postponed the time until treatment with levodopa was needed. However, no difference in the deterioration between the selegiline and placebo groups was noted during an eight-week "washout" phase. Pålhagen *et al.* interpreted the data as consistent with a neuroprotective effect. The studies of selegiline have been confounded by the symptomatic effect of selegiline, and a neuroprotective effect has not been unequivocally demonstrated.

Anticholinergic drugs

Anticholinergic drugs were discovered by serendipity to be beneficial in PD in the nineteenth century by Charcot, when he administered *Atropa belladonna* to control the excessive salivation in PD patients. Cantello *et al.* (1986) compared bornaprine to placebo in a randomized, double blind, crossover trial. They found the most substantial benefit to be in reduction of tremor, but they also noted benefit for bradykinesia and rigidity. This pattern reflects the general clinical experience with anticholinergic drugs. Unfortunately, anticholinergic drugs commonly have peripheral side effects such as blurred vision, urinary retention, nausea, constipation, and dry mouth. The central side effects can be more limiting and include memory impairment, confusion hallucinations and delirium.

Amantadine

Amantadine is another drug that was discovered by serendipity to be beneficial in PD, when Schwab *et al.* (1969) used it for influenza prophylaxis in Parkinsonian patients. The mechanism of action of amantadine is complex but it appears to enhance the release of dopamine from presynaptic terminals, an effect on postsynaptic dopaminergic receptors, an anticholinergic action and an antagonist to the NMDA glutamate receptor. Butzer *et al.* (1975) carried out a double-blind, placebo-controlled, crossover study and found a modest (12%) but statistically significant improvement in the clinical assessments of PD. Side effects of amantadine include peripheral edema, livido reticularis, rash and confusion.

More recently amantadine has been reported to reduce dyskinesia. Three studies have reported that treatment with amantadine at doses of up to 300 or 400 mg/day were able to reduce dyskinesia induced by intravenous levodopa or oral levodopa or as measured as cumulative dyskinesia recorded in diaries (Verhagen *et al.*, 1999; Luginger *et al.*, 2000; Snow *et al.*, 2000).

Treatments of cognitive and psychiatric complications

The prevalence of dementia in PD is approximately 25% and increases with advancing disease (Aarsland *et al.*,

2003), and approximately 15% of patients will develop hallucinations.

Aarsland and colleagues (2002) reported that treatment with donepezil statistically significantly but modestly improved the score on the mini-mental state examination in cognitively impaired PD patients.

Typical antipsychotic drugs, such as haloperidol, worsen parkinsonism and should be avoided in PD patients. Friedman and colleagues in the Parkinson Study Group (1999) reported that clozapine significantly improved drug-induced psychosis in PD patients without worsening of parkinsonism. Unfortunately, patients on clozapine can develop agranulocytosis, as well as seizures and myocarditis, and complete blood count must be monitored closely. Other atypical antipsychotic drugs have been studied in PD. Unfortunately, olanzapine worsens the parkinsonian features (Goetz *et al.*, 2000). Risperidone may also worsen parkinsonism and has recently been reported to be associated with an increase in the incidence of stroke when used in elderly, demented patients. Although controlled, randomized, prospective studies of quetiapine for the treatment of psychosis in PD have not been reported, it has been reported to reduce psychosis in PD patients without clinically significant worsening of parkinsonism

Intervention in the malfunctioning circuitry

Three regions have been targeted for surgical interventions in PD – the thalamus, globus pallidus interna (GPi) and subthalamic nucleus (STN). Ablative procedures, e.g. thalamotomy, were initially employed but recently have been largely supplanted by deep brain stimulation (DBS). For excellent overviews of these therapies please see the reviews of Hallett and Litvan (1999) and Lang (2000).

Thalamotomy has been employed for management of PD tremor since the middle of the previous century. Ablative lesions, usually of the ventral intermediate nucleus, can strikingly reduce tremor in the contralateral arm but have little effect on the other signs of PD. Bilateral lesions typically lead to impairment in speech and swallowing and are avoided. DBS of the thalamus has the advantage that permanent complications are less common. In a randomized, prospective study, Schuurman *et al.* (2000) compared thalamotomy to DBS in patients with PD (45), essential tremor (13) and multiple sclerosis (10) and used videotapes to achieve blinded assessment of tremor. They concluded that both were equally effective in suppression of tremor, which was not adequately responsive to drug treatment, but that DBS had fewer adverse effects and resulted in greater functional improvement.

In the early 1990s, pallidal surgery for PD was revived by Laitinen *et al.* (1992). Most of the reports of pallidotomy for PD have not been prospective, randomized or blinded. De Bie *et al.* (1999) reported on a series of 37 cases of PD, which could not be managed satisfactorily with medical therapy. The patients were randomly assigned to receive unilateral pallidotomy or medical therapy and were assessed after 6 months. An assessor, who was blinded to the treatment, evaluated the patients. The primary response variable was the median change in the score on the motor portion of the UPDRS during a clinically defined off period, and the patients who underwent pallidotomy improved (47 to 32.5, 31%) and the medically treated group worsened slightly (52.5 to 56.5), and the difference was highly significant. Pallidotomy patients also had less dyskinesia and improvement in activities of daily living. However, two pallidotomy patients had major, persistent adverse events. These changes are similar to those reported in unblinded studies (for review see Lang, 2000). Unfortunately, bilateral pallidotomy is often accompanied by serious adverse events, most frequently impairments of speech and cognition (de Bie *et al.*, 2002).

DBS of the GPi or STN have largely supplanted unilateral pallidotomy because of ability to manipulate the circuitry bilaterally and a lower likelihood of permanent adverse events. DBS of the STN for PD was pioneered by Benabid and colleagues (Limousin *et al.*, 1998). Investigators have been reluctant to perform ablative procedures of the STN because of the possibility of causing hemiballismus. Burchiel *et al.* (1999) reported on a pilot study in which 10 PD patients were randomized to either bilateral GPi stimulation or bilateral STN stimulation and had data sufficient to report on four patients with pallidal stimulation and five patients with STN stimulation. They found that the improvement in the UPDRS motor scores during a clinically defined off period was equivalent at 12 months. Patients who received STN stimulation, but not those with pallidal stimulation, were able to reduce the dosages of their dopaminergic medications, and the patients with pallidal stimulation had greater improvement in bradykinesia. Both groups had reduction of dyskinesia, but the effect in this small, pilot study only reached significance for the STN group, which also had reduction in dosage of dopaminergic therapy.

The Deep-Brain Stimulation for Parkinson's Disease Study Group (2001) carried out a study in which 18 centers enrolled 143 PD patients and implanted bilateral electrodes in either the GPi (38) or STN (96) according to the experience and preference of the investigators at each site in 134 patients. At six months the patients were assessed with the motor portion of the UPDRS after medication and stimulation had been discontinued overnight. Ninety-six of the patients were randomly evaluated in a crossover design with the stimulator either on or off with neither the evaluator nor patient informed as to whether the stimulator was on or off. Significant improvement was noted in both patients who received STN stimulation (51%) and GPi stimulation (33%). Home diaries indicated improvement in on time without dyskinesia. However, there were seven intracranial hemorrhages and two infections requiring removal of electrodes in the 143 patients.

The data suggest that in patients with advanced PD, who cannot be managed satisfactorily medically, DBS of either the GPi or STN can improve motor function and reduce dyskinesia. However, as with pallidotomy, there is the risk of intracranial hemorrhage and neuropsychological changes (Trepanier *et al.*, 2000) and the additional risks of infection and hardware failure (Oh *et al.*, 2002). The better site for DBS, GPi or STN, is uncertain, but the Dept. of Veterans Affairs is carrying out a prospective, randomized trial to address this question.

Regeneration

In the past decade considerable research has been directed to the development of therapies to induce regeneration of the nigrostriatal dopaminergic system in PD (Isacson, 2002). Much of this work has been directed to identification of trophic factors that can protect and/or induce regeneration of this system, and a number of trophic factors that have an effect on the nigrostriatal system have been identified, with the most promising being glial cell line-derived neurotrophic factor (GDNF) and other members of this family (Shults, 1998). This work led to a clinical trial of intraventricular infusion of GDNF in patients with PD, and the results of this study have been recently published (Nutt *et al.*, 2003). One report of a patient who came to autopsy indicated no improvement or signs of regeneration and adverse events (L'hermitte's sign and intermittent hallucinations) (Kordower *et al.*, 1999). This report underscores the needs for delivery of the trophic factor to the appropriate target, e.g. the striatum, and for delivery of the trophic factor in a controlled fashion. A recent, preliminary study suggests that direct delivery into the putamen may be beneficial (Gill *et al.*, 2003). Alternative delivery strategies, such as viral vectors, have been studied in MPTP-treated monkeys (Kordower *et al.*, 2000).

Neuroimmunophilin ligands, e.g. GPI-1046, have also been reported to promote regeneration of the injured nigrostriatal dopaminergic system, but this remains controversial (Zhang *et al.*, 2001; Eberling *et al.*, 2002). GPI-1046 has been studied in PD patients but the results have been disappointing (Gold & Nutt, 2002).

Replacement

During the past two decades, considerable effort has been directed to developing cells that can be implanted into the striatum of PD patients and serve as a source of dopamine. Fetal mesencephalic cells are the cells that have been studied most extensively (Björklund, 2000; Lindvall & Hagell, 2001). Studies in preclinical animal models of PD, mostly rodent models, have demonstrated that the dopaminergic cells can survive, form connections with striatal neurons and attenuate abnormal, parkinsonian behavior. Pilot studies in PD patients, which were not blinded and lacked control cases, suggested that transplantation of fetal, mesencephalic cells into the striatum in PD patients could reduce the need for dopaminergic therapy and improve function.

Transplantation of fetal mesencephalic cells in PD patients has been studied in two prospective, randomized, sham operation-controlled trials in PD patients (Freed *et al.*, 2000, Olanow *et al.*, 2003) Fluorodopa PET imaging in the patients indicated that the implanted cells had survived and were biochemically functional. Unfortunately, the primary analysis in both studies indicated that the implanted patients were not functionally improved by the procedure. Some of the patients developed disabling dyskinesia, which could not be controlled by adjustment of medication.

These studies underscore the need for properly conducted clinical trials in assessment of the usefulness of all new therapies in PD. It also appears that in the future cell replacement therapies should first be studied in non-human primate models of PD in which the animals have previously been exposed to levodopa and thereby primed for the development of dyskinesias. The previous studies also point out the challenges that will need to be met in cell replacement therapy in PD. The cells will need to survive and become somewhat integrated into targeted region (typically the striatum) so that they deliver dopamine to the denervated region of implantation in a fashion that approximates the normal, physiological delivery of dopamine. In addition, previous studies of transplantation of fetal cells have targeted the striatum because of the large projection of dopaminergic axons from the substantia nigra to the striatum and the profound depletion of dopamine in the striatum in PD patients. However, the mesencephalic dopaminergic neurons project to other regions, e.g. the globus pallidus and neocortex, and restitution of dopaminergic input in regions other than the stria-

tum may be necessary for improved function without side effects.

Recent research effort has been directed to development of stem cells as a source of dopamine producing cells for replacement. These efforts resulted in part from ethical and logistical concerns regarding procurement of the number of human embryos needed to provide enough fetal dopaminergic cells to adequately re-innervate the striatum in PD patients (some groups have used up to four fetuses per striatum). Although stem cells may provide an adequate supply of cells that can produce dopamine, use of stem cells will face the additional challenge that the stem cells must be differentiated into a phenotype similar to that of a dopaminergic neuron.

REFERENCES

Aarsland, D., Laake, K., Larsen, J. P. & Janvin, C. (2002). Donepezil for cognitive impairment in Parkinson's disease: a randomised controlled study. *J. Neurol., Neurosurg. Psychiatry*, **72**, 708–12.

Aarsland, D., Andersen, K., Larsen, J. P., Lolk, A. & Kragh-Sorensen, P. (2003). Prevalence and characteristics of dementia in Parkinson disease: an 8-year prospective study. *Arch. Neurol.*, **60**, 387 92.

Adler, C. H., Singer, C., O'Brien, C. *et al.* (1998). Randomized, placebo-controlled study of tolcapone in patients with fluctuating Parkinson disease treated with levodopacarbidopa. Tolcapone Fluctuator Study Group III. *Arch. Neurol.*, **55**, 1089–95.

Alam, Z. I., Daniel, S. E., Lees, A. J. *et al.* (1997). A generalized increase in protein carbonyls in the brain in Parkinson's but not incidental Lewy body disease. *J. Neurochemi.*, **69** (3), 1326–9.

Andersen, J. K. (2001). Does neuronal loss in Parkinson's disease involve programmed cell death? *Bioessays*, **23** (7), 640–6.

Barone, P., Bravi, D., Bermejo-Pareja, F. *et al.* (1999). Pergolide monotherapy in the treatment of early PD. A randomized controlled study. *Neurology*, **53**, 573–9.

Beal, M. F. (2002). Oxidatively modified proteins in aging and disease. *Free Radic. Biol. Med.*, **32** (9), 797–803.

Björklund, A. (2000). Cell replacement strategies for neurodegenerative disorders. *Novartis Foundation Symposium*, **231**, 7–15; discussion 16–20.

Braak, H. & Braak, E. (2000). Pathoanatomy of Parkinson's disease. *J. Neurol.*, **247** (2), II3–10.

Brooks, D. J., Abbott, R. J., Lees, A. J. *et al.* (1998). A placebo-controlled evaluation of ropinirole, a novel D2 agonist, as sole dopaminergic therapy in Parkinson's disease. *Clin. Neuropharmacol.*, **21**, 101–7.

Burchiel, K. J., Anderson, V. C., Favre, J. *et al.* (1999). Comparison of pallidal and subthalamic nucleus deep brain stimulation for advanced Parkinson's disease: results of a randomized, blinded pilot study. *Neurosurgery*, **45** (6), 1375–82.

Butzer, J. F., Silver, D. E. & Sans, A. L. (1975). Amantadine in Parkinson's disease. A double-blind, placebo-controlled, crossover study with long-term follow-up. *Neurology*, **25**, 603–6.

Calne, D. B., Techenne, P. F., Claveria, L. E. *et al.* (1974). Bromocriptine in Parkinsonism. *Br. Med. J.*, **4**, 442–4.

Cantello, R., Riccio, A., Gilli, M. *et al.* (1986). Bornaprine vs placebo in Parkinson disease: double-blind controlled cross-over trial in 30 patients. *Ital. J. Neurol. Sci.*, **7**, 139–43.

Chung, K. K., Dawson, V. L. & Dawson, T. M. (2001). The role of the ubiquitin-proteasomal pathway in Parkinson's disease and other neurodegenerative disorders. *Trends Neurosci.*, **24** (11 Suppl), S7–14.

Cotzias, G. C., Papavasiliou, P. S. & Gellene, R. (1969). Modification of Parkinsonism-chronic treatment with L-dopa. *N. Engl. J. Med.*, **280**, 337–45.

de Bie, R. M., de Haan, R. J., Nijssen, P. C. *et al.* (1999). Unilateral pallidotomy in Parkinson's disease: a randomised, single-blind, multicentre trial. *Lancet*, **354** (9191), 1665–9.

de Bie, R. M., de Haan, R. J., Schuurman, P. R. *et al.* (2002). Morbidity and mortality following pallidotomy in Parkinson's disease: a systematic review. *Neurology*, **58** (7), 1008–12.

Dexter, D. T., Carter, C. J., Wells, F. R. *et al.* (1989). Basal lipid peroxidation in substantia nigra is increased in Parkinson's disease. *J. Neurochem.*, **52** (2), 381–9.

Drukarch, B. & van Muiswinkel, F. L. (2000). Drug treatment of Parkinson's disease. Time for phase II. *Biochem. Pharmacol.*, **59** (9), 1023–31.

Du, Y., Ma, Z., Lin, S. *et al.* (2001). Minocycline prevents nigrostriatal dopaminergic neurodegeneration in the MPTP model of Parkinson's disease. *Proc. Natl Acad. Sci. USA*, **98** (25), 14669–74.

Dupont, E., Anderson, A., Boqs, J. *et al.* (1996). Sustained-release Madopar HBS compared with standard Madopar in the long-term treatment of de novo parkinsonian patients. *Acta Neurol. Scand.*, **93**, 14–20.

Eberling, J. L., Pivirotto, P., Bringas, J. *et al.* (2002). The immunophilin ligand GPI-1046 does not have neuroregenerative effects in MPTP-treated monkeys. *Exp. Neurol.*, **178** (2), 236–42.

Etminan, M., Samii, A., Takkouche, B. *et al.* (2001). Increased risk of somnolence with the new dopamine agonists in patients with Parkinson's disease: a meta-analysis of randomised controlled trials. *Drug Safety*, **24** (11), 863–8.

Freed, C. R., Greene, P. E., Breeze, R. E. *et al.* (2001). Transplantation of embryonic dopamine neurons for severe Parkinson's disease. *New Engl. J. Med.*, **344** (10), 710–19.

Furukawa, Y., Vigouroux, S., Wong, H. *et al.* (2002). Brain proteasomal function in sporadic Parkinson's disease and related disorders. *Ann. Neurol.*, **51** (6), 779–82.

Galvin, J. E., Lee, V. M., Schmidt, M. L. *et al.* (1999). Pathobiology of the Lewy body. *Adv. Neurol.*, **80**, 313–24.

Giasson, B. I. & Lee, V. M. (2001). Parkin and the molecular pathways of Parkinson's disease. *Neuron*, **31** (6), 885–8.

Giasson, B. I., Duda, J. E., Murray, I. V. *et al.* (2000). Oxidative damage linked to neurodegeneration by selective alpha-synuclein nitration in synucleinopathy lesions. *Science*, **290** (5493), 985–9.

Gill, S. S., Patel, N. K., Hotton, G. R., O'Sullivan, K. *et al.* (2003). Direct brain infusion of glial cell line-derived neurotrophic factor in Parkinson disease. *Nat. Med.*, **9** (5), 589–95.

Goetz, C. G., Blasucci, L. M., Leurgans, S. & Pappert, E. J. (2000). Olanzapine and clozapine: comparative effects on motor function in hallucinating PD patients. *Neurology*, **55**, 789–94.

Gold, B. G. & Nutt, J. G. (2002). Neuroimmunophilin ligands in the treatment of Parkinson's disease. *Curr. Opin. Pharmacol.*, **2** (1), 82–6.

Guttman, M. and the International Pramipexole-Bromocriptine Study Group (1997). Double-blind comparison of pramipexole and bromocriptine treatment with placebo in advanced Parkinson's disease. *Neurology*, **49**, 1060–5.

Haas, R. H., Nasirian, F., Nakano, K., Ward, D. *et al.* (1995). Low platelet mitochondrial Complex I and Complex II/III activity in early untreated Parkinson's disease. *Ann. Neurol.*, **37**, 714–22.

Hallett, M. & Litvan, I. (1999). Evaluation of surgery for Parkinson's disease: a report of the Therapeutics and Technology Assessment Subcommittee of the American Academy of Neurology. The Task Force on Surgery for Parkinson's Disease. *Neurology*, **53** (9), 1910–21.

Halliwell, B. (2001). Role of free radicals in the neurodegenerative diseases: therapeutic implications for antioxidant treatment. *Drugs Aging*, **18** (9), 685–716.

Hely, M. A., Morris, J. G. L. & Reid, W. G. J. (1994). The Sydney multicentre study of Parkinson's disease: a randomized, prospective five year study comparing low dose bromocriptine with low dose levodopa-carbidopa. *J. Neurol., Neurosurg., Psychiatry*, **57**, 903–10.

Hirsch, E. C., Hunot, S., Damier, P. *et al.* (1998). Glial cells and inflammation in Parkinson's disease: a role in neurodegeneration? *Ann. Neurol.*, **44** (3 Suppl 1), S115–20.

Hornykiewicz, O. (2002). Dopamine miracle: from brain homogenate to dopamine replacement. *Movement Disord.*, **17** (3), 501–8.

Hutton, J. T., Morris, J. L., Bush, D. F. *et al.* (1989). Multicenter controlled study of Sinemet CR vs Sinemet (25/100) in advanced Parkinson's disease. *Neurology*, **39**, 67–72.

Isacson, O. (2002). Models of repair mechanisms for future treatment modalities of Parkinson's disease. *Brain Res. Bull.*, **57** (6), 839–46.

Kingsbury, A. E., Mardsen, C. D. & Foster, O. J. (1998). DNA fragmentation in human substantia nigra: apoptosis or perimortem effect? *Movement Disord.*, **13** (6), 877–84.

Kitada, T., Asakawa, S., Hattori, N. *et al.* (1998). Mutations in the parkin gene cause autosomal recessive juvenile parkinsonism. *Nature*, **392**, 605–8.

Koller, W. C., Hutton, J. T., Tolosa, E. *et al.* (1999). Immediate-release and controlled-release carbidopa/levodopa in PD: a 5-year randomized multicenter study. *Neurology*, **53**, 1012–19.

Kordower, J. H., Palfi, S., Chen, E. Y. *et al.* (1999). Clinicopathological findings following intraventricular glial-derived neurotrophic factor treatment in a patient with Parkinson's disease. *Ann. Neurol.*, **46** (3), 419–24.

Kordower, J. H., Emborg, M. E., Bloch, J. *et al.* (2000). Neurodegeneration prevented by lentiviral vector delivery of GDNF in primate models of Parkinson's disease. *Science*, **290** (5492), 767–73.

Kumar, S., Bhatia, M. & Behari, M. (2002). Sleep disorders in Parkinson's disease. *Movement Disord.*, **17** (4), 775–81.

Laitinen, L. V., Bergenheim, A. T. & Hariz, M. I. (1992). Leksell's posteroventral pallidotomy in the treatment of Parkinson's disease. *J. Neurosurg.*, **76** (1), 53–61.

Lang, A. E. (2000). Surgery for Parkinson disease: A critical evaluation of the state of the art. *Arch. Neurol.*, **57** (8), 1118–25.

Lang, A. E. & Lozano, A. M. (1998). Parkinson's disease. First of two parts. *N. Engl. J. Med.*, **339** (15), 1044–53.

Langston, J. W., Ballard, P., Tetrud, J. W. & Irwin, I. (1983). Chronic parkinsonism in humans due to a product of meperidine-analog synthesis. *Science*, **219**, 979–80.

Langston, J. W., Forno, L. S., Tetrud, J. *et al.* (1999). Evidence of active nerve cell degeneration in the substantia nigra of humans years after 1-methyl-4-phenyl-1,2,3,6-tetrahydropyridine exposure. *Ann. Neurol.*, **46** (4), 598–605.

Lieberman, A., Ranhosky, A. & Korts, D. (1997). Clinical evaluation of pramipexole in advanced Parkinson's disease: results of a double-blind, placebo controlled, parallel-group study. *Neurology*, **49**, 162–8.

Limousin, P., Krack, P., Pollak, P. *et al.* (1998). Electrical stimulation of the subthalamic nucleus in advanced Parkinson's disease. *N. Engl. J. Med.*, **339** (16), 1105–11.

Lindvall, O. & Hagell, P. (2001). Cell therapy and transplantation in Parkinson's disease. *Clin. Chem. Laborat. Med.*, **39** (4), 356–61.

Luginger, E., Wenning, G. K., Bosch, S. & Poewe, W. (2000). Beneficial effects of amantadine on L-dopa-induced dyskinesias in Parkinson's disease. *Movement Disord.*, **15**, 873–8.

Matthews, R. T., Klivenyi, P., Mueller, G. *et al.* (1999). Novel free radical spin traps protect against malonate and MPTP neurotoxicity. *Exp. Neurol.*, **157** (1), 120–6.

McGeer, E. G. & McGeer, P. L. (1997). The role of the immune system in neurodegenerative disorders. *Movement Disord.*, **12** (6), 855–8.

McNaught, K. S., Olanow, C. W., Halliwell, B. *et al.* (2001). Failure of the ubiquitin-proteasome system in Parkinson's disease. *Nat. Rev. Neurosci.*, **2** (8), 589–94.

Mizuno, Y., Hattori, N., Mori, H. *et al.* (2001). Parkin and Parkinson's disease. *Curr. Opin. Neurol.*, **14** (4), 477–82.

Montastruc, J. L., Rascol, O., Senard, J. M. & Rascol, A. (1994). A randomized controlled study comparing bromocriptine to which levodopa was later added, with levodopa alone in previously untreated patients with Parkinson's disease: a five year follow-up. *J. Neurol., Neurosurg. Psychiatry*, **57**, 1034–8.

Nijhawan, D., Honarpour, N. & Wang, X. (2000). Apoptosis in neural development and disease. *Ann. Rev. Neurosci.*, **23**, 73–87.

Nutt, J. G., Burchiel, K. J., Comella, C. L. *et al.* and ICV GDNF Study Group (2003). Implanted intracerebroventricular glial cell line-derived neurotrophic factor. Randomized, double-blind trial of glial cell line-derived neurotrophic factor (GDNF) in PD. *Neurology*, **60**, 69–73 .

Oh, M. Y., Abosch, A., Kim, S. H. *et al.* (2002). Long-term hardware-related complications of deep brain stimulation. *Neurosurgery*, **50** (6), 1268–74; discussion 1274–6.

Olanow, C. W., Fahn, S., Muenter, M. *et al.* (1994). A muticenter double-blind placebo-controlled trial of pergolide as an adjunct to Sinemet in Parkinson's disease. *Movement Disord.*, **9**, 40–7.

Olanow, C. W., Hauser, R. A., Gauger, L. *et al.* (1995). The effect of deprenyl and levodopa on the progression of Parkinson's disease. *Ann. Neurol.*, **38**, 771–7.

Olanow, C. W., Goetz, C. G., Kordower, J. H. *et al.* (2003). A double-blind controlled trial of bilateral fetal nigral transplantation in Parkinson's disease. *Ann Neurol.*, **54**, 403–14.

Pålhagen, S., Heinonan, E. H., Hagglund, J. *et al.* (1998). Selegiline delays the onset of disability in de novo parkinsonian patients. Swedish Parkinson Study Group. *Neurology*, **51**, 520–5.

Parkinson Disease Research Group in the United Kingdom (1993). Comparisons of therapeutic effects of levodopa, levodopa and selegiline, and bromocriptine in patients with early, mild Parkinson's disease: three-year interim report. *Br. Med. J.*, **307**, 469–72.

Parkinson Study Group. (1993). Effects of tocopherol and deprenyl on the progression of disability in early Parkinson's disease. *N. Engl. J. Med.*, **328**, 176–83.

(1997a). Safety and efficacy of pramipexole in early Parkinson disease. A randomized dose-ranging study. Parkinson Study Group. *J. Am. Med. Assoc.*, **278** (2), 125–30.

(1997b). Entacapone improves motor fluctuations in levodopa-treated Parkinson's disease patients. *Ann. Neurol.*, **42** (5), 747–55.

(1999). Low-dose clozapine for the treatment of drug-induced psychoses in Parkinson's disease. *N. Engl. J. Med.*, **340**, 757–63.

(2000). Pramipexole vs. levodopa as initial treatment for Parkinson's disease: a randomized controlled trial. *J. Am. Med. Assoc.*, **284**, 1931–8.

Polymeropoulos, M. H., Lavedan, C., Leroy, E. *et al.* (1997). Mutation in the α-synuclein gene identified in families with Parkinson's disease. *Science*, **276**, 2045–7.

Przedborski, S. & Jackson-Lewis, V. (1998). Mechanisms of MPTP toxicity. *Movement Disord.*, **13** Suppl 1, 35–8.

Rajput, A. H., Martin, W., Saint-Hilaire, M. H. *et al.* (1997). Tolcapone improves motor function in Parkinsonian patients with the "wearing-off" phenomenon: a double-blind, placebo-controlled, multicenter trial. *Neurology*, **49**, 1066–71.

Rascol, O., Brooks, D. J., Korczyn, A. D. *et al.* (2000). A five-year study of the incidence of dyskinesia in patients with early Parkinson's disease who were treated with ropinirole or levodopa. *N. Engl. J. Med.*, **342**, 1484–91.

Reed, J. C. (2002). Apoptosis-based therapies. *Nat. Rev. Drug Discovery*, **1** (2), 111–21.

Rinne, U. K., Larsen, J. P., Siden, A. *et al.* (1998). Entacapone enhances the response to levodopa in parkinsonian patients with motor fluctuations. *Neurology*, **51**, 1309–14.

Riopelle, R. J. (1987). Bromocriptine and the clinical spectrum of Parkinson's disease. *Can. J. Neurol. Sci.*, **14**, 455–9.

Sanchez-Ramos, J. R., Övervik, E. & Ames, B. N. (1994). A marker of oxyradical-mediated DNA damage (8-hydroxy-2'deoxyguanosine) is increased in nigro-striatum of Parkinson's disease brain. *Neurodegeneration*, **3**, 197–204.

Schapira, A. H. V., Mann, V. M., Cooper, J. M. *et al.* (1990). Anatomic disease specificity of NADH CoQ1 reductase complex I deficiency in Parkinson's disease. *J. Neurochem.*, **55**, 2142–5.

Schuurman, P. R., Bosch, D. A., Bossuyt, P. M. *et al.* (2000). A comparison of continuous thalamic stimulation and thalamotomy for suppression of severe tremor. *N. Engl. J. Med.*, **342** (7), 461–8.

Schwab, R. S., England, A. C. Jr., Poskancer, D. C. *et al.* (1969). Amantadine in the treatment of Parkinson's disease. *J. Am. Med. Assoc.*, **208**, 1168–70.

Shimura, H., Hattori, N., Kubo, S. *et al.* (2000). Familial Parkinson disease gene product, parkin, is a ubiquitin-protein ligase. *Nat. Genet.*, **25**, 302–5.

Shults, C. W. (1998). Neurotrophic factors in neurodegenerative disorder. In *Parkinson's Disease and Movement Disorders*, ed. J. Jankovic and E. Tolosa, pp. 105–18. 3rd edn. Williams and Wilkins.

Shults, C. W., Haas, R. H., Passov, D. & Beal, M. F. (1997). Coenzyme Q_{10} levels correlate with the activities of complexes I and II/III in mitochondria from parkinsonian and nonparkinsonian subjects. *Ann. Neurol.*, **42**, 261–4.

Shults, C. W., Oakes, D., Kieburtz, K. *et al.* (2002). Effects of coenzyme Q10 in early Parkinson disease-Evidence of slowing of the functional decline. *Arch. Neurol.*, **59**, 1541–50.

Sian, J., Dexter, D. T., Lees, A. J. *et al.* (1994). Alterations in glutathione levels in Parkinson's disease and other neurodegenerative disorders affecting basal ganglia. *Ann. Neurol.*, **36** (3), 348–55.

Snow, B. J., MacDonald, L., Mcauley, D. *et al.* (2000). The effect of amantadine on levodopa-induced dyskinesias in Parkinson's disease: a double-blind, placebo-controlled study. *Clin. Neuropharmacol.*, **23**, 82–5.

Spillantini, M. G., Schmidt, M. L., Lee, V. M. *et al.* (1997). Alpha-synuclein in Lewy bodies. *Nature*, **388** (6645), 839–40.

Takeda, A., Mallory, M., Sundsmo, M. *et al.* (1998). Abnormal accumulation of NACP/alpha-synuclein in neurodegenerative disorders. *Am. J. Pathol.*, **152** (2), 367–72.

Tan, E. K., Lum, S. Y., Fook-Chong, S. M. *et al.* (2002). Evaluation of somnolence in Parkinson's disease: comparison with age- and sex-matched controls. *Neurology*, **58** (3), 465–8.

Tarnopolsky, M. A. & Beal, M. F. (2001). Potential for creatine and other therapies targeting cellular energy dysfunction in neurological disorders. *Ann. Neurol.*, **49** (5), 561–74.

Teismann, P. & Ferger, B. (2001). Inhibition of the cyclooxygenase isoenzymes COX-1 and COX-2 provide neuroprotection in the MPTP-mouse model of Parkinson's disease. *Synapse*, **39** (2), 167–74.

The Deep-Brain Stimulation for Parkinson's Disease Study Group (2001). Deep-brain stimulation of the subthalamic nucleus or the pars interna of the globus pallidus in Parkinson's disease. *N. Engl. J. Med.*, **345**, 956–63.

The Parkinson Study Group (1999). Low-dose clozapine for the treatment of drug-induced psychosis in Parkinson's disease. *N. Engl. J. Med.*, **1340**, 757–63.

Trepanier, L. L., Kumar, R., Lozano, A. M. *et al.* (2000). Neuropsychological outcome of GPi pallidotomy and GPi or STN deep brain stimulation in Parkinson's disease. *Brain Cogn.*, **42** (3), 324–47.

Verhagen Metman, L. V., Del Dotto, P., LePoole, K. *et al.* (1999). Amantadine for levodopa-induced dyskinesias. A 1-year follow-up study. *Arch. Neurol.*, **56**, 1383–6.

Wakabayashi, K., Matsumoto, K., Takayama, K. *et al.* (1997). NACP, a presynaptic protein, immunoreactivity in Lewy bodies in Parkinson's disease. *Neurosci. Lett.*, **239** (1), 45–8.

Wermuth, L. and the Danish Pramipexole Study Group (1998). A double-blind, placebo-controlled, randomized, multi-center study of pramipexole in advanced Parkinson's disease. *Eur. J. Neurol.*, **5**, 235–44.

Wolters, E. C., Tesselaar, H. J. M. and the International (NL and UK) Sinemet CR Study Group (1996). International (NL–UK) double-blind study of Sinemet CR and standard Sinemet (25/100) in 170 patients with fluctuating Parkinson's disease. *J. Neurol.*, **243**, 235–40.

Wu, D. C., Jackson-Lewis, V., Vila, M. *et al.* (2002). Blockade of microglial activation is neuroprotective in the 1-methyl-4-phenyl-1,2,3,6-tetrahydropyridine mouse model of Parkinson disease. *J. Neurosci.*, **22** (5), 1763–71.

Zhang, C., Steiner, J. P., Hamilton, G. S. *et al.* (2001). Regeneration of dopaminergic function in 6-hydroxydopamine-lesioned rats by neuroimmunophilin ligand treatment. *J. Neurosci.*, **21** (15), RC156.

Zimmermann, K. C., Bonzon, C. & Green, D. R. (2001). The machinery of programmed cell death. *Pharmacol. Therap.*, **92** (1), 57–70.

43

Multiple system atrophy

Felix Geser,[1] Carlo Colosimo[2] and Gregor K. Wenning[1]

[1]Clinical Department of Neurology, Innsbruck Medical University, Austria
[2]Department of Neurology, University "La Sapienza" Rome, Italy

Historical review

The term multiple system atrophy (MSA) was introduced by Graham and Oppenheimer in 1969 to denote a neurodegenerative disease characterized clinically by various combinations of autonomic, parkinsonian, cerebellar or pyramidal symptoms and signs and pathologically by cell loss and gliosis in some or all of the following structures: putamen, caudate nucleus, globus pallidus, substantia nigra, locus ceruleus, inferior olives, pontine nuclei, cerebellar Purkinje cells, intermediolateral cell columns and Onuf's nucleus of the spinal cord.

Previously, cases of MSA were reported under the rubrics of olivopontocerebellar atrophy (OPCA), idiopathic orthostatic hypotension (IOH) or progressive autonomic failure (PAF), Shy–Drager syndrome (SDS) and striatonigral degeneration (SND). Although Dejerine and Thomas were the first to introduce the term OPCA in 1900 reporting two sporadic cases of late-onset ataxia, the case of Stauffenberg in 1918, diagnosed in life as OPCA, was the first to associate cerebellar, parkinsonian and autonomic features with identified pathological lesions not only of olives, pons and cerebellum, but also of basal ganglia pigmentation and atrophy of putamen, with additional cell loss in caudate and globus pallidus (Quinn, 1994).

The term SND was introduced in 1960 by van der Eecken, Adams and van Bogaert (van der Eecken et al., 1960; Adams et al., 1961, 1964) who noted pronounced shrinkage and brownish discoloration of the putamen and pallidum as well as depigmentation of the substantia nigra in three patients with progressive and severe parkinsonism associated with cerebellar, pyramidal and autonomic features. Earlier reports of SND include those of Fleischhacker (1924) and Scherer (1933a,b) (Berciano et al., 1998; Wenning et al., 2000b). In 1960 Shy and Drager reported two cases with marked autonomic failure, slurred speech, ataxia, parkinsonian features, pyramidal signs and distal muscle wasting. Postmortem examination of case 2 demonstrated pathological lesions consistent with MSA, including involvement of the intermediolateral cell column. Subsequently, the term SDS was erroneously widened to include cases of Parkinson's disease (PD) and autonomic failure. Its further use has therefore been discouraged (Quinn et al., 1995). In 1989 Papp and colleagues reported glial cytoplasmic inclusions (GCIs) in the brains of patients with MSA regardless of presentation (SND, OPCA and SDS). GCIs were not present in a large series of patients with other neurodegenerative disorders. The abundant presence of GCIs in all clinical subtypes of MSA introduced grounds for considering SDS, SND and sporadic OPCA as one disease entity characterized by neuronal multisystem degeneration based on unique oligodendroglial inclusion pathology. Subsequently, neuronal and axonal inclusions were also identified in MSA brains, however, they were less numerous compared to GCIs (Papp & Lantos, 1992, 1994). In the late 1990s α-synuclein immunostaining was recognized as the most sensitive marker of inclusion pathology in MSA, being superior to ubiquitin immunostaining that was previously used (Wakabayashi et al., 1998c; Spillantini et al., 1998). In parallel, the clinical recognition greatly improved following the introduction of diagnostic criteria. Quinn first proposed in 1989 a list of diagnostic criteria for MSA (Quinn, 1989b). The criteria were revised in 1994 to include sphincter EMG evidence (Table 43.5) (Quinn, 1994). In the late 1990s a number of pitfalls associated with the Quinn criteria were identified and Consensus diagnostic criteria were therefore developed in 1998 (Tables 43.6, 43.7 and 43.8) (Gilman et al., 1998, 1999). The Consensus conference criteria have since been widely established in the research community as well as movement disorders clinics.

Table 43.1. Main pathological abnormalities (cell loss and/or gliosis) in 203 MSA cases

	SN	Put	Caud	Pall	Inf Oli	Pons	PCs	Dentate	ILCC	AHC	Pyr
Normal	8.6%	14.6%	45.2%	25.5%	22.1%	30.2%	16.9%	68.8%	31.7%	51.9%	45.2%
Mild	6.5%	6.7%	24.5%	36.6%	17.7%	9.5%	22.4%	16.1%	6.9%	16.0%	26.9%
Moderate	29.6%	16.3%	27.7%	30.4%	21.5%	21.9%	30.1%	11.6%	34.7%	28.3%	25.8%
Severe	55.4%	62.4%	2.6%	7.5%	38.7%	38.5%	30.6%	3.6%	26.7%	3.8%	2.2%
Total *n*	*n* = 186	*n* = 178	*n* = 155	*n* = 161	*n* = 181	*n* = 169	*n* = 183	*n* = 112	*n* = 101	*n* = 106	*n* = 93

Key: SN-substantia nigra, Put-putamen, Caud-caudate nucleus, Pall-globus pallidus, Inf Oli-inferior olive, Pons-pontine nuclei, PCs-Purkinje cells, Dentate-dentate nucleus, ILCC-intermediolateral cell column, AHC-anterior horn cells, Pyr-spinal cord pyramidal tracts. Reproduced with kind permission from Wiley-Liss, Inc., a subsidiary of John Wiley & Sons, Inc.: Wenning *et al.* (1997b).

Table 43.2. Other pathological abnormalities in 203 MSA cases

	Cortex	Thal	Luys	Cerul	Vest	DVN	Ambig	Onuf
Normal	78.4%	77.6%	59.4%	12.8%	43.6%	29.6%	58.3%	35.7%
Mild	12.7%	11.2%	18.8%	11.2%	21.8%	22.2%	25.0%	0%
Moderate	6.9%	8.4%	15.6%	45.6%	32.7%	33.3%	8.3%	14.3%
Severe	2.0%	2.8%	6.3%	30.4%	1.8%	14.8%	8.3%	50.0%
Total *n*	*n* = 102	*n* = 107	*n* = 32	*n* = 125	*n* = 55	*n* = 54	*n* = 12	*n* = 14

Key: Cortex-cerebral cortex, Thal-thalamus, Luys-subthalamic nucleus, Cerul-Locus coeruleus, Vest-vestibular nuclei, DVN-Dorsal motor nucleus X, Ambig-nucleus ambiguus, Onuf-Onuf's nucleus.
Reproduced with kind permission from Wiley-Liss, Inc., a subsidiary of John Wiley & Sons, Inc.: Wenning *et al.* 1997b (C) 1997 Movement Disorder Society.

Morphological pattern of vulnerability

In MSA-P, the striatonigral system is the main site of pathology but less severe degeneration can be widespread (Tables 43.1 and 43.2) and usually includes the olivopontocerebellar system (Wenning *et al.*, 1996c). The putamen is shrunken with grey–green discoloration (Fig. 43.1). When putaminal pathology is severe there may be a cribriform appearance. In early stages the putaminal lesion shows a distinct topographical distribution with a predilection for the caudal and dorsolateral regions (Kume *et al.*, 1993). Later on during the course of disease, the entire putamen is usually affected with the result that bundles of striatopallidal fibres are narrowed and poorly stained for myelin. Degeneration of pigmented nerve cells occurs in the substantia nigra pars compacta (SNC), while non-pigmented cells of the pars reticulata are reported as normal. The topographical patterns of neurodegeneration involving the motor neostriatum, efferent pathways, and nigral neurones, reflect their anatomical relationship and suggest a common denominator or "linked" degeneration (Kume *et al.*, 1993). In MSA-C, the brunt of pathology is in the olivopontocerebellar system while the involvement of striatum and substantia nigra is less severe. The basis pontis

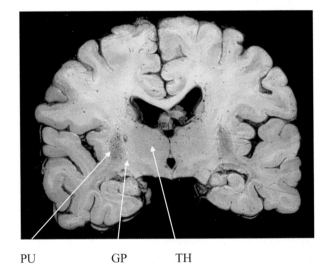

PU   GP   TH

Fig. 43.1 Coronal slice of cerebrum. The putamena are symmetrically shrunken. Pallida are atrophic. PU: Putamen, GP: Globus Pallidus, TH: Thalamus.

is atrophic (Fig. 43.2), with loss of pontine neurones and transverse pontocerebellar fibers. In sections stained for myelin, the intact descending corticospinal tracts stand out against the degenerated transverse fibers and the atrophic middle cerebellar peduncles. There is a disproportionate depletion of fibers from the middle cerebellar peduncles compared with the loss of pontine neurones, an observation consistent with a "dying back" process.

A supraspinal contribution to the autonomic failure of MSA is now well established. Cell loss is reported in dorsal motor nucleus of the vagus (Sung *et al.*, 1979) and involves catecholaminergic neurons of ventrolateral medulla (Benarroch *et al.*, 1998). It has also been described for the Edinger–Westphal nucleus and posterior hypothalamus (Shy & Drager, 1960) including the tuberomamillary nucleus (Nakamura *et al.*, 1996). Papp and Lantos (1994) have shown marked involvement of brainstem pontomedullary reticular formation with GCIs, providing a supraspinal histological counterpart for impaired visceral function. Autonomic neuronal degeneration affects the locus ceruleus, too (Wenning *et al.*, 1997b). Disordered bladder, rectal, and sexual function in MSA-P and MSA-C have also been associated with cell loss in parasympathetic preganglionic nuclei of the spinal cord. These neurons are localized rostrally in Onuf's nucleus between sacral segments S2 and S3 and more caudally in the inferior intermediolateral nucleus chiefly in the S3 to S4 segments (Konno *et al.*, 1986). Degeneration of sympathetic preganglionic neurones in the intermediolateral column of the thoracolumbar spinal cord is considered contributory to orthostatic hypotension. Most of the cells lie within the lateral horn of grey matter where they are irregularly distributed and prone to shrink according to agonal state and postmortem fixation. If one considers only those reports in which formal cell counts have been made, with very few exceptions all cases of MSA with predominant pathology in either the striatonigral or olivopontocerebellar system show loss of intermediolateral cells (Daniel, 1999). However, it is noteworthy that there is not always a strong correlation between nerve cell depletion or gliosis and the clinical degree of autonomic failure. It is estimated, that more than 50% of cells within the intermediolateral column need to decay before symptoms become evident (Oppenheimer, 1980). In the peripheral component of the autonomic nervous system, Bannister and Oppenheimer (1972) have described atrophy of the glossopharyngeal and vagus nerves.

A variety of other neuronal populations are noted to show cell depletion and gliosis with considerable differences in vulnerability from case to case. These sites are listed in Table 43.2 and only a few of the reported lesions are discussed here. Various degree abnormalities in the cerebral hemisphere, including Betz cell loss, were detected

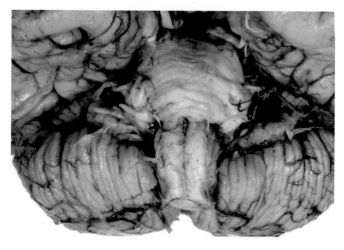

(a)

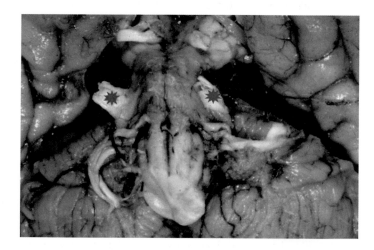

(b)

Fig. 43.2 Macroscopic appearance of the brainstem. When compared with normal (a), in MSA (b) the pons and middle cerebellar peduncles are atrophic and the trigeminal nerves (*) are prominent. (Reprinted with permission from Oxford University Press (www.oup.com), Daniel, 1999.)

in pathologically proven MSA cases (Tsuchiya *et al.*, 2000, Wakabayashi *et al.*, 1998b, Konagaya *et al.*, 1999, 2002). Fujita *et al.* (1993) demonstrated a distinct laminar astrocytosis of the motor cortices in the fifth layer in four of six sporadic OPCA cases and in none of five control cases by immunohistochemistry for glial fibrillary acidic protein. Furthermore, anterior horn cells may show some depletion but rarely to the same extent as that occurring in motor neurone disease (Konno *et al.*, 1986; Sima *et al.*, 1993). Depletion of large myelinated nerve fibers in the recurrent laryngeal nerve which innervates intrinsic laryngeal muscles has been demonstrated in MSA patients with vocal cord palsy (Hayashi *et al.*, 1997). The neuropathological background of abnormal eye movements is ill defined, although Mizutani *et al.* (1988) describe degeneration in the pathways concerned with the cerebellar fugal control of ocular movement.

From a neuropathological viewpoint, there is little cause for confusion of MSA with other neurodegenerative conditions. The GCI is the hallmark that accompanies signs of degeneration involving striatonigral and olivopontocerebellar systems. GCI are distinctly different from filamentous oligodendroglial inclusions, called coiled bodies, found in other neurodegenerative diseases, including PSP, CBD and argyrophilic grain disease (Braak & Braak, 1989; Yamada & McGeer, 1990; Arima *et al.*, 1997; Chin & Goldman, 1996). Rarely, MSA may be combined with additional pathologies. Lewy bodies (LBs) have been reported in 8–10 per cent of MSA cases and show a distribution comparable with that of PD (Wenning & Quinn, 1994). This frequency is similar to that of controls and suggests an incidental finding related to aging and/or presymptomatic PD. Isolated reports of unusual clinicopathological cases occur and include overlap of MSA with PSP and CBD (Ansorge *et al.*, 1997a, Takanashi *et al.*, 2002), MSA with Alzheimer's disease and PD (Ansorge *et al.*, 1997b), and MSA with atypical Pick's disease (Horoupian & Dickson, 1991).

The discovery of glial cytoplasmic inclusions (GCIs) in MSA brains in 1989 highlighted the unique glial pathology as biological hallmark of this disorder (Papp *et al.*, 1989). GCIs are argyrophilic and half moon, oval or conical in shape (Lantos, 1998) and are composed of 20- to 30-nm tubular filaments (Gai *et al.*, 2003). Although inclusions have been described in five cellular sites, i.e. in oligodendroglial and neuronal cytoplasm and nuclei as well as in axons (Papp & Lantos, 1992), glial cytoplasmic inclusions (GCIs) (Papp *et al.*, 1989) are most ubiquitous and appear to represent the subcellular hallmark lesion of MSA (Lantos, 1998). Their distribution selectively involves basal ganglia, supplementary and primary motor cortex, the reticular formation, basis pontis, the middle cerebellar peduncles and the cerebellar white matter (Lantos, 1998; Papp & Lantos, 1994). GCIs contain classical cytoskeletal antigens, including ubiquitin and tau (Lantos, 1998; Cairns *et al.*, 1997a). More recently, α-synuclein immunoreactivity has been recognized as the most sensitive marker of GCIs (Dickson *et al.*, 1999b) (Fig. 43.3). In fact, α-synuclein, a presynaptic protein which is affected by point mutations in some families with autosomal dominant PD (Goedert & Spillantini, 1998) and which is present in LBs (Spillantini

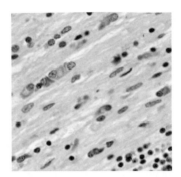

Fig. 43.3 α-Synuclein immunostaining reveals GCIs in subcortical white matter.

et al., 1997), has also been observed in both neuronal and glial cytoplasmic inclusions (Wakabayashi *et al.*, 1998a,c; Arima *et al.*, 1998; Tu *et al.*, 1998; Spillantini *et al.*, 1998) in brains of patients with MSA. GCI filaments are multilayered in structure, with alpha-synuclein oligomers forming the central core fibrils of the filaments (Gai *et al.*, 2003). The accumulation of α-synuclein into filamentous inclusions appears to play a key role not only in MSA, but also in a growing number of α-synucleinopathies such as Parkinson's disease, dementia with LBs, Down's syndrome, familial Alzheimer's disease, and sporadic AD (Trojanowski, 2002). The α-synuclein accumulation in GCIs as well as in neuronal inclusions associated with MSA precedes their ubiquitination (Gai *et al.*, 1998). Importantly, α-synuclein, but not ubiquitin, antibodies also reveal numerous degenerating neurites in the white matter of MSA cases (Gai *et al.*, 1998). This suggests that an as yet unrecognized degree of pathology may be present in the axons of MSA cases, although whether neuronal/axonal α-synuclein pathology precedes glial α-synuclein pathology has not been examined.

Biochemical/neuropharmacological findings

Biochemical findings

Neurochemical studies have shown alterations consistent with sites of major pathology. Calcineurin, a marker for medium-sized spiny neurons, is decreased in striosomes of the putamen and in the efferent pathway of the globus pallidus and substantia nigra (Goto *et al.*, 1989b). Regardless of clinical presentation, there is reduced immunoreactivity for additional markers of the striatal efferent system, including met-enkephalin, substance P, and calbindin (Ito *et al.*, 1996). In the SNC, tyrosine hydroxylase (TH) containing dopaminergic neurons are depleted. Similar neurones in the C1 and A2 regions of the medulla also showed reduced TH activity, which has been associated with orthostatic hypotension (Kato *et al.*, 1995).

Biochemical analyses have found only minor differences in reduced striatal and nigral dopamine content in MSA when compared with PD (Brücke *et al.*, 1997). However, unlike PD, mitochondrial respiratory chain function in the substantia nigra is normal in MSA (Gu *et al.*, 1997). An increase in total iron content appears to reflect sites of primary damage and occurs in both PD and MSA substantia nigra, as well as in MSA striatum (Dexter *et al.*, 1991). Decreased noradrenaline levels are reported in septal nuclei, nucleus accumbens, hypothalamus, and locus ceruleus, while a consistent deficit of choline acetyltransferase is found in red nucleus, dentate, pontine, and inferior olivary nuclei, with variable involvement of the striatum and additional areas (Spokes *et al.*, 1979). Cerebellar and, in particular, Purkinje cell damage, has been indicated by reduced levels of glutamate dehydrogenase (Plaitakis *et al.*, 1993), amino acid binding sites (Price *et al.*, 1993), and cerebrospinal fluid calbindin-D (Kiyosawa *et al.*, 1993).

The content of neurofilament (NFL) in CSF was significantly higher both in PSP and MSA compared to PD patients (Holmberg *et al.*, 1998). The high values of NFL indicate an ongoing neuronal degeneration affecting mainly the axonal compartment in PSP and MSA patients, whereas there was no difference in glial involvement as measured by GFAP in PD, PSP, and MSA patients (Holmberg *et al.*, 1998). Furthermore, CSF-NFL and levodopa tests combined with discriminant analysis may contribute even better to the differential diagnosis of parkinsonian syndromes (Holmberg *et al.*, 2001). Whereas the CSF-NFL and levodopa tests predicted 79 and 85% correct diagnoses (PD or non-PD (MSA and PSP)), respectively, the combined test predicted 90% correct diagnoses.

Kuiper *et al.* (1994) investigated nitrite and nitrate in CSF of PD, AD, and MSA patients and controls. They found for all patient groups, compared with controls, significantly decreased levels of nitrate, but not nitrite. This finding seems to indicate a decreased NO production of the central nervous system (CNS) in these neurodegenerative disorders. Alterations in neuronal NO production may play a role in the pathophysiology of PD, AD, and MSA. The biosynthesis of NO is dependent on the availability of L-arginine, the substrate for NOS, and on L-glutamate, which stimulates NO synthesis via the NMDA receptor. In this process L-citrulline is formed. A slight but statistically significant elevation of CSF L-citrulline was found

in 15 MSA patients by Kuiper *et al.* (2000) and there were no significant changes in L-arginine levels. The relation between the CSF levels of these amino acids and neuronal NO production is still unclear. Konings *et al.* (1999) measured total glutathione concentrations in the CSF of PD (non-demented or demented), MSA, and AD patients and age-matched controls. No statistically significant differences in the mean total CSF glutathione concentrations were found between groups and dopaminomimetic treatment was not found to have any effect on total CSF glutathione levels. 8-hydroxy-2′-deoxyguanosine (8-OHdG) or 8-hydroxyguanosine (8-OHG), a product of oxidized DNA or RNA, is a good marker of oxidative cellular damage. Kikuchi *et al.* (2002) measured the 8-OHdG/8-OHG levels in the serum and CSF of patients with PD and MSA. Compared to age-matched controls, the mean levels of serum 8-OHdG/8-OHG were significantly higher in PD patients. 8-OHdG/8-OHG levels in CSF were also increased significantly in patients with PD and MSA, however, their relative values were generally much lower than those in the serum.

Since idiopathic chronic autonomic dysfunction may occur as pure autonomic failure (PAF) or in association with MSA, specific studies have been carried out in both these conditions. CSF immunoreactivity to rat locus ceruleus occurred in a significantly greater number of samples from MSA patients compared to control subjects or patients with PAF (Polinsky *et al.*, 1991). Other brain regions infrequently showed immunoreactivity. These findings suggest that degeneration in MSA may release antigen(s) that induce antibodies against locus ceruleus neurons. Further studies are required to determine whether immune abnormalities play a pathogenetic role in MSA (Gahring *et al.*, 1997; Schelhaas *et al.*, 1997).

There are several studies measuring CSF content of biogenic amine metabolites/derivates, thiamine, neuropeptide Y, substance P, or corticotropin-releasing hormone in MSA patients (Gonzalez-Quevedo *et al.*, 1993; Botez *et al.*, 2001; Ichikawa *et al.*, 1986; Orozco *et al.*, 1989; Martignoni *et al.*, 1992; Nutt *et al.*, 1980; Suemaru *et al.*, 1995). Botez *et al.* (2001) measured levels of the dopamine metabolite homovanillic acid (HVA), the serotonin metabolite 5-hydroxindoleacetic acid (5HIAA) and precursor tryptophan, as well as the noradrenaline metabolite 3-methoxy-4-hydroxyphenylethylene glycol (MHPG) and thiamine in the CSF of patients with OPCA (among others), as compared with sex- and age-matched control subjects. CSF HVA, MHPG and thiamine values were markedly lower than those in control patients, whereas CSF 5HIAA values showed only a trend towards lower levels than control subjects.

Neuropharmacological findings

The combination of nigral and striatal degeneration is the core pathology underlying parkinsonism in MSA. The degenerative process affects nigrostriatal dopaminergic transmission at both pre- and post-synaptic sites (Fearnley & Lees, 1991; Kume *et al.*, 1993). Pathologically, the loss of dopaminergic neurons in MSA-P is comparable to that found in PD (Tison *et al.*, 1995a). Only few patients with MSA exhibit a presynaptic pattern with minimal putaminal changes (Tison *et al.*, 1995a; Wenning *et al.*, 1994b; Berciano *et al.*, 2002). There is a close anatomical relationship between nigral and striatal degeneration in MSA-P. Degeneration of pigmented dopaminergic neurons begins and predominantly involves the ventrolateral tier of SNC which in turn projects to the dorsolateral posterior putamen; the latter is the predominant site of striatal degeneration in MSA. Several post-mortem immunohistochemical and autoradiographical, as well as in vivo neuroimaging studies, suggest that both striatal outflow pathways are affected: encephalin-containing striatal neurons projecting to the external globus pallidus that carry dopamine D2 receptors (indirect pathway) and substance P (SP)-containing cells projecting to internal globus pallidus and substantia nigra pars reticulata (SNR) that carry D1 receptors (direct pathway) (Quik *et al.*, 1979; Cortes *et al.*, 1989; Shinotoh *et al.*, 1991, 1993; Brooks *et al.*, 1992; Churchyard *et al.*, 1993; Vogels *et al.*, 2000; Goto *et al.*, 1989a,c, 1990, 1996; Schelosky *et al.*, 1993; van Royen *et al.*, 1993; Ito *et al.*, 1996).

In accordance with the topographical projection of the putamen onto pallidal segments, the posterolateral portions of the external and internal globus pallidus, and the ventrolateral portion of the substantia nigra are deafferented from striatal projections (Brooks *et al.*, 1992). Churchyard *et al.* (1993), in a postmortem binding study of two MSA brains, found loss of putaminal D2 receptors in both, but loss of D1 receptors in only one case. Because the duration of the disease was shorter and histopathological changes were less severe in the latter case they suggested the possibility that the disease may initially affect striatal cells expressing D2 receptors (indirect pathway), and only subsequently D1 receptor expressing neurons (direct pathway). However, this assumption remains contentious. The evidence considered so far suggests that the pathology of parkinsonism in MSA-P incorporates variable combinations of loss of dopaminergic nigrostriatal transmission, and impairment of both the indirect and direct striatal outflow pathways at the striatal level, with relative preservation of subthalamic nucleus, globus pallidus and thalamus.

Progressive loss of striatal dopamine receptors and striatal output systems might explain levodopa unresponsiveness in most MSA-P patients (Tison *et al.*, 1995a; Ito *et al.*, 1996; Parati *et al.*, 1993; Rajput *et al.*, 1990). Those patients with a good initial response to levodopa would thus have less striatal damage than those with absent or poor initial response. However, there is evidence suggesting that the response to levodopa does not always depend solely on the degree of striatal cell loss (Wenning *et al.*, 1994b). In vivo PET studies by Brooks *et al.* (1992) have also failed to clearly correlate therapeutic response with striatal D2 receptor status. However, reduced D2 binding as assessed by SPECT or PET performed in levodopa-naive patients with parkinsonism may predict a lack of response to apomorphine, lack of subsequent response to chronic levodopa therapy or a clinical diagnosis of MSA-P (Schelosky *et al.*, 1993; Schwarz *et al.*, 1998). Additional loss of D1 and opiate receptors could also be an important factor underlying dopaminergic unresponsiveness in MSA-P (Shinotoh *et al.*, 1993; Burn *et al.*, 1995), as well as other changes downstream of the striatum itself.

Neurotransmitter release is modulated by presynaptic histamine H(3) receptors located on histaminergic, noradrenergic and other non-histaminergic neurons of the central and peripheral nervous system. Wiedemann *et al.* (2002) reported the determination of the structure of the human histamine H(3) receptor gene (HRH3) and the identification of a missense mutation in a patient with MSA and autonomic failure. The homozygous Ala280Val variation in the third intracellular loop of the histamine H(3) receptor may be related to the etiology of the illness due to altered norepinephrine release.

Overstimulation of alpha1B-adrenergic receptors in transgenic mice resulted in autonomic failure and motor impairment due to neuronal multisystem degeneration (Zuscik *et al.*, 2000, 2001). Whether this phenotype represents a useful model of MSA has been debated (Seppi *et al.*, 2001; Perez, 2001).

Molecular biology

α-synuclein is a 140 amino acid protein that is abundantly expressed in the brain and typically enriched at presynaptic terminals (Dickson *et al.*, 1999a; Clayton & George, 1999). α-Synuclein is exclusively expressed in the soluble fraction of the neuronal cytoplasm in normal humans. However, in MSA (oligo-)glial cytoplasmic inclusions, strongly immunoreactive for α-synuclein (Fig. 43.3), are the most distinctive neuropathological feature (Tu *et al.*, 1998), regardless of phenotypical presentation. Formation of GCIs appears to be the key pathway to selective loss of oligodendroglia and neurons in MSA. The differential distribution of α-synuclein deposits and associated neuronal pathology (SND, OPCA and spinal cord) suggests variability of pathogenetic mechanisms underlying the multifaceted disease process of MSA. α-Synuclein appears to be extensively nitrated in the cytoplasmic aggregates of PD, DLB, and MSA brains suggesting that nitration is involved in the onset and/or progression of these neurodegenerative diseases (Duda et al., 1999). Presumably, tyrosine 125 plays a critical role for alpha-synuclein dimerization under nitrative stress (Takahashi et al., 2002). Protein nitration in Lewy body diseases and MSA cases has a widespread distribution and is not only associated with the alpha-synuclein deposits (Gomez-Tortosa et al., 2002). Moreover, it has been shown that α-synuclein is phosphorylated by tyrosine kinases (Nakamura et al., 2001; Negro et al., 2002; Ellis et al., 2001), and that some of these tyrosine kinases may play an antineurodegenerative role by phosphorylating α-synuclein, thereby preventing its aggregation (Negro et al., 2002). The amino-terminal half of NAC (Non-Aβ Component of AD amyloid), as well as stretches of nine and more amino acid residues derived from this part, is able to fibrillate and to seed fibrillation of full-length α-synuclein (Uversky & Fink, 2002). It has been shown that β- and γ-synucleins may inhibit the fibrillation of α-synuclein (Uversky et al., 2002, Hashimoto et al., 2001). Accumulation of α-synuclein may require additional proteins as pathologic chaperones (Tu et al., 1998). If chaperones are involved, their nature is likely to be unique to MSA, because the morphology and array of immunoreactive components in GCIs and NCIs differ from those characterizing Lewy bodies (Spillantini et al., 1998). Engelender et al. (1999) identified an α-synuclein-associated novel protein named synphilin-1, and reported that cotransfection of both α-synuclein and synphilin-1 in mammalian cells yielded eosinophilic cytoplasmic inclusions resembling LB. More recently, it was shown that synphilin-1 immunoreactivity is present in Lewy bodies as well as in GCIs (Wakabayashi et al., 2000, 2002). Various neuronal and glial inclusions in neurodegenerative disorders other than LB disease and MSA were synphilin-1 negative. Therefore, abnormal accumulation of synphilin-1 appears to be specific for brain lesions in which α-synuclein is a major component (Wakabayashi et al., 2002). Whether the α-synuclein aggregation is induced by some other factor(s), or whether it is the primary trigger of MSA pathology is unknown. Impairment in the ability of oligodendrocytes to degrade α-synuclein which they may normally produce at low levels may also promote abnormal subcellular aggregation in MSA (Tu et al., 1998). Alternatively, selective

upregulation in the expression of α-synuclein in glial cells could occur in response to certain pathologic conditions (Arima et al., 1998). However, expression levels of α-synuclein mRNA in MSA brains are similar to those of control subjects (Ozawa et al., 2001). These results suggest that the transcriptional regulation of the α-synuclein gene is unlikely to be affected in MSA.

Pathogenesis/mechanism of disease

Recent findings support an important role for glial cells and inflammatory reactions in many neurodegenerative diseases including PD, DLB and MSA (Hirsch et al., 1998; Togo et al., 2001; Vila et al., 2001). Neuronal survival is critically dependent on glial function, which can exert both neuroprotective and neurotoxic influences. Glial cells are a primary target of cytokines and are activated in response to many cytokines, including tumor necrosis factor (TNF)-α (Allan & Rothwell, 2001). This activation can trigger further release of cytokines that might enhance or suppress local inflammatory responses and neuronal survival. These cytokines may also participate in neurodegeneration either indirectly by activating other glial cells or directly by inducing apoptosis (Boka et al., 1994; Hunot et al., 1999; Mogi et al., 1994). Several studies indicated that TNF-α is toxic for dopaminergic neurons in vitro (McGuire et al., 2001) and in vivo (Aloe & Fiore, 1997), thus supporting the potential involvement of this pro-inflammatory cytokine in the neurodegenerative processes in PD and other α-synucleinopathies. However, the relationship between intracellular α-synuclein positive inclusions and the proinflammatory response in α-synucleinopathies remains obscure. The activation of microglial cells may be the final common pathway, contributing both to demyelination and neuronal removal, irrespective of the mode of cell death. PK 11195 selectively binds to benzodiazepine sites on activated microglia. [11]C PK 11195 positron emission tomography has demonstrated activated microglia in vivo in the putamen, pallidum, substantia nigra, and pontine region in four patients with MSA (Gerhard et al., 2000).

Trophic factors have been studied in a number of neurodegenerative diseases, both for their potential pathogenetic role and also for their possible therapeutic benefit. Neurotrophic factors such as nerve growth factor (NGF), glial derived neurotrophic factor (GDNF), brain-derived neurotrophic factor (BDNF), basic fibroblast growth factor (bFGF), and platelet derived growth factor (PDGF) have been shown to exert neuroprotective and neuroregenerative effects in various neurodegenerative disorders (Olanow

& Tatton, 1999; Gash *et al.*, 1998; Lindsay *et al.*, 1994). However, until now it is not clear whether neurotrophins may have a direct influence on α-synuclein aggregation and cell death. A study by Stefanis & Cole (2001) suggested that the expression of α-synuclein may be directly regulated by neurotrophic factors such as NGF in neuronal cells, whereas another study did not confirm these findings (Satoh & Kuroda, 2001). Further, no correlation was found between synuclein expression and apoptotic death following trophic deprivation (Stefanis *et al.*, 2001). Since neurotrophic factors have a variety of biological effects including modulation of proteasomic function and apoptosis (Yuan & Yankner, 2000), it seems likely that neurotrophins could have a direct effect on the survival of neuronal and glial cells overexpressing α-synuclein. BDNF is abundantly and widely expressed in neurones of the adult mammalian brain. It has a neurotrophic effect on many neuronal types, including nigral dopaminergic and striatal neurones (Murer *et al.*, 2000). BDNF positive neurites have been shown to be more abundant in the striatum of patients with MSA than in the striatum of those with PD and normal controls. The upregulation of BDNF has been interpreted as a protective mechanism against progressive degeneration of the striatal neurones in MSA (Kawamoto *et al.*, 1999). However, it is not clear whether the upregulation has occurred in the major striatal afferents originating in the cortex or in nigral afferents, since the striatal neurones themselves are not BDNF immunoreactive (Murer *et al.*, 2000). White matter astrocytes produce PDGF, which has been shown to act as a survival factor for newly formed oligodendrocytes (Barres *et al.*, 1992). It has been demonstrated that the sensitivity of oligodendrocytes to astrocyte derived PDGF is greatly enhanced by an extracellular matrix glycoprotein, laminin-2 (Frost *et al.*, 1999), which is expressed by Purkinje cell axons (Powell *et al.*, 1998). Laminin-2 also appears to play an important part in the signaling mechanisms that stimulate oligodendrocytes to elaborate the myelin sheath (Buttery & ffrench-Constant, 1999). Neurones/axons generate several isoforms of neuregulins, which are members of a large trophic family all originating from a single gene. Some of the isoforms promote proliferation and survival of oligodendrocytes through their interaction with the erb-B family of receptors, expressed by the oligodendrocytes (Burden & Yarden, 1997). One neuregulin isoform (glial growth factor) promotes proliferation and survival of oligodendrocyte progenitors but inhibits their further differentiation (Canoll *et al.*, 1996, 1999). So far, there have been no reports of alterations in glial growth factors in patients with MSA (Burn & Jaros, 2001). Glial growth factors are derived from both astrocytes and neurones. Other isoforms (acteylcholine receptor-inducing activity protein, neu

differentiation factors (NDFα, and NDFβ)) act as morphogenes for developing oligodendrocytes by promoting the extension and complexity of their processes (Vartanian *et al.*, 1994, 1997; Raabe *et al.*, 1997). In addition to the well-documented effects of neuregulins on glial cells, there is also evidence that neuregulins have direct effects on CNS neurones (Bermingham-McDonogh *et al.*, 1996; Yang *et al.*, 1998; Ozaki *et al.*, 1997). Different groups of neuronal populations appear to use different neuregulin isoforms at successive development of stages of the CNS to support the oligodendrocytes which myelinate their axonal projections. It is conceivable that polymorphisms in certain neuregulin isoforms, which are shared by the suprasegmental motor system, the supraspinal autonomic systems, and their targets, could be a risk factor for MSA and could also underlie the system-bound distribution of the oligodendroglial and neuronal pathology in this disease (Jaros & Burn, 2000).

MSA, as reflected in its current definition, is regarded as a sporadic disease (Wenning *et al.*, 1993) and no confirmed familial cases of MSA have been described yet; notwithstanding, it is conceivable that genetic factors may play a role in the aetiology of the disease. This has, for example, been convincingly demonstrated for PSP (Baker *et al.*, 1999), another disease which, in the vast majority of cases, is a sporadic disease. However, initial screening studies for candidate genes revealed no risk factors (Bandmann *et al.*, 1997; Nicholl *et al.*, 1999; R. Krüger, personal communication). Other recent studies have further looked for polymorphisms or mutations in candidate genes, which may predispose an individual towards developing MSA. The apolipoprotein ε4 allele is not over-represented in MSA when compared with controls, and there have been conflicting reports of the association of a cytochrome P-450–2D6 polymorphism with MSA (Cairns *et al.*, 1997b; Iwahashi *et al.*, 1995; Bandmann *et al.*, 1995). No association was found between MSA and polymorphisms in other genes possibly involved in neurodegenerative diseases (CYP1A1, *N*-acetyltransferase 2, dopamine transporter and glutathione-S-transferase M1) (Nicholl *et al.*, 1999). Furthermore, there is no evidence to support an association between MSA and polymorphisms in the H5 pore region of the human homologue of the weaver mouse gene hiGIRK2, the insulin-like growth factor 1 receptor gene, or the ciliary neurotrophic factor gene (Bandmann *et al.*, 1997). No epidemiological analytical study has yet investigated the relationship between genotype and environment. The pathogenetic role of α-synuclein is still unclear. Inactivation of the α-synuclein gene by homologous recombination did not lead to a severe neurological phenotype (Abeliovich *et al.*, 2000). So, loss of function of the α-synuclein protein is unlikely to account for its role in neurodegeneration. Mice that lack α-synuclein were found to show increased release of striatal dopamine, indicating that this protein could function as an activity-dependent, negative regulator of neurotransmission in the striatum. While there is strong evidence that α-synuclein participates in the pathogenesis of some types of familial PD (Polymeropoulos *et al.*, 1997; Kruger *et al.*, 1998), no mutations have been found in the entire coding region of the α-synuclein gene in MSA (Ozawa *et al.*, 1999) nor in sporadic forms of PD and DLB (El-Agnaf *et al.*, 1998). However, mutations in the regulatory or intronic regions of the gene have not been ruled out (Burn & Jaros, 2001). Polymorphisms in the α-synuclein gene have been identified in PD (Krüger *et al.*, 1999). They may also increase the risk of developing MSA by promoting α-synuclein protein aggregation. Polymorphisms in codons 1 to 39 of the α-synuclein gene, a domain related to interaction with synphilin-1, or indeed polymorphisms in the synphilin-1 gene itself, or in the genes of other protein-interacting partners of α-synuclein may also need to be considered in the pathogenesis of MSA (Engelender *et al.*, 1999). The number of α-synuclein protein-interacting partners has expanded to include 14-3-3 protein chaperones, protein kinase C, extracellular regulated kinase, and BAD, a Bcl-2 homologue that regulates cell death (Ostrerova *et al.*, 1999). Nevertheless, association studies with genetic polymorphisms for α-synuclein, have so far been negative in MSA (Bandmann *et al.*, 1997; Morris *et al.*, 2000). Gilman *et al.* (1996) have reported a MSA-like phenotype including GCI like (α-synuclein negative) inclusions in one SCA 1 (spinocerebellar ataxia type 1) family. Other SCA mutations (except for SCA-2 (Bösch *et al.*, 2002a)) have not been reported to present with MSA-like features (Schöls *et al.*, 2000; Ranum *et al.*, 1995; Silveira *et al.*, 1996; Leggo *et al.*, 1997; Futamura *et al.*, 1998; Moseley *et al.*, 1998). Conversely, the majority of MSA-C patients do not appear to have expanded SCA1 and SCA3 alleles (Bandmann *et al.*, 1997). MSA-C appears to be a frequent form of sporadic cerebellar ataxia of late onset. 29% of sporadic adult-onset ataxia patients suffer from MSA (Abele *et al.*, 2002). This finding corresponds well to data of a study of sporadic OPCA patients who were followed 3 months to 10 years (Gilman *et al.*, 2000). Within this period, 17 out of 51 patients developed autonomic failure or parkinsonism indicating a diagnosis of MSA. Increased expression of a brain specific protein called ZNF231 in cerebellar neurones has been reported to occur in patients with MSA (Hashida *et al.*, 1998). The gene is located on chromosome 3p21 and encodes a neuronal double zinc finger protein with a nuclear targeting sequence, suggesting that it might function as a transcription regulator. The importance of this finding is as yet uncertain, but it is possible that patients with MSA differ from unaffected individuals by sequence polymorphisms within, and flanking, the putative functional motifs of the ZNF231 gene.

Clinical picture

Introduction

In a series of 100 cases of clinically probable MSA (Wenning *et al.*, 1994a; Wenning & Quinn, 1997), at the last evaluation, 97% of patients with MSA had autonomic failure, 91% had parkinsonism, 52% had cerebellar features and 61% had pyramidal features. Autonomic failure may be associated with either levodopa unresponsive parkinsonism in 80% of cases (MSA-P subtype) or with cerebellar ataxia in 20% of cases (MSA-C subtype). There is commonly clinical and subclinical evidence of autonomic failure in both MSA variants.

Presenting features

MSA patients may present with parkinsonism that usually responds poorly to levodopa. This has been identified as the most important early clinical discriminator of MSA and PD (Quinn, 1989b; Schwarz *et al.*, 1992; Schelosky *et al.*, 1993; Wenning *et al.*, 2000a), although a subgroup of MSA patients may show a good or, rarely, excellent, but usually short-lived, response to levodopa (Bösch *et al.*, 2002b; Hughes *et al.*, 1992; Parati *et al.*, 1993). Progressive ataxia may also be the presenting feature of MSA (Schulz *et al.*, 1994; Wenning *et al.*, 1997a). A cerebellar presentation of MSA appears to be more common than the parkinsonian variant in Japan compared to Western countries (Watanabe *et al.*, 2002). Autonomic failure with symptomatic orthostatic hypotension and/or urogenital disturbance may accompany the motor disorder in up to 50% of patients at disease onset.

Unusual presentations in pathologically proven cases have included stroke-like episodes evolving into parkinsonism (Lambie *et al.*, 1947), REM sleep disorder (Tison *et al.*, 1995b), pseudo-TIAs in the anterior or posterior circulation (Bannister & Oppenheimer, 1972; Klein *et al.*, 1995) as well as limb shaking attacks (Litvan, personal communication).

Features of established disease

Parkinsonism

Bradykinesia, rigidity, postural tremor as well as dysequilibrium and gait unsteadiness characterize parkinsonism associated with MSA. Jerky postural tremor and less

Table 43.3. Frequency (%) of individual clinical features in three series of MSA

	MSA 168	MSA 100	MSA 35
Sex ratio (male:female)	1.4 :1	1.9 :1	1.2:1
Mean age at onset (yrs)	54.1	52.5	55
Median survival (yrs)	6.0	9.3	7.3
Autonomic symptoms	71	97	97
Postural faintness (incl. syncope)	na	53	31
Syncope	24	15	20
Urinary incontinence	56	71	51
Urinary retention	18	27	34
Fecal incontinence	12	2	3
Impotence	43	90	62
Parkinsonism	84	91	100
Tremor	64	66	80
present at rest	40	29	34
pill-rolling	7	9	11
Cerebellar signs	59	52	34
Gait ataxia	54	37	29
Limb ataxia	51	47	31
Pyramidal signs	48	61	54
Stridor	9	34	34
Dysarthria	79	96	89
Antecollis	4	15	9
Myoclonus	na	31	29

MSA 168 refers to the series of well documented pathologically proven MSA cases reported in the literature (Wenning *et al.*, 1997b) excluding the 35 confirmed cases from the UK Parkinson's Disease Society Brain Bank that constitute MSA 35 (Wenning *et al.*, 1995). MSA 100 refers to the clinical series of 100 cases with probable MSA (Wenning *et al.*, 1994a). na: not available. (Reprinted with permission from Wenning & Quinn, 1997.)

commonly tremor at rest may be superimposed. Frequently, patients exhibit orofacial dystonia associated with a characteristic quivering high-pitched dysarthria. Postural stability is compromised early on, however, recurrent falls at disease onset are unusual in contrast to PSP. The majority of patients with MSA treated fail to show a sustained, long-term response to levodopa.

The clinical data in Table 43.3 are derived from three MSA series (Wenning & Quinn, 1997): 168 well-documented clinicopathological cases of MSA reported in the literature (Wenning *et al.*, 1997b), 100 cases of clinically probable MSA (Wenning *et al.*, 1994a), and 35 cases of pathologically confirmed MSA from the United Kingdom Parkinson's Disease Society Brain Bank (UKPDSBB) (Wenning *et al.*, 1995). The vast majority of patients in the three series (84–100%) developed parkinsonism. Pure MSA-P (parkinsonism without cerebellar signs) represented the single most common motor subtype ranging from 40% (literature) through 48% (clinical series) to 66% (UKPDSBB series). In contrast, pure MSA-C (cerebellar ataxia without parkinsonism) was absent in the UKPDSBB series, and present in 9% of patients in the clinical series, and in 16% in the literature series. It has been suggested that a symmetrical atremulous picture might distinguish MSA-P from PD (Fearnley & Lees, 1990, Albanese *et al.*, 1995; Colosimo *et al.*, 1995; Gouider-Khouja *et al.*, 1995). However, motor disturbance was asymmetrical in 74% of patients in the clinical series, and unilateral at onset in 47% of literature cases, and in many of the UKPDSBB cases. Also, some sort of tremor was present in 64% to 80% of cases, and tremor present at rest was observed in 29% to 40% of cases. Even so, a classical pill-rolling resting tremor was reported in only 7% to 9% of subjects. Therefore, the differential diagnosis of MSA-P and PD may be exceedingly difficult in the early stages due to a number of overlapping features such as rest tremor or asymmetrical akinesia and rigidity. Furthermore, levodopa induced improvement of parkinsonism may be seen in 30% of MSA-P patients, however, the benefit is transient in most of them. Levodopa-induced dyskinesia affecting orofacial and neck muscles occur in 50% of MSA-P patients, sometimes in the absence of motor benefit (Bösch *et al.*, 2002b; Hughes *et al.*, 1992). In most instances a fully developed clinical picture of MSA-P evolves within 5 years of disease onset, allowing a clinical diagnosis during follow-up (Wenning *et al.*, 2000a).

Dysautonomia

Dysautonomia is characteristic of both MSA subtypes, primarily comprising urogenital and orthostatic dysfunction.

Urinary incontinence (71%) or retention (27%), often early in the course or as presenting symptoms, are frequent (Wenning *et al.*, 1994a/1999c; Beck *et al.*, 1994; Sakakibara *et al.*, 2000a). Disorders of micturition in MSA generally occur more commonly, earlier, and to a more severe degree than in PD (Beck *et al.*, 1994). Urinary retention can be caused or exacerbated by benign prostatic hypertrophy or, in women, by perineal laxity secondary to difficult childbirth or uterine descent. In men, the urological symptoms of pollakiuria, urgency, nocturia and incontinence together with hesitancy and incomplete emptying or chronic retention may simulate those of prostatic outflow obstruction. In a series of patients with probable MSA, 43% of males had undergone futile prostatic or bladder neck surgery before the correct diagnosis was made, although more than half of them had neurological symptoms or signs at the time of the procedure (Beck *et al.*, 1994). Stress incontinence occurred in 57% of the women and of these half had undergone surgery. The results of surgery were also poor (Beck *et al.*, 1994; Chandiramani *et al.*, 1997). Fecal incontinence was much rarer (2–12%) (Wenning & Quinn, 1997), despite frequent severe denervation of the external anal sphincter, suggesting that the mechanisms of urinary and fecal continence are distinct in MSA.

Early impotence is virtually universal in men with MSA. In a series of 62 MSA patients, impotence occurred in 96% of the men and was the first symptom alone in 37% (Beck *et al.*, 1994). Reduced genital sensitivity with or without impaired libido has been recently reported in the majority of female MSA patients (Oertel *et al.*, 2003). In addition, MSA patients may note increased constipation and hypo- or anhydrosis.

Based on Shy and Drager's description (1960), recurrent syncopal attacks are commonly regarded as a typical feature of MSA. However, severe orthostatic hypotension with recurrent (more than three) syncopes was only reported in 15% of subjects whereas postural faintness was present, but only to a mild or moderate degree, in up to 53% of cases (Wenning *et al.*, 1994a,c). The analysis of a detailed questionnaire and autonomic function tests in a series of 121 patients with clinically diagnosed MSA showed that urinary symptoms (96%) were more common than orthostatic symptoms (43%) (Sakakibara *et al.*, 2000a) (see Section in Onset). Orthostatic hypotension is frequently associated with impaired or absent reflex tachycardia upon standing. Dopaminergic drugs may provoke or worsen orthostatic hypotension. Recumbent arterial hypertension, mainly due to loss of baroreflexes, may be seen in a few patients with severe cardiovascular autonomic failure (Bannister & Mathias, 1999a).

Cerebellar disorder

The cerebellar disorder comprises gait ataxia, limb kinetic ataxia and scanning dysarthria as well as cerebellar oculomotor disturbances. Cerebellar signs, most commonly manifesting as a wide-based ataxic gait developed in 34–59% of patients (Wenning & Quinn, 1997; Schulz *et al.*, 1994) (see Table 43.3). However, a subgroup of patients presented with narrow-based unsteady gait due to more marked impairment of postural reflexes (Wenning *et al.*, 1997a). Spontaneous and/or gaze-evoked nystagmus, often subtle, was detected in 23–25% of patients (Wenning *et al.*, 1994a, 1997a), and cerebellar scanning dysarthria may occur. The finding of a mixed dysarthria with combinations of hypokinetic, ataxic, and spastic components is consistent with both the overall clinical and the neuropathologic changes in MSA (Kluin *et al.*, 1996, Garratt *et al.*, 1994).

Patients with MSA-C develop additional non-cerebellar symptoms and signs, but before doing so may be indis-

tinguishable from other patients with idiopathic late onset cerebellar ataxia (ILOCA), many of whom have a disease restricted clinically to cerebellar signs and pathologically to degeneration of the cerebellum and olives (Abele *et al.*, 2002, Wenning & Geser, 2003).

Pyramidal signs

Although pyramidal signs may be elicited in up to 61% of MSA patients (Wenning & Quinn, 1997), obvious spastic paraparetic gait or significant pyramidal weakness should cast doubt upon the clinical diagnosis of MSA.

Other clinical features

Besides the poor response to levodopa, and the additional presence of pyramidal or cerebellar signs or autonomic failure as major diagnostic clues, certain other features may either raise suspicion of MSA, or at least suggest that one might not be dealing with PD (Quinn, 1989b). These features (Table 43.4), so called "red flags," often are early warning signs of MSA (Gouider-Khouja *et al.*, 1995).

Dystonia of orofacial and platysma musculature may either be present spontaneously or it may emerge in 30% of levodopa treated patients, sometimes resulting in a characteristic facial distortion particularly, but not exclusively, in MSA-P patients reminiscent of risus sardonicus of cephalic tetanus (Fig. 43.4) (Hughes *et al.*, 1992; Wenning *et al.*, 1996b, 2003a; Bösch *et al.*, 2002b).

Subacute *Pisa syndrome*, a form of severe axial dystonia, has been reported in MSA (Kan, 1978; Colosimo, 1998). However, Pisa syndrome is a non-specific feature of parkinsonism and it may also emerge in patients with otherwise classical PD.

A frequent and characteristic feature suggesting MSA is the development of a *disproportionate antecollis* (Langston, 1936; Neumann, 1977; Caplan, 1984; Quinn, 1989a; Rivest *et al.*, 1990; Bösch *et al.*, 2002b) hampering feeding, communication and vision. The pathophysiological basis remains uncertain. Botulinum toxin injections into sternocleidomastoid muscles are usually unrewarding and worsen dysphagia (Thobois *et al.*, 2001).

Other manifestations of focal dystonia are less common, but may include *hand dystonia, torticollis*, and *dystonic toe movements*. Levodopa exposure may worsen dystonic movements in the absence of antiparkinsonian benefit (Bösch *et al.*, 2002b).

Tremulous myoclonic jerks, usually affecting the fingers, of small amplitude, and often stretch-sensitive, occur in a number of patients with MSA, but are otherwise rare in non-demented parkinsonian patients (Quinn, 1989b; Salazar *et al.*, 2000).

Table 43.4. "Red flags": Warning features of MSA*

Motor Red Flags	Definition
Orofacial dystonia	Atypical spontaneous or L-Dopa induced dystonia predominantly affecting orofacial muscles, occasionally resembling risus sardonicus of cephalic tetanus.
Pisa syndrome	Subacute axial dystonia with a severe tonic lateral flexion of the trunk, head, and neck (contracted and hypertrophic paravertebral muscles may be present).
Disproportionate antecollis	Chin-on-chest, neck can only with difficulty be passively and forcibly extended to its normal position. Despite severe chronic neck flexion, flexion elsewhere is minor.
Jerky tremor	Irregular (jerky) postural or action tremor of the hands and/or fingers.
Dysarthria	Atypical quivering, irregular, severely hypophonic or slurring high-pitched dysarthria, which tends to develop earlier, be more severe and be associated with more marked dysphagia compared with **PD**.
Non-motor Red Flags	
Abnormal respiration	Nocturnal (harsh or strained, high pitched inspiratory sounds) or diurnal inspiratory stridor, involuntary deep inspiratory sighs/gasps, sleep apnoea (arrest of breathing for $\geq$10 s), and excessive snoring (increase from premorbid level, or newly arising).
REM sleep behaviour disorder	Intermittent loss of muscle atonia and appearance of elaborate motor activity (striking out with arms in sleep often with talking/shouting) associated with dream mentation.
Cold hands/feet	Coldness and color change (purple/blue) of extremities not due to drugs with blanching on pressure and poor circulatory return.
Raynaud's phenomenon	Painful "white finger," which may be provoked by ergot drugs.
Emotional incontinence	Crying inappropriately without sadness or laughing inappropriately without mirth.

* Excluding cardinal diagnostic features of MSA such as orthostatic hypotension, urinary incontinence/retention, levodopa unresponsive parkinsonism, cerebellar (ataxia) and pyramidal signs. Also excluding non-specific features suggesting atypical parkinsonism such as rapid progression or early instability and falls. (Reprinted with permission from John Wiley: Wenning & Geser, 2003b.)

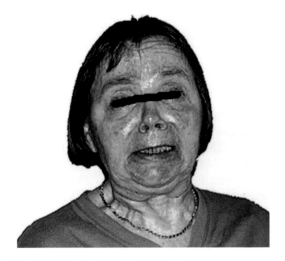

Fig. 43.4 Risus Sardonicus (RS) of a patient with MSA-P showing hypomimia, asymmetric orofacial dystonia and cervical dystonia affecting the platysma. (Reprinted with permission from John Wiley: Wenning *et al.*, 2003a.)

Speech impairment develops in virtually all MSA patients and is probably largely related to laryngeal dysfunction (Garratt *et al.*, 1994). It tends to be dominated by hypophonic monotony or a scanning quality according to clinical subtype (Kluin *et al.*, 1996). As well as the low volume monotony of parkinsonism, a quivering, irregular, severely hypophonic or slurring *dysarthria* is "often so characteristic that the diagnosis can be suggested by listening to the patient on the telephone" (Caplan, 1984). Dysarthria tends to develop earlier, be more severe and be associated with more marked dysphagia in MSA compared to PD (Müller *et al.*, 2001).

MSA patients are prone to sleep-related breathing disorders, often resulting in nighttime oxygen desaturation (Wenning & Quinn, 1997). *Nighttime respiratory stridor*, commonly attributed to vocal cord paralysis (Williams *et al.*, 1979; Hughes *et al.*, 1998) but perhaps reflecting dystonia of the vocal cords (Merlo *et al.*, 2002) is also a helpful diagnostic pointer. Nocturnal stridor has been considered a poor prognostic feature. Analysis of survival curves of 30 patients with follow-up information showed a significantly shorter survival from the sleep evaluation, but not from disease onset, for patients with stridor compared with those without (Silber & Levine, 2000). Inspiratory stridor was documented in 9–34% (Wenning & Quinn, 1997) of patients and occurred at any time point in the disease process. In fact, several cases have presented acutely with laryngeal palsy requiring tracheostomy (Kew *et al.*, 1990) or nasotracheal intubation (Flugel *et al.*, 1984). Tracheostomy in later disease stages may be more controversial. In contrast, stridor is very uncommon in PD.

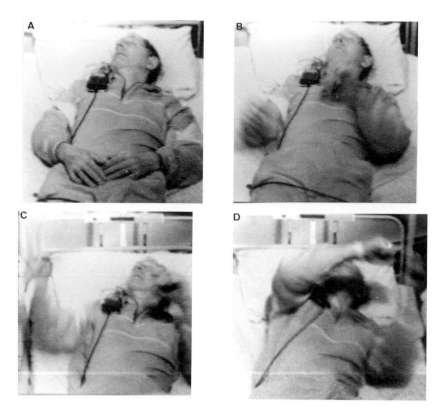

Fig. 43.5 RBD (striking out with arms in sleep often with sleep talking/shouting and recall of frightening dreams if awakened).

MSA patients also often show disrupted sleep with rapid eye movement (REM) phase alterations and may present with isolated *REM behavior disorder (RBD)* (Tison *et al.*, 1995b; Plazzi *et al.*, 1997) (Fig. 43.5). Sleep disorders are more common in patients with MSA than in those with PD after the same duration of the disease, reflecting the more diffuse underlying pathological process in MSA (Ghorayeb *et al.*, 2002c).

Patient with MSA often have cold, dusky, violaceous hands, with poor circulatory return after blanching by pressure. Changes in skin color or temperature were easily detected by Klein *et al.* (1997), and suggest a defect in neurovascular control of distal extremities. This *"cold hand sign"* is another clinical "red flag" that helps to raise the suspicion of MSA.

In MSA a large proportion report cold sensitivity or *Raynaud's phenomenon* (Santens *et al.*, 1996), with initial pallor followed by cyanosis and in some the later onset of redness, affecting both hands and feet (Mallipeddi & Mathias 1998).

Pseudobulbar crying/laughing spells may be evident in some patients; more commonly this frequent phenomenon may only be elicited by direct questioning (Quinn, 1994).

Core characteristics of the disease

The extrapyramidal features appear similar to those in PD, including bradykinesia with rigidity, postural instability, hypokinetic speech, and occasionally tremor, usually with a poor or unsustained response to chronic levodopa therapy. The signs of cerebellar dysfunction include disorders of extraocular movements, ataxic speech, and ataxia of limb movements and gait resulting in postural instability and frequent falls. Autonomic insufficiency results in orthostatic hypotension, urinary retention or incontinence, and impotence, often accompanied by constipation and decreased sweating. Extrapyramidal, cerebellar and autonomic features often occur in combination in MSA, but in some patients one or two features may predominate.

Clinical variants and their frequency

The clinical diagnosis of MSA is fraught with difficulty and there are no pathognomonic features to discriminate the common (80% of cases) parkinsonian variant (MSA-P) from PD. In a clinicopathologic study (Litvan *et al.*, 1997),

Table 43.5. Clinical diagnostic criteria for multiple system atrophy (Quinn, 1994)

SND type (predominantly parkinsonism)		OPCA type (predominantly cerebellar)
Sporadic adult onset non/poorly levodopa responsive parkinsonism[a]	Possible	Sporadic adult-onset cerebellar syndrome with parkinsonism
Above[b], plus severe symptomatic autonomic failure[c] or cerebellar signs or pyramidal signs or pathological sphincter electromyogram	Probable	Sporadic adult-onset cerebellar syndrome[a] (with or without parkinsonism or pyramidal signs) plus severe symptomatic autonomic failure[c] or pathological sphincter electromyogram
P/m confirmed	Definite	P/m confirmed

[a] Without DSM III dementia, generalized tendon areflexia, prominent supranuclear palsy for downgaze or other identifiable cause.

[b] Moderate or good, but often waning, response to levodopa may occur, in which case multiple atypical features need to be present.

[c] Postural syncope or presyncope and/or urinary incontinence or retention not due to other causes.

Sporadic: no other case of MSA among first- or second-degree relatives allowable.

Adult onset: onset age 30 years or above. (Reprinted with permission from Quinn, 1994.)

primary neurologists (who followed up the patients clinically) identified only 25% of MSA patients at the first visit (42 months after disease onset). Even at last neurological follow-up (74 months after disease onset), half of the patients were misdiagnosed and the correct diagnosis in the other half was established on average 4 years after disease onset. Mean rater sensitivity for movement disorder specialists was higher but still suboptimal at the first (56%) and last (69%) visit.

Consistent with this observation, most of the MSA patients identified in the epidemiological survey by Schrag *et al.* (1999) were only diagnosed during the study, suggesting that MSA is poorly recognized in clinical practice and is commonly mistaken for PD due to a number of overlapping features (Wenning *et al.*, 2000a). In a more recent study, the clinical diagnosis of MSA maintained until death by neurologists was incorrect in 8 (14%) of 59 cases and application of either Quinn or consensus criteria improved the clinical diagnosis of MSA at first, but not at last visit (Osaki *et al.*, 2002). In an earlier clinicopathological study, 12 of 35 MSA cases remained misdiagnosed as PD until death (Wenning *et al.*, 1995). MSA may be also confused with PSP (Wenning *et al.*, 2000a; Litvan *et al.*, 1996), and other atypical parkinsonian disorders.

In a review of the clinical and pathological diagnoses of 143 cases of parkinsonism the diagnostic accuracy for PD, MSA and PSP was higher than most previous prospective clinicopathological series and studies using the retrospective application of clinical diagnostic criteria (Hughes *et al.*, 2002). The positive predictive value of a clinical diagnosis of MSA was 85.7% (30 out of 35), and the sensitivity was 88.2% (30 out of 34). This study implies that neurologists with particular expertise in the field of movement disorders may be using a method of pattern recognition for

diagnosis which goes beyond that inherent in any formal set of diagnostic criteria.

Clinical diagnostic criteria for MSA were proposed by Quinn (1989b) and later slightly modified (Quinn, 1994). According to this schema, patients are classified as either SND or OPCA type MSA depending on the predominance of parkinsonism or cerebellar ataxia (Table 43.5). There are three levels of diagnostic probability: possible, probable and definite. Patients with sporadic adult-onset (> 30 years) poorly levodopa-responsive parkinsonism fulfil criteria for *possible* SND. The presence of other atypical features such as severe autonomic failure, cerebellar or pyramidal signs or a pathological sphincter EMG is required for a diagnosis of *probable* SND. Patients with sporadic late-onset predominant cerebellar ataxia with additional mild parkinsonism or pyramidal signs are considered *possible* OPCA type MSA. This may result in confusion since some patients with possible OPCA may also qualify for probable SND provided predominant cerebellar ataxia is accompanied by parkinsonian features. A diagnosis of *probable* OPCA type MSA requires the additional presence of severe autonomic failure or a pathological sphincter EMG. A definite diagnosis rests on neuropathological confirmation. Predominant SND or OPCA type presentations may be distinguished from pure types on the basis of associated cerebellar (predominant SND) or parkinsonian features (predominant OPCA). Since some degree of autonomic failure is present in almost all SND and OPCA type MSA patients (Wenning *et al.*, 1994a; Magalhães *et al.*, 1995) a further "autonomic" subtype (SDS) was not considered useful (Quinn *et al.*, 1995).

A number of exclusion criteria were also proposed: onset should be age 30 years or more, and in order to exclude inherited adult-onset ataxias there should be no family history of MSA. However, the chance occurrence of PD in

Table 43.6. Clinical domains, features and criteria used in the diagnosis of MSA according to Gilman *et al.* (1999)*

I. Autonomic and urinary dysfunction

A. Autonomic and urinary features

1. Orthostatic hypotension (by 20 mmHg systolic or 10 mmHg diastolic)
2. Urinary incontinence or incomplete bladder emptying

B. Criterion for autonomic failure or urinary dysfunction in MSA

Orthostatic fall in blood pressure (by 30 mmHg systolic or 15 mmHg diastolic) or urinary incontinence (persistent, involuntary partial or total bladder emptying, accompanied by erectile dysfunction in men) or both

II. Parkinsonism

A. Parkinsonian features

1. Bradykinesia (slowness of voluntary movement with progressive reduction in speed and amplitude during repetitive actions)
2. Rigidity
3. Postural instability (not caused by primary visual, vestibular, cerebellar, or proprioceptive dysfunction)
4. Tremor (postural, resting or both)

B. Criterion for Parkinsonism in MSA

Bradykinesia plus at least one of items 2 to 4

III. Cerebellar dysfunction

A. Cerebellar features

1. Gait ataxia (wide-based stance with steps of irregular length and direction)
2. Ataxic dysarthria
3. Limb ataxia
4. Sustained gaze-evoked nystagmus

B. Criterion for cerebellar dysfunction in MSA

Gait ataxia plus at least one of items 2 to 4

IV. Corticospinal tract dysfunction

A. Corticospinal tract features

1. Extensor plantar responses with hyperreflexia

B. Corticospinal tract dysfunction in MSA: no corticospinal tract features are used in defining the diagnosis of MSA

---

* A feature (A) is a characteristic of the disease and a criterion (B) is a defining feature or composite of features required for diagnosis. Reproduced with kind permission from Gilman *et al.* (1999).

Table 43.7. Diagnostic categories of MSA according to Gilman *et al.* (1999)*

I. Possible MSA

One criterion plus two features from separate other domains. When the criterion is parkinsonism, a poor levodopa response qualifies as one feature (hence only one additional feature is required).

II. Probable MSA

Criterion for autonomic failure/urinary dysfunction plus poorly levodopa-responsive parkinsonism or cerebellar dysfunction.

III. Definite MSA

Pathologically confirmed by the presence of a high density of glial cytoplasmic inclusions in association with a combination of degenerative changes in the nigrostriatal and olivopontocerebellar pathways.

---

* The features and criteria for each clinical domain are shown in Table 43.6.

Reproduced with kind permission from Gilman *et al.* (1999).

suboptimal diagnostic accuracy (Litvan *et al.*, 1998; Osaki *et al.*, 2002).

In April 1998 an International Consensus Conference was convened to develop optimized criteria for a clinical diagnosis of MSA (Gilman *et al.*, 1998, 1999). The Gilman criteria are now widely used for a clinical diagnosis of MSA. These criteria specify three diagnostic categories of increasing certainty: possible, probable and definite (Table 43.7). The diagnosis of possible and probable MSA are based on the presence of clinical features listed in Table 43.6. In addition, exclusion criteria have to be considered (Table 43.8). A definite diagnosis requires a typical neuropathological lesion pattern as well as deposition of α-synuclein-positive glial cytoplasmic inclusions (Dickson *et al.*, 1999a). A recent retrospective evaluation of the Gilman criteria showed excellent positive predictive values for both possible and probable MSA, however, sensitivity for probable MSA was poor (Osaki *et al.*, 2002). Whether the Gilman criteria will improve recognition of MSA patients especially in early disease stages needs to be investigated by prospective surveys with neuropathological confirmation in as many cases as possible.

Time course of the disease

MSA usually manifests in middle age, affects both sexes, and progresses relentlessly with a mean survival of 6–9 years (Ben-Shlomo *et al.*, 1997; Wenning *et al.*, 1994a, 1997b).

relatives is allowable. Although some limitation of upgaze and convergence can occur in both MSA and in PD, a prominent downgaze palsy with marked slowing of voluntary saccades is an exclusion criterion for a clinical diagnosis of MSA. Further exclusion criteria include dementia, optic atrophy, pigmentary retinopathy, and generalized tendon areflexia. So far, sensitivity and specificity of the Quinn criteria have never been prospectively determined. Two retrospective validation studies demonstrated

Table 43.8. Exclusion criteria for the diagnosis of MSA according to Gilman *et al.* (1999)

I. History
Symptomatic onset under 30 years of age
Family history of a similar disorder
Systemic disease or other identifiable causes for features listed in
    Table 43.6
Hallucinations unrelated to medication

II. Physical examination
DSM IV criteria for dementia
Prominent slowing of vertical saccades or vertical supranuclear
    gaze palsy[a]
Evidence of focal cortical dysfunction such as aphasia, alien limb
    syndrome and parietal dysfunction

III. Laboratory investigation
Metabolic, molecular genetic and imaging evidence of an
    alternative cause of features listed in Table 43.6

---

[a] In practice, MSA is most frequently confused with PD or PSP (PSP) (Litvan *et al.*, 1997). Mild limitation of upward gaze alone is non-specific, whereas a prominent (>50%) limitation of upward gaze or any limitation of downward gaze suggests PSP (Litvan *et al.*, 1996). Before the onset of vertical gaze limitation, a clinically obvious slowing of voluntary vertical saccades is usually easily detectable in PSP and assists in the early differentiation of these two disorders (Litvan *et al.*, 1996). Reproduced with kind permission from Gilman *et al.* (1999).

Onset

MSA is a disease that commonly causes clinical symptoms beginning in the sixth decade, although occasionally symptoms commence as early as the fourth decade (Sima *et al.*, 1993). In a series of 100 cases of MSA reported by Wenning *et al.* (1994a), the median age of onset was 53 and the range was 33 to 76 years. In a meta-analysis of 433 cases, mean age of onset was 54.2 years (range 31 to 78) (Ben Shlomo *et al.*, 1997). Latency to onset, but not duration, of symptomatic orthostatic hypotension or urinary incontinence differentiates PD from other parkinsonian syndromes, particularly MSA. Wenning *et al.* (1999c) found significant group differences for latency, but not duration, of symptomatic orthostatic hypotension and urinary incontinence: latencies to onset of either feature were short in patients with MSA, intermediate in patients with DLB, CBD, and PSP, and long in those with PD. Symptomatic orthostatic hypotension occurring within the first year after disease onset predicted MSA in 75% of cases; early urinary incontinence was less predictive for MSA (56%). It is likely that urinary dysfunction is more common

and often an earlier manifestation than orthostatic hypotension in patients with MSA, although subclinical cardiovascular abnormalities appear in the early stage of the disease (Sakakibara *et al.*, 2000a). The responsible sites seem to be central and peripheral for both dysfunctions.

Latencies to onset of falls were short in PSP patients, intermediate in MSA, DLB, and CBD, and long in PD (Wenning *et al.*, 1999a). Recurrent falls occurring within the first year after disease onset predicted PSP in 68% of the patients. Conversely, latency to onset, but not duration, of recurrent falls differentiates PD from other parkinsonian disorders.

Progression

MSA is a chronically progressive disease characterized by the gradual onset of neurological symptoms and accumulation of disability reflecting involvement of the systems initially unaffected. Thus, patients who present initially with extrapyramidal features commonly progress to develop autonomic disturbances, cerebellar disorders, or both. Conversely, patients who begin with symptoms of cerebellar dysfunction often progress to develop extrapyramidal or autonomic disorders, or both. Patients whose symptoms initially are autonomic may later develop cerebellar, extrapyramidal or both types of disorders.

The progression to different H & Y stages was evaluated in 81 pathologically confirmed patients with parkinsonism. Patients with PD showed significantly longer latencies to each H&Y stage than patients with an atypical parkinsonian disorder (APD). In fact, development of a H&Y-III within 1 year of motor onset accurately predicted an APD. However, the progression to each H&Y stage was unhelpful in distinguishing the APDs from each other. Once patients with PD and APD became wheelchair-bound, both had equally short survival times (Müller *et al.*, 2000).

In a more recent study (Watanabe *et al.*, 2002), median intervals from onset to aid-requiring walking, confinement to a wheelchair, a bedridden state and death were 3, 5, 8 and 9 years, respectively. Patients manifesting combined motor and autonomic involvement within 3 years of onset had a significantly increased risk of not only developing advanced disease stage but also shorter survival. MSA-P patients had more rapid functional deterioration than MSA-C patients, but showed similar survival.

Prognosis

MSA is a progressive disorder associated with a shortened lifespan, with death occurring on average within about

10 years of symptom onset. In one clinical study, the median survival from onset of symptoms was 9.5 years (Wenning *et al.*, 1994a), and in another 7.5 years (Testa *et al.*, 1996), whereas more recently, Tison *et al.* (2000b) showed a mean disease duration of 6.8 years. Similar average survivals were reported in two autopsy-verified series of MSA patients, 8.7 years in one (Wenning *et al.*, 1995) and 8.0 years in another (Hughes *et al.*, 1992). Schulz *et al.* (1994) found among 32 cases a median survival time after onset of motor symptoms of 4 years in SND and 9.1 years in OPCA. In a meta-analysis of 433 cases of pathologically proven MSA over a 100-year period survival showed a secular trend from a median duration of 4.9 years for publications between 1887 and 1970 to 6.8 years between 1991 and 1994 (Ben-Shlomo *et al.*, 1997). Older age of onset was associated with shorter survival; the hazard ratio for patients with onset after 60 years was 1.8 compared with patients between 31 and 49 years. Cerebellar features were associated with marginally increased survival. These results demonstrate the poor prognosis for patients with MSA but may be biased toward the worst cases.

Epidemiology

Determining the incidence and prevalence of MSA is difficult, as only a few epidemiologic studies have been reported. Estimates of the prevalence of MSA (per 100 000 in the poplution) in five studies were 1.9 (Tison *et al.*, 2000b), 2.3 (Wermuth *et al.*, 1997), 4.4 (Schrag *et al.*, 1999), 4.9 (Chio *et al.*, 1998) and 310 (in individuals older than 65 years) (Trenkwalder *et al.*, 1995). The annual incidence of MSA was estimated to be about 0.6 cases per 100 000 persons or 3.0/100 000 people over the age of 50 years (Bower *et al.*, 1997). Analytical epidemiology of MSA is even poorer: a case-control study in North America showed an increased risk of MSA associated with occupational exposure to organic solvents, plastic monomers and additives, pesticides and metals (Nee *et al.*, 1991). Another multicenter case-control study in Europe (Vanacore *et al.*, in press), showed a significantly higher risk of developing MSA in subjects having worked in agriculture. Smoking habits seem to be less frequent in MSA cases (as in PD cases) than in healthy controls. The fact that the inverse association with smoking found previously in PD is shared by MSA but not by PSP lends epidemiologic support to the notion that different smoking habits are associated with different groups of neurodegenerative disease (Vanacore *et al.*, 2000).

Investigations

Introduction

The clinical diagnosis of MSA rests largely on history and physical examination. Additional investigations are particularly helpful in excluding differential diagnoses, however, they may also support a presumptive clinical diagnosis. MSA-P patients are usually misdiagnosed as PD early in their disease. Regular follow-up is therefore required to detect development of atypical features suggestive of MSA.

Autonomic function tests

Autonomic function tests are a mandatory part of the diagnostic process and clinical follow-up in patients with MSA. Findings of severe autonomic failure early in the course of the disease make the diagnosis of MSA more likely, although the specificity in comparison to other neurodegenerative disorders is unknown in a single patient. Pathological results of autonomic function tests may account for a considerable number of symptoms in MSA patients and should prompt specific therapeutic steps to improve quality of life and prevent secondary complications like ascending urinary infections or injuries due to hypotension induced falls.

Cardiovascular function

A history of postural faintness or other evidence of orthostatic hypotension, e.g. neck ache on rising in the morning or posturally related changes of visual perception, should be sought in all patients in whom MSA is suspected. After taking a comprehensive history, testing of cardiovascular function should be performed according to consensus recommendations (Consensus statement on the definition of orthostatic hypotension, pure autonomic failure, and multiple system atrophy, 1996; Braune *et al.*, 1999a). A drop in systolic blood pressure (BP) of 20 mm Hg or more, or in diastolic BP of 10 mm Hg or more, compared with baseline within a standing time of 3 minutes is defined as orthostatic hypotension (Consensus statement on the definition of orthostatic hypotension, pure autonomic failure, and multiple system atrophy, 1996) and must lead to more specific assessment. This is based on continuous non-invasive measurement of blood pressure and heart rate during tilt table testing (Bannister & Mathias, 1999b; Braune *et al.*, 1996a, b). Although abnormal cardiovascular test results may provide evidence of sympathetic and/or parasympathetic failure, they do not differentiate autonomic failure associated with PD vs. MSA (Riley & Chelimsky, 2003).

In MSA, cardiovascular dysregulation appears to be caused by central rather than peripheral autonomic failure. During supine rest norepinephrine (noradrenaline) levels (representing postganglionic sympathethic efferent activity) are normal (Ziegler *et al.*, 1977; Polinsky *et al.*, 1981), and there is no denervation hypersensitivity, which indicates a lack of increased expression of adrenergic receptors on peripheral neurons (Polinsky *et al.*, 1981). Uptake of the norepinephrine analogue meta-iodobenzylguanedine is normal in postganglionic cardiac neurons (Braune *et al.*, 1999b; Orimo *et al.*, 1999; Takatsu *et al.*, 2000; Taki *et al.*, 2000) (see Section on functional imaging) and the response to tilt is impaired with little increase in noradrenaline. In contrast, mainly postganglionic sympathetic dysfunction is thought to account for autonomic failure associated with PD. In keeping with this assumption, both basal and tilted noradrenaline levels are low.

Neuroendocrine testing

In vivo studies in MSA, which involved testing of the endocrine component of the central autonomic nervous systems (the hypothalamopituitary axis) with a variety of challenge procedures, provided evidence of impaired humoral responses of the anterior and the posterior part of the pituitary gland with impaired secretion of adrenocorticotropic hormone (ACTH) (Polinsky *et al.*, 1987), growth hormone (Kimber *et al.*, 1997), and vasopressin/ADH (Kaufmann *et al.*, 1992), respectively. Although these observations can be made in virtually all patients in an advanced stage of the disease, their prevalence during the early course of MSA is unknown.

There is an ongoing debate about the diagnostic value of the growth-hormone response to clonidine (CGH-test), a neuropharmacological assessment of central adrenoceptor function, in PD and MSA. Clonidine is a centrally active alpha 2-adrenoceptor agonist which lowers blood pressure predominantly by reducing CNS sympathetic outflow. In an early study, there was no increase in GH levels after clonidine in patients with MSA compared to those with PD or pure autonomic failure (Zoukos *et al.*, 1993). Kimber *et al.* (1997) confirmed a normal serum GH increase in response to clonidine in 14 PD patients (without autonomic failure) and in 19 patients with pure autonomic failure, whereas there was no GH rise in 31 patients with MSA. However, these findings have been challenged subsequently (Clarke *et al.*, 1999, Tranchant *et al.*, 2000, Strijks *et al.*, 2002). After clonidine administration, GH rose in PSP subjects and controls, unlike MSA subjects (Kimber *et al.*, 2000). In PSP subjects, responses to both physiological and pharmacological tests provided evidence against widespread autonomic dysfunction; this differed markedly from MSA subjects. Stimulation of GH release with GH releasing hormone plus arginine (GHRH-Arg) rather than clonidine may differentiate MSA from IPD and ILOCA (Pellecchia *et al.*, 2001), but this hypothesis would need to be confirmed by further investigations. In normal man, clonidine reduces arginine-vasopressin (AVP) secretion, probably by presynaptic inhibition of noradrenergic neuron terminals in the supraoptic nucleus. A lesion of noradrenergic pathways in animals abolishes this response to clonidine. At postmortem in MSA there is marked loss of hypothalamic noradrenergic innervation. Following clonidine there was a significantly greater fall of AVP levels in controls than MSA suggesting that there is an abnormal AVP response to clonidine in MSA, which probably represents loss of functional noradrenergic innervation of the supraoptic nucleus (Kimber *et al.*, 1999a). More studies in well-defined patient cohorts are needed before clonidine challenge tests can be recommended as helpful diagnostic tests in patients with suspected MSA.

Hypothalamic dopaminergic pathways are involved in the regulation of growth hormone and prolactin release from the anterior pituitary. Neuroendocrine studies in patients with MSA, in whom there is a reported loss of hypothalamic dopamine, are few and contradictory. In patients with MSA, the GHRH and GH responses to levodopa were preserved and were similar to responses in age-matched control subjects in a study by Kimber *et al.* (1999b). In contrast, there was impaired dopaminergic suppression of prolactin secretion. In MSA patients this may represent a selective dysfunction, rather than generalized loss, of tubero-infundibular dopaminergic neurones.

Bladder function

Assessment of bladder function is mandatory in MSA and usually provides evidence of involvement of the autonomic nervous system already at an early stage of the disease. Following a careful history regarding frequency of voiding, difficulties in initiating or suppressing voiding and the presence and degree of urinary incontinence, a standard urine analysis should exclude an infection. Postvoid residual volume needs to be determined sonographically or via catheterization to initiate intermittent self catheterization (ISC) in due course. In some patients only cystometry can discriminate between hypocontractile detrusor function and a hyperreflexic sphincter-detrusor dyssynergy.

The nature of bladder dysfunction is different in MSA and PD. Although frequency and urgency are common in both disorders, marked urge or stress incontinence with continuous leakage is not a feature of PD apart from very advanced cases. Urodynamic studies show a characteristic pattern of abnormality in MSA patients (Kirby *et al.*, 1986). In the early stages there is often detrusor hyperreflexia, often with bladder neck incompetence due to abnormal urethral sphincter function, which result in early frequency and urgency followed by urge incontinence. Later on, the ability to initiate a voluntary micturition reflex and the strength of the hyperreflexic detrusor contractions diminish, and the bladder may become atonic, accounting for increasing postmicturition residual urine volumes.

The detrusor hyperreflexia may result from a disturbance of the pontine micturition centre (Beck *et al.*, 1994; Wenning *et al.*, 1996c). Alternatively, degeneration of substantia nigra and other regions of the basal ganglia that are important in the control of micturition, may contribute to urological symptoms. The atonic bladder in advanced MSA has been related to the progressive degeneration of the intermediolateral columns of the thoracolumbar spinal cord (Beck *et al.*, 1994); however, this remains speculative.

Sexual function

Sexual dysfunction is a frequent and early symptom of MSA, particularly in male patients. Since male MSA patients frequently develop erectile failure in their forties, and therefore experience substantial impairment of their sexual performance, expert uroneurological advice should be sought for further investigation and implementation of appropriate therapeutic intervention. The pathophysiology of impotence in MSA is unclear; however, it is likely to include central autonomic disturbance, and more rarely, peripheral factors such as venous leakage.

Thermoregulation

Abnormal sudomotor function, sympathetic skin response, impaired heat tolerance and skin temperature regulation have been described in MSA (Cohen *et al.*, 1987; Sandroni *et al.*, 1991; Kihara *et al.*, 1991; Santens *et al.*, 1996; Klein *et al.*, 1997) (see Section on other clinical features).

The thermoregulatory sweat test (TST) as a test of preganglionic sympathetic function detects sweating by a color change of an indicator after thermal stimulation, whereas the quantitative sudomotor axon reflex test (QSART) measures an axon reflex mediated by the postganglionic sympathetic sudomotor axon following stimulation of sweat glands with acetylcholine. In MSA, using TST and QSART, both pre- and postganglionic sympathetic failure has been reported (Kihara *et al.*, 1991).

Specialized autonomic units may offer tests of thermoregulatory sweating to search for evidence of central autonomic failure. However, the sensitivity and specificity of these tests in MSA is unknown and they require specialist experience and equipment.

The pathogenesis of anhidrosis associated with MSA remains unclear. This symptom may be entirely the result of central autonomic dysfunction, or due to (additional) postganglionic sympathetic dysfunction. The latter proposal is supported by tests using direct cholinergic stimulation of peripheral parasympathetic nerves (Baser *et al.*, 1991; Cohen *et al.*, 1987; Sandroni *et al.*, 1991).

Gastrointestinal function

Gastrointestinal motility in MSA has not been investigated in detail, and a single study from Stocchi and colleagues (2000) comparing anorectal function in MSA and PD demonstrated that most patients in both groups showed an abnormal straining pattern, decreased anal tone, or both dysfunctions. The authors suggested that, although bowel and anorectal dysfunctions do not differentiate MSA from PD, both abnormalities occur earlier and develop faster in MSA than in PD. In another study, in seven patients with MSA, pancreatic polypeptide response to insulin-induced hypoglycemia was impaired, indicating involvement of parasympathetic-mediated gastrointestinal function (Polinsky *et al.*, 1982).

Imaging

Magnetic resonance imaging (MRI)

MRI scanning of patients with MSA often, but not always, reveals atrophy of cerebellar vermis and, less marked, of cerebellar hemispheres (Schrag *et al.*, 2000). There is also evidence of shrinkage of pons as well as middle cerebellar peduncles (Schulz *et al.*, 1994), differentiating MSA-C from cortical cerebellar atrophy (CCA). The pattern of infratentorial atrophy visible on MRI correlates with the pathological process of OPCA affecting cerebellar vermis and hemispheres, middle cerebellar peduncles, pons, and lower brainstem (Klockgether *et al.*, 1990). The MRI changes may be indistinguishable from those of patients with autosomal dominant cerebellar ataxias (Wüllner *et al.*, 1993). MRI measures of basal ganglia pathology in MSA such as width of SNC, lentiform nucleus, head of the caudate, etc. are less well established and naked eye assessments are often unreliable. In advanced cases putaminal atrophy may be detectable and may correlate with severity of extrapyramidal symptoms (Wakai *et al.*, 1994). However, in one study MRI-based two-dimensional basal ganglia morphometry has proved unhelpful in the early differential

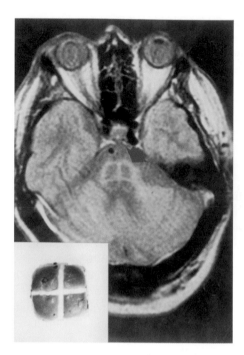

Fig. 43.6 T$_2$-weighted images (0.5 T) in a patient with pathologically proved multiple system atrophy showing infratentorial atrophy and signal change in pons (cross sign, arrow) resembling a hot cross bun (inset) baked for the last Thursday before Easter. Reproduced with kind permission from the BMJ Publishing Group: Schrag *et al.* Clinical usefulness of magnetic resonance imaging in multiple system atrophy. *Journal of Neurology, Neurosurgery and Psychiatry* 1998; **65**(1):65–71.

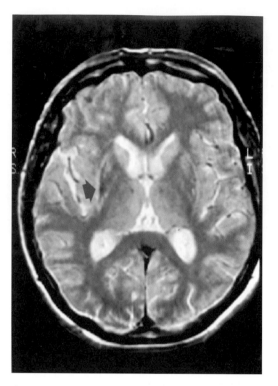

Fig. 43.7 Putaminal atrophy, hyperintense rim (arrow), and putaminal hypointensity in comparison with the globus pallidus on T$_2$ weighted images (1.5 T) in a patient with multiple system atrophy.

Reproduced with kind permission from the BMJ Publishing Group: Schrag *et al.* Clinical usefulness of magnetic resonance imaging in multiple system atrophy. *Journal of Neurology, Neurosurgery and Psychiatry* 1998; **65**(1):65–71.

diagnosis of patients with levodopa unresponsive parkinsonism (Albanese *et al.*, 1995). A significant progression of atrophy to under the normal limit was observed in the cerebrum, frontal and temporal lobes, showing the involvement of the cerebral hemisphere, especially the frontal lobe (Konagaya *et al.*, 2002). Abnormalities on MRI may include not only atrophy, but also signal abnormalities on T$_2$-weighted images within the pontocerebellar system and putamen. Signal hyperintensities sometimes seen within the pons and middle cerebellar peduncles are thought to reflect degeneration of pontocerebellar fibers and therefore, together with marked atrophy in these areas, indicate a major site of pathology in OPCA type MSA (Savoiardo *et al.*, 1990; Schulz *et al.*, 1994). The characteristic infratentorial signal change on T$_2$-weighted 1.5 tesla MRI ("hot cross bun" sign, Fig. 43.6) may also corroborate the clinical diagnosis of MSA (Schrag *et al.*, 2000). Putaminal hypointensities (Fig. 43.7) in supposedly APD were first reported in 1986 by two groups using a 1.5 tesla magnet and T$_2$-weighted images (Pastakia *et al.*, 1986; Drayer *et al.*, 1986). This change has subsequently been observed by

others in cases clinically thought to have MSA (Olanow, 1992; Wakai *et al.*, 1994; Schulz *et al.*, 1994), and in some cases with pathological confirmation (Lang *et al.*, 1994; Schwarz *et al.*, 1996; O'Brien *et al.*, 1990). A lateral to medial as well as posterior to anterior gradient is also well established with the most prominent changes in the posterolateral putamen (Pastakia *et al.*, 1986; Wakai *et al.*, 1994; Lang *et al.*, 1994). This putaminal hypointensity has been proposed as a sensitive and specific abnormality in patients with MSA, and to reflect increased iron deposition. However, similar abnormalities may occur in patients with classical PD (Stern *et al.*, 1989; Schrag *et al.*, 1998) or may represent incidental findings in patients without basal ganglia disorders (unpublished observations). The notion of increased iron deposition has been challenged by Brooks and colleagues (1989) and later by Schwarz and colleagues (1996). Recently it was shown that hypointense putaminal signal changes were more often observed in MSA than in PD patients using T$_2^*$-weighted gradient echo (GE) but not T_2-weighted fast spin echo images, indicating that T_2^*-weighted GE sequences are of diagnostic value for patients with parkinsonism (Kraft *et al.*, 2002). Increased putaminal relative to pallidal hypointensities may be seen as well as a slit-like hyperintense band lateral to the putamen (Fig. 43.7) (Schwarz *et al.*, 1996; Konagaya *et al.*, 1993, 1994; Yekhlef *et al.*, 2003). These changes are consistent with a clinical diagnosis of MSA. However, they appear to be nonspecific and have also been noted in clinically diagnosed PD and PSP (Schrag *et al.*, 1998, 2000). The pattern consisting of hypointense and hyperintense T_2 changes within the putamen is a highly specific MRI sign of MSA, while hypointensity alone remains a sensitive, but nonspecific sign of MSA (Kraft *et al.*, 1999). The hyperintense signal correlated with the most pronounced reactive microgliosis and astrogliosis or highest iron content in MRI-postmortem studies (Lang *et al.*, 1994, Schwarz *et al.*, 1996). Konagaya *et al.* (1998) reported that, in a case of MSA, the slit hyperintensity at the putaminal margin represented widened intertissue space due to a severe shrinkage and rarefaction of the putamen. However, in spite of these speculations the nature of this abnormal signal intensity remains uncertain.

Diffusion-weighted imaging (DWI) may represent a useful diagnostic tool that can provide additional support for a diagnosis of MSA-P. DWI, even if measured in the slice direction only, is able to discriminate MSA-P and both patients with PD and healthy volunteers on the basis of putaminal rADC (regional apparent diffusion coefficients) values (Fig. 43.8) (Schocke *et al.*, 2002). The increased putaminal rADC values in MSA-P are likely to reflect ongoing striatal degeneration, whereas most neuropathologic studies reveal intact striatum in PD. But, since in PSP compared to PD patients rADCs were also significantly increased in both putamen and globus pallidus (Seppi *et al.*, 2003), increased putaminal rADC values do not discriminate MSA-P from PSP.

Whether magnetic resonance volumetry will contribute to the differential diagnosis of MSA from other parkinsonian disorders remains to be confirmed. Schulz *et al.* (1999) found significant reductions in mean striatal and brainstem volumes in patients with MSA-P, MSA-C, and PSP, whereas patients with MSA-C and MSA-P also showed a reduction in cerebellar volume. Total intracranial volume-normalized magnetic resonance imaging-based volumetric measurements provide a sensitive marker to discriminate typical and atypical parkinsonism. Voxel based morphometry (VBM) confirmed previous region of interest (ROI)-based volumetric studies (Schulz *et al.*, 1999) showing basal ganglia and infratentorial volume loss in MSA-P patients (Brenneis *et al.*, 2003). These data revealed prominent cortical volume loss in MSA-P mainly

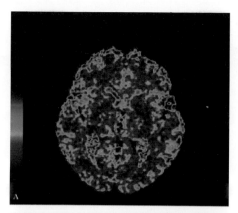
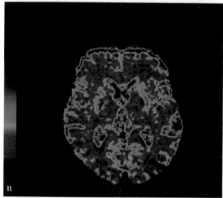
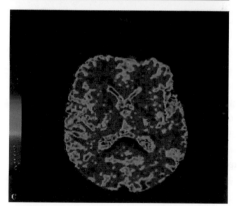

Fig. 43.8 Apparent diffusion coefficient (ADC) maps (diffusion gradient switched in slice direction) calculated by fitting over 3 b-values in PD (A), the Parkinson variant of multiple system atrophy (MSA-P) (B), and controls (C). Blue, green, red, and black represent descending regional ADC values. Note the marked difference in putaminal ADC maps between MSA-P (B) and PD (A) as well as controls (C).

Reproduced with kind permission from Lippincott Williams & Wilkins: Schocke, M., Seppi, K., Eserhammer, R., Kremser, C., Jaschke, W. *et al.* Diffusion-weighted MRI differentiates the Parkinson variant of multiple system atrophy from PD. *Neurology* 2002; **58(4)**: 575–80.

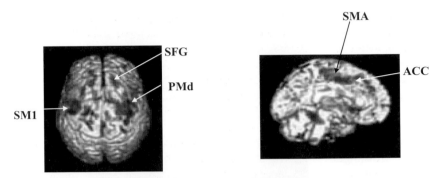

Fig. 43.9 VBM detects frontal lobe atrophy in MSA-P. SM1, primary sensorimotor cortex, PMd, dorsal premotor cortex; SMA, supplementary motor area; ACC, anterior cingulate cortex; SFG, Superior frontal gyrus. IMSA-SG (Innsbrucker MSA-Study Group) (unpublished data)

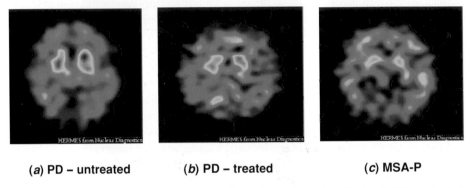

(a) PD – untreated   **(b) PD – treated**   **(c) MSA-P**

Fig. 43.10 Transverse IBZM SPECT images at the level of the striatum in patients with PD – untreated (A), PD – treated (B), and MSA-P (C). Images B and C show bilateral loss of tracer uptake (IMSA-SG). (From Colosimo *et al.*, 2004. © Elservier. Reproduced with permission.)

comprising the cortical targets of striatal projections such as the primary sensorimotor, lateral premotor cortices and the prefrontal cortex, but also the insula (Fig. 43.9). These changes are consistent with the established frontal lobe impairment of MSA patients (Robbins *et al.*, 1992).

Proton magnetic resonance spectroscopy (MRS) is a noninvasive method that provides information about the chemical pathology of disorders affecting the central nervous system. The largest peak visible with MRS is derived from *N*-acetylaspartate (NAA), an amino acid contained almost exclusively within neurons and their processes in the adult brain (Urenjak *et al.*, 1993). In general, MRS studies have generated conflicting observations of limited relevance to differential diagnosis. Davie *et al.* (1995) showed reduced NAA/Cr in the putamen in MSA compared with PD and controls. Federico *et al.* (1999) have also shown reduced NAA/Cr and NAA/Cho in MSA compared with controls and reduced NAA/Cr in MSA compared with PD. The King's College group initially found reductions in NAA/Cr and NAA/Cho in MSA compared with controls, but a similar reduction in PD (Ellis *et al.*, 1996). More recently, they

have failed to confirm this finding (Hu *et al.*, 1998). In the only study to use absolute quantitation of metabolite concentrations, NAA was unchanged in MSA patients (Clarke & Lowry, 2000).

Functional imaging

Single-photon emission tomography (SPECT) or Positron emission tomography (PET) studies of patients with MSA-P have demonstrated the combined nigral and striatal pathology using [^{123}I]β-CIT [2β-carboxymethoxy-3β-(4-iodophenyl)tropane] (SPECT) or [^{10}F]fluorodopa (PET) and a variety of postsynaptic dopamine or opiate receptor ligands such as [^{123}I]iodobenzamide (IBZM) (SPECT) (Fig. 43.10), [^{11}C]raclopride or [^{11}C]diprenorphin (PET).

The Hammersmith Cyclotron Unit, using PET found that putaminal uptake of the presynaptic dopaminergic markers [^{18}F]fluorodopa and S-[^{11}C]nomifensine (Brooks *et al.*, 1990a, b; Burn *et al.*, 1994) was similarly reduced in MSA and PD; in approximately half the MSA subjects, caudate uptake was also markedly reduced, as opposed to only moderate reduction in PD. However, discriminant function analysis of striatal [^{18}F]fluorodopa uptake separated MSA and PD patients poorly (Burn *et al.*, 1994). Patients with PD, PSP and MSA share a marked loss of fluorodopa uptake in the putamen; however, uptake in the caudate nucleus differs among the three groups, with patients who have MSA showing uptake rates intermediate between those of patients with PD (normal uptake) and with PSP (markedly reduced uptake) (Brooks *et al.*, 1990a). Measurements of striatal dopamine D2 receptor densities using raclopride and PET failed to differentiate between idiopathic and atypical parkinsonism, demonstrating a similar loss of densities in levodopa treated patients with fluctuating PD, MSA and PSP (Brooks *et al.*, 1992). PET studies using other ligands such as [^{11}C]diprenorphine (non-selective opioid receptor antagonist) (Burn *et al.*, 1995) and [^{18}F]fluorodeoxyglucose (Antonini *et al.*, 1998; de Volder 1989; Eidelberg *et al.*, 1993; Perani *et al.*, 1995) have proved more consistent in detecting striatal degeneration and in distinguishing patients with MSA-P from those with PD, particularly when combined with a dopamine D2 receptor scan (Ghaemi *et al.*, 2002). Widespread functional abnormalities in MSA-C have been demonstrated using [^{18}F]fluorodeoxyglucose and PET (Gilman *et al.*, 1994). Reduced metabolism was most marked in the brainstem and cerebellum, but other areas such as the putamen, caudate nucleus, thalamus and cerebral cortex were also involved, differentiating MSA-C from SCAs. Subclinical evidence of striatal pathology in MSA-C, in the absence of extrapyramidal features, has been demonstrated using the non-selective opioid receptor ligand diprenorphine and PET (Rinne *et al.*, 1995). Striatal opiate receptors are reduced not only in MSA-P (Burn *et al.*, 1995) but also in MSA-C with associated autonomic failure (Rinne *et al.*, 1995) supporting its nosological status as the cerebellar subtype of MSA. In another PET study using [^{18}F]fluorodeoxyglucose in comparison with normal controls, putaminal hypometabolism was absent in sporadic OPCA patients without autonomic failure and extrapyramidal features, but present in those who were classified as OPCA type MSA and therefore had autonomic dysfunction with or without parkinsonian features at the time of examination (Gilman *et al.*, 1994). Differences in cerebellar benzodiazepine receptor binding densities have also been shown in MSA-C, CCA and SCA using [^{11}C]flumazenil and PET (Gilman *et al.*, 1995). Additionally, the poor levodopa response may be related to a deficiency in striatal D1 receptor binding, as shown by PET studies in clinically diagnosed patients with MSA using the ligand [^{11}C]SCH 23390 (Shinotoh *et al.*, 1993). This is a potentially helpful observation that may aid early differentiation of MSA and PD if corroborated by other groups.

SPECT imaging studies of patients with dopa naive parkinsonism have used [^{123}I]iodobenzamide (IBZM) as D2 receptor ligand (Fig. 43.10) (Schwarz *et al.*, 1992; Schelosky *et al.*, 1993). A good response to apomorphine and subsequent benefit from chronic dopaminergic therapy was observed in subjects with normal IBZM binding whereas subjects with reduced binding failed to respond. Some of these patients developed other atypical clinical features suggestive of MSA during follow-up (Schwarz *et al.*, 1993). Other SPECT studies have also revealed significant reductions of striatal IBZM binding in clinically probable MSA subjects compared to PD patients (Brücke *et al.*, 1993; Schulz *et al.*, 1994) or controls (Brücke *et al.*, 1993; van Royen *et al.*, 1993). There has been much debate about the mechanism of levodopa-unresponsiveness in MSA. As well as loss of striatal dopamine binding sites, alterations further downstream probably also contribute (Tison *et al.*, 1995a,b). SPECT evaluation of the dopamine transporter (DAT) using [123I]beta-CIT can easily distinguish patients with essential tremor and patients with "lower body parkinsonism" due to a subcortical vascular encephalopathy. MSA and PSP cannot be separated from PD with this method alone (Brücke *et al.*, 2000). DAT SPECT may be useful in differentiating parkinsonism from controls and D2 SPECT in further differentiating MSA from PD and possibly PSP (Kim *et al.*, 2002). In another DAT SPECT study, striatal [^{123}I]beta-CIT uptake was markedly reduced in both the PD and MSA groups (Varrone *et al.*, 2001). In addition, MSA patients showed more symmetric DAT loss compared with the PD patients, consistent with the more symmetric clinical motor dysfunction observed in MSA. Since [^{123}I]beta-CIT SPECT reliably enables the visualization of the presynaptic dopaminergic lesion in patients with MSA, PSP, and CBD (Pirker *et al.*, 2000), this method was used as a label of DAT to study the progression of presynaptic dopaminergic degeneration in PD and APD by Pirker *et al.* (2002). The results of the sequential [123I]beta-CIT SPECT imaging demonstrate a rapid decline of striatal beta-CIT binding in patients with APD, exceeding the reduction in PD.

Scintigraphic visualisation of postganglionic sympathetic cardiac neurons was found to differentiate patients with MSA from patients with PD (Braune *et al.*, 1999b; Orimo *et al.*, 1999; Takatsu *et al.*, 2000; Taki *et al.*, 2000). Considering all reports published so far standard scintigraphy with [^{123}I]metaiodobenzylguanidine (MIBG), which has been used to detect pheochromocytoma cells for years, was able to correctly allocate each of about 70 patients with MSA versus more than 200 patients with PD, because all patients in the latter group showed a severely reduced cardiac uptake of the radioactive ligand. This method appears to be a highly sensitive and specific tool to discriminate between MSA and PD already within 2 years of onset of symptoms; however, the test cannot distinguish MSA from other APDs such as PSP (Yoshita, 1998).

Neurophysiology

The external anal or urethral sphincter EMG is a useful investigation in patients with suspected MSA. Due to degeneration of Onuf's nucleus both anal and urethral external sphincter muscles undergo denervation and re-innervation. Abnormality of the striated urethral sphincter EMG in MSA was first shown by Martinelli and Coccagna (1978). Subsequently, Kirby *et al.* (1986) confirmed the presence of polyphasia and abnormal prolongation of individual motor units in MSA, and also examined the potential diagnostic role of sphincter EMG in patients with MSA and PD (Eardley *et al.*, 1989). Sixteen (62%) of 26 patients with probable MSA, and only 1 (8%) of 13 with probable PD had a pathological EMG result (sensitivity 0.62, specificity 0.92). This test also helps to identify patients in whom incontinence may develop or worsen following surgery. Anal sphincter EMG is generally better tolerated, and yields identical results (Beck *et al.*, 1994). At least 80% of patients with MSA EMG of the external anal sphincter reveal signs of neuronal degeneration in Onuf's nucleus with spontaneous activity and increased polyphasia (Pramstaller *et al.*, 1995; Palace *et al.*, 1997; Tison *et al.*, 2000a). However, these findings do not reliably differentiate between MSA and other forms of APD. An abnormal anal sphincter examination was present in five of 12 (41.6%) PSP patients (Valldeoriola *et al.*, 1995). Furthermore, neurogenic changes of external anal sphincter muscle have also been demonstrated in advanced stages of PD by several investigators (Libelius & Johansson, 2000; Giladi *et al.*, 2000). Also chronic constipation, previous pelvic surgery or vaginal deliveries can be confounding factors to induce non-specific abnormalities (Colosimo *et al.*, 2000). In summary, in patients with probable MSA, abnormal sphincter EMG, as compared to control subjects, has been found in the vast majority of patients, including those who, as yet, have no urological or anorectal problems. The prevalence of abnormalities in the early stages of MSA is as yet unclear. Patients with PD as a rule do not show severe sphincter EMG abnormalities in the early stage of the disease, unless other causes for sphincter denervation are present. With such criteria, the sensitivity of the method is, however, low and, indeed, sphincter EMG does not distinguish MSA from PSP (Vodusek, 2001). For these reasons, this examination has not been eventually included in the guidelines suggested by the Consensus Conference (Gilman *et al.*, 1998).

In general, the value of evoked potential studies in the diagnosis of MSA is limited. Magnetic evoked potentials are often, but not always, normal in MSA (Wenning & Smith, 1997; Abbruzzese *et al.*, 1997). Somatosensory, visual, and acoustic evoked potentials may show prolonged latencies in up to 40% of patients, but most patients show no abnormalities of central efferent and afferent neuronal pathways (Abele *et al.*, 2000a; Delalande *et al.*, 1998; Abbruzzese *et al.*, 1997).

Some investigators (Montagna *et al.*, 1983; Cohen *et al.*, 1987) have suggested that both somatic anterior horn cells and peripheral nerves are commonly affected in MSA, and their involvement has therefore been regarded as part of the clinical spectrum of MSA. Abnormalities of nerve conduction studies seem to be more frequent in MSA-P (43%) compared to MSA-C (14%) (Abele *et al.*, 2000b) suggesting that the peripheral nervous system is differentially affected in the motor presentations of this disorder.

On electro-oculography many MSA patients show impaired ocular fixation with increased square wave jerks (Rascol *et al.*, 1991). Saccadic pursuit, gaze paretic down-beating nystagmus (Stell & Bronstein, 1994), and impaired vestibuloocular reflex (VOR) suppression may be detectable indicating the presence of concomitant cerebellar pathology (Rascol *et al.*, 1995). Marked supranuclear vertical palsy, more prominent on down- than upgaze, with slowing of voluntary saccades, was not observed in two large series studied by Wenning *et al.* (1994a and 1995) and helped to distinguish MSA from PSP in patients with APD. However, there are three (2%) pathologically proven MSA cases in the literature with documented impairment of downgaze (Gosset *et al.*, 1983 (cases 1 and 3); Jankovic *et al.*, 1993b). A laboratory-based investigation showed similar mild eye movement deficits in MSA-P and PD patients (Vidailhet *et al.*, 1994), but the authors excluded individuals with cerebellar signs.

Excessive auditory startle responses (ASR) may also help differentiate MSA both from PD and other forms of APD (Kofler *et al.*, 2001). Exaggerated ASR may reflect disinhibition of lower brainstem nuclei due to the degenerative disorder. ASR appear to be more disinhibited in MSA-P than MSA-C, and there is a lack of ASR habituation in MSA-C unlike MSA-P, suggesting involvement of different neural structures in the two MSA-subtypes (Kofler *et al.*, 2003).

Other investigations

In its early stages, MSA-C can be indistinguishable from idiopathic late-onset cerebellar ataxia. Six patients with ILOCA, that later evolved to MSA, had impaired hypoxic ventilatory response when autonomic failure was present, whereas in patients with unimpaired hypoxic ventilatory response the diagnosis remained ILOCA (Tsuda *et al.*, 2002). The demonstration of impaired hypoxic ventilatory response appears to be a good marker enabling earlier diagnosis of MSA in patients presenting with ILOCA.

Patients with MSA usually retain normal intelligence levels, but abnormalities of neuropsychological function have been described (Meco *et al.*, 1996). In a few studies, a distinctive pattern of cognitive defects was found suggesting normal intelligence but disorders of frontal lobe function (Robbins *et al.*, 1992; Brown *et al.*, 2002). These included difficulties with attentional set shifting when extradimensional shifting was required, impairment in subject-ordered tests of spatial working memory, and deficits in speed of thinking (rather than of accuracy) in the Tower of London task. Another study in patients with MSA-P demonstrated impairment on category and phonemic fluency, frontal behaviors, trail making test A and B, and free recall in the Grober and Buschke test (Pillon *et al.*, 1995). These patients were normal on the revised Wechsler Adult Intelligence Scale verbal scale, Wechsler memory scale, Raven 47 colored progressive matrices, California Verbal Learning Test, Wisconsin Card Sorting Test, and the Stroop interference condition.

Treatment

Autonomic failure

Unfortunately there is no causal therapy of autonomic dysfunction available. Therefore the therapeutic strategy is defined by clinical symptoms and impairment of quality of life in these patients. Due to the progressive course of MSA a regular review of the treatment is mandatory to adjust measures according to clinical needs.

The concept to treat symptoms of orthostatic hypotension is based on the increase of intravasal volume and the reduction of volume shift to lower body parts when changing to upright position. The selection and combination of the following options depend on the severity of symptoms and their practicability in the single patient, but not on the extent of blood pressure drop during tilt test. Non-pharmacological options include sufficient fluid intake, high salt diet, more frequent, but smaller meals per day to reduce postprandial hypotension by spreading the total carbohydrate intake and custom made elastic body garments. During night, head-up tilt increases intravasal volume up to 1 l within a week, which is particularly helpful to improve hypotension early in the morning. This approach

is successful in particular in combination with fludrocortisone, which further supports sodium retention.

The next group of drugs to consider are the sympathomimetics. These include ephedrine (with both direct and indirect effects) which is often valuable in central autonomic disorders such as MSA. With higher doses, side effects include tremulousness, loss of appetite, and urinary retention in men.

Among the large number of vasoactive agents that have been evaluated in MSA only one, the directly acting α-adrenergic agonist midodrine, meets the criteria of evidence based medicine (Jankovic *et al.*, 1993a; Low *et al.*, 1997; Wright *et al.*, 1998). Side effects are usually mild and only rarely lead to discontinuation of treatment because of urinary retention or pruritus, predominantly on the scalp. Another promising drug appears to be the norepinephrine precursor L-threo-dihydroxy-phenylserine (L-threo-DOPS), which has been used in this indication in Japan for years and efficacy of which has now been shown by a recent open, dose-finding trial (Mathias *et al.*, 2001). In case the above mentioned drugs do not produce the desired effects, selective targeting is needed. The somatostatin analogue, octreotide, is often beneficial in postprandial hypotension (Alam *et al.*, 1995), presumably because it inhibits release of vasodilatory gastrointestinal peptides (Raimbach *et al.*, 1989); importantly it does not enhance nocturnal hypertension (Alam *et al.*, 1995).

The vasopressin analogue, desmopressin, which acts on renal tubular vasopressin-2 receptors, reduces nocturnal polyuria and improves morning postural hypotension (Mathias *et al.*, 1986). The peptide erythropoietin may be beneficial in some patients by raising red cell mass, secondarily improving cerebral oxygenation (Perera *et al.*, 1995; Winkler *et al.*, 2001). A broad range of drugs (see above) have been used in the treatment of postural hypotension (Mathias & Kimber, 1999). Unfortunately, the value and side effects of many of these drugs have not been adequately determined in MSA patients using appropriate endpoints.

In the management of neurogenic bladder including residual urine, clean intermittent catheterization three to four times per day is a widely accepted approach to prevent secondary consequences of failure to micturate. It may be necessary to provide the patient with a permanent transcutaneous suprapubic catheter if mechanical obstruction in the urethra or motor symptoms of MSA prevent uncomplicated catheterisation.

Pharmacological options with anti- or pro-cholinergic drugs or –adrenergic substances are usually not successful to adequately reduce post-void residual volume in MSA, but anticholinergic agents like oxybutynin can improve symptoms of detrusor hyperreflexia or sphincter-detrusor

Table 43.9. Practical management of MSA

A.   Pharmacotherapy

I.   For akinesia-rigidity
- Levodopa up to 800–1000 mg/day, if tolerated (↔)
- Dopamine agonists as second-line antiparkinsonian drugs (dosing as for PD patients) (↔)
- Amantadine as third-line drug, 100 mg up to three times daily (↔)

II.   For focal dystonia
- Botulinum toxin A (↔)

III. For orthostatic hypotension
- Head-up tilt of bed at night (↔)
- Elastic stockings or tights (↔)
- Increased salt intake (↔)
- Fludrocortisone 0.1–0.3 mg/day (↔)
- Ephedrine 15–45 mg t.i.d (↔)
- L-threo-DOPS (300 mg b.i.d.) (↔)
- Midodrine 2.5 – 10 mg t.i.d. (↑↑)

IV.   For postprandial hypotension
- Octreotide 25–50 mcg s.c. 30 min before a meal (↔)

V.   For nocturnal polyuria
- Desmopressin (spray: 10–40 mcg/night or tablet: 100–400 mcg/night) (↔)

VI.   For bladder symptoms
- Oxybutynin for detrusor hyperreflexia (2.5–5 mg b.i.d-t.i.d.) (↔)
- Intermittent self-catheterization for retention or residual volume >100 ml (↔)

B.   Other therapies
- Physiotherapy (↔)
- Speech therapy (↔)
- Occupational therapy (↔)
- Percutaneous endoscopic gastrostomy (PEG) (rarely needed in late stage) (↔)
- Provision of wheelchair (↔)
- CPAP (↑) (rarely tracheostomy [↔]) for inspiratory stridor

(Reprinted by permission from John Wiley & Sons Inc.: Wenning & Geser, 2003b.)

dyssynergy in the early course of the disease (Beck *et al.*, 1994). Recently, α-adrenergic receptor antagonists (prazosin and moxisylyte) have been shown to improve voiding with reduction of residual volumes in MSA patients (Sakakibara *et al.*, 2000b). Urological surgery must be avoided in these patients because postoperative worsening of bladder control is most likely (Beck *et al.*, 1994).

The necessity of a specific treatment for sexual dysfunction needs to be evaluated individually in each MSA patient. Male impotence can be partially circumvented by the use of intracavernosal papaverine, prostaglandin E1 or penile implants (Colosimo & Pezzella, 2002). Preliminary evidence in PD patients (Zesiewicz *et al.*, 2000) suggests that sildenafil may also be successful in treating erectile failure in MSA: a recent trial confirmed the efficacy of this compound in MSA, but also suggested caution because of the frequent cardiovascular side-effects (Hussain *et al.*, 2001). Erectile failure in MSA may also be improved by oral yohimbine (Beck *et al.*, 1994).

Constipation can be relieved by increasing the intraluminal volume which may be achieved by using macrogol–water solution (Eichhorn & Oertel, 2001).

Inspiratory stridor develops in about 30% of patients. Continuous positive airway pressure (CPAP) may be helpful in some of these patients (Iranzo *et al.*, 2000). In only about 4% a tracheostomy is needed and performed.

Motor disorder

General approach
Because the results of drug treatment for the motor disorder of MSA are generally poor, other therapies are all the more important. Physiotherapy helps maintain mobility and prevent contractures, and speech therapy can improve speech and swallowing and provide communication aids. Dysphagia may require feeding via a nasogastric tube or even percutaneous endoscopic gastrostomy (PEG). Occupational therapy helps to limit the handicap resulting from the patient's disabilities and should include a home visit. Provision of a wheelchair is usually dictated by the liability to falls because of postural instability and gait ataxia but not by akinesia and rigidity *per se*. Psychological support for patients and partners needs to be stressed.

Parkinsonism
Parkinsonism is the predominant motor disorder in MSA and therefore represents a major target for therapeutic intervention. Although less effective than in PD and despite the lack of randomized-controlled trials, levodopa replacement represents the mainstay of antiparkinsonian therapy in MSA. Open-label studies suggest that up to 30–40% of MSA patients may derive benefit from levodopa at least transiently (Parati *et al.*, 1993, Wenning *et al.*, 1994a). Occasionally, a beneficial effect is evident only when seemingly unresponsive patients deteriorate after levodopa withdrawal (Hughes *et al.*, 1992). Pre-existing orthostatic hypotension is often unmasked or exacerbated in levodopa treated MSA patients associated with autonomic failure. In contrast, psychiatric or toxic confusional states appear to be less common than in Parkinson's disease (Wenning *et al.*, 1994a). Results with dopamine agonists have been even more disappointing (Lees, 1999).

Severe psychiatric side effects occurred in a double-blind crossover trial of six patients on lisuride, with nightmares, visual hallucinations and toxic confusional states (Lees & Bannister, 1981). Wenning *et al.* (1994a) reported a response to oral dopamine agonists only in 4 of 41 patients. None of 30 patients receiving bromocriptine improved, but three of ten who received pergolide had some benefit. Twenty-two percent of the levodopa responders had good or excellent response to at least one orally active dopamine agonist in addition. Antiparkinsonian effects were noted in 4 of 26 MSA patients treated with amantadine (Wenning *et al.*, 1994a); however, there was no significant improvement in an open study of nine patients with atypical parkinsonism, including five subjects with MSA (Colosimo *et al.*, 1996).

Blepharospasm as well as limb dystonia, but not antecollis, may respond well to local injections of botulinum toxin A.

Ablative neurosurgical procedures such as medial pallidotomy fail to improve parkinsonian motor disturbance in MSA (Lang *et al.*, 1997). However, more recently beneficial short-term and long-term effects of bilateral subthalamic nucleus high-frequency stimulation have been reported in four patients with MSA-P (Visser-Vandewalle *et al.*, 2003).

Cerebellar ataxia

There is no effective therapy for the progressive ataxia of MSA-C.

Occasional successes have been reported with cholinergic drugs, amantadine, 5-hydroxytryptophan, isoniazid, baclofen and propanolol; for the large majority of patients these drugs proved to be ineffective.

One intriguing observation is the apparent temporary exacerbation of ataxia by cigarette smoking (Graham & Oppenheimer, 1969; Johnsen & Miller, 1986). Nicotine is known to increase the release of acetylcholine in many areas of the brain and probably also releases noradrenaline, dopamine, 5-hydroxytryptophan and other neurotransmitters. Nicotinic systems may therefore play a role in cerebellar function and trials of nicotinic antagonists such as dihydro-beta-erythroidine might be worthwhile in MSA-C.

Practical therapy

Because of the small number of randomized controlled trials, the practical management of MSA is largely based on empirical evidence ($\leftrightarrow$) or single randomized studies ($\uparrow$), except for three randomized controlled studies of mido-

drine ($\uparrow\uparrow$). The present recommendations are summarized in Table 43.9.

Future therapeutic approaches

Two European research initiatives, i.e. the European MSA-Study Group (EMSA-SG) as well as the Neuroprotection and Natural History in Parkinson Plus Syndromes (NNIPPS), are presently conducting multicentre intervention trials in MSA. These trials will radically change our approach to MSA. For the first time, prospective data concerning disease progression will become available allowing us to reliably identify predictors of survival.

The need for prospective natural history studies has led the EMSA-SG to develop the Unified MSA Rating Scale (UMSARS) including a video teaching tape to standardize severity assessments in specialized clinics and research programs (Wenning *et al.*, 2002). This novel scale will also be useful in future multicenter intervention trials.

Furthermore, surrogate markers of the disease process will be identified by the EMSA-SG and NIPPS trials using structural and functional neuroimaging. These markers will allow to plan future phase III intervention trials more effectively.

Research into the etiopathogenesis and neuropathology of MSA is being conducted by EMSA-SG, NNIPPS and North American MSA-Study Group (NAMSA-SG). A number of animal models have become available as testbeds for preclinical intervention studies (Wenning *et al.*, 1996a, 1999b, 2000c; Scherfler *et al.*, 2000; Waldner *et al.*, 2001; Fernagut *et al.*, 2002; Ghorayeb *et al.*, 2000, 2002a, b, Kahle *et al.*, 2002). This work will lead to a multitude of neuroprotective candidate agents ready to be tested during the next decade.

Conclusions

During the last 15 years there have been major advances in our understanding of the cellular pathology of MSA. At the same time the first multicentre intervention trials have been launched in Europe. Although therapeutic options are limited at present, there is a real hope for a radical change of our approach to this devastating illness.

Acknowledgements

GKW received grants from the Fonds zur Förderung der wissenschaftlichen Forschung (FWF, Vienna), Nationalbank (Vienna), Bundesministerium für Bildung, Wissenschaft und Kultur (BMWK, Vienna), and the European Community (Fifth framework programme).

REFERENCES

Abbruzzese, G., Marchese, R. & Trompetto, C. (1997). Sensory and motor evoked potentials in multiple system atrophy: comparative study with Parkinson's disease. *Mov. Disord.*, **12**(3), 315–21.

Abele, M., Schulz, J. B., Burk, K., Topka, H., Dichgans, J. & Klockgether, T. (2000a). Evoked potentials in multiple system atrophy (MSA). *Acta Neurol. Scand.*, **101**(2), 111–15.

(2000b). Nerve conduction studies in multiple system atrophy. *Eur. Neurol.*, **43**(4), 221–3.

Abele, M., Burk, K., Schols, L. *et al.* (2002). The aetiology of sporadic adult-onset ataxia. *Brain*, **125**(5), 961–8.

Abeliovich, A., Schmitz, Y., Farinas, I. *et al.* (2000). Mice lacking alpha-synuclein display functional deficits in the nigrostriatal dopamine system. *Neuron*, **25**(1), 239–52.

Adams, R. D., van Bogaert, L. & van der Eecken, H. (1961). Dégénérescences nigro-striées et cérébello-nigro-striees. *Psychiat. Neurol.* **142**, 219–59.

(1964). Striato-nigral degeneration. *J. Neuropathol. Expl. Neurol.*, **23**, 584–608.

Alam, M., Smith, G., Bleasdal-Barr, K., Pavitt, D. V. & Mathias, C. J. (1995). Effects of the peptide release inhibitor, octreotide, on daytime hypotension and on nocturnal hypertension in primary autonomic failure. *J. Hypertens.*, **13**(12/2), 1664–9.

Albanese, A., Colosimo, C., Bentivoglio, A. R. *et al.* (1995). Multiple system atrophy presenting as parkinsonism: clinical features and diagnostic criteria. *J. Neurol. Neurosurg. Psychiatry*, **59**(2), 144–51.

Allan, S. M. & Rothwell, N. J. (2001). Cytokines and acute neurodegeneration. *Nat. Rev. Neurosci.*, **2**(10), 734–44.

Aloe, L. & Fiore, M. (1997). TNF-alpha expressed in the brain of transgenic mice lowers central tyroxine hydroxylase immunoreactivity and alters grooming behaviour. *Neurosci. Lett.*, **238**(1–2), 65–8.

Ansorge, O., Lees, A. J., Brooks, D. J. & Daniel, S. E. (1997a). Multiple system atrophy presenting as progressive supranuclear palsy and vice-versa: two unusual cases. *Mov. Disord.*, **12**(suppl.1), 96.

Ansorge, O., Lees, A. J. & Daniel, S. E. (1997b). Pathological overlap of Alzheimer's disease, Parkinson's disease and multiple system atrophy. *Neuropathol. Appl. Neurobiol.*, **23**, 179.

Antonini, A., Kazumata, K., Feigin, A. *et al.* (1998). Differential diagnosis of parkinsonism with [18F]fluorodeoxyglucose and PET. *Mov. Disord.*, **13**(2), 268–74.

Arima, K., Nakamura, M., Sunohara, N. *et al.* (1997). Ultrastructural characterization of the tau-immunoreactive tubules in the oligodendroglial perikarya and their inner loop processes in progressive supranuclear palsy. *Acta Neuropathol. (Berl.)*, **93**(6), 558–66.

Arima, K., Ueda, K., Sunohara, N. *et al.* (1998). NACP/alpha-synuclein immunoreactivity in fibrillary components of neuronal and oligodendroglial cytoplasmic inclusions in the pontine nuclei in multiple system atrophy. *Acta Neuropathol. (Berl.)*, **96**(5), 439–44.

Baker, M., Litvan, I., Houlden, H. *et al.* (1999). Association of an extended halotype in the tau gene with progressive supranuclear palsy. *Hum. Mol. Genet.*, **8**(4), 711–15.

Bandmann, O., Wenning, G. K., Quinn, N. P. & Harding, A. E. (1995). Arg296 to Cys296 polymorphism in exon 6 of cytochrome P-450–2D6 (CYP2D6) is not associated with multiple system atrophy. *J. Neurol. Neurosurg. Psychiatry*, **59**(5), 557.

Bandmann, O., Sweeney, M. G., Daniel, S. E. *et al.* (1997). Multiple-system atrophy is genetically distinct from identified inherited causes of spinocerebellar degeneration. *Neurology*, **49**(6), 1598–604.

Bannister, R. & Oppenheimer, D. R. (1972). Degenerative diseases of the nervous system associated with autonomic failure. *Brain*, **95**(3), 457–74.

Bannister, R. & Mathias, C. J. (1999a). Clinical features and evaluation of the primary chronic autonomic failure syndromes. In *Autonomic Failure. A Textbook of Clinical Disorders of the Autonomic Nervous System.*, ed. C. J. Mathias & R. Bannister. Oxford: Oxford University Press, pp. 307–16.

(1999b). Investigation of autonomic disorders. In *Autonomic Failure. A Textbook of Clinical Disorders of the Autonomic Nervous System*, ed. C. J. Mathias & R. Bannister. Oxford: Oxford University Press, pp. 169–95.

Barres, B. A., Hart, I. K., Coles, H. S. *et al.* (1992). Cell death and control of cell survival in the oligodendrocyte lineage. *Cell*, **70**(1), 31–46.

Baser, S. M., Meer, J., Polinsky, R. J. & Hallett, M. (1991). Sudomotor function in autonomic failure. *Neurology*, **41**(10), 1564–6.

Beck, R. O., Betts, C. D. & Fowler, C. J. (1994). Genitourinary dysfunction in multiple system atrophy: clinical features and treatment in 62 cases. *J. Urol.*, **151**(5), 1336–41.

Benarroch, E. E., Smithson, I. L., Low, P. A. & Parisi, J. E. (1998). Depletion of catecholaminergic neurons of the rostral ventrolateral medulla in multiple systems atrophy with autonomic failure. *Ann. Neurol.*, **43**(2), 156–63.

Ben-Shlomo, Y., Wenning, G. K., Tison, F. & Quinn, N. P. (1997). Survival of patients with pathologically proven multiple system atrophy: a meta-analysis. *Neurology*, **48**, 384–93.

Berciano, J., Combarros, O., Polo, J. M., Pascual, J. & Oterino, A. (1998). Who first described striatonigral degeneration? *Neurology*, **50**(suppl 4), 120.

Berciano, J., Valldeoriola, F., Ferrer, I. *et al.* (2002). Presynaptic parkinsonism in multiple system atrophy mimicking Parkinson's disease: a clinicopathological case study. *Mov. Disord.*, **17**(4), 812–16.

Bermingham-McDonogh, O., McCabe, K. L. & Reh, T. A. (1996). Effects of GGF/neuregulins on neuronal survival and neurite outgrowth correlate with erbB2/neu expression in developing rat retina. *Development*, **122**(5), 1427–38.

Bösch, S. M., Schocke, M., Seppi, K., Hollosi, P., Poewe, W. & Wenning, G. K. (2002a). Abnormal striatal dopaminergic function in SCA2 revealed by beta-CIT and IBZM SPECT. *Mov. Disord.*, **17**(Suppl 5), 311.

Bösch, S. M., Wenning, G. K., Ransmayr, G. & Poewe, W. (2002b). Dystonia in multiple system atrophy. *J. Neurol. Neurosurg. Psychiatry*, **72**(3), 300–3.

Boka, G., Anglade, P., Wallach, D., Javoy-Agid, F., Agid, Y. & Hirsch, E. C. (1994). Immunocytochemical analysis of tumor necrosis factor and its receptors in Parkinson's disease. *Neurosci. Lett.*, **172**(1–2), 151–4.

Botez, M. I. & Young, S. N. (2001). Biogenic amine metabolites and thiamine in cerebrospinal fluid in heredodegenerative ataxias. *Can. J. Neurol. Sci.*, **28**(2), 134–40.

Bower, J. H., Maraganore, D. M., McDonnell, S. K. & Rocca, W. A. (1997). Incidence of progressive supranuclear palsy and multiple system atrophy in Olmsted County, Minnesota, 1976 to 1990. *Neurology*, **49**, 1284–8.

Braak, H. & Braak, E. (1989). Cortical and subcortical argyrophilic grains characterize a disease associated with adult onset dementia. *Neuropathol. Appl. Neurobiol.*, **15**(1), 13–26.

Braune, S., Auer, A., Schulte-Mönting, J., Schwerbrock, S. & Lücking, C. H. (1996a). Cardiovascular parameters: sensitivity to detect autonomic dysfunction and influence of age and sex in normal subjects. *Clin. Auton. Res.*, **6**, 3–15.

Braune, S., Schulte-Monting, J., Schwerbrock, S. & Lucking, C. H. (1996b). Retest variation of cardiovascular parameters in autonomic testing. *J. Auton. Nerv. Syst.*, **60**(3), 103–7.

Braune, S., Elam, M., Baron, R. & Low, P. A. (1999a). Assessment of blood pressure regulation. The International Federation of Clinical Neurophysiology. *Electroencephalogr. Clin. Neurophysiol.*, Suppl **52**, 287–91.

Braune, S., Reinhardt, M., Schnitzer, R., Riedel, A. & Lücking, C. H. (1999b). Cardiac uptake of (123I)MIBG separates Parkinson's disease from multiple system atrophy. *Neurology*, **53**(5), 1020–5.

Brenneis, C., Seppi, K., Schocke, M. F. *et al.* (2003). Voxel-based morphometry detects cortical atrophy in the parkinson variant of multiple system atrophy. *Mov. Disord.*, **18**(10), 1132–8.

Brooks, D. J., Luthert, P., Gadian, D. & Marsden, C. D. (1989). Does signal-attenuation on high-field T$_2$-weighted MRI of the brain reflect regional cerebral iron deposition? Observations on the relationship between regional cerebral water proton T2-values and iron levels. *J. Neurol. Neurosurg. Psychiatry*, **52**, 108–11.

Brooks, D. J., Ibanez, V., Sawle, G. V. *et al.* (1990a). Differing patterns of striatal 18-F-Dopa uptake in Parkinson's disease, multiple system atrophy and progressive supranuclear palsy. *Ann. Neurol.*, **28**, 547–55.

Brooks, D. J., Salmon, E. P., Mathias, C. J. *et al.* (1990b). The relationship between locomotor disability, autonomic dysfunction, and the integrity of the striatal dopaminergic system in patients with multiple system atrophy, pure autonomic failure, and Parkinson's disease, studied with PET. *Brain*, **113**, 1539–52.

Brooks, D. J., Ibanez, V., Sawle, G. V. *et al.* (1992). Striatal D2 receptor status in patients with Parkinson's disease, striatonigral degeneration, and progressive supranuclear palsy, measured with 11C-raclopride and positron emission tomography. *Ann. Neurol.*, **31**(2), 184–92.

Brown, R. G., Pillon, B., Uttner, I., Payan, C. & Lacomblez, L. (2002). Members of the Neuropsychology Working Group and NNIPPS Consortium. Cognitive function in patients with Progressive Supranuclear Palsy (PSP) and Multiple System Atrophy (MSA). *Mov. Disord.*, **17**(Suppl 5), 221.

Brücke, T., Wenger, S. & Asenbaum, S. (1993). Dopamine D2 receptor imaging and measurement with SPECT. *Adv. Neurol.*, **60**, 494–500.

Brücke, T., Asenbaum, S., Pirker, W. *et al.* (1997). Measurement of the dopaminergic degeneration in Parkinson's disease with [123I] beta-CIT and SPECT. Correlation with clinical findings and comparison with multiple system atrophy and progressive supranuclear palsy. *J. Neural Transm.* Suppl., **50**, 9–24.

Brücke, T., Djamshidian, S., Bencsits, G., Pirker, W., Asenbaum, S. & Podreka, I. (2000). SPECT and PET imaging of the dopaminergic system in Parkinson's disease. *J. Neurol.*, **247**(4), IV/2–7.

Burden, S. & Yarden, Y. (1997). Neuregulins and their receptors: a versatile signaling module in organogenesis and oncogenesis. *Neuron*, **18**(6), 847–55.

Burn, D. J. & Jaros, E. (2001). Multiple system atrophy: cellular and molecular pathology. *Mol. Pathol.*, **54**(6), 419–26.

Burn, D. J., Sawle, G. V. & Brooks, D. J. (1994). Differential diagnosis of Parkinson's disease, multiple system atrophy, and Steele–Richardson–Olszewski syndrome: discriminant analysis of striatal ^{18}F-dopa PET data. *J. Neurol. Neurosurg. Psychiatry*, **57**(3), 278–84.

Burn, D. J., Rinne, J. O., Quinn, N. P., Lees, A. J., Marsden, C. D. & Brooks, D. J. (1995). Striatal opioid receptor binding in Parkinson's disease, striatonigral degeneration and Steele–Richardson–Olszewski syndrome. A [11C]diprenorphine PET study. *Brain*, **118**(4), 951–8.

Buttery, P. C. & ffrench-Constant, C. (1999). Laminin-2/integrin interactions enhance myelin membrane formation by oligodendrocytes. *Mol. Cell. Neurosci.*, **14**(3), 199–212.

Cairns, N. J., Atkinson, P. F., Hanger, D. P., Anderton, B. H., Daniel, S. E. & Lantos, P. L. (1997a). Tau protein in the glial cytoplasmic inclusions of multiple system atrophy can be distinguished from abnormal tau in Alzheimer's disease. *Neurosci. Lett.*, **230**(1), 49–52.

Cairns, N. J., Atkinson, P. F., Kovacs, T., Lees, A. J., Daniel, S. E. & Lantos, P. L. Apolipoprotein E ε4 allele frequency in patients with multiple system atrophy. *Neurosci. Lett.*, **221**(2–3), 161–4.

Canoll, P. D., Musacchio, J. M., Hardy, R., Reynolds, R., Marchionni, M. A. & Salzer, J. L. (1996). GGF/neuregulin is a neuronal signal that promotes the proliferation and survival and inhibits the differentiation of oligodendrocyte progenitors. *Neuron*, **17**(2), 229–43.

Canoll, P. D., Kraemer, R., Teng, K. K., Marchionni, M. A. & Salzer, J. L. (1999). GGF/neuregulin induces a phenotypic reversion of oligodendrocytes. *Mol. Cell. Neurosci.*, **13**(2), 79–94.

Caplan, L. R. (1984). Clinical features of sporadic (Dejerine-Thomas) olivopontocerebellar atrophy. *Adv. Neurol.*, **41**, 217–24.

Chandiramani, V. A., Palace, J. & Fowler, C. J. (1997). How to recognize patients with parkinsonism who should not have urological surgery. *Br. J. Urol.*, **80**(1), 100–4.

Chin, S. S. & Goldman, J. E. (1996). Glial inclusions in CNS degenerative diseases. *J. Neuropathol. Exp. Neurol.*, **55**(5), 499–508.

Chio, A., Magnani, C. & Schiffer, D. (1998). Prevalence of Parkinson's disease in northwestern Italy: comparison of tracer methodology and clinical ascertainment of cases. *Mov. Disord.*, **13**(3), 400–5.

Churchyard, A., Donnan, G. A., Hughes, A. *et al.* (1993). Dopa resistance in multiple-system atrophy: loss of postsynaptic D2 receptors. *Ann. Neurol.*, **34**(2), 219–26.

Clarke, C. E. & Lowry, M. (2000). Basal ganglia metabolite concentrations in idiopathic Parkinson's disease and multiple system atrophy measured by proton magnetic resonance spectroscopy. *Eur. J. Neurol.*, **7**(6), 661–5.

Clarke, C. E., Ray, P. S. & Speller, J. M. (1999). Failure of the clonidine growth hormone stimulation test to differentiate multiple system atrophy from early or advanced idiopathic Parkinson's disease. *The Lancet*, **353**, 1329–30.

Clayton, D. F. & George, J. M. (1999). Synucleins in synaptic plasticity and neurodegenerative disorders. *J. Neurosci. Res.*, **58**(1), 120–9.

Cohen, J., Low, P., Fealey, R., Sheps, S. & Jiang, N. S. (1987). Somatic and autonomic function in progressive autonomic failure and multiple system atrophy. *Ann. Neurol.*, **22**, 692–9.

Colosimo, C. (1998). Pisa syndrome in a patient with multiple system atrophy. *Mov. Disord.*, **13**(3), 607–9.

Colosimo, C. & Pezzella, F. R. (2002). The symptomatic treatment of multiple system atrophy. *Eur. J. Neurol.*, **9**(3), 195–9.

Colosimo, C., Merello, M. & Pontieri, F. E. (1996). Amantadine in parkinsonian patients unresponsive to levodopa: a pilot study. *J. Neurol.*, **243**, 422–5.

Colosimo, C., Albanese, A., Hughes, A. J., de Bruin, V. M. & Lees, A. J. (1995). Some specific clinical features differentiate multiple system atrophy (striatonigral variety) from Parkinson's disease. *Arch. Neurol.*, **52**(3), 294–8.

Colosimo, C., Inghilleri, M. & Chaudhuri, K. R. (2000). Parkinson's disease misdiagnosed as multiple system atrophy by sphincter electromyography. *J. Neurol.*, **247**, 559–61.

Colosimo, C., Geser, F. and Wenning, G. K. (2004). Clinical spectrum and pathological features of multiple system atrophy. In: *Animal Models of Movement Disorders*, ed. M. LeDoux, pp. 541–70. Amsterdam: Elsevier.

Consensus statement on the definition of orthostatic hypotension, pure autonomic failure, and multiple system atrophy. (1996). *J. Neurol. Sci.*, **144**(1–2), 218–19.

Cortes, R., Camps, M., Gueye, B., Probst, A. & Palacios, J. M. (1989). Dopamine receptors in human brain: autoradiographic distribution of D1 and D2 sites in Parkinson syndrome of different etiology. *Brain Res.*, **483**(1), 30–8.

Daniel, S. E. (1999). The neuropathology and neurochemistry of multiple system atrophy. In *Autonomic Failure. A Textbook of Clinical Disorders of the Autonomic Nervous System*, ed. C. J. Mathias & R. Bannister. Oxford: Oxford University Press, pp. 321–8.

Davie, C. A., Wenning, G. K., Barker, G. J. *et al.* (1995). Differentiation of multiple system atrophy from idiopathic Parkinson's disease using proton magnetic resonance spectroscopy. *Ann. Neurol.*, **37**, 204–10.

Dejerine, J. & Thomas, A. A. (1900). L'atrophie olivo-ponto-cérébelleuse. *Nouv. Iconogr. Salpêtrière*, **13**, 330–70.

Delalande, I., Hache, J. C., Forzy, G., Bughin, M., Benjadjali, J. & Destee, A. (1998). Do visual-evoked potentials and spatiotemporal contrast sensitivity help to distinguish idiopathic Parkinson's disease and multiple system atrophy? *Mov. Disord.*, **13**(3), 446–52.

De Volder, A. G., Francart, J., Laterre, C. *et al.* (1989). Decreased glucose utilization in the striatum and frontal lobe in probable striatonigral degeneration. *Ann. Neurol.*, **26**, 239–47.

Dexter, D. T., Carayon, A., Javoy-Agid, F. *et al.* (1991). Alterations in the levels of iron, ferritin and other trace metals in Parkinson's disease and other neurodegenerative diseases affecting the basal ganglia. *Brain*, **114**(4), 1953–75.

Dickson, D. W., Liu, W., Hardy, J. *et al.* (1999a). Widespread alterations of alpha-synuclein in multiple system atrophy. *Am. J. Pathol.*, **155**(4), 1241–51.

Dickson, D. W., Lin, W., Liu, W. K. & Yen, S. H. (1999b). Multiple system atrophy: a sporadic synucleinopathy. *Brain Pathol.*, **9**(4), 721–32.

Drayer, B. P., Olanow, W., Burger, P., Johnson, G. A., Herfkens, R. & Ricderer, S. (1986). Parkinson Plus Syndrome: diagnosis using high field MR imaging of brain iron. *Radiology*, **159**, 493–8.

Duda, J. E., Shah, U., Arnold, S. E., Lee, V. M. & Trojanowski, J. Q. (1999). The expression of alpha-, beta-, and gamma-synucleins in olfactory mucosa from patients with and without neurodegenerative diseases. *Exp. Neurol.*, **160**(2), 515–22.

Eardley, I., Quinn, N. P., Fowler, C. J. *et al.* (1989). The value of urethral sphincter electromyography in the differential diagnosis of parkinsonism. *Br. J. Urol.*, **64**, 360–2.

Eichhorn, T. E. & Oertel, W. H. (2001). Macrogol 3350/electrolyte improves constipation in Parkinson's disease and multiple system atrophy. *Mov. Disord.*, **16**(6), 1176–7.

Eidelberg, D., Takikawa, S., Moeller, J. R. *et al.* (1993). Striatal hypometabolism distinguishes striatonigral degeneration from Parkinson's disease. *Ann. Neurol.*, **33**, 518–27.

El-Agnaf, O. M., Curran, M. D., Wallace, A. *et al.* (1998). Mutation screening in exons 3 and 4 of alpha-synuclein in sporadic Parkinson's and sporadic and familial dementia with Lewy bodies cases. *Neuroreport*, **9**(17), 3925–7.

Ellis, C., Lemmens, G., Williams, S. C. R., Simmons, A., Leigh, P. N. & Chaudhuri, K. R. (1996). Striatal changes in striatonigral degeneration and Parkinson's disease: a proton magnetic resonance spectroscopy study. *Mov. Disord.*, **11**, 104.

Ellis, C. E., Schwartzberg, P. L., Grider, T. L., Fink, D. W. & Nussbaum, R. L. (2001). Alpha-synuclein is phosphorylated by members of the Src family of protein-tyrosine kinases. *J. Biol. Chem.*, **276**(6), 3879–84.

Engelender, S., Kaminsky, Z., Guo, X. *et al.* (1999). Synphilin-I associates with alpha-synuclein and promotes the formation of cytosolic inclusions. *Nat. Genet.*, **22**(1), 110–14.

Fearnley, J. M. & Lees, A. J. (1990). Striatonigral degeneration. A clinico-pathological study. *Brain*, **113**(6), 1823–42.

(1991). Ageing and Parkinson's disease: substantia nigra regional selectivity. *Brain*, **114**(5), 2283–301.

Federico, F., Simone, I. L., Lucivero, V. *et al.* (1999). Usefulness of proton magnetic resonance spectroscopy in differentiating parkinsonian syndromes. *Ital. J. Neurol. Sci.*, **20**(4), 223–9.

Fernagut, P., Diguet, E., Stefanova, N. *et al.* (2002). Subacute systemic 3-nitropropionic acid intoxication induces a distinct motor disorder in adult C57Bl/6 mice: behavioural and histopathological characterisation. *Neuroscience*, **114**(4), 1005–17.

Fleischhacker, H. (1924). Afamiliäre chronisch progressive Erkrankung des mittleren Lebensalters vom Pseudosklerosetyp. *Z. Gesamte Neurol. Psychiatrie*, **91**, 1–22.

Flugel, K. A., Mosler, T. A. & Wild, R. H. (1984). Bulbar paralytic symptoms including acute vocal cord paralysis in Shy-Drager syndrome. *Nervenarzt*, **55**(6), 293–8.

Frost, E. E., Buttery, P. C., Milner, R. & ffrench-Constant, C. (1999). Integrins mediate a neuronal survival signal for oligodendrocytes. *Curr. Biol.*, **9**(21), 1251–4.

Fujita, T., Doi, M., Ogata, T., Kanazawa, I. & Mizusawa, H. (1993). Cerebral cortical pathology of sporadic olivopontocerebellar atrophy. *J. Neurol. Sci.*, **116**(1), 41–6.

Futamura, N., Matsumura, R., Fujimoto, Y., Horikawa, H., Suzumura, A. & Takayanagi, T. (1998). CAG repeat expansions in patients with sporadic cerebellar ataxia. *Acta Neurol. Scand.*, **98**(1), 55–9.

Gahring, L. C., Rogers, S. W. & Twyman, R. E. (1997). Autoantibodies to glutamate receptor subunit GluR2 in nonfamilial olivopontocerebellar degeneration. *Neurology*, **48**(2), 494–500.

Gai, W. P., Power, J. H., Blumbergs, P. C. & Blessing, W. W. (1998). Multiple-system atrophy: a new alpha-synuclein disease? *Lancet*, **352**(9127), 547–8.

Gai, W. P., Pountney, D. L., Power, J. H. *et al.* (2003). α-Synuclein fibrils constitute the central core of oligodendroglial inclusion filaments in multiple system atrophy. *Exp. Neurol.*, **181**(1), 68–78.

Garratt, H., Wenning, G. K., Barnes, C., Howard, R. & Quinn, N. P. (1994). Speech dysfunction and levodopa response in multiple system atrophy. *N. Trends Clin. Neuropharmacol.*, 206–7.

Gash, D. M., Zhang, Z. & Gerhardt, G. (1998). Neuroprotective and neurorestorative properties of GDNF. *Ann. Neurol.*, **44**(3 Suppl 1), 121–5.

Gerhard, A., Banati, R., Cagnin, A. *et al.* (2000). In vivo imaging of activated microglia with [11C]PK11195 positron emission tomography in patients with multiple system atrophy. *Mov. Disord.*, **15**(Suppl. 3), 215–16.

Ghaemi, M., Hilker, R., Rudolf, J., Sobesky, J. & Heiss, W. D. (2002). Differentiating multiple system atrophy from Parkinson's disease: contribution of striatal and midbrain MRI volumetry and multi-tracer PET imaging. *J. Neurol. Neurosurg. Psychiatry*, **73**(5), 517–23.

Ghorayeb, I., Fernagut, P. O., Aubert, I. *et al.* (2000). Toward a primate model of L-dopa-unresponsive parkinsonism mimicking striatonigral degeneration. *Mov. Disord.*, **15**(3), 531–6.

Ghorayeb, I., Fernagut, P. O., Hervier, L., Labattu, B., Bioulac, B. & Tison, F. (2002a). A 'single toxin-double lesion' rat model of striatonigral degeneration by intrastriatal 1-methyl-4-phenylpyridinium ion injection: a motor behavioural analysis. *Neuroscience*, **115**(2), 533–46.

Ghorayeb, I., Fernagut, P. O., Stefanova, N., Wenning, G. K., Bioulac, B. & Tison, F. (2002b). Dystonia is predictive of subsequent altered dopaminergic responsiveness in a chronic 1-methyl-4-phenyl-1,2,3,6-tetrahydropyridine+3-nitropropionic acid model of striatonigral degeneration in monkeys. *Neurosci. Lett.*, **335**(1), 34–8.

Ghorayeb, I., Yekhlef, F., Chrysostome, V., Balestre, E., Bioulac, B. & Tison, F. (2002c). Sleep disorders and their determinants in multiple system atrophy. *J. Neurol. Neurosurg. Psychiatry*, **72**(6), 798–800.

Giladi, N., Simon, E. S., Korczyn, A. D. *et al.* (2000). Anal sphincter EMG does not distinguish between multiple system atrophy and Parkinson's disease. *Muscle Nerve*, **23**(5), 731–4.

Gilman, S., Koeppe, R. A., Junck, L., Kluin, K. J., Lohman, M. & St. Laurent, R. T. (1994). Patterns of cerebral glucose metabolism detected with positron emission tomography differ in multiple system atrophy and olivopontocerebellar atrophy. *Ann. Neurol.*, **36**, 166–75.

(1995). Benzodiazepine receptor binding in cerebellar degenerations studied with positron emission tomography. *Ann. Neurol.*, **38**, 176–85.

Gilman, S., Sima, A. A., Junck, L., Kluin, K. J., Koeppe, R. A. & Lohman, M. E. & Little, R. (1996). Spinocerebellar ataxia type 1 with multiple system degeneration and glial cytoplasmic inclusions. *Ann. Neurol.*, **39**(2), 241–55.

Gilman, S., Low, P., Quinn, N. *et al.* (1998). Consensus statement on the diagnosis of multiple system atrophy. American Autonomic Society and American Academy of Neurology. *Clin. Auton. Res.*, **8**(6), 359–62.

(1999). Consensus statement on the diagnosis of multiple system atrophy. *J. Neurol. Sci.*, **163**(1), 94–8.

Gilman, S., Little, R., Johanns, J. *et al.* (2000). Evolution of sporadic olivopontocerebellar atrophy into multiple system atrophy. *Neurology*, **55**(4), 527–32.

Goedert, M. & Spillantini, M. G. (1998). Lewy body diseases and multiple system atrophy as alpha-synucleinopathies. *Mol. Psychiatry*, **3**(6), 462–5.

Gomez-Tortosa, E., Gonzalo, I., Newell, K., Garcia Yebenes, J., Vonsattel, P. & Hyman, B. T. (2002). Patterns of protein nitration in dementia with Lewy bodies and striatonigral degeneration. *Acta Neuropathol. (Berl.)*, **103**(5), 495–500.

Gonzalez-Quevedo, A., Garcia, J. C., Fernandez, R. & Fernandez Cartaya, L. (1993). Monoamine metabolites in normal human cerebrospinal fluid and in degenerative diseases of the central nervous system. *Bol. Estud. Med. Biol.*, **41**(1–4), 13–19.

Gosset, A., Pellissier, J. F., Delpuech, F. & Khalil, R. (1983). Degenerescence striato-nigrique associée a une atrophie olivo-ponto-cerebelleuse. *Rev. Neurol. (Paris)*, **139**(2), 125–39.

Goto, S., Hirano, A. & Matsumoto, S. (1989a). Subdivisional involvement of nigrostriatal loop in idiopathic Parkinson's disease and striatonigral degeneration. *Ann. Neurol.*, **26**(6), 766–70.

Goto, S., Hirano, A. & Rojas-Corona, R. R. (1989b). Calcineurin immunoreactivity in striatonigral degeneration. *Acta Neuropathol. (Berl.)*, **78**(1), 65–71.

(1989c). Immunohistochemical visualization of afferent nerve terminals in human globus pallidus and its alteration in neostriatal neurodegenerative disorders. *Acta. Neuropathol. (Berl.)*, **78**(5), 543–50.

Goto, S., Hirano, A. & Matsumoto, S. (1990). Met-enkephalin immunoreactivity in the basal ganglia in Parkinson's disease and striatonigral degeneration. *Neurology*, **40**(7), 1051–6.

Goto, S., Matsumoto, S., Ushio, Y. & Hirano, A. (1996). Subregional loss of putaminal efferents to the basal ganglia output nuclei may cause parkinsonism in striatonigral degeneration. *Neurology*, **47**(4), 1032–6.

Gouider-Khouja, N., Vidailhet, M., Bonnet, A. M., Pichon, J. & Agid, Y. (1995). "Pure" striatonigral degeneration and Parkinson's disease: a comparative clinical study. *Mov. Disord.*, **10**(3), 288–94.

Graham, J. G. & Oppenheimer, D. R. (1969). Orthostatic hypotension and nicotine sensitivity in a case of multiple system atrophy. *J. Neurol. Neurosurg. Psychiatry*, **32**(1), 28–34.

Gu, M., Gash, M. T., Cooper, J. M. *et al.* (1997). Mitochondrial respiratory chain function in multiple system atrophy. *Mov. Disord.*, **12**(3), 418–22.

Hashida, H., Goto, J., Zhao, N. *et al.* (1998). Cloning and mapping of ZNF231, a novel brain-specific gene encoding neuronal double zinc finger protein whose expression is enhanced in a neurodegenerative disorder, multiple system atrophy (MSA). *Genomics*, **54**, 50–8.

Hashimoto, M., Rockenstein, E., Mante, M., Mallory, M. & Masliah, E. (2001). Beta-synuclein inhibits alpha-synuclein aggregation: a possible role as an antiparkinsonian factor. *Neuron*, **32**(2), 213–23.

Hayashi, M., Isozaki, E., Oda, M., Tanabe, H. & Kimura, J. (1997). Loss of large myelinated nerve fibres of the recurrent laryngeal nerve in patients with multiple system atrophy and vocal cord palsy. *J. Neurol. Neurosurg. Psychiatry*, **62**(3), 234–8.

Hirsch, E. C., Hunot, S., Damier, P. & Faucheux, B. (1998). Glial cells and inflammation in Parkinson's disease: a role in neurodegeneration? *Ann. Neurol.*, **44**(3 Suppl 1), 115–20.

Holmberg, B., Rosengren, L., Karlsson, J. E. & Johnels, B. (1998). Increased cerebrospinal fluid levels of neurofilament protein in progressive supranuclear palsy and multiple-system atrophy compared with Parkinson's disease. *Mov. Disord.*, **13**(1), 70–7.

Holmberg, B., Johnels, B., Ingvarsson, P., Eriksson, B. & Rosengren, L. (2001). CSF-neurofilament and levodopa tests combined with discriminant analysis may contribute to the differential diagnosis of Parkinsonian syndromes. *Parkinsonism Relat. Disord.*, **8**(1), 23–31.

Horoupian, D. S. & Dickson, D. W. (1991). Striatonigral degeneration, olivopontocerebellar atrophy and "atypical" Pick disease. *Acta Neuropathol. (Berl.)*, **81**(3), 287–95.

Hu, M. T. M., Simmons, A., Glover, A. *et al.* (1998). Proton magnetic resonance spectroscopy of the putamen in Parkinson's disease and multiple system atrophy. *Mov. Disord.*, **13**, 182.

Hughes, A. J., Colosimo, C., Kleedorfer, B., Daniel, S. E. & Lees, A. J. (1992). The dopaminergic response in multiple system atrophy. *J. Neurol. Neurosurg. Psychiatry*, **55**(11), 1009–13.

Hughes, A. J., Daniel, S. E., Ben-Shlomo, Y. & Lees, A. J. (2002). The accuracy of diagnosis of parkinsonian syndromes in a specialist movement disorder service. *Brain*, **125**(4), 861–70.

Hughes, R. G., Gibbin, K. P. & Lowe, J. (1998). Vocal fold abductor paralysis as a solitary and fatal manifestation of multiple system atrophy. *J. Laryng. Otol.*, **112**(2), 177–8.

Hunot, S., Dugas, N., Faucheux, B. *et al.* (1999). Fc-epsilon RII/CD23 is expressed in Parkinson's disease and induces, in vitro, production of nitric oxide and tumor necrosis factor-alpha in glial cells. *J. Neurosci.*, **19**(9), 3440–7.

Hussain, I. F., Brady, C. M., Swinn, M. J., Mathias, C. J. & Fowler, C. J. (2001). Treatment of erectile dysfunction with sildenafil citrate (Viagra) in parkinsonism due to Parkinson's disease or multiple system atrophy with observations on orthostatic hypotension. *J. Neurol. Neurosurg. Psychiatry*, **71**, 371–4.

Ichikawa, N. (1986). Study on monoamine metabolite contents of cerebrospinal fluid in patients with neurodegenerative diseases. *Tohoku J. Exp. Med.*, **150**(4), 435–46.

Iranzo, A., Santamaria, J. & Tolosa, E. (2000). Continuous positive air pressure eliminates nocturnal stridor in multiple system atrophy. Barcelona Multiple System Atrophy Study Group. *The Lancet*, **356**, 1329–30.

Ito, H., Kusaka, H., Matsumoto, S. & Imai, T. (1996). Striatal efferent involvement and its correlation to levodopa efficacy in patients with multiple system atrophy. *Neurology*, **47**(5), 1291–9.

Iwahashi, K., Miyatake, R., Tsuneoka, Y. *et al.* (1995). A novel cytochrome P-450IID6 (CYPIID6) mutant gene associated with multiple system atrophy. *J. Neurol. Neurosurg. Psychiatry*, **58**(2), 263–4.

Jankovic, J., Gilden, J. L., Hiner, B. C. *et al.* (1993a). Neurogenic orthostatic hypotension: a double-blind, placebo-controlled study with midodrine. *Am. J. Med.*, **95**, 38–48.

Jankovic, J., Rajput, A. H., Golbe, L. & Goodman, J. C. (1993b). What is it? Case 1. Parkinsonism, dysautonomia, and ophthalmoparesis. *Mov. Disord.*, **8**, 525–32.

Jaros, E. & Burn, D. J. (2000). The pathogenesis of multiple system atrophy: past, present and future. *Mov. Disord.*, **15**(5), 784–8.

Johnsen, J. A. & Miller, V. T. (1986). Tobacco intolerance in multiple system atrophy. *Neurology*, **36**, 986–8.

Kahle, P. J., Neumann, M., Ozmen, L. *et al.* (2002). Hyperphosphorylation and insolubility of alpha-synuclein in transgenic mouse oligodendrocytes. *EMBO Rep.*, **3**(6), 583–8.

Kan, A. E. (1978). Striatonigral degeneration. *Pathology*, **10**(1), 45–52.

Kato, S., Oda, M., Hayashi, H. *et al.* (1995). Decrease of medullary catecholaminergic neurons in multiple system atrophy and Parkinson's disease and their preservation in amyotrophic lateral sclerosis. *J. Neurol. Sci.*, **132**(2), 216–21.

Kaufmann, H., Oribe, E., Miller, M., Knott, P., Wiltshire-Clement, M. & Yahr, M. D. (1992). Hypotension-induced vasopressin release distinguishes between pure autonomic failure and multiple system atrophy with autonomic failure. *Neurology*, **42**(3), 590–3.

Kawamoto, Y., Nakamura, S., Akiguchi, I. & Kimura, J. (1999). Increased brain-derived neurotrophic factor-containing axons in the basal ganglia of patients with multiple system atrophy. *J. Neuropathol. Exp. Neurol.*, **58**(7), 765–72.

Kew, J., Gross, M. & Chapman, P. (1990). Shy–Drager syndrome presenting as isolated paralysis of vocal cord abductors. *Br. Med. J.*, **300**, 1441.

Kihara, M., Suganoya, J. & Takahashi, A. (1991). The assessment of sudomotor dysfunction in multiple system atrophy. *Clin. Auton. Res.*, **1**, 297–302.

Kikuchi, A., Takeda, A., Onodera, H. *et al.* (2002). Systemic increase of oxidative nucleic acid damage in Parkinson's disease and multiple system atrophy. *Neurobiol. Dis.*, **9**(2), 244–8.

Kim, Y. J., Ichise, M., Ballinger, J. R. *et al.* (2002). Combination of dopamine transporter and D2 receptor SPECT in the diagnostic evaluation of PD, MSA, and PSP. *Mov. Disord.*, **17**(2), 303–12.

Kimber, J. R., Watson, L. & Mathias, C. J. (1997). Distinction of idiopathic Parkinson's disease from multiple system atrophy by stimulation of growth-hormone release with clonidine. *The Lancet*, **349**, 1877–81.

Kimber, J., Watson, L. & Mathias, C. J. (1999a). Abnormal suppression of arginine-vasopressin by clonidine in multiple system atrophy. *Clin. Auton. Res.*, **9**(5), 271–4.

(1999b). Neuroendocrine responses to levodopa in multiple system atrophy (MSA). *Mov. Disord.*, **14**(6), 981–7.

Kimber, J., Mathias, C. J., Lees, A. J. *et al.* (2000). Physiological, pharmacological and neurohormonal assessment of autonomic function in progressive supranuclear palsy. *Brain*, **123**(7), 1422–30.

Kirby, R., Fowler, C. J., Gosling, J. & Bannister, R. (1986). Urethro-vesical dysfunction in progressive autonomic failure with multiple system atrophy. *J. Neurol. Neurosurg. Psychiatry*, **49**, 554–62.

Kiyosawa, K., Mokuno, K., Murakami, N. *et al.* (1993). Cerebrospinal fluid 28-kDa calbindin-D as a possible marker for Purkinje cell damage. *J. Neurol. Sci.*, **118**(1), 29–33.

Klein, C., Wenning, G. K. & Quinn, N. P. (1995). Pseudotransitory ischemic attacks as the initial symptom of multiple system atrophy. *Nervenarzt*, **66**(2), 133–5.

Klein, C., Brown, R., Wenning, G. & Quinn, N. (1997). The "cold hand sign" in multiple system atrophy. *Mov. Disord.*, **12**(4), 514–18.

Klockgether, T., Schroth, G., Diener, H. C. & Dichgans, J. (1990). Idiopathic cerebellar ataxia of late onset: natural history and MRI morphology. *J. Neurol. Neurosurg. Psychiatry*, **53**, 297–305.

Kluin, K. J., Gilman, S., Lohmann, M. & Junck, L. (1996). Characteristics of the dysarthria of multiple system atrophy. *Arch. Neurol.*, **53**, 545–8.

Kofler, M., Müller, J., Wenning, G. K. *et al.* (2001). The auditory startle reaction in parkinsonian disorders. *Mov. Disord.*, **16**(1), 62–71.

Kofler, M., Muller, J., Seppi, K. & Wenning, G. K. (2003). Exaggerated auditory startle responses in multiple system atrophy: a comparative study of parkinson and cerebellar subtypes. *Clin. Neurophysiol.*, **114**(3), 541–7.

Konagaya, M., Konagaya, Y., Honda, H. & Iida, M. (1993). A clinico-MRI study of extrapyramidal symptoms in multiple system atrophy – linear hyperintensity in the outer margin of the putamen. *No To Shinkei*, **45**(6), 509–13.

Konagaya, M., Konagaya, Y. & Iida, M. (1994). Clinical and magnetic resonance imaging study of extrapyramidal symptoms in multiple system atrophy. *J. Neurol. Neurosurg. Psychiatry*, **57**, 1528–31.

Konagaya, M., Sakai, M., Matsuoka, Y., Goto, Y., Yoshida, M. & Hashizume, Y. (1998). Patho-MR imaging study in the putaminal margin in multiple system atrophy. *No To Shinkei*, **50**(4), 383–5.

Konagaya, M., Sakai, M., Matsuoka, Y., Konagaya, Y. & Hashizume, Y. (1999). Multiple system atrophy with remarkable frontal lobe atrophy. *Acta Neuropathol. (Berl.)*, **97**(4), 423–8.

Konagaya, M., Konagaya, Y., Sakai, M., Matsuoka, Y. & Hashizume, Y. (2002). Progressive cerebral atrophy in multiple system atrophy. *J. Neurol. Sci.*, **195**(2), 123–7.

Konings, C. H., Kuiper, M. A., Teerlink, T., Mulder, C., Scheltens, P. & Wolters, E. C. (1999). Normal cerebrospinal fluid glutathione concentrations in Parkinson's disease, Alzheimer's disease and multiple system atrophy. *J. Neurol. Sci.*, **168**(2), 112–15.

Konno, H., Yamamoto, T., Iwasaki, Y. & Iizuka, H. (1986). Shy–Drager syndrome and amyotrophic lateral sclerosis. Cytoarchitectonic and morphometric studies of sacral autonomic neurons. *J. Neurol. Sci.*, **73**(2), 193–204.

Kraft, E., Schwarz, J., Trenkwalder, C., Vogl, T., Pfluger, T. & Oertel, W. H. (1999). The combination of hypointense and hyperintense signal changes on T_2-weighted magnetic resonance imaging sequences: a specific marker of multiple system atrophy? *Arch. Neurol.*, **56**(2), 225–8.

Kraft, E., Trenkwalder, C. & Auer, D. P. (2002). T_2^*-weighted MRI differentiates multiple system atrophy from Parkinson's disease. *Neurology*, **59**(8), 1265–7.

Krüger, R., Kuhn, W., Muller, T. *et al.* (1998). Ala30Pro mutation in the gene encoding alpha-synuclein in Parkinson's disease. *Nat. Genet.*, **18**(2), 106–8.

Krüger, R., Vieira-Saecker, A. M., Kuhn, W. *et al.* (1999). Increased susceptibility to sporadic Parkinson's disease by a certain combined alpha-synuclein/apolipoprotein E genotype. *Ann. Neurol.*, **45**(5), 611–17.

Kuiper, M. A., Visser, J. J., Bergmans, P. L., Scheltens, P. & Wolters, E. C. (1994). Decreased cerebrospinal fluid nitrate levels in Parkinson's disease, Alzheimer's disease and multiple system atrophy patients. *J. Neurol. Sci.*, **121**(2), 46–9.

Kuiper, M. A., Teerlink, T., Visser, J. J., Bergmans, P. L., Scheltens, P. & Wolters, E. C. (2000). L-glutamate, L-arginine and L-citrulline levels in cerebrospinal fluid of Parkinson's disease, multiple system atrophy, and Alzheimer's disease patients. *J. Neural Transm.*, **107**(2), 183–9.

Kume, A., Takahashi, A. & Hashizume, Y. (1993). Neuronal cell loss of the striatonigral system in multiple system atrophy. *J. Neurol. Sci.*, **117**(1–2), 33–40.

Lambie, C. G., Latham, O. & Mac Donald, G. L. (1947). Olivo-pontocerebellar atrophy (Marie's ataxia). *Med. J. Aust.*, **2**, 626–32.

Lang, A. E., Curran, T., Provias, J. & Bergeron, C. (1994). Striatonigral degeneration: iron deposition in putamen correlated with the slit-like void signal of magnetic resonance imaging. *Can. J. Neurol. Sci.*, **21**, 311–18.

Lang, A. E., Lozano, A., Duff, J. *et al.* (1997). Medial pallidotomy in late-stage Parkinson's disease and striatonigral degeneration. *Adv. Neurol.*, **74**, 199–211.

Langston, W. (1936). Orthostatic hypotension: report of a case. *Ann. Int. Med.*, **10**, 688–95.

Lantos, P. L. (1998). The definition of multiple system atrophy: a review of recent developments. *J. Neuropathol. Exp. Neurol.*, **57**, 1099–111.

Lees, A. J. (1999). The treatment of the motor disorders of multiple system atrophy. In *Autonomic Failure*, ed. C. J. Mathias & R. Bannister. Oxford: Oxford University Press, pp. 357–63.

Lees, A. J. & Bannister, R. (1981). The use of lisuride in the treatment of multiple system atrophy with autonomic failure (Shy Drager syndrome). *J. Neurol. Neurosurg. Psychiatry*, **44**, 347–51.

Leggo, J., Dalton, A., Morrison, P. J. *et al.* (1997). Analysis of spinocerebellar ataxia types 1,2,3, and 6, dentatorubral-pallidoluysian atrophy, and Friedreich's ataxia genes in spinocerebellar ataxia patients in the UK. *J. Med. Genet.*, **34**(12), 982–5.

Libelius, R. & Johannson, F. (2000). Quantitative electromyography of the external anal sphincter in Parkinson's disease and multiple system atrophy. *Muscle Nerve*, **23**(8), 1250–6.

Lindsay, R. M., Wiegand, S. J., Altar, C. A. & DiStefano, P. S. (1994). Neurotrophic factors: from molecule to man. *Trends Neurosci.*, **17**(5), 182–90.

Litvan, I., Agid, Y., Calne, D. *et al.* (1996). Clinical research criteria for the diagnosis of progressive supranuclear palsy (Steele–Richardson–Olszewski syndrome): report of the NINDS-SPSP international workshop. *Neurology*, **47**(1), 1–9.

Litvan, I., Goetz, C. G., Jankovic, J. *et al.* (1997). What is the accuracy of the clinical diagnosis of multiple system atrophy? A clinicopathologic study. *Arch. Neurol.*, **54**(8), 937–44.

Litvan, I., Booth, V., Wenning, G. K. *et al.* (1998). Retrospective application of a set of clinical diagnostic criteria for the diagnosis of multiple system atrophy. *J. Neural Transm.*, **105**(2–3), 217–27.

Low, P. A., Gilden, J. L., Freeman, R., Sheng, K. N. & McElligott, M. A. (1997). Efficacy of midodrine vs placebo in neurogenic orthostatic hypotension. A randomized, double-blind multicenter study. Midodrine Study Group. *J. Ann. Med. Assoc.*, **277**, 1046–51.

Magalhães, M., Wenning, G. K., Daniel, S. E. & Quinn, N. P. (1995). Autonomic dysfunction in pathologically confirmed multiple system atrophy and idiopathic Parkinson's disease – a retrospective comparison. *Acta Neurol. Scand.*, **91**, 98–102.

Mallipeddi, R. & Mathias, C. J. (1988). Raynaud's phenomenon after sympathetic denervation in patients with primary autonomic failure: questionnaire survey. *Br. Med. J.*, **316**(7129), 438–9.

Martignoni, E., Blandini, F., Petraglia, F., Pacchetti, C., Bono, G. & Nappi, G. (1992). Cerebrospinal fluid norepinephrine, 3-methoxy-4-hydroxyphenylglycol and neuropeptide Y levels in Parkinson's disease, multiple system atrophy and dementia of the Alzheimer type. *J. Neural Transm. Park Dis., Dement. Sect.*, **4**(3), 191–205.

Martinelli, P. & Coccagna, G. (1978). Etude electromyographique du sphincter strie de l'anus dans trois cas de syndrome de Shy-Drager. In *Electromyographie*, ed. L. Arbus & J. Cadilhac. Toulouse: Premières Journées Languedociènnes d'Electromyographie, 321–6.

Mathias, C. J. & Kimber, J. R. (1999). Postural hypotension: causes, clinical features, investigation, and management. *Annu. Rev. Med.*, **50**, 317–36.

Mathias, C. J., Fosbraey, P., da Costa, D. F., Thornley, A. & Bannister, R. (1986). The effect of desmopressin on nocturnal polyuria, overnight weight loss, and morning postural hypotension in patients with autonomic failure. *Br. Med. J. (Clin. Res. Ed.)*, **293**, 353–4.

Mathias, C. J., Senard, J. M., Braune, S. *et al.* (2001). L-threo-dihydroxyphenylserine (L-threo-DOPS; droxidopa) in the management of neurogenic orthostatic hypotension: a multinational, multi-center, dose-ranging study in multiple system atrophy and pure autonomic failure. *Clin. Auton. Res.*, **11**(4), 235–42.

McGuire, S. O., Ling, Z. D., Lipton, J. W., Sortwell, C. E., Collier, T. J. & Carvey, P. M. (2001). Tumor necrosis factor alpha is toxic to embryonic mesencephalic dopamine neurons. *Exp. Neurol.*, **169**(2), 219–30.

Meco, G., Gasparini, M. & Doricchi, F. (1996). Attentional functions in multiple system atrophy and Parkinson's disease. *J. Neurol. Neurosurg. Psychiatry*, **60**, 393–8.

Merlo, I. M., Occhini, A., Pacchetti, C. & Alfonsi, E. (2002). Not paralysis, but dystonia causes stridor in multiple system atrophy. *Neurology*, **58**(4), 649–52.

Mizutani, T., Satoh, J. & Morimatsu, Y. (1988). Neuropathological background of oculomotor disturbances in olivopontocerebellar atrophy with special reference to slow saccade. *Clin. Neuropathol.*, **7**(2), 53–61.

Mogi, M., Harada, M., Riederer, P., Narabayashi, H., Fujita, K. & Nagatsu, T. (1994). Tumor necrosis factor alpha (TNF-alpha) increases both in the brain and in the cerebrospinal fluid from parkinsonian patients. *Neurosci. Lett.*, **165**(1–2), 208–10.

Montagna, P., Martinelli, P., Rizzuto, N., Salviati, A., Rasi, F. & Lugaresi, E. (1983). Amyotrophy in Shy–Drager syndrome. *Acta Neurol. Belg.*, **83**, 142–57.

Morris, H. R., Vaughan, J. R., Datta, S. R. *et al.* (2000). Multiple system atrophy/progressive supranuclear palsy:

alpha-synuclein, synphilin, tau, and APOE. *Neurology*, **55**(12), 1918–20.

Moseley, M. L., Benzow, K. A., Schut, L. J. *et al.* (1998). Incidence of dominant spinocerebellar and Friedreich triplet repeats among 361 ataxia families. *Neurology*, **51**(6), 1666–71.

Müller, J., Wenning, G. K., Jellinger, K., McKee, A., Poewe, W. & Litvan, I. (2000). Progression of Hoehn and Yahr stages in parkinsonian disorders: a clinicopathologic study. *Neurology*, **55**(6), 888–91.

Müller, J., Wenning, G. K., Verny, M. *et al.* (2001). Progression of dysarthria and dysphagia in postmortem-confirmed parkinsonian disorders. *Arch. Neurol.*, **58**(2), 259–64.

Murer, M. G., Yan, Q. & Raisman-Vozari, R. (2000). Brain-derived neurotrophic factor in the control human brain, and in Alzheimer's disease and Parkinson's disease. *Prog. Neurobiol.*, **63**(1), 71–124.

Nakamura, S., Ohnishi, K., Nishimura, M. *et al.* (1996). Large neurons in the tuberomammillary nucleus in patients with Parkinson's disease and multiple system atrophy. *Neurology*, **46**(6), 1693–6.

Nakamura, T., Yamashita, H., Takahashi, T. & Nakamura, S. (2001). Activated Fyn phosphorylates alpha-synuclein at tyrosine residue 125. *Biochem. Biophys. Res. Commun.*, **280**(4), 1085–92.

Nee, L. E., Gomez, M. R., Dambrosia, J., Bale, S., Eldridge, R. & Polinsky, R. J. (1991). Environmental – occupational risk factors and familial associations in multiple system atrophy: a preliminary investigation. *Clin. Auton. Res.*, **1**(1), 9–13.

Negro, A., Brunati, A. M., Donella-Deana, A., Massimino, M. L. & Pinna, L. A. (2002). Multiple phosphorylation of alpha-synuclein by protein tyrosine kinase Syk prevents cosin-induced aggregation. *FASEB J.*, **16**(2), 210–12.

Neumann, M. A. (1977). Pontocerebellar atrophy combined with vestibular-reticular degeneration. *J. Neuropathol. Exp. Neurol.*, **36**(2), 321–37.

Nicholl, D. J., Bennett, P., Hiller, L. *et al.* (1999). A study of five candidate genes in Parkinson's disease and related neurodegenerative disorders. European Study Group on Atypical Parkinsonism. *Neurology*, **53**(7), 1415–21.

Nutt, J. G., Mrox, E. A., Leeman, S. E., Williams, A. C., Engel, W. K. & Chase, T. N. (1980). Substance P in human cerebrospinal fluid: reductions in peripheral neuropathy and autonomic dysfunction. *Neurology*, **30**(12), 1280–5.

O'Brien, C., Sung, J. H., McGeachie, R. E. & Lee, M. C. (1990). Striatonigral degeneration: clinical, MRI, and pathologic correlation. *Neurology*, **40**(4), 710–11.

Oertel, W. H., Wachter, T., Quinn, N. P., Ulm, G. & Brandstadter, D. (2003). Reduced genital sensitivity in female patients with multiple system atrophy of parkinsonian type. *Mov. Disord.*, **18**(4), 430–2.

Olanow, C. W. (1992). Magnetic resonance imaging in parkinsonism. *Neurol. Clin.*, **10**, 405–420.

Olanow, C. W. & Tatton, W. G. (1999). Etiology and pathogenesis of Parkinson's disease. *Annu. Rev. Neurosci.*, **22**, 123–44.

Oppenheimer, D. R. (1980). Lateral horn cells in progressive autonomic failure. *J. Neurol. Sci.*, **46**(3), 393–404.

Orimo, S., Ozawa, E., Nakade, S., Sugimoto, T. & Mizusawa, H. (1999). ^{123}I-metaiodobenzylguanidine myocardial scintigraphy in Parkinson's disease. *J. Neurol. Neurosurg. Psychiatry*, **67**(2), 189–94.

Orozco, G., Estrada, R., Perry, T. L. *et al.* (1989). Dominantly inherited olivopontocerebellar atrophy from eastern Cuba. Clinical, neuropathological, and biochemical findings. *J. Neurol. Sci.*, **93**(1), 37–50.

Osaki, Y., Wenning, G. K., Daniel, S. E. *et al.* (2002). Do published criteria improve clinical diagnostic accuracy in multiple system atrophy? *Neurology*, **59**(10), 1486–91.

Ostrerova, N., Petrucelli, L., Farrer, M. *et al.* (1999). alpha-synuclein shares physical and functional homology with 14-3-3 proteins. *J. Neurosci.*, **19**(14), 5782–91.

Ozaki, M., Sasner, M., Yano, R., Lu, H. S. & Buonanno, A. (1997). Neuregulin-beta induces expression of an NMDA-receptor subunit. *Nature*, **390**(6661), 691–4.

Ozawa, T., Takano, H., Onodera, O. *et al.* (1999). No mutation in the entire coding region of the alpha-synuclein gene in pathologically confirmed cases of multiple system atrophy. *Neurosci. Lett.*, **270**(2), 110–12.

Ozawa, T., Okuizumi, K., Ikeuchi, T., Wakabayashi, K., Takahashi, H. & Tsuji, S. (2001). Analysis of the expression level of alpha-synuclein mRNA using post-mortem brain samples from pathologically confirmed cases of multiple system atrophy. *Acta Neuropathol. (Berl.)*, **102**(2), 188–90.

Palace, J., Chandiramani, V. A. & Fowler, C. J. (1997). Value of sphincter electromyography in the diagnosis of multiple system atrophy. *Muscle & Nerve*, **20**(11), 1396–403.

Papp, M. I. & Lantos, P. L. (1992). Accumulation of tubular structures in oligodendroglial and neuronal cells as the basic alteration in multiple system atrophy. *J. Neurol. Sci.*, **107**(2), 172–82.

(1994). The distribution of oligodendroglial inclusions in multiple system atrophy and its relevance to clinical symptomatology. *Brain*, **117**(2), 235–43.

Papp, M. I., Kahn, J. E. & Lantos, P. L. (1989). Glial cytoplasmic inclusions in the CNS of patients with multiple system atrophy (striatonigral degeneration, olivopontocerebellar atrophy and Shy–Drager syndrome). *J. Neurol. Sci.*, **94**(1–3), 79–100.

Parati, E. A., Fetoni, V., Geminiani, G. C. *et al.* (1993). Response to L-Dopa in multiple system atrophy. *Clin. Neuropharmacol.*, **16**(2), 139–44.

Pastakia, B., Polinsky, R., Di Chiro, G. *et al.* (1989). Multiple system atrophy (Shy–Drager syndrome): MR imaging. *Radiology*, **159**, 499–502.

Pellecchia, M. T., Salvatore, E., Pivonello, R. *et al.* (2001). Stimulation of growth hormone release in multiple system atrophy, Parkinson's disease and idiopathic cerebellar ataxia. *Neurol. Sci.*, **22**(1), 79–80.

Perani, D., Bressi, S., Testa, D. *et al.* (1995). Clinical/metabolic correlations in multiple system atrophy. A fludeoxyglucose F18 Positron Emission Tomography Study. *Arch. Neurol.*, **52**, 179–85.

Perera, R., Isola, L. & Kaufmann, H. (1995). Effect of recombinant erythropoietin on anaemia and orthostatic hypotension in primary autonomic failure. *Clin. Auton. Res.*, **5**(4), 211–13.

Perez, D. (2001). Overstimulation of the alpha1B-adrenergic receptor causes a "seizure plus" syndrome. *Nat. Med.*, **7**(2), 132–3.

Pillon, B., Gouider-Khouja, N., Deweer, B. *et al.* (1995). Neuropsychological pattern of striatonigral degeneration: comparison with Parkinson's disease and progressive supranuclear palsy. *J. Neurol. Neurosurg. Psychiatry*, **58**, 174–9.

Pirker, W., Asenbaum, S., Bencsits, G. *et al.* (2000). (123I)beta-CIT SPECT in multiple system atrophy, progressive supranuclear palsy, and corticobasal degeneration. *Mov. Disord.*, **15**(6), 1158–67.

Pirker, W., Djamshidian, S., Asenbaum, S. *et al.* (2002). Progression of dopaminergic degeneration in Parkinson's disease and atypical parkinsonism: a longitudinal beta-CIT SPECT study. *Mov. Disord.*, **17**(1), 45–53.

Plaitakis, A., Flessas, P., Natsiou, A. B. & Shashidharan, P. (1993). Glutamate dehydrogenase deficiency in cerebellar degenerations: clinical, biochemical and molecular genetic aspects. *Can. J. Neurol. Sci.*, **20**(Suppl 3), S109–16.

Plazzi, G., Corsini, R. & Provini, F. (1997). REM sleep behavior disorders in multiple system atrophy. *Neurology*, **48**, 1094–7.

Polinsky, R. J., Brown, R. T., Lee, G. K. *et al.* (1987). Beta-endorphin, ACTH, and catecholamine responses in chronic autonomic failure. *Ann. Neurol.*, **21**(6), 573–7.

Polinsky, R. J., Kopin, I. J., Ebert, M. H. & Weise, V. (1981). Pharmacologic distinction of different orthostatic hypotension syndromes. *Neurology*, **31**(1), 1–7.

Polinsky, R. J., Taylor, I. L., Chew, P., Weise, V. & Kopin, L. J. (1982). Pancreatic polypeptide responses to hypoglycaemia in chronic autonomic failure. *J. Clin. Endocrinol. Metab.*, **54**(1), 48–52.

Polinsky, R. J., McRae, A., Baser, S. M. & Dahlstrom, A. (1991). Antibody in the CSF of patients with multiple system atrophy reacts specifically with rat locus ceruleus. *Neurol. Sci.*, **106**(1), 96–104.

Polymeropoulos, M. H., Lavedan, C., Leroy, E. *et al.* (1997). Mutation in the alpha-synuclein gene identified in families with Parkinson's disease. *Science*, **276**(5321), 2045–7.

Powell, S. K., Williams, C. C., Nomizu, M., Yamada, Y. & Kleinman, H. K. (1998). Laminin-like proteins are differentially regulated during cerebellar development and stimulate granule cell neurite outgrowth in vitro. *J. Neurosci. Res.*, **54**(2), 233–47.

Pramstaller, P., Wenning, G. K., Smith, S. J. M., Beck, R. O., Quinn, N. P. & Fowler, C. J. (1995). Nerve conduction studies, skeletal muscle EMG, and sphincter EMG in multiple system atrophy. *J. Neurol. Neurosurg. Psychiatry*, **58**, 618–21.

Price, R. H., Albin, R. L., Sakurai, S. Y., Polinsky, R. J., Penney, J. B. & Young, A. B. (1993). Cerebellar excitatory and inhibitory amino acid receptors in multiple system atrophy. *Neurology*, **43**(7), 1323–8.

Quik, M., Spokes, E. G., Mackay, A. V. & Bannister, R. (1979). Alterations in [3H]spiperone binding in human caudate nucleus, substantia nigra and frontal cortex in the Shy–Drager syndrome and Parkinson's disease. *J. Neurol. Sci.*, **43**(3), 429–37.

Quinn, N. (1989a). Disproportionate antecollis in multiple system atrophy. *Lancet*, **1**(8642), 844.

(1989b). Multiple system atrophy – the nature of the beast. *J. Neurol. Neurosurg. Psychiatry*, **52**(Suppl.), 78–89.

(1994). Multiple system atrophy. In *Movement Disorders 3*, ed. C. D. Marsden & S. Fahn. London: Butterworth-Heinemann, pp. 262–81.

Quinn, N. P., Wenning, G. & Marsden, C. D. (1995). The Shy–Drager syndrome. What did Shy and Drager really describe? *Arch. Neurol.*, **52**(7), 656–7.

Raabe, T. D., Suy, S., Welcher, A. & DeVries, G. H. (1997). Effect of neu differentiation factor isoforms on neonatal oligodendrocyte function. *J. Neurosci. Res.*, **50**(5), 755–68.

Raimbach, S. J., Cortelli, P., Kooner, J. S., Bannister, R., Bloom, S. R. & Mathias, C. J. (1989). Prevention of glucose-induced hypotension by the somatostatin analogue octreotide (SMS 201–995) in chronic autonomic failure: haemodynamic and hormonal changes. *Clin. Sci. (Lond.)*, **77**, 623–8.

Rajput, A. H., Rozdilsky, B., Rajput, A. & Ang, L. (1990). Levodopa efficacy and pathological basis of Parkinson syndrome. *Clin. Neuropharmacol.*, **13**(6), 553–8.

Ranum, L. P., Lundgren, J. K., Schut, L. J. *et al.* (1995). Spinocerebellar ataxia type 1 and Machado–Joseph-disease: incidence of CAG expansions among adult-onset ataxia patients from 311 families with dominant, recessive, or sporadic ataxia. *Am. J. Hum. Genet.*, **57**(3), 603–8.

Rascol, O., Sabatini, U., Simonetta-Moreau, M., Montastruc, J. L., Rascol, A. & Clanet, M. (1991). Square wave jerks in Parkinsonian syndromes. *J. Neurol. Neurosurg. Psychiatry*, **54**, 599–602.

Rascol, O., Sabatini, U., Fabre, N. *et al.* (1995). Abnormal vestibuloocular reflex cancellation in multiple system atrophy and progressive supranuclear palsy but not in Parkinson's disease. *Mov. Disord.*, **10**(2), 163–70.

Riley, D. E. & Chelimsky, T. C. (2003). Autonomic nervous system testing may not distinguish multiple system atrophy from Parkinson's disease. *J. Neurol. Neurosurg. Psychiatry*, **74**(1), 56–60.

Rinne, J. O., Burn, D. J., Mathias, C. J., Quinn, N. P., Marsden, C. D. & Brooks, D. J. (1995). Positron emission tomography studies on the dopaminergic system and striatal opioid binding in the olivopontocerebellar atrophy variant of multiple system atrophy. *Ann. Neurol.*, **37**, 568–73.

Rivest, J., Quinn, N. & Marsden, C. D. (1990). Dystonia in Parkinson's disease, multiple system atrophy, and progressive supranuclear palsy. *Neurology*, **40**, 1571–8.

Robbins, T. W., James, M., Lange, K. W., Owen, A. M., Quinn, N. P. & Marsden, C. D. (1992). Cognitive performance in multiple system atrophy. *Brain*, **115**(1), 271–91.

Sakakibara, R., Hattori, T., Uchiyama, T. *et al.* (2000a). Urinary dysfunction and orthostatic hypotension in multiple system atrophy: which is the more common and earlier manifestation? *J. Neurol. Neurosurg. Psychiatry*, **68**(1), 65–9.

Sakakibara, R., Hattori, T., Uchiyama, T. *et al.* (2000b). Are alpha-blockers involved in lower urinary tract dysfunction in multiple system atrophy? A comparison of prazosin and moxisylyte. *J. Auton. Nerv. Syst.*, **79**, 191–5.

Salazar, G., Valls-Sole, J., Marti, M. J., Chang, H. & Tolosa, E. S. (2000). Postural and action myoclonus in patients with parkinsonian type of multiple system atrophy. *Mov. Disord.*, **15**(1), 77–83.

Sandroni, P., Ahlskog, J. E., Fealy, R. D. & Low, P. A. (1991). Autonomic involvement in extrapyramidal and cerebellar disorders. *Clin. Auton. Res.*, **1**, 147–55.

Santens, P., Crevits, L. & van der Linden, C. (1996). Raynaud's phenomenon in a case of multiple system atrophy. *Mov. Disord.*, **11**, 586–8.

Satoh, J. I. & Kuroda, Y. (2001). Alpha-synuclein expression is upregulated in NTera2 cells during neuronal differentiation but unaffected by exposure to cytokines and neurotrophic features. *Parkinsonism Relat. Disord.*, **8**(1), 7–17.

Savoiardo, M., Strada, L. & Girotti, F. (1990). Olivopontocerebellar atrophy: MR diagnosis and relationship to multisystem atrophy. *Radiology*, **174**, 693–6.

Schelhaas, H. J., Hageman, G. & Post, J. G. (1997). Cerebellar ataxia, dementia, pyramidal signs, cortical cataract of the posterior pole and a raised IgG index in a patient with a sporadic form of olivopontocerebellar atrophy. *Clin. Neurol. Neurosurg.*, **99**(2), 99–101.

Schelosky, L., Hierholzer, J., Wissel, J., Cordes, M. & Poewe, W. (1993). Correlation of clinical response in apomorphine test with D2-receptor status as demonstrated by 123I IBZM-SPECT. *Mov. Disord.*, **8**(4), 453–8.

Scherer, H. J. (1933a). Beiträge zur pathologischen Anatomie des Kleinhirns. III. Mitteilung: Genuine Kleinhirnatrophien. *Z. Gesamte. Neurol. Psychiatrie*, **145**, 335–405.

(1933b). Extrapyramidale Störungen bei der olivopontocerebellären Atrophie. *Z. Gesamte. Neurol. Psychiatrie*, **145**, 406–19.

Scherfler, C., Puschban, Z., Ghorayeb, I. *et al.* (2000). Complex motor disturbances in a sequential double lesion rat model of striatonigral degeneration (multiple system atrophy). *Neuroscience*, **99**(1), 43–54.

Schocke, M., Seppi, K., Esterhammer, R. *et al.* (2002). Diffusion-weighted MRI differentiates the Parkinson variant of multiple system atrophy from PD. *Neurology*, **58**(4), 575–80.

Schöls, L., Szymanski, S., Peters, S. *et al.* (2000). Genetic background of apparently idiopathic sporadic cerebellar ataxia. *Hum. Genet.*, **107**(2), 132–7.

Schrag, A., Kingsley, D., Phatouros, C. *et al.* (1998). Clinical usefulness of magnetic resonance imaging in multiple system atrophy. *J. Neurol. Neurosurg. Psychiatry*, **65**(1), 65–71.

Schrag, A., Ben-Shlomo, Y. & Quinn, N. P. (1999). Prevalence of progressive supranuclear palsy and multiple system atrophy: a cross-sectional study. *Lancet*, **354**, 1771–5.

Schrag, A., Good, C. D., Miszkiel, K. *et al.* (2000). Differentiation of atypical parkinsonian syndromes with routine MRI. *Neurology*, **54**(3), 697–702.

Schulz, J. B., Klockgether, T., Petersen, D. *et al.* (1994). Multiple system atrophy: natural history, MRI morphology, and dopamine receptor imaging with 123IBZM-SPECT. *J. Neurol. Neurosurg. Psychiatry*, **57**(9), 1047–56.

Schulz, J. B., Skalej, M., Wedekind, D. *et al.* (1999). Magnetic resonance imaging-based volumetry differentiates idiopathic Parkinson's syndrome from multiple system atrophy and progressive supranuclear palsy. *Ann. Neurol.*, **45**, 65–74.

Schwarz, J., Tatsch, K., Arnold, G. *et al.* (1992). 123I-iodobenzamide-SPECT predicts dopaminergic responsiveness in patients with de novo parkinsonism. *Neurology*, **42**, 556–61.

Schwarz, J., Tatsch, K., Arnold, G. *et al.* (1993). 123I-iodobenzamide-SPECT in 83 patients with de novo parkinsonism. *Neurology*, **43**, 17–20.

Schwarz, J., Weis, S. & Kraft, E. (1996). Signal changes on MRI and increases in reactive microgliosis, astrogliosis, and iron in the putamen of two patients with multiple system atrophy. *J. Neurol. Neurosurg. Psychiatry*, **60**, 98–101.

Schwarz, J., Tatsch, K., Gasser, T. *et al.* (1998). 123I-IBZM binding compared with long-term clinical follow up in patients with de novo parkinsonism. *Mov. Disord.*, **13**(1), 16–19.

Seppi, K., Puschban, Z., Stefanova, N. *et al.* (2001). Overstimulation of the alpha1B-adrenergic receptor causes a "seizure plus" syndrome. *Nat. Med.*, **7**(2), 132.

Seppi, K., Schocke, M. F., Esterhammer, R. *et al.* (2003). Diffusion-weighted imaging discriminates progressive supranuclear palsy from PD, but not from the parkinson variant of multiple system atrophy. *Neurology*, **60**(6), 922–7.

Shinotoh, H., Aotsuka, A., Inoue, O. *et al.* (1991). Imaging of dopamine D1 and D2 receptors by a high resolution positron emission tomography. *Adv. Exp. Med. Biol.*, **287**, 294–53.

Shinotoh, H., Inoue, O., Hirayama, K. *et al.* (1993). Dopamine D1 receptors in Parkinson's disease and striatonigral degeneration: a positron emission tomography study. *J. Neurol. Neurosurg. Psychiatry*, **56**(5), 467–72.

Shy, G. M & Drager, G. A. (1960). A neurological syndrome associated with orthostatic hypotension. A clinicopathological study. *Arch. Neurol.*, **2**, 511–27.

Silber, M. H. & Levine, S. (2000). Stridor and death in multiple system atrophy. *Mov. Disord.*, **15**(4), 699–704.

Silveira, I., Lopes-Cendes, I., Kish, S. *et al.* (1996). Frequency of spinocerebellar ataxia type 1, dentatorubropallidoluysian atrophy, and Machado–Joseph disease mutations in a large group of spinocerebellar ataxia patients. *Neurology*, **46**(1), 214–18.

Sima, A. A. F., Caplan, M., D'Amato, C. J., Pevzner, M. & Furlong, J. W. (1993). Fulminant multiple system atrophy in a young adult presenting as motor neuron disease. *Neurology*, **43**, 2031–5.

Spillantini, M. G., Schmidt, M. L., Lee, V. M., Trojanowski, J. Q., Jakes, R. & Goedert, M. (1979). Alpha-synuclein in Lewy bodies. *Nature*, **388**(6645), 839–40.

Spillantini, M. G., Crowther, R. A., Jakes, R., Cairns, N. J., Lantos, P. L. & Goedert, M. (1998). Filamentous alpha-synuclein inclusions link multiple system atrophy with Parkinson's disease and dementia with Lewy bodies. *Neurosci. Lett.*, **251**(3), 205–8.

Spokes, E. G., Bannister, R. & Oppenheimer, D. R. (1979). Multiple system atrophy with autonomic failure: clinical, histological and neurochemical observations on four cases. *J. Neurol. Sci.*, **43**(1), 59–82.

Stauffenberg, (1918). Zur Kenntnis des extrapyramidalen motorischen Systems und Mitteilung eines Falles von sog. "Atrophie olivo-pontocérébelleuse". *Z. Gesamte. Neurol. Psychiatrie*, **39**, 1–55.

Stefanis, L., Kholodilov, N., Ridcout, H. J., Burke, R. E. & Greene, L. A. (2001). Synuclein-1 is selectively up-regulated in response to nerve growth factor treatment in PC12 cells. *J. Neurochem.*, **76**(4), 1165–76.

Stell, R. & Bronstein, A. M. (1994). Eye abnormalities in extrapyramidal diseases. In *Movement Disorders 3*, ed. C. D. Marsden & S. Fahn. London: Butterworth-Heinemann, pp. 88–113.

Stern, M. B., Braffman, B. H., Skolnick, B. E., Hurtig, H. I. & Grossman, R. I. (1989). Magnetic resonance imaging in Parkinson's disease and parkinsonian syndromes. *Neurology*, **39**, 1524–6.

Stocchi, F., Badiali, D., Vacca, L. *et al.* (2000). Anorectal function in multiple system atrophy and Parkinson's disease. *Mov. Disord.*, **15**(1), 71–6.

Strijks, E., van't Hof, M., Sweep, F., Lenders, J. W., Oyen, W. J. & Horstink, M. W. (2002). Stimulation of growth-hormone release with clonidine does not distinguish individual cases of idiopathic Parkinson's disease from those with striatonigral degeneration. *J. Neurol.*, **249**(9), 1206–10.

Suemaru, S., Suemaru, K., Kawai, K. *et al.* (1995). Cerebrospinal fluid corticotrophin-releasing hormone in neurodegenerative diseases: reduction in spinocerebellar degeneration. *Life Sci.*, **57**(24), 2231–5.

Sung, J. H., Mastri, A. R. & Segal, E. (1979). Pathology of Shy–Drager syndrome. *J. Neuropathol. Exp. Neurol.*, **38**(4), 353–68.

Takahashi, M., Ohta, S., Matsuoka, S., Mori, H. & Mizuno, Y. (2002). Mixed multiple system atrophy and progressive supranuclear palsy: a clinical and pathological report of one case. *Acta Neuropathol. (Berl.)*, **103**(1), 82–7.

Takatsu, H., Nagashima, K., Murase, M., Fujiwara, H., Nishida, H. & Matsuo, H. (2000). Differentiating Parkinson disease from multiple-system atrophy by measuring cardiac iodine-123 metaiodobenzymguanidine accumulation. *J. Am. Med. Assoc.*, **284**(1), 44–5.

Taki, J., Nakajima, K., Hwang, E. H., Matsunari, I., Komai, K. & Yoshita, M. (2000). Peripheral sympathetic dysfunction in patients with Parkinson's disease without autonomic failure is heart selective and disease specific. *Eur. J. Nucl. Med.*, **27**, 566–73.

Testa, D., Filippini, G., Farinotti, M., Palazzini, E. & Caraceni, T. (1996). Survival in multiple system atrophy: a study of prognostic factors in 59 cases. *J. Neurol.*, **243**, 401–4.

Thobois, S., Broussolle, E., Toureille, L. & Vial, C. (2001). Severe dysphagia after botulinum toxin injection for cervical dystonia in multiple system atrophy. *Mov. Disord.*, **16**, 764–5.

Tison, F., Wenning, G. K., Daniel, S. E. & Quinn, N. (1995a). The pathophysiology of parkinsonism in multiple system atrophy. *Eur. J. Neurol.*, **2**, 435–44.

Tison, F., Wenning, G. K., Quinn, N. P. & Smith, S. J. (1995b). REM sleep behaviour disorder as the presenting symptom of multiple system atrophy. *J. Neurol. Neurosurg. Psychiatry*, **58**(3), 379–80.

Tison, F., Arne, P., Sourgen, C., Chrysostome, V. & Yeklef, F. (2000a). The value of external anal sphincter electromyography for the diagnosis of multiple system atrophy. *Mov. Disord.*, **15**(6), 1148–57.

Tison, F., Yekhlef, F., Chrysostome, V. & Sourgen, C. (2000b). Prevalence of multiple system atrophy. *Lancet*, **355**(9202), 495–6.

Togo, T., Iseki, E., Marui, W., Akiyama, H., Ueda, K. & Kosaka, K. (2001). Glial involvement in the degeneration process of Lewy body-bearing neurons and the degradation process of Lewy bodies in brains of dementia with Lewy bodies. *J. Neurol. Sci.*, **184**(1), 71–5.

Tranchant, C., Guiraud-Chaumeil, C., Echaniz-Laguna, A. & Warter, J. M. (2000). Is clonidine growth hormone stimulation a good test to differentiate multiple system atrophy from idiopathic Parkinson's disease? *J. Neurol.*, **247**(11), 853–6.

Trenkwalder, C., Schwarz, J., Gebhard, J. *et al.* (1995). Starnberg trial on epidemiology of parkinsonism and hypertension in the elderly. Prevalence of Parkinson's disease and related disorders assessed by a door-to-door survey of inhabitants older than 65 years. *Arch. Neurol.*, **52**, 1017–22.

Trojanowski, J. Q. (2002). Tauists, baptists, syners, apostates, and new data. *Ann. Neurol.*, **52**(3), 263–5.

Tsuchiya, K., Ozawa, E., Haga, C. *et al.* (2000). Constant involvement of the Betz cells and pyramidal tract in multiple system atrophy: a clinicopathological study of seven autopsy cases. *Acta Neuropathol. (Berl.)*, **99**(6), 628–36.

Tsuda, T., Onodera, H., Okabe, S., Kikuchi, Y. & Itoyama, Y. (2002). Impaired chemosensitivity to hypoxia is a marker of multiple system atrophy. *Ann. Neurol.*, **52**(3), 367–71.

Tu, P. H., Galvin, J. E., Baba, M. *et al.* (1998). Glial cytoplasmatic inclusions in white matter oligodendrocytes of multiple system atrophy brains contain insoluble alpha-synuclein. *Ann. Neurol.*, **44**(3), 415–22.

Urenjak, J., Williams, S. R., Gadian, D. G. & Noble, M. (1993). Proton nuclear magnetic resonance spectroscopy unambiguously identifies different neuronal cell types. *J. Neurosci.*, **13**, 981–9.

Uversky, V. N. & Fink, A. L. (2002). Amino acid determinants of alpha-synuclein aggregation: putting together pieces of the puzzle. *FEBS Lett.*, **522**(1–3), 9–13.

Uversky, V. N., Li, J., Souillac, P. *et al.* (2002). Biophysical properties of the synucleins and their propensities to fibrillate: inhibition of alpha-synuclein assembly by beta- and gamma-synucleins. *J. Biol. Chem.*, **277**(14), 11970–8.

Valldeoriola, F., Valls-Sole, J., Tolosa, E. S. & Marti, M. J. (1995). Striated anal sphincter denervation in patients with progressive supranuclear palsy. *Mov. Disord.*, **10**(5), 550–5.

Vanacore, N., Bonifati, V., Fabbrini, G. *et al.* (2000). Smoking habits in multiple system atrophy and progressive supranuclear palsy. *Neurology*, **54**, 114–19.

Vanacore, N., Bonifati, V., Fabbrini, G. *et al*. (ESGAP) (2004). Case-control study of multiple system atrophy. *Mov. Disord.* (in press).

van der Eecken, H., Adams, R. D. & van Bogaert, L. (1960). Striopallidal-nigral degeneration. A hitherto undescribed lesion in paralysis agitans. *J. Neuropathol. Exp. Neurol.*, **19**, 159–61.

van Royen, E., Verhoeff, N. F., Speelman, J. D., Wolters, E. C., Kuiper, M. A. & Janssen, A. G. (1993). Multiple system atrophy and progressive supranuclear palsy. Diminished striatal D2 dopamine receptor activity demonstrated by 123I-IBZM single photon emission computed tomography. *Arch. Neurol.*, **50**(5), 513–16.

Varrone, A., Marek, K. L., Jennings, D., Innis, R. B. & Seibyl, J. P. (2001). (123)I-beta-CIT SPECT imaging demonstrates reduced density of striatal dopamine transporters in Parkinson's disease and multiple system atrophy. *Mov. Disord.*, **16**, 1023–32.

Vartanian, T., Corfas, G., Li, Y., Fischbach, G. D. & Stefansson, K. (1994). A role for the acetylcholine receptor-inducing protein ARIA in oligodendrocyte development. *Proc. Natl Acad. Sci., USA*, **91**(24), 11626–30.

Vartanian, T., Goodearl, A., Vichover, A. & Fischbach, G. (1997). Axonal neuregulin signals cells of the oligodendrocyte lineage through activation of HER4 and Schwann cells through HER2 and HER3. *J. Cell. Biol.*, **137**(1), 211–20.

Vidailhet, M., Rivaud, S., Gouider-Khouja, N. *et al*. (1994). Eye movements in parkinsonian syndromes. *Ann. Neurol.*, **35**, 420–6.

Vila, M., Jackson-Lewis, V., Guegan, C. *et al*. (2001). The role of glial cells in Parkinson's disease. *Curr. Opin. Neurol.*, **14**(4), 483–9.

Visser-Vandewalle, V., Temel, Y., Colle, H. & van der Linden, C. (2003). Bilateral high-frequency stimulation of the subthalamic nucleus in patients with multiple system atrophy – parkinsonism. Report of four cases. *J. Neurosurg.*, **98**(4), 882–7.

Vodusek, B. (2001). Sphincter EMG and differential diagnosis of multiple system atrophy. *Mov. Disord.*, **16**(4), 600–7.

Vogels, O. J., Veltman, J., Oyen, W. J. & Horstink, M. W. (2000). Decreased striatal dopamine D2 receptor binding in amyotrophic lateral sclerosis (ALS) and multiple system atrophy (MSA): D2 receptor down-regulation versus striatal cell degeneration. *J. Neurol. Sci.*, **180**(1–2), 62–5.

Wakabayashi, K., Hayashi, S., Kakita, A. *et al*. (1998a). Accumulation of alpha-synuclein/NACP is a cytopathological feature common to Lewy body disease and multiple system atrophy. *Acta Neuropathol. (Berl.)*, **96**(5), 445–52.

Wakabayashi, K., Ikeuchi, T., Ishikawa, A. & Takahashi, H. (1998b). Multiple system atrophy with severe involvement of the motor cortical areas and cerebral white matter. *J. Neurol. Sci.*, **156**(1), 114–17.

Wakabayashi, K., Yoshimoto, M., Tsuji, S. & Takahashi, H. (1998c). Alpha-synuclein immunoreactivity in glial cytoplasmic inclusions in multiple system atrophy. *Neurosci. Lett.*, **249**(2–3), 180–2.

Wakabayashi, K., Engelender, S., Yoshimoto, M., Tsuji, S., Ross, C. A. & Takahashi, H. (2000). Synphilin-1 is present in Lewy bodies in Parkinson's disease. *Ann. Neurol.*, **47**(4), 521–3.

Wakabayashi, K., Engelender, S., Tanaka, Y. *et al*. (2002). Immunocytochemical localization of synphilin-1, an alpha-synuclein-associated protein, in neurodegenerative disorders. *Acta Neuropathol. (Berl.)*, **103**(3), 209–14.

Wakai, M., Kume, A., Takahashi, A., Ando, T. & Hashizume, Y. (1994). A study of parkinsonism in multiple system atrophy: clinical and MRI correlation. *Acta Neurol. Scand.*, **90**, 225–31.

Waldner, R., Puschban, Z., Scherfler, C., Seppi, K., Jellinger, K. & Poewe, W. (2001). No functional effects of embryonic neuronal grafts on motor deficits in a 3-nitropropionic acid rat model of advanced striatonigral degeneration (multiple system atrophy). *Neuroscience*, **102**(3), 581–92.

Watanabe, H., Saito, Y., Terao, S. *et al*. (2002). Progression and prognosis in multiple system atrophy: an analysis of 230 Japanese patients. *Brain*, **125**, 1070–83.

Wenning, G. K., Wagner, S., Daniel, S. E. & Quinn, N. P. (1993). Multiple system atrophy: sporadic or familial? *Lancet*, **342**(8872), 681.

Wenning, G. K., Ben Shlomo, Y., Magalhaes, M., Daniel, S. E. & Quinn, N. P. (1994a). Clinical features and natural history of multiple system atrophy. An analysis of 100 cases. *Brain*, **117**(4), 835–45.

Wenning, G. K., Quinn, N., Magalhaes, M., Mathias, C. & Daniel, S. E. (1994b). "Minimal change" multiple system atrophy. *Mov. Disord.*, **9**(2), 161–6.

Wenning, G. K. & Geser, F. (2003). Atrophie multisystematisee. *Rev. Neurol. (Paris)*, **159**(5 Pt 2), 31–8.

Wenning, G. & Quinn, N. (1994). Are Lewy bodies non-specific epiphenomena of nigral damage? *Mov. Disord.*, **9**(3), 378–9.

Wenning, G. K. & Quinn, N. P. (1997a). Multiple system atrophy. In *Bailliere's Clin. Neurol.*, ed. N. P. Quinn, **6**, 187–204.

Wenning, G. K. & Smith, S. J. M. (1997b). Magnetic brain stimulation in multiple system atrophy. *Mov. Disord.*, **12**(3), 452–3.

Wenning, G. K., Ben-Shlomo, Y., Magalhaes, M., Daniel, S. E. & Quinn, N. P. (1995). Clinicopathological study of 35 cases of multiple system atrophy. *J. Neurol. Neurosurg. Psychiatry*, **58**, 160–6.

Wenning, G. K., Granata, R., Laboyrie, P. M., Quinn, N. P., Jenner, P. & Marsden, C. D. (1996a). Reversal of behavioural abnormalities by fetal allografts in a novel rat model of striatonigral degeneration. *Mov. Disord.*, **11**(5), 522–32.

Wenning, G. K., Quinn, N. P., Daniel, S. E., Garratt, H. & Marsden, C. D. (1996b). Facial dystonia in pathologically proven multiple system atrophy: a video report. *Mov. Disord.*, **11**(1), 107–9.

Wenning, G. K., Tison, F., Elliott, L., Quinn, N. P. & Daniel, S. E. (1996c). Olivopontocerebellar pathology in multiple system atrophy. *Mov. Disord.*, **11**(2), 157–62.

Wenning, G. K., Kraft, E., Beck, R. *et al*. (1997a). Cerebellar presentation of multiple system atrophy. *Mov. Disord.*, **12**(1), 115–17.

Wenning, G. K., Tison, F., Ben Shlomo, Y., Daniel, S. E. & Quinn, N. P. (1997b). Multiple system atrophy: a review of 203 pathologically proven cases. *Mov. Disord.*, **12**(2), 133–47.

Wenning, G. K., Ebersbach, G., Verny, M. *et al.* (1999a). Progression of falls in postmortem-confirmed parkinsonian disorders. *Mov. Disord.*, **14**, 947–50.

Wenning, G. K., Granata, R., Puschban, Z., Scherfler, C. & Poewe, W. (1999b). Neural transplantation in animal models of multiple system atrophy: a review. *J. Neural Transm.*, **55**, 103–13.

Wenning, G. K., Scherfler, C., Granata, R., Bösch, S., Verny, M. & Chaudhuri, K. R. (1999c). Time course of symptomatic orthostatic hypotension and urinary incontinence in patients with postmortem confirmed parkinsonian syndromes: a clinicopathological study. *J. Neurol. Neurosurg. Psychiatry*, **67**, 620–3.

Wenning, G. K., Ben-Shlomo, Y., Hughes, A., Daniel, S. E., Lees, A. J. & Quinn, N. P. (2000a). What clinical features are most useful to distinguish definite multiple system atrophy from Parkinson's disease? *J. Neurol. Neurosurg. Psychiatry*, **68**(4), 434–40.

Wenning, G. K., Jellinger, K. J., Quinn, N. P. & Poewe, W. H. (2000b). An early report of striatonigral degeneration. *Mov. Disord.*, **15**(1), 159–62.

Wenning, G. K., Tison, F., Scherfler, C. *et al.* (2000c). Towards neurotransplantation in multiple system atrophy: clinical rationale, pathophysiological basis, and preliminary experimental evidence. *Cell Transpl.*, **9**, 279–88.

Wenning, G. K., Seppi, K., Sampaio, C., Quinn, N. P., Poewe, W. & Tison, F. (2002). European Multiple System Atrophy Study Group (EMSA-SG): Validation of the Unified MSA Rating Scale (UMSARS). *Mov. Disord.*, **17**(Suppl 5), 252.

Wenning, G. K., Geser, F. & Poewe, W. (2003a). The 'risus sardonicus' of multiple system atrophy. *Mov. Disord.*, **18**(10), 1211.

Wenning, G. K., Geser, F., Stampfer-Kountchev, M. & Tison, F. (2003b). Multiple system atrophy: an update. *Mov. Disord.*, **18** (suppl. 6), S34–42.

Wermuth, L., Joensen, P., Bunger, N. & Jeune, B. (1997). High prevalence of Parkinson's disease in the Faroe Islands. *Neurology*, **49**, 426–32.

Wiedemann, P., Bonisch, H., Oerters, F. & Bruss, M. (2002). Structure of the human histamine H3 receptor gene (HRH3) and identification of naturally occurring variations. *J. Neural Transm.*, **109**(4), 443–53.

Williams, A., Hanson, D. & Calne, D. B. (1979). Vocal cord paralysis in the Shy–Drager syndrome. *J. Neurol. Neurosurg. Psychiatry*, **42**, 151–3.

Winkler, A. S., Marsden, J., Parton, M., Watkins, P. J. & Chaudhuri, K. R. (2001). Erythropoietin deficiency and anaemia in multiple system atrophy. *Mov. Disord.*, **16**, 233–9.

Wright, R. A., Kaufmann, H. C., Perera, R. *et al.* (1998). A double-blind, dose response study of midodrine in neurogenic orthostatic hypotension. *Neurology*, **51**(1), 120–4.

Wüllner, U., Klockgether, T., Petersen, D., Naegele, T. & Dichgans, J. (1993). Magnetic resonance imaging in hereditary and idiopathic ataxia. *Neurology*, **43**, 318–25.

Yamada, T. & McGeer, P. L. (1990). Oligodendroglial microtubular masses: an abnormality observed in some human neurodegenerative diseases. *Neurosci. Lett.*, **120**(2), 163–6.

Yang, X., Kuo, Y., Devay, P., Yu, C. & Role, L. (1998). A cysteine-rich isoform of neuregulin controls the level of expression of neuronal nicotinic receptor channels during synaptogenesis. *Neuron*, **20**(2), 255–70.

Yekhlef, F., Ballan, G., Macia, F., Delmer, O., Sourgen, C. & Tison, F. (2003). Routine MRI for the differential diagnosis of Parkinson's disease, MSA, PSP, and CBD. *J. Neural Transm.*, **110**(2), 151–69.

Yoshita, M. (1998). Differentiation of idiopathic Parkinson's disease from striatonigral degeneration and progressive supranuclear palsy using iodine-123 meta-iodobenzylguanidine myocardial scintigraphy. *J. Neurol. Sci.*, **155**, 60–7.

Yuan, J. & Yankner, B. A. (2000). Apoptosis in the nervous system. *Nature*, **407**(6805), 802–9.

Zesiewicz, T. A., Helal, M. & Hauser, R. A. (2002). Sildenafil citrate (Viagra) for the treatment of erectile dysfunction in men with Parkinson's disease. *Mov. Disord.*, **15**, 305–8.

Ziegler, M. G., Lake, C. R. & Kopin, I. J. (1977). The sympathetic-nervous-system defect in primary orthostatic hypotension. *N. Engl. J. Med.*, **296**(6), 293–7.

Zoukos, Y., Thomaides, T., Pavitt, D. V., Cuzner, M. L. & Mathias, C. J. (1993). Beta-adrenoceptor expression on circulating mononuclear cells of idiopathic Parkinson's disease and autonomic failure patients before and after reduction of central sympathetic outflow by clonidine. *Neurology*, **43**(6), 1181–7.

Zuscik, M. J., Sands, S., Ross, S. A. *et al.* (2000). Overexpression of the alpha1B-adrenergic receptor causes apoptotic neurodegeneration: multiple system atrophy. *Nat. Med.*, **6**(12), 1388–94.

Zuscik, M. J., Chalothorn, D., Hellard, D. *et al.* (2001). Hypotension, autonomic failure, and cardiac hypertrophy in transgenic mice overexpressing the alpha 1B-adrenergic receptor. *J. Biol. Chem.*, **276**(17), 13738–43.

44

Progressive supranuclear palsy

Lawrence I. Golbe

Department of Neurology, Robert Wood Johnson Medical School, New Brunswick, NJ, USA

Introduction

Progressive supranuclear palsy (PSP) is unusual among the neurodegenerative disorders in the variety of neural structures it involves and the complexity of the illness that results. The tau-based neurofibrillary tangles and the associated degeneration affect both neurons and glia. The damage involves systems at every level from cerebral cortex to lumbar spinal cord. It affects dopaminergic, cholinergic and GABAergic systems. Its superficial clinical resemblance to Parkinson's disease (PD) and close pathological resemblance to postencephalitic parkinsonism delayed its definitive clinicopathological description until the early 1960s. (Richardson, 1963; Olszewski, 1963; Steele *et al.*, 1964). Its full-blown, typical clinical appearance is unmistakable, but atypical forms are frequent and multiple conditions can mimic it.

The etiology of PSP is no clearer than that of most other neurodegenerative disorders but the late 1990s have brought important new insights into the molecular defects underlying neurofibrillary tangle formation. Such insights will probably prove the best route to treatment of PSP, as symptomatic palliative treatments have been disappointing.

Clinical summary

Presentation

In its full-blown, typical state, PSP will not be confused with other illnesses. There can be little diagnostic doubt in a patient with a progressive syndrome of gait instability with early falls, neck rigidity with erect posture and bradykinesia, predominantly vertical supranuclear gaze abnormality, spastic dysarthria, dangerous dysphagia, tonically contracted facies and frontal behavioral abnormalities.

Restriction of vertical gaze with preserved oculocephalic reflexes is the most specific feature of PSP and the source of its name. However, gaze restriction is often absent until the middle of the course and is only rarely the presenting symptom (Table 44.1). Gaze palsy may fail to appear during life in up to half of all autopsy-confirmed cases (Birdi, 2002). Yet many physicians fail to consider the diagnosis of PSP until vertical gaze restriction occurs.

Well over half of all patients with PSP present with gait disturbance, usually with falls in the first year of illness (Birdi, 2002; Golbe, 1988; Maher, 1986; Litvan, 1997a; Wenning, 1999). This may prompt a workup for vestibulopathy, myelopathy, basilar artery ischemia, cardiac syncope or epilepsy. In the minority of cases presenting with gaze palsy, dysarthria or dysphagia, the initial workup may embark on a search for myasthenia gravis, progressive bulbar palsy or local causes of esophageal dysmotility. Cataract extraction may be performed in an attempt to correct the non-refractible visual deficit of unrecognized supranuclear gaze fixation instability.

Cases departing from the typical picture are common. Some patients with PSP have prominent dementia suggestive of Alzheimer's disease (Milberg, 1989). Others have asymmetric apraxia or dystonia suggestive of corticobasal degeneration, and others resemble Parkinson's disease or MSA of the parkinsonian type until late in the illness, when clear vertical supranuclear gaze abnormalities finally appear. Even such findings as moderate asymmetry and mild rest tremor (Rivest, 1990; Gibb, 1989), claimed by earlier authors to virtually exclude PSP, occurred in two of 12 pathologically confirmed cases in a recent series (Collins, 1995). A few patients in the literature have "pure akinesia" without other features of PSP until very late in the course (Mizusawa, 1993; Riley, 1994).

Table 44.1. Actuarially adjusted median interval from initial symptom to onset of disease milestones in PSP (Golbe, 1988)

Milestone	Years
Initial gait difficulty	0.3
Cane or helper needed to walk	3.1
Dysarthria	3.4
Visual symptoms	3.9
Dysphagia	4.4
Confined to bed or wheelchair	8.2
Death	9.7

Atypical clinical features tend to cluster in patients with atypical pathological and molecular features that occur in Alzheimer's disease (Morris, 2002). This suggests that there may be two or more disease entities presently lumped as "PSP."

Rating scale and diagnostic criteria

A clinical disability rating scale, the "PSP Rating Scale," has been devised for use by neurologists (Golbe, 1997; Golbe, 1999). It is available at http://www.psp.org.

A set of diagnostic criteria (Golbe, 1988) has been formulated for use in settings that permit detailed examination of patients (Table 44.2). Its specificity is 96% (Litvan, 1996a). Another set (Litvan, 1996a) includes "probable" clinical criteria with the high specificity necessary to a treatment trial and "possible" criteria sufficiently sensitive for use in a prevalence study (Table 44.3).

Differential diagnosis

For a neuropathologist, the principal entities competing with PSP are only corticobasal degeneration (CBD), postencephalitic parkinsonism (PEP) and the Parkinson–dementia complex of Guam (PDC) (Hauw, 1994). The clinician must contend with not only these, but also some cases of PD, CBD, multiple system atrophy (MSA) (principally striatonigral degeneration but also olivopontocerebellar atrophy) (Robbins, 1994), progressive subcortical gliosis (Will, 1988), Creutzfeldt-Jakob disease (Bertoni, 1983), Alzheimer's disease with parkinsonism, diffuse Lewy-body disease (Fearnley, 1991), Pick's disease and the primary pallidal atrophies including dentatorubropallidoluysian atrophy (Pahwa, 1993). Lacunar states, the most common non-degenerative PSP mimic, can reproduce virtually the full range of clinical features of PSP (Tanner, 1987; Winikates and Jankovic, 1994; Dubinsky & Jankovic, 1987).

Hydrocephalus can approximate a PSP-like syndrome as well (Curran & Lang, 1994).

In patients under age 50 with a PSP-like picture, especially with a positive family history, frontotemporal dementia related to chromosome 17 (Stanford, 2000) and Niemann–Pick disease type C (Josephs, 2003) are considerations. Whipple's disease that impairs vertical gaze can be mistaken for PSP (Averbuch-Heller, 1999), as can the mitochondrial encephalomyopathies, which are protean in their presentations (Truong, 1990).

Clinical points by which PSP can be differentiated from the most common of these entities appear as Table 44.4. Perhaps the most difficult differentiation of PSP is from MSA of the parkinsonian type, particularly in the absence of specific signs such as downgaze palsy or extensor axial dystonia (Colosimo, 1995).

Clinical evaluation

A thorough clinical examination and history will generally reveal PEP, PDC, myasthenia gravis (as a cause of gaze palsy, dysarthria and dysphagia), mitochondrial myopathy (as a cause of gaze palsy), and bulbar amyotrophic lateral sclerosis. MRI or X-ray computed tomography may reveal mimics such as hydrocephalus (Curran and Lang, 1994), midbrain tumors and a multi-infarct state.

Radiologic evaluation

Positron emission tomography using ^{18}F-fluorodopa distinguished 90% of patients with clinically diagnosed PSP, where the ratio of putaminal to caudate uptake constants is close to unity, from a group with PD, where the ratio is higher (Burn, 1994). Similar results are produced by use of ^{18}F-deoxyglucose (FDG) as a marker of cortical and subcortical metabolic rate (Burn, 1994; Foster, 1988; D'Antona, 1985; Nagahama, 1997) and by comparing caudate and putamen with regard to uptake of a dopamine transporter marker (Ilgin, 1999).

Although ^{18}F-fluorodopa and ^{18}FDG PET can identify presymptomatic members of families with PSP (Piccini, 1998), the sensitivity and specificity of PET in distinguishing patients with clinically equivocal or early PSP from other conditions has not been assessed. For this reason, PET is not yet considered a standard diagnostic tool in PSP.

MRI (Table 44.5) and CT imaging are non-specific in early PSP. In the moderate to advanced stages, they may reveal thinning of the anteroposterior diameter of the midbrain tectum and tegmentum with atrophy of the colliculi and disproportionate enlargement of the sylvian fissures and posterior third ventricle (Schonfeld, 1987; Drayer, 1986; Savoiardo, 1989; Saitoh, 1987; Yuki, 1990; Stern, 1989). The

Table 44.2. *Diagnostic criteria for PSP* (proposed by Golbe, 1988)

All four of these:	Criteria for Supranuclear Gaze Palsy:
Onset at age 40 or later	
Progressive course	Either: *both of these*:
Bradykinesia	Voluntary downgaze less than 15 degrees (tested by instructing
Supranuclear gaze palsy, *per criteria at right*	patient to "look down" without presenting a specific target;
	accept the best result after several attempts).
Plus any three of these five:	
Dysarthria or dysphagia	Preserved horizontal oculocephalic reflexes (except in very
Neck rigidity (to flexion/extension) greater than limb rigidity	advanced stages)
Neck in a posture of extension	
Minimal or absent tremor	or *all three of these*:
Frequent falls or gait disturbance early in course	Slowed downward saccades (defined as slow enough for the
	examiner to perceive the movement itself)
Without any of these:	
Early or prominent cerebellar signs	Impaired opticokinetic nystagmus with the stimulus moving
Unexplained polyneuropathy	downward
Prominent noniatrogenic dysautonomia other than	
isolated postural hypotension	Poor voluntary suppression of vertical vestibulo-ocular reflex

Table 44.3. *Diagnostic criteria for PSP* (proposed by Litvan, 1996)

"Possible" PSP	"Probable" PSP
All three of these:	All five of these:
1. Gradually progressive disorder	1. Gradually progressive disorder
2. Onset at age 40 or later	2. Onset at age 40 or later
3. No evidence for competing diagnostic possibilities	3. No evidence for competing diagnostic possibilities
	4. Vertical gaze palsy
Plus either of these:	5. Slowing of vertical saccades *and* prominent postural
4. Vertical gaze palsy or	instability with falls in the first year
5. Slowing of vertical saccades *and* prominent postural instability with falls in the first year	
Criteria that would exclude PSP from consideration:	
1. Recent encephalitis	
2. Alien limb syndrome, cortical sensory defects or temporoparietal atrophy	
3. Psychosis unrelated to dopaminergic treatment	
4. Important cerebellar signs	
5. Important unexplained dysautonomia	
6. Severe, asymmetric parkinsonian signs	
7. Relevant structural abnormality of basal ganglia on neuroimaging	
8. Whipple's disease on CSF PCR, if indicated	

MRI features that are most likely to permit a differentiation of PSP from MSA are the absence (in PSP) of abnormal signal and/or atrophy in the cerebellum, middle cerebellar peduncle, pons and inferior olive. The hyperintense putamenal rim caused by iron deposition also occurs less commonly and later in PSP than MSA (Stern, 1989).

Also of undetermined utility in early, diagnostically equivocal cases is single photon emission computed tomography (SPECT) using markers of cerebral blood flow and/or metabolism. Such studies show bifrontal hypometabolism in established PSP (Timmons, 1989; Habert, 1991; Neary, 1987). However, SPECT imaging of D2 receptor sites using ^{123}I-iodobenzamide (IBZM) is promising as a means of differentiating PSP, where there is often detectable striatal D2 loss, from PD, where there is not (van Royen, 1993; Schwarz, 1992).

Magnetic resonance spectroscopy (MRS) is starting to show promise as a means of differentiating PSP from PD or other states (Davie, 1997; Abe, 2000; Clarke, 2001). The diagnostic finding is a reduction in the ratio of *N*-acetyl

Table 44.4. Clinical points differentiating PSP from some other parkinsonian disorders

	PSP	PD	MSA (SND)	CBD
Symmetry of deficit	+++	+	+++	−
Axial rigidity	+++	++	++	++
Limb dystonia	+	+	+	+++
Postural instability	+++	++	++	+
Vertical supranuclear gaze restriction	+++	+	++	++
Frontal behavior	+++	+	+	++
Dysautonomia	−	+	++	−
Levodopa response early in course	+	+++	+	−
Levodopa response late in course	−	++	+	−
Asymmetric cortical atrophy on MRI	−	−	−	++

Table 44.5. MRI features of PSP and some other conditions

	PSP	PD	MSA (OPCA)	MSA (SND)	CBGD	AD
Cortical atrophy	++	+	+/−	+	++/−	++
Putaminal atrophy	−	−	−	++	−	−
Pontine atrophy	+	−	+++	−	+/−	−
Midbrain atrophy	++	−	+	−	+/−	−
Cerebellar atrophy	−	−	++/−	−	−	−
High putaminal iron	−	−	+/−	+/−	−	−

− absent or rare; + occasional, mild or late; ++ usual, moderate; +++ usual, severe or early.

aspartate to creatine in the region of the putamen and/or pallidum. However, as for PET, the ability of this modality to distinguish the conditions during their early, clinically equivocal phases is unproven. The same caveat applies to diffusion-weighted MR imaging, where the apparent diffusion coefficient of the putamen increases in PSP but not in PD (Seppi, 2003).

Neuropathology, neurochemistry and their clinical correlates

Neurofibrillary tangles

The filaments composing the NFTs of PSP are unpaired straight filaments 15 to 18 nm in diameter composed of at least six protofilaments 2 to 5 nm in diameter (Powell, 1974; Tellez-Nagel, 1973; Tomonaga, 1977; Montpetit, 1985). A few cortical areas in PSP, or even subcortical nuclei, may display paired helical filaments of the Alzheimer type (Ghatak, 1980; Ikeda, 1994). The tangles themselves, unlike those of AD, tend to be globose rather than flame-shaped.

The immunostaining and ultrastructural properties of the filaments of PSP tangles are nearly identical to those

of CBD (Ikeda, 1994; Mori, 1994). However, the white matter tangles of CBD occur in oligodendroglia rather than in astrocytes, as in most cases of PSP (Wakabayaski *et al.*, 1994; Inagaki, 1994). These are referred to as "tufted astrocytes" (Yamada, 1993). The tau-positive "tufts" and neuropil threads are similar to those in affected neurons. Such astrocytic pathology may be unique to PSP. These changes appear to be primary rather than reactive to degeneration of the astrocytes or other cells (Togo & Dickson, 2002).

Tau protein

Cortical NFTs of PSP appear to be antigenically identical to those of AD, most notably with regard to the presence of abnormally phosphorylated tau protein (Pollock, 1986; Love, 1988; Tabaton, 1988; Yamada, 1993). PSP tau exhibits bands on Western blot of 64 and 69 kD, while AD and Down's syndrome tau exhibits those two bands plus one of 55 kD (Flament, 1991; Vermersch, 1994).

Anti-tau staining reveals neuropil threads, also known as curly fibers, in the same neurons that include NFTs and in oligodendroglia of white matter tracts connecting affected areas of subcortical gray matter (Probst, 1988; Nelson, 1989;

Iwatsubo, 1994). The NFTs of PSP stain weakly or not at all for ubiquitin (Lennox, 1988).

A mouse model of PSP has recently been described. (Lewis, 2000). It expresses one of the mutant forms of tau that causes frontotemporal dementia, but the distribution of lesions is similar to that of human PSP. *Drosophila* models of a generic tauopathy have also been reported (Wittman, 2001; Lewis, 2001). In one of these, intriguingly, adult-onset, selective neurodegeneration with accumulation of abnormal tau occurred without NFTs (Wittman *et al.*, 2001). This and other experimental evidence from many sources suggests that the toxic species is not mature NFTs, but tau in an early stage of aggregation.

Other changes

Grumose degeneration, in which eosinophilic material surrounds degenerating neurons, accompanied by spherical argentophilic components, occurs in a significant minority of cases with PSP, particularly in the cerebellar dentate nucleus (Olszewski, 1963; Arai, 1987). It appears to be composed of abnormally regenerated synaptic terminal material of Purkinje cells.

While amyloid or senile plaques do not occur in PSP, granulovacuolar degeneration, another hallmark of AD, does occur to a mild extent. In addition, swollen, achromatic neurons characteristic of CBD or Pick's disease occur in a few cases of otherwise typical PSP, generally in tegmental and inferior temporal areas (Giaccone, 1988).

Microglial activation, another pathologic change that occurs in some neurodegenerative disorders, has recently been found to be common in PSP (Ishizawa & Dickson, 2001). In the brainstem in PSP, microglial activation does not correlate well with the presence of NFTs. This suggests that neither is the direct cause of the other and that microglia may help produce the neuronal loss of PSP.

Anatomic distribution of degeneration and clinical correlates

Overview

The major areas of primary involvement in PSP are the cerebral cortex, producing cognitive and behavioral changes; the nigrostriatalpallidal area, producing rigidity, bradykinesia and postural instability; the cholinergic pontomesencephalic nuclei area, producing gaze palsies, sleep disturbances and axial motor abnormalities; and the hindbrain area, producing dysarthria and dysphagia (Hauw, 1994).

The daunting complexity of this syndrome may be the principal reason for the continuing resistance of PSP to pathophysiologic understanding and pharmacologic intervention (Table 44.6).

Dopaminergic damage in the nigrostriatal pathway and cholinergic damage in many areas are the most consistent, severe neurotransmitter-related changes in PSP (Jellinger, 1988; Kish, 1985; Ruberg, 1985). GABA-ergic function of the basal ganglia (in striatum and GPi and GPe) is moderately but widely impaired (Levy, 1995). Unlike the case in PD, the peptidergic systems and the mesolimbic and mesocortical dopaminergic systems are intact. Serotonergic receptor sites are reduced in the cortex, but unlike in PD, are normal in basal ganglia (Landwehrmeyer and Palacios, 1994). The loss of adrenoceptors is widespread (Pascual, 1993) reflecting the wide projections of the severely damaged locus ceruleus.

Cerebral cortex

Pathoanatomy

Cortical involvement in PSP differs importantly from that in AD at the gyral, laminar, cytologic, ultrastructural and biochemical levels. Central and cortical atrophy of cerebrum is only mild in PSP (Cordato, 2000). Motor strip (Area 4) and a partly ocular motor association area (Area 39) are the most important of many sites of neocortical pathology (Hauw *et al.*, 1990; Hof, 1992; Braak, 1992). PSP affects the large pyramidal and small neurons of layers V and VI, while AD affects the medium-sized neurons of layers III and V (Bergeron, 1997).

Anatomic and neurochemical changes

The prefrontal areas, which are the most obviously affected by behavioral testing and by measures of cerebral blood flow (Timmons, 1989; Habert, 1991; Neary, 1987; D'Antona, 1985; Noster, 1988; Leenders, 1988; Goffinet, 1989) display relatively little neurofibrillary pathology or neuronal loss in PSP (Verny, 1994; Hauw *et al.*, 1990). This dysfunction may therefore be secondary to subcortical pathology, as in the cholinergic nucleus basalis of Meynert and the cholinergic pedunculopontine nucleus (Tagliavini, 1984; Zweig, 1987; Jellinger, 1988).

Clinical correlates

Behavioral changes were the initial symptom of PSP in 22% of patients in one series (Birdi, 2002) and eventually produce disability in at least 80% (Golbe, 1988; Jankovic & Van der Linden, 1990). Clinical frontal lobe dysfunction in PSP is often the most disabling area of cognitive loss and

Table 44.6. Principal clinicopathological correlates in PSP

Area	Severity (+ to ++++)	Principal presumptive clinical correlate
Cerebrum		
frontal cortex	+ +	frontal behavior
precentral cortex	+ +	frontal motor phenomena
Limbic system		
amygdala	+	depression
hippocampus	+ +	memory disorder
Basal ganglia		
caudate	+ + +	
putamen	+ + +	
globus pallidus	+ +	bradykinesia, dysarthria, dystonia, postural instability
subthalamic nucleus	+ + + +	
thalamus (interlaminar nuclei)	+	
Basal forebrain		
nucleus basalis of Meynert	+ + +	dementia
hypothalamus	+	dysautonomia
Dorsal midbrain		
superior colliculus	+ + + +	coordination of head movement with gaze
rostral interstitial nucleus of the medial longitudinal fasciculus	+ + +	
periaqueductal gray	+ + + +	vertical gaze palsy
oculomotor nucleus	+ +	
interstitial nucleus of Cajal	+ +	nuchal rigidity, postural instability
Midbrain tegmentum		
substantia nigra zona compacta	+ + +	bradykinesia
SN zona reticulata	+ +	bradykinesia
ventral tegmental area	+ +	frontal behavior
red nucleus	+ + +	?motor deficit
pedunculopontine nucleus	+ + +	postural instability, dementia, sleep disorder
Pons		
locus ceruleus	+ +	gait disorder, dementia, depression, sleep disorder
nucleus of the dorsal raphe	+ + +	frontal behavior, depression, sleep disorder
nuclei basis pontis	+ +	horizontal saccadic disorder
Medulla		
vestibular nuclei	+ +	dysequilibrium, abnormal gaze
Cerebellum		
dentate nucleus	+ +	?dysarthria,?postural instability
Spinal cord		
nucleus of Onuf	+ +	dysautonomia
intermediolateral column	+ +	

can progress rapidly (Soliveri, 2000). Apathy, intellectual slowing and impairment of "executive" functions with little abnormal motor behaviors are the consistent findings (Litvan, 1996b). The executive dysfunction (Pillon, 1995) comprises difficulty with shifting mental set, sorting, problem solving, abstract thinking, motor inhibition and lexical fluency (Podoll, 1991; Rosser & Hodges, 1994). A brief but formal "Frontal Assessment Battery" is useful for bedside quantification of these deficits (Dubois, 2000).

Apraxia that is milder and less asymmetric than that of CBD is common in PSP (Bergeron, 1997) and can produce diagnostic confusion.

Hippocampus

The hippocampus, a primary site of pathology in AD, is involved in only half of cases of PSP (Agid, 1987). This probably explains the relative preservation of memory in PSP except for memory tasks requiring goal-directed searching, a frontal lobe function (Pillon & Dubois, 1992; Pillon, 1994).

Nigrostriatal system

Distribution of pathology

The most consistent abnormality in PSP is damage to the pigmented neurons of the zona compacta of the substantia nigra (Fearnley & Lees, 1991). However, in PSP, the damage is relatively uniform except for relative sparing of a small, extreme lateral portion, while in PD, both the dorsal and extreme lateral portions are affected little. The dorsal portion projects principally to the caudate, the ventral to the putamen. This probably explains the relative sparing of presynaptic caudate dopamine reuptake in PD and its involvement in PSP, as measured by ^{18}F-fluorodopa PET (Brooks, 1990; Curran & Lang, 1994). Tissue binding studies have demonstrated little or no loss of postsynaptic dopamine D1 receptors and only mild and inconsistent loss of D2 receptors (Landwehrmeyer & Palacios, 1994; Baron, 1986; Brooks, 1992).

In the striatum, the few neurons lost are mostly cholinergic interneurons (Young, 1985; Villares, 1994; Oyanaki, 1991). However, there is important loss of astrocytes (Ruberg, 1985, Probst 1993). which display the "tufted"appearance described above.

Clinical course

Postural instability is the initial symptom in approximately two-thirds of patients with PSP (Golbe, 1988; Maher & Lees, 1986). Frank falls start a median of 1.8 years into the illness (Bergeron, 1997) and are often unrelated to obstacles or antecedent sensations of imbalance. The initial or only gait abnormality may be severe gait "freezing" or "apraxia" (Matsuo, 1991; Imai, 1993), with no rigidity. In PD, by contrast, gait difficulty or postural instability is a presenting feature in only 11% (Hoehn & Yahr, 1967).

The postural instability is usually the most disabling feature of later PSP. The median intervals from initial symptom are 3.1 years until assistance is required and 8.2 years until wheelchair confinement (Golbe, 1988).

Contrary to widespread impression, rest tremor can occur in PSP, affecting 5–10% of patients, usually early in the course (Masucci, 1989; Jankovic & Van der Linden, 1990). Action or postural tremor occurs in about 25%. The limb rigidity and distal bradykinesia are mild relative to axial rigidity.

Other basal ganglia

Damage to the subthalamic nucleus ranks beside that of the substantia nigra as a constant in PSP and is far more specific to it (Olszewski, 1963). Damage to the GPi in PSP is slightly less constant, but it is sufficient to predict that stereotactic GPi lesions or its inhibition by deep-brain stimulation would be ineffective against PSP despite their efficacy against PD.

The GPi, which is GABA-ergic, projects not only to the thalamus, which is nearly intact in PSP, but also to the cholinergic pedunculopontine nucleus (PPN), which is severely affected (Zweig, 1987; Jellinger, 1988; Morizumi & Hattori, 1992). Experimental lesions of the PPN alone can cause severe postural instability (Masdeu, 1994).

There is also severe depletion of GPe neurons in PSP (Hardman & Halliday, 1999). While most of the thalamus is spared in PSP, there is pathology in the glutamatergic caudal intralaminar nuclei, which regulate caudate and putamen (Henderson, 2000).

Mesencephalic and pontine ocular motor areas

Pathoanatomy

Experimental lesions of the interstitial nucleus of Cajal in monkeys produce extensor rigidity at the neck, postural instability and vertical gaze palsy (Carpenter, 1970). However, in PSP, the last finding could also be caused by the damage to other areas of the rostral midbrain, namely the nucleus of Darkschewitsch, the rostral interstitial nucleus of the medial longitudinal fasciculus, and the mesencephalic reticular formation (Fukushima, 1987; Zweig, 1987; Juncos, 1991; Jellinger & Bancher, 1992). There also appears to be a contribution from the substantia nigra pars reticulata (Halliday, 2000) which projects to the superior colliculus. The ventral tegmental area, red nucleus and locus ceruleus are also involved in PSP (Olszewrski *et al.*, 1963) but their specific contributions to the clinical deficits are unclear.

The horizontal gaze palsy that appears eventually in most cases is attributable to degeneration of nuclei of the pontine base (Malessa, 1994). The ocular motor cranial nerve nuclei are perhaps the sole example of cholinergic nuclei to escape important involvement in PSP.

Table 44.7. Clinical ocular motor findings in PSP

Usually precede frank gaze restriction

- Hypometric saccades, particularly downward
- Disordered opticokinetic nystagmus, particularly downward
- Slowing of downward saccades (especially when starting at upgaze)
- Square-wave jerks
- Inability to voluntarily suppress the vestibulo-ocular reflex
- Hesitancy ("apraxia") on command downgaze

Occur in middle stages of illness

- Restriction of range of voluntary downgaze
- Impaired convergence
- Disordered Bell's phenomenon
- Visual grasping
- Lid retraction with reduced blink rate
- Apraxia of lid opening or closing

Tend to begin in later stages of illness

- Restriction of range of voluntary horizontal gaze
- Loss of oculocephalic reflex
- Disconjugate gaze
- Disabling blepharospasm

Clinical phenomenology

(Table 44.7) Symptomatic eye movement difficulty does not begin until a median of 3.9 years after disease onset, nearly half the clinical course (Golbe, 1988). The loss of range of downgaze, although more specific for PSP, is often exceeded by the loss of upgaze. Voluntary gaze without a specific target (i.e. "look down") is usually worse than command gaze to a target, which is worse than pursuit, and reflex gaze is by far the least affected.

Signs that can be observed with no specialized apparatus in the examining room and long precede the onset of frank visual symptoms in most patients include delay in saccade initiation, slowing of vertical saccades (Leigh, 2000), saccadic pursuit, breakdown of opticokinetic nystagmus in the vertical plane, disordered Bell's phenomenon, poor convergence and subtle square-wave jerks (SWJs) (Pfaffenbach, 1972; Chu, 1979; Troost & Daroff, 1977). The last finding has close to 100% sensitivity (Troost & Daroff, 1977; Rascol, 1991). In some patients, SWJs are seen only during fixation on a distant light source in the dark. SWJs occur in very few patients with PD, but are sufficiently common in MSA and other cerebellar conditions that they cannot differentiate them from PSP (Rascol, 1977).

The frontal defect impairs the antisaccade task, where the patient is instructed to quickly direct gaze to the examiner's hand that does *not* wave. An altitudinal visual attentional deficit (Rafal, 1988) arising from damaged tectal centers may contribute to overloading the fork, poor aim of the urinary stream, poor attention to dress and apathy for the severity of postural instability.

Reflex gaze

From the earliest stages, most patients also suffer loss of the ability to voluntarily suppress the vestibulo-ocular reflex (VOR) (Rascol, 1993). This may be tested by seating the patient in a swivel chair and asking him to extend the arms at the level of the eyes, clasp hands and fixate on one thumbnail as the examiner slowly rotates the chair and patient *en bloc*. Patients with PSP (and many other basal ganglia disorders) are unable to suppress the opticokinetic nystagmus produced by relative movement of the environment.

Eyelid movement

Eyelid movement abnormalities, particularly apraxia of eyelid opening (perhaps better termed "lid levator inhibition" (Lepore & Duvoisin, 1985)) and blepharospasm or a combination of these occurs in about one third of patients and can cause functional blindness (Dehaene, 1984; Jankovic, 1984a; Golbe, 1989). Apraxia of lid closing and the very slow blink rate of PSP, often less than 5/minute, can allow conjunctival drying with annoying exposure keratopathy and reflex lacrimation. The electrical blink reflex is severely impaired, unlike in PD, CBD or MSA (Valls-Solé, 1997), testimony to the profound brainstem pathology in PSP.

Brainstem centers controlling sleep and arousal

The prominent sleep disturbances of PSP are probably explained by damage to the (serotonergic) raphe nuclei, the (cholinergic) pedunculopontine nucleus and others, the (noradrenergic) locus ceruleus and the periaqueductal gray. The most important clinical component is a severe reduction in rapid eye movement (REM) sleep (Aldrich, 1989) with loss of sleep spindles and K-complexes. During the remaining REM-sleep, there are abnormal slow waves and absence of normal sawtooth waves (Leygonie, 1976).

Daytime hypersomnolence, often a disabling problem in PSP, is probably related to damage of dopaminergic systems that maintain wakefulness. There is a fragmentation of sleep/wake periods that culminates at the end stage of PSP in a constant sleep-like state from which the patient can be roused but briefly.

The auditory startle and auditory blink reflexes are absent or severely impaired in PSP despite normal auditory evoked potentials (Tolosa & Zeese, 1979). Startle is mediated via the lower pontine reticular formation, in particular

Table 44.8. Components of dysarthria in PSP and some related conditions

	Hypokinesia	Ataxia	Spasticity
PSP	++	+	+++
PD	+++	–	–
MSA (striatonigral degeneration)	+++	++	+
MSA (olivoponto-cerebellar atrophy)	+	+++	++

the nucleus reticularis pontis caudalis, which degenerates in PSP.

Brainstem centers controlling speech and swallowing

Dysarthria

The dysarthria of PSP is spastic, with a slow rate and a strained, strangled quality. Ataxic components are usually present, creating a combination highly specific for PSP (Kluin, 1993) (Table 44.8). Within 2 years after disease onset, 41% of patients or their families have detected dysarthria. By the fifth year, the figure is 68% (Golbe, 1988).

Dysphagia

Aspiration pneumonia is a major morbidity and mortality risk in advanced PSP (Muller, 2001) but only 18% of patients report symptomatic dysphagia within 2 years after PSP onset and 46% do so by 5 years (Golbe, 1988). In a study using objective criteria, dysphagia occurred in 26 of 27 patients with mean disease duration of 52 months (Litvan, 1997b). While the dysphagia of PSP arises from many levels of the oropharyngeal axis (Leopold, 1997; Sonies, 1992) it emphasizes oral rather than pharyngeal abnormalities, distinguishing it from the dysphagia of PD (Johnston, 1997).

It is common for patients with PSP, but not with PD, to exacerbate the effects of dysphagia by overloading the fork, probably through a combination of poor downgaze, frontal disinhibition, and vertical visual inattention (Rafal & Grimm, 1981). The retrocollis that occurs eventually in some patients with PSP may decrease the ability of the epiglottis to protect the airway.

Spinal and autonomic centers

The spinal cord involvement in PSP principally affects the motor area (lamina IX) and the intermedio-lateral column with minor gray matter tract degeneration (Jellinger & Bancher, 1992; Sakakibara, 1993; Vitaliani, 2002). There is also severe degeneration of the nucleus of Onuf in the sacral cord (Scaravilli, 2000) and brainstem autonomic nuclei (Rub, 2002). Urinary incontinence occurred in 42% of patients at some point in PSP in one series and started a mean of 3.5 years into the disease course (Gert van Dijk, 1991). Overall, however, PSP produces less dysautonomia than PD (Gert van Dijk, 1991; Skimber, 2000), a point useful in its clinical differentiation from MSA. Anal sphincter EMG reveals denervation caused by loss of Onuf's nucleus in both PSP and MSA, but its sensitivity is low (Vodusek, 2001).

Epidemiology and etiology

Descriptive epidemiology

Onset age

PSP typically begins in the late 50s to mid-60s, one in three cases starting before age 60 (Golbe, 1988). The standard deviation of the onset age is typically between 6 and 7 years, (Golbe, 1988), far less than the 11 years typical for PD. This suggests that the range of etiologies for PSP is narrower than for PD. Age-specific incidence figures are not available.

Survival

Death occurred at an actuarially corrected median of 9.7, 7.0 and 5.9 years in three studies (Maher & Lees, 1986; Golbe, 1988; Testa, 2001). Ten-year survival is approximately 30% (Testa, 2001). Death is usually related to pneumonia and other inevitable complications of immobility, but frank aspiration, head trauma due to falls, and complications of hip fracture are important preventable causes of death in PSP.

Prevalence

The prevalence ratio of previously diagnosed PSP is 1.0–1.4 per 100 000 (Golbe, 1988; Nath, 2001). The overall prevalence, comprised mostly of patients who had not received the diagnosis until researchers with a special interest in PSP examined them, was 6.4 (Schrag, 1999) and 5.0 (Nath, 2001) per 100 000.

Incidence

In Rochester, Minnesota, a study covering the years 1976 to 1990 gave an annual incidence in the population over age 49 of 5.3 per 100 000 per year. (Bower, 1997). Previous figures using indirect methods reached a similar result (Golbe, 1996a). This figure lies very close to that of some

Table 44.9. Approximate incidence rates of PSP and some other neurologic disorders (new cases per 100 000 population per year)

	Incidence Rate
Parkinson's disease	20
ALS	10–20
Guillain–Barré syndrome	10
All muscular dystrophies	7
Polymyositis	5
Tourette syndrome	5
Huntington's disease	5
PSP	**3–4**
Myasthenia gravis	3–4
Syringomyelia	3
Charcot–Marie-Tooth	2
Wilson's disease	2

better-recognized neurologic conditions such as myasthenia gravis and Huntington's disease (Kurtzke & Kurland, 1973) (Table 44.9).

Sex ratio

Most published series reveal a sex ratio (M:F) of approximately 3:2. The absence of so asymmetric a ratio in other highly referred neurodegenerative disorders is a point against gender-related referral bias as the explanation in PSP and points to an occupational toxin or X-linked mutation as an etiologic factor.

Analytic epidemiology

Two case-control studies from the same New Jersey clinic using clinic and spouse controls, respectively, gave opposite positive results regarding educational attainment of patients (Davis, 1988; Golbe, 1996b). This etiologic clue therefore awaits clarification. Other risk factors implicated in at least one other neurodegenerative disease, including occupation, smoking and head trauma, gave negative results. Attempts to transmit PSP to primates (Brown, 1994) and a search for a prion protein have proven unsuccessful (Jendroska, 1994).

Geographic clusters

Two geographic clusters of PSP-like tauopathies are known. Lytigo-bodig, or the amyotrophic lateral sclerosis–parkinsonism–dementia complex of Guam (PDC), has resisted multiple careful etiologic investigations, but its markedly declining incidence since the westernization of Guam after World War II suggests an environmental cause

(Steele, 2002). The distribution of tau isoforms is similar to that of AD and not PSP (Steele, 2002).

An unusual concentration of a PSP-like tauopathy on the Caribbean island of Guadeloupe is identical to PSP at the level of tau isoforms (Caparros-Lefebvre, 2002). A case-control survey found illness to be associated with consumption of two indigenous plants, soursop and sweetsop (*Annona muricata* and *A. squamosa*), which harbor a number of neurotoxins (Caparros-Lefebvre, 1999). The use of extracts of these plants to produce an animal model and to understand tauopathies in general is starting to be explored (Steele, 2002).

Clinical genetics

A case-control study (Davis, 1988) elicited reports of "Parkinson's disease" among parents, siblings, grandparents, aunts, uncles and first cousins 5.0 times as frequently from patients with PSP as controls. For "Alzheimer's or dementia," the ratio was 3.6. Another study found that 39% of 23 asymptomatic first-degree relatives of patients with PSP, but none of 23 controls, had abnormal scores on a battery that screens for parkinsonism (Baker & Montgomery, 2001).

Eight reports of families with more than one member with proven PSP usually with autosomal dominant transmission and no purely maternal transmission, offer hope of a clue to the cause of sporadic PSP (Ohara, 1992; Brown, 1993; Gazely & Maguire, 1994; de Yébenes, 1995; Golbe & Dickson, 1995; Tetrud, 1996; Uitti, 1999). It is intriguing that some of these families, including a Spanish family that is by far the largest, include additional members with reports of typical PD or essential tremor (Rojo, 1999; Piccini, 2001). Genetic screening of these families is negative to date.

Nuclear molecular genetics

Tau isoforms
In PSP, the ratio of the two human brain tau isoforms is at least 3:1 in favor of 4-repeat tau (Flament, 1991). Disordered regulation of exon 10 splicing may therefore explain tau aggregation into NFTs in PSP and other tauopathies.

A clue from FTD
Several mutations in and near the 5′ splice site downstream of exon 10 have been described in families with hereditary frontotemporal dementia with parkinsonism related to chromosome 17 (FTDP-17), another 4-repeat tauopathy that occasionally resembles PSP clinically (Hutton, 1998; Spillantini, 1998; Stanford 2000). These probably disrupt a stem–loop structure in the RNA transcribed at the

Table 44.10. Frequency of tau haplotypes and genotypes in PSP (Baker, 1999)

		PSP	Controls
N		64	145
Haplotypes	H1	94%	78%
		6%	22%
p			0.00013
	H1/H1	88%	63%
Genotypes	H1/H2	12%	31%
	H2/H2	0	6%
p			0.00098

downstream end of exon 10. This stem–loop regulates splicing of the exon 10 transcript, the inappropriate inclusion of which produces an excess of 4-repeat tau. The cause then, of PSP and other sporadic tauopathies may be dysfunction of the same RNA stem-loop, but from a different cause.

A *tau* allelic variant

A haplotype, "H1," spanning the *tau* gene on chromosome 17q21 is present in approximately 90% of patients with PSP but also in approximately 60% of controls (Conrad, 1997; Baker, 1999; Higgins, 1999; Molinuevo, 2000) (Table 44.10). This suggests that a genetic variation necessary but not sufficient to cause PSP is located in or near *tau*. The precise mutation is not known, but mutations in the *tau* promoter region in linkage dysequilibrium with H1 have been described (Ezquerra, 1999; de Silva, 2001).

The occurrence of PSP in sporadic rather than familial fashion must then require an additional exogenous or genetic factor. This caveat is underscored by the observation that corticobasal degeneration shares the haplotype that characterizes PSP (Di Maria, 2000; Houlden, 2001; Pastor *et al.*, 2001), as does PD to a lesser degree (Golbe, 2002). Furthermore, the presence or absence of the H1 haplotype or the H1/H1 genotype has no effect on the age of onset, clinical progression (Morris, 2001; Litvan, 2001a), the anatomical distribution of degeneration or on the biochemical features of the abnormal tau protein (Liu, 2001).

Variants in apo-E that are associated with AD and variants in α-synuclein and synphilin that are associated with PD are absent in PSP (Anouti, 1995; Tabaton, 1995; Morris, 2000).

Mitochondrial or oxidative mechanisms

Skeletal muscle mitochondrial respiratory function is reduced by about 30% in PSP. Evidence for oxidative stress in brain tissue are marked increases in levels of superoxide dismutase 1 and/or 2 activity, malondialdehyde and lipid peroxidation products specifically in areas that degenerate in PSP (Albers, 1999; Cantuti-Castelvetri, 2000; Swerdlow, 2000).

Evidence that deficiency of Complex I of mitochondrial genetic origin contributes to the cause of typical PSP is provided by the observation of low Complex I activity and mitochondrial dysfunction in cultured neuronal cells in which native mitochondria were replaced by mitochondria from patients with PSP (Swerdlow, 2000; Chirichigno, 2002).

An area of recent inquiry is the role of transglutaminases in PSP (Kim, 2002). Enzymes normally important in stabilizing protein structure, they are aberrantly activated in PSP and other neurodegenerative disorders by oxidative stress. The resulting cross-linking of tau protein could help explain the formation of NFTs or the dysfunction of other proteins and offers a promising site of action for neuroprotective therapy.

Treatment

Pharmacotherapy

As is the case for most other degenerative disorders, neurotransmitter replacement or receptor stimulation in PSP encounters little or none of the success it has with PD (Nieforth & Golbe, 1993; Kompoliti, 1998).

Dopaminergics

In two retrospective, uncontrolled studies, 51% (Jankovic, 1984b) and 38% (Nieforth & Golbe, 1993) of patients responded, most of them minimally. (The placebo response rate in PD drug trials is generally about 30%.) Only the rigidity and bradykinesia, including those components of dysarthria and dysphagia attributable to them, may respond more than would be expected from placebo. The extent and nature of the benefit of levodopa in PSP has not been adequately studied in double-blind fashion, but any benefit is nearly always mild and/or brief. Dopamine receptor agonists give similar benefit or lesser with additional risks (Nieforth & Golbe, 1993; Jankovic, 1983; Weiner, 1999).

Hyperkinetic and behavioral side effects of levodopa are very rare in PSP (Nieforth & Golbe, 1993). This prompts the use of approximately twice the levodopa/carbidopa dosages used for PD with the equivalent degree of parkinsonism.

Cholinergics and anticholinergics

Amantadine, which has anticholinergic, dopaminergic and antiglutamatergic properties, is a close second to levodopa in risk/benefit ratio for PSP (Nieforth & Golbe, 1993). A trial of amantadine starting at 100 mg daily and increasing to a maximum of 100 mg twice daily is worthwhile for most patients with PSP. It should be tapered and discontinued if symptomatic benefit is not apparent within a month. The typical "pure" anticholinergic agents give little benefit and tend to be poorly tolerated.

Trials of cholinergics have been inspired by the severe and widespread degeneration of acetylcholinergic systems in PSP. The cholinesterase inhibitor physostigmine was reported to improve PET evidence of prefrontal dysfunction, long-term verbal memory, and visuospatial attention, all very slightly (Kertzman, 1990; Litvan, 1989) but a subsequent trial by one of these groups gave negative results, with worsening of gait (Litvan, 1994). Donepezil, a commercially available cholinesterase inhibitor minimally effective in AD, has no benefit against PSP (Litvan, 2001b).

Antidepressants

Amitriptyline improved gait and rigidity in three of four patients in a small double-blind trial (Newman, 1985). In a retrospective series (Nieforth & Golbe, 1993) amitriptyline gave a risk/benefit ratio that was slightly less favorable than those of levodopa and amantadine. Amitriptyline is generally started at 10 mg at bedtime, increasing by that amount each week, given in two divided doses. If 20 mg twice daily proves ineffective, higher dosages are unlikely to do otherwise.

Botulinum toxin

Blepharospasm in PSP usually responds to botulinum A (Piccione, 1997). Torticollis or retrocollis in PSP may also respond, but the occasional occurrence of mild dysphagia after botulinum injection for idiopathic spasmodic torticollis dictates caution in the case of PSP, where slight exacerbation of dysphagia could allow aspiration. Botulinum toxin may also be useful in focal limb dystonia of PSP (Polo & Jabbari, 1994).

Nonpharmacologic therapy

Locomotory aids

The tendency of many patients with PSP to be almost anosognosic for their postural instability requires that the physician and other caregivers encourage the use of a walker early in the course. A heavy rolling model with a low basket into which bricks can be placed as a counterweight against falls often serves well. If falls occur despite the walker, the patient must be strongly encouraged to use a wheelchair and to resist the frequent temptation to arise from it without help, a tendency that may be related to the frontal motor dysinhibition of PSP.

Gaze and lid pareses

Some patients can overcome the voluntary downgaze palsy that impairs eating by using their remaining pursuit downgaze ability to follow the fork down to the plate. If downgaze palsy or inattention to the lower half of space is present, low-lying obstacles should be removed from the patient's environment. While prisms are not usually useful in correcting the patient's inability to attend to the lower half of space, they may help diplopia related to dysconjugate gaze. The chronic conjunctivitis and reactive lacrimation caused by the low blink rate may be treated by instillation of lubricants.

Physical, speech and swallowing therapy

Physical therapy seems to be of little or no benefit against the postural instability of PSP, but regular exercise has a clear psychological benefit (Sosner, 1993). Similarly, speech therapy is of little benefit, but the speech pathologist may be able to arrange adjunctive means of communication such as electronic typing devices or simple pointing boards if the visual function permits.

Dysphagia in PSP is also unlikely to respond to therapy. However, the family may be instructed in the preparation of foods of proper consistency, using a blender or cornstarch-based thickeners as necessary. A barium swallow radiograph using boluses of varying consistency will guide this advice. The speech pathologist can teach the patient safer swallowing techniques and can monitor the patient for the need for a feeding gastrostomy. Reducing the risk of aspiration may be the most effective means of prolonging the life of a patient with PSP.

Surgical implants

Fetal or porcine nigral cell striatal allografts have not been attempted in PSP, but the advanced state of degeneration of centers downstream from the striatum, contrasting with the situation in PD, suggests that such procedure is unlikely to be of benefit. This prediction is supported by the unfavorable results of a trial of adrenal medullary tissue autografts to striatum (Koller, 1989). A similar rationale predicts that deep brain stimulation would not help PSP.

Patient resources

The Society for Progressive Supranuclear Palsy (www.psp.org) is headquartered in Baltimore and serves North America. The Progressive Supranuclear Palsy

Association (www.pspeur.org) is based in the UK and serves all of Europe. They offer support meetings, lay-language literature and research funding to scientists in all countries. Smaller organizations have recently been founded in other countries.

REFERENCES

Note: PSP = progressive supranuclear palsy

Abe, K., Terakawa, H., Takanashi, M. *et al.* (2000). Proton magnetic resonance spectroscopy of patients with parkinsonism. *Brain Res. Bull.*, **52**, 589–95.

Agid, Y., Javoy-Agid, F., Ruberg, M. *et al.* (1987). PSP: anatomo-clinical and biochemical considerations. *Adv. Neurol.*, **45**, 191–206.

Albers, D. S., Augood, S. J., Martin, D. M., Standaert, D. G., Vonsattel, J. P. G. & Beal, M. F. (1999). Evidence for oxidative stress in the subthalamic nucleus in PSP. *J. Neurochem.*, **73**, 881–4.

Aldrich, M. S., Foster, N. L., White, R. F., Bluemlein, L. & Prokopowicz, G. (1989). Sleep abnormalities in PSP. *Ann. Neurol.*, **25**, 577–81.

Anouti, A., Schmidt, K., Lyons, K. E. *et al.* (1996). Normal distribution of apolipoprotein E alleles in PSP. *Neurology*, **46**, 1156–7.

Arai, N. (1987). "Grumose degeneration" of the dentate nucleus: a light and electron microscopic study in PSP and dentatorubropallidoluysian atrophy. *J. Neurol. Sci.*, **90**, 131–45.

Averbuch-Heller, L., Paulson, G. W., Daroff, R. B. & Leigh, R. J. (1999). Whipple's disease mimicking PSP: the diagnostic value of eye movement recording. *J. Neurol. Neurosurg. Psychiatry*, **66**, 532–5.

Baker, K. B. & Montgomery, E. B. Jr. (2001). Performance on the PD test battery by relatives of patients with PSP. *Neurology*, **56**, 25–30.

Baker, M., Litvan, I., Houlden, H. *et al.* (1999). Association of an extended haplotype in the tau gene with PSP. *Hum. Mol. Genet.*, **8**, 711–15.

Baron, J. C., Mazière, B., Loc'h, C. *et al.* (1986). Loss of striatal (^{76}Br)-bromospiperone binding sites demonstrated by positron emission tomography in PSP. *J. Cereb. Blood. Flow. Metab.*, **6**, 131–6.

Bergeron, C., Pollanen, M. S., Weyer, L. & Lang, A. E. (1997). Cortical degeneration in PSP: a comparison with cortical-basal ganglionic degeneration. *J. Neuropath. Exp. Neurol.*, **56**, 726–34.

Bertoni, J. N., Label, L. S., Sackellares, C. & Hicks, S. P. (1983). Supranuclear gaze palsy in familial Creutzfeldt–Jakob disease. *Arch. Neurol.*, **40**, 618–22.

Birdi, S., Rajput, A. H., Fenton, M. *et al.* (2002). PSP diagnosis and confounding features: report on 16 autopsied cases. *Mov. Disord.*, **17**, 1255–67.

Bower, J. H., Maraganore, D. M., McDonnell, S. K. & Rocca, W. A. (1997). Incdence of PSP and multiple system atrophy in Olmsted County, Minnesota, 1976 to 1990. *Neurology*, **49**, 1284–8.

Braak, H., Jellinger, K., Braak, E. & Bohl, J. (1992). Allocortical neurofibrillary changes in PSP. *Acta Neuropath.*, **84**, 478–83.

Brooks, D. J., Ibanez, V., Sawle, G. V. *et al.* (1990). Differing patterns of striatal ^{18}F-dopa uptake in Parkinson's disease, multiple system atrophy, and PSP. *Ann. Neurol.*, **28**, 547–55.

Brooks, D. J., Ibanez, V., Sawle, G. V. *et al.* (1992). Striatal D$_2$ receptor status in patients with Parkinson's disease, striatonigral degeneration, and PSP, measured with ^{11}C-raclopride and positron emission tomography. *Ann. Neurol.*, **31**, 184–92.

Brown, J., Lantos, P., Stratton, M., Roques, P. & Rossor, M. (1993). Familial PSP. *J. Neurol. Neurosurg. Psychiatry*, **56**, 473–6.

Brown, P., Gibbs, C. J., Rodgers-Johnson, P. *et al.* (1994). Human spongiform encephalopathy: the National Institutes of Health series of 300 cases of experimentally transmitted disease. *Ann. Neurol.*, **35**, 513–29.

Bueé-Scherrer, V., Bueé, L., Hof, P. R. *et al.* (1995). Neurofibrillary degeneration in amyotrophic lateral sclerosis/parkinsonism-dementia complex of Guam. Immunochemical characterisation of tau proteins. *Am. J. Pathol.*, **146**, 924–32.

Burn, D. J., Sawle, G. V. & Brooks, D. J. (1994). Differential diagnosis of Parkinson's disease, multiple system atrophy, and Steele–Richardson–Olszewski syndrome: discriminant analysis of striatal ^{18}F-dopa PET data. *J. Neurol. Neurosurg. Psychiatry*, **57**, 278–84.

Cantuti-Castelvetri, I., Keller-McGandy, C. E. & Albers, D. S. *et al.* (2002). Expression and activity of antioxidants in the brain in PSP. *Brain Res.*, **15**, 170–81.

Caparros-Lefebvre, D., Elbaz, A. and the Caribbean Parkinsonism Study Group (1999). Possible relation of atypical parkinsonism in the French West Indies with consumption of tropical plants: a case-control study. *Lancet*, **354**, 281–6.

Caparros-Lefebvre, D., Sergeant, N., Lees, A. *et al.* (2002). Guadeloupean parkinsonism: a cluster of PSP-like tauopathy. *Brain*, **125**, 801–11.

Carpenter, M. B., Harbison, J. W. & Peter, P. (1970). Accessory oculomotor nuclei in the monkey: projections and effects of discrete lesions. *J. Comp. Neurol.*, **140**, 131–47.

Chirichigno, J., Manfredi, G., Beal, M. & Albers, D. (2002). Stress-induced mitochondrial depolarization and oxidative damage in PSP hybrids. *Brain Res.*, **95**, 31–35.

Chu, F. C., Reingold, D. B., Cogan, D. G. & Williams, A. C. (1979). The eye movement disorders of PSP. *Ophthalmology*, **86**, 422–8.

Clarke, C. E. & Lowry, M. (2001). Systematic review of proton magnetic resonance spectroscopy of the striatum in parkinsonian syndromes. *Eur. J. Neurol.*, **8**, 573–7.

Collins, S. J., Ahlskog, J. E., Parisi, J. E. & Maraganore, D. M. (1995). PSP: neuropathologically based diagnostic clinical criteria. *J. Neurol. Neurosurg. Psychiatry*, **58**, 167–73.

Colosimo, C., Albanese, A., Hughes, A. J., de Bruin, V. M. & Lees, A. J. (1995). Some specific clinical features differentiate multiple system atrophy (striatonigral variety) from Parkinson's disease. *Arch. Neurol.*, **52**, 294–8.

Conrad, C., Andreadis, A., Trojanowski, J. Q. *et al.* (1997). Genetic evidence for the involvement of tau in PSP. *Ann. Neurol.*, **41**, 277–81.

Cordato, N. J., Halliday, G. M., Harding, A. J., Hely, M. A. & Morris, J. G. L. (2000). Regional brain atrophy in PSP and Lewy body disease. *Ann. Neurol.*, **47**, 718–28.

Curran, T. & Lang, A. E. (1994). Parkinsonian syndromes associated with hydrocephalus: case reports, a review of the literature, and pathophysiological hypotheses. *Mov. Disord.*, **9**, 508–20.

D'Antona, R., Baron, J. C., Sanson, Y. *et al.* (1985). Subcortical dementia: Frontal cortex hypometabolism detected by positron tomography in patients with PSP. *Brain*, **108**, 785–99.

Davie, C. A., Barker, G. J., Machado, C., Miller, D. H. & Lees, A. J. (1997). Proton magnetic resonance spectroscopy in Steele–Richardson–Olszewski syndrome. *Movement Disord.*, **12**, 767–71.

Davis, P. H., Bergeron, C. & McLachlan, D. R. (1985). Atypical presentation of PSP. *Ann. Neurol.*, **17**, 337–43.

Davis, P. H., Golbe, L. I., Duvoisin, R. C. & Schoenberg, B. S. (1988). Risk factors for PSP. *Neurology*, **38**, 1546–52.

de Silva, R., Weiler, M., Morris, H. R., Martin, E. R., Wood, N. W. & Lees, A. J. (2001). Strong association of a novel tau promoter haplotype in PSP. *Neurosci. Lett.*, **311**, 145–8.

de Yébenes, J. G., Sarasa, J. L., Daniel, S. E. & Lees, A. J. (1995). Familial PSP. Description of a pedigree and review of the literature. *Brain*, **118**, 1093–103.

Dehaene, I. (1984). Apraxia of eyelid opiening in PSP. *Neurology*, **15**, 115–16.

Di Maria, E., Tabaton, M., Vigo, T. *et al.* (2000). Corticobasal degeneration shares a common genetic background with PSP. *Ann. Neurol.*, **47**, 374–7.

Di Monte, C. A., Harati, Y., Jankovic, J., Sandy, M. S., Jewell, S. A. & Langston, J. W. (1994). Muscle mitochondrial ATP production in PSP. *J. Neurochem.*, **62**, 1631–4.

Dickson, D. W. (1997). Neurodegenerative diseases with cytoskeletal pathology: a biochemical classification. *Ann. Neurol.*, **42**, 541–4.

Drayer, B. P., Olanow, W., Burger, P., Johnson, G. A., Herfkens, R. & Riederer, S. (1986). Parkinson plus syndrome: diagnosis using high field MR imaging of brain iron. *Radiology*, **159**, 493–8.

Dubas, F., Gray, F. & Escourolle, R. (1992). Maladie de Steele–Richardson–Olszewski sans ophthalmoplégie; 6 cas anatomo-cliniques. *Rev. Neurol.*, **139**, 407–16.

Dubinsky, R. M. & Jankovic, J. (1987). PSP and a multi-infarct state. *Neurology*, **37**, 570–6.

Dubois, B., Slachevsky, A., Litvan, I. & Pillon, B. (2000). The FAB: a Frontal Assessment Battery at bedside. *Neurology*, **55**, 1621–6.

Elipe, J. G., Sanchez Pernaute, R., Sandiumenge, A. & de Yebenes, J. G. (1996). Clinical symptoms in relatives of probands with PSP. *Neurology*, **46**, A386–7.

Ezquerra, M., Pastor, P., Valldeoriola, F. *et al.* (1999). Identification of a novel polymorphism in the promoter region of the tau gene highly associated to PSP in humans. *Neurosci. Lett.*, **275**, 183–6.

Fearnley, J. M. & Lees, A. J. (1991). Ageing and Parkinson's disease: substantia nigra regional selectivity. *Brain*, **114**, 2283–301.

Fearnley, J. M., Revesz, T., Brooks, D. J., Frackowiak, R. S. J. & Lees, A. J. (1991). Diffuse Lewy body disease presenting with a supranuclear gaze palsy. *J. Neurol. Neurosurg. Psychiatry*, **54**, 159–61.

Flament, S., Delacourte, A., Verny, M., Hauw, J.-J. & Javoy-Agid, F. (1991). Abnormal tau proteins in PSP. *Acta Neuropathol. (Berl.)*, **81**, 591–6.

Foster, N. L., Gilman, S., Berent, S., Morin, E. M., Brown, M. B. & Koeppe, R. A. (1988). Cerebral hypometabolism in PSP studied with positron emission tomography. *Ann. Neurol.*, **24**, 399–406.

Fukushima-Kudo, J., Fukushima, K. & Tahiro, K. (1987). Rigidity and dorsiflexion of the neck in PSP and the interstitial nucleus of Cajal. *J. Neurol. Neurosurg. Psychiatry*, **50**, 1197–203.

Gazely, S. & Maguire, J. (1994). Familial PSP. *Brain Pathol*, **4**, 534.

Gearing, M., Olson, D. A., Watts, R. L. & Mirra, S. S. (1994). PSP: neuropathologic and clinical heterogeneity. *Neurology*, **44**, 1015–24.

Gert van Dijk, J., Haan, J., Koenderink, M. & Roos, R. A. C. (1991). Autonomic nervous function of PSP. *Arch. Neurol.*, **48**, 1083–4.

Ghatak, N. R., Nochlin, D. & Hadfield, M. G. (1980). Neurofibrillary pathology in PSP. *Acta Neuropathol. (Berl.)*, **52**, 73–6.

Giaccone, G., Tagliavini, F., Street, J. S., Ghetti, B. & Bugiani, O. (1988). PSP with hypertrophy of the olives: an immunohistochemical study of argyrophilic neurons. *Acta Neuropathol. (Berl.)*, **77**, 14–20.

Gibb, W. R. G., Luthert, P. J. & Marsden, C. D. (1989). Corticobasal degeneration. *Brain*, **112**, 1171–92.

Goffinet, A. M., De Volder, A. G., Guillain, C. *et al.* (1989). Positron tomography demonstrates frontal lobe hypometabolism in PSP. *Ann. Neurol.*, **25**, 131–9.

Golbe, L. I. The epidemiology of PSP (1996). *Adv. Neurol.*, **69**, 25–31.

Golbe, L. I. & Dickson, D. W. (1995). Familial autopsy-proven PSP. *Neurology*, **45** (Suppl 4), A255.

Golbe, L. I., Davis, P. H., Schoenberg, B. S. & Duvoisin, R. C. (1988). Prevalence and natural history of PSP. *Neurology*, **38**, 1031–4.

Golbe, L. I., Davis, P. H. & Lepore, F. E. (1989). Eyelid movement abnormalities in PSP. *Mov. Disord.*, **4**, 297–302.

Golbe, L. I., Rubin, R. S., Cody, R. P. *et al.* (1996). Follow-up study of risk factors in PSP. *Neurology*, **47**, 148–54.

Golbe, L. I. and the Medical Advisory Board of the Society for PSP (1997). A clinical rating scale and staging system for PSP. *Neurology*, **48** (suppl), A326.

Golbe, L. I., Lepore, F. E., Johnson, W. G., Belsh, J. M., Powell, A. L. & Treiman, D. M. (1999). Inter-rater reliability of the PSP rating scale. *Neurology*, **52** (suppl), A227.

Golbe, L. I., Lazzarini, A. M., Spychala, J. R. *et al.* (2001). The tau A0 allele in Parkinson's disease. *Mov. Disord.*, **16**, 442–7.

Habert, M. O., Spampinato, U., Mas, J. L. *et al.* (1991). A comparative technetium 99m hexamethylpropylene amine oxime SPECT study in different types of dementia. *Eur. J. Nucl. Med.*, **18**, 3–11.

Halliday, G. M., Hardman, C. D., Cordato, N. J., Hely, M. A. & Morris, J. G. (2000). A role for the substantia nigra pars reticulata in the gaze palsy of PSP. *Brain*, **123**, 724–32.

Hardman, C. D. & Halliday, G. M. (1999). The external globus pallidus in patients with PD and PSP. *Mov. Disord.*, **14**, 626–33.

Hauw, J.-J., Verny, M., Delaere, P., Cervera, P., He, U. & Duyckaerts, C. (1990). Constant neurofibrillary changes in the neocortex in PSP. Basic differences with Alzheimer's disease and aging. *Neurosci. Lett.*, **119**, 182–6.

Hauw, J.-J., Daniel, S. E., Dickson, D. *et al.* (1994). Preliminary NINDS neuropathologic criteria for Steele–Richardson–Olszewski syndrome (PSP). *Neurology*, **44**, 2015–19.

Henderson, J. M., Carpenter, K., Cartwright, H. & Halliday, G. M. (2000). Loss of thalamic intralaminar nuclei in PSP and PD: clinical and therapeutic implications. *Brain*, **123**, 1410–21.

Higgins, J. J., Adler, R. L. & Loveless, J. M. (1999). Mutational analysis of the tau gene in PSP. *Neurology*, **53**, 1421–4.

Hoehn, M. M. & Yahr, M. D. (1967). Parkinsonism: onset, progression, and mortality. *Neurology*, **17**, 427–42.

Hof, P. R., Delacourte, A. & Bouras, C. (1992). Distribution of cortical neurofibrillary tangles in PSP: a quantitative analysis of six cases. *Acta Neuropathol. (Berl.)*, **84**, 45–51.

Houlden, H., Baker, M., Morris, H. R. *et al.* (2001). Corticobasal degeneration and PSP share a common tau haplotype. *Neurology*, **56**, 1702–6.

Hutton, M., Lendon, C. L., Rizzu, P. *et al.* (1998). Association of missense and 5′-splice-site mutation in tau with the inherited dementia FTDP-17. *Nature*, **393**, 702–5.

Ikeda, K., Akiyama, H., Haga, C., Kondo, H., Arima, K. & Oda, T. (1994). Argyrophilic thread-like structure in corticobasal degeneration and supranuclear palsy. *Neurosci. Lett.*, **174**, 157–9.

Ilgin, N., Zubieta, J., Reich, S. G., Dannals, R. F., Ravert, H. T. & Frost, J. J. (1999). PET imaging of the dopamine transporter in PSP and PD. *Neurology*, **52**, 1221–6.

Imai, H., Nakamura, T., Kondo, T. & Narabayashi, H. (1993). Dopa-unresponsive pure akinesia or freezing: a condition with a wide spectrum of PSP? *Adv. Neurol.*, **60**, 622–5.

Inagaki, T., Ishino, H., Seno, H., Yamamori, C. & Iijima, M. (1994). An autopsy case of PSP with astrocytic inclusions. *Jap. J. Psychiatry Neurol.*, **48**, 85–9.

Ishizawa, K. & Dickson, D. W. (2001). Microglial activation parallels system degeneration in PSP and corticobasal degeneration. *J. Neuropathol. Exp. Neurol.*, **60**, 647–57.

Iwatsubo, T., Hasegawa, M. & Ihara, Y. (1994). Neuronal and glial tau-positive inclusions in diverse neurologic diseases share common phosphorylation characteristics. *Acta Neuropathol. (Berl.)*, **88**, 129–36.

Jackson, J. A., Jankovic, J. & Ford, J. (1983). PSP: Clinical features and response to treatment in 16 patients. *Ann. Neurol.*, **13**, 273–8.

Jankovic, J. (1983). Controlled trial of pergolide mesylate in Parkinson's disease and PSP. *Neurology*, **33**, 505–7.

Jankovic, J. (1984a). Apraxia of eyelid opening in PSP: Reply. *Neurology*, **15**, 116.

Jankovic, J. (1984b). PSP: Clinical and pharmacologic update. *Neurol. Clin.*, **2**, 473–86.

Jankovic, J., Beach, J., Schwartz, K. & Contant, C. (1995). Tremor and longevity in relatives of patients with Parkinson's disease, essential tremor, and control subjects. *Neurology*, **45**, 645–8.

Jankovic, J. & Friedman, D. I., Pirozzolo, F. J. & McCrary, J. A. (1990). PSP: motor, neurobehavioral, and neuro-ophthalmic findings. *Adv. Neurol.*, **53**, 293–304.

Jankovic, J. & Van der Linden, C. (1990). PSP (Steele–Richardson–Olszewski syndrome). In *Movement Disorders*, ed. S. Chokroverty, pp. 267–86. New York: PMA Publishing.

Jellinger, K. (1988). The pedunculopontine nucleus in Parkinson's disease, PSP and Alzheimer's disease. *J. Neurol. Neurosurg. Psychiatry*, **52**, 540–3.

Jellinger, K. A. & Bancher, C. (1992). Neuropathology. In PSP: *Clinical and Research Approaches*, ed. I. Litvan & Y. Agid, pp. 44–88. New York: Oxford.

Jendroska, K., Hoffmann, O., Schelosky, L., Lees, A. J., Poewe, W. & Daniel, S. (1994). Absence of disease related prion protein in neurodegenerative disorders presenting with Parkinson's syndrome. *J. Neurol. Neurosurg. Psychiatry*, **57**, 1249–51.

Johnston, B. T., Castell, J. A., Stumacher, S. *et al.* (1997). Comparison of swallowing function in PD and PSP. *Mov. Disord.*, **12**, 322–7.

Josephs, K. A., Van Gerpen, M. W. & Van Gerpen, J. A. (2003). Adult onset Niemann–Pick disease type C presenting with psychosis. *J. Neurol. Neurosurg. Psychiatry*, **74**, 528–9.

Juncos, J. L., Hirsch, E. C., Malessa, S., Duyckaerts, C., Hersh, L. B. & Agid, Y. (1991). Mesencephalic cholinergic nuclei in PSP. *Neurology*, **41**, 25–30.

Kertzman, C., Robinson, D. L. & Litvan, I. (1990). Effects of physostigmine on spatial attention in patents with PSP. *Arch. Neurol.*, **47**, 1346–50.

Kida, E., Barcikowska, M. & Niemszewska, M. (1992). Immunohistochemical study of a case with PSP without ophthalmoplegia. *Acta Neuropathol.*, **83**, 328–32.

Kim, S. Y., Jeiter, T. M. & Steinert, P. M. (2002). Transglutaminases in disease. *Neurochem. Internat.*, **40**, 85–103.

Kimber, J., Mathias, C. J., Lees, A. J. *et al.* (2000). Physiological, pharmacological and neurohormonal assessment of autonomic function in PSP. *Brain*, **123**, 1422–30.

Kluin, K. J., Foster, N. L., Berent, S. & Gilman, S. (1993). Perceptual analysis of speech disorders in PSP. *Neurology*, **43**, 563–6.

Koller, W. C., Morantz, R., Vetere-Overfield, B. & Waxman, M. (1989). Autologous adrenal medullary transplant in PSP. *Neurology*, **39**, 1066–8.

Kompoliti, K., Goetz, C. G., Litvan, I., Jellinger, K. & Verny, M. (1998). Pharmacological therapy in PSP. *Arch. Neurol.*, **55**, 1099–102.

Kurtzke, J. F. & Kurland, L. T. (1973). Neuroepidemiology: a summation. In *Epidemiology of Neurologic and Sense Organ Disorders*, ed. L. T. Kurland, J. F. Kurtzke & I. D. Goldberg, pp. 305–332. Cambridge, MA: Harvard.

Landwehrmeyer, B. & Palacios, J. M. (1994). Neurotransmitter receptors in PSP. *J. Neural. Transm.* suppl **42**, 229–46.

Lannuzel, A., Michel, P. P., Caparros-Lefebvre, D., Abaul, J., Hocquemiller, R. & Ruberg, M. (2001). Toxicity of *Annonaceae* for dopaminergic neurons: potential role in atypical parkinsonism in Guadeloupe. *Mov. Disord.*, **17**, 84–90.

Leenders, K. L., Frackowiak, R. S. J. & Lees, A. J. (1988). Steele–Richardson–Olszewski syndrome: brain energy metabolism, blood flow and fluorodopa uptake measured by positron emission tomography. *Brain*, **111**, 615–30.

Leigh, R. J. & Riley, D. E. (2000). Eye movements in parkinsonism: it's saccadic speed that counts. *Neurology*, **54**, 1018–19.

Lennox, G., Lowe, J., Morrell, K., Landon, M. & Mayer, R. J. (1988). Ubiquitin is a component of neurofibrillary tangles in a variety of neurodegenerative diseases. *Neurosci. Lett.*, **94**, 211–17.

Leopold, N. A. & Kagel, M. C. (1997). Dysphagia in PSP: radiologic features. *Dysphagia*, **12**, 140–3.

Lepore, F. E. & Duvoisin, R. C. (1985). "Apraxia" of eyelid opening: an involuntary levator inhibition. *Neurology*, **35**, 423–7.

Levy, R., Ruberg, M., Herrero, M. T. *et al.* (1995). Alterations of GABAergic neurons in the basal ganglia of patients with PSP: an *in situ* hybridization study of GAD$_{67}$ messenger RNA. *Neurology*, **45**, 127–34.

Lewis, J., McGowan, E., Rockwood, J. *et al.* (2000). Neurofibrillary tangles, amyotrophy and progressive motor disturbance in mice expressing mutant (P301L) tau protein. *Nat. Genet.*, **25**, 402–5.

Lewis, J., Dickson, D. W., Lin, W.-L. *et al.* (2001). Enhanced neurofibrillary degeneration in transgenic mice expressing mutant tau and APP. *Science*, **293**, 1487–91.

Leygonie, F., Thomas, J., Degos, J. D., Bouchareine, A. & Barbizet, J. (1976). Troubles du sommeil dans la maladie de Steele–Richardson: etude polygraphique de 3 cas. *Rev. Neurol.*, **132**, 125–36.

Litvan, I., Gomez, C., Atack, J. R. *et al.* (1989). Physostigmine treatment of PSP. *Ann. Neurol.*, **26**, 404–7.

Litvan, I., Blesa, R., Clark, K. *et al.* (1994). Pharmacological evaluation of the cholinergic system in PSP. *Ann. Neurol.*, **36**, 55–61.

Litvan, I., Agid, Y., Calne, D. *et al.* (1996a). Clinical research criteria for the diagnosis of PSP: report of the NINDS-SPSP International Workshop. *Neurology*, **47**, 1–9.

Litvan, I., Mega, M. S., Cummings, J. L. & Fairbanks, L. (1996b). Neuropsychiatric aspects of PSP. *Neurology*, **47**, 1184–9.

Litvan, I., Campbell, G., Mangone, C. A. *et al.* (1997a). Which clinical features differentiate PSP from related disorders? A clinicopathological study. *Brain*, **120**, 65–74.

Litvan, I., Sastry, N. & Sonies, B. C. (1997b). Characterizing swallowing abnormalities in PSP. *Neurology*, **48**, 1654–62.

Litvan, I., Baker, M. & Hutton, M. (2001a). Tau genotype: no effect on onset, symptom severity, or survival in PSP. *Neurology*, **57**, 138–40.

Litvan, I., Phipps, M., Pharr, V. L., Hallett, M., Grafman, J. & Salazar, A. (2001b). Randomized placebo-controlled trial of donepezil in patients with PSP. *Neurology*, **57**, 467–73.

Liu, W. K., Le, T. V., Adamson, J. *et al.* (2001). Relationship of the extended tau haplotype to tau biochemistry and neuropathology in PSP. *Ann. Neurol.*, **50**, 494–502.

Love, S., Saitoh, T., Quijada, S., Cole, G. M. & Terry, R. D. (1988). Alz-50, ubiquitin and tau immunoreactivity of neurofibrillary tangles, Pick bodies and Lewy bodies. *J. Neuropathol. Exp. Neurol.*, **47**, 393–405.

Maher, E. R. & Lees, A. J. (1986). The clinical features and natural history of the Steele–Richardson–Olszewski syndrome (PSP). *Neurology*, **36**, 1005–8.

Malessa, S., Gaymard, B., Rivaud, S. *et al.* (1994). Role of pontine nuclei damage in smooth pursuit impairment of PSP: a clinical–pathologic study. *Neurology*, **44**, 716–21.

Masdeu, J. C., Alampur, U., Cavaliere, R. & Tavoulareas, G. (1994). Astasia and gait failure with damage of the pontomesencephalic locomotor region. *Ann. Neurol.*, **35**, 619–21.

Mastaglia, F. L., Grainger, K., Kee, F., Sadka, M. & Lefroy, R. (1973). PSP (the Steele–Richardson–Olszewski syndrome): clinical and electrophysiological observations in eleven cases. *Proc. Austral. Assoc. Neurol.*, **10**, 35–44.

Masucci, E. F. & Kurtzke, J. F. (1989). Tremor in PSP. *Acta Neurol. Scand.*, **80**, 296–300.

Matsuo, H., Takashima, H., Kishikawa, M. *et al.* (1991). Pure akinesia: an atypical manifestation of PSP. *J. Neurol. Neurosurg. Psychiatry*, **54**, 397.

Milberg, W. & Albert, M. (1989). Cognitive differences between patients with PSP and Alzheimer's disease. *J. Clin. Exp. Neuropsychol.*, **11**, 605–11.

Mizusawa, H., Mochizuki, A., Ohkoshi, N., Yoshizawa, K., Kanazawa, I. & Imai, H. (1993). PSP presenting with pure akinesia. *Adv. Neurol.*, **60**, 618–21.

Molinuevo, J. L., Valldeoriola, F., Alegret, M., Oliva, R. & Tolosa, E. (2000). PSP: earlier age of onset in patients with the tau protein A0/A0 genotype. *J. Neurol.*, **247**, 206–8.

Montpetit, V., Clapin, D. R. & Guberman, A. (1985). Substructure of 20 nm filaments of PSP. *Acta Neuropathol.*, **68**, 311–18.

Mori, H., Nishimura, M., Namba, Y. & Oda, M. (1994). Corticobasal degeneration: a disease with widespread appearance of abnormal tau and neurofibrillary tangles, and its relation to PSP. *Acta Neuropathol.*, **88**, 113–21.

Moriizumi, T. & Hattori, T. (1992). Separate neuronal populations of the rat globus pallidus projecting to the subthalamic nucleus, auditory cortex and pedunculopontine tegmental area. *Neuroscience*, **46**, 701–10.

Morris, H. R., Gibb, G., Katzenschlager, R. *et al.* (2002). Pathological, clinical and genetic heterogeneity in PSP. *Brain*, **125**, 969–75.

Morris, H. R., Schrag, A., Nath, U. *et al.* (2001). Effect of ApoE and tau on age of onset of PSP and multiple system atrophy. *Neurosci. Lett.*, **312**, 118–20.

Morris, H. R., Vaughan, J. R., Datta, S. R. *et al.* (2000). Multiple system atrophy / PSP: α-synuclein, synphilin, tau, and APOE. *Neurology*, **55**, 1918–20.

Muller, J., Wenning, G. K., Verny, M. *et al.* (2001). Progression of dysarthria and dysphagia in postmortem-confirmed parkinsonian disorders. *Arch. Neurol.*, **58**, 259–64.

Nagahama, Y., Fukuyama, H., Turjanski, N. *et al.* (1997). Cerebral glucose metabolism in corticobasal degeneration: comparison with PSP and normal controls. *Mov. Disord.*, **12**, 691–6.

Nath, U., Ben-Shlomo, Y., Thomson, R. G. *et al.* (2001). The prevalence of PSP (Steele–Richardson–Olszewski syndrome) in the UK. *Brain*, **124**, 1438–49.

Neary, D., Snowdon, J. S., Shields, R. A. *et al.* (1987). Single photon emission tomography using [99]mTc-HM-PAO in the investigation of dementia. *J. Neurol. Neurosurg. Psychiatry*, **50**, 1101–9.

Nelson, S. J., Yen, S-H., Davies, P. & Dickson, D. W. (1989). Basal ganglia neuropil threads in PSP. *J. Neuropathol. Exp. Neurol.*, **48**, 324.

Newman, G. C. (1985). Treatment of PSP with tricyclic antidepressants. *Neurology*, **35**, 1189–93.

Nieforth, K. A. & Golbe, L. I. (1993). Retrospective study of drug response in 87 patients with PSP. *Clin. Neuropharmacol.*, **16**, 338–46.

Nuwer, M. R. (1981). PSP despite normal eye movements. *Arch. Neurol.*, **38**, 784.

Odetti, P., Garibaldi, S., Norese, R. *et al.* (2000). Lipoperoxidation is selectively involved in PSP. *J. Neuropath. Exp. Neurol.*, **59**, 393–7.

Ohara, S., Kondo, K., Morita, H., Maruyama, K., Ikeda, S. & Yanagisawa, N. (1992). PSP-like syndrome in two siblings of a consanguineous marriage. *Neurology*, **42**, 1009–14.

Olszewski, J., Steele, J. & Richardson, J. C. (1963). Pathological report on six cases of heterogeneous system degeneration. *J. Neuropathol. Exp. Neurol.*, **23**, 187–8.

Oyanaki, K., Takahashi, H., Wakabayashi, K. & Ikuta, F. (1991). Large neurons in the neostriatum in Alzheimer's disease and PSP: a topographic, histologic and ultrastructural investigation. *Brain Res.*, **544**, 221–6.

Pahwa, R., Koller, W. C. & Stern, M. B. (1993). Primary pallidal atrophy, In *Parkinsonian Syndromes*, ed. M. B. Stern & W. C. Koller, pp. 433–40. New York: Marcel Dekker.

Pascual, J., Berciano, J., Gonzalez, A. M., Grijalba, B., Figols, J. & Pazos, A. (1993). Autoradiographic demonstration of loss of alpha-2-adrenoceptors in PSP: preliminary report. *J. Neurol. Sci.*, **114**, 165–9.

Pastor, P., Ezquerra, M., Tolosa, E. *et al.* (2001). Further extension of the H1 haplotype associated with PSP. *Mov Disord.*, **17**, 550–556.

Pfaffenbach, D. D., Layton, D. D. & Kearns, T. P. (1972). Ocular manifestations in PSP. *Am. J. Ophthalmol.*, **74**, 1179–84.

Piccini, P., de Yebenes, J., Lees, A. J. *et al.* (2001). Familial PSP: detection of subclinical cases using 18F-dopa and 18-fluorodeoxyglucose positron emission tomography. *Arch. Neurol.*, **58**, 1846–51.

Piccione, F., Mancini, E., Tonin, P. & Bizzarini, M. (1997). Botulinum toxin treatment of apraxia of eyelid opening in PSP: report of two cases. *Arch. Phys. Med. Rehab.*, **78**, 525–9.

Pillon, B., Deweer, B., Michon, A., Malapani, C., Agid, Y. & Dubois, B. (1994). Are explicit memory disorders of PSP related to damage to striatofrontal circuits? Comparison with Alzheimer's, Parkinson's and Huntington's diseases. *Neurology*, **44**, 1264–70.

Pillon, B. & Dubois, B. (1992). Cognitive and behavioral impairments. In *PSP: Clinical and Research Approaches*, ed. I. Litvan, and Y. Agid, pp. 223–39. New York: Oxford.

Pillon, B., Gouider-Khouja, N., Deweer, B. *et al.* (1995). Neuropsychological pattern of striatonigral degeneration: comparison with Parkinson's disease and PSP. *J. Neurol. Neurosurg. Psychiatry*, **58**, 174–9.

Podoll, K., Schwarz, M. & Noth, J. (1991). Language functions in PSP. *Brain*, **114**, 1457–72.

Pollock, N. J., Mirra, S. S., Binder, L. I., Hansen, L. A. & Wood, J. G. (1986). Filamentous aggregates in Pick's disease, PSP, and Alzheimer's disease share antigenic determinants with microtubule-associated protein, tau. *Lancet*, **ii**, 1211.

Polo, K. B. & Jabbari, B. (1994). Botulinum toxin-A improves the rigidity of progressive supranculear palsy. *Ann. Neurol.*, **35**, 237–9.

Powell, H. C., London, G. W. & Lampert, P. W. (1974). Neurofibrillary tangles in PSP. *J. Neuropath. Exp. Neurol.*, **33**, 98–106.

Probst, A., Langui, D., Lautenschlager, C., Jlrich, J., Brion, J. P. & Anderton, B. H. (1988). PSP: extensive neuropil threads in addition to neurofibrillary tangles. *Acta Neuropathol. (Berl.)*, **77**, 61–8.

Probst, A., Luginbühl, M., Langui, D., Ulrich, J. & Landwehrmeyer, B. (1994). Pathology of the striatum in PSP: abnormal tau proteins in astrocytes and cholinergic interneurons. *Neurodegeneration*, **2**, 183–93.

Rafal, R. D. & Grimm, R. J. (1981). PSP: Functional analysis of the response to methysergide and antiparkinsonian agents. *Neurology*, **31**, 1507–18.

Rafal, R. D., Posner, M. I., Friedman, J. H., Inhoff, A. W. & Bernstein, E. (1988). Orienting of visual attention in PSP. *Brain*, **111**, 267–80.

Rajput, A. H., Offord, K. P., Beard, C. M. & Kurland, L. T. (1984). Epidemiology of parkinsonism: incidence, classification, and mortality. *Ann. Neurol.*, **16**, 278–82.

Rascol, O., Sabatini, U., Simonetta-Moreau, M., Montastruc, J. L., Rascol, A. & Clanet, M. (1991). Square wave jerks in parkinsonian syndromes. *J. Neurol. Neurosurg. Psychiatry*, **54**, 599–602.

Rascol, O., Clanet, M., Senard, J. M., Montastruc, J. L. & Rascol, A. (1993). Vestibulo-ocular reflex in Parkinson's disease and multiple system atrophy. *Adv. Neurol.*, **60**, 395–7.

Richardson, J. C., Steele, J. & Olszewski, J. (1963). Supranuclear ophthalmoplegia, pseudobulbar palsy, nuchal dystonia and dementia: a clinical report on eight cases of "heterogeneous system degeneration." *Trans. Am. Neurol. Assoc.*, **88**, 25–9.

Riley, D. E., Fogt, N. & Leigh, R. J. (1994). The syndrome of "pure akinesia" and its relationship to PSP. *Neurology*, **44**, 1025–9.

Rivest, J., Quinn, N. & Marsden, C. D. (1990). Dystonia in Parkinson's disease, multiple system atrophy, and PSP. *Neurology*, **40**, 1571–8.

Robbins, T. W., James, M., Owen, A. M. *et al.* (1994). Cognitive deficits in PSP, Parkinson's disease, and multiple system atrophy in tests sensitive to frontal lobe dysfunction. *J. Neurol. Neurosurg. Psychiatry*, **57**, 79–88.

Rojo, A., Pernaute, S., Fontán, A. *et al.* (1999). Clinical genetics of familial PSP. *Brain*, **122**, 1233–45.

Rosser, A. & Hodges, J. R. (1994). Initial letter and semantic category fluency in Alzheimer's disease, Huntington's disease, and PSP. *J. Neurol. Neurosurg. Psychiatry*, **57**, 1389–94.

Rub, U., Del Tredici, K., Schultz, C. *et al.* (2002). PSP: neuronal and glial cytoskeletal pathology in the higher order processing autonomic nuclei of the lower brainstem. *Neuropathol. Appl. Neurobiol.*, **28**, 12–22.

Ruberg, M., Javoy-Agid, F., Hirsch, E. *et al.* (1985). Dopaminergic and cholinergic lesions in PSP. *Ann. Neurol.*, **18**, 523–9.

Saitoh, H., Yoshii, F. & Shinohara, Y. (1987). Computed tomographic findings in PSP. *Neuroradiology*, **29**, 168–71.

Sakakibara, R., Hattori, T., Tojo, M., Yamanishi, T. & Yasuda, K. (1993). Micturitional disturbance in PSP. *J. Auton. Nerv. Syst.*, **45**, 101–6.

Savoiardo, M., Strada, L., Girotti, F. *et al.* (1989). MR imaging in PSP and Shy–Drager syndrome. *J. Comput. Assist. Tomogr.*, **13**, 555–60.

Scaravilli, T., Pramstaller, P. P., Salerno, A. *et al.* (2000). Neuronal loss in Onuf's nucleus in three patients with progressive supranuclear palsy. *Ann. Neurol.*, **48**, 97–101.

Schneider, J. A., Gearing, M., Robbins, R. S., de l'Aune, W. & Mirra, S. S. (1995). Apolipoprotein E genotype in diverse neurodegenerative disorders. *Ann. Neurol.*, **38**, 131–5.

Schonfeld, S. M., Golbe, L. I., Safer, J., Sage, J. I. & Duvoisin, R. C. (1987). Computed tomographic findings in PSP: correlation with clinical grade. *Mov. Disord.*, **2**, 263–78.

Schrag, A., Ben-Shlomo, Y. & Quinn, N. (1999). Prevalence of PSP and MSA: a cross-sectional study. *Lancet*, **354**, 1771–2.

Schwarz, J., Tatsch, K., Arnold, G. *et al.* (1992). [123]-Iodobenzamide-SPECT predicts dopaminergic responsiveness in patients with de novo parkinsonism. *Neurology*, **42**, 556–61.

Seppi, K., Schocke, M. F., Esterhammer, R. *et al.* (2003). Diffusion-weighted imaging discriminates PSP from PD, but not from the Parkinson variant of multiple system atrophy. *Neurology*, **60**, 922–7.

Shinotoh, H., Namba, H., Yamaguchi, M. *et al.* (1999). PET measurement of acetylcholinesterase activity reveals differential loss of ascending cholinergic systems in PD and PSP. *Ann. Neurol.*, **46**, 62–9.

Sonies, B. C. (1992). Swallowing and speech disturbances. In *PSP: Clinical and Research Approaches*, ed. I. Litvan & Y. Agid, pp. 240–54. New York: Oxford.

Sosner, J., Wall, G. C. & Sznajder, J. (1993). PSP: clinical presentation and rehabilitation of two patients. *Arch. Phys. Med. Rehab.*, **74**, 537–9.

Spillantini, M. G., Murrell, J. R., Goedert, M., Farlow, M. R., Klug, A. & Ghetti, B. (1998). Mutation in the tau gene in familial multiple system tauopathy with presenile dementia. *Proc. Natl Acad. Sci., USA*, **95**, 7737–41.

Stanford, P. M., Halliday, G. M., Brooks, W. S. *et al.* (2000). PSP pathology caused by a novel silent mutation in exon 10 of the tau gene: expansion of the disease phenotype caused by tau gene mutations. *Brain*, **123**, 880–93.

Steele, J. C., Richardson, J. C. & Olszewski, J. (1964). PSP: A heterogeneous degeneration involving the brain stem, basal ganglia and cerebellum, with vertical gaze and pseudobulbar palsy, nuchal dystonia and dementia. *Arch. Neurol.*, **10**, 333–59.

Steele, J. C., Caparros-Lefebvre, D., Lees, A. J. & Sacks, O. W. (2002). PSP and its relation to Pacific foci of the parkinson-dementia complex and Guadeloupean parkinsonism. *Parkinsonism Rel. Dis.*, **9**, 39–54.

Stern, M. B., Braffman, B. H., Skolnick, B. E., Hurtig, H. I. & Grossman, R. I. (1989). Magnetic resonance imaging in Parkinson's disease and parkinsonian syndromes. *Neurology*, **39**, 1524–6.

Swerdlow, R. H., Golbe, L. I., Parks, J. K. *et al.* (2000). Mitochondrial dysfunction in cybrid lines expressing mitochondrial genes from patients with PSP. *J. Neurochem.*, **75**, 1681–4.

Tabaton, M., Whitehouse, P. J., Perry, G., Davies, P., Autilio-Gambetti, L. & Gambetti, P. (1988). Alz 50 recognized abnormal filaments in Alzheimer's disease and PSP. *Ann. Neurol.*, **24**, 407–13.

Tabaton, M., Rolleri, M., Masturzo, P. *et al.* (1995). Apolipoprotein E epsilon 4 allele frequency is not increased in PSP. *Neurology*, **45**, 1764–5.

Tagliavini, F., Pilleri, G., Bouras, C. & Constantinidis, J. (1984). The basal nucleus of Meynert in patients with PSP. *Neurosci. Lett.*, **44**, 37–42.

Tanner, C. M., Goetz, C. G. & Klawans, H. L. (1987). Multi-infarct PSP. *Neurology*, **37**, 1819.

Tellez-Nagel, I. & Wisniewski, H. M. (1973). Ultrastructure of neurofibrillary tangles in Steele-Richardson-Olszewski syndrome. *Arch. Neurol.*, **29**, 324–7.

Testa, D., Monza, D., Ferrarini, M., Soliveri, P., Girotti, F. & Filippini, G. (2001). Comparison of natural histories of PSP and multiple system atrophy. *Neurol. Sci.*, **22**, 247–51.

Tetrud, J. W., Golbe, L. I., Farmer, P. M. & Forno, L. S. (1996). Autopsy-proven PSP in two siblings. *Neurology*, **46**, 931–4.

Timmons, J. H., Bonikowski, F. W. & Harshorne, M. F. (1989). Iodoamphetamine-123 brain imaging demonstrating cortical deactivation in a patient with PSP. *Clin. Nucl. Med.*, **14**, 841–2.

Togo, T. & Dickson, D. W. (2002). Tau accumulation in astrocytes in PSP is a degenerative rather than a reactive process. *Acta Neuropathol.*, **104**, 398–402.

Tolosa, E. S. & Zeese, J. A. (1979). Brainstem auditory evoked responses in PSP. *Ann. Neurol.*, **6**, 369.

Tomonaga, M. (1977). Ultrastructure of neurofibrillary tangles in PSP. *Acta Neuropathol. (Berl.)*, **37**, 1771–1781.

Troost, B. T. & Daroff, R. B. (1977). The ocular motor defects in PSP. *Ann. Neurol.*, **2**, 397–403.

Truong, D. D., Harding, A. E., Scaravilli, F., Smith, S. J. M., Morgan-Hughes, J. A. & Marsden, C. D. (1990). Movement disorders in mitochondrial myopathies: a study of nine cases with two autopsy studies. *Mov. Disord.*, **5**, 109–17.

Uitti, R., Evidente, V. G. H., Dickson, D. W. & Graff-Radford, N. (1999). A kindred with familial PSP. *Neurology*, **52**, A227.

Valls-Solé, J., Valldeoriola, F., Tolosa, E. & Marti, M. J. (1997). Distinctive abnormalities of facial reflexes in patients with PSP. *Brain*, **120**, 1877–83.

van Royen, E., Verhoeff, N. F., Speelman, J. D., Wolters, E. C., Kuiper, M. A. & Janssen, A. G. (1993). Multiple system atrophy and PSP: diminished striatal D2 dopamine receptor activity demonstrated by ^{123}I-IBZM single photon emission computed tomography. *Arch. Neurol.*, **50**, 513–16.

Vanacore, N., Bonifati, V., Fabbrini, G. *et al.* (2000). Smoking habits in multiple system atrophy and PSP. *Neurology*, **54**, 114–19.

Vermersch, P., Robitaille, Y., Bernier, L., Wattez, A., Gauvreau, D. & Delacourte, A. (1994). Biochemical mapping of neurofibrillary degeneration in a case of PSP: evidence for general cortical involvement. *Acta Neuropathol.*, **87**, 572–7.

Verny, M., Duyckaerts, C., Delaére, P., He, Y. & Hauw, J.-J. (1994). Cortical tangles in PSP. *J. Neural. Transm.*, suppl **42**, 179–88.

Vidailhet, M., Rothwell, J. C., Thompson, P. D., Lees, A. J. & Marsden, C. D. (1992). The auditory startle response in the Steele–Richardson–Olszewski syndrome and Parkinson's disease. *Brain*, **115**, 1181–92.

Villares, J., Strada, O., Faucheux, B., Javoy-Agid, F., Agid, Y. & Hirsch, E. C. (1994). Loss of striatal high affinity NGF binding sites in PSP but not in Parkinson's disease. *Neurosci. Lett.*, **182**, 59–62.

Vitaliani, R., Scaravilli, T., Egarter-Vigl, E. *et al.* (2002). The pathology of the spinal cord in PSP. *J. Neuropathol. Appl. Neurol.*, **61**, 268–74.

Vodusek, D. B. (2001). Sphincter EMG and differential diagnosis of multiple system atrophy. *Mov. Disord.*, **16**, 600–7.

Wakabayashi, K., Oyanagi, K., Makifuchi, T. *et al.* (1994). Corticobasal degeneration: etiopathological significance of the cytoskeletal alterations. *Acta Neuropathol.*, **87**, 545–53.

Weiner, W. J., Minagar, A. & Shulman, L. M. (1999). Pramipexole in PSP. *Neurology*, **52**, 873–4.

Wenning, G. K., Ebersbach, G., Verny, M. *et al.* (1999). Progression of falls in postmortem-confirmed parkinsonian disorders. *Mov. Disord.*, **14**, 947–50.

Will, R. G., Lees, A. J., Gibb, W. & Barnard, R. O. (1988). A case of progressive subcortical gliosis presenting clinically as Steele–Richardson–Olszewski syndrome. *J. Neurol. Neurosurg. Psychiatry*, **51**, 1224–7.

Winikates, J. & Jankovic, J. (1994). Vascular PSP. *J. Neural. Transm.*, **42** (suppl), 189–201.

Wittmann, C. W., Wszolek, M. F., Shulman, J. M. *et al.* (2001). Tauopathy in *Drosophila*: neurodegeneration without neurofibrillary tangles. *Science*, **293**, 711–14.

Yamada, T., Calne, D. B., Akiyama, H., McGeer, E. G. & McGeer, P. L. (1993). Further observations on Tau-positive glia in the brains with PSP. *Acta Neuropathol.*, **85**, 308–15.

Young, A. B. (1985). PSP: postmortem chemical analysis. *Neurology*, **18**, 521–2.

Yuki, N., Sato, S., Yuasa, T., Ito, J. & Miyatake, T. (1990). Computed tomographic findings of PSP compared with Parkinson's disease. *Jpn. J. Med.*, **29**, 506–11.

Zweig, R. M., Whitehouse, P. J., Casanova, M. F. *et al.* (1987). Loss of pedunculopontine neurons in PSP. *Ann. Neurol.*, **22**, 18–25.

45

Corticobasal degeneration

Kailash P. Bhatia and Anthony E. Lang

Sobell Department of Movement Neuroscience, Institute of Neurology, Queen Square, London, UK

Historical review

Dutil (1899) from the Salpêtrière may have been describing a case of corticobasal degeneration (CBD) when reporting a patient said to have the so- called "hemiplegic" form of "parkinsonism in extension," the latter being the description used by Charcot and his pupils to describe cases of parkinsonism who were atypical because of an extended posture rather than the characteristic flexed posture of paralysis agitans which they recognized. The picture of this patient shows a French woman with a hypomimic face and a rather erect posture with the right arm rigidly flexed at the elbow and perhaps is the first picture of a CBD patient (Goetz, 2000). However, the first clear description was given by Rebeiz, Kolodny, and Richardson (1968), who described three cases with a distinct clinical syndrome characterized by an asymmetric onset of slow, clumsy limb movement, accompanied by rigidity, tremor and dystonia, progressing to impairment of gait, dysarthria and dysphagia, disordered eye movement, and increasing disability. Intellectual function was said to be relatively intact. The illness led to death in 6 to 8 years. The pathological findings were distinctive. There was asymmetric frontal and parietal cortical atrophy, with extensive neuronal loss and gliosis. Some of the cortical pyramidal neurons, mainly in the third and fifth layers, had an unusual swollen hyaline appearance; the cytoplasm did not take up usual stains, except for faint eosinophilia, so such neurons were termed achromatic. No classical Pick bodies, neurofibrillary tangles, senile plaques, or Lewy bodies were found. Such changes were not evident in the hippocampal formation, occipital cortex, inferior or medial temporal cortex. Other findings included loss of pigmented neurons in the substantia nigra, changes in the subthalamic nucleus and in the dentate nucleus, and degeneration of the corticospinal pathways. Rebeiz et al. (1968) termed this entity as "corticodentatonigral degeneration with neuronal achromasia." Other terms used by different authors to describe the same pathological changes of frontal and parietal lobe atrophy associated with atrophy of the basal ganglia and other subcortical nuclei include corticonigral degeneration with neuronal achromasia (Case Records of the Massachusetts General Hospital, 1985), cortical degeneration with swollen chromatolytic neurons (Clark et al., 1986), corticobasal (CBD) (Gibb et al., 1989; Rinne et al., 1994), cortico-basal ganglionic (Watts et al., 1985) and cortical basal ganglionic (Riley et al., 1990) degeneration (CBGD). Numerous clinical case series based on the characteristic clinical picture have been reported in the literature, few with pathological verification (Rebeiz et al., 1968; Case Records of the Massachusetts General Hospital, 1985; Clark et al., 1986; Gibb et al., 1989; Watts et al., 1985, 1989; Greene et al., 1990; Lippa et al., 1990; Paulus & Selim, 1990; Riley et al., 1990; Rinne et al., 1994; Wenning et al., 1998; Kompoliti et al., 1998). Clinical features in the majority of cases reported initially with this pathology were dominated by an asymmetric extrapyramidal and frontal motor disorder with elements of apraxia, rigidity, involuntary movements, dystonia, the alien limb sign, dysarthria, and a supranuclear disorder of eye movement. Some authors have also described this clinical syndrome as progressive apraxic rigidity (Watts et al., 1985; Le Witt et al., 1989).

Most of the earlier reports thus focused on the abnormalities in motor function as that was thought to be the predominant presentation. Initial patient series suggested that this was a distinct clinical–pathological disorder that could be readily differentiated from other "Parkinson-plus" syndromes with which it was classified. However, of late a wider clinical spectrum of this disorder is being recognized, including dementia as the initial or predominant feature (Grimes et al., 1999), as well as progressive aphasia or a behavioral disorder. It has become apparent that the exact clinical manifestations depend on the topographical distribution of the pathology. Also being recognized is the fact that a variety of different pathological entities may give rise to the same clinical syndrome (Boeve *et al.*, 1999; Bhatia *et al.*, 2000).

In this regard historically the main difficulty related to the pathological overlap with Pick's disease is the severe cortical cell loss with associated gliosis of the subcortical white matter and the large swollen achromatic cells were similar to the findings in Pick's disease. Those who supported the notion that CBD was a separate disorder from Pick's used the basis that argyrophilic inclusions (Pick bodies), typical of Pick's disease, were thought to be uncommon or not found in CBD and that the distribution of atrophy was frontoparietal in CBD in contrast to the frontotemporal lobar atrophy of Pick's disease. Since then, the classification of neurodegenerations on the basis of the dominant accumulated protein and, in the case of disorders characterized by the aggregation of the microtubule-associated protein tau, the specific protein isoforms, has revolutionized our understanding of CBD and its relationship to other neurodegenerations. With advances in molecular pathology (see below) CBD is now known to be a fairly distinct lobar and basal ganglia tauopathy with selective aggregation of four repeat tau protein with characteristic antigenic and ultrastructural characteristics.

Morphological pattttern of involvement

Anatomical pathology

The macroscopic pathological findings consist of severe focal cortical atrophy centred on the peri-Rolandic posterior frontal and parietal cortex with lesser involvement of adjacent cortex, and relative sparing of the temporal and occipital regions (Fig. 45.1). Accordingly, the motor and sensory areas of the cerebral cortex are most severely affected, and there is secondary degeneration of the corticospinal tracts. The cortical atrophy tends to be asymmetric, being most marked opposite to the most affected limb. However, in the dementing or aphasic presentation more symmetric and more severe involvement of the frontal and temporal lobes may be present. In the affected cortical regions, the normal cortical architecture is destroyed, the definition of the layers of the cerebral cortex is lost, and there is intense fibrillary gliosis. The white matter beneath the affected cortical areas is atrophic and gliotic. Neuronal degeneration with nerve cell loss and gliosis are present, particularly in the third and fifth pyramidal cell layers of the cortex. Atrophy and cell loss, accompanied by gliosis, is also marked in the lateral two-thirds of the substantia

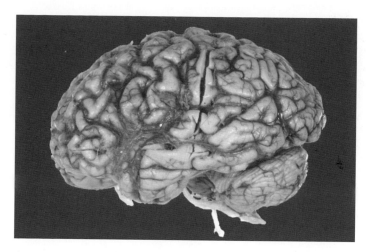

Fig. 45.1 Frontal atrophy in a case with corticobasal degeneration (courtesy Dr T. Revesz, Institute of Neurology, Queen Square, London).

nigra with loss of pigmented cells (Rebeiz *et al.*, 1968; Gibb *et al.*, 1989). The degeneration also affects the medial third of the subthalamic nucleus, the neostriatum, globus pallidus, the posterolateral thalamus, the red nucleus and other brainstem nuclei. In two of the original cases reported by Rebeiz *et al.* (1968) there was marked atrophy of the dentatorubrothalamic tract; the dentate nucleus was abnormal in these cases but the cerebellar cortex was normal. In subsequent reports, involvement of the cerebellum has been infrequent and the "dentate" component of the original description has been omitted (Case Records of the Massachusetts General Hospital, 1985). Corticospinal tract degeneration has been present in some cases (Rebeiz *et al.*, 1968; Gibb *et al.*, 1989).

Recently it has been shown that the cerebellar Purkinje cells are involved with granular accumulation of tau in about half the cases of CBD studied by Piao *et al.* (2002) using monoclonal antibodies. The spinal cord has not been reported on frequently but in the era prior to the recent advances in molecular pathology was said to have been normal.

A characteristic feature of the degeneration is the presence of large pale neurons to which the term neuronal achromasia was derived (Rebeiz *et al.*, 1968). The affected cortical neurons are medium to large pyramidal cells. They are found most frequently in those cortical regions moderately, rather than severely, affected. They are also found in subcortical and brainstem nuclei including the substantia nigra. These cells, which are indistinguishable from Pick cells, have variously been referred to as ballooned, swollen, chromatolytic-like, or achromatic cells (Gibb *et al.*, 1989) (Fig. 45.2). They are most prominent

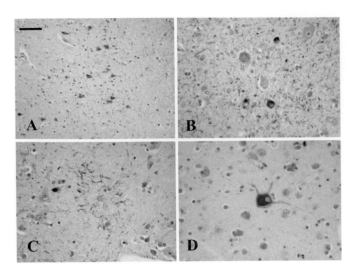

Fig. 45.2 Tau-positive intraneuronal inclusions (**A**), neuropil threads (**B**) and astrocytic plaque in the posterior frontal cortex in a case with corticobasal degeneration. Ballooned neurons are mainly present in the deeper cortical laminae (**D**). **A**, **B** and **C**: tau immunohistochemistry (antibody AT8), **D**: αB-crystallin immunohistochemistry. Bar on **A** represents 200 μm on **A** and 80 μm on **B**, **C** and **D**. (courtesy Dr T. Revesz, Institute of Neurology, Queen Square, London).

in the third, fifth, and sixth laminae of the cerebral cortex. The swollen achromatic nerve cells are filled with homogenous material which shows faint and variable eosinophilia (Rebeiz *et al.*, 1968) and argyrophilia (Clark *et al.*, 1986). The nucleus is eccentrically located and Nissl substance is not detected within the neurons, distinguishing the degeneration from that seen in central chromatolysis (Rebeiz *et al.*, 1968; Case Records of the Massachusetts General Hospital, 1985). The cytoplasm of such ballooned achromatic neurons stains positively for phosphorylated neurofilaments and beta crystalline, and variably with antibodies to ubiquitin and tau (Gibb *et al.*, 1989; Smith *et al.*, 1992; Dickson, 2000). The presence of ballooned neurons was thought to be characteristic of Pick's disease (hence called Pick cells) and CBD. However, it is clear that these are also (though less commonly) seen in progressive supranuclear palsy (PSP), Alzheimer's disease (AD), frontotemporal dementia and even Creutzfeldt–Jacob disease (CJD). Therefore, it is not the presence of the ballooned neurons alone that is important for the diagnosis. The distribution and the quantity at different sites is crucial, as well as the ultrastructural pattern of the neurofilaments (see below). Lewy bodies, granulovacuolar degeneration, extensive plaque, and neurofibrillary tangle formation have not been features of the cases reported.

Ultrastructurally, as early as 1989 (Watts *et al.*) it had been noted that the the cytoplasm of the swollen pale neurons was filled with aggregates of 10 nm intermediate filaments. The pathological filamentous inclusions of CBD are now known to be composed primarily of abnormally phosphorylated tau similar to other sporadic and familial neurodegenerative diseases, such as Alzheimer's disease, PSP, Pick's and frontotemporal dementia with parkinsonism linked to chromosome 17 (FTDP-17), collectively referred to as tauopathies. Cortical tau positive neuronal inclusions are found in pyramidal and non-pyramidal neurons and may have a characteristic perinuclear, coiled filamentous appearance. Weakly basophilic nigral neuronal inclusions were first described by Gibb *et al.* (1989), referred to as corticobasal inclusions and were initially thought to be specific for CBD. However, subsequently it has become clear that these inclusions can be morphologically heterogenous. They vary from slightly fibrillar to frankly filamentous and thus may be indistinguishable from tau-positive neurofibrillary tangles (NFTs) associated with PSP. However, cortical tau positive neuronal inclusions are more common in CBD than PSP, while in the latter disorder the neuronal inclusions are more abundant in the brainstem and deep gray matter. Thus, the distribution of the neuronal (and glial – see below) lesions is important for the pathological differentiation. Feany and Dickson (1995, 1996) and others have also detailed the cytoskeletal abnormalities by immunohistochemical methods looking at the neuropathological overlap between CBD and related conditions, particularly Pick's disease and PSP (see section below on molecular pathology). Apart from the neuronal changes there is glial tau pathology in CBD characterized by two main features, namely astrocytic plaques and coiled bodies which are tau-immunoreactive inclusions in astrocytes and oligodendrocytes in gray and white matter (Komori, 1999; Forman *et al.*, 2002). *Astrocytic plaques* is the term used to describe distinctive annular clusters of thick, short, tau positive deposits within the distal processes of cortical astrocytes (Fig. 45.2). They are thought to be more specific for CBD, than other disorders, such as PSP. These plaques are not associated with beta amyloid. In contrast, *tufted astrocytes* are characteristic of PSP. Astrocytic plaques of CBD also have to be differentiated from thorn-shaped astrocytes, which are not disease specific. The distribution of the abnormal astrocytes is somewhat different. In CBD astrocytic inclusions are more common in cortex than in the deep gray matter or brainstem. Coiled bodies, which are ubiquitin-negative, tau-immunoreactive oligodendroglial inclusions, are also common in the cortical and subcortical regions in CBD. These appear as fine bundles of filaments coiled around a nucleus and extend to the proximal part of the cell process. These inclusions are morphologically and antigenically distinct from the glial cytoplasmic inclusions seen in multiple system atrophy (MSA).

Table 45.1. Neuropathologic criteria for the diagnosis of corticobasal degeneration

Core features
- Focal cortical neuronal loss
- Substantia nigra neuronal loss
- Cortical and striatal Gallyas/tau-positive neuronal and glial lesions, especially astrocytic plaques and threads, in both white matter and gray matter

Supportive features
- Cortical atrophy, often with superficial spongiosis
- Ballooned neurons, usually numerous in atrophic cortices
- Tau-positive oligodendroglial coiled bodies

Adapted from Dickson *et al.*, 2002.

Table 45.2. Conditions characterized by the deposition of tau containing neurofibrillary tangles (tauopathies)

Progressive supranuclear palsy (PSP)
Corticobasal degeneration (CBD)
Frontotemporal dementia parkinsonism-chromosome 17 (FTDP-17)
Postencephalitic parkinsonism (encephalitis lethargica)
Post-traumatic parkinsonism (including dementia pugilistica)
Parkinson–dementia complex of Guam
Alzheimer's disease
Niemann–Pick type C
Subacute sclerosing panencephalitis(SSPE)

Adapted from Morris *et al.*, 1999.

Thin tau-immunoreactive *threads* of neuronal and glial origin are present throughout the gray and white matter and, although infrequently seen in Pick's disease, are particularly numerous in CBD. Given these nuances, it had been important that pathological diagnosis was made only by those with considerable experience in evaluating these conditions. However, recently validated neuropathologic diagnostic criteria (Dickson *et al.*, 2002, Table 45.1) will be a big help in this regard. These criteria emphasize the presence of tau-immunoreactive lesions in neurons, glia and cell processes. The minimal pathologic features for a diagnosis of CBD are the presence of cortical and striatal tau- (or Gallyas-) positive neuronal and glial lesions, especially astrocytic plaques and thread-like structures in both white matter and gray matter combined with neuronal loss both in focal cortical regions and in the substantia nigra. Although ballooned (achromatic) neurons identical to "Pick cells" were initially believed to be the pathological hallmark of the disorder, they are now considered only a supportive feature in view of rare cases lacking this abnormality but typical in every other way. These criteria provide good differentiation of CBD from other tauopathies with the one important exception being some cases of frontotemporal dementia and parkinsonism linked to specific mutations in chromosome 17. In these cases, additional clinical (particularly a positive family history) or molecular genetic information is required to make an accurate diagnosis.

Molecular pathology

Accumulation of hyperphosphorylated tau, comprising the abnormal filamentous inclusions in neurons and glia, is the characteristic feature of CBD and other tauopathies (Table 45.2). Unique antigenic, biochemical and ultrastructural features help to differentiate these different disorders.

The tau gene is located on chromosome 17 and has 13 exons. Six tau isoforms result from variable splicing of exons 2,3 and 10, and these isoforms are variably phosphorylated at specific serine and threonine residues. Three of these isoforms carry the segment specified by exon 10 and four repeats of a microtubule-binding domain called four repeat tau (4R tau). The other three isoforms lack this fourth domain and are hence called three repeat tau (3R tau). Normally 3R and 4R are in equal concentration. Tau isoforms cannot be differentiated by electrophoretic pattern alone and antibodies to exon-specific epitopes help to identify different tau-related neurodegenerative disorders. Differences in morphology and distribution of tau immunoreactivity also have to be taken in consideration when reaching a conclusion.

For example, CBD and PSP have similarity in the electrophoretic pattern of tau both having 68 and 64 kilodalton doublets. However, studies with antibodies to exon 3 tau specific epitopes show that, in contrast to PSP, the CBD inclusions typically lack exon 3 sequences. Also immunoblot studies of CBD and PSP show distinctive patterns of tau fragments suggesting differing intracellular processing of aggregated tau despite identical composition of tau isoforms (Arai *et al.*, 2001). Ultrastructurally, tau in CBD forms paired helical filaments (PHFs). On electron microscopy these have been shown to be less abundant in the double stranded form which separates into the more abundant 15 nm wide, single stranded filaments (Dickson *et al.*, 2000). Straight filaments (15 nm) are also seen in PSP and Pick's disease. However, paired wide twisted ribbons are only seen in Pick's and not in PSP. The tau profile of CBD is also distinct from that seen in AD and chromosome 17 linked dementia (Morris *et al.*, 1999). Thus, CBD is a fairly distinct lobar and basal ganglia tauopathy with selective aggregation of 4R tau, which has characteristic antigenic and ultrastructural characteristics (Feany & Dickson, 1996; Forman *et al.*, 2002).

Another disorder, which can present with dementia personality change, emotional imbalance and has a pathological overlap with CBD and PSP is the recently recognised entity called argyrophilic grain disease (AGD)(Togo et al., 2002). Spindle- or comma-shaped argyrophilic grains in the neuropil of entorhinal cortex, hippocampus, and amygdala characterize AGD. Immunohistochemistry with monoclonal antibodies specific to tau isoforms with four (4R) or three (3R) repeats in the microtubule-binding domain showed immunostaining of grains with 4R, but not 3R, tau antibodies, suggesting that AGD is a 4R tauopathy. The 4R/3R tau ratio is 1 or less for Alzheimer disease controls and more than 1 for AGD, decreasing with increasing neurofibrillary pathology and demonstrating that insoluble tau in AGD is enriched in 4R tau. The frequency of an extended tau haplotype designated H1 (see below) is increased in AGD as it is in the other sporadic 4R tauopathies, progressive supranuclear palsy (PSP) and corticobasal degeneration (CBD). Furthermore, AGD also occurs in PSP and CBD more frequently than in dementia controls, including Alzheimer's disease. These results suggest that AGD, PSP and CBD are all 4R tauopathies and share common pathologic, biochemical, and genetic characteristics (Togo et al., 2002).

Only few neurochemistry studies have been undertaken in CBD. A profound reduction (>90%) in the concentration of dopamine in the substantia nigra, caudate nucleus, and putamen was found in one patient (Riley et al., 1990), corresponding to the degeneration of the substantia nigra and loss of the nigrostriatal pathway.

Pathogenesis/mechanism of disease

The identification of an association between homozygosity for the tau haplotype H1 in PSP led to similar studies in CBD. Di Maria et al. (2000) found the same association in cases with a clinical diagnosis of CBD. Houlden et al. (2001) in an international collaborative effort also confirmed this association in 57 pathologically confirmed cases (to avoid diagnostic errors). Thus this identical association of the H1 haplotype for both CBD and PSP has led to the notion that abnormalities of the tau gene located on chromosome 17 may be responsible for both CBD and PSP. In this regard it is interesting to note that certain families with FTDP-17 with mutations located in exon 10 of the tau gene or in the 5′ exon splice site of exon 10 have been described with a phenotype similar to that of CBD (Dickson et al., 2000). However, the typical sporadic cases of CBD do not have mutations of the tau gene.

Although most cases of CBD are sporadic some familial cases have been described, mostly presenting with a dementing illness with the diagnosis of CBD being made only on pathology (Mitsuyama et al., 1992; Brown et al., 1996, 1997). For example Brown et al. (1996) described a dementing syndrome in multiple members of two families, both with an autosomal dominant inheritance, in which the brain pathological findings in one member from each family showed changes consistent with CBD. Verin et al. (1997) reported (in abstract form) two brothers with a probable diagnosis of CBD based on clinical, radiological and metabolic imaging features. Finally there has been a report of monozygotic twins, one of whom (index case) presented with clinical and imaging features of CBD. The other though clinically unaffected, had a positron emission tomography (PET) ^{18}F fluorodeoxyglucose (FDG) scan showing global hypo metabolism and neuropsychological studies suggestive of left hemispheric dysfunction suggesting presymptomatic CBD (Caselli et al., 1995). There was no mention of tau gene sequencing in any of these reports and it can be debated whether some of these families have CBD or FTDP-17. Nevertheless, these reports and those of the CBD phenotype in some families with FTDP-17 with exon 10 mutations (Bugiani et al., 1999), as well as the H1 haplotype association of CBD and PSP, leads one to reconsider the relationship between these disorders. Indeed, it is being increasingly recognised that CBD may present with a frontal lobe type of dementing illness (see clinical features below) and some cases of FTDP-17 closely resemble the more classic CBD or PSP phenotype (Bugiani et al., 1999; Lee et al., 2001).

Clinical features

Symptoms begin insidiously in the sixth to eighth decades. In the series by Rinne et al. (1994), the youngest age of onset was 40 years, and the eldest 76 years. The condition occurs sporadically and usually there is no family history of a similar disorder. Males and females are probably equally affected although some have wondered about a small female preponderance (Schneider et al., 1994).

The core clinical features are shown in Table 45.3. Although presentation with a dementing process is being recognized of late the most common mode of presentation in the cases reported so far has been that of a slowly evolving motor disorder involving the arm or the leg, particularly the arm. One important source of potential bias for this clinical presentation is that most series (generally lacking neuropathological confirmation) have originated from movement disorders clinics (where these patients present as "atypical parkinsonism") rather than behavioral neurology or dementia clinics (where patients may present with a variety of cognitive, language or behavioral problems).

One of the most striking findings in the early stages of the illness is the asymmetry of limb involvement. At the onset symptoms may be vague and related to an inexplicable loss of hand function with clumsiness, loss of dexterity of fine finger movement or stiffness. Formal testing at this time may reveal slowness in hand and finger movement, difficulty in using objects or mimicking gestures or producing sequences of movement with the affected hand consistent with an *apraxia* (limb-kinetic or ideomotor). In attempting to perform manual tasks there may be perseveration of one part of the movement. Occasional patients have presented with an akinetic–rigid syndrome, a supranuclear gaze palsy, a pseudobulbar syndrome, and alien limb, a focal movement disorder (e.g. dystonic hand), or a sensory disturbance.

In the series of 36 patients of Rinne *et al.* (1994) five types of initial presentation emerged:

(i) The most common: a "useless arm," which was either rigid, dystonic, akinetic and apractic, with or without alien limb behavior, or rigid and jerking with stimulus-sensitive and action myoclonus (20 patients);

(ii) a gait disorder due to a rigid, apraxic leg with occasional myoclonus or disequilibrium, or both (ten patients);

(iii) prominent early sensory symptoms, sometimes with severe pain (three patients) and often in combination with clumsiness;

(iv) an isolated speech disturbance with dysarthria, although this was often associated with limb symptoms (two patients);

(v) falls and a prominent behavioral disorder (one patient).

Two other large series (Wenning *et al.*, 1998; Kompoliti *et al.*, 1998) and numerous smaller ones or case reports have more or less been in agreement with the motor syndrome as mentioned in the series of Rinne *et al.* (1994). In the series of 14 pathologically proven cases of CBD reported by Wenning *et al.* (1998) the most commonly reported symptom at onset included asymmetric limb clumsiness, with or without rigidity (50%), or tremor (21%). At the first neurological visit, on average 3.0 years after symptom onset, the most often encountered extrapyramidal features included unilateral limb rigidity (79%), bradykinesia (71%), postural imbalance (45%), and unilateral limb dystonia (43%). Ideomotor apraxia (64%), and to a lesser extent cortical dementia (36%), were the most common cortical signs at that stage. During the course of the disease, virtually all patients developed asymmetric or unilateral akinetic rigid

parkinsonism and a gait disorder. Kompoliti *et al.* (1998) reported a series of 147 mostly clinically diagnosed cases of CBD (only 7 with autopsy diagnosis). Based on retrospective chart review, they found parkinsonism as the most common feature (100%) along with higher cortical dysfunction (93%). The section below details some of the major clinical features.

Once again, it should be emphasized that all of these series (including the Wenning *et al.*, 1998 pathology study) originated from movement disorders clinics and therefore suffer from referral bias with respect to the presenting clinical features.

Apraxia

The major component of the higher-order motor deficit seen in the affected limbs in CBD might best be described as limb-kinetic apraxia, although it may be difficult to ascertain this given that bradykinesia, rigidity and dystonia may coexist. Most patients fail tests for ideomotor apraxia, but they rarely exhibit ideational apraxia (Leiguarda *et al.*, 1994). Ideomotor apraxia is for both transitive and intransitive tasks. CBD patients show impairment in production of meaningless and symbolic gestures and imitation, as well as in using real objects (Spatt *et al.*, 2002). Patients are impaired at using tools, miming tool use and initiating mimes of tool use. Motor performance in the use of tools improves with tactile stimulation (holding the appropriate tool or neutral object) but is not facilitated by visual input, for example being shown a diagram of the tool or the actual tool (Graham *et al.*, 1999). Although ideomotor apraxia can also rarely occur in PSP it is clearly much more severe in CBD (Pharr *et al.*, 2001). Apraxia of the lower limb may present as difficulty walking and may be the presenting complaint. The foot may tend to stick to the floor as walking is initiated or it may drag and cause the patient to trip on uneven surfaces or if attention is diverted. Examination of the affected leg may reveal slowness of rapid alternating movements and difficulty performing sequences of leg movement when lying down. In addition to limb apraxia, it is now recognized that facial apraxia with impairment of tongue and lip movements can also occur fairly frequently in CBD (Rosser & Tyrrel, 1992; Ozsancak *et al.*, 2000). Truncal apraxia has also been recorded (Okuda *et al.*, 2001).

The neural basis of the ideomotor apraxia is uncertain. Jacobs *et al.* (1999) have suggested that the ideomotor apraxia in CBD patients is of the anterior or production type whereby these patients are able to comprehend and discriminate gestures, unlike the posterior type due to involvement of the dominant parietal lobe, which leads to gesture recognition and gesture discriminative deficits. Similarly, using three-dimensional movement analyses to compare apraxia in a patient with CBD with that seen with a left parietal stroke Merians *et al.* (1999) reported that the CBD patient showed abnormal trajectories when actually manipulating the tool and object. The post-stroke deficits were most pronounced to verbal command with some improvement (although still with overall impairment) on actual tool and object manipulation. However, Spatt *et al.* (2002) felt that, although the main feature is a breakdown of motor programming (anterior involvement), in CBD some patients also have deficits in mechanical problem solving, which has been linked to the parietal lobe. The observation that some CBD patients also have some impairment of semantic memory suggests that the apraxia may be multifactorial (Spatt *et al.*, 2002). In line with this are results of some investigative studies of apraxic CBD patients. Okuda *et al.* (1995) reported that limb kinetic apraxia in CBD arose from involvement of the perirolandic area and constructional apraxia from the opposite parietal lobe on the basis of hypo perfusion of these areas on single photon emission tomography (SPECT) scans. In another study the N20 latency was shown to be significantly prolonged following median nerve stimulation on the more apraxic side, compared with the less apraxic side, suggesting that limb apraxia is partly due to disordered somatosensory processing through the parietal cortex (Okuda *et al.*, 1998). A PET scan study showed hypo metabolism of the anterior cingulate in patients with limb apraxia versus those without apraxia (Peigneux *et al.*, 2001).

Alterations in muscle tone with either *lead-pipe rigidity* or *Gegenhalten* of the affected limbs are a common finding. The affected arm does not swing in the normal manner during walking and tends to flex at the elbow. The hand may progressively adopt a flexed, often fixed, *dystonic posture* with clenching of the fingers into a fist, often closing around the thumb, which is held adducted in the palm. Skin maceration of the palm due to the fingers digging in forcibly is often seen. Pain often accompanies dystonia. Asymmetric limb dystonia was seen in 92% of cases reported by Vanek and Jankovic (2000). Dystonia of the leg was uncommon and dystonia of the head, neck or trunk is almost never seen in CBD (Vanek & Jankovic, 2000). Whether the dystonia in CBD is due to involvement of the striatum, to degeneration of the motor cortex or even parietal cortex is unclear.

In addition to limb apraxia, other frontal lobe motor signs become more evident with progression of the disease. *Gegenhalten* is often present from an early stage, as are *frontal release signs* such as grasp reflexes in the hands and feet, sucking and rooting reflexes. Patients may complain of an inability to release objects from this grasp in addition to the loss of fine motor skills. The *alien limb phenomenon* may be one of the most striking features of the syndrome.

This refers to slow, involuntary, wandering, levitation-like movements of the arm which often are associated with a prominent grasp reflex, forced grasping and groping (Adie & Critchley, 1927), magnetic hand movements (compulsive tactile exploration) (Denny-Brown, 1958) and intermanual conflict. The wandering hand frequently grasps on to parts of the patient's own body, the bedclothes, adjacent furniture or even people next to them, and will not let go. First described in association with tumors of the corpus callosum (Brion & Jedanyk, 1972), alien limb behavior has since been reported in association with infarction of the medial frontal cortex (Goldberg *et al.*, 1981; McNabb *et al.*, 1988; Feinberg *et al.*, 1992; Trojano *et al.*, 1993). The movements are slow and may appear quasi-purposeful; the hand typically rises slowly at the side of the patient who may be unaware of the movement. The unexpected appearance of the patient's hand beside their face gave rise to the term *le signe de la main étrangère* (Brion & Jedanyk, 1972) or alien limb. Limb levitation alone does not constitute true alien limb phenomenon and is often a source of misdiagnosis with other parkinsonism disorders for instance PSP (Barclay *et al.*, 1999; Boeve *et al.*, 2003). This description encompasses both the involuntary active wandering and other behaviors of the affected arm and the patient's lack of awareness or neglect of the limb and the feeling that it is foreign (Doody & Jankovic, 1992). In addition, the apraxic difficulty in using the hand to perform even simple tasks often leads patients to describe the limb as ". . . not doing what I want it to . . . ," or to state that it ". . . has a mind of its own." Often the patient uses their relatively normal hand to restrain the alien one. Another striking feature of the alien limb is intermanual conflict in which the affected limb reaches across to interfere with the voluntary activities of the contra-lateral normal hand (see Case 2, Rebeiz *et al.*, 1968). Alien leg movements also occur, with the leg rising while the patient is seated. About 40% of CBD patients will develop the alien limb phenomenon (Kumar *et al.*, 1998).

With increasing rigidity, difficulty walking, bradykinesia and facial immobility, the clinical picture becomes one of an *akinetic–rigid syndrome*. Kompoliti *et al.* (1998) in their review of 147 cases (7 autopsy proven) reported that parkinsonism was present in all patients with rigidity being the most common feature (92%), followed by bradykinesia (80%), gait disorder (80%) and tremor (55%). With progression, disequilibrium becomes a common feature in virtually all patients with postural instability and falls. The akinesia and rigidity generally show a poor or unsustained response to dopamine replacement therapy, despite the profound nigrostriatal pathology and the demonstration of dopamine depletion in these structures.

In addition to the asymmetric akinetic–rigid dystonic syndrome there may be *involuntary movements*. Chorea, tremor, and action and stimulus sensitive myoclonus may occur with or without the alien limb movement (mentioned above). Rebeiz *et al.* (1968) (case 2) mention "whenever he moved the hand, it underwent a series of alternating athetoid movements." Case 3 reported by Gibb *et al.* (1989) noticed that her hand tended to "levitate and the fingers wandered like tentacles." Tremor and myoclonus interfere with any attempts to use the arm and hand (or leg and foot). The tremor is not the classical rest tremor of Parkinson's disease, but a more jerky irregular tremor most evident in posture or movement. The myoclonus begins at first in the affected limbs. It is typically exquisitely sensitive to cutaneous stimuli and muscle stretch. The precise origin of the reflex myoclonus is uncertain (see below). Seizures are not a feature of the illness and the electroencephalogram does not show epileptic activity.

A *supranuclear gaze palsy* may be an early and prominent sign leading to confusion with PSP. The ocular motor disorder is progressive. It may take the form of a gaze apraxia with difficulty initiating saccades but with preservation of spontaneous reflexive saccades and eye movements elicited by the oculocephalic reflex. Fixation spasm may be evident. Patients may be unable to initiate eye movements to command without using head thrusts or a blink. There also may be marked saccadic hypometria, in both horizontal and vertical directions of gaze, and slowing of voluntary saccadic eye movements (Stell & Bronstein, 1994). Gaze impersistence also has been described. Pursuit eye movements are often saccadic and jerky at an early stage but, with progression of the disease the range of voluntary smooth pursuit becomes restricted and finally all voluntary eye movements may be lost. However, even at these stages it is usually possible to demonstrate that the ocular movement disorder is supranuclear in origin. Vidhailet *et al.* (1994) have suggested that horizontal saccadic latencies are increased before vertical latencies in CBD (at least in the early stages), unlike PSP where the opposite occurs. There is also decreased saccadic amplitude in the latter, thus helping to differentiate the two conditions. In a longitudinal study it was shown that saccadic velocities are preserved in CBD while PSP patients show decreased saccadic velocity throughout the disease course (Rivaud-Pechoux *et al.*, 2000). The same authors also noted that increased unilateral saccadic latency in CBD occurred ipsilateral to the side with apraxia early on in the course of the illness. Blepharospasm and levator inhibition may produce difficulties in eye opening.

Dysarthria is usually present and becomes increasingly severe, as does dysphagia. Progressive pronunciation difficulty, loss of speech, and orofacial apraxia may be the presenting features (Lang, 1992) and a primary progressive aphasia as the sole presentation with involvement of the superior temporal gyrus has been recognized (Kertesz *et al.*, 2000).

True weakness is not a feature to begin with, but with the passage of time the limb(s) become useless because of rigidity and apraxia. In addition, *pyramidal signs* appear with hyperreflexia and extensor plantar responses.

Cortical sensory signs with symptoms of numbness or tingling may appear at an early stage. Impaired joint position sense, two point discrimination, graphesthesia and astereognosis with intact primary sensory modalities is typical of cortical sensory loss.

Cognitive changes were believed to be unusual early in the disease; in fact, some reports specifically mentioned that the intellect was generally preserved (Riley *et al.*, 1990; Rinne *et al.*, 1994). Formal psychometric assessment was said to show some impairment on tests sensitive to frontal lobe damage, but this was attributed to performance difficulties due to the profound motor deficits. Cognitive performance in everyday life was usually felt to be unimpaired. However, it was clear even in the early reports, which stressed the motor aspects of CBD, that with the passage of time, memory impairment and dysphasic speech disturbance emerged as the disease progressed. However, there were some reports of focal cortical syndromes with pathological changes similar to those of CBD in which the major symptoms were related to a disturbance of language (i.e. dysphasia) with only subtle motor signs in the limbs (Lippa *et al.*, 1990, 1991; Lang, 1992), and of cases with combinations of dysphasia and limb apraxia (Cases 1, 4, of Sawle *et al.*, 1991). It is only recently that it has been clearly recognised that CBD (proven pathologically) may manifest as a dementing disorder alone or initially with later manifestation of the motor syndrome (Grimes *et al.*, 1999; Bergeron *et al.*, 1998). In one brain bank study involving patients referred by both movement disorders and memory clinics, dementia was the commonest presenting feature (9 of 13) and occurred in all but one of 13 cases over the course of the disease (Grimes *et al.*, 1999). Importantly, the classical movement disorder presentation (a "perceptuomotor" phenotype now often termed the corticobasal syndrome or CBS –see below), encouraging a diagnosis of CBD in life, was present in only 4 of the 13 patients in this study.

CBD can present with severe cognitive deficits with frontal lobe predilection with executive dysfunction, learning difficulties easily compensated for by use of semantic cues for encoding and retrieval, and disorders of dynamic motor execution which include temporal organisation, bimanual coordination, control and inhibition

(Pillon *et al.*, 1995), a pattern different from that typically seen in Alzheimer's disease (AD). However like AD, CBD patients also have prominent deficits on tests of sustained attention/mental control and verbal fluency (Massman *et al.*, 1996). Psychomotor depression is more common and severe in CBD than AD and PSP while apathy is more common in PSP (Litvan *et al.*, 1998).

CBD-like syndromes due to other pathologies

The classical clinical phenotype of CBD has become fairly well established. However, in recent years it has become apparent that a similar clinical picture may turn out to have a different pathological cause (Boeve *et al.*, 1999; Bhatia *et al.*, 2000; Boeve, 2001). PSP is probably the commonest source of this misdiagnosis. For example, there are reports of patients with a diagnosis of PSP proven pathologically, who exhibited a fairly typical CBD phenotype (i.e. CBS) with an asymmetric akinetic–rigid syndrome with dystonia of the affected arm, an alien limb, abnormal eye movement (with normal down gaze), dysarthria and dysphagia, and an impaired gait (Case Records of the Massachusetts General Hospital, 1993; Boeve *et al.*, 1999; Oide *et al.*, 2002). Other patients presenting with a dystonic, alien hand with myoclonus, apraxia, sensory inattention, amnesia, but relatively preserved speech have had the pathology of Alzheimer's disease (Ball *et al.*, 1993; Crystal *et al.*, 1982; Boeve *et al.*, 1999; Bhatia *et al.*, 2000). Also encountered have been patients with a grossly asymmetric rigid dystonic arm, some with alien behavior and myoclonus, attributable to cerebrovascular disease. Furthermore, Pick's disease, FTD with non-specific degeneration, FTDP-17, primary progressive aphasia (all part of the so called "Pick complex"), CJD (Boeve *et al.*, 1999; Kertesz *et al.*, 2000; Anschel *et al.*, 2002), as well as pigmentary sudanophilic leucodystrophy (Bhatia *et al.*, 2000), progressive multifocal leukoencephalopathy, and even a case with Fahr's disease with basal ganglia calcification (Warren *et al.*, 2001) have been reported with a CBD-like clinical picture. Such cases of a CBS due to other pathological causes have been referred to as corticobasal "look-alikes" (Bhatia *et al.*, 2000). It would appear that the constellation of clinical features of CBD can be caused by a variety of pathologies with asymmetric parietofrontocortical (with or without basal ganglia) involvement. An updated review of this heterogeneity from one institution (Boeve *et al.*, 1999) indicated that the underlying pathology in 32 autopsied cases with clinical features of CBD were as follows: CBD, 18; Alzheimer's, 3; Picks disease, 2; PSP, 6; dementia lacking specific histology, 2; Creutzfeldt–Jakob disease, 3. Others have described dementia with Lewy bodies (Horoupian

Table 45.3. *Proposed criteria for the diagnosis of the corticobasal syndrome*

Core features

Insidious onset and progressive course

No identifiable cause (e.g tumor, infarct)

Cortical dysfunction as reflected by at least one of the following:
  Focal or asymmetrical ideomotor apraxia
  Alien limb phenomena
  Cortical sensory loss
  Visual or sensory hemineglect
  Constructional apraxia
  Focal or asymmetric myoclonus
  Apraxia of speech/nonfluent aphasia

Extrapyramidal dysfunction as reflected by one of the following:
  Focal or asymmetric appendicular rigidity lacking prominent and sustained l-dopa response
  Focal or asymmetrical appendicular dystonia

Supportive investigations
  Variable degrees of focal or lateralised cognitive dysfunction, with relative preservation of learning and memory, on neuropsychometric testing

Focal or asymmetric atrophy on CT or MRI imaging, typically in perifrontal cortex

Focal or asymmetric hypoperfusion on SPECT or PET typically maximal in parietofrontal cortex +/- basal ganglia

Adapted from Boeve *et al.*, 2003.

& Wasserstein, 1999) and motor neurone inclusion body dementia (Grimes *et al.*, 1999). Hence Boeve *et al.*, 2003 have recently suggested that the term *corticobasal syndrome* (CBS) be used to characterise the constellation of typical features initially considered the defining characteristics of corticobasal degeneration with the term corticobasal degeneration (CBD) reserved for the histopathological diagnosis. Boeve *et al.*, 2003 have also proposed criteria for the diagnosis of the corticobasal syndrome (Table 45.3).

Of all these disorders the greatest similarities are undoubtedly between PSP and CBD both with regard clinical features and pathology and hence some may question whether these two are distinct disorders or variants of the same pathophysiological process (Boeve *et al.*, 2003). Both have prominent tau pathology with the presence of 4R-tau isoforms and are associated with the H1 tau haplotype and have overlapping clinical features. On the other hand, in support of the notion that these may be distinct clinico-pathological entities is a recent report showing distinct patterns of microglial activation and tau pathology in the two disorders (Ishizawa & Dickson 2001). In this regard Lang (2003) has suggested two possible explanations as shown in Fig. 45.3. One possibility is that these are two distinct nosological entities caused by different factors (environmental/genetic) occurring in individuals with similar genetic predisposition (H1/H1 tau genotype). The second as shown in Fig. 45.3 (B) is that these are distinct phenotypes of the same disorder, occurring in individuals with similar genetic predisposition with differences secondary to differences in genetic background and/or specific differences in the etiologic triggering agent(s) (Lang, 2003). However, the jury is still out on this and further work in this area will be needed to provide the answer to this question.

Epidemiology

It is clear that CBD is a relatively rare neurodegenerative disorder, however the true incidence and prevalence of the disorder remains unknown. It would be true to say that it is the least common of the four parkinsonian disorders which clinicians typically consider in their differential diagnosis of a patient with a neurodegenerative cause of an akinetic rigid syndrome which include Parkinson's disease (PD), multiple system atrophy (MSA), PSP and CBD. In this regard in a recent community based prevalence study of parkinsonian disorders not a single case of CBD was identified vs. rates of 4 and 6/100 000 for MSA and PSP, respectively (Schrag et al., 1999). CBD is estimated to account for 0.9% of parkinsonian cases in a specialized movement disorder clinic compared to PSP which accounts for about 5%. Togasaki and Tanner (2000) have estimated CBD will develop in 4–6% of those with parkinsonism and based on the incidence of Parkinson's disease the estimated incidence rate of CBD would be 0.62–0.92/100 000 per year with a prevalence of 4.9–7.3/100 000 based on a survival rate of 7.9 years. However, this could be an overestimate with regard the motor (akinetic rigid) presentation of the disorder due to referral bias of a specialised movement disorder clinic. On the other hand, it may well be an underestimate since the dementia phenotype of CBD may be more common than is currently appreciated.

Investigations

Routine laboratory studies of blood, urine, and cerebrospinal fluid (CSF) are normal. Riley et al. (1990) noted that 4 of their 15 cases had a history of dysimmune diseases, but this has not been a general finding. Heavy metal toxic screens in urine have been negative. Watts et al. (1985) described decreased levels of somatostatin in CSF in three cases, but this has not been replicated. Increased total CSF tau protein has been reported in patients with CBD compared with normal controls and total CSF tau is said to be

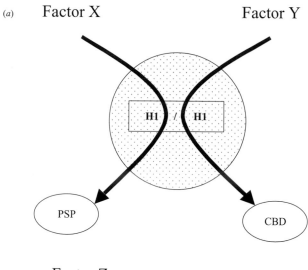

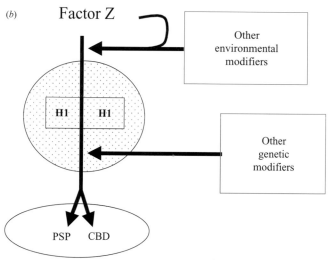

Fig. 45.3 Two possible explanations for the relationship between corticobasal degeneration (CBD) and progressive supranuclear palsy (PSP). (a) Two distinct nosological entities caused by different factors (environmental/ genetic) occurring in individuals with similar genetic predisposition (H1/H1 tau genotype). (b) Distinct phenotypes of the same disorder, occurring in individuals with similar genetic predisposition; differences secondary to differences in genetic background and/or specific differences in the etiologic triggering agent(s). (From Lang, 2003 with permission.)

higher in CBD than PSP (Mitani et al., 1998; Urakami et al., 1999, 2001).

Imaging

Computerized tomography (CT) and magnetic resonance imaging (MRI) of the brain will show localized and asymmetric frontoparietal atrophy in 50–96% of cases (Savoiardo *et al.*, 2000). Atrophy of the middle and posterior part of the corpus callosum has also been described in CBD (Yamauchi *et al.*, 1998). Hyperintense lesions of the primary motor cortex (M1), extending to the midline and possibly supplementary motor area (SMA) have been reported in two CBD cases (Winklemann *et al.*, 1999). Hyperintensity of the atrophic cortex or white matter may be seen particularly with fluid attenuated reversion recovery (FLAIR) sequences and hypointensity of the lentiform nuclei on T_2-weighted images has also been mentioned (Doi *et al.*, 1999; Savoiardo *et al.*, 2000). Atrophy tends to become more severe as the disease progresses. Early minimal cortical atrophy may be detected only by specialised three-dimensional MRI techniques (Caselli *et al.*, 1992). Reduced *N*-acetylaspartate (NAA) to choline (Cho) ratios were observed by MR spectroscopy in the right basal ganglia in one study of patients said to have the Pick complex which included patients with CBD (Kizu *et al.*, 2002). In the same study in patients with CBD low NAA/ creatine (Cr) ratios were also detected in the right perisylvian region. The explanation for the preferential involvement of the right side was not entirely clear.

Positron emission tomography (PET) has shown a typical pattern of an asymmetric reduction in the uptake of ^{18}F-6-fluorodopa in the striatum (caudate and putamen) and in the medial frontal cortex (Riley *et al.*, 1990; Sawle *et al.*, 1991; Blin *et al.*, 1992). Caudate and putamen are said to be almost equally affected, in contrast to Parkinson's disease where ^{18}F-6-fluorodopa uptake into putamen is considerably reduced, but that into caudate nucleus is relatively spared. This is consistent with the loss of nigrostriatal projections as predicted by the profound nigral cell loss demonstrated pathologically (Rebeiz *et al.*, 1968; Gibb *et al.*, 1989) and the striatal dopamine depletion in the case reported by Riley *et al.* (1990).

Characteristic patterns of asymmetric cerebral cortical hypo metabolism are seen with the greatest reductions of oxygen metabolism in the superior and posterior temporal, inferior parietal and occipital visual association cortices (Sawle *et al.*, 1991). There is also some reduction of oxygen metabolism in medial frontal regions, especially in those patients exhibiting alien limbs. Significant regional asymmetries in cerebral glucose metabolism also have been found in the thalamus, inferior parietal lobule, and hippocampus (Eidelberg *et al.*, 1991). This picture on FDG-PET can be apparent on simple visual inspection and can be present early on even before the characteristic signs appear to be able make a diagnosis on clinical grounds (Coulier *et al.*, 2003). Similar asymmetry has been found in regional blood flow using single photon emission computed tomography (SPECT) with significant reduction in the posterior

frontal and parietal cortex, as well as the caudate and thalamus (Markus *et al.*, 1995). These changes were bilateral though more pronounced on the side opposite to the more affected side (Markus *et al.*, 1995). FDG PET studies in cognitively impaired CBD patients compared to PSP patients found that the CBD group had significant hypometabolism in the parietal lobes and suggested that this played a role in the cognitive changes in CBD (Hosaka *et al.*, 2002).

PET studies attempting in vivo imaging of activated microglia. With a ligand [11C]PK11195 are said to show an increased [11C](R) PK11195 signal in the cortex, thalamus and pons contralateral to the more affected side in a few patients with CBD (A. Gerhard and D. Brooks, personal communication). Formal reports of these studies are awaited.

It should be emphasized once again both that the CBS is not specific for the pathology of CBD and the pathology of CBD may present with features other than the classical CBS (i.e., dementia, progressive aphasia, etc.). Therefore, the metabolic or blood flow imaging patterns described above, obtained in clinically diagnosed cases, correlate with a distribution of underlying pathological change (and thus with a clinical phenotype) rather than a specific type of pathology.

Electrophysiology

The electroencephalogram is usually normal initially, but may develop asymmetric slowing, maximal over the hemisphere contralateral to the most affected limbs. Nerve conduction studies and electromyography have not revealed consistent evidence of peripheral nerve involvement, although evidence for a sensorimotor polyneuropathy has been found rarely (Case Records of the Massachusetts General Hospital, 1985). Visual and brainstem-evoked potentials have been normal.

Some authors have drawn attention to the similarity of the focal stimulus sensitive myoclonus to that seen in cortical reflex myoclonus (Riley *et al.*, 1990), although there are several differences (Thompson *et al.*, 1990, 1994). Somatosensory evoked potentials (SEP) may be abnormal (Thompson *et al.*, 1990, 1994). However, unlike classical reflex myoclonus, there is no enlargement of the secondary components of the SEP (P_1–N_2 component), but instead the later parietal components are distorted. Absent or increased latency of N30 SEP frontal component has also been reported in CBD (Monza *et al.*, 2003). There is no cortical discharge preceding myoclonic jerks on back-averaging (Thompson *et al.*, 1990; Monza *et al.*, 2003), although magnetoencephalography does support a cortical origin for the myoclonus (Mima *et al.*, 1998). Median nerve stimulation in the affected arm often produces abnormal late C waves, corresponding to myoclonic jerks (Thompson *et al.*, 1990; Riley *et al.*, 1990). The latency of the reflex myoclonus following stimulation, of the order of 40 ms (Thompson *et al.*, 1994; Chen *et al.*, 1992), is shorter than the reflex latency of 50–60 ms in typical cortical reflex myoclonus (Obeso *et al.*, 1985). Reduced inhibition following magnetic stimulation of the cortex in CBD has been described (Strafella *et al.*, 1997). Similarly, significantly shortened post-motor-evoked potential (MEP) silent period has been reported in CBD (Lu *et al.*, 1998) supporting the notion that the action myoclonus is a result of pathological motor cortex hyperexcitability, probably due to loss of input from the sensory cortex.

Treatment

Unfortunately, there is no effective treatment for this condition (Kompoliti *et al.*, 1998), which is relentlessly progressive and universally fatal. Levodopa and dopamine agonists have little effect, but are tried. Kompoliti and colleagues (1998) found that 92% of the 147 cases in their international series had received dopaminergic drugs and a beneficial result was reported in only 24% with levodopa being the most effective. However, the effect if any is marginal and not sustained. Rarely, levodopa-induced dyskinesias may occur even in the absence of clinical benefit. Baclofen and/or an anticholinergic may help the rigidity a little, but they usually produce unwanted side effects. Clonazepam may dampen the myoclonus and dystonia somewhat (Kompoliti *et al.*, 1998). Other drugs such as dopamine antagonists, propranolol, dantrolene sodium, anticonvulsants including sodium valproate and serotonin agonists, are generally of no help. Botulinum toxin injections into the rigid limb muscles may be useful. Two recent studies have found that EMG activity recorded at rest and during active and passive flexion/extension movements of the finger and wrist was useful both in distinguishing between muscle contraction and underlying contractures and in determining the dosage of botulinum toxin to be used in those with a dystonic clenched fist. Some benefit could be produced which depended on the severity of the deformity and the degree of contracture (Cordivari *et al.*, 2001; Muller *et al.*, 2002). All patients had significant benefit to pain and the muscle relaxation made it possible to cleanse the palms and reduce palmar infection when present (Cordivari *et al.*, 2001). Stereotaxic thalamotomy in a single case did not help the painful arm dystonia and myoclonus (Riley *et al.*, 1990). Other functional neurosurgical procedures effective in Parkinson's disease (e.g. deep brain stimulation of the subthalamic nucleus) would not be expected

to reduce disability in CBD since the benefit closely correlates with ongoing response to levodopa. The main thrust of management is thus confined to measures to assist mobility and distress. There are important roles for physio- and occupational therapy however, the apraxia often limits the extent to which patients can benefit from these interventions. Ongoing concern for the well being of the caregiver is also a critical component of the management strategy.

REFERENCES

Adie, W. J. & Critchley, M. (1927). Forced grasping and groping. *Brain*, **50**, 142–76.

Anschel, D. J., Simon, D. K., Llinas, R. & Joseph, J. T. (2002). Spongiform encephalopathy mimicking corticobasal degeneration. *Mov. Disord.*, **17**, 606–7.

Ball, J. A., Lantos, P. L., Jackson, M., Marsden, C. D., Scadding, J. W. & Rossor, M. N. (1993). Alien hand sign in association with Alzheimer's histopathology. *J. Neurol. Neurosurg. Psychiatry*, **56**, 1020–3.

Barclay, C. L., Bergeron, C. & Lang, A. E. (1999). Arm levitation in progressive supranuclear palsy. *Neurology*, **52**, 879–82.

Benson, D. F., Davis, R. J., Snyder, J. *et al.* (1988). Progressive cortical atrophy. *Arch. Neurol.*, **45**, 789–93.

Bergeron, C., Davis, A. & Lang, A. E. (1998). Corticobasal ganglionic degeneration and progressive supranuclear palsy presenting with cognitive decline. *Brain Pathol.*, **8**, 355–65.

Bhatia, K. P., Lee, M. S., Rinne, J. O. *et al.* (2000). Corticobasal degeneration look-alikes. *Adv. Neurol.*, **82**, 169–82.

Blin, J., Baron, J. C., Dubois, B., Pillon, B., Cambon, H. & Agid, Y. (1988). PET studies of brain energy metabolism in a model of subcortical dementia: progressive supranuclear palsy. In *Senile dementia*, ed. A. Agnoli, J. Cahn, N. Lassen & R. Mayeux, pp. 73–80. Paris: John Libbey.

Blin, J., Vidailhet, M. J., Pillon, B., Dubois, B., Feve, J. R. & Agid, Y. (1992). Corticobasal degeneration: decreased and asymmetrical glucose consumption as studied with PET. *Mov. Disord.*, **7**, 348–54.

Boeve, B. F., Maraganore, D. M., Parisi, J. E. *et al.* (1999). Pathologic heterogeneity in clinically diagnosed corticobasal degeneration. *Neurology*, **53**, 795–800.

Boeve, B. F., Lang, A. E. & Litvan, I. (2003). Corticobasal degeneration and its relationship to progressive supranuclear palsy and frontotemporal dementia. *Ann. Neurol.*, **54** Suppl 5, S15–19.

Brion, S. & Jedanyk, C.-P. (1972). Trouble du transfert interhémisphérique: a propos de trois observations de tumeurs du corps calleux: le signe de la main étrangère. *Rev. Neurol.*, **126**, 257–66.

Bugiani, O., Murrell, J. R., Giaccone, G. *et al.* (1999). Frontotemporal dementia and corticobasal degeneration in a family with a P301S mutation in tau. *J. Neuropathol. Exp. Neurol.*, **58**, 667–77.

Case Records of the Massachusetts General Hospital. Case 38 (1985). Case of corticonigral degeneration with neuronal achromasia. *N. Engl. J. Med.*, **313**, 739–48.

Case Records of the Massachusetts General Hospital. Case 46 (1993). *N. Engl. J. Med.*, **329**, 1560–7.

Caselli, R. J., Jack, C. R. Jr, Petersen, R. C., Wahner, H. W. & Yanagihara, T. (1992). Asymmetric cortical degenerative syndromes: clinical and radiologic correlations. *Neurology*, **42**(8), 1462–8.

Chen, R., Ashby, P. & Lang A. E. (1992). Stimulus-sensitive myoclonus in akinetic-rigid syndromes. *Brain*, **115**, 1875–88.

Clark, A. W., Manz, H. J., White, C. L. 3rd, Lehmann, J., Miller, D. & Coyle, J. T. (1986). Cortical degeneration with swollen chromatolytic neurons: its relationship to Pick's disease. *J. Neuropath. Exp. Neurol.*, **45**, 268–84.

Cole, M., Wright, D. & Barker, B. Q. (1979). Familial aphasia due to Pick's disease. *Ann. Neurol.*, **6**, 158.

Cordivari, C., Misra, V. P., Catania, S. & Lees, A. J. (2001). Treatment of dystonic clenched fist with botulinum toxin. *Mov. Disord.*, **16**, 907–13.

Coulier, I. M. F., de Vries, J. J. & Leenders, K. L. (2003). Is FDG-PET a useful tool in clinical practice for diagnosing corticobasal ganglionic degeneration? *Mov. Disord.*, published online 29 May.

Crystal, H. A., Horoupian, D. S., Katzman, R. & Jotkowitz, S. (1982). Biopsy-proved Alzheimer disease presenting as a right parietal lobe syndrome. *Ann. Neurol.*, **12**, 186–8.

Denny-Brown, D. (1958). The nature of apraxia. *J. Nerv. Ment. Dis.*, **126**, 9–32.

Dickson, D. W., Liu, W. K., Ksiezak-Reding, H. & Yen, S. H. (2000). Neuropathologic and molecular considerations. *Adv. Neurol.*, **82**, 9–27.

Dickson, D. W., Bergeron, C., Chin, S. S. *et al.* (2002). Office of Rare Diseases of the National Institutes of Health. Office of Rare Diseases neuropathologic criteria for corticobasal degeneration. *J. Neuropathol. Exp. Neurol.*, **61**, 935–46.

Di Maria, E., Tabaton, M., Vigo, T. *et al.* (2000). Corticobasal degeneration shares a common genetic background with progressive supranuclear palsy. *Ann. Neurol.*, **47**, 374–7.

Doi, T., Iwasa, K., Makifuchi, T. & Takamori, M. (1999). White matter hyperintensities on MRI in a patient with corticobasal degeneration. *Acta Neurol. Scand.*, **99**, 199–201.

Doody, R. S. & Jankovic, J. (1992). The alien hand and related signs. *J. Neurol. Neurosurg. Psychiatry*, **55**, 806–10.

Eidelberg, D., Dhawan, V., Moeller, J. R. *et al.* (1991). The metabolic landscape of cortico-basal ganglionic degeneration: regional asymmetries studied with positron emission tomography. *J. Neurol. Neurosurg. Psychiatry*, **54**, 856–62.

Feinberg, T. E., Schindler, R. J., Flanagan, N. G. & Haber, L. D. (1992). Two alien hand syndromes. *Neurology*, **42**, 19–24.

Feany, M. B. & Dickson, D. W. (1995). Widespread cytoskeletal pathology characterizes corticobasal degeneration. *Am. J. Pathol.*, **146**, 1388–96.

(1996). Neurodegenerative disorders with extensive tau pathology: a comparative study and review. *Ann. Neurol.*, **40**, 139–48.

Forman, M. S., Zhukareva, V., Bergeron, C. *et al.* (2002). Signature tau neuropathology in gray and white matter of corticobasal degeneration. *Am. J. Pathol.*, **160**, 2045–53.

Gibb, W. R., Luthert, P. J. & Marsden, C. D. (1989). Corticobasal degeneration. *Brain*, **112**, 1171–92.

Goetz, C. G. (2000). Nineteenth century studies of atypical parkinsonism: Charcot and his Salpêtrière School. *Adv. Neurol.*, **82**, 1–8.

Goldberg, G., Mayer, N. H. & Toglia, J. U. (1981). Medial frontal cortex infarction and the alien hand sign. *Arch. Neurol.*, **38**, 683–6.

Graham, N. L., Zeman, A., Young, A. W., Patterson, K. & Hodges, J. R. (1999). Dyspraxia in a patient with corticobasal degeneration: the role of visual and tactile inputs to action. *J. Neurol. Neurosurg. Psychiatry*, **67**, 334–44.

Greene, P. E., Fahn, S., Lang, A. E., Watts, R. L., Eidelberg, D. & Powers, J. M. (1990). What is it? Case 1, 1990: progressive unilateral rigidity, bradykinesia, tremulousness, and apraxia, leading to fixed postural deformity of the involved limb. *Mov. Disord.*, **5**, 341–51.

Grimes, D. A., Lang, A. E. & Bergeron, C. B. (1999). Dementia as the most common presentation of cortical-basal ganglionic degeneration. *Neurology*, **53**, 1969–74.

Higuchi, M., Ishihara, T., Zhang, B. *et al.* (2002). Transgenic mouse model of tauopathies with glial pathology and nervous system degeneration. *Neuron*, **35**, 433–46.

Horoupian, D. S. & Wasserstein, P. H. (1999). Alzheimer's disease pathology in motor cortex in dementia with Lewy bodies clinically mimicking corticobasal degeneration. *Acta Neuropathol.*, **98**, 317–22.

Hosaka, K., Ishii, K., Sakamoto, S. *et al.* (2002). Voxel-based comparison of regional cerebral glucose metabolism between PSP and corticobasal degeneration. *J. Neurol. Sci.*, **199**, 67–71.

Houlden, H., Baker, M., Morris, H. R. *et al.* (2001). Corticobasal degeneration and progressive supranuclear palsy share a common tau haplotype. *Neurology*, **56**, 1702–6.

Ishizawa, K. & Dickson, D. W. (2001). Microglial activation parallels system degeneration in progressive supranuclear palsy and corticobasal degeneration. *J. Neuropathol. Exp. Neurol.*, **60**, 647–57.

Jacobs, D. H., Adair, J. C., Macauley, B., Gold, M., Gonzalez Rothi, L. J. & Heilman, K. M. (1999). Apraxia in corticobasal degeneration. *Brain Cogn.*, **40**(2), 336–54.

Kertesz, A., Martinez-Lage, P., Davidson, W. & Munoz, D. G. (2000). The corticobasal degeneration syndrome overlaps progressive aphasia and frontotemporal dementia. *Neurology*, **55**, 1368–75.

Komori, T. (1999). Tau-positive inclusions in progressive supranuclear palsy, corticobasal degeneration and Pick's disease. *Brain Pathol.*, **9**, 663–79.

Kompoliti, K., Goetz, C. G., Boeve, B. F. *et al.* (1998). Clinical presentation and pharmacological therapy in corticobasal degeneration. *Arch. Neurol.*, **55**(7), 957–61.

Kizu, O., Yamada, K. & Nishimura, T. (2002). Proton chemical shift imaging in pick complex. *Am. J. Neuroradiol.*, **23**, 1387–92.

Kumar, R., Bergeron, C., Pollanen & Lang, A. E. (1998). Corticobasal ganglionic degeneration. In *Parkinson's Disease and Movement Disorders*, ed. J. Jankovic & E. Tolosa, pp. 297–316, Baltimore: Williams and Wilkins.

Lang, E. (1992). Corticobasal ganglionic degeneration presenting with progressive loss of speech output and orofacial dyspraxia. *J. Neurol. Neurosurg. Psychiatry*, **55**(11), 1101.

Lang, A. E. (2003). Corticobasal degeneration: selected developments. *Mov. Disord.*, **18** (suppl 6), S51–6.

Lee, V. M., Goedert, M. & Trojanowski, J. Q. (2001). Neurodegenerative tauopathies. *Annu. Rev. Neurosci.*, **24**, 1121–59.

Lees, A. J. (1987). The Steele–Richardson–Olszewski syndrome (progressive supranuclear palsy). In *Movement Disorders*, Vol. 2, ed. C. D. Marsden & S. Fahn, pp. 272–87. London: Butterworths.

Leiguarda, R., Lees, A. J., Merello, M., Starkstein, S. & Marsden, C. D. (1994). The nature of apraxia in corticobasal degeneration. *J. Neurol. Neurosurg. Psychiatry*, **57**(4), 455–9.

Le Witt, P., Friedman, J., Nutt, J., Korczyn, A., Brogna, C. & Truong, D. (1989). Progressive rigidity with apraxia: the variety of clinical and pathological features. *Neurology*, Suppl. 1, **39**, 140.

Lippa, C. F., Smith, T. W. & Fontneau, N. (1990). Corticonigral degeneration with neuronal achromasia. A clinicopathologic study of two cases. *J. Neurol. Sci.*, **98**, 301–10.

Lippa, C. F., Cohen, R., Smith, T. W. & Drachman, D. A. (1991). Primary progressive aphasia with focal neuronal achromasia. *Neurology*, **41**(6), 882–6.

Litvan, I., Agid, Y., Goetz, C. *et al.* (1997). Accuracy of the clinical diagnosis of corticobasal degeneration: a clinicopathologic study. *Neurology*, **48**(1), 119–25.

Litvan, I., Cummings, J. L. & Mega, M. (1998). Neuropsychiatric features of corticobasal degeneration. *J. Neurol. Neurosurg. Psychiatry*, **65**, 717–21.

Litvan, I., Grimes, D. A., Lang, A. E. *et al.* (1999). Clinical features differentiating patients with postmortem confirmed progressive supranuclear palsy and corticobasal degeneration. *J. Neurol.*, **246** Suppl 2, II1–5.

Lu, C. S., Ikeda, A., Terada, K. *et al.* (1998). Electrophysiological studies of early stage corticobasal degeneration. *Mov. Disord.*, **13**, 140–6.

Markus, H. S., Lees, A. J., Lennox, G., Marsden, C. D. & Costa, D. C. (1995). Patterns of regional cerebral blood flow in corticobasal degeneration studied using HMPAO SPECT; comparison with Parkinson's disease. *Mov. Disord.*, **10**, 179–87.

Massman, P. J., Kreiter, K. T., Jankovic, J. & Doody, R. S. (1996). Neuropsychological functioning in cortical-basal ganglionic degeneration: Differentiation from Alzheimer's disease. *Neurology*, **46**, 720–6.

McNabb, A. W., Carroll, W. M. & Mastaglia, F. L. (1988). "Alien hand" and loss of bimanual coordination after dominant anterior cerebral artery territory infarction. *J. Neurol. Neurosurg. Psychiatry*, **51**, 218–22.

Merians, A. S., Clark, M., Poizner, H. *et al.* (1999). Apraxia in corticobasal degeneration and left parietal stroke: a case study. *Brain Cogn.*, **40**, 314–35.

Mima, T., Nagamine, T., Ikeda, A., Yazawa, S., Kimura, J. & Shibasaki, H. (1998). Pathogenesis of cortical myoclonus studied by magnetoencephalopathy. *Ann. Neurol.*, **43**, 598–607.

Mitani, K., Furiya, Y., Uchihara, T. *et al.* (1998). Increased CSF tau protein in corticobasal degeneration. *J. Neurol.*, **245**, 44–6.

Monza, D., Ciano, C., Scaioli, V. *et al.* (2003). Neurophysiological features in relation to clinical signs in clinically diagnosed corticobasal degeneration. *Neurol. Sci.*, **24**, 16–23.

Morris, H. R., Lees, A. J. & Wood, N. W. (1999). Neurofibrillary tangle parkinsonian disorders – tau pathology and tau genetics. *Mov. Disord.*, **14**, 731–6.

Muller, J., Wenning, G. K., Wissel, J., Seppi, K. & Poewe, W. (2002). Botulinum toxin treatment in atypical parkinsonian disorders associated with disabling focal dystonia. *J. Neurol.*, **249**, 300–4.

Obeso, J. A., Rothwell, J. C. & Marsden, C. D. (1985). The spectrum of cortical myoclonus. From focal reflex jerks to spontaneous motor epilepsy. *Brain*, **108**, 193–24.

Oide, T., Ohara, S., Yazawa, M. *et al.* (2002). Progressive supranuclear palsy with asymmetric tau pathology presenting with unilateral limb dystonia. *Acta Neuropathol.*, **104**, 209–14.

Okuda, B., Tachibana, H., Takeda, M., Kawabata, K., Sugita, M. & Fukuchi, M. (1995). Focal cortical hypoperfusion in corticobasal degeneration demonstrated by three-dimensional surface display with 123I-IMP: a possible cause of apraxia. *Neuroradiology*, **37**, 642–4.

Okuda, B., Tachibana, H., Takeda, M., Kawabata, K. & Sugita, M. (1998). Asymmetric changes in somatosensory evoked potentials correlate with limb apraxia in corticobasal degeneration. *Acta Neurol. Scand.*, **97**, 409–12.

Okuda, B., Tanaka, H., Kawabata, K., Tachibana, H. & Sugita, M. (2001). Truncal and limb apraxia in corticobasal degeneration. *Mov. Disord.*, **16**, 760–2.

Ozsancak, C., Auzou, P. & Hannequin, D. (2000). Dysarthria and orofacial apraxia in corticobasal degeneration. *Mov. Disord.*, **15**(5), 905–10.

Paulus, W. & Selim, M. (1990). Corticonigral degeneration with neuronal achromasia and basal neurofibrillary tangles. *Acta Neuropathol.*, **81**, 89–94.

Peigneux, P., Salmon, E., Garraux, G. *et al.* (2001). Neural and cognitive bases of upper limb apraxia in corticobasal degeneration. *Neurology*, **57**(7), 1259–68.

Pharr, V., Uttl, B., Stark, M., Litvan, I., Fantie, B. & Grafman, J. (2001). Comparison of apraxia in corticobasal degeneration and progressive supranuclear palsy. *Neurology*, **56** (7), 957–63.

Piao, Y. S., Hayashi, S., Wakabayashi, K. *et al.* (2002). Cerebellar cortical tau pathology in progressive supranuclear palsy and corticobasal degeneration. *Acta Neuropathol.*, **103**, 469–74.

Pillon, B., Blin, J., Vidailhet, M. *et al.* (1995). The neuropsychological pattern of corticobasal degeneration: comparison with progressive supranuclear palsy and Alzheimer's disease. *Neurology*, **45**, 1477–83.

Rebeiz, J. J., Kolodny, E. H. & Richardson, E. P. Jr. (1968). Cortico-dentatonigral degeneration with neuronal achromasia. *Arch. Neurol.*, **18**(1), 20–33.

Rivaud-Pechoux, S., Vidailhet, M., Gallouedec, G., Litvan, I., Gaymard, B. & Pierrot-Deseilligny, C. (2002). Longitudinal ocular motor study in corticobasal degeneration and progressive supranuclear palsy. *Neurology*, **54**, 1029–32.

Riley, D. E., Lang, A. E., Lewis, A. *et al.* (1990). Cortical-basal ganglionic degeneration. *Neurology*, **40**, 1203–12.

Rinne, J. O., Lee, M. S., Thompson, P. D. & Marsden, C. D. (1994). Corticobasal degeneration. A clinical study of 36 cases. *Brain*, **117**, 1183–96.

Rosser, N. & Tyrrell, P. (1992). Cortical basal ganglionic degeneration presenting with progressive loss of speech output and orofacial apraxia. *J. Neurol. Neurosurg. Psychiatry*, **55**, 1101.

Savoiardo, M., Grisoli, M. & Girotti, F. (2000). Magnetic resonance imaging in CBD, related atypical parkinsonian disorders, and dementias. *Adv. Neurol.*, **82**, 197–208.

Sawle, G. V., Brooks, D. J., Marsden, C. D. & Frackowiak, R. S. (1991). Corticobasal degeneration. A unique pattern of regional cortical oxygen hypometabolism and striatal fluorodopa uptake demonstrated by positron emission tomography. *Brain*, **114**, 541–56.

Schneider, J. A., Watts, R. L., Gearing, M., Brewer, R. P. & Mirra, S. S. (1997). Corticobasal degeneration: neuropathologic and clinical heterogeneity. *Neurology*, **48**, 959–69.

Schrag, A., Ben-Shlomo, Y. & Quinn, N. P. (1999). Prevalence of progressive supranuclear palsy and multiple system atrophy: a cross-sectional study. *Lancet*, **354**, 1771–5.

Soliveri, P., Monza, D., Paridi, D. *et al.* (1999). Cognitive and magnetic resonance imaging aspects of corticobasal degeneration and progressive supranuclear palsy. *Neurology*, **53**, 502–7.

Smith, T. W., Lippa, C. F. & de Girolami, U. (1992). Immunocytochemical study of ballooned neurons in cortical degeneration with neuronal achromasia. *Clin. Neuropathol.*, **11**, 28–35.

Spatt, J., Bak, T., Bozeat, S., Patterson, K. & Hodges, J. R. (2002). Apraxia, mechanical problem solving and semantic knowledge: contributions to object usage in corticobasal degeneration. *J. Neurol.*, **249**(5), 601–8.

Stell, R. & Bronstein, A. M. (1994). Eye movement abnormalities in extrapyramidal diseases. In *Movement disorders*, Vol. 3, ed. C. D. Marsden & S. Fahn, pp. 88–113. Oxford: Butterworth-Heinemann.

Strafella, A., Ashby, P. & Lang, A. E. (1997). Reflex myoclonus in cortical-basal ganglionic degeneration involves a transcortical pathway. *Mov. Disord.*, **12**, 360–9.

Thompson, P. D., Day, B. L., Rothwell, J. C., Brown, P., Britton, T. C. & Marsden, C. D. (1994). The myoclonus in corticobasal degeneration. Evidence for two forms of cortical reflex myoclonus. *Brain*, **117**, 1197–207.

Thompson, P. D., Day, B. L., Rothwell, J. C. & Marsden, C. D. (1990). Clinical and physiological findings in corticobasal degeneration. *Mov. Disord.*, **5** (Suppl.), 43.

Togasaki, D. M. & Tanner, C. M. (2000). Epidemiologic aspects. *Adv. Neurol.*, **82**, 53–9.

Togo, T., Sahara, N., Yen, S. H. *et al.* (2002). Argyrophilic grain disease is a sporadic 4-repeat tauopathy. *J. Neuropathol. Exp. Neurol.*, **61**(6), 547–56.

Trojano, L., Crisci, C., Lanzillo, B., Elefante, R. & Caruso, G. (1993). How many alien hand syndromes? Follow-up of a case. *Neurology*, **43**, 2710–12.

Urakami, K., Mori, M., Wada, K. *et al.* (1999). A comparison of tau protein in cerebrospinal fluid between corticobasal degeneration and progressive supranuclear palsy. *Neurosci. Lett.*, **259**, 127–9.

Urakami, K., Wada, K., Arai, H. *et al.* (2001). Diagnostic significance of tau protein in cerebrospinal fluid from patients with corticobasal degeneration or progressive supranuclear palsy. *J. Neurol. Sci.*, **183**, 95–8.

Vanek, Z. F. & Jankovic, J. (2000). Dystonia in corticobasal degeneration. *Adv. Neurol.*, **82**, 61–7.

Verin, M., Rancurel, G., Ode, M. & Edan, G. (1997). Five familial cases of corticobasal degeneration. *Mov. Disord.*, Suppl 1, **12**, 55.

Vidailhet, M., Rivaud, S., Gouider-Khouja, N. *et al.*. (1994). Eye movements in parkinsonian syndromes. *Ann. Neurol.*, **35**, 420–6.

Warren, J. D., Mummery, C. J., Al-Din, A. S., Brown, P. & Wood, N. W. (2002). Corticobasal degeneration syndrome with basal ganglia calcification: Fahr's disease as a corticobasal look-alike? *Mov. Disord.*, **17**, 563–7.

Watts, R. L., Williams, R. S., Growdon, J. V., Young, R. R., Haley, E. C. Jr. & Beal, M. F. (1985). Cortico-basal ganglionic degeneration. *Neurology*, Suppl. 1, **35**, 178.

Watts, R. L., Mirra, S. S., Young, R. R., Burger, P. C., Villier, J. A. & Heyman, A. (1989). Cortico-basal ganglionic degeneration (CBGD) with neuronal achromasia: clinical pathological study of two cases. *Neurology*, Suppl. 1, **39**, 140.

Watts, R. L., Mirra, S. S. & Richardson, E. P. (1994). Corticobasal ganglionic degeneration. In *Movement Disorders*, Vol. 3, ed. C. D. Marsden & S. Fahn, pp. 282–99. Oxford: Butterworths-Heinemann.

Wenning, G. K., Litvan, I., Jankovic, J. *et al.* (1998). Natural history and survival of 14 patients with corticobasal degeneration confirmed at postmortem examination. *J. Neurol. Neurosurg. Psychiatry*, **64**, 184–9.

Winkelmann, J., Auer, D. P., Lechner, C., Elbel, G. & Trenkwalder, C. (1999). Magnetic resonance imaging findings in corticobasal degeneration. *Mov. Disord.*, **14**, 669–73.

Yamauchi, H., Fukuyama, H., Nagahama, Y. *et al.* (1998). Atrophy of the corpus callosum, cortical hypometabolism, and cognitive impairment in corticobasal degeneration. *Arch. Neurol.*, **55**, 609–14.

Part VIII

Cerebellar degenerations

46

Approach to the patient with ataxia

Thomas Klockgether

Department of Neurology, University of Bonn, Germany

Definition and classification of ataxia

The term *ataxia* is derived from ancient Greek and literally means absence of order. In modern clinical neurology, ataxia is used to denote disturbances of coordinated muscle activity. Ataxia is caused by disorders of the cerebellum and its afferent or efferent connections. Spinal afferent pathways are often involved in ataxia disorders. Diseases of the peripheral nervous system, such as chronic idiopathic demyelinating polyneuropathy, may also cause ataxia. However, ataxia is rarely the prominent symptom in these disorders.

The afferent and efferent connections of the cerebellar cortex are topographically organized resulting in functional specialization of different parts of the cerebellum. Dysfunction of the lower vermis (vestibulocerebellum) leads to truncal ataxia. Spinocerebellar lesions (upper vermis and anterior parts of hemispheres) are characterized by unsteadiness of gait and stance which are more evident after eye closure (positive Rombergism). The most prominent symptom of neocerebellar damage (cerebellar hemispheres) is ataxia of intended limb movements. Ataxic limb movements are irregular and jerky and tend to overshoot the target (past-pointing). They are often accompanied by rhythmic side-to-side movements as the target is approached (action or intention tremor). Dysarthria characterized by slow and segmented speech with variable intonation and disturbances of ocular movements (broken-up smooth pursuit, saccadic hypermetria, gaze-evoked nystagmus) almost invariably accompany ataxia of gait and limb movements (Diener & Dichgans, 1992; Thach *et al.*, 1992).

Knowledge of the topographical organization of the cerebellum is helpful for the localisation of focal cerebellar disease. However, it is only of limited value in the differential diagnosis of non-focal cerebellar disorders such as cerebellar degenerations or cerebellar encephalitis, because these disorders are usually associated with a pancerebellar syndrome involving all aspects of ataxia.

Traditionally, classifications of ataxia were based on neuropathological criteria. Thus, Holmes (1907) distinguished between spinocerebellar degeneration, degeneration of the cerebellar cortex, and olivopontocerebellar atrophy. More recently, a clinical classification introduced by Harding (1983) gained wide acceptance. This classification distinguishes between congenital, hereditary and non-hereditary ataxias. Hereditary ataxias are further subdivided into ataxias with autosomal recessive inheritance such as Friedreich's ataxia (FRDA), and ataxias with autosomal dominant inheritance which are now usually named spinocerebellar ataxias (SCA). In recent years, the causative mutations of most hereditary ataxias have been identified allowing a rational classification of hereditary ataxias (Table 46.1). The non-hereditary ataxias comprise diseases with unknown etiology and symptomatic ataxias with a known cause.

Diagnostic approach to the patient with ataxia

Patients with ataxia may cause considerable diagnostic problems because a variety of heterogeneous diseases are associated with a widely uniform clinical picture. The diversity of disorders associated with ataxia may lead clinicians to apply extensive laboratory screening programs to each individual patient with ataxia. Although such an unspecific approach may be required in some patients, many have characteristic clinical features that allow to select and apply appropriate diagnostic tests.

A rational diagnostic approach implies a sequence of three steps. The first step is to distinguish focal and non-focal cerebellar disorders. The second step is to identify

Table 46.1. Classification of ataxia

Hereditary ataxias
  Autosomal recessive ataxias
  Autosomal dominant ataxias
    Spinocerebellar ataxias
    Episodic ataxias

Non-hereditary ataxias
  Multiple system atrophy, cerebellar type
  Sporadic adult-onset ataxia of unknown origin
  Symptomatic ataxias
    Alcoholic cerebellar degeneration
    Ataxias due to other toxic causes
    Paraneoplastic cerebellar degeneration
    Ataxia due to acquired vitamin deficiency or metabolic
      disorders
    Cerebellar encephalitis (including immune-mediated
      cerebellar degenerations other than paraneoplastic
      cerebellar degeneration)
    Ataxia due to physical causes

Table 46.2. Ataxia disorders with a highly characteristic clinical phenotype

Disorder	Phenotype	Laboratory test
Friedreich's ataxia (FRDA)	clinical diagnostic criteria (early disease onset, areflexia, dysarthria, posterior columns signs)	intronic GAA expansion of X25/FRDA gene
Ataxia telangiectasia (AT)	early disease onset, telangiectasias, immuno-deficiency	α-fetoprotein hypersensitivity of fibroblasts and lymphocytes to ionizing radiation mutation of ATM gene
Cerebrotendinous xanthomatosis	xanthomas	cholestanol
Spinocerebellar ataxia type 7 (SCA7)	autosomal dominant inheritance, retinal degeneration	CAG expansion of SCA7 gene
Multiple system atrophy (MSA)	autonomic failure	not available

disorders with a highly characteristic clinical phenotype that can be diagnosed on purely clinical grounds and to confirm the suspected diagnosis by a specific laboratory test. After these initial two steps, there is still a considerable number of patients in which the diagnosis remains unclear. The further diagnostic tests in these patients should be guided by considering the following aspects of the disease: mode of inheritance, age at disease onset, progression rate, accompanying symptoms. Thus, the initial diagnostic program in a young ataxia patient will be different from that in a patient with disease onset in late adulthood. Similarly, patients with rapid disease progression require another approach than patients with stationary or slowly progressive ataxia. Finally, presence of a specific accompanying symptom such as myoclonus will guide the further procedures in a certain direction.

Focal cerebellar disorders

The first step in the diagnosis of ataxia is to distinguish between focal cerebellar disease (tumor, abscess, ischemia, hemorrhage, focal demyelination) and non-focal disorders. In many cases, this distinction is easily made by taking the history and examining the patient. Acute disease onset, headache, vomiting and unilateral symptoms strongly argue in favor of a focal disease. A definite distinction between focal and non-focal cerebellar disorders is achieved by the use of imaging methods. Magnetic resonance imaging (MRI) is preferable to computed tomography (CT) because MRI – in contrast to CT – is capable of imaging the cerebellum and brainstem at different planes, with high resolution and without major artefacts (Wüllner et al., 1993).

Multiple sclerosis is an important differential diagnosis in the work-up of patients with ataxia. Remitting–relapsing course and multifocal involvement will raise suspicion of multiple sclerosis. To definitely establish the diagnosis of multiple sclerosis, MRI studies and cerebrospinal fluid examinations are required.

Ataxia disorders with highly characteristic phenotypes

A number of ataxia disorders have a highly characteristic clinical phenotype that allows to make a diagnosis on purely clinical grounds. In most of these disorders, laboratory tests are available that serve to confirm the suspected clinical diagnosis (Table 46.2). Friedreich's ataxia (FRDA) is an example for this type of disease. The clinical diagnostic criteria for FRDA, as defined by Geoffrey et al. (1976) and Harding (1981) include progressive ataxia with early disease onset, areflexia, dysarthria and signs of posterior column dysfunction. These criteria have an almost 100% specificity. It is important to recall that the characteristic phenotypical features that establish a diagnosis of FRDA, although being specific, lack sensitivity. In other words, a considerable number of patients who do not have the typical FRDA phenotype, may nevertheless suffer from FRDA

(Dürr *et al.*, 1996; Filla *et al.*, 1996). Demonstration of an expanded GAA repeat of the frataxin gene will confirm the clinically suspected diagnosis (Campuzani *et al.*, 1996). Table 46.2 gives a list of disorders in which a diagnosis can be made on the basis of a characteristic clinical phenotype. Most of these disorders are hereditary disorders with the notable exception of multiple system atrophy (MSA). MSA is an adult-onset sporadic disorder clinically characterized by various combinations of cerebellar ataxia, parkinsonism, pyramidal signs and autonomic failure (Quinn, 1989). In general, differential diagnosis of adult-onset sporadic ataxia disorders may be difficult and includes a wide variety of hereditary, degenerative and acquired disorders (Abele *et al.*, 2002). Autonomic failure in association with ataxia, however, occurs almost exclusively in MSA (Quinn, 1989; Wenning *et al.*, 1994; Schulz *et al.*, 1994). Demonstration of autonomic failure in a patient with sporadic adult-onset ataxia will thus establish the diagnosis of MSA without the necessity to perform a large battery of diagnostic tests.

Diagnosis in specific clinical situations

Autosomal recessive inheritance
Autosomal recessive inheritance is highly probable if there are more than one affected siblings in one generation while the parents are healthy. In addition, consanguinity of parents is a strong argument for autosomal recessive inheritance. Nevertheless, most autosomal recessive disorders manifest as sporadic diseases from non-consanguinous marriages. Typically, autosomal recessive disorders start in childhood, adolescence or early adulthood. Since acquired ataxia disorders are rare in young people, sporadic ataxia disorders with early disease onset are most often due to autosomal recessive inheritance. Thus, all diagnostic considerations that refer to autosomal recessive disorders also apply for sporadic disorders with early disease onset (see p. 00). Traditionally, early disease onset is defined as onset of symptoms before the age of 25 years (Harding, 1983). Although 25 years may serve as a general cut-off between early and late disease onset, autosomal recessive disorders may occasionally start much later, in some instances even after the age of 50 years (Dürr *et al.*, 1996; Filla *et al.*, 1996; Saviozzi *et al.*, 2002).

Table 46.3 gives a list of autosomal recessive ataxias along with the laboratory tests that allow to establish a definite diagnosis. For FRDA and autosomal recessive spastic ataxia of Charlevoix-Saguenay (ARSACS), genetic tests are established (Campuzano *et al.*, 1996; Mercier *et al.*, 2001). In abetalipoproteinemia, ataxia with isolated

Table 46.3. Laboratory tests in autosomal recessive ataxias

Disorder	Laboratory test
Friedreich's ataxia (FRDA)	intronic GAA expansion of frataxin gene
Ataxia telangiectasia (AT)	α-fetoprotein hypersensitivity of fibroblasts and lymphocytes to ionizing radiation mutation of ATM gene
Autosomal recessive ataxia with oculomotor apraxia (AOA)	albumin (?)
Abetalipoproteinemia	vitamin E lipid electrophoresis
Ataxia with isolated vitamin E deficiency (AVED)	vitamin E
Refsum's disease	phytanic acid
Autosomal recessive spastic ataxia of Charlevoix-Saguenay (ARSACS)	sacsin mutations
Cerebrotendinous xanthomatosis	cholestanol
Autosomal recessive spinocerebellar ataxia, non-Friedreich type 1 (SCAR1)	creatine kinase (?) α-fetoprotein (?)
Autosomal recessive ataxia with hearing impairment and optic atrophy	not available
Infantile-onset spinocerebellar ataxia (IOSCA)	not available
Early-onset cerebellar ataxia (EOCA)	not available

vitamin E deficiency (AVED), Refsum's disease and cerebrotendinous xanthomatosis, the affected genes are known, but – due to considerable allelic heterogeneity – the diagnosis still relies on the demonstration of characteristic biochemical abnormalities. In three other recessive ataxias, autosomal recessive non-Friedreich spinocerebellar ataxia type 1 (SCAR1), autosomal recessive ataxia with hearing impairment and optic atrophy (Bomont *et al.*, 2000), and infantile-onset spinocerebellar ataxia (IOSCA) (Lonnqvist *et al.*, 1998), the chromosomal loci are known, but the affected genes and mutations remain unidentified. In these disorders, a definite diagnosis can only be made by a linkage analysis of the family. In two disorders, autosomal recessive ataxia with oculomotor apraxia (AOA) (Moreira *et al.*, 2001; Date *et al.*, 2001) and SCAR1 (Bomont *et al.*, 2000; Nemeth *et al.*, 2000), biochemical abnormalities have been reported (decrease of albumin in AOA; increase of creatine kinase and α-fetoprotein in SCA1R), but it is not known how reliable these tests are.

A particular diagnostic problem are patients with oculomotor apraxia. Oculomotor apraxia denotes a peculiar difficulty to initiate saccades. In contrast to ophthalmoplegia,

Table 46.4. Mutations, genetic tests and clinical phenotypes of spinocerebellar ataxias (SCA)

Disorder	Mutation	Genetic test	Gene product	Clinical phenotype
SCA1	translated CAG repeat expansion	available	ataxin-1	ataxia, pyramidal signs, neuropathy, dysphagia, restless legs syndrome
SCA2	translated CAG repeat expansion	available	ataxin-2	ataxia, slow saccades, neuropathy, restless legs syndrome
SCA3 (Machado-Joseph disease)	translated CAG repeat expansion	available	ataxin-3	ataxia, pyramidal signs, ophthalmoplegia, neuropathy, dystonia, restless legs syndrome
SCA4	unknown	not available	unknown	ataxia, neuropathy
SCA5	unknown	not available	unknown	almost pure cerebellar ataxia
SCA6	translated CAG repeat expansion	available	calcium channel subunit (CACNA1A)	almost pure cerebellar ataxia
SCA7	translated CAG repeat expansion	available	ataxin-7	ataxia, ophthalmoplegia, visual loss
SCA8	untranslated CTG repeat expansion	available	unknown	almost pure cerebellar ataxia
SCA10	intronic ATTCT repeat expansion	available	unknown	ataxia, epilepsy
SCA11	unknown	not available	unknown	almost pure cerebellar ataxia
SCA12	untranslated CAG repeat expansion	available	phosphatase subunit (PP2A-PR55ß)	ataxia, tremor
SCA13	unknown	not available	unknown	ataxia, mental retardation
SCA14	unknown	not available	unknown	ataxia, myoclonus
SCA15	unknown	not available	unknown	almost pure cerebellar ataxia
SCA16	unknown	not available	unknown	almost pure cerebellar ataxia
SCA17	translated CAG repeat expansion	available	TATA binding protein	ataxia, dystonia
SCA18	unknown	not available	unknown	ataxia, neuropathy
SCA19	unknown	not available	unknown	ataxia, myoclonus, tremor

eye movements can be completed in the full range when given sufficient time. When patients intend gaze shifts, they often move their head into the desired direction causing a reflectory, tonic drift of the eyes away from the target. The target is then refixated with considerable delay. Oculomotor apraxia may occur as an isolated problem in a congenital disorder named Cogan's syndrome. It is also occurs in a number of ataxia disorders, namely AT, AOA and SCA1R. SCA2 patients with slow saccades (Table 46.4) may have similar problems when attempting to shift their gaze (Bürk *et al.*, 1999). Since reliable genetic and biochemical tests for AOA and SCA1R are not established, the diagnosis may remain uncertain in patients with ataxia and oculomotor apraxia in whom AT and SCA2 are excluded.

The diagnosis early-onset cerebellar ataxia (EOCA) should be reserved for ataxia disorders with an onset before the age of 25 years, in which a definite diagnosis cannot be made (Harding, 1981; Klockgether *et al.*, 1991).

Autosomal dominant inheritance

Presence of ataxia in subsequent generations is highly suggestive of autosomal dominant inheritance, provided that all affected family members have the same disease and that the disease is transmitted by both sexes. In cases in which other affected family members are not available for personal examination, it may be difficult to decide whether they really suffer from the same disease or from an unrelated medical problem. In patients with proven or suspected autosomal dominant mode of inheritance, molecular genetic tests for SCA mutations should be performed (Pulst *et al.*, 1996; Kawaguchi *et al.*, 1994; Zhuchenko *et al.*, 1997). Although the various SCA mutations are associated with characteristic clinical phenotypes, there is large clinical overlap between the different mutations (Bürk *et al.*, 1996; Filla *et al.*, 1996; Schöls *et al.*, 1997). Table 46.4 gives an overview of all known SCA mutations, the available genetic tests and the major features of the respective clinical phenotypes. There is large clinical overlap between the different SCA mutations precluding a definite clinical diagnosis of a particular SCA mutation. The only exception are patients from families with dominant ataxia and retinal degeneration. This clinical phenotype is almost invariably associated with the SCA7 mutation (Giunti *et al.*, 1999). Tests for the most frequent mutations, SCA1, SCA2, SCA3 and SCA6 are offered by many laboratories.

If tests for SCA mutations are negative in a patient with dominant ataxia, dentatorubral-pallidoluysian atrophy (DRPLA) (Koide *et al.*, 1994) or Gerstmann–Sträussler–Scheinker disease (GSS), a dominantly inherited transmissible spongiform encephalopathy (Hsiao *et al.*, 1989), should be considered as a differential diagnosis. Both disorders have a characteristic clinical presentation that allows to distinguish them from SCA mutations in most cases.

In approximately 30 to 40% of all dominant ataxia families, all presently available molecular tests are negative. These families probably suffer from a yet unidentified SCA mutation (Riess *et al.*, 1997; Moseley *et al.*, 1998).

Early-onset sporadic disease

As discussed earlier, most cases of early-onset sporadic ataxia are manifestations of an autosomal recessive disorder. Thus, the diagnostic tests recommended for autosomal recessive ataxias should be also applied to young patients with sporadic ataxia. In rare instances, sporadic ataxia starting in young age may be due to maternal inheritance (mitochondrial disease), X chromosomal inheritance (adrenoleukodystrophy) (Kurihara *et al.*, 1993; Takada *et al.*, 1987; Kusaka & Imai, 1992) or autosomal dominant inheritance (spinocerebellar ataxias, SCA). All these disorders may well start before the age of 25 years. Autosomal dominant ataxia may occur as a sporadic disease if it is due to a novel mutation. In addition, the family history may be uninformative, if parents died before manifestation of the disease, or fatherhood may be false.

Furthermore, early-onset sporadic ataxia may occur as an acquired disease (symptomatic ataxia) without any genetic background. The most frequent type of symptomatic ataxia in young people is cerebellar encephalitis associated with viral infections (Klockgether *et al.*, 1993). Although ataxia due to paraneoplastic cerebellar degeneration typically starts in adulthood, paraneoplastic cerebellar degeneration may affect children with neuroblastoma and young patients with malignant lymphoma. All other types of symptomatic ataxias are infrequent before the age of 25 years.

Adult-onset sporadic disease

The adult-onset sporadic ataxias can be divided into three major groups. The first group comprises the symptomatic ataxias that are due to identifiable exogenous causes. The second group includes hereditary ataxias presenting as sporadic adult-onset disorders. The third group are non-hereditary degenerative ataxias such as the cerebellar type of MSA.

Symptomatic ataxias

Symptomatic ataxia denotes all types of acquired disease in which a non-genetic cause can be identified. Usually, symptomatic ataxias start after the age of 25 years, although there are some exceptions that I have discussed above. The most frequent cause of symptomatic ataxia are chronic alcoholism (Timmann & Diener, 2000), other toxic causes (anticonvulsant drugs, antineoplastic drugs, lithium salts) (Botez *et al.*, 1988), malignant disease (paraneoplastic cerebellar degeneration) (Dalmau *et al.*, 1999), vitamin deficiency (vitamin B1, B12, E) (Harding *et al.*, 1982; Victor *et al.*, 1971), other metabolic causes (hypothyroidism) (Hammar & Regli, 1975), cerebellar encephalitis (Klockgether *et al.*, 1993; Connolly *et al.*, 1994), Miller Fisher syndrome (Berlit & Rakicky, 1992), immune-mediated cerebellar damage associated with anti-GAD (Abele *et al.*, 1999; Honnorat *et al.*, 2001), antigliadin (Hadjivassiliou *et al.*, 2002), or antithyroid antibodies (Selim & Drachman, 2001) and less frequently heat stroke. In most cases, history and clinical examination give important hints at the cause of symptomatic ataxia. Nevertheless, there are a number of diagnostic tests that are recommended in the work-up of a patient with suspected symptomatic ataxia (Table 46.5).

Genetic causes of sporadic adult-onset ataxia

Although autosomal recessive ataxias usually start before the age of 25 years, there are exceptional cases with much later disease onset. For example, age of onset is beyond 25 years in about 15% of FRDA patients (Dürr *et al.*, 1996; Filla *et al.*, 1996; Klockgether *et al.*, 1993). Since recessive ataxias occur sporadically in the majority of cases, some patients with adult-onset sporadic ataxia will suffer from an autosomal recessive ataxia with late disease onset. In a survey of 112 patients with sporadic adult-onset ataxia, we recently found 5 patients with the FRDA mutation (Abele *et al.*, 2002). Similarly, negative family history does not exclude autosomal dominant ataxia. Family history may be uninformative because an affected parent died before onset of symptoms. Not infrequently, this is the case for SCA6 because the age of onset is relatively late so that affected parents may have died before ataxia became apparent (Matsumura *et al.*, 1997; Schöls *et al.*, 1998). In addition, negative family history may be due to false fatherhood or to novel mutations. In our own study of 112 patients we

Table 46.5. Diagnostic tests in symptomatic ataxias

Disorder	Diagnostic test
Alcoholic cerebellar degeneration	liver enzymes, carbonyl-deficient transferrin, mean corpuscular volume (MCV)
Other toxic causes	serum levels of lithium/anticonvulsant drugs
Paraneoplastic cerebellar degeneration	antineuronal antibodies (anti-Hu, anti-Yo, anti-Ri, anti-TR) repeated search for occult neoplastic disease
Vitamin deficiency	vitamin B1, B12, E vitamin B12 absorption test (Schilling test)
Hypothyroidisms	thyroid hormones
Cerebellar encephalitis	CSF examination serological test for viral infections
Miller Fisher syndrome	CSF examination nerve conduction studies anti-GQ_{1B} antibodies
Other immune-mediated ataxias	anti-GAD, -gliadin, -thyroid antibodies
Heat stroke	not available

Table 46.6. Disorders that may cause ataxia and myoclonus

Disorder	Diagnostic test
Lafora disease(65)	Lafora bodies in skin, muscle and liver biopsy mutation of EPM2A gene
Progressive myoclonus epilepsy of Unverricht-Lundborg type (EPM1)	mutation of cystatin B gene
Myoclonus epilepsy with ragged red fibers (MERRF)	ragged red fibers in muscle biopsy 8344 point mutation of mitochondrial $tRNA^{Lys}$ gene
Sialidosis type 1	retinal-macular cherry-red spot sialooligosaccharides in urine neuraminidase activity in white blood cells mutation of neuraminidase gene
Neuronal ceroid lipofuscinosis (infantile, late infantile, juvenile, adult forms)(66)	ultrastructural analysis of lymphocytes and skin (eccrine sweat gland epithelial cells) different gene mutations (CLN1–3)
Dentatorubral-pallidoluysian atrophy (DRPLA)	CAG repeat expansion of DRPLA gene
Early-onset cerebellar ataxia with myoclonus (Ramsay Hunt syndrome)	not available

found SCA2 mutations in 1, SCA3 in 2 and SCA6 mutation in 7 patients (Abele *et al.*, 2002).

In our study of 112 patients, the percentage of sporadic ataxia patients with positive genetic tests was 13% (Abele *et al.*, 2002). In other studies, the frequency of positive genetic tests in apparently sporadic ataxia patients ranged from 2% to 22% (Moseley *et al.*, 1998; Matsumura *et al.*, 1997; Schöls *et al.*, 2000; Pujana *et al.*, 1999).

Sporadic degenerative ataxia disorders

After all known symptomatic and genetic causes have been ruled out a group of sporadic adult-onset ataxia patients remains in whom a sporadic neurodegenerative disease (comparable to sporadic amyotrophic lateral sclerosis or idiopathic Parkinson's disease) is assumed. In 1981, Harding reported a series of 36 patients with sporadic late-onset ataxia of unknown etiology for which she coined the term idiopathic cerebellar ataxia (IDCA) (Harding, 1981). Since then, various genetic and non-genetic causes of late-onset sporadic ataxia have been identified some of which may have been responsible for the disease in Harding's patients. In addition, it has been found that a considerable portion of IDCA patients suffered from MSA (Quinn, 1989; Wenning *et al.*, 1994). In our above mentioned study of 112 adult-onset ataxia patients there was clinical evidence of MSA in 29%, while the disease remained unexplained in 58%. For this latter group, the designations IDCA or alternatively sporadic adult-onset ataxia of unknown origin may be used. Compared with MSA, patients with sporadic adult-onset ataxia of unknown origin have a more favorable prognosis (Abele *et al.*, 2002).

Rapid disease progression

Most types of hereditary and non-hereditary ataxias are characterized by an insidious onset and continuous disease progression within years. Sudden disease onset and rapid progression are suspicious of focal cerebellar disease. Nevertheless, a number of non-focal cerebellar disorders may cause ataxia with subacute onset and rapid deterioration. These disorders include cerebellar encephalitis associated with viral infection (Klockgether *et al.*, 1993), Miller Fisher syndrome (Berlit & Rakicky, 1992), paraneoplastic cerebellar degeneration (Dalmau *et al.*, 1999), transmissible spongiform encephalopathy, Wernicke's encephalopathy (Victor *et al.*, 1971) and vitamin B12 deficiency.

Myoclonus

Myoclonus is associated with progressive ataxia in a number of disorders. Often, myoclonus and ataxia are part of a larger syndrome that is characterized by ataxia,

Table 46.7. Disorders that may cause ataxia and retinal degeneration

Disorder	Ocular disorder	Laboratory test
Abetalipoproteinemia	retinitis pigmentosa (predominantly of posterior fundus)	vitamin E lipid electrophoresis
Refsum's disease	retinitis pigmentosa posterior subcapsular cataracts	phytanic acid
Ataxia with isolated vitamin E deficiency (AVED)	retinitis pigmentosa	vitamin E
Neuronal ceroid lipofuscinosis (infantile, late infantile, juvenile, adult forms)	retinitis pigmentosa	ultrastructural analysis of lymphocytes and skin (eccrine sweat gland epithelial cells) different gene mutations (CLN1–3)
Sialidosis type 1	retinal-macular cherry-red spot	sialooligosaccharides in urine neuraminidase activity in white blood cells mutation of neuraminidase gene
Spinocerebellar ataxia type 7 (SCA7)	macular degeneration	CAG expansion of SCA7 gene
Cockayne syndrome	retinal dystrophy	not available

myoclonus, epilepsy and progressive dementia. This syndrome is known as progressive myoclonus epilepsy (PME) (Berkovic *et al.*, 1993). In patients with ataxia and accompanying myoclonus all known causes of PME should be considered, even if epilepsy and cognitive disturbances are not prominent. Table 46.6 gives a list of disorders that may cause PME along with the appropriate diagnostic tests. According to general experience, there is a substantial number of patients in whom careful diagnostic work-up will not result in a definite diagnosis. In most of these patients, epilepsy and dementia are mild or absent. These patients should be diagnosed as early-onset cerebellar ataxia with myoclonus (Harding, 1983). This descriptive term seems to be more appropriate than the traditional term Ramsay Hunt syndrome (Marseille Consensus Group, 1990).

Retinal degeneration

Symptoms of retinal degeneration include slowly progressive visual loss and poor night vision. Peripheral retinal degeneration causes constriction of visual fields to the extent of gun-barrel vision, while macular degeneration affects central vision and visual acuity. Progressive visual loss in patients with ataxia requires an ophthalmological examination with detailed fundoscopy followed by a number of ancillary investigations (fluorescein retinography, electroretinogram). Table 46.7 gives a list of disorders that may cause retinal degeneration in association with progressive ataxia.

Table 46.8. Specific treatment for ataxia disorders

Disorder	Treatment
Friedreich's ataxia (FRDA)	idebenone (?)
Abetalipoproteinemia	vitamin E supplementation
Ataxia with isolated vitamin E deficiency (AVED)	vitamin E supplementation
Refsum's disease	dietary restriction of phytanic acid
Cerebrotendinous xanthomatosis	chenodeoxycholate, simvastatin
Alcoholic cerebellar degeneration	alcohol withdrawal, treatment for alcoholism, vitamin B1
Ataxia due to other toxic causes	withdrawal of toxic compounds
Vitamin deficiency	vitamin supplementation
Hypothyroidisms	thyroid hormone supplementation
Miller Fisher syndrome	i.v. immunoglobulins

Management of ataxia patients

Although a careful diagnostic work-up allows the cause of most ataxia disorders to be identified, rational treatment approaches are not available for all. Nevertheless, there are a number of ataxia disorders for which specific therapies are available (Klockgether *et al.*, 1996). An overview of these therapies is given in Table 46.8.

In many ataxia disorders, only supportive treatment is possible. In general, it is assumed that physiotherapy and speech therapy are helpful in ataxia disorders. The goal should be to maintain the highest possible level of autonomy, to cope with physical disability and to prevent secondary complications. With progression of the disease many patients will require walking aids and a wheelchair.

It has been repeatedly claimed that drugs that increase neurotransmission at central 5-HT receptors temporarily improve cerebellar ataxia (Trouillas et al., 1995). Three recent studies investigated the antiataxic effect of the anxiolytic 5-HT$_{1A}$ receptor agonist buspirone. Results of an open-label study of 20 patients with different forms of degenerative ataxia suggested an antiataxic action of buspirone at a dose of 30–60 mg per day (Lou et al., 1995). Efficacy of buspirone was confirmed in a randomized, placebo-controlled study of 19 patients with ataxia due to cerebellar cortical atrophy (Trouillas et al., 1997). In contrast, another study did not report a favorable effect of buspirone in ataxia (Hassin-Baer et al., 2000). In my own experience, the efficacy of antiataxic drugs is low, and only very few patients really benefit from them.

There are numerous neurological and non-neurological symptoms that may occur in association with certain ataxia disorders. Well-known examples are cardiomyopathy and diabetes mellitus in FRDA and autonomic failure in MSA. These accompanying symptoms require conventional medical and neurological treatment.

REFERENCES

Abele, M., Weller, M., Mescheriakov, S., Bürk, K., Dichgans, J. & Klockgether, T. (1999). Cerebellar ataxia with glutamic acid decarboxylase autoantibodies. Neurology, 52, 857–9.

Abele, M., Bürk, K., Schols, L. et al. (2002). The aetiology of sporadic adult-onset ataxia. Brain, 125, 961–8.

Berkovic, S. F., Cochius, J., Andermann, E. & Andermann, F. (1993). Progressive myoclonus epilepsies: clinical and genetic aspects. Epilepsia, 34 Suppl 3, S19–S30.

Berlit, P. & Rakicky, J. (1992). The Miller Fisher syndrome. Review of the literature. J. Clin. Neuroophthalmol., 12, 57–63.

Bomont, P., Watanabe, M., GershoniBarush, R. et al. (2000). Homozygosity mapping of spinocerebellar ataxia with cerebellar atrophy and peripheral neuropathy to 9q33–34, and with hearing impairment and optic atrophy to 6p21–23. Eur. J. Hum. Genet., 8, 986–90.

Botez, M. I., Attig, E. & Vezina, J. L. (1998). Cerebellar atrophy in epileptic patients. Can. J. Neurol. Sci., 15, 299–303.

Bürk, K., Abele, M., Fetter, M. et al. (1996). Autosomal dominant cerebellar ataxia type I – clinical features and MRI in families with SCA1, SCA2 and SCA3. Brain, 119, 1497–505.

Bürk, K., Fetter, M., Abele, M. et al. (1999). Autosomal dominant cerebellar ataxia type I: oculomotor abnormalities in families with SCA1, SCA2, and SCA3. J. Neurol., 246, 789–97.

Campuzano, V., Montermini, L., Moltò, M. D. et al. (1996). Friedreich's ataxia: autosomal recessive disease caused by an intronic GAA triplet repeat expansion. Science, 271, 1423–7.

Connolly, A. M., Dodson, W. E., Prensky, A. L. & Rust, R. S. (1994). Course and outcome of acute cerebellar ataxia. Ann. Neurol., 35, 673–9.

Dalmau, J., Gultekin, H. S. & Posner, J. B. (1999). Paraneoplastic neurologic syndromes: pathogenesis and physiopathology. Brain Pathol., 9, 275–84.

Date, H., Onodera, O., Tanaka, H. et al. (2001). Early-onset ataxia with ocular motor apraxia and hypoalbuminemia is caused by mutations in a new HIT superfamily gene. Nat. Genet., 29, 184–8.

Diener, H. C. & Dichgans, J. (1992). Pathophysiology of cerebellar ataxia. Mov. Disord., 7, 95–109.

Dürr, A., Cossee, M., Agid, Y. et al. (1996). Clinical and genetic abnormalities in patients with Friedreich's ataxia. N. Engl. J. Med., 335, 1169–75.

Filla, A., De Michele, G., Campanella, G. et al. (1996a). Autosomal dominant cerebellar ataxia type I. Clinical and molecular study in 36 Italian families including a comparison between SCA1 and SCA2 phenotypes. J. Neurol. Sci., 142, 140–7.

Filla, A., De Michele, G., Cavalcanti, F. et al. (1996b). The relationship between trinucleotide (GAA) repeat length and clinical features in Friedreich ataxia. Am. J. Hum. Genet., 59, 554–60.

Geoffrey, G., Barbeau, A., Breton, G. et al. (1976). Clinical description and roentgenologic evaluation of patients with Friedreich's ataxia. Can. J. Neurol. Sci., 3, 279–86.

Giunti, P., Stevanin, G., Worth, P. F., David, G., Brice, A. & Wood, N. W. (1999). Molecular and clinical study of 18 families with ADCA type II: evidence for genetic heterogeneity and de novo mutation. Am. J. Hum. Genet., 64, 1594–603.

Hadjivassiliou, M., Grunewald, R. A. & Davies-Jones, G. A. B. (2002). Gluten sensitivity as a neurological illness. J. Neurol. Neurosurg. Psychiatry, 72, 560–3.

Hammar, C. H. & Regli, F. (1975). [Cerebellar ataxia due to hypothyroidism in adults (case report)]. Dtsch. Med. Wochenschr., 100, 1504–6.

Harding, A. E. (1981a). Early onset cerebellar ataxia with retained tendon reflexes: a clinical and genetic study of a disorder distinct from Friedreich's ataxia. J. Neurol. Neurosurg. Psychiatry, 44, 503–8.

Harding, A. E. (1981b). Friedreich's ataxia: a clinical and genetic study of 90 families with an analysis of early diagnostic criteria and intrafamilial clustering of clinical features. Brain, 104, 589–620.

Harding, A. E. (1981c). "Idiopathic" late onset cerebellar ataxia. A clinical and genetic study of 36 cases. J. Neurol. Sci., 51, 259–71.

Harding, A. E. (1983). Classification of the hereditary ataxias and paraplegias. Lancet, 1, 1151–5.

Harding, A. E., Muller, D. P., Thomas, P. K. & Willison, H. J. (1982). Spinocerebellar degeneration secondary to chronic intestinal malabsorption: a vitamin E deficiency syndrome. *Ann. Neurol.*, **12**, 419–24.

Hassin-Baer, S., Korczyn, A. D. & Giladi, N. (2000). An open trial of amantadine and buspirone for cerebellar ataxia: a disappointment. *J. Neural Transm.*, **107**, 1187–9.

Holmes, G. (1907). An attempt to classify cerebellar disease, with a note on Marie's hereditary cerebellar ataxia. *Brain*, **30**, 545–67.

Honnorat, J., Saiz, A., Giometto, B. *et al.* (2001). Cerebellar ataxia with anti-glutamic acid decarboxylase antibodies – Study of 14 patients. *Arch. Neurol.*, **58**, 225–30.

Hsiao, K., Baker, H. F., Crow, T. J. *et al.* (1989). Linkage of a prion protein missense variant to Gerstmann–Sträussler syndrome. *Nature*, **338**, 342–5.

Kawaguchi, Y., Okamoto, T., Taniwaki, M. *et al.* (1994). CAG expansions in a novel gene for Machado-Joseph disease at chromosome 14q32.1. *Nat. Genet.*, **8**, 221–8.

Klockgether, T. & Dichgans, J. (1996). Inherited and noninherited ataxias. In *Neurological Disorders: Course and Treatment*, ed. T. Brandt, L. R. Caplan, J. Dichgans, H. C. Diener & C. Kennard, pp. 705–13. San Diego: Academic Press.

Klockgether, T., Petersen, D., Grodd, W. & Dichgans, J. (1991). Early onset cerebellar ataxia with retained tendon reflexes. Clinical, electrophysiological and MRI observations in comparison with Friedreich's ataxia. *Brain*, **114**, 1559–73.

Klockgether, T., Doller, G., Wüllner, H., Petersen, D. & Dichgans, J. (1993). Cerebellar encephalitis in adults. *J. Neurol.*, **240**, 17–20.

Klockgether, T., Chamberlain, S., Wüllner, U. *et al.* (1993). Late-onset Friedreich's ataxia. Molecular genetics, clinical neurophysiology, and magnetic resonance imaging. *Arch. Neurol.*, **50**, 803–6.

Koide, R., Ikeuchi, T., Onodera, O. *et al.* (1994). Unstable expansion of CAG repeat in hereditary dentatorubral-pallidoluysian atrophy (DRPLA). *Nat. Genet.*, **6**, 9–13.

Kurihara, M., Kumagai, K., Yagishita, S. *et al.* (1993). Adrenoleukomyeloneuropathy presenting as cerebellar ataxia in a young child: a probable variant of adrenoleukodystrophy. *Brain Dev.*, **15**, 377–80.

Kusaka, H. & Imai, T. (1992). Ataxic variant of adrenoleukodystrophy: MRI and CT findings. *J. Neurol.*, **239**, 307–10.

Lonnqvist, T., Paetau, A., Nikali, K., von Boguslawski, K. & Pihko, H. (1998). Infantile onset spinocerebellar ataxia with sensory neuropathy (IOSCA): neuropathological features. *J. Neurol. Sci.*, **161**, 57–65.

Lou, J. S., Goldfarb, L., McShane, L., Gatev, P., Hallett, M. (1995). Use of buspirone for treatment of cerebellar ataxia – an open-label study. *Arch. Neurol.*, **52**, 982–8.

Marseille Consensus Group (1990). Classification of progressive myoclonus epilepsies and related disorders. Marseille Consensus Group. *Ann. Neurol.*, **28**, 113–16.

Matsumura, R., Futamura, N., Fujimoto, Y. *et al.* (1997). Spinocerebellar ataxia type 6 – molecular and clinical features of 35 Japanese patients including one homozygous for the CAG repeat expansion. *Neurology*, **49**, 1238–43.

Mercier, J., Prevost, C., Engert, J. C., Bouchard, J. P., Mathieu, J. & Richter, A. (2001). Rapid detection of the sacsin muta-

tions causing autosomal recessive spastic ataxia of Charlevoix-Saguenay. *Genetic Testing*, **5**, 255–9.

Moreira, M. C., Barbot, C., Tachi, N. *et al.* (2001). The gene mutated in ataxia–ocular apraxia 1 encodes the new HIT/Zn-finger protein aprataxin. *Nat. Genet.*, **29**, 189–93.

Moseley, M. L., Benzow, K. A., Schut, L. J. *et al.* (1998). Incidence of dominant spinocerebellar and Friedreich triplet repeats among 361 ataxia families. *Neurology*, **51**, 1666–71.

Nemeth, A. H., Bochukova, E., Dunne, E. *et al.* (2000). Autosomal recessive cerebellar ataxia with oculomotor apraxia (Ataxia-telangiectasia-like syndrome) is linked to chromosome 9q34. *Am. J. Hum. Genet.*, **67**, 1320–6.

Pujana, M. A., Corral, J., Gratacos, M. *et al.* (1999). Spinocerebellar ataxias in Spanish patients: genetic analysis of familial and sporadic cases. The Ataxia Study Group. *Hum. Genet.*, **104**, 516–22.

Pulst, S. M., Nechiporuk, A., Nechiporuk, T. *et al.* (1996). Moderate expansion of a normally biallelic trinucleotide repeat in spinocerebellar ataxia type 2. *Nat. Genet.*, **14**, 269–76.

Quinn, N. (1989). Multiple system atrophy – the nature of the beast. *J. Neurol. Neurosurg. Psychiatry*, Suppl, 78–89.

Riess, O., Schöls, L., Bottger, H. *et al.* (1997). SCA6 is caused by moderate CAG expansion in the alpha1A-voltage-dependent calcium channel gene. *Hum. Mol. Genet.*, **6**, 1289–93.

Saviozzi, S., Saluto, A., Taylor, A. M. R. *et al.* (2002). A late onset variant of ataxia-telangiectasia with a compound heterozygous genotype, A8030G/7481insA. *J. Med. Genet.*, **39**, 57–61.

Schöls, L., Amoiridis, G., Büttner, T., Przuntek, H., Epplen, J. T. & Riess, O. (1997). Autosomal dominant cerebellar ataxia: phenotypic differences in genetically defined subtypes? *Ann. Neurol.*, **42**, 924–32.

Schöls, L., Krüger, R., Amoiridis, G., Przuntek, H., Epplen, J. T. & Riess, O. (1998). Spinocerebellar ataxia type 6: genotype and phenotype in German kindreds. *J. Neurol. Neurosurg. Psychiatry*, **64**, 67–73.

Schöls, L., Szymanski, S., Peters, S. *et al.* (2000). Genetic background of apparently idiopathic sporadic cerebellar ataxia. *Hum. Genet.*, **107**, 132–7.

Schulz, J. B., Klockgether, T., Petersen, D. *et al.* (1994). Multiple system atrophy: natural history, MRI morphology, and dopamine receptor imaging with 123IBZM-SPECT. *J. Neurol. Neurosurg. Psychiatry*, **57**, 1047–56.

Selim, M. & Drachman, D. A. (2001). Ataxia associated with Hashimoto's disease: progressive non-familial adult onset cerebellar degeneration with autoimmune thyroiditis. *J. Neurol. Neurosurg. Psychiatry*, **71**, 81–7.

Takada, K., Onoda, K., Takahashi, K., Nakamura, H. & Taketomi, T. (1987). An adult case of adrenoleukodystrophy with features of olivo-ponto-cerebellar atrophy: I. Clinical and pathological studies. *Jpn. J. Exp. Med.*, **57**, 53–8.

Thach, W. T., Goodkin, H. P. & Keating, J. G. (1992). The cerebellum and the adaptive coordination of movement. *Annu. Rev. Neurosci.*, **15**, 403–42.

Timmann, D. & Diener, H. C. (2000). Alcoholic cerebellar degeneration (including ataxias that are due to other toxic causes). In

Handbook of Ataxia Disorders, ed. T. Klockgether, pp. 571–605. New York: Marcel Dekker.

Trouillas, P., Serratrice, G., Laplane, D. *et al.* (1995). Levorotatory form of 5-hydroxytryptophan in Friedreich's ataxia: results of a double-blind drug-placebo cooperative study. *Arch. Neurol.*, **52**, 456–60.

Trouillas, P., Xie, J., Adeleine, P. *et al.* (1997). Buspirone, a 5-hydroxytryptamine$_{1A}$ agonist, is active in cerebellar ataxia – results of a double-blind drug placebo study in patients with cerebellar cortical atrophy. *Arch. Neurol.*, **54**, 749–52.

Victor, M., Adams, R. D. & Collins, G. H. (1971). The Wernicke–Korsakoff syndrome. A clinical and pathological study of 245 patients, 82 with post-mortem examinations. *Contemp. Neurol. Ser.*, **7**, 1–206.

Wenning, G. K., Ben Shlomo, Y., Magalhaes, M., Daniel, S. E. & Quinn, N. P. (1994). Clinical features and natural history of multiple system atrophy. An analysis of 100 cases. *Brain*, **117**, 835–45.

Wüllner, U., Klockgether, T., Petersen, D., Naegele, T. & Dichgans, J. (1993). Magnetic resonance imaging in hereditary and idiopathic ataxia. *Neurology*, **43**, 318–25.

Zhuchenko, O., Bailey, J., Bonnen, P. *et al.* (1997). Autosomal dominant cerebellar ataxia (SCA6) associated with small polyglutamine expansions in the α_{1A}-voltage-dependent calcium channel. *Nat. Genet.*, **15**, 62–9.

47

Autosomal dominant cerebellar ataxia

Henry L. Paulson

Department of Neurology, University of Iowa Hospitals and Clinics, IA, USA

This review discusses clinical and genetic features of dominantly inherited ataxia. In addition, potential pathogenic mechanisms are discussed with a special focus on the polyglutamine disorders, since most is known about this group of diseases.

Classification of ADCA

Most adult onset hereditary ataxias are dominantly inherited. Harding (1993) clinically divided autosomal dominant cerebellar ataxia (ADCA) into four types, I through IV. Type I ADCA represents cerebellar disease accompanied by brainstem signs. ADCA type II is similar to type I but also includes retinopathy. ADCA type III represents later onset, "pure" cerebellar disease and ADCA type IV represents episodic ataxia.

A newer, favored classification for ADCA reflects the growing number of identified genetic loci, each of which is designated a specific spinocerebellar ataxia or SCA (Table 47.1). As SCAs are mapped to loci, they are assigned numbers – SCA1, SCA2 and so forth, currently up to 21 at the time of this writing. Most SCAs fall within Harding's ADCA type I classification. There is considerable clinical overlap among the ADCA type I group, even within families. In contrast, the sole genetic cause of ADCA type II appears to be SCA7, the only dominant ataxia routinely accompanied by retinal degeneration. Most patients with SCA6 (and several rarer SCAs for which the gene defects have not been identified) manifest as a pure cerebellar syndrome and thus fall within ADCA III. Finally, ADCA type IV currently consists of two genetically identified forms of episodic ataxia (EA), EA-1 and EA-2, caused by mutations in a potassium and calcium channel respectively. Additional, less well-characterized loci for episodic ataxia also exist.

As we learn more about the clinical, radiographic and pathological features of each genetic form of ataxia, and particularly as we move toward rational therapies based on defined molecular defects, these disorders should be identified by their SCA, not ADCA, designation.

Molecular mechanisms of ADCA

Dynamic repeat expansions cause most adult onset ataxias

Classification of late-onset ataxias was formerly confusing due to their highly variable manifestations. Adding to the confusion was the fact that many late-onset ataxias show anticipation – the trend toward worsening severity in successive generations. Anticipation and disease variability, we now know, are explained by the remarkable genetic defect underlying most late-onset ataxias: dynamic expansions of simple sequence DNA repeats (Cummings & Zoghbi, 2000). In most cases these are triplet repeat expansions, but tetranucleotide, pentanucleotide and dodecanucleotide repeat expansions have also been identified. Figure 47.1 shows a gene schematic illustrating where the nine known ataxia-causing expanded repeats reside in the gene. All but one of these, Friedreich ataxia, are dominantly inherited. As discussed below, precisely how a repeat expansion causes disease differs depending upon at least three factors: what kind of repeat it is, where it resides in the gene, and what the gene's function is. The single largest category consists of diseases caused by a polyglutamine-encoding CAG repeat.

CAG repeat/polyglutamine ataxias

At least nine diseases are due to a CAG repeat that encodes an expanded polyglutamine tract in the disease protein

Table 47.1. Polyglutamine diseases

Huntington disease
Spinobulbar muscular atrophy (Kennedy disease)
Dentatorubral-pallidoluysian atrophy
Spinocerebellar ataxia type 1
Spinocerebellar ataxia type 2
Machado-Joseph disease/Spinocerebellar ataxia type 3
Spinocerebellar ataxia type 6
Spinocerebellar ataxia type 7
Spinocerebellar ataxia type 17

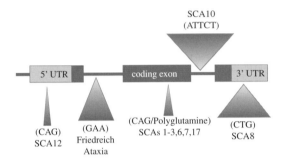

Fig. 47.1 Schematic of a gene indicating the repeat sequence for the known ataxia-causing dynamic repeats and their place of occurrence within the respective disease genes. Range of expansion size is approximated by the width of the triangle. UTR = untranslated regions. Introns and exons are denoted by lines and boxes, respectively.

(Table 47.1). These polyglutamine disorders include at least six dominantly inherited SCAs (types 1, 2, 3, 6, 7 and 17) as well as Huntington's disease (HD), DRPLA and spinobulbar muscular atrophy (SBMA) (Cummings & Zoghbi, 2000). All are progressive neurodegenerative diseases in which the disease protein apparently misfolds, resulting in the formation of abnormal protein inclusions inside neurons. Longer repeats cause more severe and typically earlier onset disease. Polyglutamine expansion thus confers upon the disease protein a novel, dominant neurotoxic property that increases in potency with longer repeats (for review see Taylor *et al.*, 2002; Zoghbi, 2000).

Precisely how expanded polyQ proteins cause neuronal dysfunction and cell death is still not known. Currently, several models of pathogenesis are supported by research: (i) perturbations in protein homeostasis; (ii) dysregulation of gene expression; and (iii) aberrant processing of proteins, leading to the production of toxic fragments of the protein. These are not mutually exclusive hypotheses. Indeed, elements of all three may contribute to disease mechanisms in different polyQ diseases.

Of these three models of pathogenesis, evidence most strongly supports the view that perturbations in protein homeostasis are central to disease. Although the hallmark protein inclusions seen in polyQ diseases may not be directly toxic, they do argue for a fundamental problem in protein folding and clearance. In many cellular and animal models, cellular components that ensure protein quality control have been implicated in polyQ diseases (for review see Bonini, 2002; Muchowski, 2002; Sherman & Goldberg, 2001). For example, heat shock protein molecular chaperones consistently turn up as suppressors of polyQ toxicity in vitro and in vivo. Chaperones capable of suppressing toxicity do so in a manner that alters the solubility of the mutant protein (Bonini, 2002; Chan *et al.*, 2000). One possibility is that suppressor chaperones directly bind abnormal polyglutamine protein and thereby inhibit the formation of toxic monomers, oligomers or protofibrils – which of these species is the actual toxic factor is unknown. The ability to model polyglutamine protein folding in the test tube now allows this to be tested experimentally.

Evidence for dysregulation of gene expression (e.g. Hughes, 2002) has started to build in the past few years. It is still too early, however, to gauge the full significance of these findings. For example, do the observed gene expression changes reflect a primary effect on specific transcription factors, an indirect effect through other cellular pathways, or both? It is clear that at least two polyQ disease proteins normally play central roles in controlling gene expression in the cell. Among the polyQ ataxias, the SCA17 disease protein, TBP, is an essential part of the basal transcription complex. In SCA17, an intrinsic defect in TBP function in transcription may well contribute to pathogenesis. In other polyQ diseases, aberrant protein interactions between the disease protein and various transcription factors or cofactors may disrupt the highly regulated expression of neuronal genes, with deleterious consequences for the neuron.

The toxic fragment hypothesis of polyQ diseases has been studied most extensively in the non-ataxia members of the group: HD, DRPLA and SBMA. For these diseases, a strong, but not foolproof, case can be made that proteolytic cleavage of the disease protein occurs as part of pathogenesis. Much of the work has focused on caspases as the culprit proteases, but recent studies in HD suggest that calpains and aspartic proteases also cleave this disease protein. Data are less well developed and convincing for the six polyQ ataxias. Indeed, in SCA1 there is no evidence that the disease protein ataxin-1 becomes cleaved.

The fact that polyQ diseases are clinically distinct disorders suggests that the individual disease proteins, dissimilar except for their polyQ tract, contribute in unique ways

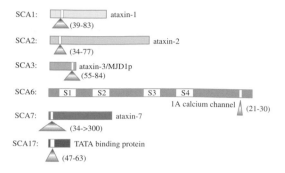

Fig. 47.2 Disease proteins in the polyglutamine ataxias are shown here as boxes proportionate to their size. Polyglutamine disease proteins differ greatly in size and sequence (here denoted by boxes of various shades of gray). The position of the polyglutamine domain (white box), and the size of the expansion differ for each protein (disease repeat range is shown in parentheses). The protein's function is well established for only two of the ataxia-causing polyglutamine proteins: the SCA17 disease protein, the TATA binding protein, is a critical component of the basal transcription machinery, and the SCA6 protein is an alpha subunit of a voltage-dependent calcium channel. These two also represent the shortest and longest proteins in this group (339 and 2320 amino acids, respectively). In SCA6, the four multi transmembrane domains are shown (S1–S4).

to pathogenesis in each disease (Fig. 47.2). Even though the diseases likely share a common pathogenesis based on biochemical properties of expanded polyglutamine, the individual proteins almost certainly have divergent functions. Likewise, they probably interact with different, though overlapping, sets of proteins. This suggests that the particular protein context surrounding polyQ dictates many of the disease-specific characteristics of neuronal dysfunction and degeneration in each disease. An extreme case is SCA6, which may differ mechanistically from other polyglutamine diseases based on the fact that the disease protein is a transmembrane, voltage-dependent calcium channel (all other polyQ disease proteins are soluble proteins). In the context of this calcium channel, expanded polyglutamine causes disease with much smaller expansions than are required for the other diseases. Direct changes in ion channel properties may contribute to the cerebellar deficits in this disorder (e.g. Piedras-Renteria *et al.*, 2001).

Researchers have begun to identify compounds and genes that suppress polyQ aggregation and/or toxicity, and the availability of animal models for most polyQ diseases should speed preclinical testing of such genes and compounds. One hopes, of course, that a protective pharmacological therapy for polyQ diseases will arise from such studies. Another direct and simple-minded approach to therapy is based on the premise that, whatever the

pathogenic mechanism may be, the mutant protein is clearly a bad player; eliminating its expression, therefore, would be therapeutically useful. The recent discovery that small interfering RNA (siRNA) can be used to silence target genes with exquisite sequence specificity raises the possibility that this new technology might be harnessed to knock down expression of polyQ disease alleles (Miller *et al.*, 2003; Xia *et al.*, 2002).

Ataxias due to noncoding repeat expansions

At least three dominant ataxias are caused by repeats that are not translated into protein. One of these, SCA8, is a CTG repeat transcribed into RNA in the brain. Similarities between the SCA8 repeat and the two repeats causing myotonic dystrophy suggest that this repeat may act in a dominant manner at the RNA level to alter mRNA processing (Ranum *et al.*, 1994). Transgenic mice containing the SCA8 mutation show abnormalities in central nervous system function and premature death (Moseley *et al.*, 2002). Further studies of this mouse model should help define the molecular mechanisms of SCA8. In SCA10, the mutation is a huge ATTCT repeat, larger than any other repeat expansion described to date (Matsuura *et al.*, 2000). The repeat resides in the ninth intron of the *E46L* gene, which is highly expressed in brain. Here, too, a dominant RNA effect is one of several possibilities for its mechanism of action. A third, much smaller repeat is the CAG expansion in SCA12, residing in the 5′ region of the *PPP2R2B* gene (Holmes *et al.*, 1999). This modest expansion has been proposed to alter the expression of the PP2R2B gene product, a regulatory subunit for protein phosphatase 2A. Changes in activity of this phosphatase may have deleterious consequences for neurons, though this is purely speculative.

The spinocerebellar ataxias

SCAs are characterized by progressive ataxia with varying degrees of bulbar dysfunction, ophthalmoparesis, pyramidal and extrapyramidal signs, optic atrophy and dementia. Pathological studies show variable spinocerebellar degeneration even in the same SCA. Three SCAs (SCA2, MJD/SCA3 and SCA6) are the most common, together accounting for approximately half of all affected families worldwide.

As of this writing, at least 19 SCAs have been mapped to chromosomal loci, and the genetic defects have been identified in at least 10 (Table 47.2). Thus far, all but one are dynamic repeat expansions. SCA14 is the sole exception, which is instead caused by point mutations

Table 47.2. Spinocerebellar ataxias

Disease	Locus	Mutation	Associated features
SCA1	6p22.3	CAG/polyQ	ophthalmoparesis, pyramidal and extrapyramidal findings
SCA2	12q24.12	CAG/polyQ	slow saccades, hyporeflexia, dementia
MJD/SCA3	14q32.12	CAG/polyQ	bulging eyes, ophthalmoparesis, spasticity, neuropathy, lingual/facial fasciculations, DOPA-responsive parkinsonism
SCA4	16q22.1	unknown	early areflexia, sensory neuropathy
SCA5	11p11–q11	unknown	milder disease than SCAs1–4
SCA6	19p13.2	CAG/PolyQ	late onset, slow course, often pure cerebellar, gaze-evoked and vertical nystagmus
SCA7	3p14.1	CAG/polyQ	retinal degeneration
SCA8	13q21.33	CTG	bulbar findings, sensory neuronopathy
SCA10	22q13	ATTCT	seizures
SCA11	chr15	unknown	mild disease
SCA12	5q32	CAG	tremor, late dementia
SCA13	19q13.3–13.4	unknown	motor dysfunction, mental retardation
SCA14	19q13.4	PKRCG gene	axial myoclonus
SCA15	undetermined	unknown	pure ataxia, mild
SCA16	8q23–24.1	unknown	head tremor
SCA17	6q27	CAG/poly	dementia, dystonia
SCA18	7q31–32	unknown	sensory/motor neuropathy with ataxia
SCA19	1p21–q21	unknown	mild, myoclonus
SCA21	7p21.3–p15.1	unknown	hyporeflexia, akinesia, rigidity

in the PRKCG gene (Chen *et al.*, 2003). As the number keeps climbing, it becomes increasingly clear that different mutations in dissimilar genes can cause a very similar, in some cases indistinguishable, clinical picture of progressive ataxia. Moreover, as is true of other repeat expansion diseases, the phenotype can vary greatly, primarily due to differences in repeat size. Because of this variability and phenotypic overlap, distinguishing the various forms of SCA is difficult on clinical grounds alone. There are, however, clues to be gained from the neurological exam. For instance, the patient with remarkably slowed saccades is most likely to have SCA2; a mild form of disease characterized by truncal ataxia and nystagmus might be SCA6; the presence of retinopathy strongly suggests SCA7; and dementia suggests that SCA2 or SCA17 may be the cause.

Here, features of each of the SCAs identified at the time of this writing will be discussed. Elsewhere in this volume, Klockgether discusses more thoroughly the diagnostic approach to ataxia. For an ataxic patient with slowly progressive disease and a positive family history, commercial testing for SCA mutations is appropriate for at least two reasons. First, a positive test result eliminates the need for other more expensive, less definitive tests. Second, knowledge of the genetic basis can be empowering to the patient and his or her family because an element of uncertainty has been removed. Undergoing genetic testing, however, is a patient's personal decision that should only be made after informed and thorough counseling by a doctor or genetic counselor.

SCA1

The first genetically identified dominant ataxia (Orr *et al.*, 1993), SCA1 is less common than several other SCAs. It is the best understood, however, due to the pioneering research of Drs. Orr, Zoghbi and colleagues (Zoghbi & Orr, 2000). Neuropathological findings include neuronal loss in the brainstem and cerebellum (principally Purkinje cells), and degeneration of spinocerebellar tracts. Atrophy is pronounced in the cerebellar cortex, ventral pons, middle cerebellar peduncles and inferior olives.

SCA1 begins as a gait disorder and evolves to severe four-limb ataxia with dysarthria. Most patients are wheelchair-bound within 15 years of onset. Dysphagia can present early and becomes life threatening. In many patients, early nystagmus and ocular dysmetria progress to ophthalmoparesis. Variable degrees of lower limb amyotrophy, spasticity and choreoathetosis may be seen. Intellect remains largely intact until late stages of disease, when behavioral changes and a frontal lobe-like syndrome may occur. As with other polyQ diseases, SCA1 shows phenotypic variability and anticipation (Ranum *et al.*, 1994).

SCA1 is caused by an expanded CAG repeat in the *SCA1* gene that encodes polyQ in the disease protein, ataxin-1. The SCA1 triplet repeat is 6 to 39 repeats long in normal individuals, with normal repeats greater than 21 being interrupted by 1–4 histidine encoding CAT repeats. In contrast, disease alleles are uninterrupted stretches of 39 to 82 CAG repeats. As with other polyglutamine diseases, longer repeats strongly correlate with earlier onset disease. Mutant ataxin-1, which is an RNA binding protein, is prone to misfold and form inclusions in the nucleus of specific neurons. Nuclear localization, but not inclusion formation, appears to be critical for pathogenesis in SCA1.

SCA2

Initially described in a large Cuban family, SCA2 is one of the most common dominant ataxias, displaying a highly variable phenotype (Cancel *et al.*, 1997). Most often it is characterized by ataxia, dysarthria, slow saccades, neuropathy and little or no corticospinal or extrapyramidal signs (though parkinsonism has been reported in some cases, Shan *et al.*, 2001). Extremely slow saccades are common but not pathognomonic. Areflexia, facial myokymia and dementia are also fairly common. Radiological and pathological studies usually show olivopontocerebellar atrophy.

Three separate groups identified the *SCA2* disease gene in 1996, confirming that, as many suspected, it is a polyQ disease (Imbert *et al.*, 1996; Pulst *et al.*, 1996; Sanpei *et al.*, 1996). Normal alleles are between 15 and 32 repeats in length, and expanded alleles are ~34 to 77 repeats in length (Geschwind *et al.*, 1997; Imbert *et al.*, 1996; Pulst *et al.*, 1996; Sanpei *et al.*, 1996; Schols *et al.*, 1997). There exists a "zone of reduced penetrance" (32–34 repeats) within which not all individuals develop signs of disease in their lifetime. Compared to most other polyQ diseases, the range of pathogenic alleles in SCA2 is shifted toward smaller repeats. The disease protein, ataxin-2, is a cytoplasmic protein that is highly conserved in evolution and has predicted RNA binding motifs. The protein is thought to play a role in development and may participate in RNA processing or distribution within neurons.

Machado-Joseph disease/ SCA3

MJD/SCA3 is probably the most common dominantly inherited ataxia in the world (Durr *et al.*, 1996; Maciel *et al.*, 1995; Matilla *et al.*, 1995; Schols *et al.*, 1995). MJD was originally described in families of Portuguese Azorean descent. Soon after the mutation in MJD was identified, scientists discovered that SCA3, a dominant ataxia characterized in French and German families, was due to the same mutation. Though the official HUGO designation is MJD, some (including this writer) prefer to call the disease MJD/SCA3.

Most often, MJD/SCA3 begins as a progressive ataxia accompanied by difficulties with eye movements, speech and swallowing. Neuropathological findings include degeneration of cerebellar afferent and efferent pathways, pontine and dentate nuclei, substantia nigra and subthalamic nucleus, globus pallidus, cranial motor nerve nuclei and anterior horn cells. The cerebral cortex, striatum, cerebellar cortex and olivary neurons tend to be spared.

As with other polyglutamine diseases, signs of MJD/SCA3 most frequently appear when patients are in their 30s or 40s, but may begin before age 10 or as late as age 60. The first symptom is usually gait ataxia. Within a few years, many younger patients show signs of progressive supranuclear ophthalmoparesis. Dysarthria, followed by dysphagia and dysphonia, occur. In somewhat less than a third of patients,

lid retraction and decreased blinking lead to characteristic "bulging eyes." Facial fasciculations are more common in MJD/SCA3 than in most other SCAs. Eventually patients are terminally bedridden, but cognitive functions remain largely intact. MJD/SCA3 progresses over a 15- to 30-year period, resulting in death.

The phenotype can vary markedly even within a family, largely due to differences in repeat size. Younger onset patients, who typically have longer repeats, are more likely to show rigidity and dystonia. This dystonic form has been called Type 1 disease. The more common, adult onset ataxic form has been called Type 2 disease. Later onset patients (after age 40) are more likely to develop milder ataxia accompanied by peripheral neuropathy and motor neuron loss (so called Type 3 disease). In addition, some patients develop parkinsonism responsive to dopamine, referred to by some as Type 4 disease. There is little utility in labeling patients as any particular type, especially since there is no clear demarcation separating the types. The most variable feature of SCA3 is the degree of peripheral involvement. Some patients will develop hyperreflexia while marked distal amyotrophy with areflexia occurs in others. Sensory disturbances occur frequently.

There are no pathognomonic MRI findings in MJD/SCA3. Abnormalities range from simple enlargement of the fourth ventricle to severe spinopontine atrophy sparing the olives. PET and SPECT have demonstrated decreased glucose metabolism and blood flow in brainstem structures, but the pattern does not reliably distinguish SCA3 from other SCAs.

In 1994, Kakizuka and colleagues identified the mutation in MJD/SCA3 as a CAG repeat expansion in the *MJD1* gene on chromosome 14 (Srivastava AK *et al.*, 2001). This results in a polyQ expansion in the disease protein, ataxin-3, which recently has been shown to be a ubiquitin binding protein (Chai *et al.*, 2003; Donaldson *et al.*, 2003). The CAG/polyglutamine repeat is 12 to 42 repeats in normal alleles and ~60 to 84 repeats in disease alleles. This gap between normal and disease repeat length is greater for MJD/SCA3 than in any other polyQ disease. Testing for the expanded repeat is highly sensitive and specific, eliminating the need for other more expensive tests. A few individuals have been identified with intermediate size alleles (Taylor *et al.*, 2002; van Alfen N *et al.*, 2001) that are associated with restless leg syndrome and polyneuropathy (van Alfen *et al.*, 2001).

SCA4

In SCA4, progressive ataxia is accompanied by a sensory axonal neuropathy and pyramidal tract signs, but eye movements are preserved (e.g. Nagaoka *et al.*, 2000). The genetic defect has not been reported.

SCA5

SCA5 is characterized by pure cerebellar ataxia and dysarthria, with minimal shortening of lifespan. The genetic defect is unknown, but in the large Lincoln kindred maps to chromosome 11.

SCA6

Together with SCA2 and MJD/SCA3, SCA6 is one of the three most common dominant ataxias. In contrast to the other two, SCA6 represents a milder form of disease often manifesting as a "pure" cerebellar ataxia (e.g. Gomez *et al.*, 1997; Ikeuchi *et al.*, 1997). Characteristic features are a slowly progressive gait and limb ataxia, dysarthria, and nystagmus. The typical age at onset is around age 50 but ranges from less than 30 to greater than 70 years of age. Noncerebellar symptoms occur less frequently and may include decreased vibration and position sense and, later in disease, spasticity and hyperreflexia. Disease progresses more slowly than other SCAs, and is usually compatible with a normal lifespan.

In some respects, SCA6 is an exception to the general rules of polyQ disorders. First, the polyglutamine expansion (Zhuchenko *et al.*, 1997) is much smaller than in the other disorders: Normal SCA6 alleles range from 3 to 17 CAG repeats, and disease alleles are expanded to between 21 and 30 repeats. Thus, pathogenic SCA6 alleles fall within a range that, in other polyQ diseases, would represent normal alleles. Second, the disease protein is a membrane protein, a voltage-dependent calcium channel, whereas all other polyglutamine proteins are soluble. And third, there is only modest evidence for protein accumulation in disease tissue. These differences all suggest that the disease mechanism in SCA6 may differ from that in other polyQ diseases. The calcium channel gene responsible for SCA6 (*CACNA1A*) is also the defective gene in episodic ataxia type 2 and familial hemiplegic migraine. In these two diseases, the causative mutations are traditional, non-repeat mutations. This emphasizes the point that clinically distinguishable disorders can arise from different mutations in the same gene.

SCA7

SCA7 is distinguished from other SCAs by the presence of retinal degeneration. In a study of molecularly confirmed SCA7, the mean age at onset of visual failure was 22 years with a range from 1 to 45 years. Decreased visual acuity occurred in 83%, blindness in 28%, optic atrophy in 69% and pigmentary retinopathy in 43% of affected individuals. In most other respects, SCA7 resembles other SCAs characterized by ataxia and brainstem findings.

The defect is an expanded CAG/polyQ repeat in the *SCA7* gene, which encodes a novel protein, ataxin-7 (David *et al.*, 1997; Holmberg *et al.*, 1998). Expanded repeat size is highly variable, ranging from 34 to greater than 200 repeats, whereas normal alleles range from 7 to 17 repeats. Germline repeat instability is a common feature of polyQ diseases but is particularly impressive in SCA7, especially with paternal transmission. In some cases, this leads to massive expansions that cause systemic disease and abnormal brain development in infancy or may manifest even as embryonic lethality.

SCA8

The genetic defect in SCA8 was identified in 1999 by Ranum and colleagues (Koob *et al.*, 1999). It seems to be a trinucleotide repeat disease but, unlike the polyQ disorders, not a disease of protein misfolding. Affected individuals have an unstable CTG repeat expansion in the *SCA8* gene that is transcribed into RNA but not translated into protein. As mentioned earlier, the mechanism of pathogenesis is still unclear. Some individuals with very large SCA8 expansions do *not* develop disease, indicating that SCA8 repeat expansions either are not fully penetrant (which seems most likely) or the actual mutation lies elsewhere in the gene and is in linkage dysequilibrium with the expansion (less likely). Commercial testing is available for the SCA8 repeat, but because of this uncertainty test results must be interpreted with caution (Sobrido *et al.*, 2001).

SCA8 clinically resembles most other SCAs: adult onset ataxia with variable brainstem signs. In a study of a seven-generation family, the main clinical symptoms were prominent gait and limb ataxia accompanied by abnormalities of swallowing, speech, and eye movements (Day *et al.*, 2000). In contrast to many other SCAs in which paternal transmission is more prone to result in further expansion of the repeat, there is marked *maternal* bias in SCA8 disease transmission. This may reflect contractions of the expanded repeat during spermatogenesis (Moseley *et al.*, 2000).

SCA10

Described in Mexican families, SCA10 is characterized by prominent cerebellar symptoms and seizures (Grewal *et al.*, 2002; Matsuura *et al.*, 2002). In 2000, Ashizawa and colleagues identified the genetic defect (Matsuura *et al.*, 2000) as a new type of dynamic repeat expansion – an extremely large expansion arising from a *penta*nucleotide (ATTCT) repeat in an intron of the *SCA10* gene, also known as *E46L*. Normally 10–22 ATTCT repeats in length, the repeat becomes grossly expanded in affected individuals, in some cases to several thousand repeats in length.

SCA10 is uncommon outside of families of Mexican descent (Matsuura *et al.*, 2002).

SCA11

This relatively mild form of ataxia, described in two British families, maps to chromosome 15. Mean age of onset is 25 but the disease is compatible with a normal life expectancy.

SCA12

Margolis and colleagues identified a CAG expansion in the 5′ untranslated region of the *PPP2R2B* gene that encodes a regulatory subunit for protein phosphatase 2A (Holmes *et al.*, 1999). This CAG repeat expansion segregates with disease in multiple families, suggesting that it is indeed the causative mutation. SCA12 may be more common in India, but is otherwise rare (Srivastava *et al.*, 2001). Age at onset of ataxia ranges from 8 to 55 years, with other symptoms including arm and head tremor, paucity of movements and abnormal eye movements. Dementia can be present in elderly patients.

SCA13

Reported in French families, SCA13 has been linked to chromosome 19 (Herman-Bert *et al.*, 2000). Age at onset is in early childhood with cerebellar symptoms, psychomotor development, mental retardation and slow progression.

SCA14

Initially described in a Japanese family, SCA14 localizes near the SCA13 locus on chromosome 19 (Yamashita *et al.*, 2000). In this family, SCA14 is characterized by prominent ataxia, occasional axial myoclonus and tremor. It is a slowly progressive disease with an age of onset between 10 and 50. As additional families were mapped to the same region (Brkanac *et al.*, 2002), the disease gene was identified this past year. Point mutations were found in the PRKCG gene encoding a gamma subunit of protein kinase C (Chen *et al.*, 2003). SCA14, thus, has broken the trend of expanded repeats as the cause of dominant ataxias.

SCA15

This SCA is a mild and late onset "pure" form of disease (Storey *et al.*, 2001) for which the locus has not been reported.

SCA 16

This ataxia, which localizes to chromosome 8, can be associated with head tremor (Miyoshi *et al.*, 2001). The genetic defect is unknown.

SCA 17

SCA17 is the most recently identified polyQ disease, caused by a glutamine-encoding CAG repeat in the TATA binding protein gene (TBP or TFIID). SCA17 typically manifests in midlife and the ataxia is accompanied by more dementia and extrapyramidal features (bradykinesia and dystonia) than most SCAs. Neurodegeneration also is more widespread in SCA17 than in most SCAs.

TBP is a critical component of the basal transcription machinery. Because of its polymorphic CAG/glutamine repeat and central role in gene expression, TBP had long been viewed as a prime candidate gene in inherited neuropsychiatric diseases. In 1999, Tsuji and colleagues identified a single patient with sporadic ataxia who proved to have a CAG/polyglutamine expansion in the TBP gene (Koide *et al.*, 1999). More recently, additional Japanese and European families showed this same expansion, confirming that SCA17 is the newest polyQ disease (e.g. Nakamura *et al.*, 2001).

SCA 18

This disorder merges clinical features of hereditary sensory neuropathy and hereditary ataxia and thus has been called autosomal dominant sensory/motor neuropathy with ataxia, or SMNA. SCA18, mapped to chromosome 7q31–q32 in a large Irish American family (Brkanac *et al.*, 2002), shows clinical variability with ataxia, sensory loss, muscle weakness and pyramidal tract signs.

SCA 19

This disorder was recently described in a large Dutch family, manifesting as mild cerebellar ataxia with occasional cognitive difficulties and myoclonus (Verbeek *et al.*, 2002). The locus maps to chromosome 1.

SCA21

This dominant ataxia shows variable onset and slow progression in the single large French family in which it has been described (Vuillaume *et al.*, 2002). In this family, hyporeflexia, akinesia and rigidity were seen in some affected persons and anticipation may have occurred, based on age of symptom onset in various generations.

Episodic ataxias

Less common than the SCAs, the episodic ataxias are also a genetically heterogeneous disorders (Baloh *et al.*, 1997). Two forms of dominantly inherited episodic ataxia have been genetically identified. EA-1, due to mutations in the potassium channel gene *KCNA1*, typically causes brief (minutes) episodes of ataxia that may be precipitated by stress or exercise. Myokymia often accompanies this condition. EA-2, which is due to mutations in the *CACNA1A* gene encoding a calcium channel, typically causes longer bouts of ataxia (hours to days) that also may be precipitated by stress, exercise or fatigue. Acetazolamide can prevent attacks in some patients, particularly those with EA-2. Thus, a trial of this medication should be offered to any patient with episodic ataxia. Two other kindreds with dominantly inherited episodic ataxia do not map to the loci for EA-1 and EA2. A North Carolinian family has been described with periodic vestibular ataxia (Damji *et al.*, 1996), and a Canadian family has been reported with episodic ataxia accompanied by vertigo, tinnitus and interictal myokymia (Steckley *et al.*, 2001). EA-3 and EA-4 are the respective designations, but the genetic loci have not been published as of this writing.

Other dominantly inherited ataxias

Nearly all ADCA represent one of the SCAs describe above. Two other conditions, however, should be considered in the ataxic patient with a dominant family history: the polyQ disorder, dentatorubral pallidoluysian atrophy (DRPLA), and the prion disorder Gerstmann–Straussler–Scheinker disease (GSS). Among the polyglutamine diseases, DRPLA most closely resembles HD yet patients often have ataxia as a primary sign (Yabe *et al.*, 2002). Rare in the USA, DRPLA is one of the more common polyglutamine diseases in Japan. GSS is a rare, dominantly inherited disease that most often presents as progressive ataxia and is due to mutations in the prion gene. Mutational screening is not commercially available but can be obtained through research laboratories. Although the 14–3–3 test may help identify sporadic cases of Creutzfeld–Jakob disease, its sensitivity and specificity for familial prion disease is uncertain. Brain biopsy in GSS reveals Kuru amyloid plaques and accumulated prion protein, and western blot analysis of brain lysate demonstrates protease-resistant prion protein.

REFERENCES

Baloh, R. W., Yue, Q., Furman, J. M. & Nelson, S. F. (1997). Familial episodic ataxia: clinical heterogeneity in four families linked to chromosome 19p. *Ann. Neurol.*, **41**(1), 8–16.

Bonini, N. M. (2002). Chaperoning brain degeneration. *Proc. Natl Acad. Sci., USA*, **99** (Suppl. 4), 16407–11.

Brkanac, Z., Bylenok, L., Fernandez, M. *et al.* (2002a). A new dominant spinocerebellar ataxia linked to chromosome 19q13.4-qter. *Arch. Neurol.*, **59**(8), 1291–5.

Brkanac, Z., Fernandez, M., Matsushita, M. *et al.* (2002b). Autosomal dominant sensory/motor neuropathy with Ataxia

(SMNA): Linkage to chromosome 7q22–q32. *Am. J. Med. Genet.*, **114**(4), 450–7.

Cancel, G., Durr, A., Didierjean, O. *et al.* (1997). Molecular and clinical correlations in spinocerebellar ataxia 2: a study of 32 families. *Hum. Mol. Genet.*, **6**(5), 709–15.

Chai, Y., Berke, S. S., Cohen, R. E. & Paulson, H. L. (2003). Polyubiquitin binding by the polyQ disease protein ataxin-3 links its normal function to protein surveillance pathways. *J. Biol. Chem.*, **279**, 3605–11.

Chan, H. Y., Warrick, J. M., Gray-Board, G. L., Paulson, H. L. & Bonini, N. M. (2000). Mechanisms of chaperone suppression of polyglutamine disease: selectivity, synergy and modulation of protein solubility in *Drosophila*. *Hum. Mol. Genet.*, **22**, **9**(19), 2811–20.

Chen, D.-H., Brkanac, Z., Verlinde, C. L. M. J. *et al.* (2003). Missense mutations in the regulatory domain of PKC-gamma: a new mechanism for dominant nonepisodic cerebellar ataxia. *Am. J. Hum. Genet.*, **72**, 839–49.

Cummings, C. J. & Zoghbi, H. Y. (2000). Trinucleotide repeats: mechanisms and pathophysiology. *Annu. Rev. Genom. Hum. Genet.*, **1**, 281–328.

Damji, K. F., Allingham, R. R., Pollock, S. C. *et al.* (1996). Periodic vestibulocerebellar ataxia, an autosomal dominant ataxia with defective smooth pursuit, is genetically distinct from other autosomal dominant ataxias. *Arch. Neurol.*, **53**, 338–44.

David, G., Abbas, N., Stevanin, G. *et al.* (1997). Cloning of the SCA7 gene reveals a highly unstable CAG repeat expansion. *Nat. Genet.*, **17**, 65–70.

Day, J. W., Schut, L. J., Moseley, M. L., Durand, A. C. & Ranum, L. P. (2000). Spinocerebellar ataxia type 8. Clinical features in a large family. *Neurology*, **55**, 649–57.

Donaldson, K. M., Li, W., Ching, K. A., Batalov, S., Tsai, C. C. & Joazeiro, C. A. (2003). Ubiquitin-mediated sequestration of normal cellular proteins into polyglutamine aggregates. *Proc. Natl Acad. Sci., USA*, **100**(15), 8892–7.

Durr, A., Stevanin, G., Cancel, G. *et al.* (1996). Spinocerebellar ataxia 3 and Machado–Joseph disease: clinical, molecular and neuropathologic features. *Ann. Neurol.*, **39**, 490–9.

Geschwind, D. H., Perlman, S., Figueroa, C. P., Yreiman, L. J. & Pulst, S. M. (1997). The prevalence and wide clinical spectrum of the spinocerebellar ataxia type 2 trinucleotide repeat in patients with autosomal dominant cerebellar ataxia. *Am. J. Hum. Genet.*, **60**, 842–50.

Gomez, C. M., Thompson, R. M., Gammack, J. T. *et al.* (1997). Spinocerebellar ataxia type 6: gaze-evoked and vertical nystagmus, Purkinje cell degeneration, and variable age of onset. *Ann. Neurol.*, **42**, 933–50.

Grewal, R. P., Achari, M., Matsuura, T. *et al.* (2002). Clinical features and ATTCT repeat expansion in spinocerebellar ataxia type 10. *Arch. Neurol.*, **59**(8), 1285–90.

Harding, A. E. (1993). Clinical features and classification of inherited ataxias. *Adv. Neurol.*, **61**, 1–14.

Herman-Bert, A., Stevanin, G., Netter, J. C. *et al.* (2000). Mapping of spinocerebellar ataxia 13 to chromosome 19q13.3–q13.4 in a family with autosomal dominant cerebellar ataxia and mental retardation. *Am. J. Hum. Genet.*, **67**, 229–35.

Holmberg, M., Duysckaerts, C., Durr, A. *et al.* (1998). Spinocerebellar ataxia type 7 (SCA7): a neurodegenerative disorder with neuronal intranuclear inclusions. *Hum. Mol. Genet.*, **7**, 913–18.

Holmes, S. E., O'Hearn, E. E., McInnis, M. G. *et al.* (1999). Expansion of a novel CAG trinucleotide repeat in the 5' region of PPP2R2B is associated with SCA12. *Nat. Genet.*, **23**, 391–2.

Hughes, R. E. (2002). Polyglutamine disease: acetyltransferases awry. *Curr. Biol.*, **12**(4), R141–3.

Ikeuchi, T., Takano, H., Koide, R. *et al.* (1997). Spinocerebellar ataxia type 6: CAG repeat expansion in a1A voltage-dependent calcium channel gene and clinical variations in Japanese population. *Ann. Neurol.*, **42**, 879–84.

Imbert, G., Sandon, F., Yvert, G. *et al.* (1996). Cloning of the gene for spinocerebellar ataxia 2 reveals a locus with high sensitivity to expanded CAG/glutamine repeats. *Nat. Genet.*, **14**, 285–91.

Koide, R., Kobayashi, S., Shimohata, T. *et al.* (1999). A neurological disease caused by an expanded CAG trinucleotide repeat in the TATA-binding protein gene: a new polyglutamine disease? *Hum. Molec. Genet.*, **8**, 2047–53.

Koob, M. D., Moseley, M. L., Schut, L. J. *et al.* (1999). An untranslated CTG expansion causes a novel form of spinocerebellar ataxia (SCA8). *Nat. Genet.*, **21**, 379–8493.

Maciel, P., Gaspas, C., De Stefano, A. L. *et al.* (1995). Correlation between CAG repeat length and clinical features in Machado–Joseph disease. *Am. J. Hum. Genet.*, **57**, 54–61.

Matilla, T., McCall, A., Subramony, S. H. & Zoghbi, H. Y. (1995). Molecular and clinical correlations in spinocerebellar ataxia type 3 and Machado–Joseph disease. *Ann. Neurol.*, **38**, 68–72.

Matsuura, T., Yamagata, T. & Burgess, D. L. (2000). Large expansion of the ATTCT pentanucleotide repeat in spinocerebellar ataxia 10. *Nat. Genet.*, **26**(2), 191–4.

Matsuura, T., Ranum, L. P., Volpini, V. *et al.* (2002). Spinocerebellar ataxia type 10 is rare in populations other than Mexicans. *Neurology*, **58**(6), 983–4.

Miller, V. M., Xia, H., Marrs, G. L. *et al.* (2003). Allele specific silencing of dominant disease genes. *Proc. Natl Acad. Sci., USA*, **100**(12), 7195–200.

Miyoshi, Y., Yamada, T., Tanimura, M. *et al.* (2001). A novel autosomal dominant spinocerebellar ataxia (SCA16) linked to chromosome 8q22.1–24.1. *Neurology*, **57**(1), 96–100.

Moseley, M. L., Schut, L. J., Bird, T. D. *et al.* (2000). SCA8 CTG repeat: en masse contractions in sperm and intergenerational sequence changes may play a role in reduced penetrance. *Nat. Genet.*, **26**(2), 191–4.

Moseley, M. L., Weatherspoon, M., Rasmussen, L., Day, J. W. & Ranum, L. P. W. (2002). SCA8 BAC transgenic mice have a progressive and lethal neurological phenotype demonstrating pathogenicity of the CTG expansion. *Am. Soc. Hum. Genet. Abstract.*

Muchowski, P. J. (2002). Protein misfolding, amyloid formation, and neurodegeneration: a critical role for molecular chaperones? *Neuron*, **35**(1), 9–12.

Nagaoka, U. Takashima, M., Ishikawa, K. *et al.* (2000). A gene on SCA4 locus causes dominantly inherited pure cerebellar ataxia. *Neurology*, **54**(10), 1971–5.

Nakamura, K., Jeong, S.-Y., Uchihara, T. *et al.* (2001). SCA17, a novel autosomal dominant cerebellar ataxia caused by an expanded polyglutamine in TATA-binding protein. *Hum. Molec. Genet.*, **10**, 1441–8.

Orr, H. T., Chung, M. Y., Banfi, S. *et al.* (1993). Expansion of an unstable trinucleotide CAG repeat in spinocerebellar ataxia type 1. *Nat. Genet.*, **4**, 221–6.

Piedras-Renteria, E. S., Watase, K., Harata, N. *et al.* (2001). Increased expression of alpha 1A Ca2+ channel currents arising from expanded trinucleotide repeats in spinocerebellar ataxia type 6. *J. Neurosci.*, **21**, 9185–93.

Pulst, S-M., Nechiporuk, A., Nechiporuk, T. *et al.* (1996). Moderate expansion of a normally biallelic trinucleotide repeat in spinocerebellar ataxia type 2. *Nat. Genet.*, **14**, 269–76.

Ranum, L. P., Chung, M. Y., Banfi, S. *et al.* (1994). Molecular and clinical correlations in spinocerebellar ataxia type 1: evidence for familial effects on the age of onset. *Am. J. Hum. Genet.*, **55**, 244–52.

Sanpei, K., Takano, H., Igarashi, S. *et al.* (1996). Identification of the spinocerebellar ataxia type 2 gene using a direct identification of repeat expansion and cloning technique, DIRECT. *Nat. Genet.*, **14**, 277–84.

Schols, L., Vieira-Saecker, A. M., Schols, S., Przuntek, H., Epplen, J. T., Riess, D. & Schols, L. (1995). Trinucleotide expansion within the MJD1 gene presents clinically as spinocerebellar ataxia and occurs most frequently in German SCA patients. *Hum. Mol. Genet.*, **4**, 1001–5.

Schols, L., Gispert, S., Vorgerd, M. *et al.* (1997). Spinocerebellar ataxia type 2. Genotype and phenotype in German kindreds. *Arch. Neurol.*, **54**(9), 1073–80.

Shan, D. E., Soong, B. W., Sun, C. M., Lee, S. J., Liao, K. K. & Liu, R. S. (2001). Spinocerebellar ataxia type 2 presenting as familial levodopa-responsive parkinsonism. *Ann. Neurol.*, **50**(6), 812–15.

Sherman, M. Y. & Goldberg, A. L. (2001). Cellular defenses against unfolded proteins: a cell biologist thinks about neurodegenerative diseases. *Neuron*, **29**(1), 15–32.

Sobrido, M. J., Cholfin, J. A., Perlman, S., Pulst, S. M. & Geschwind, D. H. (2001). SCA8 repeat expansions in ataxia: a controversial association. *Neurology*, **57**(7), 1310–12.

Srivastava, A. K., Choudhry, S., Gopinath, M. S. *et al.* (2001). Molecular and clinical correlation in five Indian families with spinocerebellar ataxia 12. *Ann. Neurol.*, **50**(6), 796–800.

Steckley, J. L., Ebers, G. C., Cader, M. Z. & McLachlan, R. S. (2001). An autosomal dominant disorder with episodic ataxia, vertigo, and tinnitus. *Neurology*, **57**, 1499–502.

Storey, E., Gardner, R. J., Knight, M. A. *et al.* (2001). A new autosomal dominant pure cerebellar ataxia. *Neurology*, **57**, 1913–15.

Taylor, J. P., Hardy, J. & Fischbeck, K. H. (2002). Toxic proteins in neurodegenerative disease. *Science*, **296**(5575), 1991–5.

van Alfen, N., Sinke, R. J., Zwarts, M. J. *et al.* (2001). Intermediate CAG repeat lengths (53,54) for MJD/SCA3 are associated with an abnormal phenotype. *Ann. Neurol.*, **49**(6), 805–7.

Verbeek, D. S., Schelhaas, J. H., Ippel, E. F., Beemer, F. A., Pearson, P. L. & Sinke, R. J. (2002). Identification of a novel SCA locus (SCA19) in a Dutch autosomal dominant cerebellar ataxia family on chromosome region 1p21–q21. *Hum. Genet.*, **111**, 388–93.

Vuillaume, I., Devos, D., Schraen-Maschke, S. *et al.* (2002). A new locus for spinocerebellar ataxia (SCA21) maps to chromosome 7p21.3–p15.1. *Ann. Neurol.* 2002 (on line)

Xia, H., Mao, Q., Paulson, H. L. & Davidson, B. L. (2002). siRNA-mediated gene silencing in vitro and in vivo. *Nat. Biotechnol.*, **20**(10), 1006–10.

Yabe, I., Sasaki, H., Kikuchi, S. *et al.* (2002). Late onset ataxia phenotype in dentatorubro-pallidoluysian atrophy (DRPLA). *J. Neurol.*, **249**, 432–6.

Yamashita, I., Sasaki, H., Yabe, I. *et al.* (2000). A novel locus for dominant cerebellar ataxia (SCA14) maps to a 10.2-cm interval flanked by D19S206 and D19S605 on chromosome 19q13.4-qter. *Ann. Neurol.* **48**(2), 156–63.

Zoghbi, H. Y. & Orr, H. T. (2000). Glutamine repeats and neurodegeneration. *Ann. Rev. Neurosci.*, **23**, 217–47, 52–3.

Zhuchenko, O., Bailey, J., Bonnen, P. *et al.* (1997). Autosomal dominant cerebellar ataxia (SCA6) associated with small polyglutamine expansions in the alpha 1A-voltage-dependent calcium channel. *Nat. Genet.*, **15**(1), 62–9.

48

Friedreich's ataxia and other autosomal recessive ataxias

Hélène Puccio and Michel Koenig

Institut de Génétique et de Biologie Moléculaire et Cellulaire (IGBMC), CNRS/INSERM/Université
Louis Pasteur, Hôpitaux Universitaires de Strasbourg, France

Autosomal recessive neurodegenerative ataxias are classified according to the major site of degeneration, which can be the cerebellum or the spinal cord. In the latter case, affection of the posterior columns and of spinocerebellar tracts leads to sensory (proprioceptive) and cerebellar ataxia. A third group of affections recently identified associates cerebellar degeneration and sensorimotor peripheral neuropathy, therefore resulting in sensory and cerebellar ataxia associated with neuromuscular weakness. The first group is dominated by ataxia-telangiectasia (A-T), where cerebellar atrophy is associated with immune deficiency and susceptibility to develop malignancies. Ataxia-telangiectasia and related disorders will be developed in the following chapter. Another member of the first group is spastic ataxia of the Charlevoix–Saguenay region (ARSACS). The second group is dominated by Friedreich's ataxia (FRDA), recognized since the XIXth century. Rare forms of spinal cord ataxias include the inherited vitamin E deficiencies (isolated vitamin E deficiency (AVED) and abetalipoproteinemia (ABL)), Refsum disease (RD), infantile onset spinocerebellar ataxia (IOSCA), and ataxia + blindness + deafness (SCABD). The group of cerebellar atrophy with sensorimotor neuropathy (third group) comprises only very recently identified conditions, such as ataxia + oculomotor apraxia, forms 1 and 2 (AOA1 and AOA2) and spinocerebellar ataxia + neuropathy (SCAN1). All advances on the delineation of the rare forms of recessive ataxias were made thanks to the development of positional cloning strategies based on homozygosity mapping of consanguineous families and on the development of the human genome project.

Friedreich's ataxia

Nicholaus Friedreich (1825–1882) described a familial form of cerebellar ataxia in 1863, clinically different from atax-ias called "locomotrices" (motor) in 1858 by Duchenne de Boulogne, for the tabès. The clinical entity emerged from the following observations: three sibships including nine patients, presented with balance difficulties in young adulthood, associated with muscular weakness and sensory loss. Scoliosis, foot deformation, and cardiac signs were frequent (Friedreich, 1863a,b). At this time, the loss of tendon reflexes was not mentioned because tendon reflexes were described by Erb only in 1875. Pathologically, the Friedreich cases showed spinocerebellar and posterior column degeneration. The clinical and pathological diagnostic criteria of Friedreich's ataxia were founded on this initial description, until the very recent discovery of the responsible gene and mutation in 1996.

Clinical and pathological features

Epidemiology
Friedreich's ataxia is the most common inherited degenerative ataxia, and accounts for half of the inherited degenerative ataxias, and for three-quarters of those with onset before age 25. FRDA affects 1:50 000 individuals with an estimated prevalence at birth of 1:29 000 due to a GAA expansion carriers frequency of 1 : 85 in the European population (Cossee *et al.*, 1997). Given the high carrier frequency, the finding of a heterozygous expansion in a caucasian patient should lead to the search for a point mutation in the other allele to confirm the involvement of the frataxin gene. The incidence of Friedreich's ataxia is rare in Finland and among black Africans, and the disease is absent in Japan.

Clinical features
Friedreich's ataxia is a progressive and unremitting mixed cerebellar-sensory ataxia with onset usually around puberty, but wide variations are observed, ranging from 2

to 50 years (mean and standard deviation are 15 ± 8 years) (Durr *et al.*, 1996; Filla *et al.*, 1996; Montermini *et al.*, 1997b; Geschwind *et al.*, 1997; Schols *et al.*, 1997; Ragno *et al.*, 1997; Gellera *et al.*, 1997). The presenting symptom is usually gait ataxia (65%) or generalized clumsiness (25%), except for scoliosis and cardiomyopathy, which can be present before the gait ataxia (5% each of cases). Speech and coordination of the upper limbs may be normal in the first five years of the disease. Decreased reflexes in the lower limbs, extensor plantar response, decreased vibration sense at the ankles, axonal neuropathy, and cardiomyopathy constitute the complete clinical picture of Friedreich's ataxia and are present in more than 70% of the Friedreich's ataxia patients. In the majority of the patients the reflexes are decreased in the upper limbs, and there is proximal weakness in the lower limbs. Scoliosis and pes cavus are present in 60% of the patients. Nystagmus is present in less than half of the patients, decreased visual acuity and hypoacousia may be present late in the course of the disease. In contrast, fixation instability, expressed as square waves when registered on ocular movement recording, are a typical finding when cerebellar ataxia is evident. Optic atrophy is a rare finding. Atypical presentation in patients homozygous for the GAA expansion are observed, such as ophthalmoplegia, dystonia, myoclonus (Durr *et al.*, 1996; Schols *et al.*, 1997), ptosis (Schols *et al.*, 1997), chorea (Hanna *et al.*, 1998), seizures, dysmorphia, and mental retardation (Durr *et al.*, 1996). The diagnostic criteria proposed by several studies before the discovery of the gene were revised by Harding to include patients with onset up to 25 years and to take into account incomplete clinical presentations in patients in whom the disease duration was less than 5 years (Harding, 1981).

Cardiomyopathy is a frequent non-neurological finding in FRDA (Pandolfo, 1997). Cardiac involvement is more often observed in patients with earlier age of onset. About 10% of FRDA patients have diabetes mellitus, and an additional 20% have carbohydrate intolerance. A detailed study of glucose and insulin metabolism in FRDA patients revealed a deficiency in arginine-stimulated insulin secretion in all cases, suggesting that beta cells are invariably affected by the primary genetic defect of FRDA (Finocchiaro *et al.*, 1988).

Pathological features

Degeneration of the posterior columns of the spinal cord is the hallmark of the disease (Friedreich, 1863a,b). This is due to an invariable loss of the large primary sensory neurons of the dorsal root ganglia (DRG) (Oppenheimer & Esiri, 1992), resulting in atrophy of the central branches of the corresponding axons causing thinning of the dorsal roots, particularly at the lumbosacral level, and atrophy of the peripheral branches causing loss of large myelinated fibers from peripheral nerves. The fine unmyelinated fibers are well preserved, and interstitial connective tissue is increased. The motor component of peripheral nerves is well preserved. Atrophy is also observed in the spinocerebellar tracts, the dorsal being more affected than the ventral. Clarke columns, where the spinocerebellar tracts originate, show severe loss of neurons. Therefore, the sensory systems providing information to the brain and cerebellum about the position and speed of body segments, particularly the lower limbs, are severely compromised in FRDA.

Motor neurons in the ventral horns are well preserved, but the corticospinal motor tracts are atrophied, explaining the pyramidal signs. The pattern of atrophy of the corticospinal tracts suggests a "dying back" process (Said *et al.*, 1986). In the brainstem, neuronal loss can be observed in the gracile and cuneate nuclei, where the dorsal column tracts terminate, and in the medial lemnisci, that continue the central sensory pathway after these nuclei (Oppenheimer & Esiri, 1992). Sensory cranial nerves also show myelin pallor and loss of fibers. The cerebellar cortex shows only mild loss of Purkinje cells late in the disease course. This pattern of involvement contrasts with other inherited degenerative ataxias (Riva & Bradac, 1995), in particular with the group of early onset ataxias with retained reflexes (EOCA), where the cerebellum is much more atrophic than the cervical spinal cord. Nevertheless, radiologic evidence of cerebellar atrophy in addition to cervical cord atrophy is observed in several patients. The deep cerebellar nuclei, where cerebellar efferents originate, are severely affected with marked neuronal loss and gliosis in the dentate nucleus (Oppenheimer & Esiri, 1992). As a consequence, the superior cerebellar pedunculi appear markedly atrophic. Other cerebral structures do not appear to be directly involved by the disease, with the exception of a loss of large pyramidal cells in the primary motor areas.

Both the heart and β cells of the pancre as are thought to be primary sitis of degeneration in FRDA patients. Enlargement of the heart is the typical finding, with thickening of ventricular walls and/or interventricular septum (Pasternac *et al.*, 1980; Gottdiener *et al.*, 1982) which is best evidenced by echocardiography (Morvan *et al.*, 1992). Connective tissue is increased, with diffuse and focal inflammatory cell infiltration, and intracellular iron deposits in cardiomyocytes are an invariable finding. The pancreas of patients with diabetes mellitus shows a loss of islet cells without sign of autoimmune inflammation (Schoenle *et al.*, 1989).

Molecular pathogenesis

FRDA gene

The human FRDA gene, positionally cloned in 1996, is localised on 9q13 and is composed of seven exons spanning 80 kb of genomic DNA (Campuzano *et al.*, 1996). Northern blot analysis in human and mouse, RNAse protection assay and cDNA cloning indicate that the 1.3 kb major transcript is made from five exons (1 to 5a). This transcript encodes a protein of 210 amino acids called frataxin. A very minor alternative transcript contains exon 5b instead of 5a, followed by the noncoding exon 6. The functional significance of this transcript, if any, is still uncertain.

The FRDA gene demonstrates tissue-specific and developmentally controlled expression by northern blot (in human and mouse tissues) and in situ hybridisation (in mouse tissues only) (Campuzano *et al.*, 1996; Jiralerspong *et al.*, 1997; Koutnikova *et al.*, 1997). The expression partially correlates with the main sites of pathology of the disease. DRGs, where the sensory cell bodies are located, are the major sites of expression in the nervous system, from embryonic day 12 until adult life. Deep sensory neuropathy and degeneration of the posterior columns therefore appear as a direct consequence of reduced frataxin level in these structures. Expression in the spinal cord is comparatively much lower, suggesting that degeneration of the spinocerebellar tracts and of the Clarke's columns (containing respectively the axons and the cell bodies of secondary neurons projecting to the cerebellum) might be secondary to degeneration of the DRG neurons. Significant frataxin expression is also observed in the granular layer of the cerebellum. Degeneration of the motor corticospinal (pyramidal) tracts might correlate with frataxin expression in mature cells of the developing forebrain (Jiralerspong *et al.*, 1997), though it was not detected in mouse adult cerebral cortex (Koutnikova *et al.*, 1997). Expression in mouse brain is mostly restricted to the periventricular zone in embryos and to the corresponding ependymal layer in adults (Koutnikova *et al.*, 1997).

The frataxin gene is also expressed in non-neuronal tissues, such as heart and pancreas, which may account for hypertrophic cardiomyopathy and the increased incidence of diabetes observed in FRDA patients (Campuzano *et al.*, 1996; Koutnikova *et al.*, 1997). Frataxin is also prominently expressed in tissues apparently not affected by the disease, such as liver, muscle, thymus and brown fat. All tissues highly expressing frataxin are rich in mitochondria, with brown fat, present in newborns, being particularly rich (Koutnikova *et al.*, 1997). The difference between non-affected and affected tissues may lie in the non-dividing nature of the latter (neurons, cardiocytes and β cells of the pancreas), implying that cells are not replaced when they die. Also, neurons and cardiocytes have an exclusive aerobic metabolism, making them more sensitive to mitochondrial defect. However, further factors must come into play to explain the specific vulnerability of specific cell types (e.g. the affected sensory system vs. the spared motor system).

FRDA mutations

FRDA is most commonly caused by a large GAA triplet repeat expansion within the first intron of the gene encoding frataxin (Campuzano *et al.*, 1996). Ninety-six per cent of patients are homozygous for GAA trinucleotide repeat expansions while the remaining 4% of cases are compound heterozygotes for a GAA expansion and a point mutation (or a deletion/insertion mutation) within the coding region of the gene (Campuzano *et al.*, 1996; Cossee *et al.*, 1999). Truncating and missense mutations are equally represented, although missense mutations are preferentially found in the second half of the protein, suggesting an important functional domain. In most cases, point mutations are found in clinically typical FRDA patients with few exceptions. The G130V missense mutation always appears associated with an atypical presentation (retained knee reflexes, often brisk, absence of dysarthria, moderate ataxia, spastic gait, and slow progression) (Cossee *et al.*, 1999; Bidichandani *et al.*, 1997; Forrest *et al.*, 1998). The G130V mutation is one of the most frequent frataxin point mutations and arose from a common founder event (Delatycki *et al.*, 1999b). Other missense mutations each represented by a single case (L106S (Campuzano *et al.*, 1996), D122Y (Cossee *et al.*, 1999), R165C and L182F (Forrest *et al.*, 1998)) also seem to be associated with mild presentation.

The clinical equivalence between the GAA intronic expansion and the truncating mutations suggests that the expansion acts by loss of function on frataxin. Indeed, RT-PCR and RNAse protection experiments revealed that frataxin mRNA levels are markedly decreased in comparison to controls or unrelated ataxias (Campuzano *et al.*, 1996; Cossee *et al.*, 1997; Bidichandani *et al.*, 1998). RNAse protection and in vitro transcription experiments suggest that the expansion acts at the transcriptional level, rather than interfere with the splicing of intron 1 (Bidichandani *et al.*, 1998; Ohshima *et al.*, 1998). Experiments using in vitro and in vivo expression systems revealed that the GAA repeat interferes with transcription in an orientation and length-dependent manner (Bidichandani *et al.*, 1998; Ohshima *et al.*, 1998). The molecular basis for these results was proposed to be the formation of a non-B DNA conformation, probably a triple helical structure. Indeed, Sakamoto *et al.* recently described a novel DNA structure, "sticky DNA," for long tracts of GAA from the frataxin gene (Sakamoto *et al.*, 1999). Sticky DNA is formed by the association of two purine–purine–pyrimidine (R–R–Y) triple helical structures under the influence of negative supercoiling, thereby inhibiting transcription (Sakamoto *et al.*, 2001). Therefore, the formation of sticky DNA in a FRDA patient would be the mechanism by which the expansion suppresses gene expression, resulting in reduced levels of frataxin.

The normal GAA repeat in the Caucasian population shows two main classes of alleles (Cossee *et al.*, 1997; Epplen *et al.*, 1997; Montermini *et al.*, 1997a). About 80% of alleles have 7–12 GAAs (the most frequent alleles carry nine repeats). A second heterogenous mode of 16–34 GAAs accounts for 17% of alleles. Heterozygote carriers of expansions >100 GAAs were found at a frequency of 1/85, predicting a disease incidence of about 1/29 000 (Cossee *et al.*, 1997). Haplotype examination strongly suggests that the expanded alleles arise from large normal alleles with the presence of a single or few initial founder events leading to a large normal allele. The fact that very similar haplotypes were found in North African and Yemenite subjects with large normal and expanded alleles suggests the founder event is very old (Cossee *et al.*, 1997).

Clinical–genetic correlation and prognosis

The direct involvement of the GAA expansion as the cause of FRDA is demonstrated by the very significant inverse correlation between the size of the smaller of the two expansions and the age of onset, the severity of the disease and the risk of occurrence of optional signs such as cardiomyopathy, scoliosis and diabetes (Montermini *et al.*, 1997b; Durr *et al.*, 1996; Filla *et al.*, 1996; Isnard *et al.*, 1997; Lamont *et al.*, 1997; Monros *et al.*, 1997). These observations suggest that some frataxin is produced from alleles carrying smaller expansions, in a length dependent manner. This was confirmed using a monoclonal antibody directed against frataxin (Campuzano *et al.*, 1997) and is in agreement with the transcript analyses. The smallest pathological expansions are in the range of 90–110 repeats, and are found in patients with late onset and atypical presentation of the disease (Cossee *et al.*, 1997; Durr *et al.*, 1996) (one exception described (Epplen *et al.*, 1997) is most likely due to the presence of an unstable premutation in one of the parents). As a consequence, the molecular definition of Friedreich's ataxia based on the presence of the GAA expansion mutation is broader than the previous clinically based definition. Patients with small expansions (<400 repeats) often show onset of the symptoms after age 25 or have retained tendon reflexes (Montermini *et al.*, 1997b; Durr *et al.*, 1996; Filla *et al.*, 1996; Lamont *et al.*, 1997; Monros *et al.*, 1997), features previously considered as exclusion criteria (Harding, 1981). Molecular diagnosis demonstrates that about 12% of cases fulfilling Harding's essential criteria of the disease are negative for GAA expansion (McCabe *et al.*, 2000), while, conversely, one-quarter of patients homozygous for GAA expansion show atypical phenotypes (Berciano *et al.*, 2002). Detection of the expansion mutation thus provides a most useful diagnostic test. The length of expansion has however little value for individual prognosis, given the large scattering of points along the correlation curve.

Frataxin function

Frataxin is a 210 amino acid protein showing no similarity with protein domains of known function. Therefore, the function of frataxin cannot be inferred from its amino acid sequence. The protein, however, shows a striking degree of evolutionary conservation, particularly in a stretch of 27 amino acids encoded by exons 4 and 5a. In the past few years, many studies have addressed the function of frataxin. Although the exact function of frataxin is still controversial, there are currently at least four predominant non-exclusive hypotheses for frataxin's physiological role: roles in (i) mitochondrial iron transport, (ii) iron–sulfur cluster biogenesis (iii) iron binding/sequestration, (iv) response to oxidative stress. In the past year, the most favored hypothesis is that frataxin has an essential role in iron–sulfur cluster biogenesis.

Frataxin mitochondrial localization

A first suggestion that frataxin could be a mitochondrial protein came from phylogenetic studies. Sequence comparisons showed the presence of more distant homologues in gram-negative (γ purple), but not in gram-positive bacteria (Gibson *et al.*, 1996). This suggests that the frataxin gene might be derived from the bacterial precursor of the mitochondrial genome which shares phylogenetic ancestry with gram-negative bacteria, and then underwent transfer to the nuclear genome. Furthermore, computer analysis predicted a mitochondrial targeting signal at the N-terminus of yeast and mouse frataxin, a domain that is absent in the bacterial homologues (Koutnikova *et al.*, 1997). Human and yeast frataxin were directly demonstrated to be mitochondrial proteins by epitope tagging experiments and colocalization with well-established mitochondrial markers (Babcock *et al.*, 1997; Koutnikova *et al.*, 1997; Priller *et al.*, 1997; Wilson & Roof, 1997). Mitochondrial localization of endogenous frataxin was demonstrated using specific monoclonal antibodies. Immunoelectron microscopy results indicate that human frataxin, that has no hydrophobic transmembrane segment, is nevertheless associated with mitochondrial membranes and crests (Campuzano *et al.*, 1997), while fractionation experiments demonstrate that yeast frataxin behaves like a soluble matrix protein (Branda *et al.*, 1999; Geissler *et al.*, 2000).

The N-terminal mitochondrial targeting sequence of both mammalian and yeast frataxin is proteolytically removed in a two-step cleavage resulting in an 18 kD mature protein (Branda *et al.*, 1999; Campuzano *et al.*, 1997; Koutnikova *et al.*, 1998), whereas the precursors of most mitochondrial matrix proteins are subjected to a single proteolytic event upon import. Both cleavage steps involve the mitochondrial processing peptidase (MPP), a dimeric protease whose β subunit binds to the N-terminus of frataxin (Branda *et al.*, 1999; Koutnikova *et al.*, 1998). MPP first cleaves the precursor to the intermediate form and subsequently converts the intermediate to mature size protein of 18 kD (Cavadini *et al.*, 2000a).

Frataxin and iron homeostasis

Yeast as a model organism proved to be an invaluable system for first insight to unravel frataxin function within the mitochondria. Deletion of the frataxin yeast homologue (YFH1) results in mutant strains that show growth defect on fermentable carbon source, accumulate mitochondrial iron and exhibit a high sensitivity to oxidative stress induced by oxidant agents such as hydrogen peroxide or iron, as well as a reduction in oxidative phosphorylation (Babcock *et al.*, 1997; Foury & Cazzalini, 1997; Koutnikova *et al.*, 1997; Radisky *et al.*, 1999; Wilson & Roof, 1997). In parallel, not only the high affinity iron import system is constitutively turned on in the ΔYFH1 mutants (Babcock *et al.*, 1997; Radisky *et al.*, 1999), but using DNA microarray hybridization analysis, Foury and Talibi found that the expression of all known members of the "iron regulon" was increased in a frataxin-deficient strain (Foury & Talibi, 2001), implying that cells are starved for cytosolic iron. Together, these observations lead to the hypothesis that frataxin is directly involved in iron homeostasis, possibly by mediating iron efflux. Therefore, the direct consequence of frataxin deficiency would be iron accumulation which likely catalyzes the formation of hydroxyl radicals via the Fenton reaction leading to an iron-induced oxidative stress provoking the loss of mitochondrial DNA and iron–sulfur proteins characteristic of the ΔYFH1 yeast (Babcock *et al.*, 1997; Foury & Cazzalini, 1997).

There are multiple evidences that mammalian and yeast frataxins are true orthologues and that human frataxin might also be involved in iron homeostasis. Human frataxin can complement the defect in ΔYfh1 cells (Cavadini *et al.*, 2000b; Wilson & Roof, 1997), and this complementation is abolished by the introduction of disease-causing missense mutations within the gene (Cavadini *et al.*, 2000b). Moreover, pathological and clinical studies show that consequences of frataxin reduction are indeed similar in human cells. Iron deposits are consistently observed on autopsy in hearts of FRDA patients (Bradley *et al.*, 2000; Lamarche *et al.*, 1993). Magnetic resonance imaging data indicate that iron also accumulates in the dentate nucleus (Waldvogel *et al.*, 1999), an affected cerebellar structure. Mitochondrial iron content of FRDA fibroblasts, an unaffected cell type in this disease, is minimally increased (Delatycki *et al.*, 1999a). Moreover, an increased serum level of transferrin receptor, the major mediator of iron uptake, has been found in FRDA patients (Wilson *et al.*, 2000) which may indicate an abnormal intracellular distribution of iron. However, a similar increase in patients with other degenerative ataxia was observed (Wilson *et al.*, 2000), suggesting that the elevated transferrin levels is a feature of several degenerative ataxias, rather than specific to FRDA.

Frataxin and the biogenesis of iron-sulfur clusters

A selective deficiency of the respiratory chain complexes I-III and of both mitochondrial and cytosolic aconitases activities in the heart biopsy and autopsy material of patients has been reported (Bradley *et al.*, 2000; Rotig *et al.*, 1997). All the deficient enzymes and complexes contain iron–sulfur (Fe–S) clusters in their active sites. Fe–S proteins are remarkably sensitive to free radicals, and their inactivation further suggests oxidative stress in FRDA affected tissues which could be a consequence of iron accumulation. However, data from FRDA mouse models (see below) demonstrate that the Fe–S protein deficiency occurs prior to iron accumulation (Puccio *et al.*, 2001), suggesting that iron accumulation might not be the primary consequence of frataxin deficiency. We cannot exclude though that deregulation of iron homeostasis without significant iron deposit or accumulation leads to iron-induced oxidative stress.

Is the Fe–S protein deficiency a cause or a consequence of mitochondrial iron accumulation? Studies in the yeast demonstrate that the presence of iron-chelator in the culture media restores normal intramitochondrial iron levels and normal oxidative respiration in ΔYfh1 yeast cells, while the activity of aconitase is not fully restored (Foury, 1999). These results suggest that the reduction in the activity of the respiratory chain complexes is a consequence of mitochondrial iron accumulation, while the reduced aconitase activity is directly linked in part to frataxin deficiency. Mitochondrial aconitase deficiency therefore does not seem to be a mere consequence of mitochondrial dysfunction. In addition, the inactivation of cytosolic aconitase in FRDA patients (yeasts do not have cytosolic aconitase), suggests that a general iron–sulfur defect is the underlying mechanism. However, it is possible that the loss of cytosolic aconitase activity observed in FRDA might also reflect a decrease of cytosolic iron content, since cytosolic aconitase loses its Fe–S cluster to acquire iron-responsive element (IRE) binding properties in response to low iron concentration (Kaptain *et al.*, 1991).

It is interesting to note that two other yeast mutants (ΔAtm1 and ΔSsq1) which specifically accumulate iron in the mitochondria are involved in Fe–S cluster biogenesis. The Atm1 gene encodes a 7 transmembrane ABC ATPase (a putative ABC transporter) which appears to be involved in export of iron-sulfur clusters from the mitochondria (Kispal *et al.*, 1997, 1999). Attempts to identify a direct functional relation between frataxin and Atm1 have failed so far. Interestingly, mutations in ABC7, the human homologue of the Atm1 gene, are responsible for a rare X-linked recessive disease, defined by spinocerebellar ataxia and anemia (Allikmets *et al.*, 1999). The Ssq1 gene, encoding a low abundance mitochondrial heat shock 70 protein (mtHsp70) (Knight *et al.*, 1998), was recently demonstrated to be required for Fe–S cluster assembly in mitochondria, together with the co-chaperone Jac1, a mitochondrial DnaJ homologue (Lutz *et al.*, 2001). Furthermore, the Fe–S cluster assembly into ferredoxin (itself involved in Fe–S assembly) requires frataxin (Lutz *et al.*, 2001). In concordance with these latter results, the phylogenetic distribution of frataxin in 56 available genomes identified an identical phylogenetic distribution with hscA, a paralogue of Ssq1 and hscB, an orthologue of Jac1 (Huynen *et al.*, 2001). Therefore, combining phylogenetic data with experimental and predicted cellular localization data supports the hypothesis that frataxin is directly involved in iron–sulfur cluster assembly. More recently, three independent groups have obtained direct evidence that frataxin promotes Fe–S center synthesis using in vitro and in vivo experiments. Frataxin was shown to be required but not indispensable for cellular Fe/S protein assembly by directly measuring the *de novo* maturation of several Fe/S proteins in yeast (Muhlenhoff *et al.*, 2002). Furthermore, inhibition of Fe–S cluster biosynthesis by absence of frataxin decreases mitochondrial iron export in the yeast (Chen *et al.*, 2002). All these studies suggest that frataxin is not indispensable for this process, but renders it more efficient.

Frataxin as an iron-storage protein

An attractive hypothesis recently put forward suggests that the function of frataxin is to bind iron and keep it in a soluble and bioavailable form (Adamec *et al.*, 2000). By gel filtration experiments and analytical ultracentrifugation, the authors demonstrated that recombinant purified yeast frataxin is a soluble monomer that contains no iron, which assembles into a high molecular weight regular spherical multimer sequestering more than 3000 atoms of iron upon titration with increasing concentration of ferrous iron. This function of frataxin is consistent with the role played by frataxin in iron export and would also account for the proposed role in Fe–S cluster assembly. Furthermore, storing uncomplexed iron should prevent iron toxicity, and therefore oxidative damage. Yeast frataxin acts as a ferroxidase in the first oligomerization steps, oxidizing the initial atoms of Fe^{2+} that are incorporated, and then, when more iron gets into the larger complexes, it oxidizes spontaneously (Park *et al.*, 2002). Accordingly, mammalian frataxins, and human frataxin in particular, forms similar complexes, although under different kinetics. Human frataxin is unable to form the ferritin-like particles, but does assemble into higher-order filamentous structures (Cavadini *et al.*, 2002). However, so far, no other group has been able to reproduce the iron binding results for human frataxin.

Analysis of the solution (Musco *et al.*, 2000) and crystal (Dhe-Paganon *et al.*, 2000; Cho *et al.*, 2000) structures of human frataxin and its bacterial Cyay homologue has revealed a compact and globular protein with a novel fold consisting of a five-stranded anti-parallel ß sheet packing against a pair of parallel α helices. Frataxin does not have any features resembling known iron-binding sites, and the structure rather suggests that it interacts with a large ligand, probably a protein. However, attempts by different groups to identify the interacting protein have been unsuccessful, possibly because the interaction might be transient. Furthermore, both the crystal and NMR study suggest that human frataxin is not an iron binding protein, under any concentration of iron tested (Dhe-Paganon *et al.*, 2000; Musco *et al.*, 2000). A comparative study using human, yeast and bacterial frataxins selected as representatives of different evolutionary steps, shows that these three proteins preserve their fold but have largely different stability, which is strongly influence by the presence of cations. Using mutagenesis, the surface involved in iron binding was identified and was shown not to be conserved among the three species. In addition, the high-molecular weight supramolecular structure and the iron binding capability of human frataxin could not be confirmed (Adinolfi *et al.*, 2002).

The different behavior of yeast vs. mammalian frataxin could possibly be explained by the recent discovery of a mitochondrial ferritin in higher eukaryotes (Levi *et al.*, 2001). Although both yeast and mamalian frataxin has the properties for the chaperone activity in Fe/S cluster biosynthesis, an additional iron storage function may have been taken up by the yeast which has no ferritins. Only the chaperone activity in Fe/S cluster biosynthesis would be needed in higher eukaryotes since they have both cystosolic and mitochondrial ferritins.

Frataxin and oxidative stress

Whether frataxin is directly involved in iron homeostasis or Fe–S cluster biogenesis, the generation of reactive oxygen species plays an important role in the pathogenesis of FRDA. Consistent with this hypothesis, vitamin E deficiency produces a disease very similar to FRDA (see below).

Although the speculation of oxidative stress involvement in FRDA has long been accepted, it is not until very recently that an increased oxidative stress has been demonstrated in individuals with FRDA. Schulz et al. reported elevated urinary concentrations of 8-hydroxy-2′-deoxyguanosine (8OH2′dG), a marker of oxidative damage to DNA, in patients with FRDA (Schulz et al., 2000). Similarly, Edmond et al. found increased levels of plasma malondialdehyde (MDA), a product of lipid peroxidation (Emond et al., 2000). More recently, Piemonte et al. demonstrated decreased free glutathione concentration in blood of patients with FRDA (Piemonte et al., 2001). Glutathione, the most abundant antioxidant in the cell, can act either as a free radical scavenger or a co-substrate for important enzymes such as glutathione peroxidase and glutathione transferases (Hayes & McLellan, 1999). These studies thus further imply a role of free radical cytotoxicity in the pathophysiology of the disease. In addition, these studies are important because they used readily available fluids, and thus the assays could provide a way to monitor disease status or treatment efficacy.

Therefore, it is unquestionable that oxidative stress plays an important role in the pathogenesis of FRDA. Could frataxin be directly involved in oxidative stress response or is this oxidative stress iron-induced? To address this question, the group of Dr. Rustin devised experimental conditions to endogenously produce superoxides in cells deficient in frataxin (FRDA fibroblasts) by inhibiting the ATP synthase with oligomycin (Chantrel-Groussard et al., 2001). This inhibition normally results in an important superoxide dismutases (SODs) induction, however FRDA cells failed to normally increase SODs activity and iron import and to decrease iron storage capacity, despite parallel loss of membrane bound iron-containing enzyme activity. Similarly, the group of Dr. Pandolfo showed that FRDA fibroblasts exposed to iron, and therefore to iron-induced oxidative stress, failed to normally upregulate the mitochondrial SOD (Jiralerspong et al., 2001). Finally, measurements of SOD enzymes activity in the heart of the conditional mouse models of FRDA (see below) show lower SODs activity than in age-match control mice (Chantrel-Groussard et al., 2001). These observations are consistent

with expression data from DNA chips experiments which show no increase in SOD transcripts in ΔYfh1 yeast (Foury & Talibi, 2001). Therefore, together, these results suggest that decreased Fe–S biosynthesis impairs early antioxidant defenses resulting in higher cell lethality in response to oxidative stress. The mechanism involved remains to be established, although one can hypothesize that it could be either a Fe–S protein acting as an oxidative damage sensor in the mitochondria or that an abnormal status of mitochondrial iron disturbs the antioxidant response system. However, the primary involvement of superoxide injury is consistent with the pathology of the disease (neurons and cardiomyocytes have limited antioxidant defenses), and the increase in oxidative stress found in FRDA.

Mouse models for FRDA

To further study the mechanism of the disease and to test pharmacological therapy, several mouse models have been generated. Our group generated a classical mouse model by constitutive inactivation of frataxin by homologous recombination (Cossee et al., 2000). Homozygous deletion of frataxin causes embryonic lethality a few days after implantation, demonstrating an important role for frataxin during early development. These results suggest that the milder phenotype in humans is due to residual frataxin expression associated with the expansion mutations. No iron accumulation was observed during embryonic resorption, suggesting that cell death might be due to a mechanism independent of iron accumulation.

To circumvent embryonic lethality, we recently generated in parallel two different conditional knockout models, based on the Cre-lox system, in which frataxin was deleted either specifically in skeletal and cardiac muscle (using a transgenic mouse expressing Cre under the muscle creatine kinase promoter) or predominantly in neuronal tissues (neuron specific enolase promoter) (Puccio et al., 2001). Both models are viable and reproduce some morphological and biochemical features observed in FRDA patients including cardiac hypertrophy without skeletal muscle involvement, large sensory neuron dysfunction without alteration of the small sensory and motor neurons, and deficient activities of complexes I–III of the respiratory chain and of the aconitases. Time course experiments reveal that the Fe–S enzyme deficiencies begin in the initial phase of the pathology, and that intramitochondrial iron accumulation occurs later. In addition, as mentioned above, the SODs are abnormally low in the diseased mouse (Chantrel-Groussard et al., 2001). These mutant mice therefore represent the first mammalian models to evaluate treatment strategies for the human disease.

More recently, the group of Dr. Pandolfo attempted to generate a mouse model by introducing a $(GAA)_{230}$ repeat within the mouse frataxin gene to mirror the chronically reduced levels of frataxin expression found in the human disease (Miranda *et al.*, 2002). Bred with the *Frda* knockout, the authors obtained animals expressing 25–36% of wild-type frataxin levels, an expression level associated to mildly affected FRDA patients. Unfortunately, these mice did not develop abnormalities of motor coordination, cardiomyopathy, or iron metabolism.

The group of Dr. Chamberlain were able to overcome the embryonic lethality of the *Frda* knockout by generating a transgenic mouse that contains the entire frataxin gene within a human YAC clone onto the null mouse background (Pook *et al.*, 2001). The human frataxin was expressed in the appropriate tissues at levels comparable to the endogenous mouse frataxin, and was correctly processed and localized to mitochondria. Biochemical analysis of heart tissue demonstrated preservation of mitochondrial respiratory chain function. Therefore, it is possible to envision the generation of a mouse model expressing low levels of frataxin by using a human YAC derived from a patient, thereby having a repeat within the first intron inhibiting the expression of frataxin. It is clearly important to generate a mouse model that molecularly mirrors the human disease in addition to the already existing models.

Therapeutic trials for FRDA

Based on the recent discoveries of the potential function of frataxin, and more specifically on the consequences of frataxin reduction, therapeutic advances can be envisioned. Whether the mitochondrial iron accumulation is a primary or a secondary effect of frataxin deficiency, all data suggest that intracellular iron imbalance and oxidative stress are involved in the pathogenesis of FRDA. This led to initial enthusiasm for iron chelators, such as desferrioxamine, as therapeutic reagents for treating the disease. However, desferrioxamine has a significant side effect profile and its effect on individuals who do not have a generalized iron overload is not well studied. FRDA patients have normal serum iron and ferritin levels (Wilson *et al.*, 1998). Moreover, Rustin *et al.* have experimental evidence suggesting that caution should be taken when using iron chelators as a therapeutic agent since it could displace rather than protect against iron-mediated toxicity (Rustin *et al.*, 1999b).

Since it has been proposed that reducing the load of free radicals will slow the progression of the disease, antioxidants which are usually devoid of side effects can be considered as potential therapeutic reagents. Rustin *et al.*

have shown by in vitro experiments that the antioxidant idebenone, a short chain analogue of coenzyme Q10, protects the membrane respiratory chain enzymes against iron-induced injury without causing a reduction in soluble aconitase activity (Rustin *et al.*, 1999a,b). In addition, the short side chain of idebenone allows it to cross membranes readily (including the blood–brain barrier). Preliminary results on the cardiomyopathy of 40 FRDA patients (Rustin *et al.*, 1999b, 2002) are promising and warrant establishing a larger clinical trial using idebenone. Furthermore, Schulz *et al.* found that 8 weeks of treatment with idebenone decreased the urine levels of 8OH2′dG by 20% (Schulz *et al.*, 2000). Finally, our unpublished results of treatment of the conditional cardiac mouse model show a statistically significant increase in the life span of the animals. Therefore, idebenone appears to have some therapeutic effect, although the neurological consequences need to be evaluated in the long term. On the other hand, treatment of FRDA patients for 6 months with the antioxidants coenzyme Q10 and vitamin E resulted in an increased in the cardiac phosphocreatine to ATP ratios and improved muscle mitochondrial ATP production (Lodi *et al.*, 2001). However, whether FRDA patients will benefit clinically from this bioenergetic improvement needs to be evaluated by appropriate trials in the future.

In conclusion, these findings contribute to the growing body of evidence that treatments aimed to enhance mitochondrial function and reduce toxic radical production are rational and may be a realistic hope for the patients and their families. The next challenge is to resolve the controversial issues as to the function of frataxin to provide solid bases for designing eagerly awaited therapeutic approaches for Friedreich's ataxia.

Other sensory and spinocerebellar ataxias

Ataxia due to isolated vitamin E deficiency (AVED)

The first case of inherited isolated vitamin E deficiency was reported in 1981 by Burck and colleagues (Burck *et al.*, 1981). For 10 years, this entity was considered as extremely rare, until the discovery of an important founding group in North Africa (Ben Hamida *et al.*, 1993a,b; Cavalier *et al.*, 1998). Age of onset is often around 10 years but ranges from 2 to 52 years in exceptional cases. In its classical form, AVED is very similar to Friedreich's ataxia but differs from it by the absence of cardiomyopathy and diabetes and by the presence of head titubation in 28% of cases and of dystonia in an additional 13% of cases (Cavalier *et al.*, 1998). In the absence of supplementation treatment, the patients will eventually become wheelchair bound after a mean 13 years of disease duration and may develop retinitis pigmentosa (Yokota *et al.*, 1997; Shimohata *et al.*, 1998; Benomar *et al.*, 2002). The pathological study of a single case revealed a severe demyelination of the posterior columns of the spinal cord and a severe atrophy of the sensory nuclei of the medulla, an important loss of cerebellar Purkinje cells and a moderate atrophy of the lateral pyramidal tracts in the spinal cord, and of the dorsal root ganglia and peripheral nerves (Larnaout *et al.*, 1997). Electrophysiologically, the sensory action potentials are altered less and later than in Friedreich's ataxia (Zouari *et al.*, 1998). Another important histological feature was widespread neuronal and muscular lipofucsin accumulation. The lipofucsin deposits were autofluorescent, electron dense, membrane bound and phosphatase acid positive, suggesting a lysosomal origin (Burck *et al.*, 1981; Laplante *et al.*, 1984; Trabert *et al.*, 1989; Stumpf *et al.*, 1987; Yokota *et al.*, 1987). These deposits are thought to represent lipoperoxidation products resulting from the absence of lipophyllic anti-oxidative properties of vitamin E. Indicators of lipid peroxidation (vulnerability of erythrocyte membranes, presence of thiobarbituric acid-reactive substances in blood) are positive (Kohlschutter *et al.*, 1988; Amiel *et al.*, 1995; Schuelke *et al.*, 1999). However, red blood cells morphology is normal and no acanthocytes are present (Burck *et al.*, 1981; Laplante *et al.*, 1984; Stumpf *et al.*, 1987; Harding *et al.*, 1985). Diagnosis of AVED is made by low serum vitamin E levels in absence of fat malabsorption. Serum vitamin E levels are well below the normal range (<2.5 mg/l, often <1 mg/l, with $6<N<15$ mg/l). Fat malabsorption should be excluded by a normal lipidogram: triglycerides, cholesterol, beta-lipoprotein and other liposoluble vitamins (A,D,K) are normal. Parents and carriers often have vitamin E values at the lower limit of the normal range (Harding *et al.*, 1985; Ben Hamida *et al.*, 1993b).

In normal subjects, vitamin E is absorbed and secreted from the intestine into plasma in chylomicrons. During chylomicron catabolism in the plasma, vitamin E is transferred to circulating lipoprotein particles (IDL, LDL, HDL), which can deliver vitamin E to tissues. The chylomicron remnants are taken up by the liver, which then selects only RRR-α-tocopherol stereoisomer from all the forms of vitamin E for secretion in nascent very low-density lipoproteins (VLDL) (Kayden, 1993). RRR-α-tocopherol represents therefore the almost exclusive form of circulating vitamin E in plasma. Other isomers and stereoisomers are eliminated, presumably through the bile. The specific transfer of vitamin E to nascent VLDL is the work of a liver specific protein, the α-tocopherol transfer protein (α-TTP) (Sato *et al.*, 1991), which is defective in AVED (Ouahchi

et al., 1995; Gotoda *et al.*, 1995). AVED patients absorb vitamin E normally, but their conservation of plasma RRR-α-tocopherol is poor due to impaired secretion of RRR-α-tocopherol in VLDL (Traber *et al.*, 1990, 1993). In the absence of recycling, the entire plasma pool of vitamin E is rapidly eliminated in a little more than a day (Traber *et al.*, 1994). The human α-TTP gene, on chromosome 8q13, is composed of five exons and encodes a 278 amino-acid protein which exhibits structural homologies with the cellular retinaldehyde-binding protein (CRALBP, present only in the retina) and the yeast Sec14 protein, involved in phosphatidylinositol and phosphatidylcholine transfer into membranes (Arita *et al.*, 1995). AVED mutations are scattered throughout all five exons. In Tunisia, AVED is as frequent as Friedreich's ataxia, due to the spreading of the founder mutation 744delA, which is also present in the other North African countries, and in Italy and France. All but one North African AVED patients were found to be homozygous for the 744delA mutation, while the 513insTT mutation is the major mutation across Europe and North America (Cavalier *et al.*, (1998) and unpublished results). The most frequent mutation in Japan is a missense change, H101Q, associated with a very mild phenotype and late onset (Gotoda *et al.*, 1995; Yokota *et al.*, 1997).

There is no limitation or difficulty with the absorption of vitamin E by the intestinal tract in AVED patients. The administration of vitamin E supplements in divided doses daily has resulted in cessation of progression of the neurologic symptoms and signs, and some amelioration of established neurologic abnormalities in a number of patients (Kohlschutter *et al.*, 1988; Martinello *et al.*, 1998). Administration to adults of 800 mg of RRR α-tocopherol given twice daily with meals containing fat, results in plasma α-tocopherol levels that are at or above the normal range (Cavalier *et al.*, 1998). The important number of new cases recently reported indicates that AVED is not so rare, stressing again the importance not to miss the diagnosis in this treatable condition and to institute therapy promptly.

Abetalipoproteinemia (ABL)

The first report of abetalipoproteinemia was published in 1950 by Bassen & Kornzweig from a consanguineous family with two affected children (Bassen & Kornzweig, 1950). In 1958, Jampel and Falls identified in this condition a deficiency in cholesterol and triglycerides associated with a deficiency of plasma lipid transport (Jampel & Falls, 1958), itself causing a deficiency of the lipophylic vitamins A, K and mostly E. Abetalipoproteinemia presents initially in the neonatal period with gastrointestinal manifestations related to malabsorption of fat, such as vomiting, diarrhea, and failure to gain weight normally (Kohlschutter, 2000). Endoscopy reveals a yellow discoloration of the duodenum and intestinal mucosa biopsies reveal vacuolization of the cytoplasm of villus cells which are fat-engorged, but otherwise morphologically normal, unlike celiac disease, with which abetalipoproteinemia is frequently confused. The intestinal symptoms tend to diminish with age, reflecting in part a striking aversion of many patients to dietary fat. In the absence of vitamin E supplementation, neurological and visual manifestations progressively appear. The neurological manifestations mimic Friedreich's ataxia, beginning with diminution of the deep tendon reflexes, followed by vibration sense and proprioception loss and finally appearance of an ataxic gait, dysarthria, pes cavus, pes equinovarus and kyphoscoliosis. The characteristic sites of the degenerative process are the large sensory neurons of the dorsal root ganglia and their myelinated axons that enter the spinal cord lateral to the posterior funiculus. The axons degenerate and lead to a secondary demyelination of the posterior columns. As in isolated vitamin E deficiency, muscle biopsy after a long disease duration reveals accumulation of ceroid and lipofuscin pigments. The most prominent ophthalmic abnormality is pigmentary retinal degeneration with involvement of the posterior fundus and loss or attenuation of the pigment epithelium. The presence of lipofuscin pigment in the retina suggests that vitamin E deficiency plays a central role in the retinopathy, although the combined deficiency of n–3 type essential fatty acids probably also contribute to its occurrence. Loss of night vision is frequently a presenting symptom and may be related to moderate vitamin A deficiency. Since the early description of abetalipoproteinemia, the abundant presence of abnormal star-shaped erythrocytes, termed acanthocytes, was noted in peripheral blood. The erythrocytes assume the acanthocytic form because of an abnormal composition of their membrane, which itself reflects the abnormal composition of the plasma lipoproteins (Kohlschutter, 2000). Severe anemia is frequent and is the consequence of the malabsorption syndrome.

Patients are virtually free of serum lipoproteins of the b group (chylomicrons, LDL and VLDL, that is all lipoproteins that contain B apolipoproteins), resulting in reduced cholesterol levels (< 500 mg/l), almost undetectable triglyceride levels (<100 mg/l) and reduced lipophylic vitamins (E, A and K) in the plasma, which when combined with acanthocytosis, establishes the diagnosis of abetalipoproteinemia. This deficiency is due to the inability of intestine and liver cells to secrete B-100 lipoproteins (Wetterau et al., 1992). However, it is not due to mutations in the Apo B gene, but to mutations in the gene encoding the large subunit of the microsomal triglyceride transfer protein (MTP) (Sharp et al., 1993; Shoulders et al., 1993). The MTP gene, located on chromosome 4q23, is composed of 18 exons and is physiologically expressed in intestinal, liver and cardiac cells. MTP can transfer triglycerides and cholesteryl esters between lipidic vesicles and is thought to promote the acquisition of non polar lipids during or just after completion of translation of apo B, at the luminal aspect of the rough ER (Kane & Havel, 2001). It is likely that Apo-B interacts physically with MTP during the initial lipidation step. In the absence of normal initiation of lipidation of Apo B-100, the latter is degraded by intraluminal protease(s) and transport of plasma lipids is supplemented by apolipoproteins E and A-II.

Treatment involves reduction of dietary fat to prevent steatorrhea and supplementation with vitamin E to prevent progression of the neurological and retinal degenerative disease (Kohlschutter, 2000). A proportion of the ingested fat can be replaced by medium-chain triglycerides, which can be absorbed without the formation of chylomicrons, supplemented with essential fatty acids. Due to the malabsorption and lipoprotein abnormalities that make transfer into the central nervous system extremely difficult, vitamin E supplementation requires the use of large oral doses, up to 150 mg of natural α-tocopherol per kg body weight per day in three divided doses. Repeated evaluation of the vitamin E status is necessary to monitor the effectiveness of the treatment. Supplementation with water-soluble preparation of vitamin A appears also reasonable, but should be carefully monitored due to its toxic effects at high doses.

The primary defect causing Friedreich's ataxia, ataxia with isolated vitamin E deficiency and abetalipoproteinemia shed light on a possible general pathological scheme that would explain the shared sites of degeneration and shared dying-back axonal neuropathy. In Friedreich's ataxia, the disease is thought to result from abnormal Fe–S assembly leading to increased production of free radicals, while in the vitamin E ataxias, the disease appears to be the consequence of reduced neuronal membrane defense against lipid peroxidation and other oxidative stress damage. The effectiveness of idebenone in the therapy of Friedreich's ataxia lends support to the hypothesis that free-radicals are central to the pathology of these and possibly other neurodegenerative diseases.

Refsum disease (RD)

In 1946, Sir Sigvald Refsum described a new neurological entity called heredopathia atactica polyneuritiformis (Refsum, 1946), which was subsequently shown to be due to phytanic acid accumulation (Klenk & Kahlke, 1963).

Refsum disease is defined by the association of retinitis pigmentosa, peripheral polyneuropathy, cerebellar and sensory ataxia, and elevated cerebrospinal fluid proteins in absence of pleocytosis (Gibberd & Wierzbicki, 2000). It usually presents between the ages of 10 and 20 years with retinitis pigmentosa, causing night blindness and restricted peripheral vision that can progress to complete blindness. Anosmia is common. Ataxia develops later, associated with neuropathy. Sensorineural deafness, myopathy and ichthyosis occur in more severe cases. Bony abnormalities may be present, and if they are, they are present early on. The most common abnormality is shortening of the terminal phalanges of the thumb. Asymmetrical shortening of the fourth metatarsal and other long bone abnormalities are also seen. In untreated patients, cardiac arrhythmia and hypertrophic cardiomyopathy may develop.

The clinical biochemical feature is raised plasma phytanic acid more than three times the upper limit of normal (i.e. more than 100 mmol/l). If untreated, phytanic acid accumulates in tissues and may represent up to 5% to 30% of total plasma free fatty acids. Phytanic acid is an isoprenoid fatty acid derived from phytol which is the alcohol anchor moiety of a molecule of chlorophyll. Only bacteria that occur in the digestive tracts of herbivores and fishes can break down chlorophyll to phytol. Hence, in humans, phytanic acid is exclusively of nutritional origin, mostly from dairy products and from fat and meat of ruminant animals and fishes. Long-term diets with food containing no phytanic acid will eventually normalize phytanic acid levels in Refsum patients. Green vegetables and many other products such as pork and poultry contain no phytanic acid. Synthetic phytanic acid free diets also exist. Ataxia, neuropathy, ichthyosis and cardiac arrhythmia are the symptoms that respond best to the lowering of phytanic acid in the blood, while others may be irreversible. Plasmapheresis or lipapheresis may be used initially to achieve efficacy rapidly for the severe cases.

Accumulation of phytanic acid is due to the deficiency of the first step of its degradation, which is an alpha-oxidation that takes place in the peroxisomes. This step yields pristanic acid, which is then degraded by beta-oxidation in the mitochondria. The first step of alpha oxidation involves an alpha-hydroxylation of phytanoyl-CoA. The cloning of the phytanoyl-CoA hydroxylase (PAHX) gene and the identification of mutations therein allowed demonstration of the role of this enzyme in Refsum disease (Jansen et al., 1997; Mihalik et al., 1997). The most common mutation is an in-frame deletion of 111 bp in the mid region of the gene (135–246del111). However, Refsum disease is genetically heterogeneous and a second locus must exist. Curiously, phytol is also the membrane anchor moiety of vitamin E

and nuclear orphan receptors that bind phytanic acid exist. Whether this may explain some of the clinical similarities between Refsum disease and vitamin E deficiencies is only speculative.

Infantile onset spinocerebellar ataxia (IOSCA)

This form of ataxia, reported in 1985 and 1994 by Kallio and Jauhiainen and by Koskinen and colleagues, respectively (Kallio & Jauhiainen, 1985; Koskinen et al., 1994), was so far found only in patients from Finland (21 patients belonging to 15 nuclear families). The disease manifests close to the age of 1 year as acute or subacute clumsiness, athetoid movements in hands and face, hypotonia and loss of deep tendon reflexes in the legs. Ophthalmoplegia and sensorineural hearing deficit are found by school age, sensory neuropathy (decreased or absent sensory action potentials) and optic atrophy by the age of 10–15 years, and female hypogonadism and epilepsy by the age of 15–20 years. Most patients are nonambulatory by the age of 20. Ten of the 21 patients have had seizures, eight of whom had one or more acute crises that progressed to a therapy-resistant status epilepticus and lasted for 2–4 weeks (Lonnqvist et al., 2000). The fact that three patients never regained consciousness and died in their third decade suggests that lifespan may not be normal. The main pathological features of the disease are sensory axonal neuropathy (with severe loss of especially the large myelinated fibres), and progressive atrophy of the spinal cord, brain stem and eventually cerebellum (Lonnqvist et al., 1998). However, athetosis and epilepsy denote an additional involvement of the cerebrum.

The gene defect of IOSCA has been localised to chromosome 10q24.1 (Nikali et al., 1995). All patients seem to share one founder mutation, as they all bear a common haplotype around the disease gene locus (Nikali et al., 1995). The smallest region of haplotype sharing, defined by a few ancient haplotype recombinations, is 150 kb and contains a single known gene, the paired-box protein 2, PAX2 (Nikali et al., 1997). However, no mutation has been found in the PAX2 gene of IOSCA patients. A disease-causing role for nucleotide changes in non-coding sequences is difficult to assess, particularly since there is no ethnically unrelated patients with linkage at the same locus, which could pinpoint to an independent mutation. The identification of the molecular defect in IOSCA may therefore prove difficult.

Ataxia + blindness + deafness (SCABD)

In 1974, van Bogaert and Martin reported a family with autosomal recessive spinocerebellar ataxia plus optic and cochleo-vestibular degeneration leading to deafness and blindness (van Bogaert & Martin, 1974). We have reported a similar family, for which we demonstrated linkage to a 17 cM region on chromosome 6p21–23 (Bomont *et al.*, 2000). In our family, an uncle and a niece, both born from consanguineous parents, started with gait ataxia at 3 years of age. The niece had no cranial nerve involvement at age 6 but showed slow responses on electroretinograms at age 14 and had impaired hearing and vision by age 17 years. The uncle was wheelchair bound and almost deaf by age 27 years. Fundus examination revealed bilateral optic atrophy. Common causes of recessive ataxia were excluded, including mitochondrial diseases. The identification of additional families linked to 6p21–23 is needed in order to delineate a precise clinical presentation and progression for this condition.

Cerebellar ataxia + peripheral neuropathy

Ataxia + oculomotor apraxia 1 (AOA1)

The first two cases of ataxia + oculomotor apraxia were reported in 1971 by Inoue *et al.* and were Japanese patients (Inoue *et al.*, 1971). The identification of the gene defective in form 1 revealed that the disease is more frequent in Japan due to the occurrence of two ancient founder mutations, but exists also worldwide, with a major Caucasian founder mutation. In 1988 Aicardi *et al.* collected reports of 14 AOA patients, 6 of them already described in the literature (Aicardi *et al.*, 1988). In 2001, Barbot *et al.* reported 22 Portuguese cases, of which 14 turned out to be defective for the AOA1 gene (Barbot *et al.*, 2001). AOA1 is defined by early onset (between 2 to 5 years of age) cerebellar ataxia, ocular apraxia and areflexia indicative of peripheral axonal neuropathy, which translates later as a clinical motor neuropathy (causing neurogenic distal muscular atrophy). Ocular apraxia is defined as the limitation of ocular movements on command dissociated from movements of pursuit. In the case of AOA1, ocular apraxia would be better defined by saccadic failure or slow (viscous) eye movements and would indicate neuronal lesion in the pons rather than in the motor cortex, as for pure ocular apraxia. The cerebellum is severely atrophic while the brainstem and spinal cord are usually preserved. Dystonia and/or athetosis may be occasionally found. Patients often have borderline intelligence. They may have a normal lifespan, although with severe motor handicap leading to loss of ambulation by age 15 years.

Localization of the defective gene to chromosome 9p13.3 in Portuguese families allowed demonstration that AOA1 is the same disorder as early onset cerebellar ataxia with hypoalbuminemia (EOCA-HA) (Moreira *et al.*, 2001a), described a few years earlier in Japan (Uekawa *et al.*, 1992). As such, both entities are characterized by reduced serum albumin and elevated cholesterol after a long disease duration (usually 15 years). These biochemical abnormalities (of hepatic and not renal origin) cannot be used for early diagnosis. The FRDA2 locus identified in 9p23-p11 (Christodoulou *et al.*, 2001) is presumably identical with AOA1. Date and colleagues and our group independently identified the AOA1 gene, which encodes for a novel HIT/Zn-finger protein named aprataxin (Date *et al.*, 2001; Moreira *et al.*, 2001b). Proteins containing a histidine triad (HIT) domain are known to have nucleotide polyphosphate hydrolase activity. We have shown in addition that the major isoform of aprataxin (long isoform) encodes an additional domain related to the N-terminal domain of polynucleotide 5′ kinase, 3′ phosphatase (PNKP) involved in base excision repair (BER) of DNA single strand breaks (SSB). Both this similarity and the nuclear localization prediction of aprataxin suggested that aprataxin might also be involved in SSB repair (Moreira *et al.*, 2001b), a conclusion also supported by the identification of a direct interaction between aprataxin and XRCC1, another component of the SSBR complex (Caldecott, 2003). AOA1 is the most frequent cause of recessive ataxia in Japan, where two founder mutations (689insT and P206L) account for the vast majority of cases (Date *et al.*, 2001; Moreira *et al.*, 2001b). The W279X mutation, found in five out of six Portuguese families (Moreira *et al.*, 2001b), is also widespread and by far the most frequent mutation in the Caucasian population (M.-C. Moreira, personal communication). The missense mutation P206L is associated with a some what later onset (around 10 years of age (Date *et al.*, 2001; Moreira *et al.*, 2001b)), and the V263G and K197Q mutations are associated with significantly milder presentations (onset at 25 and 15 years, respectively (Date *et al.*, 2001; Tranchant *et al.*, 2003)). Several DNA repair disorders, such as ataxia-telangiectasia (A-T), xeroderma pigmentosum and Cockayne syndrome, are associated with cerebellar ataxia, neoplasia and/or immunodeficiency (see following chapter). AOA1 shares with A-T early onset cerebellar ataxia and ocular apraxia, but not the extraneurologic features of A-T, suggesting that pathology related to partial BER deficiency might be restricted to postmitotic neuronal tissues. A second disease that rapidly came to support this view is SCAN1.

Spinocerebellar ataxia + neuropathy 1 (SCAN1)

SCAN1 shares with AOA1 the cerebellar atrophy and axonal sensorimotor neuropathy but not ocular apraxia. SCAN1 also shares with AOA1 the borderline low serum albumin and high cholesterol. The entity was reported in a single multigenerational, consanguineous, family with nine affected (Takashima *et al.*, 2002). Age at onset of the disease ranged from 13 to 15 years in three patients. The disease is linked to chromosome 14q31 and was shown to be due to the H493R mutation in the Tyrosyl-DNA Phosphodiesterase 1 (TDP1) gene (Takashima *et al.*, 2002). TDP1 is an enzyme that repairs stalled covalently bound topoisomerase I-DNA complexes, which lead to single strand breaks during DNA unwinding. H493 is one of the two histidines of TDP1 that act as the nucleophile that attacks the tyrosyl-DNA phosphodiester bond. DNA breaks liberated from the tyrosyl moiety by TDP1 are then repaired by the BER pathway, including intervention of PNKP (see above). It is therefore possible that AOA1 and SCAN1 pathology proceeds from the same biochemical pathway in which aprataxin plays an as yet unidentified role (Caldecott, 2003).

Ataxia + oculomotor apraxia 2 (AOA2)

The first AOA2 family was reported in 1998 by Watanabe and colleagues (Watanabe *et al.*, 1998). The four Japanese patients had cerebellar atrophy, sensory neuropathy but no oculomotor apraxia. Brainstem and spinal cord was preserved. The four patients had moderately elevated alpha-fetoprotein, immunoglobulins and creatine kinase in their blood. The defective gene was localized to 9q34 (Bomont *et al.*, 2000). At the same time, a large Pakistani family with ataxia + oculomotor apraxia was also reported to be linked to 9q34 (Nemeth *et al.*, 2000). The five patients had, however, normal levels of alpha-fetoprotein, immunoglobulins and creatine kinase. We have since then identified eight additional potentially linked families, based on homozygosity of patients born from (remotely) consanguineous parents (unpublished results). Five families had moderately elevated serum alpha-fetoprotein levels and four had oculomotor apraxia. Immunoglobulins and creatine kinase levels were normal and their elevation was presumably fortuitous in the first reported family. Age at onset for all linked families ranged from 14 to 22 years, which is significantly later than for AOA1. It is likely that the majority of the adolescent onset A-T like patients with elevated alpha-fetoprotein levels (Taylor *et al.*, 1994, 1996) do not have hypomorphic ATM mutations but rather AOA2. However, identification of the defective gene is necessary, in order to precisely delineate the clinical features of this entity.

Spastic ataxia of Charlevoix–Saguenay (ARSACS)

More than 300 ARSACS affected individuals are known to live in the Province of Québec, Canada, most of them in the region of Charlevoix-Saguenay. Molecularly proven cases of ARSACS outside Canada have so far been reported only in Tunisia, but presumably also exist elsewhere. ARSACS was first described by Bouchard and colleagues in 1978 (Bouchard *et al.*, 1978). ARSACS is defined by early and marked degeneration of both the pyramidal tracts of the spinal cord and of the superior cerebellar vermis with subsequent cerebellar hemisphere progressive atrophy (Bouchard *et al.*, 1998). Onset occurs at gait initiation (around 1–2 years). Pyramidal signs dominate the clinical presentation. Spasticity of the lower limbs is the first sign, plantar response is always abnormal, either equivocal or indifferent in youngsters and extensor thereafter. Deep tendon reflexes are increased, often with clonus at the ankles and patellae in early adulthood. Cerebellar signs are sparse at the beginning, but increase slowly from adolescence onwards. They include gait ataxia, dysarthria and nystagmus. The eye signs are most typical of the disease. These early non-progressive signs include saccadic alteration of smooth ocular pursuit and prominent myelinated fibers radiating from the optic disc and embedding part of the retinal blood vessels at fundoscopy (Bouchard *et al.*, 1978, 1998). There is, however, no visual deficit. The abnormal retinal myelinated fibers were not seen in the Tunisian patients (Mrissa *et al.*, 2000). In the mid-20s, motor axonal polyneuropathy appears, resulting in absent ankle jerks. ARSACS patients become wheelchair-bound at a mean age of 41, with a wide range of 17–57 years. The verbal IQ is usually within normal limits, but the handling of visuospatial material is poor and deteriorates with time (Bouchard *et al.*, 1979; Peyronnard *et al.*, 1979). Some patients survive into their 70s, but become bedridden by that time. ARSACS is therefore a very early onset disease with more obvious progression in teenagers and young adults and again subsequent slow progression.

The ARSACS gene was localized to 13q11 in 1999 (Richter *et al.*, 1999) and identified in 2000 (Engert *et al.*, 2000). It is a remarkable intron-less 13 kb long gene encoding for a novel 3829 residue protein named sacsin. Sacsin contains repeated heat-shock domains, suggesting a role in chaperone mediated protein folding. Ninety-six per cent of the Québec patients are homozygous for the 6594delT founder mutation and the remaining cases (two families) are compound heterozygotes for the founder mutation and a 5254C–>T nonsense mutation. Four Tunisian and two Turkish ARSACs families have been identified by linkage analysis (Mrissa *et al.*, 2000; Gucuyener *et al.*, 2001) and all four Tunisian families bear a different mutation (El Euch-Fayache *et al.*, 2003), also different from the Canadian mutations. The diversity of mutations causing ARSACS, including truncating mutations, indicates that ARSACS results from a complete loss of function of sacsin, a result that was initially unexpected given the high geographic clustering of the cases.

Conclusions

The unravelling of the molecular cause of a growing number of recessive ataxias has revealed that these often rare diseases are the consequences of a large variety of different mechanisms, even involving novel, unsuspected molecular pathways. The functions of the, sometimes novel, proteins encoded by the so far identified defective genes suggest however that the recessive ataxias involving primarily the spinal cord or the cerebellum may proceed from two distinct general pathways. On one hand, Friedreich's ataxia and the vitamin E deficiency ataxias, involving primarily the spinal cord appear to result from increased production of, or lack of protection against, free radical damage, whereas ataxia-telangiectasia, AOA1, SCAN1, as well as MRE11 partial deficiency (see following chapter) appear to result from impaired DNA single or double strand break repair. Further studies on the newly identified proteins defective in recessive ataxias and identification of the, predictably numerous, new genes involved in recessive ataxias when defective should tell whether this trend is a naïve view biased by a small number of observations, or whether it reflects general pathological neurodegenerative mechanisms, which could be amenable to therapy.

REFERENCES

Adamec, J., Rusnak, F., Owen, W. G. et al. (2000). Iron-dependent self-assembly of recombinant yeast frataxin: implications for Friedreich ataxia. Am. J. Hum. Genet., 67, 549–62.

Adinolfi, S., Trifuoggi, M., Politou, A. S., Martin, S. & Pastore, A. (2002). A structural approach to understanding the iron-binding properties of phylogenetically different frataxins. Hum. Mol. Genet., 11, 1865–77.

Aicardi, J., Barbosa, C., Andermann, E. et al. (1988). Ataxia-ocular motor apraxia: a syndrome mimicking ataxia-telangiectasia. Ann. Neurol., 24, 497–502.

Allikmets, R., Raskind, W. H., Hutchinson, A., Schueck, N. D., Dean, M. & Koeller, D. M. (1999). Mutation of a putative mitochondrial iron transporter gene (ABC7) in X-linked sideroblastic anemia and ataxia (XLSA/A). Hum. Mol. Genet., 8, 743–9.

Amiel, J., Maziere, J. C., Beucler, I. et al. (1995). Familial isolated vitamin E deficiency. Extensive study of a large family with a 5-year therapeutic follow-up. J. Inherit. Metab. Dis., 18, 333–40.

Arita, M., Sato, Y., Miyata, A. et al. (1995). Human alpha-tocopherol transfer protein: cDNA cloning, expression and chromosomal localization. Biochem. J., 306, 437–43.

Babcock, M., de Silva, D., Oaks, R. et al. (1997). Regulation of mitochondrial iron accumulation by Yfh1p, a putative homolog of frataxin. Science, 276, 1709–12.

Barbot, C., Coutinho, P., Chorao, R. et al. (2001). Recessive ataxia with ocular apraxia: review of 22 Portuguese patients. Arch. Neurol., 58, 201–5.

Bassen, F. A. & Kornzweig, A. L. (1950). Malformation of the erythrocytes in a case of atypical retinitis pigmentosa. Blood, 5, 381–7.

Ben Hamida, C., Doerflinger, N., Belal, S. et al. (1993a). Localization of Friedreich ataxia phenotype with selective vitamin E deficiency to chromosome 8q by homozygosity mapping. Nat. Genet., 5, 195–200.

Ben Hamida, M., Belal, S., Sirugo, G. et al. (1993b). Friedreich's ataxia phenotype not linked to chromosome 9 and associated with selective autosomal recessive vitamin E deficiency in two inbred Tunisian families. Neurology, 43, 2179–83.

Benomar, A., Yahyaoui, M., Meggouh, F. et al. (2002). Clinical comparison between AVED patients with 744 del A mutation and Friedreich ataxia with GAA expansion in 15 Moroccan families. J. Neurol. Sci., 198, 25–9.

Berciano, J., Mateo, I., De Pablos, C., Polo, J. M. & Combarros, O. (2002). Friedreich ataxia with minimal GAA expansion presenting as adult-onset spastic ataxia. J. Neurol. Sci., 194, 75–82.

Bidichandani, S. I., Ashizawa, T. & Patel, P. I. (1997). Atypical Friedreich ataxia caused by compound heterozygosity for a novel missense mutation and the GAA triplet-repeat expansion. Am. J. Hum. Genet., 60, 1251–6.

Bidichandani, S. I., Ashizawa, T. & Patel, P. I. (1998). The GAA triplet-repeat expansion in Friedreich ataxia interferes with transcription and may be associated with an unusual DNA structure. Am. J. Hum. Genet., 62, 111–21.

Bomont, P., Watanabe, M., Gershoni-Barush, R. et al. (2000). Homozygosity mapping of spinocerebellar ataxia with cerebellar atrophy and peripheral neuropathy to 9q33–34, and with hearing impairment and optic atrophy to 6p21–23. Eur. J. Hum. Genet., 8, 986–90.

Bouchard, J. P., Barbeau, A., Bouchard, R. & Bouchard, R. W. (1978). Autosomal recessive spastic ataxia of Charlevoix-Saguenay. Can. J. Neurol. Sci., 5, 61–9.

Bouchard, R. W., Bouchard, J. P., Bouchard, R. & Barbeau, A. (1979). Electroencephalographic findings in Friedreich's ataxia and autosomal recessive spastic ataxia of Charlevoix-Saguenay (ARSACS). Can. J. Neurol. Sci., 6, 191–4.

Bouchard, J. P., Richter, A., Mathieu, J. et al. (1998). Autosomal recessive spastic ataxia of Charlevoix-Saguenay. Neuromuscul. Disord., 8, 474–9.

Bradley, J. L., Blake, J. C., Chamberlain, S., Thomas, P. K., Cooper, J. M. & Schapira, A. H. (2000). Clinical, biochemical and molecular genetic correlations in Friedreich's ataxia. Hum. Mol. Genet., 9, 275–82.

Branda, S. S., Cavadini, P., Adamec, J., Kalousek, F., Taroni, F. & Isaya, G. (1999). Yeast and human frataxin are processed to mature form in two sequential steps by the mitochondrial processing peptidase. J. Biol. Chem., 274, 22763–9.

Burck, U., Goebel, H. H., Kuhlendahl, H. D., Meier, C. & Goebel, K. M. (1981). Neuromyopathy and vitamin E deficiency in man. *Neuropediatrics*, **12**, 267–78.

Caldecott, K. W. (2003). DNA single-strand break repair and spinocerebellar ataxia. *Cell*, **112**, 7–10.

Campuzano, V., Montermini, L., Molto, M. D. *et al.* (1996). Friedreich's ataxia: autosomal recessive disease caused by an intronic GAA triplet repeat expansion. *Science*, **271**, 1423–7.

Campuzano, V., Montermini, L., Lutz, Y. *et al.* (1997). Frataxin is reduced in Friedreich ataxia patients and is associated with mitochondrial membranes. *Hum. Mol. Genet.*, **6**, 1771–80.

Cavadini, P., Adamec, J., Taroni, F., Gakh, O. & Isaya, G. (2000a). Two-step processing of human frataxin by mitochondrial processing peptidase. Precursor and intermediate forms are cleaved at different rates. *J. Biol. Chem.*, **275**, 41469–75.

Cavadini, P., Gellera, C., Patel, P. I. & Isaya, G. (2000b). Human frataxin maintains mitochondrial iron homeostasis in *Saccharomyces cerevisiae*. *Hum. Mol. Genet.*, **9**, 2523–30.

Cavadini, P., O'Neill, H. A., Benada, O. & Isaya, G. (2002). Assembly and iron-binding properties of human frataxin, the protein deficient in Friedreich ataxia. *Hum. Mol. Genet.*, **11**, 217–27.

Cavalier, L., Ouahchi, K., Kayden, H. J. *et al.* (1998). Ataxia with isolated vitamin E deficiency: heterogeneity of mutations and phenotypic variability in a large number of families. *Am. J. Hum. Genet.*, **62**, 301–10.

Chantrel-Groussard, K., Geromel, V., Puccio, H. *et al.* (2001). Disabled early recruitment of antioxidant defenses in Friedreich's ataxia. *Hum. Mol. Genet.*, **10**, 2061–7.

Chen, O. S., Hemenway, S. & Kaplan, J. (2002). Inhibition of Fe-S cluster biosynthesis decreases mitochondrial iron export: evidence that Yfh1p affects Fe-S cluster synthesis. *Proc. Natl Acad. Sci., USA*, **99**, 12321–6.

Cho, S. J., Lee, M. G., Yang, J. K., Lee, J. Y., Song, H. K. & Suh, S. W. (2000). Crystal structure of *Escherichia coli* CyaY protein reveals a previously unidentified fold for the evolutionarily conserved frataxin family. *Proc. Natl Acad. Sci., USA*, **97**, 8932–7.

Christodoulou, K., Deymeer, F., Serdaroglu, P. *et al.* (2001). Mapping of the second Friedreich's ataxia (FRDA2) locus to chromosome 9p23–p11: evidence for further locus heterogeneity. *Neurogenetics*, **3**, 127–32.

Cossee, M., Schmitt, M., Campuzano, V. *et al.* (1997). Evolution of the Friedreich's ataxia trinucleotide repeat expansion: founder effect and premutations. *Proc. Natl Acad. Sci., USA*, **94**, 7452–7.

Cossee, M., Durr, A., Schmitt, M. *et al.* (1999). Friedreich's ataxia: point mutations and clinical presentation of compound heterozygotes. *Ann. Neurol.*, **45**, 200–6.

Cossee, M., Puccio, H., Gansmuller, A. *et al.* (2000). Inactivation of the Friedreich ataxia mouse gene leads to early embryonic lethality without iron accumulation. *Hum. Mol. Genet.*, **9**, 1219–26.

Date, H., Onodera, O., Tanaka, H. *et al.* (2001). Early-onset ataxia with ocular motor apraxia and hypoalbuminemia is caused by mutations in a new HIT superfamily gene. *Nat. Genet.*, **29**, 184–8.

Delatycki, M. B., Camakaris, J., Brooks, H. *et al.* (1999a). Direct evidence that mitochondrial iron accumulation occurs in Friedreich ataxia. *Ann. Neurol.*, **45**, 673–5.

Delatycki, M. B., Paris, D. B., Gardner, R. J. *et al.* (1999b). Clinical and genetic study of Friedreich ataxia in an Australian population. *Am. J. Med. Genet.*, **87**, 168–74.

Dhe-Paganon, S., Shigeta, R., Chi, Y. I., Ristow, M. & Shoelson, S. E. (2000). Crystal structure of human frataxin. *J. Biol. Chem.*, **275**, 30753–6.

Durr, A., Cossee, M., Agid, Y. *et al.* (1996). Clinical and genetic abnormalities in patients with Friedreich's ataxia. *N. Engl. J. Med.*, **335**, 1169–75.

El Euch-Fayache, G., Lalani, I., Amouri, R. *et al.* (2003). Phenotypic features and genetic findings in sacsin related autosomal recessive ataxia in Tunisia. *Arch. Neurol.*, **60**, 982–8.

Emond, M., Lepage, G., Vanasse, M. & Pandolfo, M. (2000). Increased levels of plasma malondialdehyde in Friedreich ataxia. *Neurology*, **55**, 1752–3.

Engert, J. C., Berube, P., Mercier, J. *et al.* (2000). ARSACS, a spastic ataxia common in northeastern Quebec, is caused by mutations in a new gene encoding an 11.5-kb ORF. *Nat. Genet.*, **24**, 120–5.

Epplen, C., Epplen, J. T., Frank, G., Miterski, B., Santos, E. J. & Schols, L. (1997). Differential stability of the (GAA)n tract in the Friedreich ataxia (STM7) gene. *Hum. Genet.*, **99**, 834–6.

Filla, A., De Michele, G., Cavalcanti, F. *et al.* (1996). The relationship between trinucleotide (GAA) repeat length and clinical features in Friedreich ataxia. *Am. J. Hum. Genet.*, **59**, 554–60.

Finocchiaro, G., Baio, G., Micossi, P., Pozza, G. & di Donato, S. (1988). Glucose metabolism alterations in Friedreich's ataxia. *Neurology*, **38**, 1292–6.

Forrest, S. M., Knight, M., Delatycki, M. B. *et al.* (1998). The correlation of clinical phenotype in Friedreich ataxia with the site of point mutations in the FRDA gene. *Neurogenetics*, **1**, 253–7.

Foury, F. (1999). Low iron concentration and aconitase deficiency in a yeast frataxin homologue deficient strain. *FEBS Lett.*, **456**, 281–4.

Foury, F. & Cazzalini, O. (1997). Deletion of the yeast homologue of the human gene associated with Friedreich's ataxia elicits iron accumulation in mitochondria. *FEBS Lett.*, **411**, 373–7.

Foury, F. & Talibi, D. (2001). Mitochondrial control of iron homeostasis. A genome wide analysis of gene expression in a yeast frataxin-deficient strain. *J. Biol. Chem.*, **276**, 7762–8.

Friedreich, N. (1863a). Über degenerative Atrophie der spinalen Hinterstränge. *Virchows Arch. Pathol. Anat.*, **26**, 433–59.

Friedreich, N. (1863b). Über degenerative Atrophie der spinalen Hinterstränge. *Virchows Arch. Pathol. Anat.*, **27**, 1–26.

Geissler, A., Krimmer, T., Schonfisch, B., Meijer, M. & Rassow, J. (2000). Biogenesis of the yeast frataxin homolog Yfh1p. Tim44-dependent transfer to mtHsp70 facilitates folding of newly imported proteins in mitochondria. *Eur. J. Biochem.*, **267**, 3167–80.

Gellera, C., Pareyson, D., Castellotti, B. *et al.* (1997). Very late onset Friedreich's ataxia without cardiomyopathy is associated with limited GAA expansion in the X25 gene. *Neurology*, **49**, 1153–5.

Geschwind, D. H., Perlman, S., Grody, W. W. *et al.* (1997). Friedreich's ataxia GAA repeat expansion in patients with recessive or sporadic ataxia. *Neurology*, **49**, 1004–9.

Gibberd, F. B. & Wierzbicki, A. S. (2000). Heredopathia atactica polyneuritiformis – Refsum disease. In *Handbook of Ataxia Disorders*, Vol. 50, ed. T. Klockgether, New York: Marcel Dekker, pp. 235–256.

Gibson, T. J., Koonin, E. V., Musco, G., Pastore, A. & Bork, P. (1996). Friedreich's ataxia protein: phylogenetic evidence for mitochondrial dysfunction. *Trends Neurosci.*, **19**, 465–8.

Gotoda, T., Arita, M., Arai, H. *et al.* (1995). Adult-onset spinocerebellar dysfunction caused by a mutation in the gene for the alpha-tocopherol-transfer protein. *N. Engl. J. Med.*, **333**, 1313–18.

Gottdiener, J. S., Hawley, R. J., Maron, B. J., Bertorini, T. F. & Engle, W. K. (1982). Characteristics of the cardiac hypertrophy in Friedreich's ataxia. *Am. Heart J.*, **103**, 525–31.

Gucuyener, K., Ozgul, K., Paternotte, C. *et al.* (2001). Autosomal recessive spastic ataxia of Charlevoix-Saguenay in two unrelated Turkish families. *Neuropediatrics*, **32**, 142–6.

Hanna, M. G., Davis, M. B., Sweeney, M. G. *et al.* (1998). Generalized chorea in two patients harboring the Friedreich's ataxia gene trinucleotide repeat expansion. *Mov. Disord.*, **13**, 339–40.

Harding, A. E. (1981). Friedreich's ataxia: a clinical and genetic study of 90 families with an analysis of early diagnostic criteria and intrafamilial clustering of clinical features. *Brain*, **104**, 589–620.

Harding, A. E., Matthews, S., Jones, S., Ellis, C. J., Booth, I. W. & Muller, D. P. (1985). Spinocerebellar degeneration associated with a selective defect of vitamin E absorption. *N. Engl. J. Med.*, **313**, 32–5.

Hayes, J. D. & McLellan, L. I. (1999). Glutathione and glutathione-dependent enzymes represent a co-ordinately regulated defence against oxidative stress. *Free Radic. Res.*, **31**, 273–300.

Huynen, M. A., Snel, B., Bork, P. & Gibson, T. J. (2001). The phylogenetic distribution of frataxin indicates a role in iron–sulfur cluster protein assembly. *Hum. Mol. Genet.*, **10**, 2463–8.

Inoue, N., Izumi, K., Mawatari, S., Shida, K. & Kuroiwa, Y. (1971). Congenital ocular motor apraxia and cerebellar degeneration – report of two cases. *Rinsho Shinkeigaku*, **11**, 855–61.

Isnard, R., Kalotka, H., Durr, A. *et al.* (1997). Correlation between left ventricular hypertrophy and GAA trinucleotide repeat length in Friedreich's ataxia. *Circulation*, **95**, 2247–9.

Jampel, R. S. & Falls, H. F. (1958). Atypical retinitis pigmentosa, acanthocytosis, and heredodegenerative neuromuscular disease. *Arch. Ophthalmol.*, **59**, 818.

Jansen, G. A., Ofman, R., Ferdinandusse, S. *et al.* (1997). Refsum disease is caused by mutations in the phytanoyl-CoA hydroxylase gene. *Nat. Genet.*, **17**, 190–3.

Jiralerspong, S., Liu, Y., Montermini, L., Stifani, S. & Pandolfo, M. (1997). Frataxin shows developmentally regulated tissue-specific expression in the mouse embryo. *Neurobiol. Dis.*, **4**, 103–13.

Jiralerspong, S., Ge, B., Hudson, T. J. & Pandolfo, M. (2001). Manganese superoxide dismutase induction by iron is impaired in Friedreich ataxia cells. *FEBS Lett.*, **509**, 101–5.

Kallio, A. K. & Jauhiainen, T. (1985). A new syndrome of ophthalmoplegia, hypoacusis, ataxia, hypotonia and athetosis (OHAHA). *Adv. Audiol.*, **3**, 84–90.

Kane, J. P. & Havel, R. J. (2001). Disorders of the biogenesis and secretion of lipoproteins containing the B apolipoproteins. In *The Metabolic and Molecular Bases of Inherited Disease*, Vol. II ed. C. Scriver, A. Beaudet, W. Sly, & D. Valle, New York: McGraw-Hill, pp. 2717–52.

Kaptain, S., Downey, W. E., Tang, C. *et al.* (1991). A regulated RNA binding protein also possesses aconitase activity. *Proc. Natl Acad. Sci., USA*, **88**, 10109–13.

Kayden, H. J. (1993). The neurologic syndrome of vitamin E deficiency: a significant cause of ataxia. *Neurology*, **43**, 2167–9.

Kispal, G., Csere, P., Guiard, B. & Lill, R. (1997). The ABC transporter Atm1p is required for mitochondrial iron homeostasis. *FEBS Lett.*, **418**, 346–50.

Kispal, G., Csere, P., Prohl, C. & Lill, R. (1999). The mitochondrial proteins Atm1p and Nfs1p are essential for biogenesis of cytosolic Fe/S proteins. *Embo J.*, **18**, 3981–9.

Klenk, E. & Kahlke, W. (1963). Uber das Vorkommen der 3.7.11.15-Tetramethyl hexadecansäure (Phytansäure) in den Cholesterinestern und anderen Lipoidfraktionen der Organe bei einem Krankheitsfall unbekannter Genese (Verdacht auf Heredopathia Atactica Polyneuritiformis Refsum Syndrome). *Hoppe-Seyler Z. Physiol. Chem.*, **333**, 133–9.

Knight, S. A., Sepuri, N. B., Pain, D. & Dancis, A. (1998). Mt-Hsp70 homolog, Ssc2p, required for maturation of yeast frataxin and mitochondrial iron homeostasis. *J. Biol. Chem.*, **273**, 18389–93.

Kohlschutter, A., Hubner, C., Jansen, W. & Lindner, S. G. (1988). A treatable familial neuromyopathy with vitamin E deficiency, normal absorption, and evidence of increased consumption of vitamin E. *J. Inherit. Metab. Dis.*, **11**, 149–52.

Kohlschutter, A. (2000). Abetalipoproteinemia. In *Handbook of Ataxia Disorders*, Vol. 50, ed. T. Klockgether, New York: Marcel Dekker, pp. 205–21.

Koskinen, T., Santavuori, P., Sainio, K., Lappi, M., Kallio, A. K. & Pihko, H. (1994). Infantile onset spinocerebellar ataxia with sensory neuropathy: a new inherited disease. *J. Neurol. Sci.*, **121**, 50–6.

Koutnikova, H., Campuzano, V., Foury, F., Dolle, P., Cazzalini, O. & Koenig, M. (1997). Studies of human, mouse and yeast homologues indicate a mitochondrial function for frataxin. *Nat. Genet.*, **16**, 345–51.

Koutnikova, H., Campuzano, V. & Koenig, M. (1998). Maturation of wild-type and mutated frataxin by the mitochondrial processing peptidase. *Hum. Mol. Genet.*, **7**, 1485–9.

Lamarche, J. B., Shapcott, D., Cote, M. & Lemieux, B. (1993). Cardiac iron deposits in Friedreich's ataxia. In *Handbook of Cerebellar Diseases*, ed. R. Lechtenberg NY: Marcel Dekker, Inc. pp. 453–8.

Lamont, P. J., Davis, M. B. & Wood, N. W. (1997). Identification and sizing of the GAA trinucleotide repeat expansion of Friedreich's ataxia in 56 patients. Clinical and genetic correlates. *Brain*, **120**, 673–80.

Laplante, P., Vanasse, M., Michaud, J., Geoffroy, G. & Brochu, P. (1984). A progressive neurological syndrome associated with an isolated vitamin E deficiency. *Can. J. Neurol. Sci.*, **11**, 561–4.

Larnaout, A., Belal, S., Zouari, M. *et al.* (1997). Friedreich's ataxia with isolated vitamin E deficiency: a neuropathological study of a Tunisian patient. *Acta Neuropathol. (Berl.)*, **93**, 633–7.

Levi, S., Corsi, B., Bosisio, M. *et al.* (2001). A human mitochondrial ferritin encoded by an intronless gene. *J. Biol. Chem.*, **276**, 24437–40.

Lodi, R., Hart, P. E., Rajagopalan, B. *et al.* (2001). Antioxidant treatment improves in vivo cardiac and skeletal muscle bioenergetics in patients with Friedreich's ataxia. *Ann. Neurol.*, **49**, 590–6.

Lonnqvist, T., Paetau, A., Nikali, K., von Boguslawski, K. & Pihko, H. (1998). Infantile onset spinocerebellar ataxia with sensory neuropathy (IOSCA): neuropathological features. *J. Neurol. Sci.*, **161**, 57–65.

Lonnqvist, T., Paetau, A., Pihko, H. & Nikali, K. (2000). Infantile-onset spinocerebellar ataxia. In *Handbook of Ataxia Disorders*, Vol. 50, ed. T. Klockgether, New York: Marcel Dekker, pp. 293–309.

Lutz, T., Westermann, B., Neupert, W. & Herrmann, J. M. (2001). The mitochondrial proteins Ssq1 and Jac1 are required for the assembly of iron sulfur clusters in mitochondria. *J. Mol. Biol.*, **307**, 815–25.

Martinello, F., Fardin, P., Ottina, M. *et al.* (1998). Supplemental therapy in isolated vitamin E deficiency improves the peripheral neuropathy and prevents the progression of ataxia. *J. Neurol. Sci.*, **156**, 177–9.

McCabe, D. J., Ryan, F., Moore, D. P. *et al.* (2000). Typical Friedreich's ataxia without GAA expansions and GAA expansion without typical Friedreich's ataxia. *J. Neurol.*, **247**, 346–55.

Mihalik, S. J., Morrell, J. C., Kim, D., Sacksteder, K. A., Watkins, P. A. & Gould, S. J. (1997). Identification of PAHX, a Refsum disease gene. *Nat. Genet.*, **17**, 185–9.

Miranda, C. J., Santos, M. M., Ohshima, K. *et al.* (2002). Frataxin knockin mouse. *FEBS Lett.*, **512**, 291–7.

Monros, E., Molto, M. D., Martinez, F. *et al.* (1997). Phenotype correlation and intergenerational dynamics of the Friedreich ataxia GAA trinucleotide repeat. *Am. J. Hum. Genet.*, **61**, 101–10.

Montermini, L., Andermann, E., Labuda, M. *et al.* (1997a). The Friedreich ataxia GAA triplet repeat: premutation and normal alleles. *Hum. Mol. Genet.*, **6**, 1261–6.

Montermini, L., Richter, A., Morgan, K. *et al.* (1997b). Phenotypic variability in Friedreich ataxia: role of the associated GAA triplet repeat expansion. *Ann. Neurol.*, **41**, 675–82.

Moreira, M. C., Barbot, C., Tachi, N. *et al.* (2001a). Homozygosity mapping of Portuguese and Japanese forms of ataxia-oculomotor apraxia to 9p13, and evidence for genetic heterogeneity. *Am. J. Hum. Genet.*, **68**, 501–8.

Moreira, M. C., Barbot, C., Tachi, N. *et al.* (2001b). The gene mutated in ataxia – ocular apraxia 1 encodes the new HIT/Zn-finger protein aprataxin. *Nat. Genet.*, **29**, 189–93.

Morvan, D., Komajda, M., Doan, L. D. *et al.* (1992). Cardiomyopathy in Friedreich's ataxia: a Doppler-echocardiographic study. *Eur. Heart J.*, **13**, 1393–8.

Mrissa, N., Belal, S., Hamida, C. B. *et al.* (2000). Linkage to chromosome 13q11–12 of an autosomal recessive cerebellar ataxia in a Tunisian family. *Neurology*, **54**, 1408–14.

Muhlenhoff, U., Richhardt, N., Ristow, M., Kispal, G. & Lill, R. (2002). The yeast frataxin homolog Yfh1p plays a specific role in the maturation of cellular Fe/S proteins. *Hum. Mol. Genet.*, **11**, 2025–36.

Musco, G., Stier, G., Kolmerer, B. *et al.* (2000). Towards a structural understanding of Friedreich's ataxia: the solution structure of frataxin. *Structure Fold Des.*, **8**, 695–707.

Nemeth, A. H., Bochukova, E., Dunne, E. *et al.* (2000). Autosomal recessive cerebellar ataxia with oculomotor apraxia (ataxia-telangiectasia-like syndrome) is linked to chromosome 9q34. *Am. J. Hum. Genet.*, **67**, 1320–6.

Nikali, K., Suomalainen, A., Terwilliger, J., Koskinen, T., Weissenbach, J. & Peltonen, L. (1995). Random search for shared chromosomal regions in four affected individuals: the assignment of a new hereditary ataxia locus. *Am. J. Hum. Genet.*, **56**, 1088–95.

Nikali, K., Isosomppi, J., Lonnqvist, T., Mao, J. I., Suomalainen, A. & Peltonen, L. (1997). Toward cloning of a novel ataxia gene: refined assignment and physical map of the IOSCA locus (SCA8) on 10q24. *Genomics*, **39**, 185–91.

Ohshima, K., Montermini, L., Wells, R. D. & Pandolfo, M. (1998). Inhibitory effects of expanded GAA.TTC triplet repeats from intron I of the Friedreich ataxia gene on transcription and replication in vivo. *J. Biol. Chem.*, **273**, 14588–95.

Oppenheimer, D. & Esiri, M. (1992). *Disease of the Basal Ganglia, Cerebellum and Motor Neurons*, ed. Adams, J. H., Corsellis, J. A. N., Duchen, L. W., London: Arnold, p. 1015.

Ouahchi, K., Arita, M., Kayden, H. *et al.* (1995). Ataxia with isolated vitamin E deficiency is caused by mutations in the alpha-tocopherol transfer protein. *Nat. Genet.*, **9**, 141–5.

Pandolfo, M. (1997). Friedreich's ataxia. *Current Neurology*, **17**, 47–78.

Park, S., Gakh, O., Mooney, S. M. & Isaya, G. (2002). The ferroxidase activity of yeast frataxin. *J. Biol. Chem.*, **277**, 38589–95.

Pasternac, A., Krol, R., Petitclerc, R., Harvey, C., Andermann, E. & Barbeau, A. (1980). Hypertrophic cardiomyopathy in Friedreich's ataxia: symmetric or asymmetric? *Can. J. Neurol. Sci.*, **7**, 379–82.

Peyronnard, J. M., Charron, L. & Barbeau, A. (1979). The neuropathy of Charlevoix-Saguenay ataxia: an electrophysiological and pathological study. *Can. J. Neurol. Sci.*, **6**, 199–203.

Piemonte, F., Pastore, A., Tozzi, G. *et al.* (2001). Glutathione in blood of patients with Friedreich's ataxia. *Eur. J. Clin. Invest.*, **31**, 1007–11.

Pook, M. A., Al-Mahdawi, S., Carroll, C. J. *et al.* (2001). Rescue of the Friedreich's ataxia knockout mouse by human YAC transgenesis. *Neurogenetics*, **3**, 185–93.

Priller, J., Scherzer, C. R., Faber, P. W., MacDonald, M. E. & Young, A. B. (1997). Frataxin gene of Friedreich's ataxia is targeted to mitochondria. *Ann. Neurol.*, **42**, 265–9.

Puccio, H., Simon, D., Cossee, M. et al. (2001). Mouse models for Friedreich ataxia exhibit cardiomyopathy, sensory nerve defect and Fe–S enzyme deficiency followed by intramitochondrial iron deposits. Nat. Genet., 27, 181–6.

Radisky, D. C., Babcock, M. C. & Kaplan, J. (1999). The yeast frataxin homologue mediates mitochondrial iron efflux. Evidence for a mitochondrial iron cycle. J. Biol. Chem., 274, 4497–9.

Ragno, M., De Michele, G., Cavalcanti, F. et al. (1997). Broadened Friedreich's ataxia phenotype after gene cloning. Minimal GAA expansion causes late-onset spastic ataxia. Neurology, 49, 1617–20.

Refsum, S. (1946). Heredopathia atactica polyneuritiformis. A familial syndrome not hitherto described. A contribution to the clinical study of the hereditary disorders of the nervous system. Acta Psychiatr. Scand., Suppl 38.

Richter, A., Rioux, J. D., Bouchard, J. P. et al. (1999). Location score and haplotype analyses of the locus for autosomal recessive spastic ataxia of Charlevoix-Saguenay, in chromosome region 13q11. Am. J. Hum. Genet., 64, 768–75.

Riva, A. & Bradac, G. B. (1995). Primary cerebellar and spinocerebellar ataxia: an MRI study on 63 cases. J. Neuroradiol., 22, 71–6.

Rotig, A., de Lonlay, P., Chretien, D. et al. (1997). Aconitase and mitochondrial iron–sulphur protein deficiency in Friedreich ataxia. Nat. Genet., 17, 215–17.

Rustin, P., Munnich, A. & Rotig, A. (1999a). Quinone analogs prevent enzymes targeted in Friedreich ataxia from iron-induced injury in vitro. Biofactors, 9, 247–51.

Rustin, P., von Kleist-Retzow, J. C., Chantrel-Groussard, K., Sidi, D., Munnich, A. & Rotig, A. (1999b). Effect of idebenone on cardiomyopathy in Friedreich's ataxia: a preliminary study. Lancet, 354, 477–9.

Rustin, P., Rotig, A., Munnich, A. & Sidi, D. (2002). Heart hypertrophy and function are improved by idebenone in Friedreich's ataxia. Free Radic. Res., 36, 467–9.

Said, G., Marion, M., Selva, J. & Jamet, C. (1986). Hypotrophic and dying-back nerve fibers in Friedreich's ataxia. Neurology, 36, 1292.

Sakamoto, N., Chastain, P. D., Parniewski, P. et al. (1999). Sticky DNA: self-association properties of long GAA.TTC repeats in R.R.Y triplex structures from Friedreich's ataxia. Mol. Cell., 3, 465–75.

Sakamoto, N., Ohshima, K., Montermini, L., Pandolfo, M. & Wells, R. D. (2001). Sticky DNA, a self-associated complex formed at long GAA*TTC repeats in intron 1 of the frataxin gene, inhibits transcription. J. Biol. Chem., 276, 27171–7.

Sato, Y., Hagiwara, K., Arai, H. & Inoue, K. (1991). Purification and characterization of the alpha-tocopherol transfer protein from rat liver. FEBS Lett., 288, 41–5.

Schoenle, E. J., Boltshauser, E. J., Baekkeskov, S., Landin Olsson, M., Torresani, T. & von Felten, A. (1989). Preclinical and manifest diabetes mellitus in young patients with Friedreich's ataxia: no evidence of immune process behind the islet cell destruction. Diabetologia, 32, 378–81.

Schols, L., Amoiridis, G., Przuntek, H., Frank, G., Epplen, J. T. & Epplen, C. (1997). Friedreich's ataxia. Revision of the phenotype according to molecular genetics. Brain, 120, 2131–40.

Schuelke, M., Mayatepek, E., Inter, M. et al. (1999). Treatment of ataxia in isolates' vitamin E deficiency caused by alpha-tocopherol transfer protein deficiency. J. Pediatr., 134, 240–4.

Schulz, J. B., Dehmer, T., Schols, L. et al. (2000). Oxidative stress in patients with Friedreich ataxia. Neurology, 55, 1719–21.

Sharp, D., Blinderman, L., Combs, K. A. et al. (1993). Cloning and gene defects in microsomal triglyceride transfer protein associated with abetalipoproteinaemia. Nature, 365, 65–9.

Shimohata, T., Date, H., Ishiguro, H. et al. (1998). Ataxia with isolated vitamin E deficiency and retinitis pigmentosa. Ann. Neurol., 43, 273.

Shoulders, C. C., Brett, D. J., Bayliss, J. D. et al. (1993). Abetalipoproteinemia is caused by defects of the gene encoding the 97 kDa subunit of a microsomal triglyceride transfer protein. Hum. Mol. Genet., 2, 2109–16.

Stumpf, D. A., Sokol, R., Bettis, D. et al. (1987). Friedreich's disease: V. Variant form with vitamin E deficiency and normal fat absorption. Neurology, 37, 68–74.

Takashima, H., Boerkoel, C. F., John, J. et al. (2002). Mutation of TDP1, encoding a topoisomerase 1-dependent DNA damage repair enzyme, in spinocerebellar ataxia with axonal neuropathy. Nat. Genet., 32, 267–72.

Taylor, A. M., McConville, C. M., Rotman, G., Shiloh, Y. & Byrd, P. J. (1994). A haplotype common to intermediate radiosensitivity variants of ataxia-telangiectasia in the UK. Int. J. Radiat. Biol., 66, S35–41.

Taylor, A. M., Metcalfe, J. A., Thick, J. & Mak, Y. F. (1996). Leukemia and lymphoma in ataxia telangiectasia. Blood, 87, 423–38.

Traber, M. G., Sokol, R. J., Burton, G. W. et al. (1990). Impaired ability of patients with familial isolated vitamin E deficiency to incorporate alpha-tocopherol into lipoproteins secreted by the liver. J. Clin. Invest., 85, 397–407.

Traber, M. G., Sokol, R. J., Kohlschutter, A. et al. (1993). Impaired discrimination between stereoisomers of alpha-tocopherol in patients with familial isolated vitamin E deficiency. J. Lipid. Res., 34, 201–10.

Traber, M. G., Ramakrishnan, R. & Kayden, H. J. (1994). Human plasma vitamin E kinetics demonstrate rapid recycling of plasma RRR-alpha-tocopherol. Proc. Natl Acad. Sci., USA, 91, 10005–8.

Trabert, W., Stober, T., Mielke, U., Heck, F. S. & Schimrigk, K. (1989). [Isolated vitamin E deficiency]. Fortschr. Neurol. Psychiatr., 57, 495–501.

Tranchant, C., Fleury, M., Moreira, M. C., Koenig, M. & Warter, J. M. (2003). Phenotypic variability of aprataxin gene mutations. Neurology, 60, 868–70.

Uekawa, K., Yuasa, T., Kawasaki, S., Makibuchi, T. & Ideta, T. (1992). [A hereditary ataxia associated with hypoalbuminemia and hyperlipidemia – a variant form of Friedreich's disease of a new clinical entity?]. Rinsho Shinkeigaku, 32, 1067–74.

van Bogaert, L. & Martin, L. (1974). Optic and cochleovestibular degenerations in the hereditary ataxias. I. Clinico-pathological and genetic aspects. *Brain*, **97**, 15–40.

Waldvogel, D., Gelderen, P. V. & Hallett, M. (1999). Increased iron in the dentate nucleus of patients with Friedreich's ataxia. *Annals in Neurology*, **46**, 123–5.

Watanabe, M., Sugai, Y., Concannon, P. *et al.* (1998). Familial spinocerebellar ataxia with cerebellar atrophy, peripheral neuropathy, and elevated level of serum creatine kinase, gamma-globulin, and alpha-fetoprotein. *Ann. Neurol.*, **44**, 265–9.

Wetterau, J. R., Aggerbeck, L. P., Bouma, M. E. *et al.* (1992). Absence of microsomal triglyceride transfer protein in individuals with abetalipoproteinemia. *Science*, **258**, 999–1001.

Wilson, R. B. & Roof, D. M. (1997). Respiratory deficiency due to loss of mitochondrial DNA in yeast lacking the frataxin homologue. *Nat. Genet.*, **16**, 352–7.

Wilson, R. B., Lynch, D. R. & Fischbeck, K. H. (1998). Normal serum iron and ferritin concentrations in patients with Friedreich's ataxia. *Ann. Neurol.*, **44**, 132–4.

Wilson, R. B., Lynch, D. R., Farmer, J. M., Brooks, D. G. & Fischbeck, K. H. (2000). Increased serum transferrin receptor concentrations in Friedreich ataxia. *Ann. Neurol.*, **47**, 659–61.

Yokota, T., Wada, Y., Furukawa, T., Tsukagoshi, H., Uchihara, T. & Watabiki, S. (1987). Adult-onset spinocerebellar syndrome with idiopathic vitamin E deficiency. *Ann. Neurol.*, **22**, 84–7.

Yokota, T., Shiojiri, T., Gotoda, T. *et al.* (1997). Friedreich-like ataxia with retinitis pigmentosa caused by the His101Gln mutation of the alpha-tocopherol transfer protein gene. *Ann. Neurol.*, **41**, 826–32.

Zouari, M., Feki, M., Ben Hamida, C. *et al.* (1998). Electrophysiology and nerve biopsy: comparative study in Friedreich's ataxia and Friedreich's ataxia phenotype with vitamin E deficiency. *Neuromuscul. Disord.*, **8**, 416–25.

49

Ataxia telangiectasia

Richard A. Gatti[1], Tom O. Crawford[2], Alan S. Mandir[2], Susan Perlman[3] and Howard T. J. Mount[4]

[1]Department of Pathology and Laboratory Medicine, David Geffen School of Medicine at UCLA, Los Angeles, CA, USA
[2]Department of Neurology, Johns Hopkins University School of Medicine, Baltimore, MD, USA
[3]Department of Neurology, David Geffen School of Medicine at UCLA, Los Angeles, CA, USA
[4]CRND, Department of Medicine, Division of Neurology, University of Toronto, Toronto, ON, Canada

Ataxia-telangiectasia (A-T) is an autosomal recessive disorder associated with abnormal function of the nervous, immune and endocrine systems. It was initially described by Syllaba and Henner (1926) and was more completely characterized by Boder and Sedgwick (1958), who also coined the name. The disorder is characterized by a progressive gait and truncal ataxia, immunodeficiency, thymic degeneration, chromosomal instability, predisposition to lymphoreticular malignancies and hypersensitivity to ionizing radiation (for review see Boder, 1985; Gatti et al., 1991; Sedgwick & Boder, 1991; Woods & Taylor, 1992; Gatti, 2002).

Early research into the genetic cause of A-T suggested the presence of as many as four different responsible genes since fusion of fibroblasts from various A-T patients were able to complement one another in radiation sensitivity assays (Jaspers et al., 1988). However, all four groups were subsequently found to have loss-of-function mutations in a single gene, named ATM (ataxia-telangiectasia mutated), located on chromosome 11q22.3 (Gatti et al., 1988; Savitsky et al., 1995).

The ATM protein is a serine/threonine kinase responsible for maintaining genomic integrity by triggering arrest of the cell cycle, increasing transcription of stress response genes, and repair of double strand breaks in DNA (Shiloh, 2003). Among the many identified substrates are p53, p53BP, MDM2, Chk2, nibrin, Mre11, H2AX, SMC1, Pin2/TRF1, FANCD2, MDC1, and BRCA1. A-T patients express a functionally deficient ATM message, with diminished or absent levels of ATM protein (Chun et al., 2003). How mutations in ATM result in radiation hypersensitivity or neuronal integrity remains unclear. The function of the ATM protein is addressed in greater detail in Chapter 10.

Neuropathogenesis

The most prominent neuropathologic hallmark of A-T is a marked loss of cerebellar Purkinje and granule neurons. Dendritic arbors of the few remaining Purkinje cells are often abnormal, with abnormal proximal branching of the primary dendrite, reduced secondary and tertiary branching, or both (Fig. 49.1). Shrinkage of the cell soma and "torpedo" formation swelling of the axons are commonly found. Purkinje cell migrational defects are suggested by an increase in the proportion of ectopic cells in the molecular and granule cell layers. However, the majority of Purkinje cells are believed to migrate correctly to the Purkinje cell layer before degenerating. This conclusion is supported by the appropriate positioning of many empty basket cell processes that cradle the Purkinje cell soma only upon its migration into the Purkinje cell layer (Vinters et al., 1985; Gatti et al., 1985). Loss of the granule cells, manifested by thinning of the densely packed granule cell layer, parallels the loss of Purkinje cells. Granule cells synapse upon the Purkinje cell dendritic arbor within the molecular layer, and the loss of either of these cell groups may represent the primary effect of the loss of ATM protein. Reduced numbers of interneurons in the molecular layer and reduced neurons in deep cerebellar nuclei are also observed. Reactive astrocytes and activated microglia have also been observed in the cerebellar white matter, implicating an immune response in the degeneration.

How mutations in ATM result in specific neurologic phenotypes remains under investigation. ATM protein recognizes DNA damage probably to signal other proteins that facilitate DNA repair. Consistent with this function, in situ hybridization has shown that ATM mRNA is confined to subpopulations of cells within highly proliferative zones

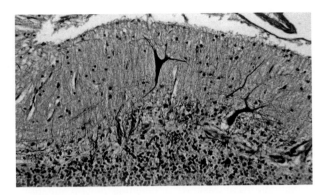

Fig. 49.1 Immunohistochemistry on A-T cerebellum shows depletion and dysmorphology of Purkinje cells, with loss of secondary and tertiary arborization. An ectopic Purkinje cell is visible in the centre of the field.

of the brain early in mouse development (Becker-Catania *et al.*, 2000). *ATM* expression is at its peak during embryonic stages during the genesis of early cerebellar and other neuronal precursors. ATM likely has the same critical role of DNA damage surveillance in these proliferating neuroepithelial cells, that later migrate throughout the brain and differentiate into multiple neuronal types. At postnatal times, however, *ATM* expression in the brain is quite low, even in the cerebellar Purkinje and granule cells where neurodegeneration is most prominent. It has yet to be demonstrated that ATM has the same function within postmitotic neurons, but some evidence has suggested that the ATM protein may play a neuroprotective role in tissues undergoing oxidative stress (Barlow *et al.*, 1999).

It is also possible that multiple isoforms of the ATM protein exist. This is suggested by the preponderance of weak splice junctions in the *ATM* gene (Eng *et al.*, 2004). Extensive alternative splicing of large genes, such as *Dscam* (with over 38 000 possible isoforms), has proved important in axonal targeting of olfactory receptor neurons (Hummel *et al.*, 2003). ATM could play a similar role in brain development, in addition to its role as a hierarchical cell signaling kinase.

Mice with targeted knockouts of the *ATM* gene (Barlow *et al.*, 1996; Elson *et al.*, 1996; Xu *et al.*, 1996; Borghesani *et al.*, 2000) exhibit a phenotype that recapitulates many aspects of the human disease, including immune system defects and predisposition to cancer. The cellular phenotype of these mice also includes radiation sensitivity and cell cycle defects. However, the *ATM* $^{-/-}$ (ATM-KO) mice exhibit no obvious neuropathological changes and only mild behavioral disturbances (Barlow *et al.*, 1996; Borghesani *et al.*, 2000; Mount *et al.*, 2004). Atm-KO cerebella display elevated markers of oxidative stress (Barlow *et al.*, 1999;

Quick & Dugan, 2001; Kamsler *et al.*, 2001), increased lysosomes (Barlow *et al.*, 2000) and subtle alteration of synaptic activity (Chiesa *et al.*, 2000), but not the extensive loss of Purkinje cells, thinning of the granule cell layer or gliosis consistently observed in postmortem A-T brain.

Reduced tyrosine hydroxylase and dopamine transporter immunolabeling in the nigrostriatal system of certain Atm-KO mice suggested that the sensorimotor phenotype might be caused by a reduction in dopaminergic transmission (Eilam *et al.*, 1998), an hypothesis consistent with clinical evidence for non-cerebellar extrapyramidal involvement in the human disease (for review see Mount *et al.*, 2002). However, L-DOPA was subsequently found to produce no short-term benefit in clinical trials and neurochemical measurements in behaviorally impaired Atm-KO mice revealed no depletion in catecholamine levels, or turnover in the striatum, ventral mesencephalon, or cerebellum (Mount *et al.*, 2004).

Alternatively, the behavioral phenotype of Atm-KO mice could arise as a consequence of changes in the peripheral nervous system. In support of this notion, *Atm* mRNA is expressed at very low levels in the CNS, but at high levels selectively in sensory neurons of the mature dorsal root ganglion (Soares *et al.*, 1998). In the *dystonia musculorum (dt)* mouse, degeneration of the dorsal root ganglion causes an ataxic condition that is due to the loss of spinocerebellar input, rather than to any direct effect on Purkinje cells (Sotelo & Guenet, 1988; Lalonde *et al.*, 1994). Peripheral neuropathy is common in A-T patients, but it appears relatively later than the other more profound motor impairments, and hence likely does not have a primary role.

Molecular genetics

A specific mutation within the *ATM* gene may confer a milder or more severe disease phenotype (McConville *et al.*, 1996; Gilad *et al.*, 1998; Stankovic *et al.*, 1998; Stewart *et al.*, 2001). The large size of the *ATM* gene along with the fact that mutations occur throughout the 62 coding exons of the gene, prevents direct sequencing as a cost-effective approach for A-T diagnosis. The additional problems of false positives that would result from polymorphisms also reduces this feasibility (Concannon & Gatti, 1997; Mitui *et al.*, 2003; Bernstein *et al.*, 2003).

A-T patients who are not from consanguineous families, carry 2 different mutations in the *ATM* gene, one from each parent. Thus, they are "compound" heterozygotes. A large majority of *ATM* mutations are null mutations resulting in undetectable ATM protein levels (Chun *et al.*, 2003; Butch *et al.*, 2004). Despite this, mRNA levels are abundant in virtually all A-T patients studied to date. Most *ATM* mutations lead to premature termination codons, or mutations that delete portions of the message (Telatar *et al.*, 1996; Teraoka *et al.*, 1999; Mitui *et al.*, 2003). Also included in this group of mutations are those that alter splicing motifs and result in the skipping of certain exons or parts of exons (Eng *et al.*, 2004). More rarely, mutations may result in psuedo-exons, (i.e. insertion of intronic regions into the mRNA). These also result in downstream frameshifts and premature termination codons (McConville *et al.*, 1996; Pagani *et al.*, 2002; Eng *et al.*, 2004).

Missense mutations that change the amino acid sequence account for less than 10% of A-T cases. However, some of these missense mutations may in fact act via exon splice enhancer (ESE) and exon splice silencer (ESS) motifs that alter preRNA splicing (Eng *et al.*, 2004; Coutinho *et al.*, 2004). Thus, the frequency of *ATM* missense mutations is likely to be lower than current estimates.

ATM mutations are mostly detected by serial testing of the DNA and RNA from lymphoblastoid cells (LCL) (Mitui *et al.*, 2003; Coutinho *et al.*, 2004). The large size of *ATM* has made screeing for mutations difficult, and several strategies are used by different laboratories. A useful approach is to first identify the *ATM* haplotype using four very informative microsatellite short tandem repeat (STR) markers: S1819, NS22, S2179 and S1818. The alleles for each marker are carefully standardized so that haplotypes are compared to a global database of affected haplotypes from more than 500 A-T patients (Mitui *et al.*, 2003) (see also www.benaroyaresearch.org/bri_investigators/atm.htm).
Further identification techniques include ascertaining SNP (single nucleotide polymorphism) haplotypes across the region of the *ATM* gene (Campbell *et al.*, 2003). Once the *ATM* haplotypes have been identified, the mutations most commonly associated with a given haplotype can be checked quickly by single stranded conformational polymorphism (SSCP)(see below). Approximately 30% of all new patients have mutations within previously defined haplotypes, a probability that increases to as high as 95% in certain well-studied ethnic groups, such as Costa Rica, Norway, Spain, Brazil, Poland or Turkey (Telatar *et al.*, 1996, 1998a,b; Mitui *et al.*, 2003; Coutinho *et al.*, 2004) and other genetically isolated populations, such as the Amish, Mennonite, or Moroccan Jews. On the other hand, the percentage of *ATM* mutations that can be identified by this haplotype-shortcut decreases as the genetic heterogeneity of a population increases. For example, the American population typifies a genetically heterogeneous population in which the identification of *ATM* mutations by standardized haplotyping is not particularly efficient (Mitui *et al.*, 2003).

If common *ATM* mutations are not identified by haplotyping, RNA is collected from the patient's LCL, converted to cDNA, and screened first by protein truncation testing (PTT). This gel-based method efficiently identifies the position of truncating mutations (i.e. those leading to premature stop codons) in fragments of approximately 1500 nucleotide length (Telatar *et al.*, 1996). Thus, by studying only eight overlapping fragments, the entire *ATM* transcript (9168 nucleotides) can be screened in a single experiment. Overall, 70% of all *ATM* mutations in A-T patients are detected by this method, although this excludes missense mutations. In contrast, when screening for *ATM* mutations in breast cancer patients, which are primarily of the missense type, PTT is not an efficient method (FitzGerald *et al.*, 1997).

SSCP is a method that detects all types of mutations in fragments of less than 300 nucleotide length. This alternate method is used when a suspected A-T patient does not demonstrate mutations by PTT screening. Screening the ATM cDNA with SSCP involves analysis of 34 overlapping fragments. Twenty patients can be screened for 3 fragments on a single gel (Castellvi-Bel *et al.*, 1999). Detection efficiency of SSCP approximates 80%.

Denatured high-performance liquid chromatography (dHPLC) uses genomic DNA and is a more automated screening method, involving capillary gel electrophoresis. However, interpretation of the resulting chromatogram for each segment requires considerable expertise, varies slightly from one apparatus to another, and is difficult to validate for clinical application. The 62 coding exons, and approximately 50 nucleotides of flanking intronic DNA are PCR-amplified and allowed to form heteroduplexes – these would arise if the patient were heterozygous for a mutation in a particular region of the gene (Thorstenson *et al.*, 2001; Bernstein *et al.*, 2003). Inclusion of flanking intronic DNA in each heteroduplex allows for the identification of splice site mutations. In those patients from consanguineous matings (who would be expected to be homozygous for an *ATM* mutation) heteroduplexes cannot form and the mutation cannot be detected by dHPLC unless additional DNA from a normal person is added to the test sample. The efficiency of dHPLC for detecting *ATM* mutations approximates 85% (Bernstein *et al.*, 2003).

When an abnormal pattern is detected by any of the above methods, the suspect region is sequenced to identify the specific genomic mutation. When all these methods are used serially, the detection efficiency approximates 95% for the *ATM* gene (Mitui *et al.*, 2003). The missing 5% reflects the fact that each of these methods depends upon PCR amplification across only exons and the immediately adjacent sequences, leaving large stretches of intron sequences or the upstream or downstream regulatory regions of the gene unamplified and unstudied. This is primarily because these regions are very large (>90% of the *ATM* gene) and the yield of mutations in these regions is low. Furthermore, limited understanding of these regions of most genes makes it difficult to interpret the functional significance of DNA changes at specific sites. Other missed *ATM* mutations involve large deletion and duplication rearrangements within the *ATM* gene that are masked by the other allele.

Correlating phenotype with specific genotype is in progress, now that both mutations have been identified in a large proportion of patients. To date, only a handful of mutations seem to correlate with phenotypic variations of the classical A-T syndrome, as defined by Boder and Sedgwick (1958). These include: IVS40+1126A>G (McConville *et al.*, 1996) and the 7271T>G (Stankovic *et al.*, 1998; Stewart *et al.*, 2001) mutations. These mutations are associated with slower progression of neurological symptoms, extended life span, and possibly less radiation sensitivity.

Clinical aspects

The onset of unsteadiness and truncal ataxia is generally detected before 3 years of age (Boder & Sedgwick, 1958; Gatti *et al.*, 1991; Gatti, 2002) and head-tilting is sometimes noted as early as 6 months. Ocular motor apraxia, which refers to an incoordination of eye and head movement with shift of gaze in the horizontal axis, generally first appears in early school years (Lewis *et al.*, 1999). Slurred speech is obvious before 5 years. However, the characteristic oculocutaneous telangiectasia are not observed until many of the neurologic symptoms are well established. Most children benefit from the assistance of a wheelchair by the age of 11. In the late teen years, the rate of neurological deterioration appears to slow: whether this is by actual slowing of the underlying pathology or by an increasing ability to cope with the progressive deficits is not clear. Impaired control of head movement and difficulties in swallowing and coughing lead to problems of aspiration, pneumonia, and sinopulmonary infections with non-opportunistic organisms. Whether immunodeficiency adds to the pathogenesis of lung disease is also unclear; pneumonia in older individuals does not appear to correlate with any other laboratory measure of immune function.

Children with A-T have poor articulation of speech, difficulty with handwriting, reading, and mobility, leading to a lifelong dependency for activities of daily living. Mental status is normal in most cases, and in some cases patients have been able to complete a university-level education. Life expectancy varies, some patients living into the sixth decade. This appears to have changed dramatically over the past 30 years, for unknown reasons. The two main causes of death are malignancy and pneumonia, with another group succumbing to a wide variety of complications. Malignancies, chiefly lymphoreticular, may arise at any age. In many cases pneumonia may be due to chronic aspiration secondary to swallowing dysfunction. A few patients have had fatal reactions to radiation therapy for their malignancies (Gotoff *et al.*, 1967; Gatti, 2002). Because the malignancy sometimes precedes any obvious neurological impairment, it is recommended that a diagnosis of A-T be considered in *all* very young cancer patients before the age when neurodegeneration is prominent, in order to prevent complications of excessive radiation.

Cancer susceptibility

Malignancies in A-T are common, affecting approximately one-third of patients (Swift *et al.*, 1976). Lymphomas and leukemias are the predominate forms of malignancy (Gatti & Good, 1971; Spector *et al.*, 1982; Su & Swift, 2000). Younger children are more likely to develop common acute lymphocytic leukemia, while older children also develop TCL-1 expressing T-prolymphocytic leukemia (formerly called T-CLL) (Chun *et al.*, 2002). Both T-cell and B-cell lymphomas occur. Older patients may also develop non-lymphoid cancers including stomach, breast, basal cell, ovarian, liver, and uterine cancers, as well as melanoma (Su & Swift, 2000). The inherent sensitivity of A-T patients to radiation therapy and chemotherapy has complicated therapy (Gotoff *et al.*, 1967; Gatti, 2002).

Whether heterozygotes for *ATM* mutations demonstrate increased propensities for malignancy is still being investigated. *ATM* heterozygotes may account for about 5% of familial breast cancer (Swift *et al.*, 1991; Gatti *et al.*, 1999), a level greater than the 1–2% that is attributable to mutations in *BRCA1* and *BRCA2* (Chevenix-Trench *et al.*, 2002). *ATM* mutation frequencies vary from 2–16% for various breast cancer cohort studies, with relative risks approximating four times that of the general population. However, estimates of risk are influenced greatly by study designs, age of onset of cancer, and penetrance estimates, and large statistical confidence intervals complicate the interpretation of such results.

The spectra of *ATM* mutations for A-T patients versus unrelated breast cancer patients appears to differ dramatically (Gatti *et al.*, 1999; Concannon 2002). The frequencies of missense and nonsense mutations in breast cancer cohort studies are 15% nonsense and 85% missense, respectively. In contrast, in A-T patients, approximately 90% of mutations are of the nonsense (null) type, while only about 10% are of the missense type. Furthermore, breast cancer patients in cohorts who are heterozygous for *ATM* mutations do not seem to have any relatives with A-T. Thus, study design biases which types of *ATM* mutations are found. It was hypothesized that heterozygosity for some missense mutations may result in a dominant negative effect (Gatti *et al.*, 1999), i.e. that the presence of mutated ATM protein may result in more serious biological consequences than the absence of protein, as is seen with null or nonsense mutations in most A-T patients. Recent studies with *Atm* knock-in mouse models strongly support a dominant negative model (see below). A dominant negative effect on cancer susceptibility is also observed when heterozygous mutations in the H2AX gene are introduced into p53-/- (apoptosis-deficient) mice (Bassing *et al.*, 2003).

When missense *Atm* mutations were introduced by knock-in approaches, an increased frequency of tumors in heterozygous (and homozygous) mice was observed (Spring *et al.*, 2002; Concannon, 2002). This was in stark contrast to the absence of tumors in previous studies using mice that were heterozygous for knock-out mutations in the *Atm* gene (Barlow *et al.*, 1996). Thus, dominant negative missense *ATM* mutations may serve to increase susceptibility to cancer in the general population. This is further supported by the mutagenesis experiments of Scott *et al.* (2002).

Taken together, these analyses of *ATM* heterozygosity in cancer cohorts suggest that the carrier frequency in the general population may exceed 5%, as compared with the previous 1% carrier frequency estimate that was based on families with A-T children (Swift *et al.*, 1986). However, carriers of missense *ATM* mutations do not appear to manifest any obvious neurological symptoms.

AT-phenocopy disorders

Several AT-related disorders have been described. However, only Mre11 deficiency (also called A-T Like Disorder) has ataxia with cerebellar degeneration, is radiosensitive in diagnostic testing, and might be misdiagnosed as A-T (Stewart *et al.*, 1999; Pitts *et al.*, 2001). Because Mre11 deficiency is very rare, it is difficult to generalize about the clinical picture or cancer risk of homozygotes or heterozygotes. Many of the neurologic features overlap with A-T, although the overall severity in the seven known kindreds resembles a somewhat milder disorder than classic A-T. Telangiectasiae have not been observed.

Since Mre11 forms a DNA repair complex with Rad50 and nibrin, and is phosphorylated by ATM in response to radiation damage, it is not surprising that the phenotypes of Mre11 deficiency and A-T overlap. When the *Mre11* gene is knocked-out in mice, the animals die before birth.

Nibrin protein is absent on conventional immunoblot of lysates from patients with Nijmegan Breakage Syndrome (NBS). Nibrin is a direct target of ATM phosphorylation as well. NBS patients are clinically identified by prominent microcephaly and do not have any of the motor difficulties or ocular telangiectasia that characterize A-T (Hiel *et al.*, 2000). NBS patients manifest both in vitro and in vivo radiosensitivity (Sun *et al.*, 2002; Bakhshi *et al.*, 2003). All three disorders manifest an increased frequency of translocations involving chromosomes 7 and 14 in peripheral blood lymphocytes. The G1/S checkpoint is also impaired in all. ATM protein levels are approximately normal in Mre11 deficiency and NBS patients. The similarities of cellular phenotypes between A-T, Mre11 deficiency, and NBS relate these disorders more closely to one another than do their clinical features (Uziel *et al.*, 2003).

The diagnosis of early onset ataxias that are not obviously of a dominant nature must also include two newly defined autosomal recessive ataxias with oculomotor apraxia (AOA1 and AOA2): AOA1 appears to be more common than A-T, NBS, or Mre11-deficiency in at least Portugal and Japan (Moreira *et al.*, 2001a). Clinically, the ataxia appears early in childhood and is not associated with telangiectasia or an elevated alphafetoprotein. Mutations in the ataxin (*APTX*) gene on chromosome 9p13 have been identified in these patients. The APTX protein is depleted or absent by immunoblotting. Cells from AOA1 patients are not sensitive to ionizing radiation; however, single strand break repair is defective and can be demonstrated by the response to hydrogen peroxide damage. The APTX protein colocalizes in nuclei with XRCC1 and poly(ADP-ribose) polymerase (PARP) (Moreira *et al.*, 2001b).

AOA2 is associated with mutations in the senataxin gene on chromosome 9q34. These patients have a later onset of ataxia and do not have telangiectasia. Serum alphafetoprotein levels are elevated, similar to A-T. Cells from AOA2 patients do not appear to be sensitive to ionizing radiation but again may be defective in single strand break repair. The protein is absent on immunoblots of cell extracts from AOA2 patients. AOA2 has helicase function (Moreira *et al.*, 2004).

Laboratory diagnosis

Three routine tests are immediately available to support a diagnosis of A-T in a young child: 1) serum alphafetoprotein

(AFP); 2) karyotyping, with special attention for translocations involving chromosomes 7 and 14; 3) and immune status of B and T cell compartments. The AFP is elevated in more than 95% of A-T patients (Chun *et al.*, 2003). False positives appear to be a diagnostic problem in children under 2 years of age, however, as the AFP descends from very high levels in the fetus at a variable rate during infancy. Serial measurements of AFP can distinguish those with slow descent of normal fetal expression. Elevated AFP is also associated with some malignancies. Karyotyping is seldom normal in A-T cells; however, mitogen-stimulated A-T lymphocytes may have to be harvested slightly later than routine in order to visualize a sufficient number of metaphases for a careful analysis. T cell levels are mildly low in most A-T patients but overlap with the wide range of normal is not uncommon. Gamma/delta T cell levels are usually elevated, probably reflecting a maturation defect in this pathway. B cell levels are normal, or slightly elevated. Serum immunoglobulin levels often reveal marked deficiencies of IgE (80% of patients), IgG2 (80%), and IgA (60%). None of these above parameters changes with age. Patients may develop monoclonal or polyclonal gammopathy, sometimes to the degree that treatment for hyperviscosity is required (Nowak-Wegrzyn *et al.*, 2004).

Radiosensitivity is also characteristic of A-T cells (Taylor *et al.*, 1975) and has been used to confirm the clinical diagnosis. The most commonly used assay is a colony survival assay (CSA)(Huo *et al.*, 1994; Sun *et al.*, 2002). This assay is performed on EBV-transformed lymphoblastoid cells (LCLs) and has a 3 month turnaround time in the laboratory. However, the same LCL can also be used for immunoblottiing, to measure ATM protein levels, as well as for testing ATM kinase function and for determining mutations in the *ATM* gene. Virtually all cell lines from A-T patients are radiosensitive (Fig. 49.2). LCLs from patients with a variety of other disorders are also radiosensitive by CSA; of these, only Mre11 deficiency manifests radiosensitivity by CSA and an ataxia of early onset that might be confused with A-T (see below). Conversely, LCLs from patients with Friedreich's ataxia or AOA1 are not radiosensitive (Huo *et al.*, 1994; Gatti, 2002; Sun *et al.*, 2002). Chromosomal breakage studies following in vitro irradiation also demonstrate this radiosensitivity; however, rigorous diagnostic ranges for such testing have not been defined (Woods & Taylor, 1992). Patients with Fanconi anemia are also radiosensitive by CSA (Sun *et al.*, 2002; Nahas *et al.*, 2005); however, these patients characteristically do not manifest ataxia.

Immunoblotting of extracts from normal cells is used to detect ATM protein (Becker-Catania *et al.*, 2000; Chun *et al.*, 2003). If performed on blood, 10–20 million cells are

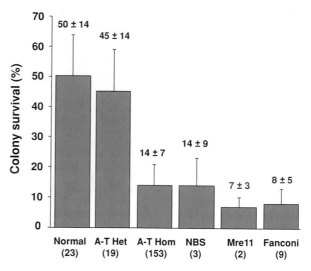

Fig. 49.2 Radiosensitivity of lymphoblastoid cells from patients with A-T, NBS, Mre11 deficiency, Fanconi anemia (6 complementation groups), as well as normal controls and A-T heterozygotes. Numbers in parenthesis represent the number of patients tested for each disorder. The Colony Survival Assay (CSA) is scored 10 days after irradiation with 1 Gray (Huo *et al.*, 1994; Sun *et al.*, 2002).

needed to obtain reliable results because ATM protein concentrations are normally low. This makes immunoblotting impractical for testing small infants unless a cell line is first established. ATM protein is absent in more than 85% of A-T patients. Very small amounts of ATM protein are seen in the remaining 15% of patients. Controls are also used to ensure equal protein representation within each lane of the gal antibodies to hMre11 can be used for this purpose. Thus, this protocol further serves to screen for patients with Mre11 deficiency (Stewart *et al.*, 1999).

In rare circumstances, an A-T phenotype may present with normal amounts of ATM protein (Stankovic *et al.*, 1998; Stewart *et al.*, 2001). The ATM protein in these cases is functionally defective. This can be demonstrated by assessing ATM kinase activity, wherein Serine or Threonine residues of known ATM substrates are phosphorylated. Either in vivo or in vitro assays of kinase activity can be used (Chun *et al.*, 2003). The most commonly tested ATM substrate is p53, which is phosphorylated by ATM on Serine 15 (Canman *et al.*, 1998; Banin *et al.*, 1998). Studies of >50 A-T patients, with or without detectable ATM protein, have shown that typical A-T cells do not phosphorylate p53, nor alternate substrates like MDM2, SMC1, or nibrin. Patients with some detectable ATM protein, or with some detectable kinase activity, may have slower neurological progression and longer survival (Gilad *et al.*, 1998; Becker-Catania *et al.*, 2000; Saviozzi *et al.*, 2002; Chun *et al.*, 2003).

Differential diagnosis and imaging

A-T is more easily diagnosed in older children once the ataxia, apraxia, telangiectasia, and dysarthria are fully expressed. By this time, the disorder will be clearly progressive and may also be apparent in other sibs, or relatives, indicating a genetic disorder of autosomal recessive pattern. Conversely, early diagnosis is often missed because of the absence of ocular telangiectasia, which is not usually apparent at the time of first concern about impaired balance and motor ability (Cabana *et al.*, 1998). It is in very young patients that laboratory diagnosis is most helpful. Early diagnosis can play a major role in family planning. It can also help to avoid years of costly diagnostic testing.

In very young infants the diagnosis can be easily confused with mild cerebral palsy, acute infectious or episodic ataxia, malignancy, or even with some other rare genetic or mitochondria disorders, such as MERFF or Leigh's Disease (Gatti, 2002). In the United States, A-T is the most common of the known monogenic autosomal recessive ataxic disorders of children before school age; the more common Friedreich's ataxia generally does not begin to manifest until later childhood, adolescence or beyond. Friedreich's ataxia can generally be distinguished from A-T by the early abnormal Romberg sign, hyporeflexia, abnormal Babinski response, and normal control of saccadic eye movements.

Cerebellar atrophy is usually not apparent by MRI in young A-T patients. In a study of MRI changes involving A-T patients of various ages, the pattern of cerebellar atrophy appeared to progress from the lateral hemispheres to the inferior and superior portions (Tavani *et al.*, 2003).

Treatment

Advances in understanding the molecular genetics of A-T have improved understanding of pathogenetic mechanisms and the accuracy and precision of diagnostic testing. Unfortunately, these advances have not yet led to the development of effective neuroprotective, or neurorestorative therapies. Thus, A-T treatment continues to focus upon the supportive care, and in particular the medical management of sinopulmonary infection and dysfunction, immmunodeficiency, malignancy and upon rehabilitative efforts in speech and swallowing, nutrition, physical and occupational therapy and the use of adaptive equipment. Occasional patients have expressed improved control of balance, incoordination and dysarthria with hydroxyphenyldil, amantadine (Botez *et al.*, 1996), buspirone (Trouillas *et al.*, 1997) and fluoxetine (Seliger *et al.*,

1989). Clonazepam and gabapentin and other anticonvulsants have been found to help with the cerebellar tremor (Faulkner *et al.*, 2003). Anti-cholinergic compounds can provide some control over drooling, and along with dopaminergic agonists, may also reduce basal ganglia dysfunction. Multiple factors, including significant placebo effects, the pleomorphic nature of movement abnormalities in A-T, tolerance effects of any one medication, rarity of the disorder and individual differences, all undermine the potential for systematic clinical trials of any one agent.

As in essential tremor, botulinum toxin injections to selected muscles have been used to control cerebellar-mediated tremor of the head or limbs. However, the complex and multifactorial nature of the movement abnormalities in A-T inhibits the development of other interventions such as deep brain ablative and stimulation procedures.

Secondary complications of progressive ataxia can include deconditioning/immobility, weight loss or gain, skin breakdown, recurrent pulmonary and urinary tract infections, aspiration, occult respiratory failure, and obstructive sleep apnea, all of which can be life-threatening. Depression in the older patient and involved family members can be encountered, as maturing patients come to realize their physical and social limitations more fully.

Symptomatic treatment can greatly improve the quality of life of these patients and prevent complications that could hasten death. Supportive interventions should always be offered – education about the disease itself, genetic counseling, individual and family counseling, referral to support groups and advocacy groups, and guidance to online resources (e.g. the A-T Children's Project: www.atcp.org).

Treatment is symptom-focused (imbalance/incoordination/dysarthria; cerebellar tremor) and may be monitored with a few, simple, reproducible, and semi-quantitative measures of performance (timing of gait, single-limb balance, hand and foot tapping, completion of a spiral maze or pegboard, reading of a standard paragraph) (Notermans *et al.*, 1994). Self-reporting of functional measures (use of aids to gait, number of falls, success at a keyboard or electronic game or carrying a cup of coffee across a room, need for assistance with dressing or personal care or eating, difficulty being understood) can also be reliable indicators (D'Ambrosio *et al.*, 1987). The use of clinical rating scales sensitive and specific for the most important features of A-T along with other objective, sensitive measure may be invaluable for future clinical trials (Crawford *et al.*, 2000).

Controlled trials of disease-modifying therapy in A-T have not yet been published. Presumed mechanisms of pathophysiology resulting from increased oxidative stress (Barzilai *et al.*, 2002) have examined antioxidant/free radical scavengers in vitro and in vivo. However, the treatment regimens in these studies do not demonstrate improvement in the neurologic features of any of the inherited ataxias (vitamin E (Marcelain *et al.*, 2002), alpha-lipoic acid (Gatei *et al.*, 2001), *N*-acetylcysteine (Edwards *et al.*, 2002), selenium (Jauslin *et al.*, 2002), idebenone/coenzyme Q10 (Artuch *et al.*, 2002)). The effects of timing in treatment initiation and dosing are unknown. Furthermore, few of these agents cross the blood–brain barrier effectively. Although many antioxidant therapies are safely tolerated, patients trying high-dose antioxidant therapies should be monitored for potential hematologic or hepatic side effects. Recently, the laboratory use of aminoglycosides to increase intracellular ATM levels (400- to 800-fold) and correct ATM function has been reported (Lai *et al.*, 2004), Suggesting that the identification of mutations in AT patients may become relevant to therapy.

REFERENCES

Artuch, R., Aracil, A., Mas, A. *et al.* (2002). Friedreich's ataxia. idebenone treatment in early stage patients. *Neuropediatrics*, **33**, 190–3.

Bakhshi, S., Cerosaletti, K. M., Concannon, P. *et al.* (2003). Medulloblastoma with adverse reaction to radiation therapy in Nijmegen Breakage Syndrome. *J. Pediat. Hematol./Oncol.*, **25**, 248–51.

Banin, S., Moyal, L., Shieh, S.-Y. *et al.* (1998). Enhanced phosphorylation of p53 by ATM in response to DNA damage. *Science*, **281**, 1675–7.

Barlow, C., Hirotsune, S., Paylor, R. *et al.* (1996). Atm-deficient mice: a paradigm of ataxia telangiectasia. *Cell*, **86**, 159–71.

Barlow, C., Dennery, P. A., Shigenaga, M. K. *et al.* (1999). Loss of the ataxia-telangiectasia gene product causes oxidative damage in target organs. *Proc. Natl Acad. Sci., USA*, **96**, 9915–19.

Barlow, C., Ribault-Barassin, C., Zwingman, T. A. *et al.* (2000). ATM is a cytoplasmic protein in mouse brain required to prevent lysosomal accumulation. *Proc. Natl Acad. Sci. USA*, **97**, 871–6.

Barzilai, A., Rotman, G. & Shiloh, Y. (2002). ATM deficiency and oxidative stress: a new dimension of defective response to DNA damage. *DNA Repair (Amsterdam)*, **1**, 3–25.

Bassing, C. H., Suh, H., Ferguson, D. O. *et al.* (2003). Histone H2AX: a dosage-dependent suppressor of oncogenic translocations and tumors. *Cell*, **114**, 359–70.

Becker-Catania, S. G., Chen, G., Hwang, M. J. *et al.* (2000). Ataxia-telangiectasia: phenotype/genotype studies of ATM protein expression, mutations, and radiosensitivity. *Mol. Genet. Metab.*, **70**, 122–33.

Bernstein, J. L., Teraoka, S., Haile, R. W. *et al.* (2003). Designing and implementing quality control for multi-center screening of mutations in the *ATM* gene among women with breast cancer. *Hum. Mutat.*, **21**, 542–50.

Boder, E. & Sedgwick, R. P. (1958). Ataxia-telangiectasia: a familial syndrome of progressive cerebellar ataxia, oculocutaneous telangiectasia and frequent pulmonary infection. *Pediatrics*, **21**, 526–54.

Boder, E. (1985). Ataxia-telangiectasia: an overview. In *Ataxia-Telangiectasia: Genetics, Neuropathology and Immunology of a Degenerative Disease of Childhood*, ed. R. A. Gatti and M. Swift. New York: Alan R Liss Inc. pp. 1–63.

Botez, M. I., Botez-Marquard, T., Elie, R., Pedraza, O. L., Goyette, K. & Lalonde, R. (1996). Amantadine hydrochloride treatment in heredodegenerative ataxias: a double blind study. *J. Neurol. Neurosurg. Psychiatry*, **61**, 259–64.

Borghesani, P. R., Alt, F. W., Bottaro, A. *et al.* (2000). Abnormal development of Purkinje cells and lymphocytes in Atm mutant mice. *Proc. Natl Acad. Sci., USA*, **97**, 3336–41.

Butch, A. W., Chun, H. H., Nahas, S. A. & Gatti, R. A. (2004). Immunoassay to measure ataxia–telangiectasia mutated protein in cellular lysates, *Clin. Chem.* **50**, 2302–8.

Cabana, M. D., Crawford, T. O., Winkelstein, J. A., Christensen, J. R. & Lederman, H. M. (1998). Consequences of delayed diagnosis of ataxia-telangiectasia. *Pediatrics*, **102**, 98–100.

Campbell, C., Mitui, M., Eng, L., Coutinho, G., Thorstenson, Y. & Gatti, R. A. (2003). ATM mutations on distinct SNP and STR haplotypes in ataxia-telangiectasia patients of differing ethnicities reveal ancestral founder effects. *Hum. Mutat.*, **21**, 80–85.

Canman, C. E., Lim, D.-S., Cimprich, K. A. *et al.* (1998). Activation of the ATM kinase by ionizing radiation and phosphorylation of p53. *Science*, **281**, 1677–9.

Castellvi-Bel, S., Sheikhavandi, S., Telatar, M. *et al.* (1999). New mutations, polymorphisms, and rare variants in the *ATM* gene detected by a novel strategy. *Hum. Mutat.*, **14**, 156–62.

Chevenix-Trench, G., Spurdle, A. B., Gatei, M. *et al.* (2002). Dominant negative *ATM* mutations in breast cancer families. *J. Natl Cancer Inst.*, **94**, 205–15.

Chiesa, N., Barlow, C., Wynshaw-Boris, A., Strata, P. & Tempia, F. (2002). Atm-deficient mice Purkinje cells show age-dependent defects in calcium spike bursts and calcium currents. *Neuroscience*, **96**, 575–83.

Chun, H. H., Castellvi-Bel, S., Wang, Z. *et al.* (2002). TCL-1, MTCP-1 and TML-1 gene expression profile in non-leukemic proliferations associated with ataxia-telangiectasia. *Int. J. Cancer*, **97**, 726–31.

Chun, H. H., Sun, X., Nahas, S. A. *et al.* (2003). Improved diagnostic testing for ataxia-telangiectasia by immunoblotting of nuclear lysates for ATM protein expression. *Mol. Genet. Metab.*, **80**, 437–43.

Concannon, P. & Gatti, R. A. (1997). Diversity of *ATM* gene mutations detected in patients with ataxia-telangiectasia. *Hum. Mutat.*, **10**, 100–7.

Concannon, P. (2002). *ATM* heterozygosity and cancer risk. *Nat. Genet.*, **32**, 89–90.

Coutinho, G., Mitui, M., Campbell, C. *et al.* (2004). Five haplotypes account for fifty-five percent of *ATM* mutations in Brazilian patients with ataxia-telangiectasia: seven new mutations. *Am. J. Med. Genet.*, **126A** (1), 33–40.

Crawford, T. O., Mandir, A. S., Lefton-Greif, M. A. *et al.* (2000). Quantitative neurologic assessment of ataxia-telangiectasia. *Neurology*, **54**, 1505–9.

D'Ambrosio, R., Leone, M., Rosso, M. G., Mittino, D. & Brignolio, F. (1987). Disability and quality of life in hereditary ataxias: a self-administered postal questionnaire. *Int. Disabil. Stud.*, **9**, 10–14.

Edwards, M. J., Hargreaves, I. P., Heales, S. J., Jones S. J., Ramachandran, V., Bhatia, K. P. & Sisodiya, S. (2002). *N*-acetylcysteine and Unverricht-Lundborg disease: variable response and possible side effects. *Neurology*, **59**, 1447–9.

Eilam, R., Peter, Y., Elson, A. *et al.* (1998). Selective loss of dopaminergic nigro-striatal neurons in brains of Atm-deficient mice. *Proc. Natl Acad. Sci., USA*, **95**, 12653–6.

Elson, A., Wang, Y., Daugherty, C. J. *et al.* (1996). Pleiotropic defects in ataxia-telangiectasia protein-deficient mice. *Proc. Natl Acad. Sci., USA*, **93**, 13084–9.

Eng, L., Coutinho, G., Nahas, S. *et al.* (2004). Non-classical splicing mutations in the coding and non-coding regions of the *ATM* gene: maximum entropy estimates of splice junction strengths. *Hum. Mutat.*, **23**, 67–76.

Faulkner, M. A., Bertoni, J. M. & Lenz, T. L. (2003). Gabapentin for the treatment of tremor. *Ann. Pharmacother.*, **37**, 282–6.

FitzGerald, M. G., Bean, J. M., Hegde, S. R. *et al.* (1997). Heterozygous *ATM* mutations do not contribute to early onset of breast cancer. *Nat. Genet.*, **15**, 307–10.

Gatei, M., Shkedy, D., Khanna, K. K. *et al.* (2001). Ataxia-telangiectasia: chronic activation of damage-responsive functions is reduced by alpha-lipoic acid. *Oncogene*, **20**, 289–94.

Gatti, R. A. (2002). Ataxia-telangiectasia. In *The Genetic Basis of Human Cancer*, ed. B. Vogelstein & K. W. Kinzler, New York: McGraw-Hill Inc. pp. 239–66.

Gatti, R. A. & Good, R. A. (1971). Occurrence of malignancy in immunodeficiency diseases. *Cancer*, **28**, 89–98.

Gatti, R. A. & Vinters, H. V. (1985). Cerebellar pathology in ataxia-telangiectasia. In *Ataxia-Telangiectasia: Genetics, Neuropathology and Immunology of a Degenerative Disease of Childhood*, ed. R. A. Gatti & M. Swift. New York: Alan R. Liss Inc. pp. 225–32.

Gatti, R. A., Berkel, I., Boder, E. *et al.* (1988). Localization of an ataxia-telangiectasia gene to chromosome 11q22–23. *Nature*, **336**, 577–80.

Gatti, R. A., Boder, E., Vinters, H. V., Sparkes, R. S., Norman, A. & Lange, K. (1991). Ataxia-telangiectasia: an interdisciplinary approach to pathogenesis. *Medicine*, **70**, 99–117.

Gatti, R. A., Tward, A. & Concannon, P. (1999). Cancer risk in *ATM* heterozygotes: a model of phenotypic and mechanistic differences between missense and truncating mutations. *Mol. Genet. Metab.*, **69**, 419–23.

Gilad, S., Chessa, L., Khosravi, R. *et al.* (1998). Genotype–phenotype relationships in ataxia-telangiectasia and variants. *Am. J. Hum. Genet.*, **62**, 551–61.

Gotoff, S. P., Amirmokri, E. & Liebner, E. J. (1967). Ataxia telangiectasia: neoplasia, untoward response to x-irradiation, and tuberous sclerosis. *Am. J. Dis. Child.*, **114**, 617–25.

Hiel, J. A., Weemaes, C., Van den Heuvel, I. P. *et al.* (2000). (International NBS Study Group). Nijmegen Breakage Syndrome. *Arch. Dis. Child.*, **82**, 400–6.

Hummel, T., Vasconcelos, M. L., Clemens, J. C., Fiswhilevich, Y., Vosshall, L. B. & Zipursky, S. L. (2003). Axonal targeting of olfactory receptor neurons in *Drosophila* is controlled by Dscam. *Neuron*, **37**, 221–31.

Huo, Y. K., Wang, Z., Hong, J.-H. *et al.* (1994). Radiosensitivity of ataxia-telangiectasia, X-linked agammaglobulinemia and related syndromes. *Cancer Res.*, **54**, 2544–7.

Jaspers, N. G. L., Gatti, R. A., Baan, C., Linssen, P. C. M. L. & Bootsma, D. (1988). Genetic complementation analysis of ataxia-telangiectasia and Nijmegen breakage syndrome: a survey of 50 patients. *Cytogenet. Cell. Genet.*, **49**, 259–63.

Jauslin, M. L., Wirth, T., Meier, T. & Schoumacher, F. (2002). A cellular model for Friedreich Ataxia reveals small-molecule glutathione peroxidase mimetics as novel treatment strategy. *Hum. Mol. Genet.*, **11**, 3055–63.

Kamsler, A., Daily, D., Hochman, A. *et al.* (2001). Increased oxidative stress in ataxia telangiectasia evidenced by alterations in redox state of brains from Atm-deficient mice. *Cancer Res.*, **61**, 1849–54.

Lai, C.-H., Chun, H. H., Nahas, S. A. *et al.* (2004). Correction of ATM gene function by aminoglycoside-induced read-through of premature termination codons. *Proc. Am. Acad. Sci.*, **101**, 15676–81.

Lalonde, R., Joyal, C. C. & Botez, M. I. (1994). Exploration and motor coordination in dystonia musculorum mutant mice. *Physiol. Behav.*, **56**, 277–80.

Lewis, R. F., Lederman, H. M. & Crawford, T. O. (1999). Oculomotor abnormalities in ataxia-telangiectasia. *Ann. Neurol.*, **46**, 287–95.

Marcelain, K., Navarrete, C. L, Bravo, M., Santos, M., Be, C. & Pincheira, J. (2002). Effect of vitamin E (DL-alpha-tocopherol) on the frequency of chromosomal damage in lymphocytes from patients with ataxia telangiectasia. *Rev. Med. Chil.*, **130**, 957–63.

McConville, C. M., Stankovic, T. *et al.* (1996). Mutations associated with variant phenotypes in ataxia-telangiectasia. *Am. J. Hum. Genet.*, **59**, 320–30.

Mitui, M., Campbell, C., Coutinho, G. *et al.* (2003). Independent mutational events are rare in the *ATM* gene: haplotype pre-screening enhances mutation detection rate. *Hum. Mutat.*, **22**, 43–50.

Moreira, M. C., Barbot, C., Tachi, N. *et al.* (2001a). Homozygosity mapping of Portuguese and Japanese forms of ataxia-oculomotor apraxia to 9q13, and evidence for genetic heterogeneity. *Am. J. hum. Genet.*, **68**, 501–8.

Moreira, M., Barbot, C., Tachi, N. *et al.* (2001b). The gene mutated in ataxia-ocular apraxia 1 encodes the new HIT/Zn-finger protein aprataxin. *Nat. Genet.*, **29**, 189–93.

Moreira, M.- C., Klur, S., Watanabe, M. *et al.* (2004). Senataxin, the ortholog of a yeast RNA helicasse, is mutant in ataxia-ocular apraxia 2. *Nat. Genetic.*, **36**, 225–7.

Mount, H. T. J., Wu, Y., Fluit, P., Bi, Q., Crawford, T. O. & Mandir, A. S. (2002). Parkinsonian features of ataxia-telangiectasia and of the Atm-deficient mouse. In *Parkinson's Disease*, ed. E. Ronken, L. Turski & G. van Scharrenburg, Amsterdam: IOS publishers, pp. 182–93.

Mount, H. T. J., Martel, J.-C., Fluit, P. *et al.* (2004). Progressive sensorimotor impairment is not associated with reduced dopamine and high energy phosphate donors in a model of ataxia-telangiectasia. *J. Neurochem.*, **88**, 1449–54.

Nahas, S. A., Lai, C.-H., Gatti, R. A. SMC1 phosphorylation is independent of the Fanconi protein complex. *Int. J. Radiat. Biol.*, in press.

Notermans, N. C., van Dijk, G. W., van der, Graaf, Y., van Gijn, J. & Wokke, J. H. (1994). Measuring ataxia: quantification based on the standard neurological examination. *J. Neurol. Neurosurg. Psychiatry*, **57**, 22–6.

Nowak-Wegrzyn, A., Winkelstein, J. A., Carson, K. A. & Lederman, H. M. (2004). Immunodeficiency and infections in ataxia telangiectasia. *J. Pediat.*, **144**, 505–11.

Pagani, F., Buratti, E., Stuani, C., Bendix, R., Dork, T. & Baralle, F. E. (2002). A new type of mutation causes a splicing defect in ATM. *Nat. Genet.*, **30**, 426–9.

Pitts, S. A., Kullar, H. S., Stankovic, T. *et al.* (2001). HMRE11: genomic structure and a null mutation identified in a transcript protected from nonsense-mediated mRNA decay. *Hum. Mol. Genet.*, **10**, 1155–62.

Quick, K. L. & Dugan, L. L. (2001). Superoxide stress identifies neurons at risk in a model of ataxia-telangiectasia. *Ann. Neurol.*, **49**, 627–35.

Saviozzi, S., Saluto, A., Taylor, A. M. R. *et al.* (2002). A late onset variant of ataxia-telangiectasia with a compound heterozygous genotype, A8030G/7481insA. *J. Med. Genet.*, **39**, 57–61.

Savitsky, K., Bar-Shira, A., Gilad, S. *et al.* (1995). A single ataxia-telangiectasia gene with a product similar to PI-3 kinase. *Science*, **268**, 1749–53.

Scott, S. P., Bendix, R., Chen, P., Clark, R., Dork, T. & Lavin, M. F. (2002). Missense mutations but not allelic variants alter the function of ATM by dominant interference in patients with breast cancer. *Proc. Natl Acad. Sci., USA*, **99**, 925–30.

Sedgwick, R. P. & Boder, E. (1991). Ataxia-telangiectasia. In *Handbook of Clinical Neurology*, Vol 16(60), *Hereditary Neuropathies and Spinocerebellar Atrophies*, ed. J. M. B. V. de Jong. Amsterdam: Elsevier, pp. 347–423.

Seliger, G. M. & Hornstein, A. (1989). Serotonin, fluoxetine, and pseudobulbar affect. *Neurology*, **39**, 1400.

Shiloh, Y. (2003). ATM and related protein kinases: safeguarding genome integrity. *Nat. Rev./Cancer*, **3**, 155–68.

Soares, H. D., Morgan, J. I. & McKinnon, P. J. (1998). *Atm* expression patterns suggest a contribution from the peripheral nervous system to the phenotype of ataxia-telangiectasia. *Neuroscience*, **86**, 1045–54.

Sotelo, C. & Guenet, J. L. (1988). Pathological changes in the CNS of *dystonia musculorum* mutant mouse: an animal model for human spinocerebellar ataxia. *Neuroscience*, **27**, 403–24.

Spector, B. D., Filipovich, A. H., Perry, G. S. & Kersey, J. H. (1982). Epidemiology of cancer in ataxia-telangiectasia. In *Ataxia-Telangiectasia – Cellular and Molecular Link Between Cancer, Neuropathology and Immune Deficiency*, ed. B. A. Bridges & D. G. Harnden. London: John Wiley, pp. 103–7.

Spring, K., Ahangari, F., Scott, S. P. *et al.* (2002). Mice heterozygous for mutation in *Atm*, the gene involved in ataxia-telangiectasia, have heightened susceptibility to cancer. *Nat. Genet.*, **32**, 185–90.

Stankovic, T., Kidd, A. M. J., Sutcliffe, A. *et al.* (1998). ATM mutations and phenotypes in ataxia-telangiectasia families in the British Isles: expression of mutant ATM and the risk of leukemia, lymphoma, and breast cancer. *Am. J. Hum. Genet.*, **62**, 334–45.

Stewart, G. S., Maser, R. S., Stankovic, T. *et al.* (1999). The DNA double-strand break repair gene hMRE11 is mutated in individuals with an ataxia-telangiectasia-like disorder. *Cell*, **99**, 577–87.

Stewart, G. S., Last, J. I. K., Stakovic, T. *et al.* (2001). Residual ataxia telangiectasia mutated protein function in cells from A-T patients, with 5762ins137 and 7271T> G mutations, showing a less severe phenotype. *J. Biol. Chem.*, **276**, 30103–41.

Su, Y. & Swift, M. (2000). Mortality rates among carriers of ataxia-telangiectasia mutant alleles. *Ann. Intern. Med.*, **133**, 770–8.

Sun, X., Becker-Catania, S. G., Chun, H. H. *et al.* (2002). Early diagnosis of ataxia-telangiectasia using radiosensitivity testing. *J. Pediat.*, **140**, 732–5.

Swift, M., Sholman, L., Perry, M. & Chase, C. (1976). Malignant neoplasms in the families of patients with ataxia-telangiectasia. *Cancer Res.*, **36**, 209–15.

Swift, M., Morrell, D., Cromartie, E., Chamberlin, A. R., Skolnick, M. H. & Bishop, D. T. (1986). The incidence and gene frequency of ataxia-telangiectasia in the United States. *Am. J. Hum. Genet.*, **39**, 573–83.

Swift, M., Morrell, D., Massey, R. B. & Chase, C. L. (1991). Incidence of cancer in 161 families affected by ataxia-telangiectasia. *N. Engl. J. Med.*, **325**, 1831–6.

Syllaba, L. & Henner, K. (1926). Contribution a l'independane de l'athetose double idiopathique et congenitale. *Rev. Neurol.*, **1**, 541–6.

Tavani, F., Zimmerman, R. A., Berry, G. T., Sullivan, K., Gatti, R. & Bingham, P. (2003). Ataxia-telangiectasia: the pattern of cerebellar atrophy on MRI. *Neuroradiology*, **45**, 315–19.

Taylor, A. M. R., Harnden, D. G., Arlett, C. F. *et al.* (1975). Ataxia-telangiectasia: a human mutation with abnormal radiation sensitivity. *Nature*, **258**, 427–9.

Telatar, M., Wang, Z., Udar, N. *et al.* (1996). Ataxia-telangiectasia: mutations in *ATM* cDNA detected by protein-truncation screening. *Am. J. Hum. Genet.*, **59**, 40–4.

Telatar, M., Wang, Z., Castellvi-Bel, S. *et al.* (1998a). A model for *ATM* heterozygote identification in a large population: four founder-effect *ATM* mutations identify most of Costa Rican patients with ataxia telangiectasia. *Mol. Genet. Metabol.*, **64**, 36–43.

Telatar, M., Teraoka, S., Wang, Z. *et al.* (1998b). Ataxia-telangiectasia: identification and detection of founder-effect mutations in the *ATM* gene in ethnic populations. *Am. J. Hum. Genet.*, **62**, 86–97.

Teraoka, S., Telatar, M., Becker-Catania, S. *et al.* (1999). Splicing defects in the ataxia-telangiectasia gene, *ATM*: underlying mutations and phenotypic consequences. *Am. J. Hum. Genet.*, **64**, 1617–31.

Thorstenson, Y. R., Shen, P., Tusher, V. G., Davis, R. W., Chu, G. & Oefner, P. J. (2001). Global analysis of *ATM* polymorphism reveals significant functional constraint. *Am. J. Hum. Genet.*, **69**, 396–412.

Trouillas, P., Xie, J., Adeleine, P. *et al.* (1997). Buspirone, a 5-hydroxytryptamine1A agonist, is active in cerebellar ataxia. Results of a double-blind drug placebo study in patients with cerebellar cortical atrophy. *Arch. Neurol.*, **54**, 749–52.

Uziel, T., Lerenthal, Y., Moyal, L., Andegeko, Y., Mittelman, L. & Shiloh, Y. (2003). Requirement of the MRN complex for ATM activation by DNA damage. *Embo J.*, **22**, 5612–21.

Vinters, H. V., Gatti, R. A. & Rakic, P. (1985). Sequence of cellular events in cerebellar ontogeny relevant to expression of neuronal abnormalities in ataxia-telangiectasia. In *Ataxia-Telangiectasia: Genetics, Neuropathology, and Immunology of a Degenerative Disease of Childhood*, ed. R. A. Gatti & M. Swift. New York: Alan R Liss Inc. pp. 233–55.

Woods, C. G. & Taylor, A. M. R. (1992). Ataxia telangiectasia in the British Isles: the clinical and laboratory features of 70 affected individuals. *Quart. J. Med. New Series*, **298**, 169–79.

Xu, Y., Ashley, T., Brainerd, E. E., Bronson, R. T., Meyn, M. S. & Baltimore, D. (1996). Targeted disruption of *ATM* leads to growth retardation, chromosomal fragmentation during meiosis, immune defects, and thymic lymphoma. *Genes Dev.*, **10**, 2411–22.

Part IX

Motor neuron diseases

50

An approach to the patient with motor neuron dysfunction

Matthew J. Parton and P. Nigel Leigh

Department of Neurology, The Institute of Psychiatry and Guy's, King's and St Thomas' School of Medicine, London, UK

Introduction

Anatomically, motor system dysfunction is defined as a derangement – either alone or in combination – of the pyramidal neurons of the corticospinal tract (upper motor neurons – UMN), brainstem motor nerve nuclei or spinal cord anterior horn cells (lower motor neurons – LMN). Both UMN and LMN lesions will cause muscle weakness, but other clinical features allow the two to be differentiated (a pyramidal pattern of weakness, spasticity and brisk reflexes follow UMN damage, whereas wasting, fasciculations and reduced or absent reflexes reflect LMN involvement).

A range of neurological conditions may cause a selective motor syndrome. Other illnesses will lead to such dysfunction, together with involvement of other body systems. Alternatively, some conditions will mimic a pure motor disorder but result from a non-selective disease process. These various diseases differ in their etiology, prognosis and management. It is therefore essential to evaluate patients presenting with motor neuron dysfunction carefully, and to make a firm diagnosis as early as possible. With early diagnosis, it is easier to organize effective care, and to keep the patient informed of likely developments in his or her condition.

In this chapter we will discuss the assessment of patients presenting with motor dysfunction and how this allows an accurate diagnosis to be made. We will also introduce and briefly review the principal disorders.

Clinical evaluation

History

The site that was first affected should be determined, as should the precise nature of the original symptom. Patients usually report a problem with function – difficulty with speech or walking, or with using tools or cutlery – and, at root, these earliest symptoms reflect muscle weakness. In those patients with long-standing problems, the history may reveal that symptoms began in childhood or early adulthood. Such individuals may have had difficulty competing in sports at school, or in passing medical examinations for military service or employment. It should be ascertained whether the original problem has progressed – and over what time – and if other sites of the body have become affected. Questioning may reveal whether the UMN or LMN is involved, for example, if there are symptoms of stiffness or jerking (reflecting spasticity) or loss of muscle bulk or fasciculations (indicating LMN damage). It is important to know if pelvic sphincter or sexual function is impaired. Direct questioning should seek evidence of involvement of other neurological systems (cognitive, sensory or cerebellar). Systemic symptoms such as malaise, weight loss and pain must be evaluated. Finally, a detailed family history should be taken, and a family tree with first- and second- degree relatives drawn. In summary, the history should assess with clarity and precision the nature of the first symptoms, their progression and functional consequences, and should seek evidence to identify or exclude other neurological and systemic disorders. The history serves therefore to propose a hypothesis about the pathological anatomy of the patient's complaint, as well as to place it in the complete medical, social and psychological context of the individual and his or her family.

Examination

A thorough neurological examination and assessment of other body systems will demarcate the sites affected and indicate other possible diagnoses. Attention should be directed as to whether the UMN, LMN or both are involved,

Table 50.1a. Signs associated with upper motor neuron damage

Sign	Comment
Emotional lability (tendency to laugh or cry inappropriately)	As observed during consultation; by reaction to emotionally charged questions
Brisk pout reflex	Tapping upper lip
Brisk facial reflexes	Tapping facial muscles at angle of mouth induces twitch of lower facial muscles
Brisk jaw jerk	Tapping slightly opened jaw causes masseter reflex
Spasticity of tongue	Stiffness and slowing of rapid tongue movements (often best demonstrated by asking patient to repeat lingual phonemes, e.g. "la la la . . .")
Spasticity of limbs	Very variable in ALS/MND
Brisk tendon reflexes in limbs:	Sometimes difficult to determine if *pathologically* brisk
• Finger jerks	Usually (but not always) a sign of UMN damage
• Positive Hoffman sign	Almost always pathologically significant
• Brisk and crossed thigh adductor jerks	Almost always pathologically significant
• Positive Babinski sign	Present in ~60% of cases of ALS/MND at some time in the disease

Table 50.1b. Signs associated with lower motor neuron damage

Sign	Comment
Fasciculation	Limbs must be warm and relaxed; fasciculations confined to calves are often innocent
Muscle wasting	Look for characteristic distribution of non-motor neuron disorders (e.g. inclusion body myositis)
Depressed or absent reflexes	LMN form of ALS/MND accounts for ~15% of all cases

and if any other neurological or medical abnormalities are present (see Tables 50.1a and 50.1b). The examination will add to that information already gained from the history, and so clinical evaluation alone will allow the construction of a differential diagnosis. Tables 50.2 and 50.3 list the principal conditions that cause motor neuron dysfunction.

Investigation

Certain investigations are required in order to arrive at a firm diagnosis (Table 50.4). In particular, electrophysi-

ological investigation of motor syndromes is mandatory. Electromyelogram (EMG) examination is directed at finding evidence of LMN damage in both clinically affected and unaffected muscles, and excluding other pathologies (such as a myopathy). Nerve conduction studies should also be undertaken to determine if there is neuropathy with or without motor nerve conduction block. Additionally, and particularly when either LMN signs are cranial to UMN involvement or when sensory symptoms complicate the presentation, MRI scanning is indicated to rule out compression or infiltration of the brainstem, spinal cord or nerve roots. T_2-weighted MRI of the brain may occasionally demonstrate increased signal along the corticospinal tracts, but this finding is non-specific (Goodin *et al.*, 1988; Ellis *et al.*, 1999). Creatine kinase may be raised up to 3–4 times normal.

For several motor syndromes – notably amyotrophic lateral sclerosis/motor neuron disease (ALS/MND) – no specific test exists. Therefore, a diagnosis must be established on clinical grounds and supported by appropriate investigations that also exclude other conditions. Research criteria for the diagnosis of ALS/MND have been adopted (World Federation of Neurology Research Group on Neuromuscular Diseases, 1994; World Federation of Neurology Research Group on Motor Neuron Diseases, 1998). The clinical and electrophysiological details are summarized in Tables 50.5 and 50.6.

In certain situations, additional investigation may be required. Muscle biopsy can be helpful when EMG changes are either equivocal or suggestive of a myopathic process. Inclusion body myositis in particular should be considered. DNA analysis will identify Kennedy's disease and antiganglioside (anti-GM1) antibody testing aids the diagnosis of multifocal motor neuropathy with conduction block (MFMN). Anti-GM1 antibodies and conduction block are often difficult to demonstrate in MFMN, but where there is reasonable suspicion of this potentially treatable disorder, a therapeutic trial of intravenous immunoglobulin (0.4 g/kg body weight daily for 5 days) may be considered. Quantitative myometry and clinical assessment before and after treatment are essential to document any response.

Management of the patient

Even before a diagnosis has been established, attention should focus on the management of the difficulties posed by the patient's condition. All progressive motor syndromes will cause increased disability over time, with variable loss of limb, bulbar and respiratory muscle function. Care should be tailored to individual needs, but we will briefly review the range of interventions and the

Table 50.2. Differential diagnosis of patients with motor neuron dysfunction

Condition	Comment
Amyotrophic lateral sclerosis (ALS) / motor neuron disease (MND)	ALS is specifically the idiopathic degeneration of both UMN and LMN, whereas progressive muscular atrophy (PMA) and primary lateral sclerosis (PLS) are respectively *sustained* isolated LMN and UMN syndromes. The term MND is broader and allows for the inclusion of all three patterns of involvement.
Spinal cord pathology (especially cervical myelopathy) or disease of the spinal roots or nerves	Clinical features should differentiate these, but they may co-exist with ALS/MND. Consider MRI if appropriate.
Multiple cerebrovascular accidents	Pure motor syndrome unlikely, consider imaging.
Inclusion body myositis	Preferential involvement of quadriceps and finger flexors. May require muscle biopsy.
Kennedy's disease (X-linked bulbar and spinal muscular atrophy)	LMN syndrome affecting males only. Family history and/or features of androgen resistance (gynaecomastia, testicular atrophy, etc.). Diagnosis by detection of trinucleotide repeat expansion in androgen receptor gene.
Multifocal motor neuropathy (MFMN)	Patchy weakness – proportionally greater than wasting; characteristic immunological and electrophysiological findings. Consider trial of IVIg.
Chronic inflammatory demyelinating neuropathy (CIDP)	Symmetrical signs, often sensory symptoms. Raised CSF protein and prolonged nerve conduction studies. Consider steroids and other immunomodulatory treatments.
Other rare CNS degenerations:	
• Adult onset spinal muscular atrophy	Isolated, usually symmetrical LMN syndrome, slowly progressive
• Progressive supranuclear palsy	Vertical gaze palsy, early falls, extrapyramidal features present
• Multi-system atrophy	Complex presentation – amyotrophy rare
• Cortico-basal degeneration	Presents with features of basal ganglia and cerebral cortex dysfunction, amyotrophy occasionally seen
• Machado–Joseph disease (spinocerebellar atrophy type 3)	Complex multi-system presentation overlaps with ALS/MND; autosomal dominant inheritance – trinucleotide repeat expansion in gene linked to chromosome 14q23
• Dementia–disinhibition–parkinsonian amyotrophy complex (DDPAC)	Mutations found in *tau* gene (microtubule associated protein – chromosome 17q); amyotrophy rare
• ALS–parkinsonian–dementia complex of Western Pacific	Geographical isolate; cause unknown

management of particular aspects of motor system dysfunction below.

It is now generally agreed that the key to effective care is regular review by a multi-disciplinary team (Table 50.7). This should seek to identify and anticipate an individual's problems as early as possible, so as to avoid crises when the patient and carers become overwhelmed. Coordination of care, which is often provided by many healthcare and social services professionals, is of prime importance.

Imparting the diagnosis

This should be done in private, but with the patient's carer(s) in attendance and with ample time for discussion. An early follow-up appointment should be offered to deal with points raised later, and to introduce members of the multi-disciplinary team. Appropriate information, with contact telephone numbers and relevant internet site addresses, should be made available.

Limb dysfunction – managing physical disability

Physiotherapists and occupational therapists play a key role in providing support and advice on mobility and appropriate aids and appliances. Additional assistance can be obtained from specialised services – regional driving assessment centres, rehabilitation units for provision of environmental control systems (giving control of doors, lighting, television, radio, and so on).

Bulbar dysfunction

Assessment of the patient by a speech therapist is desirable when either speech or swallowing become affected by disease. A variety of aids exist that can improve communication, ranging from simple pointing boards to computerised speech synthesisers. Excess salivation (sialorrhea) may be embarrassing and inconvenient, while violent yawning can be a problem, occasionally leading to jaw dislocation – standard treatments for bulbar spasticity are shown in Table 50.8.

Table 50.3. Other rare motor neuron disorders

Genetically determined forms of motor neuron disorder
Familial ALS
Brown-Vialetto-Van Laere syndrome (early onset bulbar and
  spinal ALS with sensorineural deafness)
Fazio-Londe syndrome (infantile progressive bulbar palsy)
Hexosaminidase A deficiency
Hereditary spastic paraplegia (many forms, including ALS2, ALS4)
Spinal muscular atrophy (SMA)
  Proximal childhood and later onset forms of SMA (types 1–4),
    SMN gene related
  Distal SMA (various forms)
  Adult onset proximal SMA (unrelated to SMN gene mutations)
  Juvenile or adult onset laryngeal and distal SMA (Harper Young
    syndrome)
Hereditary Motor and Sensory Neuropathy (predominantly
  motor forms)
Algrove syndrome

Apparently sporadic (idiopathic) forms of motor neuron disorder
Distal sporadic focal spinal muscular atrophy ('Hirayama
  syndrome')
Atypical juvenile onset ALS in South India ('Madras' form of ALS)
Western Pacific and other similar forms of ALS (Guam, Kii
  peninsula, New Guinea)
Motor neuron degeneration in Guadeloupe PSP-Dementia-ALS
  syndrome
Motor neuron degeneration in Multiple system atrophy
Motor neuron degeneration in Progressive supranuclear palsy
Motor neuron degeneration in Corticobasal ganglionic
  degeneration

Acquired forms of motor neuron disorder
HTLV-1 associated myelopathy (HAM)
HIV-associated ALS syndrome
Creutzfeld-Jacob disease (amyotrophic forms)
Multifocal motor neuronopathy
Acute poliomyelitis
Lead, mercury toxicity
Neurolathyrism (due to *lathyrus sativa*, containing
  β–oxalyl-L-aminoacid, BOAA)
Konzo (due to toxic cyanogenic cassava)
Radiation myelopathy (e.g., cervical and lumbo-sacral
  radiculopathy)
Post-polio progressive muscular atrophy syndrome
Autoimmune disorders (e.g., Sjögren's disease)
Endocrinopathy (Hyperthyroidism, hyperparathyroidism,
  hypoglycaemia)

Table 50.4. Investigations in patients with motor system
dysfunction

- Neurophysiological tests (seeking evidence of anterior horn
  cell damage in regions not supplied by the same nerve, root or
  segment)
- Serum creatine kinase (often elevated, but seldom > 4 ×
  normal)
- Brain and spinal cord MRI
- DNA analysis – *SOD1* mutation for ALS/MND and the
  expanded trinucleotide repeat in the androgen receptor gene
  for Kennedy's disease
- Anti-GM1 ganglioside antibodies (high titre of IgM suggests
  MFMN)
- Muscle biopsy

Table 50.5. ALS/MND (World Federation of Neurology
Research Group on Motor Neuron Diseases 1998)

Required features:
- Evidence of lower motor neuron (LMN) degeneration by
  clinical, electrophysiological or neuropathologic examination
- Evidence of upper motor neuron (UMN) degeneration by
  clinical examination
- Evidence of progressive spread of symptoms or signs within a
  region or to other regions, as determined by history or
  examination
- No electrophysiological, pathological or neuroimaging
  evidence of other disease processes that might explain
  observed signs

specific symptoms should be sought (including exertional
dyspnoea, orthopnea, disturbed sleep with possible morning headache – indicating carbon dioxide retention and/or
daytime somnolence), as early indications of respiratory
compromise, together with appropriate signs. It is our practice to refer patients for consideration of respiratory support by non-invasive positive pressure ventilation (NIPPV).
This avoids tracheostomy and has been shown to improve
survival, symptoms and quality of life (Pinto *et al.*, 1995;
Lyall *et al.*, 2001; Newsom-Davis *et al.*, 2001). Both patients
and carers should understand that respiratory support is
part of palliative care, and that the underlying disease will
progress.

Respiratory care

Motor neuron diseases usually cause death by neuromuscular respiratory failure. Earlier, weakness of the chest wall
and diaphragm can cause significant distress. A history of

Nutritional support

Even without bulbar weakness, motor neuron dysfunction
is often associated with weight loss and malnutrition. We
found that 21% of ALS/MND patients were malnourished,

Table 50.6. Electrophysiological diagnostic features of ALS/MND (World Federation of Neurology Research Group on Motor Neuron Diseases, 1998)

1. EMG features of LMN involvement: items a) and b) are required
(a) Evidence of active denervation
  • Fibrillation potentials.
  • Positive sharp waves.
(b) Evidence of chronic denervation
  • Large motor unit potentials (increased duration, increased proportion of polyphasic potentials, often increased amplitude).
  • Reduced interference pattern with firing rates > 10 Hz (unless significant UMN component, when firing rate may be < 10 Hz).
  • Unstable motor unit potentials.
(c) Fasciculation potentials
  • Characteristic and rarely absent in ALS/MND (especially if of long duration and polyphasic). Occur with normal morphology in normal subjects (benign fasciculations) and with abnormal morphology in other denervation disorders (e.g., motor neuropathies).
2. Nerve conduction studies
  • Required principally to define and exclude other disorders (peripheral nerve, neuromuscular junction and muscle); should generally be normal or near normal.
3. Electrophysiological features compatible with UMN involvement include:
  • Up to 30% increase in central motor conduction time determined by cortical magnetic stimulation.
  • Low firing rates of motor unit potentials on maximal effort.
4. Electrophysiological features suggesting disease processes other than ALS/MND include:
  • Evidence of motor conduction block.
  • Motor conduction velocities lower than 70% of normal, and/or distal motor latencies over 130% of normal.
  • Abnormal sensory nerve conduction studies (may be difficult to elicit due to peripheral neuropathies, advanced age, etc., especially in the lower limbs).
  • F-wave or H-wave latencies more than 130% of normal.
  • Decrements greater than 20% on repetitive stimulation.
  • Somatosensory evoked response latency greater than 120% of normal.
  • Full interference pattern in a clinically weak muscle.
  • Significant abnormalities in autonomic function or electronystagmography.

with no difference between bulbar-onset and limb-onset cases (Worwood & Leigh, 1998). In addition to difficulty with eating and swallowing, respiratory failure, depression and infection can contribute to poor nutrition. Management is multi-disciplinary: speech therapists assess swallowing and advise on techniques to ease eating and avoid aspiration; a dietician's review will maximise calorific intake in as easily ingested a form as possible. Despite such intervention, oral intake may well become inadequate and so enteral feeding should be considered. Percutaneous endoscopic gastrostomy (PEG) can improve survival prognosis (Mazzini *et al.*, 1995) and is more successful if it is undertaken before respiratory function deteriorates (Chio *et al.*, 1999). The American Academy of Neurology practice parameters state that PEG should be undertaken before vital capacity falls below 50% of predicted? (Miller *et al.*, 1999). More recently, radiologically inserted gastrostomy (RIG) has been advanced and is perhaps suited to patients with respiratory compromise (Thornton *et al.*, 2002). Gastrostomy placement should therefore be considered

early, but as with ventilation, intervention should be considered in the overall context of the individual's quality of life.

Psychological

Depression and anxiety should be treated appropriately, and not viewed as unavoidable consequences of a progressive disease. Emotional lability is usually associated with pseudobulbar palsy and can be eased with antidepressants particularly SSRIs (such as citalopram or fluoxetine, see Table 50.8). Carers should be supported as well, and patient support organisations can be of great help in such situations.

Other common symptoms

Cramps are a frequent early symptom and may be bothersome. Spasticity may compromise mobility, but can in fact aid weak legs to support the body. Fasciculations are

Table 50.7. Multi-professional care of motor
neuron diseases

- General practitioner and district nurse
- Physiotherapists
- Occupational therapists
- Speech and language therapists
- Dieticians
- Counsellors (for bereavement, family support, etc.)
- Specialist nurses
- Palliative care team
- Relevant medical specialities and support staff
  (gastroenterology, respiratory medicine)
- Care coordinators
- Neurologists

Table 50.8. Symptom control

Symptom	Treatment
Sialorrhea	Amitriptyline 25–150 mg o.d.
	Hyoscine patch (1mg) for three days
	Glycopyrronium bromide 200 mcg (via gastrostomy)
	Unilateral parotid gland radiotherapy
Fasciculations	Carbamazepine titrated from 200 mg b.d.
Cramps	Quinine sulphate 200 mg o.n. – 300 mg b.d.
Spasticity	Baclofen 5 mg t.d.s. initially, increasing as required
	Tizanidine 2 mg o.d. initially, increasing as required
Emotional lability	Amitriptyline 25–150 mg o.d.
	SSRI e.g. citalopram 20 mg o.d., fluoxetine 20 mg o.d., paroxetine 20 mg o.d.

seldom intrusive and often diminish as the disease progresses. Treatment of these symptoms is also outlined in
Table 50.8.

End of life

Palliative care can be important before the terminal
stages of disease. Home care teams and day centres may
offer respite care, with a parallel set of staff comple-
menting those provided elsewhere. Terminal care often
involves alleviating distress from respiratory failure. Benzodiazepines and agents to dry secretions may be helpful
and opiates can relieve dyspnoea, anxiety, pain or other
distress.

Disease-modifying drugs

At the time of writing, only one drug – riluzole for ALS/
MND – has been shown to increase survival and thus gain
a therapeutic licence. In clinical trials, 18 months' administration of riluzole prolonged life or time to ventilation by
an average of about three months (Bensimon et al., 1994;
Lacomblez et al., 1996). Patients usually tolerate the drug
well, though some experience problems with fatigue and
nausea. However, trials demonstrated no convincing effect
on functional deterioration, and no assessment was made
of quality of life. With these results (and also its relative
expense, at ∼£3000 per person per year in the UK), its use
was controversial in some countries and it was not licensed
in others (e.g. Australia).

Genetic issues

The only proven causes of ALS/MND are genetic. Mutation
of the gene encoding the enzyme copper/zinc superoxide
dismutase (SOD1) has been demonstrated in around one-
fifth of patients with a family history and 3% of sporadic
cases (Rosen et al., 1993; Shaw et al., 1998). A second gene,
ALS2 or Alsin, was identified by linkage studies in 2001, but
at present the frequency of mutation is unknown (Hadano
et al., 2001; Yang et al., 2001). Genetic counselling of presymptomatic relatives is necessary before genetic testing is
undertaken. Such individuals should be made aware that
in 75–80% of familial cases no causative mutation will be
found, and thus a negative test does not exclude inheritance of the disease-causing allele. Other rarer conditions
(e.g. Kennedy's disease) have wholly hereditary bases.

REFERENCES

Bensimon, G., Lacomblez, L. et al. (1994). A controlled trial of
riluzole in amyotrophic lateral sclerosis. ALS/Riluzole Study
Group. N. Engl. J. Med., **330**, 585–91.

Chio, A., Finocchiaro, E. et al. (1999). Safety and factors related
to survival after percutaneous endoscopic gastrostomy in
ALS. ALS Percutaneous Endoscopic Gastrostomy Study Group.
Neurology, **53**, 1123–5.

Ellis, C. M., Simmons, A. et al. (1999). Distinct hyperintense MRI signal changes in the corticospinal tracts of a patient with motor
neuron disease. Amyotrophic Lateral Sclerosis and Other Motor
Neuron Disorders, vol. 1, pp. 41–4.

Goodin, D. S., Rowley, H. A. et al. (1988). Magnetic resonance imaging in amyotrophic lateral sclerosis. Ann. Neurol., **23**, 418–20.

Hadano, S., Hand, C. K. et al. (2001). A gene encoding a putative
GTPase regulator is mutated in familial amyotrophic lateral
sclerosis 2. Nat. Genet., **29**, 166–73.

Lacomblez, L., Bensimon, G. *et al.* (1996). Dose-ranging study of riluzole in amyotrophic lateral sclerosis. *Lancet*, **347**, 1425–31.

Lyall, R. A., Donaldson, N. *et al.* (2001). A prospective study of quality of life in ALS patients treated with noninvasive ventilation. *Neurology*, **57**, 153–6.

Mazzini L., Corra T. *et al.* (1995). Percutaneous endoscopic gastrostomy and enteral nutrition in amyotrophic lateral sclerosis. *J. Neurol.*, **242**, 695–8.

Miller, R. G., Rosenberg, J. A. *et al.* (1999). Practice parameter: the care of the patient with amyotrophic lateral sclerosis (an evidence-based review): report of the Quality Standards Subcommittee of the American Academy of Neurology: ALS Practice Parameters Task Force. *Neurology*, **52**, 1311–23.

Newsom-Davis, I. C., Lyall, R. A. *et al.* (2001). The effect of non-invasive positive pressure ventilation (NIPPV) on cognitive function in amyotrophic lateral sclerosis (ALS): a prospective study. *J. Neurol., Neurosurg. Psychiatry*, **71**, 482–7.

Pinto, A. C., Evangelista, T. *et al.* (1995). Respiratory assistance with a non-invasive ventilator (Bipap) in MND/ALS patients: survival rates in a controlled trial. *J. Neurol. Sci.*, **129**, 19–26.

Rosen, D. R., Siddique, T. *et al.* (1993). Mutations in Cu/Zn superoxide dismutase gene are associated with familial amyotrophic lateral sclerosis. *Nature*, **362**, 59–62.

Shaw, C. E., Enayat, Z. E. *et al.* (1998). Mutations in all five exons of SOD-1 cause ALS. *Ann. Neurol.*, **43**, 390–4.

Thornton, F. J., Fotheringham, T. *et al.* (2002). Amyotrophic lateral sclerosis: enteral nutrition provision – endoscopic or radiologic gastrostomy? *Radiology*, **224**, 713–17.

World Federation of Neurology Research Group on Motor Neuron Diseases (1998). El Escorial revisited: Revised criteria for the diagnosis of amyotrophic lateral sclerosis. http://www.wfnals.org/Articles/elescorial1998.htm

World Federation of Neurology Research Group on Neuromuscular Diseases (1994). El Escorial World Federation of Neurology criteria for the diagnosis of amyotrophic lateral sclerosis. *J. Neurol. Sci.* **124** (Suppl), 96–107.

Worwood, A. M. & Leigh, P. N. (1998). Indicators and prevalence of malnutrition in motor neurone disease. *Eur. Neurol.*, **40**, 159–63.

Yang, Y., Hentati, A. *et al.* (2001). The gene encoding alsin, a protein with three guanine–nucleotide exchange factor domains, is mutated in a form of recessive amyotrophic lateral sclerosis. *Nat. Genet.*, **29**, 160–5.

51

The genetics of amyotrophic lateral sclerosis

Ammar Al-Chalabi[1] and Robert H. Brown, Jr.[2]

[1]Department of Neurology, Institute of Psychiatry, London, UK
[2]Cecil B. Day Neuromuscular Laboratory, Massachusetts General Hospital East, Charlestown, MA, USA

Models of inheritance

The genetics of a disease such as amyotrophic lateral sclerosis (ALS) require some flexibility in thinking about familiality compared with the genetics of isolated cases. About 10% of the time, an individual who develops ALS also has first-degree relatives who have been affected. For the remainder, the disease is said to be sporadic, but detailed investigation of the family tree may occasionally reveal that cousins or other more distant relatives have been affected. ALS can therefore be seen as a disease with an inheritance pattern that lies on a continuum from sporadic disease, to familial clustering to clear Mendelian familiality. For simplicity we have maintained the conventional separation of familial and sporadic disease, but as will become obvious, this distinction is largely artificial.

Familial ALS and the first descriptions

The concepts of genetics were coming into being at about the same time as the earliest descriptions of motor neuron diseases. Mendel presented his classic paper in 1865 (Mendel, 1865) in which he described his famous sweet pea hybridization experiments. He did not use the term gene or genetic to describe the heritable units but called them "formative elements." Cambridge Professor of Biology William Bateson coined the term "genetics" (from the Greek "to generate") in 1905 when applying for a university chair in a letter to the Cambridge zoologist, Adam Sedgwick. He wrote, "Such a word is badly wanted and if it were desirable to coin one, Genetics might do." He was not successful in his application for the chair. The term was first used at a public conference in 1906 (Bateson, 1906), and in 1908 Bateson was finally appointed to the first Chair of Genetics at Cambridge. While it might seem obvious to us now that genes are carried on particles called chromo-somes, this was not necessarily a widely held view, even by those who strongly supported Mendel, such as Bateson, who believed they were carried as waves or vibrations. This was seen as a reasonable explanation for how such heritable factors could affect the entire body.

In about 10% of cases, amyotrophic lateral sclerosis is inherited as an autosomal dominant trait with age-dependent penetrance of about 96% by the age of 70. About 20% of such families have mutations in the gene for copper/zinc superoxide dismutase, SOD1 (Rosen et al., 1993; Siddique et al., 1991). Although in general, familial ALS is dominant, it is not uncommon for cousins or more distant relatives to be affected. This pattern of familial clustering may be explained by a single gene with very low penetrance, or by more than one locus contributing to disease susceptibility. Either of these explanations could also explain sporadic disease.

Although Charcot first described ALS in 1869 (Charcot & Joffroy, 1869), a familial case of motor neuron disease had been described by the French physician Aran in 1850, in his classic paper describing progressive muscular atrophy. He reported the case of a seaman who had developed cramps in the upper limbs, with subsequent wasting that spread to involve all limbs. The patient had a sister and two maternal uncles with a similar condition.

Aran's 1850 report portrayed an individual with lower motor neuron degeneration. Because predominant lower motor neuron involvement is often the pattern in SOD1-mediated familial ALS, it is possible that this individual, although reported as having progressive muscular atrophy, in fact had SOD1-mediated familial ALS. His pedigree would be consistent with autosomal dominant inheritance with variable penetrance, concepts and language that did not yet exist.

Pedigrees with familial ALS comprise the most informative group for gene-hunting experiments. The usual

Table 51.1. Familial ALS loci

Familial ALS type	Locus	Gene	Inheritance	Pattern	Mutations	Found in sporadic disease?	References
ALS1	21q	SOD1	AD	Classical	> 105	yes	(Siddique *et al.*, 1991; Rosen *et al.*, 1993)
ALS2	2q33	ALS2	AR	Young onset, UMN	9	no	(Hentati *et al.*, 1994; Hadano *et al.*, 2001; Yang *et al.*, 2001)
ALS3	18q		AD	Classical			(Hand *et al.*, 2002)
ALS4	9q34	SETX	AD	Young onset, slow	3	unknown	(Chance *et al.*, 1998; Ying-Zhang *et al.*, 2004)
ALS5	15q15		AR	Young onset			(Hentati *et al.*, 1998)
ALS6	16q		AD	Classical and with FTD			(Sapp *et al.*, 2003; Ruddy *et al.*, 2003)
ALS7	20p		AD	Classical			(Sapp *et al.*, 2003)
ALS8	20q13.3	VAPB	AD	Classical and lower motor neuron patterns	1	unknown	(Nishimura *et al.*, 2004a, b)
ALS-X	X		X-linked	Young onset			(Siddique, 1998)
ALS-FTD	9q21		AD	With FTD			(Hosler *et al.*, 2000)

Classification of familial ALS, loci, known genes, phenotype and number of mutations reported to date. AD = autosomal dominant, AR = autosomal recessive, UMN = upper motor neuron predominant, FTD = frontotemporal dementia.

method for gene-hunting in familial diseases is the linkage study. This is a technique based on the discovery by Bateson that some heritable characters tend to be transmitted together and comprise a linkage group. The statistical foundations to utilize this for gene-hunting were developed by Morton in 1955 (Morton, 1955) and constitute the basis of the LOD score method. The ideal pedigree for a linkage study is of at least three generations, as this provides sufficient information on the recombination events to generate a LOD score. This means that it is difficult to perform in a disease such as familial ALS; by the time the diagnosis is established in mid-life in patients, parents may no longer be alive, and children are not yet at the age of risk. Despite these limitations, several successful linkage studies have been performed in ALS, leading to the initial discovery of SOD1 mutations as well as several other loci.

Linked genetic loci in familial ALS

The first locus to be linked to familial ALS was on chromosome 22q21.2, later found to be the location of the SOD1 gene (Rosen *et al.*, 1993; Siddique *et al.*, 1991). This has catalyzed a variety of new lines of investigation in ALS, including the establishment of transgenic mouse and in vitro models of the disease, and has provided insight into the molecular pathogenesis of ALS, as discussed in detail below. Table 51.1 provides a summary of loci and genes to date.

A rare autosomal recessive form of slowly progressive, juvenile-onset predominantly upper motor neuron ALS was described in consanguineous families from Tunisia. Of

the three phenotypic groups, one has been linked to chromosome 2q33 and another to 15q15 (Hentati *et al.*, 1994, 1998). As reviewed below, the chromosome 2q-linked families are now known to have mutations in a novel gene coding for a G-protein known as alsin (Hadano *et al.*, 2001; Yang *et al.*, 2001). Although the initial description of these families included a pedigree with a lower motor neuron component, no other pedigree has amyotrophy, and subsequent mutations have been found in pedigrees with various phenotypes of hereditary spastic paraparesis or primary lateral sclerosis (Eymard-Pierre *et al.*, 2002; Devon *et al.*, 2003). Nevertheless, even though it is not strictly speaking an ALS gene, we will discuss the ALS2 gene and its protein in more detail below.

Typical ALS has also been linked to chromosome 20 and to chromosome 18q (Hand *et al.*, 2002; Sapp *et al.*, 2003). Juvenile ALS with very long survival (tens of years) has been linked to 9q34 in a single large pedigree (Chance *et al.*, 1998).

Predominantly lower motor neuron ALS with tremor has recently been mapped to chromosome 20, and a missense mutation identified in the VAPB gene, involved in vesicle trafficking (Nishimura *et al.*, 2004a).

A US family with typical ALS has been linked to the chromosome X centromeric region in a single brief report presented at a conference (Siddique *et al.*, 1998a).

Recently, four families, three with typical ALS and one with ALS and frontotemporal dementia, were linked to the same region of chromosome 16 (Ruddy *et al.*, 2003; Sapp *et al.*, 2003; Abalkhail *et al.*, 2003). The inheritance of the disease in the typical families was autosomal dominant with high penetrance, but the family with frontotemporal dementia showed a markedly reduced penetrance. It may seem surprising that a family with ALS may also have individuals affected by frontotemporal dementia, but this is not unusual. The relationship between ALS and frontotemporal dementia is intriguing both pathologically and clinically. ALS with frontotemporal dementia has been linked to chromosome 9q21-q22 (Hosler *et al.*, 2000). A form of parkinsonism with dementia and amyotrophy has been linked to chromosome 17q and subsequently shown to be due to mutations in the gene for microtubule-associated protein tau (for review see (Rosso & van Swieten, 2002)).

Cytosolic Cu/Zn superoxide dismutase (SOD1)

SOD1 is a five-exon gene on the short arm of chromosome 21 that codes for a free radical scavenging enzyme, copper/zinc superoxide dismutase. Mutations in this gene are the only proven cause of typical Charcot ALS. More than 100 mutations have now been described, and rather than tending to cluster in a particular part of the gene, they are scattered throughout the coding region (Andersen *et al.*, 2003). The active site of the enzyme is coded for by exon 3 and this has the fewest reported mutations, suggesting that it is the least tolerant to variation.

The most frequent SOD1 variant worldwide is the D90A mutation, predominant in Scandinavia. In northern Sweden this mutation is present as a clinical silent polymorphism with upwards of 5% of the normal population carrying a copy; indeed, the presence of this variant was first detected by an abnormal pattern of migration of the SOD1 protein in 1968 (Beckman, 1973). In contrast, in southern Sweden, Europe and North America this mutation is rare. In the USA, the A4V variant is the most frequent, accounting for about 60% of SOD1-associated cases. Worldwide, the most common mutations are this A4V substitution and the mutation I113T. Two of these three variants, D90A and I113T, have very low penetrance, implying a low negative evolutionary selection pressure. This could account for their relative abundance in the ALS population. A4V is an aggressive variant, but it is likely that a founder effect in the US population accounts for the high frequency. The low penetrance variants are less likely to generate pedigrees that look suitable for linkage analysis, and it is possible that if these were the only mutations of SOD1 in existence, this cause of ALS would not yet have been found.

Although SOD1 mutations typically cause an autosomal dominant high penetrance ALS, the situation is not straightforward; as noted, some mutations have low penetrance. There is also evidence for a dose effect of mutant SOD1 protein in initiating motor neuron cell death.

This is illustrated by consideration of the D90A mutation (also discussed in more detail in the section on sporadic disease). In northern Sweden, where the D90A variant is common, this missense change generally does not cause ALS when present in single copy, as one would predict of a seemingly benign polymorphism. In contrast, individuals with two copies develop ascending ALS that progresses very slowly. On the other hand, in individuals from other geographic regions, presumably with distinctly different genetic backgrounds, the same mutation can cause ALS when not present in two copies. This propensity to cause ALS when present in heterozygotes is typical of the dominant mechanism of action of all of the other SOD1 missense mutations. In one family, the situation is confounded by the observation that a heterozygous D90A mutation co-exists in affected individuals with the D96N mutation (Siddique *et al.*, 1998b). Whether the disease is solely a consequence of the D96N mutation or the accumulated effects of mutant proteins from both mutant alleles is not clear. Perhaps the best evidence for a dose relationship of mutant SOD1 protein to the initiation of cell death are reports that, in two cases, unusually aggressive, early onset forms of rapidly paralytic motor neuron disease were seen in individuals homozygous for either N86S (Hayward *et al.*, 1998) and L126S (Kato *et al.*, 2001). In the former, the reported case began in early adolescence and proved lethal within only weeks.

In general, there is a poor correlation between genotype and phenotype for most SOD1 mutations, although for most mutations the number of cases on which to base phenotype studies is small (Cudkowicz *et al.*, 1997; Radunovic & Leigh, 1996). SOD1 mutations are often characterized by a predominantly lower motor neuron pattern of ALS, although in such cases the clinical phenotype is otherwise indistinguishable from non-familial ALS. Extramotor involvement (e.g. paraesthesiae or pain) is sometimes seen with SOD1-mediated ALS; the A89V mutation is associated with a sensory neuropathy (Rezania *et al.*, 2003). Bladder disturbances and autonomic dysfunction have also been reported.

The A4V mutation, which may account for up to 60% of SOD1 mutations in the USA, is associated with a poor prognosis; it is not uncommon for A4V cases to survive no more than 12 months or so. The D90A mutation causing disease in single copy is associated with typical ALS, but homozygous (recessive) D90A has a uniform slowly ascending paretic phenotype. Two other exon 4 variants that also have slow progression are G93C and E100K. Exonic position is not a good marker of prognosis, however; for example D90V and I112T are also exon 4 variants but are associated with aggressive disease, while G37R and G41D are associated with a slower progression but are not exon 4 mutations. One reasonably consistent pattern is that variants associated with lower limb onset are also associated with slow progression and ascending weakness (for example G41D, H46R, D76V, D90A recessive, and E100K). G37R and L38V are associated with an earlier age at onset of symptoms.

ALS2

A form of juvenile, predominantly upper motor neuron, slowly progressive recessive ALS was described in 17 Tunisian pedigrees in 1990 (Ben Hamida *et al.*, 1990). Three phenotypes were distinguished in the initial paper. Group 1 was characterized by corticospinal signs with weakness with wasting in the upper limbs, beginning in early–mid teen years. Two aspects distinguish this phenotype from the other two classes of recessive JALS in this series. First, although there were subtle bulbar findings, no Group 1 cases demonstrated pseudobulbar affective signs. Second, the weakness showed a proclivity to involve the hands early in the disease course, even within the first decade; moreover, the early hand weakness was sometimes unilateral for several years. This form of JALS has been genetically linked to chromosome 15q15-q22 (Hentati *et al.*, 1998) (and designated ALS5) but there is almost certainly genetic heterogeneity in the Group 1 families. Group 2 cases begin early (first or second decade onset) and are clinically characterized by peroneal atrophy with foot drop and spastic paraplegia (with absent ankle reflexes). EMG studies show denervation in all limbs, with normal nerve conduction velocities. Group 3 was defined by one large, consanguineous pedigree with a rather uniform clinical picture of early onset (less than 10 years), spastic paraplegia and prominent pseudobulbar findings. Denervational atrophy was clinically minimal although electromyography demonstrated dysfunction of lower motor neurons in six of six cases.

Group 3 juvenile ALS cases were genetically linked to chromosome 2q33 (Hentati *et al.*, 1994) (and designated ALS2). Subsequently, other recessive families with a similar phenotype and inheritance were found in Kuwait and Saudi Arabia. None had amyotrophy and it may be that this is a unique feature in the one large Tunisian family. In 2001, it was determined that all of the chromosome 2q33 linked juvenile ALS cases had loss of function mutations in a novel gene predicted to have 34 exons encoding a novel protein designated alsin (Hadano *et al.*, 2001; Yang *et al.*, 2001). The first three linked families had small deletions in this gene, predicting a frameshift and premature stop codon resulting in a truncated alsin protein. This gene is normally processed into two transcripts, short and long. Both are ubiquitously expressed, in the neurons of the central nervous system and other tissues, although the shorter transcript is the predominant form in the liver. Only the Tunisian deletion affects both the short and the long transcripts, and this was postulated as a cause of the amyotrophy seen uniquely in the Tunisian pedigree. Since then, a further deletion also affecting the shorter transcript but not associated with amyotrophy has been reported suggesting that the amyotrophy has a different cause. In the last 2 years, the ALS2 phenotype has been broadened to include infantile hereditary spastic paraplegia with bulbar involvement and mutations have now also been found in families from Algeria, France, Italy and Pakistan, bringing the number of deletions to eight (Devon *et al.*, 2003; Eymard-Pierre *et al.*, 2002). Full length alsin therefore seems necessary for normal motor neuron function, but it is not clear what phenotype if any, would result from missense mutations that do not alter transcript length. The phenotype is more akin to a juvenile hereditary spastic paraplegia with corticobulbar involvement than typical ALS.

Alsin consists of three guanine exchange factor (GEF) domains: a Ran GEF, Rho GEF and a vacuolar sorting domain motif (VP39 GEF). Guanine exchange factors are small proteins involved in cycling of GTP/GDP for GTPases and are therefore involved in cell signalling. Alsin also contains a membrane occupation and recognition nexus motif (MORN). From this homology, various functions have been proposed, including organization of vacuolar traffic, control of chromatin condensation and cytoskeletal organization.

It is generally recognized that seemingly sporadic forms of ALS might be secondary to defects in genes whose normal functions are important determinants of motor neuron viability. For example, mutations that are either weakly dominant (such as the I113T SOD1 mutation) or recessive in an outbred population could produce apparently sporadic forms of ALS. Because a recessive gene defect would thus be able to masquerade as a cause of sporadic disease, we have recently screened the ALS2 gene for mutations in sporadic ALS cases with some features (early onset, long survival) mimicking features of ALS2. In this study, the alsin gene was sequenced in twelve individuals with predominantly upper motor neuron, young onset (mean age 29, youngest seven years), slowly progressive ALS (Al-Chalabi *et al.*, 2003a). All except one individual were still alive with median survival of 8 years at time of study. Five single nucleotide polymorphisms were found in the coding region, of which all except one were conservative. The non-conservative variant (1102g>a, V368M) in blade 4 of the regulation of chromatin condensation (RCC1) propeller had already been described in the original papers and does not appear to increase the risk of ALS. (It should be noted that the sequence numbering in the original papers is different in that one starts at base 1 of the coding sequence and the other starts at base 1 of exon 1). Using a maximum likelihood approach to haplotype analysis, regions of linkage disequilibrium were mapped in the gene. Single nucleotide polymorphisms from these regions were used to look for association with ALS in 300 cases and 300 matched controls. No difference was found, suggesting that variants in the ALS2 gene are not a common cause of typical ALS, nor of predominantly upper motor neuron young onset slowly progressive ALS.

Dynactin

Within the last 2 years, another gene defect has been identified in a motor neuron disorder that is an ALS variant. This is coinherited as a dominant trait in a family whose affected members show a late childhood onset form of predominantly lower motor neuron disease with prominent bulbar features. Because it is transmitted equally from mothers and fathers to either daughters or sons, this phenotype might be described as an autosomal form of Kennedy's spinal muscular atrophy. In 2002, Puls and colleagues reported that this disease is a consequence of dominantly acting mutations in the gene that encodes a form of dynactin (Puls *et al.*, 2003). This observation is of considerable biological importance because dynactin is involved in a complex of proteins that comprise a molecular motor for axonal transport; the implication is that an inherited disorder that closely resembles ALS can arise from perturbations in axonal transport. The plausibility of this hypothesis was strengthened by the near simultaneous report that defects in another motor protein, dynein, underlie an inherited motor neuron disease in two strains of mice ("legs at odd angles" or *loa* and "cramping" or *cra*) (Hafezparast *et al.*, 2003).

ALS4

In 1998, a form of slowly progressive, young onset amyotrophic lateral sclerosis was described in a single 11-generation American family (Chance *et al.*, 1998). The phenotype was of distal limb amyotrophy and pyramidal tract signs with severe loss of motor neurons in the brainstem and spinal cord. Mapping studies localized the genetic region to 9q34 with a LOD score of 18.8 and recently, two other families linked to the same locus have allowed the gene to be identified (Ying-Zhang *et al.*, 2004). The SETX (senataxin) gene is a DNA/RNA helicase also responsible

for autosomal recessive ataxia oculomotor apraxia type 2 (AOA2)(Moreira *et al.*, 2004). While three point mutations have been identified scattered through the gene in ALS4, all the mutations identified in AOA2 have been homozygous null deletions except for one compound heterozygote.

ALS8 and VAPB

A form of ALS in which a slowly progressive, predominantly lower motor neuron weakness is associated with fasciculation, cramps and tremor, was recently mapped to the long arm of chromosome 20, in a four-generation, white, Brazilian family (Nishimura *et al.*, 2004a). This was classified as ALS8, and a missense mutation was subsequently found at a conserved amino acid in the vesicle-trafficking protein, VAPB (166c>t, P56S) (Nishimura *et al.*, 2004b). This segregated with disease, and was also found in six other families, also with Portuguese ancestry, and probably from the same founder. Two of these had late-onset, slowly progressive ALS (ALS8 phenotype), three had late-onset spinal muscular atrophy, and one had members with both aggressive, classical ALS and the less typical ALS8 phenotype. This mutation probably disrupts intracellular membrane transport and secretion, especially of the endoplasmic reticulum and Golgi apparatus.

Sporadic ALS

While there is obviously a major genetic contribution from a single gene locus to the development of ALS in Mendelian pedigrees, the situation is not so clear for families with more than a single affected individual but without a clearly Mendelian transmission pattern. The role of inheritance in the majority of cases that are seemingly sporadic is also not defined. The available epidemiological and molecular evidence is that in these cases, the liability to disease is the result of the action of several genes and environmental factors. In such a model, the individual genetic components of disease susceptibility are heritable, but disease does not develop unless a threshold of liability is exceeded. This is best understood by considering the genetics of a continuous trait that shows heritability in humans, such as height.

The distribution of height in the population is Gaussian, and tall parents tend to have tall children. It seems unlikely that there is a single gene, different alleles of which determine height, since the number of discrete alleles required would be huge, and yet height clearly shows heritability. This was the conundrum that faced geneticists in the early twentieth century and was resolved by Fisher in 1918. If a single gene has two alleles, A and a, then if A increases height by a factor of half a unit above the mean and the a allele decreases height by half a unit below the mean, then the possible combinations, AA, Aa, aA and aa result in heights that are +1, 0, 0 and −1 units around the mean, respectively. If a further locus with alleles B and b has the same effect then the possible combinations AABB, AABb, etc through to aabb result in heights that range from +2 to −2, again with the extremes being rarer than middle values. A three locus system is in fact sufficient to result in a distribution that is almost Gaussian and with the effect of variation from environmental factors, is truly Gaussian. Thus a simple genetic process can result in continuous variation in the population. What is not so clear is whether such a process could result in a tendency to disease that appears sporadic or only showing occasional familial clustering.

The model most geneticists now use to explain this is the liability threshold model. The tendency (or liability) to develop a particular disease shows a Gaussian distribution and could be described by the multilocus inheritance described above. In this model, disease only manifests at one extreme of the distribution, so that only those individuals with a liability to disease above a particular threshold will develop the condition. Under this model, the tendency to sporadic disease is heritable and in some situations this will result in familial clustering. This model also has the property that individuals normally expected to be at lower risk that do develop disease must carry a greater burden of disease-causing genes. For example, in ALS younger individuals are less at risk, so a young person with sporadic ALS would be expected to carry a higher genetic load. A similar argument could be made for females, since there is a 3:2 ratio of men to women. We can therefore believe that sporadic ALS may have a heritable genetic component in theory, but what is the evidence that this is the case?

Evidence that all ALS has a significant genetic basis

Epidemiological studies

There are a number of epidemiological study designs that can provide evidence of a genetic basis for disease. Unfortunately, to date, few of these have been carried out in ALS. The most basic study is a segregation analysis. In this method, the pedigree of everyone in a defined population (for example, those attending a specialist clinic) is used to look for patterns of inheritance. At its most basic, if 50% of family members develop ALS, this constitutes strong evidence for autosomal dominant inheritance. For recessive inheritance the situation is a little more complex. This is

because families in which both parents are carriers, but who by chance do not produce affected offspring, will be common but unknown to the researcher. A correction for ascertainment bias is therefore needed. There are now various computer programs that will analyze large sets of pedigree data for the most appropriate genetic model or combination of models to explain the data. This simple process has not been performed in ALS but could provide evidence that a mixture of dominant genes of major effect and multiple genes of minor effect do indeed produce the distribution of ALS inheritance patterns we see.

Twin studies, adoption studies and adoptive twin studies have proven difficult to carry out in ALS. This is because ALS is relatively rare, and obtaining sufficient numbers is not always possible. One UK-based twin study identified 77 twin probands in 10 872 death certificates bearing the term "motor neuron disease" (used synonymously with ALS in the UK)(Graham *et al.*, 1997). Of these, 26 were monozygotic and 51 dizygotic. Four of the monozygotic probands were concordant with the co-twin for motor neuron disease, although two came from a family with known familial ALS. Based on these figures, the heritability of ALS was estimated as between 0.38 and 0.85.

Epidemiological evidence of familial clustering is important and is used to estimate lambda S (λ_s), the risk to a sibling compared with the general population risk. For ALS, the lifetime risk can be estimated from published epidemiological studies at between 1 in 250 and 1 in 1000 by the age of 70. For those in a family showing autosomal dominant inheritance, there is a 50% chance of inheriting a disease-causing gene and (presuming high penetrance) there is therefore a 50% chance of developing ALS. To understand the risk to a sibling, we can explore a theoretical situation of two siblings adopted into the same family, one of whom develops ALS. What is the risk to the sibling, given that nothing is known about their biological family? There would be a 10% chance that they have come from a family with autosomal dominant ALS, and if so, the risk to the sibling would be 50%. The overall risk is therefore 10% of 50%, which is 5%. When compared with the population risk of 1 in 1000, this gives us lambda S as 50. This is a high figure but is estimated presuming that autosomal dominant disease has high penetrance and that sporadic disease does not increase the risk to a sibling. However, among the 90% of families without autosomal dominant, high penetrance ALS will be some with low penetrance disease. In addition, if we accept the liability threshold model for sporadic ALS, there will be an increased risk for those with no family history at all. In general, for a trait with a normally distributed liability, the risk to a first-degree relative is approximately the square root of the population risk. (This is a result of the properties

Table 51.2. Sporadic ALS candidates

Gene	Findings	References
SOD1	About 2 to 3% sporadic cases have mutations	(Jones *et al.*, 1994; Andersen *et al.*, 1997; Jackson *et al.*, 1997)
APOE	Multiple studies suggest no increased risk, no modification of age of onset. Possible effect on prognosis and presentation	(Al-Chalabi *et al.*, 1996; Moulard *et al.*, 1996; Bachus *et al.*, 1997; Siddique *et al.*, 1998b)
CNTF	Negative association studies. Anecdotal studies suggestive of age of onset modification, not shown in case-control study. Homozygous deletion not fully excluded as modifier.	(Takahashi *et al.*, 1994; Orrell *et al.*, 1995; Takahashi, 1995; Imura *et al.*, 1998; Al-Chalabi *et al.*, 2003b)
ALS2	Variants not a common cause of sporadic ALS	(Al-Chalabi *et al.*, 2003a)
Mitochondrial SOD	Possible risk factor in small studies	(Dhaliwal & Grewal, 2000; Ro *et al.*, 2003; Mawrin *et al.*, 2003)
Dynein heavy chain	No increased risk in small study of 3 exons	(Ahmad-Annuar *et al.*, 2003)
MnSOD	Contradictory results in small studies	(Tomkins *et al.*, 2001; Van Landeghem *et al.*, 1999; Parboosingh *et al.*, 1995; Tomblyn *et al.*, 1998)
SMN1	Abnormal copy number possible risk factor. Deletion not.	(Jackson *et al.*, 1996; Orrell *et al.*, 1997; Parboosingh *et al.*, 1999; Corcia *et al.*, 2002)
SMN2	Homozygous deletion possible risk factor	(Moulard *et al.*, 1998; Veldink *et al.*, 2001)
APEX nuclease	Possible risk factor	(Olkowski, 1998; Tomkins *et al.*, 2000; Hayward *et al.*, 1999)
LIF	Single small positive study	(Giess *et al.*, 2000)
NEFH	Multiple positive studies suggest possible susceptibility factor. About 1% of sporadic cases have tail domain indel mutations.	(Al-Chalabi *et al.*, 1999; Figlewicz *et al.*, 1994; Tomkins *et al.*, 1998)
VEGF	Single large multicenter study strongly suggests promoter region SNP haplotype is a risk factor	(Lambrechts *et al.*, 2003)

Candidate genes studied as possible modifiers or susceptibility factors in sporadic ALS.

of the normal distribution and the distribution of liability in the mating population.) For sporadic ALS this would therefore be the square root of 1 in 1000, which is about 1 in 30. Lambda S is therefore about 30 for sporadic ALS. Under these assumptions therefore, the risk to a first degree relative of someone with ALS is between 30 and 50 times the population risk.

Other more unusual methods are also available to provide evidence for a genetic basis of disease. One such is based on the observation that spermatogenesis in humans results in increasing numbers of meioses with increasing paternal age. Since each meiosis carries a small but significant chance of deleterious mutation, genetic disease should arise *de novo* more frequently in those with older fathers (Crow, 2000). This can be tested by inspection of birth order. Last born children will on average have older fathers than first born children, and the demonstration that ALS more commonly occurs in last born than first born individuals would constitute evidence for a genetic basis for ALS.

Another method is estimation of relatedness by isonymy (Lasker, 1968; 1977). This is based on the patrilineal inheritance of surnames in many societies, so that surname inheritance is analogous to Y-chromosome inheritance. In communities with restricted opportunities for outbreeding there is a tendency for a single surname to dominate,

such as Jones or Richards in Wales, or Chan in parts of China. Thus, a restricted set of surnames can be a marker for a genetic bottleneck. Demonstration of a reduced set of surnames in ALS would constitute evidence for increased inter-relatedness of individuals with ALS and therefore of a genetic cause. This has been tested in the UK, Ireland and Germany and has shown a restricted set of surnames for familial disease but not for sporadic disease (Al-Chalabi, personal observation). This is probably because the underlying assumptions of the test are violated sufficiently frequently to reduce its power significantly.

Although the epidemiological evidence is sparse, it does support the notion that there is a significant genetic component to all ALS including sporadic cases. Linkage studies have demonstrated the genes and loci involved in familial disease, but different methods are required in sporadic disease. Table 51.2 summarizes the studies of possible genetic factors in sporadic ALS to date.

Genetic studies – SOD1

Mutations in SOD1 are found in about 3% of apparently sporadic cases (Jackson *et al.*, 1997; Andersen *et al.*, 1997; Jones *et al.*, 1994). In only one case has this been conclusively shown to be due to new mutation (Alexander *et al.*, 2002); it is likely that, in other cases, carrier parents did not manifest disease. More than 100 SOD1 mutations exist, which suggests that mutation in this gene has not been an uncommon event in our evolutionary history. On the other hand, more than 2000 cases of sporadic ALS per year worldwide should be directly attributable to SOD1 mutation. Because in general ALS affects people after they have started a family, there is not a large negative selection pressure. If the majority of SOD1-mediated sporadic ALS were due to new mutation, the numbers with ALS should be rising rapidly. Further evidence that SOD1 is not especially prone to new mutation comes from four studies of familial ALS that have shown a single founder for two mutants (D90A (Al-Chalabi *et al.*, 1998) and R115G (Niemann *et al.*, 2004)) and two founders for A4V (one for North American cases (Rosen, 2004) and another for the small families from Sweden and Italy (P. Anderson, pers.comm.)).

Two SOD1 mutations in particular, are frequently associated with sporadic disease, I113T and D90A. New mutation is not the usual cause of sporadic cases having SOD1 mutations, and for these two SOD1 variants at least, the explanation is low penetrance. In parts of Scandinavia, D90A in single copy can be regarded as a normal polymorphism of SOD1 with up to 5% of the population carrying it (Andersen *et al.*, 1995, 1996). Individuals homozygous for D90A develop a characteristic phenotype of ALS that is slowly progressive with predominantly spastic legs. (Similar families have also been found in Canada, France, Germany, Italy, Russia and the USA and there is evidence for such a family in Australia). Outside Scandinavia, some individuals with a single copy of the D90A variant develop ALS, either as a sporadic disease or in the context of familial ALS. Such individuals and families have been found in Belgium, Belorussia France, the UK and the USA. These cases generally have a more typical ALS phenotype. Two international haplotype studies have now shown that all D90A variants are identical-by-descent from a single founder, but individuals with the form needing two copies to develop ALS are a subgroup descended from a single more recent founder. The interpretation of this data has been that the recent founder carried a protective factor tightly linked to SOD1 so that in single copy D90A could not cause ALS, whereas individuals descended from the more distant founder alone did not carry such a factor and D90A is therefore toxic in single copy (Al-Chalabi *et al.*, 1998; Parton *et al.*, 2002). An alternative explanation lies within the liability threshold model. If we postulate that the D90A variant is not very toxic but increases liability to ALS by say 51%, then one copy would not cause disease but two copies would. If an individual carries other genetic factors or is exposed to environmental factors that increase liability to ALS by more than 50%, then ALS will result even though there is a single copy of D90A. In those with a predominantly genetic cause, the other liability factors would tend to be inherited by other siblings, but only 50% of them by offspring. ALS resulting from single copies of D90A would therefore tend to occur in multiple members of the same generation but not in multiple generations, a situation that is in fact observed.

Genetic studies – candidate gene association studies

Other than examining familial genes in sporadic disease, until recently, the only way of finding genes for sporadic disease was the candidate gene association study. This technique relies on selection of a candidate for being a disease-causing gene based on *a priori* assumptions about disease causation or by analogy from animal models. The gene is then assayed for variants in large numbers of cases and controls and if a particular variant is over-represented among the cases the disease is said to be associated with that variant. Association does not imply causation. If cases are not well matched with controls, the distribution of variants between the groups may vary because there may be differences other than disease status between groups. This is known as population stratification. Nevertheless, this technique has yielded some positive results and has excluded other candidates as being important in disease causation.

One of the earliest candidate genes studied was the heavy neurofilament subunit gene, NEFH. Because neurofilament accumulations are a hallmark of the pathology of ALS, they were an obvious choice. The NEFH subunit has a repetitive motif in the tail domain that is heavily phosphorylated. This region was examined in three studies which between them genotyped about 1000 sporadic cases and 1000 controls (Al-Chalabi *et al.*, 1999; Figlewicz *et al.*, 1994; Tomkins *et al.*, 1998). Variants of the tail domain consisting primarily of whole motif deletions or insertions were found in about 1% of cases and 0.2% of controls (both below the usual age of risk, in their thirties). An NEFH deletion was also found in a familial case of ALS, but unfortunately it has not been possible to determine if the mutation segregates with disease in this family. Another study examined 117 unrelated familial cases without finding mutations (Rooke *et al.*, 1996). This suggests that NEFH deletions are susceptibility factors rather than being sufficient to cause disease alone and are therefore predominantly found in sporadic ALS rather than familial ALS.

In Alzheimer's dementia and many other neurological disorders, the 4 allele of APOE is associated with disease or poor prognosis. In ALS several studies have examined this gene. The first of these showed no association between alleles of APOE and susceptibility, age of onset or disease duration of ALS (Mui *et al.*, 1995). It was subsequently suggested that the 4 allele was associated with bulbar onset ALS (Al-Chalabi *et al.*, 1996) with a trend towards worse prognosis, but not with susceptibility. This association with bulbar onset was also found in a French study, and in that study the association with survival reached significance. In addition, the converse was true for the 2 allele, which conferred protection (Moulard *et al.*, 1996). These findings were called into doubt by subsequent studies that failed to show any association with bulbar onset (Bachus *et al.*, 1997; Siddique *et al.*, 1998a,b). This was the case, too, in a recent study, that also failed to show association with age at onset, but did show a significantly poorer survival in those with the 4 allele by Kaplan–Meier analysis and the log rank test (Drory *et al.*, 2001). It may be that this finding too would disappear if known prognostic factors were controlled for in a multivariate analysis. Finally, a further study has shown no relationship between APOE genotype and clinical presentation or survival, but did show a relationship between APOE plasma levels and survival (Lacomblez *et al.*, 2002).

While dominant mutations of SOD1 can be found in sporadic ALS, it would be reasonable to expect that a recessive mutation might be even more frequent. As discussed above, a form of recessive, juvenile, slowly progressive, predominantly upper motor neuron ALS was recently mapped to the ALS2 (*alsin*) gene on chromosome 2 (Eymard-Pierre *et al.*, 2002; Hadano *et al.*, 2001; Yang *et al.*, 2001). This was therefore a good candidate for sporadic disease and was sequenced in 12 individuals, chosen for having a predominantly upper motor neuron slowly progressive ALS and with a generally young age of onset (Al-Chalabi *et al.*, 2003a). The youngest individual was seven and the mean age of onset was 29. All except one individual were still alive at the time of the study with a median survival of eight years. Several single nucleotide polymorphisms (SNPs) were found, five of which were in the coding region. All were conservative except one, 1102g>a, V368M, which had already been described. This variation occurs in blade four of the RCC1 propeller domain and does not appear to increase the risk of ALS. A further study of 300 cases and 300 matched controls was performed, testing for association with SNP alleles. No difference in allele frequency was found between groups. These findings suggest that variants of the ALS2 gene do not commonly cause typical ALS, nor a predominantly upper motor neuron, slowly progressive form of the disease.

Occasionally, a surprising candidate gene is suggested by accident. One such was the vascular endothelial growth factor gene, VEGF. Transgenic mice with deletion of the VEGF promoter hypoxia response element were gener-ated by a research team studying the vascular response to hypoxia. Unexpectedly, these mice developed a slowly progressive motor neuron degeneration, with features suggestive of a chronic motor neuropathy or slow ALS in humans. Examination of SNPs in the equivalent region of human VEGF in more than 1900 individuals has shown an association between homozygosity for haplotype AGG or AAG at positions +2,578, −1,154, −634 and ALS. This confers an increased risk of ALS of 1.8, $P < 0.00004$ (Lambrechts *et al.*, 2003). It is known that hypoxia leads to non-specific neuronal death, but this study shows that motor neurons may be especially vulnerable. There is anecdotal evidence of an increased risk of ALS in airline pilots, and it may be that individuals with this haplotype are at risk in certain occupations. There is also an increased risk of ALS in those who exercise heavily, and this, too, may be related to the response to hypoxia. This finding also has implications for the management of respiratory failure in ALS and suggests that aggressive and early treatment may be prognostically very important.

The ciliary neurotrophic factor gene, CNTF, codes for a 200-amino acid protein that is important in the maintenance and repair of the adult nervous system. Studies in mice have shown that disruption of CNTF or its receptor leads to motor neurodegeneration. In humans there is a null allele of CNTF, generated by a G to A intronic mutation. This results in a new splice site and a shorter protein (Takahashi *et al.*, 1994). Homozygous individuals comprise up to 2.3% of the population, but are not at increased risk of neurodegeneration including ALS (Takahashi *et al.*, 1994; Orrell *et al.*, 1995; Takahashi, 1995; Imura *et al.*, 1998). Reports have suggested that CNTF null alleles may be a risk factor for ALS resulting in younger onset and rapid disease (Giess *et al.*, 1998, 2001, 2002). A study of more than 350 individuals with ALS and 167 controls showed no association of the null allele with ALS, clinical features, age of onset or prognosis (Al-Chalabi *et al.*, 2003b).

Another trophic factor, leukemia inhibitory factor, has been implicated in ALS in a single study of 104 patients and 304 controls. Four patients were found to have a 3400 g > a, V64M mutation which was not found in any controls (Giess *et al.*, 2000) (P 0.0029 two-tailed Fisher exact test).

The survival motor neuron gene, SMN, has been studied extensively in ALS because of its role in the etiology of spinal muscular atrophy. SMN is found in a duplicated region on the q arm of chromosome 5. Homozygous deletion of SMN1, the telomeric copy, results in spinal muscular atrophy, but the disease severity is modified by the lower activity centromeric copy, SMN2. No study has identified SMN1 deletion as a risk factor for ALS (Jackson *et al.*, 1996; Orrell *et al.*, 1997; Parboosingh *et al.*, 1999; Moulard *et al.*,

1998) but a single study has demonstrated an increased risk of ALS associated with an abnormal SMN1 copy number (1 or 3 copies). Twenty eight of 167 patients compared with seven of 167 controls had an abnormal copy number giving an odds ratio of 1.85 (p 0.00035) for developing ALS (Corcia *et al.*, 2002). One study demonstrated an association of ALS with SMN 2 deletion (but not SMN1) (Moulard *et al.*, 1998) while another showed that homozygous SMN2 deletion is a prognostic factor in ALS, as it is in spinal muscular atrophy (Veldink *et al.*, 2001).

Oxidative stress can lead to alkylating DNA damage. There is evidence of a reduced capacity for repair of such damage in ALS (Tandan *et al.*, 1987; Kisby *et al.*, 1997). A multifunction enzyme APEX nuclease, also known as APE/ Ref-1 has a primary function of apurinic/apyrimidinic endonuclease repair. Three studies have shown rare mutations in sporadic ALS and one suggested that an allele of a common polymorphism D148E was over-represented in ALS (Olkowski, 1998; Tomkins *et al.*, 2000; Hayward *et al.*, 1999).

Mitochondrial SOD and MnSOD have been studied as possible candidates in sporadic ALS because of the involvement of Cu/Zn superoxide dismutase. Investigation of mitochondrial SOD mutation requires special techniques because of heteroplasmy. Mitochondria have their own genome and replicate independently of the Mendelian system used by the autosomes and sex chromosomes. Three studies, all small as a result, have been performed. Two of these suggest that mutation or deletion is commoner in ALS than in controls, and another found such changes equally in cases and controls (Dhaliwal & Grewal, 2000; Ro *et al.*, 2003; Mawrin *et al.*, 2003). The studies of Mn SOD have been small and contradictory (Tomkins *et al.*, 2001; Van Landeghem *et al.*, 1999; Parboosingh *et al.*, 1995; Tomblyn *et al.*, 1998).

Genetic studies – genome-wide association studies

The studies discussed above all suffer from the shortcoming that the disease gene needs to be specified *a priori*. In a linkage study, there is no prior assumption about what the disease gene is. The genome scan generates a LOD score which, if sufficiently high, prompts further investigation by haplotyping, fine mapping and positional cloning. This can be done because the common ancestor for family studies is only a few generations back and there will have been little chance for recombination to disrupt the linkage between disease gene and marker. Markers can therefore be placed up to 14 cM apart meaning that 300–400 markers are sufficient. In addition, only family members need be typed, so typically there will be perhaps a maximum of 100 individuals to genotype. What is needed is a similar process for sporadic disease gene hunting.

Groups of apparently unrelated individuals will always have a common ancestor if we look back far enough. Because of the rapid and recent expansion of humans on earth, the effective population size is thought to be only 10 000 individuals. In other words, the six billion people on earth have the genetic diversity of just 10 000. This means that relationships between genetic markers in the genome have been preserved over larger genetic distances than one might expect. The tendency for genetic markers to be inherited together is known as linkage disequilibrium (to highlight its opposite situation of independent inheritance of two loci, or linkage equilibrium). To perform a genome-wide association study in ALS, markers would need to be spaced far closer than in a linkage study because the common ancestor is more distant and linkage disequilibrium will not extend very far in terms of genetic distance. To maximize the chance that a disease gene will be in linkage disequilibrium with a nearby marker requires that the distance between adjacent markers should be much closer than 1cM and probably tens of kilo-bases at most. This means that over 3000 markers would be needed. To have sufficient power to detect a gene of moderate effect needs at least 300 cases and 300 controls, and ideally far more. This means that using today's technology, at least 1.8 million individual genotypings would be needed, compared with, at most, 40 000 for a typical linkage study. The costs and time required mean that for the time being, this is not feasible and other solutions are needed.

One method that has been explored is DNA pooling. In this technique, the DNA from each case is combined as a single sample, and the same is done for controls. The process is carefully controlled so that each person contributes as near as possible the same number of DNA molecules. Although certain measures need to be taken to control for artefacts, this method does allow the estimation of allele frequencies and potentially reduces the workload to just 6000 genotypings. It can also be used without allele frequency estimation as a screen for relative differences between pools.

Another method that will soon be available is the whole-genome association study based on DNA microarrays. With this technology, the genotyping of for example 100 000 SNPs takes about 3 days. The main problem at present is the cost, but this will improve with time.

Conclusions

The finding of SOD1 gene defects in both familial and sporadic cases, and the clustering of ALS seen in families without clear autosomal dominant inheritance unmistakably argue that the distinction between sporadic and familial

ALS is to some extent artificial. As linkage in more low penetrance families is reported, and as the technology to find multiple genes simultaneously contributing to disease improves, the line between familial and sporadic ALS will blur still further.

In the long term, one anticipates that insights acquired through the study of gene defects that cause or predispose to ALS will facilitate the discovery of new approaches to treating this disease. It is evident, for example, that strategies to inactivate dominantly acting mutant alleles and proteins may ameliorate the associated motor neuron death. While a comprehensive view of such therapeutic directions is beyond the scope of this review, we note that multiple approaches to allele inactivation are formally possible. These include techniques using DNA–protein hybrids to correct missense mutations using site directed somatic cell mutagenesis, discovery of small molecules that inhibit the offending promoter, and strategies such as ribozymes, anti-sense oligonucleotides, and inhibitory RNA (Parekh-Olmedo *et al.*, 2002; Xiang *et al.*, 1997). At this point, two groups have reported successful generation of RNAi to inhibit SOD1, both non-specifically and in a mutant, allele-specific manner (Maxwell *et al.*, 2004; Ding *et al.*, 2003). If such molecules can be delivered to the CNS, it is conceivable that they may be beneficial at least for mutant-SOD1 mediated motor neuron disease.

Acknowledgements

AAC is an MRC Clinician Scientist Fellow. The authors wish to thank the Motor Neurone Disease Association (UK), Amyotrophic Lateral Sclerosis Association, Angel Fund, Project ALS, the Pierre L. de Bourgknecht ALS Research Foundation, the National Institutes of Health (National Institute for Neurological Diseases and Stroke and the National Institute for Aging), the Medical Research Council and the C. B. Day Foundation.

REFERENCES

Abalkhail, H., Mitchell, J., Habgood, J., Orrell, R. & De Belleroche, J. (2003). A new familial amyotrophic lateral sclerosis locus on chromosome 16q12.1–16q12.2. *Am. J. Hum. Genet.*, **73**, 383–9.

Ahmad-Annuar, A., Shah, P., Hafezparast, M. *et al.* (2003). No association with common Caucasian genotypes in exons 8, 13 and 14 of the human cytoplasmic dynein heavy chain gene (DNCHC1) and familial motor neuron disorders. *Amyotroph. Lateral Scler. Other Motor Neuron Disord.*, **4**, 150–7.

Al-Chalabi, A., Andersen, P. M., Chioza, B. *et al.* (1998). Recessive amyotrophic lateral sclerosis families with the D90A SOD1 mutation share a common founder: evidence for a linked protective factor. *Hum. Mol. Genet.*, **7**, 2045–50.

Al-Chalabi, A., Andersen, P. M., Nilsson, P. *et al.* (1999). Deletions of the heavy neurofilament subunit tail in amyotrophic lateral sclerosis. *Hum. Mol. Genet.*, **8**, 157–64.

Al-Chalabi, A., Enayat, Z. E., Bakker, M. C. *et al.* (1996). Association of apolipoprotein E epsilon 4 allele with bulbar-onset motor neuron disease. *Lancet*, **347**, 159–60.

Al-Chalabi, A., Hansen, V. K., Simpson, C. L. *et al.* (2003a). Variants in the ALS2 gene are not associated with sporadic amyotrophic lateral sclerosis. *Neurogenetics*.

Al-Chalabi, A., Scheffler, M. D., Smith, B. N. *et al.* (2003b). Ciliary neurotrophic factor genotype does not influence clinical phenotype in amyotrophic lateral sclerosis. *Ann. Neurol.*, **54**, 130–4.

Alexander, M. D., Traynor, B. J., Miller, N. *et al.* (2002). "True" sporadic ALS associated with a novel SOD-1 mutation. *Ann. Neurol.*, **52**, 680–3.

Andersen, P. M., Forsgren, L., Binzer, M. *et al.* (1996). Autosomal recessive adult-onset amyotrophic lateral sclerosis associated with homozygosity for Asp90Ala CuZn-superoxide dismutase mutation. A clinical and genealogical study of 36 patients. *Brain*, **119**, 1153–72.

Andersen, P. M., Nilsson, P., Ala-Hurula, V. *et al.* (1995). Amyotrophic lateral sclerosis associated with homozygosity for an Asp90Ala mutation in CuZn-superoxide dismutase. *Nat. Genet.*, **10**, 61–6.

Andersen, P. M., Nilsson, P., Keranen, M. L. *et al.* (1997). Phenotypic heterogeneity in motor neuron disease patients with CuZn-superoxide dismutase mutations in Scandinavia. *Brain*, **10**, 1723–37.

Andersen, P. M., Sims, K. B., Xin, W. W. *et al.* (2003). Sixteen novel mutations in the Cu/Zn superoxide dismutase gene in amyotrophic lateral sclerosis: a decade of discoveries, defects and disputes. *Amyotroph. Lateral Scler. Other Motor Neuron Disord.*, **4**, 62–73.

Bachus, R., Bader, S., Gessner, R. & Ludolph, A. C. (1997). Lack of association of apolipoprotein e epsilon 4 allele with bulbar-onset motor neuron disease. *Ann. Neurol.*, **41**, 417.

Bateson, W. (1906). Address. In *Third Conference on Hybridisation*, Cambridge, UK.

Beckman, G. (1973). Population studies in northern Sweden. VI. Polymorphism of superoxide dismutase. *Hereditas*, **73**, 305–10.

Ben Hamida, M., Hentati, F. & Ben Hamida, C. (1990). Hereditary motor system diseases (chronic juvenile amyotrophic lateral sclerosis). Conditions combining a bilateral pyramidal syndrome with limb and bulbar amyotrophy. *Brain*, **113**, 347–63.

Chance, P. F., Rabin, B. A., Ryan, S. G. *et al.* (1998). Linkage of the gene for an autosomal dominant form of juvenile amyotrophic lateral sclerosis to chromosome 9q34. *American Journal of Human Genetics*, **62**, 633–40.

Charcot, J. M. & Joffroy, A. (1869). Deux cas d'atrophie musculaire progressive avec lesions de la substance grise et des faisceaux antero-lateraux de la moelle epiniere. *Arch. Physiol., Neurol. Pathol.*, **2**, 744.

Chen, Y. Z., Beunett, C. L., Huynh, H. M. *et al.* (2004). DNA/RNA helicase gene mutations in a form of juvenile amyotrophic lateral sclerosis (ALS4). *Am. J. Hum. Genet.*, **74**(6), 1128–35.

Corcia, P., Mayeux-Portas, V., Khoris, J. *et al.* (2002). Abnormal SMN1 gene copy number is a susceptibility factor for amyotrophic lateral sclerosis. *Ann. Neurol.*, **51**, 243–6.

Crow, J. F. (2000). The origins, patterns and implications of human spontaneous mutation. *Nat. Rev. Genet.*, **1**, 40–7.

Cudkowicz, M. E., McKenna-Yasek, D., Sapp, P. E. *et al.* (1997). Epidemiology of mutations in superoxide dismutase in amyotrophic lateral sclerosis [see comments]. *Ann. Neurol.*, **41** (2), 210–21.

Devon, R., Helm, J., Rouleau, G. *et al.* (2003). The first nonsense mutation in alsin results in a homogeneous phenotype of infantile-onset ascending spastic paralysis with bulbar involvement in two siblings. *Clin. Genet.*, **64**, 210–15.

Dhaliwal, G. K. & Grewal, R. P. (2000). Mitochondrial DNA deletion mutation levels are elevated in ALS brains. *NeuroReport*, **11**, 2507–2509.

Ding, H., Schwarz, D. S., Keene, A. *et al.* (2003). Selective silencing by RNAi of a dominant allele that causes amyotrophic lateral sclerosis. *Aging Cell*, **2**, 209–17.

Drory, V. E., Birnbaum, M., Korczyn, A. D. & Chapman, J. (2001). Association of APOE varepsilon4 allele with survival in amyotrophic lateral sclerosis. *J. Neurol. Sci.*, **190**, 17–20.

Eymard-Pierre, E., Lesca, G., Dollet, S. *et al.* (2002). Infantile-onset ascending hereditary spastic paralysis is associated with mutations in the alsin gene. *Am. J. Hum. Genet.*, **71**, 518–27.

Figlewicz, D. A., Krizus, A., Martinoli, M. G. *et al.* (1994). Variants of the heavy neurofilament subunit are associated with the development of amyotrophic lateral sclerosis. *Hum. Mol. Genet.*, **3**, 1757–61.

Giess, R., Beck, M., Goetz, R., Nitsch, R. M., Toyka, K. V. & Sendtner, M. (2000). Potential role of LIF as a modifier gene in the pathogenesis of amyotrophic lateral sclerosis. *Neurology*, **54**, 1003–5.

Giess, R., Braga, M., Holtmann, B., Tokya, K. & Sendtner, M. (2001). A CNTF null mutation as a potential modifier to disease onset in familial ALS with a mutation in the SOD-1 gene and transgenic SOD-1 mutant mice. *J. Neurol.*, **248**, 41–2.

Giess, R., Goetz, R., Schrank, B., Ochs, G., Sendtner, M. & Toyka, K. (1998). Potential implications of a ciliary neurotrophic factor gene mutation in a German population of patients with motor neuron disease. *Muscle Nerve*, **21**, 236–8.

Giess, R., Holtmann, B., Braga, M. *et al.* (2002). Early onset of severe familial amyotrophic lateral sclerosis with a SOD-1 mutation: potential impact of CNTF as a candidate modifier gene. *Am. J. Hum. Genet.*, **70**, 1277–86.

Graham, A. J., Macdonald, A. M. & Hawkes, C. H. (1997). British motor neuron disease twin study. [Review] [60 refs]. *J. Neurol, Neurosurg. Psychiatry*, **62**, 562–9.

Hadano, S., Hand, C. K., Osuga, H. *et al.* (2001). A gene encoding a putative GTPase regulator is mutated in familial amyotrophic lateral sclerosis 2. *Nat. Genet.*, **29**, 166–73.

Hafezparast, M., Klocke, R., Ruhrberg, C. *et al.* (2003). Mutations in dynein link motor neuron degeneration to defects in retrograde transport. *Science*, **300**, 808–12.

Hand, C. K., Mayeux-Portas, Y., Khoris, J. *et al.* (2001). Compound heterozygous D90A and D96N SOD1 mutations in a recessive amyotrophic lateral sclerosis family. *Ann. Neurol.*, **49**(2), 267–71.

Hand, C. K., Khoris, J., Salachas, F. *et al.* (2002). A novel locus for familial amyotrophic lateral sclerosis, on chromosome 18q. *Am. J. Hum. Genet.*, **70**, 251–6.

Hayward, C., Brock, D. J., Minns, R. A. & Swingler, R. J. (1998). Homozygosity for Asn86Ser mutation in the CuZn-superoxide dismutase gene produces a severe clinical phenotype in a juvenile onset case of familial amyotrophic lateral sclerosis [letter]. *J. Med. Genet.*, **35**, 174.

Hayward, C., Colville, S., Swingler, R. J. & Brock, D. J. (1999). Molecular genetic analysis of the APEX nuclease gene in amyotrophic lateral sclerosis. *Neurology*, **52**, 1899–901.

Hentati, A., Bejaoui, K., Pericak Vance, M. A. *et al.* (1994). Linkage of recessive familial amyotrophic lateral sclerosis to chromosome 2q33–q35. *Nat. Genet.*, **7**, 425–8.

Hentati, A., Ouahchi, K., Pericak-Vance, M. A. *et al.* (1998). Linkage of a commoner form of recessive amyotrophic lateral sclerosis to chromosome 15q15–q22 markers [In Process Citation]. *Neurogenetics.*, **2**, 55–60.

Hosler, B. A., Siddique, T., Sapp, P. C. *et al.* (2000). Linkage of familial amyotrophic lateral sclerosis with frontotemporal dementia to chromosome 9q21–q22. *J. Am. Med. Assoc.*, **284**, 1664–9.

Imura, T., Shimohama, S., Kawamata, J. & Kimura, J. (1998). Genetic variation in the ciliary neurotrophic factor receptor alpha gene and familial amyotrophic lateral sclerosis [letter]. *Annals of Neurology*, **43**, 275.

Jackson, M., Al-Chalabi, A., Enayat, Z. E., Chioza, B., Leigh, P. N. & Morrison, K. E. (1997). Copper/zinc superoxide dismutase 1 and sporadic amyotrophic lateral sclerosis: analysis of 155 cases and identification of a novel insertion mutation. *Ann. Neurology*, **42**, 803–7.

Jackson, M., Morrison, K. E., Al-Chalabi, A., Bakker, M. & Leigh, P. N. (1996). Analysis of chromosome 5q13 genes in amyotrophic lateral sclerosis: homozygous NAIP deletion in a sporadic case. *Ann. Neurol.*, **39**, 796–800.

Jones, C. T., Swingler, R. J. & Brock, D. J. (1994). Identification of a novel SOD1 mutation in an apparently sporadic amyotrophic lateral sclerosis patient and the detection of Ile113Thr in three others. *Hum. Mol. Genet.*, **3**(4), 649–50.

Kato, M., Aoki, M., Ohta, M. *et al.* (2001). Marked reduction of the Cu/Zn superoxide dismutase polypeptide in a case of familial amyotrophic lateral sclerosis with the homozygous mutation. *Neurosci. Lett.*, **312**, 165–8.

Kisby, G. E., Milne, J. & Sweatt, C. (1997). Evidence of reduced DNA repair in amyotrophic lateral sclerosis brain tissue. *NeuroReport*, **8**, 1337–40.

Lacomblez, L., Doppler, V., Beucler, I. *et al.* (2002). APOE: a potential marker of disease progression in ALS. *Neurology*, **58**, 1112–14.

Lambrechts, D., Storkebaum, E., Morimoto, M. *et al.* (2003). VEGF is a modifier of amyotrophic lateral sclerosis in mice and humans and protects motoneurons against ischemic death. *Nat. Genet.*, **34**, 383–94.

Lasker, G. W. (1968). The occurrence of identical (isonymous) surnames in various relationships in pedigrees: a preliminary analysis of the relation of surname combinations to inbreeding. *Am. J. Hum. Genet.*, **20**, 250–7.

Lasker, G. W. (1977). A coefficient of relationship by isonymy: a method for estimating the genetic relationship between populations. *Hum. Biol.*, **49**, 489–93.

Mawrin, C., Kirches, E. & Dietzmann, K. (2003). Single-cell analysis of mtDNA in amyotrophic lateral sclerosis: towards the characterization of individual neurons in neurodegenerative disorders. *Pathol Res. Pract.*, **199**, 415–18.

Maxwell, M. M., Pasinelli, P., Kazantsev, A. G. & Brown, R. H., Jr. (2004). RNA interference-mediated silencing of mutant superoxide dismutase rescues cyclosporin A-induced death in cultured neuroblastoma cells. *Proc. Natl Acad. Sci. USA*, **101**, 3178–83.

Mendel, G. (1865). Versuche uber Pflanzen-Hybriden (Experiments in Plant Hybridization). In *Verhandlungen es naturforschenden Vereines in Brunn 4 (Natural History Society of Brunn 4)* Bohemia, Czechoslovakia.

Moreira, M. C., Klur, S., Watanabe, M. *et al.* (2004). Senataxin, the orthologue of a yeast RNA helicase, is mutant in ataxia-ocular apraxia 2. *Nat. Genet.*, **36**, 225–7.

Morton, N. E. (1955). Sequential tests for the detection of linkage. *Am. J. Hum. Genet.*, **7**, 277–318.

Moulard, B., Salachas, F., Chassande, B. *et al.* (1998). Association between centromeric deletions of the SMN gene and sporadic adult-onset lower motor neuron disease. *Ann. Neurol.*, **43**, 640–4.

Moulard, B., Sefiani, A., Laamri, A., Malafosse, A. & Camu, W. (1996). Apolipoprotein E genotyping in sporadic amyotrophic lateral sclerosis, evidence for a major influence on the clinical presentation and prognosis. *J. Neurol. Sci.*, **139**, 34–7.

Mui, S., Rebeck, G. W., McKenna Yasek, D., Hyman, B. T. & Brown, R. H., Jr. (1995). Apolipoprotein E epsilon 4 allele is not associated with earlier age at onset in amyotrophic lateral sclerosis. *Ann. Neurol.*, **38**, 460–3.

Niemann, S., Joos, H., Meyer, T. *et al.* (2004). Familial ALS in Germany: origin of the R115G SOD1 mutation by a founder effect. *J. Neurol. Neurosurg. Psychiatry*, **75**, 1186–8.

Nishimura, A. L., Mitne-Neto, M., Silva, H. C., Oliveira, J. R., Vainzof, M. & Zatz, M. (2004a). A novel locus for late onset amyotrophic lateral sclerosis/motor neurone disease variant at 20q13. *J. med. Genet.*, **41**, 315–20.

Nishimura, A. L., Mitne-Neto, M., Silva, H. C. *et al.* (2004b). A mutation in the vesicle-trafficking protein VAPB causes late-onset spinal muscular atrophy and amyotrophic lateral sclerosis. *Am. J. Hum. Genet.*, **75**, 822–31.

Olkowski, Z. L. (1998). Mutant AP endonuclease in patients with amyotrophic lateral sclerosis. *NeuroReport*, **9**, 239–42.

Orrell, R. W., Habgood, J. J., de Belleroche, J. S. & Lane, R. J. M. (1997). The relationship of spinal muscular atrophy to motor neuron disease: Investigation of SMN and NAIP gene deletions in sporadic and familial ALS. *J. Neurol. Sci.*, **145**, 55–61.

Orrell, R. W., King, A. W., Lane, R. J. & de Belleroche, J. S. (1995). Investigation of a null mutation of the CNTF gene in familial amyotrophic lateral sclerosis. *J. Neurol. Sci.*, **132**, 126–8.

Parboosingh, J. S., Meininger, V., McKenna-Yasek, D., Brown, R. H., Jr. & Rouleau, G. A. (1999). Deletions causing spinal muscular atrophy do not predispose to amyotrophic lateral sclerosis. *Archives of Neurology*, **56**, 710–12.

Parboosingh, J. S., Rouleau, G. A., Meninger, V., McKenna Yasek, D., Brown, R. H., Jr. & Figlewicz, D. A. (1995). Absence of mutations in the Mn superoxide dismutase or catalase genes in familial amyotrophic lateral sclerosis. *Neuromuscul. Disord.*, **5**, 7–10.

Parekh-Olmedo, H., Krainc, D. & Kmiec, E. B. (2002). Targeted gene repair and its application to neurodegenerative disorders. *Neuron*, **33**, 495–8.

Parton, M. J., Broom, W., Andersen, P. M. *et al.* (2002). D90A-SOD1 mediated amyotrophic lateral sclerosis: a single founder for all cases with evidence for a Cis-acting disease modifier in the recessive haplotype. *Hum. Mutat.*, **20**, 473.

Puls, I., Jonnakuty, C., LaMonte, B. H. *et al.* (2003). Mutant dynactin in motor neuron disease. *Nat. Genet.*, **33**, 455–6.

Radunovic, A. & Leigh, P. N. (1996). Cu/Zn superoxide dismutase gene mutations in amyotrophic lateral sclerosis: Correlation between genotype and clinical features. *J. Neurol. Neurosurg. Psychiatry*, **61**, 565–72.

Rezania, K., Yan, J., Dellefave, L. *et al.* (2003). A rare Cu/Zn superoxide dismutase mutation causing familial amyotrophic lateral sclerosis with variable age of onset, incomplete penetrance and a sensory neuropathy. *Amyotroph. Lateral Scler. Other Motor Neuron Disord.*, **4**, 162–6.

Ro, L. S., Lai, S. L., Chen, C. M. & Chen, S. T. (2003). Deleted 4977-bp mitochondrial DNA mutation is associated with sporadic amyotrophic lateral sclerosis: a hospital-based case-control study. *Muscle Nerve*, **28**, 737–43.

Rooke, K., Figlewicz, D. A., Han, F. Y. & Rouleau, G. A. (1996). Analysis of the KSP repeat of the neurofilament heavy subunit in familial amyotrophic lateral sclerosis. *Neurology*, **46**, 789–90.

Rosen, D. R. (2004). A shared chromosome-21 haplotype among amyotrophic lateral sclerosis families with the A4V SOD1 mutation. *Clin. Genet.*, **66**, 247–50.

Rosen, D. R., Siddique, T., Patterson, D. *et al.* (1993). Mutations in Cu/Zn superoxide dismutase gene are associated with familial amyotrophic lateral sclerosis [published erratum appears in Nature 1993 Jul 22;364(6435):362] [see comments]. *Nature*, **362**, 59–62.

Rosso, S. M. & van Swieten, J. C. (2002). New developments in frontotemporal dementia and parkinsonism linked to chromosome 17. *Curr. Opin. Neurol.*, **15**, 423–8.

Ruddy, D. M., Parton, M. J., Al-Chalabi, A. *et al.* (2003). Two families with familial amyotrophic lateral sclerosis are linked to a novel locus on chromosome 16q. *Am. J. Hum. Genet.*, **73**, 390–6.

Sapp, P. C., Hosler, B. A., McKenna-Yasek, D. *et al.* (2003). Identification of two novel loci for dominantly inherited familial amyotrophic lateral sclerosis. *Am. J. Hum. Genet.*, **73**, 397–403.

Siddique, T., Figlewicz, D. A., Pericak Vance, M. A. *et al.* (1991). Linkage of a gene causing familial amyotrophic lateral sclerosis to chromosome 21 and evidence of genetic-locus heterogeneity [published errata appear in N Engl J Med 1991 Jul 4;325(1):71 and 1991 Aug 15;325(7):524] [see comments]. *N. Engl. J. Med.*, **324**, 1381–4.

Siddique, T., Hong, S., Brooks, B. *et al.* (1998a). X-linked dominant locus for late-onset familial amyotrophic lateral sclerosis. *Am. J. Hum. Genet.*

Siddique, T., Pericak-Vance, M. A., Caliendo, J. *et al.* (1998b). Lack of association between apolipoprotein E genotype and sporadic amyotrophic lateral sclerosis. *Neurogenetics*, **1**, 213–16.

Takahashi, R. (1995). Deficiency of human ciliary neurotrophic factor (CNTF) is not causally related to amyotrophic lateral sclerosis (ALS). *Clin. Neurol.*, **35**, 1543–5.

Takahashi, R., Yokoji, H., Misawa, H., Hayashi, M., Hu, J. & Deguchi, T. (1994). A null mutation in the human CNTF gene is not causally related to neurological diseases. *Nat. Genet.*, **7**, 79–84.

Tandan, R., Robison, S. H., Munzer, J. S. & Bradley, W. G. (1987). Deficient DNA repair in amyotrophic lateral sclerosis cells. *J. Neurol. Sci.*, **79**, 189–203.

Tomblyn, M., Kasarskis, E. J., Xu, Y. & St Clair, D. K. (1998). Distribution of MnSOD polymorphisms in sporadic ALS patients. *J. Mol. Neurosci.*, **10**, 65–6.

Tomkins, J., Banner, S. J., McDermott, C. J. & Shaw, P. J. (2001). Mutation screening of manganese superoxide dismutase in amyotrophic lateral sclerosis. *NeuroReport*, **12**, 2319–22.

Tomkins, J., Dempster, S., Banner, S. J., Cookson, M. R. & Shaw, P. J. (2000). Screening of AP endonuclease as a candidate gene for amyotrophic lateral sclerosis (ALS). *NeuroReport*, **11**, 1695–7.

Tomkins, J., Usher, P., Slade, J. Y. *et al.* (1998). Novel insertion in the KSP region of the neurofilament heavy gene in amyotrophic lateral sclerosis (ALS). *NeuroReport*, **9**, 3967–70.

Van Landeghem, G. F., Tabatabaie, P., Beckman, G., Beckman, L. & Andersen, P. M. (1999). Manganese-containing superoxide dismutase signal sequence polymorphism associated with sporadic motor neuron disease. *Eur. J. Neurol.*, **6**, 639–44.

Veldink, J. H., van den Berg, L. H., Cobben, J. M. *et al.* (2001). Homozygous deletion of the survival motor neuron 2 gene is a prognostic factor in sporadic ALS. *Neurology*, **56**, 749–52.

Xiang, Y., Cole-Strauss, A., Yoon, K., Gryn, J. & Kmiec, E. B. (1997). Targeted gene conversion in a mammalian CD34+-enriched cell population using a chimeric RNA/DNA oligonucleotide. *J. Mol. Med.*, **75**, 829–35.

Yang, Y., Hentati, A., Deng, H. X. *et al.* (2001). The gene encoding alsin, a protein with three guanine-nucleotide exchange factor domains, is mutated in a form of recessive amyotrophic lateral sclerosis. *Nat. Genet.*, **29**, 160–5.

52

Current and potential therapeutics

Clare Wood-Allum and Pamela J. Shaw

Academic Neurology Unit, Sheffield University Medical School, UK

Introduction

This chapter will survey the research underpinning current therapeutic candidates for amyotrophic lateral sclerosis (ALS), hereditary spastic paraplegia (HSP), Kennedy's disease (SBMA) and spinal muscular atrophy (SMA). It will also review the evidence base and rationale for the use of riluzole in ALS, the only disease-modifying agent currently licensed for use in any neurodegenerative disease of the motor neuron. In the absence of effective therapies to slow disease progression, the focus of management must be on symptomatic therapies aimed at improving quality of life. Guidelines for the symptomatic management of ALS have been generated by the American Academy of Neurology (Miller *et al.*, 1999b) and a number of systematic reviews of the symptomatic management of ALS are also available from the Cochrane library – symptomatic therapies will not be further discussed here (Annane *et al.*, 2000; Langmore *et al.*, 2003). In recent years, improvements in materials science, bioinformatics and the development of exciting new techniques in molecular biology have brought about a revolution in the way that therapeutic candidates are selected and tested. The likely impact of these new techniques on drug development for disorders of motor neurons will also be discussed.

Disease modifying therapies for amyotrophic lateral sclerosis

Aims of therapy

Motor neurons are post-mitotic cells, which make numerous, complex synaptic connections. They are found in the motor cortex, the brainstem and along the entire length of the spinal cord. Even with encouraging developments in stem-cell research (Holden, 2002), it is difficult to see how motor neurons from brain to distal lumbar spine can be replaced and remake the complex synaptic connections needed for the reversal of disability – a "cure." For now, at least, the focus must realistically be on halting or slowing the loss of further motor neurons. Unfortunately, at the time of symptom onset a significant proportion of spinal motor neurons may already have been lost (Sobue *et al.*, 1983). In the absence of reliable early diagnostic markers of the disease, a firm clinical diagnosis can often only be made many months after symptom onset (World Federation of Neurology Research Committee on Motor Neuron Diseases, 1998), by which time even more motor neurons have been lost. Until a firm, early diagnosis can be made, the use of treatments to halt disease progression before significant functional impairment has occurred is unrealistic. Asymptomatic, but at-risk, members of families affected by superoxide dismutase 1-related familial ALS in whom the mutation is known may be an exception to this. At-risk people found to carry the mutant gene in pre-symptomatic genetic testing would, in theory, be excellent candidates for the pre-symptomatic institution of any new disease-halting therapy. At present, the pragmatic, if unsatisfactory, aim of new disease-modifying therapies is to halt or slow disease progression, extending patients' survival without undue compromise to quality of life.

Testing therapies in transgenic mice

The discovery in 1993 that mutations in the gene encoding copper/zinc superoxide dismutase (SOD1) cause 20% of cases of familial ALS (Rosen *et al.*, 1993), led to the development of transgenic mouse models of the disease (Doble & Kennel, 2000). Different transgenic mouse models carry different FALS-causing mutations of the human SOD1 gene in a variety of copy numbers and overproduce the mutant protein to different degrees. Different lines of SOD1 transgenic mice vary phenotypically as a result. All are born neurologically intact, but as adults go on to develop a progressive and fatal motor dysfunction very similar to that seen in human ALS. Mean survival is also dependent upon which SOD1 mutation the mice carry and the number of transgene copies.

SOD1 transgenic mice provide a system in which to investigate ALS pathogenesis and test therapeutic candidates. Unfortunately, several agents shown to have promise in trials in transgenic mice have failed to fulfil this promise when tested in patients (Table 52.2). This has prompted renewed scrutiny of the design of therapeutic trials in animal models and several potential confounding factors have been identified. A study of 2000 high copy number G93A SOD1 transgenic mice revealed differences in survival between male and female mice (Ramesh *et al.*, 2002). Differences in survival were also found between litters of mice. Thanks to the polymerase chain reaction, it is possible to identify presymptomatic transgenic mice and thereby study their entire disease course. It is not possible to identify presymptomatic human patients and is often unrealistic to follow-up trial patients until they die, 3–5 years after symptom onset. Assessment of disease progression in patients therefore tends to start later, occurs at a less well-defined stage of disease and covers a smaller proportion of the total disease course than is the case in transgenic mouse models.

In future, studies involving transgenic mice will need to control for mouse gender and, where possible, littermate controls should be used. Avoidance of these recognized confounding factors may improve the congruency of therapeutic trials in mouse models and patients.

Testing therapies in patients

Conducting clinical trials in ALS is far from straightforward (Turner & Leigh, 2003). Diagnosis is clinical, made late (problematic when testing putative neuroprotective agents) and can be difficult (Davenport *et al.*, 1996). Choosing appropriate endpoints is complicated by the effects upon survival of interventions such as PEG (percutaneous endoscopic gastrostomy) feeding and the initiation of respiratory support (Turner *et al.*, 2002). Measuring disease progression is difficult because of problems in finding reliable measures of bulbar dysfunction and muscle power. In the past these problems have made the interpretation of ALS clinical trials difficult. In recognition of this, a World Federation of Neurology committee met in 1998 to update their guidelines for the design and imple-

Table 52.1. World Federation of Neurology guidelines for trials in ALS: inclusion and exclusion criteria

1. Diagnosis should conform to WFN El Escorial/Airlie diagnostic criteria.
2. Patients with sporadic or familial ALS can be entered depending on the nature of the trial.
3. Entry should be limited to patients between the ages of 18 and 85 years.
4. There should be evidence of progression during a period of six months from onset of symptoms; but not more than 5 years.
5. Patients with significant sensory abnormalities, dementia, other neurologic diseases, uncompensated medical illness, substance abuse or psychiatric illness should be excluded.
6. The patient should not be on concurrent investigational drugs.

mentation of clinical trials in ALS (Miller *et al.*, 1999a). These are also available online at http://www.wfnals.org/ guidelines/1998airlieclintrial/airlie1998.htm. The guidelines recommend the use of the El Escorial/Airlie House diagnostic criteria (World Federation of Neurology Research Committee on Motor Neuron Diseases, 1998) and define common inclusion and exclusion criteria (Table 52.1). Primary endpoints should include survival or death/permanent continuous ventilation along with change in muscle strength. Importantly, given that the recommendations largely apply to trials of agents designed to prolong life, it was also recommended that quality of life should be included as an outcome measure in all trials. Useful guidance was also supplied about techniques for measuring disease progression, ensuring patient safety and the statistical analysis and disclosure of results. It is hoped that the application of these guidelines will improve the usefulness of future clinical trials of disease-modifying therapies in ALS.

Current and future therapies for ALS

Therapeutic candidates have been generated by chance observations in models of other neurodegenerative diseases, by systematic screening of novel agents and drugs already in use for other conditions in in vitro neuroprotection models and by theoretical extrapolation from improvements in the understanding of pathogenetic mechanisms (Table 52.3). Riluzole is the only disease-modifying agent currently licensed for use in ALS and is only modestly effective (Miller *et al.*, 2002). The need for new and more effective agents is pressing and is the focus of intense research activity. In this section we will consider the evidence base underlying the use of riluzole and survey trials of other potential therapies for ALS in models of the disease and in patients.

Table 52.2. Incongruency between therapeutic trials in mouse models and patients

Therapeutic candidate	Results in mouse models	Results in patients
Creatine monohydrate (Klivenyi et al., 1999, Mazzini et al., 2001, Groeneveld et al., 2003)	Extended survival in G93A SOD1 transgenic mice and improved motor performance	No effect on survival No slowing of motor decline
α-tocopherol (Vitamin E) (Gurney et al., 1996, Desnuelle et al., 2001)	Delayed disease onset in G93A SOD1 transgenic mice and slowed progression No effect upon survival	Not assessable No effect upon progression No effect upon survival
Brain-derived Neurotrophic Factor (BDNF) (Mitsumoto et al., 1994b, Ishiyama et al., 2002, 1999, Ochs et al., 2000)	Disease slowing in wobbler mice	No effect on disease-slowing or survival
Ciliary Neurotrophic Factor (CNTF) (Miller et al., 1996, Mitsumoto et al., 1994a, Mitsumoto et al., 1994b)	Disease slowing and prolonged survival in pmn mice. Short-term arrest of disease progression in wobbler mice (cotreatment with BDNF)	No effect on functional scores. Survival only a 2° endpoint but no beneficial effect and reduced vs. placebo in one subgroup in one trial
Gabapentin (Gurney et al., 1996, Miller et al., 2001a)	Modestly prolonged survival in one of two G93A transgenic mice strains tested	No effect on rate of decline of muscle strength of upper limb muscles in patients

Table 52.3. Theories of pathogenesis and some related therapeutic candidates

Pathogenetic mechanism	Therapy	Therapeutic candidates			
Excitotoxicity	Riluzole	Branched chain amino acids	L-threonine	ONO-2506	
Oxidative stress		Vitamin E	Tamoxifen	Selegiline	
Neuroprotective/trophic effects		CTNF	BDNF	IGF-1	Xaliproden
Mitochondrial dysfunction		Creatine monohydrate	Coenzyme Q_{10}	Gingko biloba	
Inflammation		Minocycline	COX-2 inhibition	ONO-2506	
Apoptosis		Minocycline	Caspase inhibitors		

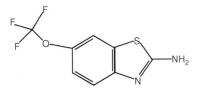

Fig. 52.1 Riluzole is a benzothiazole.

Riluzole

Excitotoxicity

Riluzole (Fig. 52.1) acts to inhibit the presynaptic release of the excitatory neurotransmitter glutamate (Doble, 1996). Several lines of evidence suggest that excessive excitatory input to motor neurons, mediated by glutamate, may contribute to motor neuron dysfunction and death (excitotoxicity) (Shaw & Ince, 1997). Excess glutamate acting at its receptors on motor neurons results in an influx of cations including calcium and over-depolarization of the cell membrane. These changes trigger a cascade of damaging reactions which may, eventually, lead to the death of the motor neuron. In support of this idea is the finding of raised glutamate in the CSF of subsets of ALS patients (Shaw et al., 1995a; Spreux-Varoquaux et al., 2002). The measurement of glutamate in CSF is technically challenging, however, and not all groups have replicated these findings. The excitatory stimulus to motor neurons is terminated by removal of glutamate from the synaptic cleft predominantly by EAAT2, an astrocytic glutamate transporter. Expression of this molecule is reduced in ALS spinal cord (Rothstein et al., 1995, Fray et al., 1998). EAAT2 has also been shown to be a target of oxidative modification by 4-hydroxynonenal (4-HNE), resulting in impaired glutamate transport (Keller et al., 1997). 4HNE is itself generated as a result of oxidative damage to lipids and is increased in the CSF of ALS patients (Smith *et al.*, 1998). No firmer evidence has yet emerged, however, that excitotoxicity is the primary insult resulting in cell death in ALS.

Mechanism of action

Riluzole (2-amino-6-(trifluoromethoxy)benzothiazole) is a benzothiazole, first developed as an antiepileptic drug. Although the initial rationale for its use in ALS was its inhibition of the presynaptic release of glutamate (Cheramy *et al.*, 1992; Martin *et al.*, 1993), riluzole is believed to exert additional neuroprotective effects through several other mechanisms including the inhibition of glutamate-gated and voltage-gated sodium channels (Ashton *et al.*, 1997; Hubert *et al.*, 1994), and the inhibition of protein kinase C (Noh *et al.*, 2000). It has also been shown to induce expression of neurotrophic factors in cultured mouse astrocytes (Mizuta *et al.*, 2001). It is likely that a combination of these potentially neuroprotective mechanisms underlies the undoubted, if modest, clinical efficacy of riluzole.

Trial data

The use of riluzole in ALS is supported by a small number of largely well-conducted clinical trials. The first, published in 1994 by Bensimon *et al.*, was a prospective, double-blinded, randomized trial of 100 mg riluzole vs placebo (Bensimon *et al.*, 1994). Outpatients aged between 20 and 75 years with a diagnosis of probable or definite ALS were eligible. Excluded were patients with evidence of other disease processes, symptoms >5 years, an FVC <60% predicted, pregnant patients, patients with a tracheostomy and those with renal or hepatic impairment or other life-threatening conditions. The primary endpoints were survival/tracheostomy and rate of change of functional status measured on a four-point scale. The main secondary endpoint was change in muscle power measured by manual power testing using the MRC scale. Analysis was performed on an intention-to-treat basis. After 12 months, 58% of the placebo group were alive compared with 74% of the riluzole-treated group ($P = 0.014$). Of patients in the bulbar-onset subgroup, 35% of the placebo group were alive at 12 months compared to 73% of the riluzole-treated group ($P = 0.014$). In patients in the limb-onset subgroup there was a trend towards increased survival but significance was not reached. At the end of the placebo-controlled period, when the analysis of the data had been completed, survival was still significantly increased in the group as a whole and in the bulbar sub-group (median follow-up 573d). Deterioration in muscle strength, the chief secondary endpoint, was also significantly slower (33.4% reduction) in patients treated with riluzole ($P = 0.028$).

Lacomblez *et al.* published a second trial in 1996. This was a multi-centre, dose-ranging, randomised, placebo-controlled, double-blinded study of 959 ALS patients (Lacomblez *et al.*, 1996). The primary endpoint was survival without tracheostomy and the secondary outcome was rate of change of a number of functional measures. Patients with clinically probable or definite ALS, of no more than 5 years' duration, aged 18–75, with an FVC of >60% predicted were eligible. Exclusions were identical to the previous trial. Follow-up was for a mean of 18 months and analysis was again done on an intention-to-treat basis. At the end of the study, 50.8% of placebo-treated and 56.8% of patients receiving 100 mg riluzole/d remained alive without tracheostomy (adjusted risk of death 0.65, $P = 0.002$). This corresponded to a decrease in the risk of death or tracheostomy of 35% for patients receiving 100 mg riluzole. Of patients receiving 50 mg and 200 mg of riluzole, 55.3% and 57.8%, respectively, were alive and without tracheostomy at the end of the study. No significant difference in any of the secondary functional measures was found between the groups. This trial included a higher proportion of bulbar-onset patients (295/959 vs 32/155) than did the Bensimon trial and unlike Bensimon, improval in survival in riluzole-treated patients was significant for both bulbar and limb-onset patient subgroups.

A systematic review of the use of riluzole in ALS has been carried out for Cochrane (Miller *et al.*, 2002). Three reports of randomized trials of riluzole in a total of 1282 patients with ALS were considered; the two trials earlier discussed and a third which included many older patients and many patients with more advanced disease. Together these constituted a total of 876 riluzole-treated patients and 406 placebo-treated patients. A fourth trial performed in Japan (Yanagisawa *et al.*, 1997) also met selection criteria but data on tracheostomy-free survival were not available so it was not included in the analysis.

The third trial was multi-centre, double-blind, parallel group, placebo-controlled, and randomized and was carried out in 168 adult patients with ALS who failed to qualify for the Lacomblez trial on the grounds of age, FVC, or disease duration. Treatment with riluzole 50 mg bd was compared to placebo. The primary outcome measure was survival without tracheostomy or endotracheal intubation. Secondary outcomes included changes in functional scales, muscle strength and respiratory function. The findings of this trial were made available to the Cochrane reviewers but have not been formally published (Meininger

Table 52.4. Conclusions of the Cochrane systematic review of the use of riluzole in ALS (Miller *et al.*, 2002)

Implications for practice

Riluzole 100 mg daily probably prolonged life by about two months in patients with probable and definite amyotrophic lateral sclerosis with symptoms less than five years, forced vital capacity greater than 60% and age less than 75 years. More studies are needed, especially to determine whether older, more advanced patients with longstanding disease derive the same benefit. Benefits are not apparent to individual patients. The most frequent side effects are nausea and asthenia. Liver function becomes altered and requires monitoring.

Implications for research

Future trials should examine the effect on quality of life and in different subgroups (for example, more severely affected compared with mildly affected patients). Data from all clinical trials should be made available to the scientific community.

Table 52.5. American Academy of Neurology guidelines for the use of riluzole (1997)

A. *ALS patients for whom class I evidence suggests riluzole may prolong survival includes those who have:*
1. Definite or probable ALS by World Federation of Neurology (WFN) criteria (other causes for progressive muscle atrophy have been excluded),
2. Symptoms present for less than 5 years,
3. FVC >60% predicted,
4. No tracheostomy.

B. *ALS patients for whom no class I evidence supports the use of riluzole but expert opinion suggests potential benefit includes those who have:*
1. Suspected or possible ALS by WFN criteria,
2. Symptoms present for more than 5 years,
3. FVC <60% predicted,
4. Tracheostomy for prevention of aspiration only (ventilator independent).

C. *Expert consensus suggests riluzole is of uncertain benefit in patients with:*
1. Tracheostomy required for ventilation,
2. Other incurable life-threatening disorders,
3. Other forms of anterior horn cell disease.

et al., 1995). There was no significant difference in percentage mortality at 12 months between riluzole-treated patients and placebo-treated patients, with a relative risk of 0.99 (95% CI 0.79 to 1.25). This lack of difference between the groups was maintained at all time points throughout the trial.

In the Cochrane meta-analysis, the Parmar method was used to compare the results of these 3 trials (Parmar *et al.*, 1998). The primary endpoint was the hazard ratio for percentage mortality at 12 months. When the first two trials were assessed there was evidence for a modest benefit of riluzole 100 mg when compared to placebo ($P = 0.039$, HR 0.80, CI 0.64–0.99). Inclusion of the third trial, however, introduced evidence of heterogeneity – unsurprising given the increased age and severity of disease of patients recruited to this trial. Once this was taken into account, statistical significance was not quite reached ($P = 0.056$, HR 0.84, CI 0.70 −1.01).

The conclusions of the Cochrane reviewers are given in Table 52.5. One important point raised was that none of the trials considered quality of life. In the dose-ranging study by Lacomblez *et al.*, patients receiving riluzole were found to remain in a combined "mild or moderate health state" for significantly longer than were the placebo-treated patients. There was no significant prolongation by riluzole of time spent in a combined "severe or terminal health state." It is an important concern that an agent which acts to slow disease progression, may theoretically result in a prolongation of the terminal stages of the disease, when quality of life of patients may be poor. For this reason, one of the recommendations of the WFN consensus guidelines on trial design (Appendix 4), is that that data must be collected on quality of life in all future clinical trials in ALS.

Prescription guidelines for riluzole

Riluzole is currently the only drug licensed in the UK and USA for slowing the progression of ALS. It is an expensive drug. In the UK, the annual cost of riluzole is ∼£3700 and the estimated cost of a quality adjusted life year (QALY) is £34 000–£43 500. Use of riluzole in the UK is governed by guidelines recently published by NICE (National Institute for Clinical Excellence, 2001), also available at http://www.nice.org.uk/pdf/RILUZOLE_full_guidance.pdf. Under this guidance riluzole should be prescribed only for patients meeting diagnostic criteria for the ALS variant of motor neuron disease (World Federation of Neurology Research Committee on Motor Neuron Diseases, 1998) and not for progressive muscular atrophy (PMA) or primary lateral sclerosis (PLS). This limitation of riluzole treatment to patients with ALS is at variance with the views of many neurologists who consider PMA, ALS and PLS as artificially demarcated subgroups of a continuous spectrum of disease. Guidelines for the use of riluzole in the USA were published by the American Academy of Neurology in 1997 (http://www.aan.com) and are summarized in Table 52.4.

Practicalities of prescribing riluzole

Data from Lacomblez *et al.* indicate that the optimal dose of riluzole is 100 mg/d, usually taken in divided doses of 50 mg (Lacomblez *et al.*, 1996). Doses over 100 mg/d did not further increase survival but did cause more drug-related adverse events. Although largely well-tolerated, recognized side effects include nausea and vomiting, loss of appetite, dizziness, weariness and increases in liver transaminases. The drug is contraindicated in patients with renal and hepatic impairment and also during pregnancy and breast-feeding. If more than one baseline liver function test (LFT) is significantly raised, the drug should not be prescribed. LFTs should be checked monthly for the first 3 months of treatment, 3-monthly for a further 9 months and annually thereafter. Trial data indicate that ~50% of patients will have at least one abnormal LFT at some point, 8% will experience elevations > three times normal and only 2% will experience elevations > five times normal. The drug should be discontinued if transaminase levels rise to five times normal and more frequent blood tests instituted if levels rise to three times normal. Gastrointestinal side effects will often diminish with a dose reduction for a few weeks after which time the full dose can often be reinstituted without recurrence. There are only very occasional reports of neutropenia associated with riluzole (Debove *et al.*, 2001) but patients should be warned to report any febrile illness to their doctor in order that a full blood count can be checked. Very recently, a well-documented single case report was published of hypersensitivity pneumonitis seemingly attributable to riluzole (Cassiman *et al.*, 2003) – the possibility of idiosyncratic drug reactions to riluzole should also be borne in mind.

Amino acids

Based on work by Plaitakis (Plaitakis *et al.*, 1980, 1984) which suggested that a deficiency of glutamate dehydrogenase (GDH) might underlie abnormal glutamate metabolism in ALS, several trials of L-leucine, L-valine and L-isoleucine (branched-chain amino acids which serve to activate GDH) were performed in the 1980s and 1990s (Gil & Neau, 1992; Testa *et al.*, 1989; Plaitakis & Sivak, 1992). A Cochrane systematic review has recently been performed of these trials, which concluded that overall no benefit was demonstrated (Parton *et al.*, 2003). L-threonine, an amino acid thought to increase levels of the inhibitory neurotransmitter glycine, has also been investigated in ALS but again, no benefit was shown (Patten & Klein, 1988; Blin *et al.*, 1992; Testa *et al.*, 1992).

Anti-oxidant drugs

Oxygen free radicals such as the superoxide ($O_2^{\bullet-}$) and hydroxyl radical ($OH^-\cdot$) and their derivatives are generated as by-products of normal metabolism (Turrens, 1997; Han *et al.*, 2001). An array of anti-oxidants within the cell serves to defend proteins, lipids and DNA from the oxidative damage they would otherwise sustain from reaction with these radicals. These include anti-oxidant enzymes such as catalase, glutathione peroxidases, peroxiredoxins and also free radical scavengers such as vitamins C and E, co-enzyme Q_{10} and others. When the quantity of free radicals generated exceeds the capacity of these anti-oxidant defences to remove them, the cell is said to be under oxidative stress. In this condition, damage to cellular components occurs, which disrupts normal cellular function and may, ultimately, lead to cell death. The discovery that mutations to SOD1 are responsible for some cases of familial ALS increased research interest in oxidative stress as a pathogenetic mechanism (Rosen *et al.*, 1993). SOD1 is an important anti-oxidant protein, which acts to convert superoxide to hydrogen peroxide. This species, itself capable of generating the even more reactive hydroxyl radical via the Fenton reaction, is then detoxified by catalase and other peroxidases.

There is good evidence for oxidative stress in ALS (Robberecht & de Jong, 2000). Protein carbonylation is a marker of oxidative damage to proteins. Increases in carbonylated proteins have been found in the spinal cords of patients with ALS (Shaw *et al.*, 1995b), and also in SOD1 transgenic mice (Andrus *et al.*, 1998). At disease onset, G93A mice were shown by Beal's group to have defective functioning of the electron transfer chain and ATP synthesis along with evidence of oxidative damage to mitochondrial proteins (increased brain and spinal cord protein carbonylation) and lipids (increased brain lipid hydroperoxides). These deficiencies were not evident in presymptomatic G93A mice nor in mice expressing normal human SOD1 (Mattiazzi *et al.*, 2002). Superoxide may also react with nitric oxide to generate another free radical, peroxinitrite ($ONOO^-\cdot$). Peroxynitrite reacts with proteins to form nitrosylated tyrosine residues. An increase in free nitrotyrosines was found by Tohgi *et al.* in the CSF of patients with ALS (Tohgi *et al.*, 1999). Oxidative damage to lipids is reflected in levels of 4-hydroxynonenal. Smith *et al.* found 4-hydroxynonenal to be increased in ALS spinal cord (Smith *et al.*, 1998). There is, additionally, some evidence for a compensatory upregulation of some anti-oxidant enzymes in ALS (Shaw *et al.*, 1997). This and other evidence has led to the investigation of anti-oxidant agents as potential therapeutic agents. A number of clinical trials have been performed and a Cochrane systematic review has been commissioned to examine the evidence they collectively provide for the efficacy of anti-oxidant treatment (Orrell et al., 2003). It is the practice of many neurologists to co-prescribe vitamins C and E along with riluzole in response to the evidence for oxidative stress in ALS. Convincing evidence for additional benefit has yet to be demonstrated for these, or any other anti-oxidant therapies, however.

Vitamin E

A study in SOD1 transgenic mice showed that whilst levels of vitamin E in homogenized spinal cord and brain increased with age in wild-type mice and those expressing normal human SOD1, there was a depletion of vitamin E in mutant SOD1 transgenic mice (Gurney et al., 1996). Supplementation of the diet of these mice with vitamin E caused both a delay in the onset of symptoms of ALS and slowed its subsequent progression. There was no effect, however, upon survival. Desnuelle et al. recently published a randomised placebo-controlled trial of 500 mg of α-tocopherol (vitamin E) in 289 patients with ALS already treated with riluzole (Desnuelle et al., 2001). Additional treatment with α-tocopherol had no effect upon the rate of deterioration (modified Norris score) nor was there any effect upon survival. Patients receiving α-tocopherol were, however, less likely to progress from a mild to a more severe ALS Health State ($P = 0.046$).

N-acetylcysteine

N-acetylcysteine is a membrane-permeant molecule, which within the cell is rapidly converted to cysteine, the rate-limiting precursor of glutathione, a natural intracellular anti-oxidant. Work in cell-culture models of SOD1-related familial ALS suggested that N-acetylcysteine could ameliorate mitochondrial dysfunction observed in the presence of mutant SOD1 (Beretta et al., 2003). Trials of the drug in mouse models of the disease, however, have produced conflicting results (Andreassen et al., 2000; Jaarsma et al., 1998). A randomized, double-blind, placebo-controlled clinical trial of subcutaneous N-acetylcysteine (50 mg/kg) in 110 patients with ALS showed no significant difference in survival or in disease progression between treated and control groups (Louwerse et al., 1995).

Selegiline

Selegiline is a monoamine oxidase B-inhibitor, which increases SOD1 and catalase activity, and probably has additional anti-oxidant properties. A 6-month, double-blind placebo-controlled study in 133 ALS patients showed no effect on the progression of the disease (Lange et al., 1998). These results support a previous, small and also negative trial of selegiline in ALS (Mitchell et al., 1995).

Tamoxifen

Tamoxifen is an established drug in the treatment of breast cancer. It has recently been found to inhibit protein kinase C (Mandlekar & Kong, 2001), a known effect of riluzole (Noh et al., 2000). Activation of protein kinase C appears to be a critical common pathway in many oxidative insults in neurons; it has therefore been suggested that part of the effectiveness of riluzole may lie in an anti-oxidant action mediated by inhibition of protein kinase C. On the basis of this and unpublished work in mice, a dose-ranging study of tamoxifen in ALS patients is under way in the USA.

Combinations of anti-oxidants

Vyth et al. published an observational study of a small group of ALS patients treated at their center over a 5-year period with a variety of anti-oxidant cocktails, which included N-acetylcysteine; vitamins C and E; N-acetylmethionine; and dithiothreitol or its isomer dithioerythritol. Whilst a modest survival benefit appeared to be gained, the methods used in this study were far from ideal and the authors themselves concluded that whilst their cocktails of anti-oxidants appeared safe, they could not be said to prolong survival (Vyth et al., 1996).

Bioenergetic modifiers

There is increasing evidence implicating mitochondrial dysfunction in the pathogenesis of ALS, but it remains to be seen whether this dysfunction is the primary cause of motor neuron death (Wood-Allum & Shaw, 2003). Mitochondria are the chief source of oxygen free radicals within the cell, producing superoxide as an unavoidable byproduct of oxidative phosphorylation. Mitochondrial morphological abnormalities have been demonstrated in several neural and non-neural tissues from patients with ALS (Nakano et al., 1987; Siklos et al., 1996) as well as in transgenic mouse (Kong & Xu, 1998) and cell-culture models of the disease (Menzies et al., 2002). Several studies have shown that the activities of electron transport chain complexes are altered in ALS (Fujita et al., 1996; Borthwick et al., 1999). Reduction in the efficiency with which the electron transport chain operates will affect the adequacy of the mitochondrial membrane potential it supports, the supply of ATP it is able to generate and will also increase the production of free radicals. Compounds known to support the bioenergetic economy of the cell have therefore become candidates for the treatment of ALS.

Creatine monohydrate

Creatine and phosphocreatine co-exist within the cell. Phosphocreatine acts as a temporal buffer of ATP supply allowing the re-phosphorylation of ADP to ATP at times of high energy demand in a reaction catalyzed by creatine kinase. It also acts as a spatial energy buffer between mitochondria and cytosol (Tarnopolsky & Beal, 2001). Exogenous creatine comes in the form of creatine monohydrate, which has been shown to be both well tolerated and safe when taken as a dietary supplement.

Klivenyi et al. administered a dietary supplement of 1% or 2% creatine monohydrate to G93A SOD1 transgenic mice (Klivenyi et al., 1999). A statistically significant, dose-dependent improvement of motor performance and improved survival resulted, along with a reduction of the loss of motor neurons at 120 days when comparison was made with control mice. Mean survival of unsupplemented mice was 143.7 ± 2.3 days compared to 157.2 ± 2.8 days for 1% creatine supplemented mice, and 169.3 ± 4.7 days for 2% supplemented mice representing an extension of survival of 13 days and 26 days, respectively. Riluzole extended survival in this model by 13 days. In unsupplemented G93A SOD1 transgenic mice, there was 95% loss of large ventral horn motor neurons when compared to non-transgenic littermate controls. In G93A SOD1 transgenic mice fed a diet supplemented by 1% creatine this loss of large ventral horn motor neurons did not seem to occur. The increase in levels of 3-nitrotyrosine usually seen in the spinal cords of G93A SOD1 transgenic mice was also not seen in G93A SOD1 transgenic mice whose diet was supplemented with 1% creatine monohydrate.

Preliminary results of a small study of creatine supplementation in 28 patients with clinically probable or definite ALS have been published (Mazzini et al., 2001). Supplementation was high dose (20 g/day) for a week, and lower dose (3 g/day) for 3 and 6 months. The maximal voluntary isometric muscular contraction (MVIC) was measured in 10 muscle groups by dynamometry. MVIC was increased significantly in knee extensors (70% patients) and elbow flexors (53% patients) after 7 days of high dose supplementation. A proportion of patients also showed reduced measures of fatigue in two muscle groups. Longer-term follow-up, however, showed a linear decline in MVIC in all muscle groups. As no untreated group was included in the study, the results do not allow assessment of whether the rate of decline was slowed by creatine supplementation. Groeneveld et al. performed a double-blind, placebo-controlled, sequential clinical trial of creatine monohydrate to assess its effects on survival and disease progression in 175 probable, probable-laboratory-supported or definite ALS patients (Groeneveld et al., 2003). Patients received either creatine monohydrate or placebo 10 g daily. Death, persistent assisted ventilation, or tracheostomy were selected as primary endpoints and the rate of decline of isometric arm muscle strength, forced vital capacity, functional status, and quality of life were included as secondary endpoints. In this trial, creatine did not affect survival (cumulative survival probability of 0.70 in the creatine group vs 0.68 in the placebo group at 12 months, and 0.52 in the creatine group vs. 0.47 in the placebo group at 16 months), or the rate of decline of functional measurements.

Coenzyme Q_{10} (CoQ_{10})

CoQ_{10}, the electron transport chain electron carrier, signalling molecule and anti-oxidant has been suggested as a potential therapy in mitochondrial disease and a number of neurodegenerative diseases, including ALS, in which mitochondrial dysfunction is believed to play a part (Strong & Pattee, 2000). Oral CoQ_{10} supplementation from 50 days of age at a dose of 200 mg/day has been carried out in a small group of G93A transgenic mice (Matthews et al., 1998). Supplementation produced a modest but statistically significant increase in survival from a mean of 135 days for unsupplemented mice to a mean of 141 days for mice receiving CoQ_{10}. A study of CoQ_{10} levels in serum from patients with ALS, however, showed them to be no different from those of controls (Molina et al., 2000). No study on the effect of CoQ_{10} in patients with ALS has yet been published although small, unpublished pilot studies have been undertaken.

Gingko biloba

Gingko biloba extract is a mixture of compounds obtained from the plant of the same name, which seems to act to reduce mitochondrial damage by reactive oxygen species. Ferrante et al. report a statistically significant prolongation of life, improvement of motor performance and protection against loss of anterior horn cells in male G93A SOD1 transgenic mice whose diet was supplemented with EGb761, a standardized extract of green Gingko biloba (Ferrante et al., 2001). These beneficial effects were not seen in their female transgenic littermates in whom only a non-statistically significant increase in survival was seen. Both male and female treated transgenic mice showed a reduction in weight loss. This substance has not yet been evaluated in ALS patients.

Neurotrophic agents

Neurotrophic agents are usually, but not always, recombinant versions of endogenous peptides with positive effects on neuronal development and viability in vitro. Unfortunately, promising trials of several neurotrophic agents in animal models have not been followed by equally positive results in patients. Cardiotrophin-1 (Bordet *et al.*, 2001) and glial-derived neurotrophic factor (Acsadi *et al.*, 2002; Manabe *et al.*, 2003) were found to be neuroprotective in transgenic mouse models of ALS, but no reports have yet been published on the use of these agents in ALS patients.

Ciliary neurotrophic factor (CNTF)

Promising work in vitro (Martinou *et al.*, 1992) and in the treatment of wobbler mice (Mitsumoto *et al.*, 1994b) with CNTF led to trials in ALS patients. No significant difference was found in a variety of functional scores between groups of ALS patients receiving either 15 µg/kg or 30 µg/kg of *sc* CNTF 3 times weekly and those receiving placebo (The ALS CNTF Treatment Study Group, 1996). A second study of over 500 ALS patients compared placebo, 0.5, 2 or 5 µg *sc* CNTF per day. The primary endpoint was a composite score of muscle scores and FVC measured monthly for only 6 months. Survival was included as a secondary endpoint. No significant benefit was demonstrated and the survival of the group receiving 5 µg of CNTF was reduced when compared to placebo (Miller *et al.*, 1996).

Human insulin-like growth factor-I (IGF-1)

IGF-1 is a naturally occurring peptide with neurotrophic effects on motor neurons, neuromuscular junctions and muscle (Lewis *et al.*, 1993). Recombinant human IGF-I has been shown to promote the survival of motor neurons in several experimental models of neuronal injury (Neff *et al.*, 1993) and IGF-1 receptors have been reported to be upregulated in postmortem ALS spinal cord (Caroni, 1993). On this basis, subcutaneous recombinant human IGF-1 has been evaluated in ALS. A recent Cochrane systematic review, however, identified only two randomized, controlled trials of IGF-1 (Mitchell *et al.*, 2002). The US trial indicated that 0.1 mg/kg/d *sc* rhIGF-1 taken for 9 months slowed the rate of progression of ALS measured using the Appel ALS Rating Score (AALSRS) by 26% compared to placebo (Lai *et al.*, 1997). The lower dose of 0.05 mg/kg/d showed

only a trend towards progression slowing which did not reach significance. The European trial also used a dose of 0.1 mg/kg/d and showed only a trend towards disease-slowing, again measured using the AALSRS score (Borasio *et al.*, 1998). Unfortunately the methodology used in both of these trials was deemed to be sufficiently problematic that the Cochrane review's authors (one also the main author of the European trial), felt that a reliable assessment of the efficacy of IGF-1 in ALS could not be made from their results. In particular, neither used survival as an endpoint. It was recommended rather that further trials of rhIGF-1 be carried out and such trials are underway.

Brain-derived neurotrophic factor (BDNF)

As a result of reports of in vitro neurotrophic effects on developing motor neurons, BDNF was tested in the wobbler mouse. Two trials, one of BDNF alone and the other of co-administration of BDNF and CNTF, showed statistically significant slowing of disease progression (Mitsumoto *et al.*, 1994b). A further, more recent, study confirmed the positive effects of BDNF in wobbler mice (Ishiyama *et al.*, 2002). The first randomized, controlled trial in patients compared 25 µg or 100 µg of *sc* recombinant methionyl BDNF with placebo in 1135 ALS patients (The BDNF Study Group, 1999). No significant difference was found in the primary endpoints of survival at 9 months and 6-months % change from baseline FVC. A higher than expected 9-month survival of patients in the trial at 85% may have masked any positive effects of BDNF in this study. Further trials of *sc* BDNF have been carried out but were negative and they remain unpublished. The authors of a small study of the safety and feasibility of intrathecal BDNF concluded that the drug may safely be administered by this route, although there were CNS side-effects at higher doses (Ochs *et al.*, 2000). A further, placebo-controlled, randomized trial of intrathecal BDNF was terminated early because of a higher incidence of adverse events, including death, in the treated group (unpublished).

Xaliproden

This compound is an orally administered agent believed to act at 5HT$_{1A}$ receptors with neurotrophic effects in models of neurodegeneration. A phase II study of this drug has been completed but is yet to report. Buspirone, in established use as an anxiolytic, also has a high affinity for 5HT$_{1A}$ receptors. It is also thought to stimulate endogenous neurotrophins. Trials in transgenic mice and patients are underway.

Viral vector-mediated delivery of neurotrophic factors

In response to concerns that delivery to motor neurons of intact neurotrophic factors administered orally or subcutaneously is poor and that this may underlie the to-date disappointing results of trials in patients, efforts have been made to find innovative ways of more efficiently delivering active drug to motor neurons. The discovery that adeno-associated virus (AAV) injected into skeletal muscle is taken up by motor neuron terminals and moved by retrograde axonal transport up the axon to the nucleus of the motor neuron opened up the possibility of delivering neurotrophic factors to motor neurons by viral vector (Davidson et al., 2000). Kaspar et al. injected AAV-IGF-1 or AAV-GDNF into skeletal muscle of G93A SOD1 transgenic mice at 60 days, some 30 days before the usual onset of symptoms. Symptom onset was delayed by a mean of 31 and 16 days respectively and survival increased by a mean of 37 and 11 days respectively. Perhaps more powerfully, AAV-IGF injected at 90 days, when symptoms first begin – more realistically modeling the situation for patients – also prolonged life, albeit to a lesser extent (Kaspar et al., 2003). This approach is clearly promising but there is much work still to be done to assess its feasibility and safety in patients.

Anti-inflammatory agents

Histopathology of the spinal cords of patients with ALS and SOD1 transgenic mice indicates that there is significant gliosis in the grey matter of the spinal cord, suggestive of an inflammatory component to the pathological process. This and much other evidence of inflammation in the spinal cord in ALS, reviewed elsewhere (McGeer & McGeer, 2002), has led to interest in anti-inflammatory drugs as potential therapeutic agents.

Minocycline

Minocycline is a second-generation tetracycline with a proven safety record and good blood-brain penetrance. It has been shown to have neuroprotective effects in a number of models of neurodegeneration; effects which appear to be mediated by an inhibition of transcriptional upregulation and activation of caspases 1 and 3 and inhibition of microglial activation (Fournier et al., 1993). Evidence suggesting that motor neuron death in ALS occurs at least partially via an apoptotic route and that microglial activation may be responsible for the spread between contiguous spinal cord segments which characterizes disease progression, prompted testing of minocycline in models of ALS.

Minocycline protects cultured spinal motor neurons from the toxic effects of CSF from patients with D90A ALS, non-SOD1 familial ALS and sporadic ALS (Tikka et al., 2002). Minocycline also delayed disease onset and extended survival of G93A mice in a dose-dependent fashion (Van Den Bosch et al., 2002). At 120 days of age, minocycline protected mice from the loss of motor neurons and vacuolisation observed in untreated mice. In a second study, Kriz et al. randomized late pre-symptomatic G37R SOD1 transgenic mice and non-transgenic littermate controls to a diet supplemented with 1g/kg minocycline or an unsupplemented diet (Kriz et al., 2002). Minocycline slowed loss of motor performance but did not prevent eventual paralysis. The average lifespan of treated G37R mice was ~3 weeks longer than that of untreated mice. Axon-counting at 46 weeks (early symptomatic phase) of the L4 and L5 ventral spinal roots showed that minocycline treatment delayed, but did not prevent, the massive loss of motor axons observed in untreated mice. Immunohistochemistry of spinal cord sections showed attenuation of Mac-2 and p-p38 immunoreactivity, both markers of microglial activation, in minocycline-treated transgenic mice compared with untreated transgenics. These findings were reproduced and extended by Zhu et al. (2002) who randomised G93A SOD1 transgenic mice to injections of either 10 mg/kg/d minocycline or saline from 5 weeks of age. Onset of impaired motor performance in minocycline-treated mice was delayed and survival extended. Minocycline is currently in phase III clinical trials in patients with ALS.

Celecoxib

Cyclo-oxygenase 2 (COX2) is a rate-limiting enzyme in the synthesis of prostaglandins, which are mediators of the inflammatory response. Prostaglandins generated by COX2 have been shown to cause astrocytic release of glutamate. In a study of spinal cord homogenates of 11 ALS cases and 27 neurological and healthy controls, Yasojima et al. demonstrated that there was an over seven-fold upregulation of COX-2 mRNA in the ALS cases compared to controls ($P < 0.0001$). Western blotting for COX-2 showed upregulation of protein expression by 3.79-fold compared with non-ALS spinal cord (Yasojima et al., 2001). These findings were borne out by a further study by Almer et al. who found increases in COX2 mRNA, COX2 protein expression and prostaglandin E2 (a pro-inflammatory COX2 product) in spinal cord homogenates of symptomatic G93A SOD1 transgenic mice when compared to levels in age-matched non-transgenic mice (Almer et al., 2001). Levels of PGE2 were also found to be significantly elevated in postmortem spinal cord homogenates from ALS patients when compared to controls.

In the light of this evidence of increased expression of COX2 in relevant areas of the CNS in SOD1 transgenic mice and ALS patients, COX2 inhibitors became potential therapeutic candidates. Drachman *et al.* used an in vitro model of excitotoxicity to test the COX2 inhibitor SC236 (Drachman & Rothstein, 2000). Rat organotypic spinal cord cultures challenged with THA, an inhibitor of astroglial glutamate uptake, undergo a gradual loss of motor neurons attributable to an excess of extracellular glutamate. Treatment of these cultures with SC236 significantly reduced the loss of motor neurons. In a second study, G93A mice treated with celecoxib, another selective COX2 inhibitor, had reduced spinal cord PGE2, delayed onset of weakness and weight loss and a 25% increase in survival compared to controls. Histology of the spinal cords of treated G93A mice showed preservation of motor neurons and a reduction of astrogliosis and activation of microglial activation compared to untreated mice (Drachman *et al.*, 2002).

The Northeast ALS consortium in the USA is currently conducting a multi-centre, double-blinded, randomized, controlled clinical trial of celecoxib in 300 ALS patients.

Immunomodulators

An autoimmune basis for ALS has long been sought and some supportive evidence has been found (Appel *et al.*, 2000). In response to this evidence (and possibly also because neurologists are familiar with their use in other neurological conditions) several immunomodulatory therapies have been tried in ALS. These include IVIG (intravenous pooled donor immunoglobulin) (Meucci *et al.*, 1996), plasmapheresis (Kelemen *et al.*, 1983), interferon-α (Mora *et al.*, 1986) and -β (Westarp *et al.*, 1992), cyclophosphamide $\pm$ steroids (Brown *et al.*, 1986), azathioprine (Werdelin *et al.*, 1990) and levamisole (Olarte and Shafer, 1985). Unfortunately none has been shown to be of benefit.

Pentoxifylline

Pentoxifylline (Trental®) is a drug already in use for the symptomatic relief of peripheral vascular disease. It is a phosphodiesterase 4B (PDE4B) inhibitor and also modulates the production of pro- and anti-inflammatory cytokines. PDE4B was identified as a potential therapeutic target for ALS through screening in transgenic mice. Encouraging neuroprotective properties were found in vitro. The drug is currently being tested in ALS patients

as add-on therapy with riluzole in a randomized, double-blind multi-centre, placebo-controlled trial.

ONO-2506

This novel agent is believed to modify astrocytic activation, in addition to upregulating expression at the gene level of astrocytic glutamate transporters. A multi-centre, double-blind placebo-controlled study of ONO-2506 as add-on therapy with riluzole is currently being undertaken in 400 ALS patients drawn from several European centres.

The drug-cocktail approach

In the presence of evidence supportive of several different pathogenetic mechanisms, no one of which can explain all the known facts and in the absence of any one therapeutic agent conferring dramatic benefit in either disease models or in patients, investigators have, rationally, turned their attention to cocktails of possible neuroprotective agents. The hope is that agents acting on complementary molecular pathways which when given alone confer only a modest benefit may produce additional benefits when administered together. On this principle, reports of several therapeutic trials employing combination therapies in mouse models of ALS have recently been published. These include combinations of minocycline, riluzole and nimodipine (Kriz *et al.*, 2003); creatine and riluzole (Snow *et al.*, 2003); creatine and minocycline (Zhang *et al.*, 2003); and creatine and rofecoxib (Klivenyi *et al.*, 2004). Most, but not all, of these trials have reported additional survival benefits from combination therapies, suggesting that this may well be a productive approach to the treatment of patients.

Disease-modifying agents for other motor neuron disorders

Under the guidelines issued by NICE, riluzole may not be prescribed for primary lateral sclerosis or progressive muscular atrophy in the UK, nor does the AAN practice advisory committee (Miller *et al.*, 1999b) recommend its use in these patients in the presence of only uncertain benefit. There are no other disease-modifying agents for hereditary spastic paraplegia, spinal muscular atrophy, or Kennedy's disease in use at present. As pathogenetic mechanisms are clarified, this situation may change but until then only symptomatic therapies are available. Prenatal and pre-implantation diagnosis is possible in some of these disorders (Hedera *et al.*, 2001, Matthijs *et al.*, 1998).

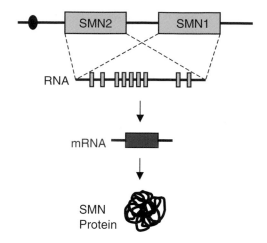

Fig. 52.2 The SMA locus on chromosome 5q13.

SMA

SMA is a progressive disease, in which anterior horn cells degenerate producing a symmetrical and predominantly proximal lower motor neuron weakness and atrophy. The commonest type of SMA is autosomal recessive and is associated with abnormalities of the SMN (survival motor neuron) gene. Three main forms are recognized, the severity of which is inversely related to the amount of SMN protein present in anterior horn cells. The most severe form causes death in infancy, the least severe is compatible with life into adulthood but continues to be slowly progressive and is accompanied by considerable disability.

The pathogenetic mechanisms underlying SMA are increasingly well understood, perhaps as a consequence of its largely autosomal recessive etiology, but despite this, very few clinical trials have yet been performed (Merlini *et al.*, 2002). The genes which code for SMN protein form part of a rather complex genetic locus at 5q13 (Fig. 52.2) in which there are two copies of the SMN gene; a telomeric version, *SMN1*, which codes for a full-length SMN protein and a second, more centromeric version, *SMN2*. *SMN2* differs from *SMN1* by only one nucleotide, which acts to alter the activity of a splicing enhancer in exon 7. As a result, mRNA transcripts from *SMN2* frequently lack exons 3, 5 or 7 and very little full-length protein is generated. Loss-of-function mutations to both copies of the *SMN1* gene result in the development of an SMA phenotype. The SMN protein has a role in pre-mRNA splicing, small ribonuclear protein synthesis and the regulation of transcription (Wirth, 2002). The small amount of full-length *SMN2* gene product produced acts to modify disease severity in dose-dependent fashion but cannot completely ameliorate a lack of full length SMN from *SMN1*.

As all SMA patients have at least one copy of *SMN2*, upregulation of this gene has been identified as a therapeutic target. More recently, SR-(serine–arginine-rich)-like splicing factor Htra2-beta 1 has been shown to correct the aberrant splicing of *SMN2*, thereby increasing production of full-length SMN protein (Hofmann *et al.*, 2000). In consequence, upregulation of SR-like splicing factor Htra2-beta 1 has also become a therapeutic goal. Exciting new biotechnologies aimed at manipulating splicing events to increase expression of full-length SMA protein from *SMA2* include the use of targeted peptide-nucleic acid (PNA) mimetics (Cartegni & Krainer, 2003), and bifunctional antisense oligonucleotides (Skordis *et al.*, 2003). These techniques, which have been recently reviewed (Khoo *et al.*, 2003), remain at an early stage of development and as in the therapy of ALS, effective delivery of these agents to the motor neuron is far from straightforward. In addition to this practical caveat, there remain concerns that the less specifically targeted of these agents may have widespread, and potentially deleterious, effects on the splicing of genes other than *SMN2*.

A number of different SMA transgenic mouse models have been made in which the single murine *SMN* gene (equivalent to *SMN1*) is knocked out and the phenotype SMN1 rescued by expression of human *SMN2* in varying amounts (Monani *et al.*, 2000; Hsieh-Li *et al.*, 2000). These mice are being used to test candidate therapeutic agents in SMA.

Sodium butyrate

Chang *et al.* generated lines of immortalized lymphoid cells by transforming lymphocytes obtained from SMA patients with Epstein–Barr virus (Chang *et al.*, 2001). These cells were exposed to candidate drugs and reverse transcriptase PCR performed to establish whether the production of full length *SMN2* mRNA had been increased. Sodium butyrate increased *SMN2* transcription and also increased the inclusion of exon 7 in *SMN2* transcripts, thereby increasing the production of full-length *SMA2* mRNA. A corresponding increase in SMN protein was also seen. Phenylbutyrate has also been reported to increase the in vitro production of SMN protein in cultured fibroblasts obtained from SMA patients (Andreassi *et al.*, 2004). The Chang group went on to expose small numbers of their transgenic SMA II and III mice to sodium butyrate. SMN II mice whose drinking water was supplemented with sodium butyrate for 1–12 weeks lived 4–5 days longer than did untreated mice. The histopathology of the tail muscles of treated SMA II and III mice was much less abnormal than that of untreated SMA mice and immunohistochemistry was used to demonstrate an increased expression of exon 7-containing SMN protein in a number of tissues of treated mice, including spinal motor neurons. Chang then went on to treat *Smn+/− SMN2* intercrossed pregnant mice with sodium butyrate. These mice give birth to types I, II and III SMA pups along with unaffected pups, in varying proportions. Pregnant mice treated with sodium butyrate gave birth to a higher proportion of less severely affected pups than did untreated pregnant mice.

Sodium butyrate and similarly acting drugs have been evaluated for the treatment of the thalassemias and sickle cell anaemia (Sher *et al.*, 1995, Collins *et al.*, 1995) and are relatively well tolerated. A short pilot trial of oral phenylbutyrate has been carried out in 10 SMA II patients (Mercuri *et al.*, 2004). The drug was well tolerated and some improvement in the Hammersmith functional motor scale of patients was observed.

Aclarubicin

A similar approach was adopted by Andreassi *et al.* who used in vitro cell culture models of SMA to screen drugs for the ability to increase the amount of full length *SMN2* mRNA transcribed (Andreassi *et al.*, 2001). Aclarubicin induced incorporation of exon 7 into *SMN2* transcripts in fibroblasts obtained from patients with SMA type I and increased their expression of the SMN protein back to normal levels. Unfortunately, aclarubicin is a chemotherapeutic agent with potentially serious side effects, including cardiomyopathy, which make it a poor candidate for the treatment of children with SMA.

Sodium valproate

Brichta *et al.* (2003) showed that in fibroblast cultures derived from SMA patients, treatment with therapeutic doses of valproic acid could increase the level of full-length *SMN2* mRNA/protein. Brichta *et al.* (2003) showed that, in fibroblast cultures derived from SMA patients, treatment with therapeutic doses of valproic acid could increase the level of full-length SMN2 mRNA/protein. They attributed this increase to raised levels of Htra2-beta 1 and increased correct splicing of *SMN2* as well as to activation of SMN gene transcription. An increase in SMN protein levels through transcriptional activation was also found in rat organotypic hippocampal brain slices. This work was confirmed by another group in cultured fibroblasts obtained from patients with type I SMA (Sumner *et al.*, 2003). The fact that sodium valproate has been used safely for many years in the treatment of epilepsy, including in children, makes

it a particularly attractive candidate for the treatment of patients with SMA.

Thyrotropin-releasing hormone (TRH)

A small randomized, double-blind 5-week trial of protirelin (a synthetic TRH) vs placebo was carried out in six SMA patients and three controls by Tzeng *et al.* (2000). Protirelin or placebo was delivered intravenously at a dose of 0.1 mg/kg (in 50 ml of normal saline) for a total of 29 days. Dynamometry improved modestly in the six treated subjects ($P = 0.02$) but not in control subjects. A further, larger study is needed before the efficacy of TRH in SMA can be assessed.

Gabapentin

A randomized, double-blind, multi-centre trial of gabapentin 1200 mg *tds* vs placebo was recently completed in the USA (Miller *et al.*, 2001b). The drug or placebo was administered to 84 patients with type II or III SMA for 12 months. The primary outcome measure was percentage change in a composite of the strength of elbow flexion and hand grip bilaterally. Secondary outcome measures included FVC, a functional rating scale and a quality of life scale. No significant differences were found in either the primary outcome measure or any of the secondary outcome measures between patients given gabapentin or placebo.

Riluzole

The proven benefits of riluzole to patients with ALS prompted investigators to trial it in SMA mutant mice and in patients. Haddad *et al.* reported an increase in median survival of SMA mutant mice treated with riluzole (Haddad *et al.*, 2003) but a pilot trial in patients was unfortunately cut short for administrative reasons (Russman *et al.*, 2003). This pilot, a phase I trial, was as a result underpowered (only seven children treated with riluzole, three with placebo) and the question of whether riluzole may be helpful in SMA remains unanswered.

Neurotrophic factors

Lesbordes *et al.* injected SMA mice intramuscularly with an adenoviral vector expressing cardiotrophin-1 (CT-1), and found that it improved median survival, delayed onset of motor dysfunction and seemed to be protective against the loss of proximal motor axons and aberrant cytoskeletal organization of motor synaptic terminals (Lesbordes *et al.*, 2003). The use of an adeno-associated viral vector to carry extra copies of *SMN1* or *2* into motor neurons to increase expression of the SMN protein has not thus far been reported.

Kennedy's disease (X-linked spinobulbar muscular atrophy)

Kennedy's disease is the result of a CAG repeat expansion within exon 1 of the androgen receptor gene on the X chromosome. It is inherited in an X-linked recessive fashion and affects male carriers. Most female carriers are phenotypically normal although raised creatine kinase and abnormalities on electromyography can be seen. In common with other triplet repeat disorders, the expanded region is unstable between generations and anticipation occurs. Affected males develop a progressive proximal weakness accompanied by wasting and fasciculation and dysarthria and may also have gynaecomastia, reduced fertility, and testicular atrophy; signs of androgen insensitivity. Onset is usually in the third to fifth decade and the disease may reduce life expectancy. Weakness is the result of the loss of anterior horn cells from spinal cord and brainstem. The expanded CAG repeat in the androgen receptor gene codes for repeated glutamine residues in the translated protein, which give the protein a tendency to form high molecular weight aggregates. These can be seen by immunohistochemistry as androgen-receptor-immunoreactive nuclear inclusions in motor neurons and some other tissues, for example testis. It seems increasingly likely that these protein aggregates may be responsible for the pathogenicity of the mutation but this remains a subject of debate and ongoing research (Gallo, 2001; Wood *et al.*, 2003).

Development of a transgenic mouse model of Kennedy's disease was far from straightforward as the choice of promoter appeared to affect the neurological phenotype. Abel *et al.* described a transgenic mouse generated from a 5′ truncated, much expanded (112 CAG repeats) androgen receptor gene driven by a neurofilament light promoter (Abel *et al.*, 2001). Unlike SOD1 transgenic mouse models of ALS, whose phenotype closely mirrors that of the related human disease, these Kennedy's mice did not develop the neurogenic muscle atrophy that characterizes human disease. They did, however, develop a gait disturbance and adult-onset hind-limb weakness and display the neuronal intranuclear inclusions (NII), which characterize triplet repeat disorders. More recently, transgenic mouse models whose disease better resembles human SBMA have been developed. One such model, expressing a full-length human androgen receptor gene with expanded CAG repeats and controlled by a CMV enhancer and chicken β-actin promoter, exhibits muscle wasting and weakness, markedly worse in males and rescued by castration (Katsuno *et al.*, 2002). The luteinizing hormone-releasing hormone agonist leuprorelin, which acts to reduce testosterone release by the testes, has recently been shown to rescue the phenotype of these mice (Katsuno *et al.*, 2003) raising the possibility of anti-androgen therapy in patients with SBMA. Androgen-receptor antagonists which bind the receptor and allow or even encourage its nuclear translocation exert no such beneficial effect (Takeyama *et al.*, 2002; Katsuno *et al.*, 2003).

The expanded androgen receptor co-localizes in nuclear aggregates with molecular chaperones, 26S proteasome components and ubiquitin. Overexpression of various heat shock proteins (HSPs) in cell-culture models of SBMA reduced androgen receptor aggregation and cell death by an increase in the solubility of the expanded androgen receptor and its degradation by the proteasome (Ishihara *et al.*, 2003; Kobayashi *et al.*, 2000; Bailey *et al.*, 2002). Sobue *et al.* went on to look at the effect of overexpression of chaperones in SBMA transgenic mice by creating dual transgenics. Their dual transgenic SBMA mice also expressed inducible, human HSP70. Overexpression of HSP70 ameliorated the motor phenotype of the mice and also reduced the nuclear accumulation of androgen receptor (Adachi *et al.*, 2003). It is likely that this line of enquiry may identify new therapeutic candidates as well as clarifying the pathogenetic mechanism underlying SBMA.

Hereditary spastic paraplegia (HSP)

Hereditary spastic paraplegia is characterized by progressive disability due to lower limb spasticity and weakness. In uncomplicated HSP this may be accompanied by urinary sphincter disturbance and mild impairment of vibration sense in the distal lower limbs. A spastic paraparesis that begins after childhood is usually insidiously progressive. Complicated HSP is defined by the presence of additional features including seizures, dementia, cataracts, extrapyramidal deficits and amyotrophy (Fink, 2002b). HSP is an inherited condition but shows marked genetic heterogeneity. Thus far there are 20 known HSP loci; 10 with autosomal dominant inheritance, 7 with autosomal recessive inheritance and 3 of which are X-linked recessive. These loci are labelled SPG1–21 in order of their discovery. Of these, 10 HSP genes and the proteins they code have been identified: spastin (SPG4), paraplegin (SPG6), atlastin (SPG3A), heat shock protein 60, proteolipid protein, L1 cell adhesion molecule (Fink, 2002a), spartin (Patel *et al.*, 2002), KIF5A (Reid *et al.*, 2002), (SPG21) maspardin (Simpson *et al.*, 2003), and NIPA1 (Rainier *et al.*, 2003). The multiple genes and diverse functions of the proteins they code make the prospect of a disease-modifying therapy based on the underlying pathophysiology of the disease and applicable to all HSP a remote one. Therapies tailored to particular, genetically defined, HSP variants or which target a common final pathogenic pathway may be a more realistic goal. At present, research efforts are focussed on defining more clearly the molecular basis of the disease and on the development of a transgenic HSP mouse model. Once disease pathogenesis is better understood, therapeutic candidates will surely follow. In the meantime, management of HSP is symptomatic and predominantly involves the use of spasmolytic agents. Prenatal diagnosis is increasingly possible although there are ethical considerations to be taken into account in this condition which may be phenotypically mild and which is not associated with a reduced life expectancy.

Future directions

Earlier diagnosis of ALS

For patients to benefit from newly developed neuroprotective agents at a time when most of their motor neurons are still salvageable, there needs to be earlier, and reliable, diagnosis of ALS. Currently diagnosis is late, clinical and on occasion incorrect (Davenport *et al.*, 1996). A simple diagnostic test which could be performed at the time of first presentation (when patients are unlikely to have disease sufficiently advanced to meet current diagnostic criteria) would allow the earlier institution of neuroprotective therapy. Where to look for such an early diagnostic marker? CSF bathes the motor roots and spinal cord and as such may be expected to reflect the extracellular milieu of motor neurons and their supporting glia. Several biochemical changes have been found in the CSF of ALS patients, reviewed elsewhere (Shaw, 2001), but none, regrettably, is sensitive or specific enough to be of practical use in the early diagnosis of ALS. Attention has recently shifted to changes in the level and post-translational modifications of proteins within CSF. New advances in the separation and subsequent identification of components of complex protein mixtures from biological samples are being applied to this problem, techniques collectively known as proteomics (Banks *et al.*, 2000). The 14–3–3 proteins which contribute to the diagnosis of Creutzfeldt–Jacob disease were discovered using such a proteomic approach (Harrington *et al.*,

1986). It is hoped that ALS-specific protein changes within CSF may be identified using these new proteomic techniques which might provide the basis of the sought-after early diagnostic test.

Clarification of subgroups with differing responses to therapy

It has long been suspected that the generally poor overall response of ALS patients in clinical trials of neuroprotective agents may be due to the masking of a strongly positive response in a subset of patients by a lack of response in the remainder. Subgroups with different responses to a therapy may be identified by the enrolment of adequate numbers of patients with different (and clearly defined) clinical features or "effect modifiers" (e.g. bulbar onset, slowly progressive disease, LMN at onset, UMN at onset) to allow meaningful subgroup analysis (Miller *et al.*, 1999a). Better definition of the response of patient subgroups to therapeutic candidates may allow recognition of the neuroprotective effects of a therapy useful to at least a subset of ALS patients which might otherwise be overlooked.

Candidate approach via clarification of molecular biology

Drug development in motor neuron disorders is hampered by an incomplete understanding of disease pathogenesis. Despite the discovery of SOD1 gene mutations in 20% of cases of familial ALS in 1993, it still remains unclear exactly how mutant SOD1 brings about motor neuron death. It is even less clear what insult underlies the death of motor neurons in the often clinically indistinguishable sporadic form of the disease. The precise pathogenetic mechanisms which underly the dying-back axonopathy of HSP are unknown, as are the molecular pathways which cause lower motor neurons in SMA to die whilst sparing cortical motor neurons. Clarification of these mechanisms at a molecular level will inevitably generate new therapeutic targets and new therapeutic candidates. The relatively recent discovery of a mutation to the gene coding a novel protein called alsin, which causes the childhood onset of a PLS-like syndrome, is one such advance in the field of ALS (Yang *et al.*, 2001; Hadano *et al.*, 2001). Another is the fortuitous finding that mutation of the gene for a protein known as vascular endothelial growth factor (VEGF) in mice results in a motor neuron-like phenotype (Oosthuyse *et al.*, 2001).

High throughput screening approaches

New developments in proteomics and DNA microarray technology have made possible the large-scale screening of therapeutic candidates. Advances in the understanding of disease pathogenesis are first used to identify molecular targets, for example, an increase in the transcription of full-length SMN in SMA. Thousands of candidate drugs can then be screened for the ability to bring about the desired alteration to cellular biochemistry (detected by analysis of changes in gene expression or of protein expression) in in vitro models of motor neuron disorders. Successful candidates may then progress to trials in animal models and ultimately in patients. High throughput screening approaches may also be used to generate therapeutic targets. By using microarray technology, the levels of mRNAs coding tens of thousands of proteins can be measured (Luo & Geschwind, 2001). Powerful data analysis and statistics software can then be used to compare such data obtained from wild-type and from transgenic mouse models of a motor neuron disorder. Those mRNAs whose levels differ between disease and non-disease models may then be investigated further. One drug currently being evaluated in ALS patients was selected as a therapeutic candidate on the basis of high-throughput microarray screening for differences in mRNA splicing between transgenic and wild-type ALS mice.

Stem cell therapy

Given the current problems with early diagnosis and the fact that at diagnosis ALS patients have already lost considerable numbers of their motor neurons, consideration of therapies aimed at replacing dead and dying motor neurons is rational. The discovery that there are pluripotent stem cells present in the adult CNS, capable of differentiating into hippocampal, olfactory bulb and neocortical cells, has made this approach seem more achievable although there are still formidable hurdles to be overcome (Nakatomi et al., 2002). Exogenous sources of cells able to differentiate into neurons under consideration for this role include fetal spinal progenitor cells, umbilical cord blood cells, human fibroblasts, fetal brain stem cells, murine neural stem cells and porcine fetal neurons (Holden, 2002). Unlike Parkinson's disease, in which the site of neuronal loss is highly localized to the substantia nigra of the basal ganglia, motor neuronal loss in ALS and indeed in SMA and SBMA occurs over a wide anatomical area. Replacement stem cells therefore need to migrate long distances from cerebral cortex to spinal cord; this ability tends to be lost as cells become more differentiated. Interesting work done on chimeric transgenic/non-transgenic SOD1 mice

(Clement et al., 2003), moreover, indicates that that the provision of a healthy neighborhood around motor neurons may be protective even when those motor neurons express mutant SOD1. This work raises the possibility that stem cell therapy might also beneficially be used to supply healthy non-neuronal cells to the spinal cord to support motor neurons.

Rejection remains a concern, although as an immunologically privileged site, this may be a less prominent problem in the CNS than elsewhere in the body. There are also dangers of introducing poorly differentiated cells into an adult CNS. Uncontrolled overgrowth of introduced stem cells may ultimately generate a mass of cells big enough to cause problems of space occupation clinically. Synaptic connections made by newly differentiated neurons settling in the wrong location or even aberrant connections made by correctly located cells may also produce unwanted side effects.

Despite these difficulties, and significant ethical and political barriers to research on stem cells, some progress has nevertheless been made. As part of a systematic evaluation of the characteristics of different embryoid body stem cells, derived from the germ cells of aborted fetuses, Gearhart et al. injected laboratory-sprouted intermediate-stage embryonic body stem cells into a rat model of SMA. Some mobility was restored to animals previously paralyzed, offering a tantalising glimpse of the possible therapeutic benefits of stem-cell therapy (Vastag, 2001). This work remains at a very early stage and it remains to be seen whether its early promise is borne out in real benefits for patients with motor neuron disorders.

REFERENCES

Abel, A., Walcott, J., Woods, J., Duda, J. & Merry, D. E. (2001). Expression of expanded repeat androgen receptor produces neurologic disease in transgenic mice. *Hum. Mol. Genet.*, **10**, 107–16.

Acsadi, G., Anguelov, R. A., Yang, H. *et al.* (2002). Increased survival and function of SOD1 mice after glial cell-derived neurotrophic factor gene therapy. *Hum. Gene. Ther.*, **13**, 1047–59.

Adachi, H., Katsuno, M., Minamiyama, M. *et al.* (2003). Heat shock protein 70 chaperone overexpression ameliorates phenotypes of the spinal and bulbar muscular atrophy transgenic mouse model by reducing nuclear-localized mutant androgen receptor protein. *J. Neurosci.*, **23**, 2203–11.

Almer, G., Guegan, C., Teismann, P. *et al.* (2001). Increased expression of the pro-inflammatory enzyme cyclooxygenase-2 in amyotrophic lateral sclerosis. *Ann. Neurol.*, **49**, 176–85.

Andreassen, O. A., Dedeoglu, A., Klivenyi, P., Beal, M. F. & Bush, A. I. (2000). *N*-acetyl-L-cysteine improves survival and preserves motor performance in an animal model of familial amyotrophic lateral sclerosis. *Neuroreport*, **11**, 2491–3.

Andreassi, C., Jarecki, J., Zhou, J. *et al.* (2001). Aclarubicin treatment restores SMN levels to cells derived from type I spinal muscular atrophy patients. *Hum. Mol. Genet.*, **10**, 2841–9.

Andreassi, C., Angelozzi, C., Tiziano, F. D. *et al.* (2004). Phenylbutyrate increases SMN expression in vitro: relevance for treatment of spinal muscular atrophy. *Eur. J. Hum. Genet.*, **12**, 59–65.

Andrus, P. K., Fleck, T. J., Gurney, M. E. & Hall, E. D. (1998). Protein oxidative damage in a transgenic mouse model of familial amyotrophic lateral sclerosis. *J. Neurochem.*, **71**, 2041–8.

Annane, D., Chevrolet, J. C., Chevret, S. & Raphael, J. C. (2000). Nocturnal mechanical ventilation for chronic hypoventilation in patients with neuromuscular and chest wall disorders. *Cochrane Database Syst Rev.*, CD001941.

Appel, S. H., Alexianu, M., Engelhardt, J. I. *et al.* (2000). Involvement of immune factors in motor neuron cell injury in amyotrophic lateral sclerosis. In *Amyotrophic Lateral Sclerosis*, ed. R. H. Brown, V. Meininger & M. Swash, pp. 309–26. London, UK: Martin Dunitz.

Ashton, D., Willems, R., Wynants, J. *et al.* (1997). Altered Na(+)-channel function as an in vitro model of the ischemic penumbra: action of lubeluzole and other neuroprotective drugs. *Brain Res.*, **745**, 210–21.

Bailey, C. K., Andriola, I. F., Kampinga, H. H. & Merry, D. E. (2002). Molecular chaperones enhance the degradation of expanded polyglutamine repeat androgen receptor in a cellular model of spinal and bulbar muscular atrophy. *Hum. Mol. Genet.*, **11**, 515–23.

Banks, R. E., Dunn, M. J., Hochstrasser, D. F. *et al.* (2000). Proteomics: new perspectives, new biomedical opportunities. *Lancet*, **356**, 1749–56.

Bensimon, G., Lacomblez, L. & Meininger, V. (1994). A controlled trial of riluzole in amyotrophic lateral sclerosis. ALS/Riluzole Study Group. *N. Engl. J. Med.*, **330**, 585–91.

Beretta, S., Sala, G., Mattavelli, L. *et al.* (2003). Mitochondrial dysfunction due to mutant copper/zinc superoxide dismutase associated with amyotrophic lateral sclerosis is reversed by *N*-acetylcysteine. *Neurobiol. Dis.*, **13**, 213–21.

Blin, O., Pouget, J., Aubrespy, G. *et al.* (1992). A double-blind placebo-controlled trial of L-threonine in amyotrophic lateral sclerosis. *J. Neurol.*, **239**, 79–81.

Borasio, G. D., Robberecht, W., Leigh, P. N. *et al.* (1998). A placebo-controlled trial of insulin-like growth factor-I in amyotrophic lateral sclerosis. European ALS/IGF-I Study Group. *Neurology*, **51**, 583–6.

Bordet, T., Lesbordes, J. C., Rouhani, S. *et al.* (2001). Protective effects of cardiotrophin-1 adenoviral gene transfer on neuromuscular degeneration in transgenic ALS mice. *Hum. Mol. Genet.*, **10**, 1925–33.

Borthwick, G. M., Johnson, M. A., Ince, P. G., Shaw, P. J. & Turnbull, D. M. (1999). Mitochondrial enzyme activity in amyotrophic lateral sclerosis: implications for the role of mitochondria in neuronal cell death. *Ann. Neurol.*, **46**, 787–90.

Brichta, L., Hofmann, Y., Hahnen, E. *et al.* (2003). Valproic acid increases the SMN2 protein level: a well-known drug as a potential therapy for spinal muscular atrophy. *Hum. Mol. Genet.*, **12**, 2481–9.

Brown, R. H., Jr., Hauser, S. L., Harrington, H. & Weiner, H. L. (1986). Failure of immunosuppression with a ten- to 14-day course of high-dose intravenous cyclophosphamide to alter the progression of amyotrophic lateral sclerosis. *Arch. Neurol.*, **43**, 383–4.

Caroni, P. (1993). Activity-sensitive signaling by muscle-derived insulin-like growth factors in the developing and regenerating of neuromuscular system. *Ann. NY Acad. Sci.*, **692**, 209–22.

Cartegni, L. & Krainer, A. R. (2003). Correction of disease-associated exon skipping by synthetic exon-specific activators. *Nat. Struct. Biol.*, **10**, 120–5.

Cassiman, D., Thomeer, M., Verbeken, E. & Robberecht, W. (2003). Hypersensitivity pneumonitis possibly caused by riluzole therapy in ALS. *Neurology*, **61**, 1150–1.

Chang, J. G., Hsieh-Li, H. M., Jong, Y. J. *et al.* (2001). Treatment of spinal muscular atrophy by sodium butyrate. *Proc. Natl Acad. Sci., USA*, **98**, 9808–13.

Cheramy, A., Barbeito, L., Godeheu, G. & Glowinski, J. (1992). Riluzole inhibits the release of glutamate in the caudate nucleus of the cat in vivo. *Neurosci. Lett.*, **147**, 209–12.

Clement, A. M., Nguyen, M. D., Roberts, E. A. *et al.* (2003). Wild-type nonneuronal cells extend survival of SOD1 mutant motor neurons in ALS mice. *Science*, **302**, 113–17.

Collins, A. F., Pearson, H. A., Giardina, P. *et al.* (1995). Oral sodium phenylbutyrate therapy in homozygous beta thalassemia: a clinical trial. *Blood*, **85**, 43–9.

Davenport, R. J., Swingler, R. J., Chancellor, A. M. & Warlow, C. P. (1996). Avoiding false positive diagnoses of motor neuron disease: lessons from the Scottish Motor Neuron Disease Register. *J. Neurol. Neurosurg. Psychiatry*, **60**, 147–51.

Davidson, B. L., Stein, C. S., Heth, J. A. *et al.* (2000). Recombinant adeno-associated virus type 2, 4, and 5 vectors: transduction of variant cell types and regions in the mammalian central nervous system. *Proc. Natl Acad. Sci., USA*, **97**, 3428–32.

Debove, C., Zeisser, P., Salzman, P. M., Powe, L. K. & Truffinet, P. (2001). The Rilutek (riluzole) Global Early Access Programme: an open-label safety evaluation in the treatment of amyotrophic lateral sclerosis. *Amyotroph. Lateral Scler. Other Motor Neuron Disord.*, **2**, 153–8.

Desnuelle, C., Dib, M., Garrel, C. & Favier, A. (2001). A double-blind, placebo-controlled randomized clinical trial of alpha-tocopherol (vitamin E) in the treatment of amyotrophic lateral sclerosis. ALS riluzole-tocopherol Study Group. *Amyotroph. Lateral Scler. Other Motor Neuron Disord.*, **2**, 9–18.

Doble, A. (1996). The pharmacology and mechanism of action of riluzole. *Neurology*, **47**, S233–41.

Doble, A. & Kennel, P. (2000). Animal models of amyotrophic lateral sclerosis. *Amyotroph. Lateral Scler. Other Motor Neuron Disord.*, **1**, 301–12.

Drachman, D. B., Frank, K., Dykes-Hoberg, M. *et al.* (2002). Cyclooxygenase 2 inhibition protects motor neurons and prolongs survival in a transgenic mouse model of ALS. *Ann. Neurol.*, **52**, 771–8.

Drachman, D. B. & Rothstein, J. D. (2000). Inhibition of cyclooxygenase-2 protects motor neurons in an organotypic model of amyotrophic lateral sclerosis. *Ann. Neurol.*, **48**, 792–5.

Ferrante, R. J., Klein, A. M., Dedeoglu, A. & Beal, M. F. (2001). Therapeutic efficacy of EGb761 (*Gingko biloba* extract) in a transgenic mouse model of amyotrophic lateral sclerosis. *J. Mol. Neurosci.*, **17**, 89–96.

Fink, J. K. (2002a). Hereditary spastic paraplegia. *Neurol. Clin.*, **20**, 711–26.

Fink, J. K. (2002b). Hereditary spastic paraplegia: the pace quickens. *Ann. Neurol.*, **51**, 669–72.

Fournier, J., Steinberg, R., Gauthier, T. *et al.* (1993). Protective effects of SR 57746A in central and peripheral models of neurodegenerative disorders in rodents and primates. *Neuroscience*, **55**, 629–41.

Fray, A. E., Ince, P. G., Banner, S. J. *et al.* (1998). The expression of the glial glutamate transporter protein EAAT2 in motor neuron disease: an immunohistochemical study. *Eur. J. Neurosci.*, **10**, 2481–9.

Fujita, K., Yamauchi, M., Shibayama, K. *et al.* (1996). Decreased cytochrome c oxidase activity but unchanged superoxide dismutase and glutathione peroxidase activities in the spinal cords of patients with amyotrophic lateral sclerosis. *J. Neurosci. Res.*, **45**, 276–81.

Gallo, J. M. (2001). Kennedy's disease: a triplet repeat disorder or a motor neuron disease? *Brain Res. Bull.*, **56**, 209–14.

Gil, R. & Neau, J. P. (1992). A double-blind placebo-controlled study of branched chain amino acids and L-threonine for the short-term treatment of signs and symptoms of amyotrophic lateral sclerosis. *La semaine des (Paris)*, **68**, 1472–5.

Groeneveld, G. J., Veldink, J. H., van der Tweel, I. *et al.* (2003). A randomized sequential trial of creatine in amyotrophic lateral sclerosis. *Ann. Neurol.*, **53**, 437–45.

Gurney, M. E., Cutting, F. B., Zhai, P. *et al.* (1996). Benefit of vitamin E, riluzole, and gabapentin in a transgenic model of familial amyotrophic lateral sclerosis. *Ann. Neurol.*, **39**, 147–57.

Hadano, S., Hand, C. K., Osuga, H. *et al.* (2001). A gene encoding a putative GTPase regulator is mutated in familial amyotrophic lateral sclerosis 2. *Nat. Genet.*, **29**, 166–73.

Haddad, H., Cifuentes-Diaz, C., Miroglio, A. *et al.* (2003). Riluzole attenuates spinal muscular atrophy disease progression in a mouse model. *Muscle Nerve*, **28**, 432–7.

Han, D., Williams, E. & Cadenas, E. (2001). Mitochondrial respiratory chain-dependent generation of superoxide anion and its release into the intermembrane space. *Biochem. J.*, **353**, 411–16.

Harrington, M. G., Merril, C. R., Asher, D. M. & Gajdusek, D. C. (1986). Abnormal proteins in the cerebrospinal fluid of patients with Creutzfeldt–Jakob disease. *N. Engl. J. Med.*, **315**, 279–83.

Hedera, P., Williamson, J. A., Rainier, S. *et al.* (2001). Prenatal diagnosis of hereditary spastic paraplegia. *Prenat. Diagn.*, **21**, 202–6.

Hofmann, Y., Lorson, C. L., Stamm, S., Androphy, E. J. & Wirth, B. (2000). Htra2-beta 1 stimulates an exonic splicing enhancer and can restore full-length SMN expression to survival motor neuron 2 (SMN2). *Proc. Natl Acad. Sci., USA*, **97**, 9618–23.

Holden, C. (2002). Neuroscience. Versatile cells against intractable diseases. *Science*, **297**, 500–2.

Hsieh-Li, H. M., Chang, J. G., Jong, Y. J. *et al.* (2000). A mouse model for spinal muscular atrophy. *Nat. Genet.*, **24**, 66–70.

Hubert, J. P., Delumeau, J. C., Glowinski, J., Premont, J. & Doble, A. (1994). Antagonism by riluzole of entry of calcium evoked by NMDA and veratridine in rat cultured granule cells: evidence for a dual mechanism of action. *Br. J. Pharmacol.*, **113**, 261–7.

Ishihara, K., Yamagishi, N., Saito, Y. *et al.* (2003). Hsp105 alpha suppresses the aggregation of truncated androgen receptor with expanded CAG repeats and cell toxicity. *J. Biol. Chem.*, **278**, 25143–50.

Ishiyama, T., Ogo, H., Wong, V. *et al.* (2002). Methionine-free brain-derived neurotrophic factor in wobbler mouse motor neuron disease: dose-related effects and comparison with the methionyl form. *Brain Res.*, **944**, 195–9.

Jaarsma, D., Guchelaar, H. J., Haasdijk, E., de Jong, J. M. & Holstege, J. C. (1998). The anti-oxidant *N*-acetylcysteine does not delay disease onset and death in a transgenic mouse model of amyotrophic lateral sclerosis. *Ann. Neurol.*, **44**, 293.

Kaspar, B. K., Llado, J., Sherkat, N., Rothstein, J. D. & Gage, F. H. (2003). Retrograde viral delivery of IGF-1 prolongs survival in a mouse ALS model. *Science*, **301**, 839–42.

Katsuno, M., Adachi, H., Kume, A. *et al.* (2002). Testosterone reduction prevents phenotypic expression in a transgenic mouse model of spinal and bulbar muscular atrophy. *Neuron*, **35**, 843–54.

Katsuno, M., Adachi, H., Doyu, M. *et al.* (2003). Leuprorelin rescues polyglutamine-dependent phenotypes in a transgenic mouse model of spinal and bulbar muscular atrophy. *Nat. Med.*, **9**, 768–73.

Kelemen, J., Hedlund, W., Orlin, J. B., Berkman, E. M. & Munsat, T. L. (1983). Plasmapheresis with immunosuppression in amyotrophic lateral sclerosis. *Arch. Neurol.*, **40**, 752–3.

Keller, J. N., Mark, R. J., Bruce, A. J. *et al.* (1997). 4-Hydroxynonenal, an aldehydic product of membrane lipid peroxidation, impairs glutamate transport and mitochondrial function in synaptosomes. *Neuroscience*, **80**, 685–96.

Khoo, B., Akker, S. A. & Chew, S. L. (2003). Putting some spine into alternative splicing. *Trends Biotechnol.*, **21**, 328–30.

Klivenyi, P., Ferrante, R. J., Matthews, R. T. *et al.* (1999). Neuroprotective effects of creatine in a transgenic animal model of amyotrophic lateral sclerosis. *Nat. Med.*, **5**, 347–50.

Klivenyi, P., Kiaei, M., Gardian, G., Calingasan, N. Y. & Beal, M. F. (2004). Additive neuroprotective effects of creatine and cyclooxygenase 2 inhibitors in a transgenic mouse model of amyotrophic lateral sclerosis. *J. Neurochem.*, **88**, 576–82.

Kobayashi, Y., Kume, A., Li, M. *et al.* (2000). Chaperones Hsp70 and Hsp40 suppress aggregate formation and apoptosis in cultured neuronal cells expressing truncated androgen receptor protein with expanded polyglutamine tract. *J. Biol. Chem.*, **275**, 8772–8.

Kong, J. & Xu, Z. (1998). Massive mitochondrial degeneration in motor neurons triggers the onset of amyotrophic lateral sclerosis in mice expressing a mutant SOD1. *J. Neurosci.*, **18**, 3241–50.

Kriz, J., Gowing, G. & Julien, J. P. (2003). Efficient three-drug cocktail for disease induced by mutant superoxide dismutase. *Ann. Neurol.*, **53**, 429–36.

Kriz, J., Nguyen, M. D. & Julien, J. P. (2002). Minocycline slows disease progression in a mouse model of amyotrophic lateral sclerosis. *Neurobiol. Dis.*, **10**, 268–78.

Lacomblez, L., Bensimon, G., Leigh, P. N., Guillet, P. & Meininger, V. (1996). Dose-ranging study of riluzole in amyotrophic lateral sclerosis. Amyotrophic Lateral Sclerosis/Riluzole Study Group II. *Lancet*, **347**, 1425–31.

Lai, E. C., Felice, K. J., Festoff, B. W. *et al.* (1997). Effect of recombinant human insulin-like growth factor-I on progression of ALS. A placebo-controlled study. The North America ALS/IGF-I Study Group. *Neurology*, **49**, 1621–30.

Lange, D. J., Murphy, P. L., Diamond, B. *et al.* (1998). Selegiline is ineffective in a collaborative double-blind, placebo-controlled trial for treatment of amyotrophic lateral sclerosis. *Arch. Neurol.*, **55**, 93–6.

Langmore, S. E., Kasarskis, E. J. K., Manca, M. L. & Olney, R. O. (2003). Enteral feeding for amyotrophic lateral sclerosis/motor neuron disease (Protocol). *Cochrane Database Syst. Rev.*, 3.

Lesbordes, J. C., Cifuentes-Diaz, C., Miroglio, A. *et al.* (2003). Therapeutic benefits of cardiotrophin-1 gene transfer in a mouse model of spinal muscular atrophy. *Hum. Mol. Genet.*, **12**, 1233–9.

Lewis, M. E., Neff, N. T., Contreras, P. C. *et al.* (1993). Insulin-like growth factor-I: potential for treatment of motor neuronal disorders. *Exp. Neurol.*, **124**, 73–88.

Louwerse, E. S., Weverling, G. J., Bossuyt, P. M., Meyjes, F. E. & de Jong, J. M. (1995). Randomized, double-blind, controlled trial of acetylcysteine in amyotrophic lateral sclerosis. *Arch. Neurol.*, **52**, 559–64.

Luo, Z. & Geschwind, D. H. (2001). Microarray applications in neuroscience. *Neurobiol. Dis.*, **8**, 183–93.

Manabe, Y., Nagano, I., Gazi, M. S. *et al.* (2003). Glial cell line-derived neurotrophic factor protein prevents motor neuron loss of transgenic model mice for amyotrophic lateral sclerosis. *Neurol. Res.*, **25**, 195–200.

Mandlekar, S. & Kong, A. N. (2001). Mechanisms of tamoxifen-induced apoptosis. *Apoptosis*, **6**, 469–77.

Martin, D., Thompson, M. A. & Nadler, J. V. (1993). The neuroprotective agent riluzole inhibits release of glutamate and aspartate from slices of hippocampal area CA1. *Eur. J. Pharmacol.*, **250**, 473–6.

Martinou, J. C., Martinou, I. & Kato, A. C. (1992). Cholinergic differentiation factor (CDF/LIF) promotes survival of isolated rat embryonic motoneurons in vitro. *Neuron*, **8**, 737–44.

Matthews, R. T., Yang, L., Browne, S., Baik, M. & Beal, M. F. (1998). Coenzyme Q10 administration increases brain mitochondrial concentrations and exerts neuroprotective effects. *Proc. Natl Acad. Sci., USA*, **95**, 8892–7.

Matthijs, G., Devriendt, K. & Fryns, J. P. (1998). The prenatal diagnosis of spinal muscular atrophy. *Prenat. Diagn.*, **18**, 607–10.

Mattiazzi, M., D'Aurelio, M., Gajewski, C. D. *et al.* (2002). Mutated human SOD1 causes dysfunction of oxidative phosphorylation in mitochondria of transgenic mice. *J. Biol. Chem.*, **277**, 29626–33.

Mazzini, L., Balzarini, C., Colombo, R. *et al.* (2001). Effects of creatine supplementation on exercise performance and muscular strength in amyotrophic lateral sclerosis: preliminary results. *J. Neurol. Sci.*, **191**, 139–44.

McGeer, P. L. & McGeer, E. G. (2002). Inflammatory processes in amyotrophic lateral sclerosis. *Muscle Nerve*, **26**, 459–70.

Meininger, V., Lacomblez, L. & Bensimon, G. (1995). Unpublished report: controlled trial of riluzole in patients with advanced ALS. RP 54272–302.

Menzies, F. M., Cookson, M. R., Taylor, R. W. *et al.* (2002). Mitochondrial dysfunction in a cell culture model of familial amyotrophic lateral sclerosis. *Brain*, **125**, 1522–33.

Mercuri, E., Bertini, E., Messina, S. *et al.* (2004). Pilot trial of phenylbutyrate in spinal muscular atrophy. *Neuromuscul. Disord.*, **14**, 130–5.

Merlini, L., Estournet-Mathiaud, B., Iannaccone, S. *et al.* (2002). 90th ENMC international workshop: European Spinal Muscular Atrophy Randomised Trial (EuroSMART) 9–10 February 2001, Naarden, The Netherlands. *Neuromuscul. Disord.*, **12**, 201–10.

Meucci, N., Nobile-Orazio, E. & Scarlato, G. (1996). Intravenous immunoglobulin therapy in amyotrophic lateral sclerosis. *J. Neurol.*, **243**, 117–20.

Miller, R. G., Bryan, W. W., Dietz, M. A. *et al.* (1996). Toxicity and tolerability of recombinant human ciliary neurotrophic factor in patients with amyotrophic lateral sclerosis. *Neurology*, **47**, 1329–31.

Miller, R. G., Munsat, T. L., Swash, M. & Brooks, B. R. (1999a). Consensus guidelines for the design and implementation of clinical trials in ALS. World Federation of Neurology Committee on Research. *J. Neurol. Sci.*, **169**, 2–12.

Miller, R. G., Rosenberg, J. A., Gelinas, D. F. *et al.* (1999b). Practice parameter: the care of the patient with amyotrophic lateral sclerosis (an evidence-based review): report of the Quality Standards Subcommittee of the American Academy of Neurology: ALS Practice Parameters Task Force. *Neurology*, **52**, 1311–23.

Miller, R. G., Moore, D. H., 2nd, Gelinas, D. F. *et al.* (2001a). Phase III randomized trial of gabapentin in patients with amyotrophic lateral sclerosis. *Neurology*, **56**, 843–8.

Miller, R. G., Moore, D. H., Dronsky, V. *et al.* (2001b). A placebo-controlled trial of gabapentin in spinal muscular atrophy. *J. Neurol. Sci.*, **191**, 127–31.

Miller, R. G., Mitchell, J. D., Lyon, M. & Moore, D. H. (2002). Riluzole for amyotrophic lateral sclerosis (ALS)/motor neuron disease (MND). *Cochrane Database Syst. Rev.*, CD001447.

Mitchell, J. D., Houghton, E., Rostron, G. *et al.* (1995). Serial studies of free radical and anti-oxidant activity in motor neurone disease and the effect of selegiline. *Neurodegeneration*, **4**, 233–5.

Mitchell, J. D., Wokke, J. H. & Borasio, G. D. (2002). Recombinant human insulin-like growth factor I (rhIGF-I) for amyotrophic lateral sclerosis/motor neuron disease. *Cochrane Database Syst. Rev.*, CD002064.

Mitsumoto, H., Ikeda, K., Holmlund, T. *et al.* (1994a). The effects of ciliary neurotrophic factor on motor dysfunction in wobbler mouse motor neuron disease. *Ann. Neurol.*, **36**, 142–8.

Mitsumoto, H., Ikeda, K., Klinkosz, B. *et al.* (1994b). Arrest of motor neuron disease in wobbler mice cotreated with CNTF and BDNF. *Science*, **265**, 1107–10.

Mizuta, I., Ohta, M., Ohta, K. *et al.* (2001). Riluzole stimulates nerve growth factor, brain-derived neurotrophic factor and glial cell line-derived neurotrophic factor synthesis in cultured mouse astrocytes. *Neurosci. Lett.*, **310**, 117–20.

Molina, J. A., de Bustos, F., Jimenez-Jimenez, F. J. *et al.* (2000). Serum levels of coenzyme Q10 in patients with amyotrophic lateral sclerosis. *J. Neural Transm.*, **107**, 1021–6.

Monani, U. R., Coovert, D. D. & Burghes, A. H. (2000). Animal models of spinal muscular atrophy. *Hum. Mol. Genet.*, **9**, 2451–7.

Mora, J. S., Munsat, T. L., Kao, K. P. *et al.* (1986). Intrathecal administration of natural human interferon alpha in amyotrophic lateral sclerosis. *Neurology*, **36**, 1137–40.

Nakano, Y., Hirayama, K. & Terao, K. (1987). Hepatic ultrastructural changes and liver dysfunction in amyotrophic lateral sclerosis. *Arch. Neurol.*, **44**, 103–6.

Nakatomi, H., Kuriu, T., Okabe, S. *et al.* (2002). Regeneration of hippocampal pyramidal neurons after ischemic brain injury by recruitment of endogenous neural progenitors. *Cell*, **110**, 429–41.

National Institute for Clinical Excellence (2001). Guidance on the use of riluzole (Rilutek) for the treatment of motor neurone disease. *Technology Appraisal Guidance*, 20.

Neff, N. T., Prevette, D., Houenou, L. J. *et al.* (1993). Insulin-like growth factors: putative muscle-derived trophic agents that promote motoneuron survival. *J. Neurobiol.*, **24**, 1578–88.

Noh, K. M., Hwang, J. Y., Shin, H. C. & Koh, J. Y. (2000). A novel neuroprotective mechanism of riluzole: direct inhibition of protein kinase C. *Neurobiol. Dis.*, **7**, 375–83.

Ochs, G., Penn, R. D., York, M. *et al.* (2000). A phase I/II trial of recombinant methionyl human brain derived neurotrophic factor administered by intrathecal infusion to patients with amyotrophic lateral sclerosis. *Amyotroph. Lateral Scler. Other Motor Neuron Disord.*, **1**, 201–6.

Olarte, M. R. & Shafer, S. Q. (1985). Levamisole is ineffective in the treatment of amyotrophic lateral sclerosis. *Neurology*, **35**, 1063–6.

Oosthuyse, B., Moons, L., Storkebaum, E. *et al.* (2001). Deletion of the hypoxia-response element in the vascular endothelial growth factor promoter causes motor neuron degeneration. *Nat. Genet.*, **28**, 131–8.

Orrell, R. W., Lane, R. J. M. & Ross, M. (2003). Anti-oxidant treatment for amyotrophic lateral sclerosis/motor neuron disease (Protocol). *Cochrane Database Syst. Rev.*, 3.

Parmar, M. K., Torri, V. & Stewart, L. (1998). Extracting summary statistics to perform meta-analyses of the published literature for survival endpoints. *Stat. Med.*, **17**, 2815–34.

Parton, M., Mitsumoto, H. & Leigh, P. (2003). Amino acids for amyotrophic lateral sclerosis/motor neuron disease. *Cochrane Database Syst. Rev.*, **4**, CD003457.

Patel, H., Cross, H., Proukakis, C. *et al.* (2002). SPG20 is mutated in Troyer syndrome, an hereditary spastic paraplegia. *Nat. Genet.*, **31**, 347–8.

Patten, B. M. & Klein, L. M. (1988). L-Threonine and the modification of ALS. *Neurology*, **38**, 354–5.

Plaitakis, A. & Sivak, M. (1992). Treatment of amyotrophic lateral sclerosis with branched chain amino acids (BCAA): results of a second study. *Neurology*, **42**, 454.

Plaitakis, A., Nicklas, W. J. & Desnick, R. J. (1980). Glutamate dehydrogenase deficiency in three patients with spinocerebellar syndrome. *Ann. Neurol.*, **7**, 297–303.

Plaitakis, A., Berl, S. & Yahr, M. D. (1984). Neurological disorders associated with deficiency of glutamate dehydrogenase. *Ann. Neurol.*, **15**, 144–53.

Quality Standards Subcommittee of the American Academy of Neurology (1997). Practice advisory on the treatment of amyotrophic lateral sclerosis with riluzole: report of the Quality Standards Subcommittee of the American Academy of Neurology. *Neurology*, **49**, 657–9.

Rainier, S., Chai, J. H., Tokarz, D., Nicholls, R. D. & Fink, J. K. (2003). NIPA1 gene mutations cause autosomal dominant hereditary spastic paraplegia (SPG6). *Am. J. Hum. Genet.*, **73**, 967–71.

Ramesh, T. M., Buradagunta, S., Thompson, K. *et al.* (2002). Analysis of critical parameters for preclinical drug screening in the SOD1 G93A mouse model for amyotrophic lateral sclerosis (abstract). *Amytroph. Lateral Scler. Other Motor Neuron Disord.*, **3**, 5.

Reid, E., Kloos, M., Ashley-Koch, A. *et al.* (2002). A kinesin heavy chain (KIF5A) mutation in hereditary spastic paraplegia (SPG10). *Am. J. Hum. Genet.*, **71**, 1189–94.

Robberecht, W. L. & de Jong, J. M. B. V. (2000). Oxidative stress in amyotrophic lateral sclerosis: pathogenic mechanism or epiphenomenona? In *Amyotrophic Lateral Sclerosis*, ed. R. H., Brown, V. Meininger, & M. Swash, pp. 211–22. London, UK: Martin Dunitz.

Rosen, D. R., Siddique, T., Patterson, D. *et al.* (1993). Mutations in Cu/Zn superoxide dismutase gene are associated with familial amyotrophic lateral sclerosis. *Nature*, **362**, 59–62.

Rothstein, J. D., Van Kammen, M., Levey, A. I., Martin, L. J. & Kuncl, R. W. (1995). Selective loss of glial glutamate transporter GLT-1 in amyotrophic lateral sclerosis. *Ann. Neurol.*, **38**, 73–84.

Russman, B. S., Iannaccone, S. T. & Samaha, F. J. (2003). A phase 1 trial of riluzole in spinal muscular atrophy. *Arch. Neurol.*, **60**, 1601–3.

Shaw, P. J. (2001). Mechanisms of cell death and treatment prospects in motor neuron disease. *Hong Kong Med. J.*, **7**, 267–80.

Shaw, P. J. & Ince, P. G. (1997). Glutamate, excitotoxicity and amyotrophic lateral sclerosis. *J. Neurol.*, **244 Suppl 2**, S3–14.

Shaw, P. J., Forrest, V., Ince, P. G., Richardson, J. P. & Wastell, H. J. (1995a). CSF and plasma amino acid levels in motor neuron disease: elevation of CSF glutamate in a subset of patients. *Neurodegeneration*, **4**, 209–16.

Shaw, P. J., Ince, P. G., Falkous, G. & Mantle, D. (1995b). Oxidative damage to protein in sporadic motor neuron disease spinal cord. *Ann. Neurol.*, **38**, 691–5.

Shaw, P. J., Chinnery, R. M., Thagesen, H., Borthwick, G. M. & Ince, P. G. (1997). Immunocytochemical study of the distribution of the free radical scavenging enzymes Cu/Zn superoxide dismutase (SOD1) MN superoxide dismutase (MN SOD) and catalase in the normal human spinal cord and in motor neuron disease. *J. Neurol. Sci.*, **147**, 115–25.

Sher, G. D., Ginder, G. D., Little, J. *et al.* (1995). Extended therapy with intravenous arginine butyrate in patients with beta-hemoglobinopathies. *N. Engl. J. Med.*, **332**, 1606–10.

Siklos, L., Engelhardt, J., Harati, Y. *et al.* (1996). Ultrastructural evidence for altered calcium in motor nerve terminals in amyotrophic lateral sclerosis. *Ann. Neurol.*, **39**, 203–16.

Simpson, M. A., Cross, H., Proukakis, C. *et al.* (2003). Maspardin is mutated in mast syndrome, a complicated form of hereditary spastic paraplegia associated with dementia. *Am. J. Hum. Genet.*, **73**, 1147–56.

Skordis, L. A., Dunckley, M. G., Yue, B., Eperon, I. C. & Muntoni, F. (2003). Bifunctional antisense oligonucleotides provide a trans-acting splicing enhancer that stimulates SMN2 gene expression in patient fibroblasts. *Proc. Natl Acad. Sci., USA*, **100**, 4114–19.

Smith, R. G., Henry, Y. K., Mattson, M. P. & Appel, S. H. (1998). Presence of 4-hydroxynonenal in cerebrospinal fluid of patients with sporadic amyotrophic lateral sclerosis. *Ann. Neurol.*, **44**, 696–9.

Snow, R. J., Turnbull, J., da Silva, S., Jiang, F. & Tarnopolsky, M. A. (2003). Creatine supplementation and riluzole treatment provide similar beneficial effects in copper, zinc superoxide dismutase (G93A) transgenic mice. *Neuroscience*, **119**, 661–7.

Sobue, G., Sahashi, K., Takahashi, A. *et al.* (1983). Degenerating compartment and functioning compartment of motor neurons in ALS: possible process of motor neuron loss. *Neurology*, **33**, 654–7.

Spreux-Varoquaux, O., Bensimon, G., Lacomblez, L. *et al.* (2002). Glutamate levels in cerebrospinal fluid in amyotrophic lateral sclerosis: a reappraisal using a new HPLC method with coulometric detection in a large cohort of patients. *J. Neurol. Sci.*, **193**, 73–8.

Strong, M. J. & Pattee, G. L. (2000). Creatine and coenzyme Q10 in the treatment of ALS. *Amyotroph. Lateral Scler. Other Motor Neuron Disord.*, **1 Suppl 4**, 17–20.

Sumner, C. J., Huynh, T. N., Markowitz, J. A. *et al.* (2003). Valproic acid increases SMN levels in spinal muscular atrophy patient cells. *Ann. Neurol.*, **54**, 647–54.

Takeyama, K., Ito, S., Yamamoto, A. *et al.* (2002). Androgen-dependent neurodegeneration by polyglutamine-expanded human androgen receptor in *Drosophila*. *Neuron*, **35**, 855–64.

Tarnopolsky, M. A. & Beal, M. F. (2001). Potential for creatine and other therapies targeting cellular energy dysfunction in neurological disorders. *Ann. Neurol.*, **49**, 561–74.

Testa, D., Caraceni, T. & Fetoni, V. (1989). Branched-chain amino acids in the treatment of amyotrophic lateral sclerosis. *J. Neurol.*, **236**, 445–7.

Testa, D., Caraceni, T., Fetoni, V. & Girotti, F. (1992). Chronic treatment with L-threonine in amyotrophic lateral sclerosis: a pilot study. *Clin. Neurol. Neurosurg.*, **94**, 7–9.

The ALS CNTF Treatment Study Group (1996). A double-blind placebo-controlled clinical trial of subcutaneous recombinant human ciliary neurotrophic factor (rHCNTF) in amyotrophic lateral sclerosis. *Neurology*, **46**, 1244–9.

The BDNF Study Group (1999). A controlled trial of recombinant methionyl human BDNF in ALS: the BDNF Study Group (Phase III). *Neurology*, **52**, 1427–33.

Tikka, T. M., Vartiainen, N. E., Goldsteins, G. *et al.* (2002). Minocycline prevents neurotoxicity induced by cerebrospinal fluid from patients with motor neurone disease. *Brain*, **125**, 722–31.

Tohgi, H., Abe, T., Yamazaki, K. *et al.* (1999). Remarkable increase in cerebrospinal fluid 3-nitrotyrosine in patients with sporadic amyotrophic lateral sclerosis. *Ann. Neurol.*, **46**, 129–31.

Turner, M. R. & Leigh, P. N. (2003). Disease-modifying therapies in motor neuron disorders: the present position and potential future developments. In *Blue Books of Practical Neurology: Motor Neuron Disorders*, ed. P. J. Shaw & M. J. Strong, Woburn, UK: Butterworth-Heinemann.

Turner, M. R., Bakker, M., Sham, P. *et al.* (2002). Prognostic modelling of therapeutic interventions in amyotrophic lateral sclerosis. *Amyotroph. Lateral Scler. Other Motor Neuron. Disord.*, **3**, 15–21.

Turrens, J. F. (1997). Superoxide production by the mitochondrial respiratory chain. *Biosci. Rep.*, **17**, 3–8.

Tzeng, A. C., Cheng, J., Fryczynski, H. *et al.* (2000). A study of thyrotropin-releasing hormone for the treatment of spinal muscular atrophy: a preliminary report. *Am. J. Phys. Med. Rehabil.*, **79**, 435–40.

Van Den Bosch, L., Tilkin, P., Lemmens, G. & Robberecht, W. (2002). Minocycline delays disease onset and mortality in a transgenic model of ALS. *Neuroreport*, **13**, 1067–70.

Vastag, B. (2001). Stem cells step closer to the clinic: paralysis partially reversed in rats with ALS-like disease. *J. Am. Med. Assoc.*, **285**, 1691–3.

Vyth, A., Timmer, J. G., Bossuyt, P. M., Louwerse, E. S. & de Jong, J. M. (1996). Survival in patients with amyotrophic lateral sclerosis, treated with an array of anti-oxidants. *J. Neurol. Sci.*, **139 Suppl**, 99–103.

Werdelin, L., Boysen, G., Jensen, T. S. & Mogensen, P. (1990). Immunosuppressive treatment of patients with amyotrophic lateral sclerosis. *Acta. Neurol. Scand.*, **82**, 132–4.

Westarp, M. E., Westphal, K. P., Kolde, G. *et al.* (1992). Dermal, serological and CSF changes in amyotrophic lateral sclerosis with and without intrathecal interferon beta treatment. *Int. J. Clin. Pharmacol. Ther. Toxicol.*, **30**, 81–93.

Wirth, B. (2002). Spinal muscular atrophy: state-of-the-art and therapeutic perspectives. *Amyotroph. Lateral Scler. Other Motor Neuron Disord.*, **3**, 87–95.

Wood, J. D., Beaujeux, T. P. & Shaw, P. J. (2003). Protein aggregation in motor neurone disorders. *Neuropathol. Appl. Neurobiol.*, **29**, 529–45.

Wood-Allum, C. A. & Shaw, P. J. (2003). Mitochondrial dysfunction in amyotrophic lateral sclerosis (ALS). In *Blue Books of Practical Neurology: Motor Neuron Disorders*, ed. P. J. Shaw & M. J. Strong, Woburn, UK: Butterworth-Heinemann.

World Federation of Neurology Research Committee on Motor Neuron Diseases (1998). Revised criteria for the diagnosis of amyotrophic lateral sclerosis. http://wfnals.org/Articles/elescorial1998criteria.htm.

Yanagisawa, N., Tashiro, K., Tohgi, H. *et al.* (1997). Efficacy and safety of riluzole in patients with amyotrophic lateral sclerosis: double-blind placebo-controlled study in Japan. *Igakuno Ayumi.*, **182**, 851–66.

Yang, Y., Hentati, A., Deng, H. X. *et al.* (2001). The gene encoding alsin, a protein with three guanine-nucleotide exchange factor domains, is mutated in a form of recessive amyotrophic lateral sclerosis. *Nat. Genet.*, **29**, 160–5.

Yasojima, K., Tourtellotte, W. W., McGeer, E. G. & McGeer, P. L. (2001). Marked increase in cyclooxygenase-2 in ALS spinal cord: implications for therapy. *Neurology*, **57**, 952–6.

Zhang, W., Narayanan, M. & Friedlander, R. M. (2003). Additive neuroprotective effects of minocycline with creatine in a mouse model of ALS. *Ann. Neurol.*, **53**, 267–70.

Zhu, S., Stavrovskaya, I. G., Drozda, M. *et al.* (2002). Minocycline inhibits cytochrome c release and delays progression of amyotrophic lateral sclerosis in mice. *Nature*, **417**, 74–8.

53

The hereditary spastic paraplegias

John K. Fink

Department of Neurology, University of Michigan and Geriatric Research Education and Care Center,
Ann Arbor Veterans Affairs Medical Center, MI, USA

Introduction and classification

Inherited disorders in which the predominant clinical syndrome is gait disturbance due to lower extremity spastic weakness are referred to collectively as the hereditary spastic paraplegias (HSPs). The various types of HSP are classified clinically according to the mode of inheritance (dominant, recessive, and X-linked); and whether lower extremity spasticity and weakness and often urinary urgency and subtle dorsal column impairment occur alone ("uncomplicated HSP"), or are accompanied by additional neurologic or systemic symptoms for which alternative causes are excluded ("complicated HSP") (Harding, 1983).

There are at least 20 genetically distinct types of HSP (Table 53.1) including ten dominant, seven recessive, and three X-linked HSP syndromes. Eight of these HSP syndromes are "uncomplicated;" eight of these are "complicated" by the presence of additional neurologic signs; and four of these may present as either "uncomplicated" or "complicated" HSP syndromes. For some of these latter syndromes, both "uncomplicated" and "complicated" HSP phenotypes may coexist even in the same family (Table 53.1).

It is important to recognize that the HSPs are classified clinically, rather than on the basis of subclinical involvement or neuropathologic findings. Certainly, lower extremity spastic weakness may be an important feature of many other disorders, both inherited and apparently sporadic including such diverse disorders as amyotrophic lateral sclerosis, Friedreich's ataxia (Berciano *et al.*, 2002; Ragno *et al.*, 1977), Machado Joseph disease (spinocerebellar ataxia type 3), Charlevoix–Sanguenay syndrome (Engert *et al.*, 2000), primary lateral sclerosis, and familial Alzheimer's disease due to presenilin 1 mutation (Brooks *et al.*, 2003; Assini *et al.*, 2003; Tabira *et al.*, 2002).

The HSP group of disorders is distinguished from these and other conditions by the limitation of symptoms to spastic gait and urinary urgency; and by clinical or laboratory evidence (gene analysis) that the condition is inherited. Clearly, the distinctions between HSP and other causes of lower extremity spastic weakness are somewhat arbitrary. For example, HSP is not considered a lower "motor neuron disorder" despite the fact that minor loss of anterior horn cells may occur in "uncomplicated HSP." This is because HSP is classified on the basis of signs and symptoms and because anterior horn cell loss is variable, subclinical, and below the threshold of electromyographic detection. On the other hand, the "HSP group disorders" includes some conditions with marked upper extremity or lower motor neuron involvement. For example, even though some complicated HSP syndromes (Troyer (SPG20) and Silver (SPG17) syndromes, and those linked to SPG7, SPG9, SPG10, SPG14, and SPG15 loci; Table 53.1) are associated with motor neuronopathy and distal muscle wasting, they are included in the HSP family of disorders because the predominant syndrome remains progressive spastic gait.

Though imperfect and somewhat arbitrary, clinical classification of HSPs is an important tool for identifying homogeneous kindreds for genetic research; and offers some guidance for long-term prognosis. As discussed below, a molecular classification of the HSPs is emerging as HSP genes are discovered.

Clinical signs and symptoms of uncomplicated HSP

Each of the more than 20 known types of HSP represents a separate, genetically distinct disorder. Generalizations can be made only about "uncomplicated" forms of HSP, which are typically so similar that they may not be distinguished

Table 53.1.

Spastic gait (SPG) locus	Chromosome	Gene/Protein: function	HSP syndrome
Autosomal dominant HSP			
SPG4	2p22	SPG4/Spastin: Cytosolic protein, with AAA domain that binds to microtubules	Uncomplicated
SPG13	2q24–34	Heat shock protein 60 (Hsp60), mitochondrial chaperonin (Cpn60)	Uncomplicated
SPG8	8q23–q24		Uncomplicated
SPG9	10q23.3–q24.2		Complicated: spastic paraplegia associated with cataracts and gastroesophageal reflux, and motor neuronopathy
SPG17	11q12–q14		Complicated: spastic paraplegia associated with amyotrophy of hand muscles (Silver Syndrome)
SPG10	12q13	Kinesin heavy chain (KIF5A): molecular motor involved in axonal transport	Uncomplicated or complicated by distal atrophy
SPG3A	14q11–q21	SPG3A/atlastin: Predicted to be GTPase similar to dynamins	Uncomplicated
SPG6	15q11.1	NIPA1: neuron specific membrane protein of unknown function	Uncomplicated
SPG12	19q13		Uncomplicated
SPG19	9q33–q34		Uncomplicated
Autosomal recessive HSP			
SPG14	3q27–28		Complicated: spastic paraplegia associated with mental retardation and distal motor neuropathy
SPG5	8q		Uncomplicated
SPG11	15q		Uncomplicated or complicated: variably associated with HSP associated with thin corpus callosum, mental retardation, upper extremity weakness, dysarthria, and nystagmus
SPG7	16q	SPG6/paraplegin: mitochondrial protein	Uncomplicated or complicated: variably associated with mitochondrial abnormalities on skeletal muscle biopsy and dysarthria, dysphagia, optic disc pallor, axonal neuropathy, and evidence of "vascular lesions", cerebellar atrophy, or cerebral atrophy on cranial MRI
SPG15	14q		Complicated: spastic paraplegia associated with pigmented maculopathy, distal amyotrophy, dysarthria, mental retardation, and further intellectual deterioration.
SPG20	13q	SPG20/spartin: N-terminal region similar to spastin; homologous to proteins involved in the morphology and membrane trafficking of endosomes.	Complicated: spastic paraplegia associated with distal muscle wasting (Troyer syndrome)
	13q14		Childhood onset HSP variably complicated by spastic dysarthria and pseudobulbar signs 59
X-linked HSP			
SPG1	Xq28	L1 cell adhesion molecule (L1CAM)	Complicated: associated with mental retardation, and variably, hydrocephalus, aphasia, and adducted thumbs
SPG2	Xq21	Proteolipid protein (PLP): intrinsic myelin protein	Complicated: variably associated with MRI evidence of CNS white matter abnormality
SPG16	Xq11.2		Complicated: associated with motor aphasia, reduced vision, mild mental retardation, and dysfunction of the bowel and bladder

from each other by clinical signs and symptoms. In contrast, various "complicated" types of HSP often have distinctive clinical signs (such as distal muscle wasting or optic atrophy; Table 53.1) that suggest one or more specific types of HSP.

The hallmark of uncomplicated HSP is gait disturbance due to lower extremity spasticity and weakness. Symptoms may be first evident at any age, from infancy through senescence. Early symptoms of leg muscle tightness, particularly at night, and ankle and knee clonus are followed by stumbling and tripping, particularly when ascending stairs, crossing curbs, or walking rapidly. Over time, gait becomes more functionally impaired, with short strides due to limited flexion of the thigh and difficulty fully dorsiflexing the feet; circumduction; and a tendency to maintain the legs partially flexed (knees bent) due to hamstring muscle spasticity. Hyperlordosis is common.

Progressive vs. non-progressive symptoms

When HSP symptoms begin in very early childhood, developmental milestones of rolling over, sitting up, crawling, and standing, typically are not delayed. The first steps of walking may be abnormal because of toe-walking which is persistent. When symptoms begin in late infancy and early childhood, there may be very little worsening even over many years. In contrast, symptoms that begin after adolescence typically progress insidiously over many years. In part, the relative "progressive" nature of later-onset HSP versus the relatively "static" nature of early-onset HSP may reflect both different genetic types of HSP; as well as the ability of the developing nervous system to compensate for slowly progressive neurodegeneration.

Variable severity

The degree of gait impairment in uncomplicated HSP may be quite variable and range from subtle disturbance that is of no functional consequence; to frank spastic diplegia requiring full-time use of a wheel chair. Severity may be quite variable even within a given family in which all subjects have precisely the same HSP gene mutation.

Urinary urgency

This is very common in subjects with HSP. This typically follows gait impairment by at least several years. For some subjects, however, urinary urgency may be an early sign of HSP. Fecal urgency is less common although may occur. Sexual disturbances are not infrequent in HSP subjects and include erectile dysfunction; and exacerbation of lower extremity clonus and spasm. A systematic investigation of sexual and autonomic symptoms in HSP has not been reported.

Sensory symptoms

Lower extremity paresthesia are reported in many subjects with uncomplicated HSP. Limitation of paresthesia to one limb or dermatome, spinal sensory level, or loss of light touch or pinprick sensation are not features of uncomplicated HSP, however.

Subclinical cognitive disturbance and late-onset dementia

These have been described in some patients with the most common form of dominantly inherited HSP (due to *SPG4* mutations, described below); as well as in some subjects in these families shown to have inherited the mutant SPG4 allele but whose gait was as-yet unaffected (Heinzlef *et al.*, 1998; Lizcano-Gil *et al.*, 1997; Webb *et al.*, 1998; Byrne *et al.*, 1998; Reid *et al.*, 1999; Tedeschi *et al.*, 1991). The frequency of cognitive impairment in this and other forms of HSP is not known.

Neurologic examination

Neurologic examination of subjects with uncomplicated HSP shows spasticity and weakness in bilateral lower extremities particularly in tibialis anterior, hamstring, and iliopsoas muscles. Pathologic hyperreflexia in the lower extremities and ankle (and often knee clonus) is present in virtually all subjects with uncomplicated HSP except those in which significant contractures limit joint range of motion. Plantar responses are extensor in the vast majority of HSP subjects. Pes cavus is common.

The relative amounts of spasticity versus weakness are variable. Some patients have prominent weakness, particularly involving tibialis anterior, hamstrings, and iliopsoas muscles. For other patients, however, there may be no significant weakness, with gait impairment due largely to lower extremity spasticity. The relative amount of spasticity-versus-weakness influences the choice (and functional benefit) of using spasticity-reducing medication.

Subtle impairment of vibration sensation in the distal lower extremities is very common in HSP although often not an early sign. Impaired vibration sensation in the toes, when present, not associated with peripheral neuropathy, and not attributed to other causes, is a helpful diagnostic sign in distinguishing lower extremity spasticity in HSP from early stages of amyotrophic lateral sclerosis and primary lateral sclerosis (Fink, 2001).

Although upper extremity deep tendon reflexes are often brisk, there is no evidence of upper extremity weakness, spasticity, or impaired dexterity. Finger tapping is normal and there is no pronator drift in uncomplicated HSP.

Muscle bulk is usually preserved in uncomplicated HSP. However, it is not uncommon for subjects to have mildly decreased muscle bulk in their shins. The presence of significant muscle wasting should prompt electrophysiologic analysis and consideration of motor neuron disease or co-existing myopathy or peripheral neuropathy. HSP subjects with lower motor neuron deficits for which no other cause can be identified are classified as having a form of "complicated" HSP. There are a number of such HSP syndromes (Table 53.1) that include significant muscle wasting and evidence of motor neuronopathy. For example, Silver syndrome and Troyer syndrome are, respectively, autosomal dominant and autosomal recessive complicated HSP syndromes in which lower extremity spasticity is associated with distal atrophy in the hands and feet (Cross & McKusick, 1967; Farag et al., 1994; Silver, 1966).

Laboratory, neuroimaging, and neurophysiologic analysis

Analysis of HSP subjects are important in excluding other disorders. Routine laboratory studies including cerebrospinal fluid examinations are normal in subjects with uncomplicated HSP.

Muscle biopsy of some subjects with autosomal recessive HSP due to paraplegin (SPG7) gene mutation have shown ragged red fibers and cytochrome C oxidase deficient fibers (Casari et al., 1998). Muscle biopsy of subjects with autosomal dominant uncomplicated HSP have been normal, however (Hedera et al., 2000).

Magnetic resonance imaging (MRI) of the spinal cord in subjects with uncomplicated HSP may show atrophy particularly in the thoracic region. MRI of the brain in subjects with uncomplicated HSP is normal. Thin corpus callosum may be observed in subjects with autosomal recessive HSP linked to chromosome 15q (Nakamura et al., 1995; Ohnishi et al., 2001). Many of these subjects have mental retardation.

Electromyography (EMG) and nerve conduction studies (NCS) are usually normal in subjects with uncomplicated HSP (McLeod et al., 1993). Note, however, that EMG and NCS may be abnormal in types of complicated HSP that have peripheral neuropathy, motor neuronopathy, or distal muscle wasting.

Somatosensory evoked potentials (SSEP) from the lower extremities may show conduction delay (Pelosi et al., 1991; Pedersen & Trojaborg, 1981). When present, this finding is helpful in distinguishing HSP from primary lateral sclerosis and amyotrophic lateral sclerosis, disorders that do not involve dorsal columns. SSEP from the upper extremities are typically normal in uncomplicated HSP.

Central motor conduction velocity can be measured by cortico-evoked potentials. Typically, cortical evoked potentials recorded from the lower extremities show reduced conduction velocity and amplitude of the evoked potential. Cortical evoked potentials recorded from cervical spinal segments are usually normal or show only mildly reduced conduction velocity (Pelosi et al., 1991; Claus & Jaspert, 1995; Claus et al., 1990; Polo et al., 1993; Schady et al., 1991).

Pathology

Knowledge of HSP's pathology is based on very few autopsies (Schwarz, 1992; Schwarz & Liu, 1956). The pathology of HSP can be characterized predominantly by distal axonopathy affecting the terminal portions of the longest motor and sensory fibers in the central nervous system. Axonal degeneration is maximal in the distal portions of corticospinal tracts; and to a lesser extent, in the distal portions of fasciculus gracilus fibers. Spinocerebellar fibers are involved to a lesser extent. Myelin loss occurs in neurons whose axons are degenerating. Myelin loss in uncomplicated HSP is consistent with the degree of axonal degeneration and is not considered to represent a primary demyelinating process. Dorsal root ganglia, posterior roots and peripheral nerves are normal in uncomplicated HSP (Harding, 1993). Although usually normal, decreased numbers of cortical motor neurons and anterior horn cells have been reported (Harding, 1993; Behan & Maia, 1974).

Treatment

Presently, there is no treatment that prevents HSP in presymptomatic subjects; or retards the rate of progression in affected subjects. Treatment is symptomatic and directed toward reducing muscle spasm, reducing urinary urgency, and improving muscle strength and gait.

Lioresal is helpful in reducing muscle spasticity in HSP subjects. The dosage must be individualized as there is significant interindividual variation in the degree of spasticity. Intrathecal baclofen has benefited individuals with particularly severe spasticity. Additional medical approaches to reduce spasticity include tizanidine, dantrolene, and botulinum injections.

We recommend that HSP subjects undergo daily physical therapy including lower extremity muscle stretching, muscle strengthening, cardiovascular conditioning, and gait training. This recommendation is based not on well-controlled prospective studies but on the nearly unanimous beneficial reports of more than 200 HSP subjects; the importance of maintaining cardiovascular conditioning in subjects with paraplegia; and the potential value of gait training on spinal cord neuroplasticity.

Ankle foot orthotics are often helpful in reducing the tendency to catch the toes and stumble. Generally, however, subjects with significant plantar flexion will require reduction of spasticity with medication and physical therapy prior to using ankle-foot orthotic devices.

Prognosis and genetic counseling

Subjects in whom HSP symptoms begin after adolescence, usually experience gait disturbance that gets slowly worse over many years. As noted previously, many subjects with early childhood onset of HSP symptoms do not appear to worsen even over many years.

It is important to recognize the often significant variation in symptom severity when providing genetic counseling. Age of symptom onset, rate of worsening, and degree of disability may be either uniform or highly variable within a given family in which all subjects share precisely the same HSP gene mutation. Such phenotypic differences are attributed to differences in modifying genes and potentially to environmental factors. Whereas the risk of inheriting or transmitting HSP can be estimated from pedigree analysis (or determined accurately in cases where the HSP gene has been identified), it is usually not possible to determine the age at which symptoms will begin (childhood versus adulthood) and whether symptoms will be severe or not functionally disabling.

Genetic analysis of the HSPs

Twenty different genetic forms of HSP have been defined by their linkage to different genetic loci. HSP loci (and the respective types of HSP) are designated Spastic Gait (SPG) loci 1 through 20 in order of their discovery. Thus far, ten

autosomal dominant, seven autosomal recessive, and three X-linked HSP loci have been discovered (Table 53.1).

Whereas various types of "complicated" HSP can sometimes be recognized by their associated signs (Table 53.1), clinical and neuroimaging parameters can not reliably distinguish one genetic form of "uncomplicated" HSP from another. There are differences in the average age at which symptoms first appear however. Gait disturbance generally begins in childhood for subjects with HSP linked to chromosomes 12 (SPG10), 14 (SPG3), and 19 (SPG12) (for review see Fink & Hedera, 1999); and after age 20 in subjects with autosomal dominant uncomplicated HSP linked to chromosomes 2p (SPG4), 2q (SPG13), 8 (SPG8), and 15(SPG6). There is significant overlap in the range of ages at which symptoms begin between the various forms of uncomplicated HSP. This limits the accuracy of predicting the genetic type of uncomplicated HSP from the age of symptom onset.

The most common types of autosomal dominant uncomplicated HSP are those linked to chromosome 2p (SPG4/spastin gene) and chromosome 14q (SPG3A/ atlastin gene), representing approximately 40% and 10% of such families, respectively (Fink et al., 1996). Each of the other types of autosomal dominant HSP are rare and have been reported in only one to several kindreds.

It is estimated that 50% of autosomal recessive HSP kindreds are linked to the SPG11 locus (Martinez-Murillo et al., 1999; Shibaski et al., 2000) on chromosome 15q13–q15. Each of the other types of autosomal recessive HSP have been described in only a few kindreds.

HSP genes

Nine HSP genes have been identified (Table 53.1). Little is known about the function of most of these proteins because they are novel and have only recently been discovered.

SPG4 gene (spastin protein) mutations are the single most common cause of autosomal dominant uncomplicated HSP. SPG4 mutations cause approximately 40% of autosomal dominant HSP (Hazan et al., 1999). SPG4 gene analysis is available commercially (Athena Diagnostics, Boston) and can be used for confirmation of diagnosis and for prenatal diagnosis.

More than 80 SPG4 mutations have been identified (see Hazan et al., 1999; Hentati et al., 2000; Lindsey et al., 2000; Fonknecten et al., 2000; Svenson et al., 2000; Wang et al., 2002). These are almost always unique to the family in which they are discovered. Most, if not all SPG4 mutations are considered to be pathogenic through haploinsufficiency (insufficient abundance of sequence-normal spastin) (Hazan et al., 1999; Charvin et al., 2002) rather than through a dominant negative mechanism.

SPG4 is widely expressed (Charvin *et al.*, 2002). The function of SPG4's encoded protein ("spastin") is not known. Spastin contains an *A*TPase associated with diverse cellular *a*ctivities (AAA) domain (Hazan *et al.*, 1999), and may interact with microtubules (Azim *et al.*, 2000; Errico *et al.*, 2002). Spastin's intracellular distribution is uncertain as both nuclear (Hazan *et al.*, 1999) and cytoplasmic (Errico *et al.*, 2002) localization have been observed.

SPG3A gene ("atlastin" protein) mutations cause approximately 10% of autosomal dominant HSP (Fink *et al.*, 1996; Zhao *et al.*, 2001). SPG3 ADHSP typically begins in childhood. One studied observed *SPG3A* mutations in 25% of autosomal dominant HSP kindreds in which all affected subjects developed symptoms in childhood (Alvarado *et al.*, 2001).

Atlastin's function and the mechanisms by which atlastin mutations cause HSP are not known. Atlastin contains conserved motifs for GTP binding and hydrolysis (Zhao *et al.*, 2001), and bears structural homology to guanylate binding protein 1 (GBP1), a member of the dynamin family of large GTPases (Zhao *et al.*, 2001). The occurrence of an HSP specific mutation in atlastin's GTPase motif indicates the likely significance of this domain (Muglia *et al.*, 2002).

Mutations in kinesin heavy chain (KIF5A) cause either uncomplicated autosomal dominant HSP; or ADHSP associated with distal muscle atrophy (Pericak-Vance *et al.*, 2002). KIF5A is a molecular motor that participates in the intracellular movement of organelles and macromolecules along microtubules. Disturbance in this axonal transport could cause distal axonal degeneration in this and possibly other forms of HSP (Crosby & Proukakis, 2002).

Mutations in mitochondrial chaperonin 60 (also known as heat shock protein 60) cause uncomplicated ADHSP (Hansen *et al.*, 2002). The mechanisms by which disturbance in this mitochondrial protein cause HSP are not known.

SPG7/araplegin gene mutations cause a rare form of autosomal recessive HSP (De Michele *et al.*, 1998). Subjects with paraplegin mutations exhibit either uncomplicated HSP; or HSP associated with dysarthria, dysphagia, optic disc pallor, axonal neuropathy, and evidence of "vascular lesions," cerebellar atrophy, or cerebral atrophy on cranial MRI.

Like chaperonin 60, paraplegin is a mitochondrial chaperone protein (DeMichele *et al.*, 1998). Muscle biopsy in some (but not all) HSP patients with *SPG7* gene mutations showed ragged-red and cytochrome oxidase negative fibers and abnormal mitochondrial structure typical of mitochondriopathy (DeMichele *et al.*, 1998).

Troyer syndrome, a complicated form of autosomal recessive HSP associated with distal muscle wasting is due to mutations in a novel gene designated Spartin

(Spastin-related autosomal recessive Troyer protein) (Patel *et al.*, 2002). Spartin's amino-terminal region is similar to spastin's. Spartin's function is unknown although homology to proteins involved in the endosome morphology and membrane trafficking suggest these possible actions.

Mutations in a novel non-imprinted Prader–Willi/ Angleman gene (*NIPA1*) were recently identified as the cause of ADHSP linked to chromosome 15q (Rainier *et al.*, 2003). NIPA1 is a neuron-specific protein of unknown function. Analysis of NIPA1's predicted secondary structure suggests that it is a membrane protein.

Proteolipid protein (PLP) gene mutations (duplications and point mutations) cause Pelizeaus-Merzbacher disease, an infantile-onset, progressive leukodystrophy; and a slowly progressive form of X-linked HSP (Cambi *et al.*, 1995; Dube *et al.*, 1997). PLP is an integral myelin protein. MRI evidence of CNS leukodystrophy is present in some but not all X-linked HSP patients with PLP mutations.

Neuronal cell adhesion molecule L1 (L1CAM) gene mutations cause a variety of X-linked developmental neurologic disorders including complicated X-linked spastic paraplegia, X-linked hydrocephalus, and X-linked mental retardation aphasia, shuffling gait, and adducted thumbs (MASA) syndrome (Fransen *et al.*, 1996). L1CAM is an integral membrane glycoprotein and a member of immunoglobulin superfamily of cell adhesion molecules that mediate cell-to-cell attachment. L1CAM functions include guidance of neurite outgrowth during development, neuronal cell migration, and neuronal cell survival (Kenwrick *et al.*, 2000).

Conclusions

HSP is a genetically and clinically heterogeneous group of disorders. At least 20 types of HSP have been genetically defined. Although core symptoms of spastic gait are shared with all types of HSP, whether gait disturbance is progressive or static, early or late onset, or associated with muscle wasting, mental retardation, or other neurologic impairments may vary from one genetic type of HSP to another. Furthermore, variation in age of symptom onset and degree of severity within a given family limits the ability to predict accurately the ultimate degree of disability for an individual at risk of developing HSP. A cautious "wait and see" approach is advised.

It is essential to carefully consider the differential diagnosis (for review, see Fink *et al.*, 1996) for subjects with progressive spastic gait, even if there is a strong family history. Alternate disorders (such as multiple sclerosis) or co-existent disorders (such as peripheral neuropathy) may occur in subjects with strong family history of HSP. Laboratory, neuroimaging, and electrodiagnostic studies are helpful in this regard.

It is perhaps not surprising that as causes of HSP have been discovered, they have proven to be molecularly diverse. The distal ends of extremely long fibers (corticospinal tracts and dorsal column fibers subserving the lower extremities) appear to be quite vulnerable to a number of distinct biochemical disturbances. It will be interesting to learn whether some of these disparate primary biochemical disturbances converge into one or more common pathways.

Over time, the HSPs will be classified by their molecular basis and not simply by mode of inheritance and clinical features. An emerging molecular classification might include a) HSP due to mitochondrial abnormality (including SPG13 due to chaperonin 60 mutation and SPG7 due to paraplegin mutation); b) HSP due to axonal transport abnormality (including SPG10 due to kinesin heavy chain mutation and possibly SPG3A (atlastin mutation) and SPG4 (spastin mutation); c) HSP due to primary myelin disturbance (SPG2 due to PLP mutation); and d) HSP due to embryonic development of corticospinal tract neurons (SPG1 due to L1CAM mutation).

Discovery of HSP genes permits laboratory-based diagnoses. Already, commercially available analysis of *SPG4*/spastin and *SPG3A*/atlastin genes will diagnose more than 50% of autosomal dominant HSP. Moreover, discovery and analysis of HSP genes is the primary method for learning the molecular basis of the HSPs, information that is essential for developing treatments for these disabling conditions.

Acknowledgements

This research is supported by grants from the Veterans Affairs Merit Review and the National Institutes of Health (NINDS R01NS33645, R01NS36177 and R01NS38713) to J.K.F. We gratefully acknowledge the expert secretarial assistance of Ms. Lynette Girbach.

REFERENCES

Alvarado, D. M., Ming, L., Hedera, P. *et al.* (2001). Atlastin gene analysis in early onset hereditary spastic paraplegia. *Am. J. Hum. Genet.*, **69**, 597(Abstract).

Assini, A., Terreni, L., Borghi, R. *et al.* (2003). Pure spastic paraparesis associated with a novel presenilin 1 R278K mutation. *Neurology*, **60**, 150.

Azim, A. C., Hentati, A., Haque, M. F. U., Hirano, M., Ouachi, K. & Siddique, T. (2000). Spastin, a new AAA protein, binds to α and β tubulins. *Am. J. Hum. Genet.* (Suppl.), **67**, 197.

Behan, W. & Maia, M. (1974). Strumpell's familial spastic paraplegia: genetics and neuropathology. *J. Neurol. Neurosurg. Psychiatry*, **37**, 8–20.

Berciano, J., Mateo, I., DePablos, C., Polo, J. M. & Combarros, O. (2002). Friedreich ataxia with minimal GAA expression presenting as adult-onset spastic ataxia. *J. Neurol. Sci.*, **194**, 75–82.

Brooks, W. S., Kwok, J. B., Kril, J. J. *et al.* (2003). Alzheimer's disease with spastic paraparesis and "cotton wool" plaques: two pedigrees with PS-1 exon 9 deletions. *Brain*, **126**, 783–91.

Byrne, P. C., Webb, S., McSweeney, F., Burke, T., Hutchinson, M., & Parfrey, N. (1998). Linkage of AD HSP and cognitive impairment to chromosome 2p: haplotype and phenotype analysis indicates variable expression and low or delayed penetrance. *Eur. J. Hum. Genet.*, **6**, 275–82.

Cambi, F., Tartaglino, L., Lublin, F. D. & McCarren, D. (1995). X-linked pure familial spastic paraparesis: characterization of a large kindred with magnetic resonance imaging studies. *Arch. Neurol.*, **52**, 665–9.

Casari, G., Fusco, M., Ciarmatori, S. *et al.* (1998). Spastic paraplegia and OXPHOS impairment caused by mutations in paraplegin, a nuclear-encoded mitochondrial metalloprotease. *Cell*, **93**, 973–83.

Charvin, D., Fonknechten, N., Cifuentes-Diaz, C. *et al.* (2002). Mutations in SPG4 are responsible for a loss of function of spastin, an abundant neuronal protein localized to the nucleus. *Am. J. Hum. Genet.*, **71**, 516 (Abstract).

Claus, D. & Jaspert, A. (1995). Central motor conduction in hereditary spastic paraparesis (Strumpell's disease) and tropical spastic paraparesis. *Neurol. Croatica*, **44**, 23–31.

Claus, D., Waddy, H. M. & Harding, A. E. (1990). Hereditary motor and sensory neuropathies and hereditary spastic paraplegia: a magnetic stimulation study. *Ann. Neurol.*, **28**, 43–9.

Crosby, A. H. & Proukakis, C. (2002). Is the transportation highway the right road for hereditary spastic paraplegia? *Am. J. Hum. Genet.*, **71**, 1009–16.

Cross, H. E. & McKusick, V. A. (1967). The Troyer syndrome. A recessive form of spastic paraplegia with distal muscle wasting. *Arch. Neurol.* **16**, 473–85.

DeMichele, G., DeFusco, M., Cavalcanti, F. *et al.* (1998). A new locus for autosomal recessive hereditary spastic paraplegia maps to chromosome 16q24.3. *Am. J. Hum. Genet.*, **63**, 135–9.

Dube, M.-P., Boutros, M., Figlewicz, D. A. & Rouleau, G. A. (1997). A new pure hereditary spastic paraplegia kindred maps to the proteolipid protein gene locus. *Am. J. Hum. Genet.*, **61**, A169 (Abstract).

Engert, J. C., Berube, P., Mercier, J. *et al.* (2000). ARSACS, a spastic ataxia common in northeastern Quebec, is caused by mutations in a new gene encoding an 11.5-kb ORF. *Nat. Genet.*, **24**, 120–5.

Errico, A., Ballabio, A. & Rugarli, E. (2002). Spastin, the protein mutated in autosomal dominant hereditary spastic paraplegia, is involved in microtubule dynamics. *Hum. Mol. Genet.*, **15**, 153–63.

Farag, T. I., El-badramany, M. H. & Al-Sharkawy, S. (1994). Troyer Syndrome: report of the first "non-Amish" sibship and review. *Am. J. Med. Genet.*, **52**, 383–5.

Fink, J. K. (2001). Progressive spastic paraparesis: hereditary spastic paraplegia and its relation to primary and amyotrophic lateral sclerosis. *Semin. Neurol.*, **21**, 199–208.

Fink, J. K. & Hedera, P. (1999). Hereditary spastic paraplegia: genetic heterogeneity and genotype–phenotype correlation. *Semin. Neurol.*, **19**, 301–10.

Fink, J. K., Heiman-Patterson, T., Bird, T. *et al.* (1996). Hereditary spastic paraplegia: advances in genetic research. *Neurology*, **46**, 1507–14.

Fonknecten, N., Mavel, D., Byrne, P. *et al.* (2000). Spectrum of SPG4 mutations in autosomal dominant spastic paraplegia. *Hum. Mol. Genet.*, **9**, 637–44.

Fransen, E., Vits, L., VanCamp, G. & Willems, P. J. (1996). The clinical spectrum of mutations in L1, a neuronal cell adhesion molecule. *Am. J. Med. Genet.*, **64**, 73–7.

Hansen, J. J., Durr, A., Cournu-Rebeix, I. *et al.* (2002). Hereditary spastic paraplegia SPG13 is associated with a mutation in the gene encoding the mitochondrial chaperonin Hsp60. *Am. J. Hum. Genet.*, **70**, 000–000.

Harding, A. E. (1983). Classification of the hereditary ataxias and paraplegias. *Lancet*, **1**, 1151–5.

Harding, A. E. (1993). Hereditary spastic paraplegias. *Semin. Neurol.*, **13**, 333–6.

Hazan, J., Fonknechten, N., Mavel, D. *et al.* (1999). Spastin, a new AAA protein, is altered in the most frequent form of autosomal dominant spastic paraplegia. *Nat. Genet.*, **23**, 296–303.

Hedera, P., DiMauro, S., Bonilla, E., Wald, J. J. & Fink, J. K. (2000). Mitochondrial analysis in autosomal dominant hereditary spastic paraplegia. *Neurology*, **55**, 1591–2.

Heinzlef, O., Paternotte, C., Mahieux, F. *et al.* (1998). Mapping of a complicated familial spastic paraplegia to locus SPG4 on chromosome 2p. *J. Med. Genet.*, **35**, 89–93.

Hentati, A., Deng, H. X., Zhai, B. A. *et al.* (2000). Novel mutations in spastin gene and absence of correlation with age at onset of symptoms. *Neurology*, **55**, 1388–90.

Hodgkinson, C. A., Bohlega, S., Abu-Amero, S. N. *et al.* (2002). A novel form of autosomal recessive pure hereditary spastic paraplegia maps to chromosome 13q14. *Neurology*, **59**, 1905–9.

Kenwrick, S., Watkins, A. & De Angelis, E. *et al.* (2000). Neural cell recognition molecule L1: relating biological complexity to human disease mutations. *Hum. Mol. Genet.*, **9**, 879–86.

Lindsey, J. C., Lusher, M. E., McDermott, C. J. *et al.* (2000). Mutation analysis of the spastin gene (SPG4) in patients with hereditary spastic paraparesis. *J. Med. Genet.*, **37**, 759–65.

Lizcano-Gil, L. A., Garcia-Cruz, D., Bernal-Beltran, M. D. P. & Hernandez, A. (1997). Association of late onset spastic paraparesis and dementia: probably an autosomal dominant form of complicated paraplegia. *Am. J. Med. Genet.* **68**, 1–6.

McLeod, J. G., Morgan, J. A. & Reye, C. (1993). Electrophysiological studies in familial spastic paraplegia. *Neurol. Neurosurg. Psychiatry*, **40**, 611–15.

Martinez-Murillo, F. M., Kobayashi, H., Pegoraro, E. *et al.* (1999). Genetic localization of a new locus for recessive familial spastic paraparesis to 15q13–15. *Neurology*, **53**, 50–6.

Muglia, M., Magariello, A., Nicoletti, G. *et al.* (2002). Further evidence that SPG3A gene mutations cause autosomal dominant hereditary spastic paraplegia. *Ann. Neurol.*, in press.

Nakamura, A., Izumi, K., Umehara, F. *et al.* (1995). Familial spastic paraplegia with mental impairment and thin corpus callosum. *J. Neurol. Sci.*, **131**, 35–42.

Ohnishi, J., Tomoda, Y. & Yokoyama, K. (2001). Neuroradiological findings in hereditary spastic paraplegia with a thin corpus callosum. *Acta. Neurol. Scand.*, **104**, 191–2.

Patel, H., Cross, H., Proukakis, C. *et al.* (2002). SPG20 is mutated in Troyer syndrome, an hereditary spastic paraplegia. *Nat. Genet.*, **31**, 347–8.

Pedersen, L. & Trojaborg, W. (1981). Visual, auditory and somatosensory pathway involvement in hereditary cerebellar ataxia, Friedreich's ataxia and familial spastic paraplegia. *Electroencephalogr. Clin. Neurophys.*, **52**, 283–97.

Pelosi, L., Lanzillo, B. & Perretti, A. (1991). Motor and somatosensory evoked potentials in hereditary spastic paraplegia. *J. Neurol. Neurosurg. Psychiatry*, **54**, 1099–102.

Pericak-Vance, M. A., Kloos, M. T., Reid, E. *et al.* (2002). A kinesin heavy chain (K1F5A) mutation in Hereditary Spastic Paraplegia (SPG10). *Am. J. Hum. Genet.*, **71**, 165 (Abstract).

Polo, J. M., Calleja, J., Combarris, O. & Berciano, J. (1993). Hereditary "pure" spastic paraplegia: a study of nine families. *J. Neurol. Neurosurg. Psychiatry*, **56**, 175–81.

Ragno, M., DeMichele, G., Cavalcanti, F. *et al.* (1997). Broadened Friedreich's ataxia phenotype after gene cloning. *Neurology*, **49**, 1617–20.

Rainier, S., Chai, J.-H., Tokarz, D., Nicholls, R. D. & Fink, J. K. (2003). NIPA1 gene mutations cause autosomal dominant hereditary spastic paraplegia (SPG6). *Nat. Genet.*, submitted:

Reid, E., Grayson, C., Rubinsztein, D. C., Rogers, M. T. & Rubinsztein, J. S. (1999). Subclinical cognitive impairment in autosomal dominant 'pure' hereditary spastic paraplegia. *J. Med. Genet.*, **36**, 797–8.

Schady, W., Dick, J. P., Sheard, A. & Crampton, S. (1991). Central motor conduction studies in hereditary spastic paraplegia. *J. Neurol. Neurosurg. Psychiatry*, **54**, 775–9.

Schwarz, G. A. (1952). Hereditary (familial) spastic paraplegia. AMA *Arch. Neurol. Psychiatry*, **68**, 655–82.

Schwarz, G. A. & Liu, C.-N. (1956). Hereditary (familial) spastic paraplegia. Further clinical and pathologic observations. *Arch. Neurol. Psychiatry*, **75**, 144–62.

Shibaski, Y., Tanaka, H., Iwabuchi, K. *et al.* (2000). Linkage of autosomal recessive hereditary spastic paraplegia with mental impairment and thin corpus callosum to chromosome 15q13–15. *Ann. Neurol.*, **48**, 108–12.

Silver, J. R. (1966). Familial spastic paraplegia with amyotrophy of the hands. *Ann. Hum. Genet.*, **30**, 69–73.

Svenson, I. K., Ashley-Koch, A. E., Gaskell, P. C. *et al.* (2000). Mutation analysis of the spastin gene in hereditary spastic paraplegia type 4 – evidence of aberrant transcript splicing caused by mutations in concanonical splice site sequences. *Am. J. Hum. Genet.*, **67** (suppl. 2), 375.

Tabira, T., Chui, D., Nakayama, H., Kuroda, S. & Shibuya, M. (2002). Alzheimer's disease with spastic paresis and cotton wool type plaques. *J. Neurosci. Res.*, **70**, 367–72.

Tedeschi, G., Allocca, S., DiCostanzo, A. *et al.* (1991). Multisystem involvement of the central nervous system in Strumpell's disease. A neurophysiological and neuropsychological study. *J. Neurol. Sci.*, **103**, 55–60.

Wang, J., Hennigan, A. N., Morini, A., Ananth, U. & Seltzer, W. K. (2002). Molecular diagnostic testing for autosomal dominant hereditary spastic paraplegia: identification of novel mutations in the SPG4 gene. *Am. J. Hum. Genet.*, **71**, 386 (Abstract).

Webb, S., Coleman, D., Byrne, P. *et al.* (1998). Autosomal dominant hereditary spastic paraparesis with cognitive loss linked to chromosome 2p. *Brain*, **121**, 601–9.

Zhao, X., Alvarado, D., Rainier, S. *et al.* (2001). Mutations in a novel GTPase cause autosomal dominant hereditary spastic paraplegia. *Nat. Genet.*, **29**, 326–31.

54

Spinal and bulbar muscular atrophy (Kennedy's disease): a sex-limited, polyglutamine repeat expansion disorder

Patrick S. Thomas, Jr.[1] and Albert R. La Spada[2]

[1]Department of Laboratory Medicine and Center for Neurogenetics and Neurotherapeutics,
[2]Department of Laboratory Medicine, Medicine and Neurology and Center for Neurogenetics and Neurotherapeutics
University of Washington Medical Center, Seattle, WA, USA

Clinical background

In 1968, William Kennedy and co-workers described a slowly progressive neuromuscular disease in male members of two families (Kennedy *et al.*, 1968). The "Kennedy's disease" syndrome that they reported was most consistent with a spinal muscular atrophy, but exhibited rather unique genetic and clinical features that differentiated it from other well-described motor neuron diseases at that time (Table 54.1). A number of other case reports describing patients with similar findings soon followed, establishing "Kennedy's disease" as a single specific genetic entity. Further work supported the classification of Kennedy's disease as a sex-linked form of spinal muscular atrophy that involved the bulbar musculature (Harding *et al.*, 1982; Ringel *et al.*, 1978; Stefanis *et al.*, 1975). Because of the bulbar involvement, the disorder also came to be known as spinal and bulbar muscular atrophy, and "SBMA" was selected as its official genetic designation. While much has been learned about the pathogenesis and molecular basis of SBMA in the last 35 years, the original description provided by Dr. Kennedy and his colleagues remains an accurate clinical and laboratory vignette of what we now know as Kennedy's disease or SBMA.

SBMA is a slowly progressive motor neuronopathy that shows an X-linked pattern of inheritance, fully affecting only males. Dysfunction followed by gradual loss of motor neurons occurs in the anterior horn of the spinal cord and in the bulbar nuclei of the brainstem, while upper motor neurons are spared. Most SBMA patients display proximal girdle muscle weakness with striking fasciculations of the tongue or chin. Chin and tongue twitching is a particularly common finding in SBMA, whereas it is not often seen in other motor neuron diseases (Harding *et al.*, 1982). Onset of SBMA in affected individuals usually occurs in the fourth or fifth decade of life, although earlier onset has been reported

(Antonini *et al.*, 2000). Even in the earliest occurrences of the disease, the first signs are seen in late puberty or early adulthood (Andrew *et al.*, 1997) – there are no cases of SBMA presenting in infants or children. Early symptoms include shoulder and pelvic girdle muscle weakness, which may present as problems lifting objects and walking. Most patients report muscle cramps, many times occurring as early as 15–25 years before complaints of muscle weakness (Harding *et al.*, 1982). In most cases, the condition of SBMA patients worsens over a period of 10–30 years. One-third of patients require a wheel chair about 20 years after symptom onset. Proximal muscle weakness is typically accompanied by a much milder distal muscle weakness. SBMA patients seldom have sensory complaints, as sensory involvement is minimal and often only revealed by physical exam or electrodiagnostic testing (Antonini *et al.*, 2000; Ferrante & Wilbourn, 1997; Harding *et al.*, 1982; Ringel *et al.*, 1978). As the disease progresses, bulbar muscles can become affected, leading to dysarthria and dysphagia. Although the bulbar weakness does not prevent the patient from acquiring adequate nutrition, it does cause significant morbidity as it places the patient at risk for asphyxiation and aspiration pneumonia. These complications are the only causes of mortality directly related to motor neuron degeneration in Kennedy's disease, and occur in no more than 10% of affected patients. Thus, despite the disability incurred by their disease, the majority of SBMA patients can expect to have a normal life-span. On physical exam, SBMA patients will demonstrate signs typical of lower motor neuron pathology – namely muscle weakness, flaccidity, and atrophy. This pathology is apparent in the proximal muscles, but is sometimes noted in the distal muscles as well (Fig. 54.1). No signs of upper motor neuron disease, such as hyperreflexia or spasticity, are evident, although cramping and tremor may be elicited upon strength testing and intention movement, respectively (Arbizu *et al.*, 1983;

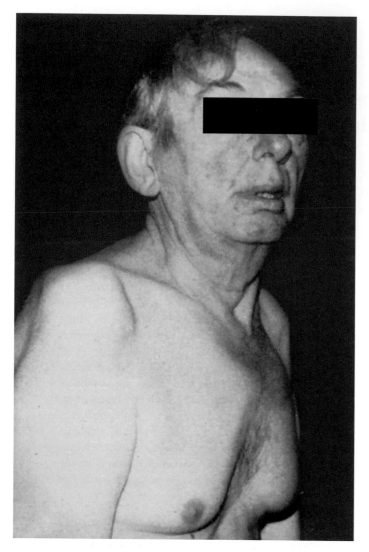

Fig. 54.1 Patient with SBMA. Note the atrophy of the proximal upper limb musculature and the presence of gynecomastia.

Table 54.1. Findings in Kennedy's disease/spinal and bulbar muscular atrophy

---

Neurological

Prominent signs of lower motor neuron disease in spinal cord and brainstem

    Muscle weakness and muscle atrophy (proximal > distal)

    Hypo-reflexia

    Fasciculations

    Late bulbar involvement (dysphagia and dysarthria)

Minimal signs of sensory tract involvement

    Decreased sensation on physical exam seen occasionally

    Reduced to absent sensory nerve action potentials

Absence of upper motor neuron disease findings

    No spasticity or hyper-reflexia

Endocrinological

Prominent signs of androgen insensitivity

    Gynecomastia

    Testicular atrophy

    Reduced fertility

Genetic

X-linked inheritance pattern

    Sex-limited penetrance with only males fully affected

Racial/population group distribution

    Caucasians and Asians (never reported in Africans or Aborigines)

    1/50 000–1/100 000 males are affected in most population groups

    Highest prevalence is among Japanese due to founder effect

Laboratory

Bio-markers

    Moderate elevations of creatine phosphokinase (CPK)

Harding *et al.*, 1982; Stefanis *et al.*, 1975). Deep tendon reflexes are either decreased or absent, depending on where the patient is in the progression of his disease. Examination of patient sensation is initially unremarkable, although decreased distal sensation on provocative testing emerges as the disease progresses. This sensory impairment, however, usually remains subclinical.

A prominent feature of Kennedy's disease / SBMA that permits its clinical differentiation from other spinal muscular atrophies and predicted its molecular delineation is the presence of striking androgen insensitivity in affected patients (Arbizu *et al.*, 1983). Most SBMA patients will display obvious gynecomastia (Fig. 54.1), and this finding is

often the initial presentation of the disease in post-pubertal teenagers who are yet to develop neuromuscular signs. Decreased testicular size and reduced fertility accompany the gynecomastia, although there is considerable variability in this triad of findings in affected patients. Despite the prominence of these findings in certain patients, no SBMA patients have failed to fully develop normal male genitalia, either externally or internally. Indeed, SBMA patients generally have normal sexual function, though some report impotence in the later stages of the disease, difficulty conceiving children, and an inability to grow thick facial hair. Thus, a thorough evaluation of male patients with onset of lower motor neuron findings demands that the clinician take a complete history and perform a full examination to document the possible coexistence of androgen insensitivity. This is extremely important as SBMA can be confused with disorders such as amyotrophic lateral sclerosis (ALS), autosomal spinal muscular atrophy type IV, spinocerebellar ataxia type 3, Friedrich's ataxia, adult-onset Tay–Sachs disease, or even the adrenomyeloneuropathy variant of adrenoleukodystrophy. ALS is most often confused with SBMA – so much so that one series found that as many as 5% of SBMA cases are misdiagnosed as ALS (Parboosingh *et al.*, 1997).

Neuropathology studies of SBMA demonstrate marked reduction in the number of anterior horn cells at all levels of the spinal cord (Amato *et al.*, 1993; Kennedy *et al.*, 1968; Ogata *et al.*, 1994). Bulbar motor neuron loss is also evident, and even dorsal root ganglia can be decreased in size and number in elderly patients at autopsy (Olney *et al.*, 1991; Sobue *et al.*, 1981). The pathology of SBMA seems to be restricted to the neurons themselves, as there is no evidence of concomitant white matter disease or corticospinal tract involvement. Muscle biopsies from several studies are consistent with denervation atrophy, although an element of myopathy can not be excluded and may be suggested by moderate elevations in serum creatine phosphokinase (CPK). Electrodiagnostic studies including electromyography (EMG) and nerve conduction velocity (NCV) testing reveal findings suggestive of denervation atrophy (Ferrante & Wilbourn, 1997; Guidetti *et al.*, 1996; Olney *et al.*, 1991). Specifically, EMGs are remarkable for large amplitude, long duration motor unit action potentials, typical of chronic denervation with reinnervation. NCVs are typically slow in all nerves, and sensory synaptic nerve action potentials (SNAPs) are reduced or absent. However, as noted above, this lack of SNAPs does not usually produce symptoms. While electrodiagnostic studies may assist in the diagnosis of SBMA, the discovery of a specific molecular defect in SBMA has made electrodiagnostic testing no longer necessary, except in atypical cases.

Other available clinical laboratory tests are of marginal utility in supporting the diagnosis of SBMA. Endocrinology tests for luteinizing hormone, follicle stimulating hormone, and testosterone yield normal results for most SBMA patients. However, serum CPK is elevated in the majority of SBMA patients at levels that exceed what one would expect for a pure motor neuronopathy. Finally, while many workers have considered the possibility that SBMA patients are at increased risk for type II diabetes mellitus, there is no clear evidence to date that the prevalence of diabetes or impaired glucose tolerance is any higher in SBMA patients than in the general population.

Genetics and molecular biology

SBMA fully affects only men, but does so rarely with a prevalence of less than 1/50 000 males (Tanaka *et al.*, 1996). The disease is observed in individuals of Caucasian and Asian racial background, but never in Africans or Aborigines. Almost all Caucasian population groups are affected, as patients of English, Irish, Belgian, Danish, Dutch, French, Italian, Finnish, German, Greek, Polish, Spanish, Swiss, Moroccan, and Turkish ancestry have been ascertained. Chinese, Japanese, Korean, and Vietnamese cases have been reported, suggesting that various Asian population groups exhibit SBMA. Of all population groups, the Japanese have the highest prevalence of SBMA by far, and this appears due to a founder effect (Tanaka *et al.*, 1996). A founder effect has also been reported in the Scandinavian population (Lund *et al.*, 2000), but is not present across other Caucasian or Asian population groups.

The X-linked inheritance pattern of SBMA allowed researchers to focus their efforts upon the X chromosome in the search for the causal SBMA gene defect and thereby take what was then called a "reverse genetics" (now positional cloning) approach to identifying the cause of this disorder. Linkage analysis of SBMA families permitted localization of the SBMA gene to the proximal long arm of the X chromosome (Fischbeck *et al.*, 1986). At around the same time, the gene for the androgen receptor (AR) was cloned and mapped to Xq11-12, an overlapping region of the X chromosome (Brown *et al.*, 1989; Lubahn *et al.*, 1988). Given the signs of the androgen insensitivity in SBMA patients and the localization of the AR gene and SBMA defect to overlapping regions of the X chromosome, the AR gene emerged as a candidate gene for SBMA. Sequencing of the AR gene in SBMA patients yielded no differences in its amino acid composition, except for an alteration in the length of a normally highly polymorphic glutamine tract in the aminoterminal region (La Spada *et al.*, 1991). The basis of this polymorphism is a CAG trinucleotide repeat in the first exon of the AR gene, and analysis of affected SBMA patients and obligate carriers indicated that expansions of the CAG tract were present in all SBMA patients or carriers (Fig. 54.2). This finding of a CAG trinucleotide repeat expansion as the cause of a human genetic disease was the first one of its kind, and occurred at the same time that another inherited disorder, the fragile X syndrome of mental retardation, was shown to be due to (what would turn out to be) a noncoding CGG repeat expansion (Verkerk *et al.*, 1991). In the case of SBMA, normal individuals possess anywhere from 5 to 36 CAG repeats in their AR genes, while affected SBMA patients and carriers have 38 to 70 CAG repeats. It is important to note that CAG repeat expansion is the only mutational cause of SBMA identified to date – thus, all SBMA affected males show a CAG repeat expansion. At the same time, the mutation appears fully penetrant – thus, no male individuals who are clinically normal have ever been shown to possess a CAG repeat expansion in their AR gene.

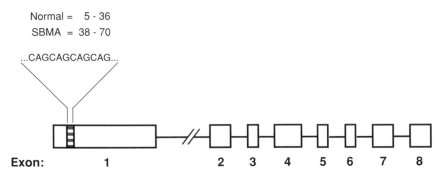

Fig. 54.2 CAG repeat expansion in the first exon of the androgen receptor (AR) gene is the cause of SBMA. The AR gene is composed of eight exons. A polymorphic CAG repeat that encodes the amino acid glutamine resides in the first exon. CAG repeat size ranges are shown for both normal individuals and for SBMA patients / carriers.

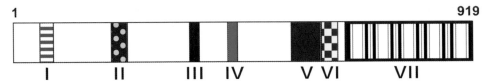

Fig. 54.3 The androgen receptor protein contains a number of functional domains. I = polyglutamine tract; II = activation function domain; III = polyproline tract; IV = polyglycine tract; V = DNA-binding (zinc finger motif) domain; VI = bipartite nuclear localization signal; and VII = ligand-binding domain.

One unique feature displayed by the CAG repeat expansion mutations seen in SBMA patients and carriers is genetic instability. When a SBMA repeat allele is transmitted from parent to offspring, it often changes in size (Biancalana *et al.*, 1992; La Spada *et al.*, 1992). The likelihood of repeat length change and of repeat expansion is significantly greater when the sex of the transmitting parent is male. This repeat instability occurs rarely in alleles of normal size (Zhang *et al.*, 1994). The genetic instability of expanded CAG repeats has yielded a wide range of allele sizes in the SBMA patient population, and a genotype–phenotype correlation of SBMA disease severity with CAG repeat length found a significant relationship between allele size and certain clinical landmarks in SBMA patients (Doyu *et al.*, 1992; La Spada *et al.*, 1992). In particular, age of onset of clinical symptoms and age of onset of difficulty climbing stairs were shown to inversely correlate with the size of the expanded CAG repeats – thus, the longer the CAG repeat expansion, the earlier the age of onset of each of these events in SBMA patients. While a significant correlation was found, it was not very strong, leading to the conclusion that other factors – genetic, environmental, or random – account for the variability in disease natural history in most SBMA patients. The tendency of CAG repeats to expand, however, is an important feature of related trinucleotide repeat diseases (see below), and is now known to

account for the phenomenon of anticipation (Harper *et al.*, 1992), which may be defined as worsening clinical severity in successive generations of a family pedigree segregating an inherited disorder.

The AR gene encodes a protein that is a well-known and well-studied member of the steroid/thyroid receptor superfamily, with a domain structure that typifies that protein family (O'Malley, 1990). The AR gene spans ∼ 150 kb, contains 8 exons, and has an ORF that codes for a 919 amino acid protein. AR has a number of functionally important domains (Fig. 54.3), including a DNA binding domain, comprised by amino acids 556–616 and composed of two zinc finger motifs. There is a bipartite nuclear localization signal at residues 617–633 (Zhou *et al.*, 1994). AR also has a ligand-binding domain at amino acid position 666–919, the carboxy-terminal one-third of the protein. These three domains are highly conserved across a wide range of mammalian and avian species (Thornton & Kelley, 1998). The large amino-terminal region, on the other hand, is mostly a poorly conserved region possessing few recognizable domains with one notable exception. Since the amino-terminal region is required for the transcription activation function of AR, a so-called "activation function" (AF) domain is contained within this portion of the protein. In addition, there are three poly-amino acid tracts. The polyglutamine tract, which expands to cause SBMA, begins at amino acid 58, and has an average length of about 21 amino acids in humans (Edwards *et al.*, 1992). The glutamine tract motif is commonly seen in transcription factors and has been shown to be important for transcription activation function. Thus, the large amino-terminal region of AR is believed to be involved in mediating transactivation via protein–protein interactions with other transcription cofactors and coregulators. AR's transactivation function is modulated by ligand binding. Unliganded AR is normally located in the cytoplasm and sequestered by heat shock proteins and chaperones (Caplan *et al.*, 1995). Upon binding to its ligands, testosterone or 5-dihydrotestosterone, AR undergoes a conformational change, dissociates from the heat shock protein / chaperone complex, and translocates to the nucleus. There it forms a complex with co-activators and other components of the transcriptional machinery, and this complex binds to specific promoter DNA sequences known as androgen response elements (ARE's), thereby producing androgen-responsive gene expression (Gelmann, 2002). Ligand binding yields a functional AR by causing an intramolecular interaction between the C-terminal and N-terminal domains, which then permits an intermolecular interaction to occur in the nucleus, resulting in an AR homodimer. Dimerization of AR is required for its transcriptional function (Langley *et al.*, 1995).

Polyglutamine expansion: a common cause of neurodegeneration

About two years after a polyglutamine expansion was found to be the cause of SBMA, an international team of researchers from multiple institutions reported that Huntington's disease (HD) is caused by the identical type of mutation – a polyglutamine expansion (Huntington's disease CRG, 1993). Over the last decade, a number of other inherited neurodegenerative disorders were found to be caused by polyglutamine expansions. In addition to SBMA and HD, dentatorubral-pallidoluysian atrophy (DRPLA) and six types of spinocerebellar ataxia (namely, SCA1, 2, 3, 6, 7, and 17) are now all known to be due to polyglutamine tract expansions within their respective proteins (Nakamura *et al.*, 2001; Zoghbi & Orr, 2000). The CAG / polyglutamine repeat diseases thus form a distinct category of neurodegenerative disorders sharing the common feature of having an unstable CAG trinucleotide repeat encoding an elongated run of glutamines as their mutational basis. For most of these diseases, a strong correlation between polyglutamine repeat length and disease severity exists, and vertical transmission of larger repeat expansions

produces childhood onset cases, a phenomenon known as anticipation (Harper *et al.*, 1992). A number of lines of evidence support the conclusion that the polyglutamine tract expansion is a gain-of-function mutation that imparts a novel activity or action to the mutant proteins within which they reside. Importantly, studies have shown that the mutant proteins are transcribed and translated (Zoghbi & Orr, 2000), and expression of the polyglutamine expansion at the protein level appears necessary for production of the full phenotype (Goldberg *et al.*, 1996). Further evidence for gain-of-function comes from the observation that loss-of-function of the different disease proteins does not cause the expected phenotypes. Among the best examples of this are SBMA and HD, which have human examples of disease protein loss of expression for their respective genes. Deletion of the AR gene (that causes SBMA) results in complete androgen insensitivity or testicular feminization, a phenotype not characterized by neuromuscular disease (Brown *et al.*, 1988). Loss of the tip of the short arm of chromosome 4 yields Wolf-Hirschhorn syndrome in humans, a multisystem disorder, but one not noted for striatal degeneration (Wilson *et al.*, 1981). To corroborate that loss-of-function does not equate with disease phenotype, certain groups have knocked out the various polyglutamine disease genes in mice, and have not reproduced the same phenotype (Duyao *et al.*, 1995; Matilla *et al.*, 1998; Nasir *et al.*, 1995; Zeitlin *et al.*, 1995). (However, as we will discuss below, a role for loss-of-function as a contributory factor in disease pathogenesis is now supported by recent findings.)

Molecular basis of polyglutamine neurotoxicity

A discussion on how gain-of-function of the polyglutamine-expanded AR leads to motor neuron pathology in SBMA requires that we consider the results of work done on all the polyglutamine diseases. Much of the earlier work on polyglutamine neurotoxicity focused upon how an expanded polyglutamine tract could be neurotoxic. Max Perutz hypothesized that expanded polyglutamine tracts would form novel structures, and he demonstrated that elongated runs of glutamine can form beta-pleated sheets by folding back on themselves (the so-called "polar zipper") and, once in this conformation, could bind with other proteins with unusually high affinities and form aggregates (Perutz *et al.*, 1994). The notion of an altered conformation as the crux of polyglutamine neurotoxicity was further advanced by the production of an antibody (1C2) that specifically recognized polyglutamine expansions (Trottier *et al.*, 1995). Once in an abnormal conformation, the expanded polyglutamine tracts were then found to be resistant to turnover and degradation by the ubiquitin-proteasome system (Bence et al., 2001; Sherman & Goldberg, 2001), suggesting that they would accumulate and thereby be able to interfere with cellular processes.

A key turning point in the polyglutamine disease field came when Gillian Bates' group identified aggregates of proteins in the nuclei of neurons from the brains of a transgenic mouse model of HD, and Hank Paulson's group detected such intraneuronal nuclear inclusions (NIs) in the brains of patients with SCA3 (Davies et al., 1997; Paulson et al., 1997). These findings led to the "aggregate" hypothesis of polyglutamine neurodegeneration that postulates that the aggregates themselves are the toxic moiety giving rise to neuronal dysfunction, degeneration, and cell death in the polyglutamine repeat diseases. Subsequent studies of a SCA1 mouse model and an HD primary striatal neuron model disconnected aggregate formation from neurodegeneration, arguing that the aggregates are not the key cause of cellular pathology in the polyglutamine diseases (Klement et al., 1998; Saudou et al., 1998). Further studies in the SCA1 mouse model showed that crossing onto a ubiquitin-protein ligase null background prevented aggregate formation but worsened the disease phenotype of SCA1 transgenic mice, suggesting that aggregation could very well be a protective mechanism in the polyglutamine diseases (Cummings et al., 1999). While the pathway by which expanded polyglutamine tracts cause neurotoxicity remains unresolved, all of these studies have established that polyglutamine expansions are intrinsically toxic. Perhaps the best illustration of this is that expression of an expanded polyglutamine tract alone, out of context of the protein within which it normally resides, is sufficient to cause neurotoxicity in a wide range of model organisms (i.e. yeast, fruitflies, worms, and mice) (Hughes et al., 2001; Marsh et al., 2000; Ordway et al., 1997; Sipione & Cattaneo, 2001). Most striking among these studies was the insertion of a polyglutamine expansion into the hypoxanthine phosphoribosyltransferase (HPRT) gene in mouse embryonic stem cells, yielding a mouse that developed a neurodegenerative phenotype with characteristic NIs due to production of a chimeric HPRT protein with an ~ 150 glutamine repeat tract (Ordway et al., 1997).

Given that all expanded polyglutamine tracts are toxic based upon their ability to form abnormal structures and adopt aberrant non-degradable conformations, the question arises: Why do the polyglutamine diseases differ in their clinical phenotypes? While one might think that the explanation would simply be different patterns of expression of the various disease genes, this is not at all the case. Most of the polyglutamine disease gene products show overlapping expression throughout the central nervous system. For example, the mutant huntingtin protein (that causes HD) is expressed highly in cerebellum, while a number of the mutant ataxin proteins (that cause the SCAs) are highly expressed in the basal ganglia. Nonetheless, classic HD patients are not ataxic, and typical SCA patients do not display choreiform movements. Thus, a key question in the polyglutamine field is how is the common pathological property of polyglutamine expansion modulated to produce selective patterns of cell-type specific neurodegeneration in the different diseases? Much of the work performed over the last decade suggests that it is the amino acid context of the protein within which the polyglutamine expansion resides that determines the pattern of pathology. Amino acid context is responsible for specifying disease pattern based upon its role in regulating protein-protein interaction. In the case of huntingtin, a long list of interacting proteins has been compiled (Jones, 1999; Kalchman et al., 1997; Li et al., 1995). For SCA7, it appears that the retinal degeneration phenotype is a reflection of a specific interaction with a protein known as the cone-rod homeobox protein (CRX) (La Spada et al., 2001). For SCA1, interaction with leucine-rich acidic nuclear protein (LANP) or polyglutamine binding protein 1 (PQBP-1) may explain the pattern of pathology seen in this disorder (Matilla et al., 1997; Okazawa et al., 2002). In each case, it is the expression pattern of the interacting protein that mirrors the pattern of at-risk neuron cell populations and thus accounts for the cell-type specificity, if this model is correct.

Molecular basis of motor neuron degeneration in SBMA

With this background in mind, we will now consider how the polyglutamine-expanded AR produces a lower motor neuron disease phenotype in patients with SBMA. As noted above, many lines of evidence support the conclusion that all polyglutamine-expanded proteins adopt an abnormal conformation and that this misfolding is the initial event in the pathogenic cascade. This also appears to be the case for the polyglutamine-expanded AR in SBMA, as immunohistochemical studies of SBMA patients material have shown that AR-containing aggregates are present in the nuclei of neurons destined to degenerate (Li et al., 1998a,b). However, in addition to detecting NIs in the remaining anterior horn cells of the spinal cord in SBMA patients, these studies also found NIs in a wide range of other nervous system tissues and non-neuronal organs (Li et al., 1998a). NIs occur in CNS tissues not affected in SBMA (such as cerebellum and cortex), as well as in skin, testes, kidney, heart and glia. While this pattern of NI formation suggests that NIs form in all tissues where AR is expressed, no NIs are found in muscle, a tissue where high-level AR expression occurs. As no studies of NI distribution have been carried out in presymptomatic or early symptomatic SBMA patients, the presence of NIs throughout the body in SBMA may be a late stage event preceded by more localized NI formation OR may be a general feature of this disorder. In one mouse model of SBMA, pure polyglutamine expansions of 239 residues were placed under the regulatory control of a promoter fragment from the human AR gene and yielded a non-specific neurological phenotype with NIs identified in a wide range of neural and non-neural tissues (Adachi et al., 2001). It would thus appear that high-level or long-term expression of polyglutamine expansion products is capable of producing NIs in a variety of cell types – even those that are not pathologically affected in the disease of interest.

One feature of SBMA that makes it unique among the polyglutamine repeat diseases is its X-linked inheritance, as all of the other polyglutamine expansion mutations show autosomal dominant inheritance. Although SBMA differs from the rest of the polyglutamine diseases in this way, the polyglutamine expansion in AR acts as a dominant, gain-of-function mutation. Despite the dominant action of the AR mutation in SBMA, female carriers seldom show appreciable findings, and to date, there have been no examples of severely affected female patients who lost mobility and ended up wheelchair-bound. In most X-linked diseases, occasional females are seriously affected due to unfavorable lyonization when random inactivation of the X chromosome bearing the normal gene in the relevant cell lineage occurs. This does not appear to happen in SBMA. Rather, female SBMA carriers seldom have symptoms, and instead are "protected," suggesting that SBMA shows sex-limited inheritance. Why is it then that female SBMA carriers are protected if the AR polyglutamine mutation is dominant in action? Although non-random X-inactivation due to selection against the X chromosome bearing the mutant AR in precursor cells could explain this, a much more attractive hypothesis has been that females are protected by virtue of the fact that their serum testosterone levels are much lower than what is seen in males. As noted above, translocation of AR from the cytoplasm and into the nucleus is strongly favored by ligand binding (Zhou et al., 1994). Confirmation of this hypothesis as the basis of sex-limited inheritance in SBMA was recently achieved by developing a mouse model of AR polyglutamine neurotoxicity using the entire AR protein. In this study, male mice and female mice widely expressed full-length AR protein containing 97 glutamines, but only the males developed the full neurological phenotype, as is seen in SBMA (Katsuno et al., 2002). Moreover, when male mice were castrated, they no longer developed neuromuscular disease, and, when female mice received testosterone injections, they became symptomatic. Similar results showing the importance of androgen binding in modulating subcellular localization and producing neurotoxicity were also generated in an elegant Drosophila model of AR polyglutamine disease (Takeyama et al., 2002). Independent corroboration of the "androgen-dependent" nature of the SBMA gene mutation also comes from a clinical study of a woman homozygous for CAG / polyglutamine repeat expansion in her AR gene (Schmidt et al., 2002). Despite having two mutant AR genes with disease-causing CAG repeat expansions, she was basically unaffected in middle age, supporting the conclusion that appreciable testosterone levels are required for phenotypic expression. Thus, the dual findings of prominent NIs in SBMA patient material and the dependence of the SBMA disease phenotype upon androgen binding to the mutant AR support a model in which nuclear localization of polyglutamine-expanded AR is required for neurotoxicity (Fig. 54.4). Such a model appears to apply to most, but not all, of the polyglutamine repeat diseases (Huynh et al., 2000; Ishikawa et al., 1999).

Another feature of androgen receptor biology that appears important for its toxicity in SBMA is proteolytic processing (Fig. 54.4). The immunohistochemical studies of SBMA patient material described above also were notable for their observation that NIs failed to label with antibodies directed against the middle portion or carboxy-terminal region of AR, suggesting that the NIs contained only amino-terminal truncation products of AR (Li et al., 1998a). Cell culture models have shown that amino-terminal truncation products are considerably more toxic that their full-length counterparts (Brooks et al., 1997; Merry et al., 1998). Furthermore, amino-terminal truncated versions of AR with 112 glutamines have been used to derive mouse models of SBMA by directing expression throughout the CNS with heterologous promoters (Abel et al., 2001). Such mouse models have recapitulated certain features of the SBMA phenotype (such as prominent motor dysfunction and NIs), but have lacked other features (namely, gender difference and motor neuron degeneration). The rationale for using truncated versions of the AR for cellular and organismal studies is biologically based. In addition to the evidence for amino-terminal truncations in patient material, numerous cell culture studies have detected amino-terminal truncations of the polyglutamine-expanded AR (Butler et al., 1998; Ellerby et al., 1999; Kobayashi et al., 1998; Merry et al., 1998). Furthermore, such amino-terminal truncations are observed in mouse models and Drosophila

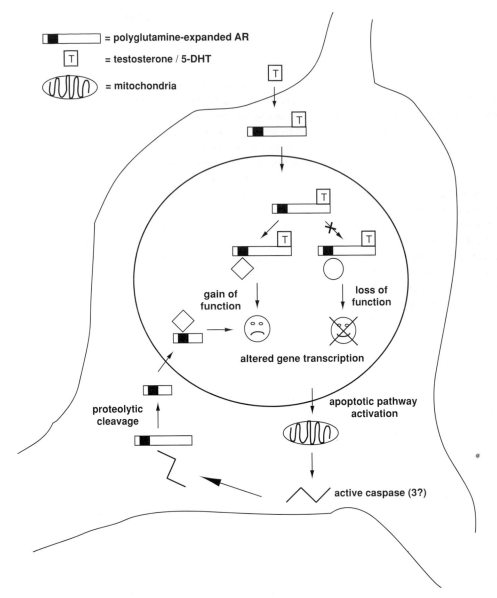

Fig. 54.4 Model for androgen receptor (AR) polyglutamine neurotoxicity in SBMA motor neurons. The polyglutamine-expanded AR is present in the cytosol, and upon ligand-binding to testosterone (T), the ligand-receptor complex translocates into the nucleus. Once in the nucleus, ligand-bound full-length polyglutamine-expanded AR may interact inappropriately with certain transcription factors and/or complexes (symbolized as a diamond), owing to its altered conformation. These aberrant and/or novel interactions represent the gain-of-function pathway of action of the mutant AR, and yield changes in gene expression that are detrimental to the neuron. Transcription interference with CBP-mediated gene expression may be one example of such aberrant interaction. At the same time, ligand-bound AR would be expected to normally interact with transcription factors and co-regulators (shown as a circle) to promote androgen-responsive gene transcription that is trophic in nature. However, the polyglutamine-expanded AR may no longer be able to perform such normal androgen-responsive transcription activation, resulting in the loss of expression of gene products important for cellular survival and homeostasis. Thus, the polyglutamine-expanded AR protein may produce altered gene transcription effects that reflect a combination of gain-of-function and loss-of-function events. These gene expression alterations likely place the neuron under stress, culminating in activation of apoptotic pathways, a process that typically involves depolarization of the outer mitochondrial membrane and yields active caspases. The polyglutamine-expanded AR has been shown to be a substrate for active caspases (such as caspase-3), and caspase cleavage may yield a proteolytic fragment(s) of the mutant AR. (The proteolytic processing is shown to occur in the cytosol, but it may take place in the nucleus and could involve a different protease.) An amino-terminal truncated version of the polyglutamine-expanded AR ends up accumulating in the nucleus where it can potently interfere with normal gene transcription, again through aberrant, perhaps now more avid, interactions with transcription factors and co-regulators (shown as a diamond). This results in further transcription dysregulation and accelerates the process of neuronal dysfunction. Ultimately, the neuronal dysfunction becomes so severe that the motor neuron begins to show degenerative changes that eventually so impair the cell that recovery is no longer possible, so the neuron dies.

models of SBMA that utilize the full-length AR cDNA in their respective expression constructs (Katsuno *et al.*, 2002; Takeyama *et al.*, 2002). The *Drosophila* study is particularly noteworthy in this regard, as it reported the production of an amino-terminal truncation fragment only when AR with 52 glutamines translocated to the nucleus upon treatment with the androgen 5-dihydrotestosterone (Takeyama *et al.*, 2002). Much of the work on AR proteolytic cleavage has focused upon the ability of AR to be cleaved by caspase-3, one of the executioner enzymes of the programmed cell death pathway (Kobayashi *et al.*, 1998; Wellington *et al.*, 1998). After demonstrating that AR is a substrate for caspase-3, one group established that the site of cleavage is at the aspartic acid residue at position 146 and went on to show that mutation of this cleavage site abolished mutant AR's ability to produce cellular toxicity and apoptotic cell death in vitro (Ellerby *et al.*, 1999). Despite these advances, the relationship between proteolytic cleavage, caspase activation, programmed cell death pathways, and AR polyglutamine neurotoxicity in SBMA remains unclear (Fig. 54.4).

Regardless of what length(s) of AR protein ends up in the nucleus (and when), it does seem likely that key events in SBMA pathogenesis do play out there. Given AR's well-known role as a nuclear transcription factor, much effort has focused upon understanding how the polyglutamine-expanded AR protein (or a fragment thereof) might interfere with normal processes of transcription regulation and gene expression. A number of findings have suggested that polyglutamine-expanded proteins may interact inappropriately with other transcription factors or co-regulators that contain glutamine tracts or glutamine-rich regions. The protein kinase A / cyclic AMP gene expression pathway involves the coordinated interaction of transcription factors and co-factors that converge upon so-called cAMP response elements (CREs) in promoters and activate gene expression (Shaywitz & Greenberg, 1999). Among the components of this transcriptional machinery is CREB-binding protein (CBP), a transcriptional co-regulator with histone acetylase activity. Recruitment of CBP favors histone acetylation that results in chromatin remodeling to an open DNA configuration that is permissive of gene transcription. CBP contains a glutamine stretch, and was initially implicated in the polyglutamine diseases when it was found that polyglutamine-expanded AR could impair CREB-mediated transcription and NIs from HD and SBMA patient material and mouse models contain CBP (McCampbell *et al.*, 2000; Steffan *et al.*, 2000). Subsequent studies, that have been performed in primary cortical neuron and *Drosophila* models, indicated that CBP loss-of-function due to aberrant interaction with polyglutamine-expanded proteins

(such as huntingtin) might underlie polyglutamine neurotoxicity (Nucifora *et al.*, 2001; Steffan *et al.*, 2001). The *Drosophila* work pinpointed CBP's acetylation function as a key potential factor, as degenerating photoreceptor cells poisoned by polyglutamine-expansion tracts could be rescued by feeding the flies drugs known as histone deacetylase inhibitors, thereby supposedly compensating for the acetylation defect (Steffan *et al.*, 2001). While the CBP connection to polyglutamine neurotoxicity and to the mutant AR is provocative and intriguing, the CBP transcription interference model can not account for the cell type specificity seen in the different polyglutamine repeat diseases, as CBP is ubiquitously expressed. In the case of SBMA, however, the basis of cell type specificity may be less complicated as the CNS regions of highest AR expression do parallel the disease phenotype (Sar & Stumpf, 1977), making a primary role for CBP interference in SBMA more feasible (Fig. 54.4).

When considering the hypothesis of transcription dysregulation as the primary event in SBMA molecular pathology, it is important to consider the possibility that polyglutamine expansions within the AR protein could be preventing AR from carrying out its normal function in motor neurons. Indeed, partial loss of AR function in SBMA males is responsible for their well described features of androgen insensitivity. At present, two competing hypotheses (that are not mutually exclusive) have been put forward to explain this partial loss of AR function. Two independent studies have argued that the transactivation competence of AR decreases with increasing glutamine length (Chamberlain *et al.*, 1994; Mhatre *et al.*, 1993). In other words, as the glutamine stretch lengthens, the AR protein is less effective in mediating transcription activation at AREs. It is relevant here to point out that within the normal range of glutamine lengths, strong data have emerged showing that shorter glutamine runs in AR are the most potent activators of transcription (Gerber *et al.*, 1994). This correlation actually underlies many independent epidemiological observations that AR CAG repeat length is a significant factor in modulating the severity and natural history of prostate cancer progression, so that individuals with the shortest glutamine tracts tend to have more aggressive tumors (Giovannucci *et al.*, 1997; Nam *et al.*, 2000; Nelson & Witte, 2002; Stanford *et al.*, 1997). However, other studies of polyglutamine-expanded AR in cell culture models have noted that less AR protein is generated from disease-length alleles (Brooks *et al.*, 1997; Choong *et al.*, 1996). The decrease in AR protein levels could be due to decreased transcription, decreased RNA stability, decreased translational efficiency, or increased protein degradation (or some combination of these!). Thus, the other possible explanation for partial loss of AR function in SBMA is decreased levels of AR protein. Studies of AR protein levels in scrotal skin fibroblasts from SBMA patients did show decreased AR levels by Scatchard analysis in a subset of cases (Warner *et al.*, 1992), and one recent in vitro study has suggested that this occurs in MN-1 motor neuron-like cells because of increased degradation by the ubiquitin-proteasome pathway (Lieberman *et al.*, 2002).

Although complete loss of AR function does not appear detrimental to motor neurons in patients with testicular feminization (tfm), partial loss of function in the context of polyglutamine neurotoxic insult could render motor neurons more susceptible to degeneration (Fig. 54.4). In support of this theory are numerous studies showing that AR is actually a trophic factor in the CNS and its absence accounts for loss of motor neurons that normally innervate the bulbocavernosus muscles in tfm rats (Breedlove & Arnold, 1980; Breedlove & Arnold, 1981; Forger *et al.*, 1992). Androgen administration can facilitate recovery from nerve transection injury and can rescue the bulbocavernosus-innervating neurons (al-Shamma & Arnold, 1995; Nordeen *et al.*, 1985; Sengelaub & Arnold, 1989; Sengelaub *et al.*, 1989a,b). In the MN-1 motor neuron-like cells, alterations in the expression of androgen-responsive genes are observed in cells expressing polyglutamine-expanded AR (Lieberman *et al.*, 2002). Such changes could tie into pathways relevant to the gain-of-function pathology. In the case of HD, a number of lines of evidence do support a role for loss-of-function in the pathogenesis of striatal degeneration. Huntingtin may function as a transcription factor and drive expression of brain-derived neurotrophic factor in cortical neurons that project to the striatum (Zuccato *et al.*, 2001). Upon polyglutamine expansion, this transcriptional function may be impaired. Even more compelling is the observation that postnatal loss of huntingtin expression from the forebrain of gene-targeted mice produces neurological phenotypes and neurodegenerative changes reminiscent of HD (Dragatsis *et al.*, 2000). Our own work on SBMA has focused upon generating a truly representative model of AR polyglutamine neurotoxicity in mice so that the roles of gain-of-function and loss-of-function may be teased out and their molecular bases determined. To do this, we have taken a transgenic approach using yeast artificial chromosomes (YACs) that contain the entire human AR gene. We have used recombination to derive a human AR YAC containing 100 CAG repeats, and have now generated transgenic mice that carry the entire human AR gene with either 20 CAGs or 100 CAGs (Sopher *et al.*, 2002). The AR YAC CAG100 mice produce the polyglutamine-expanded AR protein and develop a neurological phenotype that closely recapitulates the neuromuscular phenotype of SBMA, as severe disease is restricted to males and is characterized by denervation atrophy with motor neuron degeneration. To evaluate the role of AR's normal function in contributing to the disease phenotype, we are crossing the AR YAC CAG100 mice onto an AR null background by mating them with tfm carrier females. Ultimately, this work should allow us to assess whether or not AR's normal function modulates the gain-of-function pathway of polyglutamine neurotoxicity in an in vivo setting.

Towards therapy

Given the pace of research in the polyglutamine field and the progress on SBMA, it is now time to consider how one might go about developing and testing therapies for this disorder. A key factor to the success of this endeavor will be the availability of representative mouse models of SBMA motor neuronopathy. Numerous mouse models have been generated, including truncation fragment mice and now full-length polyglutamine-expanded AR mice driven by different heterologous promoters (Abel *et al.*, 2001; Katsuno *et al.*, 2002; McManamny *et al.*, 2002). Together with our own AR YAC CAG100 mouse model (Sopher *et al.*, 2002), it is clear that ample models are now available to move forward with testing of therapy. Based upon the recent results from the Sobue and Kato groups (Katsuno *et al.*, 2002; Takeyama *et al.*, 2002), it appears that androgen ablation could be an effective therapy. While very promising, this therapy incurs substantial unpleasant side effects and likely should only be reserved for severe or end-stage cases. Thus, it would make sense to now test if androgen ablation can reverse significant neurological dysfunction in the mouse models as a prelude to its consideration in people. Another area of focus should be transcriptional dysregulation. As explained above, feeding fruitflies histone deacetylase inhibitors (HDAC Is) prevented polyglutamine neurotoxicity, raising the question of whether such a therapy could be applied to people. In this regard, it is important to note that certain HDAC I's are entering Phase II and Phase III trials for the treatment of certain malignancies and therefore represent very viable options for polyglutamine disease patients. Again, much work needs to be done in mice, but this avenue of therapy should be pursued. Other approaches warranting consideration are those that would enhance the heat shock protein response, an evolutionarily conserved molecular process whereby chaperone proteins are elevated to counter aberrant protein misfolding induced by an increase in temperature (Hartl, 1996). Much data on the polyglutamine diseases indicate that protein misfolding is a key early event and that protection or rescue is possible by over-expression of heat shock proteins (Hsps) (Cummings *et al.*, 2001; Sherman & Goldberg, 2001; Warrick *et al.*, 1999). Studies of polyglutamine-expanded AR in cell culture have corroborated the protective role of Hsp70 and its co-chaperone Hsp40 in preventing toxicity (Kobayashi *et al.*, 2000). More recently, it has been shown that Hsp70 with Hsp40 can increase the solubility of polyglutamine-expanded AR and enhance its proteasomal degradation (Bailey *et al.*, 2002). At least one drug, geldanamycin, is effective in inducing the heat shock response and has been shown to be effective in treating Parkinson's disease in *Drosophila* (Auluck & Bonini, 2002). Clearly, combinatorial approaches to produce more effective and less toxic derivatives of geldanamycin are now warranted. Many other compounds are also being identified by high throughput drug screens, such as one large multi-institutional endeavor recently sponsored by the National Institute of Neurological Disorders and Stroke (Abbott, 2002). As we look towards therapy, it seems reasonable to be cautiously optimistic since the identification, testing, and development of one or more drugs to treat neurodegenerative disorders such as SBMA are well underway.

REFERENCES

Abbott, A. (2002). Neurologists strike gold in drug screen effort. *Nature*, **417**, 109.

Abel, A., Walcott, J., Woods, J., Duda, J. & Merry, D. E. (2001). Expression of expanded repeat androgen receptor produces neurologic disease in transgenic mice. *Hum. Mol. Genet.*, **10**, 107–16.

Adachi, H., Kume, A., Li, M. *et al.* (2001). Transgenic mice with an expanded CAG repeat controlled by the human AR promoter show polyglutamine nuclear inclusions and neuronal dysfunction without neuronal cell death. *Hum. Mol. Genet.*, **10**, 1039–48.

al-Shamma, H. A. & Arnold, A. P. (1995). Importance of target innervation in recovery from axotomy-induced loss of androgen receptor in rat perineal motoneurons. *J. Neurobiol.*, **28**, 341–53.

Amato, A. A., Prior, T. W., Barohn, R. J., Snyder, P., Papp, A. & Mendell, J. R. (1993). Kennedy's disease: a clinicopathologic correlation with mutations in the androgen receptor gene. *Neurology*, **43**, 791–4.

Andrew, S. E., Goldberg, Y. P. & Hayden, M. R. (1997). Rethinking genotype and phenotype correlations in polyglutamine expansion disorders. *Hum. Molec. Genet.*, **6**, 2005–10.

Antonini, G., Gragnani, F., Romaniello, A. *et al.* (2000). Sensory involvement in spinal-bulbar muscular atrophy (Kennedy's disease). *Muscle Nerve*, **23**, 252–8.

Arbizu, T., Santamaria, J., Gomez, J. M., Quilez, A. & Serra, J. P. (1983). A family with adult spinal and bulbar muscular atrophy, X-linked inheritance and associated testicular failure. *J. Neurol. Sci.*, **59**, 371–82.

Auluck, P. K. & Bonini, N. M. (2002). Pharmacological prevention of Parkinson disease in *Drosophila*. *Nat. Med.*, **8**, 1185–6.

Bailey, C. K., Andriola, I. F., Kampinga, H. H. & Merry, D. E. (2002). Molecular chaperones enhance the degradation of expanded polyglutamine repeat androgen receptor in a cellular model of spinal and bulbar muscular atrophy. *Hum. Mol. Genet.*, **11**, 515–23.

Bence, N. F., Sampat, R. M. & Kopito, R. R. (2001). Impairment of the ubiquitin-proteasome system by protein aggregation. *Science*, **292**, 1552–5.

Biancalana, V., Serville, F., Pommier, J., Julien, J., Hanauer, A. & Mandel, J. L. (1992). Moderate instability of the trinucleotide repeat in spino bulbar muscular atrophy. *Hum. Mol. Genet.*, **1**, 255–8.

Breedlove, S. M. & Arnold, A. P. (1980). Hormone accumulation in a sexually dimorphic motor nucleus of the rat spinal cord. *Science*, **210**, 564–6.

Breedlove, S. M. & Arnold, A. P. (1981). Sexually dimorphic motor nucleus in the rat lumbar spinal cord: response to adult hormone manipulation, absence in androgen-insensitive rats. *Brain Res.*, **225**, 297–307.

Brooks, B. P., Paulson, H. L., Merry, D. E. *et al.* (1997). Characterization of an expanded glutamine repeat androgen receptor in a neuronal cell culture system. *Neurobiol. Dis.*, **3**, 313–23.

Brown, C. J., Goss, S. J., Lubahn, D. B. *et al.* (1989). Androgen receptor locus on the human X chromosome: regional localization to Xq11–12 and description of a DNA polymorphism. *Am. J. Hum. Genet.*, **44**, 264–9.

Brown, T. R., Lubahn, D. B., Wilson, E. M., Joseph, D. R., French, F. S. & Migeon, C. J. (1988). Deletion of the steroid-binding domain of the human androgen receptor gene in one family with complete androgen insensitivity syndrome: evidence for further genetic heterogeneity in this syndrome. *Proc. Natl Acad. Sci. USA*, **85**, 8151–5.

Butler, R., Leigh, P. N., McPhaul, M. J. & Gallo, J. M. (1998). Truncated forms of the androgen receptor are associated with polyglutamine expansion in X-linked spinal and bulbar muscular atrophy. *Hum. Mol. Genet.*, **7**, 121–7.

Caplan, A. J., Langley, E., Wilson, E. M. & Vidal, J. (1995). Hormone-dependent transactivation by the human androgen receptor is regulated by a dnaJ protein. *J. Biol. Chem.*, **270**, 5251–7.

Chamberlain, N. L., Driver, E. D. & Miesfeld, R. L. (1994). The length and location of CAG trinucleotide repeats in the androgen receptor N-terminal domain affect transactivation function. *Nucl. Acids Res.*, **22**, 3181–6.

Choong, C. S., Kemppainen, J. A., Zhou, Z. X. & Wilson, E. M. (1996). Reduced androgen receptor gene expression with first exon CAG repeat expansion. *Mol. Endocrinol.*, **10**, 1527–35.

Cummings, C. J., Reinstein, E., Sun, Y. *et al.* (1999). Mutation of the E6-AP ubiquitin ligase reduces nuclear inclusion frequency while accelerating polyglutamine-induced pathology in SCA1 mice. *Neuron*, **24**, 879–92.

Cummings, C. J., Sun, Y., Opal, P. *et al.* (2001). Over-expression of inducible HSP70 chaperone suppresses neuropathology and improves motor function in SCA1 mice. *Hum. Mol. Genet.*, **10**, 1511–18.

Davies, S. W., Turmaine, M., Cozens, B. A. *et al.* (1997). Formation of neuronal intranuclear inclusions underlies the neurological dysfunction in mice transgenic for the HD mutation. *Cell*, **90**, 537–48.

Doyu, M., Sobue, G., Mukai, E. *et al.* (1992). Severity of X-linked recessive bulbospinal neuronopathy correlates with size of the tandem CAG repeat in androgen receptor gene. *Ann. Neurol.*, **32**, 707–10.

Dragatsis, I., Levine, M. S. & Zeitlin, S. (2000). Inactivation of Hdh in the brain and testis results in progressive neurodegeneration and sterility in mice. *Nat Genet.*, **26**, 300–6.

Duyao, M. P., Auerbach, A. B., Ryan, A. *et al.* (1995). Inactivation of the mouse Huntington's disease gene homolog Hdh. *Science*, **269**, 407–10.

Edwards, A., Hammond, H. A., Jin, L., Caskey, C. T. & Chakraborty, R. (1992). Genetic variation at five trimeric and tetrameric tandem repeat loci in four human population groups. *Genomics*, **12**, 241–53.

Ellerby, L. M., Hackam, A. S., Propp, S. S. *et al.* (1999). Kennedy's disease: caspase cleavage of the androgen receptor is a crucial event in cytotoxicity. *J. Neurochem.*, **72**, 185–95.

Ferrante, M. A. & Wilbourn, A. J. (1997). The characteristic electrodiagnostic features of Kennedy's disease. *Muscle Nerve*, **20**, 323–9.

Fischbeck, K. H., Ionasescu, V., Ritter, A. W. *et al.* (1986). Localization of the gene for X-linked spinal muscular atrophy. *Neurology*, **36**, 1595–8.

Forger, N. G., Hodges, L. L., Roberts, S. L. & Breedlove, S. M. (1992). Regulation of motoneuron death in the spinal nucleus of the bulbocavernosus. *J. Neurobiol.*, **23**, 1192–203.

Gelmann, E. P. (2002). Molecular biology of the androgen receptor. *J. Clin. Oncol.*, **20**, 3001–15.

Gerber, H. P., Seipel, K., Georgiev, O. *et al.* (1994). Transcriptional activation modulated by homopolymeric glutamine and proline stretches. *Science*, **263**, 808–11.

Giovannucci, E., Stampfer, M. J., Krithivas, K. *et al.* (1997). The CAG repeat within the androgen receptor gene and its relationship to prostate cancer. *Proc. Natl Acad. Sci., USA*, **94**, 3320–3.

Goldberg, Y. P., Kalchman, M. A., Metzler, M. *et al.* (1996). Absence of disease phenotype and intergenerational stability of the CAG repeat in transgenic mice expressing the human Huntington disease transcript. *Hum. Mol. Genet.*, **5**, 177–85.

Guidetti, D., Vescovini, E., Motti, L. *et al.* (1996). X-linked bulbar and spinal muscular atrophy, or Kennedy disease: clinical, neurophysiological, neuropathological, neuropsychological and molecular study of a large family. *J. Neurol. Sci.*, **135**, 140–8.

Harding, A. E., Thomas, P. K., Baraitser, M., Bradbury, P. G., Morgan-Hughes, J. A. & Ponsford, J. R. (1982). X-linked recessive bulbospinal neuronopathy: a report of ten cases. *J. Neurol. Neurosurg. Psychiatry*, **45**, 1012–19.

Harper, P. S., Harley, H. G., Reardon, W. & Shaw, D. J. (1992). Anticipation in myotonic dystrophy: new light on an old problem. *Am. J. Hum. Genet.*, **51**, 10–16.

Hartl, F. U. (1996). Molecular chaperones in cellular protein folding. *Nature*, **381**, 571–9.

Hughes, R. E., Lo, R. S., Davis, C. *et al.* (2001). Altered transcription in yeast expressing expanded polyglutamine. *Proc. Natl Acad. Sci., USA*, **98**, 13201–6.

Huntington's Disease Collaborative Research Group. (1993). A novel gene containing a trinucleotide repeat that is expanded and unstable on Huntington's disease chromosomes. *Cell*, **72**, 971–83.

Huynh, D. P., Figueroa, K., Hoang, N. & Pulst, S. M. (2000). Nuclear localization or inclusion body formation of ataxin-2 are not necessary for SCA2 pathogenesis in mouse or human. *Nat. Genet.*, **26**, 44–50.

Ishikawa, K., Fujigasaki, H., Saegusa, H. *et al.* (1999). Abundant expression and cytoplasmic aggregations of [alpha]1A voltage-dependent calcium channel protein associated with neurodegeneration in spinocerebellar ataxia type 6. *Hum. Mol. Genet.*, **8**, 1185–93.

Jones, A. L. (1999). The localization and interactions of huntingtin. *Phil. Trans. R. Soc. Lond. B Biol. Sci.*, **354**, 1021–7.

Kalchman, M. A., Koide, H. B., McCutcheon, K. *et al.* (1997). HIP1, a human homologue of *S. cerevisiae* Sla2p, interacts with membrane-associated huntingtin in the brain. *Nat. Genet.*, **16**, 44–53.

Katsuno, M., Adachi, H., Kume, A. *et al.* (2002). Testosterone reduction prevents phenotypic expression in a transgenic mouse model of spinal and bulbar muscular atrophy. *Neuron*, **35**, 843–54.

Kennedy, W. R., Alter, M. & Sung, J. H. (1968). Progressive proximal spinal and bulbar muscular atrophy of late onset. A sex-linked recessive trait. *Neurology*, **18**, 671–80.

Klement, I. A., Skinner, P. J., Kaytor, M. D. *et al.* (1998). Ataxin-1 nuclear localization and aggregation: role in polyglutamine-induced disease in SCA1 transgenic mice. *Cell*, **95**, 41–53.

Kobayashi, Y., Kume, A., Li, M. *et al.* (2000). Chaperones Hsp70 and Hsp40 suppress aggregate formation and apoptosis in cultured neuronal cells expressing truncated androgen receptor protein with expanded polyglutamine tract. *J. Biol. Chem.*, **275**, 8772–8.

Kobayashi, Y., Miwa, S., Merry, D. E. *et al.* (1998). Caspase-3 cleaves the expanded androgen receptor protein of spinal and bulbar muscular atrophy in a polyglutamine repeat length-dependent manner. *Biochem. Biophys. Res. Commun.*, **252**, 145–50.

La Spada, A. R., Fu, Y., Sopher, B. L. *et al.* (2001). Polyglutamine-expanded ataxin-7 antagonizes CRX function and induces cone-rod dystrophy in a mouse model of SCA7. *Neuron*, **31**, 913–27.

La Spada, A. R., Roling, D. B., Harding, A. E. *et al.* (1992). Meiotic stability and genotype-phenotype correlation of the trinucleotide repeat in X-linked spinal and bulbar muscular atrophy. *Nat. Genet.*, **2**, 301–4.

La Spada, A. R., Wilson, E. M., Lubahn, D. B., Harding, A. E. & Fischbeck, K. H. (1991). Androgen receptor gene mutations in X-linked spinal and bulbar muscular atrophy. *Nature*, **352**, 77–9.

Langley, E., Zhou, Z. X. & Wilson, E. M. (1995). Evidence for an anti-parallel orientation of the ligand-activated human androgen receptor dimer. *J. Biol. Chem.*, **270**, 29983–90.

Li, X. J., Li, S. H., Sharp, A. H. *et al.* (1995). A huntingtin-associated protein enriched in brain with implications for pathology. *Nature*, **378**, 398–402.

Li, M., Miwa, S., Kobayashi, Y. *et al.* (1998a). Nuclear inclusions of the androgen receptor protein in spinal and bulbar muscular atrophy. *Ann. Neurol.*, **44**, 249–54.

Li, M., Nakagomi, Y., Kobayashi, Y. *et al.*, (1998b). Nonneural nuclear inclusions of androgen receptor protein in spinal and bulbar muscular atrophy. *Am. J. Pathol.*, **153**, 695–701.

Lieberman, A. P., Harmison, G., Strand, A. D., Olson, J. M. & Fischbeck, K. H. (2002). Altered transcriptional regulation in cells expressing the expanded polyglutamine androgen receptor. *Hum. Mol. Genet.*, **11**, 1967–76.

Lubahn, D. B., Joseph, D. R., Sar, M. *et al.* (1988). The human androgen receptor: complementary deoxyribonucleic acid cloning, sequence analysis and gene expression in prostate. *Mol. Endocrinol.*, **2**, 1265–75.

Lund, A., Udd, B., Juvonen, V. *et al.* (2000). Founder effect in spinal and bulbar muscular atrophy (SBMA) in Scandinavia. *Eur. J. Hum. Genet.*, **8**, 631–6.

Marsh, J. L., Walker, H., Theisen, H. *et al.* (2000). Expanded polyglutamine peptides alone are intrinsically cytotoxic and cause neurodegeneration in *Drosophila*. *Hum. Mol. Genet.*, **9**, 13–25.

Matilla, A., Koshy, B. T., Cummings, C. J., Isobe, T., Orr, H. T. & Zoghbi, H. Y. (1997). The cerebellar leucine-rich acidic nuclear protein interacts with ataxin-1. *Nature*, **389**, 974–8.

Matilla, A., Roberson, E. D., Banfi, S. *et al.* (1998). Mice lacking ataxin-1 display learning deficits and decreased hippocampal paired-pulse facilitation. *J. Neurosci.*, **18**, 5508–16.

McCampbell, A., Taylor, J. P., Taye, A. A. *et al.* (2000). CREB-binding protein sequestration by expanded polyglutamine. *Hum. Mol. Genet.*, **9**, 2197–202.

McManamny, P., Chy, H. S., Finkelstein, D. I. *et al.* (2002). A mouse model of spinal and bulbar muscular atrophy. *Hum. Mol. Genet.*, **11**, 2103–11.

Merry, D. E., Kobayashi, Y., Bailey, C. K., Taye, A. A. & Fischbeck, K. H. (1998). Cleavage, aggregation and toxicity of the expanded androgen receptor in spinal and bulbar muscular atrophy. *Hum. Mol. Genet.*, **7**, 693–701.

Mhatre, A. N., Trifiro, M. A., Kaufman, M. *et al.* (1993). Reduced transcriptional regulatory competence of the androgen receptor in X-linked spinal and bulbar muscular atrophy. *Nat. Genet.*, **5**, 184–8.

Nakamura, K., Jeong, S. Y., Uchihara, T. *et al.* (2001). SCA17, a novel autosomal dominant cerebellar ataxia caused by an expanded polyglutamine in TATA-binding protein. *Hum. Mol. Genet.*, **10**, 1441–8.

Nam, R. K., Elhaji, Y., Krahn, M. D. *et al.* (2000). Significance of the CAG repeat polymorphism of the androgen receptor gene in prostate cancer progression. *J. Urol.*, **164**, 567–72.

Nasir, J., Floresco, S. B., O'Kusky, J. R. *et al.* (1995). Targeted disruption of the Huntington's disease gene results in embryonic lethality and behavioral and morphological changes in heterozygotes. *Cell*, **81**, 811–23.

Nelson, K. A. & Witte, J. S. (2002). Androgen receptor CAG repeats and prostate cancer. *Am. J. Epidemiol.*, **155**, 883–90.

Nordeen, E. J., Nordeen, K. W., Sengelaub, D. R. & Arnold, A. P. (1985). Androgens prevent normally occurring cell death in a sexually dimorphic spinal nucleus. *Science*, **229**, 671–3.

Nucifora, F. C., Jr., Sasaki, M., Peters, M. F. *et al.* (2001). Interference by huntingtin and atrophin-1 with cbp-mediated transcription leading to cellular toxicity. *Science*, **291**, 2423–8.

O'Malley, B. (1990). The steroid receptor superfamily: more excitement predicted for the future. *Mol. Endocrinol.*, **4**, 363–9.

Ogata, A., Matsuura, T., Tashiro, K. *et al.* (1994). Expression of androgen receptor in X-linked spinal and bulbar muscular atrophy and amyotrophic lateral sclerosis. *J. Neurol. Neurosurg. Psychiatry*, **57**, 1274–5.

Okazawa, H., Rich, T., Chang, A. *et al.* (2002). Interaction between mutant ataxin-1 and PQBP-1 affects transcription and cell death. *Neuron*, **34**, 701–13.

Olney, R. K., Aminoff, M. J. & So, Y. T. (1991). Clinical and electrodiagnostic features of X-linked recessive bulbospinal neuronopathy. *Neurology*, **41**, 823–8.

Ordway, J. M., Tallaksen-Greene, S., Gutekunst, C. A. *et al.* (1997). Ectopically expressed CAG repeats cause intranuclear inclusions and a progressive late onset neurological phenotype in the mouse. *Cell*, **91**, 753–63.

Parboosingh, J. S., Figlewicz, D. A., Krizus, A. *et al.* (1997). Spinobulbar muscular atrophy can mimic ALS: the importance of genetic testing in male patients with atypical ALS. *Neurology*, **49**, 568–72.

Paulson, H. L., Perez, M. K., Trottier, Y. *et al.* (1997). Intranuclear inclusions of expanded polyglutamine protein in spinocerebellar ataxia type 3. *Neuron*, **19**, 333–44.

Perutz, M. F., Johnson, T., Suzuki, M. & Finch, J. T. (1994). Glutamine repeats as polar zippers: their possible role in inherited neurodegenerative diseases. *Proc. Natl Acad. Sci., USA*, **91**, 5355–8.

Ringel, S. P., Lava, N. S., Treihaft, M. M., Lubs, M. L. & Lubs, H. A. (1978). Late-onset X-linked recessive spinal and bulbar muscular atrophy. *Muscle Nerve*, **1**, 297–307.

Sar, M. & Stumpf, W. E. (1977). Androgen concentration in motor neurons of cranial nerves and spinal cord. *Science*, **197**, 77–9.

Saudou, F., Finkbeiner, S., Devys, D. & Greenberg, M. E. (1998). Huntingtin acts in the nucleus to induce apoptosis but death does not correlate with the formation of intranuclear inclusions. *Cell*, **95**, 55–66.

Schmidt, B. J., Greenberg, C. R., Allingham-Hawkins, D. J. & Spriggs, E. L. (2002). Expression of X-linked bulbospinal muscular atrophy (Kennedy disease) in two homozygous women. *Neurology*, **59**, 770–2.

Sengelaub, D. R. & Arnold, A. P. (1989). Hormonal control of neuron number in sexually dimorphic spinal nuclei of the rat: I.

Testosterone- regulated death in the dorsolateral nucleus. *J. Comp. Neurol.*, **280**, 622–9.

Sengelaub, D. R., Jordan, C. L., Kurz, E. M. & Arnold, A. P. (1989a). Hormonal control of neuron number in sexually dimorphic spinal nuclei of the rat: II. Development of the spinal nucleus of the bulbocavernosus in androgen-insensitive (Tfm) rats. *J. Comp. Neurol.*, **280**, 630–6.

Sengelaub, D. R., Nordeen, E. J., Nordeen, K. W. & Arnold, A. P. (1989b). Hormonal control of neuron number in sexually dimorphic spinal nuclei of the rat: III. Differential effects of the androgen dihydrotestosterone. *J. Comp. Neurol.*, **280**, 637–44.

Shaywitz, A. J. & Greenberg, M. E. (1999). CREB: a stimulus-induced transcription factor activated by a diverse array of extracellular signals. *Annu. Rev. Biochem.*, **68**, 821–61.

Sherman, M. Y. & Goldberg, A. L. (2001). Cellular defenses against unfolded proteins: a cell biologist thinks about neurodegenerative diseases. *Neuron*, **29**, 15–32.

Sipione, S. & Cattaneo, E. (2001). Modeling Huntington's disease in cells, flies, and mice. *Mol. Neurobiol.*, **23**, 21–51.

Sobue, G., Matsuoka, Y., Mukai, E., Takayanagi, T., Sobue, I. & Hashizume, Y. (1981). Spinal and cranial motor nerve roots in amyotrophic lateral sclerosis and X-linked recessive bulbospinal muscular atrophy: morphometric and teased-fiber study. *Acta Neuropathol.*, **55**, 227–35.

Sopher, B. L., Martinez, R. A., Holm, I. E. *et al.* (2002). SBMA motor neuronopathy in AR YAC CAG100 transgenic mice. *Am. J. Hum. Genet.*, **71**, A62 {Abstract}.

Stanford, J. L., Just, J. J., Gibbs, M. *et al.* (1997). Polymorphic repeats in the androgen receptor gene: molecular markers of prostate cancer risk. *Cancer Res.*, **57**, 1194–8.

Stefanis, C., Papapetropoulos, T., Scarpalezos, S., Lygidakis, G. & Panayiotopoulos, C. P. (1975). X-linked spinal and bulbar muscular atrophy of late onset. A separate type of motor neuron disease? *J. Neurol. Sci.*, **24**, 493–503.

Steffan, J. S., Bodai, L., Pallos, J. *et al.* (2001). Histone deacetylase inhibitors arrest polyglutamine-dependent neurodegeneration in *Drosophila. Nature*, **413**, 739–43.

Steffan, J. S., Kazantsev, A., Spasic-Boskovic, O. *et al.* (2000). The Huntington's disease protein interacts with p53 and CREB-binding protein and represses transcription. *Proc. Natl Acad. Sci., USA*, **97**, 6763–8.

Takeyama, K., Ito, S., Yamamoto, A. *et al.* (2002). Androgen-dependent neurodegeneration by polyglutamine-expanded human androgen receptor in *Drosophila. Neuron*, **35**, 855–64.

Tanaka, F., Doyu, M., Ito, Y. *et al.* (1996). Founder effect in spinal and bulbar muscular atrophy (SBMA). *Hum. Mol. Genet.*, **5**, 1253–7.

Thornton, J. W. & Kelley, D. B. (1998). Evolution of the androgen receptor: structure-function implications. *Bioessays*, **20**, 860–9.

Trottier, Y., Lutz, Y., Stevanin, G. *et al.* (1995). Polyglutamine expansion as a pathological epitope in Huntington's disease and four dominant cerebellar ataxias. *Nature*, **378**, 403–6.

Verkerk, A. J., Pieretti, M., Sutcliffe, J. S. *et al.* (1991). Identification of a gene (FMR-1) containing a CGG repeat coincident with a breakpoint cluster region exhibiting length variation in fragile X syndrome. *Cell*, **65**, 905–14.

Warner, C. L., Griffin, J. E., Wilson, J. D. *et al.* (1992). X-linked spinomuscular atrophy: a kindred with associated abnormal androgen receptor binding. *Neurology*, **42**, 2181–4.

Warrick, J. M., Chan, H. Y., Gray-Board, G. L., Chai, Y., Paulson, H. L. & Bonini, N. M. (1999). Suppression of polyglutamine-mediated neurodegeneration in *Drosophila* by the molecular chaperone HSP70. *Nat. Genet.*, **23**, 425–8.

Wellington, C. L., Ellerby, L. M., Hackam, A. S. *et al.* (1998). Caspase cleavage of gene products associated with triplet expansion disorders generates truncated fragments containing the polyglutamine tract. *J. Biol. Chem.*, **273**, 9158–67.

Wilson, M. G., Towner, J. W., Coffin, G. S., Ebbin, A. J., Siris, E. & Brager, P. (1981). Genetic and clinical studies in 13 patients with the Wolf-Hirschhorn syndrome [del(4p)]. *Hum. Genet.*, **59**, 297–307.

Zeitlin, S., Liu, J. P., Chapman, D. L., Papaioannou, V. E. & Efstratiadis, A. (1995). Increased apoptosis and early embryonic lethality in mice nullizygous for the Huntington's disease gene homologue. *Nat. Genet.*, **11**, 155–63.

Zhang, L., Leeflang, E. P., Yu, J. & Arnheim, N. (1994). Studying human mutations by sperm typing: instability of CAG trinucleotide repeats in the human androgen receptor gene. *Nat. Genet.*, **7**, 531–5.

Zhou, Z. X., Sar, M., Simental, J. A., Lane, M. V. & Wilson, E. M. (1994). A ligand-dependent bipartite nuclear targeting signal in the human androgen receptor. Requirement for the DNA-binding domain and modulation by NH2-terminal and carboxyl-terminal sequences. *J. Biol. Chem.*, **269**, 13115–23.

Zoghbi, H. Y. & Orr, H. T. (2000). Glutamine repeats and neurodegeneration. *Annu. Rev. Neurosci.*, **23**, 217–47.

Zuccato, C., Ciammola, A., Rigamonti, D. *et al.* (2001). Loss of huntingtin-mediated BDNF gene transcription in Huntington's disease. *Science*, **293**, 493–8.

55

Spinal muscular atrophies

Klaus Zerres and Sabine Rudnik-Schöneborn

Institute for Human Genetics, University of Technology, Aachen, Germany

Definition

The term spinal muscular atrophy (SMA) comprises a clinically and genetically heterogeneous group of diseases characterized by degeneration and loss of the anterior horn cells in the spinal cord, and – depending on type and severity – sometimes also in the brainstem nuclei, resulting in muscle weakness and atrophy. The sensory neurons are always clinically spared, and there are no signs of upper motor neuron (pyramidal tract) involvement (Emery, 1971).

The subdivision of the SMAs into separate genetic and clinical entities (Table 55.1) is still controversial unless biochemical or molecular genetic criteria are available to define distinct pathomechanisms. The criteria used are age of onset, severity (progression, age of death), distribution of weakness, the inclusion of additional features, and different modes of inheritance.

Epidemiology

Autosomal recessive proximal SMA is one of the most common inherited diseases leading to death in early infancy. According to a rough estimate, less than 2% of cases with an onset before 10 years of age show a parent-to-child transmission (Emery, 1971). While vertical transmission of childhood-onset proximal SMA is an exception, autosomal dominant transmission can be found in about two-thirds of the adult-onset proximal SMA families (Pearn, 1978a). Assuming an incidence of about 1:10 000 for all types of autosomal recessive SMA, it has been estimated that adult SMA accounts for 8% of all SMA cases, with a prevalence of 0.32 per 100 000 of the population (Pearn, 1978b). Distal SMA accounts for about 10% of all SMAs (Pearn & Hudgson, 1979).

Proximal SMA

Clinical picture

The clinical picture of proximal SMA is highly variable, indicating a continuous spectrum with ages of onset from before birth to adulthood rather than clearly separable subgroups (Table 55.2a). A major problem of existing classifications is that the prognosis of SMA patients is often better than stated in the defined subtype (Russman et al., 1992; Zerres & Rudnik-Schöneborn, 1995) so that a "reclassification," for example, from the severe type I to the intermediate type II or even type III might be necessary if life span exceeds the designated age of death. Therefore, it is more reasonable to define SMA types I–IV by achieved motor functions and age of onset without given limitations for prognostic considerations (Table 55.2b).

The clinical signs of the most severe SMA type, which is also called Werdnig–Hoffmann disease or acute SMA, are evident from birth or soon after with a median age of onset of 1 month (Fig. 55.1). Nearly all patients present by 6 months of age, and in one-third, even abnormal fetal movements are reported. Symptoms are profound hypotonia and generalized weakness. The diaphragm and the extraocular muscles tend to be spared and distinguishes classical SMA from SMA plus forms. A certain percentage of infants show mild joint limitations from birth (limited hip abduction or knee and elbow extension, ulnar deviation of the hands), which is much less severe than in arthrogryposis multiplex congenita. In the final stage the child is practically immobile, has a nasogastric tube for feeding, a bell-shaped chest with paradoxic breathing, and is tachypneic indicating imminent respiratory insufficiency. Life-span is short with death occurring at a median age of 8 months in patients with onset in the first 6 months due to weakness affecting both bulbar and respiratory muscles.

Table 55.1. Classification of spinal muscular atrophies

1. *Proximal SMA (80–90%)*
    Infantile and juvenile SMA (SMA I–III) (a.r., a.d)
    Adult SMA (SMA IV) (a.r, a.d., mostly sporadic)
2. *Non-proximal SMA*
2.1 Distal SMA (a.d., a.r., X-linked, sporadic), predominantly of
    the legs, of the hands or both
    – segmental SMA or benign monomelic amyotrophy
       (mostly sporadic)
2.2 Scapuloperoneal SMA (a.d., a.r.)
3. *Bulbar palsy*
3.1 Progressive bulbar palsy of childhood type Fazio–Londe
    (a.r.)
    – bulbar palsy with deafness (Brown–Vialetto–van Laere
       syndrome) (a.r.)
3.2 Adult onset bulbar palsy (a.d.)
4. *Spinobulbar neuronopathy type Kennedy (X.l.)*
5. *Variants of SMA*
    Variants of infantile *SMA*
    – diaphragmatic SMA (a.r.)
    – SMA plus pontocerebellar hypoplasia (a.r.)
    – SMA plus arthogryposis and bone fractures (a.r., X.l.)
    – SMA with myoclonus epilepsy (a.r.)
    Variants of adult SMA
    – distal SMA with vocal cord paralysis (a.d.)
    – (SMA with cardiomyopathy)
    (a.r.: autosomal recessive, a.d.:autosomal dominant, X.l.:
    X-linked)

According to our studies, only 8% of patients were alive beyond the age of 10 years (Table 55.2b). However, it is important to recognize long-standing disease courses with an early onset of generalized weakness but survival into adulthood (Borkowska *et al.*, 2002). Based on molecular genetic findings, there is now strong evidence that a "congenital" type of infantile SMA exists. Major findings include severe neonatal onset with respiratory insufficiency, congenital contractures, external ophthalmoplegia and facial weakness, and severe peripheral (sensory and motor) nerve involvement (Korinthenberg *et al.*, 1997).

The clinical course of SMA type II (Fig. 55.2a,b) is marked by periods of apparent arrest in the clinical progression. The age of onset and presenting signs may be indistinguishable from SMA type I, although median age of onset is generally later (8 months). The children fail to pass motor milestones because of proximal weakness and hypotonia within the first 18 months of life. For practical purposes, this group is defined by the ability to sit independently, as the children never learn to stand or walk unaided. Hand tremor (polyminimyoclonus) and fasciculations (in 50% of the cases) are characteristic features. Pronounced weakness of trunk muscles in the nonambulatory patients give rise to spine deformities. Contractures develop early in all major joints as a result of synergist-antagonist imbalance. Fifty percent of the SMA II patients could sit independently after age 14 years (Russman *et al.*, 1996) but sitting function is not a prognostic predictor of life-span (Zerres *et al.*, 1997).

A mild form of childhood and juvenile SMA-type III is known as Kugelberg–Welander disease and shows a wide range of clinical onset from the first year of life until the third decade. Patients with SMA type III learn to walk without support, which distinguishes them from those with SMA type II. For prognostic reasons, this group can be separated into types IIIa and IIIb (Table 55.2a). In SMA type IIIa, onset is in the first 3 years of life, the children have early walking difficulties and often fail to pass further motor milestones. Since many patients are non-ambulatory by school age (50% are confined to a wheelchair 14 years after onset, Table 55.2b), there is a considerable handicap in comparison to those who start with first walking difficulties in youth or adulthood (Zerres & Rudnik-Schöneborn, 1995). In SMA type IIIb, first signs of proximal muscle weakness occur between 3 and 30 years. Life expectancy is not much reduced, the course of the disease is characterized by slow progression with periods of arrest. As in SMA II, tremor of the outstretched arm and limb fasciculations are frequently encountered. Depending on the degree of weakness, spine deformities and contractures are frequent complications, mainly in the chairbound patients. Respiratory insufficiency may become a problem in the older, wheelchairbound SMA III patients, who require assisted ventilation late in the disease course.

Intrafamilial variability of age of onset is more marked in SMA type III than in SMA type I or II. In a series of 13 sibships with SMA type III, 3 showed discordant ages of onset ranging from 5 to 15 years within a family (Rudnik-Schöneborn *et al.*, 1994). Moreover, unaffected relatives harboring identical gene defects like the affected sibs have mostly been observed in SMA III families (Hahnen *et al.*, 1995).

SMA type IV is defined to have an onset after the age of 30 years. The condition is relatively benign with slow clinical progression, and a normal life span can be expected (Zerres & Rudnik-Schöneborn, 1995). While the majority of adult onset patients do not show deletions of the SMN1 gene (Zerres *et al.*, 1995a), there are some patients with SMN1 deletions who are not diagnosed before their 50s or 60s. These patients have a strictly proximal involvement with marked weakness of the pelvic girdle and in particular of the psoas muscle. It is believed that these patients are characterized by a large number of SMN2 gene copies, but clinical variability cannot be explained by the SMN genes alone (see genetics/molecular biology). It has to be stressed that – in contrast to SMA I–III – recurrence of SMA IV within a sibship is an exception.

Table 55.2a. Classification of proximal spinal muscular atrophy according to the International SMA Consortium[*]

SMA type	Principal synonyms	Definition	Genetics
I	Werdnig–Hoffmann disease	Sitting not achieved	Autosomal recessive (about 95% SMN1 deletions)
	Acute infantile SMA	Onset usually within the first 6 months	
II	Chronic childhood SMA	Unaided sitting possible, walking not achieved	Autosomal recessive (about 95% SMN1 deletions)
	Arrested Werdnig–Hoffmann disease	Onset usually in the first two years of life Survival > 90% by 10 years	
III	Kugelberg–Welander disease	Walking without aids achieved	Autosomal recessive (80–90% SMN1 deletions)
	Juvenile SMA	– IIIa: Onset ≤3 years	Rarely autosomal dominant inheritance
		– IIIb: Onset ≥3 years	Excess of males
IV	Adult SMA	Onset > 30 years	Mostly sporadic
			Autosomal dominant (gene defect unknown)
			Autosomal recessive (rare)

[*] Zerres and Rudnik-Schöneborn (1995); Zerres and Davies (1999).

Table 55.2b. Prognostic considerations in proximal SMA type I–III[*]

Survival probability in SMA I and II	2	4	10	20	40 years of age (%)
SMA I	32	18	8	0	0
SMA II	100	100	98	77	(no data available)
Probability of being able to walk in SMA III	**2**	**4**	**10**	**20**	**40 years after onset (%)**
SMA IIIa	98	95	73	44	34
SMA IIIb	100	100	97	89	67

[*] Zerres & Rudnik-Schöneborn (1995); Zerres et al. (1997).

Diagnostic findings

The clinical and laboratory criteria of proximal SMA (Table 55.3) were defined by the International SMA Consortium (Zerres & Davies, 1999). With the evidence of deletions in the region 5q11.2–13.3, it has become possible to confirm the diagnosis of proximal SMA with localization on chromosome 5 by direct molecular analysis, although the role of the deleted genes is not fully understood by the time of this report. Therefore, the clinical diagnostic criteria are still valid, but, in fact, deletion screening of the SMN gene has become the most important diagnostic tool. Serum creatine kinase activity (sCK) is normal in SMA I and II, and only slightly increased in juvenile onset cases. If the sCK exceeds more than five fold the upper normal limit of normal, a myopathy is more likely. However, in rare instances,

CK can be as high as in muscular dystrophy causing diagnostic difficulties (Rudnik-Schöneborn et al., 1998).

Neurogenic changes can be seen on EMG and in the muscle biopsy specimen. EMG shows abnormal spontaneous activity (fibrillations, positive sharp waves, fasciculations) as a sign of acute denervation in progressive disease courses. Spontaneous activity is therefore uncommon in chronic anterior horn cell disease. Motor unit potentials show an increased mean duration and amplitude upon voluntary contraction, reflecting re-innervation. An increased proportion of motor unit potentials is polyphasic. The interference pattern on increasing effort is reduced due to loss of motor units. However, motor and sensory nerves can reveal a reduced excitability and nerve conduction can be markedly slowed in severe SMA type I (Korinthenberg et al., 1997; Rudnik-Schöneborn et al., 2003). Conduction velocity is reduced by depletion of fast conducting large-diameter nerve fibers. In severe cases, distinction from early onset peripheral neuropathies can be very difficult.

In the muscle biopsy, large group atrophy is typical in severe SMA, while the atrophic groups of both fiber types appear to be smaller in the chronic forms. Histochemical staining gives evidence of fiber type grouping mainly in the more chronic cases as a result of reinnervation processes. In SMA I and II, hypertrophic fibers of type I can be seen distributed among the atrophic fibers. In SMA III and IV the process of re-innervation gets the overhand showing type-grouping, although there is still acute denervation, i.e. small groups of angular-sized atrophic fibers. In accordance with the diagnostic criteria, peripheral nerves are morphologically normal in the vast majority of SMA patients. If axonal

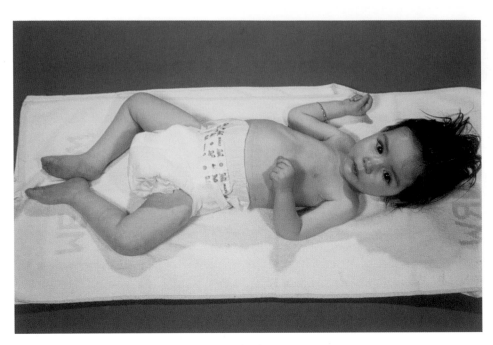

Fig. 55.1 Clinical signs of acute SMA. (Reproduced with permission.)

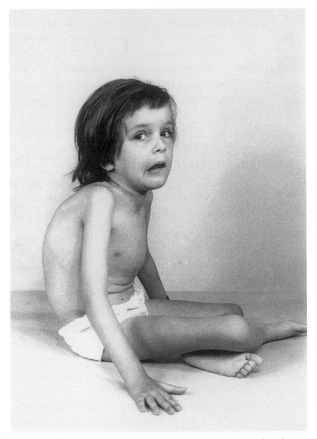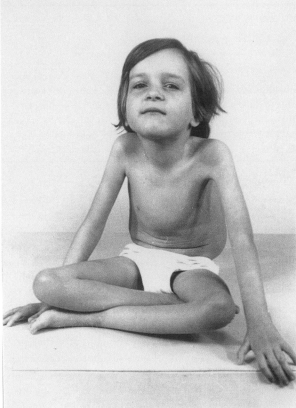

Fig. 55.2a,b Clinical course of SMA type II. (Reproduced with permission.)

Table 55.3. Diagnostic criteria of proximal spinal muscular atrophy (Zerres & Davies, 1999)

Inclusion criteria	Exclusion criteria
Symmetrical muscle weakness of trunk and limbs	Involvement of extraocular muscles, diaphragm and myocardium*
Proximal muscles > distal	Marked facial weakness* (*exceptions are rare congenital onset cases with external opthalmoplegia and facial weakness)
Lower limbs > upper limbs	CNS dysfunction
Fasciculations of tongue, tremor of hands	Arthrogryposis (but rarely seen in severe, congenital onset SMA type I)
Neurogenic changes in EMG and muscle biopsy	CK usually < 5 times the upper normal limit
Homozygous absence/mutation of the telomeric SMN gene	Reduction of motor nerve conduction velocities < 70% of lower normal limit or abnormal sensory nerve action potentials in SMA II–III (motor and sensory conduction can be markedly abnormal in SMA I)

degeneration was observed in peripheral motor nerves, this was mainly attributed to a dying forward phenomenon as a consequence of motor neuron degeneration. Meanwhile, there is increasing evidence of axonal degeneration, including reduction of myelinated fibers and dystrophic axons with shrunken and condensed axon structures, also affecting the sensory nerve system (i.e. sural nerve) at least in SMA I patients to a variable extent (Rudnik-Schöneborn et al., 2003). In the spinal cord, patho-anatomic features are gliosis of anterior horns without areas of demyelination. While the posterior roots appear to be normal, distinct demyelination can be seen in the anterior roots. The degenerated ganglion cells are small and pycnotic until an almost complete loss of anterior horn cells occurs. Since it has been reported that, in patients with severe SMA, also other parts of the central nervous system (CNS) underwent degenerative processes, the extent of pathologic abnormalities in SMA still has to be clarified.

Differential diagnosis

The differential diagnosis of acute SMA type I is given with the whole spectrum of the floppy infant syndrome. The clinical picture of the mild SMA type III is often indistinguishable from the muscular dystrophies. In many patients with limb girdle muscular dystrophy, it is now possible to classify the immunhistochemical defect in the muscle. If cardiomyopathy is seen in patients with apparent

SMA, this should prompt lamin A/C analysis and exclusion of emerin deficiency for autosomal dominant and X-linked Emery–Dreifuss muscular dystrophy, respectively. Hexosaminidase A deficiency may rarely produce a clinical picture resembling SMA type III. The most important differential diagnosis of SMA type IV is Kennedy disease and amyotrophic lateral sclerosis (ALS). Alterations of the SMN genes have been demonstrated in patients with sporadic ALS and with slowly progressive spinal muscular atrophy, suggesting that an SMN deficiency can also modify the phenotype of other motor neuron diseases (Veldink et al., 2001). Adult Pompe's disease can be misdiagnosed as SMA. In families with evidence of autosomal dominant inheritance, proximal myotonic myopathy (PROMM) has also to be considered which can display neurogenic changes in the muscle. Postpoliomyelitis muscular atrophy is supposed to be due to the progressive loss of regenerated sprouts and is a potential cause of diagnostic confusion.

Genetics/molecular biology

The proximal SMAs as well as the non-proximal SMAs are genetically heterogeneous; both autosomal recessive and autosomal dominant genes are known to cause childhood- or adult-onset SMA. The majority of cases with proximal SMA is autosomal recessively inherited but at least two autosomal dominantly inherited proximal types exist showing considerable clinical overlap (Rietschel et al., 1992). Considering the incidence of at least 1:10 000 for acute and chronic proximal SMA, the estimated heterozygosity frequency is about 1:50 in the general population. The gene responsible for most families with childhood SMA with autosomal recessive inheritance has been localized to a small region of the long arm of chromosome 5 (5q11.2–q13.3). Both the severe infantile and the chronic childhood forms were found to conform to this single gene locus at 5q (Brzustowicz et al., 1990; Gilliam et al., 1990; Melki et al., 1990a,b). Different genes and microsatellite markers have been identified in the 5q region that can be deleted in SMA patients. These are located in a complex genomic region on 5q13 that contains a large inverted duplication consisting of at least four genes (Fig. 55.3): the survival motor neuron (SMN) gene, the neuronal apoptosis inhibitory protein (NAIP) gene, the basal transcription factor subunit p44 (BTFp44), and H4F5. All genes are present in a telomeric and a centromeric copy and show homozygous deletions in SMA patients. Since deletions of the NAIP, BTFp44 and H4F5 genes can also be detected in the normal population, deletions or mutations of the telomeric copy of the SMN gene (SMN1) are disease specific. Therefore, most research has been concentrated on the SMN1 gene, as it exhibits

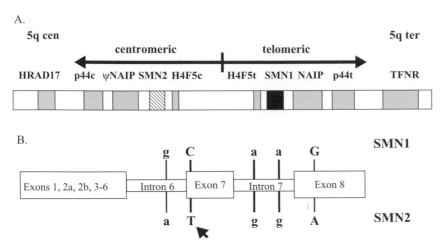

Fig. 55.3

homozygous deletions in more than 90% of SMA patients (Lefebvre *et al.*, 1995; Hahnen *et al.*, 1995). Deletions can be detected visibly by SSCA or by restriction digest of PCR products. In the vast majority of patients, exons 7 and 8 are absent, followed by a 5–10% deletion rate of exon 7 only. Moreover, isolated deletion of exon 8 has been detected in rare instances of mild SMA (Gambardella *et al.*, 1998). The proportion of clinically typical SMA patients who do not show an SMN1 deletion does not exceed 5% in severe SMA type I, but increases to 10% to 20% in mild SMA type III (Hahnen *et al.*, 1995). It has been shown that there is a correlation of SMN protein levels and SMA phenotype, with type I patients showing low SMN protein levels in particular in spinal motor neurons (Coovert *et al.*, 1997). Homozygous deletions of SMN2 genes can be detected in about 5% of the normal population and are generally not associated with a phenotype, if at least one SMN1 copy is retained.

Only in a small number of patients (approximately 3–4%) subtle mutations in the SMN gene have been identified (Parsons *et al.*, 1998; Wirth *et al.*, 1999). It is therefore tempting to speculate that other genes might be responsible for the non-deleted cases. Compound heterozygotes can be detected after PCR-based densitometric assessment of SMN-gene copy number, by pulsed field gel electrophoresis or by fluorescence-based carrier testing. More recently, quantitative analysis of SMN gene copy numbers based on real-time fluorescence polymerase chain reaction (PCR) have been developed by using a LightCycler (Feldkötter *et al.*, 2002) and TaqMan technology (Anhuf *et al.*, 2003). These quantitative methods identify patients and relatives who retain only one copy of SMN1, knowledge which can be used for further diagnostic work-up of clinically typical cases and for genetic risk calculation in affected families.

While there are deletions of variable sizes in SMA type I, gene conversion events of SMN1 to SMN2 are responsible for the reduced SMN protein transcription leading to the milder phenotype in SMA type II and III. Several studies have demonstrated chimeric SMN genes with SMN2 exon 7 fused to SMN1 exon 8 and thus increasing the number of SMN2 copies to 3–4 in milder SMA types. It was concluded that SMA I is caused by physical deletions of SMN1, while the mutations in type II and III SMA are replacements of SMN1 by SMN2. The SMN2 copy number is reflected by the copy number of the adjacent multicopy markers C212 and Ag1-CA. The number of SMN2 copies correlates with SMA subtype, age of onset and length of survival, i.e. the clinical phenotype is directed primarily by the level of functional SMN protein. However, it is not possible to predict the individual disease course on the basis of the observed deletion size or gene conversion event, as there is a wide overlap of molecular genetic findings in different SMA types.

The severity of SMA can be modulated by the number of centromeric SMN gene copies (SMN2). SMN 2 is nearly identical with the SMN1 gene except for single nucleotide differences in exon 7 and 8, yet their transcriptional products are not the same. While SMN1 predominantly produces full-length transcripts (90%), SMN2 primarily gives rise to transcripts lacking exon 7 (60%) and minor amounts of full-length transcripts (20–30%). It is believed that the SMN protein produced by the truncated transcripts is unstable and therefore less able to fulfil its role in RNA metabolism and transcription. The only critical difference between SMN1 and SMN2 is a C→T base change in exon 7, which disrupts a putative exonic splicing enhancer (ESE) and causes alternative splicing of SMN2 exon 7 (Lorson *et al.*, 1999).

It is still unclear why loss of SMN results in selective motor neuron loss, as the gene is ubiquitously expressed. This is underlined by the observation of families, primarily published as unlinked to chromosome 5q markers, in whom SMN gene deletions were found not only in the patients but also in their unaffected sibs (Hahnen et al., 1995). The 38 kDa SMN protein is found in both cytoplasm and nucleus where it is localized in structures called "gems." The SMN protein is involved in critical steps of RNA processing and acts in concert with several other proteins in the regeneration of the snRNPs and other splicing factors in the cytoplasm [for review see Sendtner, 2001; Nicole et al., 2002). Presently, it is suggested that additional factors are required to cause, or at least modify, an SMA phenotype.

Animal models

The SMN protein is transcribed by the two SMN genes that were generated by a duplication on chromosome 5q around 5 million years ago (Rochette et al., 2001), therefore no natural animal model for infantile SMA exists. Before the SMN gene was discovered, it was hoped to find a human homologue derived from the different mouse models with motor neuron degeneration (for reviews see Privoro & Mitsumoto, 1996; Monani et al., 2000b; Schmalbruch & Haase, 2001). This approach was eventually successful for the identification of the human homologue of the nmd mouse (Cox et al., 1998), which turned out to be the IGHMBP2 gene responsible for diaphragmatic SMA. As regards murine Smn and Naip genes, the number of Naip genes is increased but there is only one Smn copy. The replacement of murine Smn by human SMN2 genes resulted in transgenic mice corresponding to the human disease model (Monani et al., 2000a; Hsieh-Li et al., 2000; Jablonka et al., 2000). These mice show a reduction of motor neurons in the spinal cord without displaying any pathology in other parts of the CNS or in the dorsal ganglia. However, the morphological alterations in the spinal cord suggest that not the numerical reduction of neurons but the loss of function is important for the pathomechanism. In the transgenic mouse model created by the French group (Frugier et al., 2000) exon 7 of the murine Smn gene has been removed on both mouse chromosomes in a tissue specific manner by using the Cre/loxP recombination system. While mice with SMN deficiency restricted to the spinal cord (neuronal mutant) develop an SMA like phenotype, the situation is different in mice where SMN was deficient in the muscle. These muscular mutants developed a severe muscular dystrophy with partial dystrophin deficiency not at all connected with the SMA like phenotype (Cifuentes-Diaz et al., 2001). This sheds a new light on SMN function in different tissues.

Management perspectives

A curative treatment of the different SMAs is not available, and so far no therapy is known that has a positive long-term effect on the disease course (Zerres et al., 1995b).

As a high number of SMN2 copies is able to partly compensate motor neuron loss in transgenic mice, this finding has stimulated the planning of therapeutical trials in SMA with proven SMN deficiency where it is hoped to increase the protein transcription of SMN2, e.g. by specific splice enhancers (Hofmann et al., 2000). Transgenic mice which were fed with sodium butyrate had a longer life-span and a significantly milder phenotype compared with litter mates without treatment (Chang et al., 2001). First clinical trials have been initiated with phenylbutyrate and showed a benefit in a small number of SMA type II patients in an open study design (Mercuri et al., 2004). However, many studies on protein expression, interactions and therapeutic effects in animals are required before a causal treatment of SMA 5q is on the horizon. At present, electrical stimulation cannot be recommended as a therapeutic tool. No drug treatment can be recommended.

Non-proximal SMA

Distal SMA (Table 55.4) accounts for about 10% of all SMA cases (Pearn & Hudgson, 1979), and comprises a group of genetically and clinically heterogeneous disorders, demonstrating a broad spectrum of clinical manifestations. Both autosomal dominant and recessive genes cause childhood- and adult-onset forms, which normally have a chronic and benign course. The early childhood form of distal SMA starts soon after birth with distal hypotonia and wasting and leads to pes planus and sometimes scoliosis within the first years of life. It is rarely dominantly inherited (Adams et al., 1998). Distal SMA is also denoted as distal hereditary motor neuronopathies (HNM) which are frequently listed among the Charcot–Marie–Tooth diseases. The HMNs are currently classified into types I–VII according to age at onset, mode of inheritance and predominantly involved muscle groups (De Jonghe et al., 1998), but this purely clinical classification will probably not hold when all genes have been identified (Irobi et al., 2004). By 2004 eight autosomal dominant entities have been assigned to genetic loci and six of them identified (Zerres & Rudnik-Schöneborn, 2005). A proportion of the CMT-like patients becomes wheelchair bound in due course and some even develop respiratory insufficiency necessitating artificial ventilation. Apart from exceptional families who fit well into the entities described (Irobi et al., 2004), genetic testing is not available to

Table 55.4. Non-proximal spinal muscular atrophies*

Name	Principal synonyms	Clinical features	Inheritance	Gene defect
Distal SMA	Peroneal muscular atrophy Distal hereditary motor neuronopathy (HMN)	Distal weakness (lower or upper limb predominance) with normal conduction velocities and normal sensory findings. Sometimes pyramidal features Onset birth–adulthood	A.r. (~75%) A.d. (~25%) X-linked (rare)	Eight gene loci and six identified genes. (For details see Irobi *et al.*, 2004.)
Segmental SMA	Monomelic juvenile SMA type Hirayama Benign monomelic amyotrophy	Asymmetrical involvement confined to upper (lower) extremities Onset 2nd decade, benign course (arrest usually after 2–4 years) Male predominance	Mostly non-genetic Few a.d. cases	Unknown
Distal SMA with myoclonus epilepsy		Myoclonus epilepsy, atactic movements, muscular hypotonia and generalized weakness, normal intelligence Onset mostly in childhood	A.r. A.d.	Unknown
Distal SMA with vocal cord paralysis	Hereditary motor neuronopathy type VII	Progressive distal wasting, hoarseness of voice, no bulbar palsy Onset in adulthood	A.d.	2q14 (a.d.)
Scapulo-peroneal muscular atrophy	Scapuloperoneal atrophy type Stark–Kaeser (dominant form)	Variable weakness of foot and toe extensors, shoulder girdle and upper arms, rarely with cardiopathy Onset in youth or adulthood	A.d. A.r. (X-linked)	12q23–24 (a.d.)
Spinobulbar neuronopathy	Kennedy disease	Proximal/distal weakness mostly in adulthood, gynecomastia, bulbar palsy, sensory disturbances	X-linked	Xq13.1 (CAG repeat expansion of the androgen receptor gene)
SMA with respiratory distress	Diaphragmatic SMA	Distal SMA with respiratory distress due to diaphragmatic palsy	A.r.	11q13–q21 IGHMBP2 gene

diagnose distal SMA. The genetic defects of most autosomal recessive forms of distal SMAs remain to be determined. A chronic distal SMA with early onset but late diaphragmatic dysfunction has been assigned to the same genetic region on chromosome 11q13 like diaphragmatic SMA (Viollet *et al.*, 2002).

For other entities see Table 55.4 and detailed reviews (Zerres & Rudnik-Schöneborn, 2002; Rudnik-Schöneborn *et al.*, 1996).

Future prospects

While dramatic progress has been made in the disclosure of the molecular mechanisms of infantile SMA with localization on chromosome 5q, little is known about the pathogenesis of other SMAs. The identification of other genes involved in motor neuron degeneration will help to differentiate entities and will provide further insight into the pathogenetic pathway of motor neuron degeneration. The SMN protein is involved in critical steps of messenger RNA transcription and processing, which indicates that the SMN protein fulfils an important cellular role that is not limited to motor neurons. Hence, it is still unclear while SMN deficiency specifically affects motor neuron function. The recently identified IGHMBP2 gene is believed to have a similar function in the RNA metabolism like SMN, but further studies are needed to confirm this. The knowledge of the genetic defect in SMA 5q is helpful in diagnostication and genetic risk calculation; however, at present its value for causal treatment is limited. As a high number of SMN2 copies might be able to partly compensate motor neuron loss, it is hoped to find pharmaceutically active substances that can increase the protein transcription of SMN2.

Therapeutic strategies include the search for compounds that can upregulate SMN2 gene expression, prevention of exon 7 skipping or stabilization of truncated SMN transcripts. One has to be aware of the fact that any drug treatment will most likely not be able to re-activate motor neurons that are already degenerated. This assumption has major implications for future therapeutic studies in infantile SMA. Hence, non-targeted therapeutics, which can prevent neurodegeneration, or neuron or muscle replacement by pluripotent cells are other therapeutic approaches (Nicole et al., 2002). It can be expected that many studies on protein expression, interactions and therapeutic effects in animals are required before a causal treatment of motor neuron degeneration is on the horizon.

REFERENCES

Adams, C., Suchowersky, O. & Lowry, R. B. (1998). Congenital autosomal dominant distal spinal muscular atrophy. *Neuromusc. Disord.*, **8**, 405–8.

Anhuf, D., Eggermann, T., Rudnik-Schöneborn, S. et al. (2003). Determination of SMN1 and SMN2 copy number using TaqMan™ technology. *Hum. Mutat.*

Borkowska, J., Rudnik-Schoneborn, S., Hausmanowa-Petrusewicz et al. (2002). Early infantile form of spinal muscular atrophy (Werdnig-Hoffmann disease) with prolonged survival. *Folia Neuropathol.*, **40**, 19–26.

Brzustowicz, L. M., Lehner, T., Castilla, L. H. et al. (1990). Genetic mapping of chronic childhood-onset spinal muscular atrophy to chromosome 5q11.2–13.3. *Nature*, **344**, 540–1.

Chang, J. G., Hsieh-Li, H. M., Jong, Y. J. et al. (2001). Treatment of spinal muscular atrophy by sodium butyrate. *Proc. Natl Acad. Sci., USA*, **98**, 9808–13.

Cifuentes-Diaz, C., Frugier, T., Tiziano, F. D. et al. (2001). Deletion of murine SMN exon 7 directed to skeletal muscle leads to severe muscular dystrophy. *J. Cell Biol.*, **5**, 1107–14.

Cox, G. A., Mahaffey, C. L. & Frankel, W. N. (1998). Identification of the mouse neuromuscular degeneration gene and mapping of a second site suppressor allele. *Neuron*, **21**, 1327–37.

Coovert, D. D., Le, T. T., McAndrew, P. E. et al. (1997). The survival motor neuron protein in spinal muscular atrophy. *Hum. Mol. Genet.*, **6**, 1205–14.

De Jonghe, P., Timmerman, V. & van Broeckhoven, C. (1998). 2nd workshop of the European CMT Consortium. *Neuromusc. Disord.*, **8**, 426.

Emery, A. E. H. (1971). The nosology of the spinal muscular atrophies. *J. Med. Genet.*, **8**, 481–95.

Emery, A. E. H., Davie, A. M., Holloway, S. et al. (1976). International collaborative study of the spinal muscular atrophies. Part II: Analysis of genetic data. *J. Neurol. Sci.*, **30**, 375–84.

Feldkötter, M., Schwarzer, V. & Wirth, R. (2002). Quantitative analyses of SMN1 and SMN2 based on real-time LightCycler PCR: fast and highly reliable carrier testing and prediction of severity of spinal muscular atrophy. *Am. J. Hum. Genet.*, **70**, 358–68.

Frugier, T., Tiziano, F. D., Cifuentes-Diaz, C. et al. (2000). Nuclear targeting of SMN lacking the C-terminus in a mouse model of spinal muscular atrophy. *Hum. Mol. Genet.*, **9**, 849–58.

Gambardella, A., Mazzei, R., Toscano, A. et al. (1998). Spinal muscular atrophy due to an isolated deletion of exon 8 of the telomeric survival motor neuron gene. *Ann. Neurol.*, **44**, 836–9.

Gilliam, T. C., Brzustowicz, L. M., Castilla, L. H. et al. (1990). Genetic homogeneity between acute and chronic forms of spinal muscular atrophy. *Nature*, **345**, 823–5.

Hahnen, E., Forkert, R., Marke, C. et al. (1995). Molecular analysis of candidate genes on chromosome 5q13 in autosomal recessive spinal muscular atrophy: evidence of homozygous deletions of the SMN gene in unaffected individuals. *Hum. Mol. Genet.*, **4**, 1927–33.

Hofmann, Y., Lorson, C. L., Stamm, S. et al. (2000). Htra2-beta 1 stimulates an exonic splicing enhancer and can restore full-length SMN expression to survival motor neuron 2 (SMN2). *Proc. Natl Acad. Sci., USA*, **15**, 9618–23.

Hsieh-Li, H., Chang, J. G., Jong, Y. J. et al. (2000). A mouse model for spinal muscular atrophy. *Nat. Genet.*, **24**, 66–70.

Irobi, J., DeJonghe, P. & Timmerman, V. (2004). Molecular genetics of distal hereditary motor neuropathies. *Hum. Mol. Genet.*, **13**, R195–R202.

Jablonka, S., Schrank, B., Kralewski, M. et al. (2000). Reduced survival motor neuron (smn) dose in mice leads to motor neuron degeneration: an animal model for spinal muscular atrophy type III. *Hum. Mol. Genet.*, **9**, 341–6.

Korinthenberg, R., Sauer, M., Ketelsen, U. P. et al. (1997). Congenital axonal neuropathy caused by deletions in the spinal muscular atrophy region. *Ann. Neurol.*, **42**, 364–8.

Lefebvre, S., Bürglen, L., Reboullet, S. et al. (1995). Identification and characterization of a spinal muscular atrophy-determining gene. *Cell*, **80**, 155–65.

Lorson, C. L., Hahnen, E., Androphy, E. J. et al. (1999). A single nucleotide in the SMN gene regulates splicing and is responsible for spinal muscular atrophy. *Proc. Natl Acad. Sci., USA*, **96**, 6307–11.

McLeod, J. G. & Prineas, J. W. (1971). Distal type of chronic spinal muscular atrophy. *Brain*, **94**, 703–14.

Melki, J., Abdelhak, S., Sheth, P. et al. (1990a). Gene for chronic spinal muscular atrophies maps to chromosome 5q. *Nature*, **344**, 767–8.

Melki, J., Sheth, P., Abdelhak, S. et al. (1990b). Mapping of acute (type 1) spinal muscular atrophy to chromosome 5q12–q14. *Lancet*, **336**, 271–3.

Mercuri, E., Bertini, E., Messina, S. et al. (2004). Pilot trial of phenylbutyrate in spinal muscular atrophy. *Neuromusc. Disord.* **14**, 130–5.

Monani, U. R., Sendtner, M., Coovert, D. D. et al. (2000a). The human centromeric survival motor neuron gene (SMN2) rescues embryonic lethality in Smn -/- mice and results in a mouse with spinal muscular atrophy. *Hum. Mol. Genet.*, **9**, 333–9.

Monani, U. R., Coovert, D. D., Burghes, A. H. M. (2000b). Animal models of spinal muscular atrophy. *Hum. Mol. Genet.*, **9**, 2451–7.

Nicole, S., Cifuentes-Diaz, C., Frugier, T. *et al.* (2002). Spinal muscular atrophy: recent advances and future prospects. *Muscle Nerve*, **26**, 4–13.

Parsons, D. W., McAndrew, P. E., Iannaconne, S. T. *et al.* (1998). Intragenic telSMN mutations: frequency, distribution, evidence of a founder effect, and modifications of the spinal muscular atrophy phenotype by cenSMN copy number. *Am. J. Hum. Genet.*, **63**, 1712–23.

Pearn, J. (1978a). Autosomal dominant spinal muscular atrophy. *J. Neurol. Sci.*, **38**, 263–75.

Pearn, J. (1978b). Incidence, prevalence, and gene frequency studies of chronic childhood spinal muscular atrophy. *J. Med. Genet.*, **15**, 409–13.

Pearn, J. & Hudgson, P. (1979). Distal spinal muscular atrophy: a clinical and genetic study of eight kindreds. *J. Neurol. Sci.*, **43**, 183–91.

Pioro, E. P. & Mitsumoto, H. (1996). Animal models of ALS. *Clin. Neurosci.*, **3**, 375–85.

Rietschel, M., Rudnik-Schöneborn, S. & Zerres, K. (1992). Clinical variability of autosomal dominant spinal muscular atrophy. *J. Neurol. Sci.*, **107**, 65–73.

Rochette, C. F., Gilbert, N. & Simard, L. R. (2001). SMN gene duplication and the emergence of the SMN2 gene occurred in distinct hominids: SMN2 is unique to *Homo sapiens*. *Hum. Genet.*, **108**, 255–66.

Rudnik-Schöneborn, S., Morgan, G., Röhrig, D. *et al.* (1994). Autosomal recessive proximal spinal muscular atrophy in 101 sibs out of 48 families: clinical picture, influence of gender and genetic implications. *Am. J. Med. Genet.*, **51**, 70–6.

Rudnik-Schöneborn, S., Forkert, R., Hahnen, E. *et al.* (1996). Clinical spectrum and diagnostic criteria of infantile spinal muscular atrophy: further delineation on the basis of SMN gene deletion findings. *Neuropediatrics*, **27**, 8–15.

Rudnik-Schöneborn, S., Lützenrath, S., Borkowska, J. *et al.* (1998). Analysis of creatine kinase activity in 504 patients with proximal spinal muscular atrophy types I–II from the point of view of progression and severity. *Eur. Neurol.*, **39**, 154–62.

Rudnik-Schöneborn, S., Goebel, H. H., Schlote, W. *et al.* (2003). Classical infantile spinal muscular atrophy with SMN deficiency causes sensory neuronopathy. *Neurology*, (in press)

Russman, B. S., Iannacone, S. T., Buncher, C. R. *et al.* (1992). Spinal muscular atrophy: new thoughts on the pathogenesis and classification schema. *J. Child Neurol.*, **7**, 347–53.

Russman, B. S., Buncher, C. R., White, M. *et al.* (1996). Function changes in spinal muscular atrophy II and III. The DCN/SMA Group. *Neurology*, **47**, 973–6.

Schmalbruch, H. & Haase, G. (2001). Spinal muscular atrophy: present state. *Brain Pathol.*, **11**, 231–74.

Sendtner, M. (2001). Molecular mechanisms in spinal muscular atrophy: models and perspectives. *Curr. Opin. Neurol.*, **14**, 629–34.

Veldink, J. H., van den Berg, L. H., Cobben, J. M. *et al.* (2001). Homozygous deletion of the survival motor neuron 2 gene is a prognostic factor in sporadic ALS. *Neurology*, **56**, 749–52.

Viollet, L., Barois, A., Rebeiz, J. G. *et al.* (2002). Mapping of autosomal recessive chronic distal spinal muscular atrophy to chromosome 11q13. *Ann. Neurol.*, **51**, 585–92.

Wirth, B., Herz, M., Wetter, A. *et al.* (1999). Quantitative analysis of SMN copies: identification of subtle SMNt mutations in SMA patients, genotype-phenotype correlation and implications for genetic counseling. *Am. J. Hum. Genet.*, **64**, 1340–56.

Zerres, K. & Davies, K. (1999). 59th ENMC International workshop: Spinal muscular atrophy. Recent progress and revised diagnostic criteria. *Neuromusc. Disord.*, **9**, 272–8.

Zerres, K. & Rudnik-Schöneborn, S. (1995). Natural history in proximal spinal muscular atrophy (SMA): clinical analysis of 445 patients and suggestions for a modification of existing classifications. *Arch. Neurol.*, **52**, 518.

(2005). Spinal muscular atrophies. In *Emery and Rimoin's Principles and Practice of Medical Genetics*, 5th edn. ed. D. L. Rimoin, J. M. Connor, R. E. Pyritz & B. R. Korf (in press).

Zerres, K., Rudnik-Schöneborn, S., Forkert, R. *et al.* (1995a). Genetic basis of adult-onset spinal muscular atrophy. *Lancet*, **346**, 741–2.

Zerres, K., Rudnik-Schöneborn, S., Dubowitz, V. *et al.* (1995b). Guidelines for symptomatic therapy in spinal muscular atrophy SMA. *Acta Cardiomiol.*, **7**, 61–6.

Zerres, K., Rudnik-Schöneborn, S., Forrest, E. *et al.* (1997). A collaborative study on the natural history of childhood and juvenile onset proximal spinal muscular atrophy (type II and III SMA): 569 patients. *J. Neurol. Sci.*, **146**, 67–72.

56

Western Pacific ALS/parkinsonism–dementia complex

Daniel P. Perl[1] and Patrick R. Hof[2]

[1] Department of Pathology, Neuropathology Division
[1, 2] Fishberg Research Center for Neurobiology
[2] Kastor Neurobiology of Aging Laboratories
[2] Department of Geriatrics and Adult Development, Mount Sinai School of Medicine, One Gustave L. Levy Place, New York, NY 10029

Introduction

Guam, the southernmost of the Marianas, an archipelago consisting of a chain of 15 islands, is the largest island in the western Pacific. The Marianas are part of Micronesia, a group of Pacific islands that, in addition to the Marianas, consists of the Carolines, the Marshalls, and the Gilberts. Guam is a relatively small island measuring approximately 20 miles long and from 4 to 9 miles wide (total area, 212 square miles). Located at 13 degrees north of the equator, Guam is approximately 3500 miles west of Hawaii, 1500 miles south of Tokyo and 1500 east of Manila. Guam was obtained by the United States as a territorial possession in 1898, as part of the settlement of the Spanish–American War. In the early portion of the twentieth century, Guam served as valuable stopping off place for coal-burning steamships needing to take on fresh water and other vital supplies during their long ocean-going voyages. From a military perspective, Guam's strategic central location in the western Pacific was also important and the United States Navy administered the island from 1898 until 1950 (with the exception of the Japanese occupation during World War II). In 1950, the Organic Act of Guam was passed by the US Congress and gave the inhabitants of Guam United States citizenship. This law also gave the inhabitants of Guam the right to elect a local governor and island legislature, and to send a non-voting representative to the US Congress. The people of Guam vote in American presidency elections, serve in the US military and pay Federal taxes (collected federal tax revenues remain on the island for local use).

In 2000, the population of Guam was 154 805, of which 57 297 (37%) identified themselves as Chamorros, 40 729 (26.3%) as Filipinos, 10 592 (%) as Caucasians (mostly migrants from the mainland USA) and 11 094 (7.2%) as other Micronesians. The Chamorros are an indigenous population who have continuously inhabited Guam since approximately 1500 BC, when they are believed to have originated from the Malay Archipelago. In 1521, the Portuguese explorer Ferdinand Magellan first encountered the Chamorros of Guam when some of his crew landed near the southern village of Umatac. Magellan and his crew were in the process of circumnavigating the world and this apparently represents the first encounter of the inhabitants of Micronesia with western Europeans. Magellan's crew stopped briefly on Guam to take on supplies after their long sojourn across the Pacific. Following leaving Guam, Magellan took his fleet to the Philippines, where he was killed in a violent dispute with local natives.

The presence of a high incidence focus of neurodegenerative disease on Guam was first brought to medical attention in 1945 by Dr. Harry M. Zimmerman, a pathologist who was assigned to Guam by the United States Navy. On December 8, 1941, the day after the Japanese attack on Pearl Harbor, Japanese forces also occupied Guam. For most of World War II, the Japanese military held Guam in a rather brutal occupation. However, in the summer of 1944, United States military forces retook the island from the Japanese. Owing to the island's relatively large size and strategic position, Guam served as a major staging area and supply site for bombing attacks of the major cities of Japan.

In the final year of World War II, large numbers of military personnel to support these operations were assigned to Guam, including Dr. Zimmerman. During his stay on Guam, Zimmerman identified a number of cases of amyotrophic lateral sclerosis among the native population being cared for in the local hospital, summarizing his findings in a report to his naval supervisors in Washington, DC, including the following: "During the past few months there were admitted to the medical wards of the Civilian Hospital 7 or 8 patients with a full-blown clinical picture of amyotrophic lateral sclerosis. This was surprising in view of the infrequency with which this neurologic disorder is encountered in the States. Two of the patients died during the month of May and the diagnosis was confirmed at autopsy. It is now planned to investigate the hereditary background of all these patients in an effort to throw some light on the factors concerned in the etiology of obscure malady." (Zimmerman, 1945)

Following the end of the war, Zimmerman's message was noted and a group of clinicians and epidemiologists were sent to Guam to investigate the situation further. These investigators confirmed Dr. Zimmerman's observations of a high prevalence of cases of amyotrophic lateral sclerosis among the native Chamorro population (Koerner, 1952; Arnold *et al.*, 1953). Moreover, in performing door-to-door surveys of neurologic disease on the island a second form of neurodegenerative disease was noted to be highly prevalent among the natives, characterized by parkinsonism with accompanying severe dementia. This other disorder was subsequently called parkinsonism–dementia complex of Guam. Remarkably, within this relatively small population, living in the middle of the Western Pacific, large numbers of natives showed clinical manifestations consisting of the key features of the three major age-related neurodegenerative disorders, namely, Parkinson's disease, Alzheimer's disease and amyotrophic lateral sclerosis (ALS). Although progress has been made in characterizing and understanding the focus, the reasons for this unique phenomenon have baffled numerous investigators for over 50 years and Guam remains a rich, yet perplexing opportunity to explore basic etiologic and pathogenetic mechanisms for neurodegeneration, as seen elsewhere in the world.

Clinical features

Amyotrophic lateral sclerosis of Guam (or the Marianas form of ALS)

Experts on the clinical features of ALS have repeatedly indicated that the disease, as it is seen in the inhabitants of Guam, is virtually indistinguishable from the sporadic form of the disease, as encountered elsewhere in the world (Kurland & Mulder, 1954; Kurland *et al.*, 1956). On Guam, the disease typically begins in an insidious fashion with complaints of weakness, clumsiness and/or an unexplained weight loss. Early clinical signs may include muscle weakness, or atrophy accompanied by prominent muscular fasciculations and hyperreflexia. The disease inexorably progresses and within approximately a year prominent muscular atrophy, weakness and a flaccid paralysis are notable. In approximately 10–15% of cases,

spasticity, in the absence of identifiable muscular wasting, is noted early in the course of the illness. In later stages, prominent dysphagia and dysarthria are seen as the level of paralysis proceeds in a classic ascending fashion. As will be discussed below, despite the fact that such patients show a rather widespread and extensive distribution of neurofibrillary tangle (NFT) formation, dementia has been noted clinically in only about 10% of ALS cases seen on Guam. Death is typically the result of aspiration and/or hypostatic pneumonia. Affected individuals generally survive for approximately 2–4 years following initial diagnosis. As with the sporadic disease seen elsewhere in the world, occasional patients are encountered with more rapid progression of the illness while others have been followed with unusually prolonged periods of survival (Uebayashi, 1984; Rogers-Johnson *et al.*, 1986). Those patients with prolonged survival will typically progress in a slower fashion and their disease progression may actually plateau over a period of many years without further deterioration in their neurologic deficits. Indeed, rare individuals with the Guamanian form of ALS, verified neuropathologically at autopsy, have been followed clinically for over 15 years.

Parkinsonism–dementia complex of Guam

Parkinsonism-dementia complex of Guam was first described clinically by Kurland and Mulder and was subsequently defined as a clinicopathologic entity in the seminal papers by Hirano and colleagues (Hirano *et al.*, 1961a, b). Apparently, an earlier account of the disorder had been published in 1936 (Yase *et al.*, 1978). The major features of the disease combine parkinsonism with severe progressive loss of cognitive function. Parkinsonian features include rigidity, bradykinesia and gait disturbance. While a 4–7 Hz pill-rolling at rest "parkinsonian" tremor of the hands may be noted in some patients, it is rarely incapacitating or as prominent a feature as occurs in idiopathic Parkinson's disease. Some patients show an impairment of ocular motility which is reminiscent of patients with progressive supranuclear palsy (Lepore *et al.*, 1988). As the disease progresses, the bradykinesia and rigidity increase in severity and become a major cause of disability.

The dementia accompanying the disorder includes severe memory impairment, disorientation and difficulty with reasoning and simple calculations. In about 30% of cases, the dementia precedes the parkinsonian features which are then encountered somewhat later in the course of the disease (Elizan *et al.*, 1966). Severe personality changes, in the form of agitation, apathy, irritability and occasionally prominent aggressiveness, may be encountered in the illness and are noted somewhere in the disease course in approximately one third of cases. It is an unremittingly progressive and invariably fatal disorder and typically leads to death within 4–6 years after the initial diagnosis. Although initial therapy with levodopa may produce some modest improvement in the parkinsonian features (Schnur et al., 1971), the Guam patients soon become refractory to its effects.

Marianas dementia

More recent door-to-door surveys of neurologic disease on Guam have identified Chamorro patients suffering from dementia, in the absence of overt accompanying signs of amyotrophy or extrapyramidal features. Such individuals have been mostly women who live in the southern villages of the island and some have shown onset of symptoms in their 60s. A small number of these patients have now been followed longitudinally. Some have gone on to develop parkinsonian features indicative of parkinsonism–dementia complex of Guam. This is not surprising since many years ago Elizan and coworkers noted that 30% of parkinsonism dementia complex present with dementia (Elizan et al., 1966). However, others have shown a course with progressive cognitive loss in the absence of any superimposed parkinsonian signs or motor weakness. We have tentatively referred to this entity as "Marianas dementia," pending more detailed clinical, neuropsychological and neuropathological characterization. A limited number of autopsies have been performed on such patients and neuropathologic examination and some have revealed the typical changes associated with ALS/parkinsonism–dementia complex (Perl et al., 1994; Galasko et al., 2002). Others have shown changes of Alzheimer's disease. The cases with ALS/parkinsonism–dementia complex changes suggest that the outbreak of neurodegenerative disease on Guam may also have a form featuring an onset and clinical course consisting of a purely progressive dementing syndrome, in the absence of amyotrophy and/or parkinsonism. This may thus represent an additional clinical profile for this disorder.

Neuropathologic features of ALS/parkinsonism–dementia complex

Grossly visible features

Almost invariably, brain specimens derived from patients with either ALS or parkinsonism–dementia complex show some degree (usually prominent) of generalized cerebral atrophy accompanied by severely dilated lateral ventricles.

The brain weights of severely affected end-stage cases are frequently less than 1000 g and brains that weigh less than 900 g have been observed. In patients with parkinsonism–dementia complex the pigmented nuclei of the brainstem, the substantia nigra and locus coeruleus, are notably pale upon gross inspection. Patients with ALS often show a subtle discoloration of the lateral columns of the spinal cord that is visible with the naked eye. Atrophy of the ventral spinal roots (particularly when compared to the dorsal roots) is also easily recognized.

Microscopic features

Neurofibrillary tangles

The microscopic hallmark of both the Guamanian form of ALS and of parkinsonism–dementia complex is the presence of severe and widespread NFT formation. It was Nathan Malamud who first noted their presence in ALS cases from Guam (Malamud et al., 1961). They were further characterized in the seminal papers of Hirano and colleagues (Malamud et al., 1961; Hirano & Zimmerman, 1962; Hirano et al., 1967a). Severe NFT involvement is typically seen in the hippocampus, entorhinal cortex, amygdala and neocortex. In some cases the CA1 region of the hippocampus can show virtually complete involvement of every pyramidal neuron by NFTs. Such cases are generally accompanied by extensive neuronal loss in the hippocampus and the appearance of many extracellular "ghost" tangles with a prominent reactive glial response.

Curiously, patients with Guamanian ALS may show rather extensive hippocampal NFT formation at autopsy, yet during life had been considered to possess intact cognitive function. Clearly, in the later stages of ALS patients may have severe dysphonia, bordering on aphonia, and this inability to communicate may prevent proper assessment of cognitive function. Nevertheless, such patients appear, within their obvious physical limitations, to be able to follow and carry out commands. Such observations appear to suggest that severe involvement of the CA1 of the hippocampus by NFTs may not be associated with severe cognitive losses, particularly involving recent memory processing, as has been assumed to be operative in cases of Alzheimer's disease.

Patients demonstrating prominent extrapyramidal features show extensive NFT formation in brainstem regions, including the periaqueductal gray matter, substantia nigra and locus coeruleus. In such regions the NFTs have a globoid appearance reflecting the rounded shape of the soma, as opposed to the flame-shaped configuration seen in pyramidal neurons with NFTs. Cases with particularly severe NFT formation may display NFTs in the dentate nucleus of the cerebellum, inferior olivary nuclei and anterior horn cells.

Based on immunohistochemical and electron microscopic studies, the NFTs of patients with ALS/parkinsonism–dementia complex are virtually identical to those encountered in cases of Alzheimer's disease seen elsewhere in the world (Hirano et al., 1968; Hirano, 1973; Shankar et al., 1989). Ultrastructural studies have shown that while the NFTs of the Guam cases contain paired-helical filaments, they also commonly show admixed additional straight filaments. The NFTs of the Guam cases react with antibodies directed against abnormally phosphorylated tau protein (Buée-Scherrer et al., 1995a; Buée-Scherrer et al., 1995b), apolipoprotein E (Buée et al., 1996), lactotransferrin (Leveugle et al., 1994), beta-amyloid peptide (Ito et al., 1991) and ubiquitin, all of which parallel findings seen in the NFTs of Alzheimer's disease. Buée-Scherrer and coworkers (Buée-Scherrer et al., 1995a,b) have demonstrated that PHF-tau derived from cases of ALS/parkinsonism–dementia complex are abnormally phosphorylated and have biochemical and immunological properties that are virtually identical to the PHF-tau of Alzheimer's disease. The six isoform pattern of tau is formed in an identical fashion to that seen in cases of Alzheimer's disease. Recent studies have shown that PHF-tau associated with ALS/parkinsonism–dementia complex is phosphorylated at the identical amino acid residues as is Alzheimer's disease-related PHF-tau (Mawal-Dewan et al., 1996).

The pattern of neocortical involvement by NFTs in cases of ALS/parkinsonism–dementia complex differs significantly from what is seen in cases of Alzheimer's disease (Hof et al., 1991). In ALS/parkinsonism–dementia complex, the neocortical NFTs are most densely situated in layers II–III, when compared to the extent of involvement in layer V. This pattern of involvement differs from what is seen in cases of Alzheimer's disease, where NFT formation is more severe in the deeper layer (layer V), when compared to more superficial aspects of the cortex (layers II–III). As a general rule, parkinsonism-dementia complex cases are more severely affected by NFTs than are cases of ALS (Hof et al., 1994). Both ALS and parkinsonism–dementia complex of Guam show relatively severe involvement of the primary motor cortex by NFTs, as opposed to cases of Alzheimer's disease where such involvement is not encountered (Hof & Perl, 2002). The pattern of neocortical NFT formation demonstrated in cases of ALS/parkinsonism–dementia complex is also a characteristic feature of cases of postencephalitic parkinsonism (Hof et al., 1992b), post-traumatic dementia (dementia pugalistica) (Hof et al.,

1992a), and progressive supranuclear palsy (Hof et al., 1992c). In ALS/parkinsonism–dementia complex neurons containing the calcium-binding proteins calbindin, calretinin and parvalbumin tend to be spared from involvement in NFT formation (Hof et al., 1994), a finding that is identical to that seen in cases of Alzheimer's disease.

Beta amyloid accumulation in ALS/parkinsonism-dementia Complex of Guam

The classic neuropathologic descriptions of ALS and parkinsonism–dementia complex by Hirano make specific note of the lack of senile plaque formation in these cases, despite the presence of large numbers of NFTs. Subsequently, Guam cases considered to be senile plaque-free based on silver staining methods have been shown to be free of parenchymal amyloid accumulation by more sensitive immunohistochemical methods (Gentleman et al., 1991). More recently, about one third of autopsied cases demonstrate some degree of parenchymal amyloid accumulation. Such cases contain amyloid deposits in the form of diffuse plaques lacking any accompanying dystrophic neuritic changes. Neuritic plaques may be encountered in some cases of ALS/parkinsonism–dementia complex of Guam, however, the density of plaques seen in such cases is typically rather small. Vascular amyloid deposition (congophilic angiopathy) is notably uncommon in Guam-derived brain specimens. When present, such vascular deposits are typically scanty and the explanation for the paucity of vascular involvement remains unclear.

Eosinophilic rod-like inclusions (Hirano bodies)

Hirano's original descriptions of the neuropathologic features of ALS/parkinsonism–dementia complex included reference to eosinophilic rod-like inclusion bodies noted in the CA1 region of the hippocampus. These prominently stained inclusions are encountered immediately adjacent to the pyramidal neurons and had not apparently been previously described. They were initially considered to be unique and specific for the Guam disease but were subsequently noted in relatively small numbers in the hippocampus of some cases of Alzheimer's disease, Pick's disease and Creutzfeldt–Jakob disease. When seen in these settings the number of such inclusions was typically much smaller than is usually encountered in the Guam cases. Rare examples of the rod-like inclusions may also be encountered in the brains of elderly non-demented controls elsewhere in the world (Gibson & Tomlinson, 1977; Hirano, 1994).

The small number of such inclusions is the likely reason that, over the decades, neuropathologists failed to recognize them. It was only when Hirano encountered numerous eosinophilic rod-like inclusions in the specimens he examined on Guam that they were readily identified and thus characterized. Hirano later showed their unique "herring-bone" ultrastructural appearance. Immunohistochemical studies revealed that they contain actin and actin-associated proteins (Goldman, 1983; Galloway et al., 1987a), tau (Galloway et al., 1987b) and the middle molecular weight neurofilament protein (Schmidt et al., 1989). These eosinophilic rod-like inclusions are now referred to by most neuropathologists as "Hirano bodies" in honor of his contributions in first characterizing this lesion. The Hirano body represents an example of how, through the presence of a high density of lesions, as occurs in Guam ALS/parkinsonism–dementia complex, important insights may be gained in our understanding of Alzheimer's disease and related conditions.

Granulovacuolar degeneration

Granulovacuolar degeneration is a poorly understood alteration encountered in the hippocampus of cases of Alzheimer's disease and the normal elderly. This lesion consists of multiple vacuoles, each with a single internal deeply basophilic granule, present within the perikaryal cytoplasm of pyramidal neurons in the boundary zone of the H1 and H2 regions of the hippocampus. In the normal elderly they are seen in relatively small numbers but when present in relatively large numbers, especially in the posterior portion of the hippocampus, they correlate highly with a diagnosis of Alzheimer's disease (Tomlinson & Kitchener, 1972; Ball & Lo, 1977). Granulovacuolar degeneration is extremely prominent in the hippocampus of cases of ALS/parkinsonism–dementia complex. Although there are no specific quantitative data available, it is our impression that in Guam cases one sees larger numbers of involved neurons and within each involved neuron the number of vacuoles present is greater. The size of the individual granules also appears to be larger.

Lewy bodies and other alpha-synuclein immunoreactive inclusions

Those cases with prominent parkinsonian clinical manifestations may show a severe degree of cell loss in the substantia nigra and locus coeruleus with accompanying gliosis, incontinent neuromelanin pigment and phagocytosed neuromelanin granules within local macrophages. Rare remaining pigmented neurons will typically contain globoid-shaped NFTs. In end-stage cases the extent of nigral degeneration can be so complete that it may be difficult to identify any remaining intact pigmented neurons. Lewy bodies are rarely encountered in cases

of parkinsonism-dementia complex. A large retrospective study of Guam cases reported that approximately 10% showed evidence of Lewy bodies in either the substantia nigra or the locus coeruleus (Rogers-Johnson et al., 1986). Our experience has been quite similar. Whenever nigral or locus coeruleus Lewy bodies are identified in the Guam cases they are usually few in number and other adjacent intact pigmented neurons will show globoid tangles. The Lewy bodies in Guam cases found in these locations react immunohistochemically to ubiquitin and α-synuclein. It is of interest that, despite autopsy examination of the majority of patients from Guam who had suffered from parkinsonian symptoms over a period of over 40 years, examples of Lewy body Parkinson's disease in Chamorros have been extremely rare. Indeed, the authors are aware of only a single such case being documented at autopsy in a Chamorro native from Guam. The explanation for this absence of what is a relatively common disorder, elsewhere in the world, remains unknown.

We and others have reported evidence of α-synuclein-immunoreactive inclusion bodies occurring in the amygdala of cases of ALS/parkinsonism–dementia complex (Yamazaki et al., 2000; Forman et al., 2002). In our recent report on the findings in a series of 30 Chamorro brain specimens (Forman et al., 2002), 37% of patients with parkinsonism–dementia complex showed evidence of α-synuclein pathology but this was not detected in any Chamorros with ALS or Alzheimer's disease. Most amygdala α-synuclein aggregates occurred within neurons that also were harboring a NFT. This suggested to us that there was a possible interaction between the two proteins. Other than the presence of parkinsonism–dementia complex, there was no particular clinical manifestation that distinguished the cases with α-synuclein pathology.

Other microscopic features

Neuropil threads, a prominent feature of AD, are rarely encountered in cases of ALS/parkinsonism–dementia complex (Wakayama et al., 1993). On the other hand, similar thread-like structures have been reported in the white matter of the spinal cord, especially in patients who exhibit more prominent amyotrophic features (Umahara et al., 1994).

Using antibodies raised against the protein core of heparin sulfate proteoglycans, severe abnormalities of the cerebral microvasculature were noted in brain specimens of parkinsonism–dementia complex patients (Buée et al., 1994). The pattern of distribution of these vascular lesions suggests a spatial association between the microvascular abnormalities and a high density of NFT formation. Similar lesions have been seen in cases of Alzheimer's disease where they were thought to be related to local vascular and/or parenchymal beta-amyloid deposition. The Guam cases, with their absence of amyloid deposition, provide an opportunity to demonstrate that amyloid deposition is not required for the formation of these vascular abnormalities.

In cases of Guamanian ALS there is prominent loss of anterior horn cells, similar to that seen in the disease elsewhere in the world. Surviving anterior horn cells may show a shrunken soma with a pyknotic nucleus, or else the cell may be swollen with perikaryal accumulations of phosphorylated neurofilaments. As in classic ALS, intervening anterior horn cells may possess a normal histologic appearance. In some Guam patients with ALS, the remaining anterior horn cells may display small eosinophilic inclusions in their cytoplasm. These were first described by Bunina (1962) and are frequently referred to as "Bunina bodies." Similar to cases of sporadic ALS seen elsewhere in the world (Mourelatos et al., 1990), Guam ALS cases show fragmentation of the Golgi apparatus (Mourelatos et al., 1994). Upper motor neuron involvement is virtually always present in the Guam cases and results in prominent myelin loss in both the lateral and anterior corticospinal tracts. In contrast to some cases of familial ALS (Hirano et al., 1967b), the posterior columns of the cases of Guam ALS remain intact.

Neuropathologic studies of Chamorros of Guam with intact neurologic function

In 1979, Anderson and co-workers (1979) reported on the extent and distribution of NFT formation encountered in the brains of Chamorros living on Guam who, during life, had shown no evidence of neurological disease. Specifically, this autopsy-based study was conducted on individuals who died between 1968 and 1974 and, based on their clinical histories and autopsy reports, were considered to be free of evidence of dementia, parkinsonism or amyotrophy. Their study showed that a remarkably high percentage of relatively young Chamorro "controls" living on Guam displayed evidence of prominent NFT formation. The authors noted that when extensive NFT occurred, the overall brain distribution approached that described in full-blown diagnosed cases of ALS/parkinsonism–dementia complex. Although not overtly stated in their report, these findings suggest that Chamorros subjects who demonstrated a prominent degree of NFT formation represented unrecognized preclinical cases of ALS/parkinsonism–dementia complex. The implication was that had the subjects identified with these neuropathologic features survived to a more advanced age they would have accumulated a sufficient extent of pathologic damage to attract clinical attention and ultimately a specific neurologic diagnosis.

We had an opportunity to re-examine the microscopic slides used for the Anderson et al. study and to compare the extent of NFT formation seen in those specimens to that obtained from a new series of Chamorros without a diagnosis of neurologic disease who had died between 1988 and 1996 (Perl et al., 2003). Both sets of cases were compared to a group of brain specimens derived from age-matched subjects, free of neurologic dysfunction in life, who were autopsied at the Mount Sinai Hospital in New York, thus representing examples of normal aging in a non-Guamanian setting. We were particularly interested to see if neurologically intact Chamorros living on Guam continue to demonstrate prominent NFT formation. Furthermore, we were interested in whether the age at which such neurodegenerative changes became manifested would increase in parallel to that seen in newly diagnosed cases of ALS and PDC.

We found that a sizeable proportion of neurologically intact Guamanian Chamorros in the general population continue to show evidence of extensive NFT formation. There was not an appreciable change in the tendency of the Guamanian Chamorro to develop severe entorhinal and hippocampal NFTs, although the data suggested that it is less frequently seen among those under age 50. Of Guamanian Chamorros between the ages 50 and 64 years, 67% displayed greater than 6 NFTs/mm^2 in the CAl region of the hippocampus, a severe rating using the CERAD neuropathology protocol for Alzheimer's disease (Mirra et al., 1991), and 22% had greater than 40 NFTs/mm^2. Although these patients had not received formal neuropsychological evaluations during life, these findings raise important questions regarding the clinical significance of hippocampal involvement by NFTs, in general.

Studies of this type indicate that the Chamorro population of Guam continues to demonstrate an extent of NFT formation that is unprecedented and far in excess of what has been reported in populations elsewhere in the world. Further, it is clear that whatever is responsible for the remarkable outbreak of neurodegenerative disease on Guam is still demonstrating its effects on the local native population. These findings are well beyond those encountered in association with normal aging and the pattern of NFT formation in the neocortex, substantia nigra and locus coeruleus was not consistent with this interpretation. This was further reinforced by the lack of accompanying beta-amyloid accumulation in the form of senile plaques and vascular amyloid deposition. We believe that the Guam natives we have identified with evidence of prominent NFT formation do represent early stages of ALS/parkinsonism–dementia complex in individuals who have yet to develop a burden of neurodegenerative lesions sufficient to manifest overt neurologic symptomatology, a conclusion that was shared by Anderson and his coworkers in their 1979 report (Anderson *et al.*, 1979).

Like Alzheimer's disease, ALS/parkinsonism–dementia complex develops slowly and it is to be expected that it would take many years for a sufficient degree of neuropathologic damage to accumulate before there is a sufficient functional impairment for a clinical diagnosis to be entertained. The non-overtly impaired individuals identified by us and by Anderson in all likelihood represent preclinical ALS/parkinsonism–dementia complex patients who have died prematurely of other causes. Had they survived longer we believe these individuals would have gone on to show clinically recognizable features of ALS/parkinsonism–dementia complex. On the other hand, whether they were truly asymptomatic, as Anderson and coworkers suggested, is more difficult to speculate upon. It is more likely that had the individuals harboring these examples of rather severe NFT formation in their brains been carefully evaluated, subtle (and perhaps, not so subtle) functional deficits would have been detected on neuropsychological testing. Nevertheless, it is clear that, despite the extent of pathology documented at autopsy, the clinicians responsible for their medical care and their families were not sufficiently aware of these deficits to seek further neurologic evaluation.

Epidemiology

Over the years, many epidemiologic studies of the extent and distribution of neurologic disease among the inhabitants of Guam and its neighboring islands have been carried out. These studies were initiated in the 1950s and have continued, of and on, until the present day. Earlier studies established that the incidence of ALS on Guam was 50 to 100 times greater than was seen in the continental US and in certain of the small villages in the southern part of Guam, considerably higher rates were noted. A high incidence of the disease was also seen in the next nearest island, Rota, also populated by Chamorros. For the period 1947–1953, the average annual incidence rate of ALS for Chamorros living on Guam was twice as high for men when compared to women (85 and 40 per 100 000, respectively) with a mean age of onset of 44 years in both sexes. ALS accounted for approximately 10% of all deaths on the island, a figure that was 50 times greater than reported for the continental USA. Subsequent studies comparing rates over the period of 1945–1972 indicated a steady decline in the age-adjusted incidence rate for ALS on Guam. These data included rates for men of 67/100 000 population in 1950–1954 to 21/100 000 in 1970–1972 and of 43 and 12/100 000 for women. Finally, in 1980–1982, Garutto and coworkers

(1985) found the age-adjusted incidence rates of ALS on Guam to be less than 5/100 000 for both men and women.

In 1961, with the identification of parkinsonism–dementia complex of Guam as a distinct clinicopathologic entity, epidemiologic studies were also initiated for this condition. In 1962, Lessel and colleagues (1962) reported a prevalence for parkinsonism–dementia complex of 118/100 000 with a mean age of onset of 50 years and a male/female ratio of 2.5:1. The average annual mortality rate for the condition was 28/100 000 with a median survival of 3.5 years. Based on door-to-door surveys Reed *et al.* (1966) reported the average annual incidence per 100 000 population of parkinsonism-dementia complex to be 33 for men and 6 for women. Again, in 1985, Garruto *et al.* reported a significant decline in age-adjusted incidence rates for men and women with parkinsonism-dementia complex. Based on these reports it was widely reported that the neurodegenerative diseases on Guam were declining at a rate that suggested that before long the unique opportunity to identify important etiologic clues would be lost which might represent avenues for understanding comparable diseases elsewhere in the world (Stone, 1993). In 1990, with funding from the National Institute on Aging, the Micronesian Health Study Registry, initially directed by Dr. W. C. Wiederholt and now led by Dr. Douglas Galasko, was begun. Data from this registry indicates that parkinsonism–dementia complex is not disappearing and during 1980–1989 there was an average annual incidence of about 10 cases/100 000 population. Of interest is that the age of onset of this disorder had increased to 68.1 years (Wiederholt, 1999; Galasko *et al.*, 2000, 2002).

Other foci of ALS/parkinsonism–dementia complex

In addition to the focus of ALS/parkinsonism–dementia complex identified and extensively studied on Guam, two similar foci of endemic neurodegenerative disease have been reported, namely in the Kii Peninsula of Japan and among the Auyu and Jakai people of the Irian Jaya region of southwestern New Guinea. Kinnosuke Miura, a pupil of Charcot, published the first clinical description of a case of ALS in Japan (Miura, 1902). He subsequently claimed that ALS was more common among the Japanese than was seen in Europe and noted the unusually high incidence of the disease in the Kii Peninsula, a remote area on the southern coast of the Japanese island of Honshu (Miura, 1911). Subsequent studies indicated that the high prevalence of ALS was mostly confined to two isolated districts in the Kii Peninsula, Kozagawa and Hobara (Shiraki & Yase, 1975; Shiraki & Yase, 1991). Surveys indicated the annual incidence of ALS was 15 cases per 100 000 population in Kozagawa and 55 cases per 100 000 in Hobara.

Neuropathologic studies of ALS cases from the Kii Peninsula revealed a pattern of neuropathologic changes that is virtually identical to that seen on Guam (Shiraki & Yase, 1975, 1991). In cases from the Japanese foci, widespread NFT formation in a pattern that parallels closely what is seen in the Guam cases has been documented. Over the past 30 years the number of cases of ALS encountered in the Kii Peninsula has diminished dramatically, similar to what has been seen on Guam. Until recently cases of parkinsonism–dementia complex from the Kii Peninsula had not been reported. However, Kuzuhara and colleagues (Kokubo *et al.*, 2000; Kuzuhara *et al.*, 2001; Itoh *et al.*, 2003) have now described such cases both clinically and at autopsy. These cases have shown neuropathologic features that are virtually identical to those encountered on Guam.

The focus in the Irian Jaya region of southwestern New Guinea was first identified by Gajdusek, who described a high incidence of ALS based on brief clinical observations while passing through this extremely remote and primitive region (Gajdusek, 1963). It should be noted that this was completely separate and not related to the highland region of New Guinea where he had studied kuru among the Fore natives (Gajdusek, 1977). Gajdusek subsequently returned to the area where he had noted the ALS cases and surveyed the population more thoroughly for all forms of neurologic disease (Gajdusek & Salazar, 1980). They reported an average annual incidence of ALS for the period 1974–1980 of 147 per 1 000 000 (almost 150 times greater than is seen in the continental USA). In the same population the incidence of parkinsonism, both with and without dementia, was 79 per 100 000 population. The mean age of onset in the population for ALS and parkinsonism was 33 and 43 years, respectively, both substantially younger than was seen on Guam, even in the immediate post-World War II era. Unfortunately, although the clinical features of these patients appear quite similar to the disorder seen on Guam, no neuropathologic studies have ever been carried out on the cases from this extremely remote region.

Considerations of etiology

Nature vs. nurture

Dating from the earliest observations of Dr. Zimmerman, the inordinately high prevalence of neurodegenerative diseases among the Chamorro population of Guam has offered the promise of providing insights into etiologic factors responsible for the three analogous disorders seen elsewhere in the world, namely, ALS, Parkinson's disease and Alzheimer's disease. Zimmerman considered Guam to be an example of an island-bound genetic isolate and naturally assumed the focus to be hereditary in nature. However, a number of studies have shown that, if genetic factors are present, and they most certainly are, they are clearly not etiologic in nature and likely serve only as modifying factors related to relative susceptibility to an, as yet, unidentified environmental etiologic agent (or agents).

One of the major pieces of evidence implicating environmental factors in the etiology of the neurodegenerative disorders encountered on Guam has been the appearance of significant numbers of cases of ALS and parkinsonism–dementia complex among Filipino migrants to Guam who have had long-term residence on the island. Since the 1950s to the present time, there has been a sizable migration of individuals born and raised in the Philippines who have moved and settled permanently on Guam. These migrants do not originate from any one village or region in the Philippines and represent a rather broad spectrum of locations within this large and rather diverse nation. These immigrants have almost entirely been male and now make up a community of approximately 40 000 stable residents on Guam. Many of the Filipino migrants have married native Chamorro women and have adopted, more or less, a Guamanian way of life. However, most Filipino migrants do not eat cycad-based products and they do not eat flying foxes (see discussion of environmental agents, below). Among this Filipino migrant community, many cases of ALS have been documented. Reed and Brody first noted such cases (Reed & Brody, 1975) and Garruto *et al.* (1981) further documented nine cases of ALS and two with parkinsonism-dementia complex. Except for three cases of ALS that had developed within 3 years of their arrival on Guam, the onset of disease was at least 13 years after moving to the island. A small number of autopsies have been performed on the Filipino migrant ALS cases and NFTs have been documented in the brain specimens of half of these cases. The extent of NFT involvement was not as dramatic and widespread as is typically encountered in the native Chamorro cases, but this finding clearly separates them from sporadic ALS, as seen elsewhere in the world, since NFTs are not a recognized neuropathologic feature of ALS, especially among relatively young patients. We wonder if, in the Filipino migrant ALS cases reported as being without NFTs, the search for such lesions had been sufficiently thorough to consider them to be truly negative.

Additional cases of ALS continue to be identified among the Filipino migrant community living on Guam. Neuropathologic examination of these cases show motor neuron degeneration accompanied by mild to moderate involvement by NFTs, fitting the distribution pattern of

Guam neurodegeneration. This indicates that they are not merely incidental cases of sporadic ALS among this population but an extension of the outbreak of neurodegeneration among inhabitants of Guam. Importantly, encountering cases of parkinsonism-dementia complex among this Filipino migrant population on Guam further reinforces the concept that long-term residence on the island underlies the cause of the outbreak of neurodegenerative disease. ALS is a disease that has been seen throughout the world, yet parkinsonism–dementia complex is a disorder that has not been encountered outside the three foci of the western Pacific discussed above.

Garruto *et al.* (1981) reported clinical evaluation of a single case of parkinsonism-dementia complex in a Filipino migrant to Guam, however, no autopsy was performed on this individual. We have had the opportunity to examine the brains of two patients with parkinsonism accompanied by dementia occurring in Filipino migrants following more than 25 years of residence on Guam (Purohit *et al.*, 1992). Both cases showed the characteristic neuropathologic features of parkinsonism–dementia complex and were virtually identical to what we commonly encounter in the native Chamorro cases. In both, there was widespread, rather severe NFT formation in the hippocampus, entorhinal cortex and neocortex, in the absence of parenchymal amyloid deposition. The NFTs were predominant in the superficial cortical layers. There was severe loss of pigmented neurons in the substantia nigra and locus coeruleus with globoid forms of NFTs being seen in several remaining neurons in these nuclei. Lewy bodies were not encountered in either the pigmented neurons or the neocortex. An additional autopsy-confirmed case of parkinsonism–dementia complex in a Filipino migrant to Guam was reported by Chen *et al.* (1982). These three autopsy-proven cases represent important evidence that ALS/parkinsonism–dementia complex is not a disorder that is unique to the Chamorro population, but may also be seen in Filipinos who have lived on Guam for many years. Unless there is a hitherto unrecognized focus of ALS/parkinsonism–dementia complex in the Philippine islands, then these findings strongly support the concept that long-term exposure to a putative environmental agent present on Guam is responsible for the epidemic.

Migration studies of the Chamorros of Guam

If there is a putative environmental agent responsible for ALS/parkinsonism–dementia complex of Guam then there must be a considerable period of latency between initial exposure to such an agent and the eventual onset of neurodegenerative disease. The primary evidence for this has been studies of the large number of Chamorros of Guam who have migrated off the island. In 1950, the inhabitants of Guam were finally granted full American citizenship and from then on were allowed to travel freely and resettle anywhere they wished in the continental United States. This newly gained freedom prompted an extensive outmigration of Guamanian Chamorros to selected locations along the west coast, such as Chula Vista, San Jose and Oakland, California as well as Bremerton, Washington. In 1957, a survey of 165 adult Guamanians who had migrated to California revealed two patients with ALS. Although the sample was small, this was equivalent to a rate for the disease that was equal to what was then present on Guam (Torres *et al.*, 1957). As part of the survey activities, the investigators also learned of five additional cases of ALS among this migrant population who had died prior to the initiation of the survey. A follow-up study in 1966–1967 by Eldridge *et al.* (1969) found that of 321 Guamanians over age 40 who were then living in California, two were suffering from ALS and another two had parkinsonism–dementia complex.

Garruto *et al.* (1980) subsequently attempted to identify all Guamanian Chamorros who had migrated from the island and eventually developed ALS. They found a total of 28 cases (some of whom were included in the two prior published surveys). Of these, 21 cases had developed ALS while living in the continental United States, three had their onset in other countries (Japan, Germany and Korea) and four became ill following returning to Guam but only after long-term residence on the United States mainland. Ten of these cases had undergone postmortem studies and these showed evidence of widespread NFT formation, confirming these to be examples of the Guamanian form of the disease. In Garutto's migration study, the mean age at migration from Guam was 29.4 years (range, 18 to 63 years) with an average number of years living off Guam prior to the onset of disease of 13.6 years (range, 1 to 34 years). The mean age of onset of ALS was 48.8 years which, at that time, was 4 years younger than was being seen among Chamorros who had never left Guam. Some of these cases had developed more than 20 years after migrating from Guam.

Using the above data, Garruto and Yanigihara (1991) estimated that ALS mortality rates for Chamorros living on Guam were three times greater than for Chamorros who had migrated to the west coast, suggesting that outmigration had significantly lowered their subsequent risk of developing the disease. Nevertheless, Chamorros living off Guam still showed a five to tenfold increased risk of developing ALS, when compared to the non-Guamanian population of the mainland United States. In addition, Guamanians migrating to the continental United States were at risk of developing parkinsonism–dementia complex, a disease that has no direct counterpart in populations elsewhere in the world. Review of all of the migration studies suggests that the enhanced risk of developing ALS/parkinsonism–dementia complex is attained within the first 18 years of life and then may be retained for many decades and may even be life-long. Inherent in such considerations is the concept that whatever putative environmental agent is responsible for the development of ALS/parkinsonism–dementia complex is present on Guam but not available to those of Guamanian descent who live off the island. This assumption may or may not be correct. People tend to bring with them many aspects of their culture, native foods, festivals, etc. and this may represent an opportunity for exposure to potential environmental agents among an outmigrated community. The Guamanians have a strong attachment to their island culture and items such as diet have accompanied them in their travels and continue to be enjoyed whenever available. Further, with the ready availability of air travel, return trips to Guam are common among this migrant community.

Evidence that the putative etiologic agent has long existed on Guam

In the early 1960s when ALS and parkinsonism-dementia complex were first being characterized by researchers visiting the island, the Chamorros referred to the two maladies in their native Chamorro language as "lytico" and "bodig," respectively. The term "lytico" is said to originate from the Spanish "paralytico," referring to the progressive paralysis associated with anterior horn cell degeneration in ALS. The origin of the term "bodig" is more obscure but is loosely defined as "slow" or "lazy" and refers to the parkinsonism–dementia form of the disorder. This suggests that this society had been familiar with the disorders for many years. Furthermore, archival death certificate records had been maintained by US Navy personnel since the beginning of the twentieth century and these documents survived the extensive destruction of facilities on Guam during the hostilities of World War II. These meticulously detailed records carefully document virtually every adult death from that era and contain numerous entries with diagnoses of amyotrophic lateral sclerosis as well as other entries with "presenile degeneration of the brain and spinal cord." Finally, folklore accounts suggest that the disease had been present on Guam from at least as early as the beginning of the nineteenth century. Based on this evidence, it is clear that whatever causes this remarkable outbreak of neurodegenerative diseases had been present on Guam for hundreds of years and preceded the arrival of the myriad aspects of Western industrialized society to the island. Accordingly, a large number of potential etiologic agents related to the current presence of a highly technologic way of life on Guam (e.g. fast food restaurants, nuclear weapons, synthetic petrochemical toxins, etc.) can be eliminated as possible explanations for this outbreak.

Environmental agents

Infectious organisms

It was parkinsonism–dementia complex, rather than ALS, that raised concerns for a possible postinfectious etiology of the outbreak of neurodegenerative disease on Guam. Parkinsonism–dementia complex patients show many similarities with postencephalitic parkinsonism patients who survived the epidemic of encephalitis lethargica in the early part of the twentieth century. Postencephalitic parkinsonism patients displayed a latency period between the initial episode of encephalitis and the onset of parkinsonian symptoms. This latency could last as long as a decade or more (although 6 months to a year was, by far, more common) (Yahr, 1968). Patients with postencephalitic parkinsonism may show all of the signs and symptoms of idiopathic Parkinson's disease and are said to characteristically demonstrate oculogyric crises. Clinical studies of Guamanian cases of parkinsonism–dementia complex failed to demonstrate oculogyric crises (Elizan et al., 1966), although the significance of this negative clinical observation remains unclear. The neuropathologic features of postencephalitic parkinsonism include several features encountered in parkinsonism–dementia complex of Guam, namely NFTs in remaining neurons of the substantia nigra, in the absence of Lewy bodies and the finding of neocortical NFTs predominating in superficial layers (layer II/III) (Hof et al., 1992b).

Despite these similarities, studies of both serum and postmortem brain tissues have failed to show any consistent evidence of a preceding CNS infection. Archival death certificates through the first half of the twentieth century fail to document any major outbreaks of encephalitis in the community and interviews with knowledgeable elders in the community failed to provide anecdotal accounts of any notable episodes of encephalitis on Guam. Restricted outbreaks of Japanese B encephalitis and mumps did occur on Guam in December, 1947 and April, 1948 but subsequent interviews with patients suffering from ALS/parkinsonism–dementia complex and their families have failed to confirm a prior history of encephalitis in such cases.

Further, Guam is the southernmost of four closely situated islands which are inhabited by significant populations (i.e. Guam, Rota, Tinian and Saipan). Ongoing traffic between these four islands has always been extensive, as they are close enough to be within direct visual sighting of each other. This proximity would provide a ready means for the sharing of any infectious disease-carrying vectors. The two neighboring islands of Guam and Rota have continued to show a high incidence of ALS/parkinsonism–dementia complex among their inhabitants. However, this is in sharp contrast to the populations living on Tinian and Saipan where such cases have never been documented. It is highly unlikely that an infectious agent could remain restricted to the two southernmost islands and yet never extend to the other two nearby islands.

The possibility that Guam ALS/parkinsonism–dementia complex represents an example of a prion-related disorder has also been considered. Gibbs and Gajdusek (1982) carried out numerous attempts to transmit neurodegenerative disease through intracerebral inoculation of Guam-derived brain tissues into non-human primates and other susceptible species. All such attempts were negative, including other efforts to recover a transmissible agent through inoculation of affected brain specimens into a variety of tissue culture systems. In the face of this extensive amount of negative evidence it is difficult to consider further a possible infectious etiology for the outbreak.

Cycad

In 1964, Dr. Marjory White first suggested the presence of a putative neurotoxin in the cycad seed of the false sago palm, *Cycas circinalis* (Whiting, 1964). Cycad trees are an important indigenous plant of Guam and its fleshy seed has served as a food source for the Chamorros. The seeds do contain a potent hepatotoxin, making them rapidly fatal unless thoroughly washed prior to eating. The seeds must be soaked in many changes of water over a period of a week or more before they may be safely eaten. The natives then dry the washed seeds and grind them into a flour which is used to prepare tortillas, porridge, doughnuts and to thicken soups. Whiting proposed that a neurotoxin might be present in the seeds and be responsible for the onset of neurodegenerative disease. This gave rise to extensive research to find experimental evidence of a neurotoxin in the plant. The results of these toxicologic studies were published in a series of six cycad conferences which were held under the auspices of the National Institutes of Health (Cycads, 1964; Whiting, 1988). The detailed reports from these conferences provide extensive documentation on numerous studies that were carried out in which a wide range of animals (including non-human primates) were exposed to high doses of either raw cycad seeds obtained on Guam or their purified constituents.

Among the findings of these toxicologic studies was the identification of cycasin (methylmethoxymethanol β-D-glucosidase), a very potent alkylating agent which comprises 2–4%, by weight, of cycad seeds and is a potent carcinogen. Cycasin represents one of the strongest naturally occurring carcinogens and many of the cycad-exposed animals eventually developed a wide variety of cancers mostly involving the lungs, kidneys, and liver. Importantly, despite being exposed to high doses of cycad seed or its derivatives, the wide range of animals failed to show any evidence of neurotoxicity in these experiments. Based on this entirely negative evidence, support for the cycad hypothesis as the etiology of the Guam outbreak of neurodegeneration waned for many years.

However, in 1987, Spencer and colleagues reported clinical observations of extrapyramidal dysfunction and motor weakness in cynomologus monkeys fed large oral doses of an "unusual" amino acid present in small amounts in the cycad seed, namely β-*N*-methyl-amino-L-alanine (BMAA) (Spencer *et al.*, 1987). BMAA shares chemical similarities with β-*N*-oxalylamino-L-alanine (BOAA), which had been implicated in neural larthyrism, a disease characterized by non-progressive spastic paraparesis. In this experiment, for up to 13 weeks each monkey was fed a large daily dose of BMAA by way of gastric gavage. The BMAA was chemically synthesized by a laboratory chemist and had not been derived from cycad seeds themselves. The monkeys were reported to develop muscular weakness, masked facies and a loss of aggressiveness and the authors suggested this was similar to the clinical features of ALS/parkinsonism-dementia complex in man. However, this experiment has been questioned on a number of grounds. The doses of BMAA were extremely high (100–300 mg BMAA/kg body weight/day). Duncan *et al.* reported that BMAA is present in very small concentrations in raw cycad seed (0.1% or less, by weight) and is readily removed by even brief washing (Duncan *et al.*, 1990; Duncan, 1991). Indeed, they calculated that an adult human would have to ingest approximately 7 kg of highly toxic unwashed raw seed per day to receive a dose that was comparable to that given to the exposed animals. Since the normal practice is to wash the seeds repeatedly before being safely eaten, most of the BMAA would have been readily removed. Accordingly, a comparable dose of washed cycad seeds would require ingestion of approximately 70 kg of cycad flour per day. Additional studies have questioned whether BMAA crosses the blood brain barrier (Duncan *et al.*, 1990, 1991). Duncan and colleagues (1992) also reported the presence of significant levels of zinc, a potential neurotoxin, within samples of cycad flour provided from Chamorro sources on Guam.

Importantly, despite reporting motor weakness, evidence of actual motor neuron loss was not demonstrated in any of the BMAA-exposed monkeys. Furthermore, neither a striatal dopaminergic deficit (indicative of nigral degeneration) or denervation atrophy (suggesting anterior horn cell pathology) was documented in the exposed animals and it remains unclear why these monkeys displayed any of the reported neurologic signs. In addition, evidence of tau pathology, indicative of NFT formation was not demonstrated. Finally, the experiment, as reported, failed to compare BMAA-fed animals to controls. Spencer and colleagues (Spencer et al., 1993) has subsequently written that "the changes [induced in monkeys fed synthetic BMAA] fall short of a model of the human disease."

Nevertheless, discussion of BMAA as an etiologic factor has recently reemerged in the literature. In 2002, Cox and Sacks hypothesized that exposure of the native population to putative neurotoxins could have occurred through the local custom of consumption of flying foxes that had existed on Guam but had more recently been hunted to extinction (Cox & Sacks, 2002). The concept proposed was that flying foxes eat cycad seeds and thus could serve as a conduit for unprocessed constituents of the fruit. Banack and Cox (2003) then published data indicating a high concentration of BMAA within three dried skin specimens of Guamanian flying fox that had been preserved in a museum collection for 50 years. BMAA levels were determined by high-performance liquid chromatography (HPLC) of amino acid extracts of the rehydrated samples. Finally, this group has now indicated that cyanobacteria produce relatively small amounts of BMAA but that it is then concentrated first in the cycad tree, where the bacteria grow symbiotically in the root system and then further concentrated in flying foxes who feed on the cycad seed (Cox et al., 2003). The final step would be consumption of the BMAA through the local practice of the Guam native to boil and eat flying foxes. They also report measuring a mean free BMAA level of 6 μg/g in frontal cortex of the brains of six Chamorro patients with ALS/parkinsonism–dementia complex and a mean of 6.6 μg/g of BMAA from 2 of 13 Canadian patients who died of Alzheimer's disease.

It is difficult to know how to interpret these results or this hypothesis. The authors have not addressed many of the problems that have remained since Spencer and colleagues first announced their results following extensive dosing of monkeys. There is little evidence that BMAA is a neurotoxin, especially a toxin that is specific to motor neurons or neurons of the substantia nigra. Even if small amounts of this "false" amino acid can be detected in brain

tissues of affected patients or in flying foxes, this may have little to do with what causes ALS/parkinsonism–dementia complex of Guam. It certainly does not explain the well-documented examples of the disease among the Filipino migrants to Guam or the inhabitants of the Kii peninsula.

Shaw's laboratory has recently also pursued possible cycad-related etiologic hypotheses (Khabazian et al., 2002; Wilson et al., 2002; Shaw & Wilson, 2003). They have identified a series of sterol β-D-glycosides from washed cycad flour with potential neurotoxic properties. Feeding male CD-1 mice washed cycad flour, this group has reported evidence of progressive motor and cognitive dysfunction accompanied by rather widespread TUNEL and caspase-3 labeling of neurons as evidence of neurodegeneration. Other studies indicated that β-sitosterol β-D-glycoside represented the most potent toxic metabolite in the flour. Their work continues in the development and characterization of what they feel is an animal model of ALS/parkinsonism–dementia.

Toxic metals

Yase first suggested that neurodegeneration seen on Guam and the Kii peninsula might be related to exposure to potentially neurotoxic metals (Yase, 1972). He noted that manganese and aluminum were present in significant amounts in the soils of Guam and the Kii peninsula. Manganese poisoning is well documented to produce a parkinsonian syndrome, however, this metal produces degeneration of the striatum with sparing of the substantia nigra and pars compacta (Olanow et al., 1994). Aluminum, on the other hand, had been experimentally linked to neurofibrillary degeneration through the induction of tangle-like lesions in rabbits following direct exposure to aluminum-containing compounds (Klatzo et al., 1965; Terry & Pena, 1965).

In 1980, using the techniques of electron probe microanalysis, Perl and Brody first demonstrated evidence of aluminum accumulation in the NFT-bearing neurons of Alzheimer's disease (Perl & Brody, 1980). Using a similar microprobe approach on unstained tissue sections, Perl and colleagues then showed evidence of dramatic aluminum accumulation in the tangle bearing neurons of patients with ALS and parkinsonism–dementia complex of Guam (Perl et al., 1982). Additional studies indicated that the concentration of aluminum in the tangle-bearing neurons of the Guam cases was approximately ten times greater than that of Alzheimer's disease (Good & Perl, 1994). Although the association of aluminum and Alzheimer's disease continues to remain controversial, the finding of excess aluminum in tangles encountered in the Guam cases has now been confirmed in a number of different laboratories using five different physical methods (Garruto *et al.*, 1984; Linton *et al.*, 1987; Piccardo *et al.*, 1988; Good & Perl, 1993).

The environmental source of these dramatic intraneuronal accumulations of aluminum remains unclear. It had been hypothesized that a deficiency in environmental sources of calcium and magnesium, physiologically essential ionic constituents, could lead to increased aluminum uptake as an alternative dietary source of cations. However, search for evidence of calcium deficiency among Guamanians did not reveal consistent alterations (Steele *et al.*, 1990; Ashkog *et al.*, 1994) and other alternative explanations must be sought. Guam is partially a volcanic island with an aluminum-rich bauxite soil. One study indicates that the soils of Guam contain 42 times the amount of elutable aluminum when compared to two other bauxite islands, namely, Jamaica and Palau (McLachlan *et al.*, 1989). This suggested that Guam soil may contain a great deal more bioavailable aluminum when compared to other volcanic islands. However, a recent evaluation of Guam soil has failed to confirm these soil findings (Miller & Sanzolone, 2003).

Subsequent microprobe studies using laser microprobe mass analysis demonstrated that the NFTs of Guam cases contained accumulations of iron, as well as aluminum, a finding that parallels that obtained using this technique with cases of Alzheimer's disease. Iron and aluminum excess has also been detected in the neuromelanin granules and Lewy bodies of cases of idiopathic Parkinson's disease (Hirsch *et al.*, 1991; Good *et al.*, 1992). Iron, through the Fenton reaction, is a powerful prooxidant and is capable of catalyzing the production of the highly reactive hydroxyl radical from hydrogen peroxide, a byproduct of normal dopamine metabolism. We have suggested (Olanow & Perl, 1994) that the combination of iron and aluminum may place a neuron in a state of oxidative stress because of aluminum's apparent ability to increase iron's capacity to induce lipid peroxidation (Gutteridge *et al.*, 1985). Recent findings of mutations in the Cu/Zn superoxide dismutase gene in cases of familial ALS (Rosen *et al.*, 1993) as well as the production of transgenic models of motor neuron disease through the introduction of such mutations may have relevance to Guam neurodegeneration (Gurney *et al.*, 1994). Cu/Zn superoxide dismutase plays a role in the balancing of the production of oxygen radicals through energy utilization and the body's natural defenses against the potentially damaging effects of such radical production. In some way that is still not yet understood, altering this critical balance may induce progressive neuronal degeneration in the form of similar neurodegenerative disorders. Whether the striking aluminum and iron accumu-

lations identified in target neurons for neurodegeneration in cases of ALS/parkinsonism–dementia complex of Guam are truly etiologic in nature, remains unknown. The source of these deposits and the mechanism by which they occur also remains to be elucidated.

General comments

It is a mistake to dismiss ALS/parkinsonism–dementia complex of Guam as a unique and completely separate disorder that is without implications for relevant diseases seen elsewhere in the world. Guam represents a rich laboratory in which to explore the dual interactions between environmental factors and genetic factors in the induction of the cardinal features of the age-related neurodegenerative disorders. On Guam, the strongest factor appears to be environmental in nature. Through the study of genetically based familial outbreaks of disease, critical insights into underlying hereditary factors can be gained. However, in a unique geographic isolate, such a Guam, environmentally based aspects may more easily be addressed. Despite extensive research over several decades, the mystery of the etiology of the remarkable concentration of neurodegeneration on the island of Guam remains unsolved. Despite this, Guam still remains the richest resource yet to be identified in which to unravel those critical environmental factors of importance to an understanding of both the disorders seen on Guam but also the analogous disorders encountered throughout the world.

Acknowledgement

The authors would like to all our collaborators in the Micronesian Health Study. This work has been supported by NIH grant AG014382.

REFERENCES

Anderson, F. H., Richardson, E. P., Okazaki, H. & Brody, J. A. (1979). Neurofibrillary degeneration on Guam. Frequency in Chamorros and non-Chamorros with no known neurological disease. *Brain*, **102**, 65–77.

Arnold, A., Edgren, D. C. & Palladino, V. S. (1953). Amyotrophic lateral sclerosis. Fifty cases observed on Guam. *J. Nerv. Ment. Dis.*, **117**, 135–9.

Ashkog, J. E., Waring, S. C., Petersen, R. C. *et al.* (1994). Guamanian neurodegenerative disease: failure to find abnormal calcium metabolism. *Neurology*, **44**, **S**2, 193–9.

Ball, M. J. & Lo, L. (1977). Granulovacuolar degeneration in the ageing brain and in dementia. *J. Neuropathol. Exp. Neurol.*, **36**, 474–87.

Banack, S. A. & Cox, P. A. (2003). Biomagnification of cycad neurotoxins in flying foxes: implications for ALS–PDC in Guam. *Neurology*, **61**, 387–9.

Buée, L., Hof, P. R., Bouras, C. *et al.* (1994). Pathological alterations of the cerebral microvasculature in Alzheimer's disease and related dementing disorders. *Acta Neuropathologica, Berlin*, **87**, 469–80.

Buée, L., Perez-Tur, J., Leveugle, B. *et al.* (1996). Apolipoprotein E in Guamanian amyotrophic lateral sclerosis/parkinsonism-dementia complex: genotype analysis and relationships to neuropathologic changes. *Acta Neuropathol. (Berl.)*, **91**, 247–53.

Buée-Scherrer, V., Buée, L., Hof, P. R. *et al.* (1995a). Neurofibrillary degeneration in amyotrophic lateral sclerosis/parkinsonism-dementia complex of Guam: immunochemical characterization of tau proteins. *Am. J. Pathol.*, **68**, 924–32.

Buée-Scherrer, V., Buée, L., Hof, P. R. *et al.* (1995b). Tau variants in aging and neurodegenerative disease. *Alzheimer's Disease: Lessons from Cell Biology*, ed. K. S. Kosik, pp. 132–49. Berlin, Springer-Verlag.

Bunina, T. L. (1962). On intracellular inclusions in familial amyotrophic lateral sclerosis. *Korsakov J. Neuropath. Psychiatry*, **62**, 1293–9.

Chen, K. M., Makifuchi, T., Garruto, R. M. & Gajdusek, D. C. (1982). Parkinsonism-dementia in a Filipino migrant: a clinicopathologic case report. *Neurology*, **32**, 1221–6.

Cox, P. A., Banack, S. A. & Murch, S. J. (2003). Biomagnification of cyanobacterial neurotoxins and neurodegenerative disease among the Chamorro people of Guam. *Proc. Natl Acad. Sci., USA*, **100**, 13380–3.

Cox, P. A. & Sacks, O. W. (2002). Cycad neurotoxins, consumption of flying foxes, and ALS-PDC disease in Guam. *Neurology*, **58**, 956–9.

Duncan, M. W. (1991). Role of the cycad neurotoxin BMAA in the amyotrophic lateral sclerosis–parkinsonism dementia complex of the western Pacific. *Adv. Neurol.*, **56**, 301–10.

Duncan, M. W., Steele, J. C., Kopin, I. J. & Markey, S. P. (1990). 2-Amino-3-(methylamino)-propanoic acid (BMAA) in cycad flour: an unlikely cause of amyotrophic lateral sclerosis and parkinsonism–dementia of Guam. *Neurology*, **40**, 767–72.

Duncan, M. W., Villacreses, N. E., Pearson, P. G. *et al.* (1991). 2-amino-3-(methylamino)-propanoic acid (BMAA) pharmacokinetics and blood–brain-barrier permeability in the rat. *J. Pharmacol. Exp. Ther.*, **258**, 27–35.

Duncan, M. W., Marini, A. M., Watters, R., Kopin, I. J. & Markey, S. P. (1992). Zinc, a neurotoxin to cultured neurons, contaminates cycad flour prepared by traditional guamanian methods. *J. Neurosci.*, **12**, 1523–37.

Eldridge, R., Ryan, E., Rosario, J. & Brody, J. A. (1969). Amyotrophic lateral sclerosis and parkinsonism–dementia in a migrant population from Guam. *Neurology*, **19**, 1029–37.

Elizan, T. S., Hirano, A., Abrams, B. M., Need, R. L., Van Nuis, C. & Kurland, L. T. (1966). Amyotrophic lateral sclerosis and parkinsonism–dementia complex of Guam. Neurological reevaluation. *Arch. Neurol.*, **14**, 356–68.

Forman, M. S., Schmidt, M. L., Kasturi, S., Perl, D. P., Lee, V. M. & Trojanowski, J. Q. (2002). Tau and alpha-synuclein pathology in amygdala of Parkinsonism–dementia complex patients of Guam. *Am. J. Pathol.*, **160**, 1725–31.

Gajdusek, D. C. (1963). Motor neuron disease in natives of New Guinea. *N. Engl. J. Med.*, **268**, 474–6.

Gajdusek, D. C. (1977). Unconventional viruses and the origin and disappearance of kuru. *Science*, **197**, 943–60.

Gajdusek, D. C. & Salazar, A. M. (1980). Amyotrophic lateral sclerosis and parkinsonian syndromes in high incidence among the Auyu and Jakai people in West New Guinea. *Neurology*, **32**, 107–26.

Galasko, D., Salmon, D., Craig, U. K. & Wiederholt, W. (2000). The clinical spectrum of Guam ALS and Parkinson–dementia complex: 1997–1999. *Ann. NY Acad. Sci.*, **920**, 120–5.

Galasko, D., Salmon, D. P., Craig, U. K., Thal, L. J., Schellenberg, G. & Wiederholt, W. (2002). Clinical features and changing patterns of neurodegenerative disorders on Guam, 1997–2000. *Neurology*, **58**, 90–7.

Galloway, P. G., Perry, G. & Gambetti, P. (1987a). Hirano bodies contain actin and actin-associated proteins. *J. Neuropath. Exp. Neurol.*, **46**, 185–99.

Galloway, P. G., Perry, G., Kosik, K. & Gambetti, P. (1987b). Hirano bodies contain tau protein. *Brain Res.*, **403**, 337–40.

Garruto, R. M., Fukatsu, R., Yanagihara, R., Gajdusek, D. C., Hook, G. & Fiori, C. (1984). Imaging of calcium and aluminum in neurofibrillary tangle-bearing neurons in parkinsonism–dementia of Guam. *Proc. Natl Acad. Sci., USA*, **81**, 1875–9.

Garruto, R. M., Gajdusek, D. C. & Chen, K. M. (1980). Amyotrophic lateral sclerosis among Chamorro migrants from Guam. *Neurology*, **8**, 612–19.

Garruto, R. M., Gajdusek, D. C. & Chen, K. M. (1981). Amyotrophic lateral sclerosis and parkinsonism–dementia among Filipino migrants to Guam. *Ann. Neurol.*, **10**, 341–50.

Garruto, R. M. & Yanagihara, R. (1991). Amyotrophic lateral sclerosis in the Marianas Islands. *Handbook of Clinical Neurology, Vol. 15 (59), Diseases of the Motor System*, ed. J. M. B. V. deJung, pp. 253–71. Amsterdam: Elsevier Scientific Publishers.

Garruto, R. M., Yanagihara, R. & Gajdusek, D. C. (1985). Disappearance of high-incidence amyotrophic lateral sclerosis and parkinsonism–dementia on Guam. *Neurology*, **35**, 193–8.

Gentleman, S. M., Perl, D., Allsop, D., Clinton, J., Royston, M. C. & Roberts, G. W. (1991). Beta (A4)-amyloid protein and parkinsonian dementia complex of Guam. *Lancet*, **337**, 55–6.

Gibbs, C. J., Jr. & Gajdusek, D. C. (1982). An update on long-term in vivo and in vitro studies designed to identify a virus as the cause of amyotrophic lateral sclerosis, parkinsonism dementia and Parkinson's disease. *Adv. Neurol.*, **36**, 343–53.

Gibson, P. H. & Tomlinson, B. E. (1977). Numbers of Hirano bodies in the hippocampus of normal and demented people with Alzheimer's disease. *J. Neurol. Sci.*, **33**, 199–206.

Goldman, J. E. (1983). The association of actin with Hirano bodies. *J. Neuropath. Exp. Neurol.*, **42**, 146–52.

Good, P. F., Olanow, C. W. & Perl, D. P. (1992). Neuromelanin-containing neurons of the substantia nigra accumulate iron and aluminum in Parkinson's disease: a LAMMA study. *Brain Res.*, **593**, 343–6.

Good, P. F. & Perl, D. P. (1993). Aluminium in Alzheimer's? *Nature*, **362**, 418.

Good, P. F. & Perl, D. P. (1994). A quantitative comparison of aluminum concentration in neurofibrillary tangles of Alzheimer's disease and parkinsonian dementia complex of Guam by laser microprobe mass analysis. *Neurobiol. Aging*, **15**, S28–30.

Gurney, M. E., Pu, H., Chiu, A. Y. *et al.* (1994). Motor neuron degeneration in mice that express a human Cu,Zn superoxide dismutase mutation. *Science*, **264**, 1772–5.

Gutteridge, J. M., Quinlan, G. J., Clark, I. & Halliwell, B. (1985). Aluminum salts accelerate peroxidation of membrane lipids stimulated by iron salts. *Biochem. Biophys. Acta*, **835**, 441–7.

Hirano, A. (1973). Progress in the pathology of motor neuron diseases. *Prog. Neuropath.*, **2**, 181–215.

Hirano, A. (1994). Hirano bodies and related neuronal inclusions. *Neuropath. Appl. Neurobiol.*, **20**, 3–11.

Hirano, A., Arumugasamy, N. & Zimmerman, H. M. (1967a). Amyotrophic lateral sclerosis. A comparison of Guam and classical cases. *Arch. Neurol.*, **16**, 357–63.

Hirano, A., Dembitzer, H. M., Kurland, L. T. & Zimmerman, H. M. (1968). The fine structure of some intraganglionic alterations. Neurofibrillary tangles, granulovacuolar bodies and "rod-like" structures as seen in Guam amyotrophic lateral sclerosis and parkinsonism–dementia complex. *J. Neuropathol. Exp. Neurol.*, **27**, 167–82.

Hirano, A., Kurland, L. T., Krooth, R. S. & Lessell, S. (1961a). Parkinsonism–dementia complex, an endemic disease on the island of Guam I. Clinical features. *Brain*, **84**, 642–61.

Hirano, A., Kurland, L. T. & Sayre, G. P. (1967b). Familial amyotrophic lateral sclerosis: a subgroup characterized by posterior and spinocerebellar tract involvement and hyaline inclusions in the anterior horns. *Arch. Neurol.*, **16**, 232–43.

Hirano, A., Malamud, N. & Kurland, L. T. (1961b). Parkinsonism–dementia complex, an endemic disease on the island of Guam II. Pathological features. *Brain*, **84**, 662–79.

Hirano, A. & Zimmerman, H. M. (1962). Alzheimer's neurofibrillary changes. A topographic study. *Neurology*, **7**, 227–42.

Hirsch, E. C., Brandel, J. P., Galle, P., Javoy-Agid, F. & Agid, Y. (1991). Iron and aluminum increase in the substantia nigra of patients with Parkinson's disease: an X-ray microanalysis. *J. Neurochem.*, **56**, 446–51.

Hof, P. R., Bouras, C., Buée, L., Delacourte, A., Perl, D. P. & Morrison, J. H. (1992a). Differential distribution of neurofibrillary tangles in the cerebral cortex of dementia pugilistica and Alzheimer's disease cases. *Acta Neuropathol. Berl.*, **85**, 23–30.

Hof, P. R., Charpiot, A., Delacourte, A. *et al.* (1992b). Distribution of neurofibrillary tangles and senile plaques in the cerebral cortex in postencephalitic parkinsonism. *Neurosci. Lett.*, **139**, 10–14.

Hof, P. R., Delacourte, A. & Bouras, C. (1992c). Distribution of cortical neurofibrillary tangles in progressive supranuclear palsy: a quantitative analysis of six cases. *Acta Neuropathol. Berl.*, **84**, 45–51.

Hof, P. R. & Perl, D. P. (2002). Neurofibrillary tangles in the primary motor cortex in Guamanian amyotrophic lateral sclerosis/parkinsonism–dementia complex. *Neurosci. Lett.*, **328**, 294–8.

Hof, P. R., Perl, D. P., Loerzel, A. J. & Morrison, J. H. (1991). Neurofibrillary tangle distribution in the cerebral cortex of parkinsonism–dementia cases from Guam: differences with Alzheimer's disease. *Brain Res.*, **564**, 306–13.

Hof, P. R., Perl, D. P., Loerzel, A. J., Steele, J. C. & Morrison, J. H. (1994). Amyotrophic lateral sclerosis and parkinsonism–dementia from Guam: differences in neurofibrillary tangle distribution and density in the hippocampal formation and neocortex. *Brain Res.*, **650**, 107–16.

Ito, H., Goto, S., Hirano, A. & Yen, S. H. (1991). Immunohistochemical study of the hippocampus in parkinsonism-dementia complex on Guam. *J. Geriat. Psychiatry & Neurol.*, **4**, 134–42.

Itoh, N., Ishiguro, K., Arai, H. *et al.* (2003). Biochemical and ultrastructural study of neurofibrillary tangles in amyotrophic lateral sclerosis/parkinsonism–dementia complex in the Kii peninsula of Japan. *J. Neuropathol. Exp. Neurol.*, **62**, 791–8.

Khabazian, I., Bains, J. S., Williams, D. E. *et al.* (2002). Isolation of various forms of sterol beta-D-glucoside from the seed of *Cycas circinalis*: neurotoxicity and implications for ALS-parkinsonism dementia complex. *J. Neurochem.*, **82**, 516–28.

Klatzo, I., Wisniewski, H. & Streicher, E. (1965). Experimental production of neurofibrillary pathology: I. Light microscopic observations. *J. Neuropathol. Exp. Neurol.*, **24**, 187–99.

Koerner, D. R. (1952). Amyotrophic lateral sclerosis on Guam: a clinical study and review of the literature. *Ann. Int. Med.*, **37**, 1204–20.

Kokubo, Y., Kuzuhara, S. & Narita, Y. (2000). Geographical distribution of amyotrophic lateral sclerosis with neurofibrillary tangles in the Kii Peninsula of Japan. *J. Neurol.*, **247**, 850–2.

Kurland, L. T. & Mulder, D. W. (1954). Epidemiologic investigations of amyotrophic lateral sclerosis. 1. Preliminary report on geographic distribution, with special reference to the Mariana Islands, including clinical and pathologic observations. *Neurology*, **4**, 355–78, 438–48.

Kurland, L. T., Mulder, D. W., Sayre, G. P. *et al.* (1956). Amyotrophic lateral sclerosis in the Marianas Islands. *Arch. Neurol. Psychiatry*, **75**, 435–41.

Kuzuhara, S., Kokubo, Y., Sasaki, R. *et al.* (2001). Familial amyotrophic lateral sclerosis and parkinsonism–dementia complex of the Kii Peninsula of Japan: clinical and neuropathological study and tau analysis. *Ann. Neurol.*, **49**, 501–11.

Lepore, F. E., Steele, J. C., Cox, T. A. *et al.* (1988). Supranuclear disturbances of ocular motility in Lytico-Bodig. *Neurology*, **38**, 1849–53.

Lessel, S., Hirano, A., Torres, J. & Kurland, L. T. (1962). Parkinsonism–dementia complex, epidemiologic considerations in the

Chamorros of the Marianas islands, including clinical and pathologic observations. *Arch. Neurology*, **7**, 377–85.

Leveugle, B., Spik, G., Perl, D. P., Bouras, C., Fillit, H. M. & Hof, P. R. (1994). The iron-binding protein lactoferrin is present in pathologic lesions in a variety of neurodegenerative disorders: a comparative immunohistochemical analysis. *Brain Res.*, **650**, 20–31.

Linton, R. W., Bryan, S. R., Cox, X. B. *et al.* (1987). Digital imaging studies of aluminum and calcium in neurofibrillary tangle-bearing neurons using SIMS (secondary ion mass spectrometry). *Trace Elements in Med.*, **4**, 99–104.

Malamud, N., Hirano, A. & Kurland, L. T. (1961). Pathoanatomic changes in amyotrophic lateral sclerosis on Guam. *Neurology*, **5**, 401–14.

Mawal-Dewan, M., Schmidt, L., Balin, B., Perl, D. P., Lee, V. M. Y. & Trojanowski, J. Q. (1996). Identification of phosphorylation sites in PHF-tau from patients with Guam amyotrophic lateral sclerosis/parkinsonism–dementia complex. *J. Neuropathol. Exp. Neurol.*, **55**, 1051–9.

McLachlan, D. R., McLachlan, C. D., Krishnan, B., Krishnan, S. S., Dalton, A. J. & Steele, J. C. (1989). Aluminum and calcium in soil and food from Guam, Palau and Jamaica: implications for amyotrophic lateral sclerosis and parkinsonism–dementia syndromes of Guam. *Environm. Geochem. Hlth.*, **11**, 45–53.

Miller, W. R. & Sanzolone, R. F. (2003). Investigation of the possible connection of rock and soil geochemistry to the occurrence of high rates of neurodegenerative diseases on Guam and a hypothesis for the cause of the diseases. Denver, CO, US Department of the Interior, US Geological Survey: 1–44.

Miura, K. (1902). Uber die amyotrophische lateralskerlose. *Neurology Japonica* **1**, 1–15.

(1911). Amyotrophische lateralsklerose unter dem blide von sog. bulbarparalyse. *Neurology Japonica*, **10**, 366–369.

Mirra, S. S., Heyman, A., McKeel, D. *et al.* (1991). The consortium to establish a registry for Alzheimer's disease (CERAD). Part II. Standardization of the neuropathologic assessment of Alzheimer's disease. *Neurology*, **41**, 479–86.

Mourelatos, Z., Adler, H., Hirano, A., Donnenfeld, H., Gonatas, J. O. & Gonatas, N. K. (1990). Fragmentation of the Golgi apparatus of motor neurons in amyotrophic lateral sclerosis revealed by organelle-specific antibodies. *Proc. Natl Acad. Sci., USA*, **87**, 4393–5.

Mourelatos, Z., Hirano, A., Rosenquist, A. & Gonatas, N. (1994). Fragmentation of the Golgi apparatus of motor neurons in amyotrophic lateral sclerosis (ALS). Clinical studies in ALS of Guam and experimental studies in deafferented neurons and in beta,beta-iminodipropionitrile axonopathy. *Am. J. Pathol.*, **144**, 1288–300.

Olanow, C. W., Calne, D. B., Chu, N. S. & Perl, D. P. (1994). Manganese-induced neurotoxicity. *Advances in Research on Neurodegeneration. Volume II. Etiopathogenesis*, ed. Y. Mizuno, D. B. Calne & R. Horowski, pp. 53–62. Boston: Birkhauser.

Olanow, C. W. & Perl, D. P. (1994). Free radicals and neurodegeneration. *Trends Neurosci.*, **17**, 193–4.

Perl, D. P. & Brody, A. R. (1980). Alzheimer's Disease: X-ray spectrographic evidence of aluminum accumulation in neurofibrillary tangle-bearing neurons. *Science*, **208**, 297–9.

Perl, D. P., Gajdusek, D. C., Garruto, R. M., Yanagihara, R. T. & Gibbs, C. J., Jr. (1982). Intraneuronal aluminum accumulation in amyotrophic lateral sclerosis and parkinsonism–dementia of Guam. *Science*, **217**, 1053–5.

Perl, D. P., Hof, P. R., Purohit, D. P., Loerzel, A. J. & Kakulas, B. A. (2003). Hippocampal and entorhinal cortex neurofibrillary tangle formation in Guamanian Chamorros free of overt neurologic dysfunction. *J. Neuropathol. Exp. Neurol.*, **62**, 381–8.

Perl, D. P., Hof, P. R., Steele, J. C. *et al.* (1994). Marianas dementia: a purely dementing form of ALS/parkinsonism–dementia complex of Guam. *Soc. Neurosci. Abst.*, **20**, 1649–50.

Piccardo, P., Yanagihara, R., Garruto, R. M., Gibbs, C. J., Jr. & Gajdusek, D. C. (1988). Histochemical and X-ray microanalytical localization of aluminum in amyotrophic lateral sclerosis and parkinsonism-dementia of Guam. *Acta Neuropathol. Berl.*, **77**, 1–4.

Purohit, D. P., Perl, D. P. & Steele, J. C. (1992). ALS/parkinsonism–dementia complex among Filipino migrants to Guam: report of two cases with parkinsonian features. *J. Neuropathol. Exp. Neurol.*, **51**, 323–30.

Reed, D., Plato, C., Elizan, T. & Kurland, L. T. (1966). The amyotrophic lateral sclerosis/parkinsonism–dementia complex: a ten-year follow-up on Guam. Part I. Epidemiologic studies. *Am. J. Epidemiol.*, **83**, 54–73.

Reed, D. M. and Brody, J. A. (1975). Amyotrophic lateral sclerosis and parkinsonism–dementia of Guam, 1945–1972. I. Descriptive epidemiology. *Am. J. Epidemiol.*, **101**, 287–301.

Rogers-Johnson, P., Garruto, R. M., Yanagihara, R., Chen, K., Gajdusek, D. C. & Gibbs, C. J., Jr. (1986). Amyotrophic lateral sclerosis and parkinsonism-dementia on Guam: a 30-year evaluation of clinical and neuropathologic trends. *Neurology*, **36**, 7–13.

Rosen, D. R., Siddique, T., Patterson, D. *et al.* (1993). Mutations in Cu/Zn superoxide dismutase gene are associated with familial amyotrophic lateral sclerosis. *Nature*, **362**, 59–62.

Schmidt, M. L., Lee, V. M.-Y. & Trojanowski, J. Q. (1989). Analysis of epitopes shared by Hirano bodies and neurofilament proteins in normal and Alzheimer's disease hippocampus. *Laborat. Invest.*, **60**, 513–22.

Schnur, J. A., Chase, T. N. & Brody, J. A. (1971). Parkinsonism–dementia of Guam: treatment with L-dopa. *Neurology*, **21**, 1236–42.

Shankar, S. K., Yanagihara, R., Garruto, R. M., Grundke-Iqbal, I., Kosik, K. S. & Gajdusek, D. C. (1989). Immunocytochemical characterization of neurofibrillary tangles in amyotrophic lateral sclerosis and parkinsonism–dementia of Guam. *Ann. Neurol.*, **25**, 146–151.

Shaw, C. A. & Wilson, J. M. (2003). Analysis of neurological disease in four dimensions: insight from ALS-PDC epidemiology and animal models. *Neurosci. Biobehav. Rev.*, **27**, 493–505.

Shiraki, H. & Yase, Y. (1975). Amyotrophic lateral sclerosis in Japan. *Handbook of Clinical Neurology*, Volume 22, ed. P. J. Vinken & G. W. Bruyn, pp. 353–419. New York, Elsevier.

Shiraki, H. & Yase, Y. (1991). Amyotrophic lateral sclerosis and parkinsonism–dementia in the Kii Peninsula: comparison with the same disorders in Guam and with Alzheimer's disease. *Handbook of Clinical Neurology*, Vol. 15 (59), *Diseases of the Motor System*, ed. J. M. B. V. deJung, pp. 273–300. Amsterdam: Elsevier Scientific Publishing.

Spencer, P. S., Kisby, G. E., Ross, S. M. *et al.* (1993). Guam ALS–PDC: possible causes. *Science*, **262**, 825–6.

Spencer, P. S., Nunn, P. B., Hugon, J. *et al.* (1987). Guam amyotrophic lateral sclerosis–parkinsonism–dementia linked to a plant excitant neurotoxin. *Science*, **237**, 517–22.

Steele, J. C., Guzman, T. Q. & Driver, M. G. (1990). Nutritional factors in amyotrophic lateral sclerosis on Guam: observations from Umatac. *Amyotrophic Lateral Sclerosis: Concepts in Pathogenesis and Etiology*, ed. A. J. Hudson, pp. 193–223. Toronto: Univ. of Toronto Press.

Stone, R. (1993). Guam: deadly disease dying out. *Science*, **261**, 424–6.

Terry, R. D. & Pena, C. (1965). Experimental production of neurofibrillary pathology: electron microscopy, phosphate histochemistry and electron probe analysis. *J. Neuropathol. Exp. Neurol.*, **24**, 200–10.

Tomlinson, B. E. & Kitchener, D. (1972). Granulovacuolar degeneration of hippocampal pyramidal cells. *J. Pathol.*, **106**, 165–85.

Torres, J., Iriarte, L. L. & Kurland, L. T. (1957). Amyotrophic lateral sclerosis among Guamanians in California. *California Med.*, **4**, 385–8.

Uebayashi, Y. (1984). Long survival cases of motor neuron disease in the Kii peninsula and Guam. *Amyotrophic Lateral Sclerosis in Asia and Oceania*, ed. K. M. Chen & Y. Yase, pp. 43–64. Taiwan: National Taiwan University.

Umahara, T., Hirano, A., Kato, S., Shibata, N. & Yen, S. H. (1994). Demonstration of neurofibrillary tangles and neuropil thread-like structures in spinal cord white matter in parkinsonism–dementia complex on Guam and in Guamanian amyotrophic lateral sclerosis. *Acta Neuropathol. Berl.*, **88**, 180–4.

Wakayama, I., Kihira, T., Yoshida, S. & Garruto, R. M. (1993). Rare neuropil threads in amyotrophic lateral sclerosis and parkinsonism–dementia on Guam and in the Kii Peninsula of Japan. *Dementia*, **4**, 75–80.

Whiting, M. (1964). Toxicity of cycads. *Econ. Botany*, **17**, 64–71.

Whiting, M. (1988). *Toxicity of Cycads: Implications for Neurodegenerative Diseases and Cancer. Transcripts of Four Cycad Conferences*. New York: Third World Medical Research Foundation.

Wiederholt, W. C. (1999). Neuroepidemiologic research initiative on Guam: past and present. *Neuroepidemiology*, **18**, 279–91.

Wilson, J. M., Khabazian, I., Wong, M. C. *et al.* (2002). Behavioral and neurological correlates of ALS–parkinsonism dementia complex in adult mice fed washed cycad flour. *Neuromolec. Med.*, **1**, 207–21.

Yahr, M. D. (1968). Encephalitis lethargica (Von Economo's disease, epidemic encephalitis). *Handbook of Clinical Neurology*, Volume 34. ed. P. J. Vinken & G. W. Bruyn. Amsterdam: Elsevier/North-Holland. pp. 451–7.

Yamazaki, M., Arai, Y., Baba, M. *et al.* (2000). Alpha-synuclein inclusions in amygdala in the brains of patients with the parkinsonism–dementia complex of Guam. *J. Neuropathol. Exp. Neurol.*, **59**, 585–91.

Yase, Y. (1972). The pathogenesis of amyotrophic lateral sclerosis. *Lancet*, **2**, 292–6.

Yase, Y., Chen, K. M., Brody, J. A. & Toyokura, Y. (1978). An historical note on the parkinsonism–dementia complex of Guam. *Neurol. Med.*, **8**, 583–9.

Zimmerman, H. M. (1945). Monthly report to Medical Officer in Command. *US Naval Medical Research Unit No.2.*

Part X

Other neurodegenerative diseases

57

Huntington's disease

Christoph M. Kosinski[1] and Bernhard Landwehrmeyer[2]

[1]Department of Neurology, University Hospital Aachen, Germany
[2]Department of Neurology, University of Ulm, Germany

Introduction

The description by George Huntington in 1872 of the disease that has subsequently borne his name is remarkable for its clarity and comprehensiveness (Huntington, 1872). It was not the first description of the disorder (see, for instance, Charles Oscar Waters, 1842, and Johan Christian Lund, 1860) (Waters, 1842; Lund, 1860), but it stands out as the first full delineation of the condition as a specific disease entity, quite separate from other forms of chorea. Huntington's paper was given at Middleport, Ohio, and published later in the Philadelphia journal, *The Medical and Surgical Reporter*. One can do no better than quote it here:

The hereditary chorea, as I shall call it, is confined to certain and fortunately a few families, and has been transmitted to them, an heirloom from generations away back in the dim past. It is spoken of by those in whose veins the seeds of the disease are known to exist, with a kind of horror, and not at all alluded to except through dire necessity, when it is mentioned as 'that disorder'. It is attended generally by all the symptoms of common chorea, only in an aggravated degree hardly ever manifesting itself until adult or middle life, and then coming on gradually but surely, increasing by degrees, and often occupying years in its development, until the hapless sufferer is but a quivering wreck of his former self. (. . .) There are three marked peculiarities in this disease: 1. Its hereditary nature. 2. A tendency to insanity and suicide. 3. Its manifesting itself as a grave disease only in adult life. (. . .) When either or both the parents have shown manifestations of the disease, and more especially when these manifestations have been of a serious nature, one or more of the offspring almost invariably suffer from the disease, if they live to adult age. But if by any chance these children go through life without it, the thread is broken and the grandchildren and great-grandchildren of the original shakers may rest assured that they are free from the disease. (. . .) The tendency to insanity, and sometimes that form of insanity which leads to suicide, is marked. I know of several instances of suicide of people suffering from this form of chorea. As the disease progresses the mind becomes more or less

impaired, in many amounting to insanity, while in others mind and body both gradually fail until death relieves them of their sufferings (. . .). It begins as an ordinary chorea might begin, by the irregular and spasmodic action of certain muscles, as of the face, arms, etc. These movements gradually increase, when muscles hitherto unaffected take on the spasmodic action, until every muscle in the body becomes affected (excepting the involuntary ones), and the poor patient presents a spectacle which is anything but pleasing to witness. (. . .) They are suffering from chorea to such an extent that they can hardly walk, and would be thought, by a stranger, to be intoxicated. (. . .) I have never known a recovery or even an amelioration of symptoms in this form of chorea; when once it begins it clings to the bitter end. No treatment seems to be of any avail.

All the cardinal features of Huntington's disease (HD) are recognized in this description: the adult onset, the progressive course and eventually fatal outcome, the choreic movements combined with mental impairment, even the pattern of inheritance; George Huntington's role as a family doctor, following his father and grandfather to give a 78-year total period of observation, gave him an unique perspective to appreciate the hereditary nature and the clinical features of HD.

The recognition of juvenile HD (Hoffmann, 1888) led to the realization that chorea was not the only motor disorder in HD, and that some patients show a predominance of rigidity and hypokinesia ('Westphal variant' (Westphal, 1883)) usually in young adults or children, but occurring in the same families as cases with chorea as the presenting feature.

It was no earlier than the 1920s that there was general agreement that the neuropathological abnormalities in HD were primarily degenerative and atrophic, despite Jelgersma's description in 1908 (Jelgersma, 1908) reporting generalized shrinkage of the HD brain and atrophy of the caudate nucleus (reduced to one-third of its original volume).

HD as a Mendelian disorder

HD displays an autosomal dominant pattern of inheritance: equal sex incidence, equal transmission by both sexes, a 50% proportion of affected offspring born to an affected parent, and lack of transmission by unaffected family members, are all features that are evident from any large HD pedigree. The HD gene was mapped to chromosome 4 in a classic study of RFLP positional cloning using the anonymous G8 marker (Gusella *et al.*, 1983). In 1985, studies of chromosome 4 of Wolf–Hirschhorn syndrome patients allowed to place the HD gene on the short (p) arm of chromosome 4 (Gusella *et al.*, 1985). Ten years after the mapping of the HD gene to chromosome 4, a gene in the critical region, named 'interesting transcript 15' (IT15), proved to contain a CAG repeat in its first exon, which was expanded in HD patients (Huntington's Group, 1993). The CAG expansion appears to vary and expansions of more than 36 CAG repeats are associated with the HD phenotype. There are quite distinct peaks (at 40 and 16 repeats, respectively), but the tails of the two curves approach each other closely. There is a narrow region of overlap, even though few individuals are represented in this borderline region; therefore there is no absolute separation between the normal and the pathological range – a conclusion of practical importance when the information is being used diagnostically. Generally, repeat size is determined by PCR; it should be kept in mind that another (CCG) repeat existed immediately 3' to the CAG repeat, which was variable in the normal population (7–12 repeats) and could thus confuse the sizing of the CAG repeats close to the borderline of normal and abnormal (Rubinsztein *et al.*, 1993; Barron *et al.*, 1994; Andrew *et al.*, 1994b); most laboratories therefore use primers 3' to the CCG repeat. There are also reports of a polymorphism at the 3' end of the CAG repeat usually containing a CAACAG sequence, but in a few people, the CAA codon does not occur and thus primers which overlap with this end of the repeat will fail to amplify. Thus, this rare polymorphism may lead to an erroneous diagnostic result (Gellera *et al.*, 1996). Overall, the CAG expansion can be considered as the mutation accounting for all patients with true HD. Sample mix-up or misclassification are the most common causes for the apparent absence of the mutation (Andrew *et al.*, 1994a).

The CAG repeat expansion is unstable on meiotic transmission; one of the key consequences of genetic instability in HD is that different individuals carrying the mutation will have different degrees of expansion in the CAG repeat sequence. A strong inverse correlation between repeat number and age at onset was demonstrated (Duyao *et al.*, 1993; Andrew *et al.*, 1993; MacMillan *et al.*, 1993; Snell *et al.*, 1993; Zuhlke *et al.*, 1993; Claes *et al.*, 1995). The CAG repeat length appears to account for 47–73% of the variance in age of onset in studies of various HD populations (Ranen *et al.*, 1995; Brinkman *et al.*, 1997; Rosenblatt *et al.*, 2001), although it was estimated to account for only 7% of this variance in late-onset cases (Goldberg *et al.*, 1993). A range of onset can be established for each specific repeat number (Brinkman *et al.*, 1997). However, it is important to note the considerable variation for each repeat number. For example, with a repeat number of 41 ($n = 98$), onset ranged from 35–75 years, with a cumulative probability of 0.38 by age 50 (95% confidence intervals 0.48–0.26) and 0.88 by age 65 (0.94–0.76). The strength of the correlation was greatest for the largest repeats, which are frequently associated with juvenile onset of disease, and was weakest in the lower part of the abnormal range, corresponding to the vast majority of adult-onset HD cases.

In contrast to the clear relationship between CAG repeat number and age of disease onset, there is little evidence for a similar correlation with rate of disease progression (Kieburtz *et al.*, 1994; Ashizawa *et al.*, 1994; Brandt *et al.*, 1996). In conclusion, the number of repeats in a HD mutation carrier is strongly correlated with age at onset of disease, especially for large repeat expansions; it is also correlated with severity of brain pathology (Penney, Jr. *et al.*, 1997), but not with the development of psychiatric features or rate of decline. In vitro studies are also demonstrating a relationship between CAG repeat number and formation of protein aggregates (Chen *et al.*, 2002).

Most juvenile and early-onset cases of HD are paternally transmitted; in addition, there appeared to be 'anticipation', i.e. progressively earlier onset in successive generations, in male-transmitted cases. Until 1993, these observations were unexplained. Although the concept of anticipation in HD is an old one, the disorder for which most evidence existed has been myotonic dystrophy (McComas *et al.*, 1978; Mahadevan *et al.*, 1992). The correlation of age at onset with the extent of the mutational defect, already discussed, was the first important fact, with juvenile and other early-onset cases showing the largest expansions. Next, two-generation data showed clearly that the anticipation seen in individual families was closely paralleled by an increased number of CAG repeats (Huntington's Group, 1993; Duyao *et al.*, 1993; Andrew *et al.*, 1993). In a series of 254 parent–child pairs with HD (Kremer *et al.*, 1995), expansion was seen in 70% of meioses. Although small increases in repeat number (up to seven repeats) were seen in transmission by both sexes (47.1% of males and 37.8% of females), large increases (more than seven repeats) were seen almost exclusively in the offspring of males (21.0% vs. 0.7% in the offspring of females). The largest increases were particularly likely to occur in individuals who themselves had the largest expansions (Trottier *et al.*, 1994; Ranen *et al.*,

1995), confirming a size-dependent instability. Analysis of single sperm (Leeflang *et al.*, 1995; Chong *et al.*, 1997) gives a clear picture of the distribution of sperm with different repeat numbers generated at male meiosis, confirming a high frequency (>90%) of increased repeat number for alleles in the pathological range. For an intermediate allele carrier (for definition of 'intermediate allele' see above) this figure was still over 50%, with 8% in the clinically significant range. Large series of sporadic cases showed in most clinically typical cases the HD mutation (MacMillan *et al.*, 1993; Davis *et al.*, 1994; Mandich *et al.*, 1996). When parents of such patients were studied, it became clear that while the clinical phenotype of HD might arise *de novo*, the molecular defect did not, with one parent invariably showing an expanded allele, usually in the 30–38 repeat range, but not associated with evidence of clinical disease, even at an advanced age (Goldberg *et al.*, 1993; Myers *et al.*, 1993). In all six cases in the series of Goldberg *et al.* where parental origin could be determined, the father was the one with the intermediate allele. The recognition of intermediate allele carriers has led to an assessment of penetrance of the HD phenotype in this borderline repeat range. A multicentre study (Rubinsztein *et al.*, 1996) re-analysed 178 individuals with a CAG repeat in the 30–39 range in a single laboratory and estimated the penetrance of the HD phenotype at different points in this range. The finding of six clinically normal individuals aged 75 to over 90 in the 36–39 repeat range is a clear indication of incomplete penetrance in this range, while no individuals with 35 repeats or less were found to have HD.

One of the questions that arose from a study of HD and other diseases caused by trinucleotide repeat expansions is the molecular mechanism by which those expansions occurred in the first place; the same mechanism is likely involved in the generation of intermediate alleles and in their expansion into the HD range as well. DNA undergoes a number of processes during which size changes in repeats could possibly occur. These include replication, recombination, transcription, and repair. The best evidence for the mechanism of instability is that the HD transgenic R6/1 models when crossed with $Msh2^{-/-}$ mice have no expansion of the HD mutation in germ cells (Kovtun & McMurray, 2001); this almost certainly reflects a loss of gap repair function rather than DNA strand slippage.

Defining the borderline of the normal and abnormal ranges has received considerable attention since it became clear that they were so close as to give the possibility of overlap. Fortunately, the steep curves of both normal and HD distributions, and the wide separation of the peaks, means that results in the borderline range occur rarely (2–3%) of the total, but it is essential that a clear policy is available for anticipating and handling them. Assuming that a method is used that excludes the CCG repeat, there is now general agreement that a result of 39 repeats or more in a clinically symptomatic individual is likely to indicate HD; no unequivocal results in this range have been reported in the normal population, though penetrance may be less than complete for 39 repeats. Likewise, a result of 34 or less is almost certainly normal in terms of clinical disease, though not in terms of consequences for the next generation. Thus the problem lies with the very small number of patients lying in the 34–38 repeat range, although many diagnostic laboratories have the policy of repeating all in the range 31–39, to allow for any PCR error or difficulty in reading through stutter bands. Rubinzstein *et al.* (1996) have produced a combined analysis of samples and data from different centres falling in this borderline range; out of 178 individuals with a repeat number of 30–40, seven affected had 36 repeats, while six healthy elderly individuals were found with 36–39 repeats. When such an intermediate result is found in a clinically abnormal individual, there are several approaches to resolving uncertainty. First, the test should be repeated, using a second sample if necessary. Second, if a family history of HD exists, then samples from parents should be taken where possible, to determine whether the borderline result has been transmitted from the HD or unaffected side of the family; in a number of cases it has turned out that the smaller allele has come from the affected parent, allowing a confident prediction of normality, whereas if a borderline result is also present in the affected parent and is the allele that has been transmitted, it is more likely to be associated with the disease. If the result is confirmed as being in the equivocal range, its interpretation will depend on the context; thus it will be unlikely to be relevant if the clinical situation is suspected juvenile HD, but more likely to be so if the picture is of mild disease in later life. It is thus clear that molecular analysis is of considerable value in confirming whether what appears to be typical HD is actually this disorder, as well as providing confirmation in cases where either the whole family or one particular individual is atypical. Another consideration, even more important, is the situation where a family history of HD exists, but the symptoms are not typical; in such a situation careful consideration should be given to whether the individual should be handled through a protocol appropriate for presymptomatic testing or indeed whether testing is appropriate at all. If the mutation is detected in such a person (usually at 50% risk), there is no guarantee that its presence is necessarily related to the symptoms that the patient has, and an unwanted and potentially harmful predictive test result may have been generated inadvertently.

Quality control schemes have now been set up Europewide (Losekoot *et al.*, 1999). It is clear that there remains room for improvement since the latter study showed a 1.3% rate of misdiagnosis. In the USA, laboratory guidelines have also been produced (Nance, 1998) giving not only recommended laboratory procedures but also interpretation of the ranges of results, including intermediate alleles.

Three genetic modifiers of the HD gene have been reported, each probably accounting for only a small proportion of the variance in age of onset of HD. A non-coding TAA repeat polymorphism in the 3′ UTR of the kainate receptor (GluR6) gene was reported to account for varying amounts of the residual age at onset variation in HD (Pickering *et al.*, 1993; Rubinsztein *et al.*, 1997). *APOE* genotype had a small but significant effect with the $\epsilon 2 \epsilon 3$ genotype associated with an earlier onset in males than females (Kehoe *et al.*, 1999). *APOE* genotype is the only robust genetic risk factor associated with late onset AD (Panas *et al.*, 1999), where it does have an influence on age at onset. Yet another genetic variation detected as influencing age of onset in HD is a length polymorphism in a polyglutamine tract encoded in the CA150 gene, a transcription factor of unknown function, which interacts directly with huntingtin (Holbert *et al.*, 2001). A recent 10-cM density genomewide scan in 629 affected sibling pairs provides suggestive evidence for linkage at 4p16, 6p21–23 and 6q24–26 (Li *et al.*, 2003).

Differential diagnosis

It seems there is a group of rare cases, which may or may not show atypical symptoms, which are not due to an expansion in the HD gene (Vuillaume *et al.*, 2000). Some of these disorders are rare autosomal dominant diseases, which look like HD and some of these have now had genes associated with them. An HD-like disease in a single pedigree was mapped to chromosome 20p12 (Moore *et al.*, 2001), the site of the prion protein PrP gene, and found to segregate with a 192 nucleotide insertion in the PrP gene, encoding eight octapeptide repeats. This disease was called HD-like 1 (HDL1). Margolis *et al.* (2001) reported an HD-like disease (HDL2), with very similar symptoms and pathology to HD, almost certainly associated with an expanded polyglutamine tract, as an antibody which detects only expanded polyglutamine-containing inclusions found such inclusions in postmortem brain from a member of this family. A consanguineous family affected by an autosomal recessive, progressive neurodegenerative HD-like disorder was recently described in Saudi Arabia (Kambouris *et al.*, 2000). The disease manifests at approximately 3–4 years and is characterized by both pyramidal and extrapyramidal abnormalities, including chorea, dystonia, ataxia, gait instability, spasticity, seizures, mutism,

and intellectual impairment. Linkage with a LOD score of 3.03 was initially achieved with a marker at 4p15.3 (Kambouris *et al.*, 2000).

Finally, a late-onset basal ganglia disease first detected in families in the north of England was associated with an insertion in the ferritin light-chain gene and is called neuroferritinopathy (Curtis *et al.*, 2001). Related polyglutamine diseases like DRPLA, SCA3 and SCA17 may mimic HD (Quinn & Schrag, 1998; Bauer *et al.*, 2004). In addition, neurological conditions associated with acanthocytes may resemble HD (Hardie *et al.*, 1991; Danek *et al.*, 2001). Choreo-acanthocytosis, or neuroacanthocytosis, is one of a heterogeneous group of neurological disorders associated with irregular spiny erythrocytes, or acanthocytes, that can be detected in a peripheral blood smear. Among the neurological disorders with acanthocytes, two groups may be distinguished. The first may additionally be characterized by low serum betalipoproteins and includes Bassen Kornzweig disease (abetalipoproteinemia; a recessive disease with vitamin E dependent polyneuropathy and ataxia); a form of hypobetalipoproteinemia (Mars *et al.*, 1969); and the HARP syndrome – hypoprebetalipoproteinemia, acanthocytosis, retinitis pigmentosa, and pallidal degeneration (Higgins *et al.*, 1992). A second group comprises those with normal serum betalipoproteins and, apart from a few patients with Hallervorden–Spatz-like disease, includes patients with neuromuscular and basal ganglia disease with or without the McLeod bloodgroup phenotype. This latter group is known as chorea-acanthocytosis, neuroacanthocytosis, familial amyotrophic chorea with acanthocytosis, or the Levine–Critchley syndrome (Critchley *et al.*, 1967). Choreo-acanthocytosis is a slowly progressive neurodegenerative disorder that affects the basal ganglia, peripheral nerves, and muscle. In a review of 19 sporadic and familial British cases, as well as 26 cases from the literature, Hardie and co-authors found onset varying between 8 and 62 years, with a mean of about 32.5 years. Of these 45, 8 were reported to have died between 7 and 24 years after onset of the disease (mean 13.9 years) (Hardie *et al.*, 1991). The clinical manifestations may resemble those of HD, and often patients with this disorder have first been diagnosed as having HD. Mild cognitive impairment and psychiatric symptoms may manifest early in the disease. Dementia will develop in most patients, but early in the disease frontal lobe dysfunction dominates. Personality changes, impulsive and distractable behavior, mood disorder, paranoid delusions, and obsessive-compulsive features may necessitate psychiatric help. In contrast to adult patients with HD, epilepsy occurs much more frequently than in the general population, with about half of the reported cases affected. Choreic movements of the limbs and face are present in almost all cases: they usually start in the legs. Orofacial dyskinesia may lead to tongue and lip biting and offer a strong clue to diagnosis. Orofacial dyskinesia may cause severe problems with speaking and swallowing. Apart from chorea, dystonia, parkinsonism and tics may occur in the course of the disease. Vocalizations and, rarely, coprolalia may resemble that seen in Tourette's disease. CT or MRI studies of the brain may reveal atrophy of the caudate nucleus. In addition, in a number of cases focal symmetrical abnormalities can be demonstrated in various parts of the basal ganglia that consist of hyperintense lesions in T_2-weighted sequences. These lesions can be found in the caudate, putamen, or globus pallidus, where they may resemble the "eye of the tiger" sign in Hallervorden–Spatz disease. The clinical feature that distinguishes neuroacanthocytosis from HD is the presence of neuromuscular abnormalities, consisting of hypo- or areflexia of tendon reflexes and distal amyotrophy. Serum CK activity is elevated in the majority of cases, while nerve conduction studies reveal reduced sensory action potentials in about 50% of cases. In contrast, motor nerve conduction studies are generally uninformative, and electromyography reveals denervation only in a minority of cases (Hardie *et al.*, 1991).

Senile chorea, or chorea of late onset in the elderly person without a family history of other affected individuals may clinically resemble HD or any of the aforementioned disorders (Shinotoh *et al.*, 1994; Garcia Ruiz *et al.*, 1997). Senile chorea, of unknown origin, and late-onset HD may be clinically indistinguishable, requiring CAG repeat length assessment to produce a diagnosis (Garcia Ruiz *et al.*, 1997). The cause of non-HD senile chorea is a clinical diagnostic challenge. All of the non-inherited causes that are discussed in the previous paragraph should be considered.

Huntington's disease – the clinical phenotype

Clinically, Huntington's disease is characterized by a triad of symptoms and signs: (i) a prominent movement disorder (in adult onset patients chorea), (ii) behavioral and emotional alterations and (iii) a cognitive decline.

Onset of symptoms and signs

A consensus exists among clinicians that a clinical diagnosis of Huntington's disease should only be made with certainty in the presence of a motor disorder. Thus, defining the clinical onset of Huntington's disease as the onset of the motor disorder yields a more or less reproducible way to conduct, for example, onset age surveys or genotype–phenotype correlation studies. However, it should be realized that the onset of motor abnormalities is neither a

sensitive measure of disease onset nor a specific and reliable measure since even well-trained motor raters may over-interpret and over-diagnose mild motor abnormalities resulting in poor inter-observer agreement in assessing the presence of motor signs (de Boo *et al.*, 1998). Prior to motor manifestations mood disorders and cognitive deficits disclosed by neuropsychological testing may be present, accompanied or followed by non-specific, minor motor abnormalities (e.g. general restlessness, abnormal eye movements or impaired optokinetic nystagmus, hyper-reflexia, impaired finger tapping or rapid alternating hand movements, etc.) (Penney, Jr. *et al.*, 1990) which eventually evolve into a recognizable extrapyramidal syndrome. In one series of 171 so-called presymptomatic carriers, mutation carriers performed significantly worse than non-carriers on neuropsychological tests such as the digit symbol test, picture arrangement, and arithmetic; mild impairment was noticed on reaction time tasks and various timed movement paradigms (Kirkwood *et al.*, 2000).

The classic phenotype

On neurological examination Huntington's disease is characterized by both extrapyramidal motor abnormalities and an impairment of voluntary movements affecting gait, speech, and swallowing. Chorea is the major motor sign of Huntington's disease, hence the designation "Huntington's chorea". Choreic movements are excessive movements, involuntary, abrupt, irregularly timed, and randomly distributed typically though with some distal (finger and toes) accentuation. Choreic movements are continuously present during waking hours and worsen during stress. Mild and intermittent choreic movements often go unnoticed by patients, while observers tend to describe them as "nervousness." Severity may vary from restlessness, fidgeting movements of the hands, unstable, dance-like gait to a continuous flow of exhausting and severely disabling, violent movements. Chorea is a sign in most patients suffering from Huntington's disease and tends to increase in severity during the first phase (~10 years) of the patients' illness. Muscle tone is typically decreased. However, rigidity and dystonia are often found in patients in advanced stages of Huntington's disease. As the disease advances, the severity of chorea tends to decrease and chorea tends to be replaced by the more disabling bradykinesia, rigidity and dystonia discussed below (Young *et al.*, 1986).

Bradykinesia and rigidity, best known as core features in Parkinson's disease, appear gradually and often dominate the final stages of Huntington's disease (Young *et al.*, 1986; Penney, Jr. *et al.*, 1990). Early in the illness, bradykinesia alone may contribute to impairment in voluntary motor performance; some patients display a significant decrease in overall daytime motor activity, suggestive of hypokinesia, or paucity of movements (van Vugt *et al.*, 1996). The use of neuroleptic drugs, intended to suppress choreic movements, may aggravate any existing bradykinesia and rigidity.

Dystonia, characterized by slow, abnormal twisting movements and abnormal posturing with increased muscle tone, may become a prominent feature towards the later stages of Huntington's disease (Young *et al.*, 1986). In a recent study of patients who attended a Huntington's disease speciality clinic, the prevalence of dystonia of any severity was found to be 95%, while in seven of 42 patients (17%) the dystonia was severe and constant although most patients did not complain and appeared hardly bothered (Louis *et al.*, 1999). Dystonia is particularly prominent in juvenile onset patients and in patients with late stage disease. The dystonia-predominant adult-onset form of the disease was recently reported to constitute 11.8% of an adult population seen at an HD speciality clinic (Louis *et al.*, 2000). Oculomotor disturbances are among the earliest signs and are present in the vast majority of affected patients (Schubotz *et al.*, 1976; Lasker & Zee, 1997). Saccadic eye movements are primarily disturbed with inability to suppress reflexive glances to suddenly appearing novel stimuli, and delayed initiation of voluntary saccades (Lasker & Zee, 1997). Later in the disease, slowing of saccades may be seen in up to 75% of symptomatic individuals, especially in early-onset cases, affecting vertical more than horizontal movements (Oepen *et al.*, 1981; Beenen *et al.*, 1986; Lasker *et al.*, 1988; Lasker & Zee, 1997). Impaired pursuit with saccadic intrusions, impairment of gaze fixation due to distractibility, slowing of optokinetic nystagmus and inability to suppress blinking during saccades may also occur (Oepen *et al.*, 1981; Beenen *et al.*, 1986; Penney, Jr. *et al.*, 1990; Tian *et al.*, 1991; Lasker & Zee, 1997). Voluntary motor function is impaired early (Folstein *et al.*, 1983; Hefter *et al.*, 1987; Thompson *et al.*, 1988). Patients and their families describe clumsiness in common daily activities. Disturbances in motor speed, fine motor control and gait correlate with disease progression and appear to be better measures of duration of illness than chorea (Folstein *et al.*, 1983). Mechanisms proposed to underly the slowing of voluntary motor activities include impaired internal motor cueing (Thompson *et al.*, 1988; Phillips *et al.*, 1996; Curra *et al.*, 2000), impairment in constructing and refining internal representations of movement (Georgiou *et al.*, 1997), or a reduced ability to process relevant afferent input (Schwarz *et al.*, 2001). Gait disturbances ultimately result in severe disability. Patients experience frequent falls and are ultimately confined to a wheelchair. Neuroleptic treatment that suppresses choreic movements does not improve the gait disturbance (Koller & Trimble, 1985). Most patients display speech abnormalities and dysphagia most prominently in later stages of Huntington's disease. Choking with aspiration secondary to dysphagia is a common cause of morbidity.

The final years of most Huntington's disease patients are dominated by loss of independence, severe restrictions in functioning and dependence upon others for activities of daily living. During this phase most patients live in nursing homes.

In advanced stages of the disease, speech is often severely dysarthric and may impair communication to a great extent. Swallowing is equally impaired, which requires very careful assistance by the nursing staff during meals, or, alternatively, feeding through a nasogastric tube or a percutaneous endoscopic gastrostomy (PEG) tube. Patients lose independent gait and spend their days in a chair, a wheelchair, or in bed. An increase in muscle tone which often develops in late stages of Huntington's disease may result in secondary joint contractures, while immobility increases the risk of pressure sores. Reflexes tend to be brisk but hyporeflexia is also often seen. However, in patients in whom weight loss is prominent, it may be hard to judge whether lower motor neuron pathology with muscle atrophy is present, or just plain malnourishment.

Weight loss and striking emaciation are features of late-stage Huntington's disease (Kremer & Roos, 1992). This weight loss may occur in conjunction with adequate dietary intake or even increased carbohydrate intake (Sanberg *et al.*, 1981; Farrer, 1985; Morales *et al.*, 1989). Sedentary energy expenditure is higher than in controls in proportion to the severity of the movement disorder. Total free-living energy expenditure is not higher, however, because patients with HD appear to engage in less voluntary physical activity (Pratley *et al.*, 2000). Intriguingly, a relationship has been found between weight at initial examination and rate of progress of the disease (Myers *et al.*, 1991). The leading causes of death in persons with HD are pneumonia (33%) and – reportedly – heart disease (24%) (Haines & Conneally, 1986; Lanska *et al.*, 1988). Pneumonia occurs five times more commonly in Huntington's disease than in controls and is likely to be secondary to the significant dysphagia, which results in choking and aspiration pneumonia.

Assessment of neurological and functional decline

Although clinical deterioration may be well documented in a qualitative way in the patient's file, long-term follow-up studies and the advent of experimental therapeutics made a more quantitative description of disease progression necessary. Early attempts at measuring progression focused upon the severity of the motor disorder, but investigators soon turned to the assessment of functional status as a relevant, reliable and reproducible indicator of disease progression. The Total Functional Capacity (TFC) scale introduced by Shoulson and Fahn in 1979 (Shoulson & Fahn, 1979; Shoulson, 1981) has been extensively used. This rating scale with a range from 0 (minimal) to 13 (maximal) is simple to score, more or less linear in its downward slope over the early and mid stages of the disease, and correlates strongly with various other clinical parameters of disease progression (Young et al., 1986; Shoulson et al., 1989; Penney, Jr. et al., 1990; Kremer et al., 1999). During early and mid-disease stages the average annual deterioration is about 0.6 to 0.7 points per year, irrespective of age at onset of HD, body weight, gender of affected parent, or history of neuroleptic use (Feigin et al., 1995; Marder et al., 2000). However, decline slows down, in terms of TFC score, in later disease stages (Marder et al., 2000). This phenomenon represents a floor effect of the scale. Apart from quantitative functional capacity assessments, pure motor assessment scales specifically developed for HD are available, e.g. the Quantified Neurological Examination, first described in 1983 (Folstein et al., 1983). This rating instrument has provided the model for the motor section of the UHDRS. In order to provide a comprehensive assessment of the clinical status of a HD patient, the Unified Huntington's Disease Rating Scale (UHDRS) was developed by the US based Huntington Study Group in 1994 (Huntington Study Group, 1996); the UHDRS is widely used for quantifying progression in natural history and interventional studies.

Non-motor signs and symptoms

Although the motor symptoms are most immediately evident, there is little doubt that it is the non-motor symptoms that have great impact on patients' daily lives, and contribute prominently to patients' loss of independence. The cognitive changes in Huntington's disease have traditionally been referred to as a dementia, an appropriate descriptor when used to indicate that changes are (a) progressive and (b) affect more than one area of cognitive function. In the past, the term dementia has carried the notion of a generalized intellectual impairment affecting all aspects of cognition in a diffuse, undifferentiated way. This is not an accurate portrayal of degenerative brain disorders in general; it is particularly inaccurate in the case of HD. People with HD have specific and characteristic cognitive difficulties, with other aspects of cognitive function remaining well preserved. Cognitive

deficits lie particularly in the realm of executive functions, which include the ability to plan, organize and monitor behavior, to show mental flexibility and switch from one way of responding to another (mental set shifting) (Butters et al., 1986; Bylsma et al., 1991). In addition, procedural memory and psychomotor skills are impaired. Primary tools of cognition, such as language, are relatively preserved. In their daily lives, people with Huntington's disease often exhibit poor planning and judgement. They may appear impulsive and show an absence of forethought, their actions being governed by immediate rather than long-term considerations. Actions are disorganized, a feature that contributes to early occupational and domestic inefficiency. People with Huntington's disease have difficulty coping with multiple tasks simultaneously, suggesting difficulty in the allocation and switching of attention. Difficulty with simultaneous tasks may extend to activities such as talking and walking: Huntington's disease patients are often noted to stop walking in order to answer a question, suggesting that overload of attentional resources may contribute to the multiple-task difficulty. People with Huntington's disease show impaired ability to self-monitor and often fail to notice errors that are apparent to others, sometimes creating a false impression of indolence. People with Huntington's disease are often reported by relatives to be inflexible, rigid in their thinking, with difficulty seeing another's point of view. They are poorly adaptable to altered circumstances and may prefer routine. Cognitive functioning declines over the course of the disease. Nevertheless, the rate of decline is variable so that duration of illness per se is a relatively poor indicator of cognitive performance (Brandt et al., 1984). Moreover, different domains of cognitive function do not decline in a uniform fashion (Bamford et al., 1995; Snowden et al., 2001). Bamford et al. showed most significant and consistent decline over time in psychomotor skills. Snowden et al. showed that, over a 1-year period, significant decline could be detected on low level psychomotor tasks, object recall and verbal fluency. By contrast, there was no change in performance even over 3 years on a test of executive function (Wisconsin Card Sorting Test) and egocentric spatial function (Road map test). It is worth emphasizing that HD is slowly progressive and cognitive changes over one year are typically relatively small. Therapeutic trials that seek to slow the natural course of disease will need to evaluate performance over years rather than months in order to demonstrate efficacy.

Psychiatric changes are distressing for patients and carers alike, but many changes are amenable to symptomatic treatment, so that early detection is vital. Behavioral problems in Huntington's disease are, however, complex. The factors underlying patients' altered behavior need to be assessed individually to improve patient care.

Huntington's disease – the neuropathological phenotype

Gross pathology

Macroscopic inspection of the brain of advanced HD patients at autopsy found that HD brains weigh less than brains of age-matched controls with the weight being reduced about 10–20%. Reduction in size occurs in the cerebral hemispheres, the diencephalon, the cerebellum and also the brainstem and the spinal cord (Forno & Norville, 1979). The most striking neuropathological feature is the shrunken appearance of the neostriatum with gross atrophy of the caudate nucleus and putamen with the caudate nucleus reduced to a thin rim of tissue. Reduction in the size of the caudate is accompanied by secondary enlargement of the lateral ventricles. Another notable feature is the reduced amount of white matter under the cortical mantel.

Microscopic pathology

Neostriatum

At the microscopic level, the atrophied neostriatum shows marked neuronal loss and astrogliosis which has been the topic of many quantitative analyses (Bruyn, 1979; Vonsattel *et al.*, 1985; Roos *et al.*, 1985; Myers *et al.*, 1988; Heinsen *et al.*, 1994). Striatal pathology likely underlies involuntary movements (chorea and dystonia), disordered planning, impulsive behaviors, and diminished emotional control as well as some other symptoms of HD (Crossman, 1987; Reiner *et al.*, 1988; Albin *et al.*, 1989). The extent of gross and microscopic striatal pathology provides a basis for dividing the severity of HD pathology into five grades (0 to 4) of increasing pathologic severity, which correlate with clinical progression (Vonsattel *et al.*, 1985; Myers *et al.*, 1988). Grade 0 cases have a strong clinical and familial history suggesting Huntington's disease but no detectable histological neuropathology at autopsy. In grade 1 cases, neuropathological changes can be detected microscopically with as much as 50% depletion of striatal neurons but without visible gross atrophy. In more severe grades (2–4), gross atrophy, neuronal depletion, and gliosis are progressively more pronounced, and pallidal pathology becomes evident. In the most severe grade (4), more than 90% of striatal neurons are lost, and microscopic studies predominantly reveal the remaining astrocytes. There is a dorsal to ventral, anterior to posterior, and medial to lateral progression of neuronal death with the dorsomedial striatum affected earliest and relative sparing of the ventral striatum and nucleus accumbens (Bots & Bruyn, 1981; Vonsattel *et al.*, 1985; Roos *et al.*, 1985).

The Huntington's disease gene, the Huntington's disease protein ("Huntingtin") and the Huntington's disease mutation

The Huntington's disease gene contains 67 exons (Huntington's Group, 1993) and encodes a 350 kDa protein, named huntingtin. The CAG repeat is located within the first exon and is translated into a polyglutamine tract. Huntingtin is ubiquitously expressed not only throughout the brain but also in many other tissues like muscle, liver, or lymphocytes and its expression pattern cannot account for the regional selectivity of neurodegeneration (Li *et al.*, 1993; Landwehrmeyer *et al.*, 1995; Sharp *et al.*, 1995; Schilling *et al.*, 1995). It is of note that, when the gene was cloned, it had no identifying homologies in the databases and to a very large extent this remains true today. Since the cloning of the HD gene, several other genes with expanded CAG repeats have been isolated (for review, see Cummings & Zoghbi, 2000). All lead to neurodegeneration, have similar sizes of disease causing repeats, and contain expanded glutamine tracts in their cognate proteins.

Whereas neurodegeneration occurs in different brain regions in all these CAG repeat disorders, another similarity between these diseases is that the CAG repeat is always located within the coding region of the protein so that the disease-causing proteins share a region with an expanded polyglutamine repeat.

It was Max Perutz who first hypothesized that instability in the chemical properties of polyglutamines might account for a conformational change above a certain threshold length of the polylglutamine stretch which might, in turn, be related to disease occurrence: *"Poly-L-glutamines form pleated sheets of beta-strands held together by hydrogen bonds between their amides. Incorporation of glutamine repeats into a small protein of known structure made it associate irreversibly into oligomers. That association took place during the folding of the protein molecules and led to their becoming firmly interlocked by either strand- or domain-swapping. Thermodynamic considerations suggest that elongation of glutamine repeats beyond a certain length may lead to a phase change from random coils to hydrogen-bonded hairpins (Perutz, 1996)."* A length-dependent oligomerization of polyglutamines into amyloid-like aggregates was demonstrated in vitro and in vivo shortly afterwards (Scherzinger *et al.*, 1997). The polyglutamine length above which oligomerization takes place is exactly in the range between 30 and 40 repeats which in Huntington's disease and other CAG triplet disorders delineates a normal from a disease gene. For the first time a plausible explanation for this threshold effect could be given.

Further pending questions were whether such polyglutamine oligomers are, in fact, present in Huntington's disease brains and how these might possibly cause neurodegeneration. In fact, amyloid-like aggregates had already been described by Roizin et al. in 1979 predominantly in neuronal nuclei when electron microscopy studies were applied to examine brain biopsies from Huntington's disease patients. Without the knowledge about the Huntington's disease gene defect and a possible role of polyglutamine aggregates, however, the significance of this finding could not be acknowledged at that time.

First clear evidence for the development of amyloid-like aggregates in Huntington's disease, which are formed from a polyglutamine containing fragment of the Huntington's disease protein came from the development of Huntington's disease transgenic mice. Gill Bates group was the first who developed a transgenic mouse which expressed only exon 1 of the human Huntington's disease gene with a massively expanded polyglutamine (around 150 repeats) (Mangiarini et al., 1996). This exon 1 was not only sufficient to cause a neurodegenerative disease in mice but also they described as the most prominent neuropathological finding amyloid like aggregates which were ubiquitinated and could be stained with antibodies against N'-terminal huntingtin. Because of their predominant localization in nuclei and absence in glial cells, these aggregates were named "neuronal nuclear inclusions" (NII). Meanwhile polyglutamine containing amyloid-like aggregates which are highly ubiquitinated have also been described in postmortem Huntington's disease brains where they were not only found in neuronal nuclei but also in dystrophic neurites (DiFiglia et al., 1997).

While the presence of polylgutamine containing ubiquitinated aggregates is widely accepted as a key feature of CAG triplet disorders (Davies et al., 1997), it is still disputed what their exact pathophysiological role is and how important their presence is for the process of neuronal degeneration.

From more detailed analyses of NII in Huntington's disease it is known that these aggregates do not contain the entire huntingtin protein but only a N'-terminal fragment including the polyglutamine chain. In a number of Huntington's disease disease models cleavage of the polyglutamine containing fragment from the rest of the protein can be induced in a length dependent manner by activation of proteinases such as caspases 1 (Wellington et al., 1997). Cleavage seems to be a precondition for the translocation of the polyglutamine containing fragment from the usual cytoplasm localization of the normal huntingtin protein into the nucleus. In turn, blockade of this cleavage process by caspase inhibition can reduce disease progression in Huntington's disease disease models.

These experiments not only demonstrate that cleavage of huntingtin is a pathophysiological key step but they also emphasize the importance of nuclear localization of expanded polyglutamine oligomers for disease development. This fact has been supported also by Saudou et al. who showed very elegantly in genetically modified cellular models of Huntington's disease that nuclear localization of the expanded polyglutamine is necessary to induce cell death (Saudou et al., 1998). This notion is also supported by studies in which normal cell cultures were exposed to chemically synthesized polyglutamine peptides which were readily taken up by the cells into the cytoplasm. Those polyglutamines only became toxic to the cells when they also contained a nuclear localization signal and did thus enter the nucleus (Yang et al., 2002).

To further elucidate the function of huntingtin and how the expanded polyglutamines may cause cell death yeast two hybrid systems and immunoprecipitation assays were developed to screen for interacting protein partners and abnormal protein interactions. Within this screen a number of transcription factors (Sp1, TAFII130, N-CoR, mSin3, p53, CREB binding protein, Gln-Ala repeat transcriptional activator CA150) were identified which interact with mutant huntingtin in a polyglutamine length dependent manner, i.e. increasing aggregation with expansion of the polyglutamine (Steffan et al., 2000; Holbert et al., 2001; Dunah et al., 2002; Li et al., 2002; Boutell et al., 2004). This is not very surprising since it is well known that many transcription factors contain polyglutamine rich regions themselves. Also a number of transcription factors like CREB binding protein (CBP) and P53 were identified as components of neuronal nuclear inclusions in Huntington's disease (Steffan et al., 2000; Nucifora, Jr. et al., 2001). Cell nuclei were depleted of these transcription factors not only in various disease models but also in HD brain tissue and compensation for CBP loss through CBP overexpression could rescue cells from polyglutamine induced neuronal toxicity in vitro (Steffan et al., 2000; Nucifora, Jr. et al., 2001).

The expected consequence of nuclear transcription factor inactivation through interaction with polyglutamines from mutant huntingtin protein is a change in the transcriptional activity of the affected cell. In fact, early and very specific changes in the mRNA expression pattern were first demonstrated in Huntington's disease transgenic mouse models for various neurotransmitter receptors (Cha et al., 1998, 1999). Meanwhile this concept has been largely expanded through mRNA expression profiling applying microchip array techniques. A characteristic pattern of reduced mRNA expression was found for encoding components of neurotransmitter systems, proteins involved in calcium homeostasis and also the retinoid signaling pathways. Similar changes were observed in different HD transgenic mouse models which are known to be critical to neuronal function. Time-course studies also revealed that mRNA changes develop in parallel with pathologic and behavioral deterioration in these animals.

Thus transcriptional dysregulation due to interaction of misfolded mutant polyglutamines in cell nuclei with transcription factors is now thought to be a key feature of HD pathology (Cha, 2000). As a consequence, neuronal dysfunction may occur in parallel at many different cell sites which are all in itself essential for cell survival. A number of well described examples which may thus be all understood as rather late events in the cascade of molecular events are glutamate related excitotoxicity, mitochondrial dysfunction and deficits in energy metabolism, as well as induction of the apoptotic signaling pathway (Beal, 1995; Koroshetz et al., 1997; Browne et al., 1999; Schapira, 1999; Cepeda et al., 2001; Zeron et al., 2002; Behrens et al., 2002; Panov et al., 2002; Ross, 2002; Friedlander, 2003; Hickey & Chesselet, 2003). More than 10 years after the gene defect in HD has been identified there is still a number of unsolved problems in our understanding of the molecular disease mechanisms. Examples are the exact function of the normal huntingtin protein and the regional selectivity of neurodegeneration. But it should be emphasized that our current understanding offers entirely new opportunities for therapeutic approaches. A number of these approaches have already been successfully tested in HD transgenic mouse models. Most promising for a therapeutic intervention in Huntington's disease patients are obviously results with drugs which are already approved by the FDA for diseases or which do not need approval since they are understood as natural food supplements. Examples are inhibition of caspase 1 activity with minocycline (Chen et al., 2000); inhibition of nuclear polyglutamine aggregation with the disaccharide trehalose (Tanaka et al., 2004); compensation for loss of CBP dependent transcriptional activity through treatment with the histone deacetylase inhibitors SAHA (suberoylanilide hydroxamic acid) or sodium butyrate (Steffan et al., 2001; Hockly et al., 2003; Ferrante et al., 2004); improvement of mitochondrial energy metabolism through treatment with creatine (Ferrante et al., 2000; Dedeoglu et al., 2003).

REFERENCES

Albin, R. L., Young, A. B. & Penney, J. B. (1989). The functional anatomy of basal ganglia disorders. *Trends Neurosci.*, **12**, 366–75.

Andrew, S. E., Goldberg, Y. P., Kremer, B. *et al.* (1993). The relationship between trinucleotide (CAG) repeat length and clinical features of Huntington's disease. *Nat. Genet.*, **4**, 398–403.

Andrew, S. E., Goldberg, Y. P., Kremer, B. *et al.* (1994a). Huntington disease without CAG expansion: phenocopies or errors in assignment? *Am. J. Hum. Genet.*, **54**, 852–63.

Andrew, S. E., Goldberg, Y. P., Theilmann, J., Zeisler, J. & Hayden, M. R. (1994b). A CCG repeat polymorphism adjacent to the CAG repeat in the Huntington disease gene: implications for diagnostic accuracy and predictive testing. *Hum. Mol. Genet.*, **3**, 65–7.

Ashizawa, T., Wong, L. J., Richards, C. S., Caskey, C. T. & Jankovic, J. (1994). CAG repeat size and clinical presentation in Huntington's disease. *Neurology*, **44**, 1137–43.

Bamford, K. A., Caine, E. D., Kido, D. K., Cox, C. & Shoulson, I. (1995). A prospective evaluation of cognitive decline in early Huntington's disease: functional and radiographic correlates. *Neurology*, **45**, 1867–73.

Barron, L. H., Rae, A., Holloway, S., Brock, D. J. & Warner, J. P. (1994). A single allele from the polymorphic CCG rich sequence immediately 3′ to the unstable CAG trinucleotide in the IT15 cDNA shows almost complete disequilibrium with Huntington's disease chromosomes in the Scottish population. *Hum. Mol. Genet.*, **3**, 173–5.

Bauer, P., Laccone, F., Rolfs, A. *et al.* (2004). Trinucleotide repeat expansion in SCA17/TBP in white patients with Huntington's disease-like phenotype. *J. Med. Genet.*, **41**, 230–2.

Beal, M. F. (1995). Aging, energy, and oxidative stress in neurodegenerative diseases. *Ann. Neurol.*, **38**, 357–66.

Beenen, N., Buttner, U. & Lange, H. W. (1986). The diagnostic value of eye movement recordings in patients with Huntington's disease and their offspring. *Electroencephalogr. Clin. Neurophysiol.*, **63**, 119–27.

Behrens, P. F., Franz, P., Woodman, B., Lindenberg, K. S. & Landwehrmeyer, G. B. (2002). Impaired glutamate transport and glutamate-glutamine cycling: downstream effects of the Huntington mutation. *Brain*, **125**, 1908–22.

Bots, G. T. & Bruyn, G. W. (1981). Neuropathological changes of the nucleus accumbens in Huntington's chorea. *Acta Neuropathol. (Berl.)*, **55**, 21–2.

Boutell, J. M., Thomas, P., Neal, J. W. *et al.* (2004). Aberrant interactions of transcriptional repressor proteins with the Huntington's disease gene product, huntingtin. *Hum. Mol. Genet.*, **1999**, 1647.

Brandt, J., Strauss, M. E., Larus, J., Jensen, B., Folstein, S. E. & Folstein, M. F. (1984). Clinical correlates of dementia and disability in Huntington's disease. *J. Clin. Neuropsychol.*, **6**, 401–12.

Brandt, J., Bylsma, F., Gross, R., Stine, O., Ranen, N. & Ross, C. (1996). Trinucleotide repeat length and clinical progression in Huntington's disease. *Neurology*, **46**, 531–5.

Brinkman, R. R., Mezei, M. M., Theilmann, J., Almqvist, E. & Hayden, M. R. (1997). The likelihood of being affected with Huntington disease by a particular age, for a specific CAG size. *Am. J. Hum. Genet.*, **60**, 1202–10.

Browne, S. E., Ferrante, R. J. & Beal, M. F. (1999). Oxidative stress in Huntington's disease. *Brain Pathol.*, **9**, 147–63.

Bruyn, G. W. (1979). [Huntington's chorea]. *Tijdschr. Ziekenverpl.*, **32**, 101–5.

Butters, N., Wolfe, J., Granholm, E. & Martone, M. (1986). An assessment of verbal recall, recognition and fluency abilities in patients with Huntington's disease. *Cortex*, **22**, 11–32.

Bylsma, F. W., Rebok, G. W. & Brandt, J. (1991). Long-term retention of implicit learning in Huntington's disease. *Neuropsychologia*, **29**, 1213–21.

Cepeda, C., Ariano, M. A., Calvert, C. R. *et al.* (2001). NMDA receptor function in mouse models of Huntington disease. *J. Neurosci. Res.*, **66**, 525–39.

Cha, J. H.. (2000). Transcriptional dysregulation in Huntington's disease. *Trends Neurosci.*, **23**, 387–92.

Cha, J. H., Kosinski, C. M., Kerner, J. A. *et al.* (1998). Altered brain neurotransmitter receptors in transgenic mice expressing a portion of an abnormal human huntington disease gene. *Proc. Natl Acad. Sci. USA*, **95**(11), 6480–5.

Cha, J. H., Frey, A. S., Alsdorf, S. A. *et al.* (1999). Altered neurotransmitter receptor expression in transgenic mouse models of Huntington's disease. *Phil. Trans. R. Soc. Lond. B Biol. Sci.*, **354**, 981–9.

Chen, M., Ona, V. O., Li, M. *et al.* (2000). Minocycline inhibits caspase-1 and caspase-3 expression and delays mortality in a transgenic mouse model of huntington disease. *Nat. Med.*, **6**, 797–801.

Chen, S., Ferrone, F. A. & Wetzel, R. (2002). Huntington's disease age-of-onset linked to polyglutamine aggregation nucleation. *Proc. Natl Acad. Sci., USA*, **99**, 11884–9.

Chong, S. S., Almqvist, E., Telenius, H. *et al.* (1997). Contribution of DNA sequence and CAG size to mutation frequencies of intermediate alleles for Huntington disease: evidence from single sperm analyses. *Hum. Mol. Genet.*, **6**, 301–9.

Claes, S., Van Zand, K., Legius, E. *et al.* (1995). Correlations between triplet repeat expansion and clinical features in Huntington's disease. *Arch. Neurol.*, **52**, 749–53.

Critchley, E. M., Clark, D. B. & Wikler, A. (1967). An adult form of acanthocytosis. *Trans. Am. Neurol. Assoc.*, **92**, 132–7.

Crossman, A. R.. (1987). Primate models of dyskinesia: the experimental approach to the study of basal ganglia-related involuntary movement disorders. *Neuroscience*, **21**, 1–40.

Cummings, C. J. & Zoghbi, H. Y. (2000). Trinucleotide repeats: mechanisms and pathophysiology. *Annu. Rev. Genom. Hum. Genet.*, **1**, 281–328.

Curra, A., Agostino, R., Galizia, P., Fittipaldi, F., Manfredi, M. & Berardelli, A. (2000). Sub-movement cueing and motor sequence execution in patients with Huntington's disease. *Clin. Neurophysiol.*, **111**, 1184–90.

Curtis, A. R., Fey, C., Morris, C. M. *et al.* (2001). Mutation in the gene encoding ferritin light polypeptide causes dominant adult-onset basal ganglia disease. *Nat. Genet.*, **28**, 350–4.

Danek, A., Tison, F., Rubio, J., Oechsner, M., Kalckreuth, W. & Monaco, A. P. (2001). The chorea of McLeod syndrome. *Mov. Disord.*, **16**, 882–9.

Davies, S., Turmaine, M., Cozens, B. *et al.* (1997). Formation of neuronal intranuclear inclusions (NII) underlies the neurological dysfunction in mice transgenic for the HD mutation. *Cell*, **90**, 537–48.

Davis, M. B., Bateman, D., Quinn, N. P., Marsden, C. D. & Harding, A. E. (1994). Mutation analysis in patients with possible but apparently sporadic Huntington's disease. *Lancet*, **344**, 714–17.

de Boo, G., Tibben, A., Hermans, J., Maat, A. & Roos, R. A. (1998). Subtle involuntary movements are not reliable indicators of incipient Huntington's disease. *Mov. Disord.*, **13**, 96–9.

Dedeoglu, A., Kubilus, J. K., Yang, L. *et al.* (2003). Creatine therapy provides neuroprotection after onset of clinical symptoms in Huntington's disease transgenic mice. *J. Neurochem.*, **85**, 1359–67.

DiFiglia, M., Sapp, E., Chase, K. *et al.* (1997). Aggregation of huntingtin in neuronal intranuclear inclusions and dystrophic neurites in brain. *Science*, **277**, 1990–3.

Dunah, A. W., Jeong, H., Griffin, A. *et al.* (2002). Sp1 and TAFII130 transcriptional activity disrupted in early Huntington's disease. *Science*, **296**, 2238–43.

Duyao, M., Ambrose, C. & Myers, R. (1993). Trinucleotide repeat length instability and age of onset in Huntington's disease. *Nat. Genet.*, **4**, 387–92.

Farrer, L. A. (1985). Diabetes mellitus in Huntington disease. *Clin. Genet.*, **27**(1), 62–7.

Feigin, A., Kieburtz, K., Bordwell, K. *et al.* (1995). Functional decline in Huntington's disease. *Mov. Disord.*, **10**, 211–14.

Ferrante, R. J., Andreassen, O. A., Jenkins, B. G. *et al.* (2000). Neuroprotective effects of creatine in a transgenic mouse model of Huntington's disease. *J. Neurosci.*, **20**, 4389–97.

Ferrante, R. J., Kubilus, J. K., Lee, J. *et al.* (2004). Histone deacetylase inhibition by sodium butyrate chemotherapy ameliorates the neurodegenerative phenotype in Huntington's disease mice. *J. Neurosci.*, **23**, 9418–27.

Folstein, S. E., Jensen, B., Leigh, R. J. & Folstein, M. F. (1983). The measurement of abnormal movement: methods developed for Huntington's disease. *Neurobehav. Toxicol. Teratol.*, **5**, 605–9.

Forno, L. S. & Norville, R. L. (1979). Ultrastructure of the neostriatum in Huntington's and Parkinson's disease. *Adv. Neurol.*, **23**, 123–39.

Friedlander, R. M. (2003). Apoptosis and caspases in neurodegenerative diseases. *N. Engl. J. Med.*, **348**, 1365–75.

Garcia Ruiz, P. J., Gomez-Tortosa, E., del Barrio, A. *et al.* (1997). Senile chorea: a multicenter prospective study. *Acta Neurol. Scand.*, **95**, 180–3.

Gellera, C., Meoni, C., Castellotti, B. *et al.* (1996). Errors in Huntington disease diagnostic test caused by trinucleotide deletion in the IT15 gene. *Am. J. Hum. Genet.*, **59**, 475–7.

Georgiou, N., Phillips, J. G., Bradshaw, J. L., Cunnington, R. & Chiu, E. (1997). Impairments of movement kinematics in patients with Huntington's disease: a comparison with and without a concurrent task. *Mov. Disord.*, **12**, 386–96.

Goldberg, Y. P., Andrew, S. E., Theilmann, J. *et al.* (1993). Familial predisposition to recurrent mutations causing Huntington's disease: genetic risk to sibs of sporadic cases. *J. Med. Genet.*, **30**, 987–90.

Gusella, J. F., Wexler, N. S., Conneally, P. M. *et al.* (1983). A polymorphic DNA marker genetically linked to Huntington's disease. *Nature*, **306**, 234–8.

Gusella, J. F., Tanzi, R. E., Bader, P. I. *et al.* (1985). Deletion of Huntington's disease-linked G8 (D4S10) locus in Wolf–Hirschhorn syndrome. *Nature*, **318**, 75–8.

Haines, J. L. & Conneally, P. M. (1986). Causes of death in Huntington disease as reported on death certificates. *Genet. Epidemiol.*, **3**, 417–23.

Hardie, R. J., Pullon, H. W., Harding, A. E. *et al.* (1991). Neuroacanthocytosis. A clinical, haematological and pathological study of 19 cases. *Brain*, **114**(Pt 1A), 13–49.

Hefter, H., Homberg, V., Lange, H. W. & Freund, H. J. (1987). Impairment of rapid movement in Huntington's disease. *Brain*, **110**(3), 585–612.

Heinsen, H., Strik, M., Bauer, M. *et al.* (1994). Cortical and striatal neurone number in Huntington's disease. *Acta Neuropathol.*, **88**, 320–33.

Hickey, M. A. & Chesselet, M.-F. (2003). Apoptosis in Huntington's disease. *Prog. Neuropsychopharmacol. Biol. Psychiatry*, **27**, 255–65.

Higgins, J. J., Patterson, M. C., Papadopoulos, N. M., Brady, R. O., Pentchev, P. G. & Barton, N. W. (1992). Hypoprebetalipoproteinemia, acanthocytosis, retinitis pigmentosa, and pallidal degeneration (HARP syndrome). *Neurology*, **42**, 194–8.

Hockly, E., Richon, V. M., Woodman, B., *et al.* (2003). Suberoylanilide hydroxamic acid, a histone deacetylase inhibitor, ameliorates motor deficits in a mouse model of Huntington's disease. *Proc. Natl Acad. Sci., USA*, **100**, 2041–6.

Hoffmann, J. (1888). Über Chorea chronica progressiva (Huntingtonsche Chorea, Chorea hereditaria). *Virchow's Archiv für Pathol. Anat.*, **111**, 513–48.

Holbert, S., Denghien, I., Kiechle, T. *et al.* (2001). The Gln-Ala repeat transcriptional activator CA150 interacts with huntingtin: neuropathologic and genetic evidence for a role in Huntington's disease pathogenesis. *Proc. Natl Acad. Sci., USA*, **98**, 1811–16.

Huntington, G. (1872). On chorea. *Med. Surg. Rep.*, **26**, 317–21.

Huntington Study Group (1996). Unified Huntington's Disease Rating Scale: reliability and consistency. *Mov. Disord.*, **11**, 136–42.

Huntington's Disease Collaborative Research Group (1993). A novel gene containing a trinucleotide repeat that is expanded and unstable on Huntington's disease chromosomes. *Cell*, **72**, 971–83.

Jelgersma, G. (1908). Die anatomischen Veränderungen bei Paralysis agitans und chronischer Chorea. *Verh. Ges. Dtsch. Naturforsch. Ärzte*, **2**, 383–8.

Kambouris, M., Bohlega, S., Al Tahan, A. & Meyer, B. F. (2000). Localization of the gene for a novel autosomal recessive neurodegenerative Huntington-like disorder to 4p15.3. *Am. J. Hum. Genet.*, **66**, 445–52.

Kehoe, P., Krawczak, M., Harper, P. S., Owen, M. J. & Jones, A. L. (1999). Age of onset in Huntington disease: sex specific influence of apolipoprotein E genotype and normal CAG repeat length. *J. Med. Genet.*, **36**, 108–11.

Kieburtz, K., MacDonald, M., Shih, C. *et al.* (1994). Trinucleotide repeat length and progression of illness in Huntington's disease. *J. Med. Genet.*, **31**, 872–4.

Kirkwood, S. C., Siemers, E., Hodes, M.E., Conneally, P. M., Christian, J. C. & Foroud, T. (2000). Subtle changes among presymptomatic carriers of the Huntington's disease gene. *J. Neurol. Neurosurg. Psychiatry*, **69**, 773–9.

Koller, W. C. & Trimble, J. (1985). The gait abnormality of Huntington's disease. *Neurology*, **35**, 1450–4.

Koroshetz, W. J., Jenkins, B. G., Rosen, B. R. & Beal, M. F. (1997). Energy metabolism defects in Huntington's disease and effects of coenzyme Q10. *Ann. Neurol.*, **41**, 160–5.

Kovtun, I. V. & McMurray, C. T. (2001). Trinucleotide expansion in haploid germ cells by gap repair. *Nat. Genet.*, **27**, 407–11.

Kremer, B., Almqvist, E., Theilmann, J. *et al.* (1995). Sex-dependent mechanisms for expansions and contractions of the CAG repeat on affected Huntington disease chromosomes. *Am. J. Hum. Genet.*, **57**, 343–50.

Kremer, B., Clark, C. M., Almqvist, E. W. *et al.* (1999). Influence of lamotrigine on progression of early Huntington disease: a randomized clinical trial. *Neurology*, **53**, 1000–11.

Kremer, H. P. & Roos, R. A. (1992). Weight loss in Huntington's disease. *Arch. Neurol.*, **49**, 349.

Landwehrmeyer, G. B., McNeil, S. M., Dure, L. S. *et al.* (1995). Huntington's Disease Gene: regional and cellular expression in brain of normal and affected individuals. *Ann. Neurol.*, **37**, 218–30.

Lanska, D. J., Lanska, M. J., Lavine, L. & Schoenberg, B. S. (1988). Conditions associated with Huntington's disease at death. A case-control study. *Arch. Neurol.*, **45**, 878–80.

Lasker, A. G. & Zee, D. S. (1997). Ocular motor abnormalities in Huntington's disease. *Vision Res.*, **37**, 3639–45.

Lasker, A. G., Zee, D. S., Hain, T. C., Folstein, S. E. & Singer, H. S. (1998). Saccades in Huntington's disease: slowing and dysmetria. *Neurology*, **38**, 427–31.

Leeflang, E. P., Zhang, L., Tavare, S. *et al.* (1995). Single sperm analysis of the trinucleotide repeats in the Huntington's disease gene: quantification of the mutation frequency spectrum. *Hum. Molec. Genet.*, **4**, 1519–26.

Li, J. L., Hayden, M. R., Almqvist, E. W. *et al.* (2003). A genome scan for modifiers of age at onset in Huntington disease: The HD MAPS study. *Am. J. Hum. Genet.*, **73**, 682–7.

Li, S. H., Schilling, G., Young, W.3 *et al.* (1993). Huntington's disease gene (IT15) is widely expressed in human and rat tissues. *Neuron*, **11**, 985–93.

Li, S. H., Cheng, A. L., Zhou, H. *et al.* (2002). Interaction of Huntington disease protein with transcriptional activator Sp1. *Mol. Cell. Biol.*, **22**, 1277–87.

Losekoot, M., Bakker, B., Laccone, F., Stenhouse, S. & Elles, R. (1999). A European pilot quality assessment scheme for molecular diagnosis of Huntington's disease. *Eur. J. Hum. Genet.*, **7**, 217–22.

Louis, E. D., Marder, K., Moskowitz, C. & Greene, P. (1999). Arm elevation in Huntington's disease: dystonia or levitation? *Mov. Disord.*, **14**, 1035–8.

Louis, E. D., Anderson, K. E., Moskowitz, C., Thorne, D. Z. & Marder, K. (2000). Dystonia-predominant adult-onset Huntington disease: association between motor phenotype and age of onset in adults. *Arch. Neurol.*, **57**, 1326–30.

Lund, J. C. (1860). Chorea St Vitus Dance in Saetersdalen. In *Quoted by Orbeck 1*, ed. p. 137.

MacMillan, J. C., Snell, R. G., Tyler, A. *et al.* (1993). Molecular analysis and clinical correlations of the Huntington's disease mutation. *Lancet*, **342**, 954–958.

Mahadevan, M., Tsilfidis, C., Sabourin, L. *et al.* (1992). Myotonic dystrophy mutation: an unstable CTG repeat in the 3′ untranslated region of the gene. *Science*, **255**, 1253–5.

Mandich, P., Di Maria, E., Bellone, E., Ajmar, F. & Abbruzzese, G. (1996). Molecular analysis of the IT15 gene in patients with apparently 'sporadic' Huntington's disease. *Eur. Neurol.*, **36**, 348–52.

Mangiarini, L., Sathasivam, K., Seller, M. *et al.* (1996). Exon 1 of the HD gene with an expanded CAG repeat is sufficient to cause a progressive neurological phenotype in transgenic mice. *Cell*, **87**, 493–506.

Marder, K., Zhao, H., Myers, R. H. *et al.* (2000). Rate of functional decline in Huntington's disease. Huntington Study Group. *Neurology*, **54**, 452–58.

Margolis, R. L., O'Hearn, E., Rosenblatt, A. *et al.* (2001). A disorder similar to Huntington's disease is associated with a novel CAG repeat expansion. *Ann. Neurol.*, **50**, 373–80.

Mars, H., Lewis, L. A., Robertson, A. L., Jr., Butkus, A. & Williams, G. H., Jr. (1969). Familial hypo-beta-lipoproteinemia: a genetic disorder of lipid metabolism with nervous system involvement. *Am. J. Med.*, **46**, 886–900.

McComas, A. J., Sica, R. E. & Toyonaga, K. (1978). Incidence, severity, and time-course of motoneurone dysfunction in myotonic dystrophy: their significance for an understanding of anticipation. *J. Neurol. Neurosurg. Psychiatry*, **41**, 882–93.

Moore, R. C., Xiang, F., Monaghan, J. *et al.* (2001). Huntington disease phenocopy is a familial prion disease. *Am. J. Hum. Genet.*, **69**, 1385–8.

Morales, L. M., Estevez, J., Suarez, H., Villalobos, R., Chacin, D. B. & Bonilla, E. (1989). Nutritional evaluation of Huntington disease patients. *Am. J. Clin. Nutr.*, **50**, 145–50.

Myers, R. H., Vonsattel, J. P., Stevens, T. J. *et al.* (1988). Clinical and neuropathologic assessment of severity in Huntington's disease. *Neurology*, **38**, 341–7.

Myers, R. H., Sax, D. S., Koroshetz, W. J. *et al.* (1991). Factors associated with slow progression in Huntington's disease. *Arch. Neurol.*, **48**, 800–4.

Myers, R. H., MacDonald, M. E., Koroshetz, W. J. *et al.* (1993). De novo expansion of a (CAG)n repeat in sporadic Huntington's disease. *Nat. Genet.*, **5**, 168–73.

Nance, M. A. (1998). Huntington disease: clinical, genetic, and social aspects. *J. Geriatr. Psychiatry Neurol.*, **11**, 61–70.

Nucifora, F. C., Jr., Sasaki, M., Peters, M. F. *et al.* (2001). Interference by huntingtin and atrophin-1 with cbp-mediated transcription leading to cellular toxicity. *Science*, **291**, 2423–8.

Oepen, G., Clarenbach, P. & Thoden, U. (1981). Disturbance of eye movements in Huntington's chorea. *Arch. Psychiatr. Nervenkr.*, **229**, 205–13.

Panas, M., Avramopoulos, D., Karadima, G., Petersen, M. B. & Vassilopoulos, D. (1999). Apolipoprotein E and presenilin-1 genotypes in Huntington's disease. *J. Neurol.*, **246**, 574–7.

Panov, A. V., Gutekunst, C.-A., Leavitt, B. *et al.* (2002). Early mitochondrial calcium defects in Huntington's disease are a direct effect of polyglutamines. *Nat. Neurosci.*, **5**, 731–6.

Penney, J. B., Jr., Young, A. B., Shoulson, I. *et al.* (1990). Huntington's disease in Venezuela: 7 years of follow-up on symptomatic and asymptomatic individuals. *Mov. Disord.*, **5**, 93–9.

Penney, J. B., Jr., Vonsattel, J. P., MacDonald, M. E., Gusella, J. F. & Myers, R. H. (1997). CAG repeat number governs the development rate of pathology in Huntington's disease. *Ann. Neurol.*, **41**, 689–92.

Perutz, M. (1996). Glutamine repeats and inherited neurodegenerative diseases: molecular aspects. *Curr. Opin. Struct. Biol.*, **6**, 848–58.

Phillips, J. G., Bradshaw, J. L., Chiu, E., Teasdale, N., Iansek, R. & Bradshaw, J. A. (1996). Bradykinesia and movement precision in Huntington's disease. *Neuropsychologia*, **34**, 1241–45.

Pickering, D. S., Thomsen, C., Suzdak, P. D. *et al.* (1993). A comparison of two alternatively spliced forms of a metabotropic glutamate receptor coupled to phosphoinositide turnover. *J. Neurochem.*, **61**, 85–92.

Pratley, R. E., Salbe, A. D., Ravussin, E. & Caviness, J. N. (2000). Higher sedentary energy expenditure in patients with Huntington's disease. *Ann. Neurol.*, **47**, 64–70.

Quinn, N. & Schrag, A. (1998). Huntington's disease and other choreas. *J. Neurol.*, **245**, 709–16.

Ranen, N., Stine, O., Abbot, M. *et al.* (1995). Anticipation and instability of IT-15 (CAG)n repeats in parent-offspring pairs with Huntington disease. *Am. J. Hum. Genet.*, **57**, 593–602.

Reiner, A., Albin, R. L., Anderson, K. D., D'Amato, C. J., Penney, J. B. & Young, A. B. (1988). Differential loss of striatal projection neurons in Huntington disease. *Proc. Natl Acad. Sci., USA*, **85**, 5733–7.

Roizin, L., Stellar, S., & Liu, J. (1979). Neuronal nuclear-cytoplasmic changes in Huntingtons chorea: electron microscope investigations. In *Advance in Neurology, Huntington's Disease*, ed. N. Wexler & A. Barbeau, New York: Raven Press. pp. 195–22.

Roos, R. A., Pruyt, J. F., de Vries, J. & Bots, G. T. (1985). Neuronal distribution in the putamen in Huntington's disease. *J. Neurol. Neurosurg. Psychiatry*, **48**, 422–5.

Rosenblatt, A., Brinkman, R. R., Liang, K. Y. (2001). Familial influence on age of onset among siblings with Huntington disease. *Am. J. Med. Genet.*, **105**, 399–403.

Ross, C. A. (2002). Polyglutamine pathogenesis: emergence of unifying mechanisms for Huntington's disease and related disorders. *Neuron*, **35**, 819–22.

Rubinsztein, D. C., Leggo, J., Barton, D. E. & Ferguson-Smith, M. A. (1993). Site of (CCG) polymorphism in the HD gene. *Nat. Genet.*, **5**, 214–15.

Rubinsztein, D. C., Leggo, J., Coles, R. *et al.* (1996). Phenotypic characterization of individuals with 30–40 CAG repeats in the Huntington disease (HD) gene reveals HD cases with 36 repeats and apparently normal elderly individuals with 36–39 repeats. *Am. J. Hum. Genet.*, **59**, 16–22.

Rubinsztein, D. C., Leggo, J., Chiano, M. *et al.* (1997). Genotypes at the GluR6 kainate receptor locus are associated with variation in the age of onset of Huntington disease. *Proc. Natl Acad. Sci., USA*, **94**, 3872–6.

Sanberg, P. R., Fibiger, H. C. & Mark, R. F. (1981). Body weight and dietary factors in Huntington's disease patients compared with matched controls. *Med. J. Aust.* **1**, 407–9.

Saudou, F., Finkbeiner, S., Devys, D. & Greenberg, M. (1998). Huntingtin acts in the nucleus to induce apoptosis but death does not correlate with the formation of intranuclear inclusions. *Cell*, **95**, 55–66.

Schapira, A. H. (1999). Mitochondrial involvement in Parkinson's, Huntington's disease, hereditary spastic paraplegia and Friedreich's ataxia. *Biochem. Biophys. Acta*, **1410**, 99–102.

Scherzinger, E., Lurz, R., Turmaine, M. *et al.* (1997). Huntingtin-encoded polyglutamine expansions form amyloid-like protein aggregates in vitro and in vivo. *Cell*, **90**, 549–58.

Schilling, G., Sharp, A. H., Loev, S. J. *et al.* (1995). Expression of the Huntington's disease (IT15) protein product in HD patients. *Hum. Mol. Genet.*, **4**, 1365–71.

Schubotz, R., Hausmann, L., Kaffarnik, H., Zehner, J. & Oepen, H. (1976). Fatty acid patterns and glucose tolerance in Huntington's chorea. *Res. Exp. Med. (Berl.)*, **167**(3), 203–15.

Schwarz, M., Fellows, S. J., Schaffrath, C. & Noth, J. (2001). Deficits in sensorimotor control during precise hand movements in Huntington's disease. *Clin. Neurophysiol.*, **112**, 95–106.

Sharp, A. H., Loev, S. J., Schilling, G. *et al.* (1995). Widespread expression of Huntington's disease gene (IT15) protein product. *Neuron*, **14**, 1065–74.

Shinotoh, H., Calne, D. B., Snow, B. *et al.* (1994). Normal CAG repeat length in the Huntington's disease gene in senile chorea. *Neurology*, **44**, 2183–4.

Shoulson, I. (1981). Huntington disease: functional capacities in patients treated with neuroleptic and antidepressant drugs. *Neurology*, **31**, 1333–5.

Shoulson, I. & Fahn, S. (1979). Huntington disease: clinical care and evaluation. *Neurology*, **29**, 1–3.

Shoulson, I., Odoroff, C., Oakes, D. *et al.* (1989). A controlled clinical trial of baclofen as protective therapy in early Huntington's disease. *Ann. Neurol.*, **25**, 252–9.

Snell, R. G., MacMillan, J. C., Cheadle, J. P. *et al.* (1993). Relationship between trinucleotide repeat expansion and phenotypic variation in Huntington's disease. *Nat. Genet.*, **4**, 393–7.

Snowden, J., Craufurd, D., Griffiths, H., Thompson, J. & Neary, D. (2001). Longitudinal evaluation of cognitive disorder in Huntington's disease. *J. Int. Neuropsychol. Soc.*, **7**, 33–44.

Steffan, J. S., Kazantsev, A., Spasic-Boskovic, O. *et al.* (2000). The Huntington's disease protein interacts with p53 and CREB-binding protein and represses transcription. *Proc. Natl Acad. Sci., USA*, **97**, 6763–8.

Steffan, J. S., Bodai, L., Pallos, J. *et al.* (2001). Histone deacetylase inhibitors arrest polyglutamine-dependent neurodegeneration in *Drosophila*. *Nature*, **413**, 739–43.

Tanaka, M., Machida, Y., Niu, S. *et al.* (2004). Trehalose alleviates polyglutamine-mediated pathology in a mouse model of Huntington disease. *Nat. Med.*, **10**, 148–54.

Thompson, P. D., Berardelli, A., Rothwell, J. C. *et al.* (1988). The coexistence of bradykinesia and chorea in Huntington's disease and its implications for theories of basal ganglia control of movement. *Brain*, **111**(2), 223–44.

Tian, J. R., Zee, D. S., Lasker, A. G. & Folstein, S. E. (1991). Saccades in Huntington's disease: predictive tracking and interaction between release of fixation and initiation of saccades. *Neurology*, **41**, 875–81.

Trottier, Y., Biancalana, V. & Mandel, J. L. (1994). Instability of CAG repeats in Huntington's disease: relation to parental transmission and age of onset. *J. Med. Genet.*, **31**, 377–82.

van Vugt, J. P., van Hilten, B. J. & Roos, R. A. (1996). Hypokinesia in Huntington's disease. *Mov. Disord.*, **11**, 384–88.

Vonsattel, J. P., Myers, R. H., Stevens, T. J., Ferrante, R. J., Bird, E. D. & Richardson, E., Jr. (1985). Neuropathological classification of Huntington's disease. *J. Neuropathol. Exp. Neurol.*, **44**, 559–77.

Vuillaume, I., Meynieu, P., Schraen-Maschke, S., Destee, A. & Sablonniere, B. (2000). Absence of unidentified CAG repeat expansion in patients with Huntington's disease-like phenotype. *J. Neurol. Neurosurg. Psychiatry*, **68**, 672–5.

Waters, C. O. (1842). In *Practice in Medicine*, ed. R. Dunglison. Philadelphia: Lee and Blanchard. p. 312.

Wellington, C. L., Brinkman, R. R., Kusky, J. & Hayden, M. R. (1997). Toward understanding the molecular pathology of Huntington's disease. *Brain Pathol.*, **7**, 979–1002.

Westphal, C. (1883). Über eine dem Bilde der cerebrospinalen grauen Degeneration ähnlichen Erkrankung des centralen Nervensystems ohne anatomischen Befund, nebst einigen Bemerkungen über paradoxe Contractionen. *Arch. Psychiatr. Nervenkr.*, **14**, 187–94.

Yang, W., Dunlap, J. R., Andrews, R. B. & Wetzel, R. (2002). Aggregated polyglutamine peptides delivered to nuclei are toxic to mammalian cells. *Hum. Mol. Genet.*, **11**, 2905–17.

Young, A. B., Shoulson, I., Penney, J. B. *et al.* (1986). Huntington's disease in Venezuela: neurologic features and functional decline. *Neurology*, **36**, 244–9.

Zeron, M. M., Hansson, O., Chen, N. *et al.* (2002). Increased sensitivity to *N*-methyl-D-aspartate receptor-mediated excitotoxicity in a mouse model of Huntington's disease. *Neuron*, **33**, 849–60.

Zuhlke, C., Riess, O., Schroder, K. *et al.* (1993). Expansion of the (CAG)n repeat causing Huntington's disease in 352 patients of German origin. *Hum. Mol. Genet*, **2**, 1467–9.

58

Dentatorubral-pallidoluysian atrophy (DRPLA): model for Huntington's disease and other polyglutamine diseases

Christopher A. Ross,[1] Lisa M. Ellerby,[2] Jonathan D. Wood[3] and Federick C. Nucifora Jr.[1]

[1]Division of Neurobiology, Department of Psychiatry, Johns Hopkins University School of Medicine, Baltimore, MD, USA
[2]Buck Institute for Research in Aging 8001 Redwood Blvd, Novato, CA, USA
[3]The University of Sheffield Academic Neurology Unit, Medical School, Sheffield, UK

First description and historical review

Dentatorubral-pallidoluysian atrophy (DRPLA) was first reported by J. K. Smith in 1958, in a detailed clinical description of a single case (Smith *et al.*, 1958). The disorder is rare in the western hemisphere, but in Japan is approximately as prevalent as Huntington's disease (HD). Like HD, DRPLA is inherited as an autosomal dominant, and shows a wide range of age of onset, with anticipation caused by instability of the triplet repeat expansion (Naito & Oyanagi, 1982; Takahashi *et al.*, 1988; Iizuka *et al.*, 1984; Goto *et al.*, 1982). The triplet repeat expansion mutation which causes DRPLA was identified as part of a program to find genes with triplet repeats as candidates for neuropsychiatric disorders with anticipation (Li *et al.*, 1993; Ross *et al.*, 1993). Two Japanese groups independently used the primers for amplifying the CAG repeat to determine that it is expanded in DRPLA and identify the gene in which this expanded repeat is located, termed atrophin-1 (Koide *et al.*, 1994; Nagafuchi *et al.*, 1994; Margolis *et al.*, 1996). The availability of a genetic test for DRPLA then made it possible to identify other families with DRPLA, some of whom had previously been diagnosed as having HD.

Morphological pattern of pathology

Among the polyglutamine neurodegenerative diseases, the pathology of DRPLA is most similar to that of HD (Ross, 1995). The areas most severely affected are given in the name of the disease. The dentate nucleus of the cerebellum has the greatest degeneration. The red nucleus, the globus pallidus, and the subthalamic nucleus are also significantly affected. The pathology of DRPLA involves neu-ronal loss and white matter degeneration (Becher *et al.*, 1997b, Yamada *et al.*, 2000). Like the other polyglutamine disorders, DRPLA involves aggregation of the gene protein product, in this case atrophin-1, into inclusion bodies in neuronal nuclei, especially in areas with degeneration, and also in more widespread areas (Becher *et al.*, 1997a, b, 1998; Becher & Ross, 1998). There are no intranuclear inclusions in the cerebellar Purkinje cells. However it appears to be a common feature of many polyglutamine disorders that Purkinje cells are not sites of intranuclear inclusion formation (Koyano *et al.*, 2002). Atrophin-1 protein also accumulates with an apparently diffuse localization within nuclei in widespread areas of the brain, including cerebral cortex, basal ganglia and many brainstem regions (Yamada *et al.*, 2001b).

Biochemical and neuropharmacological models

There has been little work aimed at devising a pharmacological or toxicological model of DRPLA. Biochemical and genetic studies are described below.

Molecular biology

Atrophin-1 encodes a protein of 1184 amino acids (Yazawa *et al.*, 1995; Margolis *et al.*, 1996). Immunohistochemical and immunocytochemical studies have demonstrated that atrophin-1 is localized to the cytoplasm and nucleus of neuronal and non-neuronal cells (Yazawa *et al.*, 1995; Wood *et al.*, 2000b). Atrophin-1 contains an amino-terminal nuclear localization signal (NLS) and a carboxy-terminal nuclear export signal (NES), and has been hypothesized to shuttle between the cytoplasm and nucleus as part of its normal cellular function (Schilling *et al.*, 1999). Its major cellular function may be that of a general transcriptional co-repressor.

The first suggestion that atrophin-1 may function in transcriptional regulation came as a result of yeast two-hybrid screens with the amino-terminus of the protein (Wood *et al.*, 2000a, b). Atrophin-1 was shown to interact with ETO/MTG8, a known transcriptional co-repressor, and repress transcription of a luciferase reporter gene in cultured cells (Wood *et al.*, 2000b). However, the physiological relevance of reporter gene assays in cultured cells transiently transfected with naked plasmid DNA is often uncertain. It has since been demonstrated that *Drosophila melanogaster* atrophin interacts with the transcription repressor Even-skipped and is necessary for its repressive function in vivo (Zhang *et al.*, 2002a). Both the *Drosophila* and human atrophin proteins repressed expression of a genomic reporter gene in vivo (Zhang *et al.*, 2002b)), and the repressive function of *Drosophila* atrophin was shown to be essential for embryonic patterning (Zhang *et al.*, 2002a; Erkner *et al.*, 2002). Hence there is now strong evidence that atrophin-1 does indeed function as a transcriptional co-repressor.

A protein called RERE is one other known nuclear atrophin-1 interacting protein (Yanagisawa *et al.*, 2000). Atrophin-1 and RERE interact through their arginine-glutamic acid dipeptide repeats, and are probably capable of forming homo- and hetero-dimers (Yanagisawa *et al.*, 2000). Yeast two-hybrid screening with the carboxy-terminal portion of atrophin-1 containing the ER repeats pulled out numerous clones of RERE and atrophin-1, all of which contained the respective ER repeats (J. D. Wood, unpublished data). RERE is localized to nuclear promyelocytic leukaemia (PML) oncogenic domains (PODs) and enhances apoptosis (Waerner *et al.*, 2001). Immunohistochemical studies have demonstrated an association of PML protein with nuclear inclusions in DRPLA (Yamada *et al.*, 2001a, b), while atrophin-1 over-expression in cultured cells apparently disassembles PODs (Wood *et al.*, 2000b).

The function of cytoplasmic atrophin-1 is less well understood. Similarly, the factors that regulate its nuclear trafficking are unknown. What clues there are have again come from yeast two-hybrid screens. Atrophin-1 contains five PY motifs and these appear to modulate interactions with two families of WW domain-containing proteins (Wood *et al.*, 1998). MAGI-1 and MAGI-2 (previously referred to as AIP3 and AIP1 respectively) are large membrane-associated guanylate kinases (MAGUKs) with an inverted arrangement of protein-protein interaction domains. (Dobrosotskaya *et al.*, 1997). MAGI proteins appear to be impor-

tant for the assembly of signalling complexes at synapses and tight cell junctions. WWP1, WWP2 and Itch (previously referred to as AIP5, AIP2 and AIP4, respectively) are highly homologous E3 ubiquitin ligase enzymes, which may be involved in atrophin-1 turnover. At least one of these E3s appears capable of ubiquitinating atrophin-1 in a cell transfection based assay (J. D. Wood, unpublished data).

A proline-rich region in atrophin-1 binds to the SH3 domain of the L and S isoforms of the insulin receptor substrate of 53 kDa protein (IRSp53) (Okamura-Oho *et al.*, 1999, 2001). IRSp53 is a substrate for the insulin/IGF-1 receptor tyrosine kinase and may be involved in post-synaptic insulin signaling in the brain (Abbott *et al.*, 1999). A yeast two-hybrid screen with the PDZ domains of MAGI-2 pulled out the S isoform of IRSp53, which has a C-terminal PDZ domain-binding motif (J. D. Wood, unpublished data). This suggests that atrophin-1, MAGI-2 and IRSp53S have the potential to form a trimeric complex in brain. IRSp53 is known to activate actin polymerization and membrane ruffling through interaction with Rac and WAVE (Miki *et al.*, 2000). Atrophin-1 has not been demonstrated to influence actin polymerization.

Pathogenesis

Our understanding of DRPLA pathogenesis has been advanced by cell model and mouse model studies. Cell model studies have indicated that atrophin-1 with an expanded repeat can be directly toxic to cells. Shorter fragments appear to be more toxic than the full-length protein; the possible role of proteolytic processing will be discussed below. In addition, cell model studies have indicated a role for nuclear localization; fragments small enough to diffuse passively into the nucleus are toxic (Igarashi *et al.*, 1998). Furthermore, we have recently shown in studies involving mutations of putative endogenous nuclear export signal and nuclear localization signal that these localization signals are functional, and that deleting the nuclear localization signal substantially decreases toxicity, while deleting the nuclear export signal substantially enhances toxicity (Wood *et al.*, 2000b; Nucifora, Jr. *et al.*, 2003). These studies strongly suggest that, at least in vitro, nuclear localization enhances toxicity. These data, taken together with data indicating that nuclear atrophin-1 leads to alterations of normal nuclear protein such as PML, CBP and Sp1 (Yamada *et al.*, 2001a, b), indicate that abnormalities of nuclear proteins may contribute to atrophin-1 mediated toxicity.

The cell model studies have also shown that atrophin-1 with an expanded polyglutamine repeat will aggregate in cells (Igarashi *et al.*, 1998; Nucifora, Jr. *et al.*, 2003; Wood *et al.*, 2000b; Toyoshima *et al.*, 2002). However aggregation is not correlated with toxicity, and in cell model studies, there can be toxicity due to expression of mutant atrophin-1, with no aggregates of atrophin-1 visible in the light microscope (Nucifora *et al.*, 2002). These results are also comparable to those for HD, in which toxicity is enhanced by nuclear localization, but not dependent on visible aggregates. Aggregation and formation of an "aggresome" may be part of the cellular response to misfolded proteins (Kopito, 2000; Shimohata *et al.*, 2002).

Mouse model studies have contributed greatly to our understanding of the pathogenesis of DRPLA. Several mouse models have been made (Schilling *et al.*, 1999, 2001; Sato *et al.*, 1999a, b). The transgenic mouse model made in our laboratory has reproduced many of the features of DRPLA. This model was made using the prion promotor to drive atrophin-1 expression throughout the brain (except in cerebellar Purkinje cells) as well as at lower levels in some peripheral tissues. This is a strategy we have also successfully used for modeling HD (Schilling *et al.*, 1999). For DRPLA, the construct encoded full-length atrophin-1 with either a normal polyglutamine repeat or 65 consecutive glutamines, which would yield juvenile onset in human patients. Control transgenic mice were indistinguishable from non-transgenic litter mates. Mice expressing the 65-glutamine protein (at approximately two to three times the level of endogenous atrophin-1) developed a neurological phenotype resembling the human disease including ataxia, tremors, abnormal movements, and in some mice seizures. The movement disorder progressed to early death (Schilling *et al.*, 1999; Andreassen *et al.*, 2001). Neuropathologic examination of these mice revealed both intranuclear inclusions and diffuse-appearing nuclear reactivity for atrophin-1, similar to human postmortem brain material from DRPLA patients.

Western blot analysis of these mice indicated that the full-length atrophin-1 was expressed throughout the brain and was predominantly cytoplasmic. However, when a nuclear fraction was prepared, a substantial amount of a smaller species was visible. This ran at approximately 120 kDa, compared to endogenous of 200–220 kDa for full-length atrophin-1. Comparison to nuclear extracts prepared from 1-month-old and 11-month-old transgenic mice demonstrated that the 120 kDa fragments accumulated with time. Nuclear extracts from human post mortem brain material showed an almost identical-appearing species at about 120 kDa (running as a closely spaced doublet). Thus we believe there is nuclear accumulation of a fragment of mutant atrophin-1, contributing to pathogenesis. This is comparable to the toxic fragment model for Huntington's disease (Ross, 2002).

Proteolytic processing of atrophin-1

A number of lines of evidence suggest that proteolytic cleavage of mutant atrophin-1 modulate its cellular localization and may be critical for pathogenesis (Nucifora, Jr. *et al.*, 2003; Schilling *et al.*, 1999). For both DRPLA and HD, accumulation of nuclear fragments may be critical to the pathogenic mechanism, since truncation and nuclear localization of either of these proteins enhances cellular dysfunction and toxicity (Nucifora, Jr. *et al.*, 2003; Saudou *et al.*, 1998; Peters *et al.*, 1999). The signals that control cellular localization for atrophin-1 are better understood than for huntingtin, so that DRPLA may provide a model for understanding some aspects of the cellular pathogenesis of HD. Conversely, more is known about the proteases involved in cleaving huntingtin in vivo than atrophin-1, and some of the proteolytic cleavage events found in DRPLA may differ from HD. The polyglutamine tract lies near the middle of the atrophin-1 protein, while in huntingtin it is found near the N-terminus of the protein. The atrophin-1 protein contains an NLS in the N-terminus (Nucifora, Jr. *et al.*, 2003), while huntingtin does not appear to contain a functional NLS. Both proteins contain a C-terminal NES (Nucifora, Jr. *et al.*, 2003; Lo *et al.*, 2003)

Many studies in vitro and in vivo are consistent with caspase as well as calpain cleavage of huntingtin (Goldberg *et al.*, 1996; Wellington *et al.*, 1998, 2000; Holbert *et al.*, 2001; Gafni & Ellerby, 2002; Kim *et al.*, 2001). In addition, further truncation of Htt may be produced by an unknown aspartyl protease (Lunkes *et al.*, 2002). Huntingtin may be transported into the nucleus via interactions with an NLS-containing shuttle protein. (Alternatively, if cleavage takes place in the cytoplasm, it is conceivable that fragments could diffuse passively into the nucleus.) Unlike HD, in which truncation leads to small N-terminal polyQ containing products, cleavage of atrophin-1 found in mouse models and human postmortem tissue leads to the generation of a large nuclear N-terminal polyQ containing fragment of atrophin-1 containing the NLS (Schilling *et al.*, 1999).

Similar to huntingtin, atrophin-1 can be cleaved by caspases, and caspase cleavage can modulate atrophin-1 cell toxicity in vitro (Ellerby *et al.*, 1999; Miyashita *et al.*, 1997, 1998). Cleavage of atrophin-1 by caspases occurs at D109. Cleavage at this site would generate a very short fragment containing the N-terminus, and a longer fragment missing the N-terminus but containing the polyglutamine repeat. However, evidence for these products in vivo is lacking. The large N-terminal nuclear 120 kDa fragment present in the DRPLA transgenic mouse model and post-mortem tissue is immunoreactive to an N-terminal atrophin-1 antibody (Nucifora, Jr. *et al.*, 2003) and therefore cannot be caspase-derived. Indeed, the relevant fragment of atrophin-1 localized in the nucleus is not generated by any of the currently known caspases (Ellerby *et al.*, 1999; Nucifora, Jr. *et al.*, 2003). Further, calpains, which frequently have cleavage sites clustered in the same region of proteins as caspase sites, do not generate the large N-terminal nuclear 120 kDa atrophin-1 product (L. M. Ellerby, unpublished data).

The locations of the NLS and the NES in the atrophin-1 sequence suggest that truncation in vivo would delete the NES, with the shuttling of the mutant atrophin-1 fragment into the nucleus by the NLS unopposed by export pathways. Subsequent nuclear accumulation could then enhance cellular toxicity. As discussed above, expression of a mutant atrophin-1 construct, with an N-terminal fragment of similar size to the truncation product found in vivo, and lacking the NES, showed enhanced nuclear localization and cell toxicity when compared to the full-length mutant atrophin-1 protein containing the NES (Nucifora *et al.*, 2003). The proteases responsible for generating the large N-terminal nuclear 120 kDa atrophin-1 fragment found in vivo are not known, and therefore it will be important to determine the exact cleavage site in the atrophin-1 protein. This will allow studies to be directed at identifying the protease responsible for generating this cleavage product. Whether the in vitro studies suggesting the involvement of an aspartyl protease in huntingtin truncation (Lunkes *et al.*, 2002) are relevant to DRPLA proteolysis is currently not known.

Mechanisms of cell death

Based on the evidence described above, we believe that nuclear localization and proteolytic processing of mutant atrophin-1 contribute to cell toxicity. What might be the mechanisms of cell dysfunction and cell death? Disruption of gene transcription is a likely candidate. Studies have shown that mutant atrophin-1 can interfere with gene transcription when assayed in several different ways. Mutant atrophin-1, as well as mutant huntingtin, may interact with the transcription factor CBP (Nucifora, Jr. *et al.*, 2001). This effect may be mediated by a direct interaction between mutant polyglutamine in atrophin-1 and a short polyglutamine stretch normally present in CBP. The hypothesis that abnormal polyglutamine interactions might be relevant for polyglutamine diseases was first put forward by Max Perutz (Perutz, 1994, 1996), and subsequently studied by David Housman's group (Kazantsev *et al.*, 1999; Preisinger *et al.*, 1999). Elegant data have also been provided for interactions of CBP with the androgen receptor, which undergoes polyglutamine expansion in the disease spinal and bulbar muscular atrophy (SBMA) (McCampbell *et al.*, 2000; McCampbell & Fischbeck, 2001).

Abnormal phosphorylation of atrophin-1 may contribute to pathogenesis (Okamura-Oho *et al.*, 2003). Modifications by ubiquitination and especially SUMOylation may also be relevant (Terashima *et al.*, 2002; Ueda *et al.*, 2002).

Other mechanisms have been proposed as well, which may be relevant for HD, or DRPLA. Interactions with p53, or interactions with CBP not dependent on direct polyglutamine interactions have also been proposed (Steffan *et al.*, 2000). Other transcriptional mechanisms may be relevant as well. Atrophin-1 has been reported to interfere with transcription mediated via TAFII130 (Shimohata *et al.*, 2000). Another possible mechanism resulting in transcriptional disregulation, which has been proposed for HD, and might also be relevant for DRPLA, would involve interference with the interaction between Sp1 and TAFII130 (Dunah *et al.*, 2002; Jiang *et al.*, 2003). Taken together, there appears to be substantial evidence for disruption of gene transcription as at least one important mechanism for pathogenesis of DRPLA, though the exact molecular interactions are still not completely clear. One puzzle is that, unlike for huntingtin, substantial amounts of full-length atrophin-1 are present in the nucleus normally. The truncation, removing the NES, would presumably just increase levels further. However the mutant protein, especially after truncation, may interact abnormally with proteins in the nucleus, such as CBP or others, and possibly may do so in subcompartments of the nucleus different from normal.

A more difficult question is the identification of the downstream genes whose transcription might be altered. A gene expression array experiment has found changes in expression levels of a substantial number of genes in DRPLA transgenic mice (Luthi-Carter *et al.*, 2002). There is overlap between the genes changed in the DRPLA model and those changed in HD models (Luthi-Carter *et al.*, 2002; Luthi-Carter *et al.*, 2000). Some of these changes may involve genes coding for proteins involved in neuronal signaling. However, which of them, if any, are involved in pathogenesis is still unknown.

Clinical picture

The nature of the clinical presentation depends greatly on the age of onset and the length of the CAG repeat. Cases with adult onset often have a clinical presentation virtually indistinguishable from that of Huntington's diseases. Motor disorders include chorea, dystonia and voluntary movement abnormalities including incoordination and ataxia. Cognitive dysfunction includes features similar to those of HD with slowed thinking, loss of retrieval of information and difficulty in sequencing tasks initially, progressing to more severe dementia later on. In addition, a variety of emotional features can be present, including affective disorder and psychosis (Adachi *et al.*, 2001; Tsuji, 1999, 2000; Ross *et al.*, 1997b; Smith *et al.*, 1958; Smith *et al.*, 1958; Smith, 1975; Naito & Oyanagi, 1982; Takahashi *et al.*, 1988). Cerebellar ataxia can be prominent (Yabe *et al.*, 2002) head tremor can also be present (Ohizumi *et al.*, 2002). All of these features are progressive. The illness is invariably fatal except in cases with sufficiently late onset in which patients may die of other illnesses (Ross *et al.*, 1997b).

The clinical presentation of patients with early onset associated with large expansions of the CAG repeat is quite different with cognitive deterioration, incoordination, and progressive myoclonic epilepsy, or other forms of epilepsy, being quite prominent, and considerably less chorea, dystonia, or other involuntary movements (Iizuka *et al.*, 1984; Tomoda *et al.*, 1991). In some cases, features similar to those seen in autism may be present (Licht & Lynch, 2002). This is also a progressive fatal form of the illness, and because of the relatively early onset, individuals may die in early adulthood or even in childhood.

Clinical variants

DRPLA has been most carefully studied in Japan, as mentioned above, but has also been described in North America, Europe and China (Ross *et al.*, 1997b; Potter *et al.*, 1995; Warner *et al.*, 1995; Norremolle *et al.*, 1995; Le *et al.*, 2003; Lee *et al.*, 2001; Villani *et al.*, 1998; Nielsen *et al.*, 1996). While there have been some differences observed, the clinical features all seem fairly comparable. In addition, the neuropathological changes are generally similar.

A family with the clinical features of DRPLA was found in the United States prior to the discovery of the DRPLA gene. The syndrome was named the "Haw River syndrome" after the location of the pedigree in North Carolina. The syndrome in this family was subsequently shown to be caused by expansion in the atrophin-1 gene (Burke *et al.*, 1994). We have seen several families who have moved to Baltimore from this part of North Carolina, and likely represent branches of this extended pedigree. These patients and the patients described from North Carolina appear to have fairly characteristic DRPLA.

Time course

As noted above, DRPLA is invariably fatal, except in the cases in which onset is sufficiently late that affected individuals die from competing causes of illness. As has been described for Huntington's disease, there is some clinical

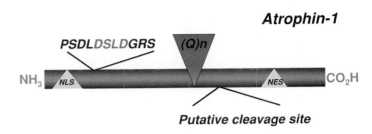

Fig. 58.1 Model for DRPLA pathogenesis. Atrophin-1 normally shuttles in and out of the nucleus, where it has a role in transcriptional regulation. After removal of the NES, it cannot be exported from the nucleus, and accumulates. Abnormal interactions with transcriptional regulators, such as CBP, contribute to toxicity. See text for details.

impression that the progression of the illness is more rapid in individuals with early onset. However, quantitative studies to document this have not yet been performed. The features that appear to be most clearly progressive are the motor disorder and the cognitive disorder. Emotional features, including affective disorder and psychotic features, are more variable, and may present at different points in the course. In patients with juvenile onset, the epilepsy tends to become more severe as the illness progresses, making management difficult.

Epidemiology

The greater prevalence in Japan compared to other regions of the world has an interesting explanation (Deka *et al.*, 1995; Masuda *et al.*, 1995; Watkins *et al.*, 1995; Yanagisawa *et al.*, 1996; Squitieri *et al.*, 1994). In the Japanese population distribution of the atrophin-1 CAG repeat length is slightly longer than in Europe and the United States, and is skewed toward more of the rare alleles at the higher end of the normal range, or, as has been described for HD, intermediate alleles. Some of these alleles toward the high end of the normal range presumably are slightly unstable, and may occasionally expand, establishing new pedigrees with DRPLA. This is the converse of the situation for HD, in which there are fewer alleles at the high end of normal in Japan, and thus fewer pedigrees with HD in Japan compared to Europe and North America.

Investigations

The major diagnostic test is the genetic test for the presence of the expanded repeat in Atrophin-1. While DRPLA is present in all populations, it is relatively rare in

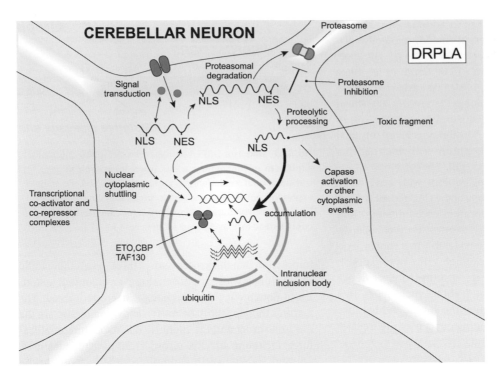

Fig. 58.2 Primary structure of atrophin-1, which contains 1184 amino acids. There is an NLS in the N-terminal region (16–32) of the protein, and an NES in the C-terminal region (1033–1041). The expanding polyglutamine stretch (indicated as (Q)n) is located at amino acid 484 of atrophin-1 and the caspase consensus site (DSLD) is at amino acids 106–109. The putative cleavage site that would release the NES is noted.

populations from European ancestry, and in those cases may be tested after a diagnostic test for HD has come back negative. MRI scans or other brain imaging can also help establish the diagnosis. The extent of cerebellar compared to cortical and other brain atrophy is somewhat variable, in part relating to age of onset of the illness. In addition to these changes, diffuse high-intensity signals are often evident in cerebral white matter on T_2-weighted MRI, particularly in adults with fewer than 65 repeats (Koide *et al.*, 1997). High-intensity signals may also be found in the brainstem, globus pallidus and thalamus on T_2-weighted and flare imaging. As in HD, there have been studies suggesting that there is abnormal cellular metabolism in DRPLA, including evidence of abnormal energy metabolism in skeletal muscle (Lodi *et al.*, 2000). Neuropathology continues to be of use in confirming the diagnosis (Yamada *et al.*, 2000, 2002; Ross *et al.*, 1997a; Becher *et al.*, 1997b).

Treatment

As with other polyglutamine neurodegenerative disorders, there are no treatments known which can delay the onset or slow the progression of the illness. However, studies in mouse models have recently begun to provide some candidate agents. A number of therapeutic studies of HD models have been done recently, based on current understanding of pathogenesis (Ferrante *et al.*, 2002; Feigin & Zgaljardic, 2002; Jankowsky *et al.*, 2002; Tarnopolsky & Beal, 2001; Steffan *et al.*, 2001; McCampbell *et al.*, 2001). Some of these approaches include designing agents to compensate for the hypothesized abnormal gene transcription caused by the polyglutamine expansion or counteract downstream effects of polyglutamine toxicity, such as increases in free radicals or excitotoxicity.

In cell models of DRPLA, it has been reported that cystamine may provide some neuroprotection (Igarashi *et al.*, 1998). Cystamine can be a transglutamase inhibitor. However it may have other effects, including effects on oxidative metabolism. The dose used in this study was relatively high, so the mechanism is uncertain. However, cystamine is one of the agents being studied for HD and if it is applicable for HD it may well be useful for DRPLA as well.

There has been little systematic therapeutic trial research in DRPLA. A large study in Huntington's disease called the CARE-HD study showed no effect of a glutamate receptor antagonist, and a possible modest effect of an anti-oxidant, Co-enzyme Q10 (Huntington Study Group, 2001). It is possible that combinations of agents acting via different mechanisms may have the best chance of success (Figs. 58.1, 58.2).

REFERENCES

Abbott, M. A., Wells, D. G. & Fallon, J. R. (1999). The insulin receptor tyrosine kinase substrate p58/53 and the insulin receptor are components of CNS synapses. *J. Neurosci.*, **19**, 7300–8.

Adachi, N., Arima, K., Asada, T. *et al.* (2001). Dentatorubral-pallidoluysian atrophy (DRPLA) presenting with psychosis. *J. Neuropsychiatry Clin. Neurosci.*, **13**, 258–60.

Andreassen, O. A., Dedeoglu, A., Ferrante, R. J. *et al.* (2001). Creatine increases survival and delays motor symptoms in a transgenic animal model of Huntington's disease. *Neurobiol. Dis.*, **8**, 479–91.

Becher, M. W., Kotzuk, J. A., Sharp, A. H. *et al.* (1997a). Intranuclear neuronal inclusions in Huntington's disease and dentatorubral and pallidoluysian atrophy: correlation between the density of inclusions and IT15 CAG triplet repeat length. *Neurobiol. Dis.*, **4**, 387–97.

Becher, M. W., Kotzuk, J. A., Sharp, A. H. *et al.* (1998). Intranuclear neuronal inclusions in Huntington's disease and dentatorubral and pallidoluysian atrophy: correlation between the density of inclusions and IT15 CAG triplet repeat length. *Neurobiol. Dis.*, **4**, 387–97.

Becher, M. W. & Ross, C. A. (1998). Intranuclear neuronal inclusions in DRPLA [letter; comment]. *Mov. Disord.*, **13**, 852–3.

Becher, M. W., Rubinsztein, D. C., Leggo, J. *et al.* (1997b). Dentatorubral and pallidoluysian atrophy (DRPLA). Clinical and neuropathological findings in genetically confirmed North American and European pedigrees. *Mov. Disord.*, **12**, 519–30.

Burke, J. R., Wingfield, M. S., Lewis, K. E. *et al.* (1994). The Haw River syndrome: dentato-rubropallidoluysian atrophy (DRPLA) in an African-American family. *Nat. Genet.*, **7**, 521–4.

Deka, R., Miki, T., Yin, S.-J. *et al.* (1995). Normal CAG repeat variation at the DRPLA locus in world populations. *Am. J. Hum. Genet.*, **57**, 508–11.

Dobrosotskaya, I., Guy, R. K. & James, G. L. (1997). MAGI-1, a membrane-associated guanylate kinase with a unique arrangement of protein-protein interaction domains. *J. Biol. Chem.*, **272**, 31589–97.

Dunah, A. W., Jeong, H., Griffin, A. *et al.* (2002). Sp1 and TAFII130 transcriptional activity disrupted in early Huntington's disease. *Science*, **296**, 2238–43.

Ellerby, L. M., Andrusiak, R. L., Wellington, C. L. *et al.* (1999). Cleavage of atrophin-1 at caspase site aspartic acid 109 modulates cytotoxicity. *J. Biol. Chem.*, **274**, 8730–6.

Erkner, A., Roure, A., Charroux, B. *et al.* (2002). Grunge, related to human Atrophin-like proteins, has multiple functions in *Drosophila* development. *Development*, **129**, 1119–29.

Feigin, A. & Zgaljardic, D. (2002). Recent advances in Huntington's disease: implications for experimental therapeutics. *Curr. Opin. Neurol.*, **15**, 483–9.

Ferrante, R. J., Andreassen, O. A., Dedeoglu, A. *et al.* (2002). Therapeutic effects of coenzyme Q10 and remacemide in transgenic mouse models of Huntington's disease. *J. Neurosci.*, **22**, 1592–9.

Gafni, J. & Ellerby, L. M. (2002). Calpain activation in Huntington's disease. *J. Neurosci.*, **22**, 4842–9.

Goldberg, Y. P., Nicholson, D. W., Rasper, D. M. *et al.* (1996). Cleavage of huntingtin by apopain, a proapoptotic cysteine protease, is modulated by the polyglutamine tract. *Nat. Genet.*, **13**, 442–9.

Goto, I., Tobimatsu, S., Ohta, M., Hosokawa, S., Shibasaki, H. & Kuroiwa, Y. (1982). Dentatorubropallidoluysian degeneration: clinical, neuro-ophthalmologic, biochemical, and pathologic studies on autosomal dominant form. *Neurology*, **32**, 1395–9.

Holbert, S., Denghien, I., Kiechle, T. *et al.* (2001). The Gln–Ala repeat transcriptional activator CA150 interacts with huntingtin: neuropathologic and genetic evidence for a role in Huntington's disease pathogenesis. *Proc. Natl Acad. Sci., USA*, **98**, 1811–16.

Huntington Study Group, T. (2001). A randomized, placebo-controlled trial of coenzyme Q10 and remacemide in Huntington's disease. *Neurology*, **57**, 397–404.

Igarashi, S., Koide, R., Shimohata, T. *et al.* (1998). Suppression of aggregate formation and apoptosis by transglutaminase inhibitors in cells expressing truncated DRPLA protein with an expanded polyglutamine stretch. *Nat. Genet.*, **18**, 111–17.

Iizuka, R., Hirayama, K. & Maehara, K. (1984). Dentato-rubro-pallido-luysian atrophy: a clinco-pathological study. *J. Neurol. Neurosurg. Psychiatry*, **47**, 1288–98.

Jankowsky, J. L., Savonenko, A., Schilling, G., Wang, J., Xu, G. & Borchelt, D. R. (2002). Transgenic mouse models of neurodegenerative disease: opportunities for therapeutic development. *Curr. Neurol. Neurosci. Rep.*, **2**, 457–64.

Jiang, H., Nucifora, F. C., Jr., Ross, C. A. & DeFranco, D. B. (2003). Cell death triggered by polyglutamine-expanded huntingtin in a neuronal cell line is associated with degradation of CREB-binding protein. *Hum. Mol. Genet.*, **12**, 1–12.

Kazantsev, A., Preisinger, E., Dranovsky, A., Goldgaber, D. & Housman, D. (1999). Insoluble detergent-resistant aggregates form between pathological and nonpathological lengths of polyglutamine in mammalian cells. *Proc. Natl Acad. Sci., USA*, **96**, 11404–9.

Kim, Y. J., Yi, Y., Sapp, E. *et al.* (2001). Caspase 3-cleaved N-terminal fragments of wild-type and mutant huntingtin are present in normal and Huntington's disease brains, associate with membranes, and undergo calpain-dependent proteolysis. *Proc. Natl Acad. Sci., USA*, **98**, 12784–9.

Koide, O., Ikeuchi, T., Onodera, O. *et al.* (1994). Unstable expansion of CAG repeat in hereditary dentatorubral-pallidoluysian atrophy (DRPLA). *Nat. Genet.*, **6**, 9–13.

Koide, R., Onodera, O., Ikeuchi, T. *et al.* (1997). Atrophy of the cerebellum and brainstem in dentatorubral pallidoluysian atrophy. Influence of CAG repeat size on MRI findings. *Neurology*, **49** (6), 1605–12.

Kopito, R. R. (2000). Aggresomes, inclusion bodies and protein aggregation. *Trends Cell Biol.*, **10**, 524–30.

Koyano, S., Iwabuchi, K., Yagishita, S., Kuroiwa, Y. & Uchihara, T. (2002). Paradoxical absence of nuclear inclusion in cerebellar Purkinje cells of hereditary ataxias linked to CAG expansion. *J. Neurol. Neurosurg. Psychiatry*, **73**, 450–2.

Le, B. I., Camuzat, A., Castelnovo, G. *et al.* (2003). Prevalence of dentatorubral-pallidoluysian atrophy in a large series of white patients with cerebellar ataxia. *Arch. Neurol.*, **60**, 1097–9.

Lee, I. H., Soong, B. W., Lu, Y. C. & Chang, Y. C. (2001). Dentatorubropallidoluysian atrophy in Chinese. *Arch. Neurol.*, **58**, 1905–8.

Li, S.-H., McInnis, M. G., Margolis, R. L., Antonarakis, S. E. & Ross, C. A. (1993). Novel triplet repeat containing genes in human brain: cloning, expression, and length polymorphisms. *Genomics*, **16**, 572–9.

Licht, D. J. & Lynch, D. R. (2002). Juvenile dentatorubralpallidoluysian atrophy: new clinical features. *Pediatr. Neurol.*, **26**, 51–4.

Lodi, R., Schapira, A. H., Manners, D. *et al.* (2000). Abnormal in vivo skeletal muscle energy metabolism in Huntington's disease and dentatorubropallidoluysian atrophy. *Ann. Neurol.*, **48**, 72–6.

Lunkes, A., Lindenberg, K. S., Ben Haiem, L. *et al.* (2002). Proteases acting on mutant huntingtin generate cleaved products that differentially build up cytoplasmic and nuclear inclusions. *Mol. Cell*, **10**, 259–69.

Luthi-Carter, R., Strand, A., Peters, N. L. *et al.* (2000). Decreased expression of striatal signaling genes in a mouse model of Huntington's disease. *Hum. Mol. Genet.*, **9**, 1259–71.

Luthi-Carter, R., Strand, A. D., Hanson, S. A. *et al.* (2002). Polyglutamine and transcription: gene expression changes shared by DRPLA and Huntington's disease mouse models reveal context-independent effects. *Hum. Mol. Genet.*, **11**, 1927–37.

Margolis, R. L., Li, S.-H., Young, W. S. *et al.* (1996). DRPLA gene (Atrophin-1) sequence and mRNA expression in human brain. *Mol. Brain Res.*, **36**, 219–26.

Masuda, N., Goto, J., Murayama, N., Watanabe, M., Kondo, I. & Kanazawa, I. (1995). Analysis of triplet repeats in the huntingtin gene in Japanese families affected with Huntington disease. *J. Med. Genet.*, **32**, 701–5.

McCampbell, A. & Fischbeck, K. H. (2001). Polyglutamine and CBP: fatal attraction? *Nat. Med.*, **7**, 528–30.

McCampbell, A., Taye, A. A., Whitty, L., Penney, E., Steffan, J. S. & Fischbeck, K. H. (2001). Histone deacetylase inhibitors reduce polyglutamine toxicity. *Proc. Natl Acad. Sci., USA*, **98**, 15179–84.

McCampbell, A., Taylor, J. P., Taye, A. A. *et al.* (2000). CREB-binding protein sequestration by expanded polyglutamine. *Hum. Mol. Genet.*, **9**, 2197–202.

Miki, H., Yamaguchi, H., Suetsugu, S. & Takenawa, T. (2000). IRSp53 is an essential intermediate between Rac and WAVE in the regulation of membrane ruffling. *Nature*, **408**, 732–5.

Miyashita, T., Nagao, K., Ohmi, K., Yanagisawa, H., Okamura-Oho, Y. & Yamada, M. (1998). Intracellular aggregate formation of dentatorubral-pallidoluysian atrophy (DRPLA) protein with the extended polyglutamine. *Biochem. Biophys. Res. Commun.*, **249**, 96–102.

Miyashita, T., Okamura-Oho, Y., Mito, Y., Nagafuchi, S. & Yamada, M. (1997). Dentatorubral pallidoluysian atrophy (DRPLA) protein is cleaved by caspase-3 during apoptosis. *J. Biol. Chem.*, **272**, 29238–42.

Nagafuchi, S., Yanagisawa, H., Ohsaki, E. *et al.* (1994). Structure and expression of the gene responsible for the triplet repeat disorder, dentatorubral and pallidoluysian atrophy (DRPLA). *Nat. Genet.*, **8**, 177–82.

Naito, H. & Oyanagi, S. (1982). Familial myoclonus epilepsy and choreoathetosis: Hereditary dentatorubral-pallidoluysian atrophy. *Neurology*, **32**, 798–807.

Nielsen, J. E., Sorensen, S. A., Hasholt, L. & Norremolle, A. (1996). Dentatorubral-pallidoluysian atrophy. Clinical features of a five-generation Danish family. *Mov. Disord.*, **11**, 533–41.

Norremolle, A., Nielsen, J. E., Sorensen, S. A. & Hasholt, E. (1995). Elongated CAG repeats of the B37 gene in a Danish family with dentato-rubral-pallido-luysian atrophy. *Hum. Genet.*, **95**, 313–18.

Nucifora, F. C., Jr., Ellerby, L. M., Wellington, C. L. *et al.* (2003). Nuclear localization of a non-caspase truncation product of atrophin-1, with an expanded polyglutamine repeat, increases cellular toxicity. *J. Biol. Chem.*, **278**, 13047–55.

Nucifora, F. C., Jr., Sasaki, M., Peters, M. F. *et al.* (2001). Interference by huntingtin and atrophin-1 with cbp-mediated transcription leading to cellular toxicity1. *Science*, **291**, 2423–8.

Ohizumi, H., Okuma, Y., Fukae, J., Fujishima, K., Goto, K. & Mizuno, Y. (2002). Head tremor in dentatorubral-pallidoluysian atrophy. *Acta Neurol. Scand.*, **106**, 319–21.

Okamura-Oho, Y., Miyashita, T., Ohmi, K. & Yamada, M. (1999). Dentatorubral-pallidoluysian atrophy protein interacts through a proline-rich region near polyglutamine with the SH3 domain of an insulin receptor tyrosine kinase substrate. *Hum. Mol. Genet.*, **8**, 947–57.

Okamura-Oho, Y., Miyashita, T. & Yamada, M. (2001). Distinctive tissue distribution and phosphorylation of IRSp53 isoforms. *Biochem. Biophys. Res. Commun.*, **289**, 957–60.

Okamura-Oho, Y., Miyashita, T., Nagao, K. *et al.* (2003). Dentatorubral-pallidoluysian atrophy protein is phosphorylated by c-Jun NH$_2$-terminal kinase. *Hum. Mol. Genet.*, **12**, 1535–42.

Perutz, M. (1994). Polar zippers: their role in human disease. In *Protein Science*, London: Cambridge University Press, pp. 1629–37.

Perutz, M. F. (1996). Glutamine repeats and inherited neurodegenerative diseases: molecular aspects. *Curr. Opini. Struct. Biol.*, **6**, 848–58.

Peters, M. F., Nucifora, F. C., Jr., Kushi, J. *et al.* (1999). Nuclear targeting of mutant Huntingtin increases toxicity 3. *Mol. Cell Neurosci.*, **14**, 121–8.

Potter, N. T., Meyer, M. A., Zimmerman, A. W., Eisenstadt, M. L. & Anderson, I. J. (1995). Molecular and clinical findings in a family with dentatorubral-pallidoluysian atrophy. *Ann. Neurol.*, **37**, 273–7.

Preisinger, E., Jordan, B. M., Kazantsev, A. & Housman, D. (1999). Evidence for a recruitment and sequestration mechanism in Huntington's disease. *Phil. Trans. Roy. Soc. Lond B Biol. Sci.*, **354**, 1029–34.

Ross, C. A. (1995). When more is less: pathogenesis of glutamine repeat neurodegenerative diseases. *Neuron*, **15**, 493–6.

Ross, C. A. (2002). Polyglutamine pathogenesis: emergence of unifying mechanisms for Huntington's disease and related disorders. *Neuron*, **35**, 819–22.

Ross, C. A., Becher, M. W., Colomer, V., Engelender, S., Wood, J. D. & Sharp, A. H. (1997a). Huntington's disease and dentatorubral-pallidoluysian atrophy: proteins, pathogenesis, and pathology. *Brain Pathol.*, **7**, 1003–16.

Ross, C. A., Margolis, R. L., Rosenblatt, A., Ranen, N. G., Becher, M. W. & Aylward, E. (1997b). Reviews in molecular medicine: Huntington disease and the related disorder, dentatorubral-pallidoluysian atrophy (DRPLA). *Medicine*, **76**, 305–38.

Ross, C. A., McInnis, M. G., Margolis, R. L. & Li, S.-H. (1993). Genes with triplet repeats: candidate mediators of neuropsychiatric disorders. *Trends Neurosci.*, **16**, 254–60.

Sato, A., Shimohata, T., Koide, R. *et al.* (1999a). Adenovirus-mediated expression of mutant DRPLA proteins with expanded polyglutamine stretches in neuronally differentiated PC12 cells. Preferential intranuclear aggregate formation and apoptosis. *Hum. Mol. Genet.*, **8**, 997–1006.

Sato, T., Oyake, M., Nakamura, K. *et al.* (1999b). Transgenic mice harboring a full-length human mutant DRPLA gene exhibit age-dependent intergenerational and somatic instabilities of CAG repeats comparable with those in DRPLA patients. *Hum. Mol. Genet.*, **8**, 99–106.

Saudou, F., Finkbeiner, S., Devys, D. & Greenberg, M. E. (1998). Huntingtin acts in the nucleus to induce apoptosis but death does not correlate with the formation of intranuclear inclusions. *Cell*, **95**, 55–66.

Schilling, G., Wood, J. D., Duan, K. *et al.* (1999). Nuclear accumulation of truncated atrophin-1 fragments in a transgenic mouse model of DRPLA. *Neuron*, **24**, 275–286.

Schilling, G., Jinnah, H. A., Gonzales, V. *et al.* (2001). Distinct behavioral and neuropathological abnormalities in transgenic mouse models of hd and drpla. *Neurobiol. Dis.*, **8**, 405–18.

Shimohata, T., Nakajima, T., Yamada, M. *et al.* (2000). Expanded polyglutamine stretches interact with TAFII130, interfering with CREB-dependent transcription. *Nat. Genet.*, **26**, 29–36.

Shimohata, T., Sato, A., Burke, J. R., Strittmatter, W. J., Tsuji, S. & Onodera, O. (2002). Expanded polyglutamine stretches form an "aggresome." *Neurosci. Lett.*, **323**, 215–18.

Smith, J. K. (1975). Dentatorubropallidoluysian atrophy. In *Handbook of Clinical Neurology*, Vol. **21**, 519–34.

Smith, J. K., Gonda, V. E. & Malamud, N. (1958). Unusual form of cerebellar ataxia; combined dentato-rubral and pallido-Luysian degeneration. *Neurology*, **8**, 205–9.

Squitieri, F., Andrew, S. E., Goldberg, Y. P. *et al.* (1994). DNA haplotype analysis of Huntington disease reveals clues to the origins and mechanisms of CAG expansion and reasons for geographic variations of prevalence. *Hum. Mol. Genet.*, **3**, 2103–14.

Steffan, J. S., Bodai, L., Pallos, J. *et al.* (2001). Histone deacetylase inhibitors arrest polyglutamine-dependent neurodegeneration in *Drosophila*. *Nature*, **413**, 739–43.

Steffan, J. S., Kazantsev, A., Spasic-Boskovic, O. *et al.* (2000). The Huntington's disease protein interacts with p53 and CREB-binding protein and represses transcription. *Proc. Natl Acad. Sci., USA*, **97**, 6763–8.

Takahashi, H., Ohama, E., Naito, H. *et al.* (1988). Hereditary dentatorubral-pallidoluysian atrophy: clinical and pathologic variants in a family. *Neurology*, **38**, 1065–70.

Tarnopolsky, M. A. & Beal, M. F. (2001). Potential for creatine and other therapies targeting cellular energy dysfunction in neurological disorders. *Ann. Neurol.*, **49**, 561–74.

Terashima, T., Kawai, H., Fujitani, M., Maeda, K. & Yasuda, H. (2002). SUMO-1 co-localized with mutant atrophin-1 with expanded polyglutamines accelerates intranuclear aggregation and cell death. *Neuroreport*, **13**, 2359–64.

Tomoda, A., Ikezawa M., Ohtani Y., Miike, T. & Kumamoto, T. (1991). Progressive myoclonus epilepsy: dentato-rubro-pallido-luysian atrophy (DRPLA) in childhood. *Brain Dev.*, **13**, 266–9.

Toyoshima, I., Sugawara, M., Kato, K. *et al.* (2002). Time course of polyglutamine aggregate body formation and cell death: enhanced growth in nucleus and an interval for cell death. *J. Neurosci. Res.*, **68**, 442–8.

Tsuji, S. (1999). Dentatorubral-pallidoluysian atrophy (DRPLA): clinical features and molecular genetics. *Adv. Neurol.*, **79**, 399–409.

Tsuji, S. (2000). Dentatorubral-pallidoluysian atrophy (DRPLA). *J. Neural. Transm. Suppl.*, 167–80.

Ueda, H., Goto, J., Hashida, H. *et al.* (2002). Enhanced SUMOylation in polyglutamine diseases. *Biochem. Biophys. Res. Commun.*, **293**, 307–13.

Villani, F., Gellera, C., Spreafico, R. *et al.* (1998). Clinical and molecular findings in the first identified Italian family with dentatorubral-pallidoluysian atrophy. *Acta Neurol. Scand.*, **98**, 324–7.

Waerner, T., Gardellin, P., Pfizenmaier, K., Weith, A. & Kraut, N. (2001). Human rere is localized to nuclear promyelocytic leukemia oncogenic domains and enhances apoptosis. *Cell Growth Differ.*, **12**, 201–10.

Warner, T. T., Williams, L. D., Walker, R. W. *et al.* (1995). A clinical and molecular genetic study of dentatorubropallidoluysian atrophy in four European families. *Ann. Neurol.*, **37**, 452–9.

Watkins, W. S., Bamshad, M. & Jorde, L. B. (1995). Population genetics of trinucleotide repeat polymorphisms. *Hum. Mol. Genet.*, **4**, 1485–91.

Wellington, C. L., Ellerby, L. M., Hackam, A. S. *et al.* (1998). Caspase cleavage of gene products associated with triplet expansion disorders generates truncated fragments containing the polyglutamine tract. *J. Biol. Chem.*, **273**, 9158–67.

Wellington, C. L., Leavitt, B. R. & Hayden, M. R. (2000). Huntington disease: new insights on the role of huntingtin cleavage 6. *J. Neural. Transm. Suppl.*, 1–17.

Wood, J. D., Yuan, J., Margolis, R. L. *et al.* (1998). Atrophin-1, the DRPLA gene product, interacts with two families of WW domain-containing proteins. *Mol. Cell Neurosci.*, **11**, 149–60.

Wood, J. D., Nucifora F. C., Jr., Wang, J. *et al.* (2000a). Pathogenesis of dentatorubral and pallidoluysianatrophy (DRPLA): comparison to Huntington's disease (HD). *Neurosci. News*, **3**, 73–9.

Wood, J. D., Nucifora, F. C., Jr., Duan, K. *et al.* (2000b). Atrophin-1, the dentato-rubral and pallido-luysian atrophy gene product, interacts with ETO/MTG8 in the nuclear matrix and represses transcription. *J. Cell Biol.*, **150**, 939–48.

Yabe, I., Sasaki, H., Kikuchi, S. *et al.* (2002). Late onset ataxia phenotype in dentatorubro-pallidoluysian atrophy (DRPLA). *J. Neurol.*, **249**, 432–6.

Yamada, M., Tsuji, S. & Takahashi, H. (2000). Pathology of CAG repeat diseases. *Neuropathology*, **20**, 319–25.

Yamada, M., Sato, T., Shimohata, T. *et al.* (2001a). Interaction between neuronal intranuclear inclusions and promyelocytic leukemia protein nuclear and coiled bodies in CAG repeat diseases. *Am. J. Pathol.*, **159**, 1785–95.

Yamada, M., Tsuji, S. & Takahashi, H. (2002). Genotype-phenotype correlation in CAG-repeat diseases. *Neuropathology*, **22**, 317–22.

Yamada, M., Wood, J. D., Shimohata, T. *et al.* (2001b). Widespread occurrence of intranuclear atrophin-1 accumulation in the central nervous system neurons of patients with dentatorubral-pallidoluysian atrophy. *Ann. Neurol.*, **49**, 14–23.

Yanagisawa, H., Fujii, K., Nagafuchi, S. *et al.* (1996). A unique origin and multistep process for the generation of expanded DRPLA triplet repeats. *Hum. Mol. Genet.*, **5**, 373–9.

Yanagisawa, H., Bundo, M., Miyashita, T. *et al.* (2000). Protein binding of a DRPLA family through arginine-glutamic acid dipeptide repeats is enhanced by extended polyglutamine. *Hum. Mol. Genet.*, **9**, 1433–42.

Yazawa, I., Nukina, N., Hashida, H., Goto, J., Yamada, M. & Kanazawa, I. (1995). Abnormal gene product identified in hereditary dentatorubral-pallidoluysian atrophy (DRPLA) brain. *Nat. Genet.* **10**, 99–103.

Zhang, S., Xu, L., Lee, J. & Xu, T. (2002a). *Drosophila* atrophin homolog functions as a transcriptional corepressor in multiple developmental processes. *Cell*, **108**, 45–56.

Zhang, S., Zhang, H. B. & Liu, D. P. (2002b). Screening regulatory sequences from bacterial artificial chromosome DNA of alpha- and beta-globin gene clusters. *Biochem. Cell Biol.*, **80**, 415–20.

59

Neuroacanthocytosis syndromes

Alexander Storch

Department of Neurology, Technical University of Dresden, Germany

Acanthocytes (*acanthos* = thorny or spiny in Greek language) are mature red blood cells with multiple protrusions or spicules, often with terminal bulbs, which are irregular in shape, orientation, and distribution. Consequently, acanthocytosis is defined as an increased amount of such misshaped erythrocytes in peripheral blood. Acanthocytes should not be present in the peripheral blood, but in some general and neurological conditions, such as uremia, advanced hepatic disease, post-splenomegaly, advanced malnutrition or spur cell anemia, significant elevations of acanthocyte levels are reported (Brin, 1993; Stevenson & Hardie, 2001). The association of acanthocytosis with neurological syndromes is found in at least three hereditary neurological disorders that are generally referred to as neuroacanthocytosis syndromes (Table 59.1). The first recognized association was that of "malformation of the erythrocyte" in a sporadic case of progressive ataxia and pigmentary retinopathy by Bassen and Kornzweig in 1950 (Bassen & Kornzweig, 1950), but the underlying inherited metabolic abnormality of abetalipoproteinemia with secondary vitamin E deficiency was established years ago. Since then two other fairly distinct syndromes have emerged: the McLeod syndrome and autosomal recessive chorea-acanthocytosis.

Chorea-acanthocytosis (ChAc)

Chorea-acanthocytosis (ChAc; also referred to as Critchley–Levine syndrome; OMIM #200150) is a multisystem degenerative neurological disorder associated with acanthocytosis in the absence of any lipid abnormalities. ChAc was first described in the late 1960s by Estes and co-workers (1967) as well as by Critchley *et al.* (1968) and Levine *et al.* (1968) in two American kindreds with very similar features. ChAc is a very rare disease, but seems to be particularly common in the Japanese population (Oshima *et al.*, 1985). The mean age of onset is around 32 years, but it can occur between the first and the seventh decade (Hardie *et al.*, 1991; Rampoldi *et al.*, 2001). The clinical symptoms include a hyperkinetic movement disorder, epileptic seizures, psychiatric symptoms and elevated serum creatine kinase. A full spectrum of movement disorders may be observed including tics, dystonia, akinetic-rigid syndrome and, most typical, chorea affecting the limbs (predominantly the legs) that resembles that seen in Huntington's disease (Bohlega *et al.*, 2003; Bostantjopoulou *et al.*, 2000; Hardie *et al.*, 1991; Spitz *et al.*, 1985). The characteristic and sometimes predominant orofacial and lingual movement abnormalities may cause vocalizations, dysarthria, dysphagia with feeding problems and severe orofacial self mutilations (Hardie *et al.*, 1991). Epileptic seizures have been reported in about half of the cases (Hardie *et al.*, 1991; Kazis *et al.*, 1995). Chronic axonal polyneuropathy with secondary demyelination with predominant involvement of the large diameter myelinated fibers in nerve biopsy studies have also been reported (Spencer *et al.*, 1987). Personality and behavioral changes as well as cognitive impairment with dementia in the late stages are common (Danek *et al.*, 2001; Hardie *et al.*, 1991; Kartsounis & Hardie, 1996). Psychiatric symptoms can comprise paranoia, depression, anxiety and emotional instability (Kartsounis & Hardie, 1996). In all cases there are signs of frontal lobe impairment. Biochemical findings include elevated creatine kinase levels in nearly all patients (Hardie *et al.*, 1991) as well as elevated liver enzymes and signs for an intravascular hemolysis in some cases. Serum lipid electrophoresis findings are normal.

Neuroimaging studies using computed tomography and magnetic resonance tomography in ChAc revealed caudate and generalised cerebral atrophy as well as hyperintensive signal changes in T$_2$-weighted images in the caudate and

Table 59.1. Neuroacanthocytosis syndromes

Syndrome	Gene	Locus	Protein	Inheritance	Reference
Chorea-acanthocytosis (ChAc)	CHAC	9q21	Chorein	autosomal recessive	Rampoldi et al., 2001; Rubio et al., 1997; Ueno et al., 2001
Autosomal-dominant ChAc	CHAC	9q21	Chorein	Autosomal dominant	Saiki et al., 2003
McLeod syndrome	XK	Xp21	Kx membrane transport protein	X-linked recessive	Bertelson et al., 1999; Danek et al., 2001; Ho et al., 1994
Dyslipoproteinemias					
Abetalipoproteinemia	MTP	4q22–24	Microsomal triglyceride transfer protein (MTP)	autosomal recessive	Sharp et al., 1993; Shoulders et al., 1993
Familial hypobetalipoproteinemia	APOB	2p22–23	Apolipoprotein B	autosomal dominant	Ross et al., 1988; Young et al., 1987
	unknown	3p21.1–22	unknown	autosomal dominant	Yuan et al., 2000
Pantothenate-kinase associated neurodegeneration (PKAN)	PANK2	20p13–p12.3	Pantothenate kinase 2	autosomal recessive	Zhou et al., 2001
HARP syndrome	PANK2	20p13–p12.3	Pantothenate kinase 2	single case reports	Ching et al., 2002

putamen in most cases (Hardie *et al.*, 1991; Okamoto *et al.*, 1997; Spitz *et al.*, 1985; Sorrentino *et al.*, 1999; Tanaka *et al.*, 1998). Positron-emission tomography (PET) studies have shown reduced blood flow and oxygen consumption in all brain areas, but particularly in the caudate nucleus, putamen and frontal cortex (Delecluse *et al.*, 1991; Dubinsky *et al.*, 1989; Tanaka *et al.*, 1998). Studies using ^{18}F-dopa, ^{11}C-raclopride and PET scans demonstrated presynaptic dysfunction only in the posterior putamen, similar to the findings in patients with Parkinson's disease, and a marked reduction of dopamine D2-receptor binding sites in the putamen and caudate nucleus (Brooks *et al.*, 1991). These observations are consistent with neuropathological data (Bird *et al.*, 1978; Hardie *et al.*, 1991; de Yebenes *et al.*, 1988; Rinne *et al.*, 1994). Consistently, in postmortem studies the most consistent neuropathological finding is an extensive neuronal loss and gliosis in the caudate and putamen, pallidum and *substantia nigra* and milder loss in the thalamus (Rinne *et al.*, 1994). The subthalamic nucleus, cerebral cortex, pons and cerebellum seem to be spared (Hardie *et al.*, 1991; Rinne *et al.*, 1994).

In a linkage study in 11 families of different geographical origin the ChAc locus was mapped to chromosome 9q21 (Rubio *et al.*, 1997). Recently two research groups have identified a novel gene mapping in this region (named *CHAC* gene) and found mutations in ChAc patients (Rampoldi *et al.*, 2001; Ueno *et al.*, 2001). The *CHAC* gene is organized in 73 exons over a chromosomal region of 250 kb.

CHAC expression could be detected in all tissues investigated, in particular in those tissues that are mainly affected in ChAc, such as brain, skeletal muscle, liver and erythroid precursors. Seventy-one mutations in the CHAC gene have been reported so far in patients with autosomal recessive ChAc (Rampoldi *et al.*, 2001; Ueno *et al.*, 2001; Dobson-Stone *et al.*, 2002) including deletions or insertions leading to frameshifts, splice-site mutations as well as nonsense/missense mutations. All mutations may lead to degradation of the corresponding mRNA through nonsense-mediated mRNA decay or to production of a truncated protein. These results implicate a loss of function as the pathophysiological mechanism making it difficult to establish any genotype–phenotype correlation. Although most cases of ChAc are transmitted as an autosomal recessive trait, some cases with similar clinical features have been reported to be inherited as an autosomal dominant trait (Hardie *et al.*, 1991; Marson *et al.*, 2003; Saiki *et al.*, 2003). Saiki and co-workers reported a single heterozygous mutation in the last nucleotide of exon 57 of the *CHAC* gene in autosomal dominant ChAc, most likely leading to skipping of the exon (Saiki *et al.*, 2003).

The *CHAC* gene product was named chorein (Ueno *et al.*, 2001), but its function is currently unclear. Amino acid sequence analysis does not reveal conserved domains, motifs or identifiable structural features. However, hints for understanding the function of chorein come from functional studies of its homologue in *Dictyostelium* (TipC) and *Saccharomyces cervisiae* (Vps13). Both proteins most likely play important roles in proper intracellular trafficking of different proteins between subcellular structures, such as the trans-Golgi network and the pre-vacuolar compartment, corresponding to the late endosome in animal cells (Raymond *et al.*, 1992; Stege *et al.*, 1999; Nakayama, 1997). Thus, chorein might control the cycling of proteins through the trans-Golgi networks and the late endosome, lysosomes and the plasma membrane. However, analysis of the function of the chorein molecule in mammalian cells is warranted to establish its physiological roles as well as the pathophysiological mechanisms leading to ChAc.

Acanthocytosis is observed in all patients with ChAc and is one of the hallmarks of this disorder (Hardie *et al.*, 1991; Brin, 1993; Feinberg *et al.*, 1991), but in some cases it can occur late during the course of the disease (Sorrentino *et al.*, 1999). The percentage of acanthocytes in the blood of ChAc patients is highly variable, usually between 5% and 70%, and does not seem to correlate with the severity of the disease. Furthermore, the percentage of acanthocytes markedly depends on the method by which red blood cell morphology is investigated. Due to experimental artefact and the occurrence of echinocytes, normal levels of acanthocytes in fresh blood samples using standard dry blood smears could be up to 3% in adult peripheral blood (Hardie *et al.*, 1991; Storch *et al.*, 1998; Storch & Schwarz, 2003). However, this method seems to be not efficient enough to detect acanthocytosis in all patients with ChAc (Feinberg *et al.*, 1991; Storch *et al.*, 2003; Storch & Schwarz, 2003). Feinberg and co-workers (1991) introduced a method utilizing the phenomenon that acanthocytes show a dramatic increase in their sensitivity to echinocytic stress of isotonic dilution of the blood sample (Feinberg *et al.*, 1991; Morrow & Andersen, 1986). Using a similar method, Storch and co-workers were able to detect significant acanthocytosis (between 10.5 and 72% of red blood cells) in all genetically confirmed ChAc patients tested (Storch *et al.*, 2003). To date, only two cases have been reported to have typical neurological symptoms of CHAC in the absence of significant acanthocytosis (Malandrini *et al.*, 1993; O'Brien *et al.*, 1990). However, it is not known whether the authors performed sensitive methods to detect acanthocytosis in these cases, such as the method by Feinberg and co-workers (1991). The mechanism of acanthocyte formation in ChAc is not known, but available data suggest that the protein content of the erythrocyte membrane is responsible for the morphological changes (Asano *et al.*, 1985; Clark *et al.*, 1989; Oshima *et al.*, 1985; Sakai *et al.*, 1991; Ueno *et al.*, 1982). It is hypothesized that impaired intracellular trafficking of membrane proteins, such as band 3 protein or furin-like proteases, to the plasma membrane due to the lack of

chorein function leads to reduced membrane fluidity and destabilization of its structure with subsequent acanthocyte formation.

McLeod syndrome

The McLeod syndrome (OMIM #314850), first described in 1961 and named after the proband (Allen *et al.*, 1961), is a rare X-linked recessive abnormality of the Kell blood group system of erythrocyte antigens in which red blood cells have no detectable Kx and all Kell antigens are expressed weakly. It is characterized by choreic movements, myopathy, cardiomyopathy, peripheral neuropathy, elevated creatine kinase levels, permanent hemolysis and acanthocytosis (Danek *et al.*, 1994, 2001; Malandrini *et al.*, 1994; Wimer *et al.*, 1977). These features can be very similar to those seen in ChAc, but severe orofacial dystonia and self-mutilations seem to be rare. However, the neurological phenotype is heterogenous and the incidence of neurological abnormalities in McLeod syndrome is unknown. The mean age of onset is in the fifth decade of life, but it can occur between the second and seventh decade (Danek *et al.*, 2001). The neurological features of genetically confirmed McLeod patients and an extensive genotype–phenotype correlation was reported by Danek and co-workers in 2001 (Danek *et al.*, 2001). Chorea of arms and legs occurs in all patients with McLeod syndrome, whereas dystonia and epileptic seizure are reported only in some patients. Cognitive impairment and psychological disturbances are found in about half of the patients in the late stage of the disease (Danek *et al.*, 1994). Muscle weakness and muscular atrophy as well as cardiomyopathy are reported in two-thirds of the patients. Consistently, muscle biopsy studies showed myopathic changes mainly of type 2 fibers without changes of dystrophin expression (Danek *et al.*, 1990; Carter *et al.*, 1990). Areflexia showing involvement of peripheral nerves is common in McLeod syndrome. Electrophysiological and nerve biopsy studies demonstrated primary axonal degeneration (Danek *et al.*, 2001; Witt *et al.*, 1992). Serum creatine kinase is usually slightly elevated. Female carriers are usually asymptomatic, but can show mild symptoms according to the degree of inactivation of the X chromosome carrying the mutant *XK* gene.

Neuroimaging studies using computed tomography and magnetic resonance tomography revealed atrophy of the caudate nucleus and hyperintensive signals in T_2-weighted images in the lateral putamen in the majority of patients (Danek *et al.*, 1994; Malandrini *et al.*, 1994). Dopamine D_2-receptor single-photon computed tomography (SPECT) studies showed diffuse reduction in dopamine

D_2-receptor binding in caudate and putamen, suggesting a cell loss in these brain regions (Danek *et al.*, 1994). PET analysis demonstrated absent metabolism in the basal ganglia and hypometabolism in the frontal and parietal cortex (Dotti *et al.*, 2000; Jung *et al.*, 2001).

The McLeod locus was mapped to chromosome Xp21 in 1988 (Bertelson *et al.*, 1988; Ho *et al.*, 1992). Subsequently, Ho and co-workers found mutations in the *XK* gene encoding for Kx in McLeod patients (Ho *et al.*, 1994; Khamlichi *et al.*, 1995). To date, over 20 mutations including deletions, splice-site mutations and missense mutations have been reported (Danek *et al.*, 2001; Dotti *et al.*, 2000; Ho *et al.*, 1994, 1996; Jung *et al.*, 2001). They seem to be distributed throughout the *XK* gene. Since all gene defects lead to a loss of *XK* gene function, there is no relevant genotype–phenotype correlation (Danek *et al.*, 2001). There is one report of McLeod phenotype caused by a *XK* missense mutation (E327K), but without hematologic (that means without acanthocytosis), neuromuscular or cerebral involvement (Jung *et al.*, 2003). So far, a single female patient with complete absence of Kx antigen expression has been reported (Hardie *et al.*, 1991; Ho *et al.*, 1996). Molecular biology and biochemistry studies demonstrate a tight linkage between the Kx and the Kell protein suggesting a disulfide bridge-bounded Kell–Kx–protein complex (Branch *et al.*, 1985; Khamlichi *et al.*, 1995). However, there are controversial results whether this linkage is needed for the localisation of both proteins on the plasma membrane (Branch *et al.*, 1985; Khamlichi *et al.*, 1995; Russo *et al.*, 1994, 1999). The exact functions of the Kell and Kx protein are not completely known. The Kell protein share homology and structural similarities with M13 metalloproteases, a subtype of zinc endopeptidases (Lee *et al.*, 1999). M13 proteases usually activate bioactive peptides by proteolytic cleavage and indeed, the Kell protein preferentially cleaves large endothelin-3 into the active peptide endothelin-3 (Lee *et al.*, 1999). The Kx protein has sequence homology with the CED-8 protein from *C. elegans*, which is mainly involved in the regulation of apoptosis (Stanfield *et al.*, 2000). The Kx and Kell protein are expressed in tissues that are mainly affected in McLeod syndrome, namely brain, skeletal muscle and cardiac muscle (Russo *et al.*, 2000). However, the pathophysiological mechanisms by which the mutations in the *XK* gene lead to the clinical spectrum of the McLeod phenotype are presently unclear.

Acanthocytosis is found in the majority of patients with McLeod syndrome with levels ranging from 3 to 40% (Danek *et al.*, 2001; Wimer *et al.*, 1977). Ultrastructural studies of red blood cell membranes showed a similar result as those found in ChAc erythrocytes suggesting some membrane instability and impaired membrane fluidity (Terada *et al.*,

1999). These changes are most likely due to the lack of both the XK protein and the Kell antigens, which are associated with the membrane cytoskeleton.

Hypolipoproteinemias

Abetalipoproteinemia (OMIM #200100) is an autosomal recessive disorder characterised by fat malabsorption, pigmentary retinal degeneration, progressive ataxia, neuropathy and acanthocytosis (Bassen & Kornzweig, 1950). Age of onset is usually in the first few years of life. Serum lipoproteins containing apolipoprotein B, low-density lipoproteins (LDL) and very low-density lipoproteins (VLDLs), are absent, which leads to severe impairment of both fat absorption and transport from the intestine. This results in very low serum levels of triglycerides, cholesterol and the fat-soluble vitamin E. The clinical spectrum is heterogeneous and includes steatorrhoea and failure to thrive due to fat malabsorption in childhood as well as spinocerebellar degeneration with ataxia, neuropathy and visual loss due to retinal degeneration in young adults. The neurological symptoms are related to the deficiency of vitamin E (Kayden & Traber, 1993) and can indeed be reversed by vitamin E supplementation (Muller *et al.*, 1985). Neuropathological studies demonstrate degeneration of the posterior columns of the spinal cord and spinocerebellar tracts, but the cerebellum seems to be spared (Harding, 1987; Nelson *et al.*, 1981). These pathological changes are similar to those seen in vitamin E deficient mammals. In contrast, the retinal pigmentary degeneration is thought to be caused by combined deficiency of vitamin A and E. Consistently, vitamin A treatment is able to restore retinal function only in the early stages of the disease, but combined treatment with both vitamin A and E has been shown to slow down retinal degeneration in the long run (Bishara *et al.*, 1982).

Abetalipoproteinemia is caused by mutations in the *MTP* gene encoding for the microsomal triglyceride transfer protein (MTP; Sharp *et al.*, 1993; Shoulders *et al.*, 1993). The *MTP* gene is localized on chromosome 4q22–24 and organized in 18 exons (Sharp *et al.*, 1993). It is expressed in enterocytes and hepatocytes and to a lower extent in kidney and cardiac muscle (Wetterau *et al.*, 1992). Over twenty mutations in the *MTP* gene have been reported in abetalipoproteinemia, which seem to be mainly clustered in the middle and C-terminal regions of the protein (Ohashi *et al.*, 2000; Sharp *et al.*, 1993; Shoulders *et al.*, 1993). These reported mutations are single-base insertions or deletions, slicing mutations and nonsense mutations as well as mutations in the non-coding highly conserved promotor region of the *MTP* gene. The MTP protein is involved in the translocation of apolipoprotein B across the endoplasmatic reticulum membrane and its assembly with lipids (Liang & Ginsberg, 2001; Jamil *et al.*, 1998). Thus, the assembly and secretion of apolipoprotein B-containing lipoproteins in hepatocytes is impaired leading to complete absence of these lipoproteins as well as reduction of vitamin E in the serum of abetalipoproteinemia patients.

Familial hypobetalipoproteinemia (OMIM #107730) is a genetically distinct condition, which is an autosomal codominant disorder characterized by extremely low serum levels of apolipoprotein B (Kayden & Traber, 1993; Linton *et al.*, 1993). Homozygotes are clinically indistinguishable from patients with abetalipoproteinemia, but the neurological involvement is usually less severe. As in abetalipoproteinemia, the clinical spectrum is most likely related to intestinal malabsorption of vitamin E and can therefore be prevented by vitamin E supplementation (Harding, 1987; Kayden & Traber, 1993; Linton *et al.*, 1993). Heterozygotes are normally asymptomatic without acanthocytosis, and serum concentrations of triglycerides, LDL cholesterol and VLDLs are all low but detectable.

In most cases, hypobetalipoproteinemia is caused by mutations in the *APOB* gene on chromosome 2p23–24 encoding for apolipoprotein B, the main apolipoprotein of chylomicrons and LDLs (Ross *et al.*, 1988). Since the first description of the gene defect causing hypobetalipoproteinemia by Young and co-workers (1987, 1988), more than 40 different mutations have been reported. Most of these are nonsense or frameshift mutations resulting in the production of truncated forms of apolipoprotein B (Linton *et al.*, 1993; Farese *et al.*, 1992; Ross *et al.*, 1988). Other defects affecting the rate of synthesis or removal of lipoproteins are emerging (Welty *et al.*, 1998; Wu *et al.*, 1999; Yuan *et al.*, 2000).

Significant acanthocytosis of between 50 and 90% of the red blood cells is commonly observed in hypobetalipoproteinemias and is most likely due to altered lipid composition of the plasma membrane. Indeed, biochemical studies in both conditions showed an increase of sphingomyelin levels and the sphingomyelin/lecithin ratio as well as a decrease of linoleic acid content of the erythrocyte membrane (Cooper *et al.*, 1977; Iida *et al.*, 1984). These alterations are known to affect the fluidity of lipid bilayers such as cell membranes.

Other rare neuroacanthocytosis syndromes

Panthothenate kinase-associated neurodegeneration (PKAN; also referred to as Hallervorden–Spatz disease or late infantile neuroaxonal dystrophy; OMIM #234200) is characterized by a progressive neurodegenerative syndrome including generalized dystonia with predominance of oromandibular muscles, rigidity, choreic and/or athetoid involuntary movements, behavioral changes followed by dementia and retinal pigmental degeneration (Hayflick, 2003). PKAN has been found to be associated with acanthocytosis in several patients (Köhler, 1989; Luckenbach *et al.*, 1983; Malandrini *et al.*, 1996; Orrell *et al.*, 1995; Roth *et al.*, 1971; Swisher *et al.*, 1972). All of these patients had normal serum lipoproteins, but six had pigmentary retinopathy. Zhou and co-workers identified causative deletions, missense and null mutations in the pantothenate kinase gene *PANK2* in patients with classical and atypical Hallervorden–Spatz disease (Zhou *et al.*, 2001). A point mutation (R371X) in the same gene causes the allelic disorder HARP syndrome (hypoprebetalipoproteinemia, acanthocytosis, retinitis pigmentosa and pallidal degeneration; OMIM #607236; Higgins *et al.*, 1992; Orrell *et al.*, 1995; Ching *et al.*, 2002).

Walker *et al.* (2002) reported a kindred with an autosomal-dominant inherited progressive neurodegenerative syndrome including chorea, dementia, parkinsonism and acanthocytosis. Autopsy in one patient revealed inclusion bodies immunoreactive to ubiquitin, polyglutamine repeats and torsinA in several areas of the cerebral cortex. Subsequent molecular genetic analysis identified repeat extensions in the *JPH3/HDL2* gene encoding junctophilin-3 as shown for Huntington's disease-like type 2 (HDL2; Holmes *et al.*, 2001; Walker *et al.*, 2003). Since investigations of red blood cell morphology in other HDL2 families did not show acanthocytosis (Walker *et al.*, 2003), it is currently unclear whether the HDL2 phenotype does not necessarily include acanthocytosis or whether acanthocytosis is a feature independent from HDL2 genotype in the kindred reported by Walker and co-workers (2002).

Wolman's disease is a fatal disorder characterized by the absence of lysosomal acid lipase activity and accumulation of cholesteryl esters and triacylglycerols caused by mutations in the gene encoding for the lysosomal acid lipase (Wolman, 1995). Eto and Kitagawa (1970) described a disorder with features of malabsorption of lipids, vomiting, growth failure, and adrenal calcification. Hypolipoproteinemia and acanthocytosis suggest this is an entity distinct from Wolman's disease, but might be related to the dyslipoproteinemias (OMIM #278100; Eto & Kitagawa, 1970).

Lerche and co-workers recently described one kindred with a novel autosomal dominant neuroacanthocytosis syndrome with exertion-induced paroxysmal dyskinesias and epileptic seizures (Lerche *et al.*, 2000). The onset is during young childhood without relevant progression.

All affected family members had normal neurological examination, normal serum lipoproteins and the McLeod phenotype was absent. The causative gene defect is unknown.

REFERENCES

Allen, F. H., Krabbe, S. M. R. & Corcoran, P. A. (1961). A new phenotype (McLeod) in the Kell blood-group system. *Vox Sang*, **6**, 555–60.

Asano, K., Osawa, Y., Yanagisawa, N., Takahashi, Y. & Oshima, M. (1985). Erythrocyte abnormalities in patients with amyotrophic chorea with acanthocytosis. Part II. Abnormalities of membrane proteins. *J. Neurol. Sci.*, **68**, 161–73.

Bassen, F. A. & Kornzweig, A. L. (1950). Malformation of the erythrocytes in a case of atypical retinitis pigmentosa. *Blood*, **5**, 381–7.

Bertelson, C. J., Pogo, A. O., Chaudhuri, A. *et al.* (1988). Localization of the McLeod locus (XK) within Xp21 by deletion analysis. *Am. J. Hum. Genet.*, **42**(5), 703–11.

Bird, T. B., Cederbaum, S., Valpey, R. W. & Stahl, W. L. (1978). Familial degeneration of the basal ganglia with acanthocytosis: a clinical, neuropathological and neurochemical study. *Ann. Neurol.*, **3**, 253–8.

Bishara, S., Merin, S., Cooper, M., Azizi, E., Delpre, G. & Deckelbaum, R. J. (1982). Combined vitamin A and E therapy prevents retinal electrophysiological deterioration in abetalipoproteinaemia. *Br. J. Ophthalmol.*, **66**(12), 767–70.

Bohlega, S., Al-Jishi, A., Dobson-Stone, C. *et al.* (2003). Choreaacanthocytosis: clinical and genetic findings in three families from the Arabian peninsula. *Mov. Disord.*, **18**(4), 403–7.

Bostantjopoulou, S., Katsarou, Z., Kazis, A. & Vadikolia, C. (2000). Neuroacanthocytosis presenting as parkinsonism. *Mov. Disord.*, **15**, 1271–2.

Branch, D. R., Sy Siok Hian, A. L. & Petz, L. D. (1985). Unmasking of Kx antigen by reduction of disulphide bonds on normal and McLeod red cells. *Br. J. Haematol.*, **59**(3), 505–12.

Brin, M. F. (1993). Acanthocytosis. In *Handbook of Clinical Neurology*, Vol. **19**(63), ed. C. G. Goetz, C. M. Tanner & M. J. Aminoff, Amsterdam: Elsevier, pp. 271–99.

Brooks, D. J., Ibanez, V., Playford, E. D. *et al.* (1991). Presynaptic and postsynaptic striatal dopaminergic function in neuroacanthocytosis: A positron emssion tomographic study. *Ann. Neurol.*, **30**, 166–71.

Ching, K. H. L., Westaway, S. K., Gitschier, J., Higgins, J. J. & Hayflick, S. J. (2002). HARP syndrome is allelic with pantothenate kinase-associated neurodegeneration. *Neurology*, **58**, 1673–4.

Clark, M. R., Aminoff, M. J., Chiu, D. T., Kuypers, F. A. & Friend, D. S. (1989). Red cell deformability and lipid composition in two forms of acanthocytosis: enrichment of acanthocytic populations by density gradient centrifugation. *J. Lab. Clin. Med.*, **113**(4), 469–81.

Carter, N. D., Morgan, J. E., Monaco, A. P., Schwartz, M. S. & Jeffery, S. (1990). Dystrophin expression and genotypic analysis of

two cases of benign X linked myopathy (McLeod's syndrome). *J. Med. Genet.*, **27**(6), 345–7.

Cooper, R. A., Durocher, J. R. & Leslie, M. H. (1977). Decreased fluidity of red cell membrane lipids in abetalipoproteinemia. *J. Clin. Invest.*, **60**(1), 115–21.

Critchley, E. M. R., Clark, D. B. & Wikler, A. (1968). Acanthocytosis and neurological disorder without abetalipoproteinemia. *Arch. Neurol.*, **18**, 134–40.

Danek, A., Rubio, J. P., Rampoldi, L. *et al.* (2001). McLeod neuroacanthocytosis: genotype and phenotype. *Ann. Neurol.*, **50**(6), 755–64.

Danek, A., Witt, T. N., Stockmann, H. B., Weiss, B. J., Schotland, D. L. & Fischbeck, K. H. (1990). Normal dystrophin in McLeod myopathy. *Ann. Neurol.*, **28**(5), 720–2.

Danek, A., Uttner, U., Vogl, T., Tatsch, K. & Witt, T. N. (1994). Cerebral involvement in McLeod syndrome. *Neurology*, **44**, 117–20.

Danek, A., Tierney, M., Sheesley, L. & Grafman, J. (2001). Cognitive findings in patients with chorea-acanthocytosis. *Mov. Disord.*, **16**(Suppl 1), S30.

Delecluse, F., Deleval, J., Gerard, J. M., Michotte, A. & Zegers de Beyl, D. (1991). Frontal impairment and hypoperfusion in neuroacanthocytosis. *Arch. Neurol.*, **48**(2), 232–4.

Dexter, D. T., Brooks, D. J., Harding, A. E. *et al.* (1994). Nigrostriatal function in vitamin E deficiency: clinical, experimental, and positron emission tomographic studies. *Ann. Neurol.*, **35**(3), 298–303.

de Yebenes, J. G., Brin, M. F., Mena, M. A. *et al.* (1988). Neurochemical findings in Neuroacanthocytosis. *Mov. Disord.*, **3**, 300–12.

Dobson-Stone, C., Danek, C., Rampoldi, L. *et al.* (2002). Mutational spectrum of the *CHAC* gene in patients with choreaacanthocytosis. *Eur. J. Hum. Genet.*, **10**(11), 773–81.

Dotti, M. T., Battisti, C., Malandrini, A. *et al.* (2000). McLeod syndrome and neuroacanthocytosis with a novel mutation in the XK gene. *Mov. Disord.*, **15**(6), 1282–4.

Dubinsky, R. M., Hallett, M., Levey, R. & Di Chiro, G. (1989). Regional brain glucose metabolism in neuroacanthocytosis. *Neurology*, **39**(9), 1253–5.

Estes, J. W., Morley, T. J., Levine, I. M. & Emerson, C. P. (1967). A new hereditary acanthocytosis syndrome. *Am. J. Med.*, **42**, 868–88.

Eto, Y. & Kitagawa, T. (1970). Wolman's disease with hypolipoproteinemia and acanthocytosis: clinical and biochemical observations. *J. Pediat.*, **77**, 862–7.

Farese, R. V., Garg, A., Peirotti, V. R., Veega, G. L. & Young, S. G. (1992). A truncated species of apolipoprotein B, B-83, associated with hypolipoproteinemia. *J. Lipid Res.*, **33**, 569–77.

Feinberg, T. E., Cianci, C. D., Morrow, J. S. *et al.* (1991). Koroshetz W. J. Diagnostic test for choreoacanthocytosis. *Neurology*, **41**, 1000–6.

Hardie, R. J., Pullon, H. W., Harding, A. E. *et al.* (1991). Neuroacanthocytosis: a clinical, hematological and pathological study of 19 cases. *Brain*, **114**, 13–49.

Harding, A. E. (1987). Vitamin E and the nervous system. *Crit. Rev. Neurobiol.*, **3**, 89–103.

Hayflick, S. J. (2003). Pantothenate kinase-associated neurodegeneration (formerly Hallervorden-Spatz syndrome). *J. Neurol. Sci.*, **207**, 106–7.

Higgins, J. J., Patterson, M. C., Papadopoulos, N. M., Brady, R. O., Pentchev, P. G. & Barton, N. W. (1992). Hypoprebetalipoproteinemia, acanthocytosis, retinitis pigmentosa and pallidal degeneration (HARP syndrome). *Neurology*, **42**, 194–8.

Ho, M. F., Monaco, A. P., Blonden, L. A. *et al.* (1992). Fine mapping of the McLeod locus (XK) to a 150–380-kb region in Xp21. *Am. J. Hum. Genet.*, **50**(2), 317–30.

Ho, M., Chelly, J., Carter, N., Danek, A., Crocker, P. & Monaco, A. P. (1994). Isolation of the gene for McLeod syndrome that encodes a novel membrane transport protein. *Cell*, **77**(6), 869–80.

Ho, M. F., Chalmers, R. M., Davis, M. B., Harding, A. E. & Monaco, A. P. (1996). A novel point mutation in the McLeod syndrome gene in neuroacanthocytosis. *Ann. Neurol.*, **39**(5), 672–5.

Holmes, S. E., O'Hearn, E., Rosenblatt, A. *et al.* (2001). A repeat expansion in the gene encoding junctophilin-3 is associated with Huntington disease-like 2. *Nat. Genet.*, **29**(4), 377–8.

Iida, H., Takashima, Y., Maeda, S. *et al.* (1984). Alterations in erythrocyte membrane lipids in abetalipoproteinemia: phospholipid and fatty acyl composition. *Biochem. Med.*, **32**(1), 79–87.

Jamil, H., Chu, C. H., Dickson, J. K. Jr. *et al.* (1998). Evidence that microsomal triglyceride transfer protein is limiting in the production of apolipoprotein B-containing lipoproteins in hepatic cells. *J. Lipid Res.*, **39**(7), 1448–54.

Jung, H. H., Hergersberg, M., Kneifel, S. *et al.* (2001). McLeod syndrome: a novel mutation, predominant psychiatric manifestations, and distinct striatal imaging findings. *Ann. Neurol.*, **49**(3), 384–92.

Jung, H. H., Hergersberg, M., Vogt, M. *et al.* (2003). Kollias, S. S., Russo, D. & Frey, B. M. (2003). McLeod phenotype associated with a XK missense mutation without hematologic, neuromuscular, or cerebral involvement. *Transfusion*, **43**, 923–8.

Kartsounis, L. D. & Hardie, R. J. (1996). The pattern of cognitive impairments in neuroacanthocytosis. *Arch. Neurol.*, **53**, 77–80.

Kayden, H. J. & Traber, M. G. (1993). Absorption, lipoprotein transport, and regulation of plasma concentrations of vitamin E in humans. *J. Lipid Res.*, **43**, 343–58.

Kazis, A., Kimiskidis, V., Georgiadis, G. & Voloudaki, E. (1995). Neuroacanthocytosis presenting with epilepsy. *J. Neurol.*, **242**, 415–17.

Khamlichi, S., Bailly, P., Blanchard, D., Goossens, D., Cartron, J. P. & Bertrand, O. (1995). Purification and partial characterization of the erythrocyte Kx protein deficient in McLeod patients. *Eur. J. Biochem.*, **228**(3), 931–4.

Köhler, B. (1989). Hallervorden–Spatz syndrome with acanthocytosis. *Monatsschr. Kinderheilkunde*, **137**, 616–19.

Lee, S., Lin, M., Mele, A. *et al.* (1999). Proteolytic processing of big endothelin-3 by the kell blood group protein. *Blood*, **94**(4), 1440–50.

Lerche, H., Storch, A., Pekrun, A. *et al.* (2000). A novel form of autosomal dominant neuroacanthocytosis with exertion-induced paroxysmal dyskinesias. *J. Neurol.*, **247**(Suppl 1), S43.

Levine, I. M., Estes, J. W. & Looney, J. M. (1968). Hereditary neurological disease with acanthocytosis. *Arch. Neurol.*, **19**, 403–9.

Liang, J. & Ginsberg, H. N. (2001). Microsomal triglyceride transfer protein binding and lipid transfer activities are independent of each other, but both are required for secretion of apolipoprotein B lipoproteins from liver cells. *J. Biol. Chem.*, **276**(30), 28606–12.

Linton, M. F., Farese, R. V. & Young, S. G. (1993). Familial hypobetalipoproteinemia. *J. Lipid Res.*, **34**, 521–41.

Luckenbach, M. W., Green, W. R., Miller, N. R., Moser, H. W., Clark, A. W. & Tennekoon, G. (1983). Ocular clinicopathologic correlation of Hallervorden–Spatz syndrome with acanthocytosis and pigmentary retinopathy. *Am. J. Ophthalmol.*, **95**, 369–82.

Malandrini, A., Fabrizi, G. M., Palmeri, S. (1993). Choreoacanthocytosis like phenotype without acanthocytes: clinicopathological case report. A contribution to the knowledge of the functional pathology of the caudate nucleus. *Acta Neuropathol. (Berl.)*, **86**(6), 651–8.

Malandrini, A., Fabrizi, G. M., Truschi, F. *et al.* (1994). Atypical McLeod syndrome manifested as X-linked choreaacanthocytosis, neuromyopathy and dilated cardiomyopathy: report of a family. *J. Neurol. Sci.*, **124**(1), 89–94.

Malandrini, A., Cesaretti, S., Mulinari, M. *et al.* (1996). Acanthocytosis, retinitis pigmentosa, pallidal degeneration. Report of two cases without serum lipid abnormalities. *J. Neurol. Sci.*, **140**, 129–31.

Marson, A. M., Bucciantini, E., Gentile, E. & Geda, C. (2003). Neuroacanthocytosis: clinical, radiological, and neurophysiological findings in an Italian family. *Neurol. Sci.*, **24**(3), 188–9.

Morrow, J. & Andersen, R. (1986). Shaping the too fluid bilayer. *Lab. Invest.*, **54**, 237–9.

Muller, D. P., Lloyd, J. K. & Wolff, O. H. (1985). The role of vitamin E in the treatment of the neurological features of abetalipoproteinaemia and other disorders of fat absorption. *J. Inherit. Metab. Dis.*, **8**(Suppl 1), 88–92.

Nakayama, K. (1997). Furin: a mammalian subtilisin/Kex2p-like endoprotease involved in processing of a wide variety of precursor proteins. *Biochem. J.*, **327**, 625–35.

Nelson, J. S., Fitch, C. D., Fischer, V. W., Broun, G. O. Jr. & Chou, A. C. (1981). Progressive neuropathologic lesions in vitamin E-deficient rhesus monkeys. *J. Neuropathol. Exp. Neurol.*, **40**(2), 166–86.

O'Brien, C. F., Schwartz, H. & Kurlan, R. (1990). Neuroacanthocytosis without acanthocytes. *Mov. Disord.*, **5**(Suppl 1), 98.

Ohashi, K., Ishibashi, S., Osuga, J. *et al.* (2000). Novel mutations in the microsomal triglyceride transfer protein gene causing abetalipoproteinemia. *J. Lipid Res.*, **41**(8), 1199–204.

Okamoto, K., Ito, J., Furusawa, T. *et al.* (1997). CT and MR findings of neuroacanthocytosis. *J. Comput. Assist. Tomogr.*, **21**(2), 221–2.

Orrell, R. W., Amrolia, P. J., Heald, A. *et al.* (1995). Acanthocytosis, retinitis pigmentosa, and pallidal degeneration: a report of three cases, including the second reported case with hypopre-betalipoproteinemia (HARP syndrome). *Neurology*, **45**, 487–92.

Oshima, M., Osawa, Y., Asano, K. & Saito, T. (1985). Erythrocyte membrane abnormalities in patients with amyotrophic chorea with acanthocytosis. I. Spin labeling studies and lipid analyses. *J. Neurol. Sci.*, **68**, 147–60.

Rampoldi, L., Dobson-Stone, C., Rubio, J. P. *et al.* (2001). A conserved sorting-associated protein is mutant in chorea-acanthocytosis. *Nat. Genet.*, **28**(2), 119–20.

Raymond, C. K., Howald-Stevenson, I., Vater, C. A. & Stevens, T. H. (1992). Morphological classification of the yeast vacuolar protein sorting mutants: evidence for a prevacuolar compartment in class E vps mutants. *Mol. Biol. Cell*, **3**(12), 1389–402.

Rinne, J. O., Daniel, S. E., Scaravilli, F., Pires, M., Harding, A. E. & Marsden, C. D. (1994). The neuropathological features of neuroacanthocytosis. *Mov. Disord.*, **9**, 297–304.

Ross, R. S., Gregg, R. E., Law, S. W. *et al.* (1988). Homozygous hypobe-talipoproteinemia: a disease distinct from abetalipoproteine-mia at the molecular level. *J. Clin. Invest.*, **81**, 590–5.

Roth, A. M., Helper, R. S., Mukoyama, M., Cancilla, P. A. & Foos, R. Y. (1971). Pigmentary retinal dystrophy in Hallervorden–Spatz disease. Clinicopathological report of a case. *Surv. Ophthalmol.*, **16**, 24–35.

Rubio, J. P., Danek, A., Stone, C. *et al.* (1997). Chorea-acanthocytosis: genetic linkage to chromosome 9q21. *Am. J. Hum. Genet.*, **61**, 899–908.

Russo, D. C., Lee, S., Reid, M. & Redman, C. M. (1994). Topology of Kell blood group protein and the expression of multiple antigens by transfected cells. *Blood*, **84**(10), 3518–23.

Russo, D. C., Lee, S. & Redman, C. M. (1999). Intracellular assembly of Kell and XK blood group proteins. *Biochim. Biophys. Acta*, **1461**(1), 10–18.

Russo, D., Wu, X., Redman, C. M. & Lee, S. (2000). Expression of Kell blood group protein in nonerythroid tissues. *Blood*, **96**(1), 340–6.

Saiki, S., Sakai, K., Kitagawa, Y., Saiki, M., Kataoka, S. & Hirose, G. (2003). Mutation in the CHAC gene in a family of autosomal dominant chorea-acanthocytosis. *Neurology*, **61**, 1614–6.

Sakai, T., Antoku, Y., Iwashita, H., Goto, I., Nagamatsu, K. & Shii, H. (1991). Chorea-acanthocytosis: abnormal composition of covalently bound fatty acids of erythrocyte membrane proteins. *Ann. Neurol.*, **29**, 664–9.

Sharp, D., Blinderman, L., Combs, K. A. *et al.* (1993). Cloning and gene defects in microsomal triglyceride transfer protein associated with abetalipoproteinaemia. *Nature*, **365**, 65–9.

Shoulders, C. C., Brett, D. J., Bayliss, J. D. *et al.* (1993). Abetalipoproteinemia is caused by defects of the gene encoding the 97 kDa subunit of a microsomal triglyceride transfer protein. *Hum. Mol. Genet.*, **2**, 2109–16.

Sorrentino, G., De Renzo, A., Miniello, S., Nori, O. & Bonavita, V. (1999). Late appearance of acanthocytes during the course of chorea-acanthocytosis. *J. Neurol. Sci.*, **163**, 175–8.

Spencer, S. E., Walker, F. O. & Moore, S. A. (1987). Chorea-amyotrophy with chronic hemolytic anemia. A variant of chorea-amyotrophy with acanthocytosis. *Neurology*, **37**, 645–9.

Spitz, M. C., Jankovic, J. & Killian, J. M. (1985). Familial tic disorder, parkinsonism, motor neuron disease and acanthocytosis: a new syndrome. *Neurology*, **35**, 366–70.

Stanfield, G. M. & Horvitz, H. R. (2000). The ced-8 gene controls the timing of programmed cell deaths in *C. elegans. Mol. Cell*, **5**(3), 423–3.

Stege, J. T., Laub, M. T. & Loomis, W. F. (1999). tip genes act in parallel pathways of early *Dictyostelium* development. *Dev. Genet.*, **25**(1), 64–77.

Stevenson, V. L. & Hardie, R. J. (2001). Acanthocytosis and neurological disorders. *J. Neurol.*, **248**, 87–94.

Storch, A., Kornhass, M. & Schwarz, J. (2004). Testing for acanthocytosis: a prospective reader-blinded study in movement disorder patients. *J. Neurol.*, in press.

Storch, A., Ludolph, A. C. & Schwarz, J. (1998). The importance of standardized blood investigations for acanthocytosis in patients with unusual movement disorders. *Neurology*, **50**(Suppl 4), A252.

Storch, A. & Schwarz, J. Diagnostic test for neuroacanthocytosis: quantitative measurement of red cell morphology. In *Neuroacanthocytosis Syndromes*, ed. A. Danek, New York: Kluwer Academic Press, pp. 71–8

Swisher, C. N., Menkes, J. H., Cancilla, P. A. & Dodge, P. R. (1972). Co-existence of Hallervorden-Spatz disease with acanthocytosis. *Trans. Am. Neurol. Assoc.*, **97**, 212–16.

Tanaka, M., Hirai, S., Kondo, S. *et al.* (1998). Cerebral hypoperfusion and hypometabolism with altered striatal signal intensity in chorea-acanthocytosis: a combined PET and MRI study. *Mov. Disord.*, **13**(1), 100–7.

Terada, N., Fujii, Y., Ueda, H. *et al.* (1999). Ultrastructural changes of erythrocyte membrane skeletons in chorea-acanthocytosis and McLeod syndrome revealed by the quick-freezing and deep-etching method. *Acta Haematol.*, **101**(1), 25–31.

Ueno, S., Maruki, Y., Nakamura, M. *et al.* (2001). The gene encoding a newly discovered protein, chorein, is mutated in chorea-acanthocytosis. *Nat. Genet.*, **28**(2), 121–2.

Ueno, E., Oguchi, K. & Yanagisawa, N. (1982). Morphological abnormalities of erythrocyte membrane in the hereditary neurological disease with chorea, areflexia and acanthocytosis. *J. Neurol. Sci.*, **56**(1), 89–97.

Walker, R. H., Morgello, S., Davidoff-Feldman, B. *et al.* (2002). Autosomal dominant chorea-acanthocytosis with polyglutamine-containing neuronal inclusions. *Neurology*, **58**(7), 1031–7.

Walker, R. H., Davidoff-Feldman, B., Rudnicki, D., Holmes, S. E. & Margolis, R. L. (2003). Huntington's disease-like type 2 with and without acanthocytosis. *Neurology*, **60**(Suppl 1), A287.

Welty, F. K., Lahoz, C., Tucker, K. L., Ordovas, J. M., Wilson, P. W. & Schaefer, E. J. (1998). Frequency of ApoB and ApoE gene mutations as causes of hypobetalipoproteinemia in the Framingham offspring population. *Arterioscler. Thromb. Vasc. Biol.*, **18**(11), 1745–51.

Wetterau, J. R., Aggerbeck, L. P., Bouma, M. E. *et al.* (1992). Absence of microsomal triglyceride transfer protein in individuals with abetalipoproteinemia. *Science*, **258**, 999–1001.

Wimer, B. M., Marsh, W. L., Taswell, H. F. & Galey, W. R. (1977). Haematological changes associated with the McLeod phenotype of the Kell blood group system. *Br. J. Haematol.*, **36**(2), 219–24.

Witt, T. N., Danek, A., Reiter, M., Heim, M. U., Dirschinger, J. & Olsen, E. G. (1992). McLeod syndrome: a distinct form of neuroacanthocytosis. Report of two cases and literature review with emphasis on neuromuscular manifestations. *J. Neurol.*, **239**(6), 302–6.

Wolman, M. (1995). Wolman disease and its treatment. *Clin. Pediatr.*, **34**(4), 207–12.

Wu, J., Kim, J., Li, Q. *et al.* (1999). Known mutations of apoB account for only a small minority of hypobetalipoproteinemia. *J. Lipid Res.*, **40**(5), 955–9.

Young, S. G., Berties, S. J., Curtiss, L. K. & Witztum, J. L. (1987). Characterisation of an abnormal species of apolipoprotein B, apolipoprotein B-37, associated with familial hypobetalipoproteinemia. *J. Clin. Invest.*, **79**, 1831–41.

Young, S. G., Narthey, S. T. & McCarthy, B. J. (1988). Low plasma cholesterol levels caused by a short deletion in the apolipoprotein B gene. *Science*, **241**, 591–3.

Yuan, B., Neuman, R., Duan, S. H. *et al.* (2000). Linkage of a gene for familial hypobetalipoproteinemia to chromosome 3p21.1–22. *Am. J. Hum. Genet.*, **66**(5), 1699–704.

Zhou, B., Westaway, S. K., Levinson, B., Johnson, M. A., Gitschier, J. & Hayflick, S. J. (2001). A novel pantothenate kinase gene (PANK2) is defective in Hallervorden-Spatz syndrome. *Nat. Genet.*, **28**, 345–9.

60

Brain iron disorders

Satoshi Kono,[1] Hiroaki Miyajima[2] and Jonathan D. Gitlin[1]

[1] Edward Mallinckrodt Department of Pediatrics, Washington University School of Medicine, St. Louis, MO, USA
[2] First Department of Medicine, Hamamatsu University School of Medicine, Hamamatsu, Japan

Introduction

Iron is an essential transition metal required for the binding and activation of dioxygen in a series of critical transport and redox reactions. The facile electron chemistry of iron also accounts for the toxicity of this metal and therefore intricate pathways have evolved to allow for the transport, trafficking and compartmentalization of iron within cells (Kaplan, 2002a). These pathways prevent the formation of iron-induced reactive oxygen intermediates that contribute to the pathogenesis of tissue injury in inherited disorders of iron homeostasis such as hemochromatosis with resultant cirrhosis, diabetes and cardiac failure (Lee *et al.*, 2002). Within the central nervous system, iron is required for critical, diverse processes including neurotransmitter biosynthesis, myelin formation and nitric oxide signaling, as well as oxidative phosphorylation essential for sustaining brain energy requirements (Sipe *et al.*, 2002). Despite this critical role of iron in brain function, the molecular and cellular details of iron metabolism within the human central nervous system remain poorly understood.

Iron uptake into the brain is dependent upon plasma transferrin and transferrin receptors localized to the microvasculature. Although both the apical membrane divalent iron transporter DMT1 and the basolateral transporter ferroportin are expressed within the central nervous system, the precise role of these proteins in brain iron homeostasis is currently unknown (Sipe *et al.*, 2002). The intracellular iron binding protein ferritin is abundantly expressed in neurons and glia and presumably serves as the major source of iron storage within these cells. Iron deficiency in the developing human has been clearly established as a causative factor in long-term developmental and cognitive impairment. In contrast, while several prominent neurodegenerative disorders including Alzheimer's disease and Parkinson's disease have been reported to be associated with excessive iron accumulation in specific brain regions the relationship of this accumulation to the disease pathogenesis is far from clear. The recent molecular characterization of two inherited neurodegenerative disorders with impaired iron metabolism, neuroferritinopathy and aceruloplasminemia, as well as the elucidation of the molecular genetic basis of a third neurodegenerative disease, Hallervorden–Spatz syndrome, with evidence of excess brain iron, has now provided new insights into the pathways of brain iron metabolism and the role of iron accumulation in brain pathology.

Neuroferritinopathy

Neuroferritinopathy is an adult-onset, autosomal dominant neurodegenerative disorder resulting from a mutation in the gene encoding the light chain of the iron storage protein ferritin (Curtis *et al.*, 2001; Crompton *et al.*, 2002). Recognition of this disorder as a unique neurodegenerative disease emerged from careful clinical observations of patients in the Cumbrian Lake District of northwest England. The proband was noted to have bradykinesia and dystonia and was originally considered to have Huntington's disease based upon a strong family history of affected individuals with choreiform movement abnormalities (Crompton *et al.*, 2002). Of note, her cognitive functions were entirely preserved and extensive review of the pedigree revealed chorea, dystonia and Parkinsonian features appearing in multiple family members in the fourth or fifth decade of life in a pattern consistent with autosomal dominant inheritance. Extensive genome linkage analysis eventually localized the affected region to chromosome 19q13.3 and analysis of candidate genes within this region resulted in the detection of a mutation in exon 4 of the ferritin light chain gene (Curtis *et al.*, 2001). The mutation is a single base pair insertion that alters the reading frame, replacing the carboxyl-terminal 22 amino acids with a novel sequence of 26 amino acids observed only in affected family members. Further analysis of patients from Northern England and France has identified this same mutation in a dozen additional cases. Haplotype analysis suggests that in each case these affected families have arisen from a common distant founder.

As noted above, neuroferritinopathy is a movement disorder that usually presents in the fourth or fifth decade, although some patients have been identified clinically in adolescence. Unlike aceruloplasminemia (see below) there are no systemic signs or symptoms and the abnormalities of the clinical exam are entirely confined to the central nervous system. All patients identified thus far have presented with chorea, dystonia or bradykinesia and the movement disorders are most predominant in the face and upper extremities, often asymmetrical (Crompton *et al.*, 2002). Biochemical analysis of affected patients reveals a reduced serum ferritin concentration (usually <200 µg/dl) but otherwise normal iron parameters and no evidence of anemia or other hematological abnormalities. Neuropathological examination of brain tissue reveals extracellular iron accumulation in the basal ganglia, forebrain and cerebellum with cystic axonal degeneration. Consistent with these observations, magnetic resonance imaging reveals increased T_2 signal in the basal ganglia. Conventional neurological treatments aimed at reducing bradykinesia and choreiform movements have been minimally effective and most patients show rapid progression from onset of symptoms. Trials of iron depletion with chelation and phlebotomy are currently under way with the hope of ameliorating disease progression in affected patients or preventing symptom development in genetically identified presymptomatic individuals.

The molecular pathogenesis of neuronal injury in neuroferritinopathy has not been elucidated but is undoubtedly related to the critical role of ferritin in cellular iron storage (Torti & Torti, 2002). Ferritin is a heteropolymer consisting of both H and L ferritin chains and it seems possible that the acquired change in the L chain carboxyl terminus must interfere with the ability of the polymer to collect, store and release iron under the appropriate physiological signals. As noted above, free iron in the presence of oxygen will catalyze the production of tissue-damaging free radicals and at the present time this is the most likely mechanism for neurodegeneration in affected individuals. While the molecular characterization of this disease clearly reveals the critical role for ferritin in central nervous system iron homeostasis, further work will be needed to define the molecular details

of how this mutation leads to the observed pathological changes. Nevertheless, the striking similarities to both the clinical and pathological findings in patients with aceruloplasminemia, reinforces the concept that this rare disorder will be of fundamental importance in our elucidation of the normal mechanisms of brain iron metabolism and the role of this metal in the pathogenesis of neurodegenerative diseases.

Aceruloplasminemia

Aceruloplasminemia is an autosomal recessive disorder of iron homeostasis due to loss-of-function mutations in the gene encoding ceruloplasmin. Clinical presentation is in adulthood with neurologic features of dystonia, dementia and dysarthria accompanied by diabetes and retinal degeneration. Laboratory findings include microcytic anemia, marked elevation in serum ferritin and absent serum ceruloplasmin ferroxidase activity. Consistent with the neurological features, iron accumulation is observed as a low-intensity signal within the basal ganglia on T_1- and T_2-weighted magnetic resonance imaging and histological studies reveal abundant iron within astrocytes and neurons in these regions (Nittis & Gitlin, 2002). Elucidation of the molecular pathogenesis of this disease has revealed an essential role for ceruloplasmin in iron homeostasis and provided new insights into the mechanisms of brain iron metabolism.

Ceruloplasmin

Ceruloplasmin is a member of the evolutionarily conserved multicopper oxidase enzyme family characterized by three types of spectroscopically distinct copper. This protein functions as a ferroxidase, utilizing the electron chemistry of bound copper ions to couple the oxidation of Fe^{2+} to the reduction of oxygen bound to a trinuclear copper cluster (Calabrese *et al.*, 1989). Ceruloplasmin is synthesized predominantly in hepatocytes where copper is incorporated into the apoprotein late in the secretory pathway prior to secretion of the holoprotein into the plasma (Sato & Gitlin, 1991; Hellman *et al.*, 2002a). The mature holoprotein has a half-life of greater than five days in the plasma and metabolic studies indicate little or no exchange of the bound copper following secretion (Hellman & Gitlin, 2002). While the availability of copper within hepatocytes has no direct effect on the rate of ceruloplasmin synthesis or secretion, impairment of copper incorporation during synthesis results in secretion of an apoceruloplasmin moiety that is rapidly degraded in the plasma and lacks any ferroxidase

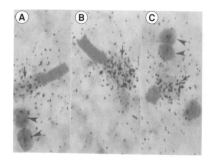
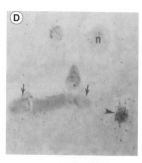

Ceruloplasmin   **Transferrin**

Fig. 60.1 (A)–(C). In situ hybridization of ceruloplasmin mRNA expression within the human brain. Arrows reveal astrocytes surrounding brain microvasculature with abundant ceruloplasmin expression. Arrowheads indicate oligodendrocytes. (D) *In situ* hybridization of transferrin mRNA in these same sections revealing transferrin gene expression within oligodendrocytes (arrowhead) but not the astrocytes shown to express ceruloplasmin (arrows). Modified and reproduced with permission (Klomp & Gitlin, 1996).

activity. As a result, any genetic or metabolic condition that impairs copper availability to the hepatocyte secretory pathway, as occurs in Wilson disease and nutritional copper deficiency, will result in a substantial decrease in the concentration of serum ceruloplasmin.

Although hepatocyte synthesis and secretion accounts for the majority of ceruloplasmin detected in the plasma, this protein is also synthesized in other cell types, including macrophages, present in extrahepatic tissues (Klomp *et al.*, 1996). Within the human central nervous system, ceruloplasmin is synthesized by astrocytes in multiple locations including the brain microvasculature, the basal ganglia and Müller glial cells of the retina (Fig. 60.1) (Klomp & Gitlin, 1996). Astrocytes have been shown to synthesize a distinct isoform of ceruloplasmin containing a glycophosphatidylinositol (GPI) membrane anchor arising from an alternative splicing event and accounting for the majority of ceruloplasmin present in the central nervous system (Patel & David, 1997; Patel *et al.*, 2000; Hellman *et al.*, 2002b). Although the precise role of this isoform in brain iron homeostasis is not established, recent studies indicate that GPI-linked ceruloplasmin is directly associated on the astrocyte plasma membrane with the ferrous iron export protein ferroportin suggesting that the coordinated action of these two proteins is essential for Fe^{2+} efflux from these cells (Jeong & David, 2003). This GPI-linked isoform of ceruloplasmin is also detected in the Sertoli cells of the testis, a finding that may indicate a role for membrane anchored ceruloplasmin in the oxidation and mobilization of iron

at the blood–brain and blood–testis barriers (Fortna *et al.*, 1999).

As noted above, multicopper oxidases utilize the facile electron chemistry of bound copper ions to couple substrate oxidation to the four-electron reduction of dioxygen. These enzymes have been characterized from bacteria, fungi, yeast, worms and mammals where the specific substrates include manganese, iron, nitrate, bilirubin, phenols and ascorbate (Hellman & Gitlin, 2002). While ceruloplasmin is capable of oxidizing multiple different substrates in vitro, critical biochemical studies by Frieden showed that serum ceruloplasmin has a ferroxidase activity required to mobilize iron from the liver with subsequent incorporation of ferric iron into apotransferrin (Osaki *et al.*, 1966, 1971). The biological role of ceruloplasmin as a ferroxidase was demonstrated by Cartwright and colleagues in nutritional experiments using pigs. These investigators showed that copper deficiency results in a marked diminution in circulating serum ceruloplasmin in association with iron accumulation in parenchymal tissues and that administration of ceruloplasmin under these circumstances results in the prompt release of tissue iron with subsequent incorporation into circulating transferrin (Lee *et al.*, 1968; Roeser *et al.*, 1970).

Further support for the role of ceruloplasmin as a ferroxidase comes from genetic and functional studies of homologous multicopper oxidases. In *Saccharomyces cerevisiae* high-affinity iron uptake requires the ferroxidase activity of a plasma membrane multicopper oxidase termed Fet 3 with significant amino acid similarity to ceruloplasmin (Askwith *et al.*, 1994). The *sla* mouse, anemic at birth due to impaired iron uptake across the placenta and gastrointestinal tract, contains a deletion in the gene encoding the multicopper oxidase hephaestin (Vulpe *et al.*, 1999). Hephaestin is highly homologous to ceruloplasmin and is believed to be required for the oxidation of ferrous iron prior to transport of this metal across the basolateral surface of the enterocyte. Definitive proof of a physiological role for ceruloplasmin in iron homeostasis came with the elucidation of the molecular defect in patients with aceruloplasminemia (Yoshida *et al.*, 1995; Harris *et al.*, 1995).

Aceruloplasminemia: genetics

In 1987, Miyajima and colleagues reported the case of a 52-year-old woman from Hamamatsu who presented to their clinic with dystonia and dysarthria. Subsequent evaluation revealed the presence of diabetes, peripheral retinal degeneration, significant iron accumulation in the basal ganglia on MRI and a complete absence of serum ceruloplasmin (Miyajima *et al.*, 1987). Careful family studies in this original case revealed that the absent serum ceruloplasmin was inherited in an autosomal recessive fashion. These findings were subsequently confirmed in a second case report of a similarly affected Japanese family as well as in two brothers from Belfast, Ireland who presented predominantly with signs of dementia (Logan *et al.*, 1994; Morita *et al.*, 1995). Given the proposed role of ceruloplasmin as a plasma ferroxidase, a direct connection was hypothesized between the absence of this protein and the iron accumulation in these patients. This concept was subsequently confirmed by molecular genetic analysis of these three original families, revealing loss-of-function mutations in the ceruloplasmin gene and leading to the characterization of this disorder as aceruloplasminemia (Yoshida *et al.*, 1995; Harris *et al.*, 1995, 1996). Although epidemiological studies in Japan suggest that this is a rare disease with an incidence of 1:500 000 in that country (Miyajima *et al.*, 1999), subsequent studies have now identified 26 distinct mutations in more than 30 affected families from around the world (Fig. 60.2) (Daimon *et al.*, 1995a, Hellman *et al.*, 2000, 2002a,b; Kohno *et al.*, 2000; Miyajima *et al.*, 1999; Okamoto *et al.*, 1996; Takahashi *et al.*, 1996; Yazaki *et al.*, 1998; Yonekawa *et al.*, 1999; Loreal *et al.*, 2002; Bosio *et al.*, 2002; Takeuchi *et al.*, 2002).

As anticipated for a rare disease, almost all mutations detected thus far are private to specific families where there is often a history of consanguinity. The ferroxidase activity of ceruloplasmin is dependent upon the trinuclear copper cluster, the ligands for which are encoded in part by exon 19 and thus each of the mutations identified thus far would be anticipated to result in complete loss-of-function (Fig. 60.2). Consistent with this concept, the clinical phenotype in affected patients shows little variation regardless of the specific mutation, a finding that also suggests minimal overriding influence of other genetic or environmental factors on the clinical outcome. While almost all patients have a complete absence of serum ceruloplasmin, a novel missense mutation at one of the type I copper binding sites (H978Q) has recently been reported to be associated with normal serum concentration of a ceruloplasmin moiety devoid of ferroxidase activity (Takeuchi *et al.*, 2002). This finding has important diagnostic implications, indicating that the presence of a normal serum ceruloplasmin concentration in a patient with otherwise typical clinical features of aceruloplasminemia requires assessment of ceruloplasmin oxidase activity before the diagnosis can be ruled out. While no mutations have been reported in exon 20, the alternative splice region resulting in GPI-linked ceruloplasmin and the predominate expression of this isoform only within the central nervous system suggests that such a mutation could result in the typi-

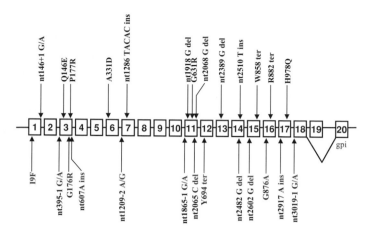

Fig. 60.2 Genetic mutations characterized in patients with aceruloplasminemia or family members. The structure of the human ceruloplasmin gene is shown with 20 exons as previously characterized (Daimon *et al.*, 1995b; Hellman *et al.*, 2002b). Alternative splicing at exon 18 allows for the secreted or GPI-linked ceruloplasmin isoforms as indicated. Mutations indicated are referenced in the text. Modified and reproduced with permission (Nittis & Gitlin, 2002).

cal neurologic features of aceruloplasminemia in a patient with normal serum ceruloplasmin oxidase activity and no evidence of diabetes (Fig. 60.2). Ceruloplasmin is a single copy gene in the human genome; however, the presence of a processed pseudogene on chromosome 8 encoding the carboxyl-terminal 563 amino acids of this protein must be taken into account in the development of strategies for molecular diagnostic testing (Koschinsky *et al.*, 1987).

Aceruloplasminemia: clinical features

Affected individuals present in the fourth or fifth decade of life with neurological signs and symptoms suggestive of basal ganglia disease, including subcortical dementia, dysarthria and dystonia (Gitlin, 1998; Miyajima *et al.*, 2003). These neurologic features are usually rapidly progressive and at the time of diagnosis invariably associated with evidence of brain iron accumulation within the basal ganglia on magnetic resonance imaging (Fig. 60.3). Cerebrospinal fluid analysis reveals no pleocytosis and normal glucose content with elevated protein and iron concentrations (Miyajima *et al.*, 1998). Opthalmologic examination will usually reveal evidence of peripheral retinal degeneration secondary to iron accumulation and photoreceptor cell loss (Fig. 60.4). At autopsy the cut surface of the brain demonstrates dark pigmentation within the nuclei of the basal ganglia with cavitary degeneration in these regions (Fig. 60.4). Consistent with these findings, biochemical

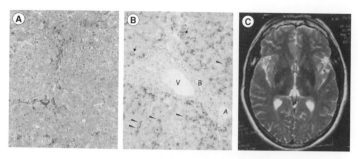

Fig. 60.3 Histological and radiological analysis of a 52-year-old male with dysarthria, diabetes, elevated serum ferritin, absent serum ceruloplasmin and molecular genetic evidence of homozygosity for a single base pair insertion in exon 14 of the ceruloplasmin gene. (A) Normal liver histology on biopsy with no evidence of cirrhosis or fibrosis. (B) Perl's stain of liver biopsy section reveals marked iron accumulation within hepatocytes (arrowheads) and Küppfer cells (arrows). (C) Magnetic resonance imaging at the time of diagnosis reveals signal attenuation in the basal ganglia consistent with iron accumulation. Modified and reproduced with permission (Hellman et al., 2000).

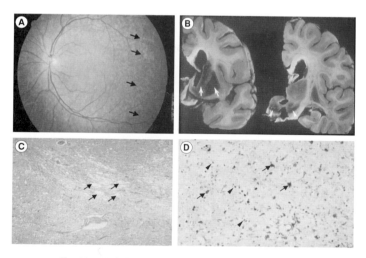

Fig. 60.4 Ophthalmoscopic and autopsy findings in aceruloplasminemia. (A) Retinal examination with normal fundus and retinal vessels but peripheral retinal degeneration (arrows). (B) Coronal section of brain from affected patient indicating brown pigmentation of basal ganglia with cavitary degeneration of caudate nucleus and putamen (arrows) and subthalamic nuclei (arrowheads). (C) Histological analysis of putamen reveals regions of neuronal loss (arrows) without gliosis or inflammation. (D) Perl's stain from section of caudate nucleus revealing iron accumulation within microglia (arrowheads) and neurons (arrows). (B) Modified and reproduced with permission (Morita et al., 1995).

studies reveal normal content of copper and zinc but marked elevation in the concentration of iron throughout the brain with the most significant increases (greater than ten-fold) within the basal ganglia (Morita et al., 1995). Histological analysis of the central nervous system at autopsy illustrates areas of neuronal dropout with spongiform degeneration without evidence of gliosis or inflammatory cell infiltrate. Analysis of sections from the basal ganglia by Perl's stain indicates abundant iron accumulation within both glia and neurons with no extracellular metal accumulation (Fig. 60.4). Taken together, these pathological findings are consistent with a primary disorder of iron homeostasis resulting in iron accumulation and subsequent cellular injury and correlate with the signs and symptoms observed in affected patients. In accord with this model of cellular injury, brain tissue from affected patients demonstrates increased lipid peroxidation and impaired fatty acid oxidation (Kaneko et al., 2002; Miyajima et al., 2002).

Although the neurologic features dominate the clinical picture in most patients, all individuals will have evidence of systemic iron overload at the time of diagnosis. In some cases, patients have been initially recognized prior to the onset of neurologic symptoms due to biochemical abnormalities indicating abnormal iron metabolism. These laboratory findings include microcytic anemia, decreased serum iron content and increased serum ferritin concentration, usually greater than 1000 ng/ml (Miyajima et al., 2003; Morita et al., 1995). Liver biopsy samples reveal normal hepatic architecture and histology with no evidence of cirrhosis or fibrosis but invariably demonstrate excess iron accumulation within both hepatocytes and reticuloendothelial cells (Fig. 60.3). Although hepatic iron content is often elevated into the range observed hemochromatosis (>1500 µg/ gram dry weight), individuals with aceruloplasminemia never evidence hepatic dysfunction or cirrhosis, a finding that may reflect the marked accumulation of reticuloendothelial iron that is not observed in hemochromatosis. Aceruloplasminemia also results in insulin-dependent diabetes mellitus and patients will most often have overt diabetes or evidence of abnormal glucose tolerance with elevated hemoglobin A_{1c} at diagnosis. Autopsy examination has revealed significant iron accumulation within the endocrine portion of the pancreas with marked diminution in the β cell population within the islets of Langerhans (Kato et al., 1997; Morita et al., 1995).

The findings of absent serum ceruloplasmin and neurologic features of basal ganglia disease may lead to diagnostic confusion with Wilson disease. In such cases, the finding of half-normal serum ceruloplasmin in the parents or siblings in conjunction with decreased serum iron, elevated serum ferritin, the presence of diabetes and MRI evidence of brain iron accumulation is useful in establishing the diagnosis of aceruloplasminemia. If patients with aceruloplasminemia are detected with abnormal parameters of iron metabolism prior to the onset of neurologic disease, diagnostic confusion with hemochromatosis may arise (Hellman *et al.*, 2000). In such circumstances the measurement of serum transferrin saturation is often useful as this will be elevated in all cases of hemochromatosis but decreased in aceruloplasminemia. Distinguishing between these conditions is important as phlebotomy, the primary treatment for iron overload in hemochromatosis, is ineffective in aceruloplasminemia and will eventually exacerbate the anemia as such individuals are unable to mobilize reticuloendothelial cell iron stores in response to blood loss. As noted previously, autosomal dominant inheritance of an insertional mutation in the gene encoding ferritin light chain results in a neuroferritinopathy characterized by basal ganglia symptoms and brain iron accumulation similar to that observed in aceruloplasminemia (Crompton *et al.*, 2002). Such patients present at a similar age as those with aceruloplasminemia but are distinguishable by the pattern of inheritance as well as decreased serum ferritin and the lack of diabetes or systemic iron overload. Genetic studies reported thus far have not revealed any evidence of ceruloplasmin gene polymorphisms or heteroallelic mutations influencing the outcome of more common disorders of iron homeostasis (Lee *et al.*, 2002). Although reports have identified neurologic abnormalities in several elderly individuals heterozygous for ceruloplasmin gene mutations, the relationship of this genetic finding to the underlying disease pathology has not been established (Daimon *et al.*, 1999; Miyajima *et al.*, 2001).

Aceruloplasminemia: pathogenesis

The distinct abnormalities of iron homeostasis observed in patients with aceruloplasminemia are most easily understood by considering the cellular physiology of systemic iron metabolism. Only a very small amount of the total iron utilized each day is derived from absorption, the overwhelming portion arising from recycling of heme iron as aging red blood cells are turned over within the reticuloendothelial system (Kaplan, 2002b). Iron recycled in this fashion is released from reticuloendothelial cells in the liver and spleen, bound to plasma transferrin and returned to the bone marrow for erythropoeisis. Ceruloplasmin functions as a critical factor in this cycle by establishing a rate of iron oxidation sufficient for sustaining iron release and uptake by transferrin. The lack of ceruloplasmin ferroxidase activity in patients with aceruloplasminemia results

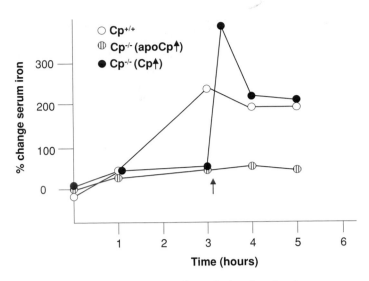

Fig. 60.5 Plasma iron in wild-type and aceruloplasminemic mice following the administration of iron in the form of heat-damaged red blood cells. Arrow illustrates the time point of administration of human ceruloplasmin to aceruloplasminemic mice (apo or holo) as a single intraperitoneal dose calculated to increase the serum ceruloplasmin concentration by approximately 25%. Modified and reproduced with permission (Harris *et al.*, 1999).

in the slow but consistent accumulation of iron within compartments where this metal is normally made available for release following the turnover of red blood cells. This concept can be readily appreciated by examining the iron cycle in a murine model of aceruloplasminemia (Fig. 60.5). When iron is administered to wild-type mice in the form of heat-damaged red blood cells, these cells are rapidly catabolized within the spleen and the heme-bound iron is released and returned to the plasma. Aceruloplasminemic mice are incapable of raising the serum iron content under these circumstances as the iron remains trapped within the reticuloendothelial system. This defect is directly due to the lack of circulating ceruloplasmin ferroxidase activity as the administration of holo, but not apo, ceruloplasmin to these mice results in the prompt release of this stored iron as reflected by increase in plasma iron content equivalent to that observed in control animals (Harris *et al.*, 1999). Similar observations have been made upon the administration of fresh frozen plasma containing ceruloplasmin to affected patients (Logan *et al.*, 1994; Yonekawa *et al.*, 1999). This impairment in the rate of reticuloendothelial cell iron release results in microcytic anemia in affected patients and illustrates the reason for the ineffectiveness and potential dangers of phlebotomy. The lack of severe anemia in patients with aceruloplasminemia indicates that sufficient iron release can occur to permit some degree of erythropoeisis, most likely due to alternative sources of ferroxidase activity such as citrate present in the plasma.

As noted above, iron also accumulates within hepatocytes, pancreatic endocrine cells and other systemic tissues in patients with aceruloplasminemia. Under these circumstances, the lack of plasma ferroxidase activity results in increased ferrous (Fe^{2+}) iron within the plasma that is then rapidly taken up from the circulation by hepatocytes and other cell types. This mechanism of iron accumulation has been well documented in atransferrinemia where serum transferrin binding capacity is absent and in hemochromatosis where the binding capacity is exceeded (Craven et al., 1987). Fe^{2+} is transported into cells in a non-transferrin dependent manner by the cation transporter DMT1 that is expressed in most tissues and it is this protein that is most likely responsible for nonreticuloendothelial cell iron accumulation observed in aceruloplasminemia (Andrews, 2002). The mechanism of iron release from most cells, including those of the reticuloendothelial system, involves the basolateral transporter ferroportin (Donovan et al., 2000; Abboud & Haile, 2000; McKie et al., 2000). As noted above, this protein is associated with GPI-linked ceruloplasmin on astrocytes and is believed to function in conjunction with this ferroxidase in the transport of Fe^{2+} into the plasma with subsequent oxidation to Fe^{3+} for incorporation into transferrin (Jeong and David, 2003). Consistent with this model, mutations in the gene encoding ferroportin result in a syndrome of iron overload with increased reticuloendothelial cell iron, decreased transferrin saturation and intolerance to phlebotomy (Montosi et al., 2001; Njajou et al., 2001).

From a clinical perspective, the most striking and important feature of aceruloplasminemia is the accumulation of iron within the central nervous system. Indeed, with the exception of neuroferritinopathy, this is the only disorder of iron homeostasis that results in brain iron accumulation and neurodegeneration (Harris et al., 1998). In contrast to the mechanisms of tissue iron overload in systemic tissues, this accumulation of iron in the central nervous system does not arise from the increased plasma ferrous iron, as brain iron is not increased in other disorders with a similar elevation in ferrous iron such as atransferrinemia and hemochromatosis. Likewise, the absence of plasma ceruloplasmin is not related to the pathogenesis of brain iron accumulation as this protein does not cross the blood–brain barrier. The abundant expression of ceruloplasmin by astrocytes, predominantly as the GPI-linked isoform, taken together with the known function of ceruloplasmin in the systemic circulation suggests that this isoform functions in an analogous fashion in the central nervous system to maintain a sufficient rate of iron release from storage cells with the retina and brain. This model of pathogenesis

implies the presence of a cycle of iron storage and reutilization within the central nervous system that is similar to but distinct from that in the systemic circulation that may be critical in minimizing the effects of systemic iron deficiency on brain function.

The mechanisms of neurodegeneration in aceruloplasminemia have not been defined but presumably are secondary to the slow but consistent accumulation of iron within neurons and glia. The excess glial iron could result in oxidative damage to this cell type with subsequent loss of glial-derived growth factors critical for neuronal survival. Alternatively, neuronal cell injury may result more directly from iron-mediated oxidation or from selective effects of iron deficiency in regions where glial cell iron can not be mobilized for uptake into neurons. A direct role of iron in oxidant-mediated neuronal injury is supported by findings of increased lipid peroxidation in the tissues of affected patients and in brain tissue and cells from a murine model of aceruloplasminemia as well as by studies that demonstrate some amelioration of neurologic symptoms following reduction of brain iron stores with systemic chelation therapy (Miyajima et al., 2002; Miyajima et al., 1997; Patel et al., 2002). Specific mutations that result in impaired ceruloplasmin trafficking with retention of misfolded protein within the endoplasmic reticulum may also contribute to pathology within the central nervous system through conformation-induced cellular injury (Hellman et al., 2002b). Effective therapy aimed at preventing neuronal injury in asymptomatic patients and ameliorating symptoms in those affected must await a more critical understanding of the molecular mechanisms of iron homeostasis within the central nervous system and the precise mechanisms of neurodegeneration in this disorder.

Hallervorden–Spatz syndrome

Hallervorden–Spatz syndrome is an autosomal recessive disorder due to mutations in the pantothenate kinase 2 gene and associated with marked basal ganglia iron accumulation (Zhou et al., 2001; Hayflick et al., 2003). The disorder encompasses a spectrum of presentations including the classic childhood form with dystonia, dysarthria and rigidity that is progressive and fatal as well as more atypical presentations with the onset of extrapyramidal symptoms later in life and a much less aggressive course. In all cases, iron deposition in the basal ganglia is detectable by magnetic resonance imaging. In the classical form of the disease, signs and symptoms of neurodegeneration usually occur within the first 5 years of life with the predominant features being dysarthria, dystonia, rigidity and choreoathetosis. Dystonia often presents in the cranial and limb muscles and later progresses to axial involvement. Cognitive decline and retinopathy are also present as the disease progresses and despite some variation in the rate of deterioration most affected individuals are nonambulatory by early in the second decade. In all cases T_2 magnetic resonance imaging will reveal bilateral hyperintensity within an area of hypointense signal in the medial globus pallidus, the so-called "eye of the tiger" pattern. This specific image is highly diagnostic for Hallervorden–Spatz syndrome and appears to result from tissue necrosis and edema within a region of iron accumulation in the basal ganglia.

Molecular genetic analysis in a series of affected patients localized the gene to chromosome 20p13 and identified mutations in a novel pantothenate kinase (*PANK2*), proposed to be a key regulatory enzyme in the pathway of coenzyme A biosynthesis (Zhou *et al.*, 2001). All patients with the classical presentation of the disease analyzed thus far have mutations in the *PANK2* gene. A detailed clinical and molecular analysis of patients with the more atypical presentations noted above found mutations in *PANK2* in a subset of these individuals where speech disorders and psychiatric symptoms predominated (Hayflick *et al.*, 2003). Importantly, regardless of the clinical presentation, this analysis revealed complete correlation between the radiographic findings of the eye-of-the-tiger on magnetic resonance imaging of the brain and the presence of mutations in the *PANK2* gene. This finding is of diagnostic significance to clinicians and suggests a direct relationship between the alterations in pantothenate kinase function and the iron accumulation associated with the radiographic findings. Most patients with an atypical presentation were found to have missense mutations, raising the possibility that the delay in symptoms in such individuals arises from residual kinase activity. This finding raises the important therapeutic possibility that dietary availability of pantothenate as vitamin B_5 may prevent or ameliorate disease onset or neurodegeneration.

In contrast to neuroferritinopathy and aceruloplasminemia, clues to the pathogenesis of iron accumulation in Hallervorden–Spatz syndrome are not directly apparent from the molecular defect. Furthermore, given the very early age of onset with the classical disease compared to that observed in all other known metal storage diseases with tissue injury, and the presence of symptoms in some patients with an atypical presentation and normal brain iron content, arguments for any direct role of iron in the neurodegenerative process remain less persuasive. Nevertheless, pantothenate kinase deficiency is predicted to lead to abnormalities in brain citrate metabolism and it is possible that this metabolite may serve to inap-

propriately sequester iron within affected neurons (Zhou *et al.*, 2001). Obviously further metabolic studies and the development of appropriate animal models will permit a more direct analysis of the role of pantothenate kinase in brain iron metabolism. Despite some similarities of brain iron accumulation to those observed in patients with neuroferritinopathy and aceruloplasminemia, individuals with Hallervorden–Spatz syndrome may be differentiated by presentation in early childhood and the lack of any biochemical evidence of perturbation in systemic iron homeostasis.

Conclusions

Elucidation of the molecular genetic basis of these three neurodegenerative diseases has provided new insight into the function of ferritin and ceruloplasmin in brain iron homeostasis. Future efforts in this area are clearly warranted given the well recognized role of iron in early cognitive development as well as recent studies that implicate brain iron accumulation in the pathogenesis of neurodegeneration observed in Parkinson's, disease and Alzheimer's disease (Andrews, 2000; Kaur *et al.*, 2003). Specific research efforts must now focus on a critical understanding of the role of the basal ganglia in brain iron metabolism as well as the mechanisms underlying the unique susceptibility of this brain region to iron-mediated neurodegeneration. Careful analysis of human genetic diseases of iron metabolism will undoubtedly continue to provide answers and permit new insights into the neurobiology, pathogenesis and treatment of neurodegenerative diseases.

Acknowledgement

We gratefully acknowledge the contributions of our many colleagues around the world who have generously referred patients and shared ideas, including James Kushner, Fernando Perez-Aguilar, Grazia Mancini, Clara Camaschella, Wolfgang Stremmel, Massimo Pandolfo, John Logan and Hiroshi Morita as well as the numerous families and patients who have contributed to this work. Work from the author's laboratory reported in this review was supported in part by National Institute of Health Grant DK 61763.

REFERENCES

Abboud, S. & Haile, D. J. (2000). A novel mammalian iron-regulated protein involved in intracellular iron metabolism. *J. Biol. Chem.* **275**, 19906–12.

Andrews, N. C. (2000). Iron metabolism: iron deficiency and iron overload. *Annu. Rev. Genom. Hum. Genet.*, **1**, 75–98.

Andrews, N. C. (2002). A genetic view of iron homeostasis. *Semin. Hematol.* **39**, 227–34.

Askwith, C. D., Eide, A., Van Ho, P. S. *et al.* (1994). The FET3 gene of *S. cerevisiae* encodes a multicopper oxidase required for ferrous iron uptake. *Cell*, **76**, 403–10.

Bosio, S., De Gobbi, M., Roetto, A. *et al.* (2002). Anemia and iron overload due to compound heterozygosity for novel ceruloplasmin mutations. *Blood*, **100**, 2246–8.

Calabrese, L., Carbonaro, M. & Musci, G. (1989). Presence of coupled trinuclear copper cluster in mammalian ceruloplasmin is essential for efficient electron transfer to oxygen. *J. Biol. Chem.*, **264**, 6183–7.

Craven, C. M., Alexander, J., Eldridge, M. Kushner, J. P. Bernstein, S. & Kaplan, J. (1987). Tissue distribution and clearance kinetics of non-transferrin-bound iron in the hypotransferrinemic mouse: a rodent model for hemochromatosis. *Proc. Natl Acad. Sci., USA*, **84**, 3457–61.

Crompton, D. E., Chinnery, P. F., Fey, C. *et al.* (2002). Neuroferritinopathy: a window on the role of iron in neurodegeneration. *Blood Cells Mol. Dis.*, **29**, 522–31.

Curtis, A. R., Fey, C., Morris, C. M. *et al.* (2001). Mutation in the gene encoding ferritin light polypeptide causes dominant adult-onset basal ganglia disease. *Nat. Genet.*, **28**, 350–4.

Daimon, M., Kato, T., Kawanami, T. *et al.* (1995a). A nonsense mutation of the ceruloplasmin gene in hereditary ceruloplasmin deficiency with diabetes mellitus. *Biochem. Biophys. Res. Commun.*, **217**, 89–95.

Daimon, M., Yamatani, K., Igarashi, M. *et al.* (1995b). Fine structure of the human ceruloplasmin gene. *Biochem. Biophys. Res. Commun.*, **208**, 1028–35.

Daimon, M., Moriai, S., Susa, S., Yamatani, K., Hosoya, T. & Kato, T. (1999). Hypocaeruloplasminaemia with heteroallelic caeruloplasmin gene mutation: MRI of the brain. *Neuroradiology*, **41**, 185–7.

Daimon, M., Susa, S., Ohizumi, T. *et al.* (2000). A novel mutation of the ceruloplasmin gene in a patient with heteroallelic ceruloplasmin gene mutation (HypoCPGM). *Tohoku J. Exp. Med.*, **191**, 119–25.

Donovan, A., Brownlie, A., Zhou, Y. *et al.* (2000). Positional cloning of zebrafish ferroportin1 identifies a conserved vertebrate iron exporter. *Nature*, **403**, 776–81.

Fortna, R. R., Watson, H. A. & Nyquist, S. E. (1999). Glycosyl phosphatidylinositol-anchored ceruloplasmin is expressed by rat Sertoli cells and is concentrated in detergent-insoluble membrane fractions. *Biol. Reprod.*, **61**, 1042–9.

Gitlin, J. D. (1998). Aceruloplasminemia. *Pediatr. Res.*, **44**, 271–6.

Harris, Z. L., Durley, A. P., Man, T. K. & Gitlin, J. D. (1999). Targeted gene disruption reveals an essential role for ceruloplasmin in cellular iron efflux. *Proc. Natl Acad. Sci., USA*, **96**, 10812–17.

Harris, Z. L., Takahashi, Y., Miyajima, H., Serizawa, M., MacGillivray, R. T. & Gitlin, J. D. (1995). Aceruloplasminemia: molecular characterization of this disorder of iron metabolism. *Proc. Natl Acad. Sci., USA*, **92**, 2539–43.

Harris, Z. L., Migas, M. C., Hughes, A. E., Logan, J. L. & Gitlin, J. D. (1996). Familial dementia due to a frameshift mutation in the caeruloplasmin gene. *Quart. J. Med.*, **89**, 355–9.

Harris, Z. L., Klomp, L. W. & Gitlin, J. D. (1998). Aceruloplasminemia: an inherited neurodegenerative disease with impairment of iron homeostasis. *Am. J. Clin. Nutr.*, **67**, 972S–7S.

Hayflick, S. J., Westaway, S. K., Levinson, B. *et al.* (2003). Genetic, clinical, and radiographic delineation of Hallervorden–Spatz syndrome. *N. Engl. J. Med.*, **348**, 33–40.

Hellman, N. E. & Gitlin, J. D. (2002). Ceruloplasmin metabolism and function. *Annu. Rev. Nutr.*, **22**, 439–58.

Hellman, N. E., Schaefer, M., Gehrke, S. *et al.* (2000). Hepatic iron overload in aceruloplasminaemia. *Gut*, **47**, 858–60.

Hellman, N. E., Kono, S., Mancini, G. M., Hoogeboom, A. J., De Jong, G. J. & Gitlin, J. D. (2002a). Mechanisms of copper incorporation into human ceruloplasmin. *J. Biol. Chem.*, **277**, 46632–8.

Hellman, N. E., Kono, S., Miyajima, H. & Gitlin, J. D. (2002b). Biochemical analysis of a missense mutation in aceruloplasminemia. *J. Biol. Chem.*, **277**, 1375–80.

Jeong, S. Y. & David, S. (2003). GPI-anchored ceruloplasmin is required for iron efflux from cells in the central nervous system. *J. Biol. Chem.*

Kaneko, K., Yoshida, K., Arima, K. *et al.* (2002). Astrocytic deformity and globular structures are characteristic of the brains of patients with aceruloplasminemia. *J. Neuropathol. Exp. Neurol.*, **61**, 1069–77.

Kaplan, J. (2002a). Mechanisms of cellular iron acquisition: another iron in the fire. *Cell*, **111**, 603–6.

Kaplan, J. (2002b). Strategy and tactics in the evolution of iron acquisition. *Semin. Hematol.*, **39**, 219–26.

Kato, T., Daimon, M., Kawanami, T., Ikezawa, Y., Sasaki, H. & Maeda, K. (1997). Islet changes in hereditary ceruloplasmin deficiency. *Hum. Pathol.*, **28**, 499–502.

Kaur, D., Yantiri, F., Rajagopalan, S. *et al.* (2003). Genetic or pharmacological iron chelation prevents MPTP-induced neurotoxicity in vivo: a novel therapy for Parkinson's disease. *Neuron*, **37**, 899–909.

Klomp, L. W. & Gitlin, J. D. (1996). Expression of the ceruloplasmin gene in the human retina and brain: implications for a pathogenic model in aceruloplasminemia. *Hum. Mol. Genet.*, **5**, 1989–96.

Klomp, L. W., Farhangrazi, Z. S., Dugan, L. L. & Gitlin, J. D. (1996). Ceruloplasmin gene expression in the murine central nervous system. *J. Clin. Invest.*, **98**, 207–15.

Kohno, S., Miyajima, H., Takahashi, Y. & Inoue, Y. (2000). Aceruloplasminemia with a novel mutation associated with parkinsonism. *Neurogenetics*, **2**, 237–8.

Koschinsky, M. L., Chow, B. K., Schwartz, J., Hamerton, J. L. & MacGillivray, R. T. (1987). Isolation and characterization of a processed gene for human ceruloplasmin. *Biochemistry*, **26**, 7760–7.

Lee, G. R., Nacht, S., Lukens, J. N. & Cartwright, G. E. (1968). Iron metabolism in copper-deficient swine. *J. Clin. Invest.*, **47**, 2058–69.

Lee, P., Gelbart, T., West, C., Halloran, C. & Beutler, E. (2002). Seeking candidate mutations that affect iron homeostasis. *Blood Cells Mol. Dis.*, **29**, 471–87.

Logan, J. I., Harveyson, K. B., Wisdom, G. B., Hughes, A. E. & Archbold, G. P. (1994). Hereditary caeruloplasmin deficiency, dementia and diabetes mellitus. *Quart. J. Med.*, **87**, 663–70.

Loreal, O., Turlin, B., Pigeon, C. *et al.* (2002). Aceruloplasminemia: new clinical, pathophysiological and therapeutic insights. *J. Hepatol.*, **36**, 851–6.

McKie, A. T., Marciani, P., Rolfs, A. *et al.* (2000). A novel duodenal iron-regulated transporter, IREG1, implicated in the basolateral transfer of iron to the circulation. *Mol. Cell*, **5**, 299–309.

Miyajima, H., Nishimura, Y., Mizoguchi, K., Sakamoto, M., Shimizu, T. & Honda, N. (1987). Familial apoceruloplasmin deficiency associated with blepharospasm and retinal degeneration. *Neurology*, **37**, 761–7.

Miyajima, H., Takahashi, Y., Kamata, T., Shimizu, H., Sakai, N. & Gitlin, J. D. (1997). Use of desferrioxamine in the treatment of aceruloplasminemia. *Ann. Neurol.*, **41**, 404–7.

Miyajima, H., Fujimoto, M., Kohno, S., Kaneko, E. & Gitlin, J. D. (1998). CSF abnormalities in patients with aceruloplasminemia. *Neurology*, **51**, 1188–90.

Miyajima, H., Kohno, S., Takahashi, Y., Yonekawa, O. & Kanno, T. (1999). Estimation of the gene frequency of aceruloplasminemia in Japan. *Neurology*, **53**, 617–19.

Miyajima, H., Kono, S., Takahashi, Y., Sugimoto, M., Sakamoto, M. & Sakai, N. (2001). Cerebellar ataxia associated with heteroallelic ceruloplasmin gene mutation. *Neurology*, **57**, 2205–10.

Miyajima, H., Kono, S., Takahashi, Y. & Sugimoto, M. (2002). Increased lipid peroxidation and mitochondrial dysfunction in aceruloplasminemia brains. *Blood Cells Mol. Dis.*, **29**, 433–8.

Miyajima, H., Takahashi, Y. & Kono, S. (2003). Aceruloplasminemia, an inherited disorder of iron metabolism. *Biometals*, **16**, 205–13.

Montosi, G., Donovan, A., Totaro, A. *et al.* (2001). Autosomal-dominant hemochromatosis is associated with a mutation in the ferroportin (SLC11A3) gene. *J. Clin. Invest.*, **108**, 619–23.

Morita, H., Ikeda, S., Yamamoto, K. *et al.* (1995). Hereditary ceruloplasmin deficiency with hemosiderosis: a clinicopathological study of a Japanese family. *Ann. Neurol.*, **37**, 646–56.

Nittis, T. & Gitlin, J. D. (2002). The copper-iron connection: hereditary aceruloplasminemia. *Semin. Hematol.*, **39**, 282–9.

Njajou, O. T., Vaessen, N., Joosse, M. *et al.* (2001). A mutation in SLC11A3 is associated with autosomal dominant hemochromatosis. *Nat. Genet.*, **28**, 213–14.

Okamoto, N., Wada, S., Oga, T. *et al.* (1996). Hereditary ceruloplasmin deficiency with hemosiderosis. *Hum. Genet.*, **97**, 755–8.

Osaki, S., Johnson, D. A. & Frieden, E. (1966). The possible significance of the ferrous oxidase activity of ceruloplasmin in normal human serum. *J. Biol. Chem.*, **241**, 2746–51.

Osaki, S., Johnson, D. A. & Frieden, E. (1971). The mobilization of iron from the perfused mammalian liver by a serum copper enzyme, ferroxidase I. *J. Biol. Chem.*, **246**, 3018–23.

Patel, B. N. & David, S. (1997). A novel glycosylphosphatidylinositol-anchored form of ceruloplasmin is expressed by mammalian astrocytes. *J. Biol. Chem.*, **272**, 20185–90.

Patel, B. N., Dunn, R. J. & David, S. (2000). Alternative RNA splicing generates a glycosylphosphatidylinositol-anchored form of ceruloplasmin in mammalian brain. *J. Biol. Chem.*, **275**, 4305–10.

Patel, B. N., Dunn, R. J., Jeong, S. Y., Zhu, Q., Julien, J. P. & David, S. (2002). Ceruloplasmin regulates iron levels in the CNS and prevents free radical injury. *J. Neurosci.*, **22**, 6578–86.

Roeser, H. P., Lee, G. R., Nacht, S. & Cartwright, G. E. (1970). The role of ceruloplasmin in iron metabolism. *J. Clin. Invest.*, **49**, 2408–17.

Sato, M. & Gitlin, J. D. (1991). Mechanisms of copper incorporation during the biosynthesis of human ceruloplasmin. *J. Biol. Chem.*, **266**, 5128–34.

Sipe, J. C., Lee, P. & Beutler, E. (2002). Brain iron metabolism and neurodegenerative disorders. *Dev. Neurosci.*, **24**, 188–96.

Takahashi, Y., Miyajima, H., Shirabe, S., Nagataki, S., Suenaga, A. & Gitlin, J. D. (1996). Characterization of a nonsense mutation in the ceruloplasmin gene resulting in diabetes and neurodegenerative disease. *Hum. Mol. Genet.*, **5**, 81–4.

Takeuchi, Y., Yoshikawa, M., Tsujino, T., *et al.* (2002). A case of aceruloplasminaemia: abnormal serum ceruloplasmin protein without ferroxidase activity. *J. Neurol. Neurosurg. Psychiatry*, **72**, 543–5.

Torti, F. M. & Torti, S. V. (2002). Regulation of ferritin genes and protein. *Blood*, **99**, 3505–16.

Vulpe, C. D., Kuo, Y. M., Murphy, T. L. *et al.* (1999). Hephaestin, a ceruloplasmin homologue implicated in intestinal iron transport, is defective in the sla mouse. *Nat. Genet.*, **21**, 195–9.

Yazaki, M., Yoshida, K., Nakamura, A. *et al.* (1998). A novel splicing mutation in the ceruloplasmin gene responsible for hereditary ceruloplasmin deficiency with hemosiderosis. *J. Neurol. Sci.*, **156**, 30–4.

Yonekawa, M., Okabe, T., Asamoto, Y. & Ohta, M. (1999). A case of hereditary ceruloplasmin deficiency with iron deposition in the brain associated with chorea, dementia, diabetes mellitus and retinal pigmentation: administration of fresh-frozen human plasma. *Eur. Neurol.*, **42**, 157–62.

Yoshida, K., Furihata, K., Takeda, S. *et al.* (1995). A mutation in the ceruloplasmin gene is associated with systemic hemosiderosis in humans. *Nat. Genet.*, **9**, 267–72.

Zhou, B., Westaway, S. K., Levinson, B., Johnson, M. A., Gitschier, J. & Hayflick, S. J. (2001). A novel pantothenate kinase gene (PANK2) is defective in Hallervorden–Spatz syndrome. *Nat. Genet.*, **28**, 345–9.

61

Neurological aspects of Wilson's disease

Peter A. LeWitt[1] and George J. Brewer[2]

[1]Departments of Neurology, Psychiatry and Behavioral Neuroscience, Wayne State University School of Medicine, and The Clinical Neuroscience Program, Southfield, MI, USA
[2]Department of Human Genetics and Department of Internal Medicine, University of Michigan School of Medicine, Ann Arbor, MI, USA

Introduction

As a trace metal with several critical metabolic roles, copper is present throughout the brain (Warren *et al.*, 1960) and other organs as an essential element needed for maintaining health. This vital mineral enters the body as a dietary component readily absorbed in the small intestine. The body's load of copper is largely stored in the liver and other visceral organs. Systemic organ load of copper is normally regulated by the ability of the biliary system to excrete excess quantities (Frommer, 1974; Gibbs & Walshe, 1980). A failure of the body's mechanisms for eliminating copper is the characteristic feature of an uncommon but distinctive systemic disorder originally termed progressive hepatolenticular degeneration, or Wilson's disease (WD). The latter eponym, now widely used for this disorder, credits the man who discovered much of what we know today and helps to avoid a mistaken notion that excess copper deposition affects only the liver and brain. WD's manifestations throughout the body can be variable from patient to patient, and can include features listed in Table 61.1. In nearly all cases, the liver is a major target of WD. Death from hepatic WD is usually inevitable unless decoppering therapy is instituted early enough. Other systemic manifestations of WD, including its propensity for neurological involvement, can vary greatly among patients. In the pediatric population, hepatic damage is often a presenting feature of the disorder, while neurological impairment becomes increasingly more common with onset in the second or third decades of life.

The pathophysiology of WD is linked to failure in copper transport. Though vital for life in trace amounts, copper in excess quantities is toxic. Normally, ingested copper is excreted into the bile (Cartwright & Wintrobe, 1964). WD arises from an inability to accomplish adequate removal of copper, leading to massive, toxic tissue deposition (O'Reilly *et al.*, 1971; Frommer, 1974; Gibbs & Walshe, 1980). While the defect in copper excretion in WD is likely a problem of protein complexing, all aspects of WD pathophysiology have not been worked out.

When first described in 1912 by the American–British neurologist Samuel Alexander Kinnier Wilson, WD was not known to have the massive tissue copper deposition that was finally recognized more than 30 years later (Cumings, 1948). Further investigation showed WD to be a direct consequence of the greatly enhanced copper concentrations in tissues. Normally, mechanisms are operative to exclude all but minute quantities of copper from all tissues of the body. In WD, tracer studies with radiolabelled copper have shown that regions correlated to WD symptomatology are at locations where the most of this trace metal has been deposited (Walshe & Potter, 1977). Prior to the development of effective decoppering agents, WD was incurable and progressive to death (Lichtenstein & Gore, 1955). Several treatment options have been devised in the past five decades that can dramatically reverse the natural history of this disease. It is now typical for WD patients to achieve at least a partial reversal of their neurological symptomatology as well as protection against further damage to the liver and other affected organs. The range of treatment options is discussed below, along with the diagnosis and pathophysiology of this disorder. WD is caused by one or more mutations in a copper transporting P-type ATPase called ATP7B, situated on chromosome 13q14.3 (Bull *et al.*, 1993; Yamaguchi *et al.*, 1993; Tanzi *et al.*, 1993). This location differs from the site for the structural gene of ceruloplasmin (CP), a liver-derived copper-binding protein whose serum concentrations are usually decreased in WD. While CP provides a useful screening marker for WD (see below), its deficiency does not appear to be involved in the pathophysiology of WD.

Table 61.1. A Survey of WD systemic manifestations (adapted from LeWitt and Pfeiffer, 2002)

Hematopoietic system: acute hemolytic anemia, Heinz body anemia, thrombocytopenia, splenomegaly (Deiss *et al.*, 1970; Goldman & Ali, 1991; Prella *et al.*, 2001)

Bone and connective tissue: Rickets, osteoarthritis, recurrent arthritis, bone fragmentation, chondrocalcinosis, osteoporosis, spinal degeneration, spontaneous fractures, spontaneous rupture of Achilles tendon (Kabra *et al.*, 1990; Dobyns *et al.*, 1979; Golding & Walshe, 1977; Feller & Schumacher, 1972; Hu, 1994; Menerey *et al.*, 1988; Olsen *et al.*, 1996; Balint & Szebenyi, 2000)

Kidney: Renal lithiasis, hematuria, hypercalcuria, nephrocalcinosis (Laufer *et al.*, 1992; Hoppe *et al.*, 1993)

Heart: Cardiomyopathy, left ventricular thickening, extrasystolic beats, supraventricular tachycardia (Hlubocka *et al.*, 2002)

Brain: Atrophy, necrosis, gliosis, demyelination, central pontine myelinolysis (see below)

Liver: Cirrhosis, acute hepatitis, ascites, cholelithiasis (Wilson, 1912; Goswami *et al.*, 2001)

Eye: Corneal (Kayser–Fleischer) rings; lens cataract ("star-burst" or "sunflower" appearance) (Heckmann *et al.*, 2000; Goyal & Tripathi, 2000; Patel & Bozdech, 2001; Deguti *et al.*, 2002)

Endocrine: Hypoparathyroidism, amenorrhea, diabetes (Erkan *et al.*, 2002); Pancreatic exocrine impairment (Owen, 1981)

Iron metabolism: Hemosiderosis (Knisely, 2001)

Spleenic rupture (Ahmed & Feller, 1996)

Skeletal muscle: Acute rhabdomyolysis (Propst *et al.*, 1995)

Autonomic nervous system: Peripheral and central dysfunction (Meenakshi-Sundaram *et al.*, 2002; Bhattacharya *et al.*, 2002)

Excessive copper deposition exerts damage to brain, liver, and other organs. However, removing the excess quantities of this metal offers some recovery from organ damage and can be lifesaving for the patient with WD. Even with massive copper deposition, reversal of liver and brain damage manifestations is possible if decoppering treatment is instituted early enough. For this reason, the challenge posed by this rare, genetically determined disorder is strong diagnostic suspicion and adequate screening studies (Shale *et al.*, 1987). The protean features of WD include clinical syndromes that can closely mimic other disorders, including several neurological conditions much more benign than WD.

Effective treatment began a half-century ago once there was recognition of massive tissue copper deposition in WD. This finding led to medications for extracting systemic copper, a search that continues. These investigations have been augmented with the discovery of a genetic animal homologue of the human disorder, the Long-Evans Cinnamon rat (Sasaki *et al.*, 1994; Yamaguchi *et al.*, 1994). Several drugs

are now available to prevent intestinal absorption of copper, to enhance its urinary excretion, or to act by additional mechanisms to produce an anticopper effect. By creating a negative systemic copper balance, WD can be arrested from its otherwise inevitable progression. In the best of circumstances, much of the liver damage, neurological impairments, and other systemic features can be reversed if treatment is started early enough. Occasionally, almost complete recovery can be achieved. In general, certain neurological problems tend to persist, such as dystonic postures, dysarthria, and behavioral disturbances (Pellecchia *et al.*, 2003). With instances of rapid progression or hepatic failure, liver transplantation can be life-saving and can lead to recovery of severe neurological manifestations (Suzuki *et al.*, 2003). The range of therapeutic options is described in a later section.

Neurological manifestations of WD

In Western countries, neurological manifestations of WD most commonly appear in the second or third decades of life (Sternlieb *et al.*, 1985; Walshe & Yealland, 1992). In India and probably in other Eastern countries, the disease tends to occur in earlier age groups (Dastur *et al.*, 1968; Bhave *et al.*, 1994, 1987). In general, neurological involvement tends to develop at a later age than cases of purely hepatic disease. Despite these generalizations, there is great variability reported in the age of onset for WD presenting with neurological impairments (from less than 5 years to greater than 50 (Fitzgerald *et al.*, 1975; Czlonkowska & Rodo, 1981; Ross *et al.*, 1985; Madden *et al.*, 1985; Pilloni *et al.*, 2000)). The presenting neurological features of WD are typically one or more types of movement disorder often with an additional type of neurological deficit (Stremmel *et al.*, 1991). Some patients develop predominantly dystonic or Parkinsonian features, while others are affected more with bulbar dysfunction and a coarse, proximal action tremor. This type of tremor can be associated with other cerebellar dysfunction such as ataxic speech. Since this pattern of neurological WD resembles some common manifestations of multiple sclerosis, this category of WD was referred to as "pseudosclerosis" in the nineteenth century literature on WD (Westphal, 1883). In a more recent series, Walshe and Yealland (1992) found one-quarter of their patients had a "pseudosclerotic" syndrome, while Parkinsonian signs affected almost one-half and the remainder presented with primarily choreic or dystonic features.

In the original descriptions of Kinnier Wilson, this disorder presented insidiously with the problems of tremor, dystonia, rigidity, dysarthria, drooling, dysphagia, unsteady gait, and mental deterioration (Wilson, 1912). The damaged structures Wilson found in the basal ganglia and elsewhere in the brain provided a correlation to the observed neurological deficits. In one series of 44 neurological WD cases, 12 presented primarily with impairments related to basal ganglia damage, 6 had cerebellar dysfunction, and 17 had a combination of these features (Dobyns *et al.*, 1979). The disruption of dopaminergic neurotransmission in striatal structures, as demonstrated in neuroimaging studies, probably contributes to the development of Parkinsonian features, dystonia, and dyskinesia in WD (Barthel *et al.*, 2001). Rarely, WD can be superimposed on another movement disorder such as essential tremor (Quinn *et al.*, 1986). This hereditary disorder can be a potentially confounding diagnostic feature in a family also affected with WD (Nicholl *et al.*, 2001). One of the curious features of WD is the considerable heterogeneity that can be observed among its manifestations in a family with several involved members. WD has a propensity for asymmetrical or focal deficits, despite neuropathological observations that virtually all cases of WD possess bilateral damage to the lenticular nuclei and other structures. As described below, there can also be extensive pathology found beyond the boundaries of the basal ganglia.

Of all the types of movement disorders that can evolve in neurological WD, tremor involving the hand is usually the first (Walshe, 1976, 1986). The tremor can be unilateral or bilateral, intermittent or continuous, or initiated only during specific motor tasks. Other locations for tremor include the head, trunk, or the tongue (Wilson, 1955; Topaloglu *et al.*, 1990). All categories of tremor (rest, postural maintenance, and action) have been observed in WD, sometimes in combination. The action tremor of WD can be similar to cerebellar disease. However, other typical signs of cerebellar dysfunction (such as dysdiadochokinesis, nystagmus, or the Holmes rebound sign) are generally lacking in the WD patient. Many observers have highlighted a characteristic pattern of tremor in WD, a coarse, irregular to-and-fro movement during action. With the arms held forward and flexed at the elbows, this maneuver can bring out a proximal tremor sometimes described as "wing-beating."

In addition to tremor, another common presentation of neurological WD is motor dysfunction involving the bulbar musculature. Illustrated in Wilson's 1912 report was a dystonic alteration of the lower face, a fixed, "sardonic" smile with retracted lips and opened jaw. One series found bulbar motor impairment to be more common than tremor as an early feature of neurological WD (Starosta-Rubenstein *et al.*, 1987). Typical features of WD include drooling, dysarthria, various focal and segmental features of cranial dystonia, and pharyngeal dysmotility (Gulyas & Salazar-Grueso, 1988). In addition, patients can exhibit facial grimacing, involuntary closure of the eyes (blepharospasm), and tongue dyskinesia (Liao *et al.*, 1991). With increasing rigidity of the oral musculature, patients can become unable to close their mouth. The sustained rigid states of cranial musculature can also exhibit spasmodic or jerking movements.

A progressive disturbance of speech is characteristic of WD. These problems include indistinct articulation, defective consonant production, "whispering dysphonia" (Parker, 1985), and slowed cadence of speech (Purdon Martin, 1968; Berry *et al.*, 1974). In its most severe form, the outcome can be complete loss of speaking capability (anarthria). The various elements of dysarthria arise from multiple regional disturbances in the control of facial and oropharyngeal musculature.

The varieties of motor impairment in WD sometimes can be difficult to categorize. Clumsiness and slowness of movement can have a major impact on everyday activities such as handwriting. The source of impaired dexterity obvious in most cases of WD (Hermann *et al.*, 2003) could arise from a number of CNS locations. Clinical testing, such as finger tapping (Davis & Goldstein, 1974), can bring out the extent of motor deficit even in early neurological WD. Other changes commonly seen in WD include trunk titubation, altered posture, and a disturbance of gait. Muscle cramping can be experienced (Golding & Walshe, 1977).

One of the challenges posed in the diagnosis of neurological WD is its duplication of other neurological disorders unrelated to excessive copper deposition. For example, some cases of WD have presented with a unilateral or bilateral Parkinsonian syndrome, including resting tremor, cogwheel rigidity, facial masking, bradykinesia, and other typical features. Ataxia has been described as the only clinical manifestation in a chronic case of WD (Madden *et al.*, 1985). These, and other instances, illustrate that clinical varieties of neurological WD can be sufficiently atypical so as to halt the search for this rare but potentially curable disorder. WD can present with neurological features of other disorders of unknown etiology, such as dystonia. Early presentations of WD have included unusual task-specific difficulties, such as inability to maintain a particular head posture, or to protrude the tongue (Purdon Martin, 1968). Many series have shown that sustained, abnormal postures characteristic of dystonia are common in WD. The varieties of dystonia in WD include generalized, segmental, or multifocal patterns, such as bilateral foot dystonia (Svetel *et al.*, 2001).

Why WD can take on such clinical heterogeneity in its presenting features has long been a mystery (Denny-Brown, 1964). For this reason, WD merits a high level of suspicion with respect to any number of categories of movement disorder. Impairment of the extrapyramidal and cerebellar systems, and bulbar dysfunction are highly typical. Other patterns of neurological damage may be intermingled. Spasticity of the limbs is not a common finding although hyper-reflexia and Babinski signs can be part of the examination. Behavioral manifestations such as pseudobulbar palsy with involuntary crying or laughter can accompany the earliest findings and can persist as a major disability (Mingazzini, 1928). The latter problems, when advanced, can be highly disabling. Certain other types of movement disorders, such as tics and myoclonus, are generally not observed. However, in one case of WD that presented as a tremor disorder, several additional types of motor impairment were reported, including episodic truncal myoclonus, priapism, and seminal ejaculation that occurred several times per day (Nair & Pillai, 1990).

Neurological WD can be picked up on a screening MRI scan even in patients lacking evidence for this disorder on clinical examination. Patients have been described with Kayser–Fleischer rings but without concurrent neurological signs or symptoms of the disease. Kayser–Fleischer rings can be difficult to recognize without magnification, or in patients with dark irises. A formal slit lamp examination by an experienced ophthalmologist is necessary to exclude the possibility of Kayser–Fleischer rings.

Psychiatric and behavioral disorders in WD

Studies of cognition, psychiatric manifestations, and behavior have demonstrated that a range of problems can evolve for patients with WD (Akil et al., 1991). While those without movement disorders or other types of neurological involvement can be spared, patients with basal ganglia lesions or more extensive pathology have shown mild impairments in all realms of cognitive functioning including frontal-executive ability, aspects of memory and visuospatial processing (Seniow et al., 2002). These neuropsychological deficits do not appear to be correlated to the extent of copper toxicity in either symptomatic or asymptomatic WD patients (Rathbun, 1996). Even early in the course some WD patients have shown a decline in memory or other types of cognitive abilities (Knehr & Beam, 1956; Goldstein et al., 1968; Scheinberg & Sternlieb, 1984). Other functions, such as the rate of information processing, may be spared (Littman et al., 1995). With more extensive brain pathology (or concomitant liver failure from hepatic copper deposition), an irreversible dementia can be the outcome. Psychiatric presentations of WD are rare but need to be considered among the "organic" causes of psychosis and mood disorders (Stiller et al., 2002).

Beyond the problems of cognitive functioning, patients with WD can experience a wide range of psychiatric and behavioral disturbances. The initial presentation of WD can be depression or other psychiatric disturbances (Keller et al., 1999; Medalia & Scheinberg, 1989; Jackson et al., 1994). Although original reports by Wilson minimized these problems, patients commonly have shown problems of anxiety, mood alteration, impulsivity, and other psychiatric disorders. Early on, children and adults with WD can manifest disturbances of school performance, altered personality traits, and behavioral indiscretions. Prominent abnormalities on the MMPI and other evaluations of personality traits may be found (Portala et al., 2001). In the latter study of 25 adult patients, these changes were not related to disease duration, age, or when WD began.

Patients with WD have a substantial incidence of moderate to severe depression and related problems (Portala et al., 2000; Akil & Brewer, 1995). In one study, 17 of 34 patients had received psychiatric treatment for various disorders (including schizophrenia, depression, and anxiety) prior to the diagnosis of WD (Rathbun, 1996). When there is clear brain abnormality on neuroimaging or in the form of a movement disorder, the likelihood of a behavioral disorder is much increased. These include aggressiveness, a low anger threshold, impulsiveness, irritability, self-injurious behaviors, suicidal ideation, sexual preoccupations, and childishness (Dening, 1985). As a result, WD is commonly associated with decline in schoolwork or work performance (Akil & Brewer, 1995), and antisocial or criminal behavior can occur (Kaul & McMahon, 1993). Rare associations with WD include reports of anorexia nervosa (Gwirtsman et al., 1993), hypersomnia (Firneisz et al., 2001) and catatonia (Davis & Borde, 1993).

The range of psychiatric disturbance in WD includes schizophreniform or paranoid features. Sometimes hallucinations or delusional thinking can be prominent (Dening, 1985; Scheinberg et al., 1968). Non-psychotic manifestations include medication-unresponsive depression, mood swings, unexplained lethargy, nightmares, disinhibited behavior (such as inappropriate laughter), or loss of insight (Scheinberg & Sternlieb, 1984; Brewer & Yuzbasiyan-Gurkan, 1992; Hawkes et al., 2001). Disordered sleep is another consequence of neurological WD, as shown by findings of increased nocturnal awakening frequency (Portala et al., 2002).

Epilepsy in WD

As recognized by Kinnier Wilson (1912), epilepsy is an uncommon occurrence in WD whether or not there is other evidence of neurological involvement. Seizures occur at an incidence approximately tenfold greater than in the general population (6.2% in the WD patient group in one large series) (Dening *et al.*, 1988). They can be focal or major motor in classification, and can occur either early or late in the course of this disorder, especially in the younger patient (Smith & Mattson, 1967; Chu, 1989). In some instances, the first occurrence of convulsions coincided with the start of decoppering treatment.

Copper deposition in the eye in WD

Copper deposition in the periphery of the cornea is characteristic of WD when it involves the CNS (Heckmann *et al.*, 2000; Patel & Bozdech, 2001). Although not recognized by Wilson in his 1912 monograph, these opaque bands of corneal pigmentation were known prior to the recognition of hepatolenticular degeneration. Reports by both Kayser (1902) and by Fleischer (1903, 1912) led to the eponym applied to these distinctive cornea signs of copper deposition. With further study of neurological WD cases, clinicians came to realize that Kayser–Fleischer (KF) rings in the cornea are nearly always present. KF rings can be the initial clinical feature of WD (Liu *et al.*, 2002) and only rarely are absent in otherwise typical cases (Ross *et al.*, 1985; Heckmann & Saffer, 1988; Walshe & Yealland, 1992). In one reported instance, KF rings developed the first time penicillamine was started in a patient with otherwise highly typical neurological WD (Willeit & Kiechl, 1991). KF rings can be confused with other peripheral corneal opacifications, such as arcus senilis. Other disorders, such as cirrhosis and other forms of biliary obstruction, can produce corneal deposits of similar appearance to KF rings (Frommer *et al.*, 1977; Fleming *et al.*, 1977).

KF rings are caused by minute copper-containing granules deposited primarily in Descemet's membrane of the cornea. Due to their copper content, KF rings have a brownish or greenish tint and are readily seen without magnification or special illumination. Most KF rings are uniformly concentric around the cornea. Sometimes there is increased prominence of a KF ring at the upper pole of the cornea, which requires lifting of the eyelid for easy recognition. In exceptional circumstances KF rings can be unilateral (Madden *et al.*, 1985; Innes *et al.*, 1979). The definitive means for detecting (or excluding) KF rings, however, is a careful ophthalmologic slit lamp examination by an ophthalmologist. The slit lamp examination also permits recognition of another characteristic finding in WD, a lens opacification with the appearance of a sunflower (Goyal & Tripathi, 2000). "Sunflower" cataracts, also caused by copper deposition, are a less common finding in WD than the KF ring but have the same significance (Wiebers *et al.*, 1977; Deguti *et al.*, 2002). For both the KF ring and the "sunflower"

cataract, Scheimpflug photography can be used to document the clinical course of corneal and lens opacification (Obara *et al.*, 1995).

In most instances, the KF ring and the "sunflower" cataract arise simultaneously when neurological manifestations of WD begin (Wiebers *et al.*, 1977). Sequential analysis of KF rings has shown that they tend to diminish with continued decoppering therapy (Sussman & Sternlieb, 1969; Esmaeli *et al.*, 1996) or after liver transplantation (Song *et al.*, 1992). With chronic therapy, KF rings can disappear. However, the usual situation is the chronic persistence of KF rings at a reduced level of intensity.

Visual and eye movement disorders in WD

Unique presentations of neurological WD include progressive visual loss (Gow *et al.*, 2001) and oculogyric crises (Lee *et al.*, 1999). Patients with neurological WD may be impaired in their reading abilities early on in the disorder (Hyman & Phuapradit, 1979). The original observations by Wilson (1912) of gaze distractability and difficulty in visual fixation have been confirmed by others (Lennox & Jones, 1989). Among the reported abnormalities of eye movements are defects of supranuclear accommodation (Klinqele *et al.*, 1980), impaired smooth pursuit, nystagmus, episodic diplopia, slowed saccadic pursuit (Kirkham & Kamin, 1974), impaired convergence (Sternlieb *et al.*, 1985; Walshe & Yealland, 1992) and apraxia of eyelid-opening (Keane, 1988).

Abnormalities of clinical neurophysiology in WD

Though peripheral nerve function is spared in WD, the damage in this disorder to central conduction pathways and neuronal circuitry is associated with neurophysiological changes representing the extent of pathology. WD does not have pathognomonic findings on electroencephalography (EEG) or evoked responses (EPs), though testing can be useful in demonstrating evidence of nervous system involvement or improvement (Chu, 1986). The EEG in WD is non-specifically abnormal, with generalized slowing and sometimes focal abnormalities (Giagheddu *et al.*, 2001). Spectral analysis and topographic mapping can enhance the recognition of slowing or epileptiform activity found in most patients with WD (Chu *et al.*, 1991). Similarly, most WD patients with neurological involvement have evidence for one or more types of prolonged EPs. EPs can serve as a tool for detecting sub-clinical WD affecting the CNS, as emphasized by a study showing abnormal EPs in almost half of those lacking other evidence of neurological impairment (Grimm et al., 1990). Brainstem auditory and somatosensory EPs may also show changes in response to therapy for WD (Grimm et al., 1992). Abnormalities of pattern-reversal visual evoked responses and flash electroretinograms can undergo improvement with treatment of WD (Satishchandra & Ravishankar, 2000).

Several patterns for delayed conduction of sensory EPs have been demonstrated (Giagheddu et al., 2001) and the general consensus is that EPs can be highly sensitive to brain or spinal cord involvement by WD. However, the several publications on this topic disagree as to the varieties of abnormality in WD. For example, several studies have reported that abnormal visual EPs are common in WD, especially with respect to the P100 waveforms (Aiello et al., 1992; Butinar et al., 1990; Satishchandra & Swamy, 1989). In a comparison of all three types of EP, brainstem auditory and somatosensory pathways were more likely to be delayed than visual EPs (Grimm et al., 1991). Other investigators testing brainstem auditory EPs have shown no abnormality (Butinar et al., 1990). In one report, prolongation of auditory EPs was unrelated to the duration or severity of the disease (Satishchandra & Swamy, 1989). Another series of patients with WD found prolongation of one or more types of EP when severe or moderately severe features of the neurological disorder were present (Grimm et al., 1991). When only mild features of neurological WD were evident, there was an abnormal EP in more than half, and 17% of cases without evidence for neurological features of WD also had one or more EP abnormalities.

In addition to evoked responses, the technique of magnetic stimulation of the motor cortex has been useful for studying damage to central conduction pathways in WD (Perretti et al., 2001). Cortically evoked motor responses can be diminished or absent in subjects with various patterns of neurological WD (Chu, 1990; Meyer et al., 1991a; Berardelli et al., 1990). In one reported case of neurological WD, the abnormal electromyographic response evoked by transcranial magnetic brain stimulation was the only electrophysiological disturbance, and this abnormality reverted to normal with effective decoppering therapy (Meyer et al., 1991b).

Neuropathological changes in WD

Kinnier Wilson's 214-page monograph on the brain's changes in hepatolenticular degeneration provided a wealth of detailed description. The most common target of pathological change is the lenticular nuclei. The cut brain in WD generally shows cavitary or cystic degeneration, sometimes with massive necrosis in this region (Schulman, 1968; Shiraki, 1968; Dastur & Manghani, 1977). The severity of change in the lenticular nuclei can vary greatly from case to case, but there is usually symmetrical involvement in each affected brain. Atrophy of the caudate nuclei and lateral putamen are typical. The putamen may be tinted brown, red, or yellow from the copper content. In the pallidum, discoloration may be present, but usually this region is spared gross degenerative change.

In about 10% of WD cases, atrophic or degenerative changes extend beyond the lenticular nuclei (Schulman, 1968). There can be cystic or cavitary necrosis in structures such as claustrum, extreme capsule, thalamus, subthalamic nucleus, and red nucleus (Dastur & Manghani, 1977; Owen, 1981; Duchen & Jacobs, 1984). Additionally, the brain in WD can show dilation of the lateral ventricles and generalized atrophy. Atypical patterns of brain involvement in WD include degenerative changes primarily in cerebral cortical gray and white matter (Schulman & Barbeau, 1963; Richter, 1948; Ishino et al., 1972; Miyakawa & Murayama, 1976). In such instances, the greatest extent tends to be most prominent in the superior and middle frontal gyri, or in the temporal and parietal cortex.

The "pseudosclerotic" clinical phenotype of WD appears to have a correlate in some unusual cases (Hedera et al., 2002). Several reports have documented an extensive loss of deep white matter so extensive as to suggest the picture of demyelinating disease (Ishino et al., 1972; Miyakawa & Murayama, 1976; Schulman & Barbeau, 1963). In another variant of WD's cerebral pathology, atrophy in the brainstem and cerebellar folia have been described (Miskolczy, 1932). With cerebellar involvement, atrophy has a predilection for superior vermis and the dentate nucleus (Bielschowsky & Hallervorden, 1931). The appearance of central pontine myelinolysis has been described in otherwise typical cases of WD (Popoff et al., 1965; Seitelberger, 1973; Horoupian et al., 1988; Shiraki, 1968), including one instance in which this picture developed after liver transplantation (Lui et al., 2000).

Microscopic pathological change in WD tends to be more widespread than would be suspected from inspection of the cut brain. Sometimes the deeper layers of cerebral cortex and adjacent white matter are the most affected regions. In the lenticular nuclei and elsewhere, prominent changes include capillary endothelial swelling and proliferation of glia (especially those of the Alzheimer Type II type) (Schulman, 1968; Scheinberg & Sternlieb, 1984). Gliosis is most abundant in the putamen and can also affect globus pallidus and caudate nuclei. Eventually, WD evolves to extensive damage to myelinated fibers in association with Alzheimer Type II gliosis diffusely throughout cerebral white matter. Among the patterns of pathological involvement in white matter are spongiform changes (Schulman, 1968).

The Alzheimer Type II glia is a distinctive change in WD, though it is not entirely specific to this disorder. However, when Type II glia arise in the context of other forms of chronic liver disease with encephalopathy, they may not be as prominently localized to the lenticular nuclei as in typical WD. Together with Alzheimer Type II glia in most cases of WD is the Opalski cell. These are large, rounded cells with irregularly shaped nuclei and PAS-positive staining for cytoplasmic granules. Opalski cells are most commonly situated in cerebral cortex cells and in the boundaries of lenticular nuclei cavitary. The finding of Opalski cells with Alzheimer Type II glia is almost pathognomonic for WD. Alzheimer Type I glia can also be found. Their presence was highly correlated to the extent of reactive astrogliosis, and inversely proportional to the severity of Alzheimer Type II changes in one study (Ma et al., 1988). Opalski cells and both Alzheimer Type I and Type II glia may be involved in a copper detoxification process, since they express the copper binding protein metallothionein (Bertrand et al., 2001).

The degenerative changes in neurons and glia can be prominent throughout the brain. In the cerebellum, pathological change is most prominent to the white matter surrounding the dentate nuclei and to Purkinje cells (Scheinberg & Sternlieb, 1984). Electron microscopy has been used to study cerebral cortex in two cases of WD (Foncin, 1970; Anzil et al., 1974). The findings included typical degenerative changes of neurons, myelin, glia, and axons; there were also Hirano bodies and protoplasmic astrocytes (probably Alzheimer Type II). Degenerative changes in cortical neurons included prominent spheroid bodies. Similar changes have appeared in the lower brainstem sensory nuclei in WD (Jellinger, 1973).

The impact of copper chelation therapy was assessed in a series of eleven WD brains taken from subjects chronically treated with penicillamine (Horoupian et al., 1988). For five of the patients, all neurological features of WD had resolved, while the remaining six patients were markedly improved. Despite continued copper chelation therapy, measurement of brain copper content showed values greatly increased over controls in 8 of the 9 brains studied in this manner. The neuropathological changes of WD were prominent in each of the penicillamine-treated cases in spite of their good neurological outcomes from decoppering therapy. These results are important clues that removing copper systemically does not fully remove abnormally high brain content of copper, nor does it avert either the gross or microscopic pathology associated with CNS WD. In this study, there was only a weak correlation between the severity of neuropathological change and regional cerebral copper content.

One confounding factor in the analysis of changes produced by WD is the effect of concomitant liver failure. In distinction to neuropathological changes found in WD, hepatic encephalopathy usually is characterized by a pseudoulegyric pattern of distribution in neuronal loss. Hepatic encephalopathy also tends to lack the necrotic changes in the putamen or frontal gyri as found in neurological WD (Shiraki, 1968).

Making the diagnosis of WD

As important as any diagnostic test for WD is the need for a high index of suspicion for the disorder, given its protean manifestations. Even with the obvious concerns that would accompany the development of CNS involvement, WD can be a late diagnosis for many affected individuals. In a review from the United Kingdom (Walshe & Yealland, 1992), symptoms referable to WD were present for 9 to 40 years (mean, 16 years). At presentation to a physician, only one-third were correctly diagnosed, and the delay in correct diagnosis for the others averaged more than 1 year. Making the best use of diagnostic options requires an understanding of their benefits and limitations. It also is important to remember that WD can arise in the context of other illness or movement disorders (Quinn et al., 1986).

Patients from 4 to 60 years old (but with the highest incidence in the second and third decades of life in Western countries) can present in roughly equal proportions with the hepatic, neurological, and psychiatric forms of WD (Brewer & Yuzbasiyan-Gurkan, 1992; Danks, 1989; Scheinberg & Sternlieb, 1984; Brewer, 2000, 2001, 2003). When WD presents as a hepatic disorder, the clinical picture closely resembles that in other primary forms of liver disease. In such instances, chronic active hepatitis may be the first diagnosis, or if the patient regularly consumes alcoholic beverages, the cirrhosis found may be incorrectly attributed to this behavior rather than to WD. Sometimes, a hepatic presentation of WD can be quite nonspecific, consisting of little more than mild hepatic failure, reduced serum albumin, ascites, and jaundice. In other instances, patients can become acutely and desperately ill with fulminant liver failure. In each of these clinical scenarios, it is incumbent on physicians to consider the possibility of WD to facilitate treatment. Once the diagnosis has been considered, one or more of the following investigations can be used to confirm or exclude the possibility of WD.

The most often used laboratory test for screening for WD is serum CP. Although one of the characteristic features of WD is a reduction in concentration of CP, it is a relatively insensitive and non-specific test, and other tests are better. Approximately 85% of patients with neurological presentations of WD have low CP levels (Brewer & Yuzbasiyan-Gurkan, 1992). However, CP levels cannot be used to confirm or exclude WD. In approximately 80% of all patients with WD, serum CP will be very low, but for 20%, concentrations can be low or midnormal (Brewer & Yuzbasiyan-Gurkan, 1992; Scheinberg & Sternlieb, 1984; Brewer, 2000, 2001, 2003). The use of CP for diagnostic purposes can be especially problematic if the patient also has an inflammatory disorder (i.e. hepatitis) or is receiving oral contraceptives. CP is an acute phase reactant, and even patients with WD can respond to stimuli increasing its production, thereby masking the low concentration they maintain at baseline. Approximately 20% of heterozygotes carrying the gene for WD manifest an intermediate or low CP level despite their freedom from copper pathology in all of their organ systems.

The measurement of urinary copper excretion over 24 hours (especially when conducted on two occasions) is an excellent way to assess whether WD is present (Brewer & Yuzbasiyan-Gurkan, 1992; Brewer, 2000, 2001, 2003). Although there are few biological reasons for false-negative or -positive results to occur, there can be several technical drawbacks to studies of urinary copper excretion. One is a practical matter involving the potential unreliability of collecting urine over 24 hours, or the copper contamination of the specimen from collection materials or other sources. Many laboratories encounter difficulties in conducting an accurate assessment of low copper concentrations in urine. Nevertheless, if conducted reliably, determinations of urinary copper output provide important information regarding the diagnosis of WD. The measurement of serum copper concentration is not a substitute for this test because blood concentrations are highly correlated to serum CP concentrations. Patients who are symptomatic with some form of WD almost always have 24-hour urine copper outputs of more than 100 μg (normal range, 20 to 50 μg). In addition to WD, there are only two known physiological mechanisms for increased urinary copper excretion. One is obstructive liver disease. When liver failure impairs the ability of copper to be excreted into the bile, hepatic copper content tends to increase, and the urinary excretion of copper is enhanced. Thus, when a patient has obstructive liver disease, the reliability of urinary copper excretion declines. Second, during an episode of hepatitis, enough copper may be released by hepatocytes, even in the absence of WD, to elevate urine copper.

Another ambiguity for diagnosing WD can arise in the evaluation of an affected patient's siblings. Each has a 25% chance of carrying two abnormal WD genes, and there is an additional 50% risk of being a heterozygous carrier. Despite their lack of other WD manifestations, heterozygous carriers can have mildly elevated urinary copper excretion with a decrease in serum CP concentration. Rates of copper excretion of 50 to 85 μg/24 h are not uncommon among WD heterozygotes (Yuzbasiyan-Gurkan *et al.*, 1991). A similar range in copper excretion rates can be encountered in WD homozygotes that are presymptomatic for clinical manifestations. In the experience of one of the authors (G. J. Brewer), the lowest rate in a presymptomatic patient has been 65 μg/24 h. The substantial overlap in 24-hour rates of urinary copper excretion among presymptomatic patients and heterozygous carriers of the gene limits the usefulness of urine copper excretion in differentiating these possibilities.

The "gold standard" for diagnosis continues to be biopsied liver tissue with quantitative assay of copper content. An accurate diagnosis requires certain skills in carrying out the analysis. Histochemical staining for copper is unreliable for diagnostic purposes. The presence of positive findings from copper stains is dependent on the sequestration of copper at high concentrations within hepatic cells. When the distribution of copper is diffuse throughout the cytoplasm, the results of staining for copper can be negative despite a very high tissue copper concentration. In general, the concentration of hepatic copper provides an unequivocal answer as to the possibility of WD (Brewer & Yuzbasiyan-Gurkan, 1992; Brewer, 2000, 2001, 2003). Concentrations of copper in WD exceed 200 μg/g tissue (dry weight); the normal range is 15–50 μg/g tissue. Heterozygote carriers can have a mild elevation of hepatic copper, but usually not more than 100 μg/g tissue. A possible ambiguity can arise in patients with obstructive liver disease because tissue concentrations of hepatic copper can increase to the range encountered in WD.

Radioisotope copper tracer tests have not been particularly reliable for the diagnosis of WD, although they can provide clues to copper handling in WD as compared to controls (Walshe & Potter, 1977; Brewer & Yuzbasiyan-Gurkan, 1992). Although these tests can reveal clear differences between normal and homozygous WD patients in the way that copper is handled, there can be substantial overlap between homozygotes and heterozygotes for the WD gene (Houwen *et al.*, 1989; Brewer & Yuzbasiyan-Gurkan, 1992).

The so-called "penicillamine provocative test" is also not a useful procedure for diagnosing WD. In this test, a dose of penicillamine is given and the urinary copper response is measured. The test has never been evaluated in terms of differentiating heterozygous carriers from homozygous affected, and there is likely strong overlap. The straight-forward basal 24-hour excretion of copper provides more reliable data.

The gene for WD, ATP7B, has been cloned (Bull *et al.*, 1993; Tanzi *et al.*, 1993; Yamaguchi *et al.*, 1993). There are already over 200 known mutations in ATP7B that disable the gene and cause WD (Cox & Roberts). In general, no single mutation, or small group of mutations, predominate as a cause of WD in any population. Hence, mutation screening as a diagnostic tool is not practical at this moment. Once a patient is diagnosed by conventional means, full siblings can be evaluated by haplotype analysis, which involves typing polymorphic markers that are close to the WD locus (Thomas *et al.*, 1995). If markers on both chromosomes match between the affected patient and a sibling, that sibling is affected with WD. If there is a single match, the sibling is a carrier, and if without matches, the sibling is homozygous normal.

There are several cases in the literature describing abnormal copper metabolism coinciding with movement disorders and other types of neurological and systemic abnormalities (Willvonseder *et al.*, 1973; Pall *et al.*, 1987). Whether these are "forme frustes" of WD or represent other types of copper pathophysiology remains to be determined.

Neuroimaging of WD: CT, MRI, PET, and SPECT

In most patients with neurological impairments with WD, one or more abnormalities can be detected by magnetic resonance imaging (MRI) (Aisen *et al.*, 1985; Prayer *et al.*, 1990; Thuomas *et al.*, 1993; Roh *et al.*, 1994; Brugieres *et al.*, 1992; Giagheddu *et al.*, 2001). Computerized tomography using X-ray also shows abnormalities (Nelson *et al.*, 1979; Harik & Post, 1981; Kendall *et al.*, 1981; Williams & Walshe, 1981; Dettori *et al.*, 1984; Chu, 1989), but is probably not as sensitive (Metzer & Angtuaco, 1986). The most common sites for abnormal MRI findings are the basal ganglia structures and the midbrain region (Starosta-Rubinstein *et al.*, 1987; Magalhaes *et al.*, 1994; Hitoshi *et al.*, 1991; Imiya *et al.*, 1992). Especially useful for detecting abnormalities are diffusion MRI (Sener, 1993) and T_2-weighted images, in which patches of increased signal intensity are characteristically found with a central core of decreased signal intensity. Other typical findings of WD are features described as the "face of the panda" sign in the midbrain (Hitoshi *et al.*, 1991) and the "bright claustrum" sign (Sener, 1993). The various abnormalities on MRI sometimes improve or recover completely following decoppering therapy (Alanen *et al.*, 1999;

Stefano Zagami & Boers, 2001). Other neuroimaging techniques useful for demonstrating the regional abnormalities of WD include positron emission tomography with fluorodopa (Snow *et al.*, 1991) and deoxyglucose (Kuwert *et al.*, 1992), and single photon emission computed tomography (SPECT) (Tatsch *et al.*, 1991; Schwarz *et al.*, 1992; Giagheddu *et al.*, 2001; Barthel *et al.*, 2001). SPECT findings in neurological WD have typically shown decreased striatal binding of the tracer, implying diminished dopaminergic projections (Barthel *et al.*, 2001). However, there can be considerable hetereogeneity in neurological WD, and despite the presence of akinesia, rigidity, and substantia nigra lesions on MRI, some patients have had normal striatal findings with SPECT using ligands for the dopamine transporter (Huang *et al.*, 2003).

Genetics and pathophysiology of WD

WD is inherited as an autosomal recessive disorder (Bearn, 1960), which means that carriers of the gene never develop the disease. Most evidence supports a conclusion that the gene is fully penetrant, so all homozygotes ultimately should develop the disease sometime during their lifetime. For this reason, each sibling of a newly diagnosed patient has a 25% risk for WD. Because there are several highly effective therapeutic options for WD, it is essential to screen siblings of affected probands to determine whether they also are affected with the disease.

The frequency of WD has been estimated to be approximately 1 per 40 000 births (Scheinberg & Sternlieb, 1984; Brewer, 2001). An attempt to refine this number for the United States led to an estimate of 1 per 55 000 births but with a wide confidence interval (Olivarez *et al.*, 2001). If we use 1 in 40 000 in the United States, this frequency means that the number of homozygotes is 5000 to 6000. Assuming this incidence figure, the carrier frequency can be calculated as approximately 1% of the population. From this estimation, the a priori risks for relatives of an affected patient can be calculated as 1 in 200 for offspring, 1 in 600 for nieces and nephews, and 1 in 800 for first cousins. The actual risk of any individual in such families developing WD is age dependent. Once an individual has passed through the age range of maximal presentation, the odds of remaining free of the disorder increase.

The gene for WD (ATP7B), a copper binding, membrane bound, ATPase shows considerable homology to the gene for Menkes disease, called ATP7A (Vulpe *et al.*, 1993; Chelly *et al.*, 1993; Mercer *et al.*, 1993). The genes show quite dissimilar expression patterns: ATP7B is primarily expressed in the liver, while ATP7A shows a

generally ubiquitous expression pattern (although with little expression in the liver). Because of the large number
of mutations, most patients with WD in most populations are compound heterozygotes. This situation ham-
pers attempts at genotype-phenotype correlation. There
has been an impression among researchers that complete
gene knockouts tend to lead to an expression of liver disease earlier in life, while missense mutations (which might
provide some low level of ATP7B protein expression) tend
to generate a neurological presentation later in life.

Although clinical manifestations can be widespread
throughout the body, the primary defect of copper
metabolism clearly is a function of the liver. The normal
mechanism for controlling copper balance involves the
excretion of excessive copper into the bile (Ravestyn, 1944;
Cartwright & Wintrobe, 1964). The failure of this mechanism leads to WD (Bush *et al.*, 1955; Frommer, 1974; O'Reilly
et al., 1971; Gibbs & Walshe, 1980). For this reason, hepatic
transplantation can cure the underlying copper disorder.
ATP7B functions in the hepatic transport of copper into
the bile in an as yet undefined manner. When both copies
of the gene are disabled, as in WD, excess copper is not
excreted, and accumulates in the liver. At some point, the
excessive copper cannot be adequately stored and begins
to cause liver damage. In some patients, this process probably begins as early as 3 years of age. Later on, excessive
circulating copper leads to accumulation in other organs,
especially in the brain where centers involved in motor control are particularly susceptible to copper accumulation.

A primary role for the copper-containing serum protein CP in the pathogenesis of WD originally was proposed
after the discovery that most patients manifest a low serum
concentration (Bearn & Kunkel, 1952; Scheinberg & Gitlin,
1952). Although CP can serve as a marker for the disease,
the structural gene for CP is found on chromosome 3, while
ATP7B is on chromosome 13. It appears that one of the functions of ATP7B in the liver is to facilitate the acquisition of
copper by CP. When both copies of ATP7B are disabled, as
in WD, the acquisition of copper by hepatic apoCP is sub-
normal. Thus, defects in ATP7B produce both inadequate
hepatic biliary excretion of copper, and inadequate hepatic
secretion of mature, copper containing, CP into the blood,
generally leading to a low blood CP level.

The toxicity of copper

All studies indicate that copper is the agent that produces
tissue damage in WD. This conclusion is established by
the complete correlation between disease manifestations
and the presence of excessive amounts of copper in tissue.

Furthermore, the remarkable recovery of patients with WD
after copper-removing therapy provides additional proof.
It is most likely that copper toxicity is pro-oxidant in nature.
The best support for this concept comes from studies
of red blood cells that show excess copper producing an
increase in oxidant radicals (Hochstein *et al.*, 1980; Metz &
Sagone, 1972; Rifkind, 1974). Copper-damaged red blood
cells exhibit Heinz bodies, which are markers in red blood
cells of oxidative damage to cell membranes (Deiss *et al.*,
1970; Ishmael *et al.*, 1972; Metz, 1969). These cells also show
an accelerated loss of reduced glutathione, a molecule that
is important for protecting against damage from oxidant
stress (Deiss *et al.*, 1970; Mital *et al.*, 1966). In some tissues, the outcome of oxidant damage involves lipid peroxidation (especially membrane peroxidation), whereas in
other cells, oxidative damage to other components may
be more important (Hochstein *et al.*, 1980; Sokol *et al.*,
1989).

The occurrence of liver damage in WD can be explained
by the extremely high concentrations of copper accumulating in this organ. The liver is capable of storing relatively
large amounts, primarily by synthesizing metallothionein,
which complexes copper for storage. However, copper is
not the best stimulus for inducing production of metallothionein. At some level of copper load, hepatic concentrations of this metal may exceed the amount that can
be complexed effectively with metallothionein. When this
occurs, hepatic cellular damage begins to develop. Ultimately, the progressive damage to the liver results in a lowering of its storage capacity, and the accumulating excess
copper reaches the point at which escape into the blood can
increase, thereby permitting its deposition in other organs
such as the brain.

Why the CNS is such a prominent target for WD involvement is not known. The concentrations of copper that accumulate in the brain are not much greater than those in other
organs, nor do the specific regions of the brain tending to
be affected (e.g. the basal ganglia) accumulate more copper
than other sites (Scheinberg & Sternlieb, 1984; Owen, 1981).
The most tenable explanation for the heightened occurrence of copper toxicity is that some sites of the brain have
a decreased resistance to the ability of copper to produce
oxidant damage. One possibility is that the specific regions
most likely to be involved are less capable of inducing
metallothionein as a protectant mechanism. Alternatively,
it is possible that enzymatic mechanisms for antioxidant
protection are diminished regionally. Although the neurotoxicity of copper is not duplicated by excess administration of other metals such as manganese (Pentschew *et al.*,
1963), there are some similarities based on pro-oxidant
effects.

Table 61.2. Recommendations for medical therapy of Wilson's disease

Clinical situation	Therapy choices	Comments
Initial treatment		
Hepatic presentation	First: trien and zinc	Best drug or combination not well established
	Second: penicillamine and zinc	
Neurological presentation	First: tetrathiomolybdate	Not generally available yet
	Second: zinc	Slow in action
	Third: trien	May precipitate neurological worsening
Maintenance treatment	First: zinc	Excellent efficacy, no toxicity
	Second: trien	Efficacious but long-term toxicities unknown
	Third: penicillamine	Efficacious but a very toxic drug
Presymptomatic treatment	Same as for maintenance treatment	Same as for maintenance treatment
Pregnancy treatment	First: zinc	Non-teratogenic in animals
	Second: trien	Teratogenic in animals

Treatment of WD

Classifications of the current treatments of WD are given in Table 61.2. The following sections provide greater details.

Initial treatment

The initial treatment of WD must be considered apart from the later strategies because there are objective differences and different therapeutic alternatives. For a patient presenting with liver disease (other than acute fulminant failure), the use of both a chelating agent and zinc can be recommended. At present, the best choice for chelation is trien because this compound is less toxic than penicillamine and appears to be just as effective. The objective for the use of a chelating agent is to mobilize copper rapidly to achieve a large negative copper balance. Administration of zinc provides a major stimulus for the synthesis of hepatic metallothionein, which sequesters copper in the hepatocyte and renders it nontoxic. This combination therapy has proved to be quite successful for the treatment of hepatic disease (Askari *et al.*, 2003). The only difficulty we have encountered has been the induction of proteinuria in a few

patients; when trien is stopped, this problem resolves. We recommend the use of this combination for 4 to 6 months followed by discontinuation of the trien. Zinc maintenance therapy provides long-term protection against recurrence of symptomatic WD.

For the patient presenting with acute fulminant hepatic failure, there is a high risk for a fatal outcome. The only effective means of avoiding progression to death in such circumstances has been through hepatic transplantation (Schilsky *et al.*, 1994). This procedure has become used on a widespread basis. An index has been developed by Nazer and colleagues (1986) to help in the differentiation of patients requiring hepatic transplantation from those who can be salvaged by medical therapy. This prognostic algorithm, which is computed from the prothrombin time and the serum concentrations of bilirubin and serum glutamic-pyruvic transaminase, has proved to be quite useful in decision-making regarding hepatic transplantation (Brewer, 2001). One issue in the use of this prognostic index formula is that bilirubin can be elevated from red blood cell destruction as well as from liver disease. Because hemolysis can be a feature of WD, the bilirubin concentration becomes a less reliable factor in the decision-making process because the elevation is derived from a cause more benign than liver disease.

For patients presenting with acute neurological illness, the situation can be quite precarious. Conventional treatments for chronic management of WD can result in significant and irreversible worsening due to mobilization of hepatic copper that can then enter the brain. The administration of chelators such as penicillamine (and probably trien as well) may cause substantial neurological deterioration. In almost 50 percent of patients, some worsening of neurological signs occurs when such therapy is instituted, and for almost 25 percent of patients, the loss of neurological function will be permanent (Brewer *et al.*, 1987b). We cannot highly recommend the use of zinc in this situation because its effect at achieving a negative copper balance is slow and progression of neurological deficits can occur during its initial use.

Because of the limitations of current therapy with respect to neurological WD, a new type of drug is under development at the University of Michigan. This drug, ammonium tetrathiomolybdate (TM), acts by promoting the complexing of copper to protein, an effect that has two advantages (Bremner *et al.*, 1982; Gooneratne *et al.*, 1981; Mills *et al.*, 1981a,b). When administered with meals, TM blocks absorption of both dietary and endogenously secreted copper, thereby achieving an immediate negative copper balance. When taken between meals, TM is absorbed and reacts with the blood-borne copper to complex with albumin (Brewer *et al.*, 1991a). This protein-linked copper becomes unavailable for cellular uptake and therefore is not toxic. With TM, it has been possible to decrease progressively the concentration of free copper in the bloodstream (Brewer *et al.*, 1991a). By this means, TM can prevent shifts of copper into the CNS that are the result of chelator therapy. Strategies for the optimal use of TM (Brewer *et al.*, 1991a, 2003) have evolved into a regimen in which the drug is administered four times per day, three doses with meals and one dose at bedtime away from food. This regimen is carried out for 8 weeks, after which a switch to zinc is undertaken as a maintenance therapy. Fifty-five patients have been treated in this manner, and they have recovered with only two instances of neurological deterioration (Brewer *et al.*, 2003), compared to the estimated 50% frequency of worsening with penicillamine (Brewer *et al.*, 1987b).

Maintenance therapy

Experience at the University of Michigan and in the Netherlands suggests that chronic maintenance therapy with zinc can be recommended. The United States Food and Drug Administration has given approval for this indication. Extensive research with zinc has shown it to be fully effective, and it has virtually no toxicity (Brewer *et al.*, 1983, 1987a, 1987c, 1989, 1990, 1991b, 1993a, 1993b, 1994, 1997, 1998, 2001; Hill *et al.*, 1986, 1987; Yuzbasiyan-Gurkan *et al.*, 1989, 1992; Brewer & Yuzbasiyan-Gurkan, 1992; Askari *et al.*, 2003; Hoogenraad *et al.*, 1978, 1979, 1987). Occasionally, patients exhibit mild discomfort related to stomach upset from zinc. This problem usually results from the first morning dose. Therefore, administration of the first dose between breakfast and lunch can lessen the risk of this problem. Studies with zinc have shown that it can bring copper toxicity under control by preventing re-accumulation of hepatic copper in patients previously treated with chelation. With zinc treatment, plasma and urinary copper concentrations are reduced, as can be confirmed by monitoring the results of 24-hour urinary excretion of copper and zinc. Patients receiving adequate therapy with zinc usually excrete at least 2 mg zinc every 24 hours (Brewer *et al.*, 1990, 1998). Incomplete compliance in drug intake will be shown by reduced quantities of zinc excretion. Urinary copper output also can be useful in guiding therapy because in the absence of chelators, urinary output of copper is proportional to the body load of copper. Thus, with adequate zinc therapy, output should be less than 125 μg every 24 hours when measured during maintenance therapy (Brewer *et al.*, 1998). When the urinary output of copper is more than 125 μg every 24 hours

(after a period of adequate control), the most likely conclusion is inadequate compliance in the regular use of zinc.

Treatment of the presymptomatic patient

Because the ideal time for treatment for the disorder is in the presymptomatic phase (during which most of the body's load of copper will be deposited), it is of vital importance to pursue the diagnostic workup to a definitive level, which may include liver biopsy, in each at-risk individual such as a WD patient's sibling. Institution of prophylactic treatment against WD appears to be served adequately by the same strategy for maintenance therapy with zinc. Thirty patients have been treated at the University of Michigan with zinc therapy alone, and results have been excellent (Brewer *et al.*, 1998, and unpublished results).

Treatment of the pregnant patient

During pregnancy, WD can present special management challenges. Both penicillamine and trien are teratogenic in animals (Keen *et al.*, 1982), although zinc is not (Food and Drug Administration, 1973). For this reason, zinc appears to be the drug of choice during pregnancy, and trien can be a second choice. At the University of Michigan, 19 women have been treated through 25 pregnancies using zinc with no significant problems for the mothers and only two fetal abnormalities noted (Brewer *et al.*, 2000). The medical literature on WD indicates that features of this disorder can progress or recur during pregnancy when medication is discontinued; hence, it is important for effective decoppering treatments to be continued.

REFERENCES

Ahmed, A. & Feller, E. R. (1996). Rupture of the spleen as the initial manifestation of Wilson's disease. *Am. J. Gastroenterol.*, **91**, 1454–5.

Aiello, I., Sau, G. F., Cacciotto, R. *et al.* (1992). Evoked potentials in patients with non-neurological Wilson's disease. *J. Neurol.*, **239**, 65–8.

Aisen, A. M., Martell, W., Gabrielsen, T. O. *et al.* (1985). Wilson's disease of the brain: MR imaging. *Radiology*, **157**, 137–41.

Akil, M. & Brewer, G. J. (1995). Psychiatric and behavioral abnormalities in Wilson's disease. In *Advances in Neurology*, Vol. 65: *Behavioral Neurology of Movement Disorders*. ed. W. J. Weiner, & A. E. Lang, pp. 171–8. New York: Raven Press.

Akil, M., Schwartz, J. A., Dutchak, D. *et al.* (1991). The psychiatric presentations of Wilson's disease. *J. Neuropsychiatry*, **3**, 377–82.

Alanen, A., Komu, M., Penttinen, M. & Leino, R. (1999). Magnetic resonance imaging and proton MR spectroscopy in Wilson's disease. *Br. J. Radiol.*, **72**, 749–56.

Anzil, A. P., Herrlinger, H., Blinzinger, K. & Heldrich, A. (1974). Ultrastructure of brain and nerve biopsy tissue in Wilson disease. *Arch. Neurol.*, **31**, 94–100.

Askari, F. K., Greenson, J., Dick, R. D. *et al.* (2003). Treatment of Wilson's disease with zinc XVIII. Intial treatment of the hepatic decompensation presentation with trientine and zinc. *J. Lab. Clin. Med.* **142**, 385–90.

Balint, G. & Szebenyi, B. (2000). Hereditary disorders mimicking and/or causing premature osteoarthritis. *Bailliere's Best Pract. Res. Clin. Rheumatol.*, **14**, 219–50.

Barthel, H., Sorger, D., Kuhn, H. J., Wagner, A., Kluge, R. & Hermann, W. (2001). Differential alteration of the nigrostriatal dopaminergic system in Wilson's disease investigated with [123I] ß-CIT and high-resolution SPET. *Eur. J. Nucl. Med.*, **28**, 1656–63.

Bearn, A. G. (1960). A genetical analysis of thirty families with Wilson's disease (hepatolenticular degeneration). *Ann. Hum. Genet.*, **24**, 33–43.

Bearn, A. G. & Kunkel H. G. (1952). Biochemical abnormalities in Wilson's disease. *J. Clin. Invest.*, **31**, 616.

Berardelli, A., Inghilleri, M., Priori, A. *et al.* (1990). Involvement of corticospinal tract in Wilson's disease: a study of three cases with transcranial stimulation. *Mov. Disord.*, **5**, 334–7.

Berry, W. R., Darley, F. L., Aronson, A. E. & Goldstein, N. P. (1974). Dysarthria in Wilson's disease. *J. Speech Hearing Res.*, **17**, 169–83.

Bertrand, E., Lewandowska, E., Szpak, G. M. *et al.* (2001). Neuropathological analysis of pathological forms of astroglia in Wilson's disease. *Folia Neuropathol.*, **39**, 73–9.

Bhattacharya, K., Velickovic, M., Schilsky, M. & Kaufmann, H. (2002). Autonomic cardiovascular reflexes in Wilson's disease. *Clin. Auton. Res.*, **12**, 190–2.

Bhave, S. A., Purohit, G. M., Pradhan, A. V. & Pandit, A. N. (1987). Hepatic presentation of Wilson's disease. *Ind. Pediat.*, **24**, 385–93.

Bhave, S., Bavdekar, A. & Pandit, A. (1994). Changing pattern of chronic liver disease (CLD) in India. *Ind. J. Pediat.*, **61**, 675–82.

Bielschowsky, M. & Hallervorden, J. (1931). Symmetrische Einschmelzungsherde in Stirnhirn beim Wilson Pseudosklerose Komplex. *J. Psych. Neurol.*, **42**, 177–89.

Bremner, I., Mills, C. F. & Young, B. W. (1982). Copper metabolism in rats given dior trithiomolybdates. *J. Inorg. Biochem.*, **16**, 109–19.

Brewer, G. J. (2000). Recognition, diagnosis, and management of Wilson's disease. *PSEBM*, **223**(1), 39–49.

(2001). *Wilson's disease: A Clinician's Guide to Recognition, Diagnosis, and Management.* Boston: Kluwer Academic Publishers.

(2003). Wilson's disease. In *Harrison's Principles of Internal Medicine.* ed. D. L. Kasper, E. Braunward, A. S. Fauci, S. L. Hauser, D. L. Longo, & J. L. Jameson. Inc. New York: McGraw-Hill Companies.

Brewer, G. J. & Yuzbasiyan-Gurkan, V. (1992). Wilson disease. *Medicine*, **71**, 139–64.

Brewer, G. J., Hill, G. M., Prasad, A. S. *et al.* (1983). Oral zinc therapy for Wilson's disease. *Ann. Intern. Med.*, **99**, 314–20.

Brewer, G. J., Hill, G. M., Dick, R. D. *et al.* (1987a). Treatment of Wilson's disease with zinc: III. Prevention of reaccumulation of hepatic copper. *J. Lab. Clin. Med.*, **109**, 526–31.

Brewer, G. J., Terry, C. A., Aisen, A. M. & Hill, G. M. (1987b). Worsening of neurologic syndrome in patients with Wilson's disease with initial penicillamine therapy. *Arch. Neurol.*, **44**, 490–3.

Brewer, G. J., Hill, G. M., Prasad, A. S. & Dick, R. D. (1987c). Treatment of Wilson's disease with zinc: IV. Efficacy monitoring using urine and plasma copper. *Proc. Soc. Exp. Biol. Med.*, **7**, 446–55.

Brewer, G. J., Yuzbasiyan-Gurkan, V., Lee, D.-Y., & Appelman, H. (1989). Treatment of Wilson's disease with zinc: VI. Initial treatment studies. *J. Lab. Clin. Med.*, **114**, 663–8.

Brewer, G. J., Yuzbasiyan-Gurkan, V. & Dick, R. (1990). Zinc therapy of Wilson's disease: VIII. Dose response studies. *S. Trace Elem. Exp. Med.*, E, 227–34.

Brewer, G. J., Dick, R. D., Yuzbasiyan-Gurkan, V. *et al.* (1991a). Initial therapy of Wilson's disease patients with tetrathiomolybdate. *Arch. Neurol.*, **48**, 42–7.

Brewer, G. J., Yuzbasiyan-Gurkan, V. & Johnson, V. (1991b). Treatment of Wilson's disease with zinc: IX. Response of serum lipids. *J. Lab. Clin. Med.*, **118**, 466–70.

Brewer, G. J., Yuzbasiyan-Gurkan, V., Johnson, V. *et al.* (1993a). Treatment of Wilson's disease with zinc: XI. Interaction with other anticopper agents. *J. Am. Coll. Nutrit.*, **12**, 26–30.

Brewer, G. J., Yuzbasiyan-Gurkan, V., Johnson, V. *et al.* (1993b). Treatment of Wilson's disease with zinc: XII. Dose regimen requirements. *Am. J. Med. Sci.*, **305**, 199–202.

Brewer, G. J., Dick, R. D., Yuzbasiyan-Gurkan, V. *et al.* (1994). Treatment of Wilson's disease with zinc: XIII. Therapy with zinc in presymptomatic patients from the time of diagnosis. *J. Lab. Clin. Med.*, **123**, 849–58.

Brewer, G. J., Johnson, V. & Kaplan, J. (1997). Treatment of Wilson's disease with zinc: XIV. Studies of the effect of zinc on lymphocyte function. *J. Lab. Clin. Med.*, **129**, 649–652.

Brewer, G. J., Dick, R. D., Johnson, V. *et al.* (1998). Treatment of Wilson's disease with zinc: XV. Long-term follow-up studies. *J. Lab. Clin. Med.*, **132**, 264–78.

Brewer, G. J., Dick, R. D., Johnson, V. *et al.* (2001). Treatment of Wilson's disease with zinc: XVI. Treatment during the pediatric years. *J. Lab. Clin. Med.*, **137**, 191–8.

Brewer, G. J., Johnson, V. D., Dick, R. D. *et al.* (2000). Treatment of Wilson's disease with zinc XVII: treatment during pregnancy. *Hepatology*, **31**, 364–70.

Brewer, G. J., Hedera, P., Kluin, K. J. *et al.* (2003). Treatment of Wilson's disease with tetrathiomolybdate III. Initial therapy in a total of 55 neurologically affected patients and follow-up with zinc therapy. *Arch. Neurol.*, **60**, 378–85.

Brugieres, P., Combes, C., Ricolfi, F. *et al.* (1992). A typical MR presentation of Wilson disease: a possible consequence of paramagnetic effect of copper? *Neuroradiology*, **34**, 222–4.

Bull, P. C., Thomas, G. R., Rommens, J. M. *et al.* (1993). The Wilson's disease gene is a putative copper transporting P-type ATPase similar to the Menkes gene. *Nat. Genet.*, **5**, 327–37.

Bush, J. A., Mahoney, J. P., Markowitz, H. *et al.* (1955). Studies on copper metabolism: XVI. Radioactive copper studies in normal subjects and in patients with hepatolenticular degeneration. *J. Clin. Invest.*, **34**, 1766–78.

Butinar, D., Trontelj, J. V., Khuraibet, A. J. *et al.* (1990). Brainstem auditory evoked potentials in Wilson's disease *J. Neurol. Sci.*, **95**, 163–9.

Cartwright, G. E. & Wintrobe, M. M. (1964). Copper metabolism in normal subjects. *Am. J. Clin. Nutr.*, **14**, 224–32.

Chelly, J., Tumer, Z., Tonnesen, T. *et al.* (1993). Isolation of a candidate gene for Menkes disease that encodes a potential heavy metal binding protein. *Nat. Genet.*, **3**, 14–19.

Chu, N.-S. (1986). Sensory evoked potentials in Wilson's disease. *Brain*, **109**, 491–506.

(1989). Clinical, CT and evoked potential manifestations in Wilson's disease with cerebral white matter involvement. *Clin. Neurol. Neurosurg.*, **91**, 45–51.

(1990). Motor evoked potentials in Wilson's disease: Early and late motor responses. *J. Neurol. Sci.*, **99**, 259–69.

Chu, N.-S., Chu, C. C., Tu, S. C. & Huang, C. C. (1991). EEG spectral analysis and topographic mapping in Wilson's disease. *J. Neurol. Sci.*, **106**, 1–9.

Cumings, J. N. (1948). The copper and iron content of brain and liver in the normal and in hepatolenticular degeneration. *Brain*, **71**, 410–15.

Czlonkowska, A. & Rodo, M. (1981). Late onset Wilson's disease. *Arch. Neurol.*, **38**, 729–30.

Danks, D. M. (1989). Disorders of copper transport. In *Metabolic Basis of Inherited Diseases*, 6th edn, vol. I, ed. C. R. Scriver, A. L. Beaudet, W. S. Sly & D. Valle, pp. 1411–31. New York: McGraw-Hill.

Dastur, D. K., Manghani, D. K. & Wadia, N. H. (1968). Wilson's disease in India I. Geographic, genetic, and clinical aspects in 16 families. *Neurology*, **18**, 21–31.

Dastur, D. K. & Manghani, D. K. (1977). Wilson's disease: inherited cuprogenic disorder of liver, brain, kidney. In *Scientific Foundations of Neurology*, ed. E. Goldensohn & S. H. Appel, chap. 64, pp. 1033–51. Philadelphia: Lea & Febiger.

Davis, E. J. & Borde, M. (1993). Wilson's disease and catatonia. *Br. J. Psychiatry*, **162**, 256–9.

Davis, L. J. & Goldstein, N. P. (1974). Psychologic investigation of Wilson's disease. *Mayo Clin. Proc.*, **49**, 409–99.

Deguti, M. M., Tietge, U. J., Barbosa, E. R. & Cancado, E. L. (2002). The eye in Wilson's disease: sunflower cataract associated with Kayser–Fleischer ring. *J. Hepatol.*, **37**, 700.

Deiss, A., Lee, G. R. & Cartwright, G. E. (1970). Hemolytic anemia in Wilson's disease. *Ann. Intern. Med.*, **73**, 413–18.

Dening, T. R. (1985). Psychiatric aspects of Wilson's disease. *Br. J. Psychiatry*, **147**, 677–82.

Dening, T. R., Berrios, G. E. & Walshe, J. M. (1988). Wilson's disease and epilepsy. *Brain*, **111**, 1139–55.

Denny-Brown, D. (1964). Hepato-lenticular degeneration (Wilson's disease). *N. Engl. J. Med.*, **270**, 1149–56.

Dettori, P., Rochelle, M. B., Demalia, L. *et al.* (1984). Computerized cranial tomography in presymptomatic and hepatic form of Wilson's disease. *Eur. Neurol.*, **23**, 56–63.

Dobyns, W. B., Goldstein, N. P. & Gordon, H. (1979). Clinical spectrum of Wilson's disease (hepatolenticular degeneration). *Mayo Clin. Proc.*, **54**, 35–42.

Duchen, L. W. & Jacobs, J. M. (1984). Nutritional deficiencies and metabolic disorders. In *Greenfield's Neuropathology*, 4th edn., ed. J. H. Adams, J. A. N. Corsellis & L. W. Duchen, pp. 595–9. New York: John Wiley.

Erkan, T., Aktuglu, C., Gulcan, E. M. *et al.* (2002). Wilson disease manifested primarily as amenorrhea and accompanying thrombocytopenia. *J. Adolesc. Hlth.*, **31**, 378–80.

Esmaeli, B., Burnstine, M., Martyonyi, C., Sugar, A., Johnson V., Brewer, G. Regression of Kayser–Fleischer rings during oral zinc therapy: correlation with systemic manifestations of Wilson's disease. *Cornea*, **15**, 582–8.

Feller, E. R. & Schumacher, H. R. (1972). Osteoarticular changes in Wilson's disease. *Arthritis Rheum.*, **15**, 259–66.

Firneisz, G., Szalay, F., Halasz, P. & Komoly, S. (2001). Hypersomnia in Wilson's disease: an unusual symptom in an unusual case. *Acta Neurol. Scand.*, **101**, 286–8.

Fitzgerald, M., Gross, J. B., Goldstein, N. P. *et al.* (1975). Wilson's disease of late adult onset. *Mayo Clin. Proc.*, **50**, 438–42.

Fleischer, B. (1903). Zwei weitere Fälle von grünliche Verfarbung der Kornea. *Klin. Mbl Augenheilk*, **41**, 489–91.

Fleischer, B. (1912). Uber eine der "Pseudosklerose" nahestehende bisher unbekannte Krankheit (gekenn zeichnet durch Tremor, psychische Störungen, braunliche Pigmententierung, bestimmter Gewebe, insobesondere suh der Hornhautperipherie, Lebercirrhose). *Deutsch Z. Nerv.*, **44**, 179–201.

Fleming, C. R., Dickson, E. R., Wahner, H. W. *et al.* (1977). Pigmented corneal rings in non-Wilsonian liver disease. *Ann. Intern. Med.*, **86**, 285–8.

Foncin, J. F. (1970). Pathologic ultrastructurale de la glie chez l'homme. *Proc. 6th Int. Congr. Neuropathol*, Paris, Masson et Cie, pp. 377–90.

Food and Drug Administration: (1974). Teratologic Evaluation of FDA 71–49 (Zinc Sulfate). Food and Drug Research Laboratories, Inc. (prepared for Food and Drug Administration, United States Department of Commerce), publication No. Parkinson's disease-221–805, February 1973, and PB-267.

Frommer, D. J. (1974). Defective biliary excretion of copper in Wilson's disease. *Gut*, **15**, 125–9.

Frommer, D., Morris, J., Sherlock, S. *et al.* (1977). Kayser–Fleischer-like rings in patients without Wilson's disease. *Gastroenterology*, **72**, 1331–5.

Giagheddu, M., Tamburini, G., Piga, M. *et al.* (2001). Comparison of MRI, EEG, EPs and ECD-SPECT in Wilson's disease. *Acta Neurol. Scand.*, **103**, 71–81.

Gibbs, K. & Walshe, J. M. (1980). Biliary excretion of copper in Wilson's disease. *Lancet*, **ii**, 538–9.

Golding, D. N. & Walshe, J. M. (1977). Arthropathy of Wilson's disease: study of clinical and radiological features in 32 patients. *Ann. Rheum. Dis.*, **36**, 99–111.

Goldman, M. & Ali, M. (1991). Wilson's disease presenting as Heinz-body hemolytic anemia. *Can. Med. Assoc. J.*, **145**, 971–2.

Goldstein, N. P., Ewert, J. C., Randall, R. V. & Gross, J. B. (1968). Psychiatric aspects of Wilson's disease (hepatolenticular degeneration): results of psychometric tests during long-term therapy. *Am. J. Psychiatry*, **124**, 1555–61.

Gooneratne, S. R., Howell, J. M. & Gawthorne, J. M. (1981). An investigation of the effects of intravenous administration of thiomolybdate on copper metabolism in chronic Cu-poisoned sheep. *Br. J. Nutr.* **46**, 469–80.

Goswami, R. P., Banerjee, D. & Shah, D. (2001). Cholelithiasis in a child – an unusual presentation of Wilson's disease. *J. Assoc. Phys. India*, **49**, 1118–19.

Gow, P. J., Peacock, S. E. & Chapman, R. W. (2001). Wilson's disease presenting with rapidly progressive visual loss: another neurologic manifestation of Wilson's disease? *J. Gastroenterol. Hepatol.*, **16**, 699–701.

Goyal, V. & Tripathi, M. (2000). Sunflower cataract in Wilson's disease. *J. Neurol. Neurosurg. Psychiatry*, **69**, 133.

Grimm, G., Oder, W., Prayer, L. *et al.* (1990). Evoked potentials in assessment and follow-up of patients with Wilson's disease. *Lancet*, **336**, 963–4.

Grimm, G., Prayer, L., Oder, W. *et al.* (1991). Comparison of functional and structural brain disturbances in Wilson's disease. *Neurology*, **41**, 272–6.

Grimm, G., Madi, C., Katzenschlager, R. *et al.* (1992). Detailed evaluation of evoked potentials in Wilson's disease. *EEG Clin. Neurophysiol.*, **82**, 119–24.

Gwirtsman, H. E., Prager, J. & Henkin, R. (1993). Case report of anorexia nervosa associated with Wilson's disease. *Int. J. Eating Disord.*, **13**, 241–4.

Gulyas, A. E. & Salazar-Grueso, E. F. (1988). Pharyngeal dysmotility in a patient with Wilson's disease. *Dysphagia*, **2**, 230–4.

Harik, S. I. & Post, J. D. (1981). Computerized tomography in Wilson's disease. *Neurology*, **31**, 107–10.

Hawkes, N. D., Mutimer, D. & Thomas, G. A. (2001). Generalised oedema, lethargy, personality disturbance, and recurring nightmares in a young girl. *Postgrad. Med. J.*, **77**, 529, 537–9.

Heckmann, J. & Saffer, D. (1988). Abnormal copper metabolism: another "non-Wilson's" case. *Neurology*, **38**, 1493–1594.

Heckmann, J. G., Lang, C. J., Neundorfer, B. & Kuchle, M. (2000). Neuro/Images. Kayser–Fleischer corneal ring. *Neurology*, **54**, 1839.

Hedera, P., Brewer, G. J. & Fink, J. K. (2002). White matter changes in Wilson disease. *Arch. Neurol.*, **59**, 866–7.

Hermann, W., Villmann, T., Grahmann, F., Kuhn, H. J. & Wagner, A. (2003). Investigation of fine-motor disturbances in Wilson's disease. *Neurol. Sci.*, **23**, 279–85.

Hill, G. M., Brewer, G. J., Juni, J. E. *et al.* (1986). Treatment of Wilson's disease with zinc: II. Validation of oral copper with copper balance. *Am. J. Med. Sci.*, **12**, 344–9.

Hill, G. M., Brewer, G. J., Prasad, A. S. *et al.* (1987). Treatment of Wilson's disease with zinc: I. Oral zinc therapy regimens. *Hepatology*, **7**, 522–8.

Hitoshi, S., Iwata, M. & Yoshikawa, K. (1991). Mid-brain pathology of Wilson's disease: MRI analysis of three cases. *J. Neurol. Neurosurg. Psychiatry*, **54**, 624–6.

Hlubocka, Z., Marecek, Z., Linhart, A. *et al.* (2002) Cardiac involvement in Wilson disease. *J. Inherit. Metab. Dis.*, **25**, 269–77.

Hochstein, P., Kumar, K. S. & Forman, S. J. (1980). Lipid peroxidation and the cytotoxicity of copper. *Ann. NY Acad. Sci.*, **355**, 240–8.

Hoogenraad, T. U., Van den Hamer, C. J. A., Koevoet, R., De Ruyter Korver, E. G. W. M. (1978). Oral zinc in Wilson's disease. *Lancet*, **ii**, 1262–3.

Hoogenraad, T. U., Loevoet, R., De Ruyter Korver, E. G. W. M. (1979). Oral zinc sulfate as long-term treatment in Wilson's disease (hepatolenticular degeneration). *Eur. Neurol.*, **18**, 205–11.

Hoogenraad, T. U., Van Hattum, J. & Van den Hamer, C. J. A. (1987). Management of Wilson's disease with zinc sulfate: experience in a series of 27 patients. *J. Neurol. Sci.*, **77**, 137–46.

Hoppe, B., Neuhaus, T., Superti-Furga, A., Forster, I. & Leumann, E. (1993). Hypercalciuria and nephrocalcinosis, a feature of Wilson's disease. *Nephron*, **65**, 460–2.

Horoupian, D. S., Sternlieb, I. & Scheinberg, I. H. (1988). Neuropathological findings in pencillamine-treated patients with Wilson's disease. *Clin. Neuropathol.*, **7**, 62–7.

Hu, R. (1994). Severe spinal degeneration in Wilson's disease. *Spine*, **19**, 372–5.

Huang, C. C., Chu, N. S., Yen, T. C., Wai, Y. Y. & Lu, C. S. (2003). Dopamine transporter binding in Wilson's disease. *Can. J. Neurol. Sci.*, **30**, 163–7.

Hyman, N. M. & Phuapradit, P. (1979). Reading difficulty as a presenting symptom in Wilson's disease. *J. Neurol. Neurosurg. Psychiatry*, **42**, 478–80.

Imiya, M., Ichikawa, K., Matsushima, H. *et al.* (1992). MR of the base of the pons in Wilson disease. *Am. J. Neuroradiol.*, **13**, 1009–12.

Innes, J. R., Strachan, I. M. & Triger, D. R. (1979). Unilateral Kayser–Fleischer ring. *Br. J. Ophthalmol.*, **70**, 469–70.

Ishino, H., Mii, T., Hayashi, Y. *et al.* (1972). A case of Wilson's disease with enormous cavity formation of cerebral white matter. *Neurology*, **22**, 905–9.

Ishmael, J., Gopinath, C. & Howell, J. M. C. (1972). Experimental chronic copper toxicity in sheep: biochemical and haematological studies during the development of lesions in the liver. *Res. Vet. Sci.*, **13**, 22–9.

Jackson, G. H., Meyer, A. & Lippmann, S. (1994). Wilson's disease. Psychiatric manifestations may be the clinical presentation. *Postgrad. Med.*, **95**, 135–8.

Jellinger, K. (1973). Neuroaxonal dystrophy: its natural history and related disorders. In *Progress in Neuropathology*, vol. 2. ed. H. M. Zimmerman, pp. 129–80. New York: Grune & Stratton.

Kabra, S. K., Bagga, A. & Malkani, I. (1990). Wilson's disease presenting with refractory rickets. *Ind. Pediatr.*, **27**, 395–7.

Kaul, A. & McMahon, D. (1993). Wilson's disease and offending behaviour – a case report. *Med. Sci. Law*, **33**, 353–8.

Kayser, B. (1902). Über einen Fall von angeborener grünlicher Verfarbung der Cornea. *Klin. Monatsb. Augenheilk.*, **40**, 22–5.

Keane, J. R. (1988). Lid-opening apraxia in Wilson's disease. *J. Clin. Neuroophthalmol.*, **8**, 31–3.

Keen, C. L., Lonnerdal, B. & Hurley, L. S. (1982). Teratogenic effect of copper deficiency and excess. In *Inflammatory Diseases and*

Copper, ed. J. R. Sorenson pp. 109–21. Clifton, NJ: Humana Press.

Keller, R., Torta, R., Lagget, M., Crasto, S. & Bergamasco, B. (1999). Psychiatric symptoms as late onset of Wilson's disease: neuroradiological findings, clinical features and treatment. *Ital. J. Neurol. Sci.*, **20**, 49–54.

Kendall, B. E., Pollock, S. S., Bass, N. M. & Valentine, A. R. (1981). Wilson's disease: Clinical correlation with cranial computed tomography. *Neuroradiology*, **22**, 1–5.

Kirkham, T. H. & Kamin, D. F. (1974). Slow saccadic eye movements in Wilson's disease. *J. Neurol. Neurosurg. Psychiatry*, **37**, 191–4.

Klinqele, T. G., Newman, S. A. & Burde, R. M. (1980). Accommodation defect in Wilson's disease. *Am. J. Ophthalmol.*, **90**, 22–4.

Knehr, C. A. & Beam, A. G. (1956). Psychological impairment in Wilson's disease. *J. Nerv. Ment. Dis.*, **124**, 251–5.

Knisely, A. (2001). Massive haemosiderosis in Wilson's disease. *Histopathology*, **39**, 323.

Kuwert, T., Hefter, H., Scholz, D. *et al.* (1992). Regional cerebral glucose consumption measured by positron emission tomography in patients with Wilson's disease. *Eur. J. Nucl. Med.*, **19**, 96–101.

Laufer, J., Passwell, J., Lotan, D. & Boichis, H. (1992). Screening for Wilson's disease in the investigation of hematuria. *Isr. J. Med. Sci.*, **28**, 367–9.

Lee, M. S., Kim, Y. D. & Lyoo, C. H. (1999). Oculogyric crisis as an initial manifestation of Wilson's disease. *Neurology*, **52**, 1714–15.

Lennox, G. & Jones, R. (1989). Gaze distractibility in Wilson's disease. *Ann. Neurol.*, **25**, 415–17.

LeWitt, P. A. & Pfeiffer, R. (2002). Neurological aspects of Wilson's disease: clinical and treatment considerations. In *Parkinson's Disease and Related Movement Disorders*, 4th edn., ed. J. Jankovic & E. Tolosa, Chap. 17, pp. 240–55.

Liao, K. K., Wang, S. J., Kwan, S. Y. *et al.* (1991). Tongue dyskinesia as an early manifestation of Wilson disease. *Brain Dev.*, **13**, 451–3.

Lichtenstein, B. W. & Gore, I. (1955). Wilson's disease – chronic form. *Arch. Neurol. Psychiatry*, **73**, 13–21.

Littman, E., Medalia, A., Senior, G. & Scheinberg, I. H. (1995). Rate of information processing in patients with Wilson's disease. *J. Neuropsychiatr. Clin. Neurosci.*, **7**, 68–71.

Lui, C. C., Chen, C. L., Chang, Y. F., Lee, T. Y., Chuang, Y. C. & Hsu, S. P. (2000). Subclinical central pontine myelinolysis after liver transplantation. *Transpl. Proc.*, **32**, 2215–16.

Liu, M., Cohen, E. J., Brewer, G. J. & Laibson, P. R. (2002). Kayser–Fleischer ring as the presenting sign of Wilson disease. *Am. J. Ophthalmol.*, **133**, 832–4.

Ma, K. G., Ye, Z. R., Fang, J. & Wu, J. V. (1988). Glial fibrillary acidic protein immunohistochemical study of Alzheimer I and II astrogliosis in Wilson's disease. *Acta Neurol. Scand.*, **78**, 290–6.

Madden, J. W., Ironside, J. W., Triger, D. R. & Bradshaw, J. P. (1985). An unusual case of Wilson's disease. *Q. J. Med.*, **55**, 63–73.

Magalhaes, A. C., Caramelli, P., Menezes, J. R. *et al.* (1994). Wilson's disease: MRI with clinical correlation. *Neuroradiology*, **36**, 97–100.

Medalia, A. & Scheinberg, I. H. (1989). Psychopathology in patients with Wilson's disease. *Am. J. Psychiatry*, **146**, 662–4.

Meenakshi-Sundaram, S., Taly, A. B., Kamath, V., Arunodaya, G. R., Rao, S. & Swamy, H. S. (2002). Autonomic dysfunction in Wilson's disease – a clinical and electrophysiological study. *Clin. Auton. Res.* **12**, 185–9.

Menerey, K. A., Eider, W., Brewer, G. J. *et al.* (1988). The arthropathy of Wilson's disease: clinical and pathologic features. *J. Rheumatol.*, **15**, 331–7.

Mercer, J. F., Livingston, J., Hall, B. *et al.* (1993). Isolation of a partial candidate gene for Menkes disease by positional cloning. *Nat. Genet.*, **3**, 20–5.

Metz, E. N. (1969). Mechanism of hemolysis by excess copper. *Clin. Res.*, **17**, 32.

Metz, E. N. & Sagone, A. L. (1972). The effect of copper on the erythrocyte hexose monophosphate shunt pathway. *J. Lab. Clin. Med.*, **80**, 405–13.

Metzer, W. S. & Angtuaco, E. (1986). Long-term follow-up computed tomography and magnetic resonance imaging findings in hepatolenticular degeneration. *Mov. Disord.*, **1**, 145–9.

Meyer, B. U., Britton, T. C. & Benecke, R. (1991a). Wilson's disease: normalisation of cortically evoked motor responses with treatment. *J. Neurol.*, **238**, 327–30.

Meyer, B. U., Britton, T. C., Bischoff, C. *et al.* (1991b). Abnormal conduction in corticospinal pathways in Wilson's disease: investigation of nine cases with magnetic brain stimulation. *Mov. Disord.*, **6**, 320–3.

Mills, C. F., El-Gallad, T. T., Bremner, I. (1981a). Effects of molybdate, sulfide, and tetrathiomolybdate on copper metabolism in rats. *J. Inorg. Biochem.*, **14**, 189–207.

Mills, C. F., El-Gallad, T. T. & Bremner, I. & Weham, G. (1981b). Copper and molybdenum absorption by rats given ammonium tetrathiomolybdate. *J. Inorg. Biochem.*, **14**, 163–75.

Mingazzini, G. (1928). Über das Zwangsweinen und -lachen. *Klin. Wochenschr. (Wien)*, **41**, 998–1002.

Miskolczy, D. (1932). Wilson'sche Krankheit und Kleinhirn. *Arch. Psych. Nervenkrankheit.*, **97**, 27–63.

Mital, V. P., Wahal, P. K. & Bansal, O. P. (1966). A study of erythrocyte glutathione in acute copper sulphate poisoning. *Ind. J. Pathol. Bact.*, **9**, 156–62.

Miyakawa, T. & Murayama, E. (1976). An autopsy case of the "demyelinating type" of Wilson's disease. *Acta Neuropathol.*, **35**, 235–41.

Nair, K. R. & Pillai, P. G. (1990). Trunkal myoclonus with spontaneous priapism and seminal ejaculation in Wilson's disease. *J. Neurol. Neurosurg. Psychiatry*, **53**, 174.

Nazer, H., Ede, R. J., Mowat, A. P. & Williams, R. (1986). Wilson's disease: clinical presentation and use of prognostic index. *Gut*, **27**, 1377–81.

Nelson, R. F., Guzman, D. A., Grahovac, Z. & Howse, D. C. N. (1979). Computerized tomography in Wilson's disease. *Neurology*, **29**, 866–8.

Nicholl, D. J., Ferenci, P., Polli, C., Burdon, M. B. & Pall, H. S. (2001). Wilson's disease presenting in a family with an apparent dominant history of tremor. *J. Neurol. Neurosurg. Psychiatry*, **70**, 514–16.

Obara, H., Ikoma, N., Sasaki, K. & Tachi, K. (1995). Usefulness of Scheimpflug photography to follow up Wilson's disease. *Ophth. Res.*, **27** [suppl 1], 100–3.

Olivarez, L., Caggana, M., Pass, K. A. *et al.* (2001). Estimate of the frequency of Wilson's disease in the US Caucasian population: a mutation analysis approach. *Ann. Human. Genet.*, **64**, 459–63.

Olsen, B. S., Helin, P. & Mortensen, H. B. (1996). Recurrent arthritis in a child. A rare manifestation of Wilson's disease. *Ugeskr Laeger*, **158**, 4305–6.

O'Reilly, S., Weber, P. M., Oswald, M. & Shipley, L. (1971). Abnormalities of the physiology of copper in Wilson's disease: III. The excretion of copper. *Arch. Neurol.* **25**, 28–32.

Owen, C. A. Jr. (1981). *Wilson's Disease. The Etiology, Clinical Aspects, and Treatment of Inherited Toxicosis*, pp. 1–215. Park Ridge, NJ: Noyes Publications.

Pall, H. S., Williams, A. C., Blake, D. R. *et al.* (1987). Movement disorder associated with abnormal copper metabolism and decreased blood anti-oxidants. *J. Neurol. Neurosurg. Psychiatry*, **50**, 1234–5.

Parker, N. (1985). Hereditary whispering dysphonia. *J. Neurol. Neurosurg. Psychiatry*, **48**, 218–24.

Patel, A. D. & Bozdech, M. (2001). Wilson disease. *Arch. Ophthalmol.*, **119**, 1556–7.

Pellecchia, M. T., Criscuolo, C., Longo, K., Campanella, G., Filla, A. & Barone, P. (2003). Clinical presentation and treatment of Wilson's disease: a single-centre experience. *Eur. Neurol.* **50**, 48–52.

Pentschew, A., Ebner, F. F. & Kovatch, R. M. (1963). Experimental manganese encephalopathy in monkeys: preliminary report. *J. Neuropath. Exp. Neuropathol.*, **22**, 488–99.

Perretti, A., Pellecchia, M. T., Lanzillo, B., Campanella, G. & Santoro, L. (2001). Excitatory and inhibitory mechanisms in Wilson's disease: investigation with magnetic motor cortex stimulation. *J. Neurol. Sci.*, **192**, 35–40.

Pilloni, L., Lecca, S., Coni, P. *et al.* (2000). Wilson's disease with late onset. *Dig. Liver Dis.*, **32**, 180.

Popoff, N. Budzilovich, G., Goodgold, A. & Faigin, I. (1965). Hepatocerebral degeneration: its occurrence in the presence and in the absence of abnormal copper metabolism. *Neurology*, **15**, 919–30.

Portala, K., Westermark, K., von Knorring, L. & Ekselius, L. (2000). Psychopathology in treated Wilson's disease determined by means of CPRS expert and self-ratings. *Acta. Psychiatr. Scand.*, **101**, 85–6, and **101**, 104–9.

Portala, K., Westermark, K., Ekselius, L. & von Knorring, L. (2001). Personality traits in treated Wilson's disease determined by means of the Karolinska Scales of Personality (KSP). *Eur. Psychiatry*, **16**, 362–71.

Portala, K., Westermark, K., Ekselius, L. & Broman, J. E. (2002). Sleep in patients with treated Wilson's disease. A questionnaire study. *Nord. J. Psychiatry*, **56**, 291–7.

Prayer, L., Wimberger, D., Kramer, J. *et al.* (1990). Cranial MRI in Wilson's disease. *Neuroradiology*, **32**, 211–14.

Prella, M., Baccala, R., Horisberger, J. D. *et al.* (2001). Haemolytic onset of Wilson disease in a patient with homozygous truncation of ATP7B at Arg1319. *Br. J. Haematol.*, **114**, 230–2.

Propst, A., Propst, T., Feichtinger, H., Judmaier, G., Willeit, J. & Vogel, W. (1995). Copper-induced acute rhabdomyolysis in Wilson's disease. *Gastroenterology*, **108**, 885–7.

Purdon, M. J. (1968). Wilson's disease. In *Handbook of Clinical Neurology*, vol. 6, ed. P. J. Vinken, G. W. Bruyn & N. L. Klawans, pp. 267–78. New York: American Elsevier.

Quinn, N. P. & Marsden, C. D. (1986). Coincidence of Wilson's disease with other movement disorders in the same family. *J. Neurol. Neurosurg. Psychiatry*, **49**, 221–2.

Rathbun, J. K. (1996). Neuropsychological aspects of Wilson's disease. *Int. J. Neurosci.*, **85**, 221–9.

Ravestyn, A. H. (1944). Metabolism of copper in man. *Acta Med. Scand.*, **118**, 163–96.

Richter, R. B. (1948). Pallidal component in hepatolenticular degeneration. *J. Neuropath. Exp. Neurol.*, **7**, 1–18.

Rifkind, J. M. (1974). Copper and the autoxidation of hemoglobin. *Biochemistry*, **13**, 2475–81.

Roberts, E. A. & Cox, D. W. (1998). Wilson disease. *Ballières Clin. Gastroenterol.*, **12**, 237–56.

Roh, J. K., Lee, T. G., Wie, B. A., Lee, S. B., Park, S. H. & Chang, K. H. (1994). Initial and follow-up brain MRI findings and correlation with the clinical course in Wilson's disease. *Neurology*, **44**, 1064–8.

Ross, M. E., Jacobson, I. M., Dienstag, J. L. & Martin, J. B. (1985). Late onset Wilson's disease with neurologic involvement in the absence of Kayser–Fleischer rings. *Ann. Neurol.*, **17**, 411–13.

Sasaki, N., Hayashizaki, Y., Muramatsu, M. *et al.* (1994). The gene responsible for LEC hepatitis, located on rat chromosome 16, is the homolog to the human Wilson disease gene. *Biochem. Biophys. Res. Commun.*, **202**, 512–18.

Satishchandra, P. & Ravishankar Naik, K. (2000). Visual pathway abnormalities in Wilson's disease: an electrophysiological study using electroretinography and visual evoked potentials. *J. Neurol. Sci.*, **176**, 13–20.

Satishchandra, P. & Swamy, H. S. (1989). Visual and brain stem auditory evoked responses in Wilson's disease. *Acta Neurol. Scand.*, **79**, 108–13.

Scheinberg, I. H. & Gitlin, D. (1952). Deficiency of ceruloplasmin in patients with hepatolenticular degeneration (Wilson's disease). *Science*, **116**, 484–5.

Scheinberg, I. H. & Sternlieb, I. (1984). *Wilson's Disease: Major Problems in Internal Medicine*, vol. 23. Philadelphia: W. B. Saunders.

Scheinberg, I. H., Sternlieb, I. & Richman, J. (1968). Psychiatric manifestations of Wilson's disease. *Birth Defects Orig. Art Ser.*, **4**, 85–6.

Schilsky, M. L., Scheinberg, I. H. & Sternlieb, I. (1994). Liver transplantation for Wilson's disease: Indications and outcome. *Hepatology*, **19**, 583–7.

Schulman, S. (1968). Wilson's disease. In *Pathology of the Nervous System*, vol. I, ed. J. Minkler, pp. 1139–51. New York: McGraw-Hill.

Schulman, S. & Barbeau, A. (1963). Wilson's disease: a case with almost total loss of cerebral white matter. *J. Neuropath. Exp. Neurol.*, **22**, 105–19.

Schwarz, J., Tatsch, K., Vogi, T. *et al.* (1992). Marked reduction of striatal dopamine D2 receptors as detected by IBZM-SPECT in a Wilson's disease patient with generalized dystonia. *Mov. Disord.*, **7**, 58–61.

Seitelberger, F. (1973). Zentrale pontin Myelinolyse. *Schweiz. Arch. Neurol. Neurochir. Psych.*, **112**, 285–97.

Sener, R. N. (1993). Diffusion MRI findings in Wilson's disease. *Comput. Med. Imaging Graph.*, **27**, 17–21.

Seniow, J., Bak, T., Gajda, J., Poniatowska, R. & Czlonkowska, A. (2002). Cognitive functioning in neurologically symptomatic and asymptomatic forms of Wilson's disease. *Mov. Disord.*, **17**, 1077–83.

Shale, H., Fahn, S., Roller, W. C. & Lang, A. E. (1987). Case 1, 1987: Unusual tremors, bradykinesia, and cerebral lucencies. *Mov. Disord.*, **2**, 321–38.

Shiraki, H. (1968). Comparative neuropathologic study of Wilson's disease and other types of hepatocerebral disease. In *Wilson's Disease*, vol. IV *Birth Defects*, original article series, ed. D. Bergsma, I. H. Scheinberg & I. Sternlieb, pp. 64–73. New York, The National Foundation–March of Dimes.

Smith, C. K. & Mattson, R. H. (1967). Seizures in Wilson's disease. *Neurology*, **17**, 1121–3.

Snow, B. J., Bhatt, M., Martin, W. R. *et al.* (1991). The nigrostriatal dopaminergic pathway in Wilson's disease studied with positron emission tomography. *J .Neurol. Neurosurg. Psychiatry*, **54**, 12–17.

Sokol, R. J., Devereaux, M. W., Traber, M. G. & Shikes, R. H. (1989). Copper toxicity and lipid peroxidation in isolated rat hepatocytes: effect of vitamin E$_l$. *Pediatr. Res.*, **25**, 55–62.

Song, H. S., Ku, W. C. & Chen, C. L. (1992). Disappearance of Kayser–Fleischer rings following liver transplantation. *Transpl. Proc.*, **24**, 1483–5.

Starosta-Rubinstein, S., Young, A. B., Kluin, K. *et al.* (1987). Clinical assessment of 31 patients with Wilson's disease: correlations with structural changes on magnetic resonance imaging. *Arch. Neurol.*, **44**, 365–70.

Stefano Zagami, A. & Boers, P. M. (2001). Disappearing "face of the giant panda". *Neurology*, **56**, 665.

Sternlieb, I., Giblin, D. R. & Scheinberg, I. H. (1985). Wilson's disease. In *Movement Disorders*, ed. C. D. Marsden & S. Fahn, pp. 288–302. New York: Butterworth.

Stiller, P., Kassubek, J., Schonfeldt-Lecuona, C. & Connemann, B. J. (2002). Wilson's disease in psychiatric patients. *Psychiatry Clin. Neurosci.*, **56**, 649.

Stremmel, W. & Meyerrose, K.-W., Niederau, K. *et al.* (1991). Wilson disease: clinical presentation, treatment, and survival. *Ann. Intern. Med.*, **115**, 720–6.

Sussman, W. & Sternlieb, I. H. (1969). Disappearance of Kayser–Fleischer rings. *Arch. Ophthal.*, **82**, 738–41.

Suzuki, S., Sato, Y., Ichida, T. & Hatakeyama, K. (2003). Recovery of severe neurologic manifestations of Wilson's disease after living-related liver transplantation: a case report. *Transpl. Proc.*, **35**, 385–6.

Svetel, M., Kozic, D., Stefanova, E., Semnic, R., Dragasevic, N. & Kostic, V. S. (2001). Dystonia in Wilson's disease. *Mov. Disord.*, **16**, 719–23.

Tanzi, R. E., Petrukhin, K., Chernov, I. *et al.* (1993). The Wilson disease gene is a copper transporting ATPase with homology to the Menkes disease gene. *Nat. Genet.*, **5**, 44–50.

Tatsch, K., Schwarz, J., Oertel, W. H. & Kirsch, C. M. (1991). SPECT imaging of dopamine D2 receptors with ^{123}I-IBZM: initial experience in controls and patients with Parkinson's syndrome and Wilson's disease. *Nucl. Med. Commun.*, **12**, 699–707.

Thomas, G. R., Roberts, E. A., Walshe, J. M. & Cox, D. W. (1995). Haplotypes and mutations in Wilson disease. *Am. J. Hum. Genet.*, **56**, 1315–19.

Thuomas, K. A., Aquilonius, S. M., Bergstrom, K. & Westermark, K. (1993). Magnetic resonance imaging of the brain in Wilson's disease. *Neuroradiology*, **35**(2), 134–41.

Topaloglu, H., Gucuyener, K., Orkun, C. & Renda, Y. (1990). Tremor of tongue and dysarthria as the sole manifestation of Wilson's disease. *Clin. Neurol. Neurosurg.*, **92**, 295–6.

Vulpe, C., Levinson, B., Whiney, S. *et al.* (1993). Isolation of a candidate gene for Menkes disease and evidence that it encodes a copper-transporting ATP-ase. *Nat. Genet.*, **3**, 7–13.

Walshe, J. M. (1976). Wilson's disease (hepatolenticular degeneration). In *Handbook of Clinical Neurology*, vol. 27, ed. P. J. Vinken, G. W. Bruyn & H. L. Klawans, pp. 379–414. New York: American Elsevier.

Walshe, J. M. (1986). Wilson's disease. In *Handbook of Clinical Neurology*, vol. 5, ed. P. J. Vinken, G. W. Bruyn & H. L. Klawans, pp. 223–38. New York: American Elsevier.

Walshe, J. M. & Potter, G. (1977). The pattern of whole body distribution of radioactive copper (^{67}Cu, ^{64}Cu) in Wilson's disease and various control groups. *Q. J. Med.*, **46**, 445–62.

Walshe, J. M. & Yealland, M. (1992). Wilson's disease: the problem of delayed diagnosis. *J. Neurol. Neurosurg. Psychiatry*, **55**, 692–6.

Warren, P. J., Earl, C. J. & Thompson, R. H. S. (1960). The distribution of copper in human brain. *Brain*, **83**, 709–17.

Westphal, C. (1883). Ueber eine dem Bilde der cerebrospinalen grauen Degeneration ähnliche Erkrankung des centralen Nervensystems ohne anatomischen Befund, nebst einigen Bermerkungen über paradoxe Contraction. *Arch. Psychiatr. Nerv.*, **14**, 87–134.

Wiebers, D. O., Hollenhorst, R. W. & Goldstein, N. P. (1977). The ophthalmologic manifestations of Wilson's disease. *Mayo Clin. Proc.*, **52**, 409–16.

Willeit, J. & Kiechl, S. G. (1991). Wilson's disease with neurological impairments but no Kayser–Fleischer rings. *Lancet*, **337**, 1426.

Williams, F. J. B. & Walshe, J. M. (1981). Wilson's disease. An analysis of the cranial computerized tomographic appearances found in 60 patients and the changes in response to treatment with chelating agents. *Brain*, **104**, 735–52.

Willvonseder, R., Goldstein, N. P., McCall, J. T. *et al.* (1973). A hereditary disorder with dementia, spastic dysarthria, vertical eye movement paresis, gait disturbance, splenomegaly, and abnormal copper metabolism. *Neurology*, **23**, 1039–49.

Wilson, S. A. K. (1912). Progressive lenticular degeneration: a familial nervous disease associated with cirrhosis of the liver. *Brain*, **34**, 295–509.

(1955). Progressive lenticular degeneration (hepatolenticular degeneration, Wilson's disease). In *Neurology*, 2nd edn, vol. 2, ed. A. N. Bruce, pp. 941–67. Baltimore, Williams & Wilkins.

Yamaguchi, Y., Heiny, M. E. & Gitlin, J. D. (1993). Isolation and characterization of a human liver cDNA as a candidate gene for Wilson disease. *Biochem. Biophys. Res. Commun.*, **197**, 271–7.

Yamaguchi, Y., Heiny, M. E., Shimizu, N., Aoki, T. & Gitlin, J. D. (1994). Expression of the Wilson disease gene is deficient in the Long-Evans Cinnamon rat. *Biochem. J.*, **301**(1), 1–4.

Yuzbasiyan-Gurkan, V., Brewer, G. J., Abrams, G. D. *et al.* (1989). Treatment of Wilson's disease with zinc: V. Changes in serum levels of lipase, amylase and alkaline phosphatase in Wilson's disease patients. *J. Lab. Clin. Med.*, **114**, 520–6.

Yuzbasiyan-Gurkan, V., Johnson, V. & Brewer, G. J. (1991). Diagnosis and characteristics of presymptomatic patients with Wilson's disease and the use of molecular genetics to aid in the diagnosis. *J. Lab. Clin. Med.*, **118**, 45–6.

Yuzbasiyan-Gurkan, V., Grider, A., Nostrant, T. *et al.* (1992). Treatment of Wilson's disease with zinc: X: Intestinal metallothionein induction. *J. Lab. Clin. Med.*, **120**, 380–6.

62

Disorders of the mitochondrial respiratory chain

Anthony H. V. Schapira

Royal Free and University College Medical School, and Institute of Neurology, University College London, UK

Introduction

Mitochondria are ubiquitous and present in all mammalian cells. They are host to a range of biochemical pathways including oxidative phosphorylation, β-oxidation and the urea cycle. Mitochondria are also important in mediating a variety of intracellular triggers for apoptotic cell death. This chapter will focus on defects of the mitochondrial respiratory chain and specifically those that are related to human diseases; toxin induced mitochondrial defects will be considered elsewhere.

The mitochondrial respiratory chain and oxidative phosphorylation system comprises five multisubunit proteins, which are embedded within the inner mitochondrial membrane. The first four complexes are connected in functional terms by coenzyme Q, and cytochrome c. Electrons are transferred from NADH and $FADH_2$ and result in the reduction of oxygen to water. This process also involves the shuttling of protons across the inner membrane to the internal membranous space, and this provides the proton motive force for the generation of ATP from ADP by complex V (ATPase).

Complexes I–V comprise approximately 82 different subunits, of which 13 are encoded by mitochondrial DNA. The remainder are encoded by nuclear genes and imported into the mitochondrium often by way of specific targeting sequences and import machinery. Mitochondrial DNA is a 16.5 kb double-stranded circular molecule, which lies in the matrix attached near its D-loop to the inner mitochondrial membrane. Mitochondrial DNA encodes 2 ribosomal RNAs, 22 transfer RNAs and 13 proteins (Table 62.1 and Fig. 62.1). It is dependent upon nuclear enzymes for transcription, translation, replication and repair.

Mitochondrial DNA is inherited virtually exclusively from the female line. There may be some paternal linkage, but this is either not replicated or is diluted beyond detection. The pattern of inheritance of mitochondrial DNA has been valuable in ethnic and migration studies. Mutations of mitochondrial DNA also result in the phenomenon of maternally inherited diseases. Over 100 different mutations of mitochondrial DNA have now been associated with human pathology. These include micro- and macro- deletions, point mutations and insertions affecting ribosomal or transfer RNA genes or protein coding genes. A quantitative defect of mitochondrial DNA (mitochondrial DNA depletion) has also been identified, although this latter phenomenon is associated with mutations of nuclear genes encoding enzymes responsible for mitochondrial DNA replication. Mitochondrial DNA mutations have a tendency to be heteroplasmic, i.e. to exist concomitantly with wild-type mitochondrial DNA at least within the same cell, and probably within the same mitochondrion. This results in a variation of mutation load between tissues and between affected individuals. There is also a relatively high carrier state associated with mitochondrial DNA mutations.

The clinical expression of disorders related to defects of the mitochondrial respiratory chain is very broad, and may include virtually any system or tissue. Those areas most commonly affected are the brain and muscle, as these tissues are probably the most dependent upon oxidative phosphorylation. Common symptoms include proximal myopathy and external ophthalmoplegia, CNS features may include seizures, dementia, ataxia and deafness, retinitis pigmentosa and diabetes mellitus. The basis to the considerable variation in clinical phenotype, even caused by the same mutation, is thought to be related to the variation in mutation load that may exist between tissues and patients. However, this is likely to be an over-simplification, and there may well be a number of other factors both genetic and environmental that might influence the expression of mitochondrial DNA mutations.

Table 62.1. Respiratory chain components

Complex	Enzyme	Subunits	MtDNA encoded subunits
I	NADH CoQ, reductase	~42	ND1–6, ND4L
II	Succinate dehydrogenase	4	–
III	Ubiquinone cytochrome c reductase	11	Cytocrome b
IV	Cytochrome oxidase	13	COI, COII, COIII
V	ATPase	15	ATPase 6 and 8

The classification of mitochondrial disorders of the respiratory chain is challenging, and none is universally accepted. Much of this difficulty is the result of only an approximate correlation of genotype and phenotype. For instance, mitochondrial DNA deletions most frequently result in chronic progressive external ophthalmoplegia (CPEO) or Kearns–Sayre syndrome (KSS). These same mutations, however, may result in isolated proximal myopathy or encephalopathy or a combination of features that might, for instance, fall within other mitochondrial phenotypes including MELAS (myopathy encephalopathy, lactic acidosis and stroke-like episodes) or isolated syndromes such as cardiomyopathy or diabetes mellitus. Similarly, the A3243G mutation in the transfer RNA for lysine, which is most commonly associated with MELAS, can also result in CPEO, pure myopathy, isolated diabetes, isolated deafness, etc. In view of this complexity, this review has taken a pragmatic approach, and will describe the major mitochondrial phenotypes caused by mutations of mitochondrial DNA. There is a second group of primary respiratory chain disorders caused by mutations of nuclear genes encoding subunits of complexes 1–V and, together, these are often referred to as the primary respiratory chain disorders.

CPEO and KSS

CPEO may manifest any time from adolescence to late adulthood, although usually, before the age of 30. Patients develop symmetric or asymmetric, slowly progressive, non-fatiguable ptosis in association with external ophthalmoplegia. Diplopia does occur, but is present only in the minority, given that the ophthalmoplegia is usually symmetrical. There may be an associated pigmentary retinopathy of the salt and pepper type, and/or a proximal myopathy. Additional complications are relatively uncommon, and the great majority of patients are never significantly disabled, and usually have a normal lifespan. Onset of CPEO in late adulthood is well recorded.

Creatine kinase is usually normal, electromyography may be normal or show some mild non-specific myopathic features. Serum lactate may be elevated at rest, and exercise may induce a significant and sustained increase. Definitive diagnosis requires a muscle biopsy, and this will show the morphological features characteristic of the mitochondrial myopathies. These include the presence of ragged red fibers on the Gomori trichrome stain. This pattern reflects the subsarcolemmal accumulation of mitochondria, often associated with increased lipid and glycogen. The ragged red fibers usually stain negative for cytochrome oxidase, and positive for succinate dehydrogenase (see Fig. 62.2). At the ultrastructural level, the mitochondria are often enlarged with aberrant crystal configuration. The matrix may be vacuolated, and para-crystalline inclusions may be present in the intra-membranous space. Although characteristic of mitochondrial myopathies, these light and electron microscopic findings are not specific. For instance, ragged red, COX negative, SDH positive fibers may be present in inflammatory myopathies. Furthermore, mitochondrial abnormalities accumulate with age, and up to 5% of fibers may be abnormal over the age of 50 (Muller-Hocker, 1990). The combination of ragged red, SDH positive, COX negative fibers is relatively typical of mitochondrial DNA deletions. *In situ* hybridization studies show that the highest percentage of mutant mtDNA is present in these fibers (Hammans *et al.*, 1993; Moraes *et al.*, 1991, 1992; Shoubridge *et al.*, 1990).

The most common mutation found in patients with CPEO is the mitochondrial DNA deletion, being found in 70% of those with CPEO (Holt *et al.*, 1988, 1989; Moraes *et al.*, 1989). The deletions are single, i.e. affecting the same segment of the mtDNA molecule in all tissues, but the proportion of deleted molecules varies from one to another. For instance, it is extremely rare to find the deletions in blood. DNA confirmation is therefore dependent on providing a tissue sample, i.e. skeletal muscle. It appears that the proportion of deleted mitochondrial DNA is stable over time. One particular mtDNA deletion is the 4977 base pair deletion, referred to as the "common deletion," and spans the region from the ATPase 8 gene to the nd5 gene. This occurs in approximately 30% of patients with CPEO or KSS (see below) (Schon *et al.*, 1989; Mita *et al.*, 1990).

KSS is defined by CPEO and pigmentary retinopathy together with either complete heart block, a cerebrospinal fluid protein level > 1 g/liter and ataxia. Onset is before the age of 20, although later-onset cases may occasionally occur. Furthermore, there may be an associated proximal limb weakness. Taken together with CPEO, ptosis may

(a)

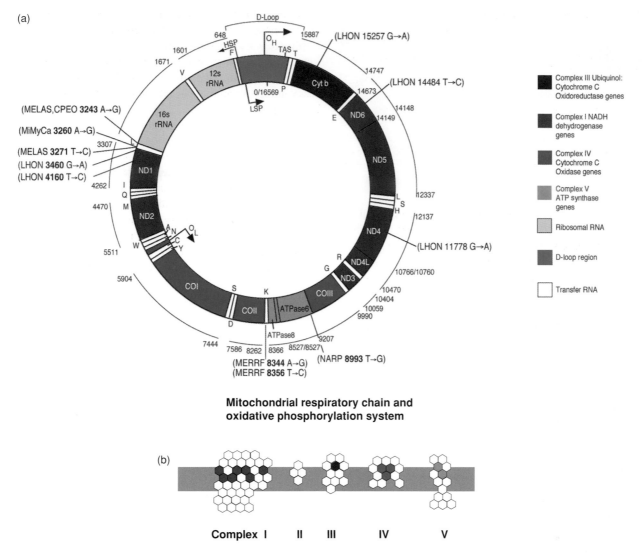

**Mitochondrial respiratory chain and
oxidative phosphorylation system**

(b)

Complex I   II   III   IV   V

Fig. 62.1 The human mtDNA genome (a). The protein coding genes are colour coded to the subunits in the respiratory chain cartoon (b). The location of some of the more common point mutations are shown in (a).

be asymmetrical in 58% or unilateral in 8%. Dysconjugate eye movements occur in 35% with transient or persistent diplopia in 36%. The ophthalmoplegia may be severe, and in 62% of patients, gaze is limited to less than 10% of normal in any direction (Petty *et al.*, 1986). Mitochondrial DNA deletions are also the most common cause of KSS being found in 80% of patients (Holt *et al.*, 1988, 1989; Moraes *et al.*, 1989). Mitochondrial DNA duplications may also be found, although in low abundance, and may be an intermediate step to deletion (Holt *et al.*, 1997) duplications of mitochondrial DNA are not necessarily pathogenic (Holt *et al.*, 1997; Tang *et al.*, 2000). In both CPEO and KSS, mitochondrial DNA deletions are present in highest proportion in the COX negative ragged red fibers.

The majority of patients with CPEO or KSS have no family history. This is thought to be due to the mitochondrial DNA deletions arising *de novo* in maternal oocytes. Duplicated mtDNA molecules have been identified with a maternal inheritance pattern such as in cases in renal tubular dysfunction ataxia and diabetes mellitus (Rotig *et al.*, 1992), CPEO, myopathy and diabetes mellitus (Dunbar *et al.*, 1993). More often, maternal inherited CPEO is due to a point mutation of mtDNA rather than a rearrangement, e.g. the A3243G mutation in tRNA (Moraes *et al.*, 1993). Several other tRNA mutations have also been associated with maternally inherited CPEO. Muscle biopsies in these patients show the typical CPEO pattern of COX negative fibers, rather

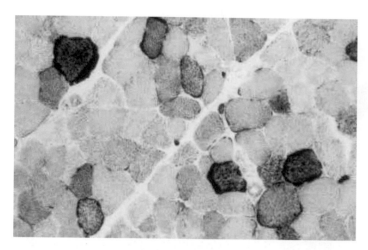

Fig. 62.2(a) Succinate dehydrogenase (SDH) stain of a muscle biopsy showing SDH positive fibers corresponding to ragged red fibers.

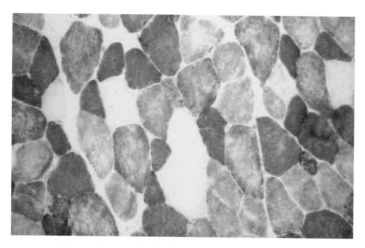

Fig. 62.2(b) Cytochrome oxidase negative fibers.

than the usual COX positive fibers associated with tRNA mutations.

CPEO may also exhibit autosomal dominant or recessive inheritance. The first description of autosomal dominant CPEO was in an Italian pedigree with onset in early adulthood of ptosis, dysarthria, dysphasia, facial and proximal limb weakness with cataracts and early death (Servidei *et al.*, 1991). Other pedigrees have been described with additional features such cardiomyopathy, endocrine abnormalities, ataxia, rhabdomyolysis and peripheral neuropathy (Melberg *et al.*, 1996, 1998). Patients often exhibit lactic acidosis and muscle biopsy shows the usual features of ragged red fibers. At least three chromosomal loci have been identified in autosomal dominant CPEO including chromosome 4 (Kaukonen *et al.*, 1999), and a mutation has

recently been identified in the gene for adenine nucleotide translocator 1 (Kaukonen *et al.*, 2000). The other locus is on chromosome 10 (Li *et al.*, 1999; Suomalainen *et al.*, 1995). There are likely to be additional loci that are not linked to either chromosome 4 or 10. Autosomal dominant CPEO is associated with multiple deletions in the same patient and as in sporadic CPEO and KSS, the deletions are not present in mitotically active cells, e.g. lymphocytes and fibroblasts.

Myopathy encephalopathy lactic acidosis and stroke-like episodes

This phenotype is characterized by growth retardation, focal and generalized seizures and recurrent stroke-like episodes, particularly hemianopia and hemiplegia. Additional features may include diabetes, deafness, dementia, ataxia and myopathy. Pigmentary retinopathy is relatively uncommon. Onset is usually in adolescence, although patients may manifest later, and MELAS remains an important differential diagnosis in patients with stroke under the age of 40. Clinical progression is usual, but at a variable rate. Many patients develop features of migraine with aura and recurrent episodes of lactic acidosis associated with nausea and vomiting. The stroke-like episodes maybe transitory or result in permanent neurological deficit. Imaging in patients with MELAS usually reveals low-density areas affecting grey and white matter, which typically do not conform to vascular territories, and most often affect the parietal occipital regions (Pavlakis *et al.*, 1984; Allard *et al.*, 1988). Elevation of CSF lactate is invariable in patients with encephalopathy.

Skeletal muscle morphology in patients with MELAS usually demonstrates ragged red and SDH positive fibers. In contrast to those with mitochondrial DNA deletions, the cytochrome oxidase fibers are usually strongly positive. Histochemical analysis of cerebral vessels also demonstrate strong SDH reactivity suggesting that angiopathy is a significant component of the pathogenesis of MELAS associated strokes (Kuriyama *et al.*, 1984). Basal ganglia calcification is also a common radiological feature of MELAS (Sue *et al.*, 1998). This most commonly affects the globus pallidus but can also include the striatum, thalamus and internal capsules.

Eighty per cent of patients meeting the clinical criteria for MELAS are positive for the A3243G mutation in the tRNA for leucine (Hammans *et al.*, 1991; Goto *et al.*, 1990; Kobayashi *et al.*, 1990). Analysis of the effects of this mutation in cybrids has shown a reduction in global protein synthesis due to abnormalities of an aminoacylation and post-transcriptional modifications of the tRNA (Borner *et al.*, 2000; Chomyn *et al.*, 1991; Helm *et al.*, 1999). There is also evidence that a partially processed polycistonic transcript (RNA19) which is composed of a segment of RNA, the tRNA leucine(UUR) stop signal and ND1 is significantly increased in cybrids (King *et al.*, 1992). This maybe incorporated into ribosomes and interfere with translation (Schon *et al.*, 1992).

Other mutations have been associated with the MELAS phenotype including four different mutations within the tRNA leucine (UUR) gene, and in numerous other tRNAs.

Cybrid analysis using the A3243G mutation showed that this particular base change was recessive in the sense that 5–10% of wild-type mitochondrial DNA was sufficient to compensate biochemically for the mutation; whether these data from cybrids can be translated to the in vivo situation is not known.

Myoclonic epilepsy and ragged red fibers (MERRF)

The core features of this syndrome are myoclonus, ataxia and seizures. Patients often manifest with myoclonic epilepsy which may be stimulation sensitive. Additional seizure types may also occur including drop attacks, tonic–clonic seizures and focal seizures (Hammans *et al.*, 1993; Berkovic *et al.*, 1989). The myopathy is usually relatively mild, and involves proximal upper and lower limb weakness. Additional clinical features may include hearing loss, neuropathy, dementia and growth retardation (Silvestri *et al.*, 1993). Some patients have been recoded with ophthalmoplegia, ptosis, optic atrophy, and cervical lipomas (Berkovic *et al.*, 1989; Fukuhara *et al.*, 1980; Truong *et al.*, 1990; Tulinius *et al.*, 1991). The clinical causes are variable, but usually progressive.

The presence of lipomas is an interesting phenomenon in MERRF patients, and as indicated, usually comprises multiple symmetrical cervical lipomas (Larsson *et al.*, 1995). In some patients, this may be the only manifestation of MERRF (Holme *et al.*, 1993). The lipomas comprise brown adipose tissue expressing mitochondrial uncoupling proteins (Vila *et al.*, 2000).

Phenotypic variation as suggested by the above range of clinical features can be substantial even within the same family (Graf *et al.*, 1993). For instance, in one family, some patients presented with Leigh syndrome, others with spinal cerebellar degeneration or a form of motor and sensory neuropathy (Howell *et al.*, 1996).

The electroencephalogram may be abnormal in MERRF patients (So *et al.*, 1989) but the changes are not specific. Plasma and CSF lactate levels may be elevated. Muscle

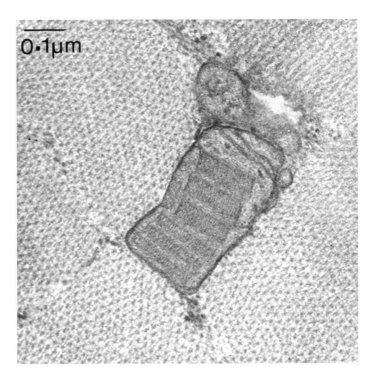

Fig. 62.2(c) Electron micrograph shows mitochondrial paracrystalline inclusions.

biopsy shows ragged red fibers, which are SDH positive, and COX negative.

The most common mutation detected in MERRF is the A8344G mutation, which is present in 80% of patients (Hammans *et al.*, 1991; Shoffner *et al.*, 1990; Zeviani *et al.*, 1991). The tRNA lysine gene may also harbor other mutations which can result in the MERRF phenotype. Likewise, single base changes in other tRNAs for leucine or serine, may also produce a phenotype with features of MERRF (Moraes *et al.*, 1993; Folgero *et al.*, 1995; Nakamura *et al.*, 1995). The MERRF mutations in cybrids result in reduced protein synthesis of certain protein translation products (Chomyn, 1998; Enriquez *et al.*, 1995; Hao & Moraes, 1996; Masucci *et al.*, 1995). There are some suggestions that the mutant load in the muscle or blood, the age of onset and certain clinical parameters may give some indication for prognosis (Hammans *et al.*, 1993; Shoffner *et al.*, 1991).

Neurogenic muscle weakness ataxia and retinitis pigmentosa (NARP)

The key features of this syndrome are myopathy, peripheral neuropathy, ataxia, seizures, dementia and retinitis pigmentosa (Holt *et al.*, 1990). They may also include migraine and mental retardation (Tsairis *et al.*, 1973; Ortiz *et al.*, 1993; Fryer *et al.*, 1994; Makela-Bengs *et al.*, 1995; Puddu *et al.*, 1993).

The most common cause of this phenotype is the T8893G mutation in the ATPase 6 gene. This mutation is heteroplasmic and, when present at around 70%, is associated with a NARP phenotype, and when present at >90%, is associated with maternal inherited Leigh syndrome (Holt *et al.*, 1990; Santorelli *et al.*, 1994). T8993C mutation has also been associated with NARP (65), and one patient with Leigh syndrome (Santorelli *et al.*, 1994). The mutations affect the region of ATPase associated with the proton channel and may result in impairment of the electrochemical gradient required to synthesize ATP (Tatuch *et al.*, 1992). Alternatively, the mutations may impair the efficiency of the coupling of proton flow to the rotation of the ATPase subcomplex in the inner membrane (Schon, 2000; Schon *et al.*, 1997).

Ragged red fibers and other morphological abnormalities are usually absent in the muscle biopsies from patients with NARP (Holt *et al.*, 1990). Biochemical analysis may also be normal unless ATPase activity is assessed specifically. Blood levels of citrulline have been found to be low in some patients with NARP and it has been suggested that it is the surrogate marker of this phenotype (Parfait *et al.*, 1999).

Additional phenotypes

Approximately 1–2% of all non-insulin dependent diabetic mellitus is thought to be related to the presence of the A3243G mutation (Kadowaki *et al.*, 1993; Gerbitz *et al.*, 1995), and this may occur as the only clinical manifestation of this mutation in some patients (Gerbitz *et al.*, 1993; Reardon *et al.*, 1992), or be present with associated sensory neural deafness (Kadowaki *et al.*, 1993; van den Ouweland *et al.*, 1992).

Sensory neural hearing loss may occur as an isolated phenomenon with mutations in the tRNA for serine (Guan *et al.*, 1998).

Cardiomyopathy which may be either dilated or hypertrophic has been reported with a number of mitochondrial DNA mutations including rRNA genes (Santorelli *et al.*, 1999). A number of cases have also been described with pure myopathy (Hudgson *et al.*, 1972; Kamieniecka, 1977). These patients usually have fatigue and exercise intolerance (Petty *et al.*, 1986), and some patients with recurrent myoglobinuria and exercise intolerance, have mitochondrial DNA deletions (Ohno *et al.*, 1991; Andreu *et al.*, 1999). Cytochrome oxidase gene mutations have also been associated with myopathy and myoglobinuria (Keightley

et al., 1996). Mutations in mitochondrial DNA COX genes have been associated with a variety of clinical presentations including motor neurone disease (amyotrophic lateral sclerosis), and sideroblastic anemia (Comi *et al.*, 1998; Gattermann *et al.*, 1997).

Leber's hereditary optic neuropathy (LHON)

This is a maternally inherited disorder characterized by acute or subacute bilateral sequential painless visual failure. The mean age of onset is in the early 20s and 90% of patients are affected by age 45; 85% are men. In most cases the visual loss is severe, and permanent, although this is dependent upon the underlying mutation.

Three mitochondrial DNA mutations are considered primary, and all are located within mitochondrial DNA complex I genes. These are the G11778A mutation in ND4, which is found in 50–70% of LHON patients, the G3460A mutation in 15–25%, and the T14484C mutation in ND6. The latter is relatively uncommon, but is associated with visual recovery in 70% (Wallace *et al.*, 1988; Howell *et al.*, 1991; Johns *et al.*, 1992; Mackey & Howell, 1992).

The mutations are detectable in blood, and are usually homoplasmic. There is evidence for a complex I defect in muscle and platelets of patients (Smith *et al.*, 1994; Larsson *et al.*, 1991), and this has been confirmed in cybrid studies. Only 15% of women who carry one of the primary mutations are clinically affected. This initially led to the suggestion of x-linked susceptibility, but no evidence has yet been found to support this (Chalmers *et al.*, 1996). Autoimmune involvement (Smith *et al.*, 1995) or alternatively some influence of nuclear expression have also been suggested to influence disease expression. Furthermore, a number of secondary mitochondrial DNA mutations have also been proposed to influence expression, and may act synergistically with a primary mutation (Howell, 1997).

Some families exhibiting features of LHON may have additional features such as dystonia or striatal degeneration, and these have also been found to be related to mutations in mitochondrial DNA complex I genes (Jun *et al.*, 1994; De Vries *et al.*, 1996), although dystonia has also been seen in some patients with the 3460 and 11778 mutations (Meire *et al.*, 1995; Nikoskelainen *et al.*, 1995; Thobois *et al.*, 1997).

Myo-neuro-gastrointestinal encephalopathy (MNGIE)

The diagnostic criteria for this phenotype include peripheral neuropathy, CPEO and gastrointestinal dysmotility.

Patient's skeletal muscle has the typical morphological features of mitochondrial myopathy. The gastrointestinal disease usually includes nausea, vomiting and diarrhoea. MR imaging may demonstrate a leukodystrophy. The peripheral neuropathy is sensory motor in type (Hirano *et al.*, 1994). The average age of onset is usually in adolescence, and most patients are dead by 40 years (Nishino *et al.*, 2000).

Southern blotting demonstrates multiple mitochondrial DNA deletions and depletion of mitochondrial DNA (Nishino *et al.*, 2000). Inheritance is autosomal recessive and mutations in thymidine phosphorylase have been identified in those patients that map to chromosome 22 (Nishino *et al.*, 1999). Thymidine phosphorylase activity is severely reduced in patients, and plasma thymidine levels are high.

Leigh syndrome

This is a subacute narcotizing encephalomyelopathy (Leigh, 1951). The clinical features are wide, and include psychomotor retardation, respiratory abnormalities, oculomotor disturbance, optic atrophy, seizures and lactic acidosis. Onset is usually in the first few months of life, or during childhood. This syndrome might be caused by a variety of biochemical abnormalities including respiratory chain defects (Di Mauro & De Vivo, 1996; Van Erven *et al.*, 1987; Willems *et al.*, 1977; Van Coster *et al.*, 199), pyruvate dehydrogenate deficiency (Kretzschmar *et al.*, 1987) or biotinidase deficiency (Baumgartner *et al.*, 1989). Respiratory chain defects include those patients with mutations of nuclear genes encoding subunits of complexes I or II (Loeffen *et al.*, 1998; Bourgeron *et al.*, 1995). Deficiency of complex IV in patients with Leigh syndrome may be associated with mutations of the SURF gene which is responsible for assembly and maintenance of complex IV (Tiranti *et al.*, 1998; Zhu *et al.*, 1998). As indicated above, approximately 20% of Leigh syndrome patients have an ATPase 6 mutation with mutant loads 90% or greater. The MELAS or MERF mutations have also been associated with a Leigh syndrome phenotype (Rahman *et al.*, 1996; Koga *et al.*, 1998).

Neurodegenerative diseases

As can be seen from the review of primary mitochondrial disorders noted above, defects of the mitochondrial respiratory chain due to mutations of mitochondrial DNA or mutations of nuclear genes encoding subunits of the respiratory chain or components required for its construc-

tion or maintenance, result in a variety of features that include progressive neurological features. The following section covers mitochondrial involvement in archetypal neurodegenerative diseases:

Parkinson's disease

Since the first report of mitochondrial dysfunction in Parkinson's disease (PD) (Schapira *et al.*, 1989), there has been considerable interest in mitochondrial dysfunction in this disorder. In the CNS the defect appears to be confined to the substantia nigra (Schapira *et al.*, 2000a,b), and there is some indication of a reduction of complex I subunits in dopaminergic neurons of this region (Hattori *et al.*, 1991). Other neurodegenerative disorders simulating Parkinson's disease, such as multiple system atrophy do not have any evidence of respiratory chain defect in the substantia nigra (Gu *et al.*, 1997). However, numerous reports have identified a complex I defect in platelets from a proportion of patients with PD (Schapira, 1994).

On a group-to-group analysis, the substantia nigra defect in PD is approximately 35%, i.e. 65% residual complex I activity. A defect of this level is likely to result in an increase in free radical release and oxidative stress in the nigra. The substantia nigra is already a site of increased iron and dopamine auto-oxidation (Dexter *et al.*, 1989; Hirsch *et al.*, 1991), and there is evidence for a decrease in reduced glutathione and increase in malonaldehyde as indicators of free-radical mediated oxidative stress and damage (Dexter *et al.*, 1994; Alam *et al.*, 1997a,b). The respiratory chain proteins are also susceptible to damage from free radicals, and this therefore has the potential to exacerbate the underlying respiratory chain defect.

The potential relevance of complex I deficiency to Parkinson's disease has been underlined by the fact that environmental toxins that are complex I inhibitors are capable of producing models of Parkinson's disease. The first of these was MPTP produced as a contaminant of a meperidine designer drug (Langston & Ballard, 1984). MPTP is first oxidized to MPP^+ by monoamine oxidase B which is found in high concentration in glia. MPP^+ is then taken up by the dopamine transporter and so is concentrated within nigra dopaminergic neurons (Chiba *et al.*, 1985; Javitch & Snyder, 1984). Because of its positive charge, MPP^+ is further concentrated several hundredfold into mitochondria, where it is an inhibitor of complex I (Ramsay *et al.*, 1986; Nicklas *et al.*, 1985). MPTP also induces increased free radical generation (Rossetti *et al.*, 1988). It is of note that transgenic mice overexpressing SOD1 are resistant to MPTP toxicity (Przedborski *et al.*, 1992). Likewise, MPTP toxicity in primates can be blocked with the neuronal nitric oxide synthase inhibitor, 7-nitroindazole (Hantraye *et al.*, 1996). A similar effect is seen in mice (Schulz *et al.*, 1995), and in neuronal nitric oxide synthase (nNOS) knockout mice (Przedborski *et al.*, 1996). Infusion of rotenone, another specific inhibitor complex I, induces nigral cell death in rodents together with the production of inclusions similar to Lewy bodies (Betarbet *et al.*, 2000). Further analysis of this model suggests that neurodegeneration is not confined to the substantia nigra, and this model may more resemble, a model of progressive supranuclear palsy (Hoglinger *et al.*, 2003).

There are also overlaps between some of the recently identified causes of familial Parkinson's disease. For instance, alpha synuclein has in some studies been associated with a decrease in mitochondrial function (Elkon *et al.*, 2002). The ubiquitin proteasomal pathway is now considered to be an important area in the pathogenesis of Parkinson's disease. Alpha synuclein is a significant component of Lewy bodies in sporadic Parkinson's disease. Over expression of this protein as well as its expression in mutant form leads to familial autosomal dominant Parkinson's disease (Singleton *et al.*, 2003). Activity of the ubiquitin proteasomal system is dependent upon ATPases, and a decrease in complex I activity impairs function of the system. Furthermore, a decrease in complex I activity results in an increase in proteins damaged by free radicals that are dependent upon the ubiquitin proteasomal system, for metabolism. A concomitant genetically determined defect of the ubiquitin proteasomal system, such as might be caused by parkin mutations, might act synergistically with a complex I defect to impair cell metabolism, and enhance cell death. Alternatively, environmental agents that impair the proteasomal pathway would have a similar effect.

At present, it is not known whether the complex I defect is a consequence of a genetic abnormality or is environmentally induced. If the latter, this could be a consequence of either exogenous or endogenous toxins. Several studies have sequenced mitochondrial DNA in patients with Parkinson's disease, but none has identified a consistent mutation. To some degree, this might be a consequence of the failure to select patients with complex I deficiency, which probably only affects a proportion of Parkinson's disease cases. Cybrid analysis of patients with complex I deficiency has shown that the defect may be transferred from the platelets of patients with Parkinson's disease to cybrid cells. This involves the passage only of mitochondrial DNA from the platelets to the cybrid cells, and therefore indicates that the complex I defect is determined by mitochondrial DNA (Gu *et al.*, 1998; Swerdlow *et al.*, 1996). What is not known is whether the complex I defect alone can induce nigral cell death or whether it is necessary for

this abnormality to be in combination with either another concomitant genetic defect or to work in synergy with an environmental agent.

Huntington's disease

Huntington's disease is an autosomal dominant disorder caused by an abnormal CAG extension in the N-terminal region of the huntingtin gene. This encodes a polyglutamine stretch. Pathology comprises severe atrophy of the caudate, and to a lesser extent the putamen with selective loss of the medium spiny neurons. The function of huntingtin is not known, but it is highly conserved and widely expressed in neural and non-neural tissues (Strong *et al.*, 1993). Cultured cells expressing mutant huntingtin developed intranuclear aggregates (Cooper *et al.*, 1998; Li & Li, 1998; Martindale *et al.*, 1998) including myoblasts from a transgenic mouse model (Orth *et al.*, 2003).

Excitotoxicity is thought to play an important role in the pathogenesis of Huntington's disease. For instance, intrastriatal injections of kainate results in striatal lesions are similar to HD (Beal, 1992; Coyle & Schwarcz, 1976; McGeer & McGeer, 1976). Quinolinic acid also results in lesions similar to HD in association with chorea (Schwarcz *et al.*, 1983; Beal *et al.*, 1986, 1989).

There is evidence of significant mitochondrial dysfunction in HD brain tissue (Mann *et al.*, 1990). This amounts to a 56% decrease in complex II and complex III activity, and a 33% defect in complex IV activity (Gu *et al.*, 1996; Browne *et al.*, 1997). There is also evidence of a defect of aconitase activity which parallels the neuropathology (Tabrizi *et al.*, 1999). Respiratory chain activities were normal in HD cerebellum and fibroblasts (Schapira, 1999). These observations are of interest, in that they parallel the biochemical defect induced by 3-nitropropionic acid (3-NP) which is an irreversible inhibitor of complex II, and infusion of this agent induces lesions that mimic those found in HD (Brouillet *et al.*, 1993; Beal *et al.*, 1993). The 3-NP induced lesions are dependent upon excitotoxicity through glutamatergic input (Weller & Paul, 1993) that is unlikely to be the only mechanism by which this toxin acts (Weller & Paul, 1993).

3-NP induces encephalopathy and coma with dystonia and chorea in human survivors (Ludolph *et al.*, 1991). The CT scans of those exposed to 3-NP show bilateral hypodensities in the putamen and global pallidus (Ludolph *et al.*, 1991). Thus, complex II inhibition can produce a biochemical and pathological picture which mimics HD.

Given that mutant huntingtin is expressed in skeletal muscle, it is of interest that phosphorus magnetic resonance spectroscopy of skeletal muscle in HD patients has demonstrated a decrease in ATP synthesis, the severity of which is dependent upon the CAG repeat (Lodi *et al.*, 2000). A similar, but milder, defect was present in pre-symptomatic patients in this study. Proton spectroscopy of HD brains has demonstrated increased lactate levels in the occipital cortex in the basal ganglia (Kuwert *et al.*, 1990; Jenkins *et al.*, 1993, 1998), although this has not been found in all studies (Hoang *et al.*, 1998). One study has also shown a decrease in cortical lactate with CoQ10 (Koroshetz *et al.*, 1997).

The mitochondrial defect present in HD brain and muscle extends to the R62 transgenic mouse model of HD, where in the striatum there is evidence of a significant reduction of complex IV and aconitase with a decrease in complex IV in cerebral cortex (Tabrizi *et al.*, 2000). These changes were accompanied by an increase in immunostaining for inducible nitric oxide synthase.

These abnormalities suggest involvement of excitoxic mechanisms, in particular, the generation of nitric oxide and peroxynitrite. The early defect of complex IV activity is supported by similar findings in HD lymphoblasts (Sawa *et al.*, 1999). This defect might initiate a chain of events resulting in excess free-radical production, complex II/III and aconitase inhibition.

The relevance of these mitochondrial abnormalities to the pathogenesis of HD remains uncertain. Importantly, their relationship to the huntingtin mutation is not known, but the correlation of the mitochondrial defect with the degree of polyglutamine expansion suggests some direct relationship between the two. Creatine supplementation prolongs the survival of the R62 transgenic mouse (Ferrante *et al.*, 2000), although creatine supplementation in HD does not appear to result in benefit at least over a 12-month period (Tabrizi *et al.*, 2003). CoQ10 has also been tried in HD patients and, whilst there was no significant improvement in the clinical features of HD, there was a trend towards benefit (Huntington Study Group, 2001).

Alzheimer's disease

Several groups have found a reduction in complex IV activity in the brain and sometimes in the platelets of patients with Alzheimer's disease (Kish *et al.*, 1992; Parker *et al.*, 1994a,b; Mutisya *et al.*, 1994). Histochemical stains have also shown a decrease in cytochrome oxidase in the dentate gyrus and hippocampus of AD (Simonian & Hyman, 1993), and there is a reduction in the mRNA for subunit II of cytochrome oxidase (Simonian & Hyman, 1993). No mutations of mitochondrial DNA have been identified in AD patients. The cytochrome oxidase defects may be the result of increased oxidative stress in AD (Bonilla *et al.*, 1999), and thus represent a secondary phenomenon. There is also evidence of microglial activation in AD, and this too could contribute to the complex IV defect.

Friedreich's ataxia

Friedreich's ataxia is an autosomal recessive disorder characterized by onset usually at adolescence with progressive limb and gait ataxia, areflexia, peripheral neuropathy and hypertrophic cardiomyopathy in association with skeletal abnormalities (Durr *et al.*, 1996). In over 95% of patients this disease is caused by GAA triplet repeat in intron I of the gene for frataxin (Campuzano *et al.*, 1996). The remaining patients are compound heterozygous with a GAA expansion in one allele and a point mutation in the other (Pook *et al.*, 2000).

The length of the GAA repeat determines the level of residual frataxin (Bidichandani *et al.*, 1998; Wong *et al.*, 1997; Campuzaro *et al.*, 1997). The physiological function of frataxin is not known, although it is a mitochondrial protein, likely involved in iron homeostasis, and probably in iron–sulphur protein construction (Lill *et al.*, 1999; Kispal *et al.*, 1999).

The yeast frataxin homologue knockout model of human frataxin deficiency results in mitochondrial abnormalities including impaired respiratory chain function, iron accumulation, decreased mitochondrial DNA levels, and increased oxidative stress. Based upon these observations, severe deficiencies of complexes I,II and III and aconitase were identified in cardiac muscle from FRDA patients (Rotig *et al.*, 1997; Bradley *et al.*, 2001). These enzymes all contain iron–sulphur clusters. The decrease in respiratory chain activities precede iron accumulation in the conditional frataxin knockout transgenic mouse model of FRDA (Puccio *et al.*, 2001), and so it appears likely that failure of construction of these iron–sulphur proteins is an early event, which may then be followed by secondary free-radical mediated damage.

The respiratory chain defect in patients can be detected by phosphorus magnetic resonance spectroscopy in vivo in skeletal muscle. The defect in ATP synthesis (V_{max}) correlated with the length of the GAA repeat (Lodi *et al.*, 1999, 2001). In addition to evidence for mitochondrial dysfunction, there is also additional evidence of free-radical mediated damage including elevated malondialdehyde levels (Emond *et al.*, 2000), and urine 8-hydroxy-2′-deoxyguanosine levels. Free glutathione is also decreased in blood from FRDA patients (Piemonte *et al.*, 2001). Fibroblast culture from FRDA patients show increased sensitivity to hydrogen peroxide (Wong *et al.*, 1999).

The evidence for mitochondrial dysfunction and free-radical damage in FRDA patients prompted therapeutic intervention with antioxidants such as idebenone and co-enzyme Q10 with vitamin E. A variety of markers for disease severity have been used in FRDA including echocardiography (Lodi *et al.*, 2001; Hausse *et al.*, 2002), phosphorus MR spectroscopy (Lodi *et al.*, 2001) and urine 8-hydroxy-2′-deoxyguanosine (Schols *et al.*, 2001).

Idebenone has shown improvement in cardiac hypertrophy as determined by echocardiography, in some, but not all patients (Hausse *et al.*, 2002). This compound failed to improve phosphorus magnetic resonance spectroscopy or echocardiography in another study (Schols *et al.*, 2001). Treatment with a combination of coenzyme Q10, 400 mg a day and vitamin E, 2100 international units a day improved MRS data in heart and skeletal muscle after 6 months (Lodi *et al.*, 2001). Four-year follow-up has shown that this benefit is maintained and is also associated with some clinical improvement (Hart & Schapira, 2004).

Motor neurone disease (amyotrophic lateral sclerosis)

Motor neurone disease (MND) or amyotrophic lateral sclerosis (ALS) is characterized by degeneration of anterior horn cells, spinal cord and motor cortex. Ten per cent of cases are familial and, in 25% of these, there are mutations in the gene encoding cytosolic copper, zinc, superoxide dismutase (Rosen *et al.*, 1993; Cudkowicz *et al.*, 1997). These mutations may produce toxicity by mechanisms involving increased peroxide nitrite formation (Moncada *et al.*, 1989; Crow *et al.*, 1997; Estevez *et al.*, 1999). There is evidence for oxidative stress and damage in ALS tissue including motor cortex (Ferrante *et al.*, 1997; Bowling *et al.*, 1993) and the spinal cord (Shaw *et al.*, 1995) and levels of 8-hydroxy-2′-deoxyguanosine (8OH2′dG) are increased in the cortex, cord (Ferrante *et al.*, 1997; Fitzmaurice *et al.*, 1996) and in urine plasma and CSF (Bogdanov *et al.*, 2000).

Several studies have demonstrated defects of the respiratory chain in tissues from MND patients. For instance, a defect in complex I activity has been found in skeletal muscle (Wiedemann *et al.*, 1998). Reduced cytochrome oxidase activity has been found in anterior horn cells (Borthwick *et al.*, 1999). Multiple mitochondrial DNA mutations have been found in ALS patients (Vielhaber *et al.*, 2000). A mutation in subunit I of complex IV with reduced cytochrome oxidase activity was identified in one patient with MND (Comi *et al.*, 1998).

The transgenic mice with an SOD1 mutation show morphological changes in the mitochondria (Kong & Xu, 1998). Creatine supplementation improves survival in these animals (Klivenyi *et al.*, 1999), but has not yet been used in patients.

REFERENCES

Alam, Z. I., Daniel, S. E., Lees, A. J., Marsden, D. C., Jenner, P. & Halliwell, B. (1997a). A generalised increase in protein carbonyls in the brain in Parkinson's but not incidental Lewy body disease. *J. Neurochem.*, **69**, 1326–9.

Alam, Z. I., Jenner, A., Daniel, S. E. *et al.* (1997b). Oxidative DNA damage in the parkinsonian brain: an apparent selective increase in 8-hydroxyguanine levels in substantia nigra. *J. Neurochem.*, **69**, 196–203.

Allard, J. C., Tilak, S., Carter, A. P. (1988). CT and MR of MELAS syndrome. *Am. J. Neuroradiol.*, **9**, 1234–8.

Andreu, A. L., Hanna, M. G., Reichmann, H., S. *et al.* (1999). Exercise intolerance due to mutations in the cytochrome b gene of mitochondrial DNA. *N. Engl. J. Med.*, **341**, 1037–44.

Baumgartner, E. R., Suormala, T. M., Wick, H. *et al.* (1989). Biotinidase deficiency: a cause of subacute necrotizing encephalomyelopathy (Leigh syndrome). Report of a case with lethal outcome. *Pediatr. Res.*, **26**, 260–6.

Beal, M. F. (1992). Does impairment of energy metabolism result in excitotoxic neuronal death in neurodegenerative illnesses? *Ann. Neurol.*, **31**, 119–30.

Beal, M. F., Kowell, N. W., Ellison, D. W. *et al.* (1986). Replication of the neurochemical characteristics of Huntington's disease by Quinolinic acid. *Nature*, **321**, 168–171.

Beal, M. F., Kowall, N. W., Ferrante, R. J. & Cippolloni, P. B. (1989). Quinolinic acid striatal lesions in primates as a model of Huntington's disease. *Ann. Neurol.*, **26**, 137.

Beal, M. F., Brouillet, E., Jenkins, B. G. *et al.* (1993). Neurochemical and histologic characterization of striatal excitotoxic lesions produced by the mitochondrial toxin 3-nitropropionic acid. *J. Neurosci.*, **13**, 4181–92.

Berkovic, S. F., Carpenter, S., Evans, A. *et al.* (1989). Myoclonus epilepsy and ragged-red fibres (MERRF). 1. A clinical, pathological, biochemical, magnetic resonance spectrographic and positron emission tomographic study. *Brain*, **112**, 1231–60.

Betarbet, R., Sherer, T. B., MacKenzie, G., Garcia-Osuna, M., Panov, A. V. & Greenamyre, J. T. (2000). Chronic systemic pesticide exposure reproduces features of Parkinson's disease. *Nat. Neurosci.*, **3**, 1301–6.

Bidichandani, S. I., Ashizawa, T. & Patel, P. I. (1998). The GAA triplet-repeat expansion Friedreich's ataxia interferes with transcription and may be associated with an unusual DNA structure. *Am. J. Hum. Genet.*, **62**, 111–12.

Bogdanov, M., Brown, R. H., Matson, W. *et al.* (2000). Increased oxidative damage to DNA in ALS patients. *Free. Radic. Biol. Med.*, **29**, 652–8.

Bonilla, E., Tanji, K., Hirano, M., Vu, T. H., DiMauro, S., Schon, E. A. (1999). Mitochondrial involvement in Alzheimer's disease. *Biochim. Biophys. Acta.*, **1410**, 171–82.

Borner, G. V., Zeviani, M., Tiranti, V. *et al.* (2000). Decreased aminoacylation of mutant tRNAs in MELAS but not in MERRF patients. *Hum. Mol. Genet.*, **9**, 467–75.

Borthwick, G. M., Johnson, M. A., Ince, P. G., Shaw, P. J. & Turnbull, D. M. (1999). Mitochondrial enzyme activity in amyotrophic lateral sclerosis: implications for the role of mitochondria in neuronal cell death. *Ann. Neurol.*, **46**, 787–90.

Bourgeron, T., Rustin, P., Chretien, D. *et al.* (1995). Mutation of a nuclear succinate dehydrogenase gene results in mitochondrial respiratory chain deficiency. *Nat. Genet.*, **11**, 144–9.

Bowling, A. C., Schulz, J. B., Brown, R. H., Jr. & Beal, M. F. (1993). Superoxide dismutase activity, oxidative damage, and mitochondrial energy metabolism in familial and sporadic amyotrophic lateral sclerosis. *J. Neurochem.*, **61**, 2322–5.

Bradley, J. L., Blake, J. C., Chamberlain, S., Thomas, P. K., Cooper, J. M. & Schapira, A. H. (2000). Clinical, biochemical and molecular genetic correlations in Friedreich's ataxia. *Hum. Mol. Genet.*, **9**, 275–82.

Brouillet, E., Jenkins, B. G., Hyman, B. T. *et al.* (1993). Age-dependent vulnerability of the striatum to the mitochondrial toxin 3-nitropropionic acid. *J. Neurochem.*, **60**, 356–9.

Browne, S. E., Bowling, A. C., MacGarvey, U. *et al.* (1997). Oxidative damage and metabolic dysfunction in Huntington's disease: selective vulnerability of the basal ganglia. *Ann. Neurol.*, **41**, 646–53.

Campuzano, V., Montermini, L., Molto, M. D. *et al.* (1996). Friedreich's ataxia: autosomal recessive disease caused by an intronic GAA triplet repeat expansion. *Science*, **8**(271), 1423–7.

Campuzano, V., Montermini, L., Lutz, Y. *et al.* (1997). Frataxin is reduced in Freidreich's ataxia patients and is associated with mitochondrial membranes. *Hum. Mol. Genet.*, **6**, 1771–80.

Chalmers, R. M., Davis, M. B., Sweeney, M. G., Wood, N. W. & Harding, A. E. (1996). Evidence against an X-linked visual loss susceptibility locus in Leber hereditary optic neuropathy. *Am. J. Hum. Genet.*, **59**, 103–8.

Chiba, K., Trevor, A. J. & Castagnoli, N. Jr. (1985). Active uptake of MPP+, a metabolite of MPTP, by brain synaptosomes. *Biochem. Biophys. Res. Commun.*, **128**, 1228–32.

Chomyn, A. (1998). The myoclonic epilepsy and ragged-red fiber mutation provides new insights into human mitochondrial function and genetics. *Am. J. Hum. Genet.*, **62**, 745–51.

Chomyn, A., Meola, G., Bresolin, N., Lai S. T., Scarlato, G. & Attardi, G. (1991). In vitro genetic transfer of protein synthesis and respiration defects to mitochondrial DNA-less cells with myopathy-patient mitochondria. *Mol. Cell. Biol.*, **11**, 2236–44.

Comi, G. P., Bordoni, A., Salani, S. *et al.* (1998). Cytochrome c oxidase subunit I microdeletion in a patient with motor neuron disease. *Ann. Neurol.*, **43**, 110–16.

Cooper, J. K., Schilling, G., Peters, M. F. *et al.* (1998). Truncated N-terminal fragments of huntingtin with expanded glutamine repeats form nuclear and cytoplasmic aggregates in cell culture. *Hum. Mol. Genet.*, **7**, 783–90.

Coyle, J. T. & Schwarcz, R. (1976). Lesion of striatal neurones with kainic acid provides a model for Huntington's chorea. *Nature*, **263**, 244–6.

Crow, J. P., Sampson, J. B., Zhuang, Y., Thompson, J. A. & Beckman, J. S. (1997). Decreased zinc affinity of amyotrophic lateral sclerosis-associated superoxide dismutase mutants leads to enhanced catalysis of tyrosine nitration by peroxynitrite. *J. Neurochem.*, **69**, 1936–44.

Cudkowicz, M. E., McKenna-Yasek, D., Sapp, P. E. *et al.* (1997). Epidemiology of mutations in superoxide dismutase in amyotrophic lateral sclerosis. *Ann. Neurol.*, **41**, 210–21.

de Vries, D. D., van Engelen, B. G., Gabreels, F. J., Ruitenbeek, W. K. & van Oost, B. A. (1993). A second missense mutation in the mitochondrial ATPase 6 gene in Leigh's syndrome. *Ann. Neurol.*, **34**, 410–12.

De Vries, D. D., Went, L. N., Bruyn, G. W. *et al.* (1996). Genetic and biochemical impairment of mitochondrial complex I activity in a family with Leber hereditary optic neuropathy and hereditary spastic dystonia. *Am. J. Hum. Genet.*, **58**, 703–11.

Dexter, D. T., Wells, F. R., Lees, A. J. *et al.* (1989). Increased nigral iron content and alterations in other metal ions occurring in brain in Parkinson's disease. *J. Neurochem.*, **52**, 1830–6.

Dexter, D. T., Holley, A. E., Flitter, W. D. *et al.* (1994). Increased levels of lipid hydroperoxides in the parkinsonian substantia nigra: an HPLC and ESR study. *Mov. Disord.*, **9**(1), 92–7. Erratum in: *Mov. Disord*, 1994 May, 9–380.

Dunbar, D. R., Moonie, P. A., Swingler, R. J., Davidson, D., Roberts, R. & Holt, I. J. (1993). Maternally transmitted partial direct tandem duplication of mitochondrial DNA associated with diabetes mellitus. *Hum. Mol. Genet.*, **2**, 1619–24.

Durr, A., Cossee, M., Agid, Y. *et al.* (1996). Clinical and genetic abnormalities in patients with Friedreich's ataxia. *N. Engl. J. Med.*, **335**, 1169–75.

Elkon, H., Don, J., Melamed, E., Ziv, I., Shirvan, A. & Offen, D. (2002). Mutant and wild-type alpha-synuclein interact with mitochondrial cytochrome C oxidase. *J. Mol. Neurosci.*, **18**, 229–38.

Emond, M., Lepage, G., Vanasse, M. & Pandolfo, M. (2000). Increased levels of plasma malondialdehyde in Friedreich ataxia. *Neurology*, **55**, 1752–3.

Enriquez, J. A., Chomyn, A. & Attardi, G. (1995). mtDNA mutation in MERRF syndrome causes defective aminoacylation of tRNA(Lys) and premature translation termination. *Nat. Genet.*, **10**, 47–55.

Estevez, A. G., Crow, J. P., Sampson, J. B. *et al.* (1999). Induction of nitric oxide-dependent apoptosis in motor neurons by zinc-deficient superoxide dismutase. *Science*, **286**, 2498–500.

Ferrante, R. J., Browne, S. E., Shinobu, L. A. *et al.* (1997). Evidence of increased oxidative damage in both sporadic and familial amyotrophic lateral sclerosis. *J. Neurochem.*, **69**, 2064–74.

Ferrante, R. J., Shinobu, L. A., Schulz, J. B. *et al.* (1997). Increased 3-nitrotyrosine and oxidative damage in mice with a human copper/zinc superoxide dismutase mutation. *Ann. Neurol.*, **42**, 326–34.

Ferrante, R. J., Andreassen, O. A., Jenkins, B. G. *et al.* (2000). Neuroprotective effects of creatine in a transgenic mouse model of Huntington's disease. *J. Neurosci.*, **20**, 4389–97.

Fitzmaurice, P. S., Shaw, I. C., Kleiner, H. E. et al. (1996). Evidence for DNA damage in amyotrophic lateral sclerosis. Muscle Nerve, 19, 797–8.

Folgero, T., Torbergsen, T. & Oian, P. (1995). The 3243 MELAS mutation in a pedigree with MERRF. Eur. Neurol., 35, 168–71.

Fryer, A., Appleton, R., Sweeney, M. G., Rosenbloom, L. & Harding, A. E. (1994). Mitochondrial DNA 8993 (NARP) mutation presenting with a heterogeneous phenotype including 'cerebral palsy'. Arch. Dis. Child., 71, 419–22.

Fukuhara, N., Tokiguchi, S., Shirakawa, K. & Tsubaki, T. (1980). Myoclonus epilepsy associated with ragged-red fibres (mitochondrial abnormalities): disease entity or a syndrome? Light- and electron-microscopic studies of two cases and review of literature. J. Neurol. Sci., 47, 117–33.

Gattermann, N., Retzlaff, S., Wang, Y. L. et al. (1997). Heteroplasmic point mutations of mitochondrial DNA affecting subunit I of cytochrome c oxidase in two patients with acquired idiopathic sideroblastic anemia. Blood, 90, 4961–72.

Gerbitz, K. D., Paprotta, A., Jaksch, M., Zierz, S. & Drechsel, J. (1993). Diabetes mellitus is one of the heterogeneous phenotypic features of a mitochondrial DNA point mutation within the tRNALeu(UUR) gene. FEBS Lett., 321, 194–6.

Gerbitz, K. D., van den Ouweland, J. M., Maassen, J. A. & Jaksch, M. (1995). Mitochondrial diabetes mellitus: a review. Biochim. Biophys. Acta, 1271, 253–60.

Goto, Y., Nonaka, I. & Horai, S. (1990). A mutation in the tRNA(Leu)(UUR) gene associated with the MELAS subgroup of mitochondrial encephalomyopathies. Nature, 348, 651–3.

Graf, W. D., Sumi, S. M., Copass, M. K. et al. (1993). Phenotypic heterogeneity in families with the myoclonic epilepsy and ragged-red fiber disease point mutation in mitochondrial DNA. Ann. Neurol., 33, 640–5.

Gu, M., Gash, M. T., Mann, V. M. Javoy-Agid F., Cooper J. M. & Schapira, A. H. (1996). Mitochondrial defect in Huntington's disease caudate nucleus. Ann. Neurol., 39, 385–9.

Gu, M., Gash, M. T., Cooper, J. M. et al. (1997). Mitochondrial respiratory chain function in multiple system atrophy. Mov. Disord., 12, 418–22.

Gu, M., Cooper, J. M., Taanman, J. W. & Schapira, A. H. (1998). Mitochondrial DNA transmission of the mitochondrial defect in Parkinson's disease. Ann. Neurol., 44, 177–86.

Guan, M. X., Enriquez, J. A., Fischel-Ghodsian, N. et al. (1998). The deafness-associated mitochondrial DNA mutation at position 7445, which affects tRNASer(UCN) precursor processing, has long-range effects on NADH dehydrogenase subunit ND6 gene expression. Mol. Cell. Biol., 18, 5868–79.

Hammans, S. R., Sweeney, M. G., Brockington, M., Morgan-Hughes, J. A. & Harding, A. E. (1991). Mitochondrial encephalopathies: molecular genetic diagnosis from blood samples. Lancet, 337, 1311–13.

Hammans, S. R., Sweeney, M. G., Brockington, M. et al. (1993). The mitochondrial DNA transfer RNA(Lys)A–>G(8344) mutation and the syndrome of myoclonic epilepsy with ragged red fibres (MERRF). Relationship of clinical phenotype to proportion of mutant mitochondrial DNA. Brain, 116, 617–32.

Hantraye, P., Brouillet, E., Ferrante, R. et al. (1996). Inhibition of neuronal nitric oxide synthase prevents MPTP-induced parkinsonism in baboons. Nat. Med., 2, 1017–21.

Hao, H. & Moraes, C. T. (1996). Functional and molecular mitochondrial abnormalities associated with a C -> T transition at position 3256 of the human mitochondrial genome. The effects of a pathogenic mitochondrial tRNA point mutation in organelle translation and RNA processing. J. Biol. Chem., 26, 271, 2347–52.

Hart, P. E. & Schapira, A. H. V. (2004). Antioxidant treatment of patients with Friedreich's ataxia: 4-year follow up. Arch. Neurol. (in press).

Hattori, N., Tanaka, M., Ozawa, T. & Mizuno, Y. (1991). Immunohistochemical studies on complexes I, II, III, and IV of mitochondria in Parkinson's disease. Ann. Neurol., 30, 563–71.

Hausse, A. O., Aggoun, Y., Bonnet, D. et al. (2002). Idebenone and reduced cardiac hypertrophy in Friedreich's ataxia. Heart, 87, 346–9.

Helm, M., Florentz, C., Chomyn, A. & Attardi, G. (1999). Search for differences in post-transcriptional modification patterns of mitochondrial DNA-encoded wild-type and mutant human tRNALys and tRNALeu(UUR). Nucl. Acids Res., 27, 756–63.

Hirano, M., Silvestri, G., Blake, D. M. et al. (1994). Mitochondrial neurogastrointestinal encephalomyopathy (MNGIE): clinical, biochemical, and genetic features of an autosomal recessive mitochondrial disorder. Neurology, 44, 721–7.

Hirsch, E. C., Brandel, J. P., Galle, P., Javoy-Agid, F. & Agid, Y. (1991). Iron and aluminum increase in the substantia nigra of patients with Parkinson's disease: an X-ray microanalysis. J. Neurochem., 56, 446–51.

Hoang, T. Q., Bluml, S., Dubowitz, D. J. et al. (1998). Quantitative proton-decoupled ^{31}P MRS and ^{1}H MRS in the evaluation of Huntington's and Parkinson's diseases. Neurology, 50, 1033–40.

Hoglinger, G. U., Feger, J., Prigent, A. et al. (2003). Chronic systemic complex I inhibition induces a hypokinetic multisystem degeneration in rats. J. Neurochem., 84, 491–502.

Holme, E., Larsson, N. G., Oldfors, A., Tulinius, M., Sahlin, P. & Stenman, G. (1993). Multiple symmetric lipomas with high levels of mtDNA with the tRNA(Lys)A–>G(8344) mutation as the only manifestation of disease in a carrier of myoclonus epilepsy and ragged-red fibers (MERRF) syndrome. Am. J. Hum. Genet., 52(3), 551–6.

Holt, I. J., Harding, A. E. & Morgan-Hughes, J. A (1988). Deletions of muscle mitochondrial DNA in patients with mitochondrial myopathies. Nature, 331, 717–19.

Holt, I. J., Harding, A. E., Cooper, J. M. et al. (1989). Mitochondrial myopathies: clinical and biochemical features of 30 patients with major deletions of muscle mitochondrial DNA. Ann. Neurol., 26, 699–708.

Holt, I. J., Harding, A. E., Petty, R. K. & Morgan-Hughes, J. A. (1990). A new mitochondrial disease associated with mitochondrial DNA heteroplasmy. Am. J. Hum. Genet., 46, 428–33.

Holt, I. J., Dunbar, D. R. & Jacobs, H. T. (1997). Behaviour of a population of partially duplicated mitochondrial DNA molecules in cell culture: segregation, maintenance and recombination dependent upon nuclear background. *Hum. Mol. Genet.*, **6**, 1251–60.

Howell, N. (1997). Leber hereditary optic neuropathy: how do mitochondrial DNA mutations cause degeneration of the optic nerve? *J. Bioenerg. Biomembr.*, **29**, 165–73.

Howell, N., Bindoff, L. A., McCullough, D. A. *et al.* (1991). Leber hereditary optic neuropathy: identification of the same mitochondrial ND1 mutation in six pedigrees. *Am. J. Hum. Genet.*, **49**, 939–50.

Howell, N., Kubacka, I., Smith, R., Frerman, F., Parks, J. K. & Parker, W. D. Jr. (1996). Association of the mitochondrial 8344 MERRF mutation with maternally inherited spinocerebellar degeneration and Leigh disease. *Neurology*, **46**, 219–22.

Hudgson, P., Bradley, W. G. & Jenkison, M. (1972). Familial "mitochondrial" myopathy. A myopathy associated with disordered oxidative metabolism in muscle fibres. 1. Clinical, electrophysiological and pathological findings. *J. Neurol. Sci.*, **16**, 343–70.

Huntington Study Group. (2001). A randomized, placebo-controlled trial of coenzyme Q10 and remacemide in Huntington's disease. *Neurology*, **57**, 397–404.

Javitch, J. A. & Snyder, S. H. (1984). Uptake of MPP(+) by dopamine neurons explains selectivity of parkinsonism-inducing neurotoxin, MPTP. *Eur. J. Pharmacol.*, **106**, 455–6.

Jenkins, B. G., Koroshetz, W. J., Beal, M. F. & Rosen, D. R. (1993). Evidence for impairment of energy metabolism in vivo in Huntington's disease using localized ^{1}H NMR spectroscopy. *Neurology*, **43**, 2689–95.

Jenkins, B. G., Rosas, H. D., Chen, Y. C. *et al.* (1998). ^{1}H NMR spectroscopy studies of Huntington's disease: correlations with CAG repeat numbers. *Neurology*, **50**, 1357–65.

Johns, D. R., Neufeld, M. J. & Park, R. D. (1992). An ND-6 mitochondrial DNA mutation associated with Leber hereditary optic neuropathy. *Biochem. Biophys. Res. Commun.*, **187**, 1551–7.

Jun, A. S., Brown, M. D. & Wallace, D. C. (1994). A mitochondrial DNA mutation at nucleotide pair 14459 of the NADH dehydrogenase subunit 6 gene associated with maternally inherited Leber hereditary optic neuropathy and dystonia. *Proc. Natl Acad. Sci., USA*, **21**(91), 6206–10.

Kadowaki, H., Tobe, K., Mori, Y. *et al.* (1993). Mitochondrial gene mutation and insulin-deficient type of diabetes mellitus. *Lancet*, **341**, 893–4.

Kamieniecka, Z. (1977). Myopathies with abnormal mitochondria. A clinical, histological, and electrophysiological study. *Acta. Neurol. Scand.*, **55**, 57–75.

Kaukonen, J., Zeviani, M., Comi, G. P., Piscaglia, M. G., Peltonen, L. & Suomalainen, A. (1999). A third locus predisposing to multiple deletions of mtDNA in autosomal dominant progressive external ophthalmoplegia. *Am. J. Hum. Genet.*, **65**, 256–61.

Kaukonen, J., Juselius, J. K., Tiranti, V. *et al.* (2000). Role of adenine nucleotide translocator 1 in mtDNA maintenance. *Science*, **289**, 782–5.

Keightley, J. A., Hoffbuhr, K. C., Burton, M. D. *et al.* (1996). A microdeletion in cytochrome c oxidase (COX) subunit III associated with COX deficiency and recurrent myoglobinuria. *Nat. Genet.*, **12**, 410–6.

King, M. P., Koga, Y., Davidson, M. & Schon, E. A. (1992). Defects in mitochondrial protein synthesis and respiratory chain activity segregate with the tRNA(Leu(UUR)) mutation associated with mitochondrial myopathy, encephalopathy, lactic acidosis, and stroke-like episodes. *Mol. Cell. Biol.*, **12**, 480–90.

Kish, S. J., Bergeron, C., Rajput, A. *et al.* (1992). Brain cytochrome oxidase in Alzheimer's disease. *J. Neurochem.*, **59**, 776–9.

Kispal, G., Csere, P., Prohl, C. & Lill, R. (1999). The mitochondrial proteins Atm1p and Nfs1p are essential for biogenesis of cytosolic Fe/S proteins. *EMBO J.*, **18**, 3981–9.

Klivenyi, P., Ferrante, R. J., Matthews, R. T. *et al.* (1999). Neuroprotective effects of creatine in a transgenic animal model of amyotrophic lateral sclerosis. *Nat. Med.*, **5**, 347–50.

Kobayashi, Y., Momoi, M. Y., Tominaga, K. *et al.* (1990). A point mutation in the mitochondrial tRNA(Leu)(UUR) gene in MELAS (mitochondrial myopathy, encephalopathy, lactic acidosis and stroke-like episodes). *Biochem. Biophys. Res. Commun.*, **173**, 816–22.

Koga, Y., Yoshino, M. & Kato, H. (1998). MELAS exhibits dominant negative effects on mitochondrial RNA processing. *Ann. Neurol.*, **43**, 835.

Kong, J. & Xu, Z. (1998). Massive mitochondrial degeneration in motor neurons triggers the onset of amyotrophic lateral sclerosis in mice expressing a mutant SOD1. *J. Neurosci.*, **18**, 3241–50.

Koroshetz, W. J., Jenkins, B. G., Rosen, B. R. & Beal, M. F. (1997). Energy metabolism defects in Huntington's disease and effects of coenzyme Q10. *Ann. Neurol.*, **41**, 160–5.

Kretzschmar, H. A., DeArmond, S. J., Koch, T. K. *et al.* (1987). Pyruvate dehydrogenase complex deficiency as a cause of subacute necrotizing encephalopathy (Leigh disease). *Pediatrics*, **79**, 370–3.

Kuriyama, M., Umezaki, H., Fukuda, Y. *et al.* (1984). Mitochondrial encephalomyopathy with lactate-pyruvate elevation and brain infarctions. *Neurology*, **34**, 72–7.

Kuwert, T., Lange, H. W., Langen, K. J., Herzog, H., Aulich, A. & Feinendegen, L. E. (1990). Cortical and subcortical glucose consumption measured by PET in patients with Huntington's disease. *Brain*, **113**, 1405–23.

Langston, J. W. & Ballard, P. (1984). Parkinsonism induced by 1-methyl-4-phenyl-1,2,3,6-tetrahydropyridine (MPTP): implications for treatment and the pathogenesis of Parkinson's disease. *Can. J. Neurol. Sci.*, **11**, 160–5.

Larsson, N. G., Andersen, O., Holme, E., Oldfors, A. & Wahlstrom, J. (1991). Leber's hereditary optic neuropathy and complex I deficiency in muscle. *Ann. Neurol.*, **30**, 701–8.

Larsson, N. G., Tulinius, M. H., Holme, E. & Oldfors, A. (1995). Pathogenetic aspects of the A8344G mutation of mitochondrial DNA associated with MERRF syndrome and multiple symmetric lipomas. *Muscle Nerve*, **3**, S102–6.

Leigh, D. (1951). Subacute necrotizing encephalomyelopathy in an infant. *J. Neurochem.*, **14**, 216–21.

Li, F. Y., Tariq, M., Croxen, R. *et al.* (1999). Mapping of autosomal dominant progressive external ophthalmoplegia to a 7-cM critical region on 10q24. *Neurology*, **53**, 1265–71.

Li, S. H. & Li, X. J. (1998). Aggregation of N-terminal huntingtin is dependent on the length of its glutamine repeats. *Hum. Mol. Genet.*, **7**, 777–82.

Lill, R., Diekert, K., Kaut, A. *et al.* (1999). The essential role of mitochondria in the biogenesis of cellular iron-sulfur proteins. *Biol. Chem.*, **380**, 1157–66.

Lodi, R., Cooper, J. M., Bradley, J. L. *et al.* (1999). Deficit of in vivo mitochondrial ATP production in patients with Friedreich ataxia. *Proc. Natl Acad. Sci., USA*, **96**, 11492–5.

Lodi, R., Schapira, A. H., Manners, D. *et al.* (2000). Abnormal in vivo skeletal muscle energy metabolism in Huntington's disease and dentatorubropallidoluysian atrophy. *Ann. Neurol.*, **48**, 72–6.

Lodi, R., Hart, P. E., Rajagopalan, B. *et al.* (2001). Antioxidant treatment improves in vivo cardiac and skeletal muscle bioenergetics in patients with Friedreich's ataxia. *Ann. Neurol.*, **49**, 590–6.

Lodi, R., Rajagopalan, B., Blamire, A. M. *et al.* (2001). Cardiac energetics are abnormal in Friedreich ataxia patients in the absence of cardiac dysfunction and hypertrophy: an in vivo 31P magnetic resonance spectroscopy study. *Cardiovasc. Res.* **52**, 111–19.

Loeffen, J., Smeitink, J., Triepels, R. *et al.* (1998). The first nuclear-encoded complex I mutation in a patient with Leigh syndrome. *Am. J. Hum. Genet.*, **63**, 1598–608.

Ludolph, A. C., He, F., Spencer, P. S., Hammerstad, J. & Sabri, M. (1991). 3-Nitropropionic acid exogenous animal neurotoxin and possible human striatal toxin. *Can. J. Neurol. Sci.*, **18**, 492–8.

Mackey, D. & Howell, N. (1992). A variant of Leber hereditary optic neuropathy characterized by recovery of vision and by an unusual mitochondrial genetic etiology. *Am. J. Hum. Genet.*, **51**, 1218–28.

Makela-Bengs, P., Suomalainen, A., Majander, A. *et al.* (1995). Correlation between the clinical symptoms and the proportion of mitochondrial DNA carrying the 8993 point mutation in the NARP syndrome. *Pediatr. Res.*, **37**, 634–9.

Mann, V. M., Cooper, J. M., Javoy-Agid, F., Agid, Y., Jenner, P. & Schapira, A. H. (1990). Mitochondrial function and parental sex effect in Huntington's disease. *Lancet*, **336**, 749.

Martindale, D., Hackam, A., Wieczorek, A. *et al.* (1998). Length of huntingtin and its polyglutamine tract influences localization and frequency of intracellular aggregates. *Nat. Genet.*, **18**, 150–4.

Masucci, J. P., Davidson, M., Koga, Y., Schon, E. A. & King, M. P. (1995). In vitro analysis of mutations causing myoclonus epilepsy with ragged-red fibers in the mitochondrial tRNA(Lys)gene: two genotypes produce similar phenotypes. *Mol. Cell. Biol.*, **15**, 2872–81.

McGeer, E. G. & McGeer, P. L. (1976). Duplication of biochemical changes of Huntington's chorea by intrastriatal injections of glutamic and kainic acids. *Nature*, **263**, 517–19.

Meire, F. M., Van Coster, R., Cochaux, P., Obermaier-Kusser, B., Candaele, C. & Martin, J. J. (1995). Neurological disorders in members of families with Leber's hereditary optic neuropathy (LHON) caused by different mitochondrial mutations. *Ophth. Genet.*, **16**, 119–26.

Melberg, A., Lundberg, P. O., Henriksson, K. G., Olsson, Y. & Stalberg, E. (1996). Muscle-nerve involvement in autosomal dominant progressive external ophthalmoplegia with hypogonadism. *Muscle Nerve*, **19**, 751–7.

Melberg, A., Holme, E., Oldfors, A. & Lundberg, P. O. (1998). Rhabdomyolysis in autosomal dominant progressive external ophthalmoplegia. *Neurology*, **50**, 299–300.

Mita, S., Rizzuto, R., Moraes, C. T. *et al.* (1990). Recombination via flanking direct repeats is a major cause of large-scale deletions of human mitochondrial DNA. *Nucleic. Acids Res.*, **18**, 561–7.

Moncada, S., Palmer, R. M. & Higgs, E. A. (1989). The biological significance of nitric oxide formation from L-arginine. *Biochem. Soc. Trans.*, **17**, 642–4.

Moraes, C. T., DiMauro, S., Zeviani, M. *et al.* (1989). Mitochondrial DNA deletions in progressive external ophthalmoplegia and Kearns-Sayre syndrome. *N. Engl. J. Med.*, **320**, 1293–9.

Moraes, C. T., Andreetta, F., Bonilla, E., Shanske, S., DiMauro, S. & Schon, E. A. (1991). Replication-competent human mitochondrial DNA lacking the heavy-strand promoter region. *Mol. Cell. Biol.*, **11**, 1631–7.

Moraes, C. T., Ricci, E., Petruzzella, V. *et al.* (1992). Molecular analysis of the muscle pathology associated with mitochondrial DNA deletions. *Nat. Genet.*, **1**, 359–67.

Moraes, C. T., Ciacci, F., Bonilla, E. *et al.* (1993). Two novel pathogenic mitochondrial DNA mutations affecting organelle number and protein synthesis. Is the tRNA(Leu(UUR)) gene an etiologic hot spot? *J. Clin. Invest.*, **92**, 2906–15.

Moraes, C. T., Ciacci, F., Silvestri, G. *et al.* (1993). Atypical clinical presentations associated with the MELAS mutation at position 3243 of human mitochondrial DNA. *Neuromuscul. Disord.*, **3**, 43–50.

Muller-Hocker, J. (1990). Cytochrome c oxidase deficient fibres in the limb muscle and diaphragm of man without muscular disease: an age-related alteration. *J. Neurol. Sci.*, **100**, 14–21.

Mutisya, E. M., Bowling, A. C. & Beal, M. F. (1994). Cortical cytochrome oxidase activity is reduced in Alzheimer's disease. *J. Neurochem.*, **63**, 2179–84.

Nakamura, M., Nakano, S., Goto, Y. *et al.* (1995). A novel point mutation in the mitochondrial tRNA(Ser(UCN)) gene detected in a family with MERRF/MELAS overlap syndrome. *Biochem. Biophys. Res. Commun.*, **214**, 86–93.

Nicklas, W. J., Vyas, I. & Heikkila, R. E. (1985). Inhibition of NADH-linked oxidation in brain mitochondria by 1-methyl-4-phenylpyridine, a metabolite of the neurotoxin, 1-methyl-4-phenyl-1,2,5,6-tetrahydropyridine. *Life Sci.*, **36**, 2503–8.

Nikoskelainen, E. K., Marttila, R. J., Huoponen, K. *et al.* (1995). Leber's "plus": neurological abnormalities in patients with Leber's hereditary optic neuropathy. *J. Neurol. Neurosurg. Psychiatry.*, **59**, 160–4.

Nishino, I., Spinazzola, A. & Hirano, M. (1999). Thymidine phosphorylase gene mutations in MNGIE, a human mitochondrial disorder. *Science*, **29**(283), 689–92.

Nishino, I., Spinazzola, A. & Papadimitriou, A. *et al.* (2000). Mitochondrial neurogastrointestinal encephalomyopathy: an autosomal recessive disorder due to thymidine phosphorylase mutations. *Ann. Neurol.*, **47**, 792–800.

Ohno, K., Tanaka, M., Sahashi, K. *et al.* (1991). Mitochondrial DNA deletions in inherited recurrent myoglobinuria. *Ann. Neurol.*, **29**, 364–9.

Orth, M., Cooper, J. M., Bates, G. P. & Schapira, A. H. (2003). Inclusion formation in Huntington's disease R6/2 mouse muscle cultures. *J. Neurochem.*, **87**, 1–6.

Ortiz, R. G., Newman, N. J., Shoffner, J. M., Kaufman, A. E., Koontz, D. A. & Wallace, D. C. (1993). Variable retinal and neurologic manifestations in patients harboring the mitochondrial DNA 8993 mutation. *Arch. Ophthalmol.*, **111**, 1525–30.

Parfait, B., de Lonlay, P., von Kleist-Retzow, J. C. *et al.* (1999). The neurogenic weakness, ataxia and retinitis pigmentosa (NARP) syndrome mtDNA mutation (T8993G) triggers muscle ATPase deficiency and hypocitrullinaemia. *Eur. J. Pediatr.*, **158**, 55–8.

Parker, W. D. Jr., Mahr, N. J., Filley, C. M. *et al.* (1994). Reduced platelet cytochrome c oxidase activity in Alzheimer's disease. *Neurology*, **44**, 1086–90.

Parker, W. D. Jr., Parks, J., Filley, C. M. & Kleinschmidt-DeMasters, B. K. (1994). Electron transport chain defects in Alzheimer's disease brain. *Neurology*, **44**, 1090–6.

Pavlakis, S. G., Phillips, P. C., DiMauro, S., De Vivo, D. C. & Rowland, L. P. (1984). Mitochondrial myopathy, encephalopathy, lactic acidosis, and stroke-like episodes: a distinctive clinical syndrome. *Ann. Neurol.* **16**, 481–8.

Petty, R. K., Harding, A. E. & Morgan-Hughes, J. A. (1986). The clinical features of mitochondrial myopathy. *Brain*, **109**, 915–38.

Piemonte, F., Pastore, A., Tozzi, G. *et al.* (2001). Glutathione in blood of patients with Friedreich's ataxia. *Eur. J. Clin. Invest.*, **31**, 1007–11.

Pook, M. A., Al-Mahdawi, S. A., Thomas, N. H. *et al.* (2000). Identification of three novel frameshift mutations in patients with Friedreich's ataxia. *J. Med. Genet.*, **37**.

Przedborski, S., Kostic, V., Jackson-Lewis, V. *et al.* (1992). Transgenic mice with increased Cu/Zn-superoxide dismutase activity are resistant to *N*-methyl-4-phenyl-1,2,3,6-tetrahydropyridine-induced neurotoxicity. *J. Neurosci.*, **12**, 1658–67.

Przedborski, S., Jackson-Lewis, V., Yokoyama, R., Shibata, T., Dawson, V. L. & Dawson, T. M. (1996). Role of neuronal nitric oxide in 1-methyl-4-phenyl-1,2,3,6-tetrahydropyridine (MPTP)-induced dopaminergic neurotoxicity. *Proc. Natl Acad. Sci., USA*, **93**, 4565–71.

Puccio, H., Simon, D., Cossee, M. *et al.* (2001). Mouse models for Friedreich ataxia exhibit cardiomyopathy, sensory nerve defect and Fe–S enzyme deficiency followed by intramitochondrial iron deposits. *Nat. Genet.*, **27**, 181–6.

Puddu, P., Barboni, P., Mantovani, V. *et al.* (1993). Retinitis pigmentosa, ataxia, and mental retardation associated with mitochondrial DNA mutation in an Italian family. *Br. J. Ophthalmol.*, **77**, 84–8.

Rahman, S., Blok, R. B., Dahl, H. H. *et al.* (1996). Leigh syndrome: clinical features and biochemical and DNA abnormalities. *Ann. Neurol.*, **39**, 343–51.

Ramsay, R. R., Salach, J. I. & Singer, T. P. (1986). Uptake of the neurotoxin 1-methyl-4-phenylpyridine (MPP+) by mitochondria and its relation to the inhibition of the mitochondrial oxidation of NAD+-linked substrates by MPP+. *Biochem. Biophys. Res. Commun.*, **134**, 743–8.

Reardon, W., Ross, R. J., Sweeney, M. G. *et al.* (1992). Diabetes mellitus associated with a pathogenic point mutation in mitochondrial DNA. *Lancet*, **340**, 1376–9.

Rosen, D. R., Siddique, T., Patterson, D. *et al.* (1993). Mutations in Cu/Zn superoxide dismutase gene are associated with familial amyotrophic lateral sclerosis. *Nature*, **362**, 59–62. Erratum in: *Nature*, **364** (6435), 362.

Rossetti, Z. L., Sotgiu, A., Sharp, D. E., Hadjiconstantinou, M. & Neff, N. H. (1988). 1-Methyl-4-phenyl-1,2,3,6-tetrahydropyridine (MPTP) and free radicals in vitro. *Biochem. Pharmacol.*, **37**, 4573–4.

Rotig, A., Bessis, J. L., Romero, N. *et al.* (1992). Maternally inherited duplication of the mitochondrial genome in a syndrome of proximal tubulopathy, diabetes mellitus, and cerebellar ataxia. *Am. J. Hum. Genet.*, **50**, 364–70.

Rotig, A., de Lonlay, P., Chretien, D. *et al.* (1997). Aconitase and mitochondrial iron–sulphur protein efficiency in Friedreich ataxia. *Nat. Genet.*, **17**, 215–17.

Santorelli, F. M., Shanske, S., Jain, K. D., Tick, D., Schon, E. A. & DiMauro, S. (1994). A T–>C mutation at nt 8993 of mitochondrial DNA in a child with Leigh syndrome. *Neurology*, **44**, 972–4.

Santorelli, F. M., Tanji, K., Manta, P. *et al.* (1999). Maternally inherited cardiomyopathy: an atypical presentation of the mtDNA 12S rRNA gene A1555G mutation. *Am. J. Hum. Genet.*, **64**, 295–300.

Sawa, A., Wiegand, G. W., Cooper, J. *et al.* (1999). Increased apoptosis of Huntington disease lymphoblasts associated with repeat length-dependent mitochondrial depolarization. *Nat. Med.*, **5**, 1194–8.

Schapira, A. H., Cooper, J. M., Dexter, D., Jenner, P., Clark. J. B. & Marsden, C. D. (1989). Mitochondrial complex I deficiency in Parkinson's disease. *Lancet*, **1**, 1269.

Schapira, A. H., Cooper, J. M., Dexter, D., Clark, J. B., Jenner, P. & Marsden, C. D. (1990). Mitochondrial complex I deficiency in Parkinson's disease. *J. Neurochem.*, **54**, 823–7.

Schapira, A. H., Mann, V. M., Cooper, J. M. *et al.* (1990). Anatomic and disease specificity of NADH CoQ1 reductase (complex I) deficiency in Parkinson's disease. *J. Neurochem.*, **55**, 2142–5.

Schapira, A. H. V. (1994). Mitochondrial dysfunction in neurodegenerative disorders and ageing. In *Mitochondrial Disorders in Neurology*, ed. A. H. V. Schapira. & S. DiMauro, pp. 227–44, Oxford UK: Butterworth Heinemann.

Schols, L., Vorgerd, M., Schillings, M., Skipka, G. & Zange, J. (2001). Idebenone in patients with Friedreich ataxia. *Neurosci. Lett.*, **29**(306), 169–72.

Schon, E. A. (2000). Mitochondrial genetics and disease. *Trends. Biochem. Sci.*, **25**, 555–60.

Schon, E. A., Rizzuto, R., Moraes, C. T., Nakase, H., Zeviani, M. & DiMauro, S. (1989). A direct repeat is a hotspot for large-scale deletion of human mitochondrial DNA. *Science*, **244**, 346–9.

Schon, E. A., Koga, Y., Davidson, M., Moraes, C. T. & King, M. P. (1992). The mitochondrial tRNA(Leu)(UUR)) mutation in MELAS: a model for pathogenesis. *Biochim. Biophys. Acta*, **1101**, 206–9.

Schon, E. A., Bonilla, E. & DiMauro, S. (1997). Mitochondrial DNA mutations and pathogenesis. *J. Bioenerg. Biomembr.*, **29**, 131–49.

Shoubridge, E. A., Karpati, G. & Hastings, K. E. (1990). Deletion mutants are functionally dominant over wild-type mitochondrial genomes in skeletal muscle fiber segments in mitochondrial disease. *Cell*, **62**, 43–9.

Schulz, J. B., Matthews, R. T., Muqit, M. M., Browne, S. E. & Beal, M. F. (1995). Inhibition of neuronal nitric oxide synthase by 7-nitroindazole protects against MPTP-induced neurotoxicity in mice. *J. Neurochem.*, **64**, 936–9.

Schwarcz, R., Whetsell, W. O. Jr. & Mangano, R. M. (1983). Quinolinic acid: an endogenous metabolite that produces axon-sparing lesions in rat brain. *Science*, **219**, 316–18.

Servidei, S., Zeviani M., Manfredi, G. *et al.* (1991). Dominantly inherited mitochondrial myopathy with multiple deletions of mitochondrial DNA: clinical, morphologic, and biochemical studies. *Neurology*, **41**, 1053–9.

Shaw, P. J., Ince, P. G., Falkous, G. & Mantle, D. (1995). Oxidative damage to protein in sporadic motor neuron disease spinal cord. *Ann. Neurol.*, **38**, 691–5.

Shoffner, J. M., Lott, M. T., Lezza, A. M., Seibel, P., Ballinger, S. W. & Wallace, D. C. (1990). Myoclonic epilepsy and ragged-red fiber disease (MERRF) is associated with a mitochondrial DNA tRNA(Lys) mutation. *Cell*, **61**, 931–7.

Shoffner, J. M., Lott, M. T. & Wallace, D. C. (1991). MERRF: a model disease for understanding the principles of mitochondrial genetics. *Rev. Neurol. (Paris)*, **147**, 431–5.

Silvestri, G., Ciafaloni, E., Santorelli, F. M. *et al.* (1993). Clinical features associated with the A–>G transition at nucleotide 8344 of mtDNA ("MERRF mutation"). *Neurology*, **43**, 1200–6.

Simonian, N. A. & Hyman, B. T. (1993). Functional alterations in Alzheimer's disease: diminution of cytochrome oxidase in the hippocampal formation. *J. Neuropathol. Exp. Neurol.*, **52**, 580–5.

Singleton, A. B., Farrer, M., Johnson, J. *et al.* (2003). Alpha-Synuclein locus triplication causes Parkinson's disease. *Science*, **302**, 841.

Smith, P. R., Cooper, J. M., Govan, G. G., Harding, A. E. & Schapira, A. H. (1994). Platelet mitochondrial function in Leber's hereditary optic neuropathy. *J. Neurol. Sci.*, **122**, 80–3.

Smith, P. R., Cooper, J. M., Govan, G. G., Riordan-Eva, P., Harding, A. E. & Schapira, A. H. (1995). Antibodies to human optic nerve in Leber's hereditary optic neuropathy. *J. Neurol. Sci.*, **130**, 134–8.

So, N., Berkovic, S., Andermann, F., Kuzniecky, R., Gendron, D. & Quesney, L. F. (1989). Myoclonus epilepsy and ragged-red

fibres (MERRF). 2. Electrophysiological studies and comparison with other progressive myoclonus epilepsies. *Brain*, **112**, 1261–76.

Strong, T. V., Tagle, D. A., Valdes, J. M. *et al.* (1993). Widespread expression of the human and rat Huntington's disease gene in brain and nonneural tissues. *Nat. Genet.*, **5**, 259–65.

Sue, C. M., Crimmins, D. S., Soo, Y. S. *et al.* (1998). Neuroradiological features of six kindreds with MELAS tRNA(Leu) A2343G point mutation: implications for pathogenesis. *J. Neurol. Neurosurg. Psychiatry*, **65**, 233–40.

Sue, C. M., Karadimas, C., Checcarelli, N. *et al.* (2000). Differential features of patients with mutations in two COX assembly genes, SURF-1 and SCO2. *Ann. Neurol.*, **47**, 589–95.

Suomalainen, A., Kaukonen, J., Amati, P. *et al.* (1995). An autosomal locus predisposing to deletions of mitochondrial DNA. *Nat. Genet.*, **9**, 146–51.

Swerdlow, R. H., Parks, J. K., Miller, S. W. *et al.* (1996). Origin and functional consequences of the complex I defect in Parkinson's disease. *Ann. Neurol.*, **40**, 663–71.

Tabrizi, S. J., Cleeter, M. W., Xuereb, J., Taanman, J. W., Cooper, J. M. & Schapira, A. H. (1999). Biochemical abnormalities and excitotoxicity in Huntington's disease brain. *Ann. Neurol.*, **45**, 25–32.

Tabrizi, S. J., Workman, J., Hart, P. E. *et al.* (2000). Mitochondrial dysfunction and free radical damage in the Huntington R6/2 transgenic mouse. *Ann. Neurol.*, **47**, 80–6.

Tabrizi, S. J., Blamire, A. M., Manners, D. N. *et al.* (2003). Creatine therapy for Huntington's disease: clinical and MRS findings in a 1-year pilot study. *Neurology*, **8**(61), 141–2.

Tang, Y., Schon, E. A., Wilichowski, E., Vazquez-Memije, M. E., Davidson, E. & King, M. P. (2000). Rearrangements of human mitochondrial DNA (mtDNA): new insights into the regulation of mtDNA copy number and gene expression. *Mol. Biol. Cell*, **11**, 1471–85.

Tatuch, Y., Christodoulou, J., Feigenbaum, A. *et al.* (1992). Heteroplasmic mtDNA mutation (T–G) at 8993 can cause Leigh disease when the percentage of abnormal mtDNA is high. *Am. J. Hum. Genet.*, **50**, 852–8.

Thobois, S., Vighetto, A., Grochowicki, M., Godinot, C., Broussolle, E. & Aimard, G. (1997). Leber "plus" disease: optic neuropathy, parkinsonian syndrome and supranuclear ophthalmoplegia. *Rev. Neurol. (Paris)*, **153**, 595–8.

Tiranti, V., Hoertnagel, K., Carrozzo, R. *et al.* (1998). Mutations of SURF-1 in Leigh disease associated with cytochrome c oxidase deficiency. *Am. J. Hum. Genet.*, **63**, 1609–21.

Truong, D. D., Harding, A. E., Scaravilli, F., Smith, S. J., Morgan-Hughes, J. A. & Marsden, C. D. (1990). Movement disorders in mitochondrial myopathies. A study of nine cases with two autopsy studies. *Mov. Disord.*, **5**, 109–17.

Tsairis, P., Engel, W. K. & Kark, P. (1973). Familial myoclonic epilepsy syndrome associated with skeletal muscle mitochondrial abnormalities. *Neurology*, **23**, 408.

Tulinius, M. H., Holme, E., Kristiansson, B., Larsson, N. G. & Oldfors, A. (1991). Mitochondrial encephalomyopathies in childhood. II. Clinical manifestations and syndromes. *J. Pediatr.*, **199**, 251–9.

Van Coster, R., Lombres, A., De Vivo, D. C. *et al.* (199). Cytochrome c oxidase-associated Leigh syndrome: phenotypic features and pathogenetic speculations. *J. Neurol. Sci.*, **104**, 97–111.

van den Ouweland, J. M., Lemkes, H. H., Ruitenbeek, W. *et al.* (1992). Mutation in mitochondrial tRNA(Leu)(UUR) gene in a large pedigree with maternally transmitted type II diabetes mellitus and deafness. *Nat. Genet.*, **1**, 368–71.

van Erven, P. M., Gabreels, F. J., Ruitenbeek, W., Renier, W. O. & Fischer, J. C. (1987). Mitochondrial encephalomyopathy. Association with an NADH dehydrogenase deficiency. *Arch. Neurol.*, **44**, 775–8.

Vielhaber, S., Kunz, D., Winkler, K. *et al.* (2000). Mitochondrial DNA abnormalities in skeletal muscle of patients with sporadic amyotrophic lateral sclerosis. *Brain*, **123**, 1339–48.

Vila, M. R., Gamez, J., Solano, A. *et al.* (2000). Uncoupling protein-1 mRNA expression in lipomas from patients bearing pathogenic mitochondrial DNA mutations. *Biochem. Biophys. Res. Commun.*, **278**(3), 800–2.

Wallace, D. C., Singh, G., Lott, M. T. *et al.* (1988). Mitochondrial DNA mutation associated with Leber's hereditary optic neuropathy. *Science*, **242**, 1427–30.

Weller, M. & Paul, S. M. (1993). 3-Nitropropionic acid is an indirect excitotoxin to cultured cerebellar granule neurons. *Eur. J. Pharmacol.*, **248**, 223–8.

Wiedemann, F. R., Winkler, K., Kuznetsov, A. V. *et al.* (1998). Impairment of mitochondrial function in skeletal muscle of patients with amyotrophic lateral sclerosis. *J. Neurol. Sci.*, **156**, 65–72.

Willems, J. L., Monnens, L. A., Trijbels, J. M. *et al.* (1977). Leigh's encephalomyelopathy in a patient with cytochrome c oxidase deficiency in muscle tissue. *Pediatr.*, **60**, 850–7.

Wong, A., Yang, J., Cavadini, P. *et al.* (1999). The Freidreich's ataxia mutation confers cellular sensitivity to oxidative stress which is rescued by chelators of iron and calcium and inhibitors of apoptotis. *Hum. Mol. Genet.*, **8**, 425–30.

Zeviani, M., Amati, P., Bresolin, N. *et al.* (1991). Rapid detection of the A–G(8344) mutation of mtDNA in Italian families with myoclonus epilepsy and ragged-red fibers (MERRF). *Am. J. Hum. Genet.*, **48**, 203–11.

Zhu, Z., Yao, J., Johns, T. *et al.* (1998). SURF1, encoding a factor involved in the biogenesis of cytochrome c oxidase, is mutated in Leigh syndrome. *Nat. Genet.*, **20**, 337–43.

Index